PEDIATRIC HYPERTENSION

CLINICAL HYPERTENSION AND VASCULAR DISEASES

WILLIAM B. WHITE, MD
SERIES EDITOR

PEDIATRIC HYPERTENSION

Second Edition

Edited by

JOSEPH T. FLYNN, MD, MS

Division of Nephrology,
Seattle Children's Hospital,
Seattle, WA, USA

JULIE R. INGELFINGER, MD

Pediatric Nephrology Unit, Department of Pediatrics,
Harvard Medical School and MassGeneral Hospital
for Children at Massachusetts General Hospital,
Boston, MA, USA

RONALD J. PORTMAN, MD

Pediatric Drug Development Program,
Bristol-Myers Squibb,
Princeton, NJ, USA

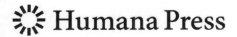 Humana Press

Editors
Joseph T. Flynn, MD, MS
Division of Nephrology
Seattle Children's Hospital
4800 Sand Point Way NE
Seattle, WA 98105, USA
joseph.flynn@seattlechildrens.org

Julie R. Ingelfinger, MD
Massachusetts General Hospital and
   Harvard Medical School
55 Fruit St.
Boston, MA 02114, USA
jingelfinger@partners.org

Ronald J. Portman, MD
Bristol-Myers Squibb
Global Clinical Research
Route 206 & Provinceline Road
Princeton, NJ 08543, USA

ISBN 978-1-60327-823-2   e-ISBN 978-1-60327-824-9
DOI 10.1007/978-1-60327-824-9
Springer New York Dordrecht Heidelberg London

Foreword

While hypertension in children and adolescents has a significant impact on adult cardiovascular disease as it transitions into adulthood, it also directly causes target organ damage and is associated with early atherosclerosis in children. The second edition of *Pediatric Hypertension* is an excellent reference textbook for any clinician or clinical researcher interested in this area as it provides a thorough review of what is known about childhood blood pressure based on the evidence from clinical studies, trials, and outcome research. The new edition has been substantially updated from the first edition of the book that was published in 2004—there are several new chapters and some old chapters have been modified or replaced. The second edition of *Pediatric Hypertension* is now a comprehensive textbook in 32 chapters that remain divided into 4 broad themes: (I) regulation of blood pressure and pathophysiology of hypertension in children; (II) assessment of blood pressure including measurement, normative data, and epidemiology; (III) definitions, predictors, risk factors, and comorbid conditions in childhood hypertension; and (IV) evaluation and treatment of hypertension in neonates and children.

As in the first edition of the book, the chapters are written by experts in their respective fields and remain nicely organized and easy to read and understand. The first section has been enlarged substantially and now includes chapters on vasoactive peptides, ion transport, and inflammatory mediators of vascular function. An excellent genomics chapter that was in edition 1 of the book has been moved into this section as well. The second section of the book now focuses not only on the epidemiology of hypertension in children but on cardiovascular diseases in general as well as on important comorbidities of obesity, diabetes, and metabolic syndromes in children and adolescents. The third section has also been expanded to encompass more in-depth discussion of perinatal programming, cardiovascular reactivity, and social environments as well as important clinical subpopulations of chronic and end-stage renal diseases and obstructive sleep apnea. In this second edition, there are also discrete new chapters on the impact of exercise on blood pressure and the utility of ambulatory blood pressure monitoring in assessing children with elevated blood pressure. The material in each chapter is presented in a logical manner, with clearly interpreted results and extensive referencing. Clinical applications are given so that the clinician can better incorporate this material into their understanding of the pathophysiology of hypertension in neonates, children, and adolescents.

It is pleasing to see the detail given in the section of the book on the management and treatment of hypertension in children. These chapters are destined to be very helpful for trainees in pediatrics and its subspecialties as well as practicing clinicians due to their pragmatic nature. The updated chapter on pediatric antihypertensive trials (Chapter 33) is particularly unique as it differentiates the issues of clinical trials for new antihypertensive medications in children versus adults and provides summary information from the US FDA.

As series editor of *Clinical Hypertension and Vascular Diseases*, I am highly enthusiastic about the second edition of *Pediatric Hypertension,* which I view as an extremely useful book that provides the most up-to-date and comprehensive review available on this important topic. I expect that pediatricians, family medicine doctors, and all physicians with an interest in basic and clinical aspects of hypertension and its complications will find *Pediatric Hypertension* a valuable addition to their medical library.

William B. White, MD
Professor of Medicine and Chief
Division of Hypertension and Clinical Pharmacology
Pat and Jim Calhoun Cardiology Center
University of Connecticut School of Medicine, Farmington
Series Editor, *Clinical Hypertension and Vascular Diseases*

Preface to the Second Edition

Interest in pediatric hypertension dates back nearly half a century, when it was first recognized that a small percentage of children and adolescents had elevated blood pressures—and in those days, the same normal values for adult blood pressure were utilized in children! The many advances since that time have led to a much clearer understanding of how to identify, evaluate, and treat hypertensive children and adolescents. At the same time, many questions remain: What causes hypertension in children without underlying systemic conditions? What are the long-term consequences of high blood pressure in the young? What is the optimal therapy of childhood hypertension? and Does such treatment benefit the affected child or adolescent? Can we identify children at risk of developing hypertension and intervene to prevent its occurrence? Readers conversant with the history of hypertension in the young will recognize that these questions were being asked decades ago and may still be unanswered for many years to come.

The first text focusing on pediatric hypertension was published in 1982. The book you are about to read is a direct descendant of that first effort to summarize what is known about hypertension in the young. We are fortunate to have been given the first opportunity to produce a second edition of such a text, which reflects the increased interest in hypertension in the young that has developed since the publication of the first edition of *Pediatric Hypertension*. Many chapters from the first edition have been revised and updated by their original authors; others have been written by new authors. New chapters on topics of recent interest in pediatric hypertension such as the metabolic syndrome and sleep disorders have been added. We hope that the reader will find this new edition of *Pediatric Hypertension* to be an up-to-date, clinically useful reference as well as a stimulus to further research in the field.

It is also our hope that the advances summarized in this text will ultimately lead to increased efforts toward the prevention of hypertension in the young, which, in turn, should ameliorate the burden of cardiovascular disease in adults. We thank our many colleagues who have taken time from their busy schedules to contribute to this text—and we are sure that you will agree with us that their combined efforts have resulted in a valuable reference to those interested in hypertension in the young.

Joseph T. Flynn
Seattle, Washington

Julie R. Ingelfinger
Boston, Massachusetts

Ronald J. Portman
Princeton, New Jersey

Contents

Contributors

ALISA A. ACOSTA, MD, MPH • *Pediatric Nephrology, Children's Hospital at Scott and White, Texas A&M College of Medicine, 2401 South 31st Street, Temple, TX, USA*

BRUCE S. ALPERT, MD • *LeBonheur Children's Medical Center, University of Tennessee Health Science Center, Memphis, TN, USA*

CRAIG W. BELSHA, MD • *Department of Pediatrics, SSM Cardinal Glennon Children's Medical Center, Saint Louis University, St. Louis, MO, USA*

DANIEL K. BENJAMIN, Jr., MD, PhD, MPH • *Pediatrics and Duke Clinical Research Institute, Duke University, Durham, NC, USA*

GERALD S. BERENSON, MD • *Department of Epidemiology, Tulane Center for Health, New Orleans, LA, USA*

DOUGLAS L. BLOWEY, MD • *Department of Pediatrics, Children's Mercy Hospital and Clinics, University of Missouri-Kansas City School of Medicine, Kansas City, MO, USA*

LAVJAY BUTANI, MD • *University of California Davis, Sacramento, CA, USA*

R. THOMAS COLLINS, II, MD • *Assistant Professor of Pediatrics, University of Arkansas for Medical Sciences, College of Medicine, Division of Cardiology, Arkansas Children's Hospital, Little Rock, AR, USA*

SANDRA COULON, BS • *Department of Psychology, Barnwell College, University of South Carolina, Columbia, SC, USA*

BONITA FALKNER, MD • *Department of Medicine, Thomas Jefferson University, Philadelphia, PA, USA*

WENDE N. FEDDER, RN, BSN, MBA • *Department of Neuroscience, Neuroscience Institute, Alexian Brothers Hospital Network, Elk Grove Village, IL, USA*

DANIEL I. FEIG, MD, PhD, MS • *Renal Section, Department of Pediatrics, Baylor College of Medicine, Texas Children's Hospital, Houston, TX, USA*

JOSEPH T. FLYNN, MD, MS • *Division of Nephrology, Seattle Children's Hospital, Seattle, WA, USA; Department of Pediatrics, University of Washington School of Medicine, Seattle, WA, USA*

SAMUEL S. GIDDING, MD • *Nemours Cardiac Center, Alfred I. DuPont Hospital for Children, Wilmington, DE, USA; Jefferson Medical College, Wilmington, DE, USA*

GREGORY A. HARSHFIELD, PhD • *Department of Pediatrics, Medical College of Georgia, The Georgia Prevention Institute, Augusta, GA, USA*

JULIE R. INGELFINGER, MD • *Pediatric Nephrology Unit, Department of Pediatrics, Harvard Medical School and MassGeneral Hospital for Children at Massachusetts General Hospital, Boston, MA, USA*

JOHN E. JONES, PhD • *Children's Research Institute, Center for Molecular Physiology Research, Children's National Medical Center, Washington, DC, USA*

PEDRO A. JOSE, MD, PhD • *Center for Molecular Physiology Research, Children's National Medical Center, Washington, DC, USA; George Washington School of Medicine & Public Health, Washington, DC, USA*

GAURAV KAPUR, MD • *Department of Pediatric Nephrology, Children's Hospital of Michigan, Wayne State University School of Medicine, Detroit, MI, USA*

RAE-ELLEN W. KAVEY, MD, MPH • *Division of Pediatric Cardiology, University of Rochester Medical Center, Rochester, NY, USA*

VERA H. KOCH, MD • *Department of Pediatrics, Instituto da Criança, Hospital das Clínicas da Faculdade de Medicina, Universidade de São Paulo (USP), São Paulo, SP, Brazil*

JENNIFER S. LI, MD, MHS • *Department of Pediatrics, Duke University Medical Center, Durham, NC, USA*

EMPAR LURBE, MD, PhD • *Pediatric Nephrology Department, Department of Pediatrics, Consorcio Hospital General Universitario de Valencia, University of Valenica, Spain; CIBERobn, Instituto de Salud Carlas III, Spain*

TEJ K. MATTOO, MD, DCH, FRCP (UK), FAAP • *Pediatric Nephrology, Department of Pediatrics, Children's Hospital of Michigan, Detroit, MI, USA*

MARK M. MITSNEFES, MD, MS • *Division of Nephrology, Department of Pediatrics, Cincinnati Children's Hospital and Medical Center, Cincinnati, OH, USA*

BRUCE Z. MORGENSTERN, MD • *University of Arizona College of Medicine,, Phoenix, AZ, USA; Mayo Clinic, College of Medicine, Phoenix, AZ, USA; Division of Nephrology, Phoenix Children's Hospital, Phoenix, AZ, USA*

ARUNA R. NATARAJAN, MD, DCh, PhD • *Department of Pediatrics, Division of Critical Care, Georgetown University Hospital, Washington, DC, USA*

RONALD J. PORTMAN, MD • *Pediatric Drug Development Program, Bristol-Myers Squibb, Princeton, NJ, USA*

JOSEP REDON, MD, PhD, FAHA • *Department of Internal Medicine, Hospital Clinico Universitario de Valencia, University of Valencia, Spain*

KAREN MCNIECE REDWINE, MD, MPH • *Department of Pediatric Nephrology, University of Arkansas for Medical Sciences and Arkansas Children's Hospital, Little Rock, AR, USA*

ALBERT P. ROCCHINI, MD • *Professor of Pediatrics, University of Michigan Medical School, Director, Pediatric Cardiology, C.S. Mott Children's Hospital, Ann Arbor, MI, USA*

FRANZ SCHAEFER, MD • *Division of Paediatric Nephrology, Center for Paediatric and Adolescent Medicine, University of Heidelberg, Im Neuenheimer Feld 151, 69120 Heidelberg, Germany*

TOMÁŠ SEEMAN, MD, PhD • *Department of Pediatrics, University Hospital Motol, Charles University Prague, 2nd Faculty of Medicine, Prague, Czech Republic*

JEFFREY L. SEGAR, MD • *Department of Pediatrics, Division of Neonatology, University of Iowa Carver College of Medicine, Iowa City, IA, USA*

THOMAS SEVERIN, MD • *Director, Pediatric Policy, Clinical Development and Medical Affairs, Novartis Pharma AG, Basel, Switzerland*

HAROLD SNIEDER, PhD • *Unit of Genetic Epidemiology & Bioinformatics, Department of Epidemiology, University Medical Center Groningen, University of Groningen, Groningen, The Netherlands*

SATHANUR R. SRINIVASAN, PhD • *Department of Epidemiology, Tulane University School of Public Health and Tropical Medicine, New Orleans, LA, USA*

RITA D. SWINFORD, MD • *Division of Pediatric Nephrology and Hypertension, Department of Pediatrics, University of Texas at Houston, Houston, TX, USA*

AVRAM Z. TRAUM, MD • *Pediatric Nephrology Unit, Harvard Medical School, Massachusetts General Hospital, Boston, MA, USA*

KJELL TULLUS, MD, PhD, FRCPCH • *Department of Nephrology, Great Ormond Street Hospital for Children, London, UK*

ELAINE M. URBINA, MD, MS • *Preventive Cardiology, Department of Pediatrics, Cincinnati Children's Hospital Medical Center, Cincinnati, OH, USA*

XIAOLING WANG, MD, PhD • *Department of Pediatrics, Georgia Prevention Institute, Medical College of Georgia, Augusta, GA, USA*

DONALD J. WEAVER, Jr., MD, PhD • *Division of Nephrology and Hypertension, Department of Pediatrics, Levine Children's Hospital at Carolinas Medical Center, Charlotte, NC, USA*

DAWN K. WILSON, PhD • *Department of Psychology, Barnwell College, University of South Carolina, Columbia, SC, USA*

ELKE WÜHL, MD • *Division of Pediatric Nephrology, Center of Pediatrics and Adolescent Medicine, University Hospital Heidelberg, Heidelberg, Germany*

IHOR V. YOSYPIV, MD • *Section of Pediatric Nephrology, Department of Pediatrics, Tulane Hospital for Children, New Orleans, LA, USA*

I

REGULATION OF BLOOD PRESSURE IN CHILDREN

1

Neurohumoral Regulation of Blood Pressure in Early Development

Jeffrey L. Segar, MD

CONTENTS

INTRODUCTION

Cardiovascular homeostasis is mediated through interacting neural, hormonal, and metabolic mechanisms that act both locally and systemically. These basic physiological mechanisms, which have been extensively studied in the adult, are functional in the fetus and newborn, although differential rates of maturation of these systems influence their ability to maintain blood pressure and delivery of oxygen and nutrients. This chapter focuses primarily on autonomic control of the fetal and newborn cardiovascular system and how hormonal and/or endocrine factors influence these systems.

Baroreceptor and chemoreceptor responses are vital for maintaining circulatory function. These neural pathways are modulated by a number of endocrine and paracrine factors, including angiotensin II (ANG II), arginine vasopressin (AVP), and corticosteroids. Understanding the neurohumoral mechanisms participating in cardiovascular regulation during the fetal and postnatal periods, particularly as they relate to the physiological adaptations occurring with the transition from fetal to newborn life, may ultimately result in new strategies to prevent complications during the perinatal period.

J.L. Segar (✉)
Department of Pediatrics, Division of Neonatology, University of Iowa Carver College of Medicine, Iowa City, IA, USA
e-mail: jeffrey-segar@uiowa.edu

From: *Clinical Hypertension and Vascular Diseases: Pediatric Hypertension*
Edited by: J. T. Flynn et al. DOI 10.1007/978-1-60327-824-9_1
© Springer Science+Business Media, LLC 2011

OVERVIEW OF AUTONOMIC FUNCTION

Blood pressure is regulated through interacting neural, hormonal, and metabolic mechanisms acting within the brain, the end organs, and the vasculature. The central nervous system is critical for cardiovascular homeostasis, as cardiac and vasculature autonomic tone is continuously modulated by an array of peripheral sensors, including arterial baroreceptors and chemoreceptors (1). Cardiovascular centers within the brain located between afferent and efferent pathways of the reflex arc integrate a variety of visceral and behavioral inputs, permitting a wide range of modulation of autonomic, cardiovascular, and endocrine responses. Developmentally regulated maturation of these basic systems in the fetus and newborn modulate the ability to maintain blood pressure and organ blood flow.

The contribution of the autonomic nervous system to cardiovascular homeostasis changes during development. Both α-adrenergic and ganglionic blockade, which inhibit sympathetic transmission at the ganglia and end organ, respectively, produce greater decreases in blood pressure in term fetal sheep than in preterm fetal sheep or newborn lambs, suggesting that fetal sympathetic tone is high late in gestation (2,3). The influence of the parasympathetic system on resting heart rate also appears to increase with maturation (4). Cholinergic blockade produces no consistent effect of heart rate in premature fetal sheep, a slight increase in heart rate in term fetuses, and the greatest effect in lambs beyond the first week of life (3,5,6).

Arterial pressure displays natural oscillations within a physiological range, the degree of which is similar in fetal and postnatal life (7–10). In the adult, ganglionic blockade increases arterial pressure variability (7,11), suggesting that a component of arterial pressure lability is peripheral or humoral in origin and is buffered by autonomic functions. In contrast, ganglionic blockade in term fetal sheep significantly slows heart rate and attenuates arterial pressure variability (9). Changes in fetal renal sympathetic nerve activity appear to correlate positively with fluctuations in heart rate and arterial pressure (9). Although fetal electrocortical and sympathetic activity have not been recorded simultaneously, fetal heart rate, arterial pressure, and catecholamine levels are highest during periods of high-voltage, low-frequency electrocortical activity, suggesting that oscillations in sympathetic tone are related to changes in the behavioral state of the fetus (12–15). Other physiological parameters, including organ blood flows, regional vascular resistance, and cerebral oxygen consumption, are also dependent on electrocortical state and likely reflect changes in autonomic activity (12,16,17).

ARTERIAL BAROREFLEX

Arterial baroreceptors, major sensing elements of the cardiovascular regulatory system, are essential in short-term control of blood pressure. Acute changes in vascular stretch related to alterations in blood pressure modify the discharge of afferent baroreceptor fibers located in the carotid sinus and aortic arch. This increase in afferent nerve traffic, in turn, results in alterations in efferent parasympathetic and sympathetic nerve activities that influence heart rate and peripheral vascular resistance, serving to buffer changes in arterial pressure (Fig. 1) (18,19). Baroreflex control of heart rate is dominated by changes in cardiac vagal tone, although integrity of the reflex is dependent upon both sympathetic and parasympathetic pathways (20). Studies in animals demonstrate that the arterial baroreflex is functional during fetal and early postnatal life (4,10,21,22). The observation that sinoaortic denervation produces marked fluctuations in fetal arterial pressure and heart rate further suggests important contributions of the baroreflex to cardiovascular homeostasis (10,22).

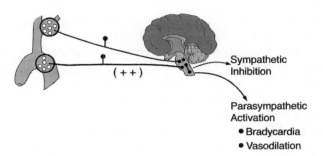

Fig. 1. Schematic representation of the arterial baroreflex, depicting how an increase in blood pressure modifies the discharge of afferent baroreceptor fibers located in the carotid sinus and aortic arch, which, in turn, results in alterations in efferent sympathetic and parasympathetic nerve activities that influence heart rate and peripheral vascular resistance, serving to buffer changes in arterial pressure.

Single-fiber recordings of baroreceptor afferents *(23–27)* in fetal and newborn animals demonstrate that carotid sinus nerve activity is phasic and pulse synchronous, and that activity increases with a rise in arterial or carotid sinus pressure *(24–26)*. Basal discharge of baroreceptor afferents does not change during fetal and postnatal maturation, despite a considerable increase in mean arterial pressure during this time, indicating that baroreceptors reset during development, continuing to function within the physiological range for arterial pressure *(24,27)*. The sensitivity of carotid baroreceptors to increases in carotid sinus pressure is greater in fetal than in newborn and 1-month-old lambs *(24)* and in newborn as compared to adult rabbits *(27)*. These findings suggest that any reduced heart rate responses to changes in arterial pressure during fetal life (as discussed below) are not due to underdeveloped afferent activity of baroreceptors but rather to differences in central integration and efferent pathways. The mechanisms regulating the changes in sensitivity of the baroreceptors early in development have not been investigated, but may be related to changes in the degree of mechanical deformation of nerve endings and thus may strain sensitivity, ionic mechanisms that operate at the receptor membrane to cause hyperpolarization, or substances released from the endothelium, including prostacyclin and nitric oxide, that modulate baroreceptor activity *(28–33)*.

Many but not all studies in fetal and newborn animals describe baroreflex sensitivity, determined by the heart rate response to alterations in blood pressure, as being decreased early in development *(34–38)*. Using reflex bradycardia in response to increased blood pressure induced by balloon inflation, Shinebourne et al. *(36)* observed that cardiac baroreflex activity is present as early as 85 days of gestation (~0.6 of the length of gestation) in fetal lambs, and that the sensitivity of the reflex increased up to term. Heart rate responses to changes in blood pressure in the premature sheep fetus also appear to be asymmetric and are more sensitive to an increase than to a decrease in blood pressure *(39)*. In contrast to findings in sheep, the sensitivity of the cardiac baroreflex is greater in the horse fetus at 0.6 of the length of gestation than at near term (0.9 of gestation) *(40)*.

Developmental changes in the cardiac baroreflex continue postnatally. Heart rate responses to pharmacologically induced changes in blood pressure in fetal (135 ± 2 days of gestation (term=145 days)), newborn, and 4–6-week-old sheep demonstrated a trend for the sensitivity of the baroreflex control of heart rate to decrease with maturation *(41)*. However, further studies in sheep *(37)* and other species *(42,43)* reported increasing cardiac baroreflex sensitivity with postnatal age. Reflex bradycardia in response to carotid sinus stimulation is absent in the newborn piglet, although vagal efferents exert a tonic action on the heart at this stage of development *(42)*. Age-related changes in heart rate in response to phenylephrine are also greater in 2-month-old piglets than in 1-day-old animals *(43)*. Differences in species, experimental conditions, and developmental changes in the innervation and functional contributions of the two arms of the autonomic nervous system (sympathetic and parasympathetic) likely contribute to these reported differences.

Baroreflex control of central sympathetic outflow, primarily measured as renal sympathetic nerve activity (RSNA), has been assessed as well. Booth et al. demonstrated in the preterm fetal sheep (at ~100 days or 0.7 of gestation) that baroreflex control of RSNA was absent although pulse synchronous bursts of RSNA were present *(39)*. Studies of the RSNA baroreflux function curve in late-gestation fetal (135 ±2 days gestation), newborn, and 4–6-week-old sheep indicated greatest sensitivity in the fetus and decreasing sensitivity during the postnatal period *(41)*. Interestingly, studies in aging animals have shown that baroreflex control of heart rate and sympathetic nerve activity is impaired with senescence *(44)*. Thus, the sensitivity of the baroreflex likely assumes an inverted "U" shape, increasing with early maturation, reaching a maximum sensitivity occurring during some developmental period, then decreasing with advancing age, an effect that may contribute to the development of hypertension.

Resetting of the Arterial Baroreflex

Resetting of the arterial baroreflex is defined as a change in the relation between arterial pressure and heart rate or between pressure and sympathetic and parasympathetic nerve activities *(29,30)*. As already noted, studies indicate that the sensitivity of the baroreflex changes with maturation. With sustained changes in blood pressure, the operating range of the baroreceptors also shifts, or resets, in the direction of the prevailing arterial pressure. This shift in the range of blood pressure over which the baroreflex remains functional occurs during fetal life, is present immediately after birth, and continues with postnatal maturation, paralleling the naturally occurring increase in blood pressure *(45)*. The mechanisms regulating developmental changes in baroreflex sensitivity and controlling the resetting of the baroreflex are poorly understood. Changes in the relationship between arterial pressure and sympathetic activity or heart rate occur at the level of the baroreceptor itself (peripheral resetting), from altered coupling within the central nervous system of afferent impulses from baroreceptors to efferent sympathetic or parasympathetic activity (central resetting) and at the end organ *(29)*. Locally produced factors, such as nitric oxide, and circulating hormones and neuropeptides, such as ANG II and AVP, activate additional neural reflex pathways that may modulate the changes in arterial baroreflex during development *(46)*.

Autonomic Function in the Developing Human

In the human infant, neural control of the circulation has been assessed most often by analysis of heart rate indices at rest and in response to postural changes. While some investigators have been unable to demonstrate a consistent response of heart rate to tilting, and concluded that the heart rate component of the baroreflex is poorly developed during the neonatal period, others have demonstrated in healthy preterm and term infants that unloading arterial baroreceptor by head-up tilting produces a significant heart rate response *(47–49)*. Using venous occlusion plethysmography, Waldman et al. *(49)* observed that healthy preterm and term infants subjected to 45° head-up tilting did not develop significant tachycardia, although, on average, a 25% decrease in limb blood flow occurred, suggestive of an increase in peripheral vascular resistance. In contrast, Myers et al. reported that 1–2-day-old healthy, term newborns display changes in heart rate with head-up and head-down tilt similar to those observed in the adults *(50)*. However, at 2–4 months of age the increase in heart rate to unloading of baroreceptors (head-up tilt) is lost *(50,51)*. One may speculate that this change may represent a vulnerable period of autonomic dysfunction and contribute to the risk for sudden infant death syndrome. Using noninvasive measurement of blood pressure sequences of spontaneous changes in blood pressure and heart rate in both premature and term infants (24 weeks gestational age to term), Gournay et al. reported that baroreflex sensitivity increased with gestational age and noted that sensitivity increased in premature infants (<32 weeks gestation), with postnatal age *(52)*.

Small, spontaneous beat-by-beat variations in heart rate may be analyzed as linear heart rate variability in both time and frequency domains and have been used in both infants *(53–55)* and fetuses *(56–58)* to evaluate the contribution of the autonomic nervous system in maintaining cardiovascular homeostasis. While the interpretation is considered somewhat subjective, analysis of fetal electrocardiogram tracings suggests differential development of the sympathetic and parasympathetic branches and progressive maturation of sympathovagal balance *(56–58)*. An increase in sympathetic tone appears around 32 weeks (0.8 of gestation), followed by moderation of sympathetic outflow related to the establishment of fetal behavioral states *(56)*.

Power spectral analysis is a technique used to characterize sympathetic and parasympathetic components of the heart rate, reported as a ratio of low-frequency (LF) to high-frequency (HF) components. In human infants, there is a progressive decline in the ratio of the low-frequency (LF) to high-frequency (HF) components with increasing postnatal and gestational age, indicating an increase in parasympathetic contribution to control of resting HR with maturation. In a small study of 24 sleeping infants, aged 31–41 weeks of conceptional age in which the babies were analyzed as 31–36-week, 37–38–week, and 39–41-week groups, Clairambault et al. *(55)* observed that changes in the HF component of the spectrum were greatest at 37–38 weeks, suggesting a steep increase in vagal tone at this age. Power spectral analysis has also been used to characterize developmental changes in sympathovagal balance in response to arterial baroreceptor unloading in preterm infants beginning at 28–30 weeks postconceptional age *(59)*. Longitudinal spectral analysis *(59)* indicated that the LF/HF ratio did not change with head-up postural change in infants at 28–30 weeks, whereas with increasing postnatal age the LF component of the spectrum increased with head-up tilt. In an elegant cross-sectional study of 1-week-old infants with postmenstrual ages ranging from 28 to 42 weeks, Andriessen observed increases in R–R interval, low- and high-frequency spectral powers, and baroreflex sensitivity with postmenstrual age *(53)*. Taken together, these observations suggest that neural regulation of cardiac function, particularly parasympathetic modulation, undergoes maturational change and becomes more functional with postnatal development.

CARDIOPULMONARY REFLEX

Cardiopulmonary receptors are sensory nerve endings located in the four cardiac chambers, in the great veins, and in the lungs *(60)*. In the adult, volume sensors mediating reflex changes in cardiovascular and renal function are believed to be primarily those residing in the atria *(61,62)* and the ventricles *(60)*. The ventricular receptors appear to be particularly important during decreases in cardiopulmonary pressures *(60,63,64)*. The majority of ventricular receptor vagal afferents are chemosensitive and mechanosensitive (activated by changes in pressure or strength) unmyelinated C-fibers *(65,66)*. These receptors have a low basal discharge rate that exerts a tonic inhibitory influence on sympathetic outflow and vascular resistance *(60)* and regulates plasma AVP concentration *(67)*. Interruption of the basal activity of the vagal afferent receptors increases heart rate, blood pressure, and sympathetic nerve activity, whereas activation of cardiopulmonary receptors causes reflex bradycardia, vasodilation, and sympathoinhibition *(60)*.

Characterization of the cardiopulmonary reflex during the perinatal and neonatal periods was initially performed by stimulation of chemosensitive cardiopulmonary receptors *(43,68,69)*. Those studies demonstrated that the heart rate, blood pressure, and regional blood flow responses to stimulation of chemosensitive cardiac receptors were smaller early during development than later in life, and absent in premature fetal lambs *(68)* and in piglets under 1 week old *(69)*. Stimulation of cardiopulmonary receptors by volume expansion had no effect on basal renal nerve activity in the fetus, but significantly reduced RSNA in newborn and 8-week-old sheep *(70,71)*. However, the decrease in RSNA in response to volume expansion was totally abolished in sinoaortic-denervated (SAD) newborn lambs but was not affected by SAD in 6–8-week-old sheep *(72)*. These results indicate that cardiopulmonary reflexes are not fully mature early in life and that stimulation of sinoaortic baroreceptors plays a greater role than cardiopulmonary mechanoreceptors in regulating changes in sympathetic activity in response to expansion of vascular volume early during development.

Cardiopulmonary mechanoreceptors also respond to reductions in blood volume by eliciting reflexes that influence systemic hemodynamics. Gomez et al. observed that hemorrhage produced a significant decrease in arterial blood pressure without accompanying changes in heart rate in fetal sheep less than 120 days gestation, whereas blood pressure remained stable and heart rate increased in near-term fetuses *(73)*. However, other investigators *(74,75)* reported that the hemodynamic response to hemorrhage was similar in immature and near-term fetuses, with reductions in both heart rate and blood pressure. Inhibition of vagal afferents during slow, nonhypotensive hemorrhage blocked the normal rise in plasma AVP but did not alter the rise in plasma renin activity in near-term fetal sheep *(74)*. When input from cardiopulmonary receptors is removed by sectioning the cervical vagosympathetic trunks, the decrease in fetal blood pressure in response to hemorrhage is similar to that in intact fetuses *(76)*, whereas vagotomy with SAD enhances the decrease in blood pressure *(74)*. Therefore, it is likely that activation of fibers from the carotid sinus (arterial baroreceptors and chemoreceptors) but not vagal afferents (cardiopulmonary baroreceptors and chemoreceptors) is involved in the maintenance of blood pressure homeostasis during fetal hemorrhage. Cardiopulmonary receptors also appear to have a diminished role in early postnatal life as reflex changes in RSNA in newborn lamb during nonhypotensive and hypotensive hemorrhage are dependent upon the integrity of arterial baroreceptors but not cardiopulmonary receptors *(77)*. In addition, the cardiovascular responses in newborn lambs to hemorrhage are dependent upon intact renal nerves that, in turn, modulate release of AVP *(78)*.

The RSNA responses to vagal afferent nerve stimulation are similar in sinoaortic-denervated fetal and postnatal lambs *(79)*, suggesting that delayed maturation of the cardiopulmonary reflex is not secondary to incomplete central integration of vagal afferent input. On the other hand, the decreased sensitivity of the cardiopulmonary reflex early in development in the face of a sensitive arterial baroreflex response (as outlined above) is intriguing. One may suggest that there is an occlusive interaction between these two reflexes during development. In support of this hypothesis, studies in adults *(80,81)* have shown that activation of arterial baroreceptors may impair the reflex responses to activation of cardiopulmonary receptors.

PERIPHERAL CHEMOREFLEX

Peripheral chemoreceptors located in the aortic arch and carotid bodies are functional during fetal and early postnatal life and participate in cardiovascular regulation *(82–84)*. Acute hypoxemia evokes integrated cardiovascular, metabolic, and endocrine responses in the fetus that result in transient bradycardia, increased arterial blood pressure and peripheral vascular resistance, and a redistribution of blood flow *(83,85)*. Oxygen sensing in the carotid body is transduced by glomus cells, which are specialized sensory neurons that respond to hypoxia at higher PaO_2 levels than other cell types. It is believed that in states of low O_2, oxygen-sensitive K^+ currents are inhibited, resulting in depolarization, an influx of Ca^{2+} and the release of neurotransmitters and neuromodulators that generate an action potential in the carotid sinus nerve *(86)*. The bradycardia associated with hypoxemia is mediated by parasympathetic efferents, while the initial vasoconstriction results from increased sympathetic tone *(84,87)*. The release of circulating factors such as AVP and catecholamines serves to maintain peripheral vasoconstriction, while heart rate returns toward basal levels.

The ontogeny of fetal chemoreflex-mediated cardiovascular responses to acute hypoxemia has primarily been assessed by studies in sheep via either umbilical cord occlusion or administration of subambient oxygen to the ewe *(84,88–91)*. Responses to moderate hypoxemia appear attenuated in preterm fetuses, possibly related to lower aerobic requirements. However, responses to prolonged asphyxia, induced by umbilical cord occlusion, are comparable in preterm, mid-term, and near-term fetuses, although the rapidity and intensity of peripheral vasoconstriction were attenuated in the younger animals *(91)*. The cardiovascular response to acute fetal hypoxemia depends upon the intrauterine milieu *(85, 92–94)*. For example, in fetal sheep, mild, acute acidemia (pH 7.29 ± 0.01), which often accompanies fetal hypoxemia, has no effects on basal cardiovascular function but markedly enhances peripheral vasoconstriction and endocrine responses to acute hypoxemia *(94)*. Such strong responses likely resulted from acidemia-mediated sensitization of the carotid body, increased sympathetic outflow and stimulation, catecholamine secretion. To examine the effects of prevailing hypoxemia on responses to acute hypoxemia, Gardner et al. *(85)* studied chronically instrumented fetal sheep, which were grouped according to PaO_2. Functional chemoreflex analysis during early hypoxemia, performed by plotting the change in PaO_2 against the change in heart rate and femoral vascular resistance, demonstrated that the slopes of the cardiac and vasoconstrictor chemoreflex curves were enhanced in hypoxic fetuses relative to control fetuses. Additional evidence suggests that exposure to hypoxia for a limited periods of time (hours to days) has a sensitizing effect on the chemoreflex, whereas more sustained hypoxia (days to weeks) may have a desensitizing effect *(93)*. The mechanisms regulating this alteration in response are unclear. In the chick embryo, hypoxia increases sympathetic nerve fiber density and neuronal capacity for norepinephrine synthesis *(95)*. Thus, augmented efferent pathways may contribute to the enhanced responses. On the other hand, recordings from carotid chemoreceptors in chronically hypoxic kittens demonstrate blunted responses to acute decreases in PaO_2 relative to control animals *(96)*. It is therefore possible that with prolonged hypoxia, blunting of the chemoreflex responses may be related to afferent mechanisms.

Although chemoreceptors are active and responsive in the fetus and newborn, studies in sheep and human infants suggest that chemoreceptor sensitivity and activity is reduced immediately after birth *(97,98)*. This decreased sensitivity persists for several days until the chemoreceptors adapt and reset after emerging from the low oxygen tension of the fetus to the higher levels seen postnatally *(98,99)*. The mechanisms involved with this resetting are not known, although the postnatal rise in PaO_2 appears crucial, since raising fetal PaO_2 produces a rightward shift in the response curve of carotid baroreceptors to differing oxygen tension *(100)*. Potential mechanisms within the glomus cells regulating developmental changes in O_2 transduction and chemoreceptor responses include, but are not limited to, anatomic maturation, developmental changes in oxygen-sensitive K^+ currents, adenosine responsiveness *(101,102)*, dopamine and catecholamine turnover within the carotid body *(103)*, and differences in intracellular calcium mobilization during hypoxia *(86,104)*.

SYMPATHETIC ACTIVITY AT BIRTH

The transition from fetal to newborn life is associated with numerous hemodynamic adjustments, including changes in heart rate and peripheral vascular resistance and a redistribution of blood flow *(105,106)*. Activation of the sympathetic nervous system appears to be important in this adaptive process and is associated with marked increases in circulating catecholamines *(107,108)*. Arterial pressure, heart rate, and cardiac output are all depressed by ganglionic blockade in newborn (1–3 days) but this does not occur in older lambs, suggesting that sympathetic tone is high during the immediate postnatal period *(109)*. Our group has demonstrated that renal sympathetic nerve activity increases nearly 250% following delivery of term fetal sheep by cesarean section and parallels the rise in arterial pressure and heart rate *(45)*. Delivery appears to produce near-maximal stimulation of renal sympathetic outflow, since further increases cannot be elicited by unloading of arterial baroreceptors *(45)*. Furthermore, reflex inhibition of this increase in RSNA could not be achieved by arterial baroreceptor stimulation, as seen in fetal and 3–7-day-old lambs *(41)*, suggesting that central influences can override the arterial baroreflex and that the maintenance of a high sympathetic tone is vital during this transition period. A similar pattern of baroreceptor reflex inhibition has been well described in adult animals as part of the defense reaction *(110)*.

The factors that mediate the increase in sympathetic outflow at birth are incompletely understood. In utero ventilation studies of fetal sheep have shown that rhythmic lung inflation increases plasma catecholamine concentrations, although there are no consistent effects on blood pressure or heart rate *(111,112)*. Fetal RSNA increases only 50% during in utero ventilation, while oxygenation and removal of the placental circulation by umbilical cord occlusion produce no additional effect *(113)*, suggesting that lung inflation and an increase in arterial oxygen tension contribute little to the sympathoexcitation process. The increases in heart rate, mean arterial blood pressure, and RSNA following delivery are similar in intact and in fetal lambs that have undergone both sinoaortic denervation and vagotomy *(114)*, demonstrating that afferent input from peripheral chemoreceptors and mechanoreceptors also contributes little to the hemodynamic and sympathetic responses at delivery.

The change in environmental temperature at birth may play an important role in the sympathoexcitatory response at birth. Cooling of the near-term fetus either in utero or in exteriorized preparations results in an increase in heart rate, blood pressure, and norepinephrine concentrations, consistent with sympathoexcitation *(115,116)*.

In contrast, exteriorization of the near-term lamb fetus into a warm water bath does not produce the alterations in systemic hemodynamics or catecholamine values typically seen at birth *(116)*. Fetal cooling, but not ventilation or umbilical cord occlusion, initiates nonshivering thermogenesis via neurally mediated sympathetic stimulation of brown adipose tissue *(117)*. In utero cooling of fetal lambs also produces an increase in RSNA of similar magnitude to that seen at delivery by cesarean section *(49)*, suggesting that cold-stress plays a role in the activation of the sympathetic nervous system at birth. These changes occur before a decrease in core temperature occurs, and are reversible with rewarming, suggesting that sensory input from cutaneous cold-sensitive thermoreceptors rather than a response to a change in core temperature is mediating the response.

Studies in adults suggest that multiple brain centers are involved in autonomic control of the systemic circulation. Sympathetic outflow is controlled not only by the medulla oblongata *(118)*, but also by higher centers, especially the hypothalamus *(119–121)*, allowing for a wide range of modulation. Neuroanatomic studies have shown that nuclei within the hypothalamus project directly to a number of areas in the hindbrain containing preganglionic sympathetic and parasympathetic neurons, including the rostral and caudal ventrolateral medulla, the intermediolateral cell column, and the dorsal motor nucleus of the vagus *(119–121)*. How the supramedullary regions influence cardiovascular function in developing animals is unclear. In fetal sheep, electrical stimulation of the hypothalamus evokes tachycardia and a pressor response, both of which are attenuated by α-adrenoreceptor blockade *(122)*. Stimulation of the dorsolateral medulla and lateral hypothalamus in the newborn piglet similarly increases blood pressure and femoral blood flow *(43)*. Since the responses to hypothalamic stimulation are lost during stress (hypoxia, hypercapnia, hemorrhage), while those elicited from the medulla are not, some investigators have proposed that the hypothalamus exerts little influence of cardiovascular function until later in postnatal development *(43)*. However, other studies suggest that forebrain structures are vital for normal physiological adaptation following the transition from fetal to newborn life. The increases in heart rate, mean arterial blood pressure, and RSNA that normally occur at birth are absent in animals subjected to transection of the brain stem at the level of the rostral pons prior to delivery *(113)*. Ablation of the paraventricular nucleus of the hypothalamus in fetal sheep attenuates the postnatal increase in sympathetic outflow and alters baroreflex function *(123)*. Thus, supramedullary structures appear intimately involved in the regulation of circulatory and autonomic functions during the transition from fetal to newborn life.

The hemodynamic and sympathetic responses at birth are markedly different in prematurely delivered lambs (0.85 of gestation (about 123 days)) compared to those delivered at term *(124)*. Postnatal increases in heart rate and blood pressure are attenuated, and the sympathoexcitatory response, as measured by RSNA, is absent *(124)*. This impaired response occurs despite the fact that the descending pathways of the sympathetic nervous system are intact and functional at this stage of development, as demonstrated by a large pressor and sympathoexcitatory response to in utero cooling *(124)*. Antenatal administration of glucocorticoids, which has been shown to improve both postnatal cardiovascular and pulmonary functions, augments sympathetic activity at birth in premature lambs and decreases the sensitivity of the cardiac baroreflex *(124)*. The mechanisms through which antenatal glucocorticoid administration augments cardiovascular and sympathetic responses at birth are unclear, although stimulation of the peripheral renin–angiotensin system and activation of peripheral angiotensin receptors appear not to be involved *(125)*.

HUMORAL FACTORS

Renin–Angiotensin System in the Fetus and Neonate

The renin–angiotensin system is active in the fetal and perinatal periods *(126–128)*. During embryonic and early fetal life, the primary function of the renin–angiotensin system may be to regulate cellular and organ growth as well as vascular proliferation *(129)*. Only later during fetal development does the renin–angiotensin system become involved in modulating cardiovascular function and renal hemodynamics. A large number of studies report that administration of inhibitors of ANG II, including angiotensin-converting enzyme inhibitors (ACEi's) and angiotensin II subtype 1 receptor blockers (AT_1 blockers, or ARBs), decreases fetal and newborn arterial blood pressure *(127,130–132)*. In normal children, plasma renin activity is high during the newborn period, declines rapidly in the first year of life, and then continues with a gradual decline until adulthood *(133,134)*. In preterm infants, plasma renin activity is markedly elevated and has close inverse relationship to postconceptual age *(135)*.

Fetal plasma renin activity and plasma ANG II concentration increase after aortic constriction, hypotension, and blood volume reduction *(126)*. Conversely, a rise in arterial blood pressure and volume expansion reduce plasma renin activity in fetal and newborn animals *(136)*. The vasopressor response and renal vascular reactivity to exogenous ANG II are less in fetal lambs than in adult sheep *(137)*. Factors explaining the higher activity of the renin–angiotensin system early in development but decreased sensitivity to ANG II have not been explored in detail. One may speculate that differences in the localization and expression of the ANG II receptor subtypes contribute to this effect.

While baroreceptors and chemoreceptors regulate the release of vasoactive hormones, such as ANG II *(46,138)*, changes in the levels of these circulating hormones, in turn, influence neural regulation of cardiovascular function. For example, in the sheep fetus, a rise in arterial blood pressure produced by ANG II administration produces little or no cardiac slowing *(137,139)*, although others have reported dose-dependent decreases in heart rate *(140,141)*. The bradycardic and sympathoinhibitory responses to a given increase in blood pressure are less for ANG II than for other vasoconstrictor agents *(142)*. In the adult ANG II facilitates activation of sympathetic ganglia and enhances the release of norepinephrine at the neuroeffector junction *(143)*. Within the central nervous system, ANG II stimulates sympathetic outflow and alters baroreceptor reflexes by acting on AT_1 receptors located within the hypothalamus, medulla, and circumventricular organs *(144–146)*. In the sheep fetus, endogenous brain ANG II appears to contribute little to basal arterial pressure. However, lateral ventricle injection of ANG II increases blood pressure, an effect blocked by AT_1 receptor antagonists *(147–149)*. Increased blood pressure via activation of angiotensin receptors was associated with elevated c-fos expression (a marker of neuronal activation) in numerous cardiovascular areas known to be AT_1 receptor abundant *(147–149)*. Lateral ventricle administration of an AT_1 but not an ANG II receptor subtype 2 (AT_2) receptor antagonist also lowers blood pressure and resets the baroreflex toward lower pressure in newborn and 8-week-old sheep at doses that have no effect when given systemically *(150)*.

Endogenous circulating ANG II participates in regulating arterial baroreflex responses early during development. The absence of rebound tachycardia after reduction in blood pressure by ACEi is well described in fetal and postnatal animals *(130)*, as well as in human adults and infants *(54)*. In the newborn lamb, angiotensin-converting enzyme inhibition or AT_1 receptor blockade decreases RSNA and heart rate, and resets the baroreflex toward lower pressure *(142,150)*. Resetting of the reflex is independent of changes in prevailing blood pressure.

Arginine Vasopressin in the Fetus and Neonate

Several lines of evidence suggest that arginine vasopressin (AVP) plays an important role in maintaining cardiovascular homeostasis during fetal and postnatal development. Plasma AVP concentrations in the fetus are increased by multiple stimuli, including hypotension, hemorrhage, hypoxemia, acidemia, and hyperosmolality *(138, 151–153)*. Vasopressin responses to hypotension are partially mediated by arterial baroreceptors, whereas the contribution of carotid or aortic chemoreceptors appears to play little role in the AVP response to hypoxia *(154,155)*. Infusion of AVP increases fetal blood pressure and decreases fetal heart rate in a dose-dependent manner *(156,157)*, although AVP appears to have little impact on basal fetal circulatory regulation. Blockade of AVP receptors in fetal sheep has no measurable effects on arterial blood pressure, heart rate, or renal sympathetic nerve activity in fetal sheep or newborn lambs *(158,159)*. However, AVP receptor inhibition impairs the ability of the fetus to maintain blood pressure during hypotensive hemorrhage and reduces the catecholamine response *(160)*.

In several adult mammalian species, AVP modulates parasympathetic and sympathetic tone and baroreflex function *(46,159,161,162)*. Administration of AVP evokes more sympathoinhibition and bradycardia than other vasoconstrictors at a comparable increase in blood pressure *(46,162)*. It has been thought that such baroreflex modulation by AVP is due to enhanced baroreflex gain and resetting of the baroreflex to a lower pressure *(46,162)*. However, in fetal and newborn sheep, sequential increases in plasma AVP do not alter heart rate or RSNA baroreflex responses to acute changes in blood pressure *(159)*.

Endogenous AVP also appears to have little effect on baroreflex function early during development. For instance, peripheral intravenous administration of a V_1-receptor antagonist has no measurable effects on resting hemodynamics in fetal sheep or on basal arterial blood pressure *(158)*, heart rate, RSNA, or baroreflex response in newborn lambs *(159)*. This lack of baroreflex modulation by AVP may facilitate the observed pressor response to AVP in fetuses and newborns during stressful situations such as hypoxia and hemorrhage. Such responses suggest that AVP could play a particularly important role in maintaining arterial pressures during stressful states in early development.

The role of AVP within the central nervous system in maintaining hemodynamic homeostasis in the developing animal has not been extensively studied. Under basal conditions fetal AVP levels are tenfold higher in the cerebrospinal fluid than in plasma, suggesting that AVP contributes to the central regulation of autonomic function (163). Intracerebroventricular infusion of AVP produces significant decreases in mean arterial blood pressure and heart rate in newborn lambs without reflex changes in RSNA *(164)*. In contrast, intracerebroventricular administration of AVP increases RSNA in 8-week-old sheep, demonstrating that the role of AVP receptors within the CNS in regulation of autonomic function is developmentally regulated *(164)*. The changes in blood pressure and heart rate are completely inhibited by administration of a V_1 antagonist, demonstrating that the central cardiovascular effects of AVP are mediated by V_1 receptors, as has been reported in mature animals *(165)*.

Corticosteroids in the Fetus and Neonate

The prepartum surge in fetal cortisol levels, observed in all mammalian species, is vital for normal physiological development. Fetal adrenalectomy attenuates the normal gestational age-dependent increase in blood pressure that occurs in late gestation, while cortisol replacement produces a sustained increase in fetal blood pressure *(166,167)*. Antenatal exposure to exogenous glucocorticoids increases fetal and postnatal arterial blood pressure by enhancing peripheral vascular resistance and cardiac output without altering heart rate *(168–170)*. The effectiveness of hydrocortisone for treatment of hypotension in preterm and term neonates is well described *(171,172)*. However, the mechanisms by which glucocorticoids increase blood pressure and vascular resistance in this age group are not clear. In the adult, administration of hydrocortisone or dexamethasone suppresses resting and stimulated muscle sympathetic nerve activity, suggesting little role for augmented sympathetic tone *(173,174)*. On the other hand, glucocorticoids enhance pressor responsiveness and vascular reactivity to norepinephrine and ANG II *(175,176)*, in part by increasing α_1-adrenergic and AT_1 receptor levels and potentiating ANG II- and AVP-induced inositol triphosphate production *(177,178)*. Glucocorticoids also reduce the activity of depressor systems, including vasodilator prostaglandins and nitric oxide, and have been shown to decrease serum $NO2^-/NO3^-$, endothelial nitric oxide synthase mRNA stability, and protein levels *(179)*.

In the sheep fetus, cortisol infusion increases blood pressure, as well as the hypertensive response to intravenous ANG II but not to norepinephrine *(166)*. However, infusions of synthetic glucocorticoids, which also increase arterial blood pressure, do not alter the pressor response to phenylephrine, ANG II, or AVP *(180)*. Furthermore, the increase in blood pressure is not inhibited by blockade of the renin–angiotensin system *(125)*. In vitro studies demonstrate that fetal treatment with betamethasone enhances the contractile response of femoral arteries to depolarizing potassium solutions, supporting a role for enhanced calcium channel activation *(181)*. Glucocorticoid exposure enhances in vitro responses of peripheral arteries to vasoconstrictors, including norepinephrine and endothelin 1, while attenuating vasodilator effects of forskolin and bradykinin and nitric oxide production *(181–184)*.

In addition to peripheral effects on vascular reactivity, antenatal glucocorticoids also modify autonomic and endocrine functions. Increases in fetal blood pressure and vascular resistance following betamethasone treatment occur despite marked suppression of circulating vasoconstrictors, including catecholamines, ANG II, and AVP *(124,168,185)*. Circulating neuropeptide Y concentration, which may provide an index of peripheral sympathetic activity, is increased following fetal exposure to dexamethasone *(186)*. Glucocorticoid treatment accelerates postnatal maturation of brain catecholaminergic signaling pathways in rats and enhances renal sympathetic nerve activity in prematurely delivered lambs *(71,187,188)*.

Endogenous production of cortisol is important for normal maturational changes in autonomic reflex function. Adrenalectomized fetal sheep fail to display the normal postnatal increase in RSNA, while the response is restored by cortisol replacement *(189)*. Restoring circulating cortisol levels to the prepartum physiological range shifts the fetal and immediate postnatal heart rate and RSNA baroreflex curves toward higher pressure without altering the slope of the curves *(189)*. Antenatal administration of betamethasone decreases the sensitivity of baroreflex-mediated changes in heart rate in preterm fetuses and premature lambs *(124)*. Antenatal glucocorticoid exposure also alters baroreflex and chemoreflex function in fetal and newborn animals *(180,187)*. Baroreflex control of heart rate and RSNA are reset toward higher pressures in steroid-exposed animals. In response to acute hypoxia, fetuses exposed to exogenous corticosteroids display prolonged bradycardia and attenuated plasma catecholamine and AVP responses *(186)*. Consistent with this finding, ovine fetuses at >140 days gestation (term 145 days) and with naturally elevated cortisol levels displayed greater heart rate, vasoconstrictor, and neuroendocrine responses to hypoxemia than fetuses at 125–140 days gestation *(92)*. At all gestational ages the responses to hypoxemia correlated with the prevailing cortisol concentration. Taken together, these findings indicate that corticosteroids modify autonomic and endocrine control of cardiovascular function during development. These effects may even persist well after cessation of exposure *(186)*.

Nitric Oxide in the Fetus and Neonate

Nitric oxide (NO) plays an important role in the control of systemic hemodynamics early in development. Nitric oxide regulates fetal vascular tone, blood pressure, and organ-specific vascular resistance. Inhibition of NO production causes an immediate rise in blood pressure and umbilicoplacental resistance, and decreases in heart rate, renal blood flow velocity, and plasma renin concentration *(190–192)*. These cardiovascular effects are significantly attenuated by prolonged or repeated exposure to NO synthesis inhibition, indicating that other vasodilatory regulatory mechanisms are functioning during fetal life *(190)*. Nitric oxide also functions as a neurotransmitter and acts centrally to regulate fetal arterial blood pressure. Administration of the NO donor, nitroglycerin, into the fourth cerebral ventricle of the ovine fetus decreases mean arterial pressure, whereas blocking NO synthase in the fourth ventricle increases fetal blood pressure *(193)*. Inhibition of endogenously produced NO also increases blood pressure in 1- and 6-week-old lambs to similar extents, although the concomitant decreases in heart rate are greater in the young lamb *(194)*. Endogenous nitric oxide regulates arterial baroreflex control of heart rate in 1-week-old but not 6-week-old lambs and may contribute to developmental changes in baroreflex function during this period *(194)*.

CONCLUSIONS

Understanding the mechanisms regulating cardiovascular function in the fetal and post-natal periods, particularly as they relate to the transition from fetal to newborn life, is important. Failure to regulate arterial pressure, peripheral resistance, and organ blood flow may lead to significant variations in substrate delivery, resulting in ischemic or hemorrhagic injury. Autonomic regulatory mechanisms, including baroreceptors and chemoreceptors, are important modulators of blood pressure and circulatory function early in life. Humoral and endocrine factors, not only those discussed above, but others such as opioids, natriuretic peptides, and prostanoids, act directly and indirectly to regulate vascular tone and cardiac function. A more complete understanding of neurohumoral control of cardiovascular function early in life may potentially lead to the development of new therapeutic strategies to prevent complications during the perinatal period.

REFERENCES

1. Spyer KM. Central nervous mechanisms contributing to cardiovascular control. J Physiol. 1994;474:1–19.
2. Tabsh K, Nuwayhid B, Ushioda E, Erkkola R, Brinkman CR, Assali NS. Circulatory effects of chemical sympathectomy in fetal, neonatal and adult sheep. Am J Physiol. 1982;243:H113–H122.

3. Vapaavouri EK, Shinebourne EA, Williams RL, Heymann MA, Rudolph AM. Development of cardiovascular responses to autonomic blockade in intact fetal and neonatal lambs. Biol Neonate. 1973;22:177–188.

4. Walker AM, Cannata J, Dowling MH, Ritchie B, Maloney JE. Sympathetic and parasympathetic control of heart rate in unanaesthetized fetal and newborn lambs. Biol Neonate. 1978;33:135–143.

5. Nuwayhid B, Brinkman CR, Bevan JA, Assali NS. Development of autonomic control of fetal circulation. Am J Physiol. 1975;228:237–344.

6. Woods JR, Dandavino A, Murayama K, Brinkman CR, Assali NS. Autonomic control of cardiovascular functions during neonatal development and in adult sheep. Circ Res. 1977;40:401–407.

7. Alper RH, Jacob JH, Brody MJ. Regulation of arterial pressure lability in rats with chronic sinoaortic deafferentation. Am J Physiol. 1987;253:H466–H474.

8. Barres C, Lewis SJ, Jacob HJ, Brody MJ. Arterial pressure lability and renal sympathetic nerve activity are disassociated in SAD rats. Am J Physiol. 1992;263:R639–R646.

9. Segar JL, Merrill DC, Smith BA, Robillard JE. Role of sympathetic activity in the generation of heart rate and arterial pressure variability in fetal sheep. Pediatr Res. 1994;35:250–254.

10. Yardly RW, Bowes G, Wilkinson M, et al. Increased arterial pressure variability after arterial baroreceptor denervation in fetal lambs. Circ Res. 1983;52:580–588.

11. Robillard JE, Nakamura KT, DiBona GF. Effects of renal denervation on renal responses to hypoxemia in fetal lambs. Am J Physiol. 1986;250(2 Pt 2):F294–F301.

12. Clapp JF, Szeto HH, Abrams R, Mann LI. Physiologic variability and fetal electrocortical activity. Am J Obstet Gynecol. 1980;136:1045–1050.

13. Mann LI, Duchin S, Weiss RR. Fetal EEG sleep stages and physiologic variability. Am J Obstet Gynecol. 1974;119:533–538.

14. Reid DL, Jensen A, Phernetton TM, Rankin JHG. Relationship between plasma catecholamine levels and electrocortical state in the mature fetal lamb. J Dev Physiol. 1990;13:75–79.

15. Wakatsuki A, Murata Y, Ninomoya Y, Masaoka N, Tyner JG, Kutty KK. Physiologic baroreceptor activity in the fetal lamb. Am J Obstet Gynecol. 1992;167:820–827.

16. Jensen A, Bamford OS, Dawes GS, Hofmeyr G, Parkes MJ. Changes in organ blood flow between high and low voltage electrocortical activity in fetal sheep. J Dev Physiol. 1986;8:187–194.

17. Richardson BS, Patrick JE, Abduljabbar H. Cerebral oxidative metabolism in the fetal lamb: relationship to electrocortical state. Am J Obstet Gynecol. 1985;153:426–431.

18. Abboud F, Thames M. Interaction of cardiovascular reflexes in circulatory control. In: Shepherd JT, Abboud FM, eds. Handbook of Physiology, Section 2, Vol III, Part 2. Bethesda, MD: American Physiological Society; 1983:675–753.

19. Persson PB, Ehmke H, Kirchheim HR. Cardiopulmonary-arterial baroreceptor interaction in control of blood pressure. NIPS. 1989;4:56–59.

20. Yu ZY, Lumbers ER. Measurement of baroreceptor-mediated effects on heart rate variability in fetal sheep. Pediatr Res. 2000;47:233–239.

21. Brinkman CRI, Ladner C, Weston P, Assali NS. Baroreceptor functions in the fetal lamb. Am J Physiol. 1969;217:1346–1351.

22. Itskovitz J, LaGamma EF, Rudolph AM. Baroreflex control of the circulation in chronically instrumented fetal lambs. Circ Res. 1983;52:589–596.

23. Biscoe TJ, Purves MJ, Sampson SR. Types of nervous activity which may be recorded from the carotid sinus nerve in the sheep foetus. J Physiol. 1969;202:1–23.

24. Blanco CE, Dawes GS, Hanson MA, McCooke HB. Carotid baroreceptors in fetal and newborn sheep. Pediatr Res. 1988;24:342–346.

25. Downing SE. Baroreceptor reflexes in new-born rabbits. J Physiol. 1960; 150:201–213.

26. Ponte J, Purves MJ. Types of afferent nervous activity which may be measured in the vagus nerve of the sheep foetus. J Physiol. 1973;229:51–76.

27. Tomomatsu E, Nishi K. Comparison of carotid sinus baroreceptor sensitivity in newborn and adult rabbits. Am J Physiol. 1982;243:H546–H550.

28. Andresen MC. Short and long-term determinants of baroreceptor function in aged normotensive and spontaneously hypertensive rats. Circ Res. 1984;54:750–759.

29. Chapleau MW, Hajduczok G, Abboud FM. Mechanisms of resetting of arterial baroreceptors: an overview. Am J Med Sci. 1988;295:327–334.

30. Chapleau MW, Hajduczok G, Abboud FM. Resetting of the arterial baroreflex: peripheral and central mechanisms. In: Zucker IH, Gilmore JP, eds. Reflex Control of the Circulation. Boca Raton, FL: CRC Press; 1991:165–194.

31. Heesch CM, Abboud FM, Thames MD. Acute resetting of carotid sinus baroreceptors. II. Possible involvement of electrogenic Na+ pump. Am J Physiol. 1984;247:H833–H839.

32. Jimbo M, Suzuki H, Ichikawa M, Kumagai K, Nishizawa M, Saruta T. Role of nitric oxide in regulation of baroreceptor reflex. J Auton Nerv Syst. 1994;50:209–219.

33. Matsuda T, Bates JN, Lewis SJ, Abboud FM, Chapleau MW. Modulation of baroreceptor activity by nitric oxide and S-nitrosocysteine. Circ Res. 1995;76(3):426–433.

34. Bauer DJ. Vagal reflexes appearing in the rabbit at different ages. J Physiol. 1939;95:187–202.

35. Dawes GS, Johnston BM, Walker DW. Relationship of arterial pressure and heart rate in fetal, new-born and adult sheep. J Physiol. 1980;309:405–417.

36. Shinebourne EA, Vapaavuori EK, Williams RL, Heymann MA, Rudolph AM. Development of baroreflex activity in unanesthetized fetal and neonatal lambs. Circ Res. 1972;31:710–718.

37. Vatner SF, Manders WT. Depressed responsiveness of the carotid sinus reflex in conscious newborn animals. Am J Physiol. 1979;237:H40–H43.

38. Young M. Responses of the systemic circulation of the new-born infant. Br Med Bull. 1966;22:70–72.

39. Booth LC, Malpas SC, Barrett CJ, Guild SJ, Gunn AJ, Bennet L. Is baroreflex control of sympathetic activity and heart rate active in the preterm fetal sheep? Am J Physiol Regul Integr Comp Physiol. 2009;296(3):R603–R609.

40. O'Connor SJ, Ousey JC, Gardner DS, Fowden AL, Giussani DA. Development of baroreflex function and hind limb vascular reactivity in the horse fetus. J Physiol. 2006;572(Pt 1):155–164.

41. Segar JL, Hajduczok G, Smith BA, Robillard JE. Ontogeny of baroreflex control of renal sympathetic nerve activity and heart rate. Am J Physiol. 1992;263:H1819–H1826.

42. Buckley NM, Gootman PM, Gootman GD, Reddy LC, Weaver LC, Crane LA. Age-dependent cardiovascular effects of afferent stimulation in neonatal pigs. Biol Neonate. 1976;30:268–279.

43. Gootman PM. Developmental aspects of reflex control of the circulation. In: Zucker IH, Gilmore JP, eds. Reflex Control of the Circulation. Boca Raton, FL: CRC Press; 1991:965–1027.

44. Hajduczok G, Chapleau MW, Johnson SL, Abboud FM. Increase in sympathetic activity with age. I. Role of impairment of arterial baroreflexes. Am J Physiol. 1991;260:H1113–H1120.

45. Segar JL, Mazursky JE, Robillard JE. Changes in ovine renal sympathetic nerve activity and baroreflex function at birth. Am J Physiol. 1994;267:H1824–H1832.

46. Bishop VS, Haywood JR. Hormonal control of cardiovascular reflexes. In: Zucker IH, Gilmore JP, eds. Reflex Control of the Circulation. Boca Raton, FL: CRC Press; 1991:253–271.

47. Picton-Warlow CG, Mayer FE. Cardiovascular responses to postural changes in the neonate. Arch Dis Child. 1970;45:354–359.

48. Thoresen M, Cowan F, Walløe L. Cardiovascular responses to tilting in healthy newborn babies. Early Hum Dev. 1991;26:213–222.

49. Waldman S, Krauss AN, Auld PAM. Baroreceptors in preterm infants: their relationship to maturity and disease. Dev Med Child Neurol. 1979;21:714–722.

50. Myers MM, Gomez-Gribben E, Smith KS, Tseng A, Fifer WP. Developmental changes in infant heart rate responses to head-up tilting. Acta Paediatr. Jan 2006;95(1):77–81.

51. Fifer WP, Greene M, Hurtado A, Myers MM. Cardiorespiratory responses to bidirectional tilts in infants. Early Hum Dev. Jul 1999;55(3):265–279.

52. Gournay V, Drouin E, Roze JC. Development of baroreflex control of heart rate in preterm and full term infants. Arch Dis Child Fetal Neonatal Ed. May 2002;86(3):F151–F154.

53. Andriessen P, Oetomo SB, Peters C, Vermeulen B, Wijn PF, Blanco CE. Baroreceptor reflex sensitivity in human neonates: the effect of postmenstrual age. J Physiol. Oct 1 2005;568(Pt 1):333–341.

54. Chatow U, Davidson S, Reichman BL, Akselrod S. Development and maturation of the autonomic nervous system in premature and full-term infants using spectral analysis of heart rate fluctuations. Pediatr Res. 1995;37:294–302.

55. Clairambault J, Curzi-Dascalova L, Kauffmann F, Médigue C, Leffler C. Heart rate variability in normal sleeping full-term and preterm neonates. Early Human Dev. 1992;28:169–183.

56. David M, Hirsch M, Karin J, Toledo E, Akselrod S. An estimate of fetal autonomic state by time-frequency analysis of fetal heart rate variability. J Appl Physiol. Mar 2007;102(3):1057–1064.

57. Karin J, Hirsch M, Akselrod S. An estimate of fetal autonomic state by spectral analysis of fetal heart rate fluctuations. Pediatr Res. Aug 1993;34(2):134–138.

58. Schneider U, Schleussner E, Fiedler A, et al. Fetal heart rate variability reveals differential dynamics in the intrauterine development of the sympathetic and parasympathetic branches of the autonomic nervous system. Physiol Meas. Feb 2009;30(2):215–226.

59. Mazursky JE, Birkett CL, Bedell KA, Ben-Haim SA, Segar JL. Development of baroreflex influences on heart rate variability in preterm infants. Early Hum Dev. 1998;53:37–52.

60. Minisi AJ, Thames MD. Reflexes from ventricular receptors with vagal afferents. In: Zucker IH, Gilmore JP, eds. Reflex Control of the Circulation. Boca Raton, FL: CRC Press; 1991:359.

61. Goetz KL, Madwed JB, Leadley RJJ. Atrial receptors: reflex effects in quadripeds. In: Zucker IH, Gilmore JP, eds. Reflex Control of the Circulation. Boca Raton, FL: CRC Press; 1991:291.
62. Hainsworth R. Reflexes from the heart. Physiol Rev. 1991;71:617–658.
63. Togashi H, Yoshioka M, Tochihara M, Matsumoto M, Saito H. Differential effects of hemorrhage on adrenal and renal nerve activity in anesthetized rats. Am J Physiol. 1990;259:H1134–H1141.
64. Victor RG, Thoren PN, Morgan DA, Mark AL. Differential control of adrenal and renal sympathetic nerve activity during hemorrhagic hypertension in rats. Circ Res. 1989;64:686–694.
65. Baker DG, Coleridge HM, Coleridge JCG. Vagal afferent C fibers from the ventricle. In: Hainsworth R, Kidd C, Linden RJ, eds. Cardiac Receptors. Cambridge: Cambridge University Press; 1979:117.
66. Gupta BN, Thames MD. Behavior of left ventricular mechanoreceptors with myelinated and nonmyelinated afferent vagal fibers in cats. Circ Res. 1983;52:291–301.
67. Thames MD, Donald SE, Shepherd JT. Stimulation of cardiac receptors with veratrum alkaloids inhibits ADH secretion. Am J Physiol. 1980;239:H784–H788.
68. Assali NS, Brinkman CR, Wood R Jr, Danavino A, Nuwayhid B. Ontogenesis of the autonomic control of cardiovascular function in the sheep. In: Longo LD, Reneau DD, eds. Fetal and Newborn Cardiovascular Physiology. New York, NY: Garland STPM Press; 1978:47–91.
69. Gootman PM, Buckley BJ, DiRusso SM, et al. Age-related responses to stimulation of cardiopulmonary receptors in swine. Am J Physiol. 1986;251:H748–H755.
70. Merrill DC, Segar JL, McWeeny OJ, Smith BA, Robillard JE. Cardiopulmonary and arterial baroreflex responses to acute volume expansion during fetal and postnatal development. Am J Physiol. 1994;267:H1467–H1475.
71. Smith F, Klinkefus J, Robillard J. Effects on volume expansion on renal sympathetic nerve activity and cardiovascular and renal function in lambs. Am J Physiol. 1992;262:R651–R658.
72. Merrill DC, McWeeny OJ, Segar JL, Robillard JE. Impairment of cardiopulmonary baroreflexes during the newborn period. Am J Physiol. 1995;268:H1343–H1351.
73. Gomez RA, Meernik JG, Kuehl WD, Robillard JE. Developmental aspects of the renal response to hemorrhage during fetal life. Pediatr Res. 1984;18:40–46.
74. Chen H-G, Wood CE, Bell ME. Reflex control of fetal arterial pressure and hormonal responses to slow hemorrhage. Am J Physiol. 1992;262:H225–H233.
75. Toubas PL, Silverman NH, Heymann MA, Rudolph AM. Cardiovascular effects of acute hemorrhage in fetal lambs. Am J Physiol. 1981;240:H45–H48.
76. Wood CE, Chen H-G, Bell ME. Role of vagosympathetic fibers in the control of adrenocorticotropic hormone, vasopressin, and renin responses to hemorrhage in fetal sheep. Circ Res. 1989;64:515–523.
77. O'Mara MS, Merrill DC, McWeeny OJ, Robillard JE. Ontogeny and regulation of arterial and cardiopulmonary baroreflex control of renal sympathetic nerve activity (RSNA) in response to hypotensive (NH) and hypotensive hemorrhage (HH) postnatally. Pediatr Res. 1995;37:31A.
78. Smith FG, Abu-Amarah I. Renal denervation alters cardiovascular and endocrine responses to hemorrhage in conscious newborn lambs. Am J Physiol. 1998;275:H285–H291.
79. Merrill DC, Segar JL, McWeeny OJ, Robillard JE. Sympathetic responses to cardiopulmonary vagal afferent stimulation during development. Am J Physiol. 1999;277:H1311–H1316.
80. Cornish KG, Barazanji MW, Yong T, Gilmore JP. Volume expansion attenuates baroreflex sensitivity in the conscious nonhuman primate. Am J Physiol. 1989;257:R595–R598.
81. Hajduczok G, Chapleau MW, Abboud FM. Increase in sympathetic activity with age: II. Role of impairment of cardiopulmonary baroreflexes. Am J Physiol. 1991;260:H1121–H1127.
82. Bishop VS, Hasser EM, Nair UC. Baroreflex control of renal nerve activity in conscious animals. Circ Res. 1987;61:I76–I81.
83. Cohn HE, Sacks EJ, Heymann MA, Rudolph AM. Cardiovascular responses to hypoxemia and acidemia in fetal lambs. Am J Obstet Gynecol. 1974;120(6):817–824.
84. Giussani DA, Spencer JAD, Moore PJ, Bennet L, Hanson MA. Afferent and efferent components of the cardiovascular reflex responses to acute hypoxia in term fetal sheep. J Physiol. 1993;461:431–449.
85. Gardner DS, Fletcher JW, Bloomfield MR, Fowden AL, Giussani DA. Effects of prevailing hypoxaemia, acidaemia or hypoglycaemia upon the cardiovascular, endocrine and metabolic responses to acute hypoxaemia in the ovine fetus. J Physiol. 2002;540:351–366.
86. Carroll JL, Kim I. Postnatal development of carotid body glomus cell O2 sensitivity. Respir Physiol Neurobiol. 2005;149(1–3):201–215.
87. Iwamota HS, Rudolph AM, Mirkin BL, Keil LC. Circulatory and humoral responses of sympathectomized fetal sheep to hypoxemia. Am J Physiol. 1983;245:H767–H772.
88. Bennet L, Rossenrode S, Gunning MI, Gluckman PD, Gunn AJ. The cardiovascular and cerebrovascular responses of the immature fetal sheep to acute umbilical cord occlusion. J Physiol. May 15 1999;517(Pt 1):247–257.

89. Iwamoto HS, Kaufman T, Keil LC, Rudolph AM. Responses to acute hypoxemia in fetal sheep at 0.6–0.7 gestation. Am J Physiol. Mar 1989;256(3 Pt 2):H613–H620.

90. Szymonowicz W, Walker AM, Yu VY, Stewart ML, Cannata J, Cussen L. Regional cerebral blood flow after hemorrhagic hypotension in the preterm, near-term, and newborn lamb. Pediatr Res. Oct 1990;28(4):361–366.

91. Wassink G, Bennet L, Booth LC, et al. The ontogeny of hemodynamic responses to prolonged umbilical cord occlusion in fetal sheep. J Appl Physiol. Oct 2007;103(4):1311–1317.

92. Fletcher AJ, Gardner DS, Edwards CM, Fowden AL, Giussani DA. Development of the ovine fetal cardiovascular defense to hypoxemia towards full term. Am J Physiol Heart Circ Physiol. Dec 2006;291(6):H3023–H3034.

93. Hanson MA. Role of chemoreceptors in effects of chronic hypoxia. Comp Biochem Physiol. 1997;119A:695–703.

94. Thakor AS, Giussani DA. Effects of acute acidemia on the fetal cardiovascular defense to acute hypoxemia. Am J Physiol Regul Integr Comp Physiol. Jan 2009;296(1):R90–R99.

95. Ruijtenbeek K, LeNoble FA, Janssen GM, et al. Chronic hypoxia stimulates periarterial sympathetic nerve development in chicken embryo. Circulation. 2000;102:2892–2897.

96. Hanson MA, Kumar P, Williams BA. The effect of chronic hypoxia upon the development of respiratory chemoreflexes in the newborn kitten. J Physiol. Apr 1989;411:563–574.

97. Blanco CE, Dawes GS, Hanson MA, McCooke HB. The response to hypoxia of arterial chemoreceptors in fetal sheep and newborn lambs. J Physiol. 1984;351:25–37.

98. Hertzberg T, Lagercrantz H. Postnatal sensitivity of the peripheral chemoreceptors in newborn infants. Arch Dis Child. 1987;62:1238–1241.

99. Kumar P, Hanson MA. Re-setting of the hypoxic sensitivity of aortic chemoreceptors in the new-born lamb. J Dev Physiol. 1989;11:199–206.

100. Blanco CE, Hanson MA, McCooke HB. Effects on carotid chemoreceptor resetting of pulmonary ventilation in the fetal lamb in utero. J Dev Physiol. Apr 1988;10(2):167–174.

101. Koos BJ, Chau A, Ogunyemi D. Adenosine mediates metabolic and cardiovascular responses to hypoxia in fetal sheep. J Physiol (Lond). 1995;488:761–766.

102. Koos BJ, Maeda T. Adenosine A2A receptors mediate cardiovascular responses to hypoxia in fetal sheep. Am J Physiol. 2001;280:H83–H89.

103. Hertzberg T, Hellstrom S, Holgert H, Lagercrantz H, Pequignot JM. Ventilatory response to hyperoxia in newborn rats born in hypoxia—possible relationship to carotid body dopamine. J Physiol. Oct 1992;456:645–654.

104. Sterni LM, Bamford OS, Tomares SM, Montrose MH, Carroll JL. Developmental changes in intracellular Ca2+ response of carotid chemoreceptor cells to hypoxia. Am J Physiol. 1995;268:L801–L808.

105. Dawes GS. Changes in the circulation at birth. Br Med Bull. 1961;17:148–153.

106. Padbury JF, Martinez AM. Sympathoadrenal system activity at birth: integration of postnatal adaptation. Semin Perinatol. 1988;12:163–172.

107. Lagercrantz H, Bistoletti P. Catecholamine release in the newborn at birth. Pediatr Res. 1973;11:889–893.

108. Padbury JF, Diakomanolis ES, Hobel CJ, Perlman A, Fisher DA. Neonatal adaptation: sympatho-adrenal response to umbilical cord cutting. Pediatr Res. 1981;15:1483–1487.

109. Minoura S, Gilbert RD. Postnatal changes of cardiac function in lambs: effects of ganglionic block and afterload. J Dev Physiol. 1986;9:123–135.

110. Hilton SM. The defense-arousal system and its relevance for circulatory and respiratory control. J Exp Biol. 1982;100:159–174.

111. Ogundipe OA, Kullama LK, Stein H, et al. Fetal endocrine and renal responses to in utero ventilation and umbilical cord occlusion. Am J Obstet Gynecol. 1993;169:1479–1486.

112. Smith FG, Smith BA, Segar JL, Robillard JE. Endocrine effects of ventilation, oxygenation and cord occlusion in near-term fetal sheep. J Dev Physiol. 1991;15:133–138.

113. Mazursky JE, Segar JL, Nuyt A-M, Smith BA, Robillard JE. Regulation of renal sympathetic nerve activity at birth. Am J Physiol. 1996;270:R86–R93.

114. Segar JL, Smith OJ, Holley AT. Mechano- and chemoreceptor modulation of renal sympathetic nerve activity at birth in fetal sheep. Am J Physiol. 1999;276:R1295–R1301.

115. Gunn TR, Johnston BM, Iwamoto HS, Fraser M, Nicholls MG, Gluckman PD. Haemodynamic and catecholamine responses to hypothermia in the fetal sheep in utero. J Dev Physiol. 1985;7:241–249.

116. Van Bel F, Roman C, Iwamoto HS, Rudolph AM. Sympathoadrenal, metabolic, and regional blood flow responses to cold in fetal sheep. Pediatr Res. 1993;34:47–50.

117. Gunn TR, Ball KT, Power GG, Gluckman PD. Factors influencing the initiation of nonshivering thermogenesis. Am J Obstet Gynecol. 1991;164:210–217.

118. Calaresu FR, Yardley CP. Medullary basal sympathetic tone. Ann Rev Physiol. 1988;50:511–524.

119. Gebber GL. Central determinants of sympathetic nerve discharge. In: Loewy AD, Spyer KM, eds. Central Regulation of Autonomic Function. New York, NY: Oxford University Press; 1990:126–144.

120. Strack AM, Sawyer WB, Platt KB, Loewy AD. CNS cell groups regulating the sympathetic outflow to adrenal gland as revealed by transneuronal cell body labeling with pseudorabies virus. Brain Res. Jul 10 1989;491(2):274–296.

121. Swanson LW, Sawchenko PE. Hypothalamic integration: organization of the paraventricular and supraoptic nuclei. Annu Rev Neurosci. 1983;6:269–324.

122. Williams RL, Hof RP, Heymann MA, Rudolph AM. Cardiovascular effects of electrical stimulation of the forebrain in the fetal lamb. Pediatr Res. 1976;10:40–45.

123. Segar JL, Ellsbury DL, Smith OM. Inhibition of sympathetic responses at birth in sheep by lesion of the paraventricular nucleus. Am J Physiol. 2002;283:R1395–R1403.

124. Segar JL, Lumbers ER, Nuyt AM, Smith OJ, Robillard JE. Effect of antenatal glucocorticoids on sympathetic nerve activity at birth in preterm sheep. Am J Physiol. 1998;274:R160–R167.

125. Segar JL, Bedell KA, Smith OJ. Glucocorticoid modulation of cardiovascular and autonomic function in preterm lambs: role of ANG II. Am J Physiol. 2001;280:R646–R654.

126. Guillery EN, Robillard JE. The renin-angiotensin system and blood pressure regulation during infancy and childhood. In: Rocchini AP, ed. The Pediatric Clinics of North America: Childhood Hypertension. Philadelphia, PA: W.B. Saunders; 1993:61–77.

127. Iwamota HS, Rudolph AM. Effects of endogenous angiotensin II on the fetal circulation. J Dev Physiol. 1979;1:283–293.

128. Lumbers ER. Functions of the renin-angiotensin system during development. Clin Exp Pharmacol Physiol. 1995;22:499–505.

129. Kim S, Iwao H. Molecular and cellular mechanisms of angiotensin II-mediated cardiovascular and renal diseases. Pharmacol Rev. 2001;52:11–34.

130. Robillard JE, Weismann DN, Gomez RA, Ayres NA, Lawton WJ, VanOrden DE. Renal and adrenal responses to converting-enzyme inhibition in fetal and newborn life. Am J Physiol. 1983;244:R249–R256.

131. Scroop GC, Stankewytsch-Janusch B, Marker JD. Renin-angiotensin and automatic mechanisms in cardiovascular homeostasis during hemorrhage in fetal and neonatal sheep. J Dev Physiol. 1992;18:25–33.

132. Weismann DN, Herrig JE, McWeeny OJ, Ayres NA, Robillard JE. Renal and adrenal responses to hypoxemia during angiotensin-converting enzyme inhibition in lambs. Circ Res. 1983;52:179–187.

133. Bartunek J, Weinberg EO, Tajima M, Rohrbach S, Lorell BH. Angiotensin II type 2 receptor blockade amplifies the early signals of cardiac growth response to angiotensin II in hypertrophied hearts. Circulation. 1999;99:22–25.

134. Stalker HB, Holland NH, Kotchen JM, Kotchen TA. Plasma renin activity in healthy children. J Pediatr. 1976;89:256–258.

135. Richer C, Hornych H, Amiel-Tison C, Relier JP, Giudicelli JF. Plasma renin activity and its postnatal development in preterm infants. Preliminary report. Biol Neonate. 1977;31:301–304.

136. Robillard JE, Weitzman RE. Developmental aspects of the fetal renal response to exogenous arginine vasopressin. Am J Physiol. 1980;238:F407–F414.

137. Robillard JE, Gomez RA, VanOrden D, Smith FG Jr. Comparison of the adrenal and renal responses to angiotensin II in fetal lambs and adult sheep. Circ Res. 1982;50:140–147.

138. Wood CE. Baroreflex and chemoreflex control of fetal hormone secretion. Reprod, Fertil Dev. 1995;7:479–489.

139. Jones III OW, Cheung CY, Brace RA. Dose-dependent effects of angiotensin II on the ovine fetal cardiovascular system. Am J Obstet Gynecol. 1991;165:1524–1533.

140. Ismay MJ, Lumbers ER, Stevens AD. The action of angiotensin II on the baroreflex response of the conscious ewe and the conscious fetus. J Physiol. 1979;288:467–479.

141. Scroop GC, Marker JD, Stankewytsch B, Seamark RF. Angiotensin I and II in the assessment of baroreceptor function in fetal and neonatal sheep. J Dev Physiol. 1986;8:123–137.

142. Segar JL, Merrill DC, Smith BA, Robillard JE. Role of endogenous angiotensin II on resetting of the arterial baroreflex during development. Am J Physiol. 1994;266:H52–H59.

143. Reid IA. Interactions between ANG II, sympathetic nervous system and baroreceptor reflex in regulation of blood pressure. Am J Physiol. 1992;262:E763–E778.

144. Bunnemann B, Fuxe K, Ganten D. The renin-angiotensin system in the brain: an update 1993. Regul Pept. 1993;46:487–509.

145. Head GA, Mayorov DN. Central angiotensin and baroreceptor control of circulation. Ann N Y Acad Sci. 2001;940:361–379.

146. Toney GM, Porter JP. Effects of blockade of AT1 and AT2 receptors in brain on the central angiotensin II pressor response in conscious spontaneously hypertensive rats. Neuropharmacology. 1993;32:581–589.

147. Shi L, Mao C, Thornton SN, et al. Effects of intracerebroventricular losartan on angiotensin II-mediated pressor responses and c-fos expression in near-term ovine fetus. J Comp Neurol. Dec 26 2005;493(4):571–579.

148. Xu Z, Shi L, Hu F, White R, Stewart L, Yao J. In utero development of central ANG-stimulated pressor response and hypothalamic fos expression. Brain Res Dev Brain Res. Nov 12 2003;145(2):169–176.

149. Xu Z, Shi L, Yao J. Central angiotensin II-induced pressor responses and neural activity in utero and hypothalamic angiotensin receptors in preterm ovine fetus. Am J Physiol Heart Circ Physiol. Apr 2004;286(4):H1507–H1514.

150. Segar JL, Minnick A, Nuyt AM, Robillard JE. Role of endogenous ANG II and AT1 receptors in regulating arterial baroreflex responses in newborn lambs. Am J Physiol. 1997;272:R1862–R1873.

151. Robillard JE, Weitzman RE, Fisher DA, Smith FG Jr. The dynamics of vasopressin release and blood volume regulation during fetal hemorrhage in the lamb fetus. Pediatr Res. 1979;13:606–610.

152. Weitzman RE, Fisher DA, Robillard J, Erenberg A, Kennedy R, Smith F. Arginine vasopressin response to an osmotic stimulus in the fetal sheep. Pediatr Res. 1978;12:35–38.

153. Wood CE, Chen HG. Acidemia stimulates ACTH, vasopressin, and heart rate responses in fetal sheep. Am J Physiol. 1989;257:R344–R349.

154. Giussani DA, McGarrigle HHG, Spencer JAD, Moore PJ, Bennet L, Hanson MA. Effect of carotid denervation on plasma vasopressin levels during acute hypoxia in the late-gestation sheep fetus. J Physiol. 1994;477:81–87.

155. Raff H, Kane CW, Wood CE. Arginine vasopressin responses to hypoxia and hypercapnia in late-gestation fetal sheep. Am J Physiol. 1991;260:R1077–R1081.

156. Irion GL, Mack CE, Clark KE. Fetal hemodynamic and fetoplacental vasopressin response to exogenous arginine vasopressin. Am J Obstet Gynecol. 1990;162:115–120.

157. Tomita H, Brace RA, Cheung CY, Longo LD. Vasopressin dose-response effects on fetal vascular pressures, heart rate, and blood volume. Am J Physiol. 1985;249:H974–H980.

158. Ervin MG, Ross MG, Leake RD, Fisher DA. V1 and V2-receptor contributions to ovine fetal renal and cardiovascular responses to vasopressin. Am J Physiol. 1992;262:R636–R643.

159. Nuyt A-M, Segar JL, Holley AT, O'Mara MS, Chapleau MW, Robillard JE. Arginine vasopressin modulation of arterial baroreflex responses in fetal and newborn sheep. Am J Physiol. 1996;271:R1643–R1653.

160. Kelly RT, Rose JC, Meis PJ, Hargrave BY, Morris M. Vasopressin is important for restoring cardiovascular homeostasis in fetal lambs subjected to hemorrhage. Am J Obstet Gynecol. 1983;146:807–812.

161. Berecek KH, Swords BH. Central role for vasopressin in cardiovascular regulation and the pathogenesis of hypertension. Hypertension. 1990;16:213–224.

162. Luk J, Ajaelo I, Wong V, et al. Role of V1 receptors in the action of vasopressin on the baroreflex control of heart rate. Am J Physiol. 1993;265:R524–R529.

163. Stark RI, Daniel SS, Husain MK, Tropper PJ, James LS. Cerebrospinal fluid and plasma vasopressin in the fetal lamb: basal concentration and the effect of hypoxia. Endocrinology. 1985;116:65–72.

164. Segar JL, Minnick A, Nuyt A-M, Robillard JE. Developmental changes in central vasopressin regulation of cardiovascular function. Pediatr Res. 1995;37:34A.

165. Unger T, Rohmeiss P, Demmert G, Ganten D, Lang RE, Luft F. Opposing cardiovascular effects of brain and plasma AVP: role of V1- and V2-AVP receptors. In: Buckley JP, Ferrario CM, eds. Brain Peptides and Catecholamines in Cardiovascular Regulation. New York, NY: Raven Press; 1987:393–401.

166. Tangalakis T, Lumbers ER, Moritz KM, Towstoless MK, Wintour EM. Effect of cortisol on blood pressure and vascular reactivity in the ovine fetus. Exp Physiol. 1992;77:709–717.

167. Unno N, Wong CH, Jenkins SL, et al. Blood pressure and heart rate in the ovine fetus: ontogenic changes and effects of fetal adrenalectomy. Am J Physiol. 1999;276:H248–H256.

168. Derks JB, Giussani DA, Jenkins SL, et al. A comparative study of cardiovascular, endocrine and behavioural effects of betamethasone and dexamethasone administration to fetal sheep. J Physiol. 1997;499:217–226.

169. Padbury JF, Polk DH, Ervin G, Berry LM, Ikegami M, Jobe AH. Postnatal cardiovascular and metabolic responses to a single intramuscular dose of betamethasone in fetal sheep born prematurely by cesarean section. Pediatr Res. 1995;38:709–715.

170. Stein HM, Oyama K, Martinez A, et al. Effects of corticosteroids in preterm sheep on adaptation and sympathoadrenal mechanisms at birth. Am J Physiol. 1993;264:E763–E769.

171. Ng PC, Lee CH, Bnur FL, et al. A double-blind, randomized, controlled study of a "stress dose" of hydrocortisone for rescue treatment of refractory hypotension in preterm infants. Pediatrics. Feb 2006;117(2):367–375.

172. Seri I, Tan R, Evans J. Cardiovascular effects of hydrocortisone in preterm infants with pressor-resistant hypotension. Pediatrics. May 2001;107(5):1070–1074.

173. Dodt C, Keyser B, Molle M, Fehm HL, Elam M. Acute suppression of muscle sympathetic nerve activity by hydrocortisone in humans. Hypertension. 2000;35:758–763.

174. Macefield VG, Williamson PM, Wilson LR, Kelly JJ, Gandevia SC, Whitworth JA. Muscle sympathetic vasoconstrictor activity in hydrocortisone-induced hypertension in humans. Blood Press. 1998;7: 215–222.

175. Grünfeld JP, Eloy L. Glucocorticoids modulate vascular reactivity in the rat. Hypertension. 1987;10: 608–618.

176. Grünfled JP. Glucocorticoids in blood pressure regulation. Horm Res. 1990;34:111–113.

177. Provencher PH, Saltis J, Funder JW. Glucocorticoids but not mineralocorticoids modulate endothelin-1 and angiotensin II binding in SHR vascular smooth muscle cells. J Steroid Biochem Mol Biol. 1995;52:219–225.

178. Sato A, Suzuki H, Iwaita Y, Nakazato Y, Kato H, Saruta T. Potentiation of inositol trisphosphate production by dexamethasone. Hypertension. 1992;19:109–115.

179. Wallerath T, Witte K, Schäfer SC, et al. Down-regulation of the expression of endothelial NO synthase is likely to contribute to glucocorticoid-mediated hypertension. PNAS. 1999;96:13357–13362.

180. Fletcher AJW, McGarrigle HHG, Edwards CMB, Fowden AL. Effects of low dose dexamethasone treatment on basal cardiovascular and endocrine function in fetal sheep during late gestation. J Physiol. 2002;545:649–660.

181. Anwar MA, Schwab M, Poston L, Nathanielsz PW. Betamethasone-mediated vascular dysfunction and changes in hematological profile in the ovine fetus. Am J Physiol. 1999;276:H1137–H1143.

182. Docherty CC, Kalmar-Nagy J. Development of fetal vascular responses to endothelin-1 and acetylcholine in the sheep. Am J Physiol. 2001;280:R554–R562.

183. Docherty CC, Kalmar-Nagy J, Engelen M, et al. Effect of in vivo fetal infusion of dexamethasone at 0.75 GA on fetal ovine resistance artery responses to ET-1. Am J Physiol. 2001;281:R261–R268.

184. Molnar J, Nijland M, Howe DC, Nathanelsz PW. Evidence for microvascular dysfunction after prenatal dexamethasone at 0.7, 0.75, and 0.8 gestation in sheep. Am J Physiol. 2002;283:R561–R567.

185. Ervin MG, Padbury JF, Polk DH, Ikegami M, Berry LM, Jobe AH. Antenatal glucocorticoids alter premature newborn lamb neuroendocrine and endocrine responses to hypoxia. Am J Physiol. 2000;279: R830–R838.

186. Fletcher AJ, Gardner DG, Edwards CMB, Fowden AL, Giussani DA. Cardiovascular and endocrine responses to acute hypoxaemia during and following dexamethasone infusion in the ovine fetus. J Physiol. 2003;15:283–291.

187. Semenza GL. HIF-1: mediator of physiological and pathophysiological responses to hypoxia. J Appl Physiol. 2000;88:1474–1480.

188. Slotkin TA, Lappi SE, McCook EC, Tayyeb MI, Eylers JP, Seidler FJ. Glucocorticoids and the development of neuronal function: effects of prenatal dexamethasone exposure on central noradrenergic activity. Biol Neonate. 1992;61:326–336.

189. Segar JL, Van Natta T, Smith OJ. Effects of fetal ovine adrenalectomy on sympathetic and baroreflex responses at birth. Am J Physiol. 2002;283:R460–R467.

190. Chlorakos A, Langille BL, Adamson SL. Cardiovascular responses attenuate with repeated NO synthesis inhibition in conscious fetal sheep. Am J Physiol. 1998;274:H1472–H1480.

191. Sanhueza EM, Riquelme RA, Herrera EA, et al. Vasodilator tone in the llama fetus: the role of nitric oxide during normoxemia and hypoxemia. Am J Physiol Regul Integr Comp Physiol. Sep 2005;289(3): R776–R783.

192. Yu ZY, Lumbers ER, Simonetta G. The cardiovascular and renal effects of acute and chronic inhibition of nitric oxide production in fetal sheep. Exp Physiol. 2002;87:343–351.

193. Ma SX, Fang Q, Morgan B, Ross MG, Chao CR. Cardiovascular regulation and expressions of NO synthase-tyrosine hydroxylase in nucleus tractus solitarius of ovine fetus. Am J Physiol Heart Circ Physiol. Apr 2003;284(4):H1057–H1063.

194. McDonald TJ, Le WW, Hoffman GE. Brainstem catecholaminergic neurons activated by hypoxemia express GR and are coordinately activated with fetal sheep hypothalamic paraventricular CRH neurons. Brain Res. 2000;885:70–78.

2

Vasoactive Factors and Blood Pressure in Children

Ihor V. Yosypiv, MD

CONTENTS

INTRODUCTION

Vasoactive peptide systems play a critical role in the regulation of arterial blood pressure (BP). Inappropriate stimulation or deregulation of cross talk between diverse vasomotor factors contributes in a major way to the development of hypertension, cardiovascular disease, and renal disease in children. Understanding how derangements in vasoactive factor systems may lead to these health problems might potentially prevent disease from occurring. This chapter will review new advances in physiology, biochemistry, pathophysiology,

I.V. Yosypiv (✉)
Section of Pediatric Nephrology, Department of Pediatrics, Tulane Hospital for Children, New Orleans, LA, USA
e-mail: iiosipi@tulane.edu

From: *Clinical Hypertension and Vascular Diseases: Pediatric Hypertension*
Edited by: J. T. Flynn et al. DOI 10.1007/978-1-60327-824-9_2
© Springer Science+Business Media, LLC 2011

and function of the renal and systemic vasoactive systems with special emphasis on their role in the pathogenesis of hypertension in children.

THE RENIN–ANGIOTENSIN SYSTEM

The renin–angiotensin system (RAS) plays a fundamental role in the regulation of arterial BP. Emerging evidence suggests that many tissues have a local tissue-specific RAS, which is of major importance in the regulation of the angiotensin (Ang) levels within many organs *(1, 2)*. The RAS includes multiple components. The enzyme renin cleaves the substrate, angiotensinogen (AGT), to generate Ang I [Ang-(1–10)] (Fig. 1). Ang I is converted to Ang II [Ang-(1–8)] by angiotensin-converting enzyme (ACE). ACE expression on endothelial cells of many vascular beds including those in the kidney, heart, and lung allows systemic formation of Ang II, the most powerful effector peptide hormone of the RAS, throughout the circulation *(3–5)*. Most of hypertensinogenic actions of Ang II are attributed to the AT_1 receptor (AT_1R) *(6)*. Additionally, there are further pathways by which angiotensins may be formed—Ang II via chymase in tissues and Ang II metabolites via ACE2, as well as via endopeptidases.

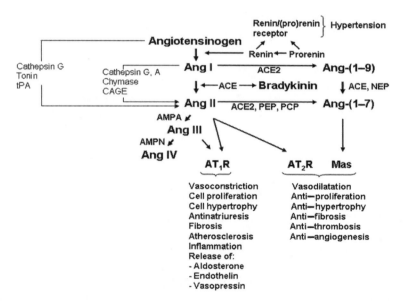

Fig. 1. Renin-Angiotensin System, with focus on target effects of Angiotensin II and alternate pathways of Angiotensin metabolism.

ANGIOTENSINOGEN

Angiotensinogen (AGT) is formed and constitutively secreted into the circulation by the hepatocytes *(7)*. In addition, AGT mRNA and protein are expressed in kidney proximal tubules, central nervous system, heart, adrenal gland, and other tissues *(8,9)*. Although AGT is the only substrate for renin, other enzymes can cleave AGT to form Ang I or Ang II (Fig. 1) *(10,11)*. Expression of the AGT gene is induced by Ang II, glucocorticoids, estrogens, thyroxine, and sodium depletion *(9,12,13)*.

A number of AGT polymorphisms appear to influence BP level. For example, an A/G polymorphism at −217 in the promoter of the AGT gene may play an important role in hypertension in African-Americans *(14)*.

PRORENIN, RENIN, AND (PRO)RENIN RECEPTOR

The major site of renin synthesis is in the juxtaglomerular cells of the afferent arterioles of the kidney, first as preprorenin *(15)*. The human renin gene, which encodes preprorenin, is located on chromosome 1 *(16)*. Cleavage of a 23-amino acid signal peptide at carboxyl terminus of preprorenin generates prorenin. Prorenin is then converted to active renin by cleavage of 43-amino acid N-terminal prosegment by proteases *(5,17)*. The kidney secretes both renin and prorenin into the peripheral circulation. Plasma levels of prorenin are approximately tenfold higher than those of renin *(18)*. Renin release is controlled relatively rapidly by baroreceptors in the afferent arterioles, chloride-sensitive receptors in the macula densa (MD) and juxtaglomerular apparatus, and renal sympathetic nerve activity in response to changes in posture or effective circulating fluid volume (Fig. 2) *(19–22)*. Inhibition of renin secretion in response to an increase in NaCl at the MD is adenosine dependent, whereas stimulation of renin release by a low perfusion pressure depends on cyclooxygenase-2 and neuronal nitric oxide (NO) synthase (NOS) *(23–25)*. In contrast, changes in AGT synthesis occur relatively slowly and thus are less responsible for the dynamic regulation of plasma Ang I and Ang II than changes in renin *(3,26)*. In addition, the circulating concentrations of AGT are more than 1000 times greater than the plasma Ang I and Ang II levels *(1)*. Therefore, renin activity is the rate-limiting factor in Ang I formation from AGT *(5)*. Although Ang II can be generated from AGT or Ang I via renin/ACE-independent pathways *(10,11)*, the circulating levels of Ang II reflect primarily the consequences of the action of renin on AGT *(27)*.

Recently, the renin/prorenin–(pro)renin receptor complex has emerged as a newly recognized pathway for tissue Ang II generation. In addition to proteolytic activation, prorenin may be activated by binding to (pro)renin receptor *(28)*.

The (pro)renin receptor is expressed on mesangial and vascular smooth muscle cells and binds both prorenin and renin *(29)*. Binding of renin or prorenin to (pro)renin receptor induces a conformational change of prorenin, facilitating catalytic activity and the conversion of AGT to Ang I *(28)*. A direct pathological role of the (pro)renin receptor in hypertension is suggested by the findings of elevated blood pressure in rats with transgenic overexpression of the human (pro)renin receptor *(30)*.

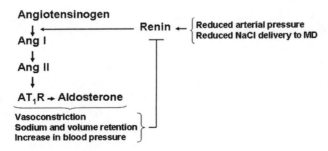

Fig. 2. Feedback loop between renin secretion and end-effects of the renin-nagiotensin-aldosterone system.

ANGIOTENSIN-CONVERTING ENZYME

Angiotensin-converting enzyme (ACE) is involved in the posttranslational processing of many polypeptides, the most notable of which are Ang I and bradykinin (BK) (Figs. 1 and 3). There are two ACE isozymes, somatic and testicular, transcribed from a single gene by differential utilization of two distinct promoters *(31)*. Human somatic ACE contains 1,306 amino acids and has a molecular weight of 140–160 kilodaltons (kDa). In the kidney, ACE is present as an ectoenzyme in glomerular vascular endothelial and proximal tubular cells *(32)*. ACE localized in glomerular endothelium may regulate intraglomerular blood flow, whereas ACE expressed in the proximal tubular epithelia and postglomerular vascular endothelium may play an important role in the regulation of tubular function and postglomerular circulation. Polymorphisms in the ACE gene appear to be important in blood pressure regulation. In particular, an insertion/deletion (I/D) polymorphism of 287 base pairs in exon 16 is associated with hypertension *(33)*. Persons with the D allele have higher plasma ACE levels and higher rates of hypertension.

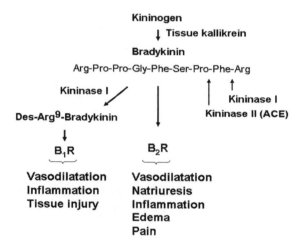

Fig. 3. Bradykinin-kinase system with focus on end-effects of bradykinin and its degredation products.

ANGIOTENSIN II RECEPTORS

Ang II acts via two major types of G-protein-coupled receptors (GPCRs): AT_1R and AT_2R. In rodents, AT_1R has two distinct subtypes, AT_{1A} and AT_{1B}, with greater than 95% amino acid sequence homology *(34)*. In the kidney, AT_1R mRNA has been localized to proximal tubules, the thick ascending limb of the loop of Henle, glomeruli, arterial vasculature, vasa recta, arcuate arteries, and juxtaglomerular cells *(35)*. Activation of Ang II binding to the AT_1R increases BP by (1) direct vasoconstriction and increase in peripheral vascular resistance; (2) stimulation of Na reabsorption via the sodium hydrogen exchanger 3 (NHE3) at the proximal nephron and by NHE3 and bumetanide-sensitive cotransporter 1 (BSC-1) at the medullary thick ascending limb of the loop of Henle, and (3) stimulation of aldosterone biosynthesis and secretion by the adrenal zona glomerulosa (Fig. 2) *(36–38)*. AT_1R activation also stimulates vasopressin and endothelin secretion and stimulates the sympathetic nervous system, and the proliferation of vascular smooth muscle and mesangial cells *(39–41)*. The AT_2R has 34% homology with AT_{1A} or AT_{1B} receptors *(42)*. The AT_2R is expressed in the glomerular epithelial cells, proximal tubules, collecting ducts, and parts of the renal vasculature of the adult rat *(43)*. In contrast to the AT_1R, the AT_2R elicits vasodilation by increasing the production of nitric oxide (NO) and cyclic guanosine monophosphate (cGMP) either by stimulating formation of bradykinin or by direct activation of NO production *(44–46)*. In addition, the AT_2R promotes renal sodium excretion and inhibits proliferation in mesangial cells *(44,47,48)*. Thus, the AT_2R generally appears to oppose AT_1R-mediated effects on blood pressure, cardiovascular and renal growth, fibrosis, and remodeling, as well as RBF, fibrosis, and sodium excretion.

ANGIOTENSIN-CONVERTING ENZYME 2

ACE2 is a homologue of ACE that is abundantly expressed in the kidney and acts to counterbalance ACE activity by promoting Ang II degradation to the vasodilator peptide Ang-(1–7) *(49,50)*. Ang-(1–7) acts via the GPCR Mas encoded by the *Mas* protooncogene and counteracts Ang II–AT1R-mediated effects *(51,52)*. An important role for ACE2 in the regulation of BP is suggested by the findings of a decreased ACE2 expression in the kidney of hypertensive rats and reduction of BP following genetic overexpression of ACE2 in their vasculature *(53,54)*. Although ACE2-null mice are normotensive and have normal cardiac structure and function, they exhibit enhanced susceptibility to Ang II-induced hypertension *(55)*. Moreover, Mas-deficient mice exhibit increased blood pressure, endothelial dysfunction, and an imbalance between NO and reactive oxygen species *(56)*. Other major degradation products of Ang II include Ang III [Ang-*(2–8)*] and Ang IV [Ang-*(3–8)*]. These peptides have biological activity, but their plasma levels are much lower than those of Ang II or Ang-(1–7) *(57)*.

DEVELOPMENTAL ASPECTS OF THE RAS

The developing metanephric kidney expresses all the components of the RAS (Table 1). The activity of the renal RAS is high during fetal and neonatal life and declines during postnatal maturation *(58,59)*. Immunoreactive Ang II levels are higher in the fetal and newborn than in adult rat kidney *(59)*. The ontogeny of AT_1R and AT_2R mRNA in the kidney differs—AT_2R is expressed earlier than AT_1R, peaks during fetal metanephrogenesis, and rapidly declines postnatally *(60,61)*. AT_1R mRNA expression increases during gestation, peaks perinatally, and declines gradually thereafter *(60–62)*. ACE mRNA and enzymatic activity are expressed in the developing rat kidney, where they are subject to regulation by endogenous Ang II and bradykinin *(59,62)*. In addition, the developing kidney expresses considerable ACE-independent Ang II-generating activity *(63)*, which may compensate for the low ACE levels in the early metanephros *(59)*. The role of the ACE2–Ang-(1–7)–Mas axis and the (pro)renin receptor in developmental origins of hypertension remains to be determined. Functionally, Ang II, acting via the AT_1R, counteracts the vasodilator actions of bradykinin on the renal microvasculature of the developing rat kidney *(64)*. Premature infants exhibit markedly elevated PRA levels, a finding that is inversely related to postconceptual age *(65)*. In healthy children, plasma renin activity (PRA) is high during the newborn period and declines gradually toward adulthood *(66)*.

Pharmacologic or genetic interruption of the RAS during development alters BP phenotype and causes a spectrum of congenital abnormalities of the kidney and urinary tract (CAKUT) in rodents and renal tubular dysgenesis (RTD) in humans (Table 2) *(67,68)*.

Table 1

Expression of the Renin–Angiotensin System Components During Metanephric Kidney Development

	E12	E14	E15	E16	E19	References
AGT	Mouse: UB, SM	UB, SM, PT			PT	(155)
			Rat: UB, SM	UB, SM, PT		(156)
Renin	Mouse: precursor cells present M of entire kidney M, close to V and G V, G					(157)
			Rat: V	V		(58)
ACE				Rat: PT, G, CD	V	(158)
AT$_1$	Mouse: UB, M	UB, G	UB, V	PT, UB, SM, G	PT, DT	(155)
			Rat: G, UB, SM	SM		(62)
AT$_2$	Mouse: MM	MM SM			PT, CD, G	(60)
		Rat: MM		Medullary SM,under renal capsule		(62)
				Condensed M Medulla, G, V		(60)

AGT, angiotensinogen; ACE, angiotensin-converting enzyme; AT$_1$/AT$_2$, angiotensin II receptors; UB, ureteric bud; M, mesenchyme; SM, stromal mesenchyme; PT, proximal tubule; G, glomeruli; V, renal vessels; CD, collecting duct.

Adapted from (159), with permission from Springer.

Table 2
Renal and Blood Pressure Phenotypic Effects of Genetic Inactivation of the
Renin–Angiotensin System Genes in Mice

Gene	Gene Function of gene	Renal phenotype	Blood pressure	References
AGT	Renin substrate	Vascular thickening	Very low	(160)
		Interstitial fibrosis		(161)
		Delayed glomerular maturation		(162)
		Hypoplastic papilla		
		Hydronephrosis		
		Reduced ability to concentrate urine		
Renin	Enzyme that generates ANG I from AGT	Arterial wall thickening	Very low	(163)
		Interstitial fibrosis		
		Glomerulosclerosis		
		Hypoplastic papilla		
		Hydronephrosis		
ACE	Enzyme which generates ANG II from ANG I	Arterial wall thickening	Very low	(164)
		Hypoplastic papilla and medulla		
		Hydronephrosis		
		Reduced ability to concentrate urine		
$AT_{1A/B}$	Ang II receptor	Decreased kidney weight	Very low	(165)
		Delayed glomerular maturation		(166)
		Arterial wall thickening		
		Interstitial fibrosis		
		Tubular atrophy		
		Hypoplastic papilla and medulla		
		Hydronephrosis		
		Reduced ability to concentrate urine		
AT_{1A}	Ang II receptor	Normal or mild papillary hypoplasia	Moderately low	(6)
AT_{1B}	Ang II receptor	Normal	Normal	(167)
AT_2	Ang II receptor	Duplicated ureters	High	(168)
		Hydronephrosis		(169)

Therefore, RAS inhibitors should not be used during pregnancy and should not be used postnatally until nephrogenesis is completed. Beyond these periods of life, high activity of the RAS coupled with persistent expression of the renal AT_1R provide the foundation for the use of the classical RAS inhibitors (ACE inhibitors and AT_1R antagonists) in the treatment of children with RAS-dependent hypertension (e.g., renovascular hypertension). In addition, both ACE inhibitors and angiotensin receptor blockers may be beneficial in children with primary hypertension, particularly in obese adolescents, who exhibit elevated plasma renin activity *(69)*. Recent availability of aliskiren, the first direct inhibitor of (pro)renin receptor, offers new possibilities in antihypertensive therapy in children that remain to be explored.

ALDOSTERONE

Ang II, acting via the AT_1R, stimulates an increase in transcription and expression of the rate-limiting enzyme in the biosynthesis of aldosterone, CYP 11B2 (aldosterone synthase) in the zona glomerulosa of the adrenal glands *(36)*. Aldosterone stimulates reabsorption of Na^+ and secretion of potassium by principal cells in the collecting duct. In turn, the retained Na^+ is responsible for increased extracellular fluid volume that increases BP. Secretion of aldosterone is stimulated by high plasma potassium concentration and adrenocorticotropic hormone (ACTH), and inhibited by atrial natriuretic peptide (ANP) *(70–72)*. Aldosterone-dependent Na^+ reabsorption is due to upregulation of epithelial Na^+ channel-α (alfa) (ENaCα) subunit gene expression and increased apical density of ENaC channels due to serum- and glucocorticoid-induced kinase-1 (Sgk1)-induced disinhibition of Nedd4-2-triggered internalization and degradation of ENaC *(73)*. Aldosterone downregulates the expression of histone H3 methyltransferase Dot1a and the DNA-binding protein Af9 complexed with chromatin within the ENaCα (alfa) 5′-flanking region *(74)*. In addition, aldosterone-induced Sgk1 phosphorylates Ser435 of Af9, causing disruption of the protein–protein interactions of Dot1a, a histone H3 lysine 79 (H3K79) methyltransferase, and Af9. This results in hypomethylation of histone H3 Lys79 and release of transcriptional repression of the ENaCα (alfa) gene. The important role of aldosterone in childhood hypertension is underscored by the ability of mineralocorticoid receptor antagonists not only to reduce elevated BP due to hyperaldosteronism (e.g., adrenal hyperplasia) effectively, but also to offer survival benefits in heart failure and augment potential for renal protection in proteinuric chronic kidney disease.

GLUCOCORTICOIDS

Glucocorticoids are vital for normal development and control of hemodynamic homeostasis. Cortisol or dexamethasone infusion increases BP in the fetal sheep *(75,76)*. Dexamethasone increases BP in $Sgk1^{+/+}$ but not in $Sgk1^{-/-}$ mice *(77)*, indicating that hypertensinogenic effects of glucocorticoids on BP are mediated in part via Sgk1. A higher ratio of cortisol to cortisone in venous cord blood is associated with higher systolic blood pressure later in life in humans *(78)*, suggesting that increased fetal glucocorticoid exposure may account for higher systolic blood pressure in childhood. However, no differences in BP and cardiovascular function are detected at school age in children treated neonatally with glucocorticoids for chronic lung disease *(79)*. It is possible that the functional consequences of glucocorticoid therapy during neonatal life may manifest only later in life. However, deleterious effects of excess glucocorticoids on childhood BP are apparent, for example, in conditions such as Cushing's syndrome or glucocorticoid-remediable aldosteronism.

KALLIKREIN–KININ SYSTEM

The kallikrein–kinin system (KKS) plays an important role in the regulation of blood pressure. Kinins, including bradykinin (BK), are formed from kininogen by kininogenase tissue kallikrein *(80)* (Fig. 3). Bradykinin is degraded by ACE, which is also called kininase II *(81)*. Kinins act by binding to the bradykinin receptors B1 (B_1R) and B2 (B_2R). The B_1R is activated by Des-Arg^9-BK produced from BK by kininase I, which mediates tissue injury and inflammation *(82)*. The renal and cardiovascular effects of BK are mediated predominantly through the B_2R. During development kininogen is expressed in the ureteric bud and stromal interstitial cells of the E15 metanephros in the rat and, presumably, in other mammals *(83)*. Following completion of nephrogenesis, kininogen is localized in the collecting duct. The main kininogenase, true tissue kallikrein, is encoded by the *KLK1* gene *(84)*. Transcription of *KLK1* gene is regulated by salt and protein intake, insulin, and mineralocorticoids. Expression of the *KLK1* gene within the kidney is suppressed in chronic phase of renovascular hypertension *(83)*.

In the developing rat kidney, kallikrein mRNA and immunoreactivity are present in the connecting tubule *(85)*. In the mature kidney, tissue kallikrein mRNA is expressed in the distal tubule and glomeruli *(86)*. Thus, BK can be generated intraluminally from kininogen present in the collecting duct or in the interstitium. BK generated intraluminally causes natriuresis, whereas interstitial BK may regulate medullary blood flow *(87)*. The proximity of the distal tubule to the afferent arteriole may allow kallikrein or BK to diffuse from the distal tubular cells and act in a paracrine manner on the preglomerular microvessels *(88)*. The human B_1R and B_2R genes are located on chromosome 14 and demonstrate 36% genomic sequence homology *(89)*. Both B_1R and B_2R are members of the seven-transmembrane GPCR family. During metanephrogenesis, B_2R is expressed in both luminal and basolateral aspects of collecting ducts, suggesting that activation of B_2R is important for tubular growth and acquisition of function *(90)*. The expression of B_1R is inducible rather than constitutive. In contrast to B_2R, B_1R is not expressed in significant levels in normal tissues *(82)*. Although BK does not appear to be a primary mediator of the maturational rise in RBF in the rat, its vasodilatory effects in the developing kidney are tonically antagonized by Ang II AT_1R *(65)*. Stimulation of the B_2R during adult life stimulates production of nitric oxide and prostaglandins resulting in vasodilation and natriuresis *(91)*. The importance of the KKS in the regulation of BP is underscored by the finding of elevated BP in mice that lack the B_2R *(92)*. Moreover, B_2R-null mice are prone to early onset of salt-sensitive hypertension *(93)*. Interestingly, B_1R receptor blockade in B_2R-null mice produces a significant hypertensive response *(94)*, indicating that both receptors participate in the development of hypertension. In keeping with this hypothesis, single-nucleotide polymorphisms in the promoters of both *B_1R* and *B_2R* genes are associated with hypertension in African-Americans, indicating that the two receptors play a role in BP homeostasis in humans *(95)*. The direct potential role of the KKS in childhood hypertension is further highlighted by studies showing that endogenous bradykinin contributes to the beneficial effects of ACE inhibition on BP in humans *(96)*.

ARGININE VASOPRESSIN

Arginine vasopressin (AVP), also known as antidiuretic hormone (ADH), is synthesized in the hypothalamus and released in response to increased plasma osmolality, decreased arterial pressure, and reductions in circulating blood volume. Three subtypes of vasopressin receptors, V_1R, V_2R, and V_3R, mediate vasoconstriction, water reabsorption, and central nervous system effects, respectively. In addition, stimulation of the V_2R induces endothelial NOS expression and promotes NO production in the renal medulla, which attenuates the V_1R-mediated vasoconstrictor effects (97). In adult species, AVP supports arterial BP when both the sympathetic system and the RAS are impaired by sympathetic blockade (98). Treatment with a V_1R antagonist has no effect on arterial BP in fetal sheep (99,100). In contrast, antagonism of V_1R during hypotensive hemorrhage impairs the ability of the fetus to maintain BP (101). Thus, endogenous AVP has little impact on basal hemodynamic homeostasis of the fetus, but plays an important role in vasopressor response to acute stress such as hemorrhage.

ENDOTHELIUM-DERIVED VASOACTIVE FACTORS

Nitric Oxide

Hypertension is associated with abnormal endothelial function in the peripheral, coronary, and renal vasculatures. Nitric oxide (NO) is an important mediator of endothelium-dependent vasodilation. NO enhances arterial compliance, reduces peripheral vascular resistance, and inhibits proliferation of vascular smooth muscle cells (102). The major source of NO production in the rat kidney is the renal medulla where NO regulates medullary blood flow, natriuresis, and dieresis (103,104). NO promotes pressure natriuresis via cGMP (105). The effects of Ang II or AVP on medullary blood flow are buffered by the increased production of NO (103), indicating that endogenous NO tonically counteracts the effects of vasoconstrictors within the renal medullary circulation. Interestingly, endothelial dysfunction is not only a consequence of hypertension, but may predispose to the development of hypertension. In this regard, impaired endothelium-dependent vasodilation has been observed in normotensive children of patients with essential hypertension compared with those without a family history of hypertension (106), demonstrating that an impairment in NO production precedes the onset of essential hypertension. Acute antagonism of NO generation leads to an increase in BP and decreases RBF in the fetal sheep (107). In fetal rat kidneys, endothelial NO synthase (eNOS) immunoreactivity is first detected in the endothelial cells of the intrarenal capillaries on E14 (108). These findings suggest that eNOS may play a role in regulating renal hemodynamics during fetal life. Moreover, eNOS-knockout mice exhibit abnormal aortic valves, congenital atrial defects, and ventricular septal defects, indicating that eNOS-derived NO plays an important role in the development of the circulatory system (109). The effect of intrarenal infusion of NO antagonist L-NAME on decreases in RBF and GFR is more pronounced in the newborn than adult kidney (110). These effects of NO may act to oppose high RAS activity present in the developing kidney.

Asymmetrical Dimethylarginine

Asymmetric dimethylarginine (ADMA) is an endogenous inhibitor of eNOS (111). Infusion of ADMA increases BP and renal vascular resistance, and decreases renal plasma flow during adulthood (112). ADMA levels in fetal umbilical venous plasma are higher than in maternal plasma (113). However, low resistance to umbilical blood flow is maintained despite substantially higher fetal ADMA levels. It is therefore conceivable that NO is a key modulator of fetal vascular tone. Hypertensive children have higher plasma ADMA levels compared with normotensive subjects (114). In contrast, plasma ADMA levels do not differ between normotensive and hypertensive young adults (115). Moreover, plasma ADMA correlate negatively with vascular resistance *(115)*, suggesting that in a physiological setting ADMA levels in subjects with elevated vascular tone may be lowered to compensate for inappropriately high resistance.

Endothelins

Endothelins (ETs) are vasoconstrictor peptides produced by endothelial cells *(116,117)*. Three ETs were described: endothelin-1 (ET-1), -2 (ET-2), and -3 (ET-3). The hemodynamic effects of ET-1 are mediated by ET_A and ET_B GPCRs. In the kidney, ET-1 mRNA is expressed in the glomeruli and medullary collecting ducts *(118,119)*. ET receptors are located in podocytes, glomeruli, afferent and efferent arterioles, proximal tubules, medullary thick ascending limbs, and collecting ducts *(120)*. The ET_B receptor activation causes natriuresis and vasodilation via release of NO and PGE_2, whereas renal vasoconstriction is mediated by the ET_A receptor *(121)*. In the fetal lamb, the ET_A and ET_B receptors expressed on vascular smooth muscle cells mediate vasoconstriction, whereas ET_B receptors located on endothelial cells mediate vasodilation *(122,123)*. In the renal circulation of fetal sheep, ET-1, acting via the ET_B receptor, causes vasodilation *(124)*. However, ET_A receptor-mediated vasoconstriction also contributes to the regulation of the fetal renal vascular tone *(125)*. The critical role for the renal ET-1 and ET_A/ET_B receptors in the regulation of systemic BP is demonstrated by the finding of increased BP in mice with collecting duct-specific genetic inactivation of either ET-1 or both ET_A and ET_B receptors *(126,127)*. Moreover, BP increases further with high salt intake, indicating that combined ET_A/ET_B receptor deficiency causes salt-sensitive hypertension.

NATRIURETIC PEPTIDES

Natriuretic peptides include atrial natriuretic peptide (ANP), brain natriuretic peptide (BNP), C-type natriuretic peptide (CNP), urodilatin, and Dendroaspis-type natriuretic peptide (DNP) *(128–131)*. Natriuretic peptides act by binding to three guanylyl cyclase-linked receptors: NPR-A, NPR-B, and NPR-C *(132)*. In the adult heart, ANP and BNP are stored in atrial and ventricular myocytes, respectively, released in response to atrial stretch, increased BP, atrial tachycardia, or increased osmolality *(132,133)*, and are rapidly degraded in the lung and kidney by neutral endopeptidase *(134)*. ANP and BNP reduce secretion of renin and aldosterone, and antagonize the effects of Ang II on vascular tone and renal tubular reabsorption to cause natriuresis, diuresis, a decrease in BP, and intravascular fluid volume *(135)*. ANP and BNP peptide levels are higher in fetal than adult ventricles, indicating that the relative contribution of ventricular ANP is greater during embryonic than adult life *(136–138)*. ANP and BNP mRNAs are expressed on E8 in the mouse and increase during gestation, suggesting that both ANP and BNP play a role in the formation of the developing heart. Circulating ANP levels are higher in the fetal than adult rat or sheep *(137,139)*. Infusion of ANP into the circulation of fetal sheep decreases BP and causes diuresis *(140)*. ANP secretion during postnatal development is stimulated in response to similar physiological stimuli as in the adult animal and can be induced by Ang II, volume loading, hypoxia, or increase in osmolality *(139,141)*. Plasma levels of ANP are higher in preterm than term infants *(142)*. In the full-term infants, circulating ANP levels increase during the first week of life and decrease thereafter *(143)*. The initial postnatal increase in ANP may mediate diuresis during the transition to extrauterine life. Subsequent decrease in plasma ANP may serve to conserve sodium required for rapid growth. Although BP remains normal in BNP-null mice *(144)*, ANP-null mice develop hypertension later in life *(145)*. Mice lacking NPR-A receptor exhibit cardiac hypertrophy and have elevated BP, indicating that the ANP and BNP play an important role in the regulation of myocyte growth and BP homeostasis during development *(146,147)*.

VASOACTIVE FACTORS AND DEVELOPMENTAL PROGRAMMING OF HYPERTENSION

An inverse relationship between birth weight or maternal undernutrition and adult BP led to the concept of developmental programming of hypertension *(147)*. Brain RAS is activated by low protein (LP) diet and hypertensive adult offspring of LP-fed dams have increased pressor response to Ang II *(148,149)*. Thus, inappropriate activation of the RAS may link fetal life to childhood and adult hypertension. Interestingly, LP maternal diet has been reported to result in decreased methylation of the promoter region of $AT_{1B}R$ in the offspring *(150)*. It is conceivable that epigenetic modifications of the $AT_{1B}R$ gene may represent one of the mechanisms implicated in developmental programming of hypertension by an aberrant RAS. LP diet or caloric restriction during gestation causes a decrease in the renal kallikrein activity, blunted vasorelaxation to NO infusion, an increase in vascular superoxide anion concentration, and a decrease in superoxide dismutase activity in offspring of dams with such restricted diets *(151–153)*. In addition, heterozygous eNOS offspring born to eNOS-null mothers exhibit impaired endothelium-dependent vasodilation compared to heterozygous pups born to $eNOS^{+/+}$ mothers *(154)*. These observations indicate that impairment in endothelium-dependent vascular function is associated with developmentally programmed hypertension and that the eNOS maternal genotype modulates a genetic predisposition to hypertension. Further studies are needed to establish the mechanisms by which alterations in the antenatal environment impact vasoactive factor systems and their interplay to program hypertension during postnatal life.

SUMMARY

Many vasoactive substances regulate cardiovascular homeostasis during development, and more are discovered each year. Many cardiovascular factors exert pleiotropic actions both systemically and within diverse organ systems. Continued discovery of new vasoactive substances and more complete knowledge of their role during development will increase our understanding of the developmental origin of hypertension and cardiovascular disease and should help in the development of strategies that will minimize the impact of these substances on hypertension Further work is needed to define more precisely the role of emerging cardiovascular regulatory factors and to understand their growing relevance to a number of conditions in animal models of human disease and in human diseases including hypertension.

REFERENCES

1. Navar LG, Harrison-Bernard LM, Nishiyama A, et al. Regulation of intrarenal angiotensin II in hypertension. Hypertension. 2002;39:316–322.
2. Kobori H, Ozawa Y, Suzaki Y, et al. Young scholars award lecture: intratubular angiotensinogen in hypertension and kidney diseases. Am J Hypertens. 2006;19:541–550.

3. Brasier AR, Li J. Mechanisms for inducible control of angiotensinogen gene transcription. Hypertension. 1996;27:465–475.
4. Navar LG. The kidney in blood pressure regulation and development of hypertension. Med Clin North Am. 1997;81:1165–1198.
5. Paul M, Mehr AP, Kreutz R. Physiology of local renin-angiotensin systems. Physiol Rev. 2006;86:747–803.
6. Ito M, Oliverio MI, Mannon PJ, Best CF, Maeda N, Smithies O, Coffman TM. Regulation of blood pressure by the type 1A angiotensin II receptor gene. Proc Natl Acad Sci USA. 1995;92:3521–3525.
7. Fukamizu A, Takahashi S, Seo MS, et al. Structure and expression of the human angiotensinogen gene. Identification of a unique and highly active promoter. J Biol Chem. 1990;265:7576–7582.
8. Ingelfinger JR, Zuo WM, Fon EA, et al. In situ hybridization evidence for angiotensinogen messenger RNA in the rat proximal tubule. An hypothesis for the intrarenal renin angiotensin system. J Clin Invest. 1990;85:417–423.
9. Lynch KR, Peach MJ. Molecular biology of angiotensinogen. Hypertension. 1991;17:263–269.
10. Yosypiv IV, el-Dahr SS. Activation of angiotensin-generating systems in the developing rat kidney. Hypertension. 1996;27:281–286.
11. Miyazaki M, Takai S. Local angiotensin II-generating system in vascular tissues: the roles of chymase. Hypertens Res. 2001;24:189–193.
12. Schunkert H, Ingelfinger JR, Jacob H, et al. Reciprocal feedback regulation of kidney angiotensinogen and renin mRNA expressions by angiotensin II. Am J Physiol. 1992;263:E863–E869.
13. Kobori H, Nangaku M, Navar LG, et al. The intrarenal renin-angiotensin system: from physiology to the pathobiology of hypertension and kidney disease. Pharmacol Rev. 2007;59:251–287.
14. Jain S, Tang X, Chittampalli SN, et al. Angiotensinogen gene polymorphism at −217 affects basal promoter activity and is associated with hypertension in African-Americans. J Biol Chem. 2002;277:36889–36896.
15. Hackenthal E, Paul M, Ganten D, et al. Morphology, physiology, and molecular biology of renin secretion. Physiol Rev. 1990;70:1067–1116.
16. Miyazaki H, Fukamizu A, Hirose S, et al. Structure of the human renin gene. Proc Natl Acad Sci USA. 1984;81:5999–6003.
17. Schweda F, Friis U, Wagner C, et al. Renin release. Physiology (Bethesda). 2007;22:310–319.
18. Danser AH, Derkx FH, Schalekamp MA, et al. Determinants of interindividual variation of renin and prorenin concentrations: evidence for a sexual dimorphism of (pro)renin levels in humans. J Hypertens. 1998;16:853–862.
19. Lorenz JN, Greenberg SG, Briggs JP. The macula densa mechanism for control of renin secretion. Semin Nephrol. 1993;13:531–542.
20. Davis JO, Freeman RH. Mechanisms regulating renin release. Physiol Rev. 1976;56:1–56.
21. Burns KD, Homma T, Harris RC. The intrarenal renin-angiotensin system. Semin Nephrol. 1993;13:13–30.
22. Handa RK, Johns EJ. Interaction of the renin-angiotensin system and the renal nerves in the regulation of rat kidney function. J Physiol. 1985;369:311–321.
23. Kim SM, Mizel D, Huang YG, et al. Adenosine as a mediator of macula densa-dependent inhibition of renin secretion. Am J Physiol Renal Physiol. 2006;290:F1016–F1023.
24. Zhou MS, Schulman IH, Raij L. Nitric oxide, angiotensin II, and hypertension. Semin Nephrol. 2004;24:366–378.
25. Touyz RM, Schiffrin EL. Signal transduction mechanisms mediating the physiological and pathophysiological actions of angiotensin II in vascular smooth muscle cells. Pharmacol Rev. 2000;52:639–672.
26. Deschepper CF. Angiotensinogen: hormonal regulation and relative importance in the generation of angiotensin II. Kidney Int. 1994;46:1561–1563.
27. Erdös EG, Skidgel RA. Renal metabolism of angiotensin I and II. Kidney Int. 1990;30:S24–S27.
28. Nguyen G, Delarue F, Burcklé C, et al. Pivotal role of the renin/prorenin receptor in angiotensin II production and cellular responses to renin. J Clin Invest. 2002;109:1417–1427.
29. Batenburg WW, Krop M, Garrelds IM, et al. Prorenin is the endogenous agonist of the (pro)renin receptor. Binding kinetics of renin and prorenin in rat vascular smooth muscle cells overexpressing the human (pro)renin receptor. J Hypertens. 2007;25:2441–2453.
30. Burcklé CA, Danser AHJ, Müller DN, et al. Elevated blood pressure and heart rate in human renin receptor transgenic rats. Hypertension. 2006;47:552–556.
31. Kumar RS, Thekkumkara TJ, Sen GC. The mRNAs encoding the two angiotensin-converting isozymes are transcribed from the same gene by a tissue-specific choice of alternative transcription initiation sites. J Biol Chem. 1991; 266:3854–3862.

32. Ramchandran R, Sen GC, Misono K, Sen I. Regulated cleavage-secretion of the membrane-bound angiotensin-converting enzyme. J Biol Chem. 1994;269:2125–2130.

33. Jiang X, Sheng H, Li J, et al. Association between renin-angiotensin system gene polymorphism and essential hypertension: a community-based study. J Hum Hypertens. 2009;23:176–181.

34. Iwai N, Inagami T. Identification of two subtypes in the rat type I angiotensin II receptor. FEBS Lett. 1992;298:257–260.

35. Tufro-McReddie A, Gomez RA. Ontogeny of the renin-angiotensin system. Semin Nephrol. 1993;13:519–530.

36. Holland OB, Carr B, Brasier AR. Aldosterone synthase gene regulation by angiotensin. Endocr Res. 1995;21:455–462.

37. Morganti A, Lopez-Ovejero JA, Pickering TG, et al. Role of the sympathetic nervous system in mediating the renin response to head-up tilt. Their possible synergism in defending blood pressure against postural changes during sodium deprivation. Am J Cardiol. 1979;43:600–604.

38. Goodfriend TL, Elliott ME, Catt KJ. Angiotensin receptors and their antagonists. N Engl J Med. 1996;334:1649–1654.

39. Gasparo M, et al. International Union of Pharmacology XXIII. The angiotensin II receptors. Pharmacol Rev. 2000;52:415–472.

40. Berry C, Touyz R, Dominiczak AF, et al. Angiotensin receptors: signaling, vascular pathophysiology, and interactions with ceramide. Am J Physiol. 2001;281:H2337–H2365.

41. Wolf G, Haberstroh U, Neilson EG. Angiotensin II stimulates the proliferation and biosynthesis of type I collagen in cultured murine mesangial cells. Am J Pathol. 1992;140:95–107.

42. Inagami T, Iwai N, Sasaki K, et al. Angiotensin II receptors: cloning and regulation. Arzneimittelforschung. 1993;43:226–228.

43. Miyata N, Park F, Li XF, et al. Distribution of angiotensin AT1 and AT2 receptor subtypes in the rat kidney. Am J Physiol. 1999;277:F437–F446.

44. Siragy HM, Carey RM. The subtype-2 (AT2) angiotensin receptor mediates renal production of nitric oxide in conscious rats. J Clin Invest. 1997;100:264–269.

45. Tsutsumi Y, et al. Angiotensin II type 2 receptor overexpression activates the vascular kinin system and causes vasodilation. J Clin Invest. 1999;104:925–935.

46. Abadir PM, et al. Angiotensin AT2 receptors directly stimulate renal nitric oxide in bradykinin B2-receptor-null mice. Hypertension. 2003;42:600–604.

47. Goto M, Mukoyama M, Suga S, Matsumoto T, Nakagawa M, Ishibashi R, Kasahara M, Sugawara A, Tanaka I, Nakao K. Growth-dependent induction of angiotensin II type 2 receptor in rat mesangial cells. Hypertension. 1997;30:358–362.

48. Gross V, Schunck WH, Honeck H, et al. Inhibition of pressure natriuresis in mice lacking the AT2 receptor. Kidney Int. 2000;57:191–202.

49. Donoghue M, Hsieh F, Baronas RE, et al. A novel angiotensin-converting enzyme-related carboxypeptidase (ACE2) converts angiotensin I to angiotensin 1-9. Circ Res. 2000;87:E1–E9.

50. Brosnihan KB, Li P, Ferrario CM. Angiotensin-(1-7) dilates canine coronary arteries through kinins and nitric oxide. Hypertension. 1996;27:523–528.

51. Santos RA, Simoes Silva AC, Maric C, et al. Angiotensin-(1-7) is an endogenous ligand for the G protein-coupled receptor Mas. Proc Natl Acad Sci U S A. 2003;100:8258–8263.

52. Santos RA, Ferreira AJ. Angiotensin-(1-7) and the renin-angiotensin system. Curr Opin Nephrol Hypertens. 2007;16:122–128.

53. Zhong JC, Huang DY, Yang YM, et al. Upregulation of angiotensin-converting enzyme 2 by all-trans retinoic acid in spontaneously hypertensive rats. Hypertension. 2004;44:907–912.

54. Rentzsch B, Todiras M, Iliescu R, et al. Transgenic angiotensin-converting enzyme 2 overexpression in vessels of SHRSP rats reduces blood pressure and improves endothelial function. Hypertension. 2008;52:967–973.

55. Gurley SB, Allred A, et al. Altered blood pressure responses and normal cardiac phenotype in ACE2-null mice. J Clin Invest. 2006;116:2218–2225.

56. Xu P, Costa-Goncalves AC, Todiras M, et al. Endothelial dysfunction and elevated blood pressure in MAS gene-deleted mice. Hypertension. 2008;51:574–580.

57. Haulica I, Bild W, Serban DN. Angiotensin peptides and their pleiotropic actions. J Renin Angiotensin Aldosterone Syst. 2005;6:121–131.

58. Gomez RA, Lynch KR, Sturgill BC, Elwood JP, Chevalier RL, Carey RM, Peach MJ. Distribution of renin mRNA and its protein in the developing kidney. Am J Physiol. 1989;257:F850–F858.

59. Yosypiv IV, Dipp S, El-Dahr SS. Ontogeny of somatic angiotensin-converting enzyme. Hypertension. 1994;23:369–374.

60. Norwood VF, Craig MR, Harris JM, et al. Differential expression of angiotensin II receptors during early renal morphogenesis. Am J Physiol. 1997;272:R662–R668.
61. Garcia-Villalba P, Denkers ND, Wittwer CT, et al. Real-time PCR quantification of AT1 and AT2 angiotensin receptor mRNA expression in the developing rat kidney. Nephron Exp Nephrol. 2003;94:e154–e159.
62. Kakuchi J, Ichiki T, Kiyama S, et al. Developmental expression of renal angiotensin II receptor genes in the mouse. Kidney Int. 1995;47:140–147.
63. Yosypiv IV, el-Dahr SS. Activation of angiotensin-generating systems in the developing rat kidney. Hypertension. 1996;27:281–286.
64. el-Dahr SS, Yosypiv IV, Lewis L, et al. Role of bradykinin B2 receptors in the developmental changes of renal hemodynamics in the neonatal rat. Am J Physiol. 1995;269:F786–F792.
65. Richer C, Hornych H, Amiel-Tison C, et al. Plasma renin activity and its postnatal development in preterm infants. Preliminary report. Biol Neonate. 1977;31:301–304.
66. Stalker HP, Holland NH, Kotchen JM, et al. Plasma renin activity in healthy children. J Pediatr. 1976;89:256–258.
67. Sánchez SI, Seltzer AM, Fuentes LB, et al. Inhibition of angiotensin II receptors during pregnancy induces malformations in developing rat kidney. Eur J Pharmacol. 2008;588:114–123.
68. Gribouval O, Gonzales M, Neuhaus T, et al. Mutations in genes in the renin-angiotensin system are associated with autosomal recessive renal tubular dysgenesis. Nat Genet. 2005;37:964–968.
69. Flynn JT, Alderman MH. Characteristics of children with primary hypertension seen at a referral center. Pediatr Nephrol. 2005;20:961–966.
70. Vinson GP, Laird SM, Whitehouse BJ, et al. The biosynthesis of aldosterone. J Steroid Biochem Mol Biol. 1991;39:851–858.
71. Himathongkam T, Dluhy RG, Williams GH. Potassim-aldosterone-renin interrelationships. J Clin Endocrinol Metab. 1975;41:153–159.
72. Chartier L, Schiffrin EL. Role of calcium in effects of atrial natriuretic peptide on aldosterone production in adrenal glomerulosa cells. Am J Physiol. 1987;252:E485–E491.
73. Debonneville C, Flores SY, Kamynina E, et al. Phosphorylation of Nedd4-2 by Sgk1 regulates epithelial Na(+) channel cell surface expression. EMBO J. 2001;20:7052–7059.
74. Zhang W, Xia X, Reisenauer MR, et al. Aldosterone-induced Sgk1 relieves Dot1a–Af9-mediated transcriptional repression of epithelial Na$^+$ channel alpha. J Clin Invest. 2007;117:773–783.
75. Tangalakis K, Lumbers ER, Moritz KM, Towsloless MK, Wintour EM. Effect of cortisol on blood pressure and vascular reactivity in the ovine fetus. Exp Physiol. 1992;77(5):709–717.
76. Fletcher AJ, McGarrigle HH, Edwards CM, Fowden AL, Giussani DA. Effects of low dose dexamethasone treatment on basal cardiovascular and endocrine function in fetal sheep during late gestation. J Physiol. 2002;545:649–660.
77. Boini KM, Nammi S, Grahammer F, et al. Role of serum- and glucocorticoid-inducible kinase SGK1 in glucocorticoid regulation of renal electrolyte excretion and blood pressure. Kidney Blood Press Res. 2008;31:280–289.
78. Huh SY, Andrew R, Rich-Edwards JW, Kleinman KP, Seckl JR, Gillman MW. Association between umbilical cord glucocorticoids and blood pressure at age 3 years. BMC Med. 2008;6:25–28.
79. de Vries WB, Karemaker R, Mooy NF, et al. Cardiovascular follow-up at school age after perinatal glucocorticoid exposure in prematurely born children: perinatal glucocorticoid therapy and cardiovascular follow-up. Arch Pediatr Adolesc Med. 2008;162:738–744.
80. Pesquero JB, Bader M. Molecular biology of the kallikrein-kinin system: from structure to function. Braz J Med Biol Res. 1998;31:197–203.
81. Erdös EG, Oshima G. The angiotensin I converting enzyme of the lung and kidney. Acta Physiol Lat Am. 1974;24:507–514.
82. Marceau F, Hess JF, Bachvarov DR. The B1 receptors for kinins. Pharmacol Rev. 1998;50:357–386.
83. el-Dahr SS, Dipp S, Guan S, et al. Renin, angiotensinogen, and kallikrein gene expression in two-kidney Goldblatt hypertensive rats. Am J Hypertens. 1993;6:914–919.
84. Clements JA. The human kallikrein gene family: a diversity of expression and function. Mol Cell Endocrinol. 1994;99:C1–C6.
85. El-Dahr SS, Dipp S, Yosypiv IV, et al. Activation of kininogen expression during distal nephron differentiation. Am J Physiol. 1998;275:F173–F182.
86. Xiong W, Chao L, Chao J. Renal kallikrein mRNA localization by in situ hybridization. Kidney Int. 1989;35:1324–1329.
87. Siragy HM. Evidence that intrarenal bradykinin plays a role in regulation of renal function. Am J Physiol. 1993;265:E648–E654.

88. Beierwaltes WH, Prada J, Carretero OA. Effect of glandular kallikrein on renin release in isolated rat glomeruli. Hypertension. 1985;7:27–31.

89. McEachern AE, Shelton ER, Bhakta S, Obernolte R, Bach C, Zuppan P, Fujisaki J, Aldrich RW, Jarnagin K. Expression cloning of a rat B2 bradykinin receptor. Proc Natl Acad Sci U S A. 1991;88:7724–7728.

90. el-Dahr SS, Figueroa CD, Gonzalez CB, et al. Ontogeny of bradykinin B2 receptors in the rat kidney: implications for segmental nephron maturation. Kidney Int. 1997;51:739–749.

91. Bhoola KD, Figueroa CD, Worthy K. Bioregulation of kinins: kallikreins, kininogens, and kininases. Pharmacol Rev. 1992;44:1–80.

92. Emanueli C, Angioni GR, Anania V, et al. Blood pressure responses to acute or chronic captopril in mice with disruption of bradykinin B2-receptor gene. J Hypertens. 1997;15:1701–1706.

93. Cervenka L, Harrison-Bernard LM, Dipp S, et al. Early onset salt-sensitive hypertension in bradykinin B(2) receptor null mice. Hypertension. 1999;34:176–180.

94. Duka I, Duka A, Kintsurashvili E, et al. Mechanisms mediating the vasoactive effects of the B_1 receptors of bradykinin. Hypertension. 2003;42:1021–1025.

95. Cui J, Melista E, Chazaro I, et al. Sequence variation of bradykinin receptors B1 and B2 and association with hypertension. J Hypertens. 2005;23:55–62.

96. Gainer JV, Morrow JD, Loveland A, et al. Effect of bradykinin-receptor blockade on the response to angiotensin-converting-enzyme inhibitor in normotensive and hypertensive subjects. N Engl J Med. 1998;339:1285–1292.

97. Szentivanyi M Jr, Park F, Maeda CY, et al. Nitric oxide in the renal medulla protects from vasopressin-induced hypertension. Hypertension. 2000;35:740–745.

98. Peters J, Schlaghecke R, Thouet H, et al. Endogenous vasopressin supports blood pressure and prevents severe hypotension during epidural anesthesia in conscious dogs. Anesthesiology. 1990;73:694–702.

99. Ervin MG, Ross MG, Leake RD, et al. V1- and V2-receptor contributions to ovine fetal renal and cardiovascular responses to vasopressin. Am J Physiol. 1992;262:R636–R643.

100. Tomita H, Brace RA, Cheung CY, et al. Vasopressin dose-response effects on fetal vascular pressures, heart rate, and blood volume. Am J Physiol. 1985;249:H974–H980.

101. Kelly RT, Rose JC, Meis PJ, et al. Vasopressin is important for restoring cardiovascular homeostasis in fetal lambs subjected to hemorrhage. Am J Obstet Gynecol. 1983;146:807–812.

102. Kielstein JT, Zoccali C. Asymmetric dimethylarginine: a cardiovascular risk factor and a uremic toxin coming of age? Am J Kidney Dis. 2005;46:186–202.

103. Cowley AW Jr, Mori T, Mattson D, Zou AP. Role of renal NO production in the regulation of medullary blood flow. Am J Physiol. 2003;284:R1355–R1369.

104. Goldblatt H, Lynch R, Hanzai R. Studies on experimental: production of persistent elevation of systolic blood pressure by means of renal ischemia. J Exp Med. 1934;59:347–350.

105. Jin XH, McGrath HE, Gildea JJ, et al. Renal interstitial guanosine cyclic 3′,5′-monophosphate mediates pressure-natriuresis via protein kinase G. Hypertension. 2004;43:1133–1139.

106. Taddei S, Virdis A, Mattei P, et al. Defective L-arginine–nitric oxide pathway in offspring of essential hypertensive patients. Circulation. 1996;94:1298–1303.

107. Yu ZY, Lumbers ER, Simonetta G. The cardiovascular and renal effects of acute and chronic inhibition of nitric oxide production in fetal sheep. Exp Physiol. 2002;87:343–351.

108. Han KH, Lim JM, Kim WY, et al. Expression of endothelial nitric oxide synthase in developing rat kidney. Am J Physiol. 2005;288:F694–F702.

109. Teichert AM, Scott JA, Robb GB, et al. Endothelial nitric oxide synthase gene expression during murine embryogenesis: commencement of expression in the embryo occurs with the establishment of a unidirectional circulatory system. Circ Res. 2008;103:24–33.

110. Solhaug MJ, Ballèvre LD, Guignard JP, et al. Nitric oxide in the developing kidney. Pediatr Nephrol. 1996;10:529–533.

111. Zager PG, Nikolic J, Brown RH, et al. U-Curve association of blood pressure and mortality in hemodialysis patients. Kidney Int. 1998;54:561–569.

112. Kielstein JT, Impraim B, Simmel S, et al. Cardiovascular effects of systemic nitric oxide synthase inhibition with asymmetrical dimethylarginine in humans. Circulation. 2004;109:172–177.

113. Maeda T, Yoshimura T, Okamura H. Asymmetric dimethylarginine, an endogenous inhibitor of nitric oxide synthase, in maternal and fetal circulation. J Soc Gynecol Investig. 2003;10:2–4.

114. Goonasekera CD, Shah V, Rees DD, et al. Vascular endothelial cell activation associated with increased plasma asymmetric dimethyl arginine in children and young adults with hypertension: a basis for atheroma? Blood Press. 2000;9:16–21.

115. Päivä H, Kähönen M, Lehtimäki T, et al. Asymmetric dimethylarginine (ADMA) has a role in regulating systemic vascular tone in young healthy subjects: the cardiovascular risk in Young Finns study. Am J Hypertens. 2008;21:873–878.

116. Yanagisawa M, Kurihara H, Kimura S, Goto K, Masaki T. A novel peptide vasoconstrictor, endothelin, is produced by vascular endothelium and modulates smooth muscle Ca2+ channels. J Hypertens Suppl. 1988;6:S188–S191.

117. Lüscher TF, Boulanger CM, Dohi Y, et al. Endothelium-derived contracting factors. Hypertension. 1992;19:117–130.

118. Kohan DE. Endothelin synthesis by rabbit renal tubule cells. Am J Physiol. 1991;261:F221–F226.

119. Ujiie K, Terada Y, Nonoguchi H, et al. Messenger RNA expression and synthesis of endothelin-1 along rat nephron segments. J Clin Invest. 1992;90:1043–1048.

120. Yamamoto T, Hirohama T, Uemura H. Endothelin B receptor-like immunoreactivity in podocytes of the rat kidney. Arch Histol Cytol. 2002;65:245–250.

121. Hirata Y, Emori T, Eguchi S, et al. Endothelin receptor subtype B mediates synthesis of nitric oxide by cultured bovine endothelial cells. J Clin Invest. 1993;91:1367–1373.

122. Arai H, Hori S, Aramori I, et al. Cloning and expression of a cDNA encoding an endothelin receptor. Nature. 1990;348:730–732.

123. Wong J, Vanderford PA, Winters J, et al. Endothelin b receptor agonists produce pulmonary vasodilation in intact newborn lambs with pulmonary hypertension. J Cardiovasc Pharmacol. 1995;25:207–215.

124. Fujimori K, Honda S, Sanpei M, Sato A. Effects of exogenous big endothelin-1 on regional blood flow in fetal lambs. Obstet Gynecol. 2005;106:818–823.

125. Fineman JR, Wong J, Morin FC, et al. Chronic nitric oxide inhibition in utero produces persistent pulmonary hypertension in newborn lambs. J Clin Invest. 1994;93:2675–2683.

126. Ahn D, Ge Y, Stricklett PK, et al. Collecting duct-specific knockout of endothelin-1 causes hypertension and sodium retention. J Clin Invest. 2004;114:504–511.

127. Ge Y, Bagnall AJ, Stricklett PK, et al. Combined knockout of collecting duct endothelin A and B receptors causes hypertension and sodium retention. Am J Physiol. 2008;295:F1635–F1640.

128. Sudoh T, Minamino N, Kangawa K, et al. C-type natriuretic peptide (NP): a new member of natriuretic peptide family identified in porcine brain. Biochem Biophys Res Commun. 1990;168:863–870.

129. Schweitz H, Vigne P, Moinier D, et al. A new member of the natriuretic peptide family is present in the venom of the Green Mamba (Dendroaspis angusticeps). J Biol Chem. 1992;267:13928–13932.

130. Hirsch JR, Meyer M, Forssmann WG. ANP and urodilatin: who is who in the kidney. Eur J Med Res. 2006;11:447–454.

131. de Bold AJ, Borenstein HB, Veress AT, et al. A rapid and potent natriuretic response to intravenous injection of atrial myocardial extract in rats. Life Sci. 1981;28:89–94.

132. Levin ER, Gardner DG, Samson WK. Natriuretic peptides. N Engl J Med. 1998;339:321–328.

133. Brenner BM, Stein JH. Atrial Natriuretic Peptides. New York, NY: Churchill Livingstone; 1989.

134. Roques BP, Noble F, Dauge V, et al. Neutral endopeptidase 24.11: structure, inhibition, and experimental and clinical pharmacology. Pharmacol Rev. 1993;45:87–146.

135. Hunt PJ, Espiner EA, Nicholls MG, et al. Differing biological effects of equimolar atrial and brain natriuretic peptide infusions in normal man. J Clin Endocrinol Metab. 1996;81:3871–3876.

136. Zeller R, Bloch KD, Williams BS, et al. Localized expression of the atrial natriuretic factor gene during cardiac embryogenesis. Genes Dev. 1987;1:693–698.

137. Wei Y, Rodi CP, Day ML, et al. Developmental changes in the rat atriopeptin hormonal system. J Clin Invest. 1987;79:1325–1329.

138. Hersey R, Nazir M, Whitney K, et al. Atrial natriuretic peptide in heart and specific binding in organs from fetal and newborn rats. Cell Biochem Funct. 1987;7:35–41.

139. Cheung C, Gibbs D, Brace R. Atrial natriuretic factor in maternal and fetal sheep. Am J Physiol. 1987;252:E279–E282.

140. Cheung C. Regulation of atrial natriuretic factor secretion and expression in the ovine fetus. Neurosci Behav Rev. 1995;19:159–164.

141. Rosenfeld CR, Samson WK, Roy TA, et al. Vasoconstrictor-induced secretion of ANP in fetal sheep. Am J Physiol. 1992;263:E526–E533.

142. Bierd TM, Kattwinkel J, Chevalier RL, et al. Interrelationship of atrial natriuretic peptide, atrial volume, and renal function in premature infants. J Pediatr. 1990;116:753–759.

143. Weil J, Bidlingmaier F, Döhlemann C, et al. Comparison of plasma atrial natriuretic peptide levels in healthy children from birth to adolescence and in children with cardiac diseases. Pediatr Res. 1986;20:1328–1331.

144. Tamura N, Ogawa Y, Chusho H, et al. Cardiac fibrosis in mice lacking brain natriuretic peptide. Proc Natl Acad Sci U S A. 2000;97:4239–4244.

145. John SWM, Krege JH, Oliver PM, et al. Genetic decreases in atrial natriuretic peptide and salt-sensitive hypertension. Science. 1995;267:679–681.

146. Knowles J, Esposito G, Mao L, et al. Pressure independent enhancement of cardiac hypertrophy in natriuretic peptide receptor A deficient mice. J Clin Invest. 2001;107:975–984.

147. Barker DJ, Bagby SP. Developmental antecedents of cardiovascular disease: a historical perspective. J Am Soc Nephrol. 2005;16:2537–2544.

148. Pladys P, Lahaie I, Cambonie G, et al. Role of brain and peripheral angiotensin II in hypertension and altered arterial baroreflex programmed during fetal life in rat. Pediatr Res. 2004;55:1042–1049.

149. Edwards LJ, Simonetta G, Owens JA, et al. Restriction of placental and fetal growth in sheep alters fetal blood pressure responses to angiotensin II and captopril. J Physiol. 1999;515:897–904.

150. Bogdarina I, Welham S, King PJ, et al. Epigenetic modification of the renin-angiotensin system in the fetal programming of hypertension. Circ Res. 2007;100:520–526.

151. Yosypiv IV, Dipp S, el-Dahr SS. Role of bradykinin B2 receptors in neonatal kidney growth. J Am Soc Nephrol. 1997;8:920–928.

152. Brawley L, Itoh S, Torrens C, et al. Dietary protein restriction in pregnancy induces hypertension and vascular defects in rat male offspring. Pediatr Res. 2003;54:83–90.

153. Franco Mdo C, Dantas AP, Akamine EH, et al. Enhanced oxidative stress as a potential mechanism underlying the programming of hypertension in utero. J Cardiovasc Pharmacol. 2002;40:501–519.

154. Longo M, Jain V, Vedernikov YP, et al. Fetal origins of adult vascular dysfunction in mice lacking endothelial nitric oxide synthase. Am J Physiol. 2005;288:R1114–R1121.

155. Iosipiv IV, Schroeder M. A role for angiotensin II AT1 receptors in ureteric bud cell branching. Am J Physiol. 2003;285:F199–F207.

156. Prieto M, Dipp S, Meleg-Smith S, et al. Ureteric bud derivatives express angiotensinogen and AT1 receptors. Physiol Genomics. 2001;6:29–37.

157. Lopez ML, Pentz ES, Robert B, Abrahamson DR, Gomez RA. Embryonic origin and lineage of juxtaglomerular cells. Am J Physiol. 2001;281:F345–F356.

158. Jung FF, Bouyounes B, Barrio R, et al. Angiotensin converting enzyme in renal ontogeny: hypothesis for multiple roles. Pediatr Nephrol. 1993;7:834–840.

159. Yosypiv IV, El-Dahr SS. Role of the renin-angiotensin system in the development of the ureteric bud and renal collecting system. Pediatr Nephrol. 2005;20:1219–1229.

160. Niimura F, Labosky PA, Kakuchi J, Okubo S, Yoshida H, Oikawa T, Ichiki T, Naftilan AJ, Fogo A, Inagami T. Gene targeting in mice reveals a requirement for angiotensin in the development and maintenance of kidney morphology and growth factor regulation. J Clin Invest. 1995;96:2947–2954.

161. Nagata M, Tanimoto K, Fukamizu A, Kon Y, Sugiyama F, Yagami K, Murakami K, Watanabe T. Nephrogenesis and renovascular development in angiotensinogen-deficient mice. Lab Invest. 1996;75:745–753.

162. Tanimoto K, Sugiyama F, Goto Y, et al. Angiotensinogen-deficient mice with hypotension. J Biol Chem. 1994;269:31334–31337.

163. Takahashi N, Lopez ML, Cowhig JE Jr, et al. Ren1c homozygous null mice are hypotensive and polyuric, but heterozygotes are indistinguishable from wild-type. J Am Soc Nephrol. 2005;16:125–132.

164. Esther CR Jr, Howard TE, Marino EM, et al. Mice lacking angiotensin-converting enzyme have low blood pressure, renal pathology, and reduced male fertility. Lab Invest. 1996;7:953–965.

165. Oliverio MI, Kim HS, Ito M, et al. Reduced growth, abnormal kidney structure, and type 2 (AT$_2$) angiotensin receptor-mediated blood pressure regulation in mice lacking both AT$_{1A}$ and AT$_{1B}$ receptors for angiotensin II. Proc Natl Acad Sci U S A. 1998;95:15496–15501.

166. Tsuchida S, Matsusaka T, Chen X, et al. Murine double nullizygotes of the angiotensin type 1A and 1B receptor genes duplicate severe abnormal phenotypes of angiotensinogen nullizygotes. J Clin Invest. 1998;101:755–760.

167. Chen X, Li W, Yoshida H, et al. Targeting deletion of angiotensin type 1B receptor gene in the mouse. Am J Physiol. 1997;272:F299–F304.

168. Oshima K, Miyazaki Y, Brock JW, et al. Angiotensin type II receptor expression and ureteral budding. J Urol. 2001;166:1848–1852.

169. Hein L, Barsh GS, Pratt RE, et al. Behavioural and cardiovascular effects of disrupting the angiotensin II type-2 receptor in mice. Nature. 1995;377:744–747.

3

Cardiovascular and Autonomic Influences on Blood Pressure

John E. Jones, PhD, Aruna R. Natarajan, MD, DCh, PhD, and Pedro A. Jose, MD, PhD

CONTENTS

The cardiovascular system provides appropriate organ and tissue perfusion at rest and at times of stress by regulation of blood pressure. The arterial pressure level reflects the composite activities of the heart and the peripheral circulation.

CONTROL OF BLOOD PRESSURE

Although the relationship between pressure and flow through the vascular tree is not linear, blood pressure can be expressed as the product of cardiac output (CO) and peripheral resistance *(1)* (Table 1). These variables are closely intertwined, and the control

J.E. Jones (✉)
Children's Research Institute, Center for Molecular Physiology Research, Children's National Medical Center, Washington, DC, USA
e-mail: jnjones@cnmc.org

From: *Clinical Hypertension and Vascular Diseases: Pediatric Hypertension*
Edited by: J. T. Flynn et al. DOI 10.1007/978-1-60327-824-9_3
© Springer Science+Business Media, LLC 2011

Table 1
Factors Influencing Arterial Pressure as the Product of Cardiac Output and Peripheral Resistance

Cardiac output
Heart rate
Stroke volume
　Venous return
　Myocardial contractility
Blood volume

Peripheral resistance
Adrenergic nerves
Circulating catecholamines
Other vasoactive substances
　Acetylcholine
　Angiotensin II (angiotensin 1–7, angiotensin 2–8)
　Calcitonin gene-related peptide (intermedin, adrenomedullin 2)
　Carbon monoxide
　Endothelium-derived contracting factor
　Hydrogen sulfide
　Kinins
　Neuropeptides (neurotensin, NPY, substance P)
　Nitric oxide
　Oxytocin
　Prostanoids (prostaglandins, HETEs, leukotrienes, thromboxanes)
　Serotonin
　Substance P
　Vasopressin
Ions and cellular regulations (e.g., calcium, sodium, chloride, potassium, magnesium,
　manganese, and trace metals, pH)
Hematocrit (viscosity)
Reactive oxygen species

mechanisms for pressure regulation involve more than simply a direct change in either CO or peripheral resistance *(2)*. The major determinant of blood pressure at rest is arteriolar resistance; during exercise, CO assumes a more important role.

Cardiac Output

CO is defined as the volume of blood pumped by the left ventricle of the heart into the aorta and thence to the circulation. In general CO is expressed in liters/minute. It represents the circulatory status of the organism and plays a critical role in maintenance of blood pressure in health and disease. Blood pressure is determined by the product of CO and systemic vascular resistance.

CO varies widely depending on metabolic and physical activity, age, and size of the body. In healthy young males, resting cardiac output is 5.6 L/min and is about 20% lower in females. As this value varies consistently with the body surface area (BSA), it is also expressed as cardiac index, which is the cardiac output per square meter BSA. This value is about 3 L/min/m *(2)*. Babies have a higher cardiac index at 5.5 L/min/m^2 which is even higher in preterm babies.

CO is tightly regulated to meet the body's rapidly changing metabolic needs. Primary and secondary mechanisms govern CO: primary mechanisms operate quickly for acute regulation, and secondary mechanisms have a slower onset and regulate long-term aspects of cardiac function. CO is derived from the product of stroke volume (volume represented by the volume of blood pumped by the heart in one beat) and the heart rate (HR) per minute. In infancy and early childhood, CO is increased mainly by an increase in HR because the capacity of the cardiac muscle to increase stroke volume during this period is limited.

Stroke Volume

Stroke volume depends on three primary factors, all of which are interrelated and not mutually exclusive.

1. *Preload* reflects venous filling of the right ventricle which subsequently determines the volume of blood available to be pumped to the circulation by the left ventricle. Preload is classically compromised in dehydration and hemorrhage.
2. *Afterload* is caused by peripheral arterial resistance and intrinsic ventricular wall stress. Afterload determines diastolic pressure and thus has a significant impact on mean arterial pressure and resulting tissue perfusion. Afterload is decreased due to vasoplegia in septic shock and increased due to vasoconstriction in hypothermia.
3. *Myocardial contractility* reflects the inherent capacity of the cardiac muscle to pump blood. This function is compromised in myocarditis and some forms of cardiomyopathy. These primary factors could be altered by secondary factors in response to the physiological state of the individual.

PRELOAD

CO output is determined primarily by the volume of venous blood that fills the ventricle during diastole, the preload or end-diastolic volume. The adult heart can pump up to 15 L of blood per minute, although the usual resting CO is only 5.6 L/min. The Frank–Starling law describes the inherent ability of the heart to regulate its output in the face of a rapidly changing preload. Increasing preload increases the end-diastolic volume which results in the stretch of the muscle fibers. Hence, increased volume at the end of diastole leads to increased stroke volume by an immediate, increased, and effective ejection during systole. This ensures that even when end-diastolic volume or filling is increased, the end-systolic volume or the volume of blood left in the ventricle at the end of systole does not increase, as all of the extra volume is pumped out. However, this process does not continue indefinitely. The energy output of a heart muscle fiber increases with increasing fiber length up to a point, beyond which further extension of the fiber results in a decrease in its contractile force, causing a reduction in stroke volume. An important aspect of the Frank–Starling law is that a change in the afterload (or outflow resistance) has almost no influence on cardiac output. Preload-dependent regulation of stroke volume is also called *heterometric regulation*. Stretching of the ventricle stretches the sinus node in the wall of the right atrium, which increases its rate of firing and increases the heart rate by 10–15%. The stretched right atrium also initiates a reflex called the Bainbridge reflex which increases heart rate in euvolemic states. In summary, increasing preload increases stroke volume and heart rate, and thus preload is a major player in enhancing cardiac output.

AFTERLOAD

Afterload is the force that opposes or resists ventricular emptying. After the ventricle has ejected its contents, the resulting increase in aortic pressure closes the aortic valve and maintains a back pressure that the next cycle of systole has to overcome. Components of the aortic back pressure include the tension developed in the aortic walls, peripheral vascular resistance, the reflected pressure waves within the ventricle, and its distribution throughout the ventricular wall. Thus ventricular pressure, myocardial thickness, and peripheral resistance all contribute to systolic wall stress, which together determine afterload. Mean arterial pressure (calculated as 2 × diastolic plus 1 × systolic BP divided by 3), which is related to CO and peripheral resistance, serves as an indication of afterload. Mean afterload is normally kept constant by central cardiovascular and autonomic control.

Because the afterload does not allow the ventricle to empty completely, a percentage of the original venous return remains in the heart. The term *ejection fraction* (EF) describes the amount of blood ejected from the ventricle during one systolic wave (stroke volume, SV) divided by the amount of blood in the ventricle at the end of diastole (left ventricular end-diastolic volume, LVEDV).

$$EF = SV/LVEDV$$

This is quantified with echocardiography by measuring the shortening fraction (SF) which is given by measuring the diameters, rather than volumes, of the left ventricle during systole and at the end of diastole, i.e., SF = LV end-diastolic diameter − LV end-systolic diameter, LV end-diastolic diameter of the muscle fiber, which correlates directly with contractility. Typically the EF for a normal adult is 0.50–0.75, while the EF is 0.18–0.42, with levels >0.3 being considered "normal" and EF of 0.26–0.30 considered to be indicative of a mild decrease in contractile function. A decrease in SF generally precedes a detectable decrease in EF. While left and right ventricular diastolic volumes do increase with gestational and postnatal age *(3)*, the EF remains the same.

MYOCARDIAL CONTRACTILITY

Myocardial contractility accounts for the increases in contractile force of a muscle fiber without an accompanying change in fiber length. This property of cardiac muscle is called *homeotropic regulation*. The heart is richly supplied with autonomic nerves, both sympathetic and parasympathetic, that have profound effects on heart rate and contractility. The resting normal sympathetic tone maintains cardiac contractility at 20% greater than that in the denervated heart. Increased sympathetic input to the heart can significantly increase both heart rate and contractile force, up to 100%. Parasympathetic innervation, on the other hand, reduces heart rate and contractile force through nerve fibers predominantly supplying the atria. In addition, intracardiac parasympathetic ganglia exert selective inhibitory effects on left ventricular contractility *(4)*. However, contractility can only be decreased by about 20%. Parasympathetic effects are mediated by the release of acetylcholine activity.

Table 2
Some Drugs Showing Selectivity for Adrenergic and Dopamine Receptor Subtypes *(19)*

Drug name	Agonists	Antagonists
Nonselective	Norepinephrine	Phentolamine
α_1	Methoxamine	Prazosin
α_{1A}	NS-49	(+) Niguldipine, 5-methyl urapidil,
	A-61603	KMD-3213
α_{1B}		
α_{1D}	Naftopidil	BMY-7378
α_2	14304	Idazoxan
		Rauwolscine
		Yohimbine
$\alpha_{2A/D}$		BRL 48962
α_{2B}		BRL 41992
α_{2C}		WB 4101
β-Adrenoceptor		
Nonselective	Isoproterenol	Propranolol
		Pindolol
β_1	Prenalterol	Metoprolol
	(-) Ro-363	Atenolol
		ICI 89,406
		CGP20712A
β_2	Salbutamol	Butoxamine
	Terbutaline	ICI 118,551 (inverse agonist)
	Zinterol	
β_3	BRL 37344	SR-59230
	CL 316243	(not blocked by propranolol)
Dopamine receptor		
Nonselective	Dopamine	
D_1-like	Fenoldopam[a]	SCH 23390[a]
D_1	A 68930	
D_5	SKF 82958	4-Chloro-3-hydroxy-7-methyl-5,6,7,8,9,14-hexahydro-dibenz[d,g]azecine
D_2-like	LY 171555	YM 09151
	SKF103376	Domperidone
D_2	U91356A	L741,626
	U95666	
D_3	PD128907	Nafadotride
	7-hydroxyPIPAT	U-99,194A
D_4	PD168077	U-101958

[a]Selective for D_1-like receptors but cannot distinguish between D_1 and D_5 receptors.

Only muscarinic m2 receptors have been thought to be expressed in the heart. However, m1 and m3 muscarinic receptors may also be present in cardiac myocytes *(5).* Sympathetic enhancement of cardiac contractility is mediated by norepinephrine from the cardiac sympathetic nerves. Norepinephrine causes an increase in shortening of the muscle fiber with a constant preload and total load resulting in increased stroke volume. This effect is mediated by the stimulation of β-adrenergic receptors, mainly of the β_1 subtype (see Table 2) on the cardiac membranes leading to an increase in cyclic AMP. cAMP increases phosphorylase B activity, which stimulates glycogen metabolism, and increases the energy needed for enhanced contractility. The combined effects of sympathetic stimulation on HR and contractility can cause a two- to threefold increase in cardiac output. Neurotrophins, including nerve growth factor, are important in cardiac sympathetic innervation, acting through the tropomyosin-related tyrosine kinase receptor to a greater extent than p75 receptor *(6).* Neurturin, a member of the glial-cell-derived neurotrophic factor, is important in the development of cardiac parasympathetic neurons *(7).*

Calcium is necessary for effective contraction of cardiac muscle. Action potential causes release of calcium into the sarcoplasm of the muscle. Instantaneously, calcium ions diffuse into the myofibrils and catalyze the chemical reactions that promote sliding of actin and myosin filaments along one another, producing muscle contraction. Because muscle sarcoplasm does not have a large store of calcium, large amounts of extracellular calcium are needed to diffuse into the T-tubules, where they are bound to glycoproteins, and released as needed to enhance contractility. In atrial cells that do not have T-tubules, calcium release may be limited to peripheral junctions on the cell surface but calcium may also arise from sarcoplasmic reticulum and the mitochondria *(8).* In the adult heart, excitation–contraction coupling caused by calcium-induced calcium release (CICR) is mediated by L-type Ca^{2+} channels while this is mediated by the reverse-mode Na^+–Ca^{2+} exchanger (NCX) activity in the developing heart *(9).*

HEART RATE AND RHYTHM

Factors affecting heart rate do so by altering the electric properties of the cardiac pacemaker cells, which have an intrinsic rate that is age dependent, being higher in infancy and decreasing with age. The autonomic nervous system exerts the most profound influence on heart rate. The sympathetic and parasympathetic systems act by changing the rate of spontaneous depolarization of the resting potential in the cardiac pacemaker cells. While sympathetic stimulation causes an increase in heart rate, parasympathetic stimulation causes a decrease in heart rate. These reflexes are immediate and represent critical survival mechanisms. During periods of tachycardia, peak ejection velocity is increased. The net effect of the tachycardia is an increased cardiac output. However, outside the normal physiologic range, large increases or decreases in heart rate result in a decrease in the net cardiac output. For example, in the adult, tachycardia of 170 beats/min or greater allows too little time for ventricular filling, and therefore stroke volume. The decreased stroke volume may not be overcome by the increased heart rate. Lower than normal heart rate, or bradycardia, causes a decreased cardiac output because stroke volume does not increase sufficiently to meet the requirements of the individual to sustain CO. At heart rates below 40 beats/min (in the adult), the increase in preload due to increased filling time is limited because major ventricular filling, which occurs early in diastole, is not maintained throughout the extent of the diastolic period.

Heart rate is one of the most important determinants of myocardial energy consumption. Generally it is more energy efficient to increase cardiac output by increasing stroke volume, rather than by increasing heart rate. Infants and children are more likely to increase their heart rate and thus expend more energy in increasing their cardiac output during stress.

PRIMARY REGULATION OF CARDIAC OUTPUT DURING DEVELOPMENT

Effective circulation is necessary in very early embryonic development and parallels structural development of the heart *(10)*. As early as 5 weeks postconception in humans, the basic circulatory parameter, heart rate, is present at about 100 beats/min. Recent advances have elucidated the genetic control of embryonic differentiation of cardiac pacemaker cells and have implicated genes in the establishment of heart rate. Shox2 homeodomain transcription factor is essential for the development of the sinoatrial node and pacemaker by repressing Nkx2-5 *(11)*.

CO is very dependent on heart rate and, after formation of the four-chambered heart, on atrioventricular synchrony. Systolic function of the heart and, consequently, CO increases with gestational age. The ejection fraction of the embryonic ventricle is roughly 30–50%, similar to adults. The fetal heart, however, has a limited ability to increase work following stretch, so the Frank–Starling curve is limited compared to adults. The lower wall stress in the embryo, due to a smaller ventricular size and lower pressures, reduces the total afterload and enhances cardiac output in the face of a high peripheral resistance. Afterload due to wall stress increases as gestation progresses, reflecting the increase in ventricular size and transmural pressures even while peripheral vascular resistance decreases.

SECONDARY REGULATION OF CARDIAC OUTPUT

A variety of factors operate in the normal individual to regulate CO over the long term. These secondary control mechanisms do not have as great an influence on the heart as the components previously described. Secondary controls include cardiovascular reflexes and hormonal influences. Cardiopulmonary receptors, which are sensory nerve endings in the atria, ventricles, coronary vessels, and lungs, have chemo- and mechanosensitive properties. The activity of these receptors is relayed to the nucleus of the tractus solitarius via vagal afferents and spinal sympathetic afferent fibers. Stimulation of these receptors evokes responses similar to those noted with arterial baroreceptors (see below). Thus, an increase in distension of the atria results in a decrease in circulating levels of vasopressin, aldosterone, and renin, among other hormones, but causes an increase in the natriuretic factors synthesized by the atrium and the ventricles (atrial natriuretic peptide, brain natriuretic peptide, C-type natriuretic peptide). Circulating atrial natriuretic peptide levels decrease with gestational and postnatal age *(12)*. Depressor reflexes in the heart originating mainly from the inferoposterior wall of the left ventricle promote bradycardia, vasodilatation, and hypotension (Bezold–Jarisch reflex) *(13)*. These are mediated by increased parasympathetic and decreased sympathetic activity. Left ventricular mechanoreceptor stimulation can also attenuate arterial baroreflex control of heart rate. Decreased activity of cardiac vagal afferents results in enhanced sympathetic activity and increased vascular resistance, renin release, and vasopressin secretion. Alterations in extracellular fluid volume influence CO via changes in preload and blood pressure. In fetal and newborn animals cardiopulmonary receptors have minimal influence in the regulation of cardiovascular and autonomic responses to changes in blood pressure or blood volume *(14)*.

Peripheral Resistance

Blood flow through a vessel is determined by two primary factors: the amount of pressure forcing the blood through the vessel and the resistance to flow. The resistance to flow in a blood vessel is best described as impedance because this takes into account inertial properties and viscosity of blood elastic properties of blood vessels and the variable geometries of blood vessels during phasic flow. One of the most important factors influencing the flow through the arteries is the vessel diameter, since the conductance is proportional to the fourth power of the diameter. Therefore, flow is influenced more by changes in vascular resistance than by pressure changes. The different variables influencing peripheral resistance are listed in Table 1.

CONTROL MECHANISMS FOR BLOOD PRESSURE REGULATION

The short-term adjustment and long-term control of blood pressure are supplied by a hierarchy of pressure controls *(2)*. The cardiovascular reflexes are the most rapidly acting pressure control mechanisms. They are activated within seconds, and the effects may last from a few minutes to a few days. The pressure controls acting with intermediate rapidity include capillary fluid shifts, stress relaxation, and hormonal control that include the angiotensin and vasopressin systems. These systems, like the cardiovascular reflexes, function to buffer acute changes in pressure. Long-term control is afforded by long-term regulation of body fluids *(2)*.

ARTERIAL BARORECEPTORS

The degree of arteriolar constriction is determined by a balance between tonic output from the pressor areas of the cardiovascular center and the degree of inhibition from the baroreceptors. The arterial baroreceptors are the major fast reacting, slowly adapting feedback elements to the central neural cardiovascular regulatory system and operate to limit sudden changes in blood pressure. Their mechanosensitive nerve endings are located at the medial–adventitial border of blood vessels with elastic structure, mainly at the aortic arch and carotid sinuses. The receptors respond to deformation of the vessel in any direction, i.e., circumferential and longitudinal stretch. This results in the stimulation of mechanosensitive channels that contain degenerin/epithelial sodium channel (DEG/ENaC) *(15,16)*. The pressure–diameter relationship is concave with the greatest distensibility at about 120–140 mmHg. There are two types of receptors in the carotid sinus: type I receptors are thin myelinated fibers and type II receptors are thick myelinated fibers with fine end branches terminating in neurofibrillar end plates. The latter receptors are also seen in the aortic arch. Postnatal hypoxemia is associated with an increased sensitivity of peripheral chemoreceptors that may be related to increased expression and activity of angiotensin type 1 receptors *(17)*.

An increase in blood pressure stimulates the mechanosensitive receptors in the baroreceptors and causes inhibition of the sympathetic nervous system and activation of the parasympathetic nervous system. This results in a decrease in heart rate, myocardial contractility, peripheral vascular resistance, and venous return. A decrease in blood pressure decreases mechanosensitive stimulation of the baroreceptors and causes inhibition of the parasympathetic nervous system and the activation of the sympathetic nervous system. This results in an increase in heart rate, myocardial contractility, peripheral vascular resistance, and venous return *(18)*. Changes in osmotic pressure affect other homeostatic mechanisms such as thirst and vasopressin release by the activation of ion channels *(19)*. Shear stress resulting from increased blood pressure also sets into motion the generation of endogenous vasodilators such as nitric oxide which cause vasodilatation to oppose the increase in blood pressure.

Sensory innervation of the aortic arch is derived from the vagus while the carotid sinus nerve originates from the glossopharyngeal nerve. The majority of the afferent nerves are myelinated type A fibers. These fibers have large and intermediate spikes of 40–120 μV corresponding to the high distensibility region. At normal pressure levels, these fibers transmit mainly the dynamic components of blood pressure, pulse pressure (dp/dt), and pulse frequency. The receptor sensitivity is highest at the lower end (60–100 mmHg) of the high distensibility region of the blood vessel. There are a few nonmyelinated type C fibers, located mainly in the carotid sinus nerve. The spikes are small (5–10 μV), have a higher static threshold (120–150 mmHg), correspond to the low distensibility region, and mainly transmit mean pressure. The type C fibers can be activated independently by sympathetic stimuli.

The arterial baroreceptors are more effective in compensating for a fall rather than a rise in mean arterial pressure. The interaction between mean and pulsatile components can be of considerable importance in the hemodynamic response to hemorrhage. For example, the initial response to moderate hemorrhage results in a decrease in pulse pressure with maintenance of mean arterial pressure. Decreasing pulse pressure results in a redistribution of CO to the mesenteric and cardiac circulations with no effect on the renal circulation.

Information carried by the afferent limb of the reflex arc from the baroreceptors is relayed to the lower brain stem via the vagus and glossopharyngeal nerves. Most secondary neurons are located at the nucleus of the tractus solitarius, and projections are directed to various regions of the brain stem. The effectors of the baroreceptors include systems that have an immediate but short-term effect on circulatory function and those that have delayed but long-term effects. Examples of the former are resistance vessels—arterioles throughout the systemic circulation—the capacitance vessels—veins and arteries—and the heart. An example of a system with a long-term effect is the kidney. In addition, neural reflexes may influence circulating levels of several hormones (e.g., renin, vasopressin) with short- and long-term effects on cardiovascular regulation. The effect of neural reflexes on the kidneys may be direct, through renal sympathetic nerve activity, or indirect, through circulating catecholamines.

Norepinephrine-containing nerve endings are found in the carotid sinus and aortic arch and may influence the sensitivity of the sinus reflex. Norepinephrine, given intravenously, decreases the distensibility of the sinus at low pressures but increases the distensibility at high pressure. In the conscious dog, sinus hypotension induces a reflex tachycardia and sympathetic vasoconstriction of the skeletal resistance vessels. The changes in the renal and mesenteric beds (45% of total peripheral resistance) seem to be solely due to autoregulation. In the anesthetized dog, sinus hypotension induces a greater magnitude and a more generalized pattern of sympathetic vasoconstriction and may include both resistance and capacitance vessels. Several paracrine factors that affect the sensitivity of arterial baroreceptors have been reported, including prostanoids and nitric oxide. In general, vasoconstrictors decrease baroreceptor sensitivity while vasodilators have the converse effect.

However, nitric oxide decreases baroreceptor sensitivity independent of its vasodilator action. Reactive oxygen species (ROS) also decrease baroreceptor sensitivity, a mechanism that may contribute to the increase in systemic blood pressure caused by ROS *(20)*. Reduction in ROS decreases central sympathetic nerve activity *(21)*.

ADAPTATION OF THE BARORECEPTORS

The baroreceptors exert a tonic inhibitory influence on peripheral sympathetic activity. Baroreceptor nerves interact by mutual inhibitory addition; with a decrease in pressure, there is less reflex inhibition and a resultant increase in sympathetic outflow. While transient baroreceptor-induced changes in heart rate are primarily mediated by the parasympathetic nervous system, steady-state responses are due to a greater involvement of the sympathetic nervous system. A sudden increase in pressure (with resultant stretching of the receptors) causes an immediate increase in baroreceptor firing rate. With continued elevation of the pressure, however, there is a decrease in the rate of baroreceptor firing. Initially the decrease is rapid, and during the succeeding hours and days it slows down. This adaptation, or resetting, in response to a lower or higher pressure seems to be complete in 2 days. This adaptation can occur at the receptor and nervous signal pathway *(2)*. The resetting of the baroreflex is much more rapid in adults than in infants *(22)*.

ARTERIAL BARORECEPTORS DURING DEVELOPMENT

Studies in humans and experimental animals suggest that arterial baroreceptors are present in the fetus and undergo postnatal maturation *(22,23)*. There is an enhanced sensitivity of the efferent limb of the baroreflex in fetal life *(22)*. Neurotrophins are important in cardiac sympathetic innervation *(7)*, and brain-derived neurotrophic factor may mediate the postnatal maturation of the baroreceptor reflex *(24)*. In adults with intact arterial baroreceptors, a rapid head-up tilt is accompanied by an immediate increase in heart rate and peripheral vascular resistance with maintenance of mean arterial pressure in the upper body. Several studies have suggested that in healthy preterm and term human infants, head-up tilting also increases heart rate in proportion to the degree of tilting. However, other studies have shown that in healthy preterm infants with a postconceptional age of 28–32 weeks, a 45° head-up tilt results in an increase in peripheral resistance without any significant changes in heart rate *(14)*. The increase in heart rate with a 45° head-up tilt increases with postconceptional age. In the conscious newborn dog, the magnitude of the increase in mean arterial pressure and peripheral resistance following bilateral carotid occlusion is less than that in the adult. In addition, these changes occur without alterations in heart rate, similar to the effects noted in infants. In fetal sheep, only the increase in heart rate with a decrease in blood pressure is noted. There is no relationship of arterial pressure and heart rate variability immediately after birth, but the fetal pattern resumes a few hours later *(25)*. Recent research has suggested that the prone sleeping position impairs the development of cardiovascular reflexes, even in term infants, especially during the 2- to 3-month age group when sudden infant death syndrome (SIDS) is most prevalent *(26,27)*.

Newborn lambs exhibit the classic inverse relationship between heart rate and blood pressure, but the sensitivity is only about 50% that of the adult. The responses to small changes in blood pressure are similar in fetal and newborn lambs. However, when the change in blood pressure is greater than 15% the responses are different. In newborn lambs a progressive tachycardia accompanies the increasing hypotension, due to a combination of increased sympathetic outflow and parasympathetic withdrawal. There is no progressive tachycardia in the fetus; in fact, when the blood pressure change is greater than 50%, bradycardia occurs, apparently due to augmentation of vagal parasympathetic tone.

There are age-dependent differences in the ability of the piglet to compensate for hemorrhage and hypoxia *(28)*. Neonatal swine are able to compensate with greater facility for venous than arterial hemorrhage *(29)*. Volume expansion inhibits the sympathetic nervous system to a greater extent in older than in newborn lambs. Increasing arterial pressure by intravenous administration of vasoconstrictor agents results in smaller changes in heart rate in the newborn animal as well. Completion of sympathetic efferent pathways occurs before baroreceptor reflex activity is capable of modulating cardiac sympathetic activity. Thus, maturation of baroreceptor reflex activity may be dependent on development of baroreceptor function or of connections between baroreceptor and sympathetic efferents *(22)*. The changes in baroreflexes during development are thought to be caused by afferent, central integration, and efferent pathways. The maturation of receptors for various humoral and hormonal agents (e.g., angiotensin II, glucocorticoids, prostanoids, vasopressin) has been shown to affect baroreflex function.

Autonomic Regulation of Blood Pressure

Regulation of the distribution of CO and maintenance of blood pressure are major functions of the autonomic nervous system. The arterioles are normally in a continuous state of partial constriction, largely determined by an equilibrium between vasoconstrictor influences from the cardiovascular centers and the inhibitory input from the peripheral baroreceptors. The veins also receive autonomic innervation. Adrenergic nerves induce venous constriction with a resultant decrease in capacitance which increases venous return and CO. The effects of the adrenergic nervous system are conveyed by the neurotransmitters: norepinephrine, epinephrine, and dopamine.

Catecholamines. Epinephrine is released mainly from the adrenal medulla, while norepinephrine is released mainly in terminal nerve endings. In organs with dopaminergic nerves, a greater proportion of catecholamine released is dopamine. Norepinephrine synthesized at peripheral nerve endings is stored in subcellular granules. After a specific stimulus, it is released into the synaptic cleft where it interacts with specific receptors at the effector cell. The neurotransmitter is inactivated to a large extent by reuptake into the storage granules. This reuptake process (reuptake-1) is stereoselective, sodium dependent, and of high affinity. A presynaptic reuptake that is of low affinity and nonsodium dependent has been termed reuptake-2. There are specific amine transporters. Although the enzymatic degradation of the neurotransmitter by monoamine oxidase and catechol-*O*-methyltransferase is much less important in termination of neurotransmitter action in nervous tissue, in vascular smooth muscles this metabolism plays an important role *(30)*. More recently a third monoamine oxidase (MAOC or renalase) has been reported to degrade circulating catecholamines, especially dopamine *(31)*. The remainder of the neurotransmitter which escapes reuptake-1 and -2 is released into the circulation. Since only about 20% of the total appears in the circulating pool the plasma levels of catecholamines are merely a rough index of adrenergic activity.

Adrenergic and dopaminergic receptors. For the neurotransmitter to exert its specific effect, it must occupy a specific receptor on the cell surface. Catecholamines can occupy specific pre- and postsynaptic receptors. Each receptor has different subtypes *(32–35)*. Table 2 lists some drugs that have relative selectivity to each particular receptor subtype in the peripheral vascular bed. Occupation of presynaptic α_2-adrenergic and dopamine receptors inhibits norepinephrine release. Occupation of presynaptic β-receptors enhances norepinephrine release. At low levels of nerve stimulation, norepinephrine release is increased; at high levels of stimulation, the inhibitory effects of presynaptic α_2-adrenergic receptors predominate, acting as a short-loop feedback. The antihypertensive effects of dopamine agonists and (β-adrenergic antagonists) may be due in part to their ability to decrease release of norepinephrine at the terminal nerve endings.

α_1-**Adrenergic receptors.** Three α_1-adrenergic receptors are expressed in mammals, α_{1A} (originally designated as the α_{1C} when cloned), α_{1B}, and α_{1D}. The effects in the vascular bed are receptor subtype specific. Thus, α_{1A} may mediate contraction of renal and caudal arteries, whereas α_{1D}-adrenergic receptors may regulate the contraction of the aorta, femoral, iliac, and superior mesenteric arteries. Mice deficient of the α_{1A}-adrenergic receptor have decreased blood pressure as do mice deficient of the α_{1D}-adrenergic receptor *(35)*. The α_{1D} receptor-deficient mice are resistant to the hypertensive effect of sodium chloride. In contrast, α_{1B}-adrenergic receptors may not regulate vascular smooth muscle contraction. Mice deficient of the α_{1B}-adrenergic receptor have normal blood pressure in the basal state *(36,37)*. Neonatal cardiac myocytes hypertrophy is mediated primarily by the α_{1A}- and α_{1B}-adrenergic receptors. Aortic hypertrophy, on the other hand, is primarily due to the actions of the α_{1D}-adrenergic receptors.

α_2-**Adrenergic receptors.** There are three α_2-adrenergic receptor subtypes, $\alpha_{2A/D}$, α_{2B}, and α_{2C}. The α_{2A} class predominates and mediates most of the classical effects of α_2-adrenergic stimulation, to decrease blood pressure and heart rate, induce sedation, and consolidate working memory. In contrast, α_{2B}-adrenergic receptors, predominantly found outside of the central nervous system at extrajunctional or postsynaptic sites, produce vasoconstriction and thus counteract the hypotensive effects of α_{2A}-adrenergic receptor stimulation. α_{2B}-Adrenergic receptors are important in vascularization of the placenta. α_{2C}-Adrenergic receptors do not have cardiovascular effects but may mediate the hypothermic response to β_2-adrenergic stimulation *(38)* and feedback inhibition of adrenal catecholamine release. The effects of the α_2-adrenergic receptors are exerted in both adrenergic (autoreceptors) and nonadrenergic (heteroreceptors) cells *(33)*.

β-**Adrenergic receptors.** There are three β-adrenergic receptors, β_1, β_2, and β_3. Disruption of either the β_1-, β_2-adrenergic receptor, or both does not affect heart rate or resting blood pressure in mice. Mice lacking the β_1-adrenergic receptor are unresponsive to cardiac β-adrenergic receptor stimulation, suggesting that neither β_2- nor β_3-adrenergic receptors play a role in the inotropic or chronotropic responses in the mouse *(39)*. Indeed, the effect of the non-β-adrenergic subtype receptor agonist isoproterenol is not altered in β_2-adrenergic receptor null mice. However, the hypotensive response to isoproterenol is impaired in both β_1- and β_2-adrenergic null mice *(40,41)*. β_3-Adrenergic receptors do not have major effects on the cardiovascular system *(42)*.

Dopamine receptors. Dopamine is an important regulator of blood pressure. Presynaptic/junctional and postsynaptic/junctional or extrasynaptic dopamine receptors are found in many organs, including the heart *(43–45)* and vascular beds. Dopamine's actions on renal hemodynamics, epithelial transport, and humoral agents such as aldosterone, catecholamines, endothelin, prolactin, pro-opiomelanocortin, renin, and vasopressin place it in a central homeostatic position for the regulation of extracellular fluid volume and blood pressure. Dopamine also modulates fluid and sodium intake via its actions in the central nervous system and gastrointestinal tract and by regulation of cardiovascular centers that control the functions of the heart, arteries, and veins. Abnormalities in dopamine production and receptor function accompany a high percentage of human essential hypertension and several forms of rodent genetic hypertension. Dopamine receptor genes, as well as genes encoding their regulators, are in loci that have been linked to hypertension in humans and in rodents. Moreover, allelic variants (single nucleotide polymorphisms, SNPs) of genes that encode the regulators of the dopamine receptors, alone or in combination with variants of genes that encode proteins that regulate the renin–angiotensin system, are associated with human essential hypertension.

Dopamine receptors. Each of the five dopamine receptor subtypes (D_1, D_2, D_3, D_4, and D_5) participates in the regulation of blood pressure by mechanisms specific for the subtype *(46–48)*. Both the D_1-like dopamine receptors (D_1 and D_5) and the D_3 receptor decrease epithelial sodium transport *(46,47)*. D_4 receptors inhibit the effects of aldosterone and vasopressin in the renal cortical collecting duct *(48,49)*. D_2-like receptors (e.g., D_2 receptor) under certain circumstances may increase sodium transport *(50,51)*. Dopamine can regulate the secretion and receptors of several humoral agents (e.g., the D_1, D_3, and D_4 receptors interact with the renin–angiotensin system). The D_1-like receptors are vasodilatory, while the D_2-like receptors can mediate vasodilation or vasoconstriction depending upon the starting vascular resistance. When vascular resistance is high, D_2-like receptors are vasodilatory by inhibition of norepinephrine release. However, when vascular resistance is low, D_2-like receptors mediate vasoconstriction probably via the D_3 receptor *(51)*. The D_1 and D_5 receptors have antioxidant functions *(33,50–53)*.

Signal transduction. The signal resulting from occupation of cell membrane receptors is amplified by the intervention of other agents called second messengers. Occupation of either the β-adrenergic receptor subtype or the D_1-like class of dopamine receptor by agonists stimulates adenylyl cyclases; agonist occupancy of β$_2$-adrenergic receptors or dopamine D_2 receptors leads to inhibition of adenylyl cyclases. The changes in intracellular cyclic adenosine monophosphate levels alter the activities of certain enzymes, e.g., protein kinase A, and mediate the eventual response of the effector cell. Certain compounds (e.g., nitric oxide) exert their vasodilatory effect by stimulation of guanylate cyclase activity *(54)*. Another second messenger is associated with the phosphoinositide system. The β$_1$-adrenergic and the D_1-like dopamine receptors are linked to phospholipase C; stimulation leads to an increase in formation of inositol phosphates and diacylglycerol. Inositol phosphates increase intracellular calcium while diacylglycerol stimulates protein kinase C. Occupation of β$_1$-adrenergic and D_1 dopamine receptors may also result in the activation of phospholipase A_2 increasing the formation of biologically active arachidonate metabolites by the action of cyclooxygenases (prostaglandins, thromboxanes), lipoxygenases (leukotrienes), and cytochrome p450 monooxygenase (e.g., 20 hydroxyeicosatetraenoic acid).

Receptor regulation. Signal transduction involves "on" and "off" pathways to ensure that signaling is achieved in a precisely regulated manner *(55–57)*. One "off" pathway is receptor desensitization or loss of receptor responsiveness. Receptor desensitization is a mechanism to dampen short-term agonist effects following repeated agonist exposure. Desensitization involves several processes, including phosphorylation, sequestration/internalization, and degradation of receptor protein *(55–57)*. An initial step in the desensitization process is the phosphorylation of the receptor by a member or members of the G protein-coupled receptor kinases (GRKs) family. GRKs are serine and threonine kinases that phosphorylate G protein-coupled receptors (GPCRs) in response to agonist stimulation. The phosphorylation of GPCRs, including D_1 receptors, leads to the binding of a member or members of the arrestin family, an uncoupling of the receptor from its

G protein complex and a decrease in functional response *(55–58)*. The phosphorylation of β-arrestin 1 or β-arrestin 2 inhibits while *S*-nitrosylation of β-arrestin 2 but not of β-arrestin 1 promotes clathrin-mediated internalization of certain GPCRs (e.g., β2-adrenergic receptor). β-arrestin 2 acts as a scaffold linking endothelial NO synthase (eNOS) with β2-adrenergic receptor, a fast recycling class A receptor, and slow recycling class B receptors (e.g., AT_1 receptor). The *S*-nitrosylation of dynamin promotes scission of the endocytosed clathrin–GPCR complex, resulting in GPCR internalization. A discrete pool of eNOS *S*-nitrosylates GRK2 upon ligand stimulation and allows for the fast recycling of class A receptors *(59,60)*. The phosphorylated GPCR and arrestin complex undergoes internalization via clathrin-coated pits into an endosome where the GPCR is dephosphorylated *(61)*, facilitated by protein phosphatases, and recycled back to the plasma membrane or degraded by lysosomes and/or proteasomes *(62)*. These processes may be specific to a particular receptor. It should also be noted that the binding of certain GPCRs (protease-activated, orexin, substance P, and leukotriene B4 receptors) to arrestin is phosphorylation independent *(63)*.

Development of receptor regulation. There are developmental changes in the desensitization process. The neonatal rat heart is resistant to β-adrenergic receptor desensitization *(64)*. Rather, β-adrenergic agonists produce sensitization caused by the induction of adenylyl cyclase activity as a consequence of loss of $G\alpha_i$ protein and function, enhancement of membranous expression of $G\alpha_s$, and, in particular, the shorter but more active 45-kDa $G\alpha_s$. The role of $G\beta/\gamma$ was not determined but in the kidney we found that the decreased inhibitory effect of D_1 receptors on the sodium hydrogen exchanger type 3 is caused by increased expression and linkage of the G protein subunit $G\beta/\gamma$ *(65)*.

Catecholamines and other vasoactive agents. Catecholamines can influence blood pressure not only by direct effects on resistance vessels but also, indirectly, by modulating the secretion of other vasoactive agents such as angiotensin II (via renin), vasopressin, prostaglandins, substance P, and other neuropeptides. In addition to direct chronotropic and inotropic effects on the heart, catecholamines can modulate CO indirectly by affecting blood volume and venous return. Blood volume can be regulated by direct effects on sodium and water transport through renal nerves, by antagonizing effects of other hormones (e.g., vasopressin), and indirectly by modulating vasopressin and aldosterone secretion.

ADRENERGIC SYSTEM DURING DEVELOPMENT

The low systolic blood pressure at birth, due to low CO and peripheral resistance, increases rapidly in the first 6 weeks of life, remains at a constant level until age 6 years, and increases gradually until age 18 years. The pattern is similar for diastolic blood pressure except that there is a slight decrease in diastolic blood pressure in the first 6 months of life (relative to the blood pressure in the first week of life). The increase in blood pressure with age in preterm infants occurs as a function of postconceptional age. With advanced age (>60 years), systolic blood pressure continues to increase but diastolic blood pressure declines some, leading to an increase in pulse pressure. Increased pulse pressure plays an independent role in the pathogenesis of the complications of high blood pressure *(66)*. The increase in blood pressure with age is due to a rise in both CO and total peripheral resistance. The age-related changes in vascular resistance are selective because in the perinatal period there is a rapid fall in resistance in the lungs, small intestines, brain, and the kidney while resistance increases in the femoral vessels *(67)*. The increase in femoral resistance with age is probably related to an increase in vascular reactivity to vasoconstrictors with no differential effects of vasodilators (nitric oxide and bradykinin). The decrease in regional vascular resistance may be caused by an increase in vessel growth and changing sensitivity and reactivity to vasoconstrictor and vasodilator agents (see below). The increase in regional blood flow with age cannot be accounted for by an increase in blood pressure. Indeed, in the immediate perinatal period, the increase in regional blood flow with postnatal age is independent of blood pressure (68). In the first 6 months of life, systolic blood pressure increases but diastolic blood pressure actually decreases after the first 2 weeks of life. This transient decrease in diastolic blood pressure in the first few months of life is associated with a low intestinal vascular resistance (69). This is apparently mediated by NO. Interestingly, increased NO production, presumably from neuronal NO synthase, as well as increased expression of angiotensin type 2 receptor, in the neonatal renal arterial bed (70–72) also dampens the increased vasoconstriction afforded by angiotensin II, early in perinatal life and catecholamines later (73). NO, however, does not play an important role in cerebrovascular responses in the newborn.

The newborn infant increases its CO mainly by increasing heart rate. The high heart rate may be due to differential sympathetic and parasympathetic effects, hypersensitivity of the cardiac receptors, and peripheral vasodilatation. The low precapillary resistance and low venous capacitance are conducive to high systemic blood flow per unit body weight and provide increased tissue perfusion for growth.

Study of the role of the adrenergic nervous system in the control of cardiovascular dynamics is complicated by species differences. Some studies have suggested that pigs and dogs provide the closest model to the newborn human in terms of cardiovascular development (72,73). On the other hand, the sheep fetus is a very useful model for chronic conscious studies (74,75). These considerations are important because the changes in maternal diet or intrauterine events can affect blood pressure of the offspring as an adult (76–79).

DEVELOPMENT OF THE SYMPATHETIC NERVOUS SYSTEM

The development of the sympathetic nervous system can be divided into three stages (80). In the first stage, the neural crest cells migrate to their positions within the body tissues. In the second stage, the cell number and type are refined by cell death (apoptosis). The third stage is concerned with the maturation of synaptic connections and selection of the neurotransmitter. There are several factors that are involved in these processes and involve the interactions of several genes and growth factor families. A very important family, the neurotrophin family of growth factors, controls autonomic development, including nerve growth factor, brain-derived neurotrophic factor, and neutrophins 3 and 4 which act via high-affinity Trk receptor tyrosine kinases A, B, and C and lower affinity neurotrophin receptor p75 (81). Ventral migration of neural crest cells is controlled by neuregulin-1; neuroblast survival and differentiation by hepatocyte growth factor; neural crest cell migration and sympathetic ganglion formation by semaphorin 3A; induction of noradrenergic differentiation by bone morphogenetic protein (BMP) family members, BMP-2 and BMP-7; and the noradrenergic phenotype by transcription factors Mash1, Phox2a and b, Cash1, dHand, and GATA-3 (82,83). Cholinergic development generally takes place prior to adrenergic differentiation (83); however, transition from adrenergic to cholinergic function can also occur. The cholinergic differentiation factors remain to be identified but may include the neurotrophins, such as neurotrophin-3, and glial-cell-derived neurotrophic factors, such as neurturin and receptors, such as glial cell line-derived neurotrophic factor family receptor alpha-2 *(7,81–83)*. In the neonatal rat heart, perinatal β-adrenergics positively regulate the development of sympathetic innervation and suppress the development of m$_2$ muscarinic acetyl choline receptors *(84)*. A critical event in the development of the adrenergic nervous system is the establishment of functional innervation of the different organs. Function requires that central nervous pathways to the preganglionic neurons be established, that information be relayed to postganglionic neurons, and that neurotransmitter synthesis, release, and reuptake and postreceptor mechanisms be operative. Effector organ innervation involves the outgrowth of new axons, appearance of intense fluorescence, and differentiation of adrenergic nerve varicosities. Maturation of the nerve terminal–effector complex occurs before ganglionic transmission is fully developed and is largely independent of neural connections. In the heart, the development of β-adrenergic receptors and their responsiveness to catecholamines are not closely linked to innervation. Nonsympathetic hormonal factors appear to control early maturation of receptors and the growth and development of the nervous system.

Plasma catecholamines. Plasma norepinephrine and dopamine levels decrease gradually with advancing gestational weeks *(85)*. Birth is associated with an increase in circulating catecholamines. Umbilical arterial epinephrine and norepinephrine concentrations in infants delivered vaginally are greater than those in infants delivered by cesarean section *(86–88)*. Because there are some studies showing no difference in plasma concentrations between infants delivered vaginally and those by cesarean section *(89,90)*, stress per se may not responsible for the high catecholamine levels with vaginal delivery. Studies in the fetal sheep indicate a surge in plasma catecholamines with the onset of parturition that is accentuated by cord cutting *(91)*. The half-life of circulating catecholamines in the preterm infant may be longer than in older children, due in part to lower levels of catecholamine-degrading enzymes. However, children may metabolize catecholamines more rapidly than adults. Preterm infants have greater levels of epinephrine in umbilical arterial plasma than full-term human infants. Preterm fetal sheep also have higher circulating catecholamine levels than their full-term counterparts. The circulating levels of catecholamines decrease with maturation, but beyond 20 years of age plasma norepinephrine increases. Adrenal medullary activity is lower than adrenergic nervous activity at birth and increases with maturation. Neonatal blood pressure waves have been reported to be associated with surges of systemic norepinephrine *(92)*.

Urinary catecholamines. Urinary catecholamines are low at birth and increase with gestational and postnatal age *(93–95)*. Small-for-gestational-age babies have greater sympathoadrenal activity than babies of the same gestational age *(93)*. Newborn preterm infants excrete less norepinephrine and more dopamine than term infants; epinephrine excretion is comparable. At 2 weeks of age, urinary dopamine and metabolites are greatly increased in preterm infants. Beyond 1 year of life, the developmental patterns of adrenergic nervous and adrenal medullary activity are similar and reach mature values at 5 years of age. When expressed as a function of surface area or weight, no changes in urinary catecholamines and metabolites occur after 1 year of age. In the first 5 years of life, however, sympathoadrenal activity is less in girls than in boys. It should be kept in mind, though, that circulating and urinary levels of catecholamines are only rough indices of adrenergic activity. Preadolescent and early adolescent children, especially females, born prematurely or small for gestational age have higher circulating and urinary catecholamine levels than their term and weight appropriate for gestational-age counterparts *(96,97)*.

Catecholamines and adaptation to extrauterine life. Catecholamine secretion at birth may be important in the adaptation of the fetus to extrauterine life *(91,67)*. Complete ganglionic blockade before delivery of the lamb does not attenuate the normal postnatal rise in blood pressure, indicating that the autonomic nervous system may not play a significant role in the increase in systemic pressure after birth. However, although clamping of adrenal vessels did not alter mean blood pressure of very young puppies *(99)*, in the newborn dog adrenalectomy leads to hypotension and bradycardia. In addition, adrenergic blockade in the newborn lamb reduces systemic pressure, whereas no effect is seen in adult sheep. Other proofs for the importance of the adrenergic nervous system during the neonatal period include both impaired myocardial contractile responses to adrenergic agents and hypoxia after adrenalectomy.

The time of development of adrenergic innervation and responses to adrenergic stimulation varies not only with species but also among vessels in the same animal. Some of the reported differences in results may also be due to experimental conditions (anesthetized versus unanesthetized state, in vitro versus in vivo studies). In the heart, responses to β-adrenergic and dopamine stimulation increase with age while the response to α-adrenergic stimulation decreases with age. While the decreasing responsiveness to β-adrenergic stimulation with maturation has been linked to similar directional changes in myocardial $α_1$-adrenergic receptors, the changes in myocardial β-adrenergic receptors are not linked. For example, in the dog heart there is an increased β-adrenergic receptor density in the newborn period. The decline in cardiac β-adrenergic receptors density with age is accompanied by decreased β-adrenergic responsive adenylyl cyclase activity. Other studies, however, have shown that cardiac β-adrenergic receptors increase with age but the proportions of β-adrenergic subtypes do not.

In the mature heart, responsiveness to β-adrenergic agonists can be regulated transsynaptically by neurotransmitter concentrations in the synaptic cleft. High levels of β-adrenergic stimulation result in depressed cardiac responsiveness and reduction in receptor density (downregulation) while the converse occurs with low levels of stimulation with upregulation of receptor density. However, this does not occur during the period in which receptor numbers and cardiac sensitivity to agonists are undergoing marked developmental increases. The developmental changes in cardiac responsiveness to dopamine have not been correlated with dopamine receptor density or adenylyl cyclase activation.

Regional vascular flow and resistance during development. The development of renal and intestinal circulation is discussed in some detail because splanchnic vascular resistance contributes significantly to peripheral vascular resistance. β-Adrenergic relaxation of the aorta of rabbits increases with age, reaching a maximal level at 1 month; thereafter a decline in responsiveness occurs. In dogs, stimulation of lumbar sympathetics induces femoral vasodilatation early in life; after 2 months a greater vasoconstriction is noted. This corresponds to a marked increase in adrenergic innervation. In the piglet, the renal vascular response to β-adrenergic stimulation is also less in the immediate newborn period compared to adults but may be markedly increased some time before maturation *(99)*. These changes in renal β-adrenergic responsiveness have been correlated with β-adrenergic receptor density in the dog *(100)*. However, $β_2$-adrenergic vasodilatory effects are enhanced in the renal vascular bed of the fetal lamb *(100)*.

The maturation of blood vessel reactivity to β-adrenergic stimulation is regional bed dependent. In general, during the neonatal period there is a lesser responsiveness of the canine aorta and sheep carotid to norepinephrine compared to the adult. This occurs in spite of comparable responsiveness to KCl *(101)*. The vasoconstrictor effects of α-adrenergic drugs are also less in immature than mature animals. In the neonatal rat femoral artery, norepinephrine causes a vasodilation rather than vasoconstriction, an effect mediated by nitric oxide *(102)*. In baboons, the maximum vasoconstrictor response to norepinephrine, thromboxane mimetic, and potassium increased with gestational age, but the sensitivity to these vasoconstrictors was similar *(67)*.

Renal vascular bed. Renal blood flow increases progressively with conceptional age reaching term values by about 35 weeks postconception. Forty weeks postconception renal blood flow expressed as a function of surface area increases with postnatal age reaching middle-age adult values by 1–2 years of life. The increase in renal blood flow is associated with a fall in renal vascular resistance. Color Doppler ultrasonography has been used to determine renal resistive index, which correlates with renal vascular resistance. In general, the values obtained using clearance methods (e.g., para-aminohippurate) have correlated well by the renal resistive index *(103)*. The increase in renal blood flow with age is due to renal growth, an increase in blood pressure, and a decrease in renal vascular resistance. The high renal vascular resistance in the perinatal period has been shown to be caused by alterations in renal vascular smooth muscle reactivity and sensitivity to vasodilators and vasoconstrictors. After the immediate newborn period, the neonatal renal and cerebral circulation are more sensitive to α-adrenergic stimulation in dogs, pigs, guinea pigs, and baboons *(72,104,105)*. The isolated renal vessels of fetal lamb studied in vitro and in vivo are also more reactive to β-adrenergic stimulation than their newborn or adult counterparts *(106)*. The increased renal α_1- and α_2-adrenergic effects in fetal sheep are related to increased α-adrenergic receptor density. Competition experiments and rank adrenergic antagonist potency suggested the presence of only the α_{1B}-adrenergic receptor in fetal and adult sheep kidneys. However, α_{1B}-adrenergic receptor does not mediate vasoconstriction in adults. The α_2-adrenergic receptor that was found only in the fetal sheep had a low affinity to rauwolscine, which is unlike that described in most species for α_2-adrenergic receptors *(107)*. However, the molecular biological class of these receptors during development has not been studied.

Inherent renal vascular hypersensitivity or hyperreactivity may be masked by counter-regulatory vasodilator mechanisms. In the fetal sheep renal vascular β_2-adrenergic receptor-mediated renal vasodilatory capacity is enhanced during fetal life *(108)*. Cerebral arteries from premature and newborn baboons showed a more marked relaxation response to iso-proterenol than did arteries from adult animals *(104)*. In the piglet, the renal vasoconstrictor effects of angiotensin II are counteracted by vasodilatory action of nitric oxide *(70,71,109)*. However, the contribution of specific adrenergic receptors and regulation of nitric oxide level or availability to the development of renal circulation remain to be determined.

The neonatal renal circulation is also more responsive to the effects of renal nerve stimulation in some species *(110)*. While renal nerve transection in piglets leads to an increase in renal blood flow *(110)*, this effect is not seen in fetal sheep. Moreover, renal nerve stimulation during α-adrenergic blockade actually increases renal blood flow *(101)*. In the neonatal dog kidney, increased α-adrenergic effects are related to increased β-adrenergic receptor density *(111)*. Dopamine mainly induces a vasoconstrictor response (an β-adrenergic receptor effect) in the early neonatal period *(111)*. Even low dosages, which produce renal vasodilatation in the adult kidney, are associated with renal vasoconstriction in the newborn period. The vasodilator effects of dopamine become evident in the femoral circulation before being noted in the kidney. When β- and β-adrenergic receptors are blocked during dopamine infusion, the renal vasodilator effect of dopamine is still less in the fetus and the newborn animal compared to the adult. In contrast to the correlation between renal vascular responses and β- and β-adrenergic receptor density, no correlation is observed with dopamine receptors and the age-related changes in renal dopamine responsiveness.

The low renal blood flow in the young is due to several factors, including smaller size, decreased number of glomeruli, lower systemic pressure, and higher renal vascular resistance. The increased renal vascular resistance in the newborn is probably due to increased activity of the renin–angiotensin system as well as increased sensitivity to vasoconstrictor catecholamines. The latter is due to receptor and postadrenergic receptor mechanisms. Critical vasodilators, such as nitric oxide, may act to counterbalance these vasoconstrictor forces. The increase in renal blood flow with age presumably occurs as the vasoconstrictor influences decline. Adult growth-restricted offspring develop hypertension that may be caused by increased renal nerve activity *(112)*.

Intestinal vascular bed. Intestinal blood flow, like renal blood flow increases with gestational age, postconceptional age, and maturation *(113)*. Fetal intestinal vascular resistance is high during fetal life. In the piglet, there is a further decrease in intestinal vascular resistance in the first few days of life, only to progressively increase after the first week of life. This is in contrast with kidneys in which there is a progressive decrease in renal vascular resistance in the perinatal period. The neonatal intestinal circulation is controlled by inherent myogenic response and nitric oxide similar to that seen in the neonatal renal circulation. Like the neonatal kidney neonatal intestinal circulation may also be regulated by alterations in α-adrenergic receptor *(114)*. However, in contrast to the neonatal kidney, endothelin plays a part in the regulation of neonatal intestinal circulation. In older piglets, regulation of the intestinal circulation does not involve nitric oxide or endothelin, the responses being mainly passive in nature *(69,115)*. In contrast to importance of nitric oxide in the renal and intestinal vasodilator response in the newborn, bradykinin and prostanoids perform this role in the neonatal cerebral vascular bed *(116)*. However, with maturation nitric oxide assumes a more important role.

CONCLUSION

In summary, increase in blood pressure with age in the first few months of life is mainly due to an increase in cardiac output. Vascular resistance in many vascular beds may transiently decrease because of increased production or availability of nitric oxide, prostanoids, or increased sensitivity to β-adrenergic stimulation. The involvement of a particular agent is regional bed dependent. While the maturation of receptor classes involved in the regulation of cardiac output and vascular resistance is known, the maturation of specific receptor subtypes in different vascular beds remains to be determined.

REFERENCES

1. Tibby SM, Murdoch IA. Monitoring cardiac function in intensive care. Arch Dis Child. 2003;88:46–52.
2. Guyton AC. Arterial Pressure and Hypertension. Philadelphia, PA: Saunders; 1980.
3. Veille JC, Hanson R, Steele L, Tatum K. M-mode echocardiographic evaluation of fetal and infant hearts: longitudinal follow-up study from intrauterine life to year one. Am J Obstet Gynecol. 1996;175:922–928.
4. Dickerson LW, Rodak DJ, Fleming TJ, Gatti PJ, Massari VJ, McKenzie JC, Gillis RA. Parasympathetic neurons in the cranial medial ventricular fat pad on the dog heart selectively decrease ventricular contractility without effect on sinus rate or AV conduction. J Auton Nerv Syst. 1998;70:129–141.
5. Wang Z, Shi H, Wang H. Functional M3 muscarinic acetylcholine receptors in mammalian hearts. Br J Pharmacol. 2004;142:395–408.
6. Habecker BA, Bilimoria P, Linick C, Gritman K, Lorentz CU, Woodward W, Birren SJ. Regulation of cardiac innervation and function via the p75 neurotrophin receptor. Auton Neurosci. 2008;140:40–48.
7. Mabe AM, Hoover DB. Structural and functional cardiac cholinergic deficits in adult neurturin knockout mice. Cardiovasc Res. 2009;82:93–99.

8. Janowski E, Cleemann L, Sasse P, Morad M. Diversity of Ca2+ signaling in developing cardiac cells. Ann N Y Acad Sci. 2006;1080:154–164.

9. Lin E, Hung VH, Kashihara H, Dan P, Tibbits GF. Distribution patterns of the Na^+-Ca^{2+} exchanger and caveolin-3 in developing rabbit cardiomyocytes. Cell Calcium. 2009;45:369–383.

10. Phoon CK. Circulatory physiology in the developing embryo. Curr Opin Pediatr. 2001;13:456–464.

11. Espinoza-Lewis RA, Yu L, He F, Liu H, Tang R, Shi J, Sun X, Martin JF, Wang D, Yang J, Chen Y. Shox2 is essential for the differentiation of cardiac pacemaker cells by repressing Nkx2-5. Dev Biol. 2009;327:376–385.

12. Walther T, Schultheiss HP, Tschope C, Stepan H. Natriuretic peptide system in fetal heart and circulation. J Hypertens. 2002;20:785–791.

13. Aviado DM, Guevara Aviado D. The Bezold-Jarisch reflex. A historical perspective of cardiopulmonary reflexes. Ann N Y Acad Sci. 2001;940:48–58.

14. Mazursky JE, Birkett CL, Bedell KA, Ben-Haim SA, Segar JL. Development of baroreflex influences on heart rate variability in preterm infants. Early Hum Dev. 1998;53:37–52.

15. Tavernarakis N, Driscoll M. Degenerins. At the core of the metazoan mechanotransducer? Ann N Y Acad Sci. 2001;940:28–41.

16. Drummond HA, Welsh MJ, Abboud FM. ENaC subunits are molecular components of the arterial baroreceptor complex. Ann N Y Acad Sci. 2001;940:42–47.

17. Fung M-L, Lam SY, Dong X, Chen Y, Leung PS. Postnatal hypoxemia increases angiotensin II sensitivity and up-regulates AT1a angiotensin receptors in rat carotid body chemoreceptors. J Endocrinol. 2002;173:305–313.

18. Lanfranchi PA, Somers VK. Arterial baroreflex function and cardiovascular variability: interactions and implications. Am J Physiol Regul Integr Comp Physiol. 2002;283:R815–R826.

19. Sharif-Naeini R, Ciura S, Zhang Z, Bourque CW. Contribution of TRPV channels to osmosensory transduction, thirst, and vasopressin release. Kidney Int. 2008;73:811–815.

20. Chapleau MW, Li Z, Meyrelles SS, Ma X, Abboud FM. Mechanisms determining sensitivity of baroreceptor afferents in health and disease. Ann N Y Acad Sci. 2001;940:1–19.

21. Wei SG, Zhang ZH, Yu Y, Felder RB. Systemically administered tempol reduces neuronal activity in paraventricular nucleus of hypothalamus and rostral ventrolateral medulla in rats. J Hypertens. 2009;27: 543–550.

22. Segar JL. Ontogeny of the arterial and cardiopulmonary baroreflex during fetal and postnatal life. Am J Physiol. 1997;273:R457–R471.

23. Longin E, Gerstner T, Schaible T, Lenz T, König S. Maturation of the autonomic nervous system: differences in heart rate variability in premature vs. term infants. J Perinat Med. 2006;34:303–308.

24. Martin JL, Jenkins VK, Hsieh HY, Balkowiec A. Brain-derived neurotrophic factor in arterial baroreceptor pathways: implications for activity-dependent plasticity at baroafferent synapses. J Neurochem. 2009;108:450–464.

25. Yu ZY, Lumbers ER. Effects of birth on baroreceptor-mediated changes in heart rate variability in lambs and fetal sheep. Clin Exp Pharmacol Physiol. 2002;29:455–463.

26. Yiallourou SR, Walker AM, Horne RS. Prone sleeping impairs circulatory control during sleep in healthy term infants: implications for SIDS. Sleep. 2008;31:1139–1146.

27. Yiallourou SR, Walker AM, Horne RS. Effects of sleeping position on development of infant cardiovascular control. Arch Dis Child. 2008;93:868–872.

28. Gootman PM, Gootman N. Postnatal changes in cardiovascular regulation during hypoxia. Adv Exp Med Biol. 2000;475:539–548.

29. Buckley BJ, Gootman N, Nagelberg JS, Griswold PR, Gootman PM. Cardiovascular response to arterial and venous hemorrhage in neonatal swine. Am J Physiol. 1984;247:8626–8633.

30. Bevan JAA, Su C. Sympathetic mechanisms in blood vessels: nerve and muscle relationships. Annu Rev Pharmacol. 1973;13:269–285.

31. Li G, Xu J, Wang P, Velazquez H, Li Y, Wu Y, Desir GV. Catecholamines regulate the activity, secretion, and synthesis of renalase. Circulation. 2008;117:1277–1282.

32. Piascik MT, Perez DM. α_1-Adrenergic receptors: new insights and directions. Pharmacol Exp Ther. 2001;298:403–410.

33. Gilsbach R, Röser C, Beetz N, Brede M, Hadamek K, Haubold M, Leemhuis J, Philipp M, Schneider J, Urbanski M, Szabo B, Weinshenker D, Hein L. Genetic dissection of alpha2-adrenoceptor functions in adrenergic versus nonadrenergic cells. Mol Pharmacol. 2009;75:1160–1167.

34. Hieble JP. Subclassification and nomenclature of alpha- and beta-adrenoceptors. Curr Top Med Chem. 2007;7(2):129–134.

35. Rokosh DG, Simpson PC. Knockout of the $\alpha1A/C$-adrenergic receptor subtype: the alpha 1A/C is expressed in resistance arteries and is required to maintain arterial blood pressure. Proc Natl Acad Sci USA. 2002;99:9474–9479.

36. Daly CJ, Deighan C, McGee A, Mennie D, Ali Z, McBride M, McGrath JC. A knockout approach indicates a minor vasoconstrictor role for vascular α_{1B}-adrenoceptors in mouse. Physiol Genomics. 2002;9:85–91.

37. Tanoue A, Koshimizu TA, Tsujimoto G. Transgenic studies of α_1-adrenergic receptor subtype function. Life Sci. 2002;71:2207–2215.

38. MacDonald E, Kobilka BK, Scheinin M. Gene targeting—homing in on alpha 2-adrenoceptor-subtype function. Trends Pharmacol Sci. 1997;18:211–219.

39. Rohrer DK. Physiological consequences of beta-adrenergic receptor disruption. J Mol Med. 1998;76:764–772.

40. Chruscinski AJ, Rohrer DK, Schauble E, Desai KH, Bernstein D, Kobilka BK. Targeted disruption of the β2 adrenergic receptor gene. J Biol Chem. 1999;274:16694–16700.

41. Rohrer DK, Chruscinski A, Schauble EH, Bernstein D, Kobilka BK. Cardiovascular and metabolic alterations in mice lacking both β1- and β2-adrenergic receptors. J Biol Chem. 1999;274:16701–16708.

42. Jimenez M, Leger B, Canola K, Lehr L, Arboit P, Seydoux J, Russell AP, Giacobino JP, Muzzin P, Preitner F. $\beta_1/\beta_2/\beta_3$-adrenoceptor knockout mice are obese and cold-sensitive but have normal lipolytic responses to fasting. FEBS Lett. 2002;530:37–40.

43. Ozono R, O'Connell DP, Wang ZQ, Moore AF, Sanada H, Felder RA, Carey RM. Localization of the dopamine D1 receptor protein in the human heart and kidney. Hypertension. 1997;30:725–729.

44. Habuchi Y, Tanaka H, Nishio M, Yamamoto T, Komori T, Morikawa J, Yoshimura M. Dopamine stimulation of cardiac beta-adrenoceptors: the involvement of sympathetic amine transporters and the effect of SKF38393. Br J Pharmacol. 1997;122:1669–1678.

45. Ding G, Wiegerinck RF, Shen M, Cojoc A, Zeidenweber CM, Wagner MB. Dopamine increases L-type calcium current more in newborn than adult rabbit cardiomyocytes via D1 and β2 receptors. Am J Physiol Heart Circ Physiol. 2008;294:H2327–H2335.

46. Zeng C, Armando I, Luo Y, Eisner GM, Felder RA, Jose PA. Dysregulation of dopamine-dependent mechanisms as a determinant of hypertension: studies in dopamine receptor knockout mice. Am J Physiol Heart Circ Physiol. 2008;294(2):H551–H556.

47. Banday AA, Lokhandwala MF. Dopamine receptors and hypertension. Curr Hypertens Rep. 2008;10(4):268–275.

48. Schafer JA, Li L, Sun D. The collecting duct, dopamine and vasopressin-dependent hypertension. Acta Physiol Scand. 2000;168:239–244.

49. Saito O, Ando Y, Kusano E, Asano Y. Functional characterization of basolateral and luminal dopamine receptors in rabbit CCD. Am J Physiol Renal Physiol. 2001;281:F114–F122.

50. Jose PA, Eisner GM, Felder RA. The renal dopamine receptors in health and hypertension. Pharmacol Ther. 1998;80:149–182.

51. Narkar V, Hussain T, Lokhandwala M. Role of tyrosine kinase and p44/42 MAPK in D_2-like receptor-mediated stimulation of Na^+, K^+-ATPase in kidney. Am J Physiol Renal Physiol. 2002;282:F697–F702.

50. Yasunari K, Kohno M, Kano H, Minami M, Yoshikawa J. Dopamine as a novel antioxidative agent for rat vascular smooth muscle cells through dopamine D_1-like receptors. Circulation. 2000;101:2302–2308.

51. Han W, Li H, Villar VA, Pascua AM, Dajani MI, Wang X, Natarajan A, Quinn MT, Felder RA, Jose PA, Yu P. Lipid rafts keep NADPH oxidase in the inactive state in human renal proximal tubule cells. Hypertension. 2008;51:481–487.

52. Yang Z, Asico LD, Yu P, Wang Z, Jones JE, Escano CS, Wang X, Quinn MT, Sibley DR, Romero GG, Felder RA, Jose PA. D5 dopamine receptor regulation of reactive oxygen species production, NADPH oxidase, and blood pressure. Am J Physiol Regul Integr Comp Physiol. 2006;290:R96–R104.

53. Banday AA, Lau YS, Lokhandwala MF. Oxidative stress causes renal dopamine D1 receptor dysfunction and salt-sensitive hypertension in Sprague-Dawley rats. Hypertension. 2008;51:367–375.

54. Hogg N. The biochemistry and physiology of S-nitrosothiols. Annu Rev Pharmacol Toxicol. 2002;42:585–600.

55. Pao CS, Benovic JL. Phosphorylation-independent desensitization of G protein-coupled receptors? Sci STKE. 2002;2002:PE42.

56. Gainetdinov RR, Premont RT, Bohn LM, Lefkowitz RJ, Caron MG. Desensitization of G protein-coupled receptors and neuronal functions. Annu Rev Neurosci. 2004;27:107–144.

57. Tobin AB. G-protein-coupled receptor phosphorylation: where, when and by whom. Br J Pharmacol. 2008;153:S167–S176.

58. Felder RA, Sanada H, Xu J, Yu P-Y, Wang Z, Watanabe H, Asico LD, Wang W, Zheng S, Yamaguchi I, Williams S, Gainer J, Brown NJ, Hazen-Martin D, Wong L-J, Robillard JE, Carey RM, Eisner GM, Jose PA. G protein-coupled receptor kinase 4 gene variants in human essential hypertension. Proc Natl Acad Sci USA. 2002;99:3872–3877.

59. Ozawa K, Whalen EJ, Nelson CD, Mu Y, Hess DT, Lefkowitz RJ, Stamler JS. S-nitrosylation of beta-arrestin regulates beta-adrenergic receptor trafficking. Mol Cell. 2008;31:395–405.

60. Whalen EJ, Foster MW, Matsumoto A, Ozawa K, Violin JD, Que LG, Nelson CD, Benhar M, Keys JR, Rockman HA, Koch WJ, Daaka Y, Lefkowitz RJ, Stamler JS. Regulation of beta-adrenergic receptor signaling by S-nitrosylation of G-protein-coupled receptor kinase 2. Cell. 2007;129:511–522.

61. Yu P, Asico LD, Eisner GM, Hopfer U, Felder RA, Jose PA. Renal protein phosphatase 2A activity and spontaneous hypertension in rats. Hypertension. 2000;36:1053–1058.

62. Li H, Armando I, Yu P, Escano C, Mueller SC, Asico L, Pascua A, Lu Q, Wang X, Villar VA, Jones JE, Wang Z, Periasamy A, Lau YS, Soares-da-Silva P, Creswell K, Guillemette G, Sibley DR, Eisner G, Felder RA, Jose PA. Dopamine 5 receptor mediates Ang II type 1 receptor degradation via ubiquitin-proteasome pathway in mice and human cells. J Clin Invest. 2008;118:2180–2189.

63. Tobin AB, Butcher AJ, Kong KC. Location, location, location... site-specific GPCR phosphorylation offers a mechanism for cell-type-specific signaling. Trends Pharmacol Sci. 2008;29:413–420.

64. Auman JT, Seidler FJ, Slotkin TA. Beta-adrenoceptor control of G protein function in the neonate: determinant of desensitization or sensitization. Am J Physiol Regul Integr Comp Physiol. 2002;283:R1236–R1244.

65. Li XX, Albrecht FE, Robillard JE, Eisner GM, Jose PA. Gβ regulation of Na/H exchanger-3 activity in rat renal proximal tubules during development. Am J Physiol Regul Integr Comp Physiol. 2000;278:R931–R936.

66. Protogerou AD, Papaioannou TG, Lekakis JP, Blacher J, Safar ME. The effect of antihypertensive drugs on central blood pressure beyond peripheral blood pressure. Part I: (Patho)-physiology, rationale and perspective on pulse pressure amplification. Curr Pharm Des. 2009;15(3):267–271.

67. Anwar MA, Ju K, Docherty CC, Poston L, Nathanielsz PW. Developmental changes in reactivity of small femoral arteries in the fetal and postnatal baboon. Am J Obstet Gynecol. 2001;184:707–712.

68. Yanowitz TD, Yao AC, Pettigrew KD, Werner JC, Oh W, Stonestreet BS. Postnatal hemodynamic changes in very-low-birthweight infants. J Appl Physiol. 1999;87:370–380.

69. Reber KM, Nankervis CA, Nowicki PT. Newborn intestinal circulation. Physiology and pathophysiology. Clin Perinatol. 2002;29:23–39.

70. Simeoni U, Zhu B, Muller C, Judes C, Massfelder T, Geisert J, Helwig JJ. Postnatal development of vascular resistance of the rabbit isolated perfused kidney: modulation by nitric oxide and angiotensin II. Pediatr Res. 1997;42:550–555.

71. Solhaug MJ, Wallace MR, Granger JP. Nitric oxide and angiotensin II regulation of renal hemodynamics in the developing piglet. Pediatr Res. 1996;39:527–533.

72. Ratliff B, Rodebaugh J, Sekulic M, Dong KW, Solhaug M. Nitric oxide synthase and renin-angiotensin gene expression and NOS function in the postnatal renal resistance vasculature. Pediatr Nephrol. Feb 2009;24(2):355–365.

73. Jose P, Slotkoff L, Lilienfield L, Calcagno P, Eisner G. Sensitivity of the neonatal renal vasculature to epinephrine. Am J Physiol. 1974;226:796–799.

74. Duckles SP, Banner W Jr. Changes in vascular smooth muscle reactivity during development. Annu Rev Pharmacol Toxicol. 1984;24:65–83.

75. Nuyt AM, Segar JL, Holley AT, Robillard JE. Autonomic adjustments to severe hypotension in fetal and neonatal sheep. Pediatr Res. 2001;49:56–62.

76. Symonds ME, Stephenson T, Budge H. Early determinants of cardiovascular disease: the role of early diet in later blood pressure control. Am J Clin Nutr. May 2009;89(5):1518S–1522S.

77. Alexander BT, Hendon AE, Ferril G, Dwyer TM. Renal denervation abolishes hypertension in low-birth-weight offspring from pregnant rats with reduced uterine perfusion. Hypertension. 2005;45:754–758.

78. Dodic M, Moritz K, Koukoulas I, Wintour EM. Programmed hypertension: kidney, brain or both? Trends Endocrinol Metab. 2002;13:403–408.

79. Ingelfinger JR. Disparities in renal endowment: causes and consequences. Adv Chronic Kidney Dis. 2008;15:107–114.

80. Francis NJ, Landis SC. Cellular and molecular determinants of sympathetic neuron development. Annu Rev Neurosci. 1999;22:541–566.

81. Hildreth V, Anderson RH, Henderson DJ. Autonomic innervation of the developing heart: origins and function. Clin Anat. 2009;22:36–46.

82. Glebova NO, Ginty DD. Growth and survival signals controlling sympathetic nervous system development. Annu Rev Neurosci. 2005;28:191–222.

83. Ernsberger U. The role of GDNF family ligand signalling in the differentiation of sympathetic and dorsal root ganglion neurons. Cell Tissue Res. 2008;333:353–371.

84. Garofolo MC, Seidler FJ, Auman JT, Slotkin TA. β-Adrenergic modulation of muscarinic cholinergic receptor expression and function in developing heart. Am J Physiol Regul Integr Comp Physiol. 2002;282:R1356–R1363.

85. Wang L, Zhang W, Zhao Y. The study of maternal and fetal plasma catecholamines levels during pregnancy and delivery. J Perinat Med. 1999;27:195–198.

86. Agata Y, Hiraishi S, Misawa H, Han JH, Oguchi K, Horiguchi Y, Fujino N, Takeda N, Padbury JF. Hemodynamic adaptations at birth and neonates delivered vaginally and by cesarean section. Biol Neonate. 1995;68:404–411.

87. Hirsimaki H, Kero P, Ekblad H, Scheinin M, Saraste M, Erkkola R. Mode of delivery, plasma catecholamines and Doppler-derived cardiac output in healthy term newborn infants. Biol Neonate. 1992;61:285–293.

88. Moftaquir-Handaj A, Barbé F, Barbarino-Monnier P, Aunis D, Boutroy MJ. Circulating chromogranin A and catecholamines in human fetuses at uneventful birth. Pediatr Res. 1995;37:101–105.

89. Pohjavuori M, Rovamo L, Laatikainen T, Kariniemi V, Pettersson J. Stress of delivery and plasma endorphins and catecholamines in the newborn infant. Biol Res Pregnancy Perinatol. 1986;7:1–5.

90. Eliot RJ, Lam R, Leake RD, Hobel CJ, Fisher DA. Plasma catecholamine concentrations in infants at birth and during the first 48 hours of life. J Pediatr. 1980;96:311–315.

91. Padbury JF, Polk DH, Newham JP, Lam RW. Neonatal adaptation: greater sympathoadrenal response in preterm than full-term fetal sheep at birth. Am J Physiol. 1985;248:E443–E449.

92. Wefers B, Cunningham S, Stephen R, McIntosh N. Neonatal blood pressure waves are associated with surges of systemic noradrenaline. Arch Dis Child Fetal Neonatal Ed. 2009;94:F149–F151.

93. Dahnaz YL, Peyrin L, Dutruge J, Sann L. Neonatal pattern of adrenergic metabolites in urine of small for gestational age and preteen infants. J Neural Trans. 1980;49:151–165.

94. Nicolopoulos D, Agathopoulos A. Galanakos-Tharouniati M, Stergiopoulos C. Urinary excretion of catecholamines by full term and premature infants. Pediatrics. 1969;44:262–265.

95. Vanpee M, Herin P, Lagercrantz H, Aperia A. Effect of extreme prematurity on renal dopamine and norepinephrine excretion during the neonatal period. Pediatr Nephrol. 1997;11:46–48.

96. Franco MC, Casarini DE, Carneiro-Ramos MS, Sawaya AL, Barreto-Chaves ML, Sesso R. Circulating renin-angiotensin system and catecholamines in childhood: is there a role for birthweight? Clin Sci (Lond). 2008;114:375–380.

97. Johansson S, Norman M, Legnevall L, Dalmaz Y, Lagercrantz H, Vanpée M. Increased catecholamines and heart rate in children with low birth weight: perinatal contributions to sympathoadrenal overactivity. J Intern Med. 2007;261:480–487.

98. Heymann MA, Iwamoto HS, Rudolph AM. Factors affecting changes in the neonatal systemic circulation. Annu Rev Physiol. 1981;43:371–381.

99. Gootman N, Gootman PM. Perinatal Cardiovascular Function. New York, NY: Marcel Dekker; 1983.

100. Robillard JE, Nakamura KT. Neurohormonal regulation of renal function during development. Am J Physiol. 1988;254:F771–F779.

101. Gray SD. Reactivity of neonatal canine aortic strips. Biol Neonate. 1977;31:10–14.

102. Nishina H, Ozaki T, Hanson MA, Poston L. Mechanisms of noradrenaline-induced vasorelaxation in isolated femoral arteries of the neonatal rat. Br J Pharmacol. 1999;127:809–812.

103. Andriani G, Persico A, Tursini S, Ballone E, Cirotti D, Lelli Chiesa P. The renal-resistive index from the last 3 months of pregnancy to 6 months old. BJU Int. 2001;87:562–564.

104. Hayashi S, Park MK, Kuehl TJ. Higher sensitivity of cerebral arteries isolated from premature and newborn baboons to adrenergic and cholinergic stimulation. Life Sci. 1984;35:253–260.

105. Fildes RD, Eisner GM, Calcagno PL, Jose PA. Renal alpha-adrenoceptors and sodium excretion in the dog. Am J Physiol. 1985;248:F128–F133.

106. Guillery EN, Segar JL, Merrill DC, Nakamura KT, Jose PA, Robillard JE. Ontogenic changes in renal response to alpha 1-adrenoceptor stimulation in sheep. Am J Physiol. 1994;267:R990–R998.

107. Gitler MS, Piccio MM, Robillard JE, Jose PA. Characterization of renal alpha-adrenoceptor subtypes in sheep during development. Am J Physiol. 1991;260:R407–R412.

108. Nakamura KT, Matherne GP, Jose PA, Alden BM, Robillard JE. Ontogeny of renal β-adrenoceptor-mediated vasodilation in sheep: comparison between endogenous catecholamines. Pediatr Res. 1987;22:465–470.

109. Sener A, Smith FG. Renal hemodynamic effects of L-NAME during postnatal maturation in conscious lambs. Pediatr Nephrol. 2001;16:868–873.

110. Gootman PM, Buckley NM, Gootman N. Postnatal maturation of neural control of the circulation. In: Scarpelli EM, Cosmi EV, eds. Reviews in Perinatal Medicine, Vol. 3. New York, NY: Raven Press; 1979:1–72.

111. Felder RA, Jose PA. Development of adrenergic and dopamine receptors in the kidney. In: Strauss J, ed. Electrolytes, Nephrotoxins, and the Neonatal Kidney. Hague, the Netherlands: Martinus-Nihjoff; 1985:3–10.

112. Alexander BT, Hendon AE, Ferril G, Dwyer TM. Renal denervation abolishes hypertension in low-birth-weight offspring from pregnant rats with reduced uterine perfusion. Hypertension. 2005;45:754–758.

113. Maruyama K, Koizumi T. Superior mesenteric artery blood flow velocity in small for gestational age infants of very low birth weight during the early neonatal period. J Perinat Med. 2001;29:64–70.

114. Hoang TV, Choe EU, Lippton HL, Hyman AL, Flint LM, Ferrara JJ. Effect of maturation on alpha-adrenoceptor activity in newborn piglet mesentery. J Surg Res. 1996;61:330–338.

115. Nankervis CA, Reber KM, Nowicki PT. Age-dependent changes in the postnatal intestinal microcirculation. Microcirculation. 2001;8:377–387.

116. Willis AP, Leffler CW. Endothelial NO and prostanoid involvement in newborn and juvenile pig pial arteriolar vasomotor responses. Am J Physiol Heart Circ Physiol. 2001;281:H2366–H2377.

4

Ion and Fluid Dynamics in Hypertension

Avram Z. Traum, MD

CONTENTS

Among the many determinants of blood pressure, ion transport has played a key role in both the basic understanding and the clinical management of hypertension. For decades, clinicians have counseled their hypertensive patients to limit salt intake. This approach has been codified in clinical guidelines and forms the backbone of what has been termed therapeutic lifestyle modifications *(1,2)*. Sodium restriction has been studied in clinical trials as an effective measure for the control of moderately elevated blood pressure *(3,4)*. In addition to sodium restriction, the role of natriuresis has been translated into pharmacologic therapy as thiazide diuretics have assumed the role of first-line pharmacologic therapy for hypertension in adults *(5,6)*.

At a more basic level, an expanding list of genes has been implicated in monogenic forms of hypertension. These genes typically encode proteins that affect renal tubular sodium handling, reviewed elsewhere in this text. Moreover, mutations leading to renal salt wasting, as observed in Bartter and Gitelman syndrome, are associated with normal and low blood pressure.

While monogenic conditions associated with high or low blood pressure provide insight into the pathogenesis of hypertension, these comprise only a small fraction of the overall burden of hypertension. More broadly, however, pathogenic changes in ion transport have been implicated both in animal models and in human studies of essential hypertension, suggesting a role for altered structure and function of ion transporters that provide additional rationale for the success of such measures as salt restriction and diuretics in treating hypertension. In this chapter, we will review some of the ion channels studied in

A.Z. Traum (✉)
Pediatric Nephrology Unit, Harvard Medical School, Massachusetts General Hospital, Boston, MA, USA
e-mail: atraum@partners.org

From: *Clinical Hypertension and Vascular Diseases: Pediatric Hypertension*
Edited by: J. T. Flynn et al. DOI 10.1007/978-1-60327-824-9_4
© Springer Science+Business Media, LLC 2011

hypertension and their relevance to clinical practice. Both channel function and structure will be considered.

SODIUM CHANNELS

Given the importance of salt in the management of blood pressure, sodium channels have been extensively studied as targets both in animal models of hypertension and in clinical research.

All relevant channels expressed along the length of the tubule have been studied. These include a variety of transporters of sodium: the Na^+/H^+ exchangers (NHEs), the $Na^+-K^+-2Cl^-$ cotransporter (NKCC), the Na^+-Cl^- cotransporter (NCC), as well as the epithelial sodium cotransporter (ENaC), the sodium–potassium ATPase (Na^+/K^+ ATPase), and the sodium–phosphate transporter (NaPi II) (see Table 1).

Table 1
Sodium Channels of the Renal Tubule

Transporter	Intrarenal location	Cellular location
Na^+/H^+ exchangers (NHEs)	Proximal tubule and TAL	Apical
$Na^+-K^+-2Cl^-$ cotransporter (NKCC)	TAL	Apical
Epithelial sodium cotransporter (ENaC)	Collecting duct	Apical
Na^+Cl^- cotransporter (NCC)	Distal tubule	Apical
Sodium–potassium ATPase (Na^+/K^+ ATPase)	Multiple segments	Basolateral
Sodium–phosphate transporter (NaPi II)	Proximal tubule	Apical

NHE Transporters

Na^+/H^+ transporters have been localized throughout the body and play a major role in cell-volume regulation and the transcellular movement of sodium and osmotically driven water. There are more than four NHEs: the NHE1 transporter is ubiquitous, while NHE3 is highly expressed in the kidney. Both NHE1 and NHE3 have been the focus of much study with respect to hypertension. Specifically, the localization of NHE1 to red blood cells (RBCs) has facilitated its study in humans and in rat models, such as the spontaneous hypertensive rat (SHR).

NHE1 activity is increased in the SHR in multiple cell types, including RBCs, platelets, leukocytes, skeletal muscle, vascular smooth muscle cells, and tubular epithelial cells. This effect was not seen in RBCs or proximal tubular cells of a second rat model of essential hypertension, the Milan hypertensive strain (MHS). RBC Na^+/H^+ transport has been examined in humans as well and appears to correlate with renal sodium retention in hypertensive individuals *(7)*. The differential effect in SHR versus MHS strains aligns well with human studies, as approximately half of the patients studied had increased RBC Na^+/H^+ activity *(8,9)*. This increased Na^+/H^+ activity likely reflects a systemic effect as it has also been demonstrated in skeletal muscle both in SHR *(10)* and in humans with essential hypertension *(11)*.

In contrast to NHE1, the related NHE3 transporter has a more restricted distribution that includes the proximal tubule, and RBC expression of NHE3 has not been reported.

In SHR, NHE3 activity is increased *(12)*, though mRNA expression is not altered. However, this enhanced activity may be related to decreased expression of the NHE regulatory factor 1 (NHERF1) *(13)*, which normally inhibits the activity of NHE transporters, suggesting that NHE3 changes are unrelated to gene expression or structure per se. Kelly et al. *(14)* studied the relative contributions to sodium transport of NHE1 and NHE3 in proximal tubule cells of SHR. Their studies revealed equal activity of both proteins. While NHE1 protein expression was similar to that of normotensive wild-type controls, NHE3 expression was increased by 50% in SHR. An earlier study *(15)* of the NHE3 knockout mouse showed findings of proximal renal tubular acidosis with salt wasting, polyuria, and lower blood pressure, in spite of rise in renin expression and aldosterone levels. These mice also demonstrated diarrhea related to decreased intestinal expression of NHE3, the other major site of expression.

Human studies on NHE3 in hypertension are limited. Zhu et al. *(16)* studied polymorphisms in *SLC9A3* to determine its association with hypertension in an ethnically diverse group of 983 persons, including some with normal and others with elevated blood pressure. None of the six polymorphisms studied was associated with hypertension, although only a subset of the gene sequence was interrogated.

NKCC Transporters

The NKCC family consists of two related proteins, NKCC1 and NKCC2. The first is expressed in a wide variety of tissues, while the second is primarily found in the kidney. In many tissues, these channels are activated by shrinkage of cell volume and conversely inhibited by cell swelling.

The importance of NKCC2 is related primarily to its role in net sodium and chloride reabsorption in the thick ascending limb of the loop of Henle and its inhibition by diuretics such as furosemide. This transport system is responsible for approximately 25% of tubular sodium reabsorption. Lifton's group *(17)* reported that mutations in the gene encoding the NKCC2 protein *(SLC12A1)* cause type 1 Bartter syndrome, a severe manifestation of Bartter syndrome that has antenatal manifestations with polyhydramnios, prematurity, and postnatal electrolyte wasting and volume depletion. Biochemically, the hallmark of this disease is elevated plasma renin activity and aldosterone level with low to normal blood pressure. Perhaps more clinically relevant are studies by the same investigator group identifying mutations in genes encoding NKCC2, NCCT, and ROMK, which appeared to be protective against hypertension from subjects in the Framingham Heart Study *(18)*.

Similar to NHE transporters, NKCC has also been studied in RBCs in animal models and in humans with hypertension. There is higher activity in RBCs in MHS rats compared with controls, and these animals demonstrate a greater natriuretic response to bumetanide *(19)*. Since this strain has normal expression of NKCC2 mRNA and protein *(20)*, it seems unlikely that the increased activity is unrelated to increased gene transcription. Higher levels of NKCC1 activity have been documented in hypertensive humans, but this finding accounts for only a fraction of those with low-renin hypertension *(21–23)*. However, these patients also have an exaggerated response to furosemide *(24)*.

The NCCT

Given the widespread use and success of thiazides in treating essential hypertension, the sparse data on this transporter in both animal models and human hypertension are surprising. Capasso et al. *(20)* demonstrated increased expression of the NCCT in MHS rats, in contrast to NKCC2 and NHE3 mRNA expression. Mutations in the NCCT gene (*SLC12A3*) were also found to be protective against the development of high blood pressure in Framingham Heart Study subjects *(18)*.

ENaC

Mutations in genes encoding the epithelial sodium channel cause Liddle syndrome, probably the best known monogenic form of hypertension. The ENaC is actually a protein complex of three subunits. The regulation of ENaC has been elucidated over the past decade and includes a complex interaction of intracellular proteins including serum- and glucose-regulated kinase (SGK1) and neural precursor cell expressed, developmentally downregulated 4-2 (Nedd4-2). The putative role of ENaC has also been studied in non-genetic forms of hypertension.

The Dahl salt-sensitive rat strain has been shown to exhibit increased activity of intrarenal ENaC. Specifically, in cell cultures of collecting ducts from these strains, sodium transport was enhanced as compared to control strains and was augmented by aldosterone and dexamethasone *(25)*. In follow-up experiments to distinguish between whether the effect was due to ENaC or to Na^+/K^+ ATPase, sodium transport was unaffected by ouabain, which inhibits the Na^+/K^+ ATPase, suggesting increased ENaC activity as the cause *(26)*.

As noted, Liddle syndrome is caused by mutations in the genes encoding the β- and γ-subunits of ENaC. These mutations result in truncated proteins without the C-terminal end, a segment that is essential for intracellular regulation. The mutations leave ENaC constitutively activated and unaffected by homeostatic stimuli, such as aldosterone. Aside from this rare genetic disease, a number of studies have attempted to assess the contribution of ENaC to essential hypertension. Persu et al. *(27)* studied β-ENaC variants in hypertensive families. After determining the most common changes observed in the last exon, they assessed the frequency in a French cohort of 525 patients. Although these changes were seen in only 1% of whites, the frequency increased up to 44% in those of African ancestry. However, only a fraction of those variants led to changes in sodium flux when studied in *Xenopus* oocytes *(27)*.

A relatively common variant in β-ENaC, T594M, has been examined in a number of studies. This variant was first reported by Su et al. *(28)* and found in 6% of 231 African American subjects but in none of the 192 Caucasians studied. This variant leads to loss of protein kinase C inhibition, providing a putative mechanism for its effect *(29)*. A second study identified an association between this same variant and hypertension in 348 blacks in a study from the UK *(30)*. The frequency of this variant was 8.3% among hypertensive persons and 2.1% in those with normal blood pressure. However, a larger study (*n*=4803) that included a large black population reported no relationship between this variant and hypertension *(31)*. Moreover, administration of amiloride to those with this variant did not demonstrate any differential effect as compared to those with wild-type β-ENaC. Thus, the role of ENaC variants in essential hypertension remains to be fully elucidated.

Na^+/K^+ ATPase

This ubiquitous pump generates the driving force for a myriad of transport processes. In the renal tubule, the pump results in net sodium gain, allowing epithelial sodium reabsorption along the length of the renal tubule. Earlier studies revealed increased Na^+/K^+ ATPase activity in MHS kidney extracts as compared with controls *(32)*. This phenomenon was due to increased activity of the pump per se, as pump number was not increased, as assessed by the number of ouabain binding sites *(33)*.

In contrast to primary overactivity of this pump, Blaustein et al. *(34)* have proposed an alternative model based on an unidentified endogenous ouabain-like substance. They hypothesize that salt retention leads to production of this ouabain-like substance, which then increases vasomotor tone due to the linked effects of the Na^+/K^+ ATPase and calcium flux *(35)*. While acute administration of ouabain to rats may induce protective effects such as increased generation of nitric oxide in response to acetylcholine, chronic administration in the rat model induces hypertension that blunts the effects of acetylcholine and generates endothelial dysfunction *(36)*. An endogenous ouabain-like substance has been isolated from MHS and mammalian hypothalamus *(37)*.

CALCIUM FLUX

As noted, sodium and calcium flux are interrelated, most notably due to the effects of the Na^+/K^+ ATPase and cross talk with the Na^+/Ca^{2+} exchanger (NCX). This effect has been harnessed therapeutically with the use of digoxin to increase myocardial contractility. Inhibition of the Na^+/K^+ ATPase leads to an increase in intracellular sodium levels with secondary redistribution of calcium due to NCX *(38)*. The resulting rise in intracellular calcium improves contractility in cardiac myocytes and vascular smooth muscle cells (VSMCs). This link has been further established on a cellular compartment level with colocalization of Na^+/K^+ ATPase and NCX.

It should be noted that differing Na^+/K^+ ATPase subtypes likely mediate this effect, with α2 subtypes having the greatest affinity for endogenous ouabain and its effect on VSMCs *(39,40)*. In mice, expression of the α2 subtype with a shortened N terminus is dominant negative for expression of wild-type full-length α2 pumps *(41)*. When this dominant-negative α2 pump was expressed using a smooth muscle-specific myosin promoter, reduced pump function and elevated blood pressure were observed *(34)*. Conversely, mice that overexpress the α2 pump within smooth muscle have significantly lower blood pressure than α2 wild-type mice and mice with α1 overexpression *(42)*.

The relationship between these transporters suggests a sequence by which increased salt and water intake leads to volume expansion, followed by secondary release of endogenous ouabain *(34,43)*. The inhibition of the Na^+/K^+ ATPase attempts to prevent further sodium retention by the kidneys. Within VSMCs, this phenomenon enhances calcium exchange via NCX with a resultant increase in intracellular calcium and vasoconstriction. Furthermore, because of membrane depolarization related to Na^+/K^+ ATPase inhibition, L-type calcium channels would be activated leading to further calcium influx, resulting in a net increase in vascular tone.

The effects of ouabain on the α2 pump as described above lead to increased vascular tone. However, the α1 pump found in the renal tubular epithelium leads to net sodium retention and would theoretically be inhibited by ouabain. This discordance can be explained by the differential effects of *physiologic levels of ouabain* on the different pump isoforms. As noted, ouabain inhibits the α2 pump, leading to calcium influx into VSMCs and increased vascular tone. In contrast, ouabain may have a net stimulatory effect in the kidney at the α1 pump via stimulation of epidermal growth factor receptor and subsequent phosphorylation and activation of the α1 pump *(44,45)*. This differential effect on isoforms of the Na^+/K^+ ATPase leads to a net increase in blood pressure *(46)*.

Perhaps the most exciting outgrowth of this research is the development of an inhibitor of the Na^+/K^+ ATPase for the treatment of hypertension. Rostafuroxin (PST 2238) is a steroid compound that competitively binds to Na^+/K^+ ATPase and inhibits the effects of ouabain. In MHS rats, rostafuroxin lowered blood pressure compared to vehicle. This effect was also seen in control rats treated with ouabain, deoxycorticosterone acetate, and salt-treated rats in a remnant kidney model *(46,47)*. This effect has not yet been studied in humans *(48)*, although it presents an opportunity to link the basic research done in this model with clinical care.

REGULATION OF ION FLUX

While multiple channels have increased activity that leads to net sodium reabsorption and hypertension in both animal and human studies, the exact mechanism remains unclear. The transporters studied generally do not have increased levels of mRNA or protein, and the association studies for specific polymorphisms in these models have provided conflicting data. However, the cytoskeleton has been implicated as having a role in this altered functional activity. For example, adducin is a component of the cytoskeleton and is ubiquitously expressed. It is found in both rats and humans, and its association with salt-sensitive hypertension has been described in both.

Adducin mutations in both α- and β-subunits have been associated with hypertension in MHS rats *(49)*. A follow-up study by this group showed that in rat tubular epithelium, adducin mutations increase Na^+/K^+ ATPase activity *(50)*. They later described that MHS rats with these mutations did not have the expected endocytosis of Na^+/K^+ pumps in response to dopamine *(51)* and may reflect a broader alteration in clathrin-dependent endocytosis *(52)*. Other groups have shown that in a variety of rat models of hypertension, genes encoding adducin subunits have been found within quantitative trait loci for hypertension *(53)*. Rostafuroxin reduces blood pressure in hypertensive MHS rats with adducin mutations as well *(46,47)*.

α-Adducin polymorphisms have been described in salt-sensitive hypertension as well. In an Italian study of 936 persons, including hypertensive siblings, hypertensive individuals, and normotensive controls, the G460W polymorphism was studied, with a significant association seen in this population *(54)*. Interestingly, this relationship was not seen in a cohort of 375 Scottish patients *(55)* or 507 Japanese patients *(56)*.

CONCLUSIONS

Aberrant ion transport is a critical component in the pathogenesis of hypertension. The research presented reflects only a subset of the published data in this field. It also represents an exciting area of potential study in children and adolescents with essential hypertension, many of whom are salt sensitive. The role of rostafuroxin has yet to be established in the treatment of hypertension, but establishes a new class of agent that more directly targets essential hypertension without the complicating metabolic side effects of thiazides.

REFERENCES

1. Chobanian AV, Bakris GL, Black HR, et al. The seventh report of the joint national committee on prevention, detection, evaluation, and treatment of high blood pressure: the JNC 7 report. JAMA. May 21 2003;289(19):2560–2572.

2. National High Blood Pressure Education Program Working Group on High Blood Pressure in Children and Adolescents. The fourth report on the diagnosis, evaluation, and treatment of high blood pressure in children and adolescents. Pediatrics. Aug 2004;114(2 Suppl 4th Report):555–576.

3. Akita S, Sacks FM, Svetkey LP, Conlin PR, Kimura G. Effects of the Dietary Approaches to Stop Hypertension (DASH) diet on the pressure-natriuresis relationship. Hypertension. Jul 2003;42(1):8–13.

4. Obarzanek E, Proschan MA, Vollmer WM, et al. Individual blood pressure responses to changes in salt intake: results from the DASH-Sodium trial. Hypertension. Oct 2003;42(4):459–467.

5. ALLHAT Collaborative Research Group. Major cardiovascular events in hypertensive patients randomized to doxazosin vs chlorthalidone: the Antihypertensive and Lipid-Lowering Treatment to Prevent Heart Attack Trial (ALLHAT). JAMA. Apr 19 2000;283(15):1967–1975.

6. Diuretic versus alpha-blocker as first-step antihypertensive therapy: final results from the Antihypertensive and Lipid-Lowering Treatment to Prevent Heart Attack Trial (ALLHAT). Hypertension. Sep 2003;42(3):239–246.

7. Diez J, Alonso A, Garciandia A, et al. Association of increased erythrocyte Na+/H+ exchanger with renal Na+ retention in patients with essential hypertension. Am J Hypertens. Feb 1995;8(2):124–132.

8. Canessa M, Morgan K, Goldszer R, Moore TJ, Spalvins A. Kinetic abnormalities of the red blood cell sodium-proton exchange in hypertensive patients. Hypertension. Mar 1991;17(3):340–348.

9. Fortuno A, Tisaire J, Lopez R, Bueno J, Diez J. Angiotensin converting enzyme inhibition corrects Na+/H+ exchanger overactivity in essential hypertension. Am J Hypertens. Jan 1997;10(1):84–93.

10. Syme PD, Aronson JK, Thompson CH, Williams EM, Green Y, Radda GK. Na+/H+ and HCO3–/Cl– exchange in the control of intracellular pH in vivo in the spontaneously hypertensive rat. Clin Sci (Lond). Dec 1991;81(6):743–750.

11. Dudley CR, Taylor DJ, Ng LL, et al. Evidence for abnormal Na+/H+ antiport activity detected by phosphorus nuclear magnetic resonance spectroscopy in exercising skeletal muscle of patients with essential hypertension. Clin Sci (Lond). Nov 1990;79(5):491–497.

12. Hayashi M, Yoshida T, Monkawa T, Yamaji Y, Sato S, Saruta T. Na+/H+-exchanger 3 activity and its gene in the spontaneously hypertensive rat kidney. J Hypertens. Jan 1997;15(1):43–48.

13. Kobayashi K, Monkawa T, Hayashi M, Saruta T. Expression of the Na+/H+ exchanger regulatory protein family in genetically hypertensive rats. J Hypertens. Sep 2004;22(9):1723–1730.

14. Kelly MP, Quinn PA, Davies JE, Ng LL. Activity and expression of Na(+)-H+ exchanger isoforms 1 and 3 in kidney proximal tubules of hypertensive rats. Circ Res. Jun 1997;80(6):853–860.

15. Schultheis PJ, Clarke LL, Meneton P, et al. Renal and intestinal absorptive defects in mice lacking the NHE3 Na+/H+ exchanger. Nat Genet. Jul 1998;19(3):282–285.

16. Zhu H, Sagnella GA, Dong Y, et al. Molecular variants of the sodium/hydrogen exchanger type 3 gene and essential hypertension. J Hypertens. Jul 2004;22(7):1269–1275.

17. Simon DB, Karet FE, Hamdan JM, DiPietro A, Sanjad SA, Lifton RP. Bartter's syndrome, hypokalaemic alkalosis with hypercalciuria, is caused by mutations in the Na-K-2Cl cotransporter NKCC2. Nat Genet. Jun 1996;13(2):183–188.

18. Ji W, Foo JN, O'Roak BJ, et al. Rare independent mutations in renal salt handling genes contribute to blood pressure variation. Nat Genet. May 2008;40(5):592–599.

19. Salvati P, Ferrario RG, Bianchi G. Diuretic effect of bumetanide in isolated perfused kidneys of Milan hypertensive rats. Kidney Int. Apr 1990;37(4):1084–1089.

20. Capasso G, Rizzo M, Garavaglia ML, et al. Upregulation of apical sodium-chloride cotransporter and basolateral chloride channels is responsible for the maintenance of salt-sensitive hypertension. Am J Physiol Renal Physiol. Aug 2008;295(2):F556–F567.

21. Cacciafesta M, Ferri C, Carlomagno A, et al. Erythrocyte Na-K-Cl cotransport activity in low renin essential hypertensive patients. A 23Na nuclear magnetic resonance study. Am J Hypertens. Feb 1994;7(2):151–158.

22. Cusi D, Fossali E, Piazza A, et al. Heritability estimate of erythrocyte Na-K-Cl cotransport in normotensive and hypertensive families. Am J Hypertens. Sep 1991;4(9):725–734.

23. Cusi D, Niutta E, Barlassina C, et al. Erythrocyte Na+,K+,Cl- cotransport and kidney function in essential hypertension. J Hypertens. Aug 1993;11(8):805–813.

24. Righetti M, Cusi D, Stella P, et al. Na+,K+,Cl- cotransport is a marker of distal tubular function in essential hypertension. J Hypertens. Dec 1995;13(12 Pt 2):1775–1778.

25. Husted RF, Takahashi T, Stokes JB. IMCD cells cultured from Dahl S rats absorb more Na+ than Dahl R rats. Am J Physiol. Nov 1996;271(5 Pt 2):F1029–F1036.

26. Husted RF, Takahashi T, Stokes JB. The basis of higher Na+ transport by inner medullary collecting duct cells from Dahl salt-sensitive rats: implicating the apical membrane Na+ channel. J Membr Biol. Mar 1 1997;156(1):9–18.

27. Persu A, Barbry P, Bassilana F, et al. Genetic analysis of the beta subunit of the epithelial Na+ channel in essential hypertension. Hypertension. Jul 1998;32(1):129–137.
28. Su YR, Rutkowski MP, Klanke CA, et al. A novel variant of the beta-subunit of the amiloride-sensitive sodium channel in African Americans. J Am Soc Nephrol. Dec 1996;7(12):2543–2549.
29. Cui Y, Su YR, Rutkowski M, Reif M, Menon AG, Pun RY. Loss of protein kinase C inhibition in the beta-T594M variant of the amiloride-sensitive Na+ channel. Proc Natl Acad Sci USA. Sep 2 1997;94(18):9962–9966.
30. Baker EH, Dong YB, Sagnella GA, et al. Association of hypertension with T594M mutation in beta subunit of epithelial sodium channels in black people resident in London. Lancet. May 9 1998;351(9113):1388–1392.
31. Hollier JM, Martin DF, Bell DM, et al. Epithelial sodium channel allele T594M is not associated with blood pressure or blood pressure response to amiloride. Hypertension. Mar 2006;47(3):428–433.
32. Melzi ML, Bertorello A, Fukuda Y, Muldin I, Sereni F, Aperia A. Na,K-ATPase activity in renal tubule cells from Milan hypertensive rats. Am J Hypertens. Jul 1989;2(7):563–566.
33. Parenti P, Villa M, Hanozet GM, Ferrandi M, Ferrari P. Increased Na pump activity in the kidney cortex of the Milan hypertensive rat strain. FEBS Lett. Sep 23 1991;290(1–2):200–204.
34. Blaustein MP, Zhang J, Chen L, et al. The pump, the exchanger, and endogenous ouabain: signaling mechanisms that link salt retention to hypertension. Hypertension. Feb 2009;53(2):291–298.
35. Haupert GT Jr. Circulating inhibitors of sodium transport at the prehypertensive stage of essential hypertension. J Cardiovasc Pharmacol. 1988;12(Suppl 3):S70–S76.
36. Cao C, Payne K, Lee-Kwon W, et al. Chronic ouabain treatment induces vasa recta endothelial dysfunction in the rat. Am J Physiol Renal Physiol. Jan 2009;296(1):F98–F106.
37. Murrell JR, Randall JD, Rosoff J, et al. Endogenous ouabain: upregulation of steroidogenic genes in hypertensive hypothalamus but not adrenal. Circulation. Aug 30 2005;112(9):1301–1308.
38. Blaustein MP. Physiological effects of endogenous ouabain: control of intracellular Ca2+ stores and cell responsiveness. Am J Physiol. Jun 1993;264(6 Pt 1):C1367–C1387.
39. Ferrandi M, Minotti E, Salardi S, Florio M, Bianchi G, Ferrari P. Ouabainlike factor in Milan hypertensive rats. Am J Physiol. Oct 1992;263(4 Pt 2):F739–F748.
40. Tao QF, Hollenberg NK, Price DA, Graves SW. Sodium pump isoform specificity for the digitalis-like factor isolated from human peritoneal dialysate. Hypertension. Mar 1997;29(3):815–821.
41. Song H, Lee MY, Kinsey SP, Weber DJ, Blaustein MP. An N-terminal sequence targets and tethers Na+ pump alpha2 subunits to specialized plasma membrane microdomains. J Biol Chem. May 5 2006;281(18):12929–12940.
42. Pritchard TJ, Parvatiyar M, Bullard DP, Lynch RM, Lorenz JN, Paul RJ. Transgenic mice expressing Na+-K+-ATPase in smooth muscle decreases blood pressure. Am J Physiol Heart Circ Physiol. Aug 2007;293(2):H1172–H1182.
43. Hamlyn JM, Hamilton BP, Manunta P. Endogenous ouabain, sodium balance and blood pressure: a review and a hypothesis. J Hypertens. Feb 1996;14(2):151–167.
44. Haas M, Askari A, Xie Z. Involvement of Src and epidermal growth factor receptor in the signal-transducing function of Na+/K+-ATPase. J Biol Chem. Sep 8 2000;275(36):27832–27837.
45. Liu J, Tian J, Haas M, Shapiro JI, Askari A, Xie Z. Ouabain interaction with cardiac Na+/K+-ATPase initiates signal cascades independent of changes in intracellular Na+ and Ca2+ concentrations. J Biol Chem. Sep 8 2000;275(36):27838–27844.
46. Ferrari P, Ferrandi M, Valentini G, Bianchi G. Rostafuroxin: an ouabain antagonist that corrects renal and vascular Na+-K+-ATPase alterations in ouabain and adducin-dependent hypertension. Am J Physiol Regul Integr Comp Physiol. Mar 2006;290(3):R529–R535.
47. Ferrari P, Ferrandi M, Tripodi G, et al. PST 2238: a new antihypertensive compound that modulates Na,K-ATPase in genetic hypertension. J Pharmacol Exp Ther. Mar 1999;288(3):1074–1083.
48. Efficacy of Rostafuroxin in the Treatment of Essential Hypertension. http://clinicaltrials.gov/ct2/show/NCT00415038. [Accessed on 17 March 2009].
49. Bianchi G, Tripodi G, Casari G, et al. Two point mutations within the adducin genes are involved in blood pressure variation. Proc Natl Acad Sci USA. Apr 26 1994;91(9):3999–4003.
50. Tripodi G, Valtorta F, Torielli L, et al. Hypertension-associated point mutations in the adducin alpha and beta subunits affect actin cytoskeleton and ion transport. J Clin Invest. Jun 15 1996;97(12):2815–2822.
51. Efendiev R, Krmar RT, Ogimoto G, et al. Hypertension-linked mutation in the adducin alpha-subunit leads to higher AP2-mu2 phosphorylation and impaired Na+,K+-ATPase trafficking in response to GPCR signals and intracellular sodium. Circ Res. Nov 26 2004;95(11):1100–1108.

52. Torielli L, Tivodar S, Montella RC, et al. alpha-Adducin mutations increase Na/K pump activity in renal cells by affecting constitutive endocytosis: implications for tubular Na reabsorption. Am J Physiol Renal Physiol. Aug 2008;295(2):F478–F487.

53. Orlov SN, Adragna NC, Adarichev VA, Hamet P. Genetic and biochemical determinants of abnormal monovalent ion transport in primary hypertension. Am J Physiol. Mar 1999;276(3 Pt 1):C511–C536.

54. Cusi D, Barlassina C, Azzani T, et al. Polymorphisms of alpha-adducin and salt sensitivity in patients with essential hypertension. Lancet. May 10 1997;349(9062):1353–1357.

55. Kamitani A, Wong ZY, Fraser R, et al. Human alpha-adducin gene, blood pressure, and sodium metabolism. Hypertension. Jul 1998;32(1):138–143.

56. Kato N, Sugiyama T, Nabika T, et al. Lack of association between the alpha-adducin locus and essential hypertension in the Japanese population. Hypertension. Mar 1998;31(3):730–733.

5

CRP, Uric Acid, and Other Novel Factors in the Pathogenesis of Hypertension

Daniel I. Feig, MD, PhD, MS

CONTENTS

INTRODUCTION

Hypertension is one of the most common diseases in the world. In Western countries, it affects between 20 and 75% of the adult population, depending on age, and is not only the most important risk factor for cardiovascular and renal disease but is also the most amenable to modification with current medical therapy *(1)*. In adult populations, the vast majority of hypertension is essential hypertension, so that standard recommended practice is not to do extensive evaluation for the secondary etiologies of hypertension at the time of diagnosis *(1)*. While this practice saves money, it compromises the ability of epidemiologists to identify mechanistic risk factors, as all hypertensive populations considered as essential hypertension are contaminated with patients with secondary hypertension of various etiologies, including monogenic conditions, renal parenchymal disease, hyperaldosteronism, renovascular disease, and others.

Childhood hypertension, increasingly common, offers an opportunity to gain insights into the early pathophysiology of what is currently called essential (primary) hypertension.

D.I. Feig (✉)
Renal Section, Department of Pediatrics, Baylor College of Medicine, Texas Children's Hospital, Houston, TX, USA
e-mail: dfeig@bcm.tmc.edu

From: *Clinical Hypertension and Vascular Diseases: Pediatric Hypertension*
Edited by: J. T. Flynn et al. DOI 10.1007/978-1-60327-824-9_5
© Springer Science+Business Media, LLC 2011

Because secondary hypertension is more common among children with elevated blood pressure than in adults, the current clinical guidelines, detailed in Chapter 28, include detailed testing and evaluation to distinguish secondary from essential hypertension (2). Such evaluation results in clearer case definition of essential hypertension among children. Further, children have fewer confounding diagnoses such as diabetes, atherosclerotic heart disease, and age-related illness, making children and adolescents the ideal population in which to study the early physiological steps that initiate essential hypertension. Studies of newly hypertensive patients also allow investigators to distinguish factors involved in initiating hypertension from those caused by persistent, chronic hypertension.

This chapter describes some of the nonconventional risk factors for hypertension. For most, the data are exclusively observational and require much more laboratory and clinical study before these factors can be considered potential therapeutic targets. In a few cases, however, the data provide a more complete pathophysiological story. This chapter emphasizes the potential roles of C-reactive protein (CRP) and uric acid in the development of hypertension, not because these should be considered major risk factors for essential hypertension, but because studies of these factors are further advanced than some of the other potential risk factors, so that such studies may serve as a model for investigating other potential novel causes of the development of hypertension.

GENETIC POLYMORPHISMS ARE AN INSUFFICIENT MODEL

Several models have been developed to support the concept of hypertension as a disease of renal sodium handling. In fact, the tendency toward sodium retention and sodium sensitivity is a common aspect of hypertension in adults and children (3,4). A favored hypothesis is that hypertension results from a polygenic defect in which there are alterations in the regulation or expression in tubular transport systems involved in sodium reabsorption and excretion (5,6). The discovery that many forms of genetic hypertension are associated with enhanced sodium reabsorption has provided support for this hypothesis (5,6). However, studies using conventional genetic methods as well as others using genome-wide association methods suggest that known genetic mechanisms can only account for a minority of cases of hypertension (7,8). Furthermore, a study of 1003 identical twins found that when one twin was hypertensive, the other was hypertensive only 44% of the time (9), which strongly argues against hypertension being a typical monogenetic or polygenic defect. Even more convincing are epidemiologic data that show a dramatic increase in the prevalence of hypertension over the past 100 years. Thus, studies in the early 1900s showed a near absence of hypertension in Africa, Asia, Arabia, South America, Australia and New Zealand, and Oceania (reviewed in (10)), but now hypertension is rapidly increasing in prevalence along with the worldwide epidemic of obesity and diabetes (11). Similarly, hypertension was observed in only 10% of the population in the USA in the early 1930s (12), but is now present in over 30% of the population (13). It is difficult to explain how a purely genetic mechanism could account for this rapid change in prevalence. Finally, a genetic defect in sodium excretion as a primary mechanism for essential hypertension does not easily account for studies that show that in early hypertension blood volume and exchangeable sodium tend to be low (14–16), that early hypertension is frequently salt-resistant (i.e., is not altered by sodium intake) (17), and that salt sensitivity increases progressively with aging (17). Consequently, a model that fully explains hypertension must include the effects of peri- and postnatal life, and exposures and effectors that alter vascular physiology after organ development is complete.

PRENATAL EXPOSURES

A nongenetic prenatal or developmental predisposition to hypertension has been hypothesized for a number of years *(18)*, based on both epidemiological and experimental observations (also see Chapter 13). First, there is evidence for a 'maternal factor' in hypertension, because hypertension is inherited more commonly through the mother than the father *(19)*. Indeed, a child's risk of hypertension is increased if the mother has hypertension, preeclampsia, obesity, or malnutrition during pregnancy *(20)*, each of which increases the risk for delivering a low birth weight baby; lower birth weight is associated with increased risk of hypertension during adulthood *(20)*. Lower birth weight associated in experimental models and, possibly, in humans, with fewer nephrons owing to impaired nephrogenesis *(21)*. In support of this hypothesis is the observation that the experimental induction of malnutrition during pregnancy in rats results in pups that are born with low nephron number and later develop salt-sensitive hypertension *(22)*. Autopsy studies of young hypertensive subjects dying from traffic accidents have also verified that the kidneys have significantly fewer nephrons than those of age-matched normotensive controls *(23)*. However, while low birth weight is especially common among African-Americans *(24)*, who have the greatest risk for hypertension in the United States, available data does not support a decreased number of nephrons. Despite strong evidence for perinatal effects, most patients who develop hypertension as adolescents or adults lack obvious pre- and perinatal risk factors. Consequently, later-acting effectors must be considered.

CRP AND HYPERTENSION

Over the past two decades a great deal of interest has focused on the role of inflammation in cardiovascular disease, particularly in atherosclerosis. A variety of protein biomarkers of ongoing inflammation can be measured in the bloodstream and have been studied as potential markers or predictors of future risk of CV events. Among such biomarkers, there is substantial evidence that C-reactive protein, beyond its tracking with ongoing inflammation, may be a marker and participant in vascular disease and/or hypertension *(25)*.

Assays to measure CRP and their interpretation have evolved over time. The original tests, used for research and clinical evaluation in the early 1990s, were developed for patients with infections and inflammatory disorders and have a detection range from 3 to 20 mg/L, well above the levels expected in healthy persons. Most laboratories now use a highly sensitive C-reactive protein (hsCRP) assay that has a linear detection range down to 0.3 mg/L. Actual values that constitute an abnormal elevation are the topic of debate and can vary from lab to lab. The Centers for Disease Control (CDC) and American Heart Association (AHA) have produced consensus definitions that hsCRP values of <1, 1–3, and >3 mg/L define the population tertiles in adults and consider values >10 mg/L as abnormal in any patients *(26)*. When CRP is measured for risk screening, the optimal technique is to use the average of two tests, at least 2 weeks apart, with a mean value of >3mg/L indicating increased CV risk *(25)*.

A possible link between CRP and atherosclerotic cardiovascular disease is controversial. Animal models show that infusion of CRP increases aortic plaque area *(27)*; CRP through activation of complement *(28,29)* can exacerbate myocardial ischemic injury *(30,31)*. In a small clinical study, seven volunteers were infused with CRP, which resulted in a transient rise in IL-6, IL-8, serum amyloid A, and several procoagulation molecules *(32)*. Larger clinical and epidemiological trials less consistently support a direct role for CRP in CV disease. Among a cohort of 50,000 adults with and without history of ischemic CV disease, persons with CRP >3 mg/L had a 1.6-fold increase in relative risk of CV events as compared to those with levels <1 mg/L *(33)*. In the same study, four genetic polymorphisms of CRP accounted for more than 60% of the variability in serum levels of CRP, yet combined polymorphisms expected to confer greater risk did not. Other studies of polymorphisms considered as high risk were also unassociated with CV risk *(34–37)*. As most studies have suggested elevated CRP is associated with risk while mechanistic studies have been inconsistent, most experts consider CRP as a marker but not a mediator of cardiovascular disease *(26)*. In children several studies have correlated CRP with CV risk *(38,39)*, metabolic syndrome *(40)*, and left ventricular hypertrophy *(41)*. It has also been noted to be higher in the offspring of parents with essential hypertension *(42)*.

The central hypothesis regarding a role of CRP in the etiology of hypertension is that it induces endothelial dysfunction and increased vascular reactivity through perivascular inflammation. CRP is an acute-phase protein that is produced predominantly in the liver under transcriptional regulation directed by inflammatory cytokines. Several studies have shown the induction of production and elaboration of CRP by interleukin-1β (IL-1β), interleukin-6 (IL-6), and tumor necrosis factor-α (TNF-α) *(43,44)*. Addition of recombinant CRP to the growth medium of cultured endothelial cells results in the reduction of NO production, which could result in reduced vasodilation *(45,46)*. In cultured vascular endothelial cells, CRP induces production and elaboration of endothelin-1, a potent vasoconstrictor *(47,48)*. Finally, CRP increases the surface expression of angiotensin II type 1 receptors on vascular smooth muscle cells *(49)*, making them more responsive to the vasoconstrictive action of angiotensin II (Ang II. While all of these experimental mechanisms are plausible pathways to hypertension, none have been confirmed in humans.

The epidemiologic evidence suggesting a link between CRP and hypertension is not definitive. The strongest evidence for a link comes from the Women's Health Study, in which 20,525 women >45 years in age were followed for 10 years. The total incidence of hypertension during the follow-up period was 26%. Baseline hsCRP was linearly associated with incident hypertension as a statistically significant independent risk factor (relative risk 1.31–2.32, depending on age and other factors) *(50)*. Likewise, an analysis of the National Health and Nutrition Examination Survey II (NHANES-II) indicated that CRP was an independent risk factor for incident systolic hypertension in girls, aged 12–17 years *(51)*. A recent bivariate analysis of the NHANES-III data reported that participants with CRP >3 mg/L had higher systolic but not diastolic blood pressure as compared to those with CRP <3 mg/L. Multiple regression analysis found that this effect was independent of other CV risk factors only in black boys and was of relatively small magnitude, 4 mmHg *(52)*. A Canadian study of 2224 children also found an association between CRP and SBP, in boys and girls, but the effect was not independent of body mass index (BMI) *(53)*. Similarly, a smaller study of 325 Columbian school-age children found that CRP was linearly associated with adiposity but not independently associated with blood pressure *(54)*. It may be that CRP is not directly associated with hypertension or that the effect may be of insufficient magnitude to be detected in children.

Unfortunately, there are currently no available medications that directly act upon the production or biological activity of CRP. Several classes of medications have been found to lower CRP, including statins *(55)*, fibrates *(56)*, nicotinic acid *(57)*, thiazolidinediones *(58)*, and angiotensin receptor blockers *(59)*. These drugs, used to mitigate CV risk factors, may exert some of their effects secondarily through reduction of CRP or a lower CRP may be an unrelated side effect. All of these classes of drugs would also be expected to have impact on blood pressure for reasons other than reduction of CRP. Consequently, a clinical trial with one or more of these medications would be unlikely to resolve the mechanistic question of whether CRP is a cause or risk factor for hypertension.

OTHER INFLAMMATORY CYTOKINES AND CARDIOVASCULAR DISEASE

Several inflammatory markers, other than CRP, have been implicated in CV disease and hypertension. These include a reported association between serum IL-6 and IL-10 levels and CV risk (60), and an association between TNF-α receptor polymorphisms and hypertension risk (61); but the greatest amount of focus is on monocyte chemoattractant protein-1 (MCP-1). MCP-1 is a potent recruitment molecule specific for monocytes that has been implicated in atherosclerosis and hypertension. Produced by cytokine-activated vascular endothelial cells (62), MCP-1 causes migration of monocytes into vascular intima initiating a perivascular inflammatory cycle that can lead to atherosclerotic plaque formation (63) and/or vascular smooth muscle cell proliferation and arteriolosclerosis (64). Genetically engineered mice lacking the receptor for MCP-1 have significantly reduced atherosclerotic plaque formation (63). CRP (47), LDL-cholesterol (65), and uric acid can activate endothelial MCP-1 expression in cultured cells; thus, it is hypothesized that MCP-1 (66) may modulate several pathways leading to increased cardiovascular risk. In a cross-sectional study of 263 adults, serum MCP-1 levels correlated with coronary risk factors including hypertension, hypercholesterolemia, diabetes, and obesity (67). Single gene polymorphisms in the MCP-1 gene have also been linked to hypertension and ischemic heart disease (68), but whether MCP-1 has a direct role in hypertension and CV disease remains an open question.

URIC ACID IN CHILDHOOD HYPERTENSION

The concept that uric acid may be involved in hypertension is not new. In the 1870s, Frederick Mahomed noted that many hypertensive patients came from gouty families and hypothesized that uric acid might be integral to the development of essential hypertension (69). Ten years later, Haig (70) proposed that hyperuricemia was the underlying cause of many pathological conditions, including hypertension, diabetes, and 'rheumatism', and that low purine diets were a critical preventive measure. In 1909, Henri Huchard noted that renal arteriolosclerosis (the histological lesion of hypertension) was observed in three groups; those with gout, lead poisoning, or have a diet consisting mainly of fatty meats, all of which are associated with hyperuricemia (71). Although an association between serum uric acid level and hypertension was repeatedly reported between 1950s and 1980s (72–74), the lack of a plausible mechanism led it being largely ignored in medical practice.

In the last decade, new epidemiologic studies have rekindled an interest in the link between uric acid and hypertension (see Table 1). Three longitudinal Japanese studies showed an association between serum uric acid level and incident hypertension. Nakanishi et al. (75) showed a 1.6-fold increased risk of new hypertension over 6 years in young adult office works with serum uric acid level in the highest tertile. Taniguchi et al. (76) showed a twofold increased risk of new hypertension over 10 years associated with elevated uric acid in the Osaka Health Study. Masuo et al. (77) evaluated the linear association of serum uric acid level and systolic blood pressure, finding an average increase of 27 mmHg per 1 mg/dL increase in serum uric acid levels among nonobese young men. In an ethnically diverse population within the Bogalusa Heart Study, higher childhood and young adult serum uric acid levels were associated with incident hypertension and progressive increase

Table 1
Epidemiology of Hyperuricemia and Hypertension

Study	Year	Population	Finding	References
Israeli Heart Study	1972	10,000 men	High uric acid associated with twofold risk of hypertension at 5 years	(107)
Fessel et al.	1973	348 adults	High uric acid associated with greater increase in SBP over 4 years	(108)
Gruskin	1985	55 adolescents	Mean uric acid higher in hypertensive children	(90)
Brand et al.	1985	4,286 adults	Uric acid had linear association with change in SBP over 9 years	(74)
Moscow Children's	1985	145 children	9% Normotensive and 73% hypertensive had uric acid >8 mg/dL	(109)
Hungarian Children's	1990	17,634 children	Uric acid predicts hypertension in late adolescence	(89)
Kaiser Permanente	1990	2,062 adults	High uric acid associated with twofold risk of hypertension at 6 years	(110)
University of Utah	1991	1,482 adults	High uric acid associated with twofold risk of hypertension over 7 years	(111)
NHANES	1993	6,768 children	High uric acid predicts hypertension in boys aged 12–17 years	(112)
Olivetti Heart Study	1994	619 men	High uric acid associated with twofold risk of hypertension at 12 years	(113)

Table 1
(continued)

Study	Year	Population	Finding	References
CARDIA Study	1999	5,115 men	High uric acid associated with increased hypertension in blacks	(114)
Osaka Health	2001	6,356 men	High uric acid associated with twofold risk of hypertension at 10 years	(76)
Hawaii LA Hiroshima	2001	140 men	High uric acid associated with 3.5-fold risk of hypertension at 15 years	(115)
Feig and Johnson	2003	125 children	Uric acid >5.5 mg/dL had 89% PPV for essential hypertension	(91)
Osaka Factory	2003	433 men	Each 1 mg/dL uric acid associate with 27 mmHg rise in SBP	(77)
Osaka Health II	2003	2,310 men	High uric acid associated with 1.6-fold risk of hypertension at 6 years	(75)
Okinawa	2004	4,489 adults	High uric acid associated with 1.7-fold risk of hypertension at 13 years	(116)
Bogalusa	2005	679 children	High uric acid associate with diastolic hypertension at 10 years	(78)
Framingham	2005	3,329 adults	High uric acid associated with 1.6-fold risk of hypertension at 4 years	(79)

Table 1
(continued)

Study	Year	Population	Finding	References
Normative Aging	2006	2,062 men	High uric acid associated with 1.5-fold risk of hypertension at 21 years	*(117)*
MRFIT	2006	3,073 men	High uric acid associated with 1.8-fold risk of hypertension at 6 years	*(118)*
ARIC	2006	9,104 adults	High uric acid associated with 1.5-fold risk of hypertension at 9 years	*(119)*
Beaver Dam	2006	2,520 adults	High uric acid associated with 1.7-fold risk of hypertension at 10 years	*(120)*
Health Professionals	2006	750 elderly men	High uric acid associated with 1.1-fold risk of hypertension at 8 years	*(121)*
CARDIA	2007	2,611 adults	Change in uric acid predicts change in blood pressure in young adults over 10 years	*(122)*
Women's Health	2009	1,469 women	High uric acid associated with 1.9-fold risk of hypertension	*(123)*
Jones et al.	2009	104 children	High uric acid associated with 2.1-fold risk of ABPM diastolic hypertension	*(124)*

in blood pressure within the normal range *(78)*. A post hoc analysis from the Framingham Heart Study also suggested that a higher serum uric acid level is associated with increased risk of rising blood pressure *(79)*. Studies specifically of older and elderly patients have had variable results *(80–83)*, implying that if uric acid leads to hypertension, there may be a preferential effect in the young.

A rat model developed in the late 1990s provided a hypothetical mechanism for uric acid-mediated hypertension and significantly increased interest in this field *(84)*. The model requires that rats be fed an inhibitor of urate oxidase, oxonic acid, to increase their uric acid levels to those found in humans. Over 7 weeks of such treatment, systolic blood pressures increase an average of 22 mmHg. The increase in blood pressure can be prevented by the co-administration of the xanthine oxidase inhibitor allopurinol or by the uricosuric agent benziodarone, indicating that the rise in uric acid is the cause of the increased blood

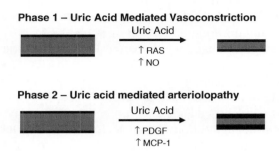

Fig. 1. Two phases of hyperuricemic hypertension: Animal model data suggest that hyperuricemia leads to hypertension in a step fashion. This is a schematic of the effects of uric acid on the blood vessels. The first phase is directly uric acid dependent and sodium independent. It occurs through the uric acid-mediated activation of the renin–angiotensin system and downregulation of endothelial nitric oxide, leading to a vasoconstricted state. The second phase, which develops over time, becomes sodium sensitive and uric acid independent. It occurs through the uric acid-mediated development of renal afferent arteriolosclerosis that induces an irreversible shift in the pressure natriuresis curve.

pressure *(84)*. After 7 weeks on a low salt diet, if the urate oxidase inhibitor, oxonic acid, is removed, the serum uric acid level decreases to normal as does the blood pressure over 3 weeks; however, if the hyperuricemic rats are then fed a high salt diet, they become hypertensive long term, even if hyperuricemia resolves *(85)*. The mechanism by which uric acid induces this change is complex and has been elucidated. Uric acid enters vascular smooth muscle cells through several biochemical steps and induces the production and elaboration of MCP-1 and platelet-derived growth factor (PDGF) *(66,84,86,87)*. This results in vascular smooth muscle proliferation and the thickening of arteriolar walls and the development of arteriolosclerosis (Fig. 1).

The two-phase development of hypertension in the rat model (phase 1, with high uric acid, and phase 2, with salt loading) provides a potential explanation for greater correlation between uric acid and hypertension in younger and prehypertensive populations. If humans follow a similar pattern, older patients would be expected to hypertension unrelated to uric acid levels. Thus, determining whether uric acid causes hypertension and to what extent, hyperuricemia ought to be managed should be approached in younger patients. Current data support this approach. In adolescents there is a close association between elevated serum uric acid level and the onset of essential hypertension. The Moscow Children's Hypertension Study reported hyperuricemia (>8.0 mg/dL) in 9.5% of children with normal blood pressure, 49% of children with borderline hypertension, and 73% of children with moderate and severe hypertension *(88)*. The Hungarian Children's Health Study followed all 17,624 children born in Budapest in 1964 for 13 years and observed elevated heart rate, early sexual maturity, and hyperuricemia were significantly associated with development of hypertension *(89)*. These two studies do not separate the hypertensive children by underlying diagnosis, so the relationship between serum uric acid level and hypertension may be skewed by ascertainment bias. In a small study, Gruskin *(90)* compared adolescents (13–18 years of age) with essential hypertension to age-matched, healthy controls with normal blood pressures. The hypertensive children had both elevated serum uric acid levels (mean >6.5 mg/dL) and higher peripheral renin activity. In a racially diverse population referred for the evaluation of hypertension, Feig and Johnson *(91)* observed that the mean serum uric acid level in children with white coat hypertension was 3.6 mg/dL, slightly higher in secondary hypertension (4.3 mg/dL) and significantly elevated in children with primary hypertension (6.7 mg/dL—tight, linear correlation between the serum uric acid levels and the systolic and diastolic blood pressures, $r=0.8$ for SBP and $r=0.6$ for DBP). Among patients referred for evaluation of hypertension, a serum uric acid level >5.5 mg/dL had an 89% positive predictive value for essential hypertension.

Results from a small very small, unblinded pilot study in children suggest that uric acid may directly contribute to the onset of hypertension in some humans. Five children, aged 14–17 years, with newly diagnosed and as yet untreated essential hypertension were treated for 1 month with allopurinol as a solitary pharmacological agent; all had a decrease in blood pressure by both casual and ambulatory monitoring and four of the five were normotensive at the end of 1 month. All also had a rebound in their blood pressures after discontinuation of the therapy *(92)*. A sample of 30 adolescents with newly diagnosed essential hypertension were treated in a randomized, double-blinded cross-over trial with allopurinol versus placebo. Sixty-seven percent of children while on allopurinol, and 91% of children who has serum uric acid level <5.5 mg/dL on treatment, had normal blood pressure, compared to 3% when children were on placebo *(93)*. While these observations should be confirmed in larger and more general population, if serum uric acid is indeed directly causing renal arteriolopathy, altered regulation of natriuresis and persistent systemic hypertension, it is a modifiable risk factor for CKD in the absence of other mechanisms.

HYPERURICEMIA ETIOLOGY

The causes of mild to moderate hyperuricemia in the young are not well established. In older patients, a variety of mechanisms, including decreased renal function, have been shown to lead to hyperuricemia. There are numerous medications that impair renal clearance of uric acid including loop and thiazide diuretics *(94)*. Genetic polymorphisms in anion transporters such as uric acid anion transporter-1 (URAT-1) may also lead to hyperuricemia *(95)*. Approximately 15% of uric acid clearance is through the GI tract, consequently small bowel disease or altered phenotype can also contribute *(96)*. Diets rich in fatty meats, seafood, and alcohol increase serum uric acid levels *(97,98)* and obesity confers a threefold increased risk of hyperuricemia *(99)*. Finally, as uric acid is the end point of the purine disposal pathway, impairment of the efficiency of purine recycling metabolism or overwhelming the recycling pathway with excessive cell death or cell turnover will increase serum uric acid levels *(100)*.

Serum uric acid levels throughout the population correlate with the rise in the obesity *(91)*, and since the introduction of high fructose corn syrup (HFCS) in the early 1970s, the intake of sweetener has increased *(101)*. Fructose increases uric acid, and it does so rapidly through activation of the fructokinase pathway in hepatocytes *(102)*. Fructokinase consumes ATP leading to an increased load of intracellular purines requiring metabolism and disposal through xanthine oxidase-mediated metabolism ending in uric acid *(102)*. Fructose-fed rats develop features of metabolic syndrome, hyperuricemia, and hypertension *(103)*, including the development of preglomerular arteriolopathy. Lowering uric acid prevents these changes despite ongoing fructose consumption *(101)*. Human studies also show that fructose loading leads to increase serum uric acid levels acutely, and that chronic increases fructose consumption leads to chronically increased serum uric acid and increases in blood pressure *(104,105)*. With the nearly universal exposure to sweetened foods and beverages in the pediatric population, it is very likely that much of the hyperuricemia, especially that associated with obesity, is dietary rather than genetic in origin *(106)*. What has not yet been proven is whether active reduction of sweetener consumption is an effective way to reduce serum uric acid levels and or blood pressure.

CONCLUSIONS AND FURTHER DIRECTIONS

The common physiological thread among the potential mediators of hypertension discussed in this chapter is the induction of an inflammatory cascade. Endothelial dysfunction, perivascular infiltration of inflammatory cells, smooth muscle proliferation, and the development of renal afferent arteriolosclerosis likely represent a common pathway to hypertension that can be engaged by a variety of stimuli (see Fig. 2). If future studies bear out some or all of these mediators as important causes of hypertension, the potential therapies may be specific to specific mediators.

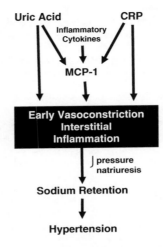

Fig. 2. A hypothetical common pathway for the development of hypertension secondary to inflammatory mediators, CRP, MCP-1 and uric acid.

REFERENCES

1. Chobanian AV, Bakris GL, Black HR, Cushman WC, Green LA, Izzo JL Jr, Jones DW, Materson BJ, Oparil S, Wright JT Jr, Roccella EJ. The seventh report of the joint national committee on prevention, detection, evaluation, and treatment of high blood pressure: the JNC 7 report. JAMA. 2003;289:2560–2572.
2. The fourth report on the diagnosis, evaluation, and treatment of high blood pressure in children and adolescents. Pediatrics. 2004;114:555–576.
3. Johnson RJ, Feig DI, Nakagawa T, Sanchez-Lozada LG, Rodriguez-Iturbe B. Pathogenesis of essential hypertension: historical paradigms and modern insights. J Hypertens. 2008;26:381–391.
4. Johnson RJ, Herrera-Acosta J, Schreiner GF, Rodriguez-Iturbe B. Subtle acquired renal injury as a mechanism of salt-sensitive hypertension. N Engl J Med. 2002;346:913–923.
5. Karet FE, Lifton RP. Mutations contributing to human blood pressure variation. Recent Prog Horm Res. 1997;52:263–276.
6. Lifton RP. Molecular genetics of human blood pressure variation. Science. 1996;272:676–680.
7. Caulfield M, Munroe P, Pembroke J, Samani N, Dominiczak A, Brown M, Benjamin N, Webster J, Ratcliffe P, O'Shea S, Papp J, Taylor E, Dobson R, Knight J, Newhouse S, Hooper J, Lee W, Brain N, Clayton D, Lathrop GM, Farrall M, Connell J. Genome-wide mapping of human loci for essential hypertension. Lancet. 2003;361:2118–2123.

8. Province MA, Kardia SL, Ranade K, Rao DC, Thiel BA, Cooper RS, Risch N, Turner ST, Cox DR, Hunt SC, Weder AB, Boerwinkle E. A meta-analysis of genome-wide linkage scans for hypertension: the National Heart, Lung and Blood Institute Family Blood Pressure Program. Am J Hypertens. 2003;16:144–147.

9. Carmelli D, Robinette D, Fabsitz R. Concordance, discordance and prevalence of hypertension in World War II male veteran twins. J Hypertens. 1994;12:323–328.

10. Johnson RJ, Titte SR, Cade JR, Rideout BA, Oliver WJ. Uric acid, primitive cultures and evolution. Semin Nephrol. 2005;25:3–8.

11. Yusuf S, Reddy S, Ounpuu S, Anand S. Global burden of cardiovascular diseases: part I: general considerations, the epidemiologic transition, risk factors, and impact of urbanization. Circulation. 2001;104:2746–2753.

12. Robinson SC, Brucer M. Range of normal blood pressure. A statistical and clinical study of 11,383 persons. Arch Intern Med. 1939;64:409–444.

13. Fields LE, Burt VL, Cutler JA, Hughes J, Roccella EJ, Sorlie P. The burden of adult hypertension in the United States 1999 to 2000: a rising tide. Hypertension. 2004;44:398–404.

14. Beretta-Piccoli C, Davies DL, Boddy K, Brown JJ, Cumming AM, East BW, Fraser R, Lever AF, Padfield PL, Semple PF, Robertson JI, Weidmann P, Williams ED. Relation of arterial pressure with body sodium, body potassium and plasma potassium in essential hypertension. Clin Sci (Lond). 1982;63:257–270.

15. Beretta-Piccoli C, Weidmann P. Circulatory volume in essential hypertension. Relationships with age, blood pressure, exchangeable sodium, renin, aldosterone and catecholamines. Miner Electrolyte Metab. 1984;10:292–300.

16. Lebel M, Grose JH, Blais R. Abnormal relation of extracellular fluid volume and exchangeable sodium with systemic arterial pressure in early borderline essential hypertension. Am J Cardiol. 1984;54:1267–1271.

17. Weinberger MH, Fineberg NS. Sodium and volume sensitivity of blood pressure. Age and pressure change over time. Hypertension. 1991;18:67–71.

18. Brenner BM, Garcia DL, Anderson S. Glomeruli and blood pressure. Less of one, more the other? Am J Hypertens. 1988;1:335–347.

19. Murakami K, Kojima S, Kimura G, Sanai T, Yoshida K, Imanishi M, Abe H, Kawamura M, Kawano Y, Ashida T, et al. The association between salt sensitivity of blood pressure and family history of hypertension. Clin Exp Pharmacol Physiol Suppl. 1992;20:61–63.

20. Barker DJ. The fetal origins of adult hypertension. J Hypertens Suppl. 1992;10:S39–S44.

21. Hughson M, Farris AB, Douglas-Denton R, Hoy WE, Bertram JF. Glomerular number and size in autopsy kidneys: the relationship to birth weight. Kidney Int. 2003;63:2113–2122.

22. Woods LL, Weeks DA, Rasch R. Programming of adult blood pressure by maternal protein restriction: role of nephrogenesis. Kidney Int. 2004;65:1339–1348.

23. Keller J, Zimmer G, Mall G, Ritz E, Amann K. Nephron number in patients with primary hypertension. N Engl J Med. 2003;348:101–118.

24. Zimanyi MA, Hoy WE, Douglas-Denton RN, Hughson MD, Holden LM, Bertram JF. Nephron number and individual glomerular volumes in male Caucasian and African American subjects. Nephrol Dial Transplant. 2009;24(8):2428–2433. Epub 2009 Mar 18.

25. Ridker PM. Clinical application of C-reactive protein for cardiovascular disease detection and prevention. Circulation. 2003;107:363–369.

26. Pearson TA, Blair SN, Daniels SR, Eckel RH, Fair JM, Fortmann SP, Franklin BA, Goldstein LB, Greenland P, Grundy SM, Hong Y, Miller NH, Lauer RM, Ockene IS, Sacco RL, Sallis JF Jr, Smith SC Jr, Stone NJ, Taubert KA. AHA guidelines for primary prevention of cardiovascular disease and stroke: 2002 update: consensus panel guide to comprehensive risk reduction for adult patients without coronary or other atherosclerotic vascular diseases. American Heart Association Science Advisory and Coordinating Committee. Circulation. 2002;106:388–391.

27. Schwedler SB, Amann K, Wernicke K, Krebs A, Nauck M, Wanner C, Potempa LA, Galle J. Native C-reactive protein increases whereas modified C-reactive protein reduces atherosclerosis in apolipoprotein E-knockout mice. Circulation. 2005;112:1016–1023.

28. Lagrand WK, Niessen HW, Wolbink GJ, Jaspars LH, Visser CA, Verheugt FW, Meijer CJ, Hack CE. C-reactive protein colocalizes with complement in human hearts during acute myocardial infarction. Circulation. 1997;95:97–103.

29. Griselli M, Herbert J, Hutchinson WL, Taylor KM, Sohail M, Krausz T, Pepys MB. C-reactive protein and complement are important mediators of tissue damage in acute myocardial infarction. J Exp Med. 1999;190:1733–1740.

30. Pepys MB, Hirschfield GM, Tennent GA, Gallimore JR, Kahan MC, Bellotti V, Hawkins PN, Myers RM, Smith MD, Polara A, Cobb AJ, Ley SV, Aquilina JA, Robinson CV, Sharif I, Gray GA, Sabin CA, Jenvey

MC, Kolstoe SE, Thompson D, Wood SP. Targeting C-reactive protein for the treatment of cardiovascular disease. Nature. 2006;440:1217–1221.

31. Kitsis RN, Jialal I. Limiting myocardial damage during acute myocardial infarction by inhibiting C-reactive protein. N Engl J Med. 2006;355:513–515.

32. Bisoendial RJ, Kastelein JJ, Levels JH, Zwaginga JJ, van den Bogaard B, Reitsma PH, Meijers JC, Hartman D, Levi M, Stroes ES. Activation of inflammation and coagulation after infusion of C-reactive protein in humans. Circ Res. 2005;96:714–716.

33. Zacho J, Tybjaerg-Hansen A, Jensen JS, Grande P, Sillesen H, Nordestgaard BG. Genetically elevated C-reactive protein and ischemic vascular disease. N Engl J Med. 2008;359:1897–1908.

34. Timpson NJ, Lawlor DA, Harbord RM, Gaunt TR, Day IN, Palmer LJ, Hattersley AT, Ebrahim S, Lowe GD, Rumley A, Davey Smith G. C-reactive protein and its role in metabolic syndrome: Mendelian randomisation study. Lancet. 2005;366:1954–1959.

35. Lange LA, Carlson CS, Hindorff LA, Lange EM, Walston J, Durda JP, Cushman M, Bis JC, Zeng D, Lin D, Kuller LH, Nickerson DA, Psaty BM, Tracy RP, Reiner AP. Association of polymorphisms in the CRP gene with circulating C-reactive protein levels and cardiovascular events. JAMA. 2006;296:2703–2711.

36. Pai JK, Mukamal KJ, Rexrode KM, Rimm EB. C-reactive protein (CRP) gene polymorphisms, CRP levels, and risk of incident coronary heart disease in two nested case-control studies. PLoS One. 2008;3:e1395.

37. Lawlor DA, Harbord RM, Timpson NJ, Lowe GD, Rumley A, Gaunt TR, Baker I, Yarnell JW, Kivimaki M, Kumari M, Norman PE, Jamrozik K, Hankey GJ, Almeida OP, Flicker L, Warrington N, Marmot MG, Ben-Shlomo Y, Palmer LJ, Day IN, Ebrahim S, Smith GD. The association of C-reactive protein and CRP genotype with coronary heart disease: findings from five studies with 4,610 cases amongst 18,637 participants. PLoS One. 2008;3:e3011.

38. Soriano-Guillen L, Hernandez-Garcia B, Pita J, Dominguez-Garrido N, Del Rio-Camacho G, Rovira A. High-sensitivity C-reactive protein is a good marker of cardiovascular risk in obese children and adolescents. Eur J Endocrinol. 2008;159:R1–R4.

39. Guran O, Akalin F, Ayabakan C, Dereli FY, Haklar G. High-sensitivity C-reactive protein in children at risk for coronary artery disease. Acta Paediatr. 2007;96:1214–1219.

40. Oliveira AC, Oliveira AM, Adan LF, Oliveira NF, Silva AM, Ladeia AM. C-reactive protein and metabolic syndrome in youth: a strong relationship? Obesity (Silver Spring). 2008;16:1094–1098.

41. Assadi F. C-reactive protein and incident left ventricular hypertrophy in essential hypertension. Pediatr Cardiol. 2007;28:280–285.

42. Diaz JJ, Arguelles J, Malaga I, Perillan C, Dieguez A, Vijande M, Malaga S. C-reactive protein is elevated in the offspring of parents with essential hypertension. Arch Dis Child. 2007;92:304–308.

43. Rader DJ. Inflammatory markers of coronary risk. N Engl J Med. 2000;343:1179–1182.

44. Wellen KE, Hotamisligil GS. Obesity-induced inflammatory changes in adipose tissue. J Clin Invest. 2003;112:1785–1788.

45. Verma S, Wang CH, Li SH, Dumont AS, Fedak PW, Badiwala MV, Dhillon B, Weisel RD, Li RK, Mickle DA, Stewart DJ. A self-fulfilling prophecy: C-reactive protein attenuates nitric oxide production and inhibits angiogenesis. Circulation. 2002;106:913–919.

46. Venugopal SK, Devaraj S, Yuhanna I, Shaul P, Jialal I. Demonstration that C-reactive protein decreases eNOS expression and bioactivity in human aortic endothelial cells. Circulation. 2002;106:1439–1441.

47. Verma S, Li SH, Badiwala MV, Weisel RD, Fedak PW, Li RK, Dhillon B, Mickle DA. Endothelin antagonism and interleukin-6 inhibition attenuate the proatherogenic effects of C-reactive protein. Circulation. 2002;105:1890–1896.

48. Devaraj S, Xu DY, Jialal I. C-reactive protein increases plasminogen activator inhibitor-1 expression and activity in human aortic endothelial cells: implications for the metabolic syndrome and atherothrombosis. Circulation. 2003;107:398–404.

49. Wang CH, Li SH, Weisel RD, Fedak PW, Dumont AS, Szmitko P, Li RK, Mickle DA, Verma S. C-reactive protein upregulates angiotensin type 1 receptors in vascular smooth muscle. Circulation. 2003;107:1783–1790.

50. Sesso HD, Buring JE, Rifai N, Blake GJ, Gaziano JM, Ridker PM. C-reactive protein and the risk of developing hypertension. JAMA. 2003;290:2945–2951.

51. Ford ES. C-reactive protein concentration and cardiovascular disease risk factors in children: findings from the National Health and Nutrition Examination Survey 1999–2000. Circulation. 2003;108:1053–1058.

52. Lande MB, Pearson TA, Vermilion RP, Auinger P, Fernandez ID. Elevated blood pressure, race/ethnicity, and C-reactive protein levels in children and adolescents. Pediatrics. 2008;122:1252–1257.

53. Lambert M, Delvin EE, Paradis G, O'Loughlin J, Hanley JA, Levy E. C-reactive protein and features of the metabolic syndrome in a population-based sample of children and adolescents. Clin Chem. 2004;50:1762–1768.

54. Lopez-Jaramillo P, Herrera E, Garcia RG, Camacho PA, Castillo VR. Inter-relationships between body mass index, C-reactive protein and blood pressure in a Hispanic pediatric population. Am J Hypertens. 2008;21:527–532.

55. Jialal I, Stein D, Balis D, Grundy SM, Adams-Huet B, Devaraj S. Effect of hydroxymethyl glutaryl coenzyme a reductase inhibitor therapy on high sensitive C-reactive protein levels. Circulation. 2001;103:1933–1935.

56. Malik J, Melenovsky V, Wichterle D, Haas T, Simek J, Ceska R, Hradec J. Both fenofibrate and atorvastatin improve vascular reactivity in combined hyperlipidaemia (fenofibrate versus atorvastatin trial—FAT). Cardiovasc Res. 2001;52:290–298.

57. Grundy SM. Statin therapy in older persons: pertinent issues. Arch Intern Med. 2002;162:1329–1331.

58. Haffner SM, Greenberg AS, Weston WM, Chen H, Williams K, Freed MI. Effect of rosiglitazone treatment on nontraditional markers of cardiovascular disease in patients with type 2 diabetes mellitus. Circulation. 2002;106:679–684.

59. Takeda T, Hoshida S, Nishino M, Tanouchi J, Otsu K, Hori M. Relationship between effects of statins, aspirin and angiotensin II modulators on high-sensitive C-reactive protein levels. Atherosclerosis. 2003;169:155–158.

60. Karpinski L, Plaksej R, Derzhko R, Orda A, Witkowska M. Serum levels of interleukin-6, interleukin-10 and C-reactive protein in patients with myocardial infarction treated with primary angioplasty during a 6-month follow-up. Pol Arch Med Wewn. 2009;119:115–121.

61. Eguchi T, Maruyama T, Ohno Y, Morii T, Hirao K, Hirose H, Kawabe H, Saito I, Hayashi M, Saruta T. Possible association of tumor necrosis factor receptor 2 gene polymorphism with severe hypertension using the extreme discordant phenotype design. Hypertens Res. 2009;32:775–779.

62. Rollins BJ, Yoshimura T, Leonard EJ, Pober JS. Cytokine-activated human endothelial cells synthesize and secrete a monocyte chemoattractant, MCP-1/JE. Am J Pathol. 1990;136:1229–1233.

63. Boring L, Gosling J, Cleary M, Charo IF. Decreased lesion formation in CCR2-/- mice reveals a role for chemokines in the initiation of atherosclerosis. Nature. 1998;394:894–897.

64. Kanellis J, Nakagawa T, Herrera-Acosta J, Schreiner GF, Rodriguez-Iturbe B, Johnson RJ. A single pathway for the development of essential hypertension. Cardiol Rev. 2003;11:180–196.

65. Cushing SD, Berliner JA, Valente AJ, Territo MC, Navab M, Parhami F, Gerrity R, Schwartz CJ, Fogelman AM. Minimally modified low density lipoprotein induces monocyte chemotactic protein 1 in human endothelial cells and smooth muscle cells. Proc Natl Acad Sci USA. 1990;87:5134–5138.

66. Kanellis J, Watanabe S, Li JH, Kang DH, Li P, Nakagawa T, Wamsley A, Sheikh-Hamad D, Lan HY, Feng L, Johnson RJ. Uric acid stimulates monocyte chemoattractant protein-1 production in vascular smooth muscle cells via mitogen-activated protein kinase and cyclooxygenase-2. Hypertension. 2003;41:1287–1293.

67. Martinovic I, Abegunewardene N, Seul M, Vosseler M, Horstick G, Buerke M, Darius H, Lindemann S. Elevated monocyte chemoattractant protein-1 serum levels in patients at risk for coronary artery disease. Circ J. 2005;69:1484–1489.

68. Bucova M, Lietava J, Penz P, Mrazek F, Petrkova J, Bernadic M, Petrek M. Association of MCP-1 -2518 A/G single nucleotide polymorphism with the serum level of CRP in Slovak patients with ischemic heart disease, angina pectoris, and hypertension. Mediators Inflamm. 2009;2009:390951.

69. Mahomed FA. On chronic Bright's disease, and its essential symptoms. Lancet. 1879;1:399–401.

70. Haig A. On uric acid and arterial tension. Br Med J. 1889;1:288–291.

71. Huchard H. Allgemeine Betrachtungen ber die Arteriosklerose. Klin Med Berlin. 1909;5:1318–1321.

72. Gertler MM, Garn SM, Levine SA. Serum uric acid in relation to age and physique in health and in coronary heart disease. Ann Int Med. 1951;34:1421–1431.

73. Breckenridge A. Hypertension and hyperuricaemia. Lancet. 1966;1:15–18.

74. Brand FN, McGee DL, Kannel WB, Stokes J 3rd, Castelli WP. Hyperuricemia as a risk factor of coronary heart disease: the Framingham Study. Am J Epidemiol. 1985;121:11–18.

75. Nakanishi N, Okamato M, Yoshida H, Matsuo Y, Suzuki K, Tatara K. Serum uric acid and the risk for development of hypertension and impaired fasting glucose or type II diabetes in Japanese male office workers. Eur J Epidemiol. 2003;18:523–530.

76. Taniguchi Y, Hayashi T, Tsumura K, Endo G, Fujii S, Okada K. Serum uric acid and the risk for hypertension and type 2 diabetes in Japanese men. The Osaka Health Survey. J Hypertens. 2001;19: 1209–1215.

77. Masuo K, Kawaguchi H, Mikami H, Ogihara T, Tuck ML. Serum uric acid and plasma norepinephrine concentrations predict subsequent weight gain and blood pressure elevation. Hypertension. 2003;42:474–480.

78. Alper AB Jr, Chen W, Yau L, Srinivasan SR, Berenson GS, Hamm LL. Childhood uric acid predicts adult blood pressure: the Bogalusa Heart Study. Hypertension. 2005;45:34–38.

79. Sundstrom J, Sullivan L, D'Agostino RB, Levy D, Kannel WB, Vasan RS. Relations of serum uric acid to longitudinal blood pressure tracking and hypertension incidence. Hypertension. 2005;45:28–33.
80. Culleton BF, Larson MG, Kannel WB, Levy D. Serum uric acid and risk for cardiovascular disease and death: the Framingham Heart Study. Ann Intern Med. 1999;131:7–13.
81. Nefzger MD, Acheson RM, Heyman A. Mortality from stroke among U.S. veterans in Georgia and 5 western states. I. Study plan and death rates. J Chronic Dis. 1973;26:393–404.
82. Saito I, Folsom AR, Brancati FL, Duncan BB, Chambless LE, McGovern PG. Nontraditional risk factors for coronary heart disease incidence among persons with diabetes: the Atherosclerosis Risk in Communities (ARIC) study. Ann Intern Med. 2000;133:81–91.
83. Staessen J. The determinants and prognostic significance of serum uric acid in elderly patients of the European Working Party on High Blood Pressure in the Elderly trial. Am J Med. 1991;90:50S–54S.
84. Mazzali M, Hughes J, Kim YG, Jefferson JA, Kang DH, Gordon KL, Lan HY, Kivlighn S, Johnson RJ. Elevated uric acid increases blood pressure in the rat by a novel crystal-independent mechanism. Hypertension. 2001;38:1101–1106.
85. Watanabe S, Kang DH, Feng L, Nakagawa T, Kanellis J, Lan HY, Johnson RJ. Uric acid hominoid evolution and the pathogenesis of salt-sensitivity. Hypertension. 2002;40:355–360.
86. Kang DH, Johnson RJ. Uric acid induces C-reactive protein expression via upregulation of angiotensin type I receptor in vascular endothelial and smooth muscle cells. J Am Soc Nephrol. 2003;F-PO336 abstract.
87. Mazzali M, Kanellis J, Han L, Feng L, Xia YY, Chen Q, Kang DH, Gordon KL, Watanabe S, Nakagawa T, Lan HY, Johnson RJ. Hyperuricemia induces a primary renal arteriolopathy in rats by a blood pressure-independent mechanism. Am J Physiol Renal Physiol. 2002;282:F991–F997.
88. Rovda Iu I, Kazakova LM, Plaksina EA. [Parameters of uric acid metabolism in healthy children and in patients with arterial hypertension]. Pediatriia. 1990;8:19–22 (in Russian).
89. Torok E, Gyarfas I, Csukas M. Factors associated with stable high blood pressure in adolescents. J Hypertens Suppl. 1985;3(Suppl 3):S389–S390.
90. Gruskin AB. The adolescent with essential hypertension. Am J Kidney Dis. 1985;6:86–90.
91. Feig DI, Johnson RJ. Hyperuricemia in childhood primary hypertension. Hypertension. 2003;42:247–252.
92. Feig DI, Nakagawa T, Karumanchi SA, Oliver WJ, Kang DH, Finch J, Johnson RJ. Hypothesis: uric acid, nephron number and the pathogenesis of essential hypertension. Kidney Int. 2004;66:281–287.
93. Feig DI, Soletsky B, Johnson RJ. Effect of allopurinol on blood pressure of adolescents with newly diagnosed essential hypertension: a randomized trial. JAMA. 2008;300:924–932.
94. Reyes AJ. The increase in serum uric acid concentration caused by diuretics might be beneficial in heart failure. Eur J Heart Fail. 2005;7:461–467.
95. Graessler J, Graessler A, Unger S, Kopprasch S, Tausche AK, Kuhlisch E, Schroeder HE. Association of the human urate transporter 1 with reduced renal uric acid excretion and hyperuricemia in a German Caucasian population. Arthritis Rheum. 2006;54:292–300.
96. Cannella AC, Mikuls TR. Understanding treatments for gout. Am J Manag Care. 2005;11: S451–S458.
97. Lee SJ, Terkeltaub RA, Kavenaugh A. Recent developments in diet and gout. Curr Opin Rheumatol. 2006;18:193–198.
98. Schlesinger N. Dietary factors and hyperuricaemia. Curr Pharm Des. 2005;11:4133–4138.
99. Hwang LC, Tsai CH, Chen TH. Overweight and obesity-related metabolic disorders in hospital employees. J Formos Med Assoc. 2006;105:56–63.
100. Masseoud D, Rott K, Liu-Bryan R, Agudelo C. Overview of hyperuricaemia and gout. Curr Pharm Des. 2005;11:4117–4124.
101. Nakagawa T, Hu H, Zharikov S, Tuttle KR, Short RA, Glushakova O, Ouyang X, Feig DI, Block ER, Herrera-Acosta J, Patel JM, Johnson RJ. A causal role for uric acid in fructose-induced metabolic syndrome. Am J Physiol Renal Physiol. 2006;290:F625–F631.
102. Fox IH, Kelley WN. Studies on the mechanism of fructose-induced hyperuricemia in man. Metabolism. 1972;21:713–721.
103. Hwang IS, Ho H, Hoffman BB, Reaven GM. Fructose-induced insulin resistance and hypertension in rats. Hypertension. 1987;10:512–516.
104. Brown CM, Dulloo AG, Yepuri G, Montani JP. Fructose ingestion acutely elevates blood pressure in healthy young humans. Am J Physiol Regul Integr Comp Physiol. 2008;294:R730–R737.
105. Brown CM, Dulloo AG, Montani JP. Sugary drinks in the pathogenesis of obesity and cardiovascular diseases. Int J Obes (Lond). 2008;32(Suppl 6):S28–S34.
106. Nguyen S, Choi H, Lustig R, Hsu C. Sugar-sweetened beverages, serum uric acid, and blood pressure in adolescents. J Pediatr. 2009;154:807–813.

107. Kahn HA, Medalie JH, Neufeld HN, et al. The incidence of hypertension and associated factors: the Israel ischemic heart study. Am Heart J. 1972;84:171–182.

108. Fessel WJ, Siegelaub AB, Johnson ES. Correlates and consequences of asymptomatic hyperuricemia. Arch Intern Med. 1993;132:44–54.

109. Rovda Iu I. [Uric acid and arterial hypertension]. Pediatriia. 1992;10–12:74–78 (in Russian).

110. Selby JV, Friedman GD, Quesenberry CP Jr. Precursors of essential hypertension: pulmonary function, heart rate, uric acid, serum cholesterol, and other serum chemistries. Am J Epidemiol. 1990;131:1017–1027.

111. Hunt SC, Stephenson SH, Hopkins PN, Williams RR. Predictors of an increased risk of future hypertension in Utah. A screening analysis. Hypertension. 1991;17:969–976.

112. Goldstein HS, Manowitz P. Relation between serum uric acid and blood pressure in adolescents. Ann Hum Biol. 1993;20:423–431.

113. Jossa F, Farinaro E, Panico S, Krogh V, Celentano E, Galasso R, Mancini M, Trevisan M. Serum uric acid and hypertension: the Olivetti heart study. J Hum Hypertens. 1994;8:677–681.

114. Dyer AR, Liu K, Walsh M, Kiefe C, Jacobs DR Jr, Bild DE. Ten-year incidence of elevated blood pressure and its predictors: the CARDIA study. Coronary Artery Risk Development in (Young) Adults. J Hum Hypertens. 1999;13:13–21.

115. Imazu M, Yamamoto H, Toyofuku M, Sumii K, Okubo M, Egusa G, Yamakido M, Kohno N. Hyperinsulinemia for the development of hypertension: data from the Hawaii-Los Angeles-Hiroshima Study. Hypertens Res. 2001;24:531–536.

116. Nagahama K, Inoue T, Iseki K, Touma T, Kinjo K, Ohya Y, Takishita S. Hyperuricemia as a predictor of hypertension in a screened cohort in Okinawa, Japan. Hypertens Res. 2004;27:835–841.

117. Perlstein TS, Gumieniak O, Williams GH, Sparrow D, Vokonas PS, Gaziano M, Weiss ST, Litonjua AA. Uric acid and the development of hypertension: the normative aging study. Hypertension. 2006;48:1031–1036.

118. Krishnan E, Kwoh CK, Schumacher HR, Kuller L. Hyperuricemia and incidence of hypertension among men without metabolic syndrome. Hypertension. 2007;49:298–303.

119. Mellen PB, Bleyer TJ, Erlinger TP, Evans GW, Nieto FJ, Wagenknecht LE, Wofford MR, Herrington DM. Serum uric acid predicts incident hypertension in a biethnic cohort: the atherosclerosis risk in communities study. Hypertension. 2006;48:1037–1042.

120. Shankar A, Klein R, Klein BE, Nieto FJ. The association between serum uric acid level and long-term incidence of hypertension: population-based cohort study. J Hum Hypertens. 2006;20:937–945.

121. Forman JP, Choi H, Curhan GC. Plasma uric acid level and risk for incident hypertension among men. J Am Soc Nephrol. 2007;18:287–292.

122. Rathmann W, Haastert B, Icks A, Giani G, Roseman JM. Ten-year change in serum uric acid and its relation to changes in other metabolic risk factors in young black and white adults: the CARDIA study. Eur J Epidemiol. 2007;22:439–445.

123. Forman JP, Choi H, Curhan GC. Uric acid and insulin sensitivity and risk of incident hypertension. Arch Intern Med. 2009;169:155–162.

124. Jones DP, Richey PA, Alpert BS. Comparison of ambulatory blood pressure reference standards in children evaluated for hypertension. Blood Press Monit. 2009;14:103–107.

6

Monogenic and Polygenic Genetic Contributions to Hypertension

Julie R. Ingelfinger, MD

CONTENTS

    INTRODUCTION
    MONOGENIC FORMS OF HUMAN HYPERTENSION
    NON-MENDELIAN, POLYGENIC HYPERTENSION
    REFERENCES

INTRODUCTION

More than 9 years have elapsed since the publications in February 2001 that provided the first maps of the human genome *(1,2)*. Increasingly, the identification of a specific gene—or genes—that causes a given disease is feasible. Indeed, genes involved in several rare, monogenic forms of familial hypertension have been identified. However, while the identification of a gene associated with Mendelian forms of hypertension is feasible, such an approach does not work as effectively for non-Mendelian forms of high blood pressure (BP), which have multiple genetic determinants. Many recently developed tools are available to reveal genes involved in primary hypertension, and studies have identified many associations with primary or essential hypertension, which is widely viewed as a polygenic disorder. This chapter discusses both monogenic and polygenic aspects of hypertension.

MONOGENIC FORMS OF HUMAN HYPERTENSION

Genes for a number of monogenic forms of human hypertension have been identified via positional cloning (in the past called "reverse genetics") *(3–5)*. In this approach large kindreds with many affected family members are phenotyped, and the mode of inheritance—autosomal recessive, autosomal dominant, sex-linked, codominant, determined. Subsequently, linkage analysis is performed using highly polymorphic genetic markers such as

J.R. Ingelfinger (✉)
Pediatric Nephrology Unit, Department of Pediatrics, Harvard Medical School and MassGeneral Hospital for Children at Massachusetts General Hospital, Boston, MA, USA
e-mail: jingelfinger@partners.org

From: *Clinical Hypertension and Vascular Diseases: Pediatric Hypertension*
Edited by: J. T. Flynn et al. DOI 10.1007/978-1-60327-824-9_6
© Springer Science+Business Media, LLC 2011

microsatellite markers that occur widely throughout the genome, evenly spaced at approximately 10 centimorgan (cM) intervals. Since most people (about 70%) are heterozygous, the inheritance of alleles can be traced through large pedigrees. In a successful linkage analysis, a specific chromosomal region in the genome linked to the trait is identified. A logarithm of the odds (LOD) score describes the presence of such a region. The generally accepted LOD score indicating linkage is greater than 3.3 (corresponding to a significance level genome-wide of 4.5×10^{-5}) *(4)*. Once linkage is identified, a search for known candidate genes in the area commences. A search using additional highly polymorphic markers may also narrow the area of interest, leading to sequences of possible genes within the area.

Most monogenic forms of hypertension identified to date are due to gain-of-function mutations *(6,7)*, most of which result in overproduction of mineralocorticoids or increased mineralocorticoid activity. Severe hypertension, often from early life—even infancy—is not unusual. Clinical hallmarks include apparent volume expansion and suppressed plasma renin activity with variable hypokalemia. An approach to evaluation of those forms of hypertension associated with hypokalemia and suppressed renin activity is shown in Fig. 1 *(8)*.

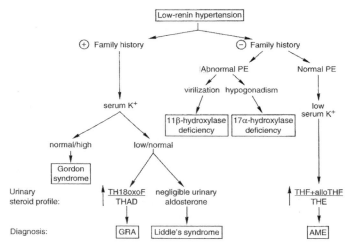

Fig. 1. Algorithm for evaluating children with low-renin hypertension. Several hypertensive syndromes share, as a common feature, very low plasma renin activity (PRA). These disorders are inherited as either an autosomal dominant (positive family history) or an autosomal recessive (negative family history) trait. Children with any of three syndromes, GRA, Liddle's syndrome, apparent mineralocorticoid excess (AME), share a clinical phenotype characterized by normal physical examinations (PEs), low PRA, and hypokalemia. These disorders are distinguishable from one another on the basis of characteristic urinary steroid profiles and genetic testing. K+, Potassium; TH18oxoF/THAD ratio of urinary 18-oxo-tetrahydrocortisol (THAD) (normal 0–0.4, GRA patients > 1); THF+ alloTHF/THE ratio of the combined urinary tetrahydrocortisol (THF) and allotetrahydrocortisol (alloTHF) to urinary tetrahydrocortisone (THE) (normal < 1.3, AME patients five- to tenfold higher; from *(8)*).

Gain-of-function mutations in transporters in the distal nephrons of the renal tubules result in hypertension via salt and water retention by the kidney *(9)*. (While mutations and polymorphisms in the genes of various components of the renin–angiotensin–aldosterone system may lead to excessive renal sodium retention, no single RAS polymorphism causes monogenic hypertension.) Clinically, most monogenic hypertension can be divided into those mutations that lead to overproduction of mineralocorticoids or increased mineralocorticoid activity and those that result in abnormalities of electrolyte transport, focusing on the role of the kidney in hypertension (Table 1) *(7)*. Additionally, some mutations in proto-oncogenes and genes that involve response to hypoxia have been linked to chromaffin tumors (Table 2) *(10)*.

Glucocorticoid-Remediable Aldosteronism or Familial Hyperaldosteronism Type 1 (OMIM #103900)

Glucocorticoid-remediable aldosteronism (GRA) or familial hyperaldosteronism type 1, an autosomal dominant disorder, is considered the most common type of monogenic hypertension and presents in early infancy in some patients *(11–15)*. GRA has been recognized since the 1960s, when Sutherland et al. *(16)* and New and Peterson *(17)* reported patients with severe hypertension accompanied by suppressed renin and increased aldosterone secretion that were found to be treatable with dexamethasone. (GRA is listed in the Online Mendelian Inheritance in Man index (OMIM) as #103900 (OMIM can be accessed at http://www.ncbi.nlm.nih.gov/Omim); note that the OMIM numbers for other Mendelian disorders will also be listed for other disorders when available.) The hypertension in GRA is moderate to severe, owing to increased aldosterone secretion driven by adrenocorticotropic hormone (ACTH).

A chimeric gene containing the 5′ regulatory sequences of 11β-hydroxylase (which confers ACTH responsiveness) fused with the distal coding sequences of aldosterone synthase causes ACTH rather than angiotensin II or potassium as the main controller of aldosterone secretion *(18,19)*. Both serum and urine aldosterone levels tend to be elevated, though not invariably. The chimeric gene product converts cortisol to 18-hydroxy and 18-oxo metabolites *(20–22)*, which can be detected in urine and are pathognomonic. The elevations of urinary cortisol metabolites TH18oxoF and 18-hydroxycortisol and an elevated ratio of TH18oxoF/THAD metabolites can be measured with a commercially available urinary steroid profile (Quest Diagnostics/Nichols Institute, San Juan Capistrano, CA) and will distinguish patients with GRA from others with AME or Liddle's syndrome *(23)*. However, specific genetic testing, which is both sensitive and specific, has largely supplanted the urinary testing when the condition is suspected.

Not all affected members of GRA families develop hypertension in childhood *(24,25)*. Dluhy et al. *(24)* assessed 20 children in 10 unrelated GRA pedigrees and observed that 16 of the 20 developed hypertension, as early as 1 month of age. However, four children were normotensive. Monotherapy using glucocorticoid suppression or aldosterone receptor and epithelial sodium channel (ENaC) antagonists was sufficient to control BP in half of the hypertensive children, though the others required polypharmacy, and three had uncontrollable hypertension *(24)*.

Cerebral hemorrhage at an early age (mean age, 32 years) is common in GRA pedigrees. And almost half of reported pedigrees (48%) and 18% of individual GRA patients have been noted to develop cerebrovascular complications *(6,7,18)*.

Familial Hyperaldosteronism Type 2 (OMIM #605635)

Familial hyperaldosteronism type 2, which appears to be autosomal dominant, is distinct from type 1 and is associated with hyperplasia of the adrenal cortex, an adenoma producing

Table 1
Forms of Monogenic Hypertension

Signs and Sx	Hormonal findings	Source	Genetics	Comment
Steroidogenic enzyme defects				
Steroid 11β-hydroxylase deficiency	⇓ PRA and aldo; high serum androgens/urine 17 ketosteroids; elevated DOC and 11-deoxycortisol	Adrenal: zona fasciculata	CYP11B1 mutation (encodes cytochrome P_{450} 11β/18 of ZF); impairs synthesis of cortisol and ZF 17-deoxysteroids	Hypertensive virilizing CAH; most patients identified by time they are hypertensive. Increased BP may also occur from medication side effects
Steroid 11α-hydroxylase/17,20-lyase deficiency	⇓ PRA and aldo; low serum/urinary 17-hydroxysteroids; decreased cortisol, ⇑ corticosterone (B), and DOC in plasma; serum androgens and estrogens very low; serum gonadotrophins very high	Adrenal: zona fasciculata; Gonadal: interstitial cells (Leydig in testis; theca in ovary)	CYP17 mutation (encodes cytochrome P_{450}C17) impairs cortisol and sex steroid production	CAH with male pseudohermaphroditism; female external genital phenotype in males; primary amenorrhea in females
Hyperaldosteronism				
Primary aldosteronism	⇓ PRA; cplasma aldosterone, 18-OH- and 18oxoF; normal 18-OH/aldo ratio	Adrenal adenoma: clear cell tumor with suppression of ipsilateral ZG	Unknown; very rare in children; female/male ratio is 2.5–3/1	Conn syndrome with aldo producing adenoma; muscle weakness and low K^+ in sodium-replete state
Adrenocortical hyperplasia	As above; source of hormone established by radiology or scans	Adrenal: focal or diffuse adrenal cortical hyperplasia	Unknown	As above

Table 1
(continued)

Signs and Sx	Hormonal findings	Source	Genetics	Comment
Idiopathic primary aldosteronism	High plasma aldo; elevated 18-OHF/aldo ratio	Adrenal: hyperactivity of ZG of adrenal cortex	Unknown	As above
Glucocorticoid-remediable aldosteronism (GRA) Familial hyperaldosteronism type 1	Plasma and urinary aldo responsive to ACTH; dexamethasone suppressible within 48 h; ⇑ urine and plasma 18OHS,18-OHF, and 18 oxoF	Adrenal: abnormal presence of enzymatic activity in adrenal ZF, allowing completion of aldo synthesis from 17-deoxy steroids	Chimeric gene that is expressed at high level in ZF (regulated like $CYP11B1$) and has 18-oxidase activity (CYP11B2 functionality)	Hypokalemia in sodium-replete state
Familial hyperaldosteronism type 2	Hyperaldosteronism. Not suppressed by dexamethasone		Unknown. A 5-Mb locus on chromosome 7p22 appears implicated	
Apparent mineralocorticoid excess (AME)	⇑ plasma ACTH and secretory rates of all corticosteroids; nl serum F (delayed plasma clearance)	⇑ plasma F bioact. in periphery (F-F→E) of bi-dir. 11β-OHSD or slow clearance by 5-α/β reduction to allo dihydro-F	Type 2 11β-OHSD mutations	Cardiac conduction changes; LVH, vessel remodeling; some calcium abnormalities; nephrocalcinosis; rickets
Mineralocorticoid receptor gain-of-function mutation	Low-renin, low-aldosterone, hypokalemia	Mineralocorticoid receptor remains active	Missense mutation—serine at amino acid 810 in the mineralocorticoid receptor is changed to leucine (S810L)	

Table 1
(continued)

Signs and Sx	Hormonal findings	Source	Genetics	Comment
Nonsteroidal defects				
Liddle's syndrome	Low plasma renin, low or normal K+; negligible urinary aldosterone	Not a disorder of steroidogenesis, but of transport	Autosomal dominant Abnormality in epithelial sodium transporter, ENaC, in which channel is constitutively active	Responds to triamterene
Pseudohypoaldosteronism II—Gordon' syndrome	Low plasma renin, normal or elevated K+	Not a disorder of steroidogenesis, but of transport	Autosomal dominant Abnormality in WNK1 or WNK4	Responds to thiazides
Brachydactyly and hypertension	No specific biochemical findings	Not a disorder of steroidogenesis	Inversion, deletion, and reinsertion at 12p12.2 to p11.2	Brachydactyly and hypertension

Adapted and expanded from New MI, Crawford C, Virdis R. Low Renin Hypertension in Childhood, in Lifshitz F (Ed.) Pediatric Endocrinology, Third Edition, Ch 53, p. 776.

Table 2
Hereditary Syndromes Associated with Pheochromocytoma

SYNDROME	CLINICAL PHENOTYPE	RISK OF PHEOCHROMOCYTOMA %	MUTATED GERM-LINE GENE
MEN-2A	Medullary carcinoma of the thyroid, hyper-parathyroidism	50	*RET* (proto-oncogene)
MEN-2B	Medullary carcinoma of the thyroid, multiple mucosal neuromas, marfanoid habitus, hyperparathyroidism	50	*RET* (proto-oncogene)
Neurofibromatosis type 1	Neurofibromas of peripheral nerves, cafe au lait spots	1	*NFI*
Von Hippel–Lindau disease (retinal cerebellar hemangioblastosis)	Retinal angioma, CNS hemangioblastoma, renal-cell carcinoma, pancreatic and renal cysts	10–20	*VHL*
Familial paraganglioma syndrome	Carotid-body tumor (chemodectoma)	20 (estimated)	*SDHS, SDHB*

MEN-2A, multiple endocrine neoplasia type 2A; MEN-2B, multiple endocrine neoplasia type 2B; CNS, central nervous system; *SDHD,* the gene for succinate dehydrogenase subunit D; and SDHB, the gene for the succinate dehydrogenase subunit B.

With permission from *(10).*

aldosterone, or both *(26–29)*. It has been estimated to be fivefold more common than GRA *(29)*. Dexamethasone fails to suppress the findings. To date, no mutation has been identified, though linkage studies have identified a 5-Mb locus on chromosome 7p22. Recently, Stowasser group *(29)* examined a number of candidate genes within 7p22, many of which involve cell growth, but have not yet definitively identified the gene responsible.

Apparent Mineralocorticoid Excess (OMIM # 218030)

Low-renin hypertension, often severe and accompanied by hypokalemia and metabolic alkalosis *(30)*, is the hallmark of apparent mineralocorticoid excess (AME), first described in 1977 by New et al. *(31,32)*. Spironolactone is often effective initially, but patients often become refractory to this drug. In AME 11β-hydroxysteroid dehydrogenase (11β-HSD) is absent, resulting in hypertension in which cortisol acts as if it were a potent mineralocorticoid. The microsomal enzyme 11β-hydroxysteroid dehydrogenase, interconverts active 11-hydroxyglucocorticoids to inactive keto-metabolites. Cortisol, as well as aldosterone, has an affinity for the mineralocorticoid receptor. Normally, 11β-HSD is protective, preventing binding of cortisol to the mineralocorticoid receptor; but in AME, the slower-than-normal metabolism of cortisol to cortisone results in cortisol acting as a potent mineralocorticoid *(31,32)*, whereas metabolism of cortisone to cortisol is normal.

Persons with classic AME usually develop symptoms in early childhood, often presenting with failure to thrive, severe hypertension, and persistent polydipsia. Affected patients appear volume expanded and respond to dietary sodium restriction. Plasma renin activity is very low. A high cortisol:cortisone ratio in plasma or an abnormal urinary ratio of tetrahydrocortisol/tetrahydrocortisone (THF/THE), in which THF predominates, makes the diagnosis.

Affected children are at high risk for cardiovascular complications, and some develop nephrocalcinosis and renal failure *(33)*; early therapy may lead to better outcome.

Several variants of AME have been reported, including a mild form in a Mennonite kindred in which there is a P227L mutation in the *HSD11B2* gene *(34,35)*; a coactivator defect with resistance to multiple steroids *(36)*; and hypertension without the characteristic findings of AME in a heterozygous father and homozygous daughter who have mutations in 11β-HSD2 *(37)*. A recent paper reported a Brazilian child with a homozygous missense mutation p.R186C in the *HSD11B2* gene *(38)*.

The hypertension in AME appears renally mediated, but recent evidence suggests that ultimately, the disorder changes from increased sodium resorption to a vascular form of hypertension *(39)*.

Mineralocorticoid Receptor Gain-of-Function Mutation

A form of monogenic hypertension due to a gain-of-function mutation in the mineralocorticoid receptor occurs due to a missense mutation that was first found in a teenage boy with hypertension, low-renin and aldosterone levels, as well as mild hypokalemia *(40)*. In toto, 11 persons in his family had this mutation. In this mutation, which influences an important binding region of the receptor, a serine at amino acid 810 in the mineralocorticoid receptor is changed to leucine (S810L).

Affected persons have refractory hypertension, and women with this mutation have severely elevated BP during pregnancy *(41,42)*. Early death due to heart failure occurred in the index family *(40)*.

It appears that the S810L mutation leads to a conformational change in the receptor that heightens the stability of steroid–receptor complexes. The mutation thus results in a steric hindrance resulting in a bending of the molecule that makes it difficult for known agonists and antagonists to act normally. Some antagonists that cannot act on the normal (wild type) receptor, work in this mutation: these include RU-486, 5-pregnane-20-one, and 4,9-androstadiene-3,17-dione *(43)*.

Steroidogenic Enzyme Defects Leading to Hypertension

Rare autosomal recessive defects in steroidogenesis associated with hypertension were well recognized before the genomic era. Cortisol is normally synthesized under the control of ACTH in the zona fasciculata, whereas aldosterone is synthesized largely under the influence of angiotensin II and potassium in the zona glomerulosa. Aldosterone synthesis is not normally controlled by ACTH, but if any of the several enzymes that are involved in cortisol biosynthesis is abnormal, the usual feedback loop is interrupted. Consequently, plasma ACTH will increase in an attempt to produce cortisol, and aberrant products will accumulate, some of which lead to hypertension.

The inherited defects of steroid biosynthesis—all autosomal recessive—are, as a group, termed congenital adrenal hyperplasia (CAH), and each results in a characteristic clinical and biochemical profile *(44–46)*. Any enzyme in the pathways of steroidogenesis may contain a mutation; the most commonly affected is 21-hydroxylase. However, mutations in 21-hydroxylase are not generally associated with hypertension. Enzyme mutations that are associated with hypertension include (in order of frequency) 11β-hydroxylase >> 3β-hydroxysteroid dehydrogenase>>> 17α-hydroxylase and cholesterol desmolase. Patients with the 11β-hydroxylase and 3β-hydroxysteroid dehydrogenase defects have a tendency to retain salt, becoming hypertensive. It is also important to remember that any person with CAH may develop hypertension owing to overzealous replacement therapy.

STEROID 11β-HYDROXYLASE DEFICIENCY

The mineralocorticoid excess in 11β-hydroxylase deficiency *(44–50)*, a form of CAH accompanied by virilization, leads to decreased sodium excretion with resultant volume expansion, renin suppression, and hypertension. Elevated BP is not invariant in

11β-hydroxylase deficiency and most often is discovered in later childhood or adolescence, often with an inconsistent correlation to the biochemical profile *(44–50)*. Hypokalemia is variable, but total body potassium may be markedly depleted in the face of normal serum or plasma potassium. Renin is generally decreased, but aldosterone is increased.

Therapy for 11β-hydroxylase deficiency should focus on normalizing steroids. Administered glucocorticoids should normalize cortisol and reduce ACTH secretion and levels to normal, thus stopping oversecretion of deoxycorticosterone (DOC). Hypertension generally resolves with such therapy *(45)*. When hypertension is severe, antihypertensive therapy should be instituted until the BP is controlled; such therapy can be tapered later.

Additional mutations can cause this syndrome. For example, a patient with 11β-hydroxylation inhibition for 17-α-hydroxylated steroids but with intact 17-deoxysteroid hydroxylation has been reported *(50)*. Multiple mutations affecting the *CYP11B1* gene have been described; these include frameshifts, point mutations, extra triplet repeats, and stop mutations *(30, 51–54)*.

STEROID 17α-HYDROXYLASE DEFICIENCY

Abnormalities in 17α-hydroxylase affect both the adrenals and gonads, since a dysfunctional 17α-hydroxylase enzyme results in decreased synthesis of both cortisol and sex steroids *(55–58)*. Affected persons appear phenotypically female (or occasionally have ambiguous genitalia), irrespective of their genetic sex, and puberty does not occur. Consequently, most cases are discovered after a girl fails to enter puberty *(57)*. An inguinal hernia is another mode of presentation. Hypertension and hypokalemia are characteristic, owing to impressive overproduction of corticosterone (compound B).

Glucocorticoid replacement is an effective therapy. However, should replacement therapy fail to control the hypertension, appropriate therapy with antihypertensive medication(s) should be instituted to control BP.

Mutations in Renal Transporters Causing Low-Renin Hypertension

PSEUDOHYPOALDOSTERONISM TYPE II—GORDON'S SYNDROME (OMIM#145260)

Pseudohypoaldosteronism type II (also known as Gordon's syndrome or familial hyperkalemia; OMIM #145260), an autosomal dominant form of hypertension associated with hyperkalemia, acidemia, and increased salt reabsorption by the kidney, is caused by mutations in the WNK1 and WNK4 kinase family *(59–63)*. Though the physiology and response to diuretics suggested a defect in renal ion transport in the presence of normal glomerular filtration rate, the genetics have only recently been delineated.

Affected persons have low-renin hypertension and improve with thiazide diuretics or with triamterene *(63)*. Aldosterone receptor antagonists do not correct the observed abnormalities.

PHAII genes have been mapped to chromosomes 17, 1, and 12 *(59,60)*. One kindred was found to have mutations in WNK1—large intronic deletions that increase WNK1 expression. Another kindred with missense mutations in WNK4, which is on chromosome 17, has been described. While WNK1 is widely expressed, WNK4 is expressed primarily in the kidney, localized to tight junctions. WNKs alter the handling of potassium and hydrogen in the collecting duct, leading to increased salt resorption and increased intravascular volume by as yet unknown means.

LIDDLE'S SYNDROME (OMIM # 177200)

In 1963 Liddle et al. *(64)* described early onset of autosomal dominant hypertension in a family in whom hypokalemia, low renin and aldosterone concentrations were noted in affected members. Inhibitors of renal epithelial sodium transport, such as triamterene, worked well in controlling hypertension, but those of the mineralocorticoid receptor did not. A general abnormality in sodium transport seemed apparent, as the red blood cell transport systems were not normal *(65)*. A major abnormality in renal salt handling seemed likely when a patient with Liddle's syndrome underwent a renal transplant, and hypertension and hypokalemia resolved post-transplant *(66)*.

While the clinical picture of Liddle's syndrome is one of aldosterone excess, aldosterone and renin levels are very low *(8)*. Hypokalemia is not invariably present. A defect in renal sodium transport is now known to cause Liddle's syndrome. The mineralocorticoid-dependent sodium transport within the renal epithelia requires activation of the epithelial sodium channel (ENaC), which is composed of at least three subunits normally regulated by aldosterone. Mutations in β and γ subunits of the ENaC have been identified (both lie on chromosome 16) *(67,68)*. Thus, the defect in Liddle's syndrome leads to constitutive activation of amiloride-sensitive epithelial sodium channels (ENaCs) in distal renal tubules, causing excess sodium reabsorption. Additionally, these gain-of-function mutations prolong the half-life of ENaCs at the renal distal tubule apical cell surface, resulting in increased channel number *(69)*.

Pheochromocytoma-Predisposing Syndromes

A variety of *RET* proto-oncogene mutations and abnormalities in tumor suppressor genes are associated with autosomal dominant inheritance of pheochromocytomas, as summarized in Table 2 *(10,70–75)*. A number of paraganglioma and pheochromocytoma susceptibility genes inherited in an autosomal dominant pattern appear to convey a propensity toward developing such tumors *(10)*. Both glomus tumors and pheochromocytomas are derived from neural-crest tissues, and the genes identified in one type of tumor may appear in the other *(76)*. For instance, germ-line mutations have been reported both in families with autosomal dominant glomus tumors and in registries with sporadic cases of pheochromocytoma *(77)*. In addition, other pheochromocytoma-susceptibility genes include the proto-oncogene *RET* (multiple endocrine neoplasia syndrome type 2 (MEN-2)), the tumor suppressor gene *VHL* observed in families with von Hippel–Lindau syndrome, and the gene that encodes succinate dehydrogenase subunit B (*SDHB*).

The genes involved in some of these tumors appear to encode proteins with a common link involving tissue oxygen metabolism *(78–80)*. In von Hippel–Lindau disease, inactivating (loss-of-function) mutations are present in the *VHL* suppressor gene, which encodes a protein integral to the degradation of other proteins—some of which, such as hypoxia-inducible factor, are involved in responding to low oxygen tension. Interestingly, the mitochondrial complex II, important in O_2 sensing and signaling, contains both SDHB (succinate dehydrogenase subunit B)and SDHD (succinate dehydrogenase subunit D). Thus, mutations in the *VHL* gene, and SDHB and SDHD might lead to increased activation of hypoxic signaling pathways leading to abnormal proliferation.

In multiple endocrinopathy-2 (MEN-2) syndromes, mutations in the *RET* proto-oncogene lead to constitutive activation (activating mutations) of the receptor tyrosine kinase. The end result is hyperplasia of adrenomedullary chromaffin cells (and in the parathyroid, calcitonin-producing parafollicular cells). In time, these cells undergo a high rate of neoplastic transformation. It now appears that apparently sporadic chromaffin tumors may also contain mutations in these genes.

Hypertension with Brachydactyly (OMIM #112410)

Hypertension with brachydactyly, also called brachydactyly, type E, with short stature and hypertension (Bilginturan syndrome) was first described in 1973 in a Turkish kindred (81). Affected persons have shortened phalanges and metacarpals, as well as hypertension. Linkage studies performed in the 1990s mapped this form of hypertension to a region on chromosome 12p, in the region 12p12.2 to p11.2 (82,83).

Patients with this form of hypertension have normal sympathetic nervous system and renin–angiotensin system responses. In 1996, some abnormal arterial loops were observed on MRI examinations of the cerebellar region. There was speculation that this abnormality could lead to compression of neurovascular bundles that would lead to hypertension (84). Another family, in Japan, also had similar findings, and a deletion in 12p was reported in that family (85).

There are several candidate genes in the region—a cyclic nucleotide phosphodiesterase (PDE3A) and a sulfonylurea receptor, SUR2, which is a subunit of an ATP-sensitive potassium channel. It was hypothesized that there could be "a chromosomal rearrangement between the candidate genes PDE3A/SUR2/KCNJ8 for hypertension and SOX5 for the skeletal phenotypes, separated by several megabases" (summarized in (86)). It then appeared, in studies using bacterial artificial chromosomes, that there was an inversion, deletion, and reinsertion in this region. It appears currently that rather than a mutation in a single gene, this form of hypertension is caused by the chromosomal rearrangement.

Other Forms of Mendelian Hypertension

In addition, there have been reports of severe insulin resistance, diabetes mellitus, and elevated BP caused by dominant-negative mutations in human PPARγ (87) There has also been a description of hypertension, hypomagnesemia, and hypercholesterolemia due to an abnormality in mitochondrial tRNA. In this case, impaired ribosomal binding is due to a missense mutation in the mitochondrial tRNA (88).

When to Suspect Monogenic Hypertension

Table 3 lists the situations in which the astute clinician should consider monogenic hypertension (7). These include both clinical and laboratory findings that should point toward further evaluation. Significant among these are a strong family history of hyper-

Table 3
When to Suspect a Hypertensive Genetic Disorder

At-risk members of kindreds with a known monogenic hypertensive disorder (e.g., multiple endocrine neoplasia, syndromes)

Hypokalemia in hypertensive children and their first-degree relatives

Juvenile onset of hypertension, particularly if plasma renin is suppressed

Physical findings suggestive of syndromes or hypertensive disorders (e.g., retinal angiomas, neck mass, hyperparathyroidism in patient with a pheochromocytoma)

Adapted from (7).

tension, particularly when the BP is difficult to control within the family. Low plasma renin activity should also point toward the possibility that a defined form of hypertension may be present.

NON-MENDELIAN, POLYGENIC HYPERTENSION

The genetic contribution to a widely prevalent condition such as essential (primary) hypertension is generally considered to involve multiple genes and is thus termed polygenic. The possibility for determining the genes involved seems far more feasible in the current genomic era, yet clear identification has proved elusive, in part because BP is a continuous variable, and the contribution of any one gene appears to be small. Relevant background for considering the genetic factors predisposing toward hypertension is described in the following sections.

Experimental Hypertension as a Tool to Investigate Polygenic Hypertension

Many studies in inbred experimental animals, mainly rats and mice, have aimed to identify genes controlling BP. In the 1980s, it was estimated that 5–10 genes control BP (89). In 2000, Rapp (90) summarized available research and estimated that 24 chromosomal regions in 19 chromosomes were associated with hypertension in various rat strains. A recent review by Delles et al. (91) notes that candidate QTLs (quantitative trait loci) have been identified on nearly every chromosome. Studies using inbred rat strains, however, did not identify polygenes and their associated alleles (92).

A large number of chromosomal regions and some candidate genes have also been suggested from experimental studies in mice. For example, targeted gene deletion studies have shown an effect on BP in more than a dozen genes, among which are endothelial nitric oxide synthase, insulin receptor substrate, the dopamine receptor, apolipoprotein E, adducin-α, the bradykinin receptor, and the angiotensin type 2 receptor, as well as other members of the renin–angiotensin system (93).

Genetic manipulation in mice has been successful in exploring contributions of various candidate genes (reviewed in (94)), most notably those of the renin–angiotensin system through two approaches, overexpression of a given gene (with "transgenic" animals (90)) and deleting gene function (with "knockouts"). An additional approach is to use gene targeting in embryonic stem (ES) cell cultures (95–97).

Inbred strains rather than transgenic or knockouts have led to important findings (97–100). A number of studies, notably those of Jacob et al. (97) and Hilbert et al. (98), found linkage in a rat model of hypertension that pointed to the angiotensin-converting enzyme (ACE) gene as important in determining hypertension. Since those reports of more nearly 20 years ago, a large number of clinical studies have suggested a link between ACE polymorphisms in humans and hypertension. See a recent commentary on the value of studies in the rat model (91,99).

Human Hypertension

A variety of studies have pointed to a link between human hypertension and genes of the renin–angiotensin system (summarized in (101,102)). However, in common diseases such as hypertension, it may be more productive to consider susceptibility alleles rather than disease alleles per se. Furthermore, some people carrying a particular susceptibility allele may not have the disease either because they do not have the environmental exposure that causes the condition to develop or because they lack another allele(s) that is needed to cause a given clinical problem. Because there are multiple potential interactions, and susceptibility alleles are generally common, following a given allele through pedigrees is difficult. In such a circumstance, segregation analysis is difficult, particularly if a given susceptibility allele has a small effect. Indeed, to date, linkage has been reported on most chromosomes in humans *(103–118)*.

Linkage analysis may still be an initial step *(3–5)*, but it is not as powerful a tool as it is in Mendelian diseases, because many people without the disease may carry the susceptibility allele. Using affected siblings (sib pairs) may be helpful to gain more understanding of the possible genetics. Siblings who are both affected with a given problem such as hypertension would be anticipated to share more than half their alleles near or at the susceptibility locus, and the chance of this occurrence is then calculated *(3–5)*. An LOD score of greater than 3.6 is taken as evidence of a linked locus, which is often very large (in the range of 20–40 cM). Once a putative linkage is confirmed in a replicate study, finer mapping can be performed to hone in on the genetic region that contains the putative gene. This is done through linkage disequilibrium or association testing between disease and genetic markers, often with single-nucleotide polymorphisms (SNPs). SNPs occur roughly every 1000 base pairs and lend themselves to automated testing. Using SNPs, a broad region (10–40 cM) can be narrowed to a far smaller region of roughly 1×10^6 base pairs *(110,111)*.

Genome-wide screens of the human genome aiming to discover hypertension genes have suggested many loci of interest *(112,113)*. These screens have included subjects with diverse phenotypes, and ethnicity; furthermore, selection criteria have varied. The numbers and composition of families have ranged from single, large pedigrees to more than 2000 sib pairs from 1500 or so families *(112)*. Using genomic scan data from four partner networks, the US Family Blood Pressure Program (FBPP) *(113)* sought to use phenotypic strategies that reflect the ethnic demography of the USA. A 140–170 cM region of chromosome 2 was linked to hypertension in several populations—Chinese sib pairs *(109)* and Finnish twins *(104)*, as well as a discordant sib-pair screen. Recently Caulfield et al. *(114)* phenotyped 2010 sib pairs drawn from 1599 families with severe hypertension as part of the BRIGHT study (Medical Research Council *BRI*tish Genetics of *Hyper*Tension) and performed a 10-cM genome-wide scan. Their linkage analysis identified a locus on chromosome 6q with an LOD score of 3.21 and genome-wide significance of 0.042. However, this locus is at the end of chromosome 6, and the end of a chromosome may generate errors; thus, caution is required in drawing conclusions from these findings. The Caulfield group also found three other loci with LOD scores above 1.57 *(114)*. One of these loci was the same as that found in the Chinese and Finnish studies *(114)*.

Within the last few years, there have been further genome-wide association studies (GWAS) concerning hypertension reported *(119,120)*. In 2007 Levy et al. *(121)* used an Affymetrix 100 K chip platform and performed a GWAS with the Framingham cohort, yet the initial analysis did not find significance for any gene. Using the Wellcome Trust Case Control Consortium (WTCCC) and an Affymetrix 500 K chip, another GWAS was reported in 2007, and it, too, did not reach genome-wide significance for any gene *(122)*. However, a study in which the subjects were from the Korean general population most recently reported genome-wide significance, though a very small effect for the ATPase, Ca^{2+} transporting, plasma membrane 1 *(ATP2B)* gene *(123)*. These rather disappointing results from GWAS studies on hypertension are discussed to indicate the complexity of primary hypertension.

Two consortiums have lately reported some more encouraging results. The Global BPgen group examined 2.5 million genotyped or imputed SNPs in 34,433 persons of European background and found 8 regions that reached genome-wide significance. These regions were associated with hypertension and lie in close proximity to genes *CYP17A1, CYP1A2, FGF5, SH2B3, MTHFR, ZNF652,* and *PLCD3* and to the chromosome 10 open-reading frame 107 (c10orf107) *(124)*. Further, the so-called CHARGE consortium *(125)* looked at 29,136 participants and studied 2.5 million genotyped or imputed SNPs; they reported significant associations with hypertension for 10 SNPs, and with systolic BP for 13 SNPs and for diastolic BP with 20 SNPs. Their findings and those of Global BPgen were then subjected to a meta-analysis, and this led to findings of genome-wide significance for a number of genes associated with elevated BP or with systolic or diastolic BP *(124)*. These included the *ATP2B* gene, as well as *CYP17A1* (steroid 17-alphamonooxygenase), *CSK-ULK3* (adjacent to c-src tyrosine kinase and unc-51-like kinase 3 loci), *TBX3-TBX5* (adjacent to T-box transcription factor TBX3 and T-box transcription factor TBX5 loci), *ULK4* (unc-51-like kinase 4), *PLEKHA7* (pleckstrin homology domain containing family A member 7), *SH2B3* (SH2B adaptor protein 3), and *CACNB2* (calcium channel, voltage-dependent, β2 subunit) *(124)*.

Candidate Genes

Another approach in assessing polygenic hypertension is to use candidate genes—which already have a known or suspected role in hypertension—that are present near the peak of observed genetic linkage. If the full sequence of the candidate gene is known, then it is relatively easier to go forward.

In the Caulfield study *(114)*, for example, there are a number of candidate genes that are within the linkage analysis-identified areas on chromosomes 2 and 9. Genes that encode serine/threonine kinases, STK39, STK17B are on chromosome 2q; PKNBETA, a protein kinase, is on chromosome 9q; G-protein-coupled receptors on chromosome 9—GPR107 on 9q 9q and GPR21 on 9q33; and on 2q24.1 there is a potassium channel, KCNJ3.

Microarrays are used to identify differential expression of expressed sequences in tissues from affected and unaffected persons. These are available either as full-length cDNAs or as expressed sequence tags (ESTs)

Candidate Susceptibility Genes

A number of genes have become candidates as susceptibility genes, particularly those of the renin–angiotensin system. A number of such genes were associated with hypertension and cardiovascular regulation in the pre-genomic era. Many associations have been described or imputed, including not only members of the renin–angiotensin system, but many other genes. For example, Izawa et al. *(117)* chose 27 candidate genes based on reviews of physiology and genetic data that looked at vascular biology, leukocyte and platelet biology, and glucose and lipid metabolism. They then also selected 33 SNPs of these genes, largely related in promoter regions, exons or spliced donor or acceptor sites in introns and looked at their relationship to hypertension in a cohort of 1940 persons. They found that polymorphisms in the CC chemokine receptor 2 gene were associated with hypertension in men and those in the *TNF-α* gene with hypertension in women *(117)*. In a GWAS in African-Americans, Adeyemo et al. *(126)* suggested that pathway and network approaches might be helpful in identifying or prioritizing various loci.

Variants or Subphenotypes

If a particular variant of a complex disease is clinically distinct, then analysis of so-called subphenotypes by positional cloning may be potentially illuminating *(3–5,118,120)*. In such an instance, there may be fewer susceptibility genes involved. However, subphenotypes may be difficult to study, as the physiology involved may be intricate. An example would be salt-sensitive hypertension *(118)*. In order to study subjects, it is necessary to perform careful metabolic studies that confirm the subphenotype (hypertension with salt sensitivity) and also are standard during testing.

Present Implications for Pediatric Hypertension

A search for monogenic forms of hypertension is clearly indicated in an infant, child, or teenager with elevated BP and history or signs compatible with one of these diagnoses. If a child is found to have one of the rare forms of monogenic hypertension, there will be specific therapy. Few data, however, exist to guide the clinician in terms of the roles polygenic hypertension in children at the present time.

REFERENCES

1. Venter JC, Adams MD, Myers EW, et al. The sequence of the human genome. Science. 2001;291: 1304–1351.
2. International Human Genome Sequencing Consortium. Initial sequencing and analysis of the human genome. Nature. 2001;409:860–921.
3. Bogardus C, Baier L, Permana P, Prochazka M, Wolford J, Hanson R. Identification of susceptibility genes for complex metabolic diseases. Ann N Y Acad Sci. 2002;967:1–6.
4. Lander E, Kruglyak L. Genetic dissection of complex traits: guidelines for interpreting and reporting linkage results. Nat Genet. 1995;11:241–247.
5. Wang DG, Fan J-B, Siao C-J, et al. Large-scale identification, mapping and genotyping of single-nucleotide polymorphisms in the human genome. Science. 1998;280:1077–1082.
6. Lifton RP, Gharavi AG, Geller DS. Molecular mechanisms of human hypertension. Cell. 2001;104: 545–556.
7. Dluhy RG. Screening for genetic causes of hypertension. Curr Hypertens Rep. 2002;4:439–444.
8. Yiu VW, Dluhy RG, Lifton RP, Guay-Woodford LM. Low peripheral plasma renin activity as a critical marker in pediatric hypertension. Pediatr Nephrol. 1997;11:343–346.
9. Wilson H, Disse-Nicodeme S, Choate K, et al. Human hypertension caused by mutations in WNK kinases. Science. 2001;293:1107–1111.
10. Dluhy RG. Pheochromocytoma: the death of an axiom. N Engl J Med. 2002;346:1486–1488.
11. Miura K, Yoshinaga K, Goto K, et al. A case of glucocorticoid-responsive hyperaldosteronism. J Clin Endocrinol Metab. 1968;28:1807.
12. New MI, Siegal EJ, Peterson RE. Dexamethasone-suppressible hyperaldosteronism. J Clin Endocrinol Metab. 1973;37:93.
13. Biebink GS, Gotlin RW, Biglieri EG, Katz FH. A kindred with familial glucocorticoid-suppressible aldosteronism. J Clin Endocrinol Metab. 1973;36:715.
14. Grim CE, Weinberger MH. Familial dexamethasone-suppressible hyperaldosteronism. Pediatrics. 1980:65:597.
15. Oberfield SE, Levine LS, Stoner E, et al. Adrenal glomerulosa function in patients with dexamethasone-suppressible normokalemic hyperaldosteronism. J Clin Endocrinol Metab. 1981;53:158.
16. Sutherland DJA, Ruse JL, Laidlaw JC. Hypertension, increased aldosterone secretion and low plasma renin activity relieved by dexamethasone. Can Med Assoc J. 1966;95:1109.
17. New MI, Peterson RE. A new form of congenital adrenal hyperplasia. J Clin Endocrinol Metab. 1967;27:300.
18. Lifton RP, Dluhy RG, Powers M, Rich GM, Cook S, Ulick S, Lalouel MA. Chimeric 11b-hydroxylase/aldosterone synthase gene causes GRA and human hypertension. Nature. 1992;355: 262–265.

19. Lifton RP, Dluhy RG, Powers M, Rich GM, Gutkin M, Fallo F, Gill JR, Feld L, Ganguly A, Laidlaw JC, Murnaghan DJ, Kaufman C, Stockigt JR, Ulick S, Lalouel MA. Hereditary hypertension caused by chimeric gene duplications and ectopic expression of aldosterone synthase. Nat Genet. 1992;2: 66–74.
20. Ulick S, Chu MD. Hypersecretion of a new corticosteroid, 18-hydroxycortisol in two types of adrenocortical hypertension. Clin Exp Hypertens. 1982;4(Suppl 9/10):1771–1777.
21. Ulick S, Chu MD, Land M. Biosynthesis of 18-oxocortisol by aldosterone-producing adrenal tissue. J Biol Chem. 1983;258:5498–5502.
22. Gomez-Sanchez CE, Montgomery M, Ganguly A, et al. Elevated urinary excretion of 18-oxocortisol in glucocorticoid-suppressible aldosteronism. J Clin Endocrinol Metab. 1984;59:1022–1024.
23. Shackleton CH. Mass spectrometry in the diagnosis of steroid-related disorders and in hypertension research. J Steroid Biochem Mol Biol. 1993;45:127–140.
24. Dluhy RG, Anderson B, Harlin B, Ingelfinger J, Lifton R. Glucocorticoid-remediable aldosteronism is associated with severe hypertension in early childhood. J Pediatr. 2001;138:715–720.
25. Fallo F, Pilon C, Williams TA, Sonino N, Morra Di Cella S, Veglio F, De Iasio R, Montanari P, Mulatero P. Coexistence of different phenotypes in a family with glucocorticoid-remediable aldosteronism. J Hum Hypertens. 2004;18:47–51.
26. Lafferty AR, Torpy DJ, Stowasser M, Taymans SE, Lin JP, Huggard P, Gordon RD, Stratakis CA. A novel genetic locus for low renin hypertension: familial hyperaldosteronism type II maps to chromosome 7 (7p22). J Med Genet. 2000;37:831–835.
27. Stowasser M, Gordon RD, Tunny TJ, Klemm SA, Finn WL, Krek AL. Familial hyperaldosteronism type II: five families with a new variety of primary aldosteronism. Clin Exp Pharm Physiol. 1992;19: 319–322.
28. Torpy DJ, Gordon RD, Lin JP, Huggard PR, Taymans SE, Stowasser M, Chrousos GP, Stratakis CA. Familial hyperaldosteronism type II: description of a large kindred and exclusion of the aldosterone synthase (CYP11B2) gene. J Clin Endocrinol Metab. 1998;83:3214–3218.
29. Jeske YW, So A, Kelemen L, Sukor N, Willys C, Bulmer B, Gordon RD, Duffy D, Stowasser M. Examination of chromosome 7p22 candidate genes RBaK, PMS2 and GNA12 in familial hyperaldosteronism type II. Clin Exp Pharmacol Physiol. 2008;35:380–385.
30. Cerame BI, New MI. Hormonal hypertension in children: 11b-hydroxylase deficiency and apparent mineralocorticoid excess. J Pediatr Endocrinol. 2000;13:1537–1547.
31. New MI, Levine LS, Biglieri EG, Pareira J, Ulick S. Evidence for an unidentified ACTH-induced steroid hormone causing hypertension. J Clin Endocrinol Metab. 1977;44:924–933.
32. New MI, Oberfield SE, Carey RM, Greig F, Ulick S, Levine LS. A genetic defect in cortisol metabolism as the basis for the syndrome of apparent mineralocorticoid excess. In: Mnatero F, Biglieri EG, Edwards CRW, eds. Endocrinology of Hypertension. Serono Symposia No. 50. New York, NY: Academic; 1982:85–101.
33. Moudgil A, Rodich G, Jordan SC, Kamil ES. Nephrocalcinosis and renal cysts associated with apparent mineralocorticoid excess syndrome. Pediatr Nephrol. 2000;15(1–2):60–62.
34. Mercado AB, Wilson RC, Chung KC, Wei J-Q, New MI. J Clin Endocrinol Metab. 1995;80:2014–2020.
35. Ugrasbul F, Wiens T, Rubinstein P, New MI, Wilson RC. Prevalence of mild apparent mineralocorticoid excess in Mennonites. J Clin Endocrinol Metab. 1999;84:4735–4738.
36. New MI, Nimkarn S, Brandon DD, Cunningham-Rundles S, Wilson RC, Newfield RS, Vandermeulen J, Barron N, Russo C, Loriaux DL, O'Malley B. Resistance to multiple steroids in two sisters. J Ster Biochem Mol Biol. 2001;76:161–166.
37. Li A, Li KXZ, Marui S, Krozowski ZS, Batista MC, Whorwood C, Arnhold IJP, Shackleton CHL, Mendonca BB, Stewart PM. Apparent mineralocorticoid excess in a Brazilian kindred: hypertension in the heterozygote state. J Hypertens. 1997;15:1397–1402.
38. Coeli FB, Ferraz LF, Lemos-Marini SH, Rigatto SZ, Belangero VM, de-Mello MP. Apparent mineralocorticoid excess syndrome in a Brazilian boy caused by the homozygous missense mutation p.R186C in the HSD11B2 gene. Arq Bras Endocrinol Metab. 2008;52:1277–1281.
39. Bailey MA, Paterson JM, Hadoke PW, Wrobel N, Bellamy CO, Brownstein DG, Seckl JR, Mullins JJ. A switch in the mechanism of hypertension in the syndrome of apparent mineralocorticoid excess. J Am Soc Nephrol. 2008;19:47–58. Epub 2007 Nov 21.
40. Geller DS, Farhi A, Pinkerton N, Fradley M, Moritz M, Spitzer A, Meinke G, Tsai FT, Sigler PB, Lifton RP. Activating mineralocorticoid receptor mutation in hypertension exacerbated by pregnancy. Science. 2000;289:119–123.
41. Rafestin-Oblin ME, Souque A, Bocchi B, Pinon G, Fagart J, Vandewalle A. The severe form of hypertension caused by the activating S810L mutation in the mineralocorticoid receptor is cortisone related. Endocrinology. 2003;144:528–533.

42. Kamide K, Yang J, Kokubo Y, Takiuchi S, Miwa Y, Horio T, Tanaka C, Banno M, Nagura J, Okayama A, Tomoike H, Kawano Y, Miyata T. A novel missense mutation, F826Y, in the mineralocorticoid receptor gene in Japanese hypertensives: its implications for clinical phenotypes. Hypertens Res. 2005;28: 703–709.

43. Pinon GM, Fagart J, Souque A, Auzou G, Vandewalle, Rafestin-Oblin ME. Identification of steroid ligands able to inactivate the mineralocorticoid receptor harboring the S810L mutation responsible for a severe form of hypertension. Mol Cell Endocrinol. 2004;217:181–188.

44. New MI, Wilson RC. Steroid disorders in children: congenital adrenal hyperplasia and apparent mineralocorticoid excess. Proc Natl Acad Sci USA. 1999;96:12790–12797.

45. New MI Seaman MP. Secretion rates of cortisol and aldosterone precursors in various forms of congenital adrenal hyperplasia. J Clin Endocrinol Metab. 1970;30:361.

46. New MI, Levine LS. Hypertension of childhood with suppressed renin. Endocrinol Rev. 1980;1:421–430.

47. New MI. Inborn errors of adrenal steroidogenesis. Mol Cell Endocrinol. 2003;211(1–2):75–83.

48. Krone N, Arlt W. Genetics of congenital adrenal hyperplasia. Best Pract Res Clin Endocrinol Metab. 2009;23:181–192.

49. Mimouni M, Kaufman H, Roitman A, Morag C, Sadan N. Hypertension in a neonate with 11 beta-hydroxylase deficiency. Eur J Pediatr. 1985;143:231–233.

50. Zachmann M, Vollmin JA, New MI, Curtius C-C, Prader A. Congenital adrenal hyperplasia due to deficiency of 11-hydroxylation of 17a-hydroxylated steroids. J Clin Endocrinol Metab. 1971;33:501.

51. White PC, Dupont J, New MI, Lieberman E, Hochberg Z, Rosler A. A mutation in CYP11B1 [Arg448His] associated with steroid 22β-hydroxylase deficiency in Jews of Moroccan origin. J Clin Invest. 1991;87:1664–1667.

52. Curnow KM, Slutker L, Vitek J, et al. Mutations in the CYP11B1 gene causing congenital adrenal hyperplasia and hypertension cluster in exons 6, 7 and 8. Proc Natl Acad Sci USA. 1993;90:4552–4556.

53. Skinner CA, Rumsby G. Steroid 11β-hydroxylase deficiency caused by a 5-base pair duplication in the CYP11B1 gene. Hum Mol Genet. 1994;3:377–378.

54. Helmberg A, Ausserer B, Kofler R. Frameshift by insertion of 2 basepairs in codon 394 of CYP11B1 causes congenital adrenal hyperplasia due to steroid 11β-hydroxylase deficiency. J Clin Endocrinol Metab. 1992;75:1278–1281.

55. Biglieri EG, Herron MA, Brust N. 17-hydroxylation deficiency. J Clin Invest. 1966;45:1946.

56. New MI. Male pseudohermaphroditism due to 17-α-hydroxylase deficiency. J Clin Invest. 1970;49:1930.

57. Mantero F, Scaroni C. Enzymatic defects of steroidogenesis: 17α-hydroxylase deficiency. Pediatr Adolesc Endocrinol. 1984;13:83–94.

58. Rosa S, Duff C, Meyer M, Lang-Muritano M, Balercia G, Boscaro M, Topaloglu AK, Mioni R, Fallo F, Zuliani L, Mantero F, Schoenle EJ, Biason-Lauber A. P450c17 deficiency: clinical and molecular characterization of six patients. J Clin Endocrinol Metab. 2007;92:1000–1007.

59. Mansfield TA, Simon DB, Farfel Z, Bia M, Tucci JR, Lebel M, Gutkin M, Vialettes B, Christofilis MA, Kauppinen-Makelin R, Mayan H, Risch N, Lifton RP. Multilocus linkage of familial hyperkalaemia and hypertension, pseudohypoaldosteronism type II, to chromosomes 1q31-42 and 17p11-q21. Nat Genet. 1997;16:202–205.

60. Wilson FH, Disse-Nicodeme S, Choate KA, Ishikawa K, Nelson-Williams C, Desitter I, Gunel M, Milford DV, Lipkin GW, Achard J-M, Feely MP, Dussol B, Berland Y, Unwin RJ, Mayan H, Simon DB, Farfel Z, Jeunemaitre X, Lifton RP. Human hypertension caused by mutations in WNK kinases. Science. 2001;293:1107–1112.

61. Wilson FH, Kahle KT, Sabath E, Lalioti MD, Rapson AK, Hoover RS, Hebert SC, Gamba G, Lifton RP. Molecular pathogenesis of inherited hypertension with hyperkalemia: the Na-Cl cotransporter is inhibited by wild-type but not mutant WNK4. Proc Natl Acad Sci USA. 2003;100:680–684.

62. Yang CL, Angell J, Mitchell R, Ellison DH. WNK kinases regulate thiazide-sensitive Na-Cl cotransport. J Clin Invest. 2003;111:1039–1045.

63. Erdogan G, Corapciolgu D, Erdogan MF, Hallioglu J, Uysal AR. Furosemide and dDAVP for the treatment of pseudohypoaldosteronism type II. J Endocrinol Invest. 1997;20:681–684.

64. Liddle GW, Bledsoe T, Coppage WS. A familial renal disorder simulating primary aldosteronism with negligible aldosterone secretion. Trans Assoc Phys. 1963;76:199–213.

65. Wang C, Chan TK, Yeung RT, Coghlan JP, Scoggins BA, Stockigt JR. The effect of triamterene and sodium intake on renin, aldosterone, and erythrocyte sodium transport in Liddle's syndrome. J Clin Endocrinol Metab. 1981;52:1027–1032.

66. Botero-Velez M, Curtis JJ, Warnock DG. Brief report: Liddle's syndrome revisited—a disorder of sodium reabsorption in the distal tubule. N Engl J Med. 1994;330:178–181.

67. Shimkets RA, Warnock DG, Bositis CM, et al. Liddle's syndrome: heritable human hypertension caused by mutations in the beta subunit of the epithelial sodium channel. Cell. 1994;79:407–414.

68. Hansson JH, Nelson-Williams C, Suzuki H, et al. Hypertension caused by a truncated epithelial sodium channel gamma subunit: genetic heterogeneity of Liddle syndrome. Nat Genet. 1995;11:76–82.

69. Rossier BC. 1996 Homer Smith Award Lecture: cum grano salis: the epithelial sodium channel and the control of blood pressure. J Am Soc Nephrol. 1997;8:980–992.

70. Eng C, Crossey PA, Milligan LM, et al. Mutations in the RET proto-oncogene and the von Hippel-Lindau disease tumour suppressor gene in sporadic and syndromic phaeochromocytomas. J Med Genet. 1995;32:934–937.

71. Erickson D, Kudva YC, Ebersold MJ, et al. Benign paragangliomas: clinical presentation and treatment outcomes in 236 patients. J Clin Endocrinol Metab. 2001;86:5210–5216.

72. Baysal BE, Ferrell RE, Willett-Brozick JE, et al. Mutations in SDHD, a mitochondrial complex II gene, in hereditary paraganglioma. Science. 2000;287:848–851.

73. Gimm O, Armanios M, Dziema H, Neumann HPH, Eng C. Somatic and occult germ-line mutations in SDHD, a mitochondrial complex II gene, in nonfamilial pheochromocytoma. Cancer Res. 2000;60: 6822–6825.

74. Aguiar RC, Cox G, Pomeroy SL, Dahia PL. Analysis of the SDHD gene, the susceptibility gene for familial paraganglioma syndrome (PGL1), in pheochromocytomas. J Clin Endocrinol Metab. 2001;86: 2890–2894.

75. Santoro M, Carlomagno F, Romano A, et al. Activation of RET as a dominant transforming gene by germline mutations of MEN2A and MEN2B. Science. 1995;267:381–383.

76. Neumann HPH, Berger DP, Sigmund G, et al. Pheochromocytomas, multiple endocrine neoplasia type 2, and von Hippel-Lindau disease. N Engl J Med. 1993;329:1531–1538.

77. Neumann HPH, Bausch B, McWhinney SR, et al. Germ-line mutations in nonsyndromic pheochromocytoma. N Engl J Med. 2002;346:1459–1466.

78. Maxwell PH, Wiesener MS, Chang GW, et al. The tumour suppressor protein VHL targets hypoxia-inducible factors for oxygen-dependent proteolysis. Nature. 1999;399:271–275.

79. Scheffler IE. Molecular genetics of succinate: quinone oxidoreductase in eukaryotes. Prog Nucleic Acid Res Mol Biol. 1998;60:267–315.

80. Ackrell BA. Progress in understanding structure-function relationships in respiratory chain complex II. FEBS Lett. 2000;466:1–5.

81. Bilginturan N, Zileli S, Karacadag S, Pirnar T. Hereditary brachydactyly associated with hypertension. J Med Genet. 1973;10:253–259.

82. Schuster H, Wienker TF, Bahring S, Bilginturan N, Toka HR, Neitzel H, Jeschke E, Toka O, Gilbert D, Lowe A, Ott J, Haller H, Luft FC. Severe autosomal dominant hypertension and brachydactyly in a unique Turkish kindred maps to human chromosome 12. Nat Genet. 1996;13:98–100.

83. Gong M, Zhang H, Schulz H, Lee AA, Sun K, Bahring S, Luft FC, Nurnberg P, Reis A, Rohde K, Ganten D, Hui R, Hubner N. Genome-wide linkage reveals a locus for human essential (primary) hypertension on chromosome 12p. Hum Mol Genet. 2003;12:1273–1277.

84. Bahring S, Schuster H, Wienker TF, Haller H, Toka H, Toka O, Naraghi R, Luft FC. Construction of a physical map and additional phenotyping in autosomal-dominant hypertension and brachydactyly, which maps to chromosome 12 (Abstract). Am J Hum Genet. 1996;59(Suppl):A55 only.

85. Nagai T, Nishimura G, Kato R, Hasegawa T, Ohashi H, Fukushima Y. Del(12)(p11.21p12.2) associated with an asphyxiating thoracic dystrophy or chondroectodermal dysplasia-like syndrome. Am J Med Genet. 1995;55:16–18.

86. Bähring S, Kann M, Neuenfeld Y, Gong M, Chitayat D, Toka HR, Toka O, Plessis G, Maass P, Rauch A, Aydin A, Luft FC. Inversion region for hypertension and brachydactyly on chromosome 12p features multiple splicing and noncoding RNA. Hypertension. 2008;51:426–431.

87. Barroso I, Gurnell M, Crowley VE, et al. Dominant negative mutations in human PPARgamma associated with severe insulin resistance, diabetes mellitus and hypertension. Nature. 1999;402: 880–883.

88. Wilson FH, Hariri A, Farhi A, et al. A cluster of metabolic defects caused by mutation in a mitochondrial tRNA. Science. 2004;306:1190–1194.

89. Harrap SB. Genetic analysis of blood pressure and sodium balance in the spontaneously hypertensive rat. Hypertension. 1986;8:572–582.

90. Rapp JP. Genetic analysis of inherited hypertension in the rat. Physiol Rev. 2000;80:135–172.

91. Delles C, McBride MW, Graham D, Padmanabhan S, Dominiczak A. Genetics of hypertension: from experimental animals to humans. Biochim Biophys Acta. Dec 24 2009. DOI:10.1016/j.bbadis.2009.12.006 (epub ahead of print).

92. Doris PA. Hypertension genetics, SNPs, and the common disease: common variant hypothesis. Hypertension. 2002;39(Pt 2):323–331.

93. Cvetkovic B, Sigmund CD. Understanding hypertension through genetic manipulation in mice. Kidney Int. 2000;57:863–874.
94. Gordon JW, Ruddle FH. Gene transfers into mouse embryos: production of transgenic mice by pronuclear integration. Methods Enzymol. 1983;101:411–433.
95. Evans MJ, Kaufman MH. Establishment in culture of pluripotential cells from mouse embryos. Nature. 1981;292:154–156.
96. Capecchi MR. Altering the genome by homologous recombination. Science. 1989;244:1288–1292.
97. Jacob HJ, Lindpaintner K, Lincoln SE, Kusumi K, Bunker RK, Mao YP, Ganten D, Dzau VJ, Lander ES. Genetic mapping of a gene causing hypertension in the stroke-prone spontaneously hypertensive rat. Cell. 1991;67:213–224.
98. Hilbert P, Lindpaintner K, Beckmann JS, Serikawa T, Soubrier F, Dubay C, Cartwright P, De Gouyon B, Julier C, Takahasi S, et al. Chromosomal mapping of two genetic loci associated with blood-pressure regulation in hereditary hypertensive rats. Nature. 1991;353:521–529.
99. Saavedra JM. Opportunities and limitations of genetic analysis of hypertensive rat strains. J Hypertens. 2009;27:1129–1133.
100. Stoll M, Kwitek-Black AE, Cowley AW, Harris EL, Happar SB, Krieger JE, Printz MP, Provoost AP, Sassard J, Jacob HJ. New target regions for human hypertension via comparative genomics. Genome Res. 2000;10:473–482.
101. Lalouel J-M, Rohrwasser A, Terreros D, Morgan T, Ward K. Angiotensinogen in essential hypertension: from genetics to nephrology. J Am Soc Nephrol. 2001;12:606–615.
102. Zhu X, Yen-Pei CC, Yan D, Weder A, Cooper R, Luke A, Kan D, Chakravarti A. Associations between hypertension and genes in the renin-angiotensin system. Hypertension. 2003;41:1027–1034.
103. Rice T, Rankinen T, Province MA, Chagnon YC, Perusse L, Borecki IB, Bouchard C, Rao DC. Genome-wide linkage analysis of systolic and diastolic blood pressure: the Quebec family study. Circulation. 2000;102:1956–1963.
104. Perola M, Kainulainen K, Pajukanta P, Terwillinger JD, Hiekkalinna T, Ellonen P, Kaprio J, Koskenvuo M, Kontula K, Peltonen L. Genome-wide scan of predisposing loci for increased diastolic blood pressure in Finnish siblings. J Hypertens. 2000;18:1579–1585.
105. Pankow JS, Rose KM, Oberman A, Hunt SC, Atwood LD, Djousse L, Province MA, Rao DC. Possible locus on chromosome 18q influencing postural systolic blood pressure changes. Hypertension. 2000;36:471–476.
106. Krushkal J, Ferrell R, Mockrin SC, Turner ST, Sing CF, Boerwinkle E. Genome-wide linkage analyses of systolic blood pressure using highly discordant siblings. Circulation. 1999;99:1407–1410.
107. Levy D, DeStefano AL, Larson MG, O'Donnell CJ, Lifton RP, Gavras H, Cupples LA, Myers RH. Evidence for a gene influencing blood pressure on chromosome 17: genome scan linkage results for longitudinal blood pressure phenotypes in subjects from the Framingham Heart Study. Hypertension. 2000;36:477–483.
108. Sharma P, Fatibene J, Ferraro F, Jia H, Monteith S, Brown C, Clyton D, O'Shaughnessy K, Brown MJ. A genome-wide search for susceptibility loci to human essential hypertension. Hypertension. 2000;35:1291–1296.
109. Xu X, Rogus JJ, Terwedow HA, Yang J, Wang Z, Chen C, Niu T, Wang B, Xu H, Weiss S, Schort NJ, Fang Z. An extreme-sib-pair genome scan for genes regulating blood pressure. Am J Hum Genet. 1999;64:1694–1701.
110. Wang DG, Fan J-B, Siao C-J, et al. Large-scale identification, mapping and genotyping of single-nucleotide polymorphisms in the human genome. Science. 1998;280:1077–1082.
111. The International SNP Map Working Group. A map of human genome sequence variation containing 1.42 million single nucleotide polymorphisms. Nature. 2001;409:928–933.
112. Harrap SB. Where are all the blood pressure genes? Lancet. 2003;361:2149–2151.
113. Province MA, Kardia SLR, Ranade K, et al. A meta-analysis of genome-wide linkage scans for hypertension: the National Heart Lung and Blood Institute Family Blood Pressure Program. Am J Hypertens. 2003;16:144–147.
114. Caulfield M, Munroe P, Pembroke J, et al. Genome-wide mapping of human loci for essential hypertension. Lancet. 2003;361:2118–2123.
115. Ehret GB, Morrison AC, O'Connor AA, Grove ML, Baird L, Schwander K, Weder A, Cooper RS, Rao DC, Hunt SC, Boerwinkle E, Chakravarti A. Replication of the Wellcome Trust genome-wide association study of essential hypertension: the Family Blood Pressure Program. Eur J Hum Genet. 2008;16: 1507–1511.
116. Hong KW, Jin HS, Cho YS, Lee JY, Lee JE, Cho NH, Shin C, Lee SH, Park HK, Oh B. Replication of the Wellcome Trust genome-wide association study on essential hypertension in a Korean population. Hypertens Res. 2009;32:570–574.

117. Izawa H, Yamada Y, Okada T, Tanaka M, Hirayama H, Yokota M. Prediction of genetic risk for hypertension. Hypertension. 2003;41:1035–1040.
118. Binder A. A review of the genetics of essential hypertension. Curr Opin Cardiol. 2007;22:176–184.
119. Hamet P, Seda O. The current status of genome-wide scanning for hypertension. Curr Opin Cardiol. 2007;22:292–297.
120. Alejandro Martinez-Aguayo a Carlos Fardella. Genetics of hypertensive syndrome. Horm Res. 2009;71:253–259.
121. Levy D, Larson MG, Benjamin EJ, et al. Framingham Heart study 100 k project: genome-wide associations for blood pressure and arterial stiffness. BMC Med Genet. 2007;8(Suppl 1):S3.
122. Wellcome Trust Case Control Consortium. Genome-wide association study of 14,000 cases of seven common diseases and 3,000 shared controls. Nature. 2007;447:661–678.
123. Cho YS, Go MJ, Kim YJ, et al. A large-scale genome-wide association study of Asian populations uncovers genetic factors influencing eight quantitative traits. Nat Genet. 2009;41:527–534.
124. Newton-Cheh-C, Johnson T, Gateva V, et al. Genome-wide association study identifies eight loci associated with blood pressure. Nat Genet. 2009;41:666–676.
125. Levy D, Ehret GB, Rice K, et al. Genome-wide association of blood pressure and hypertension. Nat Genet. 2009;41:677–687.
126. Adeyemo A, Gerry N, Guanjie Chen G, et al. A genome-wide association study of hypertension and blood pressure in African Americans. PLoS Genet. 2009;5:e1000564.

II   ASSESSMENT OF BLOOD PRESSURE IN CHILDREN: MEASUREMENT, NORMATIVE DATA, AND EPIDEMIOLOGY

7 Casual Blood Pressure Methodology

Lavjay Butani, MD
and Bruce Z. Morgenstern, MD

CONTENTS

HISTORICAL BACKGROUND

The concept of measuring blood pressure (BP) has significantly evolved over the past two centuries, overcoming the challenge posed by the well-established, but clearly subjective, art of palpation of the pulse for 'measures' other than simply determining heart rate. In the United States, the BP cuff was introduced by Cushing in Baltimore in 1901 and in Boston in 1903 *(1,2)* when he returned from a trip to Italy with a version of a Riva-Rocci mercury sphygmomanometer. Recognizing the obstacles to be overcome, Cushing noted, "The belief is more or less prevalent that the powers of observation so markedly developed in our predecessors have, to a large extent, become blunted in us, owing to the employment of instrumental aids to exactness, and the art of medicine consequently has always adopted them with considerable reluctance" *(2)*.

Cook and Briggs *(3)*, two resident house officers, quickly introduced the new cuff into clinical practice at the Johns Hopkins Hospital. They apparently had a single-sized rubber bladder covered by a canvas case that was fitted with hook and eye attachments so that it could be "fitted to any arm from that of an infant to that of a large adult". Interestingly, despite the one-size fits-all bladder, they felt that arm size was a 'very small factor' in obtaining the pressure using their device. They reported the first 'normal' values in children, systolics between 75 and 90 mmHg during the first 2 years of life and

L. Butani (✉)
University of California Davis, Sacramento, CA, USA
e-mail: lavjay.butani@ucdmc.ucdavis.edu

From: *Clinical Hypertension and Vascular Diseases: Pediatric Hypertension*
Edited by: J. T. Flynn et al. DOI 10.1007/978-1-60327-824-9_7
© Springer Science+Business Media, LLC 2011

90–110 mmHg during early childhood. This compared with their reported normal systolic BP of 130 mmHg in young adult males and 115–120 mmHg in young women. In their extensive report, they demonstrated BP responses during surgery, shock, hemorrhage, postoperative recovery, obstetrics, hypertension, and sepsis. They also documented the response of BP to pressors and volume *(3)*. It should be noted that this early technique was based upon palpation of the brachial pulse.

At roughly the same time, Korotkoff was describing sounds that could be heard by placing a stethoscope over the brachial artery at the elbow below a BP cuff as the cuff pressure was slowly released [Korotkoff NC. On methods of studying blood pressure. Izvestiia Voennomeditsinskite Akademiia. 1905;11:365, as translated in *(4)*]. The original report by Korotkoff was in fact only one paragraph long, followed by a discussion. This auscultatory method was rapidly adopted, with data in adults from the United States reported in 1910 *(5)*. The value of BP determination was quickly recognized. By 1925 reports of the association between BP and mortality among US life insurance policyholders first appeared *(6)*. Despite this, coordinated studies of BP in children were slow to be developed. The Specialized Centers of Research—Atherosclerosis (SCOR-A) studies in Bogalusa, LA; Miami, FL; and Muscatine, IA were among the earliest, starting in the late 1960s and early 1970s *(6)*. These studies were all based on the auscultatory method.

IMPORTANCE OF BP MEASUREMENT

The critical need for a 'standard' methodology for BP measurement in children stems from the recognition that both high BP and frank hypertension are pervasive problems in the present era *(7)*. The Third National Health and Nutrition Examination Survey (NHANES) showed the prevalence of frank hypertension (BP > 140/90 mmHg) in adults in the United States to be as high as 25%, with an even higher prevalence of 'suboptimal' BP *(3,7)*. While the epidemiology of childhood hypertension is less well defined, the reported prevalence of pediatric hypertension varies from a low of 0.8% *(8)* to a high of 5% *(9)*. Notwithstanding the lower prevalence of hypertension in children, the clinical impact of BP monitoring in children should by no means be considered negligible. This is based on the premise that BP 'tracks' from childhood into adulthood, and that, with intervention, the long-term adverse consequences of hypertension are almost entirely preventable. Tracking, which will be addressed in a subsequent chapter in greater detail, is defined as the tendency of an individual to maintain his or her percentile rank for a given parameter with age. While there is ongoing controversy as to how predictive childhood BP, as measured by casual methods, is for adult hypertension, it certainly appears that children who might be expected to be at greatest risk of cardiovascular complications, that is, those with persistently elevated BP readings, high body mass index, excessive weight gain, and a family history of hypertension, especially in the older age groups, have higher coefficients of tracking of BP into adulthood, and are, therefore, more likely to remain hypertensive as adults *(10–12)*. Moreover, childhood BP remains, to date, the strongest identified predictor for adult hypertension *(13)*.

Extrapolating from the adult medical literature, it has long been believed that children with hypertension are at high risk of long-term morbidity and mortality. Clearly high BP, and even less than 'optimal' BP *(14)* in adults has been shown to be a risk factor for cardiovascular morbidity (heart failure and myocardial infarction) *(15,16)*, cerebrovascular events (stroke) *(17)*, and end-stage renal disease *(18)*. Not only that, studies both in adults *(19)* and in children *(20)* have demonstrated that hypertension is an important marker since its presence is strongly associated with the coexistence of other metabolic abnormalities such as dyslipidemia, obesity, and insulin resistance, all of which compound the risk of cardio-vascular and cerebrovascular morbidity. Even if one considers the link between childhood BP and adult hypertension suspect, the more short-term adverse effects of severe hypertension, which is often clinically silent, on organ function can lead to life-threatening complications such as aortic dissection *(21)*, intracranial hemorrhage, heart failure *(22)*, and encephalopathy *(23)*. Less devastating, but possibly an equally worrisome effect of hypertension, is left ventricular hypertrophy, a major risk factor in adults for morbid cardiac events *(24)*.

When one considers that hypertension is prevalent in epidemic proportions in adults, its origins can be traced back, at least to some extent, into childhood, and it is associated with adverse short- and long- term consequences, most of which, hypothetically, can be prevented with early detection and treatment, it should come as no surprise that the periodic measurement of BP and moreover, the accurate measurement of BP, is of critical importance. Recognizing the importance of BP monitoring, the National Heart, Lung and Blood Institute and the American Academy of Pediatrics have long advocated for the routine monitoring of BP in all children above the age of 3 years on an annual basis *(25)*, or at least at the time of routine examinations. Consequently BP measurements in children have become commonplace. However, at the same time, so has the number of different devices being employed for its measurement, causing confusion and lack of uniformity in the method of BP determination. This raises important questions regarding the validity and accuracy of these devices and also highlights the need for a standardized means of testing and monitoring their performance to avoid errors in measurement that could have egregious consequences. This is even more important, when one recognizes how much more common home BP monitoring has become, both for the diagnosis and management of hypertension.

Before we discuss the individual methods for causal BP measurement in children, let us clarify the term 'casual'. The use of the term 'casual', in this chapter, refers to the more conventional practice of obtaining BP readings on an episodic or intermittent basis such as readings during an office visit, as opposed to the more 'continuous' technique of ambulatory BP monitoring, which is addressed in a more comprehensive manner in Chapter 10.

GENERAL ISSUES IN THE MEASUREMENT OF BP

There are certain general issues in the measurement of BP that apply both to children and to adults. These are discussed quite thoroughly in the American Heart Association Guidelines for the Measurement of BP *(26)* and in a review by Gillman and Cook *(27)*. Basically, these issues can be categorized into those that relate to the equipment, the patient, and the observer.

Equipment: Obviously, the equipment must be maintained, calibrated, and functional. All devices for measuring BP require ongoing maintenance. Even mercury columns can be inaccurate *(28)*.

Perhaps the most important source of error related to the equipment in the measuring process pertains to selection of the proper size cuff. This remains an area of controversy since most suggestions as to what constitutes an appropriate cuff size are based on much opinion and very limited evidence. The present viewpoint is that the 'proper' cuff is one in which the inflatable bladder either has a width that is at least 38% of the arm circumference and/or a length that encircles at least 90% if not the entire upper arm *(27)*. Similarly, the 4th Report on the Diagnosis, Evaluation and Treatment of High Blood Pressure in Children and Adolescents recommends that the bladder of the cuff have a width that is approximately 40% of the arm circumference midway between the olecranon and the acromion; this corresponds to a cuff bladder that will cover 80–100% of the arm circumference *(25)*. The British have suggested that three cuffs with bladders measuring 4×13 cm, 10×18 cm, and the adult dimensions 12×26 cm are sufficient for the range of arm sizes likely to be encountered in children from 0 to 14 years of age *(29)*. This degree of standardization of commercially available cuffs is not the case in the United States. It is interesting to note that the British cuffs have width/length ratios that (1) are variable and (2) would not allow the combination of a width/arm circumference ratio of 0.4 at the same time that they allow a length/arm circumference ratio of 0.9–1.0. It is well established that undercuffing, that is, the use of too small a cuff, leads to erroneously high BP measurements. Less well established is the converse—overcuffing. A few papers suggest that a cuff that is too large for the arm will underestimate true BP. Too large in this context generally implies widths that exceed the recommended 0.38–0.4 ratio to arm circumference. Overly long cuffs, which of necessity will overlap, do not seem to generate significant errors *(27,30)*.

The problem of cuff size selection is aggravated by the lack of standards in the United States. Although Association for the Advancement of Medical Instrumentation (AAMI) and AHA standards call for cuffs that allow a cuff width to arm circumference ratio of 0.4, and also call for a bladder length to arm circumference ratio of 0.8, they do not take the logical step of establishing a minimal bladder width to length ratio of 0.5. As a result of the lack of standards, there is a wide variability in commercially available cuffs that are designed for children. In a 1996 survey of BP cuff manufacturers by one of the authors (BZM), cuff sizes given names suggesting the population for which they were intended, were tabulated (see Table 1). The 4th Report did recommend standardization of BP cuff bladder sizes for children *(25)*.

Patient factors: Several issues relating to the patient are seemingly self-evident and therefore often overlooked. For a proper BP measurement, the subject should have sat calmly for 5 min, and not have used caffeine or tobacco products for at least 30 min (alcohol and food are also often included on this list). In addition, the use of vasoactive medications should be noted. In children this includes decongestants, while for adolescents nutritional supplements, some of which contain ephedrine or related compounds, should be kept in mind.

It has been established in adults and extrapolated to children that the proper position for the patient to be in during BP measurements is sitting with the back supported and the feet flat on the floor. Of course, for infants and toddlers, the supine posture, by necessity, is also appropriate *(27)*. The arm to be used should be elevated to heart level *(31)*. BPs also vary with time of day and ambient room temperature *(27)*.

Observer: There are many device/method-specific issues that relate to the observer. Suffice it to state that the observer needs to be trained in the proper use of the device and understand the method sufficiently to recognize valid from invalid readings. It is the observer's responsibility to determine if the patient issues listed above are in fact accounted for. The observer also needs to properly select the cuff and apply it to the upper arm. This includes making sure that the cuff is placed on the bare arm, and that no restricting clothes are placed above the cuff (e.g., a tightly rolled sleeve).

Table 1
Commercially Available BP Cuffs Available for Infants and Children in 1996

Company	Newborn/Premature Cuff (W $\times$ L)	Bladder (W $\times$ L)
WA/TYCOS	5.3 $\times$ 18.8	
BAUM	4.5 $\times$ 23	2.5 $\times$ 5
SICOA	5.2 $\times$ 18	4 $\times$ 8
GRAHAM FIELD	5.2 $\times$ 18.5	4 $\times$ 8
KOSAN/BRESCO	5.5 $\times$ 20 (prem)	4 $\times$ 9
	4 $\times$ 15 (sm prem)	2.5 $\times$ 7
K-T-K	5 $\times$ 23	
	5 $\times$ 16	
RIESTER	5 $\times$ 15.5 (NB)	3 $\times$ 5
ERKA	4.5 $\times$ 25	2.5 $\times$ 15
CREST-PYMA		2.8 $\times$ 8.4
ACCOSON		2.5 $\times$ 10.2
	Infant	
WA/TYCOS	7.4 $\times$ 26.1	5.6 $\times$ 11.9
BAUM	8 $\times$ 29	6 $\times$ 12
SICOA	7.5 $\times$ 26	5.5 $\times$ 11.5
GRAHAM FIELD	7.5 $\times$ 26.1	5.5 $\times$ 11.5
PROPPER	7.6 $\times$ 25.4	5.7 $\times$ 11.4
WINMED	7.5 $\times$ 25.4	5.7 $\times$ 11.4
K-T-K	7 $\times$ 29	
RIESTER	7.2 $\times$ 23	5 $\times$ 8
ERKA	7 $\times$ 28	5.5 $\times$ 15
CREST-MABIS		6.4 $\times$ 12.1
CREST-PYMA		5.3 $\times$ 11.4
ACCOSON		5.1 $\times$ 10.2
	Child	
WA/TYCOS	10.4 $\times$ 35.3	8.6 $\times$ 17.8
BAUM	11 $\times$ 41	9 $\times$ 18
SICOA	10.5 $\times$ 34.2	8.5 $\times$ 17
SAMMONS-PRESTON		10.2 $\times$ 17.9
GRAHAM FIELD	10.5 $\times$ 34.2	8.5 $\times$ 17
PROPPER	10.8 $\times$ 34.3	8.9 $\times$ 17.5
KOSAN/BRESCO	11 $\times$ 35 (child)	9 $\times$ 18
	8 $\times$ 26 (peds)	6 $\times$ 12
	9.5 $\times$ 30 (sm Child)	7.5 $\times$ 15

Table 1
(continued)

Company	Newborn/Premature Cuff (W × L)	Bladder (W × L)
WINMED	11 × 33.5	7.6 × 17.7
K-T-K	11 × 40	
	9.5 × 33	
RIESTER	10 × 35.5	8 × 13
ERKA	9 × 39	8 × 20
CREST-MABIS		8.3 × 17.8
CREST-PYMA		7.9 × 15.2
ACCOSON		10.2 × 19.1
		7.6 × 15.2 (young)
		8.0 × 18.0 (new)
		4 × 13 (new sm)

There is a wide range of bladder sizes for each category. Bladders that do not have a length = twice the width are unlikely to meet AAMI and AHA criteria for a width to arm circumference ratio of 0.4, while encircling 80% of the upper arm. (Data reported to Bruce Morgenstern by the manufacturers, 1996.) Dimensions are in centimeters.

METHODS OF BP MEASUREMENT

Auscultatory Methods of BP Measurement

Both mercury and aneroid devices are subject to significant observer issues. Primarily of course, the observer must be able to hear and interpret the Korotkoff sounds accurately. This requires training, which is often accomplished with taped recordings of Korotkoff sounds or stethoscopes with two sets of earpieces. The correct performance of the auscultatory method requires that the systolic pressure first be approximated by palpation. The proper bleed rate is suggested to be 2 mmHg/s, something which is even more critical when the patient's pulse rate is slow *(31)*.

Although extensive data are lacking, extant data suggest that in children, as in adults, the auscultatory method be performed with the bell of a stethoscope. The proponents of the use of the bell feel that this helps to augment the Korotkoff sounds. This brings us to yet another area of controversy with auscultation-determining which Korotkoff sound, K4 or K5, represents the diastolic BP more accurately.

In the original report of the Task Force on Blood Pressure control in children *(32)*, K4 was accepted as the measure of diastolic BP for children less than 13 years of age. In the most recent report *(25)*, this was changed to K5, since data were available to report normal K5 values in younger children, and since this obviated the step in BP values that otherwise occurred at age 13 years. However, this recommendation has not been universally accepted *(33–35)*. One study, in fact, has suggested that K4 diastolic BP measured in childhood is a better predictor of adult hypertension *(36)*.

A final and critical observer issue is observer bias. At it is simplest, this occurs when the observer has a terminal digit preference, and tends to report many BP values ending in that number (e.g., if it is zero, the majority of reported systolics and diastolics will end in zero). Also, there is the matter of whether K5, disappearance, is the last sound heard, or 2 mmHg below that value. More complex observer biases can occur when the observer has been informed of his or her digit preference and then overcompensates, avoiding reporting values with that digit. Finally, there is the bias introduced by the knowledge of a patient's previous values, described more fully in the section on random-zero sphygmomanometers (RZSs) below.

Conventional Mercury Sphygmomanometry

Mercury sphygmomanometry has been considered the 'gold standard' against which other noninvasive measures are compared. The process is straightforward, but not necessarily easy. The components of the system include the bladder and cuff, tubing, a bulb with a screw-controlled bleed valve, a mercury reservoir, and the manometer, which has a filter at the top. Regular maintenance of the tubing, the bulb, the mercury in the reservoir, and the manometer is necessary to maintain accuracy. If the filter atop the manometer becomes clogged, the mercury will not move well in the column *(28)*.

Despite its status as the gold standard, mercury manometers, when systematically evaluated, have a significant number of problems that may preclude accurate use, even if the observer and patient issues are overcome. In a study at the St George's Hospital Medical School in London, UK, of 444 devices studied, 167 (38%) had dirty columns. Ninety-five (21%) of these were due to oxidization of the mercury so that the calibration markings were obscured, making it difficult to read the level of the mercury column. In 81 (18%) the column containing the mercury had either been rotated or the markings on the columns were badly faded, again making it difficult to read the level of the mercury meniscus. In three, mercury had leaked into the metal box. One machine had so little mercury in the column that when it was inflated, air bubbled through the mercury in the column, yet it was still in use *(28)*.

In a number of other studies, between 12 and 21% of evaluated mercury sphygmomanometers were not accurate when tested, but they were still being used clinically *(37,38)*. In a systematic evaluation of sphygmomanometers in a health district in the UK, none of the 356 instruments tested met all of the standards compiled for the project (project standards) or all of the relevant British regulatory standards; 14 (39.3%) met less than half of the British standards. Only 220 (61.8%) instruments tested were accurate at all six pressure levels in a calibration check; 12 sphygmomanometers met the accuracy standard at only three pressure levels, while 13 were inaccurate at all pressure levels tested. The authors also developed health and safety standards for the use and handling of mercury manometers. Eighty-six percent of the devices studies did not meet all five health and safety related standards *(39)*.

It appears that mercury manometers are likely to be phased out over the next few years, not for reasons of inaccuracy or device failure, although these are not all that uncommon *(28)*, but more for environmental reasons. This process is already taking place to greater or lesser degree in Europe, and several states in the United States have passed regulations concerning the handling of mercury that make it far too expensive to use mercury manometers *(40)*. Although the American Heart Association has taken a position against the elimination of the mercury manometer, it remains to be seen if they can slow this movement *(41)*.

Aneroid Manometry

The aneroid manometer functions in the process of auscultatory BP measurement in essentially the same way as the mercury column. The system comprises of a metal bellows, a mechanical amplifier, springs, and a gauge that displays the pressure in the cuff and tubing of the sphygmomanometer. Aneroid devices are often felt to be less accurate than mercury columns *(42,43)*.

Aneroid manometers were evaluated in many of the same studies cited for the assessment of mercury manometers. Mion and Pierin *(38)* demonstrated that 44% of devices in the hospital and 61% of devices in outpatient settings differed by more than 3 mmHg from the standard. In the Canadian study of Vanasse, 17.7% of aneroid manometers were off by $\geq$ 5 mmHg, and 15% had at least one malfunctioning component (but 52.3% of the mercury devices did) *(37)*. Knight et al. *(39)*, as part of the same systematic study in the UK described for mercury manometers, found that none of the aneroid instruments tested met all of the project standards or all of the British regulatory standards. Seven (6.1%) of 114 devices met fewer than half of the British regulatory standards. The authors combined 14 standards against which aneroid manometers were compared for accuracy. Twenty-nine (25%) of the instruments met all 14 standards and two (1.7%) met 7 or less *(39)*.

Additional data also demonstrate that aneroid devices can be inaccurate. In one study, using the very rigid standard of ±3 mmHg concordance with the mercury standard, 35% of devices were considered 'intolerant' at two of five pressures measured *(44)*. In another assessment of accuracy, Jones et al. *(45)* found that 34% of devices were not accurate to within 4 mmHg, but only 10% were not accurate to within 8 mmHg. In a recent study, using 10 mmHg as the criteria for accuracy, 1% of mercury manometers and 10% of aneroid devices were deemed inaccurate *(46)*.

The underlying reason for this apparent inaccuracy of aneroid devices is likely the lack of a regular program of calibration and maintenance. When practitioners in Humberside and Yorkshire were surveyed in 1988, 23.5% of the 1223 respondents admitted to never servicing the sphygmomanometers in their practices over a mean of 5.75 years *(47)*. However, it has been established that with proper calibration, aneroid devices are quite accurate manometers, and therefore subject only to the errors inherent to the auscultatory method *(44,48)*. Accuracy rates with mean differences from a mercury standard of ±0.2 mmHg have been reported *(49)*. In the Mayo Clinic experience, with a program of regular maintenance and calibration, more than 99% of actively used aneroid devices remain within 3 mmHg of a digital pressure gauge standard over 6 month periods *(48)*.

Random-Zero Sphygmomanometry

The RZS was devised in 1970 as a modification of Garrow's 'zero-muddler sphygmomanometer', in an attempt to eliminate observer biases related to terminal digit preference and to previous knowledge of recorded BPs, both of which are common during conventional sphygmomanometry *(50)*. Therefore it has been considered by many to be the 'gold standard' for epidemiological studies, and has been employed in studies such as the Multiple Risk Factor Intervention Trial (MRFIT) *(51)*, and the Hypertension Prevention Trial *(52)* in adults.

The machine works on the basic principle that each time a BP reading is obtained, the observer is 'blinded' to the reading until after the measurement has been completed. This comes about as a result of the incorporation of a mercury reservoir that fills randomly and to a variable degree during each inflation of the cuff, and adds a random amount of mercury to the manometer column. The amount of mercury added to the reservoir and to the column is unknown to the person using the machine until after the BP cuff has been deflated, at which point in time this 'random-zero' number can be read and subtracted from the uncorrected systolic and diastolic readings. While experience with the RZS is more limited in children, at least one group of investigators has used it for the 'Study of Cardiovascular Risk in Young Finns' *(53).*

The RZS does indeed reduce observer bias, but it does not completely eliminate it. Both, the Hypertension Prevention Trial and the MRFIT demonstrated a marked reduction in terminal digit preference of the corrected BP readings (compared to the uncorrected measurements), and also a roughly bell-shaped distribution of the 'random-zero' values *(51,52).* Compared to conventional sphygmomanometry, use of the RZS in adults has also been shown to result in a greater intraobserver variability in BP readings *(54).* While this may seem counterproductive to some, in fact, it more likely indicates the elimination of the bias caused by observer prejudice with the conventional sphygmomanometer that artificially causes multiple BP readings by a single observer to be very close to each other due to knowledge of the prior reading. Identical findings have been reported in children, albeit in a smaller study, when the RZS was compared head to head with the conventional sphygmomanometer *(27).* While the 'Study of Cardiovascular Risk in Young Finns' did not simultaneously compare the RZS to any other casual method of BP measurement, the design of this longitudinal study was such that on the first two occasions BPs were measured, in a cohort of randomly selected children between 6 and 18 years, using a conventional sphygmomanometer. For the third survey, which was conducted on a subset of the original cohort, the RZS was used *(55).* Therefore, while the study does not allow one to comment directly on the comparability of the two methods, the results are quite interesting and are in line with the previously mentioned adult data. First of all, this study also demonstrated that, in spite of adequate training, terminal digit preference was almost universally observed in all personnel obtaining BPs (using the conventional sphygmomanometer) during the initial two surveys, while this was almost completely eliminated using the RZS in the third trial. Second, the investigators made an interesting observation that the age-related curves obtained by the two methods differed significantly, with an apparently nonlinear rise in BP (as measured by the conventional method) with age, probably related to observer bias. A more continuous rise in BP with age, as might be expected on a biological basis, was seen when the RZS data was plotted; this was especially noticeable at low BP values. Based on these findings, the study investigators concluded that BPs in children, especially in the lower ranges, are measured more accurately with the RZS compared to the conventional sphygmomanometer, and that the RZS should be the preferred instrument used for epidemiological surveys of BP in this age group.

Notwithstanding all the advantages of the RZS, especially in clinical epidemiology, several concerns have been raised about the accuracy of this instrument including its impracticality due to the bulky design, expense, extent of training needed for personnel to use it accurately, and high maintenance costs. From a practical standpoint, it also shares with the conventional sphygmomanometer the disadvantage of having mercury as an intrinsic component of its design. Many studies have also shown that the RZS, when compared to the conventional sphygmomanometer, systematically underestimates diastolic and systolic BPs, both in adults and in children *(51,55).* The degree of underestimation varies quite considerably from one study to another, with several studies demonstrating a small and consistent difference of 1–3 mmHg between the two methods *(56,57),* while others finding a much larger and significant difference *(58).* This has resulted in contentious debate among investigators; some find the instrument acceptable for use according to the guidelines of the British Hypertensive Society *(56),* while others strongly advise against its use without further study *(58).* Whether the 'underestimation' of BP by the RZS is real, or rather is due more to an 'overestimation' of BP by the conventional sphygmomanometer, is unclear. Numerous reports have emphasized that these differences can be minimized or even eliminated by rigorous attention to the details of the measurement technique, intensive training of personnel *(59)*, and meticulous maintenance of the equipment, which is prone to subtle malfunction *(57,60)*.

In conclusion, although the 'blinded' nature of BP readings using the RZS makes it an ideal candidate instrument for epidemiological studies, the limited data in children and the aforementioned contradictory findings of its accuracy among different investigators, along with the practical issues related to expense, maintenance costs, and need for intensive personnel training, make the use of the RZS very impractical, certainly for routine clinical care, and perhaps also for epidemiological studies pending further research. Ultimately, however, the demise of this instrument will probably be more due to environmental concerns rather than any issues related to its accuracy.

Oscillometric BP Measurement

Oscillometric devices have all but replaced the mercury manometer in a large number of medical centers, especially in European countries where concern about environmental contamination with mercury has been greater *(40)*. Background information on these devices and a discussion related to the advantages and disadvantages of oscillometry are discussed comprehensively in a recent review article *(61)*. In brief, development on the first commercial oscillometric device for BP measurement started in the early 1970s and resulted in the 'Dinamap', an acronym for 'device for indirect noninvasive mean arterial pressure' *(62)*. Since that time, a plethora of oscillometric devices for automated BP measurement have flooded the market, including several new modifications of the original Dinamap model 825 (Critikon division of GE Healthcare, Waukesha, WI). The basic principle underlying these devices is the same as that of other cuff-based BP measuring devices, in that compression of the arm by an inflatable cuff allows indirect determination of the intra-arterial vascular pressure. The difference between conventional sphygmomanometry and the oscillometric devices is that in the latter, cuff inflation and deflation are automated and that BP determination is made by a microprocessor using information sent to it from a pressure transducer; this potentially is tremendously advantageous by eliminating all observer biases. Only a short summary of the process of BP measurement is described herein. More details are available in the articles by Ramsey *(62)*, and Jilek and Fukushima *(63)*. In brief, the BP cuff gets automatically inflated to between 160 and 180 mmHg (or 70 and 125 mmHg in the neonatal mode), depending on the specific device, for the first BP determination and subsequently to 35 mmHg above the previously recorded systolic value. After a brief holding period, the cuff pressure is reduced in a stepwise manner in 5–10 mmHg decrements. As the cuff pressure decreases, oscillations of the arterial wall increase in amplitude and reach a maximum when the cuff pressure approaches the mean arterial pressure. With further deflation of the BP cuff, oscillations of the arterial wall diminish and eventually stop altogether. The monitor uses this information to compute and display values for the mean, systolic, and diastolic BP. The precise method of BP determination is far more complicated and is determined by a complex algorithm that varies from one device to another. It is important to point out here that systolic and diastolic BP readings in oscillometry do not correspond to the point of first appearance and disappearance, respectively, of arterial wall oscillations. The pressures displayed on the monitor, therefore, may be 'calculated' rather than actually 'measured' values, at least for some of the oscillometric devices in the market. These algorithms have been considered proprietary information and are therefore kept in confidence, making it impossible for investigators to verify the accuracy of their underlying physiological principals. In addition, since the algorithms are proprietary, the devices may not be interchangeable. Some algorithms are based on the ratio of the oscillometric waveform amplitudes, while others are based on the change in slope of the amplitude of oscillations. Supporting this observation is the finding, in one study, that two different oscillometric devices used simultaneously yielded different BP results *(64)*.

Many studies have evaluated the comparability of oscillometric readings with BP readings obtained by invasive means. Park and Menard *(65)* compared the Dinamap model 1846 and a conventional mercury sphygmomanometer with radial artery pressures in a group of infants and children admitted to the intensive care unit. While both the Dinamap model 1846 and the conventional mercury sphygmomanometer readings correlated well with intra-arterial BP measurements, the correlation coefficient was better for BP readings obtained using the Dinamap model 1846. The difference between the Dinamap model 1846 and intra-arterial BP readings was small and ranged from −7 to +7 mmHg, −9 to + 10 mmHg, and −10 to + 8 mmHg for systolic, diastolic, and mean BP, respectively. Similarly, BP readings obtained in infants using the Dinamap model 847 neonatal and Dinamap model 845 vital signs monitor were found to correlate well with BP values obtained using a central aortic catheter, with even smaller mean absolute pressure differences than seen in the previous study *(66)*, as shown in Figs. 1 and 2.

However, comparisons between BP readings using a mercury sphygmomanometer and some oscillometric devices, especially the newer models, demonstrate that the two methods are not comparable. A large single-center study evaluating the newer Dinamap model

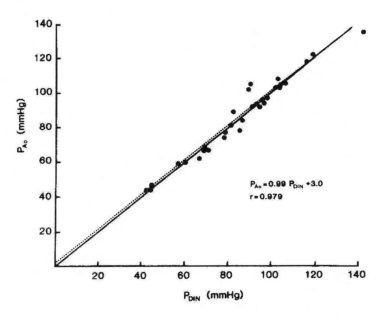

Fig. 1. The relation between central aortic (P_{AO}) and Dinamap (P_{DIN}) measurements for systolic pressure. The linear regression equation and correlation coefficient (*r*) are given. The line of identity (*solid line*) and least-squares regression line (*dotted line*) are shown. (Reproduced with permission from *(66,* figure 2.)

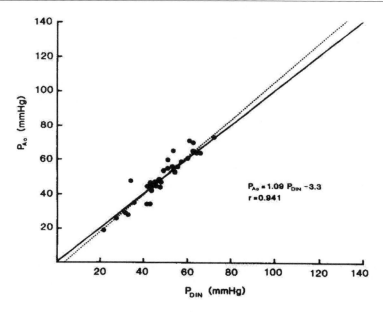

Fig. 2. The relation between central aortic (PAo) and Dinamap (PoIN) measurements for diastolic pressure. The linear regression equation, correlation coefficient, line of identity, and least-squares regression line are given as in Fig. 1. (Reproduced with permission from *(66*, figure 3.)

8100 against the conventional mercury sphygmomanometer in over 7000 children found that the mean Dinamap model 8100 readings were higher for both systolic (by 10 mmHg) and diastolic (by 5 mmHg) values. However, the 95th percentile confidence intervals for differences in systolic and diastolic BPs between the two methods were quite large and ranged from −4 to +24 mmHg and −14 to +23 mmHg, respectively, making the 'error' nonsystematic and unpredictable *(67)*. Similarly, in the Bogalusa Heart Study, significant differences were noted in BPs obtained using the Dinamap model 8100 and a conventional sphygmomanometer. While the mean systolic pressure with the Dinamap model 8100 was higher than that obtained using a conventional sphygmomanometer, similar to the study by Park et al., the mean diastolic pressure was, in fact, lower with the Dinamap model 8100 *(68)*. Moreover, an age-related difference was noted in the discrepancies between the two devices for diastolic BP. In children under 8 years of age, the Dinamap model 8100 diastolic BPs were higher compared to the conventional sphygmomanometer readings, while in children over 8 years, the Dinamap model 8100 underestimated diastolic BP.

To ensure accuracy of oscillometric BP measuring devices two different validation standards are currently in use. These are the British Hypertension Society (BHS) protocol *(69)* and the guidelines put forth by the AAMI *(70)* (Table 2). Since these two protocols can be reconciled, fulfillment of both sets of criteria should be used in validating any oscillometric device. Briefly, the BHS protocol looks at the absolute difference between BPs obtained simultaneously by the oscillometric device and a standard sphygmomanometer in different phases of use (before-use calibration, in-use phase, after-use calibration, and static validation). As the percentage of paired readings that are close to each other increases, the better is the grade assigned to the device (Grades A and B are acceptable while Grades C and D are unacceptable). The AAMI criteria, on the other hand, require that the device being tested be compared either to a standard sphygmomanometer or to direct intra-arterial

Table 2
Protocols for Assessment of the Accuracy of BP Measuring Devices

BHS grading criteria

Grade	Difference between test and 'standard' device readings (%)		
	≤5 mmHg	≤10 mmHg	≤15 mmHg
A	60	85	95
B	50	75	90
C	40	65	85
D	Worse	Worse	Worse

AAMI criteria

Grade	Mean difference between devices (mm Hg)	Standard deviation (mm Hg)
Pass	≤ 5	≤ 8
Fail	≥ 5	≥ 8

readings (especially in neonates, in whom it is often very difficult to hear the Korotkoff sounds). In order to get a passing grade from the AAMI, the test device measurements should not differ from the reference standard by a mean of >5 mmHg and a standard deviation of >8 mmHg. These standards are based upon the assumption, albeit unproven, that the physiological principles that underlie the oscillation of the arterial wall and its relation to BP are somehow identical to the Korotkoff sounds and their relation to BP. While many concerns have been raised about the reproducibility, complexity, and cumbersome nature of these two guidelines, they remain, to date the 'gold standard' for testing new devices in the market *(71)*. As environmental and other pressures increase the prominence of oscillometric devices, it is quite likely that a new set of distinct criteria will be established, much like the standards applied to direct intra-arterial measurements of BP versus auscultatory methods.

Based on the aforementioned guidelines, O'Brien et al. *(72)* recently reviewed several oscillometric devices available in the market and found that only a few fulfilled accuracy criteria for both protocols. Some of the devices that are recommended in this report for use in children are the CAS model 9010 (CAS Medical systems, Branford, CT) for in-hospital use, the Omron HEM-750CP (Omron Health Care, Inc., Vernon Hills, IL) for self-measurement and the Daypress 500 (Neural Instruments, Florence, Italy) for ambulatory BP monitoring, although only at rest. The BHS website (http://www.bhsoc.org/) also lists two other devices that have been validated in children: the Datascope Accutor Plus (Datascope Corporation, Mahwah, NJ) *(73)* and the Omron 705-IT (Omron Health Care, Inc., Vernon Hills, IL) *(74)*. The latter has not been validated in hypertensive children, nor do the data support its accuracy in obese children. Such issues, related to the need for validating devices for children with anthropometric measurements considered outside the realm of 'normal', are significant and worthy of study, considering that we are in the midst of an obesity epidemic. One of the more commonly used oscillometric devices in the United States, the Dinamap model 8100 has yielded varying results when tested for accuracy. Few pediatric studies have followed the strict guidelines of the AAMI and BHS protocols to evaluate the Dinamap model 8100. In a small study in a cohort of prepubertal children (8–13 years old), compared to the conventional sphygmomanometer, the Dinamap model 8100 was found to overestimate systolic BP and underestimate diastolic BP. These differences, however, were within the range acceptable by both the aforementioned validation standards *(75)*. The mean difference (standard deviation) between the BP readings obtained by the Dinamap model 8100 and the conventional sphygmomanometer was 4.8 (7.5) mmHg for systolic and −1.9 (7.5) mmHg for diastolic BP, making the device acceptable to the AAMI. Similarly, using the BHS criteria, the Dinamap model 8100 achieved a grade of B since more that 50% of its readings were within 5 mmHg and more than 90% were within 15 mmHg of the conventionally obtained measurements. However, other studies have not been as flattering of this device. In a study by O'Brien et al. *(76)* in 1993, the Dinamap model 8100 was evaluated for accuracy in an adult population according to the strict guidelines of the BHS protocol, and found to achieve a grading of D (unacceptable) for diastolic BP and B (acceptable) for systolic BP. Therefore, in the absence of further study in a larger group of children, the use of the Dinamap model 8100 cannot be recommended without reservation.

The 4th Report on high BP in children and adolescents recognized the practical issues related to attempting the auscultatory technique in infants and toddlers and suggested that the use of oscillometric devices in these youngest of children, that is, those less than 3 years of age, was acceptable, especially in settings when repeated measurements were felt to be necessary *(25)*. When oscillometric devices have been studied in neonates, many of the aforementioned issues become critical. One study compared three different oscillometric devices against intra-arterial measurements. Even recognizing that an oscillometric device measures a "different" pressure than a direct arterial line, the authors found significant disagreements between the devices and recommended arterial line measurements in critically ill neonates *(77)*.

Certainly there are discrepancies between auscultatory and oscillometric measurements; these discrepancies are not necessarily 'errors'. Whether the source of the discrepancy is mechanical and in the oscillometric device, or due to observer error with the conventional sphygmomanometer is, at best, speculative. It is also certainly possible that the 'error' arises from a more accurate determination of BP (especially the diastolic BP) by the oscillometric device that may be programmed to calculate values that match more closely to a 'true' intra-arterial BP, thereby eliminating the error inherent in the conventional sphygmomanometer, which necessarily has to rely on the Korotkoff sounds as an indirect and approximate surrogate indicator of true vascular pressure *(78)*. What is clear from studies comparing oscillometric devices with conventional sphygmomanometers is that these two methods of BP measurement should not be used interchangeably and that they may be measuring different biological parameters.

The potential advantage of using oscillometric devices over conventional sphygmomanometry is manifold. First and foremost, they are felt to be convenient, easy to use, and eliminate the need for highly trained personnel, although this may not really be the case *(79)*. Moreover, by avoiding terminal digit preference and bias related to prior knowledge of recorded BPs, the use of these devices, if accurate, can improve measurement precision and substantially lower the sample size required in clinical trials on hypertension. Oscillometric devices are also easier to use in younger children, neonates and infants, in whom movements of the arm may make it difficult to use auscultation to accurately hear the Korotkoff sounds; the success of oscillometric devices in obtaining BPs has been demonstrated in this age group by Park and Menard *(80)*. The use of such devices also eliminates the K4–K5 controversy mentioned previously *(36)*, since the oscillometric devices correlate very well with direct intra-arterial pressures *(65)*. However, the greatest advantage of these devices may turn out to be an ecological one. Since oscillometric devices do not use mercury, they may eventually supplant all mercury manometers due to the previously mentioned concern about the environmental hazard posed by this element *(40)*. The 4th report attempted to bridge these issues by suggesting that, in health care settings, oscillometric devices can be used, but the readings that exceed the 90th percentile norms be remeasured by an auscultatory method *(25)*.

While oscillometric devices, when correctly chosen, can greatly add to the management of patients with hypertension and improve clinical trials, their use is not without problems. As mentioned before, caution must be advised before a particular device is chosen for use, since the accuracy of many newer devices has not been tested in an unbiased manner. In addition, these are expensive pieces of equipment and also need continued upkeep and servicing to ensure optimal functioning, all of which adds to their cost. Certain drawbacks also exist in the design of these machines. While perhaps not applicable to any great extent in pediatrics, it is noteworthy that the upper limit of systolic pressure that these devices can measure is limited and varies from 240 to 280 mmHg (or about 160 mmHg in the neonatal mode) *(65,81)*.

Difficulties may also arise in BP measurements in children with cardiac arrhythmias and in those who are uncooperative and cannot hold still, leading to motion artifacts *(62)*. Moreover, the rapid rate of inflation of the cuff by the machine to a pressure of 160 mmHg may be uncomfortable and disconcerting to children, and may cause them to resist the BP measurement, leading to erroneously high readings. In fact, a 'first-reading' effect, in which the first of several BP readings is 3–5 mmHg higher than subsequent readings a few minutes later, has been noted by several investigators using oscillometric devices in children *(68,80)*. Therefore, repeat measurements of BP are important in children to avoid the overdiagnosis of hypertension. The optimal number of measurements, per patient and per visit, for oscillometric devices, may vary from machine to machine. For one particular device, the Dinamap model 845 XT, the reliability was noted to increase quite significantly when the number of BP measurements went from three to four per visit, and the number of visits went from one to two *(27)*. Finally, an issue that has irked clinical investigators for long is the knowledge that the algorithms used for determination of BP by oscillometric devices vary from one manufacturing company to another and also between different models of the same device. These algorithms have been considered to be proprietary information, and being confidential, have never been subjected to scientific scrutiny, causing health-care professionals to be somewhat skeptical of their validity *(82)*.

Users of oscillometric devices need to keep in mind a few other issues. As mentioned earlier, BPs obtained by conventional sphygmomanometry and using oscillometric devices should not be used interchangeably for study purposes, since even with the most accurate of devices, differences do exist between the two. Also, since normative data in use at present in children are based on BP measurements obtained by conventional sphygmomanometry *(25)* using these norms to determine if the BP, measured in a particular child using an oscillometric device, is normal, may not be appropriate. Having stated that, it must be noted that some normative reference data on BPs using an oscillometric device are available for children younger than 5 years of age *(80)*. It is also interesting to note that in spite of the aforementioned concerns with the use of oscillometric devices, some epidemiological studies of BP in adults and even one in children (the CATCH trial) are using such devices for BP determination *(83,84)*. Furthermore, it has recently been documented that the Dinamap has been programmed in such a way that it specifically cannot report certain values of BP *(85)*. Finally, we must all remember that, although oscillometric devices eliminate observer bias, they share with the mercury sphygmomanometer the likelihood that BP readings may be affected by environmental (e.g., ambient temperature) and patient factors (e.g., stress and arm size–cuff size discrepancy).

PROBLEMS WITH CASUAL BP MEASUREMENTS

Having reviewed the various individual methods of casual BP determination in children, we do need to recognize that these methods are not infallible and that there are many concerns related to the use of BPs obtained by such methods. Potential problems have already been discussed separately for each individual method in earlier sections of this chapter, and the reader is referred to these sections for more specific details. Suffice it so say that with meticulous attention to detail and by choosing the instrument appropriate to one's purpose, many of these problems and errors can be avoided. Table 3 compares the pros and cons of the various techniques for measuring BP in children (Table 3).

The second concern with casual BP readings is perhaps a more important and fundamental one. Although cross-sectional normative data on BP in children are routinely used in clinical management, there are no direct studies evaluating the validity of these norms in predicting the risk of adverse events in adulthood. Longitudinal epidemiological studies of BP starting in children, having commenced in the United States in the early 1970s have not had sufficient time to extend their follow-up into late adulthood to establish, if like adults, childhood hypertension or even high BP is predictive of cardiovascular and cerebrovascular morbidity and mortality. More importantly, it is not been shown for certain that early intervention is of any measurable benefit in reducing morbidity and mortality later in life. Indirectly, though, it seems biologically plausible and likely that hypertension starts in childhood and, if persistent, may be a predictor of adult onset morbidity. It would seem equally plausible that BP control in hypertensive children will reduce later morbidity. Resolution of left ventricular hypertrophy in children is seen when hypertension is treated.

The most direct evidence of a possible impact of high BP (either in of itself or by virtue of it being a surrogate marker for children with dyslipidemia, overweight, or insulin resistance) comes from the autopsy studies of the Bogalusa trial and the Pathobiological Determinants of Atherosclerosis in Youth (PDAY) trial, and also from cardiac imaging in participants in the Muscatine study. A subset of children who had participated in the Muscatine trial underwent electron beam computed tomography *(86)* to look for coronary artery calcification (CAC), which has previously been established to correlate well with the presence of atherosclerotic plaques in postmortem specimens *(87)*. An odds ratio of 3.0 (95% confidence interval 1.3–6.7) for CAC at the age of 33 years was noted for adults who were at the highest decile of body mass index in childhood. Although having high BP as a child (8–18 years) was not significantly associated with CAC, the diastolic BP as a young adult (20–34 years) certainly was, with an odds ratio of 4.2 (95% confidence interval 1.9–9.6). The same group of investigators, in a subsequent study, noted an association between CAC and carotid intimal–medial thickness, another marker of atherosclerosis, further cementing the link between BP (in young adults) and risk of future cardiovascular disease *(88)*. The Collaborative Pathology Study, a program of the Bogalusa Heart Study reported autopsy data in 93 children and young adults (2–39 years of age) who had died of traumatic causes *(89)*. These investigators found that the extent of raised fibrous plaques in the coronary arteries, which are known to be precursors of progressive atherosclerosis, correlated positively with antemortem diastolic and systolic BPs. Moreover, the greater the number of cardiovascular risk factors that were present (high body mass index, hypertension, dyslipidemia), the greater was the extent of early atherosclerosis. Finally, the PDAY study

Table 3
Comparison of the Various Methodologies for Casual BP Measurement

	Advantages	*Problems*
Conventional sphygmomanometry (CS)	Easy to use Inexpensive Commonly available Pediatric BP normative data based on it Perhaps the "gold" standard	Operation: observer biases Output: affected by technique, environmental, and mechanical factors (e.g., cuff size) Debate over use of K4 vs K5 as being representative of diastolic BP
Mercury	Minimal maintenance required to maintain calibration Portable; inexpensive Accurate	Environmental issues rehandling, spills, disposal Often not maintained Easily loses calibration
Aneroid	Measures same parameters as mercury	Gauge more subject to bias/misread than Hg column? Often not calibrated
RZS	Reduces observer biases	Design: bulky and difficult to use. Expensive. Uses mercury Operation: extensive training required for correct use Output: BP readings lower than with CS
Oscillometry	Easy to use No mercury in the instrument Frees user to allow more than one thing to be done at the same time Eliminates observer biases Easier to use in infants & young children compared to CS	Design: expensive and requires periodic maintenance Many devices in the market, few of which have been validated for use in children Output: affected by technique, environmental, and mechanical factors (e.g., cuff size) First reading effect High initial inflation pressure may cause anxiety and motion artifacts Limited normative data available for children BP reading not equivalent to CS readings

showed that hypertension augments atherosclerosis in young men and women (15–34 years of age) by accelerating the conversion of fatty streaks in the coronary arteries to raised plaques beginning in the third decade of life and that the effect of hypertension increases with age *(90)*.

So while logic and a significant body of literature would support the contention that hypertension in children, as determined by casual methods, is bad and is worthy of intervention to prevent adverse events in the future, no direct evidence to support this exists in the medical literature thus far. A second consideration, while interpreting casual BP readings obtained by any method, is the appropriateness of using such isolated and intermittent observations for making therapeutic decisions, especially those that might significantly impact on the perceived quality of life of an individual. This brings us back to the question of validity. How valid are casual, as compared to ambulatory, BP readings, in predicting adverse long-term outcomes? While this issue is discussed in greater depth in a subsequent chapter (see Chapter 10), it is important to point out here that discrepancies clearly exist in BP determinations made in an office setting to those obtained at home. A significant body of literature in adults *(91)* and some in children *(92)*, points out that a great majority of children with elevated casual BP readings, who would otherwise be classified as being hypertensive by current norms, may actually have 'white-coat' hypertension when ambulatory BP readings are used; this sub-group of children, might perhaps, be at lower or no risk of adverse outcomes, and therefore not merit extensive, expensive and invasive work-up, nor might they require long-term therapy. Preliminary studies have also shown, that like adults, hypertension in children, when determined by ambulatory methods, has a better correlation with risk factors for cardiovascular adverse outcomes such as left ventricular hypertrophy *(93)*. Home BP monitoring is an alternative to ambulatory BP monitoring that has become more prevalent in its use, even in children *(94)*. A further technological advancement in the arena of home BP monitoring relates to the development of telemonitoring systems allowing rapid and easy recording and transmission of home BP data to the health care provider's office. Readers are referred to recently published guidelines from the European Society of Hypertension, which address several issues pertaining to home BP monitoring in great detail, since these are beyond the scope of this chapter *(95)*. Suffice it to say that most studies to date suggest that home BP monitoring is at least as good, if not better than, office BP measurements in predicting adverse outcomes; coupled with its easier availability, lower cost, and convenience compared to ambulatory monitoring, home BP measurements are likely here to stay, but need to be studied in greater depth.

A final note, on the use of wrist BP devices for BP monitoring. None have been validated for use in children. Even in adults, these devices, although commercially available, are subject to errors, especially pertaining to the position of the arm in relation to the heart and are therefore not recommended. Nevertheless, the BHS website does list several such devices that, when used properly, can be used for clinical purposes in adults.

CONCLUSIONS

The concept that there is a "true" BP is probably more obfuscating that illuminating. At any given moment, each of us has a BP, but the force of that pressure will register differently as different systems are used to measure it. Moments later, the pressure is different. Korotkoff himself reported that the first sound heard (K1) appeared before the radial pulse could be palpated as the occluding cuff is deflated *(96)*. K1, on the other hand, is heard after systolic pressure is detected by an indwelling line *(97)*. Mercury and aneroid devices, as discussed earlier, when calibrated properly, agree quite closely on the pressure that they detect. Conversely, oscillometry seems to differ by device and certainly differs from the auscultatory methods, but perhaps comes closest to intra-arterial determinations.

All of these methods, if consistently applied, will correlate with the other, but they are rarely likely to be identical.

The use of casual BP measurements, when performed carefully by trained personnel using calibrated and well-maintained devices, remains the primary screening tool to assess populations for hypertension. The largest pool of normative data in children exists for values obtained by auscultatory methods (albeit the data pooled first BP readings). Auscultatory methods are accurate, but subject to many confounding issues. Oscillometric measures will likely replace auscultatory measures as the primary method of BP determination, but they do not measure the same thing that is auscultated, and they have their own unique set of confounding variables. Additional normal values based upon oscillometry are needed.

REFERENCES

1. Crenner CW. Introduction of the blood pressure cuff into U.S. medical practice: technology and skilled practice. Ann Intern Med. 1998;128:488–493.
2. Cushing H. On routine determinations of arterial tension in operating room and clinic. Boston Med Surg J. 1903;148:250–252.
3. Cook H, Briggs J. Clinical observations of blood pressure. Johns Hopkins Hosp Rep. 1903;11:451–534.
4. Lewis W. The evolution of clinical sphygmomanometry. Bull N Y Acad Med. 1941;17:87–881.
5. Gittings J. Auscultatory blood-pressure determinations. Arch Intern Med. 1910;6:196–204.
6. Labarthe DR. Overview of the history of pediatric blood pressure assessment and hypertension: an epidemiologic perspective. Blood Press Monit. 1999;4:197–203.
7. Burt VL, Whelton P, Roccella EJ, et al. Prevalence of hypertension in the US adult population. Results from the Third National Health and Nutrition Examination Survey, 1988–1991. Hypertension. 1995;25:305–313.
8. Sinaiko AR, Gomez-Marin O, Prineas RJ. Prevalence of "significant" hypertension in junior high school-aged children: the Children and Adolescent Blood Pressure Program. J Pediatr. 1989;114:664–669.
9. Mehta SK. Pediatric hypertension. A challenge for pediatricians. Am J Dis Child. 1987;141:893–894.
10. Lauer RM, Clarke WR, Mahoney LT, et al. Childhood predictors for high adult blood pressure. The Muscatine Study. Pediatr Clin North Am. 1993;40:23–40.
11. Mahoney LT, Clarke WR, Burns TL, et al. Childhood predictors of high blood pressure. Am J Hypertens. 1991;4:608S–610S.
12. Burke V, Beilin LJ, Dunbar D. Tracking of blood pressure in Australian children. J Hypertens. 2001;19:1185–1192.
13. Lauer RM, Clarke WR. Childhood risk factors for high adult blood pressure: the Muscatine Study. Pediatrics. 1989;84:633–641.
14. Vasan RS, Larson MG, Leip EP, et al. Impact of high-normal blood pressure on the risk of cardiovascular disease. N Engl J Med. 2001;345:1291–1297.
15. Stamler J, Stamler R, Neaton JD. Blood pressure, systolic and diastolic, and cardiovascular risks. US population data. Arch Intern Med. 1993;153:598–615.
16. Fiebach NH, Hebert PR, Stampfer MJ, et al. A prospective study of high blood pressure and cardiovascular disease in women. Am J Epidemiol. 1989;130:646–654.
17. Kannel WB, Wolf PA, Verter J, et al. Epidemiologic assessment of the role of blood pressure in stroke. The Framingham study. JAMA. 1970;214:301–310.
18. Klag MJ, Whelton PK, Randall BL, et al. Blood pressure and end-stage renal disease in men. N Engl J Med. 1996;334:13–18.
19. Kannel WB. Blood pressure as a cardiovascular risk factor: prevention and treatment. JAMA. 1996;275:1571–1576.
20. Srinivasan SR, Myers L, Berenson GS. Predictability of childhood adiposity and insulin for developing insulin resistance syndrome (syndrome X) in young adulthood: the Bogalusa Heart Study. Diabetes. 2002;51:204–209.
21. Vogt BA, Birk PE, Panzarino V, et al. Aortic dissection in young patients with chronic hypertension. Am J Kidney Dis. 1999;33:374–378.
22. Hari P, Bagga A, Srivastava RN. Sustained hypertension in children. Indian Pediatr. 2000;37: 268–274.
23. Cooney MJ, Bradley WG, Symko SC, et al. Hypertensive encephalopathy: complication in children treated for myeloproliferative disorders—report of three cases. Radiology. 2000;214:711–716.

24. Sorof JM, Cardwell G, Franco K, et al. Ambulatory blood pressure and left ventricular mass index in hypertensive children. Hypertension. 2002;39:903–908.

25. National High Blood Pressure Education Program Working Group on High Blood Pressure in Children and Adolescents. The fourth report on the diagnosis, evaluation, and treatment of high blood pressure in children and adolescents. Pediatrics. 2004;114:555–576.

26. Pickering TG, Hall JE, Appel LJ, et al. Recommendations for blood pressure measurement in humans and experimental animals: part 1: blood pressure measurement in humans: a statement for professionals from the Subcommittee of Professional and Public Education of the American Heart Association Council on High Blood Pressure Research. Hypertension. 2005;45:142–161.

27. Gillman MW, Cook NR. Blood pressure measurement in childhood epidemiological studies. Circulation. 1995;92:1049–1057.

28. Markandu ND, Whitcher F, Arnold A, et al. The mercury sphygmomanometer should be abandoned before it is proscribed. J Hum Hypertens. 2000;14:31–36.

29. Beevers G, Lip GY, O'Brien E. ABC of hypertension. Blood pressure measurement. Part I-sphygmomanometry: factors common to all techniques. BMJ. 2001;322:981–985.

30. Vyse TJ. Sphygmomanometer bladder length and measurement of blood pressure in children. Lancet. 1987;1:561–562.

31. Pickering TG, Hall JE, Appel LJ, et al. Recommendations for blood pressure measurement in humans and experimental animals: part 1: blood pressure measurement in humans: a statement for professionals from the Subcommittee of Professional and Public Education of the American Heart Association Council on High Blood Pressure Research. Circulation. 2005;111:697–716.

32. Blumenthal S, Epps RP, Heavenrich R, et al. Report of the task force on blood pressure control in children. Pediatrics. 1977;59:I–II, 797–820.

33. Alpert BS, Marks L, Cohen M. K5 = diastolic pressure. Pediatrics. 1996;98:1002.

34. Uhari M, Nuutinen M, Turtinen J, et al. Pulse sounds and measurement of diastolic blood pressure in children. Lancet. 1991;338:159–161.

35. Sinaiko AR, Gomez-Marin O, Prineas RJ. Diastolic fourth and fifth phase blood pressure in 10–15-year-old children. The Children and Adolescent Blood Pressure Program. Am J Epidemiol. 1990;132:647–655.

36. Elkasabany AM, Urbina EM, Daniels SR, et al. Prediction of adult hypertension by K4 and K5 diastolic blood pressure in children: the Bogalusa Heart Study. J Pediatr. 1998;132:687–692.

37. Vanasse A, Courteau J. Evaluation of sphygmomanometers used by family physicians practicing outside the hospital environment in Bas-Saint-Laurent. Can Fam Physician. 2001;47:281–286.

38. Mion D, Pierin AM. How accurate are sphygmomanometers? J Hum Hypertens. 1998;12:245–248.

39. Knight T, Leech F, Jones A, et al. Sphygmomanometers in use in general practice: an overlooked aspect of quality in patient care. J Hum Hypertens. 2001;15:681–684.

40. O'Brien E. Has conventional sphygmomanometry ended with the banning of mercury? Blood Press Monit. 2002;7:37–40.

41. Jones DW, Frohlich ED, Grim CM, et al. Mercury sphygmomanometers should not be abandoned: an advisory statement from the Council for High Blood Pressure Research, American Heart Association. Hypertension. 2001;37:185–186.

42. Perloff D, Grim C, Flack J, et al. Human blood pressure determination by sphygmomanometry. Circulation. 1993;88:2460–2470.

43. Sloan PJ, Zezulka A, Davies P, et al. Standardized methods for comparison of sphygmomanometers. J Hypertens. 1984;2:547–551.

44. Bailey RH, Knaus VL, Bauer JH. Aneroid sphygmomanometers. An assessment of accuracy at a university hospital and clinics. Arch Intern Med. 1991;151:1409–1412.

45. Jones JS, Ramsey W, Hetrick T. Accuracy of prehospital sphygmomanometers. J Emerg Med. 1987;5: 23–27.

46. Ali S, Rouse A. Practice audits: reliability of sphygmomanometers and blood pressure recording bias. J Hum Hypertens. 2002;16:359–361.

47. Hussain A, Cox JG. An audit of the use of sphygmomanometers. Br J Clin Pract. 1996;50:136–137.

48. Canzanello VJ, Jensen PL, Schwartz GL. Are aneroid sphygmomanometers accurate in hospital and clinic settings? Arch Intern Med. 2001;161:729–731.

49. Yarows SA, Qian K. Accuracy of aneroid sphygmomanometers in clinical usage: University of Michigan experience. Blood Press Monit. 2001;6:101–106.

50. Wright BM, Dore CF. A random-zero sphygmomanometer. Lancet. 1970;1:337–338.

51. Dischinger P, DuChene AG. Quality control aspects of blood pressure measurements in the Multiple Risk Factor Intervention Trial. Control Clin Trials. 1986;7:137S–157S.

52. Canner PL, Borhani NO, Oberman A, et al. The Hypertension Prevention Trial: assessment of the quality of blood pressure measurements. Am J Epidemiol. 1991;134:379–392.

53. Uhari M, Nuutinen EM, Turtinen J, et al. Blood pressure in children, adolescents and young adults. Ann Med. 1991;23:47–51.
54. Variability of blood pressure and the results of screening in the hypertension detection and follow-up program. J Chronic Dis. 1978;31:651–667.
55. Nuutinen M, Turtinen J, Uhari M. Random-zero sphygmomanometer, Rose's tape, and the accuracy of the blood pressure measurements in children. Pediatr Res. 1992;32:243–247.
56. Mackie A, Whincup P, McKinnon M. Does the Hawksley random zero sphygmomanometer underestimate blood pressure, and by how much? J Hum Hypertens. 1995 9:337–343.
57. Brown WC, Kennedy S, Inglis GC, et al. Mechanisms by which the Hawksley random zero sphygmomanometer underestimates blood pressure and produces a non-random distribution of RZ values. J Hum Hypertens. 1997;11:75–93.
58. O'Brien E, Mee F, Atkins N, et al. Inaccuracy of the Hawksley random zero sphygmomanometer. Lancet. 1990;336:1465–1468.
59. Conroy RM, Shelley E, O'Brien E, et al. Ergonomic problems with the Hawksley Random Zero Sphygmomanometer and their effect on recorded blood pressure levels. Blood Press. 1996;5:227–233.
60. McGurk C, Nugent A, McAuley D, et al. Sources of inaccuracy in the use of the Hawksley random-zero sphygmomanometer. J Hypertens. 1997;15:1379–1384.
61. Butani L, Morgenstern BZ. Are pitfalls of oxcillometric blood pressure measurements preventable in children? Pediatr Nephrol. 2003;18:313–318.
62. Ramsey M 3rd. Blood pressure monitoring: automated oscillometric devices. J Clin Monit. 1991;7:56–67.
63. Jilek J, Fukushima T. Oscillometric blood pressure measurement: the methodology, some observations, and suggestions. Biomed Instrum Technol. 2005;39:237–241.
64. Kaufmann MA, Pargger H, Drop LJ. Oscillometric blood pressure measurements by different devices are not interchangeable. Anesth Analg. 1996;82:377–381.
65. Park MK, Menard SM. Accuracy of blood pressure measurement by the Dinamap monitor in infants and children. Pediatrics. 1987;79:907–914.
66. Colan SD, Fujii A, Borow KM, et al. Noninvasive determination of systolic, diastolic and end-systolic blood pressure in neonates, infants and young children: comparison with central aortic pressure measurements. Am J Cardiol. 1983;52:867–870.
67. Park MK, Menard SW, Yuan C. Comparison of auscultatory and oscillometric blood pressures. Arch Pediatr Adolesc Med. 2001;155:50–53.
68. Wattigney WA, Webber LS, Lawrence MD, et al. Utility of an automatic instrument for blood pressure measurement in children. The Bogalusa Heart Study. Am J Hypertens. 1996;9:256–262.
69. O'Brien E, Petrie J, Littler W, et al. The British Hypertension Society protocol for the evaluation of automated and semi-automated blood pressure measuring devices with special reference to ambulatory systems. J Hypertens. 1990;8:607–619.
70. American National Standard for manual, electronic or automated sphygmomanometers. Association for the Advancement of Medical Instrumentation, Arlington, Virginia, 2002, 1–78.
71. O'Brien E. Proposals for simplifying the validation protocols of the British Hypertension Society and the Association for the Advancement of Medical Instrumentation. Blood Press Monit. 2000;5:43–45.
72. O'Brien E, Waeber B, Parati G, et al. Blood pressure measuring devices: recommendations of the European Society of Hypertension. BMJ. 2001;322:531–536.
73. Stergiou GS, Yiannes NG, Rarra VC. Validation of the Omron 705 IT oscillometric device for home blood pressure measurement in children and adolescents: the Arsakion School Study. Blood Press Monit. 2006;11:229–234.
74. Wong SN, Tz Sung RY, Leung LC. Validation of three oscillometric blood pressure devices against auscultatory mercury sphygmomanometer in children. Blood Press Monit. 2006;11:281–291.
75. Jin RZ, Donaghue KC, Fairchild J, et al. Comparison of Dinamap 8100 with sphygmomanometer blood pressure measurement in a prepubertal diabetes cohort. J Paediatr Child Health. 2001;37:545–549.
76. O'Brien E, Mee F, Atkins N, et al. Short report: accuracy of the Dinamap portable monitor, model 8100 determined by the British Hypertension Society protocol. J Hypertens. 1993;11:761–763.
77. Dannevig I, Dale HC, Liestol K, et al. Blood pressure in the neonate: three non-invasive oscillometric pressure monitors compared with invasively measured blood pressure. Acta Paediatr. 2005;94: 191–196.
78. Moss AJ, Adams FH. Index of indirect estimation of diastolic blood pressure. Am J Dis Child. 1963;106:364–367.
79. Smith GR. Devices for blood pressure measurement. Prof Nurse. 2000;15:337–340.
80. Park MK, Menard SM. Normative oscillometric blood pressure values in the first 5 years in an office setting. Am J Dis Child. 1989;143:860–864.

81. O'Brien E, Mee F, Atkins N, et al. Evaluation of three devices for self-measurement of blood pressure according to the revised British Hypertension Society Protocol: the Omron HEM-705CP, Philips HP5332, and Nissei DS-175. Blood Press Monit. 1996;1:55–61.
82. O'Brien E. Replacing the mercury sphygmomanometer. Requires clinicians to demand better automated devices. BMJ. 2000;320:815–816.
83. Kelder SH, Osganian SK, Feldman HA, et al. Tracking of physical and physiological risk variables among ethnic subgroups from third to eighth grade: the Child and Adolescent Trial for Cardiovascular Health cohort study. Prev Med. 2002;34:324–333.
84. Staessen JA, Celis H, Hond ED, et al. Comparison of conventional and automated blood pressure measurements: interim analysis of the THOP trial. Blood Press Monit. 2002;7:61–62.
85. Rose KM, Arnett DK, Ellison RC, et al. Skip patterns in DINAMAP-measured blood pressure in 3 epidemiological studies. Hypertension. 2000;35:1032–1036.
86. Mahoney LT, Burns TL, Stanford W, et al. Coronary risk factors measured in childhood and young adult life are associated with coronary artery calcification in young adults: the Muscatine Study. J Am Coll Cardiol. 1996;27:277–284.
87. Simons DB, Schwartz RS, Edwards WD, et al. Noninvasive definition of anatomic coronary artery disease by ultrafast computed tomographic scanning: a quantitative pathologic comparison study. J Am Coll Cardiol. 1992;20:1118–1126.
88. Davis PH, Dawson JD, Mahoney LT, et al. Increased carotid intimal-medial thickness and coronary calcification are related in young and middle-aged adults. The Muscatine study. Circulation. 1999;100:838–842.
89. Berenson GS, Srinivasan SR, Bao W, et al. Association between multiple cardiovascular risk factors and atherosclerosis in children and young adults. The Bogalusa Heart Study. N Engl J Med. 1998;338:1650–1656.
90. McGill HC Jr, McMahan CA, Tracy RE, et al. Relation of a postmortem renal index of hypertension to atherosclerosis and coronary artery size in young men and women. Pathobiological Determinants of Atherosclerosis in Youth (PDAY) Research Group. Arterioscler Thromb Vasc Biol. 1998;18:1108–1118.
91. Pickering TG, Coats A, Mallion JM, et al. Blood pressure monitoring. Task force V: white-coat hypertension. Blood Press Monit. 1999;4:333–341.
92. Sorof JM, Portman RJ. White coat hypertension in children with elevated casual blood pressure. J Pediatr. 2000;137:493–497.
93. Chamontin B, Amar J, Barthe P, et al. Blood pressure measurements and left ventricular mass in young adults with arterial hypertension screened at high school check-up. J Hum Hypertens. 1994;8:357–361.
94. Bald M, Hoyer PF. Measurement of blood pressure at home: survey among pediatric nephrologists. Pediatr Nephrol. 2001;16:1058–1062.
95. Parati G, Stergiou GS, Asmar R, et al. European Society of Hypertension guidelines for blood pressure monitoring at home: a summary report of the Second International Consensus Conference on Home Blood Pressure Monitoring. J Hypertens. 2008;26:1505–1526.
96. Shevchenko YL, Tsitlik JE. 90th anniversary of the development by Nikolai S. Korotkoff of the auscultatory method of measuring blood pressure. Circulation. 1996;94:116–118.
97. McAlister FA, Straus SE. Evidence based treatment of hypertension. Measurement of blood pressure: an evidence based review. BMJ. 2001;322:908–911.

8 Development of Blood Pressure Norms in Children

Bonita Falkner, MD

INTRODUCTION

Assessment of blood pressure in children and adolescents, as a measure of health status, is now part of routine clinical practice. Prior to the 1970s blood pressure was not commonly measured in very young children, due to the difficulty in obtaining reliable measurements and the general belief that hypertension was a rare problem in children *(1)*. Since measurement of blood pressure had not yet become routine, high blood pressure was detected only when significant clinical signs or symptoms were present. Due to the absence of any childhood blood pressure data on which to base an age appropriate definition of hypertension, adult criteria were the only available reference information. Based on our current knowledge on what is normal blood pressure in healthy children, we now know that the early descriptions of hypertension in the young represented only the most severe cases of childhood hypertension.

Looking back on this practice, one can understand how some beliefs in medicine develop. With regard to childhood hypertension, the belief had been that hypertension in children was always secondary to an underlying cause; and primary, or essential, hypertension did not exist in the young. With the development and understanding of reference data on blood pressure in the young, relative to physical development, this belief has changed. We now have blood pressure data and a body of clinical experience that enables clinicians to evaluate the level of blood pressure in a given child relative to age, sex, body size, and other

B. Falkner (✉)
Department of Medicine, Thomas Jefferson University, Philadelphia, PA, USA
e-mail: bonita.falkner@jefferson.edu

From: *Clinical Hypertension and Vascular Diseases: Pediatric Hypertension*
Edited by: J. T. Flynn et al. DOI 10.1007/978-1-60327-824-9_8
© Springer Science+Business Media, LLC 2011

clinical parameters. Moreover, the clinician can use the available reference blood pressure data and the clinical characteristics of the child to determine the child's health status in terms of healthy, having risk factors that warrant preventive intervention, or having a blood pressure level that warrants further evaluation. Some children, especially younger children, do indeed have hypertension secondary to an underlying disorder such as renal disease. It is now also known that essential hypertension can be detected in the young, and the value of recognizing the early phase of hypertension is the potential ability to modify the cardio-vascular outcome.

The advancement in knowledge on childhood hypertension over the past 35 years has developed from a process of accumulating, evaluating, and understanding data on blood pressure. The outcome of this process is the blood pressure normative data on which we base our current definitions of normotension and hypertension in children and adolescents. This chapter will review that process, and to a large extent, is an historical reflection on what has transpired. The questions and concerns expressed by the authors of the early reports are important to remember because those are the thoughts that moved this process forward, and provide a model to continue the forward process.

OUTCOME OF CHILDHOOD HYPERTENSION

Hypertension is a significant health problem to the extent that adverse clinical outcomes can be attributed to or associated with blood pressure levels that exceed a certain level. Little had been known about the health consequences of hypertension in childhood. Still and Cottom *(2)* provided one of the first descriptions on the outcome of severe hypertension in children by reviewing cases with sustained diastolic blood pressure greater than 120 mmHg that were treated at the Hospital for Sick Children, Great Ormond Street, UK, from 1954 to 1964. Of the 55 cases reviewed, 31 died, 18 survived with treatment that achieved a reduction in blood pressure, and 6 were cured of the hypertension following corrective surgery for an identifiable lesion (coarctation repair, unilateral nephrectomy, pheochromocytoma removal). Of the 56% of cases that died, the average duration of survival following diagnosis of the hypertension was only 14 months. The review of this sample of severe childhood hypertension indicated a 90% mortality within 1 year, a mortality rate that is the same as that of malignant hypertension in adults. While these numbers are shocking by today's standards, the message that was clearly made at that time was that severe hypertension in a child could be as deadly as it was in an adult.

The above report and others of that time period were limited to children with quite severe hypertension. In the absence of blood pressure data on normal children, the conventional adult cut point of 140/90 mmHg was generally used to define hypertension in children. This practice limited the diagnosis of hypertension in children to those with the most extreme elevations of blood pressure. In children, severe hypertension is frequently associated with renal disease or some other disorder that causes the hypertension. As a result, for some time the issue of childhood hypertension focused on the evaluation for underlying disease and search for secondary cause. Subsequent efforts to develop normative data on blood pressure in childhood were a necessary prelude for a shift from the narrow focus of secondary hypertension to a broader perspective that high levels of blood pressure could indicate an early phase of a chronic process. It was established that severe hypertension had an adverse outcome if left untreated. What was yet to be determined was how frequent did hypertension occur, and what level of blood pressure elevation in a given child conferred risk for target organ or vessel injury.

PREVALENCE OF HYPERTENSION IN CHILDHOOD

In the last half of the 20th century, hypertension was established as a significant health problem in adults, and efforts were underway, from both a public health and clinical care perspective, to improve detection and management of hypertension. To a large extent, hypertension was regarded as a component of aging and a reflection of chronic atherosclerosis. Thus, hypertension appeared to have little relevance in the young. Jennifer Loggie was one of the first to consider the possibility that "essential" hypertension could be detected in adolescents *(3)*. In a review article in 1974, Loggie discussed the available reports at that time on the prevalence of hypertension in persons 25 years or less. Of the five published reports *(4–8)* that attempted to determine the prevalence of hypertension in the young by conducting blood pressure screening on large samples of healthy individuals, the rates of hypertension in the young ranged from 1 *(8)* to 12.4% *(7)*. Table 1 summarizes these reports and denotes the differences in the criteria used to define hypertension, methods of measurement (sitting vs supine), and the age of the sample examined. These early reports, on hypertension in adolescents and young adults, defined hypertension by a set level of blood pressure, which was similar to values used for adults *(4–6,8)*. The report by Londe *(7)* was based on an examination of younger children, age 4–15 years, and used a different definition of hypertension. Londe had measured blood pressure in his own clinic and observed that blood pressure rises with age, concurrent with growth and development *(6,7)*. He then analyzed the blood pressure data to determine the range of systolic and diastolic

Table 1
Reported Prevalence of Hypertension in Persons 25 Years of Age or Less Prior to Normative Data

Authors	Subjects age (years)	Number screened	Position in which pressure was taken	Definition of hypertension (mmHg)	Prevalence (%)
Masland et al. *(4)*	"Adolescents"	1,795	Not stated	140/90	1.4
Boe et al. *(5)*	15–19	3,833	Sitting	150/90	3.01 Males 1.04 Females
Heyden et al. *(6)*	15–25	435	Sitting	140/90	11.0
Londe *(7)*	4–15	1,473	Supine	Systolic or diastolic BP >90th percentile	12.4 Males 11.6 Females
				Systolic or diastolic BP >95th percentile (repeated measures)	1.9
Wilber et al. *(8)*	15–25	799	Sitting	Systolic>160	1.0
				Diastolic>90	1.5

Adapted From Loggie *(3)*.

blood pressure stratified by age, and selected the 90th percentile for each age that defined hypertension. Thus, his reported rates of hypertension are consistent with his definition and are slightly above 10%. He also noted that on repeated measurement, there is regression toward the mean and the prevalence of persistent systolic or diastolic blood pressure greater than the 95th percentile was 1.9%. Little attention was given to Londe's work for some time. However, it is remarkable that the number of children (1.9%) with systolic or diastolic blood pressure equal to or greater than the 95 percentile on repeated measurement is very close to more contemporary data that encompasses far larger numbers of children.

DEFINITION OF HYPERTENSION IN CHILDHOOD

The fundamental problem to be resolved was what constituted normal blood pressure and what level of blood pressure defined hypertension in the young. The approach to defining abnormal blood pressure in adulthood uses, as the definition of hypertension, the approximate level of blood pressure that marks an increase in mortality that is above average. The cut-point numbers for blood pressure were largely derived from actuarial data from life insurance mortality investigations that indicated an increase in death rates when the systolic blood pressure exceeded 140 mmHg or the diastolic blood pressure exceeded 90 mmHg.

This method to define hypertension was challenged by Master et al. *(9)* in a report published in 1950. These authors argued that defining hypertension by a single number was arbitrary, because hypertension occurred far more frequently in the elderly and was commonly associated with atherosclerosis. They contended that an increase in blood pressure was a reflection of aging, and that the use of one number to define a disorder for all ages resulted in an overdiagnosis of hypertension in the elderly. They proposed a statistical definition based on the distribution of blood pressure readings around the mean, according to sex and age. Blood pressure, like most human characteristics, demonstrates a frequency distribution that yields a fairly normal curve. In a normal distribution, roughly two thirds of the observations will occur within the range of the statistical mean plus or minus one standard deviation from the mean; and 95% of the observations will be within the range of the mean plus or minus two standard deviations. They proposed that blood pressure that reached a level that was two standard deviations beyond the statistical mean, or greater than the 95th percentile, should be considered abnormal. Master et al. supported their position by examining data obtained from industrial plants in various sections of the country on about 7,400 persons who were stated to be in "average good health and able to work." Using a statistical method to define the normal range of blood pressure, they described the normal range of systolic blood pressure in males to be 105–135 mmHg at 16 years of age, and rising progressively with age to reach 115–170 mmHg at age 60–64 years. They also noted a gender difference in the normal range with females having a normal range of systolic blood pressure of 100–130 mmHg at 16 years of age, and rising to a normal range of 115–175 mmHg at age 60–64 years. The conclusion of these authors was that hypertension was overdiagnosed in adults, particularly in the elderly. Their conclusion was supported, they believed, by demonstrating that large numbers of persons with blood pressure above 140/90 mmHg were living with blood pressure at that level and were "in average good health and able to work."

A large body of subsequent epidemiological and clinical investigations on hypertension in adults has clearly dismissed the conclusion by Master et al. that hypertension is overdiagnosed because the normal range of blood pressure increases with age. Several expert panels define hypertension in adults according to the level of BP that marks an increase in cardiovascular events and mortality. This definition continues to be systolic blood pressure ≥140 mmHg or diastolic blood pressure ≥90 mmHg *(10–12)*. These numbers are the approximate blood pressure levels above which the risks for morbid events are significantly heightened and the benefits of treatment are established. It is also now recognized that the risk for cardiovascular events attributable to blood pressure level in adults does not begin only at 140/90 mmHg, but the risk is linear and begins to rise starting at a lower level of systolic blood pressure. Data derived from the Framingham Study in adults have shown that blood pressures in the 130/85 to 139/89 mmHg range have more than double the absolute risk for total cardiovascular events following 10 years, compared to blood pressure <120/80 mmHg *(13)*. In response to this emerging epidemiological data, the concept of prehypertension has been developed to designate a range of blood pressure in adults that could benefit from preventive lifestyle changes *(14)*. There are no comparable data that link a level of blood pressure in childhood with morbid events at some time later in adulthood. The original report by Master et al. is the earliest to show that the normal range of blood pressure is lower in persons age 16–19 years than that in older adults. Of most significance is that Master et al. provided a statistical method to define the normal blood pressure range; and abnormal blood pressure could then be defined in the absence of mortality or morbidity end points.

The question that remained unanswered until the early 1970s was what is the prevalence of hypertension in children and adolescents. This question could not be answered without a uniform and consistent definition of hypertension in the young. Moreover, the definition of hypertension could not be developed in the absence of knowledge about what constituted normal blood pressure in children and adolescents. There were some, but quite limited, data on blood pressure levels in normal children *(6,15–18)*. The available data indicated that the level of blood pressure was considerably lower in young children than in adults, and that there appeared to be a normal rise in blood pressure with age that was concurrent with growth *(19)*. It was also recognized that due to difficulty in measurement techniques, there was likely to be considerable variability in what data were available.

Efforts to gain a better understanding of the occurrence of hypertension in the young initially tended to focus on adolescents. Based on a careful examination of her own clinical data on cases she had evaluated for blood pressure elevation, Loggie *(3)* suggested that essential hypertension was more common in adolescents than had been previously believed. Kilcoyne et al. *(20)* made an effort to determine if asymptomatic hypertension could be detected in healthy adolescents. These investigators conducted blood pressure screening on urban high school students. They observed that female students of all races had lower systolic pressures than males. Using 140/90 mmHg as a definition of hypertension, they detected an overall prevalence of 5.4% systolic and 7.8% diastolic hypertension at the initial screening; follow-up screening of those with elevated measurements demonstrated a decline in prevalence to 1.2% systolic and 2.4% diastolic hypertension. They also noted higher rates of sustained hypertension among the black males. These investigators further examined their data by creating frequency distributions of systolic blood pressures in the males at successive age levels of 14, 16, and 18 years. These distribution curves demonstrated a progressive rightward displacement with increasing age, which, the authors suggested, indicated a transition to adult characteristics. However, they also noted that this shift in distribution did not occur in females between 14 and 19 years of age. Based on their own data, these investigators suggested that the criteria used to define blood pressure elevations in adolescents would be more meaningful if they were based on the frequency distributions of blood pressure in an adolescent sample and proposed that values exceeding one standard deviation above the statistical mean would more appropriately define hypertension. From their data, one standard deviation above the mean would be 132/85 mmHg for males and 123/82 mmHg for females. It is of note that, although one and not two standard deviations above the mean were proposed, these values are reasonably close to the numbers that Master et al. *(9)* reported to be at the top of the normal range for persons 16–19 years of age (males 135 mmHg; females 130 mmHg).

Similar efforts to investigate blood pressure in healthy adolescents were conducted by other investigators, largely in the context of high school screening projects *(21–24)*. The results of these studies also detected initial rates of hypertension, when adult criteria were used, at approximately 5%, and this rate decreased with repeat blood pressure measurements. These reports also noted lower levels of blood pressure in adolescent females compared to males. Some difference in blood pressure by race was reported, with higher levels of blood pressure and more hypertension among African Americans *(20,21)*. An effect of weight on blood pressure was also described *(21,24)*. Together, these reports emphasized a need to develop a better definition of hypertension in the young, which was based on data derived from a large sample of healthy children.

The gaps in understanding blood pressure and hypertension in childhood were recognized by the National Heart, Lung, and Blood Institute which directed the National High Blood Pressure Education Program to appoint a Task Force on Blood Pressure Control in Children. The Task Force published its first report in 1977 *(25)*. The Task Force goals were to (1) describe a standard methodology for measurement of blood pressure in the young; (2) provide blood pressure distribution curves by age and sex; (3) recommend a blood pressure level that is the upper limit of normal; and (4) provide guidelines for detection, evaluation, and treatment of children with elevated or at-risk blood pressure measurements. The blood pressure distribution curves were based on data gathered from three studies conducted in Muscatine, Iowa; Rochester, Minnesota; and Miami, Florida. The total size of the sample was 9,283 children from age 5 through 18 years, with an additional 306 children age 2–5 years (Miami). The blood pressure data were presented as percentile curves, by age, for systolic and diastolic blood pressure in males and females, similar to the standard pediatric growth curves for weight and height.

These blood pressure curves were clearly an advancement, particularly for clinicians who care for children. Although based on cross-sectional data, the curves indicate a normal increase in blood pressure level with age, which is concurrent with an increase in height and weight. The blood pressure curves also established a normative range for blood pressure in early childhood that was different than that of adults. Using a statistical definition, the 95th percentile for each age and sex was the recommended blood pressure level for ascertainment of hypertension, if verified on repeated measurement. These blood pressure curves, for the first time, provided a clear view on the levels of blood pressure that were outside of the normal range in young children. However, by age 13 years in boys, the 95th percentile had reached 140 mmHg systolic and 90 mmHg diastolic pressure. At age 18 years the 95th percentile was over 150 mmHg systolic and at 95 mmHg diastolic. These numbers seemed to indicate that by early adolescence the adult criteria to define hypertension would be appropriate. However, the 95th percentile delineated blood pressure levels that seemed to be high, particularly in view of the data that had been collected in the preceding high school screening studies. This discrepancy raised concern as to how well these distribution curves truly reflected the normative blood pressure distribution in children and adolescents.

NORMATIVE BLOOD PRESSURE DISTRIBUTION IN CHILDREN AND ADOLESCENTS

The first Task Force on Blood Pressure Control in Children and Adolescents established the importance of blood pressure in childhood as an indicator of health status. It provided a clear methodology for measurement of blood pressure in children and encouraged clinicians to measure blood pressure in the young. It also provided a definition of hypertension that could be applied to children. What was not clear was whether the blood pressure curves were an accurate reflection of the normative blood pressure distribution in healthy children. The National Heart, Lung, and Blood Institute recognized the need to obtain a larger body of data on blood pressure in the young within the context of childhood growth, and subsequently supported several epidemiological studies that prospectively investigated blood pressure and growth in children and adolescents. These projects were conducted at several sites, applied rigorous detail to the methodology of blood pressure measurement, and examined the anthropometric determinants of blood pressure level relative to physiological development.

As these data emerged, a second Task Force on Blood Pressure Control in Children and Adolescents was convened to reexamine the data on blood pressure distribution throughout childhood and prepare distribution curves of blood pressure by age accompanied by height and weight information (26). With this new information, the second Task Force also updated the guidelines for detection, evaluation, and management of hypertension in the young in its 1987 report. Table 2 provides the sites that contributed data that were used to develop the new blood pressure distribution curves. The total number of children on whom blood pressure data was available was over 60,000. This sample included an age range from infancy to 20 years with a substantial representation of different race and ethnic groups. The blood pressure percentile curves (27–40) published in the Second Task Force Report again demonstrated a progressive rise in blood pressure that was concurrent with age. Gender differences in blood pressure levels during adolescence were verified. The blood pressure in males continued to increase from age 13 through 18 years, whereas the blood pressure in females tended to plateau after age 13 years; and the normal distribution was some-

Table 2
Data Sources for the Second Task Force Report

Source	Age (years)	N
Muscatine, IA (27–29)	5–19	4,208
University of South Carolina (30)	4–20	6,657
University of Texas, Houston (31)	3–17	2,922
Bogalusa, LA (32,33)	1–20	16,442
Second National Health and Nutrition Examination Survey (34)	6–20	4,563
University of Texas, Dallas (35,36)	13–19	24,792
University of Pittsburgh (37)	Newborn–5	1,554
Providence, RI (38)	Newborn–3	3,487
Brompton, England (39,40)	Newborn–3	7,804

what higher in adolescent males compared to females. Moreover, the entire distribution was lower and consequently the 95th (and 90th) percentile delineated a level of blood pressure that was substantially lower than that described in the previous report. The Second Task Force Report applied the same definition of hypertension that was used in the First Task Force Report, which was systolic or diastolic blood pressure that was repeatedly equal to or greater than the 95th percentile. However, in consideration of how much lower the 95th percentile appeared to be at that time, along with the concern about possibly overdiagnosing hypertension in the young, this report included a classification table for *significant* and *severe* hypertension. According to age strata, the blood pressure values that approximated the 95th–99th percentiles were designated significant hypertension, and the blood pressure values that exceeded the 99th percentile were designated severe hypertension. At the time that report was developed, it could seem that the authors were hedging on the definition of hypertension in the young. However, by intention or not, the concept of staging hypertension, on the basis of degree of blood pressure elevation, was novel and had not yet been considered in the field of adult hypertension. It was not until publication of the Sixth Report of the Joint National Commission in 1998 *(10)* that hypertension stage was introduced as a method to guide in patient care and clinical management decisions in adults.

Subsequent to the 1987 Task Force Report, additional childhood blood pressure data were developed from the National Health and Nutrition Examination Survey III *(41)*. There was also reported evidence that children with elevated blood pressure in childhood often developed hypertension in early adulthood *(42)*. Based on increasing support for the concept that the origins of hypertension occurred in the young, rationale was developing for emphasis on blood pressure surveillance in the young, along with early preventive efforts. A reexamination of the national data on childhood blood pressure was necessary to provide substance to such recommendations. Therefore, a third Task Force was convened to update the normative data as well as the guidelines for management, including preventive guidelines.

The addition of the new blood pressure data and reanalysis of the entire childhood database resulted in blood pressure distribution curves that were slightly lower, but generally consistent with the findings of the second Task Force *(43)*. The third report, which was termed "Update on the 1987 Task Force Report," provided further detail on the relationship of body size to blood pressure. The contribution of body size was considered in the analysis that was conducted by the Second Task Force, as well as the analysis of the data from individual sites by the investigators who had developed the data. Analysis of that data indicated that height and body weight, as well as age, were major determinants of blood pressure. Height was considered to be the best determinant of blood pressure that was within the normal range. Therefore, it was recommended that height adjustment be applied in the evaluation of blood pressure level. To support this practice, the Second Task Force Report contained information on the 90th height percentile at the 90th percentile for blood pressure. It was assumed that pediatricians, who were accustomed to making weight for height adjustments, would be able to make the blood pressure adjustment for height. The third "Update" report expanded the presentation of the data by providing tables with the systolic and diastolic blood pressure levels at the 90th and 95th percentile for each height percentile and each age from 1 through 17 years. These tables provided a better view on the variation of blood pressure according to height as well as age.

The childhood blood pressure data were reexamined by a fourth Working Group that published expanded blood pressure percentile tables in 2004 *(44)*. These tables provide the sex, age, and height blood pressure levels for the 50th and 99th percentile as well as the 90th and 95th percentile. The intent of the Fourth Report was to provide additional guidelines in the detection and clinical management of childhood hypertension. The definition of hypertension in childhood remains the same; systolic and/or diastolic blood pressure ≥95th percentile verified on repeated measurement. This report provides additional precision in the staging of hypertension. Stage 1 hypertension is systolic or diastolic blood pressure between the 95th percentile and 5 mmHg above the 99th percentile. Stage 2 hypertension is defined as systolic or diastolic blood pressure that is greater than the 99th percentile plus 5 mmHg. The category of "high normal blood pressure" was replaced with a stage termed "prehypertension." Prehypertension is defined as systolic and/or diastolic blood pressure ≥90th percentile and <95th percentile. The definition of prehypertension in adults is systolic blood pressure between 120 and 139 mmHg or diastolic blood pressure between 80 and 89 mmHg *(14)*. In adolescence, beginning at age 12 years, the 90th percentile is higher than 120/80 mmHg. Therefore, to be consistent with the adult definition of prehypertension, prehypertension in adolescents is defined as blood pressure from 120/80 mmHg to <95th percentile. In this report, additional guidelines were provided for evaluation and treatment according to prehypertension, Stage 1 hypertension, and Stage 2 hypertension in childhood. Recommendations were also given on evaluation for other risk factors related to high blood pressure and for target organ damage.

Following publication of the Report of the Fourth Working Group, subsequent publications have reported data on the prevalence of hypertension based on these definitions. Hansen et al. *(45)* applied the above criteria for hypertension and prehypertension to electronic medical record data from well-child care visits in a cohort of over 14,000 primary care patients. With the advantage of data on repeat blood pressure measurements on separate visits, these investigators determined the prevalence of hypertension to be 3.6% and the prevalence of prehypertension to be 3.4% in children and adolescents between the age of 3 and 18 years. In a cross-sectional study limited to the adolescent age, the prevalence of prehypertension and hypertension was determined in a cohort of 6,790 high school students (11–17 years). Using the recommended repeated blood pressure measurements on those with an elevated initial blood pressure measurement, the prevalence of hypertension was 3.2% and the prevalence of prehypertension was 15.7% in adolescents *(46)*. In both reports the presence of obesity was associated with higher rates of high blood pressure. In the study on high school students by McNiece et al. *(46)*, the prevalence of hypertension and prehypertension combined was over 30% in obese boys and from 23 to 30% in obese girls depending on ethnicity.

A childhood obesity epidemic has been clearly established *(47)*. The association of overweight and obesity with higher blood pressure has been consistently demonstrated in children *(45,46,48)* as well as adults. Rosner et al. *(49)* reexamined the childhood blood pressure normative data based on normal weight children only, and found that the blood pressure percentile curves were only slightly lower, indicating that the sex-, age-, and height-adjusted percentile levels published in the Fourth Working Group report were not confounded by recent increases in the prevalence of childhood obesity. Therefore, the current criteria for high blood pressure in childhood provide important information on population trends in the prevalence of childhood hypertension. An analysis of the trends in childhood blood pressure from two sequential national cross-sectional studies identified a significant increase in both systolic and diastolic blood pressure. The blood pressure increase is most striking among minority groups that also have the highest rates of childhood obesity *(50)*. Another analysis on the same two data cohorts demonstrated an overall increase in the prevalence of hypertension from 2.7% in the 1988–1994 survey to 3.7% in the 1999–2002 survey period *(51)*. Both analyses verified that the population increase in blood pressure among children and adolescents is largely due to the increase in prevalence and severity of childhood obesity.

The current blood pressure norms are based on data that have been collected from over 70,000 children and adolescents using rigorous and quite uniform methodology. The population sample from which the data were obtained represents diverse race and ethnic groups from several areas of the USA. The analysis of this data and development of blood pressure norms provides a framework upon which to identify children and adolescents with hypertension and also to ascertain risk for future hypertension. Blood pressure reference values have also been reported in Northern Europe *(52)* and Asia *(53)*. These reports describe a slightly higher blood pressure level at the 95th percentile compared to the US data. However, all epidemiological reports on normative childhood blood pressure data demonstrate a consistent and significant relationship of blood pressure with age, height, and body weight throughout childhood.

The development of the childhood normative blood pressure data has been a process that has been underway for many years. The process has benefited by the additions of new information from other areas in the field of hypertension. The process itself has been informative. The current state of knowledge on blood pressure level and blood pressure criteria for hypertension in the young is the outcome of persistent inquiry by many thoughtful clinicians, of the clinical investigators who demanded accurate data on which to base definition, and of the skills of epidemiologists and biostatisticians who developed and analyzed the data. Consideration of the substantial progress which has occurred should provide encouragement to continue forward with the process.

REFERENCES

1. McCrory W, Nash FW. Hypertension in children: a review. Am J Med Sci. 1952;223:671–680.
2. Still JL, Cottom D. Severe hypertension in childhood. Arch Dis Child. 1967;42:34–39.
3. Loggie J. Essential hypertension in adolescents. Postgrad Med. 1974;56:133–141.
4. Masland RP Jr, Heald FP Jr, Goodale WT, Gallagher JR. Hypertensive vascular disease in adolescence. N Engl J Med. 1956;255:894–897.
5. Boe J, Humerfelt S, Wedervang F. The blood pressure in a population: blood pressure readings and height and weight determinations in the adult population of the city of Bergen. Acta Med Scand Suppl. 1957;321:1–336.
6. Heyden S, Bartel AG, Hames CG, McDonough JR. Elevated blood pressure levels in adolescents, Evans County, Georgia: seven year follow-up of 30 patients and 30 controls. JAMA. 1969;209:1683–1689.
7. Londe S. Blood pressure in children as determined under office conditions. Clin Pediatr. 1966;5:71–78.
8. Wilber JA, Millward D, Baldwin A, et al. Atlanta Community High Blood Pressure Program: methods of community hypertension screening. Circ Res. 1972;31(Suppl 2):101–109.
9. Master AM, Dublin LI, Marks HH. The normal blood pressure range and its clinical implications. JAMA. 1950;143:1464–1470.
10. Joint National Committee. The sixth report of the joint national committee on prevention, detection, evaluation and treatment of high blood pressure. Arch Intern Med. 1997;157:2413–2446.
11. McAlistar FA, Campbell NR, Zamke K, Levine M, Graham ID. The management of hypertension in Canada: a review of current guidelines, their shortcomings and implications. CMAJ. 2001;164:517–522.
12. Guidelines Subcommittee. 1999 World Health Organization—International Society of Hypertension Guidelines for the management of hypertension. J Hypertens. 1999;17:151–183.
13. Vasan RS, Larson MG, Leip MS, et al. Impact of high normal blood pressure on the risk of cardiovascular disease. N Engl J Med. 2001;345:1291–1297.
14. Chobanian AV, Bakris GL, Black HR, et al. The seventh report of the joint national committee on prevention, detection, evaluation, and treatment of high blood pressure: the JNC 7 report. JAMA. 2003;289:2560–2572.
15. Graham, AW, Hines EA, Gage RP. Blood pressures in children between the ages of five and sixteen years. Am J Dis Child. 1945;69:203.

16. Londe S. Blood pressure standards for normal children as determined under office conditions. Clin Pediatr. 1968;7:400–403.
17. U.S. Department of Health, Education, and Welfare. Public Health Service. Blood pressure levels of children 6–11 years: relationship to age, sex, race and socioeconomic status. Health and Vital Statistics. 1973;11:135.
18. Allen-Williams GM. Pulse-rate and blood pressure in infancy and early childhood. Arch Dis Child. 1945;20:125.
19. McLain LG. Hypertension in childhood: a review. Am Heart J. 1976;92:634–647.
20. Kilcoyne MM, Richter RW, Alsup PA. Adolescent hypertension. I. detection and prevalence. Circulation. 1974:50:758–764.
21. Kotchen JM, Kotchen TA, Schwertman NC, Kuller LH. Blood pressure distributions of urban adolescents. Am J Epidemiol. 1974;99:315–324.
22. Reichman LB, Cooper BM, Blumenthal S, et al. Bureau of Chronic Disease Control and Maternal and Child Health Services of the New York City Department of Health and the New York City Medical Advisory Committee on Hypertension, New York. Hypertension testing among high school students—surveillance procedures and results. J Chronic Dis. 1975;28:161–171.
23. Miller RA, Shekelle RB. Blood pressure in tenth grade students: results from the Chicago Heart Association Pediatric Heart Screening Project. Circulation. 1976;54:993–1000.
24. Garbus SB, Garbus SB, Young CJ, Hassinger G, Johnson W. Screening for hypertension in adolescents. South Med J. 1980;73:174–182.
25. NHLBI report of the task force on blood pressure control in children. Pediatrics. 1977;59(Suppl):797–820.
26. NHLBI report of the second task force on blood pressure control in children, task force on blood pressure control in children. Pediatrics. 1987;79:1–25.
27. Clarke WR, Schrott HG, Leaverton PE, Connor WE, Lauer RM. Tracking of blood lipids and blood pressure in school age children: the Muscatine study. Circulation. 1978;58:626–636.
28. Lauer RM, Clarke WR, Beaglehole R. Level, trend and variability of blood pressure during childhood: the Muscatine study. Circulation. 1984;69:242–249.
29. Lauer RM, Burns TL, Clarke WR. Assessing children's blood pressure—considerations of age and body size: the Muscatine study. Pediatrics. 1985;75:1081–1090.
30. Lackland DT, Riopel DA, Shepard DM, Wheeler FC. Blood Pressure and Anthropometric Measurement Results of the South Carolina Dental Health and Pediatric Blood Pressure Study. South Carolina Dental Health and Blood Pressure Study, January 1985.
31. Gutgesell M, Terrell G, LaBarthe DR. Pediatrics blood pressure: ethnic comparison in a primary care center. Hypertension. 1980;3:39–47.
32. Berenson GS, McMahan CA, Voors AW, et al. Cardiovascular Risk Factors in Children: The Early Natural History of Atherosclerosis and Essential Hypertension. New York, NY, Oxford University Press; 1980.
33. Voors AW, Foster TA, Frerichs RR, Webber LS, Berenson GS. Studies of blood pressure in children ages 5–14 years in a total biracial community: the Bogalusa Heart Study. Circulation. 1976;54:319–327.
34. McDowell A, Engel A, Massey J, Maurer KR. The Plan and Operation of the Second National Health and Nutrition Examination Survey, 1976–1980. Department of Health and Human Services Publication No. (PHS) 81-1317, series 1, No. 15. Government Printing Office, July 1981.
35. Fixler DE, Laird WP. Validity of mass blood pressure screening in children. Pediatrics. 1983;72:459–463.
36. Baron AE, Freyer B, Fixler DE. Longitudinal blood pressures in Blacks, Whites and Mexican Americans during adolescence and early adulthood. Am J Epidemiol. 1986;123:809–817.
37. Schachter J, Kuller LH, Perfetti C. Blood pressure during the first five years of life: relation to ethnic group (black or white) and to parental hypertension. Am J Epidemiol. 1984;119:541–553.
38. Zinner SH, Rosner B, Oh WO, Kass EH. Significance of blood pressure in infancy. Hypertension. 1985;7:411–416.
39. de Swiet M, Fayers P, Shinebourne EA. Blood pressure survey in a population of newborn Infants. Br Med J. 1976;2:9–11.
40. de Swiet M, Fayers P, Shinebourne EA. Systolic blood pressure in a population of infants in the first year of life: the Brompton study. Pediatrics. 1980;65:1028–1035.
41. Centers for Disease Control and Prevention, National Center for Health Statistics. National Health and Nutrition Survey (NHANES III), 1988–1991, Data Computed for the NHLBI. Atlanta, GA, Centers for Disease Control and Prevention.
42. Lauer RM, Clarke WR. Childhood risk factors for high adult blood pressure: the Muscatine study. Pediatrics. 1984;84:633–641.
43. Update on the 1987 Task Force Report on High Blood Pressure in Children and Adolescents: A Working Group Report from the National High Blood Pressure Education Program. Pediatrics. 1996;98:649–658.
44. National High Blood Pressure Education Program Working Group on High Blood Pressure in Children and Adolescents. The fourth report on the diagnosis, evaluation, and treatment of high blood pressure in children and adolescents. Pediatrics. 2004;114:555–576.

45. Hansen ML, Gunn PW, Kaelber DC. Underdiagnosis of hypertension in children and adolescents. JAMA. 2007;298:874–879.
46. McNiece KL, Poffenbarger TS, Turner JL, Franco KD, Sorof JM, Portman RJ. Prevalence of hypertension and pre-hypertension among adolescents. J Pediatr. 2007;150:640–644.
47. Ogden CL, Flegel KM, Carroll MD, Johnson CL. Prevalence and trends in overweight among US children and adolescents, 1999–2000. JAMA. 2002;288:1728–1732.
48. Falkner B, Gidding SS, Ramirez-Garnicia G, Armatti-Wiltrout S, West D, Rappaport EB. The relationship of body mass index with blood pressure in primary care pediatric patients. J Pediatr. 2006;148:195–200.
49. Rosner B, Cook N, Portman R, Daniels S, Falkner B. Determination of blood pressure percentiles in normal weight children: Some methodological issues. Am J Epidemiol. 2008;167:653–666.
50. Munter P, He J, Cutler JA, Wildman RP, Whelton PK. Trends in blood pressure among children and adolescents. JAMA. 2004;291:2107–2113.
51. Din-Dzietham R, Liu Y, Bielo M-V, Shamsa F. High blood pressure trends in children and adolescents in national surveys. 1963 to 2002. Circulation. 2007;116:1488–1496.
52. Munkhaugen J, Lydersen S, Wideroe T-E, Hallan S. Blood pressure reference values in adolescents: methodological aspects and suggestions for Northern Europe tables based on the Nord-Trondelag Health Study II. J Hypertens. 2008;26:1912–1918.
53. Sung RYT, Choi KC, So H-K, et al. Oscillometrically measured blood pressure in Hong Kong Chinese children and associations with anthropometric parameters. J Hypertens. 2008;26:678–684.

9 Definitions of Hypertension in Children

Karen McNiece Redwine, MD, MPH

Contents

INTRODUCTION

While noninvasive blood pressure (BP) measurement has been possible for over 100 years *(1)* and has become a routine part of clinical care for all children and adolescents, proper utilization of the information obtained by BP measurement remains an evolving process. This chapter will review a brief history of the recognition of hypertension (HTN) in children, currently accepted definitions of HTN for children and adolescents, strengths and limitations associated with these definitions, and considerations for further improving these definitions in the future.

HISTORICAL ASPECTS

As late as the 1940s, elevated BP was considered a natural response to improve circulation to major organ systems such as the heart, brain, and kidneys, and interfering with this so-called essential hypertension was believed to potentially cause more harm than

K.M. Redwine (✉)
Department of Pediatric Nephrology, University of Arkansas for Medical Sciences and Arkansas Children's
Hospital, Little Rock, AR, USA
e-mail: redwinekarenm@uams.edu

From: *Clinical Hypertension and Vascular Diseases: Pediatric Hypertension*
Edited by: J. T. Flynn et al. DOI 10.1007/978-1-60327-824-9_9
© Springer Science+Business Media, LLC 2011

good. President Franklin Delano Roosevelt who developed HTN in 1937 at the age of 55 was a typical example of those with untreated HTN during this era. He went on to develop left ventricular hypertrophy, congestive heart failure, multiple lacunar infarcts, and chronic kidney failure, ultimately dying from a cerebral hemorrhage just 8 years later *(2,3)*. While dramatic changes in the diagnosis and treatment of HTN in adults would occur over the next several decades, it was not for at least another quarter of a century that it was recognized that children might also have high BP.

One of the first investigators to be interested in childhood BP was Sol Londe, who measured BP in healthy children and noted an increase in BP relative to age, growth, and development *(4)*. He performed further analyses of the limited BP data available and described ranges of systolic and diastolic BP stratified by age as well as how children's BP tends to regress to the mean with repeated measurement. However, what was lacking at that time was a clear definition of what constituted elevated BP in children, which led to uncertainty over establishing the true prevalence of high BP in the pediatric population.

Recognizing the increased interest regarding BP in the pediatric age group, in 1977 the National Heart, Lung, and Blood Institute convened the First Task Force on Blood Pressure Control in Children *(5)* to provide specific guidelines to physicians and other healthcare providers involved in school- and community-based healthcare programs. Lacking good evidence, most of the recommendations for the diagnosis, evaluation, and management of children with elevated BP in this document were opinion based. However, this report did contain the first charts describing normal BP percentiles for children aged 2–18 years. Compiled from data collected at three centers on over 11,000 children, these charts would become the foundation for our current understanding of normal BP patterns in children. As new evidence and normative BP data have become available, these recommendations have been updated on three subsequent occasions, with the most recent report published in 2004 *(6)*. These consensus recommendations constitute the prevailing accepted criteria for diagnosing HTN in children not only in the United States but also throughout the world.

HYPERTENSION AS DEFINED BY CASUAL BLOOD PRESSURE MEASUREMENTS

Traditionally, the mainstay of the diagnosis of HTN has been based on office (or casual) BP measurements. While auscultatory methods using a mercury manometer are still considered the gold standard for BP measurement, advances in technology and environmental concerns regarding mercury toxicity have led to this procedure largely being replaced by automatic oscillometric techniques or auscultatory measurements using an aneroid sphygmomanometer. Although it is beyond the scope of this chapter to discuss the differences in these measurement techniques, it is important to keep these differences in mind when discussing definitions for childhood HTN, as the bulk of the normative BP data used to define BP in childhood were from studies that utilized mercury manometers.

Significant resources have been invested in understanding the short- and long-term effects of elevated BP, the thresholds at which significant morbidity and mortality related to high BP occur, and the benefits of therapy at various stages of this disease process in adults. This research forms the basis for the definitions used to diagnose HTN in adults and has most recently been summarized in the Seventh Report of the Joint National Committee on the Prevention, Detection, Evaluation, and Treatment of High Blood Pressure (JNC VII) *(7)*. Research attempting to define truly abnormal BP in children, however, is somewhat limited given the time that typically lapses between the development of elevated BP at a young age and morbid events such as myocardial infarction or stroke and the expense involved in conducting such a prolonged study.

Given the lack of such "hard" cardiovascular end points in children, a statistical approach *(8)* based upon the distribution of BP in childhood was adopted by Londe to define high BP in childhood. This approach was also incorporated into the first definitions of childhood HTN by the NHLBI Task Force *(5)* and has continued to be followed in all subsequent Task Force and Working Group reports. While the current consensus recommendations from the NHLBI Working Group *(6)* continue to be based on expert opinion, the normative data on childhood BP are now derived from over 83,000 measurements and therefore provide a much more stable definition of childhood HTN than had been possible in the past *(9)* (Tables 1 and 2). In the future, it may be possible to utilize the mounting evidence that elevated childhood BP is associated with early surrogate markers of target organ damage such as left ventricular hypertrophy and increased carotid artery intima–media thickness to develop evidence-based definitions of HTN in children and adolescents *(10,11)*.

Currently, children with a BP ≥95th percentile for age, gender, and height on three separate occasions should be classified as hypertensive and evaluation and management initiated as recommended (see Table 3). These measurements should be made using auscultatory methods (ideally with a mercury manometer) and Korotkoff sounds 1 and 5 used to define systolic and diastolic BP, respectively. Previous recommendations did suggest that the fourth Korotkoff sound be utilized for diastolic BP, as in some young children Kortokoff sounds can be heard down to 0 mmHg. However, to be consistent with adult recommendations, this is no longer recommended and instead an attempt should be made to repeat the BP reading using less pressure on the stethoscope. If the fifth Kortokoff sound still cannot be determined, the fourth sound should be recorded as diastolic BP for these individuals, with appropriate notation.

Elevation of either systolic or diastolic BP (or both) denotes the child as having high BP. It is also now recommended that HTN in children be staged to indicate the severity of BP elevation (Table 3). Children with a BP ≥95th percentile through the 99th percentile plus 5 mmHg should be classified as having Stage 1 HTN, while those with a BP ≥99th percentile plus 5 mmHg should be considered to have Stage 2 HTN and receive more immediate evaluation and management. It should be noted that the addition of 5 mmHg to the 99th percentile for staging was an arbitrary decision made by the most recent Working Group, who felt this would be appropriate due to the small difference (typically 7–9 mmHg) between the 95th and 99th percentiles *(6)*.

In addition, children and adolescents with a BP ≥90th percentile (or 120/80 when the 90th percentile exceeds this value) but <95th percentile should be considered prehypertensive. This is a new designation as of 2004 for the care of children with elevated BP and was not meant to be considered a diagnosis such as with HTN. Rather the goal of classifying children as prehypertensive is to identify those who may be at risk for development of HTN in the future in the hopes that lifestyle interventions might be instituted in order to prevent its development. Consequently, classifying a child as prehypertensive does not require three repeated measures across time as is required for a diagnosis of HTN.

There are a number of limitations to diagnosing HTN in this manner. First, it should be remembered that diagnosing HTN is dependent on the measurement techniques used to obtain these BP readings. Personnel must pay close attention to procedures used to measure BP to prevent misdiagnosing children with HTN based on erroneous measurements that could be obtained by using the wrong size BP cuff, improper patient positioning, and other common errors in BP measurement *(6)*. In addition, measuring BP in a clinical setting introduces the potential for a white coat effect (persistently elevated BP in a clinical setting

Table 1
Blood Pressure Levels for Boys by Age and Height Percentile[a]

Age (years)	BP Percentile ↓	Systolic BP (mmHg) ← Percentile of height →							Diastolic BP (mmHg) ← Percentile of height →						
		5th	10th	25th	50th	75th	90th	95th	5th	10th	25th	50th	75th	90th	95th
1	50th	80	81	83	85	87	88	89	34	35	36	37	38	39	39
	90th	94	95	97	99	100	102	103	49	50	51	52	53	53	54
	95th	98	99	101	103	104	106	106	54	54	55	56	57	58	58
	99th	105	106	108	110	112	113	114	61	62	63	64	65	66	66
2	50th	84	85	87	88	90	92	92	39	40	41	42	43	44	44
	90th	97	99	100	102	104	105	106	54	55	56	57	58	58	59
	95th	101	102	104	106	108	109	110	59	59	60	61	62	63	63
	99th	109	110	111	113	115	117	117	66	67	68	69	70	71	71
3	50th	86	87	89	91	93	94	95	44	44	45	46	47	48	48
	90th	100	101	103	105	107	108	109	59	59	60	61	62	63	63
	95th	104	105	107	109	110	112	113	63	63	64	65	66	67	67
	99th	111	112	114	116	118	119	120	71	71	72	73	74	75	75
4	50th	88	89	91	93	95	96	97	47	48	49	50	51	51	52
	90th	102	103	105	107	109	110	111	62	63	64	65	66	66	67
	95th	106	107	109	111	112	114	115	66	67	68	69	70	71	71
	99th	113	114	116	118	120	121	122	74	75	76	77	78	78	79
5	50th	90	91	93	95	96	98	98	50	51	52	53	54	55	55
	90th	104	105	106	108	110	111	112	65	66	67	68	69	69	70
	95th	108	109	110	112	114	115	116	69	70	71	72	73	74	74
	99th	115	116	118	120	121	123	123	77	78	79	80	81	81	82
6	50th	91	92	94	96	98	99	100	53	53	54	55	56	57	57
	90th	105	106	108	110	111	113	113	68	68	69	70	71	72	72
	95th	109	110	112	114	115	117	117	72	72	73	74	75	76	76
	99th	116	117	119	121	123	124	125	80	80	81	82	83	84	84
7	50th	92	94	95	97	99	100	101	55	55	56	57	58	59	59
	90th	106	107	109	111	113	114	115	70	70	71	72	73	74	74
	95th	110	111	113	115	117	118	119	74	74	75	76	77	78	78
	99th	117	118	120	122	124	125	126	82	82	83	84	85	86	86
8	50th	94	95	97	99	100	102	102	56	57	58	59	60	60	61
	90th	107	109	110	112	114	115	116	71	72	72	73	74	75	76
	95th	111	112	114	116	118	119	120	75	76	77	78	79	79	80
	99th	119	120	122	123	125	127	127	83	84	85	86	87	87	88
9	50th	95	96	98	100	102	103	104	57	58	59	60	61	61	62
	90th	109	110	112	114	115	117	118	72	73	74	75	76	76	77
	95th	113	114	116	118	119	121	121	76	77	78	79	80	81	81
	99th	120	121	123	125	127	128	129	84	85	86	87	88	88	89

Table 1
(continued)

Age (years)	BP Percentile ↓	Systolic BP (mmHg) ← Percentile of height →							Diastolic BP (mmHg) ← Percentile of height →						
		5th	10th	25th	50th	75th	90th	95th	5th	10th	25th	50th	75th	90th	95th
10	50th	97	98	100	102	103	105	106	58	59	60	61	61	62	63
	90th	111	112	114	115	117	119	119	73	73	74	75	76	77	78
	95th	115	116	117	119	121	122	123	77	78	79	80	81	81	82
	99th	122	123	125	127	128	130	130	85	86	86	88	88	89	90
11	50th	99	100	102	104	105	107	107	59	59	60	61	62	63	63
	90th	113	114	115	117	119	120	121	74	74	75	76	77	78	78
	95th	117	118	119	121	123	124	125	78	78	79	80	81	82	82
	99th	124	125	127	129	130	132	132	86	86	87	88	89	90	90
12	50th	101	102	104	106	108	109	110	59	60	61	62	63	63	64
	90th	115	116	118	120	121	123	123	74	75	75	76	77	78	79
	95th	119	120	122	123	125	127	127	78	79	80	81	82	82	83
	99th	126	127	129	131	133	134	135	86	87	88	89	90	90	91
13	50th	104	105	106	108	110	111	112	60	60	61	62	63	64	64
	90th	117	118	120	122	124	125	126	75	75	76	77	78	79	79
	95th	121	122	124	126	128	129	130	79	79	80	81	82	83	83
	99th	128	130	131	133	135	136	137	87	87	88	89	90	91	91
14	50th	106	107	109	111	113	114	115	60	61	62	63	64	65	65
	90th	120	121	123	125	126	128	128	75	76	77	78	79	79	80
	95th	124	125	127	128	130	132	132	80	80	81	82	83	84	84
	99th	131	132	134	136	138	139	140	87	88	89	90	91	92	92
15	50th	109	110	112	113	115	117	117	61	62	63	64	65	66	66
	90th	122	124	125	127	129	130	131	76	77	78	79	80	80	81
	95th	126	127	129	131	133	134	135	81	81	82	83	84	85	85
	99th	134	135	136	138	140	142	142	88	89	90	91	92	93	93
16	50th	111	112	114	116	118	119	120	63	63	64	65	66	67	67
	90th	125	126	128	130	131	133	134	78	78	79	80	81	82	82
	95th	129	130	132	134	135	137	137	82	83	83	84	85	86	87
	99th	136	137	139	141	143	144	145	90	90	91	92	93	94	94
17	50th	114	115	116	118	120	121	122	65	66	66	67	68	69	70
	90th	127	128	130	132	134	135	136	80	80	81	82	83	84	84
	95th	131	132	134	136	138	139	140	84	85	86	87	87	88	89
	99th	139	140	141	143	145	146	147	92	93	93	94	95	96	97

BP, blood pressure.

[a]To use the table, first plot the child's height on a standard growth curve (www.cdc.gov/growthcharts). The child's measured SBP and DBP are compared with the numbers provided in the table according to the child's age and height percentile.

Reproduced from *(6)*.

Table 2
Blood Pressure Levels for Girls by Age and Height Percentile[a]

Age (years)	BP Percentile ↓	Systolic BP (mmHg) ← Percentile of height →							Diastolic BP (mmHg) ← Percentile of height →						
		5th	10th	25th	50th	75th	90th	95th	5th	10th	25th	50th	75th	90th	95th
1	50th	83	84	85	86	88	89	90	38	39	39	40	41	41	42
	90th	97	97	98	100	101	102	103	52	53	53	54	55	55	56
	95th	100	101	102	104	105	106	107	56	57	57	58	59	59	60
	99th	108	108	109	111	112	113	114	64	64	65	65	66	67	67
2	50th	85	85	87	88	89	91	91	43	44	44	45	46	46	47
	90th	98	99	100	101	103	104	105	57	58	58	59	60	61	61
	95th	102	103	104	105	107	108	109	61	62	62	63	64	65	65
	99th	109	110	111	112	114	115	116	69	69	70	70	71	72	72
3	50th	86	87	88	89	91	92	93	47	48	48	49	50	50	51
	90th	100	100	102	103	104	106	106	61	62	62	63	64	64	65
	95th	104	104	105	107	108	109	110	65	66	66	67	68	68	69
	99th	111	111	113	114	115	116	117	73	73	74	74	75	76	76
4	50th	88	88	90	91	92	94	94	50	50	51	52	52	53	54
	90th	101	102	103	104	106	107	108	64	64	65	66	67	67	68
	95th	105	106	107	108	110	111	112	68	68	69	70	71	71	72
	99th	112	113	114	115	117	118	119	76	76	76	77	78	79	79
5	50th	89	90	91	93	94	95	96	52	53	53	54	55	55	56
	90th	103	103	105	106	107	109	109	66	67	67	68	69	69	70
	95th	107	107	108	110	111	112	113	70	71	71	72	73	73	74
	99th	114	114	116	117	118	120	120	78	78	79	79	80	81	81
6	50th	91	92	93	94	96	97	98	54	54	55	56	56	57	58
	90th	104	105	106	108	109	110	111	68	68	69	70	70	71	72
	95th	108	109	110	111	113	114	115	72	72	73	74	74	75	76
	99th	115	116	117	119	120	121	122	80	80	80	81	82	83	83
7	50th	93	93	95	96	97	99	99	55	56	56	57	58	58	59
	90th	106	107	108	109	111	112	113	69	70	70	71	72	72	73
	95th	110	111	112	113	115	116	116	73	74	74	75	76	76	77
	99th	117	118	119	120	122	123	124	81	81	82	82	83	84	84
8	50th	95	95	96	98	99	100	101	57	57	57	58	59	60	60
	90th	108	109	110	111	113	114	114	71	71	71	72	73	74	74
	95th	112	112	114	115	116	118	118	75	75	75	76	77	78	78
	99th	119	120	121	122	123	125	125	82	82	83	83	84	85	86
9	50th	96	97	98	100	101	102	103	58	58	58	59	60	61	61
	90th	110	110	112	113	114	116	116	72	72	72	73	74	75	75
	95th	114	114	115	117	118	119	120	76	76	76	77	78	79	79
	99th	121	121	123	124	125	127	127	83	83	84	84	85	86	87

Table 2
(continued)

Age (years)	BP Percentile ↓	Systolic BP (mmHg)							Diastolic BP (mmHg)						
		← Percentile of height →							← Percentile of height →						
		5th	10th	25th	50th	75th	90th	95th	5th	10th	25th	50th	75th	90th	95th
10	50th	98	99	100	102	103	104	105	59	59	59	60	61	62	62
	90th	112	112	114	115	116	118	118	73	73	73	74	75	76	76
	95th	116	116	117	119	120	121	122	77	77	77	78	79	80	80
	99th	123	123	125	126	127	129	129	84	84	85	86	86	87	88
11	50th	100	101	102	103	105	106	107	60	60	60	61	62	63	63
	90th	114	114	116	117	118	119	120	74	74	74	75	76	77	77
	95th	118	118	119	121	122	123	124	78	78	78	79	80	81	81
	99th	125	125	126	128	129	130	131	85	85	86	87	87	88	89
12	50th	102	103	104	105	107	108	109	61	61	61	62	63	64	64
	90th	116	116	117	119	120	121	122	75	75	75	76	77	78	78
	95th	119	120	121	123	124	125	126	79	79	79	80	81	82	82
	99th	127	127	128	130	131	132	133	86	86	87	88	88	89	90
13	50th	104	105	106	107	109	110	110	62	62	62	63	64	65	65
	90th	117	118	119	121	122	123	124	76	76	76	77	78	79	79
	95th	121	122	123	124	126	127	128	80	80	80	81	82	83	83
	99th	128	129	130	132	133	134	135	87	87	88	89	89	90	91
14	50th	106	106	107	109	110	111	112	63	63	63	64	65	66	66
	90th	119	120	121	122	124	125	125	77	77	77	78	79	80	80
	95th	123	123	125	126	127	129	129	81	81	81	82	83	84	84
	99th	130	131	132	133	135	136	136	88	88	89	90	90	91	92
15	50th	107	108	109	110	111	113	113	64	64	64	65	66	67	67
	90th	120	121	122	123	125	126	127	78	78	78	79	80	81	81
	95th	124	125	126	127	129	130	131	82	82	82	83	84	85	85
	99th	131	132	133	134	136	137	138	89	89	90	91	91	92	93
16	50th	108	108	110	111	112	114	114	64	64	65	66	66	67	68
	90th	121	122	123	124	126	127	128	78	78	79	80	81	81	82
	95th	125	126	127	128	130	131	132	82	82	83	84	85	85	86
	99th	132	133	134	135	137	138	139	90	90	90	91	92	93	93
17	50th	108	109	110	111	113	114	115	64	65	65	66	67	67	68
	90th	122	122	123	125	126	127	128	78	79	79	80	81	81	82
	95th	125	126	127	129	130	131	132	82	83	83	84	85	85	86
	99th	133	133	134	136	137	138	139	90	90	91	91	92	93	93

BP, blood pressure.

[a]To use the table, first plot the child's height on a standard growth curve (www.cdc.gov/growthcharts). The child's measured SBP and DBP are compared with the numbers provided in the table according to the child's age and height percentile.

Reproduced from *(6)*.

Table 3
Classification of Casual BP in Children and Adults

HTN classification	2004 Working Group (percentile)	JNC VII (mmHg)
Normotensive	<90th	<120/80
Prehypertensive	90th to <95th or if BP ≥120/80 mmHg even if <90th	120–139/80–89
Stage 1 HTN	95th–99th + 5 mmHg (at three separate visits)	140–159/90–99
Stage 2 HTN	>99th + 5 mmHg (at three separate visits)	≥160/100

HTN, Hypertension

with normal BP in other environments) and may miss children with elevated BP at other times of the day such as in the case of those with isolated nocturnal HTN which may occur with sleep apnea or other chronic medical conditions. It should also be noted that BP is a dynamic process that is constantly changing and that any one BP represents only a small snapshot of the larger process. Thus, many practitioners routinely obtain multiple readings not only across time as recommended by the Working Group but also at any one given office visit. BP readings tend to fall with this approach as a result of both an accommodation effect and a regression to the mean.

This natural variation in BP creates another challenge in defining HTN according to the Working Group guidelines. Classifying hypertensive individuals as Stage 1 or Stage 2 may be difficult as BP can shift across these categories between measurement sessions. In fact, a recent study by McNiece et al. *(12)* showed that only 56% of hypertensive students in a school-based screening had a BP that was classified in the same category on all three required visits. There are no current recommendations from the Working Group on how to address this variability when classifying patients. However, in this study, there was little difference in the ultimate classification of students with Stage 1 versus Stage 2 HTN when staged according to three different possible criteria: (1) BP stage most frequently observed across the three measurement sessions, (2) mean of all BP readings across the three measurement sessions, and (3) stage of BP at final screening.

The same variability is also present when considering BP in the prehypertensive range. Acosta et al. showed that among students in a school screening setting with a mean BP ≥90th percentile (or 120/80) on three separate visits not meeting criteria for confirmed HTN, only 35% were prehypertensives at all three visits *(13)*. The rest fell in the hypertensive range at least once. Another 151 students (out of 1,010 participating) had an elevated BP that subsequently normalized. Understanding what the variability of BP in this range means may ultimately be even more important than understanding BP variability in the hypertensive range as the risk associated with different variability patterns for the development of HTN does not appear to be equal *(14)*. In addition, there may be a subgroup of those with prehypertension who already exhibit target organ abnormalities and thus may not be appropriately classified *(15)*.

Finally, it must be remembered that the normative BP values utilized by the Working Group in forming their recommendations were generated from a population of children and adolescents from the United States and may not be representative of other populations around the world. There have been a number of additional series of "normal values" published in other populations. Some including pooled data from across Europe of 28,043 children *(16)* and another series of 11,519 Italian children *(17)* utilized auscultatory methods, while more recent surveys collected in northern Europe *(18)* and Hong

Kong Chinese children *(19)* have attempted to generate oscillometric norms. None of these series however contain sample sizes comparable to the large database utilized to generate the Working Group charts, and so they currently remain the primary reference used throughout the world, recognizing that there may be potential limitations when applied to non-American children.

HYPERTENSION AS DEFINED BY AMBULATORY BLOOD PRESSURE MEASUREMENTS

Ambulatory BP monitoring provides a technique for assessing BP that addresses many of the limitations of casual BP measurements noted above. Typically worn for 24 hours, these monitors are programmed to measure BP at regular intervals (every 15–30 min) while an individual continues to perform all of his/her normal activities. Thus, this monitoring technique gathers enough data to portray the "bigger picture" of an individual's BP allowing for a better description of BP variability within that individual's natural environment. A number of auscultatory and oscillometric ambulatory devices are available, although only a few have been independently validated in a pediatric population *(20–23)*.

Normal values for ambulatory monitoring have been generated from healthy populations of children as was done for casual measurements. The most commonly referenced are those generated from a population of 1,141 German children in 1997 *(24)*. Several years later, these data were reanalyzed to account for the non-normality of some of the BP curves likely related to the small sample size of the study *(25)*. These "LMS transformed" BP normal values are likely superior to the original normal values published by this group and have been recommended as the best currently available data for interpreting ambulatory BP monitoring studies *(26)*. Several different outcomes, including mean BP for the entire 24 h or for separate awake and sleep periods, can ultimately be assessed using ambulatory monitoring. And as with casual measurements, a mean BP ≥95th percentile is typically considered abnormal except among special at-risk populations when the 90th percentile is considered more appropriate. In addition, several other outcomes such as BP load (percentage of time BP is elevated) and percent fall in BP at night may be used by some to diagnose HTN via ambulatory monitoring. A recent consensus report on pediatric ambulatory BP monitoring from the American Heart Association has proposed standard definitions for normal and abnormal ambulatory BP *(26)* which incorporates several of these different parameters.

As with casual measurements, there are limitations in utilizing ambulatory BP monitoring to diagnose HTN. Chief among these limitations is that the most widely utilized normal ambulatory BP values were generated from a racial/ethnically nondiverse population, and may therefore not be applicable to more diverse populations. Also, substantially fewer children were included in this analysis compared to that for the normal values for casual measurements. Ambulatory normal values were generated using an oscillometric device. There is little difference noted in diastolic BP with increasing height in these BP curves as is seen for systolic BP. Whether this is related to a limitation in the monitor's ability to measure diastolic BP or an insufficient sample size to accurately define these differences is not known. In addition, whether these normal values can be applied to measurements obtained using auscultatory monitors or other oscillometric monitors, given the proprietary differences between manufacturers *(27)* for calculations used to determine systolic and diastolic BP from the mean arterial BP measured by the oscillometric monitor, is also unknown.

Although use of ambulatory monitoring in children as young as 2 years has been reported, it is typically not useful in children under 5 years of age because of their ability to comply with the procedure. Equipment is also expensive and several key parameters for interpreting ambulatory BP monitoring such as the minimal time and number of readings required for a monitoring report to be considered complete have not been standardized by experts in the field although the recent recommendations published by the American Heart Association *(26)* should help with this. For these reasons, ambulatory BP monitoring is still only recommended for routine use by experts in the field of pediatric hypertension.

Despite these limitations, ambulatory BP monitoring correlates to early target organ damage such as left ventricular hypertrophy *(28–30)* more closely than casual measurements just as it predicts long-term cardiovascular outcomes in adults *(31–34)*.

COMBINING CASUAL AND AMBULATORY BLOOD PRESSURE MEASUREMENTS

Considering both casual and ambulatory BP measurements together provides a more powerful means of diagnosing HTN. With this approach, four different diagnoses become possible (Table 4). True HTN and true normotension are conditions in which casual and ambulatory measurements agree. Alternatively, white coat HTN is a condition in which casual measurements are consistently elevated while ambulatory measurements are normal, and masked HTN is the inverse condition in which casual measurements are normal but ambulatory measurements are elevated. Recent recommendations for the clinical diagnosis of these conditions are summarized in Table 5.

White Coat Hypertension

White coat HTN is a commonly recognized condition and has a reported prevalence of 1.2–62% of children and adolescents *(35–38)*. This large variation is likely due to differences used to define abnormal BP by both casual and ambulatory means. Its true prevalence is likely closer to 20% as is seen in adult populations *(39)*. While white coat HTN was originally thought to be a benign condition, emerging evidence suggests that it may be at the least a prehypertensive state.

In adults, Verdecchia et al. *(40)* showed that the risk for stroke among adults with confirmed HTN is twice that for those with white coat HTN and normotension at 6 years. However, after 9 years, the risk for stroke among those with baseline white coat HTN exceeded those with ambulatory HTN, suggesting that many of these individuals will go

Table 4
Combining Casual and Ambulatory BP Measurements

		Casual BP measurements	
		Normal	*Elevated*
Ambulatory BP measurements	Normal	Normotension	White coat HTN
	Elevated	Masked HTN	HTN

BP, Blood pressure

Table 5
Suggested Schema for Staging of Ambulatory BP Levels in Children

Classification	Clinic BP[a] (percentile)	Mean ambulatory SBP[b] (percentile)	SBP load (%)
Normal BP	<95th	<95th	<25
White coat HTN	>95th	<95th	<25
Masked HTN	<95th	>95th	>25
Prehypertension	>95th	<95th	25–50
Ambulatory HTN	>95th	>95th	25–50
Severe ambulatory HTN (at risk for end-organ damage)	>95th	>95th	>50

Adapted from Urbina et al. *(26)*.

[a]Based on the National High Blood Pressure Education Program Task Force Standards.

[b]Based on ABPM values of Soergel et al. or the smoothed values of Wuhl.

on to develop significant hypertensive disease. Although studies in children have not consistently demonstrated a relationship between white coat HTN and target organ damage such as left ventricular hypertrophy and increased carotid artery intima–media thickness, several recent reports have reported a trend in increasing left ventricular mass index among adolescents with white coat HTN when compared to those with normal BP *(29,38,41,42)*. Thus, until further evidence is available, counseling children with white coat HTN and their parents regarding lifestyle changes to prevent the future development of HTN and closely monitoring BP, possibly with repeat ambulatory BP monitoring, is likely prudent *(11)*.

Masked Hypertension

Masked HTN was only recently described but has now been clearly documented in several pediatric populations occurring at a rate of 7.6–11% *(35,38,43)*. Adults with masked HTN have a similar risk for long-term cardiovascular morbidity as those with confirmed HTN *(44)*. In addition, children with masked HTN have a similar left ventricular mass index as their hypertensive counterparts *(29,35,38)*. Diagnosing masked HTN, though, is clearly a challenge as these children have a normal clinic BP and there are no other clearly identified characteristics of this condition to help decide which children should be screened for it. Developing approaches to identify these children, however, will likely be critical in preventing long-term cardiovascular morbidity and mortality.

FUTURE DEFINITIONS OF HYPERTENSION

As discussed above, the most significant weakness of essentially all currently accepted definitions for HTN in children is their dependence on normal values generated from a "healthy" population. In contrast, definitions for HTN in adults are based on multiple long-term studies, showing an increased risk of cardiovascular morbidity and mortality in those with an elevated BP. In children, however, these definite cardiovascular outcomes (such as myocardial infarction and stroke) do not typically occur until many years after the development of HTN. Thus, recent studies in children have focused on surrogate measures of cardiovascular morbidity such as left ventricular hypertrophy and increased carotid artery intima–media thickness, both of which are now well-established cardiovascular abnormalities seen in hypertensive adolescents. Refining definitions for HTN based on these measurable cardiovascular abnormalities will be crucial if a diagnosis of HTN in childhood is utilized to make interventions designed to reduce long-term cardiovascular morbidity and mortality. Indeed, some authors have recently advocated a more aggressive approach to childhood BP based upon the data on surrogate markers already available *(10)*.

One interesting example of an attempt to generate evidence-based interventions to reduce the sequelae of childhood HTN is the ESCAPE trial, a large multicenter study conducted in Europe on the effects of different levels of BP control on the progression of chronic kidney disease *(45)*. In this study, Wuhl et al. showed that controlling BP in a group of 3–18-year olds with chronic kidney disease to below the 50th percentile by ambulatory monitoring slowed their decline in renal function when compared to those whose BP was maintained between the 50th and 95th percentile. This goal for BP control is clearly much lower than the currently recommended target of the 90th percentile for children with chronic kidney disease *(6)*.

Similar studies are needed for defining prehypertension aimed at determining exactly which children are at risk for the more immediate development of confirmed HTN. Recent evidence suggests that current definitions for prehypertension may not be adequately identifying all those at risk. In a recent study of 1,006 adolescents *(14)*, those with a baseline mean BP that was initially ≥95th percentile but who normalized to <90th percentile on subsequent measurement sessions had a sixfold increased rate for the development of HTN when compared to those with a normal BP at baseline. These are children who are currently considered normotensive by Working Group definitions.

In conclusion, our ability to diagnose HTN and early cardiovascular disease in children has progressed substantially over the last 40 years. However, there are still many unanswered questions that must be addressed in order to achieve evidence-based definitions that will accurately identify all those with an increased risk for cardiovascular events and provide therapeutic goals which will decrease this risk.

REFERENCES

1. Booth J. A short history of blood pressure measurement. Proc R Soc Med. 1977;70:793–799.
2. Moser M. Evolution of the treatment of hypertension from the 1940s to JNC V. Am J Hypertens. 1997;10:2S–8S.
3. Messerli FH. This day 50 years ago. N Engl J Med. 1995;332:1038–1039.
4. Londe S. Blood pressure standards for normal children as determined under office conditions. Clin Pediatr (Phila). 1968;7:400–403.
5. Blumenthal S, Epps RP, Heavenrich R, et al. Report of the task force on blood pressure control in children. Pediatrics. 1977;59:797–820.
6. National High Blood Pressure Education Program Working Group on High Blood Pressure in Children and Adolescents. The fourth report on the diagnosis, evaluation, and treatment of high blood pressure in children and adolescents. National Heart, Lung, and Blood Institute, Bethesda, Maryland. National Institute of Health, NIH publication. 05:5267, 2005.
7. Chobanian AV, Bakris GL, Black HR, et al. The seventh report of the joint national committee on prevention, detection, evaluation, and treatment of high blood pressure: the JNC 7 report. JAMA. 2003;289:2560–2572.
8. Master AM, Dublin LI, Marks HH. The normal blood pressure range and its clinical implications. JAMA. 1950;143:1464–1470.

9. Falkner B. What exactly do the trends mean? Circulation. 2007;116:1437–1439.
10. Collins RT 2nd, Alpert BS. Pre-hypertension and hypertension in pediatrics: don't let the statistics hide the pathology. J Pediatr. 2009;155:165–169.
11. Flynn JT, Falkner BE. Should the current approach to the evaluation and treatment of high blood pressure in children be changed? J Pediatr. 2009;155:157–158.
12. McNiece KL, Poffenbarger TS, Turner JL, et al. Prevalence of hypertension and pre-hypertension among adolescents. J Pediatr. 2007;150:640–644.
13. Acosta AA, Samuels JA, Portma RJ, et al. Prevalence of persistent pre-hypertension in adolescents. [abstract] E-PAS. 2008:4493.3, 2008.
14. McNiece KL, Acosta AA, Poffenbarger T, et al. Incident hypertension in adolescents. [abstract] E-PAS 2008:5355.1, 2008.
15. Stabouli S, Kotsis V, Rizos Z, et al. Left ventricular mass in normotensive, prehypertensive, and hypertensive children and adolescents. Pediatr Nephrol. 2009;24:1545–1551.
16. de Man SA, Andre JL, Bachmann HJ, et al. Blood pressure in childhood: pooled findings of six European studies. J Hypertens. 1991;9:109–114.
17. Menghetti E, Virdis R, Strambi M, et al. Blood pressure in childhood and adolescence: the Italian normal standards. Study Group on Hypertension of the Italian Society of Pediatrics. J Hypertens. 1999;17: 1363–1372.
18. Munkhaugen J, Lydersen S, Widerow TE, et al. Blood pressure reference values in adolescents: methodological aspects and suggestions for Northern Europe tables based on the North Trondelag Health Study II. J Hypertens. 2008;26:1912–1918.
19. Sung RY, Choi KC, So HK, et al. Oscillometrically measured blood pressure in Hong Kong Chinese children and associations with anthropometric parameters. J Hypertens. 2008;26:678–684.
20. Belsha CW, Wells TG, Rice HB, et al. Accuracy of the Spacelabs 90207 ambulatory blood pressure monitor in children and adolescents. Blood Press Monit. 1996;1:127–133.
21. Jones DP, Richey PA, Alpert BS. Validation of the AM5600 ambulatory blood pressure monitor in children and adolescents. Blood Press Monit. 2008;13:349–351.
22. Modesti PA, Costoli A, Cecioni I, et al. Clinical evaluation of the QuietTrak blood pressure recorder according to the protocol of the British Hypertension Society. Blood Press Monit. 1996;1:63–68.
23. O'Sullivan JJ, Derrick G, Griggs PE, et al. Validation of the Takeda 2421 ambulatory blood pressure monitor in children. J Med Eng Technol. 1998;22:101–105.
24. Soergel M, Kirschstein M, Busch C, et al. Oscillometric twenty-four-hour ambulatory blood pressure values in healthy children and adolescents: a multicenter trial including 1141 subjects. J Pediatr. 1997;130:178–184.
25. Wuhl E, Witte K, Soergel M, et al. Distribution of 24-h ambulatory blood pressure in children: normalized reference values and role of body dimensions. J Hypertens. 2002;20:1995–2007.
26. Urbina E, Alpert B, Flynn J, et al. Ambulatory blood pressure monitoring in children and adolescents: recommendations for standard assessment. A scientific statement from the American Heart Association Atherosclerosis, Hypertension, and Obesity in Youth Committee of the Council on Cardiovascular Disease in the Young and the Council for High Blood Pressure Research. Hypertension. 2008;52: 433–451.
27. Butani L, Morganstern BZ. Are pitfalls of oscillometric blood pressure measurements preventable in children? Pediatr Nephrol. 2003;18:313–318.
28. Belsha CW, Wells TG, McNiece KL, et al. Influence of diurnal blood pressure variations on target organ abnormalities in adolescents with mild essential hypertension. Am J Hypertens. 1998;11:410–417.
29. McNiece KL, Gupta-Malhotra M, Samuels J, et al. Left ventricular hypertrophy in hypertensive adolescents: analysis of risk by 2004 national high blood pressure education program working group staging criteria. Hypertension. 2007;50:392–395.
30. Sorof JM, Cardwell G, Franco K, et al. Ambulatory blood pressure and left ventricular mass index in hypertensive children. Hypertension. 2002;39:903–908.
31. Verdecchia P, Porcellati C, Schillaci G, et al. Ambulatory blood pressure. An independent predictor of prognosis in essential hypertension. Hypertension. 1994;24:793–801.
32. Redon J, Campos C, Narciso ML, et al. Prognostic value of ambulatory blood pressure monitoring in refractory hypertension: a prospective study. Hypertension 1998; 21:712–718.
33. Staessen JA, Thijs L, Fagard R, et al. Predicting cardiovascular risk using conventional vs ambulatory blood pressure in older patients with systolic hypertension. Systolic Hypertension in Europe Trial Investigators. JAMA. 1999;282:539–546.
34. Metoki H, Ohtubo T, Kikuya M, et al. Prognostic significance of night-time, early morning, and daytime blood pressure on the risk for cerebrovascular and cardiovascular mortality: the Ohasama Study. J Hypertens. 2006;24:1841–1848.

35. Lurbe E, Torro I, Alvarez V, et al. Prevalence, persistence, and clinical significance of masked hypertension in youth. Hypertension. 2005;45:493–498.
36. Matsuoka S, Kawamura K, Honda M, et al. White coat effect and white coat hypertension in pediatric patients. Pediatr Nephrol. 2002;17:950–953.
37. Sorof JM, Portman RJ. White coat hypertension in children with elevated casual blood pressure. J Pediatr. 2000;137:493–497.
38. Stabouli S, Kotsis V, Toumanidis S. White-coat and masked hypertension in children: association with target-organ damage. Pediatr Nephrol. 2005;20:1151–1155.
39. O'Brien E. Is the case for ABPM as a routine investigation in clinical practice not overwhelming? Hypertension. 2007;50:284–286.
40. Verdecchia P, Reboldi GP, Angeli F, et al. Short- and long-term incidence of stroke in white-coat hypertension. Hypertension. 2005;45:203–208.
41. Kavey RE, Kveselis DA, Atallah N, Smith FC. White coat hypertension in childhood: evidence for end-organ effect. J Pediatr. 2007;150:491–497.
42. Lande MB, Meagher CC, Fisher SG, et al. Left ventricular mass index in children with white coat hypertension. J Pediatr. 2008;153:50–54.
43. Matsuoka S, Awazu M. Masked hypertension in children and young adults. Pediatr Nephrol. 2004;19: 651–654.
44. Pickering TG, Eguchi K, Kario K. Masked hypertension: a review. Hypertens Res. 2007;30:479–488.
45. Wuhl E, Trivelli A, Picca S, et al. ESCAPE Trial Group. Strict blood-pressure control and progression of renal failure in children. N Engl J Med. 2009;361:1639–1650.

10

Ambulatory Blood Pressure Monitoring Methodology and Norms in Children

Elke Wühl, MD

INTRODUCTION

In recent years ambulatory blood pressure monitoring (ABPM) has become the method of choice for the diagnosis and therapeutic monitoring of arterial hypertension in pediatric as well as in adult patients *(1–5)*. ABPM permits a more representative observation of blood pressure (BP) throughout day and night in a non-medical environment. Moreover, ABPM allows to quantify the circadian and even ultradian BP variability *(6–8)*.

While in adult patients ABPM confers a superior prognostic value for end-organ damage as compared to casual blood pressure measurements *(9–12)*, clinical endpoint assessments are still lacking for childhood-onset hypertension. Therefore, while fixed, risk-adapted cut-off levels for optimal, normal, high normal, and elevated blood pressure (BP) have been defined for the adult population *(13,14)*, pediatric targets are derived from the distribution of BP in the general pediatric population.

Although ABPM is widely used in children, there are still some open issues concerning normative data sets in infants and younger children, optimization of protocols for monitoring BP and data analysis, and appropriate validation of devices for use in the pediatric population.

E. Wühl (✉)
Division of Pediatric Nephrology, Center for Pediatrics and Adolescent Medicine, University Hospital Heidelberg,
Heidelberg, Germany
e-mail: elke.wuehl@med.uni-heidelberg.de

From: *Clinical Hypertension and Vascular Diseases: Pediatric Hypertension*
Edited by: J. T. Flynn et al. DOI 10.1007/978-1-60327-824-9_10
© Springer Science+Business Media, LLC 2011

METHODS FOR MEASURING AMBULATORY BLOOD PRESSURE

ABPM Monitors

Recommendations for the use of ABPM are included in all recent guidelines for diagnosis and treatment of high blood pressure in adults as well as in children *(13–16)*. However, some of the recommendations made for adults are not easily transferable to pediatrics.

The equipment tested and approved for adults is often not explicitly validated for use in children. The ideal device should be validated for measurements in children, lightweight, equipped with small cuff sizes starting from the infant range, and should have a robust hardware and software suitable for use in physically active children without producing too many erroneous measurements *(17)*.

As for casual BP measurements, the cuff width should cover at least 40%, and the cuff length 80–100%, of the upper arm circumference *(16)*. Cuffs are available starting from neonate size; however, validation data for this age range are missing. Standard cuff sizes for the use in infants start at 12 cm upper arm circumference. These will allow ABPM measurements from the age of 6 months onward. Measurements in infants below 2 years of age are feasible, and the number of erroneous measurements seems to be even lower than in the 3- to 5-year olds *(18,19)*, possibly due to greater physical activity and lower acceptance of the measurement procedure in preschool age. However, normative data sets for infancy are still restricted to small sample sizes *(18,19)*.

Regarding measurement technology, both auscultatory and oscillometric ABPM devices are available. The limitations of both methods are comparable to those described for casual BP devices *(16,20)*: Auscultatory ABPM devices are better graded regarding accuracy and durability according to national US (AAMI *(21)*) and British protocols (BHS *(22)*). Nevertheless, measurements are more prone to movement artifacts and the controversy which Korotkoff sound more accurately defines diastole (K4 vs. K5) has not been uniformly solved by the manufacturers. Moreover, comprehensive normative data for auscultatory ABPM devices are lacking. Oscillometric devices usually have less erroneous measurements than auscultatory devices (4 vs. 30% of measurements *(23)*) and are easier to use, although grading according to AAMI or BHS standard protocols is lower. Systole and diastole are not measured directly but are derived mathematically from mean arterial pressure by device-specific algorithms; as a result differences between oscillometric measurements and auscultatory devices used for validation are common *(20)*. However, most normative ABPM values published are oscillometric data *(3,18,19,24–26)*, and oscillometric devices are widely used in pediatric hypertension clinics.

Information on currently available ABPM monitors that have undergone independent testing and passed national standards (AAMI or BHS) is provided by the web site www.dableducational.org or the respective web sites of the national hypertension leagues (e.g., American Society of Hypertension, British Hypertension Society, Deutsche Hochdruckliga). Only devices that passed these tests should be used.

The software equipment of the monitors is variable. As a minimum requirement the frequency of measurements should be programmable and the software should allow entering pediatric 95th percentile cutoffs (*(24,25)*, see Table 1). The mean 24-h, daytime, and nighttime systolic, diastolic, and mean arterial pressure as well as BP load should be reported. Mean BP levels should be compared with normative values. In addition the nocturnal BP dipping, i.e., the percent day–night difference [(mean daytime BP – mean nighttime BP)/mean daytime BP × 100], should be determined for systolic and diastolic BP (Fig. 1).

Table 1
Ambulatory Blood Pressure Values for Healthy Caucasian Children

a. Normative ABPM values (mmHg) for boys by age (years)

BP percentile	Age (years)											
	5.0	6.0	7.0	8.0	9.0	10.0	11.0	12.0	13.0	14.0	15.0	16.0
24-h SBP												
50th	104.6	105.5	106.3	107.0	107.7	108.8	110.4	112.6	115.1	117.8	120.6	123.4
75th	109.0	110.0	111.0	111.9	112.8	114.1	115.9	118.2	120.9	123.7	126.5	129.4
90th	113.4	114.7	115.8	116.8	117.9	119.2	121.2	123.7	126.4	129.3	132.1	134.9
95th	116.4	117.7	118.9	120.0	121.1	122.5	124.6	127.1	129.9	132.7	135.5	138.2
99th	122.7	124.1	125.4	126.6	127.7	129.2	131.4	134.0	136.9	139.5	142.0	144.5
Daytime SBP												
50th	111.1	111.5	111.9	112.2	112.6	113.4	114.9	117.0	119.5	122.3	125.3	128.2
75th	115.7	116.3	116.8	117.3	117.9	118.8	120.5	122.9	125.6	128.5	131.5	134.6
90th	120.1	120.9	121.6	122.2	122.9	124.0	125.9	128.4	131.2	134.2	137.3	140.4
95th	122.9	123.8	124.6	125.3	126.1	127.3	129.3	131.8	134.7	137.7	140.8	143.9
99th	128.5	129.6	130.6	131.5	132.3	133.7	135.8	138.6	141.5	144.4	147.4	150.4
Nighttime SBP												
50th	95.0	95.5	96.1	96.7	97.3	98.1	99.4	101.2	103.4	105.8	108.3	110.9
75th	99.2	100.2	101.1	102.0	102.9	103.9	105.3	107.1	109.3	111.9	114.4	116.9
90th	103.4	104.9	106.2	107.5	108.5	109.6	111.0	112.8	115.0	117.5	120.0	122.5
95th	106.3	108.0	109.6	111.0	112.1	113.2	114.6	116.3	118.6	121.0	123.4	125.9
99th	112.3	114.6	116.7	118.4	119.6	120.7	121.9	123.4	125.5	127.8	130.1	132.3
24-h DBP												
50th	65.3	65.7	66.1	66.3	66.5	66.6	66.9	67.2	67.4	67.7	68.1	68.6
75th	68.8	69.3	69.6	69.9	70.0	70.2	70.5	70.8	71.0	71.4	71.8	72.3
90th	72.2	72.6	73.0	73.2	73.3	73.4	73.7	74.0	74.3	74.6	75.1	75.6
95th	74.4	74.8	75.1	75.2	75.3	75.4	75.7	75.9	76.2	76.6	77.0	77.5
99th	78.9	79.0	79.1	79.1	79.1	79.1	79.3	79.6	79.9	80.2	80.7	81.3
Daytime DBP												
50th	72.2	72.4	72.5	72.5	72.3	72.1	72.0	72.0	72.2	72.5	73.0	73.5
75th	75.9	76.1	76.3	76.4	76.2	76.0	76.0	76.0	76.2	76.5	77.0	77.6
90th	79.1	79.3	79.7	79.8	79.7	79.5	79.5	79.5	79.7	80.0	80.6	81.3
95th	81.0	81.3	81.6	81.8	81.7	81.5	81.5	81.6	81.7	82.1	82.8	83.5
99th	84.5	84.8	85.2	85.5	85.4	85.3	85.3	85.4	85.6	86.1	86.8	87.7
Nighttime DBP												
50th	55.0	55.3	55.5	55.7	55.8	55.8	55.9	56.0	56.3	56.5	56.8	57.1
75th	58.5	59.1	59.5	59.8	60.0	60.0	60.0	60.1	60.3	60.5	60.7	60.9
90th	62.3	63.2	63.8	64.2	64.3	64.2	64.1	64.1	64.1	64.2	64.3	64.3
95th	65.1	66.1	66.8	67.1	67.1	66.9	66.7	66.5	66.5	66.5	66.4	66.4
99th	71.6	72.7	73.5	73.5	73.2	72.6	71.9	71.4	71.1	70.8	70.6	70.3
24-h MAP												
50th	77.4	77.9	78.7	79.3	79.7	80.2	80.8	81.7	82.7	83.8	85.1	86.4
75th	81.4	81.9	82.7	83.4	83.8	84.3	85.0	85.9	86.9	88.0	89.3	90.5

Table 1
(continued)

a. Normative ABPM values (mmHg) for boys by age (years)

BP percentile	Age (years)											
	5.0	6.0	7.0	8.0	9.0	10.0	11.0	12.0	13.0	14.0	15.0	16.0
90th	85.5	86.0	86.8	87.4	87.9	88.3	88.9	89.7	90.6	91.6	92.7	93.9
95th	88.3	88.7	89.5	90.0	90.4	90.8	91.3	91.9	92.7	93.7	94.7	95.7
99th	94.3	94.6	95.1	95.4	95.6	95.7	95.8	96.2	96.7	97.3	98.1	98.9
Daytime MAP												
50th	83.5	84.1	84.5	84.8	84.9	85.0	85.3	85.9	86.8	88.0	89.4	90.8
75th	87.5	88.2	88.8	89.2	89.4	89.5	89.9	90.6	91.5	92.7	94.2	95.7
90th	91.3	92.1	92.8	93.3	93.5	93.7	94.0	94.7	95.6	96.8	98.3	99.8
95th	93.6	94.5	95.3	95.8	96.1	96.2	96.5	97.1	98.0	99.2	100.6	102.1
99th	98.2	99.2	100.1	100.7	101.0	101.0	101.2	101.6	102.4	103.4	104.7	106.1
Nighttime MAP												
50th	66.7	67.7	68.6	69.2	69.7	70.0	70.5	71.2	72.1	73.1	74.0	74.9
75th	70.5	71.7	72.8	73.5	74.1	74.5	75.0	75.6	76.4	77.2	78.0	78.6
90th	74.7	76.0	77.2	78.1	78.6	78.9	79.3	79.7	80.3	80.8	81.3	81.7
95th	77.6	79.0	80.2	81.1	81.6	81.8	82.0	82.3	82.6	82.9	83.2	83.4
99th	84.1	85.7	86.9	87.6	87.8	87.7	87.4	87.1	86.9	86.8	86.6	86.4

b. Normative ABPM values (mmHg) for boys by height (cm)

BP percentile	Height (cm)													
	120.0	125.0	130.0	135.0	140.0	145.0	150.0	155.0	160.0	165.0	170.0	175.0	180.0	185.0
24-h SBP														
50th	104.5	105.3	106.2	107.2	108.3	109.5	110.9	112.5	114.2	116.1	118.0	119.7	121.5	123.2
75th	109.2	110.1	111.1	112.1	113.3	114.6	116.1	117.7	119.5	121.4	123.2	125.0	126.6	128.2
90th	113.8	114.8	115.9	116.9	118.2	119.5	121.0	122.6	124.4	126.3	128.1	129.8	131.3	132.8
95th	116.8	117.8	118.9	120.0	121.2	122.5	124.0	125.7	127.4	129.3	131.1	132.6	134.1	135.5
99th	122.9	123.9	125.0	126.1	127.3	128.6	130.1	131.7	133.4	135.2	136.8	138.2	139.4	140.5
Daytime SBP														
50th	110.8	111.1	111.5	112.0	112.7	113.7	115.1	116.8	118.6	120.6	122.6	124.4	126.2	128.0
75th	116.2	116.5	116.9	117.4	118.0	119.0	120.4	122.1	124.2	126.4	128.4	130.3	132.2	134.1
90th	121.7	121.9	122.2	122.5	123.0	123.9	125.3	127.1	129.4	131.9	134.1	136.1	138.0	139.9
95th	125.2	125.3	125.5	125.7	126.0	126.9	128.3	130.2	132.7	135.3	137.6	139.6	141.6	143.5
99th	132.6	132.4	132.2	132.0	132.1	132.8	134.2	136.3	139.1	142.2	144.7	146.8	148.6	150.5
Nighttime SBP														
50th	93.6	94.6	95.6	96.7	97.9	99.0	100.1	101.3	102.6	104.1	105.6	107.2	108.7	110.2
75th	98.6	99.8	101.0	102.3	103.6	104.7	105.9	107.1	108.4	109.9	111.5	113.1	114.6	116.1
90th	103.3	104.8	106.3	107.8	109.3	110.6	111.8	113.0	114.3	115.7	117.2	118.8	120.3	121.8
95th	106.3	107.9	109.7	111.4	113.0	114.4	115.7	116.8	118.1	119.4	120.9	122.4	123.9	125.3
99th	112.1	114.2	116.5	118.7	120.8	122.5	123.8	124.9	126.0	127.1	128.4	129.6	131.0	132.2
24-h DBP														
50th	65.6	65.9	66.1	66.4	66.6	66.9	67.1	67.2	67.3	67.5	67.6	67.8	68.0	68.2
75th	69.7	69.9	70.2	70.4	70.6	70.8	71.0	71.1	71.2	71.3	71.5	71.7	71.8	71.9

Table 1
(continued)

b. Normative ABPM values (mmHg) for boys by height (cm)

Height (cm)

BP percentile	120.0	125.0	130.0	135.0	140.0	145.0	150.0	155.0	160.0	165.0	170.0	175.0	180.0	185.0
90th	73.9	74.1	74.2	74.4	74.5	74.7	74.8	74.8	74.9	75.1	75.3	75.4	75.5	75.6
95th	76.7	76.8	76.9	76.9	77.0	77.1	77.1	77.2	77.3	77.5	77.7	77.8	77.9	78.0
99th	82.7	82.5	82.3	82.1	81.9	81.8	81.8	81.8	81.9	82.2	82.5	82.7	82.9	83.0
Daytime DBP														
50th	72.3	72.3	72.2	72.1	72.1	72.1	72.1	72.1	72.2	72.3	72.6	72.8	73.1	73.4
75th	76.5	76.4	76.3	76.2	76.0	76.0	75.9	75.9	76.0	76.2	76.5	76.8	77.2	77.5
90th	80.2	80.1	79.9	79.7	79.5	79.4	79.3	79.3	79.4	79.7	80.0	80.5	80.9	81.3
95th	82.4	82.2	82.0	81.8	81.5	81.4	81.2	81.2	81.3	81.7	82.1	82.6	83.1	83.6
99th	86.5	86.2	85.9	85.6	85.2	85.0	84.8	84.8	85.0	85.4	86.0	86.6	87.3	87.9
Nighttime DBP														
50th	54.3	54.8	55.1	55.5	55.8	56.0	56.2	56.2	56.3	56.5	56.7	56.9	57.1	57.3
75th	57.6	58.2	58.8	59.2	59.6	59.9	60.1	60.2	60.2	60.3	60.5	60.6	60.8	60.9
90th	60.7	61.4	62.1	62.7	63.2	63.5	63.7	63.8	63.8	63.9	63.9	64.0	64.1	64.2
95th	62.6	63.4	64.2	64.8	65.4	65.8	66.0	66.0	66.0	66.0	66.1	66.1	66.1	66.2
99th	66.2	67.2	68.2	69.0	69.7	70.1	70.4	70.4	70.3	70.3	70.2	70.1	70.0	69.9
24-h MAP														
50th	77.5	78.1	78.7	79.3	79.9	80.5	81.1	81.7	82.3	83.1	83.9	84.7	85.5	86.3
75th	81.8	82.4	83.0	83.5	84.1	84.6	85.2	85.9	86.6	87.3	88.1	89.0	89.8	90.7
90th	86.3	86.7	87.2	87.6	88.0	88.5	89.1	89.7	90.3	91.1	91.9	92.7	93.5	94.3
95th	89.3	89.6	89.9	90.2	90.5	90.9	91.4	91.9	92.6	93.3	94.0	94.8	95.6	96.4
99th	95.9	95.7	95.5	95.4	95.4	95.6	95.9	96.3	96.7	97.4	98.0	98.7	99.4	100.1
Daytime MAP														
50th	83.8	84.1	84.3	84.5	84.7	85.0	85.4	85.8	86.4	87.1	88.0	89.0	90.0	91.0
75th	88.5	88.7	88.9	89.0	89.1	89.4	89.6	90.1	90.7	91.6	92.6	93.7	94.9	96.1
90th	92.9	93.0	93.1	93.1	93.1	93.2	93.4	93.8	94.5	95.4	96.5	97.7	99.0	100.3
95th	95.6	95.6	95.6	95.5	95.5	95.5	95.7	96.0	96.7	97.7	98.8	100.1	101.4	102.8
99th	101.0	100.7	100.5	100.2	99.9	99.7	99.8	100.1	100.8	101.7	102.9	104.3	105.7	107.1
Nighttime MAP														
50th	66.8	67.6	68.3	69.0	69.6	70.1	70.6	71.2	71.9	72.7	73.6	74.5	75.4	76.2
75th	71.0	71.9	72.7	73.4	73.9	74.4	74.9	75.4	76.0	76.8	77.6	78.3	79.1	79.8
90th	75.9	76.6	77.3	77.9	78.3	78.6	78.9	79.2	79.7	80.3	80.9	81.5	82.1	82.7
95th	79.5	80.0	80.5	80.9	81.2	81.3	81.4	81.5	81.9	82.3	82.8	83.3	83.8	84.3
99th	88.4	88.1	87.8	87.6	87.2	86.7	86.3	86.0	86.0	86.1	86.3	86.5	86.8	87.0

c. Normative ABPM values (mmHg) for girls by age (years)

Age (years)

BP percentile	5.0	6.0	7.0	8.0	9.0	10.0	11.0	12.0	13.0	14.0	15.0	16.0
24-h SBP												
50th	102.8	104.1	105.3	106.5	107.6	108.7	109.7	110.7	111.8	112.8	113.8	114.8
75th	107.8	109.1	110.4	111.5	112.6	113.6	114.7	115.7	116.7	117.6	118.4	119.2

Table 1
(continued)

c. Normative ABPM values (mmHg) for girls by age (years)

BP percentile	*Age (years)*											
	5.0	*6.0*	*7.0*	*8.0*	*9.0*	*10.0*	*11.0*	*12.0*	*13.0*	*14.0*	*15.0*	*16.0*
90th	112.3	113.7	115.0	116.1	117.2	118.2	119.2	120.2	121.2	121.9	122.6	123.2
95th	114.9	116.4	117.7	118.9	120.0	121.1	122.1	123.0	123.9	124.5	125.0	125.6
99th	119.9	121.5	123.0	124.3	125.5	126.5	127.5	128.4	129.0	129.5	129.7	130.0
Daytime SBP												
50th	108.4	109.5	110.6	111.5	112.4	113.3	114.2	115.3	116.4	117.5	118.6	119.6
75th	113.8	114.9	115.9	116.8	117.6	118.5	119.5	120.6	121.7	122.6	123.5	124.3
90th	118.3	119.5	120.6	121.5	122.4	123.3	124.3	125.3	126.4	127.2	127.9	128.5
95th	120.9	122.2	123.3	124.3	125.2	126.2	127.2	128.2	129.2	129.9	130.4	130.9
99th	125.6	127.1	128.4	129.6	130.6	131.7	132.7	133.7	134.5	135.0	135.2	135.4
Nighttime SBP												
50th	94.8	95.6	96.2	96.8	97.5	98.2	99.0	99.7	100.5	101.3	102.0	102.9
75th	100.2	101.1	101.8	102.5	103.2	104.0	104.7	105.2	105.8	106.3	106.8	107.3
90th	105.3	106.3	107.2	108.0	108.8	109.5	110.1	110.4	110.7	110.9	111.0	111.2
95th	108.4	109.6	110.6	111.5	112.3	113.0	113.5	113.6	113.7	113.6	113.5	113.5
99th	114.5	116.0	117.3	118.4	119.3	119.9	120.1	119.8	119.4	118.8	118.2	117.8
24-h DBP												
50th	65.5	65.6	65.8	65.9	66.0	66.2	66.4	66.6	67.0	67.2	67.5	67.7
75th	68.9	69.1	69.2	69.3	69.5	69.8	70.0	70.4	70.8	71.1	71.2	71.4
90th	72.1	72.2	72.3	72.4	72.6	72.9	73.2	73.7	74.1	74.4	74.6	74.7
95th	74.0	74.1	74.2	74.2	74.4	74.7	75.1	75.6	76.1	76.4	76.6	76.7
99th	77.6	77.6	77.6	77.6	77.7	78.0	78.4	79.1	79.7	80.1	80.4	80.5
Daytime DBP												
50th	72.6	72.6	72.4	72.2	72.0	71.8	71.8	72.1	72.4	72.8	73.2	73.5
75th	76.7	76.6	76.5	76.3	76.0	75.9	75.9	76.2	76.5	76.8	77.0	77.2
90th	80.2	80.2	80.0	79.8	79.5	79.3	79.4	79.6	80.0	80.2	80.3	80.3
95th	82.3	82.2	82.1	81.8	81.5	81.3	81.4	81.6	82.0	82.2	82.2	82.1
99th	86.1	86.0	85.8	85.5	85.2	85.0	85.0	85.3	85.6	85.7	85.6	85.4
Nighttime DBP												
50th	56.4	55.9	55.5	55.1	54.8	54.6	54.3	54.2	54.3	54.5	54.9	55.3
75th	61.1	60.6	60.1	59.7	59.4	59.2	58.9	58.7	58.7	58.7	58.8	59.1
90th	65.6	65.1	64.6	64.1	63.8	63.7	63.4	63.1	62.9	62.8	62.8	62.8
95th	68.5	67.9	67.4	66.9	66.6	66.5	66.2	65.9	65.6	65.4	65.3	65.2
99th	74.2	73.6	72.9	72.4	72.2	72.0	71.8	71.4	71.1	70.7	70.3	70.0
24-h MAP												
50th	77.5	78.0	78.4	78.8	79.2	79.6	80.2	80.9	81.5	82.2	82.7	83.0
75th	81.2	81.7	82.1	82.5	82.9	83.3	84.0	84.7	85.4	86.0	86.5	86.8
90th	84.6	85.0	85.4	85.7	86.1	86.5	87.1	87.9	88.6	89.2	89.7	89.9
95th	86.6	87.0	87.3	87.6	87.9	88.3	88.9	89.7	90.5	91.0	91.5	91.7
99th	90.5	90.8	90.9	91.0	91.2	91.6	92.2	93.0	93.7	94.2	94.6	94.8
Daytime MAP												
50th	83.7	83.9	84.0	84.1	84.2	84.4	84.7	85.2	85.9	86.5	87.1	87.7
75th	88.2	88.3	88.4	88.4	88.4	88.5	88.9	89.4	90.1	90.8	91.4	91.9

Table 1
(continued)

c. Normative ABPM values (mmHg) for girls by age (years)

Age (years)

BP percentile	5.0	6.0	7.0	8.0	9.0	10.0	11.0	12.0	13.0	14.0	15.0	16.0
90th	92.2	92.2	92.2	92.1	92.0	91.1	92.4	93.0	93.6	94.3	94.8	95.4
95th	94.6	94.5	94.4	94.2	94.1	94.2	94.4	95.0	95.6	96.2	96.8	97.3
99th	99.0	98.7	98.5	98.2	97.9	97.9	98.1	98.6	99.2	99.7	100.2	100.7
Nighttime MAP												
50th	68.7	68.8	68.8	68.8	68.9	69.1	69.3	69.6	70.1	70.6	71.2	71.8
75th	73.0	73.1	73.1	73.2	73.4	73.6	73.8	74.1	74.5	74.9	75.4	75.9
90th	76.9	77.0	77.1	77.2	77.4	77.6	77.8	78.0	78.3	78.6	78.9	79.3
95th	79.2	79.4	79.6	79.7	79.8	80.1	80.2	80.3	80.5	80.7	80.9	81.2
99th	83.8	84.1	84.2	84.3	84.5	84.6	84.7	84.6	84.6	84.6	84.6	84.7

d. Normative ABPM values (mmHg) for girls by height (cm)

Height (cm)

BP percentile	120.0	125.0	130.0	135.0	140.0	145.0	150.0	155.0	160.0	165.0	170.0	175.0
24-h SBP												
50th	104.0	105.0	106.0	106.8	107.6	108.7	109.9	111.2	112.4	113.7	115.0	116.4
75th	108.2	109.3	110.3	111.2	112.1	113.2	114.6	115.9	117.0	118.0	119.2	120.4
90th	112.0	113.2	114.3	115.3	116.2	117.4	118.7	120.0	121.0	121.8	122.8	123.8
95th	114.3	115.6	116.7	117.7	118.7	119.9	121.2	122.5	123.3	124.1	124.9	125.8
99th	118.8	120.1	121.3	122.4	123.4	124.6	126.0	127.1	127.7	128.2	128.8	129.3
Daytime SBP												
50th	110.0	110.5	111.0	111.6	112.2	113.1	114.3	115.6	117.0	118.3	119.8	121.2
75th	114.4	115.0	115.7	116.3	117.0	118.1	119.4	120.7	121.9	123.1	124.2	125.3
90th	118.2	119.0	119.7	120.4	121.3	122.5	123.9	125.2	126.4	127.3	128.1	128.9
95th	120.4	121.3	122.1	122.9	123.8	125.1	126.5	127.9	129.1	129.8	130.5	131.0
99th	124.5	125.5	126.4	127.4	128.5	129.9	131.5	133.0	134.0	134.5	134.8	135.0
Nighttime SBP												
50th	95.0	95.7	96.4	96.9	97.5	98.1	98.9	100.0	101.1	102.2	103.4	104.6
75th	99.4	100.3	101.2	101.9	102.6	103.4	104.4	105.5	106.4	107.3	108.2	109.2
90th	103.3	104.4	105.5	106.5	107.5	108.5	109.5	110.5	111.2	111.8	112.4	113.1
95th	105.6	106.9	108.1	109.3	110.4	111.6	112.7	113.6	114.1	114.4	114.8	115.3
99th	109.8	111.5	113.1	114.7	116.2	117.7	118.9	119.5	119.6	119.4	119.3	119.4
24-h DBP												
50th	65.9	65.9	66.0	66.1	66.2	66.3	66.5	66.7	67.0	67.4	68.0	68.6
75th	68.6	68.9	69.2	69.5	69.8	70.1	70.4	70.6	70.7	71.0	71.3	71.6
90th	70.9	71.4	71.9	72.4	72.9	73.4	73.8	74.0	74.1	74.2	74.4	74.5
95th	72.2	72.8	73.4	74.1	74.7	75.3	75.7	76.0	76.1	76.2	76.2	76.2
99th	74.6	75.3	76.2	77.1	77.9	78.7	79.3	79.7	79.9	79.9	79.9	79.7
Daytime DBP												
50th	73.2	72.8	72.4	72.1	71.8	71.7	71.8	72.0	72.4	73.1	73.9	74.8
75th	76.9	76.6	76.4	76.2	76.1	76.1	76.1	76.2	76.4	76.8	77.3	77.8

Table 1

(continued)

d. Normative ABPM values (mmHg) for girls by height (cm)

Height (cm)

BP percentile	120.0	125.0	130.0	135.0	140.0	145.0	150.0	155.0	160.0	165.0	170.0	175.0
90th	80.1	79.9	79.8	79.8	79.7	79.8	79.9	79.9	79.9	80.0	80.2	80.5
95th	81.9	81.8	81.8	81.8	81.9	82.0	82.0	82.0	82.0	81.9	82.0	82.0
99th	85.3	85.3	85.4	85.6	85.8	85.9	86.0	85.9	85.7	85.4	85.2	84.9
Nighttime DBP												
50th	55.4	55.3	55.1	54.8	54.6	54.4	54.3	54.4	54.6	54.9	55.1	55.4
75th	59.5	59.5	59.4	59.3	59.1	58.9	58.8	58.7	58.8	58.9	61.0	59.3
90th	63.1	63.3	63.4	63.4	63.3	63.1	63.0	62.9	62.9	62.9	66.9	63.1
95th	65.2	65.5	65.7	65.8	65.8	65.7	65.6	65.5	65.5	65.5	70.8	65.5
99th	69.1	69.6	70.1	70.4	70.6	70.8	70.8	70.7	70.7	70.6	79.0	70.4
24-h MAP												
50th	77.2	77.8	78.3	78.7	79.2	79.7	80.2	80.8	81.5	82.3	83.1	84.0
75th	80.6	81.2	81.8	82.4	82.9	83.5	84.1	84.7	85.3	85.9	86.6	87.4
90th	83.6	84.2	84.9	85.5	86.1	86.7	87.3	87.9	88.4	88.9	89.5	90.1
95th	85.3	86.0	86.7	87.4	88.0	88.6	89.2	89.7	90.2	90.6	91.1	91.7
99th	88.5	89.2	89.9	90.6	91.3	91.9	92.5	93.0	93.3	93.6	94.0	94.5
Daytime MAP												
50th	83.3	83.7	84.0	84.1	84.3	84.5	84.9	85.5	86.2	87.0	88.0	88.9
75th	87.4	87.9	88.2	88.5	88.7	88.9	89.3	89.8	90.3	90.9	91.6	92.2
90th	90.9	91.5	91.9	92.2	92.4	92.7	93.0	93.4	93.7	94.1	94.5	94.9
95th	92.9	93.6	94.0	94.4	94.6	94.9	95.1	95.4	95.6	95.8	96.1	96.4
99th	96.6	97.4	97.9	98.3	98.6	98.8	99.0	99.0	99.0	99.0	99.0	99.1
Nighttime MAP												
50th	68.0	68.2	68.4	68.5	68.7	69.0	69.3	69.8	70.4	71.2	72.0	72.8
75th	72.6	72.7	72.9	73.0	73.2	73.5	73.9	74.3	74.8	75.4	76.1	76.9
90th	76.8	76.9	77.0	77.2	77.4	77.7	78.0	78.3	78.6	79.1	79.6	80.3
95th	79.5	79.4	79.6	79.7	79.9	80.2	80.4	80.6	80.8	81.2	81.6	82.2
99th	84.6	84.4	84.5	84.6	84.8	85.0	85.0	85.0	85.0	85.0	85.3	85.6

Adapted from Wühl et al. *(25)*, with permission.

The recommended frequency for ABPM measurements is 15–20 min during daytime and 30–60 min during nighttime, resulting in at least 40–50 readings within 24 h. A low frequency of measurements is more comfortable for the patient but limits the validity of the individual profile. For analyses of blood pressure rhythmicity (ultradian rhythms) intervals of 15–20 min during daytime and of 20–30 min during nighttime are recommended *(8)*.

The ABPM recording should be edited for outliers by visual inspection of the profile. Values outside preset cutoffs (e.g., systolic BP < 60 or > 220 mmHg, diastolic BP < 35 or > 120 mmHg, heart rate < 40 or > 180 bpm, pulse pressure < 40 or > 120 mmHg) should be excluded a priori by the ABPM software program *(17)*.

All patients should be instructed to fill in a diary on physical activity, rest and sleeping times, and drug intake. This is important to account for different levels of physical activity

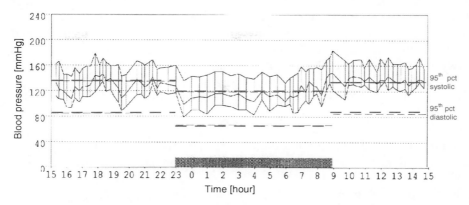

Fig. 1. Example of an ABPM profile in a child with marked systolic and diastolic hypertension. The dipping pattern is conserved (>10% difference between mean daytime and mean nighttime BP). The systolic and diastolic load (percent of BP measurements above the 95th percentile) is 100%.

during BP recording and the effect of antihypertensive medication. Daytime and nighttime (awake and sleeping periods) should be analyzed as reported in the patient's diary *(27,28)*. If information is not available alternatively the time period from 8 am to 8 pm might be chosen for daytime and from midnight to 6 am for nighttime BP evaluation. This approach discards readings obtained during transition times (i.e., 6–8 am and 10 pm to midnight) from the analysis *(24)*. Preliminary data suggest that actual sleeping and waking times determined from an actigraph, a wrist device that senses motion, may be superior to patient-initiated diary entry *(29)*.

Physical activity influences the success of BP measurements and BP itself. Simultaneous recording of activity by actigraphs shows that reliable and reproducible ABPM is feasible and that activity increases SBP and DBP by up to 10 mmHg *(2)*. It is recommended that children undergoing ABPM should continue normal activities except contact sports, vigorous exercise, and swimming. During individual measurements the arm should be held still to avoid erroneous readings.

Applying the Device

The personnel applying the ABPM monitors should be fully trained on their maintenance, application, and function. The cuffs should be laundered regularly; some manufacturers sell single-use covers for the BP cuffs. The device itself should be regularly cleaned with a wiping disinfectant.

Parents and patients should be informed how to operate the monitor (e.g., stop a reading, turn off, or restart the device). Although removal of the monitor is not recommended, if absolutely necessary, the device should be removed immediately after a reading (to reduce the number of missed readings) and reapplied as soon as possible. Contact of the electronic device with water must be avoided.

Serious adverse events have not been reported in children; however, mild sleep disturbances, petechiae, or bruises have been documented *(30)*. Contraindications to ABPM may include atrial fibrillation, coagulation disorders, and, for some brands of equipment, latex allergy.

The accuracy and precision of the devices should be checked by simultaneous measurements with a sphygmomanometer at the beginning of each test period. The average difference between the mean of three clinic and three ABPM measurements should be less than 5 mmHg to consider adequate calibration.

The cuff should be applied to the non-dominant arm, in hemodialysis patients to the non-fistula arm.

Normative Data

Comparison with appropriate normative data stratified by gender and age or height is essential for a meaningful interpretation of ABPM findings in the pediatric setting (see Table 1).

In childhood, BP is strongly influenced by body dimensions (3,16,24,26,31–34). In addition, changes in body composition during puberty have profound gender-specific effects on BP. Furthermore, the level, timing, and duration of physical activity are markedly age and gender dependent. For example, median 24-h systolic BP increases across childhood by almost 19 mmHg in boys and 12 mmHg in girls (25). Up to 11 years of age or 140 cm of height, median values are virtually identical in boys and girls. During puberty systolic BP increases more steeply in boys, resulting in a median difference of 8.4 mmHg at the age of 16 years. These differences are equally marked during daytime and nighttime (25).

In contrast to the marked increase in systolic BP, diastolic BP increases only minimally with age during childhood. The median increase in median 24-h diastolic BP over time was 3.3 and 2.2 mmHg in boys and girls, respectively (25). This finding is in contrast to reference data for casual BP measurements (32,35,36). In addition, the age-related increase in systolic BP is less marked than in casual BP reference studies. These discrepancies might be explained by a decreasing prevalence of the white coat phenomenon across childhood. However, technical artifacts, such as age-dependent differences in cuff size relative to upper arm circumference between manual and ABPM devices, cannot be completely ruled out. It is also possible that age-related differences in diastolic BP might be related to difficulties in defining diastolic BP by Korotkoff phases IV and V by auscultatory BP measurements or to the use of invalidated algorithms implemented in ABPM devices. However, even using auscultatory measurements, no systematic increase of mean diastolic BP with age was observed in a recent ABPM study assessing a large number of children aged 6–16 years, whereas systolic BP was clearly age dependent (23).

An overview on published ABPM normative data sets is given in Table 2. Up to date, few large cross-sectional ABPM studies have been performed in healthy controls. For all these studies the cutoff values for the normal range were defined by the 95th percentile of the BP distribution in healthy children. It should be recognized that ABPM BP values measured with an oscillometric device tend to be higher than resting BP values obtained by auscultation. This difference will lead to a difference in the prevalence of hypertension if the higher ambulatory norms (24,25) are used as reference compared to the lower, resting casual BP normative data (4th report). In a study by Sorof, white coat hypertension was diagnosed in only 31% of patients using the ambulatory criteria, whereas applying the lower casual BP cutoffs would result in 59% being diagnosed with white coat hypertension (37).

For casual BP a staging system was introduced (JNC7 (13) and 4th report (16)). A similar staging scheme was suggested for ABPM BP levels in children including mean ABPM levels and the calculated BP load (38) (see Table 3). BP load is defined as the percentage of valid ambulatory BP measures above a set threshold value, such as the 95th percentile of

Table 2
Published Normative ABPM Data Sets

Authors	No. of subjects	Age range studied (years)	Method	Successful exams (%)	Successful readings (%)
Harshfield et al. *(34)*	300	10–18	ausc + osc	84	85–90
Lurbe et al. *(26,64)*	333	3–18	osc	84	89.8
O'Sullivan et al. *(23)*	1121	6–16	ausc + osc	99.7	>95
Reichert et al. *(3)*	564	9–13	ausc + osc	95	64
Soergel et al. *(24)*	1245	5–21	osc	98.9	92.7
Wühl et al. *(25)*	949[a]	5–20	osc	[a]	[a]
Gellermann et al. *(19)*	61	3–6	osc	77	46–58
Varda and Gregoric *(18)*	97	0.1–2.5	osc	87	75

Osc, oscillometric device; ausc, auscultatory device.

[a]Analysis of the data set from Soergel et al. *(24)* by the LMS method *(47)*. Only complete 24-h profiles without significant gaps were eligible for this analysis.

Table 3
Staging Scheme for Ambulatory Blood Pressure Levels in Children

Staging	Clinic BP[a]	Mean ambulatory systolic BP[b]	SBP load (%)
Normal BP	<95th percentile	<95th percentile	<25
White coat hypertension	>95th percentile	<95th percentile	<25
Masked hypertension	<95th percentile	>95th percentile	>25
High normal BP	>95th percentile	<95th percentile	25–50
Ambulatory hypertension	>95th percentile	>95th percentile	25–50
Severe ambulatory hypertension (at risk for end-organ damage)	>95th percentile	>95th percentile	>50

BP, blood pressure.

[a]Based on the National High Blood Pressure Education Program data (4th report) *(16)*.

[b]Based on normative ABPM values *(24,25)*.

Modified from Lurbe et al. *(38)*, with permission.

BP for gender and age or height *(39)*. The load can be assessed for the entire 24-h period or for the awake and asleep periods separately. Loads in excess of 25–30% are considered elevated *(40)*. Loads in excess of 50% were predictive of LVH in one pediatric study *(41)*.

ABPM also allows the evaluation of nocturnal BP dipping. Normal dipping is generally defined as a nocturnal decline of mean systolic and diastolic ABPM level by at least 10%.

The non-dipping phenomenon contributes to the overall renal and cardiovascular risk of an individual *(42–44)*. The cardiovascular mortality risk attributable to non-dipping is independent of the absolute 24-h blood pressure load *(45)*. Blunted nocturnal dipping has been associated with nephropathy in patients with type 1 *(46)* and 2 diabetes mellitus *(28)* and may be an early marker for impaired renal function.

The scientific application of pediatric ABPM reference data in parametric statistical procedures is compromised by the skewed distribution of BP in childhood. This problem has been largely solved by introduction of the LMS normalization method of Cole and Green *(47)*, which transforms skewed BP values into normally distributed standard deviation scores (SDS) *(25)*. In brief, the LMS method describes the distribution of a measurement Y by its median (M), the coefficient of variation (S), and a measure of skewness (L) required to transform the data to normality. Estimates for these parameters are obtained by applying a maximum-likelihood curve-fitting algorithm to the original data plotted over the independent variable of interest, in this case either age or height. The resulting estimates of L, M, and S can be used to construct percentiles ($C_{alpha}(t)$) by the equation: $C_{alpha}(t) = M(t)[1 + L(t) \times S(t) \times z_{alpha}]^{1/L(t)}$, where $M(t)$, $L(t)$, $S(t)$, and $C_{alpha}(t)$ indicate the corresponding values of each parameter at age (or height) t. z_{alpha} is the appropriate normal equivalent deviate (e.g., for alpha = 97%, z_{alpha} = 1.88).

This equation can be rearranged to convert an individual child's BP value to an exact standard deviation score (SDS):

SDS = $[(Y/M(t))^{L(t)} - 1]/(L(t) \times S(t))$, where Y is the child's individual systolic, diastolic, mean arterial BP, or heart rate value, and $L(t)$, $M(t)$, and $S(t)$ are the gender-specific values of L, M, and S interpolated for the child's age or height.

Age-, gender-, and height-specific L, M, and S reference values for mean 24-h, daytime, and nighttime systolic, diastolic, and mean arterial pressure have been provided *(25)* (Table 4).

Advantages of ABPM vs. Home BP or Casual BP Measurements

Self-monitoring of BP (home BP) has been suggested as an alternative to ABPM in adults *(48)*. Home BP measurements appear to be a valuable addition to casual BP also in children *(49)*. Home BP measurements agree with ABPM more closely and more consistently over the whole range of BP *(50)*. The combination of home and casual BP yields a higher degree of diagnostic specificity than casual BP alone. However, the information obtained from home BP measurements cannot substitute for ABPM: in children, the maximum diagnostic sensitivity reached by combined home and casual BP is only 81%, thus one out of four children diagnosed as hypertensive by ABPM would still be missed *(50)*. Moreover, the range of agreement of home BP with ABPM, albeit narrower than that of casual BP, is unacceptably wide. Finally, alterations of nocturnal BP regulation or hypertension, which have a high prevalence in children with chronic kidney disease, cannot be assessed by any daytime BP measurement.

Variability of Blood Pressure

ABPM provides information not only on daytime and nighttime blood pressure patterns but also on BP variability. Linear analyses, such as dividing the 24-h period into day and

Table 4
LMS Reference Values of Mean 24-h, Daytime, and Nighttime Systolic, Diastolic, and Mean Arterial Pressure Relative to Age and Height in Boys and Girls

Boys

Age	N	Systolic BP 24h L	M	S	Day L	M	S	Night L	M	S	Diastolic BP 24h L	M	S	Day L	M	S	Night L	M	S	MAP 24h L	M	S	Day L	M	S	Night L	M	S
5.0	11	-2.205	104.6	0.058	-0.862	111.1	0.059	-1.929	95.0	0.062	-0.661	65.3	0.076	1.477	72.1	0.075	-2.245	55.0	0.086	-2.063	76.9	0.071	-0.132	83.5	0.069	-2.191	66.7	0.078
5.5	11	-2.066	105.1	0.059	-0.807	111.3	0.060	-1.793	95.3	0.065	-0.502	65.5	0.076	1.505	72.2	0.076	-2.065	55.1	0.089	-1.918	77.4	0.071	-0.069	83.8	0.070	-2.074	67.2	0.079
6.0	11	-1.927	105.5	0.060	-0.751	111.5	0.061	-1.658	95.5	0.067	-0.342	65.7	0.077	1.533	72.4	0.077	-1.884	55.3	0.092	-1.772	77.9	0.071	-0.007	84.1	0.071	-1.955	67.7	0.081
6.5	14	-1.786	105.9	0.061	-0.691	111.7	0.062	-1.522	95.8	0.070	-0.178	65.9	0.077	1.558	72.4	0.078	-1.702	55.4	0.095	-1.610	78.3	0.071	0.060	84.3	0.072	-1.826	68.1	0.082
7.0	15	-1.646	106.3	0.062	-0.631	111.9	0.063	-1.386	96.1	0.073	-0.014	66.1	0.077	1.583	72.5	0.079	-1.520	55.5	0.098	-1.447	78.7	0.071	0.127	84.5	0.073	-1.696	68.6	0.084
7.5	21	-1.503	106.6	0.063	-0.567	112.0	0.064	-1.251	96.4	0.076	0.144	66.2	0.077	1.599	72.5	0.080	-1.338	55.6	0.100	-1.262	79.0	0.072	0.199	84.7	0.074	-1.544	68.9	0.085
8.0	22	-1.360	107.0	0.065	-0.503	112.2	0.065	-1.116	96.6	0.078	0.301	66.3	0.078	1.614	72.5	0.081	-1.155	55.7	0.102	-1.078	79.3	0.072	0.272	84.8	0.076	-1.393	69.2	0.086
8.5	22	-1.220	107.4	0.066	-0.440	112.4	0.066	-0.984	97.0	0.080	0.441	66.4	0.078	1.620	72.4	0.082	-0.982	55.7	0.104	-0.870	79.5	0.073	0.353	84.8	0.077	-1.220	69.5	0.087
9.0	21	-1.086	107.7	0.067	-0.381	112.6	0.067	-0.856	97.3	0.081	0.574	66.5	0.078	1.622	72.3	0.083	-0.813	55.8	0.105	-0.651	79.7	0.073	0.442	84.9	0.078	-1.040	69.7	0.088
9.5	23	-0.968	108.2	0.068	-0.326	112.9	0.068	-0.733	97.7	0.082	0.688	66.5	0.079	1.621	72.1	0.083	-0.655	55.8	0.105	-0.409	79.9	0.074	0.552	84.9	0.078	-0.843	69.8	0.089
10.0	19	-0.866	108.8	0.069	-0.276	113.4	0.069	-0.616	98.1	0.083	0.786	66.6	0.079	1.614	72.1	0.083	-0.505	55.8	0.106	-0.146	80.2	0.075	0.682	85.0	0.079	-0.631	70.0	0.090
10.5	27	-0.783	109.6	0.069	-0.229	114.1	0.070	-0.503	98.7	0.083	0.865	66.7	0.079	1.598	72.0	0.083	-0.365	55.8	0.106	0.139	80.5	0.075	0.832	85.1	0.079	-0.398	70.2	0.090
11.0	25	-0.706	110.4	0.070	-0.177	114.9	0.071	-0.391	99.4	0.084	0.932	66.9	0.079	1.576	72.0	0.083	-0.229	55.9	0.105	0.443	80.8	0.076	0.998	85.3	0.080	-0.147	70.5	0.091
11.5	36	-0.627	111.5	0.071	-0.115	115.9	0.072	-0.280	100.2	0.084	0.981	67.0	0.080	1.544	72.0	0.083	-0.097	55.9	0.105	0.774	81.2	0.077	1.183	85.6	0.080	0.133	70.8	0.091
12.0	27	-0.540	112.6	0.072	-0.041	117.0	0.072	-0.171	101.2	0.084	1.017	67.2	0.080	1.505	72.0	0.083	0.031	56.0	0.104	1.119	81.7	0.077	1.378	85.9	0.081	0.437	71.2	0.091
12.5	35	-0.441	113.8	0.072	0.041	118.2	0.073	-0.065	102.3	0.084	1.044	67.3	0.080	1.460	72.1	0.083	0.154	56.1	0.104	1.470	82.1	0.078	1.569	86.3	0.081	0.761	71.6	0.090
13.0	21	-0.324	115.1	0.072	0.132	119.5	0.073	0.040	103.4	0.084	1.050	67.4	0.080	1.407	72.2	0.083	0.270	56.3	0.104	1.822	82.7	0.078	1.755	86.8	0.082	1.097	72.1	0.089
13.5	30	-0.181	116.4	0.073	0.235	120.9	0.073	0.144	104.6	0.083	1.047	67.6	0.080	1.347	72.3	0.083	0.378	56.4	0.103	2.173	83.2	0.078	1.937	87.4	0.082	1.436	72.6	0.088
14.0	16	-0.018	117.8	0.073	0.348	122.3	0.073	0.248	105.8	0.083	1.036	67.7	0.080	1.279	72.5	0.082	0.483	56.5	0.101	2.525	83.8	0.078	2.117	88.0	0.083	1.777	73.1	0.086
14.5	16	0.157	119.2	0.073	0.469	123.8	0.073	0.349	107.1	0.082	1.019	67.9	0.080	1.203	72.7	0.082	0.588	56.7	0.101	2.874	84.4	0.078	2.291	88.7	0.083	2.122	73.6	0.084
15.0	11	0.338	120.6	0.072	0.595	125.3	0.073	0.448	108.3	0.082	1.000	68.1	0.079	1.123	73.0	0.082	0.694	56.8	0.100	3.222	85.1	0.078	2.464	89.4	0.083	2.469	74.0	0.082
15.5	9	0.522	122.0	0.072	0.723	126.8	0.073	0.545	109.6	0.081	0.980	68.4	0.079	1.040	73.2	0.082	0.801	57.0	0.099	3.571	85.7	0.077	2.635	90.1	0.084	2.816	74.5	0.080
16.0	18	0.706	123.4	0.072	0.851	128.2	0.073	0.641	110.9	0.080	0.959	68.6	0.079	0.957	73.5	0.082	0.908	57.1	0.098	3.919	86.4	0.077	2.806	90.8	0.084	3.164	74.9	0.077

Girls

Height	N	Systolic BP 24h L	M	S	Day L	M	S	Night L	M	S	Diastolic BP 24h L	M	S	Day L	M	S	Night L	M	S	MAP 24h L	M	S	Day L	M	S	Night L	M	S
120	31	-1.123	104.5	0.063	-1.291	110.8	0.069	-0.053	93.6	0.077	-1.177	65.6	0.087	1.345	72.3	0.087	0.440	54.3	0.089	-1.747	77.5	0.076	0.135	83.8	0.081	-2.736	66.8	0.084
125	25	-0.991	105.3	0.064	-1.007	111.1	0.069	-0.314	94.6	0.079	-0.957	65.9	0.087	1.436	72.3	0.086	0.430	54.8	0.092	-1.352	78.1	0.076	0.368	84.1	0.080	-2.305	67.6	0.085
130	25	-0.856	106.2	0.065	-0.710	111.5	0.069	-0.570	95.6	0.080	-0.733	66.1	0.086	1.531	72.2	0.086	0.421	55.1	0.095	-0.951	78.7	0.076	0.604	84.3	0.079	-1.867	68.3	0.086
135	44	-0.709	107.2	0.066	-0.380	112.0	0.068	-0.807	96.7	0.081	-0.511	66.4	0.086	1.629	72.1	0.085	0.410	55.5	0.098	-0.547	79.3	0.075	0.844	84.5	0.078	-1.411	69.0	0.087
140	50	-0.556	108.3	0.066	-0.075	112.7	0.067	-0.997	97.9	0.082	-0.322	66.6	0.086	1.711	72.1	0.083	0.398	55.8	0.100	-0.148	79.9	0.075	1.083	84.7	0.077	-0.932	69.6	0.087
145	48	-0.406	109.5	0.067	0.117	113.7	0.067	-1.106	99.0	0.082	-0.183	66.9	0.085	1.763	72.1	0.082	0.391	56.0	0.101	0.235	80.5	0.076	1.309	85.0	0.076	-0.427	70.1	0.087
150	43	-0.275	110.9	0.067	0.125	115.1	0.067	-1.126	100.1	0.081	-0.107	67.1	0.084	1.777	72.1	0.081	0.395	56.2	0.101	0.589	81.1	0.076	1.509	85.4	0.076	0.092	70.6	0.087
155	32	-0.155	112.5	0.067	-0.031	116.8	0.066	-1.068	101.3	0.081	-0.110	67.2	0.083	1.740	72.1	0.081	0.413	56.2	0.101	0.914	81.7	0.076	1.680	85.8	0.076	0.620	71.2	0.086
160	39	-0.017	114.2	0.067	-0.251	118.6	0.067	-0.948	102.6	0.080	-0.189	67.3	0.083	1.650	72.2	0.081	0.442	56.3	0.100	1.217	82.3	0.077	1.829	86.4	0.076	1.159	71.9	0.085
165	29	0.154	116.1	0.066	-0.431	120.6	0.068	-0.795	104.1	0.079	-0.324	67.5	0.082	1.509	72.3	0.079	0.487	56.5	0.099	1.509	83.1	0.077	1.963	87.1	0.078	1.706	72.7	0.084
170	28	0.378	118.0	0.066	-0.463	122.6	0.069	-0.626	105.6	0.079	-0.479	67.6	0.081	1.329	72.6	0.079	0.556	56.7	0.097	1.805	83.9	0.077	2.092	88.0	0.080	2.269	73.6	0.082
175	31	0.651	119.7	0.064	-0.373	124.4	0.069	-0.451	107.2	0.078	-0.635	67.8	0.080	1.136	72.8	0.078	0.647	56.9	0.096	2.110	84.7	0.078	2.226	89.0	0.082	2.843	74.5	0.080
180	20	0.942	121.5	0.063	-0.244	126.2	0.069	-0.277	108.7	0.078	-0.785	68.0	0.078	0.939	73.1	0.078	0.755	57.1	0.094	2.423	85.5	0.078	2.364	90.0	0.084	3.425	75.4	0.078
185	19	1.240	123.2	0.061	-0.098	128.0	0.069	-0.100	110.2	0.078	-0.932	68.2	0.077	0.741	73.4	0.078	0.871	57.3	0.093	2.737	86.3	0.079	2.503	91.0	0.087	4.010	76.2	0.075

Table 4
(continued)

Girls

Age	N	Systolic BP 24h L	M	S	Day L	M	S	Night L	M	S	Diastolic BP 24h L	M	S	Day L	M	S	Night L	M	S	MAP 24h L	M	S	Day L	M	S	Night L	M	S
5.0	14	1.362	102.8	0.073	2.507	108.4	0.077	0.144	94.8	0.082	0.646	65.5	0.078	1.670	72.6	0.085	0.122	56.4	0.120	0.487	77.2	0.070	1.277	83.7	0.080	0.507	68.7	0.090
5.5	15	1.174	103.4	0.073	2.274	109.0	0.075	0.052	95.2	0.082	0.773	65.5	0.078	1.717	72.6	0.085	0.120	56.2	0.120	0.675	77.5	0.070	1.371	83.8	0.079	0.528	68.8	0.090
6.0	15	0.987	104.1	0.072	2.041	109.5	0.074	-0.040	95.6	0.083	0.900	65.6	0.078	1.765	72.6	0.085	0.119	55.9	0.119	0.864	77.8	0.070	1.465	83.9	0.079	0.549	68.8	0.091
6.5	17	0.811	104.7	0.071	1.819	110.1	0.073	-0.123	95.9	0.083	1.025	65.7	0.078	1.813	72.5	0.085	0.123	55.7	0.119	1.051	78.0	0.070	1.560	84.0	0.078	0.579	68.8	0.092
7.0	17	0.648	105.3	0.070	1.610	110.6	0.073	-0.194	96.2	0.083	1.148	65.8	0.078	1.861	72.4	0.085	0.129	55.5	0.119	1.239	78.2	0.071	1.656	84.0	0.078	0.617	68.8	0.092
7.5	13	0.503	105.9	0.069	1.417	111.1	0.072	-0.250	96.5	0.084	1.269	65.8	0.079	1.911	72.3	0.086	0.137	55.3	0.120	1.427	78.4	0.071	1.755	84.1	0.077	0.662	68.8	0.093
8.0	12	0.378	106.5	0.069	1.244	111.5	0.071	-0.286	96.8	0.084	1.388	65.9	0.079	1.962	72.2	0.086	0.142	55.1	0.120	1.618	78.6	0.071	1.857	84.1	0.077	0.711	68.8	0.094
8.5	12	0.278	107.0	0.067	1.096	111.9	0.070	-0.298	97.2	0.084	1.503	65.9	0.080	2.015	72.1	0.086	0.143	54.9	0.120	1.811	78.8	0.071	1.961	84.1	0.077	0.765	68.9	0.095
9.0	12	0.199	107.6	0.067	0.969	112.4	0.070	-0.289	97.5	0.084	1.611	66.0	0.080	2.066	72.0	0.086	0.141	54.8	0.121	2.001	79.0	0.071	2.066	84.2	0.076	0.824	68.9	0.095
9.5	22	0.154	108.2	0.066	0.874	112.8	0.069	-0.253	97.9	0.084	1.701	66.1	0.081	2.109	71.9	0.087	0.135	54.7	0.121	2.181	79.2	0.071	2.171	84.3	0.076	0.893	69.0	0.096
10.0	20	0.134	108.7	0.066	0.805	113.3	0.069	-0.197	98.2	0.084	1.775	66.2	0.082	2.146	71.8	0.087	0.125	54.6	0.121	2.352	79.4	0.072	2.274	84.4	0.076	0.970	69.1	0.096
10.5	37	0.151	109.2	0.066	0.775	113.7	0.068	-0.116	98.6	0.084	1.819	66.3	0.083	2.175	71.8	0.087	0.112	54.5	0.121	2.506	79.6	0.072	2.375	84.5	0.076	1.059	69.2	0.097
11.0	31	0.201	109.7	0.065	0.780	114.2	0.068	-0.015	99.0	0.084	1.832	66.4	0.084	2.195	71.8	0.087	0.096	54.3	0.121	2.640	79.9	0.073	2.474	84.7	0.076	1.160	69.3	0.097
11.5	35	0.280	110.2	0.065	0.819	114.7	0.068	0.106	99.3	0.082	1.811	66.5	0.085	2.207	71.9	0.088	0.074	54.2	0.120	2.749	80.2	0.073	2.570	84.9	0.076	1.274	69.4	0.097
12.0	31	0.378	110.7	0.065	0.878	115.3	0.068	0.241	99.7	0.081	1.757	66.6	0.086	2.210	72.1	0.087	0.043	54.2	0.119	2.836	80.5	0.073	2.663	85.2	0.076	1.399	69.6	0.097
12.5	37	0.485	111.3	0.065	0.945	115.8	0.068	0.389	100.1	0.079	1.675	66.8	0.086	2.203	72.2	0.087	0.001	54.2	0.117	2.902	80.9	0.074	2.753	85.5	0.076	1.534	69.8	0.096
13.0	31	0.599	111.8	0.064	1.020	116.4	0.067	0.549	100.5	0.078	1.571	67.0	0.087	2.192	72.4	0.087	-0.051	54.3	0.115	2.957	81.2	0.074	2.843	85.9	0.077	1.676	70.1	0.095
13.5	30	0.722	112.3	0.064	1.107	117.0	0.066	0.720	100.9	0.076	1.453	67.1	0.086	2.179	72.6	0.085	-0.110	54.4	0.112	3.008	81.5	0.074	2.933	86.2	0.076	1.825	70.3	0.094
14.0	20	0.854	112.8	0.063	1.207	117.5	0.065	0.898	101.3	0.074	1.328	67.2	0.085	2.169	72.8	0.084	-0.174	54.5	0.109	3.061	81.9	0.074	3.026	86.5	0.076	1.977	70.6	0.093
14.5	24	0.991	113.3	0.062	1.319	118.1	0.063	1.083	101.6	0.072	1.202	67.4	0.084	2.162	73.0	0.082	-0.243	54.7	0.106	3.121	82.2	0.073	3.122	86.8	0.076	2.132	70.9	0.092
15.0	16	1.129	113.8	0.061	1.435	118.6	0.062	1.269	102.0	0.069	1.075	67.5	0.082	2.158	73.2	0.080	-0.316	54.9	0.102	3.183	82.4	0.073	3.219	87.1	0.076	2.287	71.2	0.090
15.5	12	1.265	114.3	0.059	1.552	119.1	0.061	1.454	102.5	0.067	0.946	67.6	0.081	2.153	73.3	0.078	-0.391	55.1	0.099	3.243	82.7	0.072	3.317	87.4	0.075	2.440	71.5	0.089
16.0	16	1.400	114.8	0.058	1.668	119.6	0.059	1.639	102.9	0.065	0.816	67.7	0.080	2.148	73.5	0.076	-0.467	55.3	0.096	3.302	83.0	0.072	3.415	87.7	0.075	2.593	71.8	0.088

Height	N	Systolic BP 24h L	M	S	Day L	M	S	Night L	M	S	Diastolic BP 24h L	M	S	Day L	M	S	Night L	M	S	MAP 24h L	M	S	Day L	M	S	Night L	M	S
120	30	0.593	104.0	0.059	2.107	110.0	0.061	1.565	95.0	0.070	2.996	65.9	0.065	1.952	73.2	0.077	1.491	55.4	0.112	1.848	77.2	0.067	2.092	83.3	0.074	0.335	68.0	0.097
125	32	0.553	105.0	0.060	1.947	110.5	0.062	1.184	95.7	0.071	2.790	65.9	0.070	1.915	72.8	0.080	1.276	55.3	0.115	1.976	77.5	0.068	2.039	83.7	0.076	0.410	68.2	0.096
130	27	0.535	106.0	0.060	1.804	111.0	0.063	0.823	96.4	0.073	2.592	66.0	0.075	1.881	72.4	0.083	1.075	55.1	0.118	2.103	78.3	0.069	2.014	84.0	0.077	0.477	68.4	0.096
135	20	0.566	106.8	0.061	1.686	111.6	0.064	0.518	96.9	0.075	2.407	66.1	0.080	1.851	72.1	0.087	0.891	54.8	0.120	2.236	78.7	0.071	2.032	84.1	0.079	0.553	68.5	0.096
140	34	0.657	107.6	0.062	1.583	112.2	0.065	0.292	97.5	0.077	2.221	66.3	0.084	1.832	71.7	0.090	0.705	54.6	0.121	2.366	79.2	0.073	2.099	84.3	0.080	0.650	68.7	0.097
145	39	0.797	108.7	0.062	1.480	113.1	0.066	0.167	98.1	0.079	2.006	66.5	0.087	1.828	71.7	0.092	0.497	54.4	0.121	2.479	79.7	0.074	2.217	84.5	0.080	0.778	69.0	0.097
150	54	0.973	109.9	0.063	1.367	114.3	0.066	0.186	98.9	0.080	1.743	66.7	0.089	1.836	71.8	0.092	0.279	54.3	0.118	2.591	80.2	0.074	2.404	84.9	0.079	0.955	69.3	0.097
155	51	1.194	111.2	0.060	1.259	115.6	0.066	0.378	100.0	0.079	1.435	66.9	0.090	1.846	72.0	0.090	0.074	54.3	0.114	2.751	80.8	0.073	2.684	85.5	0.077	1.202	69.8	0.095
160	65	1.485	112.4	0.060	1.220	117.0	0.064	0.745	101.1	0.079	1.088	67.4	0.085	1.835	72.4	0.085	-0.091	54.6	0.110	2.967	81.5	0.072	3.042	86.2	0.074	1.514	70.4	0.093
165	53	1.834	113.7	0.058	1.261	118.3	0.060	1.272	102.2	0.073	0.700	68.0	0.077	1.799	73.1	0.077	-0.200	54.9	0.106	3.214	82.3	0.069	3.442	87.0	0.070	1.871	71.2	0.091
170	46	2.210	115.0	0.055	1.332	119.8	0.055	1.903	103.4	0.070	0.285	68.6	0.069	1.739	73.9	0.069	-0.261	55.1	0.147	3.466	83.1	0.066	3.852	88.0	0.064	2.249	72.0	0.089
175	24	2.601	116.4	0.052	1.410	121.2	0.050	2.579	104.6	0.068	-0.136	68.6	0.064	1.671	74.8	0.061	-0.296	55.4	0.099	3.728	84.0	0.064	4.268	88.9	0.059	2.638	72.8	0.087

From Wühl et al. (25), with permission.

night intervals, either arbitrarily or according to a patient diary, allow a quantification of the nocturnal BP fall, or "dipping," both in absolute and relative terms. Alternative methods include the calculation of cumulative sums *(51)*, chronobiological cosinor analysis *(52)*, and Fourier analysis, which is the simultaneous application of several cosine functions *(53)*.

Even though definitions of "non-dipping" vary, the prognostic relevance of the non-dipping phenomenon has been demonstrated in adults with renal failure *(54)* and in the general population *(45)*. Controversy persists about the physiological basis of circadian and ultradian BP rhythms. While evidence from shift workers suggests that BP rhythms are determined largely externally by physical activity, the fact that disturbances of the diurnal BP pattern are found in a variety of pathological conditions has led to the suggestion that an endogenous rhythm of autonomic nervous activity is at least partly responsible for the generation of circadian BP rhythmicity.

Fourier analysis appears to be superior to linear analysis because there is no need to define day and night intervals, which presuppose an activity-related origin of BP variations. The combination of several rhythms allows a more detailed and flexible description of the 24-h period than the original cosinor method.

Circadian cardiovascular rhythmicity is present in the majority of healthy children and adolescents with an attenuation of 24-h heart rate periodicity during puberty. In addition, ultradian rhythms are found in the majority of healthy children, with an age-related shift from 8-h to 6-h or 12-h predominant rhythmicity *(8)*. Pediatric reference ranges of ultradian rhythms have been provided *(8)*. Compared to these reference data children with chronic kidney disease show marked blunting and delay of the rhythmicity of both BP and heart rate *(55)*. Changes in ultradian and circadian rhythms were independent of each other. Also the ultradian BP amplitudes but not the circadian amplitudes or conventional dipping parameters were correlated to indices of renal function, raising the possibility that ultradian rhythms play an independent role in chronic kidney disease. Current evidence suggests that, whereas normal circadian BP variation is a positive predictor of cardiovascular outcome, ultradian BP variability is more associated with disease states. Increased BP variability has been demonstrated in obese children and is most likely related to increased sympathetic nervous system activation in obesity-related hypertension *(56)*. In adults, greater BP variability has been correlated with the development of hypertensive left ventricular hypertrophy *(57)*.

Reproducibility of ABPM

One of the key advantages of ABPM is its superior reproducibility in comparison to casual BP measurements, which has been demonstrated in adults *(58–60)* and children *(61)*. Excellent reproducibility has also been shown for the nocturnal dipping phenomenon *(62)*. Still, a certain degree of BP variability will be found even with ABPM; in children with borderline hypertension, more than one ABPM may be required to judge the consistency of elevated blood pressure *(63)*.

In view of the growing evidence for the superior quality of the information provided by ABPM, the persistent reluctance of many health-care providers, regulatory authorities, and industry researchers in accepting the primary use of this methodology in the diagnostic and therapeutic management of pediatric hypertension appears medically and ethically unjustified.

To date the vast majority of pediatric antihypertensive trials have used office BP readings to define primary study endpoints. In view of the numerous ethical and practical challenges associated with the enrollment of children in randomized, controlled antihypertensive drug trials, the superior sensitivity of ABPM in detecting treatment-induced BP changes provides a strong argument in favor of using this methodology to define primary endpoints in future clinical trials *(61)*.

Also, in the serial evaluation of blood pressure control in children receiving antihypertensive treatment the superior consistency of ABPM provides valuable qualitative and quantitative information, which is highly likely to improve blood pressure control and long-term cardiovascular outcomes.

In conclusion, with its wide availability, proven technical feasibility across the pediatric age range, availability of high-quality pediatric reference data, and superior sensitivity in diagnosing hypertension and detecting pharmacological treatment effects, ABPM should be considered the method of choice for diagnosis and follow-up in pediatric hypertension.

REFERENCES

1. Mancia G, Parati G. Experience with 24-hour ambulatory blood pressure monitoring in hypertension. Proceedings of the Annual Scientific Sessions of the American Heart Association, Anaheim, CA. 1987:1134–1140.
2. Portman RJ, Yetman RJ, West MS. Efficacy of 24-hour ambulatory blood pressure monitoring in children. J Pediatr. 1991;118:842–849.
3. Reichert H, Lindinger A, Frey O, Mortzeck J, Kiefer J, Busch C, et al. Ambulatory blood pressure monitoring in healthy school children. Pediatr Nephrol. 1995;9:282–286.
4. Flynn JT. Impact of ambulatory blood pressure monitoring on the management of hypertension in children. Blood Press Monit. 2000;5:211–216.
5. Koch VH, Colli A, Saito MI, Furusawa EA, Ignes E, Okay Y, et al. Comparison between casual blood pressure and ambulatory blood pressure monitoring parameters in healthy and hypertensive adolescents. Blood Press Monit. 2000;5:281–289.
6. Mancia G, Parati G, Pomidossi G, Grassi G, Casadei R, Zanchetti A. Alerting reaction and rise in blood pressure during measurement by physician and nurse. Hypertension. 1987;9:209–215.
7. Sorof JM, Portman RJ. White coat hypertension in children with elevated casual blood pressure. J Pediatr. 2000;137:493–497.
8. Hadtstein C, Wühl E, Soergel M, Witte K, Schaefer F. Normative values for circadian and ultradian cardiovascular rhythms in childhood. Hypertension. 2004;43:547–554.
9. Perloff D, Sokolow M, Cowan R. The prognostic value of ambulatory blood pressures. JAMA. 1989;249:2792–2798.
10. White WB, Schulman P, McCabe EJ, Dey HM. Average daily blood pressure, not office blood pressure, determines cardiac function in patients with hypertension. JAMA. 1989;261:873–877.
11. Staessen JA, Thijs L, Fagard B, O'Brien ET, Clement D, de Leeuw PW, et al. Predicting cardiovascular risk using conventional ambulatory blood pressure in older patients with systolic hypertension. JAMA. 1999;282:539–546.
12. Cuspidi C, Macca G, Sampieri L, Fusi V, Severgnini B, Michev I, et al. Target organ damage and non-dipping pattern defined by two sessions of ambulatory blood pressure monitoring in recently diagnosed essential hypertensive patients. J Hypertens. 2001;19:1539–1545.
13. Chobanian AV, Bakris GL, Black DL, Cushman WC, Green LA, Izzo JL Jr, et al. The seventh report of the joint national committee on prevention, detection, evaluation, and treatment of high blood pressure: the JNC 7 Report. JAMA. 2003;289:2560–2571.
14. 2007 Guidelines for the Management of Arterial Hypertension. The Task Force of the Management of Arterial Hypertension of the European Society of Hypertension (ESH) and the European Society of Cardiology (ESC). J Hypertens. 2007;25:1105–1187.
15. Lurbe E, Cifkova R, Cruickshank K, Dillon M, Ferreira I, Invitti C, et al. Management of high blood pressure in children and adolescents; recommendations of the European Society of Hypertension. J Hypertens. 2009;27:1719–1742.
16. National High Blood Pressure Education Program Working Group on High Blood Pressure in Children and Adolescents. The fourth report on the diagnosis, evaluation, and treatment of high blood pressure in children and adolescents. Pediatrics. 2004;114:555–576.

17. Urbina E, Alpert B, Flynn J, Hayman L, Harshfield GA, Jacobson M, et al. Ambulatory blood pressure monitoring in children and adolescents: recommendations for standard assessment. A scientific statement from the American Heart Association. Atherosclerosis, hypertension, and obesity in youth committee of the council on cardiovascular disease in the young and the council for high blood pressure research. Hypertension. 2008;52:433–451.
18. Varda NM, Gregoric A. Twenty-four-hour ambulatory blood pressure monitoring in infants and toddlers. Pediatr Nephrol. 2005;20:798–802.
19. Gellermann J, Kraft S, Ehrich JH. Twenty-four-hour ambulatory blood pressure monitoring in young children. Pediatr Nephrol. 1997;11:707–710.
20. Park MK, Menard SW, Yuang C. Comparison of auscultatory and oscillometric blood pressures. Arch Pediatr Adolesc Med. 2001;155:50–53.
21. Association for the Advancement of Medical Instrumentation/American National Standards Institute. Manual, electronic or automated spygmomanometers. Arlington, VA: ANSI/AAMI; 2002.
22. O'Brian EPJ, Little W, de Swiet M, Padfield P, Altman D, Bland M, et al. The British Hypertension Society protocol for the evaluation of blood pressure measuring devices. J Hypertens. 1993;11(Suppl 2): S43–S62.
23. O'Sullivan JJ, Derrick G, Griggs P, Foxall R, Aitkin M, Wren C. Ambulatory blood pressure in schoolchildren. Arch Dis Child. 1999;80:529–532.
24. Soergel M, Kirschstein M, Busch C, Danne T, Gellermann J, Holl R, et al. Oscillometric twenty-four-hour ambulatory blood pressure values in healthy children and adolescents: a multicenter trial including 1141 subjects. J Pediatr. 1997;130:178–184.
25. Wühl E, Witte K, Soergel M, Mehls O, Schaefer F, for the German Working Group on Pediatric Hypertension. Distribution of 24-h ambulatory blood pressure in children: normalized reference values and role of body dimensions. J Hypertens. 2002;20:1995–2007.
26. Lurbe E, Redon J, Liao Y, Tacons J, Cooper RS, Alvarez V. Ambulatory blood pressure monitoring in normotensive children. J Hypertens. 1994;12:1417–1423.
27. Flynn JT. Differentiation between primary and secondary hypertension in children using ambulatory blood pressure monitoring. Pediatrics. 2002;110:89–93.
28. Ettinger LM, Freeman K, DiMartino-Nardi JR, Flynn JT. Microalbuminuria and abnormal ambulatory blood pressure in adolescents with type 2 diabetes mellitus. J Pediatr. 2005;147:67–73.
29. Eissa MA, Poffenbarger T, Portman RJ. Comparison of the actigraph versus patients' diary information in defining circadian time periods for analyzing ambulatory blood pressure monitoring data. Blood Press Monit. 2001;6:21–25.
30. Prisant LM, Bottini PB, Carr AA. Ambulatory blood pressure monitoring: methodologic issues. Am J Nephrol. 1996;16:190–201.
31. Reusz GS, Hóbor M, Tulassay T, Sallay P, Miltény M. 24-Hour blood pressure monitoring in healthy and hypertensive children. Arch Dis Child. 1994;70:90–94.
32. de Man SA, André JL, Bachmann HJ, Grobbee DE, Ibsen KK, Laaser U, et al. Blood pressure in childhood: pooled findings of six European studies. J Hypertens. 1991;9:109–114.
33. Brotons C, Singh P, Nishio T, Labarthe DR. Blood pressure by age in childhood and adolescents: a review of 129 surveys worldwide. Int J Epidemiol. 1989;18:824–829.
34. Harshfield GA, Alpert BS, Pulliam DA, Somes GW, Wilson DK. Ambulatory blood pressure recordings in children and adolescents. Pediatrics. 1994;94:180–184.
35. National High Blood Pressure Education Programme Working Group on Hypertension Control in Children and Adolescents. Update on the 1987 task force report on high blood pressure in children and adolescents: a working group report from the national high blood pressure educational program. Pediatrics. 1996;98: 649–658.
36. Menghetti E, Virdis R, Strambi M, Patriarca V, Riccioni MA, Fossali E, et al. Blood pressure in childhood and adolescents: the Italian normal standards. J Hypertens. 1999;17:1363–1372.
37. Sorof JM, Poffenbarger T, Franco K, Portman R. Evaluation of white coat hypertension in children: importance of the definitions of normal ambulatory blood pressure and the severity of casual hypertension. Am J Hypertens. 2001;14:855–860.
38. Lurbe E, Sorof JM, Daniels SR. Clinical and research aspects of ambulatory blood pressure monitoring in children. J Pediatr. 2004;144:7–16.
39. Koshy S, Macarthur C, Luthra S, Gajaria M, Geary D. Ambulatory blood pressure monitoring: mean blood pressure and blood pressure load. Pediatr Nephrol. 2005;20:1484–1486.
40. White WB, Dey HM, Schulman P. Assessment of the daily blood pressure load as a determinant of cardiac function in patients with mild-to-moderate hypertension. Am Heart J. 1989;118:782–795.
41. Sorof JM, Cardwell G, Franco K, Portman RJ. Ambulatory blood pressure and left ventricular mass index in hypertensive children. Hypertension 2002;39:903–908.

42. Liu M, Takahashi H, Morito Y, Maruyama S, Mizuno M, Yuzawa Y, et al. Non-dipping is a potent predictor of cardiovascular mortality and is associated with autonomic dysfunction in hemodialysis patients. Nephrol Dial Transplant. 2003;18:563–569.

43. Brotman DJ, Davidson MB, Boumitri M, Vidt DG. Impaired diurnal blood pressure variation and all-cause mortality. Am J Hypertens. 2008;21:92–97.

44. Leung LC, Ng DK, Lau MW, Chan CH, Kwok KL, Chow PY, et al. Twenty-four-hour ambulatory BP in snoring children with obstructive sleep apnea syndrome. Chest. 2006;130:1009–1017.

45. Ohkubo T, Hozawa A, Yamaguchi J, Kikuya M, Ohmori K, Michima M, et al. Prognostic significance of the nocturnal decline in blood pressure in individuals with and without high 24-h blood pressure: the Ohasama study. J Hypertens. 2002;20:2183–2189.

46. Lurbe E, Redon J, Kesani A, Pascual JM, Tacons J, Alvarez V, et al. Increase in nocturnal blood pressure and progression to microalbuminuria in type 1 diabetes. N Engl J Med. 2002; 347:797–805.

47. Cole TJ, Green PJ. Smoothing reference centile curves: the LMS method and penalized likelihood. Stat Med. 1992;11:1305–1319.

48. Pickering T. Future developments in ambulatory blood pressure monitoring and self-blood pressure monitoring in clinical practice. Blood Press Monit. 2002;7:21–25.

49. Stergiou GS, Yiannes NG, Rarra VC, Panagiotakos DB. Home blood pressure normalcy in children and adolescents: the Arsakeion School Study. J Hypertens. 2007;25:1375–1379.

50. Wühl E, Hadtstein C, Mehls O, Schaefer F, ESCAPE trial group. Home, clinic, and ambulatory blood pressure monitoring in children with chronic renal failure. Pediatr Res. 2004;55:492–497.

51. Stanton A, Cox J, Atkins N, O'Malley K, O'Brian E. Cumulative sums in quantifying circadian blood pressure patterns. Hypertension. 1992;19:93–101.

52. Halberg F, Johnson EA, Nelson W, Runge W, Sothern R. Autorhythmometry: procedures for physiologic self-assessments and their analysis. Physiol Teacher. 1972;1:1–11.

53. Staessen JA, Fagard R, Thijs L, Amery A. Fourier analysis of blood pressure profiles. Am J Hypertens. 1993;6(6 Pt 2):184S–187S.

54. Liu M, Takahashi H, Morita Y, Maruyama S, Mizuno M, Yuzawa Y, et al. Non-dipping is a potent predictor of cardiovascular mortality and is associated with autonomic dysfunction in haemodialysis patients. Nephrol Dial Transplant. 2003;18:563–569.

55. Wühl E, Hadtstein C, Mehls O, Schaefer F, ESCAPE trial group. Ultradian but not circadian blood pressure rhythms correlate with renal dysfunction in children with chronic renal failure. J Am Soc Nephrol. 2005;16:746–754.

56. Sorof JM, Poffenbarger T, Franco K, Bernard L, Portman RJ. Isolated systolic hypertension, obesity and hyperkinetic hemodynamic states in children. J Pediatr. 2002;140:660–666.

57. Parati G, Faini A, Valentini M. Blood pressure variability: its measurement and significance in hypertension. Curr Hypertens Rep. 2006;8:199–204.

58. Ward A, Hansen P. Accuracy and reproducibility of ambulatory blood pressure recorder measurements during rest and exercise. New York, NY: Springer; 1984.

59. van der Steen MS, Lenders JW, Graafsma SI, den Arend J, Thien T. Reproducibility of ambulatory blood pressure monitoring in daily practice. J Hum Hypertens. 1999;13:303–308.

60. Palatini P, Mormino P, Canali C, Santonastaso M, De Venuto G, Zanata G, et al. Factors affecting ambulatory blood pressure reproducibility: results of the HARVEST Trial: hypertension and ambulatory recording Venetia study. Hypertension. 1994;23:211–216.

61. Gimpel C, Wühl E, Arbeiter K, Drozdz D, Trivelli A, Charbit M, et al. Superior consistency of ambulatory blood pressure monitoring in children: implications for clinical trials. J Hypertens. 2009;27:1568–1574.

62. Zakopoulos NA, Nanas SN, Lekakis JP, Vemmos KN, Kotsis VT, Pitiriga VC, et al. Reproducibility of ambulatory blood pressure measurements in essential hypertension. Blood Press Monit. 2001;6:41–45.

63. Rucki S, Feber J. Repeated ambulatory blood pressure monitoring in adolescents with mild hypertension. Pediatr Nephrol. 2001;16:911–915.

64. Lurbe E, Cremades B, Rodriguez C, Torro MI, Alvarez V, Redon J. Factors related to quality of ambulatory blood pressure monitoring in a pediatric population. Am J Hypertens. 1999;12:929–933.

11 Epidemiology of Essential Hypertension in Children: The Bogalusa Heart Study

Elaine M. Urbina, MD, MS, *Sathanur R. Srinivasan,* PhD, *and Gerald S. Berenson,* MD

CONTENTS

INTRODUCTION

Cardiovascular diseases including heart attack and stroke remain the leading causes of death and disability in the United States *(1)*. However, the adult heart diseases begin decades earlier *(2)*. Observations from many well-established epidemiologic studies in adults have implicated risk factors, for example, high blood pressure, hypercholesterolemia, and obesity, along with lifestyles of poor diet, smoking, and sedentary behavior, as related to the development of clinical heart disease *(3–5)*. Unfortunately, hypertension is a major public health problem involving over 30% of the adult African-American population *(6)*. Furthermore, a strong relationship has been demonstrated between cardiovascular risk factors and underlying atherosclerotic, hypertensive vascular abnormalities at autopsy both in adults and in children and adolescents *(3,4)*. The occurrence of anatomic changes at a young age is the most compelling evidence that the adverse effects of risk factors such as hypertension are not limited to adult heart disease but that hypertensive cardiovascular–renal diseases begin in childhood *(7,8)*. Epidemiologic studies at a young age now provide considerable understanding of the early natural history of high blood pressure and

E.M. Urbina (✉)
Preventive Cardiology, Department of Pediatrics, Cincinnati Children's Hospital Medical Center,
Cincinnati, OH, USA
e-mail: elaine.urbina@cchmc.org

From: *Clinical Hypertension and Vascular Diseases: Pediatric Hypertension*
Edited by: J. T. Flynn et al. DOI 10.1007/978-1-60327-824-9_11
© Springer Science+Business Media, LLC 2011

the hypertensive disease leading to clinical events. In this chapter we will summarize key findings from the Bogalusa Heart Study and other important works.

PREVALENCE OF HYPERTENSION

The prevalence of hypertension in children is influenced by the definition of what may be considered normal in growing children and methods used to obtain blood pressure levels. Indirect measurement is the accepted form, and proper cuff size is essential for valid measurements *(9–11)*. Because of considerable variation in blood pressure levels measured in childhood, replicate measures of blood pressure in the resting state best reflect an individual's blood pressure level *(11,12)*. However, the precise level defining hypertension in childhood is controversial. Early recommendations listed normal and elevated percentiles of blood pressure by gender and age *(13)*. Current guidelines improved the definition of hypertension in growing children by evaluating blood pressure levels as a function of height *(11)*. The importance of height as a determinant of blood pressure was shown in the Bogalusa Heart Study where 39% of the variability in systolic blood pressure was related to body size and not age *(14)*. Since children mature at different rates, taller children of the same age equate with a distribution at higher levels (Fig. 1). Based on this finding, it is recommended that blood pressure levels be related to height for defining abnormality.

Additional controversy exists around which gender- and height-derived percentiles are abnormally high. Current pediatric BP guidelines define hypertension as persistent BP levels above the 95th percentile for age, gender, and height *(11)*. However, anatomic changes

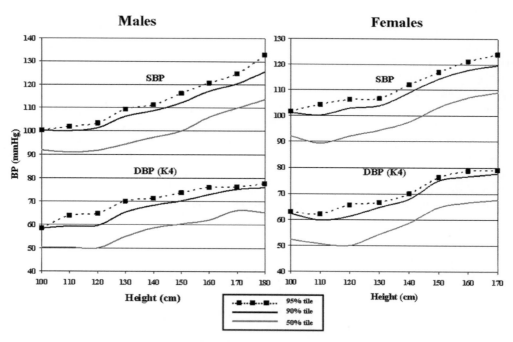

Fig. 1. Percentile levels for blood pressure by height for males and females. *The Bogalusa Heart Study* (*N*= 3352). Abbreviations: SBP, systolic blood pressure; DBP, diastolic blood pressure *(170)*.

in target organs such as development of left ventricular hypertrophy (LVH) are seen to occur at levels just above the 90th percentile *(15)* with increased left ventricular posterior wall measurements seen to occur with BP above the 80th percentile *(16)*. Furthermore, epidemiologic evidence demonstrates that presence of pre-hypertension (levels above the 90th percentile) has a sensitivity of 33.3% in predicting future adult hypertension *(17)*. Data from the National Childhood Blood Pressure database suggests that presence of pre-hypertension may predict progression to sustained hypertension in up to 12–14% of children in only 2 years of follow-up *(18)*. Bogalusa Heart Study data also indicate the importance of identifying youth crossing blood pressure percentiles since a change in blood pressure in youth was independently associated with being classified as prehypertensive or truly hypertensive as an adult *(19)*.

The definition of diastolic hypertension has also varied over time. Some have advocated abandoning diastolic blood pressure measurements in children altogether *(20)*. Others suggest reporting both K4 and K5 *(21)*, using K4 up to a certain age and then shifting to K5 *(13)* or using only K4 or K5 diastolic blood pressure measurements *(22,23)*. Although the use of K5 diastolic blood pressure would provide continuity between reporting of childhood and adult values, studies in children have demonstrated a large difference between K4 and K5 levels particularly in young children. One study found 27% of all children aged 5–8 years had at least one of six measurements of K5 near zero, a value with limited physiologically significance *(22)*. Furthermore, K4 diastolic blood pressure measurements are more reproducible in childhood and are a better predictor of adult hypertension (Fig. 2) *(24)*.

Other considerations for choice of childhood blood pressure norms exist. The most recent published guidelines for blood pressures in children base normal values on data averaged from multiple epidemiologic studies *(11)*. However, only a single measurement, often the first and only measurement, is used. The use of a single measurement to define normal blood pressure levels is markedly limited by the observed and significant within-subject variation in blood pressure levels. Replicate and serial measurements, four to six, are needed to obtain levels characteristic of a given individual or misclassification of subjects may occur *(12,25)*. Furthermore, a single blood pressure recording may be subject to the 'first

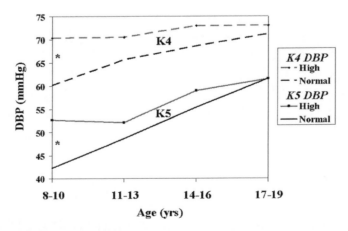

Fig. 2. Childhood K4 and K5 related to normotensive and hypertensive adults, respectively. *The Bogalusa Heart Study* (*N*=1017, *p values for difference between levels of DBP measured in childhood for normotensive and hypertensive adults are ≤0.05 for ages 8–16) *(24)*.

reading effect' both with automatic Dinamap-type devices *(12,26)* and with a mercury sphygmomanometer; the first reading may be higher than an individual's intrinsic blood pressure *(25)*. 'White coat' hypertension is a real phenomenon; however, it may be over-diagnosed with the use of a single blood pressure recording *(27,28)*. Averaging six readings of BP has led the Bogalusa Heart Study to publish blood pressure norms that are lower than national guidelines *(11)* by 5–10 mmHg for systolic blood pressure (slightly less for diastolic blood pressure) *(29)*. Circadian variation in BP levels also exists. Nighttime levels measured with 24-h ambulatory blood pressure monitoring (ABPM) dip at least 10% lower than daytime values in normal individuals. Although new guidelines are available on recommended use of ABPM in children and adolescents *(30)*, widespread use of this technique is limited by lack of availability of normative data across diverse races, genders, and ages *(31)*. Furthermore, at least two repeat 24-h ambulatory recordings are needed to account for 90% of the variability in blood pressure recordings *(32)*. Similarly, African-American children in Bogalusa have been shown to have higher resting blood pressure levels than white children *(33)*. Therefore, insufficient numbers of non-white participants in nationally published averages may make that data less readily applicable to minority populations.

Despite the difficulties in measurement, obtaining blood pressure levels can identify children needing immediate intervention and is helpful in predicting adult hypertension since blood pressure levels 'track' (remain in respective rank) over time. Tracking correlation coefficients for blood pressure range from 0.36 to 0.50 for systolic blood pressure and from 0.29 to 0.42 for diastolic blood pressure over 15 years of follow-up (Fig. 3) *(34,35)*. Children in the highest quintile for blood pressure had a nearly fourfold increase in risk of being diagnosed with clinical hypertension as an adult. Multiple elevations in blood pressure levels recorded as a child improved the ability to predict adult hypertension *(34)*.

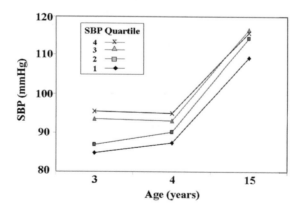

Fig. 3. Tracking of systolic blood pressure (persistence of quartiles) over 15 years of follow-up starting at the age of 2 years. *The Bogalusa Heart Study (N=185) (35)*.

CHARACTERISTICS OF THE HYPERTENSIVE CHILD

The characteristics of the hypertensive child represent the underlying determinants of hypertension.

Anthropometrics

Although height relates strongly to blood pressure levels in growing children, body fatness influences adult *(36)* and childhood blood pressure levels even after adjustment for height *(37,38)*. This relationship between obesity and blood pressure is stronger in white children than African-American, especially in African-American males *(9)*. Central body fat distribution may be even more important as it significantly relates to systolic blood pressure in children aged 5–17 years even after adjustment for peripheral body fat while the reverse is not true *(39)*. Furthermore, male children and adolescents with total body fat levels ≥25% were found to be 2.8 times more likely to have higher blood pressure levels than lean children. This remained significant even after adjusting for potential confounding factors such as age, race, and truncal fat pattern *(40)*. Data in females were similar. Which measure of adiposity relates most strongly to blood pressure levels is controversial. In one cross-sectional study, BMI for age was more powerful than waist to height ratio in identifying children with high systolic blood pressure *(41)*. With the trend toward increasing prevalence of overweight children well documented *(42–44)* obesity may be the most important, preventable cause of elevated blood pressure in young people, especially whites.

Renal Function and Electrolytes

Perturbations in renal hemodynamics have long been postulated to be an etiology for adult hypertension *(45)*. In children, a positive relation exists between 24-h sodium excretion, 24-h urine sodium to potassium ratio, and blood pressure for African-American adolescents with higher resting blood pressure levels *(46)*. Interestingly, these relationships were not seen in whites. Additional racial contrasts are seen in other renal factors related to blood pressure. African-American children, especially those with higher blood pressures for age, size, and gender, have lower plasma renin activity than white children (Table 1) *(47)*. However, renin activity correlates with blood pressure only in white youth *(48)*. White children were also more likely to demonstrate both high renin activity levels and insulin resistance as measured by post-glucose load 1-h insulin × 1-h glucose levels *(48)*. African-Americans were also found to have less urine potassium excretion and slightly lower creatinine clearance *(47)*. In a longitudinal study, baseline systolic and diastolic blood pressures were independent predictors of follow-up creatinine 7 years later in African-Americans, while the reverse was not true *(49)*. Young African-American adults also demonstrate greater natriuresis with a negative stool and urine sodium balance and a cumulative potassium balance in response to an oral potassium challenge. These results were not found for whites *(50)*. It should be noted that additional studies proved no significant difference among these two races in overall sodium to potassium dietary intake *(51)*. Unfortunately, two-thirds of these school-age children had sodium intakes above the recommended 2 g/day and 50–70% had potassium intakes below the recommended daily allowance (2 mEq/kg/day) *(52)*. It is clear that dietary modification may be an important step in preventing hypertension in genetically salt-sensitive individuals, especially in African-Americans.

Neural Mechanisms

While the hypertension in African-American adolescents from the above observations seems to be driven by renal mechanisms, elevated blood pressure in whites may have neural, specifically, sympathomimetic origins. White children demonstrate higher dopamine-β-hydroxylase levels regardless of resting blood pressure levels (Table 1) *(46)*.

Table 1

Plasma Renin Activity, Urine Potassium Excretion, and Serum Dopamine-β-Hydroxylase Levels by Blood Pressure Stratum in Children: The Bogalusa Heart Study (47) (N=272)

	Race	Gender	1 (Low BP)	2	3	4	5 (High BP)
Plasma renin activity (ng/mL/min)	White	Male	5.7 (±1.7)	7.1 (±1.7)	6.6 (±1.9)	7.6 (±2.1)	8.6 (±2.4)
		Female	7.4 (+1.1)	6.5 (+1.3)	5.9 (+1.6)	7.7 (+2.3)	8.0 (+2.4)
	African-American	Male	6.1 (±3.1)	6.9 (±2.2)	4.2 (±1.1)	4.1 (±1.3)	3.7 (±2.5)
		Female	3.5 (±2.0)	6.2 (±1.9)	5.0 (±1.2)	7.0 (±2.1)	4.5 (±1.1)
24-h urine potassium excretion (mEq/24-h)	White	No gender differences found	33.2 (±4.9)	42.0 (±5.6)	34.2 (±7.2)	44.7 (±10.2)	38.8 (±6.8)
	African-American		24.8 (± 5.7)	26.5 (±4.2)	27.4 (±4.4)	29.4 (±5.0)	29.8 (±11.6)
Serum dopamine-β-hydroxylase (mmol/min/L)	White	Male	37 (±6)	29 (±7)	32 (±8)	28 (±7)	33 (±8)
		Female	30 (±12)	25 (±8)	27 (±8)	29 (±7)	35 (±6)
	African-American	Male	26 (± 13)	23 (±5)	17 (±5)	24 (±6)	23 (±13)
		Female	17 (±7)	20 (±7)	22 (±5)	22 (±6)	19 (±18)

This suggests sympathetic predominance exits in white children *(47)*. The faster heart rates seen at higher levels of blood pressure in white children, especially boys, support this theory *(46)*. Other supportive data are found in studies of heart rate variability in adults where sympathetic predominance at rest is found as compared to age-matched controls, with the degree of abnormality correlating with severity of hypertension *(53)*. Adult hypertensives also demonstrate loss of the circadian rhythm of the low-frequency component measured by heart rate variability *(54)*. In a study using heart rate variability in children, healthy white male adolescents regardless of blood pressure level demonstrated higher sympathetic tone and lower parasympathetic tone than African-Americans. A trend for sympathetic predominance in the higher blood pressure group was noted for both races *(55)*. Again, it was hypothesized that variations in sympathetic nervous system function occur among the races in regard to initiation of essential hypertension. Studies of systolic blood pressure and heart rate show a higher 'double product' in white children also indicative of greater sympathetic tone *(56)*. However, there may be a crossover to higher sympathetic levels in African-Americans around 25 years of age accounting for the higher blood pressure and heart rate found in adults of African descent as compared to subjects of white Americans *(57)*.

Stress Responses

Not only do racial differences exist in resting autonomic tone but there are also differences demonstrated in response to stress for both children *(58)* and adults *(59)*. African-American children performing cardiovascular response tests have higher maximal stressed systolic blood pressure than whites regardless of resting blood pressure levels (Fig. 4) *(60,61)*. For the African-American adolescents with elevation of resting blood pressure, the systolic levels of blood pressure especially during orthostatic and cold pressor testing exceeded those of the other race–sex groups *(47,61)*. Peripheral vasoconstriction is also much more pronounced in African-American children in response to alpha-adrenergic stimulation such as produced by cold stress *(62,63)*, a finding that has been noted in normotensive African-American adults *(64)*. In addition, mental stress in hypertensive African-Americans results in diminished cardiac sympathomimetic tone with higher peripheral

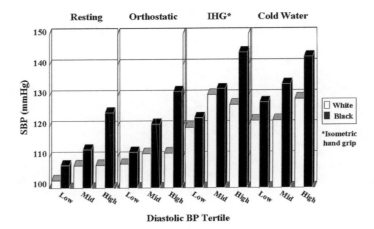

Fig. 4. Resting and maximal stress SBP levels in boys aged 7–15 years by race and resting diastolic blood pressure tertile. *The Bogalusa Heart Study* (N=136, p values for all race difference in maximal stressed SBP are ≤ 0.01) *(61)*.

vascular response *(65)*. In contrast, white males with borderline high blood pressures have a greater increase in cardiac index in response to stress *(63)* while African-American subjects exhibit increases in vascular tone *(66–68)*. Sympathetic predominance in white children has also been shown by heart rate variability data collected during reactivity testing with a trend toward sympathetic predominance in hypertensives of both races *(69)*. These data show racial differences occur in response to stress even in early borderline hypertension. There may be underlying African-American/white differences in autonomic tone or response of the nervous system to stress with different types of adrenergic receptors stimulated to different degrees. Blood pressure responses to stress may also be a marker for the individual genetically predisposed toward adult hypertension. Parker et al. found that peak blood pressure in children during orthostatic stress, isometric handgrip, and cold pressor testing helped predict future blood pressure even after adjusting for baseline blood pressure levels *(67)*. Furthermore, blood pressure reactivity has been found to be predictive of future left ventricular mass corrected for body size especially in African-Americans *(70)*. Interestingly, both blood pressure response to exercise and left ventricular mass have also been found to predict future blood pressure *(71)*. Left ventricular mass likely represents the sum of long-term effects of blood pressure both at rest and during stress *(71)*. A combination of resting and peak exercise blood pressure levels along with measurement of left ventricular mass may prove to be better predictors of adult hypertension.

Hyperdynamic Circulation

African-American/white contrasts have been demonstrated in resting measures of cardiovascular function. White children have been found to have higher resting heart rates *(61)* and higher cardiac output as measured by echocardiography (Fig. 5), and blood pressure levels were positively correlated with resting cardiac output and stroke volume *(68)*. In contrast, African-American children were found to have higher peripheral vascular resistance *(68)*. These findings in children are notable since studies in adults have suggested that a hyperdynamic state with increased cardiac output due to enhanced contractility occurs early in persons genetically susceptible to hypertension *(72)*. Later, cardiac output may

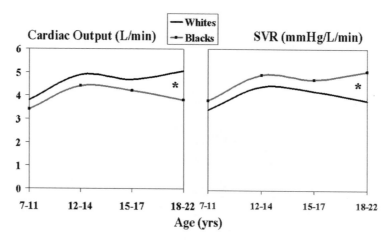

Fig. 5. Cardiac output and systemic vascular resistance (SVR) measured by echocardiography in males by race and age. *The Bogalusa Heart Study* (N=651, *p for race difference $\leq$0.01) *(68)*.

become normalized due to a sustained increase in peripheral vascular resistance occurring with a progressive downregulation of beta-receptors. This may eventually result in clinical hypertension *(63)*.

Obesity, well known to increase the risk of hypertension, may also increase risk for development of a hyperdynamic circulatory pattern. The 'double product,' or heart rate × blood pressure, has been described as a measure of hyperdynamic circulation *(56)*. Boys with obesity were found to have a higher 'double product' suggesting a link between weight and chronic cardiac stress through an effect on myocardial oxygen consumption *(56)*. Investigators have also found that obese boys (percent body fat >75th percentile) with hyperdynamic circulation (high pulse pressure and heart rate) have higher systolic blood pressure, triglyceride, VLDL cholesterol, and fasting insulin levels regardless of age and race (Fig. 6) *(73)*. These features of adult-type syndrome X persisted when the subjects were followed over 3 years ('tracking') *(73)*. These data suggest that an obesity-insulin-induced hyperdynamic circulation may be an early feature of type 2 diabetes and occurs even at young ages. The much greater frequency of pre-diabetes and metabolic syndrome reported in our nation in recent years *(74)* may impact the incidence of hypertension if obesity control measures are not promptly enacted *(75)*.

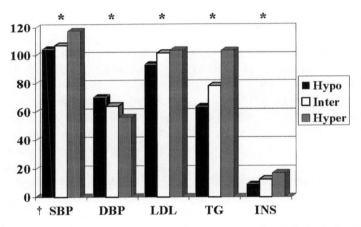

Fig. 6. Effect of hyperdynamic circulation on blood pressure, lipids, and insulin in obese boys (body fat >75%) aged 8–17 years. *The Bogalusa Heart Study* (*N*=96). (*N*=2229, *p* values for slope of linear regression of variables on hemodynamic status after adjusting for age and race are all ≤0.003). †Units are as follows: SBP and DBP, mmHg; LDL-C, HDL-C, and TG, mg/dL; insulin, μU/mL *(73)*.

Effect of Insulin on Hemodynamics

Glucose loading experiments in children have been performed to further investigate the relationships between carbohydrate metabolism and cardiovascular function. White children had higher 1-h plasma glucose levels than African-Americans, and fasting glucose levels in whites were seen to increase with each successively higher quintile of resting blood pressure (Fig. 7) *(47)*. A trend for increasing fasting insulin levels with higher levels of blood pressure was also seen in white boys even after adjusting for body weight *(47)*. When the 'peripheral insulin resistance' product was calculated for white boys (1-h glucose in mg/dL multiplied by the 1-h insulin level in μU/mL), there was a significant increase at higher levels of blood pressure. White subjects with a higher insulin resistance product demonstrated a positive relationship between fasting glucose and resting blood pressure

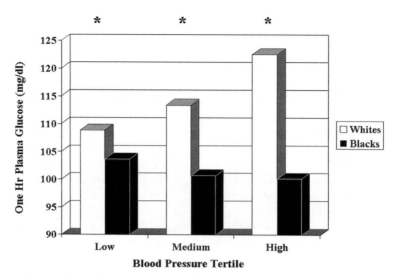

Fig. 7. One-hour plasma glucose levels by race and blood pressure level in children aged 7–15 years. *The Bogalusa Heart Study.* ($N=270$, $^*p \leq 0.05$ for the slope of the linear regression of 1-h glucose on blood pressure stratum in white subjects) *(47)*.

adjusted for body size *(76)*. Further study has confirmed racial differences in carbohydrate metabolism with African-American children demonstrating significantly higher insulin and lower glucose levels than whites *(77)*. Both race and ethnicities demonstrated a positive relationship between metabolic measures such as insulin and glucose and blood pressure levels in cross-sectional studies *(78)*; however, longitudinal analyses found that the correlation remained significant with follow-up blood pressure only in whites *(79)*. Multivariate models showed a significant relationship between fasting insulin and both systolic and diastolic blood pressure in children (5–12 years) and young adults (18–26 years) independent of glucose level and body fatness (Table 2) *(78)*. Weaker relationships were found during puberty (13–17 years) which may have been due to the complex and variable rates of change of sex hormones and growth velocity during these ages *(78)*. The stronger relationship between insulin and systolic rather than diastolic blood pressure has been postulated to be due to the effect of insulin on pulse pressure *(80)*. These studies suggest that the relationship between insulin and blood pressure may differ between individuals of different genetic/racial makeup resulting in variable alterations in sympathetic tone, sodium reabsorption by the distal renal tubules, or amount of vascular hypertrophy leading to distinct etiologies for the same manifestation (hypertension) *(78,81)*.

Regardless of ethnicity, levels of fasting insulin demonstrate tracking (persistence of relative rank over time with $r=0.23–0.36$) *(82)*. This is significant because subjects in the highest quartile of insulin at baseline demonstrated higher levels of systolic blood pressure (+7 mmHg), diastolic blood pressure (+3 mmHg), body mass index (+9 kg/m^2), triglycerides (+58 mg/dL), LDL cholesterol (+11 mg/dL), VLDL cholesterol (+8 mg/dL), and glucose (+9 mg/dL) with lower levels of HDL cholesterol (–4 mg/dL). They were 3.3 times more likely to report a parental history of diabetes and 1.2 times more likely to report a family history of hypertension *(82)*. In subjects with tracking of elevated insulin levels, the prevalence of adult hypertension was increased 2.5-fold with increased rates for obesity (3.6-fold) and dyslipidemia (3-fold) also reported *(82)*. These data introduce the concept of 'clustering' of cardiovascular risk factors where elevated levels of multiple risk factors are

Table 2
Independent Variables Associated with Blood Pressure by Age[a]: The Bogalusa Heart Study
(78)

5–8 years (N=717)	9–12 years (N=939)	13–17 years (N=1048)	18–26 years (N=814)
		Systolic blood pressure	
BMI	BMI	Age	Gender
Subscapular skinfold	Insulin	Gender	BMI
Insulin	Glucose	BMI	Insulin
Glucose		Race	Race
		Glucose	
$R^2 = 0.27$	$R^2 = 0.25$	$R^2 = 0.13$	$R^2 = 0.16$
		Diastolic blood pressure	
BMI	Subscapular skinfold	Gender	BMI
Age	Insulin	Age	Gender
Subscapular skinfold	Glucose	Glucose	Age
Race	Gender		Insulin
	BMI		
$R^2 = 0.13$	$R^2 = 0.16$	$R^2 = 0.10$	$R^2 = 0.06$

[a]Listed in order of acceptance by the stepwise regression model. BMI indicates body mass index. All $p \leq 0.05$.

found to exist together in many adults leading to a multiplicative risk of cardiovascular diseases. Clustering has also been demonstrated in children with persistently higher levels of blood pressure contributing most strongly to the prediction of multiple risk factor clustering as an adult (83). However, the adult metabolic syndrome with insulin resistance is likely the result of the eventual congruence of different physiologic processes occurring in childhood. Factor analyses of Bogalusa Heart Study data found that both metabolic (insulin resistance, dyslipidemia, obesity) and hemodynamic (insulin resistance, blood pressure) clustering in childhood may be operating as precursors of adult metabolic syndrome (84). Further analyses suggest that these clustering patterns differ by race/ethnicity. Although multivariate analyses revealed that metabolic syndrome resulted from three different factors, they differed by race. In whites, the clusters were blood pressure and adiposity; lipids and adiposity; and insulin resistance, renin levels, and adiposity. For African-American subjects, renin did not contribute (85). The importance of each of the factors (magnitude of the path analysis coefficients) in explaining metabolic syndrome was greater for whites except for the effect of age on mean arterial pressure which was stronger in blacks (85). Regardless of the pathway taken by individuals of differing genetic or race and ethnic backgrounds, it is clear that the pathophysiologic changes leading to metabolic syndrome in adults begin in childhood.

Uric Acid

Animal studies suggest a role for uric acid in the pathogenesis of hypertension (86). This may be through modulation of oxidative stress resulting in stimulation of the renin–angiotensin system or by stimulation of vascular smooth muscle proliferation (87).

Therefore, it is not surprising that a relationship was found between childhood uric acid levels and change in uric acid levels and eventual adult blood pressure *(88)*. This relationship persisted even after adjusting for traditional cardiovascular risk factors *(89)*.

Family History

Predicting and preventing adult heart and kidney diseases are the major motivations for examining children with potential hypertension. Family history is an important component of these evaluations as parental history provides a surrogate measure of future cardiovascular disease. In a study of 3,312 children aged 5–17 years, significant correlations were found between levels of risk factors in children and family history even after adjusting for age, race, and gender *(90)*. However, independent associations between childhood risk factor levels and family history were only found for combinations of parental diseases such as heart attack in the father plus high blood pressure or diabetes *(90)*. In contrast, when childhood blood pressure rank was analyzed longitudinally over 9 years, family history of hypertension alone was found to be an independent predictor of future systolic blood pressure in these children *(91)*. Similar relationships between childhood blood pressure levels and parental history of hypertension were found in the Muscatine Study *(92)*. When younger children were studied (birth to 7 years of age), the strongest relationships were found between parental and child height and weight *(93)*. However, when the parents' systolic blood pressures were related to their childrens' levels with regression coefficients, significant relationships were found which tended to increase with the child's age *(93)*. It seems logical that as parents age, they begin to develop morbidity from elevated levels of risk factors that were not apparent earlier. In fact, in a study of 8,276 subjects, the prevalence of parental cardiovascular disease was greater in subjects aged 25–31 as compared to the 5- to 10-year-old group *(94)*. This included an increase in reporting of positive family history of hypertension by up to 32% depending on race *(94)*. Furthermore, children of hypertensive parents had higher blood pressure after 10 years of age regardless of weight and also demonstrated increased prevalence of dyslipidemias *(94)*. Racial differences were also seen with white children, especially boys, demonstrating higher LDL cholesterol levels and reporting parental history of heart attack while African-Americans had higher insulin levels and were more likely to report parental hypertension *(94)*. Ambulatory blood pressure studies have also demonstrated the importance of family history of hypertension *(32)*. When ambulatory blood pressure load was calculated, the percentage of readings above the race-, gender-, and height-specific 90th percentile for systolic and diastolic blood pressure was found to be greatest in children with high resting blood pressure and a family history of hypertension. However, children with low resting blood pressure and a positive family history of hypertension also had higher ambulatory blood pressure load than normotensive children without a family history (Fig. 8) *(32)*.

Genetic Influences

Advances in genetic testing techniques have opened new avenues for evaluating the genes associated with regulation of blood pressure levels. Estimation of the heritability of longitudinal blood pressure levels (total area under the curve) was 0.66 for systolic and 0.68 for diastolic blood pressure in a sub-study using 775 white siblings *(95)*. When 357 highly polymorphic microsatellite markers were typed, linkage analyses found genes on chromosomes 2 and 18 for diastolic blood pressure and chromosome 4 for both systolic and diastolic blood pressure to be important (Fig. 9) *(95)*. Several hypertension candidate

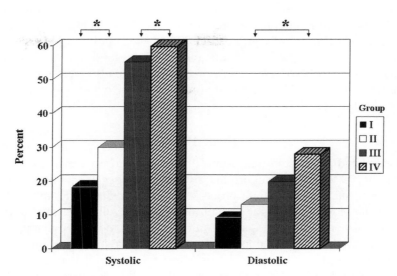

Fig. 8. Frequency of ambulatory blood pressure readings greater than the 90th percentile by blood pressure and parental history group in children aged 12–21 years. *The Bogalusa Heart Study* (*N*=57; **p* for difference between groups indicated by arrows ≤0.01). I = low blood pressure group, no parental hypertension; II = low blood pressure group, +parental hypertension; III = high blood pressure group, no parental hypertension; IV = high blood pressure group, +parental hypertension *(32)*.

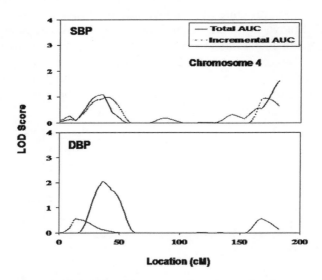

Fig. 9. Multipoint linkage results for total and incremental AUC for blood pressure in white siblings on chromosome 4. *The Bogalusa Heart Study*. LOD score peak = 2.0 for DBP at 36 cM near the marker D4S2994 (2-point LOD = 2.1) with weak linkage to SBP (total AUC LOD = 1.1 at 35 cM; SBP incremental AUC LOD = 0.99 at 39 cM). Also, SBP had total AUC LOD = 1.6 at 182 cM and incremental AUC LOD = 0.95 at 170 cM near the q-terminal of chromosome 4 2. AUC=area under the curve (mmHg) divided by the number of follow-up years. Total AUC was adjusted for age, sex, and body mass index; incremental AUC was adjusted for age, sex, body mass index, and baseline blood pressure *(95)*.

genes are located in these areas such as alpha-adducin, beta-adducin, sodium bicarbonate co-transporter, and G protein-coupled receptor kinase 4 *(95)*. Other candidate genes have also been evaluated. The non-carriers of the 894T (vs G) polymorphism of the endothelial nitric oxide synthase gene had significantly higher blood pressure especially if they were also insulin resistant *(96)*. Non-carriers of the T allele also were more likely to have a greater long-term burden of blood pressure (area under the curve) since childhood but this was only true for females *(97)*.

Birth Weight

Retrospective studies of adults have found an association between adult hypertension and low birth weight *(98,99)*. The 'fetal origins' hypothesis suggests that fetal programming by under nutrition in utero may initiate processes such as reduced numbers of nephrons in the kidney or changes in other organs, resulting in chronic diseases later in life like hypertension *(100)*. Postnatal influences, such as the increased metabolic demands imposed by the development of obesity, may amplify the effects of fetal programming *(101)*. However, data from epidemiologic studies show inconsistent relationships between birth weight and adult blood pressure levels *(102,103)*. Racial and genetic background may be influencing these results as Bogalusa Heart Study data show a stronger relationship between low birth weight and future blood pressure in whites than in African-Americans (Fig. 10) *(104)*. In fact, birth weight may be one factor accounting for race/ethnic differences in adolescent blood pressure levels *(35)*. Also, birth weight may be a better predictor of blood pressure levels when subjects are young adults *(105)* rather than during childhood *(103)* and may be better at predicting longitudinal blood pressure trends *(106)* as there has been more time to display a mature blood pressure phenotype. Additional prospective studies such as the National Children's Study (www.nationalchildrensstudy.gov) co-sponsored by the National Institute of Child Health and Human Development, the National Institute of Environmental Health Sciences, the Centers for Disease Control and Prevention, and the US Environmental Protection Agency are in progress. These studies may shed more light on this issue by factoring in influences such as gestational age *(107)*; disproportionate, head-sparing low birth weight *(98)*; and maternal factors *(108)*.

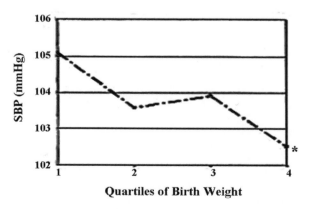

Fig. 10. Mean systolic blood pressure by quartiles of birth weight, adjusted for age, sex, ethnic group, and BMI. *The Bogalusa Heart Study* ($N=1155$, *$p \leq 0.01$ for linear trend across quartiles of birth weight) *(104)*.

SUBCLINICAL TARGET ORGAN DAMAGE, 'SILENT DISEASE'

Subclinical target organ damage occurs in children with higher levels of blood pressure and can be measured by invasive and non-invasive techniques.

Autopsy Studies

Beginning in 1978, autopsies were performed on participants in the Bogalusa Heart Study in Louisiana who died between the ages of 3 and 31 years *(2,4,109)*. Most deaths resulted from vehicular accidents, homicides, or suicides, with only 10% related to natural causes. Tissue samples collected from 85 autopsies included coronary arteries, aorta, kidney, adrenals, and blood. Aortas and coronary arteries were stained with Sudan IV and gross evaluation of fatty streaks and fibrous lesions performed according to protocols developed in the International Atherosclerosis Project *(110)*. Histological evaluations were also performed with anatomic results compared to antemortem cardiovascular risk factor data.

A consistent pattern of associations between lesions and risk factors emerged. Antemortem levels of total and LDL cholesterol were strongly related to extent of fatty streak lesion in the aorta *(2,109)*. Fatty streaks in the aorta and coronary arteries were also related to systolic blood pressure; however, after adjustment for age, the relationship was only found to be significant for the coronaries *(4)*. Importantly, fibrous plaques in coronary arteries, the type of lesions felt to be prone to progression, were also correlated with age-adjusted antemortem systolic and diastolic blood pressure levels (Fig. 11) *(4,109)*. This finding of increased prevalence of fibrous plaques in the coronary arteries of men with hypertension and other cardiovascular risk factors has been confirmed in the Pathologic Determinants of Atherosclerosis in Youth study *(3)*.

Once again race and gender differences were found. Males, especially African-Americans, demonstrated larger areas of the aorta staining for fatty streaks *(111)*. Males, in general, had more progression-prone fibrous lesions in both the aorta and the coronary arteries than females. However, this was especially true for white males *(111)*. Male subjects also demonstrated the strongest relationship between antemortem cholesterol levels and aorta fat streaks with white males showing the greatest correlation between systolic

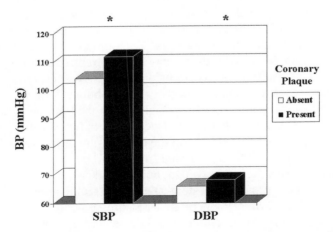

Fig. 11. Levels of blood pressure adjusted for age with and without coronary artery fibrous plaques. *The Bogalusa Heart Study (N=54, *p level for blood pressure difference is ≤ 0.04) (170).*

and diastolic blood pressure and coronary artery lesions *(111)*. In both genders, histology demonstrated greater aortic foam cell infiltration and further extent and intensity of lipid staining in subjects with higher age-adjusted blood pressure *(4)*. However, only in males, especially African-American males, were a significant correlation found between blood pressure levels and foam cell infiltration and lipid staining in the coronary arteries *(4)*. When intimal thickening of the coronary arteries was studied, a weak relationship was found with antemortem blood pressure levels. However, this coronary artery thickening did relate strongly to hyalinization of renal arterioles *(4)*.

Additional studies have been performed exploring the relationship between blood pressure and renal microvascular abnormalities. A mathematical model was developed to relate quantity of lesions found in renal arteries measuring 50–400 μm and mean blood pressure *(112)*. A linear relationship, mean BP = 1.60 × microvascular lesions +79.7, with correlation coefficient 0.698, was found for all ages *(112)*. The sample studied was from a population with a mean age of less than 20 years. These data strongly confirm that the atherosclerotic-hypertensive process begins in youth, and the degree of vascular involvement correlates with antemortem levels of cardiovascular risk factors including blood pressure levels. Furthermore, the thickening of small renal arteries is consistent with the concept of remodeling outlined by Glagov et al. *(113)* and the observations of vascular changes described by Folkow et al. *(114)* and reviewed by Mulvany *(115)*.

Cardiac Structure and Function

Even before echocardiography was in wide usage, investigators demonstrated that subtle ECG changes possibly representing early left ventricular hypertrophy were apparent in children with higher levels of blood pressure *(116)*. Later epidemiology studies measuring left ventricular thickness by M-mode analyses confirmed this hypothesis by showing a positive correlation between left ventricular wall thickness and systolic blood pressure, even after adjusting blood pressure for body size *(16)*. Other epidemiologic studies in children relating blood pressure levels to left ventricular mass, especially in males, have confirmed these relationships *(15,117–119)*. Longitudinal analyses using Bogalusa Heart Study data have also demonstrated that the cumulative burden of systolic blood pressure from childhood to adulthood is independently associated with indexed left ventricular mass in young adults *(120)*. Childhood diastolic blood pressure is also independently related to concentric left ventricular hypertrophy *(121)*, the pattern of left ventricular geometry most strongly linked to adverse cardiovascular outcomes in adults *(122)*. Although resting clinic blood pressure is clearly important, ambulatory recordings may be even more powerful than resting clinic levels in identifying youth at risk for hypertension-related left ventricular hypertrophy *(30)*. This is because there is a strong correlation between ambulatory blood pressure load *(32)*, the percentage of blood pressure recordings higher than the 95th percentile, and left ventricular mass index *(123)*. The importance of accurate characterization of blood pressure levels in children for prevention is evident in the observation of thicker left ventricular wall at levels only greater than the 80th percentile *(16)*.

Other cardiovascular risk factors may also increase the risk for development of LVH. In longitudinal studies, linear growth (i.e., height) emerged as the major determinant of heart growth in children *(124)*. Earlier, Voors et al. *(125)* stressed body mass as the major determinant of blood pressure in young children, height related in a linear fashion and weight logarithmically. However, development of obesity was shown to lead to increased left ventricular mass in children and in females with this increased mass, possibly preceding the development of high blood pressure *(124)*. Obesity in childhood was the only consistent predictor of LVM in adulthood *(120)*. Additionally, left ventricular mass was shown to demonstrate tracking through late childhood and adolescence thus confirming the importance of measuring heart size in children with blood pressure levels at the higher end of the distribution *(124)*. Exploration was also made of the relationships between obesity, metabolic syndrome, and left ventricular mass. Although no direct, independent effect of insulin on left ventricular mass was found in healthy adolescents and young adults of normal weight, in obese persons as measured by increasing subscapular skinfold thickness, increasing fasting insulin level was associated with greater heart mass (Fig. 12) *(126)*. These data suggest that the metabolic syndrome phenotype is likely to relate to target organ damage even in adolescents prior to the development of clinical type 2 diabetes. Genetic influences on left ventricular mass have also been explored. The angiotensinogen gene has been implicated in the initiation of left ventricular hypertrophy. Increasing dosage of the A(-6) allele in the gene in white and African-American subjects was associated with left ventricular mass index despite the great difference in prevalence of the allele between race/ethnicities (in whites 66.6% were carriers while in African-Americans 97% displayed the allele) *(127)*.

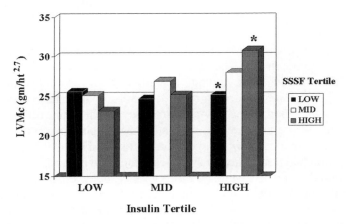

Fig. 12. Left ventricular mass by insulin and subscapular skinfold thickness in children aged 13–17 years. *The Bogalusa Heart Study (N=*216, **p ≤* 0.05 low SSSF vs high SSSF and mid-SSSF vs high SSSF. SSSF = subscapular skinfold thickness) *(126)*.

The effect of blood pressure level on cardiac function has also been examined. In a sample of children taken from across the entire blood pressure distribution, left ventricular stroke volume and cardiac output were found to be positively correlated with systolic and diastolic blood pressure while ejection fraction and peripheral vascular resistance related significantly to diastolic blood pressure levels *(68)*. With increasing systolic blood pressure and age, an increase in left ventricular output and stroke volume was seen regardless of race or gender. However, further analyses did demonstrate race–gender differences. White males as compared to African-Americans demonstrated greater cardiac output and stroke volume after adjustment for systolic blood pressure and measures of body size (1.25 L/min for ages 18–22 years and 10 mL greater). Conversely, African-American males had higher peripheral resistance (4.5 mmHg/L/min) than whites *(68)*. These findings of increased stroke volume and cardiac output and decreased peripheral vascular resistance in whites as compared to African-Americans were confirmed in a study of over 200 children in Cincinnati, Ohio *(128)*. Autonomic tone may be one factor underlying the racial difference seen in the hemodynamic mechanisms operating in the early phase of hypertension *(68)*. African-Americans demonstrate augmented muscle sympathetic nerve activity (MSNA) associated with higher blood pressures suggesting enhanced alpha-adrenergic sensitivity *(64)*. In contrast, the natural history of hypertension in whites may involve an initial increase in cardiac output followed by downregulation of beta-adrenergic receptors leading to the transition to a progressive increase in systemic vascular resistance *(129)*. Although systolic dysfunction is uncommon in youth, obesity in childhood and hypertension as a young adult were also found to be important predictors of left ventricular dilation in otherwise healthy individuals *(130)*. This suggests that early cardiac decompensation related to cardiovascular risk factors can be identified well before progression to overt left ventricular dysfunction and congestive heart failure. These observations show the importance of obesity in childhood and the burden on the CV system of higher levels of blood pressure even though not at levels considered abnormal by task force criteria.

Vascular Abnormalities

One of the earliest studies of the effect of cardiovascular risk factors on the arterial tree was conducted in the early 1980s *(131)*. In this study, ultrasounds of the carotid artery were performed to measure maximal and minimal diameters during the cardiac cycle. From these data the pressure–strain elastic modulus (E_p), a measure of stiffness that is the inverse of distensibility, was calculated. The study subjects were divided into a low- and high-risk groups based on race, gender, and age-specific tertiles for total serum cholesterol and systolic blood pressure. The high-risk group of children had stiffer carotid arteries with a mean E_p 5.1 kPa higher than in the low-risk group even after controlling for race, sex, and age *(131)*. Subjects with a positive family history for hypertension or diabetes tended to have higher E_p values than those without such a history and those with a history of parental myocardial infarction had a statistically significant increase in carotid artery stiffness *(131)*. Therefore, functional changes in great vessels can be detected in asymptomatic children and adolescents at risk for the development of adult heart disease. The importance of traditional cardiovascular risk factors in determining arterial stiffness was demonstrated in a later study using M-mode ultrasound of the common carotid artery. Systolic and diastolic blood pressure correlated with both Peterson's and Young's elastic modulus, and systolic blood pressure was an independent determinant of both stiffness measures in multivariate analyses *(132)*. Both measures increased, indicating stiffer vessels, with greater numbers of cardiovascular risk factors indicating the important effect of clustering of risk factors on arterial stiffness *(132)*. Further study revealed that candidate genes usually associated with blood pressure regulation exerted influence on carotid stiffness. In African-Americans, the presence of the T allele of the endothelial nitric oxide gene (G894T polymorphism) was associated with lower systolic blood pressure along with significantly lower carotid stiffness (Peterson and Young's elastic modulus) even after adjusting for mean arterial pressure *(133)*.

Studies of the vascular function of other portions of the vascular tree have also been conducted. Distensibility of the brachial artery was measured on 920 healthy young adults who had been followed from childhood as part of the Bogalusa Heart Study. As expected, distensibility tended to decrease with age reaching significance in females *(134)*. However, race and gender differences existed (whites > African-Americans; females > males) even after adjustment for age. When distensibility was plotted as a function of pulse pressure to control for distending pressure, subjects with higher systolic, diastolic, and mean

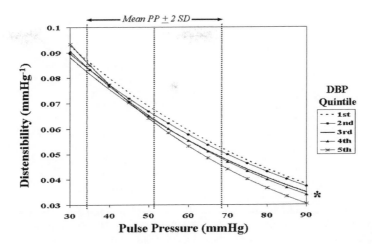

Fig. 13. Brachial artery distensibility as a function of pulse pressure by quintiles of DBP. *The Bogalusa Heart Study* (N=920, *p for distensibility decrease for the fifth as compared to the first and second quintiles ($p \leq 0.03$)) *(134)*.

arterial pressure had lower distensibility of the brachial artery (Fig. 13). The independent effect of measures of blood pressure on distensibility was confirmed in multivariate analyses *(134)*. Clustering of metabolic syndrome risk factors was also shown to predict diminished brachial artery distensibility *(135)*. Further, pediatric studies suggest that obesity and insulin resistance contribute to deterioration in brachial artery distensibility as early as the adolescent years *(136)*. Longitudinal analyses are needed to explore the effects of childhood levels of risk factors on adult measures of non-invasive subclinical vascular changes related to arteriosclerosis.

Pulse wave velocity (PWV) has also been evaluated as a measure of arterial stiffness. In hypertensive adults, the increasing PWV seen with stiffer vessels is strongly associated with presence of atherosclerosis *(137)*. Increased PWV adjusted for other cardiovascular risk factors was also the best predictor of cardiovascular mortality in this large adult study *(137)*. In asymptomatic young adults in the Bogalusa Heart Study, blood pressure is strongly related to aorto-femoral PWV (Fig. 14) *(138)* and was the first covariate to enter models exploring predictors of PWV *(139,140)*. While both systolic blood pressure and mean arterial pressure were important in explaining large and small artery compliance *(140,141)*, even more important is the observation that childhood systolic blood pressure is an independent predictor or brachial-ankle PWV as an adult *(142)*. Similar to results in carotid stiffness, candidate genes associated with blood pressure regulation appear to influence central aortic stiffness. Values for aorto-femoral PWV were significantly higher in subjects who were homozygous for the Glyc 389 polymorphism of the beta-adrenergic receptor gene even after adjustment for baseline levels of cardiovascular risk factors *(143)*. Racial differences were also apparent with the Arg 16 allele (vs glycine) associated with PWV only in African-Americans *(143)*.

In addition to abnormalities in arterial function, structural changes have been demonstrated in young, asymptomatic Bogalusa Heart Study participants. In correlation analyses, thicker intima–media thickness (IMT) of all segments of the carotid artery (common, bulb and internal) was related to higher blood pressure levels. This association retained significance in multivariate analyses for the common carotid artery and bulb *(144)*. In fact, systolic blood pressure was the first risk factor to enter models in stepwise analyses examining

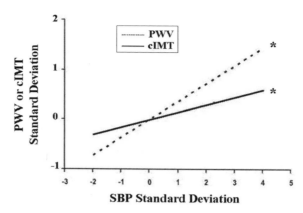

Fig. 14. Relationships of systolic blood pressure (BP) to aorto-femoral pulse wave velocity (PWV) and carotid intima–media thickness (cIMT). *The Bogalusa Heart Study* (N=900, standardized regression coefficient: PWV = 0.36, IMT = 0.15, *p for both $p \leq 0.01$) (138).

independent determinants of carotid (140) and femoral IMT (145). Systolic blood pressure measured in adult men was also a predictor of progression of a composite IMT measure in longitudinal studies after only 5.8 years of follow-up (146). The influence of blood pressure on carotid IMT may be modulated by genetic factors. Only non-carriers of the G allele for the G-6A polymorphism of the angiotensinogen gene demonstrated a significant adverse association between higher mean arterial pressure and thicker common carotid IMT (147).

Risk factor levels were also examined with subjects stratified by carotid bulb (148) or femoral (149) IMT. Subjects in the top fifth percentile for IMT were significantly more likely to be hypertensive or taking blood pressure-lowering medications compared to subjects with a normal carotid or femoral thickness (bottom fifth percentile). They also were more likely to exhibit abnormalities in other risk factors. The impact of clustering on IMT is evident as increasing numbers of CV risk factors (higher systolic blood pressure, cigarette smoking, higher total cholesterol to HDL cholesterol ratio, greater level of obesity, and higher insulin levels) or higher Framingham Risk Score was also associated with a linear increase in carotid IMT (Fig. 15) (144,150). Subjects fulfilling the criteria for a diagnosis of metabolic syndrome with either the World Health Organization or the US National Cholesterol Education Program were found to have a thicker common and internal carotid IMT than subjects without metabolic syndrome (151). Emerging data are now available relating cardiovascular risk factors such as elevated blood pressure to carotid thickness even in asymptomatic youth (152). Bogalusa data also demonstrate that childhood SBP was independently related to adult carotid IMT (153). Taken together, these data indicate the need to treat blood pressure at a young age almost as a continuous variable (rather than using a cut point) to prevent target organ damage.

Renal Dysfunction

Urine microalbumin excretion may result from increased intraglomerular pressure as a result of hypertension, thus serving as one of the best markers for subtle, asymptomatic chronic renal disease. In diabetic subjects, urine protein correlates with blood pressure levels (154). Even in healthy young individuals, there is a significant and positive relationship between urine albumin excretion and systolic and diastolic blood pressure, especially in African-Americans (Fig. 16) (155). Furthermore, in African-Americans with diagnosed

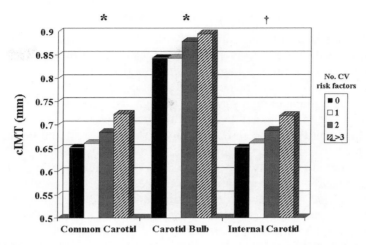

Fig. 15. The effect of multiple risk factors (total cholesterol to HDL cholesterol ratio, waist circumference, systolic blood pressure, insulin level >75th percentile specific for age, race, and gender, smoking) on carotid intima–media thickness (cIMT) in young adults. *The Bogalusa Heart Study* (N=518, $^*p \leq 0.0001$ for common and bulb, †trend for internal carotid p=0.09) *(144).*

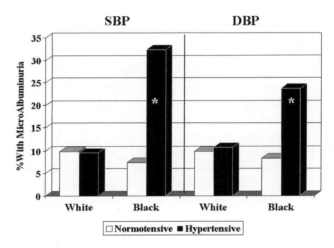

Fig. 16. Percentage of young adults with microalbuminuria by race and blood pressure classification. *The Bogalusa Heart Study* (N= 1131, $^*p$ for difference between normotensive and hypertensive African-American subjects is $\leq$0.01) *(155).*

hypertension, elevated urine albumin excretion occurs with greater frequency than those considered normotensive *(155)*. These associations were not significant in whites and it has been postulated that African-American individuals may be more susceptible to renal damage from relatively low levels of blood pressure increases *(155)*. Subclinical hypertension-related renovascular disease can also be evaluated with measures of urinary activity of N-acetyl-β-D-glucosaminidase (NAG), which is elevated even in asymptomatic young people as systolic blood pressure levels increased (4 mmHg from lowest to highest quintile) *(156)*. This effect was strongest in African-American women *(156)*. Again, these observations point to the fact that subclinical kidney damage occurs with hypertension defined by task force guideline cut points and may even occur at lower levels. Furthermore, the effects are more extensive in African-Americans.

Results of Intervention

No longer are hypertension and coronary heart disease thought of as diseases of adults. The studies described above clearly prove that hypertensive disease and atherosclerosis begin in youth. It is paramount to begin prevention efforts early to obtain maximum benefit and attempt to break the viscous cycle of developing hypertensive cardiovascular disease. Physicians should encourage screening of high-risk groups in addition to promoting a population-based approach to achieving healthy lifestyles.

Guidelines for identifying and screening high-risk families should be followed by measuring risk factor levels of all family members. Unfortunately, even if previously informed that they were hypertensive, only 64% of Bogalusa Heart Study participants were aware of their condition at follow-up 5 years later and only 25% of self-reported hypertensives were receiving treatment *(157)*. Primary care practitioners should implement both primary and secondary prevention measures at all health-care encounters *(11,158,159)*. If lifestyle modification as the initial therapy for hypertension in a child fails, behavior change combined with low-dose medication will likely prove to be both safe and effective *(11,160–162)*.

Population-based models of prevention also have been proven effective. The DASH diet in adults shows lifestyle changes can help modulate blood pressure levels in a population broadly *(163)*. The efficacy of this diet intervention in youth has now been demonstrated *(164)*. Public health approaches to prevention of heart disease also have been developed such as The Health Ahead/Heart Smart Program which was developed as an outgrowth of data collected from the Bogalusa Heart Study *(165)*. This is a coordinated and comprehensive health education program, for kindergarten through sixth grade, addressing the entire school, community, and home environment. Traditional classroom training in health-promoting behaviors is combined with education in nutrition and physical activity in a non-competitive setting. School workers are taught healthier cooking methods while parents and teachers as role models are encouraged to engage in healthy lifestyles. Family and community support are encouraged through free screenings at 'health fairs' where nutrition and exercise are promoted as family lifestyles. Studies have proven the effectiveness of these programs in changing adverse health habits in both children and adults leading to measurable decreases in blood pressure levels in parents *(166,167)*. This program of educating children to become more aware of the need to take care of their own health

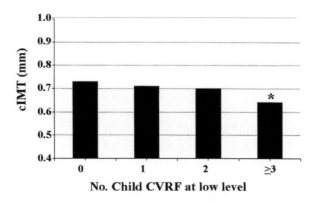

Fig. 17. Average (common, bulb, and internal) carotid intima–media thickness (cIMT) measured in adults by the number of CV risk variables at the bottom quartiles in their childhood. *The Bogalusa Heart Study* ($N = 1474$, *p for trend $= 0.013$) *(169)*.

has implications for physicians to provide leaderships to bring this message to their own communities *(168)*. The efficacy of primordial prevention (prevention of the acquisition of cardiovascular risk factors) is evident in data demonstrating lower adult carotid thickness in Bogalusa subjects who had multiple cardiovascular risk factors clustering at low levels in childhood (Fig. 17) *(169)*.

SUMMARY

It is clear that hypertension with target organ damage begins in youth. Hypertension is a complex syndrome mediated by multiple mechanisms and lifestyles. Proven methods for primary prevention should be a major goal for all health professionals along with more aggressive management of elevated blood pressure in early life.

ACKNOWLEDGMENTS

The authors wish to acknowledge the children and families in Bogalusa who made this research possible. The joint effort of the many individuals who have contributed to this study is gratefully acknowledged.

REFERENCES

1. Murray CJL, Kulkarni SC, Ezzati M. Understanding the coronary heart disease versus total cardiovascular mortality paradox: a method to enhance the comparability of cardiovascular death statistics in the United States. Circulation. 2006;113:2071–2081.
2. Berenson GS, Srinivasan SR, Bao W, Newman WP, 3rd, Tracy RE, Wattigney WA. Association between multiple cardiovascular risk factors and atherosclerosis in children and young adults. The Bogalusa Heart Study. N Engl J Med. Jun 4 1998;338:1650–1656.
3. McMahan CA, McGill HC, Gidding SS, Malcom GT, Newman WP, Tracy RE, Strong JP. PDAY risk score predicts advanced coronary artery atherosclerosis in middle-aged persons as well as youth. Atherosclerosis. Feb 2007;190:370–377.
4. Newman WP, 3rd, Wattigney W, Berenson GS. Autopsy studies in United States children and adolescents. Relationship of risk factors to atherosclerotic lesions. Ann N Y Acad Sci. 1991;623:16–25.
5. Wilson PW, Bozeman SR, Burton TM, Hoaglin DC, Ben-Joseph R, Pashos CL. Prediction of first events of coronary heart disease and stroke with consideration of adiposity. Circulation. Jul 8 2008;118:124–130.
6. Nesbitt SD. Hypertension in black patients: special issues and considerations. Curr Hypertens Rep. Aug 2005;7:244–248.
7. Berenson G, Srinivasan SR. Cardiovascular risk factors in youth with implications for aging: the Bogalusa Heart Study. Neurobiol Aging. Mar 2005;26:303–307.
8. Freedman DS, Wattigney WA, Srinivasan S, Newman WP, 3rd, Tracy RE, Byers T, Berenson GS. The relation of atherosclerotic lesions to antemortem and postmortem lipid levels: the Bogalusa Heart Study. Atherosclerosis. Dec 1993;104:37–46.
9. Voors AW, Foster TA, Frerichs RR, Webber LS, Berenson GS. Studies of blood pressures in children, ages 5–14 years, in a total biracial community: the Bogalusa Heart Study. Circulation. Aug 1976;54:319–327.
10. Chobanian AV, Bakris GL, Black HR, Cushman WC, Green LA, Izzo JL Jr, Jones DW, Materson BJ, Oparil S, Wright JT Jr, Roccella EJ. The seventh report of the joint national committee on prevention, detection, evaluation, and treatment of high blood pressure: the JNC 7 report. JAMA. May 21 2003;289:2560–2572.
11. National High Blood Pressure Education Program Working Group on High Blood Pressure in Children and Adolescents. The fourth report on the diagnosis, evaluation, and treatment of high blood pressure in children and adolescents. Pediatrics. 2004;114(Suppl 2):1–22.
12. Gillman MW, Cook NR. Blood pressure measurement in childhood epidemiological studies. Circulation. Aug 15 1995;92:1049–1057.

13. National Heart, Lung, and Blood Institute. Report of the second task force on blood pressure control in children—1987. task force on blood pressure control in children. National Heart, Lung, and Blood Institute, Bethesda, Maryland. Pediatrics. Jan 1987;79:1–25.
14. Voors AW, Webber LS, Frerichs RR, Berenson GS. Body height and body mass as determinants of basal blood pressure in children—the Bogalusa Heart Study. Am J Epidemiol. Aug 1977;106:101–108.
15. Daniels SR, Loggie JM, Khoury P, Kimball TR. Left ventricular geometry and severe left ventricular hypertrophy in children and adolescents with essential hypertension. Circulation. May 19 1998;97:1907–1911.
16. Burke GL, Arcilla RA, Culpepper WS, Webber LS, Chiang YK, Berenson GS. Blood pressure and echocardiographic measures in children: the Bogalusa Heart Study. Circulation. Jan 1987;75:106–114.
17. Shear CL, Burke GL, Freedman DS, Webber LS, Berenson GS. Designation of children with high blood pressure—considerations on percentile cut points and subsequent high blood pressure: the Bogalusa Heart Study. Am J Epidemiol. Jan 1987;125:73–84.
18. Falkner B, Gidding SS, Portman R, Rosner B. Blood pressure variability and classification of prehypertension and hypertension in adolescence. Pediatrics. Aug 2008;122:238–242.
19. Srinivasan SR, Myers L, Berenson GS. Changes in metabolic syndrome variables since childhood in prehypertensive and hypertensive subjects: the Bogalusa Heart Study. Hypertension. Jul 2006;48:33–39.
20. Weismann DN. Systolic or diastolic blood pressure significance. Pediatrics. Jul 1988;82:112–114.
21. Kirkendall WM, Burton AC, Epstein FH, Freis ED. Recommendations for human blood pressure determination by sphygmomanometers. Circulation. Dec 1967;36:980–988.
22. Hammond IW, Urbina EM, Wattigney WA, Bao W, Steinmann WC, Berenson GS. Comparison of fourth and fifth Korotkoff diastolic blood pressures in 5 to 30 year old individuals. The Bogalusa Heart Study. Am J Hypertens. Nov 1995;8:1083–1089.
23. Uhari M, Nuutinen M, Turtinen J, Pokka T. Pulse sounds and measurement of diastolic blood pressure in children. Lancet. Jul 20 1991;338:159–161.
24. Elkasabany AM, Urbina EM, Daniels SR, Berenson GS. Prediction of adult hypertension by K4 and K5 diastolic blood pressure in children: the Bogalusa Heart Study. J Pediatr. Apr 1998;132:687–692.
25. Burke GL, Webber LS, Shear CL, Zinkgraf SA, Smoak CG, Berenson GS. Sources of error in measurement of children's blood pressure in a large epidemiologic study: Bogalusa Heart Study. J Chron Dis. 1987;40:83–89.
26. Wattigney WA, Webber LS, Lawrence MD, Berenson GS. Utility of an automatic instrument for blood pressure measurement in children. The Bogalusa Heart Study. Am J Hypertens. Mar 1996;9:256–262.
27. Kouidi E, Fahadidou-Tsiligiroglou A, Tassoulas E, Deligiannis A, Coats A. White coat hypertension detected during screening of male adolescent athletes. Am J Hypertens. Feb 1999;12:223–226.
28. Sorof JM, Poffenbarger T, Franco K, Portman R. Evaluation of white coat hypertension in children: importance of the definitions of normal ambulatory blood pressure and the severity of casual hypertension. Am J Hypertens. Sep 2001;14:855–860.
29. Bronfin DR, Urbina EM. The role of the pediatrician in the promotion of cardiovascular health. Am J Med Sci. Dec 1995;310:S42–S47.
30. Urbina E, Alpert B, Flynn J, Hayman L, Harshfield GA, Jacobson M, Mahoney L, McCrindle B, Mietus-Snyder M, Steinberger J, Daniels S. Ambulatory blood pressure monitoring in children and adolescents: recommendations for standard assessment: a scientific statement from the American Heart Association Atherosclerosis, Hypertension, and Obesity in Youth Committee of the council on cardiovascular disease in the young and the council for high blood pressure research. Hypertension. Sep 2008;52:433–451.
31. Wuhl E, Witte K, Soergel M, Mehls O, Schaefer F. Distribution of 24-h ambulatory blood pressure in children: normalized reference values and role of body dimensions. J Hypertens. Oct 2002;20:1995–2007.
32. Berenson GS, Dalferes E Jr, Savage D, Webber LS, Bao W. Ambulatory blood pressure measurements in children and young adults selected by high and low casual blood pressure levels and parental history of hypertension: the Bogalusa Heart Study. Am J Med Sci. Jun 1993;305:374–382.
33. Berenson G, Srinivasan S, Chen W, Li S, Patel D. Racial (black-white) contrasts of risk for hypertensive disease in youth have implications for preventive care: the Bogalusa Heart Study. Ethn Dis. 2006;16:S4-2-9.
34. Bao W, Threefoot SA, Srinivasan SR, Berenson GS. Essential hypertension predicted by tracking of elevated blood pressure from childhood to adulthood: the Bogalusa Heart Study. Am J Hypertens. Jul 1995;8:657–665.
35. Cruickshank JK, Mzayek F, Liu L, Kieltyka L, Sherwin R, Webber LS, Srinavasan SR, Berenson GS. Origins of the "black/white" difference in blood pressure: roles of birth weight, postnatal growth, early blood pressure, and adolescent body size: the Bogalusa Heart Study. Circulation. Apr 19 2005;111:1932–1937.

36. Dyer AR, Elliott P, Shipley M, for The Intersalt Cooperative Research Group. Body mass index versus height and weight in relation to blood pressure findings for the 10,079 persons in the Intersalt Study. Am J Epidemiol. Apr 1 1990;131:589–596.

37. Lauer RM, Clarke WR. Childhood risk factors for high adult blood pressure: the Muscatine study. Pediatrics. Oct 1989;84:633–641.

38. Lurbe E, Alvarez V, Redon J. Obesity, body fat distribution, and ambulatory blood pressure in children and adolescents. J Clin Hypertens (Greenwich). Nov–Dec 2001;3:362–367.

39. Shear CL, Freedman DS, Burke GL, Harsha DW, Berenson GS. Body fat patterning and blood pressure in children and young adults. The Bogalusa Heart Study. Hypertension. Mar 1987;9:236–244.

40. Williams DP, Going SB, Lohman TG, Harsha DW, Srinivasan SR, Webber LS, Berenson GS. Body fatness and risk for elevated blood pressure, total cholesterol, and serum lipoprotein ratios in children and adolescents. Am J Public Health. Mar 1992;82:358–363.

41. Freedman DS, Kahn HS, Mei Z, Grummer-Strawn LM, Dietz WH, Srinivasan SR, Berenson GS. Relation of body mass index and waist-to-height ratio to cardiovascular disease risk factors in children and adolescents: the Bogalusa Heart Study. Am J Clin Nutr. Jul 2007;86:33–40.

42. Gidding SS, Bao W, Srinivasan SR, Berenson GS. Effects of secular trends in obesity on coronary risk factors in children: the Bogalusa Heart Study. J Pediatr. Dec 1995;127:868–874.

43. Freedman DS, Srinivasan SR, Valdez RA, Williamson DF, Berenson GS. Secular increases in relative weight and adiposity among children over two decades: the Bogalusa Heart Study. Pediatrics. Mar 1997;99:420–426.

44. Ogden CL, Flegal KM, Carroll MD, Johnson CL. Prevalence and trends in overweight among US children and adolescents, 1999–2000. JAMA. Oct 9 2002;288:1728–1732.

45. Ruilope LM, Lahera V, Rodicio JL, Carlos Romero J. Are renal hemodynamics a key factor in the development and maintenance of arterial hypertension in humans? Hypertension. Jan 1994;23:3–9.

46. Voors AW, Berenson, GS, Dalferes ER, Webber LS, Shuler SE. Racial differences in blood pressure control. Science. Jun 8 1979;204:1091–1094.

47. Berenson GS, Voors AW, Webber LS, Dalferes ER Jr, Harsha DW. Racial differences of parameters associated with blood pressure levels in children—the Bogalusa Heart Study. Metabolism. Dec 1979;28:1218–1228.

48. Chen W, Srinivasan SR, Berenson GS. Plasma renin activity and insulin resistance in African American and white children: the Bogalusa Heart Study. Am J Hypertens. Mar 2001;14:212–217.

49. Youssef AA, Srinivasan SR, Elkasabany A, Cruickshank JK, Berenson GS. Temporal relation between blood pressure and serum creatinine in young adults from a biracial community: the Bogalusa Heart Study. Am J Hypertens. Jul 2000;13:770–775.

50. Voors AW, Dalferes ER Jr, Frank GC, Aristimuno GG, Berenson GS. Relation between ingested potassium and sodium balance in young Blacks and whites. Am J Clin Nutr. Apr 1983;37:583–594.

51. Frank GC, Nicolich J, Voors AW, Webber LS, Berenson GS. A simplified inventory method for quantitating dietary sodium, potassium, and energy. Am J Clin Nutr. Sep 1983;38:474–480.

52. Frank GC, Webber LS, Nicklas TA, Berenson GS. Sodium, potassium, calcium, magnesium, and phosphorus intakes of infants and children: Bogalusa Heart Study. J Am Diet Assoc. Jul 1988;88:801–807.

53. Guzzetti S, Piccaluga E, Casati R, Cerutti S, Lombardi F, Pagani M, Malliani A. Sympathetic predominance in essential hypertension: a study employing spectral analysis of heart rate variability. J Hypertens. Sep 1988;6:711–717.

54. Guzzetti S, Dassi S, Pecis M, Casati R, Masu AM, Longoni P, Tinelli M, Cerutti S, Pagani M, Malliani A. Altered pattern of circadian neural control of heart period in mild hypertension. J Hypertens. Sep 1991;9:831–838.

55. Urbina EM, Bao W, Pickoff AS, Berenson GS. Ethnic (black-white) contrasts in twenty-four hour heart rate variability in male adolescents with high and low blood pressure: the Bogalusa Heart Study. Ann Noninvasive Electrocardiol. 2000;5:207–213.

56. Voors AW, Webber LS, Berenson GS. Resting heart rate and pressure-rate product of children in a total biracial community: the Bogalusa Heart Study. Am J Epidemiol. Aug 1982;116:276–286.

57. Osei K, Schuster DP. Effects of race and ethnicity on insulin sensitivity, blood pressure, and heart rate in three ethnic populations: comparative studies in African-Americans, African immigrants (Ghanaians), and white Americans using ambulatory blood pressure monitoring. Am J Hypertens. Dec 1996;9:1157–1164.

58. Murphy JK, Alpert BS, Walker SS. Consistency of ethnic differences in children's pressor reactivity. 1987 to 1992. Hypertension. Jan 1994;23:I152–I155.

59. Anderson NB, McNeilly M, Myers H. Autonomic reactivity and hypertension in blacks: a review and proposed model. Ethn Dis. Spring 1991;1:154–170.

60. Treiber FA, Strong WB, Arensman FW, Forrest T, Davis H, Musante L. Family history of myocardial infarction and hemodynamic responses to exercise in young black boys. Am J Dis Child. Sep 1991;145:1029–1033.

61. Voors AW, Webber LS, Berenson GS. Racial contrasts in cardiovascular response tests for children from a total community. Hypertension. Sep–Oct 1980;2:686–694.

62. Treiber FA, Musante L, Braden D, Arensman F, Strong WB, Levy M, Leverett S. Racial differences in hemodynamic responses to the cold face stimulus in children and adults. Psychosom Med. May–Jun 1990;52:286–296.

63. Sherwood A, Hinderliter AL, Light KC. Physiological determinants of hyperreactivity to stress in borderline hypertension. Hypertension. Mar 1995;25:384–390.

64. Calhoun DA, Mutinga ML, Collins AS, Wyss JM, Oparil S. Normotensive blacks have heightened sympathetic response to cold pressor test. Hypertension. Dec 1993;22:801–805.

65. Fredrikson M. Racial differences in cardiovascular reactivity to mental stress in essential hypertension. J Hypertens. Jun 1986;4:325–331.

66. Sherwood A, May CW, Siegel WC, Blumenthal JA. Ethnic differences in hemodynamic responses to stress in hypertensive men and women. Am J Hypertens. Jun 1995;8:552–557.

67. Parker FC, Croft JB, Cresanta JL, Freedman DS, Burke GL, Webber LS, Berenson GS. The association between cardiovascular response tasks and future blood pressure levels in children: Bogalusa Heart Study. Am Heart J. May 1987;113:1174–1179.

68. Soto LF, Kikuchi DA, Arcilla RA, Savage DD, Berenson GS. Echocardiographic functions and blood pressure levels in children and young adults from a biracial population: the Bogalusa Heart Study. Am J Med Sci. May 1989;297:271–279.

69. Urbina EM, Bao W, Pickoff AS, Berenson GS. Ethnic (black-white) contrasts in heart rate variability during cardiovascular reactivity testing in male adolescents with high and low blood pressure: the Bogalusa Heart Study. Am J Hypertens. Feb 1998;11:196–202.

70. Murdison KA, Treiber FA, Mensah G, Davis H, Thompson W, Strong WB. Prediction of left ventricular mass in youth with family histories of essential hypertension. Am J Med Sci. Feb 1998;315:118–123.

71. Mahoney LT, Schieken RM, Clarke WR, Lauer RM. Left ventricular mass and exercise responses predict future blood pressure. The Muscatine Study. Hypertension. Aug 1988;12:206–213.

72. Hinderliter AL, Light KC, Willis PW. Patients with borderline elevated blood pressure have enhanced left ventricular contractility. Am J Hypertens. Oct 1995;8:1040–1045.

73. Jiang X, Srinivasan SR, Urbina E, Berenson GS. Hyperdynamic circulation and cardiovascular risk in children and adolescents. The Bogalusa Heart Study. Circulation. Feb 15 1995;91:1101–1106.

74. Nguyen NT, Magno CP, Lane KT, Hinojosa MW, Lane JS. Association of hypertension, diabetes, dyslipidemia, and metabolic syndrome with obesity: findings from the National Health and Nutrition Examination Survey, 1999 to 2004. J Am Coll Surg. Dec 2008;207:928–934.

75. Nguyen QM, Srinivasan SR, Xu JH, et al. Distribution and cardiovascular risk correlates of hemoglobin A(1c) in nondiabetic younger adults: the Bogalusa Heart Study. Metabolism. Nov 2008;57:1487–1492.

76. Voors AW, Radhakrishnamurthy B, Srinivasan SR, Webber LS, Berenson GS. Plasma glucose level related to blood pressure in 272 children, ages 7–15 years, sampled from a total biracial population. Am J Epidemiol. Apr 1981;113:347–356.

77. Burke GL, Webber LS, Srinivasan SR, Radhakrishnamurthy B, Freedman DS, Berenson GS. Fasting plasma glucose and insulin levels and their relationship to cardiovascular risk factors in children: Bogalusa Heart Study. Metabolism. May 1986;35:441–446.

78. Jiang X, Srinivasan SR, Bao W, Berenson GS. Association of fasting insulin with blood pressure in young individuals. The Bogalusa Heart Study. Arch Intern Med. Feb 8 1993;153:323–328.

79. Jiang X, Srinivasan SR, Bao W, Berenson GS. Association of fasting insulin with longitudinal changes in blood pressure in children and adolescents. The Bogalusa Heart Study. Am J Hypertens. Jul 1993;6:564–569.

80. Rowe JW, Young JB, Minaker KL, Stevens AL, Pallotta J, Landsberg L. Effect of insulin and glucose infusions on sympathetic nervous system activity in normal man. Diabetes. Mar 1981;30:219–225.

81. Berenson GS, Bao W, Wattigney WA, Webber LS. Primary hypertension beginning in childhood. Cardiol Rev. 1993;1:239–249.

82. Bao W, Srinivasan SR, Berenson GS. Persistent elevation of plasma insulin levels is associated with increased cardiovascular risk in children and young adults. The Bogalusa Heart Study. Circulation. Jan 1 1996;93:54–59.

83. Myers L, Coughlin SS, Webber LS, Srinivasan SR, Berenson GS. Prediction of adult cardiovascular multifactorial risk status from childhood risk factor levels. The Bogalusa Heart Study. Am J Epidemiol. Nov 1 1995;142:918–924.

84. Chen W, Srinivasan SR, Elkasabany A, Berenson GS. Cardiovascular risk factors clustering features of insulin resistance syndrome (Syndrome X) in a biracial (Black-White) population of children, adolescents, and young adults: the Bogalusa Heart Study. Am J Epidemiol. Oct 1 1999;150:667–674.

85. Chen W, Srinivasan SR, Berenson GS. Path analysis of metabolic syndrome components in black versus white children, adolescents, and adults: the Bogalusa Heart Study. Ann Epidemiol. Feb 2008;18:85–91.

86. Kanellis J, Kang D-H. Uric acid as a mediator of endothelial dysfunction, inflammation, and vascular disease. Semin Nephrol. Jan 2005;25:39–42.

87. Corry DB, Eslami P, Yamamoto K, Nyby MD, Makino, H, Tuck ML. Uric acid stimulates vascular smooth muscle cell proliferation and oxidative stress via the vascular renin-angiotensin system. J Hypertens. Feb 2008;26:269–275.

88. Alper AB Jr, Chen W, Yau L, Srinivasan SR, Berenson GS, Hamm LL. Childhood uric acid predicts adult blood pressure: the Bogalusa Heart Study. Hypertension. Jan 2005;45:34–38.

89. Muntner P, Srinivasan S, Menke A, Patel DA, Chen W, Berenson G. Impact of childhood metabolic syndrome components on the risk of elevated uric acid in adulthood: the Bogalusa Heart Study. Am J Med Sci. May 2008;335:332–337.

90. Shear CL, Webber LS, Freedman DS, Srinivasan SR, Berenson GS. The relationship between parental history of vascular disease and cardiovascular disease risk factors in children: the Bogalusa Heart Study. Am J Epidemiol. Nov 1985;122:762–771.

91. Shear CL, Burke GL, Freedman DS, Berenson GS. Value of childhood blood pressure measurements and family history in predicting future blood pressure status: results from 8 years of follow-up in the Bogalusa Heart Study. Pediatrics. Jun 1986;77:862–869.

92. Clarke WR, Schrott HG, Burns TL, Sing CF, Lauer RM. Aggregation of blood pressure in the families of children with labile high systolic blood pressure. The Muscatine Study. Am J Epidemiol. Jan 1986;123:67–80.

93. Rosenbaum PA, Elston RC, Srinivasan SR, Webber LS, Berenson GS. Cardiovascular risk factors from birth to 7 years of age: the Bogalusa Heart Study. Predictive value of parental measures in determining cardiovascular risk factor variables in early life. Pediatrics. Nov 1987;80:807–816.

94. Bao W, Srinivasan SR, Wattigney WA, Berenson GS. The relation of parental cardiovascular disease to risk factors in children and young adults. The Bogalusa Heart Study. Circulation. Jan 15 1995;91:365–371.

95. Chen W, Li S, Srinivasan SR, Boerwinkle E, Berenson GS. Autosomal genome scan for loci linked to blood pressure levels and trends since childhood: the Bogalusa Heart Study. Hypertension. May 2005;45:954–959.

96. Chen W, Srinivasan SR, Elkasabany A, Ellsworth DL, Boerwinkle E, Berenson GS. Combined effects of endothelial nitric oxide synthase gene polymorphism (G894T) and insulin resistance status on blood pressure and familial risk of hypertension in young adults: the Bogalusa Heart Study. Am J Hypertens. Oct 2001;14:1046–1052.

97. Chen W, Srinivasan SR, Li S, Boerwinkle E, Berenson GS. Gender-specific influence of NO synthase gene on blood pressure since childhood: the Bogalusa Heart Study. Hypertension. Nov 2004;44:668–673.

98. Barker DJ, Bull AR, Osmond C, Simmonds SJ. Fetal and placental size and risk of hypertension in adult life. BMJ. Aug 4 1990;301:259–262.

99. Law CM, Shiell AW. Is blood pressure inversely related to birth weight? The strength of evidence from a systematic review of the literature. J Hypertens. 1996;14:935–941.

100. Barker DJP. Fetal origins of coronary heart disease. BMJ. 1995;311:171–174.

101. Barker DJP. Early growth and cardiovascular disease. Arch Dis Child. 1999;80:305–306.

102. Falkner B. Birth weight as a predictor of future hypertension. Am J Hypertens. Feb 2002;15:43S–45S.

103. Donker GA, Labarthe DR, Harrist RB, Selwyn BJ, Wattigney W, Berenson GS. Low birth weight and blood pressure at age 7–11 years in a biracial sample. Am J Epidemiol. Mar 1 1997;145:387–397.

104. Mzayek F, Sherwin R, Fonseca V, Valdez R, Srinivasan SR, Cruickshank JK, Berenson GS. Differential association of birth weight with cardiovascular risk variables in African-Americans and Whites: the Bogalusa heart study. Ann Epidemiol. Apr 2004;14:258–264.

105. Frontini MG, Srinivasan SR, Xu J, Berenson GS. Low birth weight and longitudinal trends of cardiovascular risk factor variables from childhood to adolescence: the Bogalusa Heart Study. BMC Pediatr. Nov 3 2004;4:22.

106. Mzayek F, Hassig S, Sherwin R, Hughes J, Chen W, Srinivasan S, Berenson G. The association of birth weight with developmental trends in blood pressure from childhood through mid-adulthood: the Bogalusa Heart study. Am J Epidemiol. Aug 15 2007;166:413–420.

107. Siewert-Delle A, Ljungman, S. The impact of birth weight and gestational age on blood pressure in adult life: a population-based study of 49-year-old men. Am J Hypertens. Aug 1998;11:946–953.

108. Shu XO, Hatch MC, Mills J, Clemens J, Susser M. Maternal smoking, alcohol drinking, caffeine consumption, and fetal growth: results from a prospective study. Epidemiology. Mar 1995;6:115–120.

109. Tracy RE, Newman WP, 3rd, Wattigney WA, Berenson GS. Risk factors and atherosclerosis in youth autopsy findings of the Bogalusa Heart Study. Am J Med Sci. Dec 1995;310 Suppl 1:S37–S41.

110. Guzman MA, McMahan CA, McGill HC Jr, Strong JP, Tejada C, Restrepo C, Eggen DA, Robertson WB, Solberg LA. Selected methodologic aspects of the International Atherosclerosis Project. Lab Invest. May 1968;18:479–497.

111. Freedman DS, Newman WP, 3rd, Tracy RE, Voors AE, Srinivasan SR, Webber LS, Restrepo C, Strong JP, Berenson GS. Black-white differences in aortic fatty streaks in adolescence and early adulthood: the Bogalusa Heart Study. Circulation. Apr 1988;77:856–864.

112. Tracy RE, Mercante DE, Moncada A, Berenson G. Quantitation of hypertensive nephrosclerosis on an objective rational scale of measure in adults and children. Am J Clin Pathol. Mar 1986;85:312–318.

113. Glagov S, Weisenberg E, Zarins CK, Stankunavicius R, Kolettis GJ. Compensatory enlargement of human atherosclerotic coronary arteries. N Engl J Med. May 28 1987;316:1371–1375.

114. Folkow B, Grimby G, Thulesius O. Adaptive structural changes of the vascular walls in hypertension and their relation to the control of the peripheral resistance. Acta Physiol Scand. Dec 15 1958;44:255–272.

115. Mulvany MJ. The fourth Sir George Pickering memorial lecture. The structure of the resistance vasculature in essential hypertension. J Hypertens. Apr 1987;5:129–136.

116. Aristimuno GG, Foster TA, Berenson GS, Akman D. Subtle electrocardiographic changes in children with high levels of blood pressure. Am J Cardiol. Dec 1 1984;54:1272–1276.

117. Schieken RM, Schwartz PF, Goble MM. Tracking of left ventricular mass in children: race and sex comparisons: the MCV Twin Study. Medical College of Virginia. Circulation. May 19 1998;97:1901–1906.

118. Janz KF, Burns TL, Mahoney LT. Predictors of left ventricular mass and resting blood pressure in children: the Muscatine Study. Med Sci Sports Exerc. Jun 1995;27:818–825.

119. Hanevold C, Waller J, Daniels S, Portman R, Sorof J, International Pediatric Hypertension A. The effects of obesity, gender, and ethnic group on left ventricular hypertrophy and geometry in hypertensive children: a collaborative study of the International Pediatric Hypertension Association. Pediatrics. Feb 2004;113:328–333.

120. Li X, Li S, Ulusoy E, Chen W, Srinivasan SR, Berenson GS. Childhood adiposity as a predictor of cardiac mass in adulthood: the Bogalusa Heart Study. Circulation. Nov 30 2004;110:3488–3492.

121. Toprak A, Wang H, Chen W, Paul T, Srinivasan S, Berenson G. Relation of childhood risk factors to left ventricular hypertrophy (eccentric or concentric) in relatively young adulthood (from the Bogalusa Heart Study). Am J Cardiol. Jun 1 2008;101:1621–1625.

122. Krumholz HM, Larson M, Levy D. Prognosis of left ventricular geometric patterns in the Framingham Heart Study. J Am Coll Cardiol. Mar 15 1995;25:879–884.

123. Sorof JM, Cardwell G, Franco K, Portman RJ. Ambulatory blood pressure and left ventricular mass index in hypertensive children. Hypertension. Apr 2002;39:903–908.

124. Urbina EM, Gidding SS, Bao W, Pickoff AS, Berdussis K, Berenson GS. Effect of body size and blood pressure on left ventricular growth in children and young adults: The Bogalusa Heart Study. Circulation. 1995;91:2400–2406.

125. Voors AW, Harsha, DW, Webber LS, Berenson GS. Relation of blood pressure to stature in healthy young adults. Am J Epidemiol. Jun 1982;115:833–840.

126. Urbina EM, Gidding SS, Bao W, Elkasabany A, Berenson GS. Association of fasting blood sugar level, insulin level, and obesity with left ventricular mass in healthy children and adolescents: The Bogalusa Heart Study. Am Heart J. Jul 1999;138:122–127.

127. Patel DA, Li S, Chen W, Srinivasan SR, Boerwinkle E, Berenson GS. G-6A polymorphism of the angiotensinogen gene and its association with left ventricular mass in asymptomatic young adults from a biethnic community: the Bogalusa Heart Study. Am J Hypertens. Nov 2005;18:1437–1441.

128. Daniels SR, Kimball TR, Khoury P, Witt S, Morrison JA. Correlates of the hemodynamic determinants of blood pressure. Hypertension. Jul 1996;28:37–41.

129. Sherwood A, Hinderliter AL. Responsiveness to alpha- and beta-adrenergic receptor agonists. Effects of race in borderline hypertensive compared to normotensive men. Am J Hypertens. Jul 1993;6:630–635.

130. Haji SA, Ulusoy RE, Patel DA, Srinivasan SR, Chen W, Delafontaine P, Berenson GS. Predictors of left ventricular dilatation in young adults (from the Bogalusa Heart Study). Am J Cardiol. Nov 1 2006;98:1234–1237.

131. Riley WA, Freedman DS, Higgs NA, Barnes RW, Zinkgraf SA, Berenson GS. Decreased arterial elasticity associated with cardiovascular disease risk factors in the young. Bogalusa Heart Study. Arteriosclerosis. Jul–Aug 1986;6:378–386.

132. Urbina EM, Srinivasan SR, Kieltyka RL, et al. Correlates of carotid artery stiffness in young adults: The Bogalusa Heart Study. Atherosclerosis. Sep 2004;176:157–164.

133. Chen W, Srinivasan SR, Bond MG, Tang R, Urbina EM, Li S, Boerwinkle E, Berenson GS. Nitric oxide synthase gene polymorphism (G894T) influences arterial stiffness in adults: The Bogalusa Heart Study. Am J Hypertens. Jul 2004;17:553–559.

134. Urbina EM, Brinton TJ, Elkasabany A, Berenson GS. Brachial artery distensibility and relation to cardiovascular risk factors in healthy young adults (The Bogalusa Heart Study). Am J Cardiol. Apr 15 2002;89:946–951.

135. Urbina EM, Kieltkya L, Tsai J, Srinivasan SR, Berenson GS. Impact of multiple cardiovascular risk factors on brachial artery distensibility in young adults: the Bogalusa Heart Study. Am J Hypertens. Jun 2005;18:767–771.

136. Urbina EM, Bean JA, Daniels SR, D'Alessio D, Dolan LM. Overweight and hyperinsulinemia provide individual contributions to compromises in brachial artery distensibility in healthy adolescents and young adults: brachial distensibility in children. J Am Soc Hypertens. Jun 2007;1:200–207.

137. Blacher J, Asmar R, Diane S, London GM, Safar ME. Aortic pulse wave velocity as a marker of cardiovascular risk in hypertensive patients. Hypertension. May 1999;33:1111–1117.

138. Chen W, Srinivasan SR, Li S, Berenson GS. Different effects of atherogenic lipoproteins and blood pressure on arterial structure and function: the Bogalusa Heart Study. J Clin Hypertens (Greenwich). May 2006;8:323–329.

139. Nguyen QM, Srinivasan SR, Xu JH, Chen W, Berenson GS. Racial (black-white) divergence in the association between adiponectin and arterial stiffness in asymptomatic young adults: the Bogalusa heart study [see comment]. Am J Hypertens. May 2008;21:553–557.

140. Bhuiyan AR, Srinivasan SR, Chen W, Paul TK, Berenson GS. Correlates of vascular structure and function measures in asymptomatic young adults: the Bogalusa Heart Study. Atherosclerosis. Nov 2006;189:1–7.

141. Bhuiyan AR, Li S, Li H, Chen W, Srinivasan SR, Berenson GS. Distribution and correlates of arterial compliance measures in asymptomatic young adults: the Bogalusa Heart Study. Am J Hypertens. May 2005;18:684–691.

142. Li S, Chen W, Srinivasan SR, Berenson GS. Childhood blood pressure as a predictor of arterial stiffness in young adults: the Bogalusa Heart Study. Hypertension. Mar 2004;43:541–546.

143. Chen W, Srinivasan SR, Boerwinkle E, Berenson GS. Beta-adrenergic receptor genes are associated with arterial stiffness in black and white adults: the Bogalusa Heart Study. Am J Hypertens. Dec 2007;20:1251–1257.

144. Urbina EM, Srinivasan SR, Tang R, Bond MG, Kieltyka L, Berenson GS. Impact of multiple coronary risk factors on the intima-media thickness of different segments of carotid artery in healthy young adults (The Bogalusa Heart Study). Am J Cardiol. Nov 1 2002;90:953–958.

145. Paul TK, Srinivasan SR, Chen W, Li S, Bond MG, Tang R, Berenson GS. Impact of multiple cardiovascular risk factors on femoral artery intima-media thickness in asymptomatic young adults (the Bogalusa Heart Study). Am J Cardiol. Feb 15 2005;95:469–473.

146. Johnson HM, Douglas PS, Srinivasan SR, Bond MG, Tang R, Li S, Chen W, Berenson GS, Stein JH. Predictors of carotid intima-media thickness progression in young adults: the Bogalusa Heart Study. Stroke. Mar 2007;38:900–905.

147. Bhuiyan AR, Chen W, Srinivasan SR, Rice J, Mock N, Tang R, Bond MG, Boerwinkle E, Berenson GS. G-6A polymorphism of angiotensinogen gene modulates the effect of blood pressure on carotid intima-media thickness. The Bogalusa Heart Study. Am J Hypertens. Oct 2007;20:1073–1078.

148. Krishnan P, Balamurugan A, Urbina E, Srinivasan SR, Bond G, Tang R, Berenson GS. Cardiovascular risk profile of asymptomatic healthy young adults with increased carotid artery intima-media thickness: the Bogalusa Heart Study. J La State Med Soc. May–Jun 2003;155:165–169.

149. Paul TK, Srinivasan SR, Wei C, Li S, Bhuiyan AR, Bond MG, Tang R, Berenson GS. Cardiovascular risk profile of asymptomatic healthy young adults with increased femoral artery intima-media thickness: The Bogalusa Heart Study. Am J Med Sci. Sep 2005;330:105–110.

150. Kieltyka L, Urbina EM, Tang R, Bond MG, Srinivasan SR, Berenson GS. Framingham risk score is related to carotid artery intima-media thickness in both white and black young adults: the Bogalusa Heart Study. Atherosclerosis. Sep 2003;170:125–130.

151. Tzou WS, Douglas PS, Srinivasan SR, Bond MG, Tang R, Chen W, Berenson GS, Stein JH. Increased subclinical atherosclerosis in young adults with metabolic syndrome: the Bogalusa Heart Study. J Am Coll Cardiol. Aug 2 2005;46:457–463.

152. Lande MB, Carson NL, Roy J, Meagher CC. Effects of childhood primary hypertension on carotid intima media thickness: a matched controlled study. Hypertension. Jul 2006;48:40–44.

153. Li S, Chen W, Srinivasan SR, Tang R, Bond, MG, Berenson GS. Race (black-white) and gender divergences in the relationship of childhood cardiovascular risk factors to carotid artery intima-media thickness in adulthood: The Bogalusa Heart Study. Atherosclerosis. 2007;194:421–425.

154. Ettinger LM, Freeman K, DiMartino-Nardi JR, Flynn JT. Microalbuminuria and abnormal ambulatory blood pressure in adolescents with type 2 diabetes mellitus. J Pediatr. Jul 2005;147:67–73.

155. Jiang X, Srinivasan SR, Radhakrishnamurthy B, Dalferes ER Jr, Bao W, Berenson GS. Microalbuminuria in young adults related to blood pressure in a biracial (black-white) population. The Bogalusa Heart Study. Am J Hypertens. Sep 1994;7:794–800.

156. Agirbasli M, Radhakrishnamurthy B, Jiang X, Bao W, Berenson GS. Urinary N-acetyl-beta-D-glucosaminidase changes in relation to age, sex, race, and diastolic and systolic blood pressure in a young adult biracial population. The Bogalusa Heart Study. Am J Hypertens. Feb 1996;9:157–161.

157. Frontini MG, Srinivasan SR, Elkasabany A, Berenson GS. Awareness of hypertension and dyslipidemia in a semirural population of young adults: the Bogalusa Heart Study. Prev Med. Apr 2003;36:398–402.

158. Daniels SR, Greer FR. Lipid screening and cardiovascular health in childhood. Pediatrics. Jul 2008;122:198–208.

159. Kavey RE, Allada V, Daniels SR, Hayman LL, McCrindle BW, Newburger JW, Parekh RS, Steinberger J. Cardiovascular risk reduction in high-risk pediatric patients: a scientific statement from the American Heart Association Expert Panel on Population and Prevention Science; the Councils on Cardiovascular Disease in the Young, Epidemiology and Prevention, Nutrition, Physical Activity and Metabolism, High Blood Pressure Research, Cardiovascular Nursing, and the Kidney in Heart Disease; and the Interdisciplinary Working Group on Quality of Care and Outcomes Research: endorsed by the American Academy of Pediatrics. Circulation. Dec 12 2006;114:2710–2738.

160. Berenson GS, Shear CL, Chiang YK, Webber LS, Voors AW. Combined low-dose medication and primary intervention over a 30-month period for sustained high blood pressure in childhood. Am J Med Sci. Feb 1990;299:79–86.

161. Farris RP, Frank, GC, Webber LS, Berenson GS. A nutrition curriculum for families with high blood pressure. J Sch Health. Mar 1985;55:110–112.

162. Cunningham RJ, Urbina EM, Hogg RJ, Sorof JM, Moxey-Mimms M, Eissa MA. A double-blind, placebo-controlled, dose escalation safety, and efficacy study of ziac in patients, ages 6–17 years, with hypertension. Am J Hypertens. 2000;13:38A–39A.

163. Sacks FM, Svetkey LP, Vollmer WM, Appel LJ, Bray GA, Harsha D, Obarzanek E, Conlin PR, Miller ER, 3rd, Simons-Morton DG, Karanja N, Lin PH. Effects on blood pressure of reduced dietary sodium and the Dietary Approaches to Stop Hypertension (DASH) diet. DASH-Sodium Collaborative Research Group. N Engl J Med. Jan 4 2001;344:3–10.

164. Couch SC, Saelens BE, Levin L, Dart K, Falciglia G, Daniels SR. The efficacy of a clinic-based behavioral nutrition intervention emphasizing a DASH-type diet for adolescents with elevated blood pressure. J Pediatr. Apr 2008;152:494–501.

165. Downey AM, Frank GC, Webber LS, Harsha DW, Virgilio SJ, Franklin FA, Berenson GS. Implementation of "Heart Smart:" a cardiovascular school health promotion program. J Sch Health. Mar 1987;57:98–104.

166. Johnson CC, Nicklas TA, Arbeit ML, et al. Cardiovascular intervention for high-risk families: the Heart Smart Program. South Med J. Nov 1991;84:1305–1312.

167. Arbeit ML, Johnson CC, Mott DS, Harsha DW, Nicklas TA, Webber LS, Berenson GS. The Heart Smart cardiovascular school health promotion: behavior correlates of risk factor change. Prev Med. Jan 1992;21:18–32.

168. Downey AM, Greenberg JS, Virgilio SJ, Berenson GS. Health promotion model for "Heart Smart": the medical school, university, and community. Health Values. Nov–Dec 1989;13:31–46.

169. Chen W, Srinivasan SR, Li S, Xu J, Berenson GS. Metabolic syndrome variables at low levels in childhood are beneficially associated with adulthood cardiovascular risk: the Bogalusa Heart Study. Diabetes Care. Jan 2005;28:126–131.

170. Urbina EM, Berenson GS. Hypertension studies in the Bogalusa Heart Study. In: McCarty RBD, Chevalier RL, eds. Development of the Hypertensive Phenotype: Basic and Clinical Studies, Vol 19. New York, NY: Elsevier; 1999:607–637.

12 Epidemiology of Cardiovascular Disease in Children

Samuel S. Gidding, MD

CONTENTS

Hypertension is one of several major risk factors for the future development of atherosclerosis and atherosclerosis-related morbidity. The additional major risk factors that precede myocardial infarction, congestive heart failure, stroke, peripheral arterial disease, and abdominal aortic aneurysm include dyslipidemia (elevated LDL cholesterol, low HDL cholesterol, and elevated triglycerides), tobacco use, and diabetes mellitus (1). Age, gender (female gender is protective), and genetic endowment are non-modifiable risk factors. Physical inactivity, obesity, family history, adverse nutrition, and low socioeconomic status function both as independent risk factors and are intimately related to the development of cardiovascular risk in adults (Table 1).

S.S. Gidding (✉)
Nemours Cardiac Center, Alfred I. DuPont Hospital for Children, Wilmington, DE,
USA; Jefferson Medical College, Wilmington, DE, USA
e-mail: sgidding@nemours.org

From: *Clinical Hypertension and Vascular Diseases: Pediatric Hypertension*
Edited by: J. T. Flynn et al. DOI 10.1007/978-1-60327-824-9_12
© Springer Science+Business Media, LLC 2011

Table 1
Risk Factors for Atherosclerosis

Major modifiable risk factors
Hypertension
Dyslipidemia (elevated LDL cholesterol, low HDL cholesterol, elevated
   triglycerides)
Tobacco use
Diabetes mellitus

Non-modifiable risk factors
Age
Gender
Genetic history

Factors that modify major risk factors and may be independent themselves
Diet
Physical activity
Family history
Obesity
Low socioeconomic status

This chapter will review the relationship of the major risk factors to atherosclerosis in childhood and to the future development of atherosclerosis in adulthood. This relationship has led to two concepts of atherosclerosis prevention in youth: primordial prevention, which is the prevention of the development of risk factors in the first place, and primary prevention, which is the identification of elevated risk and subsequent risk factor management. The epidemiology of risk factors in childhood and the development of risk as an adult will be discussed. An overview of the management of cardiovascular risk in childhood, particularly in the context of hypertension, will be provided.

ATHEROSCLEROSIS IN CHILDHOOD

That the earliest lesion of atherosclerosis, the fatty streak, is present in children and more advanced lesions may present in young adulthood has been known since the 1950s *(2)*. The landmark Pathobiological Determinants of Atherosclerosis in Youth Study (PDAY) established the relationship of the major cardiovascular risk factors to early atherosclerosis by measuring atherosclerosis directly on postmortem examination in the coronary arteries and abdominal aorta of 15- to 34-year-old men and women dying accidentally. Lesions were graded according to the standard American Heart Association classification ranging from grade I (fatty streaks) to grade V (obstructive plaques). These pathologic measurements were related to risk factors measured postmortem: height and weight, serum measures (lipids, thiocyanate, glycohemoglobin), renal artery thickness (a surrogate for blood pressure), and other physical measures such as panniculus thickness.

The major findings of the PDAY study were that atherosclerosis is present in adolescents and young adults, that the severity of atherosclerosis increases rapidly so that by early adulthood advanced lesions (American Heart Association grades IV and V) are present, that the major risk factors are strongly related to atherosclerosis at all ages, and that the

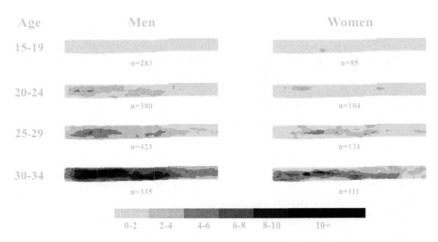

Fig. 1. Prevalence map of raised lesions of right coronary arteries by age and sex.

progression of atherosclerosis to more advanced lesions is related not only to the major risk factors but also to the presence of multiple risk factors simultaneously *(2)*. Atherosclerosis in women develops at a pace lagging about 5–10 years behind that in men (Fig. 1). Since most of the general population has at least one risk factor, the importance of public health measures and healthy behaviors in the prevention of atherosclerosis is a natural corollary of the PDAY findings. This is particularly true for children and adolescents when lesions are in the earliest and reversible phase (American Heart Association grades I and II) *(3)*.

In PDAY, hypertension was evaluated categorically as the measure of hypertension was a renal arterial thickness associated with blood pressure greater than 140/90 mmHg in adults. The presence of hypertension was significantly associated with advanced atherosclerosis in both the coronary arteries and the abdominal aorta *(4)*.

Both non-HDL cholesterol and HDL cholesterol were related to atherosclerosis, both in the coronary arteries and in the abdominal aorta. The relationship with non-HDL cholesterol is continuous and graded with each 30 mg/dl higher non-HDL cholesterol level increment associated with the equivalent of 2–3 years of vascular aging. The relationship of HDL cholesterol to atherosclerosis was less strong but significant *(5)*.

Tobacco use produced its most severe impact in the abdominal aorta; however, relationships to coronary atherosclerosis were also identified. More rapid advancement of lesions from fatty streaks to irreversible fibrous plaque was identified in smokers, particularly those with other risk factors *(6)*.

Diabetes mellitus was strongly associated with advanced atherosclerosis. It was the only risk factor to be associated with advanced lesions (American Heart Association grades IV and V) in adolescents. Obesity (body mass index > 30 kg/m^2) was related to atherosclerosis independent of other risk factors in men only *(4,7)*.

To assess the importance of multiple risk factors on atherosclerosis development, the PDAY risk score was created. Each point in the risk score was gated to the rate of change in atherosclerosis associated with 1 year of aging. Thus, a risk score of 5 indicates the presence of atherosclerosis associated with being 5 years older than chronologic age. Individuals with the highest scores had substantially more early lesions of atherosclerosis in late adolescence and substantially more advanced lesions by the first part of the fourth decade of life *(5)*. These relationships are independent of cholesterol levels, thus the presence of a threshold level of non-HDL cholesterol is not necessary for the early development of atherosclerosis *(8)*.

RISK FACTORS IN CHILDHOOD PREDICT ATHEROSCLEROSIS IN ADULTHOOD

The concept of intervention in youth to prevent atherosclerosis in adulthood is supported by observations that for many risk factors the presence of a given risk factor in youth is subsequently associated with premature cardiovascular morbidity and mortality in adulthood. For cholesterol, this evidence has been provided by genetic disorders such as familial hypercholesterolemia where in affected men, the median age of first cardiovascular event is late in the fifth decade of life and slightly older for women *(9)*. Conversely defects associated with low cholesterol are protective against future disease *(10)*. For tobacco, evidence is provided by the knowledge that tobacco is addictive, that tobacco use begins in adolescence, and that smoking cessation is associated with a dramatic reduction in future events *(11)*. For diabetes mellitus, evidence is provided by the natural history of type I diabetes mellitus with the primary cause of death in this condition being cardiovascular and also the absence of the gender protection against premature cardiovascular events. In contrast to other risk factors, female diabetics have cardiovascular events at the same age as men *(12)*.

Measures of subclinical atherosclerosis including carotid intima–media thickness (cIMT) and coronary calcium identified by CT scanning are used in longitudinal epidemiologic studies and have provided additional evidence of the relationship of risk factors in youth to future atherosclerosis. In four separate longitudinal studies conducted in various

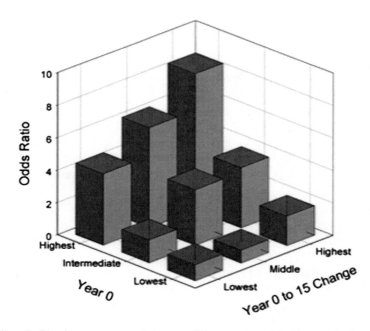

Fig. 2. The likelihood of having coronary calcium on CT scan at age 33–45 years is shown by the height of the bars. The groups are defined by tertiles of risk at baseline and change in risk over 15 years. As risk at baseline increases (higher PDAY risk score), likelihood increases. Risk change also impacts change in likelihood of future presence of coronary calcium.

populations, the Muscatine Study, the Bogalusa Heart Study, the Cardiovascular Risk in Young Finns Study, and the Coronary Risk Development in Young Adults Study (CARDIA), risk factor measures obtained in adolescence or young adulthood better predicted carotid IMT or calcium on CT scan better than risk factors measured at the time of the subclinical atherosclerosis measurement *(13–16)*. When the PDAY risk score was applied to the CARDIA and Young Finns cohorts, the PDAY risk score in adolescence or young adulthood best predicted future atherosclerosis, and change in risk score between the initial measurement and the time of subclinical atherosclerosis assessment added predictive ability *(16,17)*. Thus, improvement in risk as a young adult prevented acquisition of subclinical atherosclerosis (Fig. 2).

THE RATIONALE FOR ATHEROSCLEROSIS PREVENTION BY PRIMORDIAL AND PRIMARY STRATEGIES

Several lines of reasoning, including the information already presented in this chapter, have led to the understanding that the most effective prevention of atherosclerosis begins in youth.

Cardiovascular risk factors identified in youth track into adulthood. A recent meta-analysis has confirmed that blood pressure in childhood has a tracking correlation of about 0.4 into adulthood with the development of obesity making development of hypertension in adulthood more likely *(18)*. Cholesterol levels have a similar tracking coefficient *(19)*. By its addictive nature, tobacco use in adolescence predicts adult tobacco use. Diabetes mellitus is an unremitting disease. Thus, the child at the upper end of the risk distribution is likely to remain in that position as an adult.

Equally important is the knowledge that atherosclerosis begins in youth, and prior to adulthood is in its reversible phase. Individuals with no risk factors in the PDAY study have a low prevalence of atherosclerosis at the age of 30–34 years, and young adults with a low PDAY risk score have minimal subclinical atherosclerosis *(3,16)*. Individuals who reach the age of 50 years and have no major cardiovascular risk have a lifetime risk of cardiovascular disease up to 95 years of age of 5% *(20)*. Maintenance of a low cardiovascular risk state is highly protective against atherosclerosis-related morbidity.

Long-term adult longitudinal studies of cardiovascular disease demonstrate risk thresholds above which cardiovascular disease morbidity increases. These are LDL cholesterol levels above 100–110 mg/dl, blood pressure above 110–120/80 mmHg, absence of diabetes mellitus, and absence of tobacco use *(21,22)*. Animal models of atherosclerosis provide complementary data where the introduction of risk above threshold levels produces disease *(23)*. If one considers risk distribution of generally healthy non-obese children, the vast majority, probably greater than 90%, have risk thresholds associated with no adult cardiovascular morbidity *(24–26)*. Thus, primordial prevention, or the prevention of risk factor development, is possible beginning in youth, if those behavioral factors associated with increase in risk are addressed.

Primary prevention strategies beginning in youth, or the high-risk approach, are considered because a small percentage of children are recognized to already have severe cardiovascular risk factors and premature atherosclerosis *(1)*. For example, in heterozygous familial hypercholesterolemia, 28% of children have coronary calcium present on CT scans *(27)*. Children with end-stage renal disease, type I diabetes mellitus, and chronic severe hypertension are known to have significantly premature cardiovascular morbidity and/or measurable cardiovascular end organ injury in youth *(28,29)*. These children may benefit from aggressive risk factor reduction initiated at an early age. Although primary prevention clinical trials have not been performed in adolescents with high levels of risk, many presume that the benefit demonstrated in adult trials will also apply to this group.

DYSLIPIDEMIA

Recognition of abnormal lipid levels, particularly LDL cholesterol, has been advocated by consensus groups since the release of the 1992 NHLBI National Cholesterol Education Program Report on cholesterol and children *(30)*. Revised guidelines have been recently developed that include recommendations with regard to triglycerides, HDL cholesterol, and non-HDL cholesterol. Table 2 presents the classification of lipid levels for children from the new guideline. Triglycerides and HDL cholesterol have increased in importance because of the obesity epidemic. Non-HDL cholesterol, the difference between total and HDL cholesterol, is as useful as LDL cholesterol in the prediction of future cardiovascular risk and can be obtained in the non-fasting state *(2,31)*.

Table 2
Lipid Classification for Children and Adolescents (in mg/dl)

	Acceptable	*Borderline*	*High*
Total cholesterol	<170	170–199	≥200
Non-HDL cholesterol	<120	120–144	≥145
LDL cholesterol	<110	110–130	≥130
Triglycerides ≤ 9 years	<75	75–100	≥100
> 10 years	<90	90–130	≥130
	Acceptable	Borderline	Low
HDL cholesterol	≥45	40–44	<40

For US children, NHANES III provides a distribution of lipid levels. Fasting values are available for adolescents in that study *(26)*. There is significant variation in lipid levels by age with values increasing until about 2 years of age, remaining relatively stable until prepuberty. Cholesterol levels rise at this time, fall significantly during rapid growth, and then slowly begin to climb in males and remain relatively stable in females throughout late adolescence *(32)*. HDL cholesterol levels fall after puberty. Triglyceride levels increase during adolescence. There is a significant intrinsic variability of lipid measurements, so that unless values are extreme, repeat measures are mandatory before classifying a child as abnormal *(33)*.

Because of age-related changes and intrinsic variability in lipid levels, the prevalence of borderline dyslipidemia varies by age. In general, about 25% of children will have values for one lipid parameter considered borderline or higher. It is important to distinguish between extreme values (LDL cholesterol ≥ 160 mg/dl, non-HDL cholesterol ≥ 190 mg/dl, triglycerides ≥ 500 mg/dl) and borderline or mildly elevated levels as the latter do not require pharmacologic intervention and may improve spontaneously over time, particularly with successful behavioral intervention.

Genetic dyslipidemias are recognized by the presence of extreme values. Heterozygous familial hypercholesterolemia has a prevalence of about 1:500 in the general population and is suggested by the presence of an LDL cholesterol level above 140–160 mg/dl with a positive family history for similar dyslipidemia in a parent or history of premature coronary artery disease *(9)*. Homozygotes have total cholesterol levels in excess of 500 mg/dl, are at risk for coronary artery disease in the second and third decades of life, and require plasma-pheresis to lower lipid levels. Hypothyroidism and nephrotic syndrome must be excluded in the presence of significant elevations of LDL cholesterol.

Fasting triglyceride levels above 150 mg/dl in a lean child or above 200–250 mg/dl in an obese child suggest an inherited disorder of triglyceride metabolism or familial combined hyperlipidemia. Homozygotes with severe disorders of triglyceride metabolism have levels >1000 mg/dl and require diets with <10% fat to prevent pancreatitis *(34)*. Triglyc-erides can be transiently elevated to extreme levels with acute endothelial injury affecting lipase function; this can occur in diabetic ketoacidosis and in rare inflammatory disorders. Elevated triglycerides and other dyslipidemias may also be seen in secondary HIV chemotherapy and late after cancer chemotherapy. Triglyceride levels are highly variable so that unless a value is >500 mg/dl, a single value may not be used for classification of an abnormality.

The most prevalent dyslipidemia in the United States is the combination of elevated triglycerides and low HDL cholesterol. This is largely because of the obesity epidemic. In adults, the clustering of obesity, insulin resistance, hypertension, and dyslipidemia is called the metabolic syndrome *(21)*. No satisfactory childhood definition of this condition has been accepted; however, risk clustering is clearly present in overweight children and is likely associated with future cardiovascular morbidity *(35)*.

The initial treatment of dyslipidemia is dietary. Table 3 provides useful principles of diet management *(36,37)*. For elevated LDL and non-HDL cholesterol, a diet low in saturated fat (< 7% of total calories, < 200 mg/day of cholesterol) should be implemented in addition to the diet recommended in Table 3. Dietary fiber, particularly oat fiber, and plant sterols and stanols are also helpful in lowering LDL cholesterol. More information with regard to dietary treatment can be found in publications on the Internet from the American Heart Association, the USDA *(38)*, the National Cholesterol Education Program of the National Institutes of Health, and the American Academy of Pediatrics. For elevated triglycerides (below 750–1000 mg/dl), weight management is initial treatment. Avoidance of carbohy-drates, particularly refined sugars, is critical. Avoidance of mono- and polyunsaturated fats

Table 3
American Heart Association Pediatric Dietary Strategies for Individuals >2 Years of Age

- Balance energy intake with energy expenditure to maintain normal growth
- Engage in 60 min of moderate to vigorous physical activity daily
- Emphasize deeply colored vegetables and fruits in the diet
- Substitute vegetable fats low in saturated fat and *trans* fatty acids for most animal fats in the diet
- Limit the intake of high-sugar beverages
- Choose whole grain over refined grain products
- Use low-fat and non-fat dairy products on a regular basis
- Consume fish, especially oily fish, at least twice a week
- Reduce salt intake

is not necessary as they may be useful in maintaining or increasing associated low HDL cholesterol.

Pharmacologic treatment for elevated cholesterol is considered in children over 10 years of age with LDL cholesterol ≥190 mg/dl and failed dietary management. Statins are the initial management, and the goal of treatment is an LDL cholesterol <130 mg/dl. Liver function should be monitored and treatment is held for elevation of transaminases greater than three times normal. The presence of myalgia is an indication for witholding treatment as rhabdomyolysis can occur as a rare complication. Statins are not to be given during pregnancy or with breastfeeding. In children less than 10 years of age, statins can be considered in very high-risk settings. Randomized trials of statin treatment of up to 2 years duration have been reported (39). One randomized trial has suggested that atherosclerosis progression as assessed by carotid IMT can be slowed by statin treatment, particularly if treatment is started in adolescence but there are no trials of statin use in children demonstrating prevention of cardiovascular disease in adulthood (40,41).

In the setting of multiple risk factors, statins may be initiated at lower LDL levels. In diabetics or those with two additional significant risk factors an LDL level of 160 mg/dl (or 130 mg/dl if risk is considered significantly elevated) (42). Thus, in a patient with hypertension and an additional risk factor statins would be initiated at this lower threshold. Conversely, blood pressure treatment goals are lower in patients with elevated LDL cholesterol (43).

In childhood, pharmacologic treatment for elevated triglycerides is only considered as prevention of pancreatitis and after failed dietary management. Generally, triglyceride levels repeatedly >500–750 mg/dl are treated. Fish oil (4 g) is used initially and fibrates are considered only in severe cases; there are no clinical trials of fibrate use in childhood.

There are no indications for treatment of low HDL cholesterol in children.

TOBACCO USE

Tobacco use remains the most important preventable cardiovascular risk factor in children. In the United States, after years of decline, adolescent tobacco use spiked reaching a peak in the mid- to late 1990s. Since then, tobacco use declined until about 2002–2003, with about 15% of high school students currently describing themselves as regular smokers. The college age range has the highest tobacco use. Tobacco use rates are monitored by an annual youth behavior risk survey and are available from the Centers for Disease Control (44).

Risk factors for tobacco use are family smoking, peer group smoking, lower socioeconomic status, presence of problem or antisocial behaviors, and susceptibility to media campaigns or influences with regard to tobacco use (45). Cigarettes, because of nicotine, are highly addictive. It is estimated that smoking 100 cigarettes or less may be sufficient to become an addicted smoker. Although randomized trials suggest physicians can be effective in smoking cessation treatment, success rates are low, particularly in youth. Pharmacologic treatments are available but there is limited published experience in youth. Although adolescents frequently attempt to quit smoking, these efforts generally occur outside the setting of supervision by health-care providers or other experienced counselors. The presence of tobacco use may be an indication for intensification of management of other risk factors.

A history of tobacco use should be sought in every adolescent, particularly if a cardiovascular risk factor is present since the combination of tobacco use with another major risk factor is probably the most common and malignant setting for multiple risk *(46)*. Since most pediatric health-care providers are inexperienced in smoking cessation treatment, referral to a smoking cessation program or telephone quitline should be considered.

DIABETES MELLITUS

In adults, diabetes mellitus is considered a vascular disease equivalent *(21)*. Cardiovascular disease is the leading cause of death in diabetics. Accelerated atherogenesis is present in both type I and type II diabetes. Diabetes is the only risk factor to erase the gender protection of about 5–10 years in atherosclerosis development in women *(2)*. Studies of children with type I diabetes mellitus have shown increased carotid IMT; cardiovascular risk factors and age at onset of diabetes influence carotid IMT measurement *(47)*.

The prevalence of both type I and type II diabetes mellitus is rising, the latter because of the obesity epidemic. In adolescents type II diabetes mellitus is now almost as common as type I *(48)*.

There is currently little published experience with cardiovascular risk factor control in childhood diabetes. However, consensus recommendations consider the presence of diabetes an indication for intensification of management of cardiovascular risk factors *(42)*. Studies in adults suggest that significant cardiovascular event reduction rates, similar to those in non-diabetics, can be achieved with hypertension and lipid lowering treatment *(21)*.

OBESITY, FAMILY HISTORY, GENDER, NUTRITION, PHYSICAL ACTIVITY, SOCIOECONOMIC STATUS, ETHNIC DIVERSITY AND THE EVOLUTION OF CARDIOVASCULAR RISK

A number of factors contribute to the evolution of cardiovascular risk in childhood. Some of these, such as family history, physical inactivity, and low socioeconomic status, are also independent risk factors for cardiovascular disease. From an evidence and research standpoint it is often more difficult to directly relate these factors to cardiovascular events and intermediate measures of end organ injury. However, it is also clear that optimal health habits are critical for primordial prevention, the prevention of risk factor development in the first place.

The development of obesity is the most important pediatric public health problem today. Worsening obesity is the most important cause for the transition from the relatively low risk state of childhood to the presence of cardiovascular risk in adulthood, particularly for the development of hypertension, diabetes mellitus, and the high triglyceride/low HDL cholesterol phenotype *(49)*. These factors have been collectively termed the metabolic syndrome in adults. The presence of obesity-associated multiple risk tracks into adulthood and in one preliminary study it is associated with premature adult morbidity *(50)*. Establishing a pediatric definition has been difficult because of the dynamic nature of risk factors during youth *(35)*. Nonetheless, the prevention of obesity development in at-risk infants and children and the prevention of worsening obesity in affected children and adolescents are an important part of regular pediatric practice as at least one-third of US children are overweight or obese.

Family history remains an independent risk factor for atherosclerosis *(51)*. In adults, a positive family history increases risk even after control for potential genetic traits. Positive family history predicts risk in offspring; conversely risk in childhood predicts risk in related adults. Family history independently predicts the presence of subclinical atherosclerosis *(52,53)*. Therefore, the presence of a positive family history of atherosclerosis-related disease or risk factors should prompt evaluation of family members for both genetic and environmental risk factors for intervention.

For all risk factors, there are gender-related differences in expression. In general, atherosclerosis develops about 5–10 years later in women than men *(2)*. However, atherosclerosis-related diseases remain the leading cause of death for women. Two risk factors impact the protective relationship of gender for women: diabetic women do not have any difference in the age-related onset of atherosclerotic complications and the use of tobacco obliterates the 5- to 10-year protective effect.

Nutrition has a significant impact on the evolution of cardiovascular risk. A lifelong low cholesterol, low saturated fat diet has a small but significant effect on lipid levels and blood pressure *(54)*. A diet low in salt is associated with lower blood pressure *(55)*. Although the equivalent of the DASH study has not been performed in children, it seems reasonable to generalize the findings of that study to children as foods recommended in the DASH diet are nutrient dense and important for growth and development *(36)*. Excess caloric intake causes obesity.

Higher levels of physical fitness are associated with a small but significant effect on blood pressure and protect against the future development of obesity, hypertension, metabolic syndrome, and diabetes mellitus *(56,57)*. It is likely that an above average level of activity reduces the rate of rise of blood pressure over time *(58)*.

Socioeconomic status plays an important role in the evolution of cardiovascular disease risk, particularly with regard to behavioral factors *(59,60)*. Risk factor rates, particularly obesity-related co-morbidities and tobacco use, are much higher in groups with lower socioeconomic status. Many factors may play a role: lower educational level, less access to preventive care, lower literacy rates making comprehension of health-related messages more difficult, targeting of lower class groups for marketing of less healthy products (tobacco, fast food), less trust in physicians and health-related messages, and barriers to access to healthier nutrition.

Most data on cardiovascular disease have been acquired in Caucasian populations, particularly male. Although comparative studies across nationalities, cultural groups, and ethnic groups suggest that cardiovascular risk factors are the same in all groups, the importance of each risk factor and the expression of risk factors in relationship to environmental stress may be different. For example, factors related to the metabolic syndrome arise at different levels of body mass index in different ethnic groups *(61)*. The prevalence of specific risk factors also varies by ethnic group *(62)*. Thus, more research is necessary before cardiovascular disease prevention recommendations can be made more specific for particular cultures.

NON-TRADITIONAL RISK FACTORS

A number of factors, different from the major risk factors described above, have been identified that at least in some studies have an independent contribution to cardiovascular risk. These fall into several groups: measures of intermediate end organ injury and/or subclinical atherosclerosis, markers of inflammation, and physiologic measures that may be implicated in atherogenesis. In adults, it remains controversial whether or not these nontraditional risk factors substantially improve risk prediction beyond that provided by the major risk factors described previously in this chapter *(63)*. Although some research on these factors has been done in children, it is often cross-sectional and is insufficient to add to clinical assessment outside of a research setting.

The most important marker of end organ injury is echocardiography to assess left ventricular mass and left atrial size *(64)*. These measures are correlated with hypertension and obesity, and independent relationships to cardiovascular morbidity are well established. Subclinical atherosclerosis assessments, including CT scanning to assess for coronary calcium and cIMT, are not useful clinically in children. Calcium does not enter atherosclerotic lesions until young adulthood, and normal values for cIMT are age and operator dependent and have not been established *(64)*. Assessment of brachial reactivity using ultrasound techniques has provided insights into the presence of endothelial injury early in life, particularly with regard to tobacco exposure and the benefits of exercise; however, these studies do not yet have independent value in clinical practice beyond conventional risk factor assessment *(65,66)*.

In adults, the best studied marker of inflammation is c-reactive protein; others include various vascular adhesion molecules and inflammatory cytokines *(67)*. There are very little pediatric data on these factors and for many, pediatric levels may be different than in adults. There is no information on tracking, measurement variability, and relationship to adult intermediate endpoints. Since obesity and atherosclerosis are pro-inflammatory, it is unclear if these measures can be considered risk factors or are simply markers of ongoing physiologic processes associated with the major risk factors *(68)*.

There are diverse physiologic measures that may improve risk assessment by a small amount. Examples include urinary albumin excretion (a measure of renal vascular injury), lipoprotein (a) (a lipid particle that may have prothrombotic activity at least in some isoforms), fibrinogen (a marker of the prothrombotic state but well correlated with obesity), adiponectin and leptin (hormones associated with obesity), and homocysteine (associated with accelerated atherosclerosis when extremely elevated in genetic conditions). An additional physiologic factor under intense scrutiny is low birth weight, though the mechanisms of this relationship are beyond the scope of this review *(69)*.

SUMMARY

Atherosclerosis begins in youth. The major risk factors for the development of premature atherosclerosis are hypertension, dyslipidemia, tobacco use, and diabetes mellitus. For some individuals, genetic and other predisposing conditions may cause a high-risk state in childhood. For the general population, diet, physical activity, family history, obesity, and low socioeconomic status contribute to the development of risk factors. For most children with identified risk factors, behavioral management is critical to prevent worsening of risk. For children at extremes of the risk distribution or with multiple risk factors, pharmacologic treatment may be necessary.

REFERENCES

1. Williams CL, Hayman LL, Daniels SR, Robinson TN, Steinberger J, Paridon S, Bazzarre T. Cardiovascular health in childhood: a statement for health professionals from the Committee on Atherosclerosis, Hypertension, and Obesity in the Young (AHOY) of the Council on Cardiovascular Disease in the Young, American Heart Association. Circulation. Jul 2002;106(1):143–160.

2. McGill HC Jr, McMahan CA, Gidding SS. Preventing heart disease in the 21st century: implications of the Pathobiological Determinants of Atherosclerosis in Youth (PDAY) study. Circulation. Mar 2008;117(9):1216–1227.
3. McMahan CA, Gidding S, Malcom GT, Tracy RE, Strong JP, McGill HC Jr. PDAY risk scores are associated with early as well as advanced atherosclerosis. Pediatrics. 2006;118:1447–1455.
4. McGill HC Jr, McMahan CA, Tracy RE, Oalmann MC, Cornhill JF, Herderick EE, Strong JP. Relation of a postmortem renal index of hypertension to atherosclerosis and coronary artery size in young men and women. Pathobiological Determinants of Atherosclerosis in Youth (PDAY) Research Group. Arterioscler Thromb Vasc Biol. Jul 1998;18(7):1108–1118.
5. McMahan CA, Gidding SS, Fayad ZA, Zieske AW, Malcom GT, Tracy RE, Strong JP, McGill HC Jr. Risk scores predict atherosclerotic lesions in young people. Arch Intern Med. Apr 2005;165(8):883–890.
6. Zieske AW, McMahan CA, McGill HC Jr, Homma S, Takei H, Malcom GT, Tracy RE, Strong JP. Smoking is associated with advanced coronary atherosclerosis in youth. Atherosclerosis. May 2005;180(1):87–92.
7. McGill HC Jr, McMahan CA, Herderick EE, Zieske AW, Malcom GT, Tracy RE, Strong JP. Obesity accelerates the progression of coronary atherosclerosis in young men. Circulation. Jun 2002;105(23): 2712–2718.
8. McGill HC Jr, McMahan CA, Zieske AW, Malcom GT, Tracy RE, Strong JP. Effects of nonlipid risk factors on atherosclerosis in youth with a favorable lipoprotein profile. Circulation. Mar 2001;103(11):1546–1550.
9. Kwiterovich PO. Primary and secondary disorders of lipid metabolism in pediatrics. Pediatr Endocrinol Rev. Feb 2008;5(Suppl 2):727–738.
10. Cohen JC, Boerwinkle E, Mosley TH Jr, Hobbs HH. Sequence variations in PCSK9, low LDL, and protection against coronary heart disease. N Engl J Med. Mar 2006;354(12):1264–1272.
11. Active and passive tobacco exposure: a serious pediatric health problem. A statement from the Committee on Atherosclerosis and Hypertension in Children, Council on Cardiovascular Disease in the Young, American Heart Association. Circulation. Nov 1994;90(5):2581–2590.
12. Retnakaran R, Zinman B. Type 1 diabetes, hyperglycaemia, and the heart. Lancet. May 2008;371(9626):1790–1799.
13. Li S, Chen W, Srinivasan SR, Bond MG, Tang R, Urbina EM, Berenson GS. Childhood cardiovascular risk factors and carotid vascular changes in adulthood: the Bogalusa Heart Study. JAMA. Nov 2003;290(17):2271–2276.
14. Raitakari OT, Juonala M, Kahonen M, Taittonen L, Laitinen T, Maki-Torkko N, Jarvisalo MJ, Uhari M, Jokinen E, Ronnemaa T, Akerblom HK, Viikari JS. Cardiovascular risk factors in childhood and carotid artery intima-media thickness in adulthood: the Cardiovascular Risk in Young Finns Study. JAMA. 2003;290(17):2277–2283.
15. Mahoney LT, Burns TL, Stanford W, Thompson BH, Witt JD, Rost CA, Lauer RM. Coronary risk factors measured in childhood and young adult life are associated with coronary artery calcification in young adults: the Muscatine Study. J Am Coll Cardiol. Feb 1996;27(2):277–284.
16. Gidding SS, McMahan CA, McGill HC, Colangelo LA, Schreiner PJ, Williams OD, Liu K. Prediction of coronary artery calcium in young adults using the Pathobiological Determinants of Atherosclerosis in Youth (PDAY) risk score: the CARDIA study. Arch Intern Med. Nov 27 2006;166(21):2341–2347.
17. McMahan CA, Gidding SS, Viikari JS, Juonala M, Kahonen M, Hutri-Kahonen N, Jokinen E, Taittonen L, Pietikainen M, McGill HC Jr, Raitakari OT. Association of Pathobiologic Determinants of Atherosclerosis in Youth risk score and 15-year change in risk score with carotid artery intima-media thickness in young adults (from the Cardiovascular Risk in Young Finns Study). Am J Cardiol. Oct 1 2007;100(7): 1124–1129.
18. Chen X, Wang Y. Tracking of blood pressure from childhood to adulthood: a systematic review and meta-regression analysis. Circulation. Jun 24 2008;117(25):3171–3180.
19. Lauer RM, Clarke WR. Use of cholesterol measurements in childhood for the prediction of adult hypercholesterolemia. The Muscatine Study. JAMA. Dec 19 1990;264(23):3034–3038.
20. Lloyd-Jones DM, Leip EP, Larson MG, D'Agostino RB, Beiser A, Wilson PW, Wolf PA, Levy D. Prediction of lifetime risk for cardiovascular disease by risk factor burden at 50 years of age. Circulation. Feb 14 2006;113(6):791–798.
21. Executive summary of the third report of the National Cholesterol Education Program (NCEP) expert panel on detection, evaluation, and treatment of high blood cholesterol in adults (Adult Treatment Panel III). JAMA. May 16 2001;285(19):2486–2497.
22. Seventh report of the joint national committee on prevention, detection, evaluation and treatment of high blood pressure (JNC VII). Hypertension. 2003;42:1026.
23. Steinberg D, Gotto AM Jr. Preventing coronary artery disease by lowering cholesterol levels: fifty years from bench to bedside. JAMA. 1999;282(21):2043–2050.

24. Messiah SE, Arheart KL, Luke B, Lipshultz SE, Miller TL. Relationship between body mass index and metabolic syndrome risk factors among US 8- to 14-year-olds, 1999 to 2002. J Pediatr. Aug 2008;153(2):215–221.

25. Muntner P, He J, Cutler JA, Wildman RP, Whelton PK. Trends in blood pressure among children and adolescents. JAMA. May 5 2004;291(17):2107–2113.

26. Jolliffe CJ, Janssen I. Distribution of lipoproteins by age and gender in adolescents. Circulation. Sep 5 2006;114(10):1056–1062.

27. Gidding SS, Bookstein LC, Chomka EV. Usefulness of electron beam tomography in adolescents and young adults with heterozygous familial hypercholesterolemia. Circulation. Dec 8 1998;98(23):2580–2583.

28. Parekh RS, Gidding SS. Cardiovascular complications in pediatric end-stage renal disease. Pediatr Nephrol. Feb 2005;20(2):125–131.

29. Management of dyslipidemia in children and adolescents with diabetes. Diabetes Care. Jul 2003;26(7):2194–2197.

30. American Academy of Pediatrics. National Cholesterol Education Program: report of the expert panel on blood cholesterol levels in children and adolescents. Pediatrics. Mar 1992;89(3 Pt 2):525–584.

31. Lau JF, Smith DA. Advanced lipoprotein testing: recommendations based on current evidence. Endocrinol Metab Clin North Am. Mar 2009;38(1):1–31.

32. Labarthe DR, Nichaman MZ, Harrist RB, Grunbaum JA, Dai S. Development of cardiovascular risk factors from ages 8 to 18 in Project HeartBeat! Study design and patterns of change in plasma total cholesterol concentration. Circulation. 1997;95(12):2636–2642.

33. Gidding SS, Stone NJ, Bookstein LC, Laskarzewski PM, Stein EA. Month-to-month variability of lipids, lipoproteins, and apolipoproteins and the impact of acute infection in adolescents. J Pediatr. Aug 1998;133(2):242–246.

34. Zappalla FR, Gidding SS. Lipid management in children. Endocrinol Metab Clin North Am. Mar 2009;38(1):171–183.

35. Steinberger J, Daniels SR, Eckel RH, Hayman L, Lustig RH, McCrindle B, Mietus-Snyder ML. Progress and challenges in metabolic syndrome in children and adolescents: a scientific statement from the American Heart Association Atherosclerosis, Hypertension, and Obesity in the Young Committee of the Council on Cardiovascular Disease in the Young; Council on Cardiovascular Nursing; and Council on Nutrition, Physical Activity, and Metabolism. Circulation. Feb 3 2009;119(4):628–647.

36. Gidding SS, Dennison BA, Birch LL, Daniels SR, Gilman MW, Lichtenstein AH, Rattay KT, Steinberger J, Stettler N, Van Horn L. Dietary recommendations for children and adolescents: a guide for practitioners: consensus statement from the American Heart Association. Circulation. Sep 27 2005;112(13):2061–2075.

37. Gidding SS, Lichtenstein AH, Faith MS, Karpyn A, Mennella JA, Popkin B, Rowe J, Van Horn L, Whitsel L. Implementing American Heart Association pediatric and adult nutrition guidelines: a scientific statement from the American Heart Association Nutrition Committee of the council on nutrition, physical activity and metabolism, council on cardiovascular disease in the young, council on arteriosclerosis, thrombosis and vascular biology, council on cardiovascular nursing, council on epidemiology and prevention, and council for high blood pressure research. Circulation. Mar 3 2009;119(8):1161–1175.

38. U.S. Department of Health and Human Services, U.S. Department of Agriculture. Dietary Guidelines for Americans, 6th ed. Washington, DC: U.S. Government Printing Office; 2005.

39. McCrindle BW, Urbina EM, Dennison BA, Jacobson MS, Steinberger J, Rocchini AP, Hayman LL, Daniels SR. Drug therapy of high-risk lipid abnormalities in children and adolescents: a scientific statement from the American Heart Association Atherosclerosis, Hypertension, and Obesity in Youth Committee, Council of Cardiovascular Disease in the Young, with the Council on Cardiovascular Nursing. Circulation. Apr 10 2007;115(14):1948–1967.

40. Wiegman A, Hutten BA, de Groot E, Rodenburg J, Bakker HD, Buller HR, Sijbrands EJ, Kastelein JJ. Efficacy and safety of statin therapy in children with familial hypercholesterolemia: a randomized controlled trial. JAMA. Jul 21 2004;292(3):331–337.

41. Rodenburg J, Vissers MN, Wiegman A, van Trotsenburg AS, van der Graaf A, de Groot E, Wijburg FA, Kastelein JJ, Hutten BA. Statin treatment in children with familial hypercholesterolemia: the younger, the better. Circulation. Aug 7 2007;116(6):664–668.

42. American Diabetes Association. Management of dyslipidemia in children and adolescents with diabetes. Diabetes Care. 2003;26(7):2194–2197.

43. The fourth report on the diagnosis, evaluation, and treatment of high blood pressure in children and adolescents. Pediatrics. Aug 2004;114(2 Suppl 4th Report):555–576.

44. Morbidity and Mortality Weekly Report; Surveillance Summaries—June 9. Report. 2006;55(SS-5).

45. Elders MJ, Perry CL, Eriksen MP, Giovino GA. The report of the Surgeon General: preventing tobacco use among young people. Am J Public Health. 1994;84(4):543–547.

46. Gidding SS. Active and passive tobacco exposure. Prog Pediatr Cardiol. Jan 2001;12(2):195–198.

47. Dalla Pozza R, Bechtold S, Bonfig W, Putzker S, Kozlik-Feldmann R, Netz H, Schwarz HP. Age of onset of type 1 diabetes in children and carotid intima medial thickness. J Clin Endocrinol Metab. Jun 2007;92(6):2053–2057.

48. Dabelea D, Bell RA, D'Agostino RB Jr, Imperatore G, Johansen JM, Linder B, Liu LL, Loots B, Marcovina S, Mayer-Davis EJ, Pettitt DJ, Waitzfelder B. Incidence of diabetes in youth in the United States. JAMA. Jun 27 2007;297(24):2716–2724.

49. Steinberger J, Daniels SR. Obesity, insulin resistance, diabetes, and cardiovascular risk in children: an American Heart Association scientific statement from the Atherosclerosis, Hypertension, and Obesity in the Young Committee (Council on Cardiovascular Disease in the Young) and the Diabetes Committee (Council on Nutrition, Physical Activity, and Metabolism). Circulation. Mar 18 2003;107(10):1448–1453.

50. Morrison JA, Friedman LA, Wang P, Glueck CJ. Metabolic syndrome in childhood predicts adult metabolic syndrome and type 2 diabetes mellitus 25 to 30 years later. J Pediatr. Feb 2008;152(2):201–206.

51. O'Donnell CJ. Family history, subclinical atherosclerosis, and coronary heart disease risk: barriers and opportunities for the use of family history information in risk prediction and prevention. Circulation. Oct 12 2004;110(15):2074–2076.

52. Gaeta G, De Michele M, Cuomo S, Guarini P, Foglia MC, Bond MG, Trevisan M. Arterial abnormalities in the offspring of patients with premature myocardial infarction. N Engl J Med. Sep 21 2000;343(12): 840–846.

53. Wang TJ, Nam BH, D'Agostino RB, Wolf PA, Lloyd-Jones DM, MacRae CA, Wilson PW, Polak JF, O'Donnell CJ. Carotid intima-media thickness is associated with premature parental coronary heart disease: the Framingham Heart Study. Circulation. Aug 5 2003;108(5):572–576.

54. Niinikoski H, Lagstrom H, Jokinen E, Siltala M, Ronnemaa T, Viikari J, Raitakari OT, Jula A, Marniemi J, Nanto-Salonen K, Simell O. Impact of repeated dietary counseling between infancy and 14 years of age on dietary intakes and serum lipids and lipoproteins: the STRIP study. Circulation. Aug 28 2007;116(9): 1032–1040.

55. He FJ, MacGregor GA. Importance of salt in determining blood pressure in children: meta-analysis of controlled trials. Hypertension. Nov 2006;48(5):861–869.

56. Kelley GA, Kelley KS, Tran ZV. The effects of exercise on resting blood pressure in children and adolescents: a meta-analysis of randomized controlled trials. Prev Cardiol. Winter 2003;6(1):8–16.

57. Carnethon MR, Gidding SS, Nehgme R, Sidney S, Jacobs DR Jr, Liu K. Cardiorespiratory fitness in young adulthood and the development of cardiovascular disease risk factors. JAMA. Dec 17 2003;290(23): 3092–3100.

58. Gidding SS, Barton BA, Dorgan JA, Kimm SY, Kwiterovich PO, Lasser NL, Robson AM, Stevens VJ, Van Horn L, Simons-Morton DG. Higher self-reported physical activity is associated with lower systolic blood pressure: the Dietary Intervention Study in Childhood (DISC). Pediatrics. Dec 2006;118(6):2388–2393.

59. Lynch EB, Liu K, Kiefe CI, Greenland P. Cardiovascular disease risk factor knowledge in young adults and 10-year change in risk factors: the Coronary Artery Risk Development in Young Adults (CARDIA) Study. Am J Epidemiol. Dec 15 2006;164(12):1171–1179.

60. Lawlor DA, Sterne JA, Tynelius P, Davey Smith G, Rasmussen F. Association of childhood socioeconomic position with cause-specific mortality in a prospective record linkage study of 1,839,384 individuals. Am J Epidemiol. Nov 1 2006;164(9):907–915.

61. Razak F, Anand SS, Shannon H, Vuksan V, Davis B, Jacobs R, Teo KK, McQueen M, Yusuf S. Defining obesity cut points in a multiethnic population. Circulation. Apr 24 2007;115(16):2111–2118.

62. Winkleby MA, Robinson TN, Sundquist J, Kraemer HC. Ethnic variation in cardiovascular disease risk factors among children and young adults: findings from the Third National Health and Nutrition Examination Survey, 1988–1994. JAMA. Mar 17 1999;281(11):1006–1013.

63. Greenland P, Lloyd-Jones D. Defining a rational approach to screening for cardiovascular risk in asymptomatic patients. J Am Coll Cardiol. Jul 29 2008;52(5):330–332.

64. Gidding S. Noninvasive cardiac imaging: implications for risk assessment in adolescents and young adults. Ann Med. 2008;40:506–513.

65. Celermajer DS. Reliable endothelial function testing: at our fingertips? Circulation. May 13 2008;117(19):2428–2430.

66. Roman MJ, Naqvi TZ, Gardin JM, Gerhard-Herman M, Jaff M, Mohler E. American society of echocardiography report. Clinical application of noninvasive vascular ultrasound in cardiovascular risk stratification: a report from the American Society of Echocardiography and the Society for Vascular Medicine and Biology. Vasc Med. Nov 2006;11(3):201–211.

67. Ridker PM. Inflammatory biomarkers and risks of myocardial infarction, stroke, diabetes, and total mortality: implications for longevity. Nutr Rev. Dec 2007;65(12 Pt 2):S253–S259.
68. Rasouli N, Kern PA. Adipocytokines and the metabolic complications of obesity. J Clin Endocrinol Metab. Nov 2008;93(11 Suppl 1):S64–S73.
69. Norman M. Low birth weight and the developing vascular tree: a systematic review. Acta Paediatr. Sep 2008;97(9):1165–1172.

III HYPERTENSION IN CHILDREN: PREDICTORS, RISK FACTORS, AND SPECIAL POPULATIONS

13 Perinatal Programming and Blood Pressure

Julie R. Ingelfinger, MD

INTRODUCTION AND CONCEPTUAL BACKGROUND

Epidemiologic studies published in the late 1980s by Barker and his group *(1,2)*—and since replicated in a number of populations—provide evidence of an inverse relationship between birth weight and risk of cardiovascular disease, hypertension, renal dysfunction, and other diseases in adult life. Both clinical studies and a number of animal models have been used to investigate mechanisms underlying these observations [as cited in recent reviews *(3–6)*]. The concept that changes in the intrauterine milieu affect the growing fetus resulting in alterations in physiology and general health in later life has been termed perinatal programming or, more recently, developmental origins of health and disease (DOHaD). Yet, despite an increasingly complex literature about this phenomenon and its relationship to cardiovascular disease, the involved mechanisms remain elusive.

Nephron number is thought to influence blood pressure as well as susceptibility to renal disease in later life. Brenner et al. *(7)* were among the first to hypothesize that nephron number might influence the propensity to develop hypertension. A number of clinicopathologic observations suggest that such a relationship exists more directly. For example, Keller et al. *(8)* reported fewer nephrons in a small cohort of hypertensive adults who died in accidents as compared to the nephron number in normotensive persons who had similarly succumbed. The nephrons among the hypertensive subjects in the study were also larger than those in

J.R. Ingelfinger (✉)
Pediatric Nephrology Unit, Department of Pediatrics, Harvard Medical School and MassGeneral Hospital for
Children at Massachusetts General Hospital, Boston, MA, USA
e-mail: jingelfinger@partners.org

From: *Clinical Hypertension and Vascular Diseases: Pediatric Hypertension*
Edited by: J. T. Flynn et al. DOI 10.1007/978-1-60327-824-9_13
© Springer Science+Business Media, LLC 2011

the normotensive group. Whether these observations would hold in other studies was not known until recently, when Hoy et al. confirmed such changes in a multiracial autopsy series. Hoy et al. suggest that a relatively larger mean glomerular volume and variation in glomerular volume within a kidney are markers of "glomerular stress" *(9)*. However, there may be ethnic and racial differences in that Hughson et al. *(10)* found no relation between blood pressure and glomerular number in American blacks.

A decreased nephron number may be associated not only with hypertension but also the tendency to develop chronic kidney disease. For example, Cass et al. *(11)* reported an association between low birth weight, hypertension, and later renal disease.

A growing body of laboratory work supports the concept that perinatal programming is linked to maternal malnutrition *(3,4,12–15)*, dietary deficiencies (e.g., retinoic acid) *(16)*, or exposures to certain substances during gestation (e.g., glucocorticoids) *(17)* that result in subtle alterations that cause offspring to have a propensity to develop high blood pressure or renal dysfunction after they reach adult life (Table 1). For example, numerous studies indicate that pregnant rats or guinea pigs administered low-protein diets during gestation produce offspring with relatively low birth weights, a propensity to have elevated blood pressure at maturity and deficient nephrogenesis *(3,4,12–15,18–21)*. The hypertension in such experimental models is often observed early and appears to persist, unless treated, throughout life. This chapter focuses on human data concerning the relation between perinatal programming and hypertension in later life.

Table 1
Maternal Factors Influencing the Risk of Future Hypertension

Maternal extrinsic exposures in the perinatal period and offspring hypertension
Protein-calorie malnutrition
High-salt diet
Iron deficiency
Vitamin A deficiency
Nephrotoxic drugs

Maternal intrinsic conditions in the perinatal period and offspring hypertension
Gestational diabetes
Maternal CKD

CLINICAL OBSERVATIONS ON PROGRAMMING AND BLOOD PRESSURE IN CHILDREN

In an early study of perinatal programming Barker et al. examined BP in 9,921 ten-year-old children in whom birth weight was available and observed that systolic blood pressure was inversely related to birth weight *(22)*. Law et al. *(23)* and Whincup et al. *(24)* also reported a direct relationship between birth weight and BP in children, an effect that seems definite, if small *(25–27)*.

Renal function in later life has also been inversely associated with birth weight. For example, the Nord Trøndelag Health 2 (Hunt 2) study *(28)* reported that persons born at term with relatively low birth weights had relatively lower glomerular filtration rate (GFR) when examined at 20–30 years of age. There are also data suggesting that it is gestational age rather than birth weight per se that is important. For example, Siewert-Delle and Ljung-man *(29)* observed that gestational age rather than birth weight itself was associated with both systolic and diastolic BP in middle-aged men. Their study *(29)* suggested that middle-aged men who had been term infants had BP that related to their adult BMI, not to birth weight alone.

Evaluating the effect of birth weight on adult blood pressure has not been feasible in prospective studies that track participants from birth to adult life. However, in a systematic review of more than 444,000 male and female subjects ranging in age from infancy to 84 years of age published in 2000, Huxley and her colleagues *(30)* reviewed 80 studies and drew the conclusion, based on their analysis, that birth weight is indeed inversely related to later systolic blood pressure levels. However, they also concluded that other factors, particularly the rate of postnatal growth, are influential in determining blood pressure *(25)*.

Thus, because variables other than birth weight exert major influences on BP in children, as well as on BP in adolescents and adults, the inverse relationship between birth weight and later BP level is not evident in all studies. The effect of current weight may outstrip the effects of birth weight. However, Seidman et al. *(25)* noted that birth weight had a lesser effect as compared to present weight. In data from the Bogalusa Heart Study, children with birth weights less than 2.5 kg at birth were compared to those weighing more than 2.5 kg; no association with birth weight and later blood pressure was discerned, likely owing to the effect of present weight *(31)*. In a study in 7-year-old children, Yiu et al. *(32)* found a positive effect of birth weight on hypertension once an adjustment for present weight at the time of follow-up was introduced.

The concept that deprivation during gestation results in a "thrifty phenotype" *(33,34)* in which the fetus is poised to take advantage of limited nutritional and environmental resources helps to explain why not all people exposed to adverse in utero conditions are equally affected. When postnatal environment provides surplus nutrients, as in Westernized and emerging nations, people metabolically programmed toward "thrift" are exposed to overabundance and are at high risk to develop hypertension and other health problems. Thus, the adiposity rebound that occurs may result in metabolic syndrome and its attendant cardiovascular risks.

EFFECTS OF ADVERSE GESTATIONAL CONDITIONS

Several situations that have been associated with perinatal programming will be now discussed in more detail. These include exogenous events such as protein-calorie malnutrition, vitamin A deficiency, exposure to exogenous glucocorticoids, high-salt diet, ethanol exposure, and iron deficiency. There are many intrinsic maternal conditions that influence the intrauterine milieu; some, such as maternal diabetes and placental insufficiency, have been shown to influence later cardiovascular function of the offspring.

Protein-Calorie Malnutrition

In human beings, it is generally difficult to quantitate the amount of nutritional alteration that occurs during gestation. However, there have been a few studies that have examined offspring born during famine, during which entire populations are subjected to marked protein-calorie malnutrition. For example, the children of women who were pregnant during the Dutch Famine, which took place in the western part of the Netherlands in 1944–1945, have been a well-studied cohort. During the Dutch Famine, caloric intake per person was below 900 kcal/day for several months. The most complete reports *(35,36)* concerning the offspring of mothers subjected to this famine include 724 people (all singletons) born during the last months of World War II; they were 48–53 years old at the time of study. Interestingly, the urinary albumin excretion was increased in 12% of the cohort who had been exposed in utero to famine during mid-gestation (adjusted odds ratio 3.2, with 95% CI 1.4–7.7). These survivors had a higher likelihood of hypertension as well. Persons exposed to famine while in utero in the first and last trimesters of pregnancy had other increased risks. Thus, the time during gestation in which the famine occurred was important.

Children whose mothers were pregnant during another famine during World War II, the Siege of Leningrad, have also been studied. Yudkin et al. *(37)* studied 98 people whose mothers had been exposed to marked protein-calorie nutrition during that siege. The investigators measured microalbuminuria in these survivors and compared the results to those of 124 persons who had been infants in Leningrad during the siege but whose mothers had not been subjected to famine while pregnant and to 62 Russians of the same age who lived outside the area of the siege while it was ongoing. The investigators also compared these results to those of 236 residents of Preston, UK, who were of the same age. Only 11 people had microalbuminuria, and there were not statistically significant correlations between in utero starvation, birth weight, and microalbuminuria.

In sum, there is not strong evidence to directly or indirectly link human maternal low protein-calorie intake to hypertension. Further, there is no clear evidence that protein and calorie intake per se influence nephron number or renal size in humans.

Vitamin A Deficiency

For many years it has been known that vitamin A deficiency and a number of birth defects, including renal anomalies, are associated *(14,16,38–46)*. However, there are suggestions that mild vitamin A deficiency may be associated with subtle renal defects. While animal studies support this concept, and while retinoic acid may correct the defect in vitro *(44)*, proof in humans is difficult.

Goodyer et al. *(45)* noted that kidneys at birth are smaller in children from Bangalore, India, as compared to the kidneys of babies in Montreal. They observed that vitamin A levels in the mothers from India were lower than those of mothers in Montreal. See a recent Cochrane review for discussion of the effects of vitamin A supplementation in humans *(46)*.

Glucocorticoid Exposure

A number of studies in animal models indicate that exposure to exogenous glucocorticoids during pregnancy acts as a negative modifier of renal development, possibly resulting in higher risk for hypertension and other disease later in life *(17,47–51)*.

Glucocorticoids are used clinically, for example, to promote lung maturation in anticipated premature delivery; some follow-up data are available. One observational study of 14-year-old children who had been exposed to betamethasone in utero found higher BPs in those youngsters as compared to normal; however, the study may have been confounded by puberty, given the age of the subjects *(52)*. In another study, a small, randomized trial, systolic blood pressure was less at age 20 in young people who had been exposed to betamethasone in utero as compared to those not so exposed *(53)*.

Dalziel et al. *(54)* studied children whose mothers had taken part in a randomized study during which they had received betamethasone or placebo during pregnancy. At age 30, the now-grown children underwent examination of their blood pressure, body indices, as well as glucose tolerance, lipid status, and plasma cortisol. There were no differences in body size, BP, or cardiovascular disease in those exposed or not exposed while in utero. However, the offspring whose mothers had received betamethasone during gestation had a higher frequency of dysglycemia as measured by glucose tolerance testing.

In a multicenter study *(55)* Finken et al. evaluated 412 former premature infants (born at 32 weeks of gestation) at 19 years of age. Some participants had been born to mothers who had received two doses of betamethasone (12 mg) to induce lung maturation. There were no differences in serum lipids and insulin resistance between the groups. While estimated glomerular filtration rate (eGFR) was normal in all subjects, it was significantly lower among those subjects whose mothers had received steroids (mean ± SD = 103.5 ± 12.6 ml/min/1.73 m², betamethasone group vs. 107.0 ± 15.6 ml/min/1.73 m², control group).

High-Salt Diet

Increasing maternal salt intake can result in changes in renal structure and function quite similar to those produced by protein restriction *(56–58)*. Since increased salt intake by itself decreases fetal RAS expression, it would appear that a similar mechanism is operative.

Gestational high salt intake in animal models is associated with hypertension in offspring. Swenson et al. *(59)* observed that Sprague-Dawley rats that received a high-salt diet in the perinatal period later become hypertensive. Their work indicates that the high blood pressure is associated with increased central nervous system AT_1 receptor activation, leading to increased sympathetic nervous activity. In contrast, Vidonho et al. *(60)* reported that perinatal restriction of salt also had later adverse events.

The data concerning the perinatal effects of salt intake in humans are limited. However, Simonetti et al. *(61)* reported that children with low birth weight had increased salt sensitivity and increased responsiveness of blood pressure to changes in the salt in the diet *(62)*.

Ethanol and Renal Development

While much is known about adverse effects of ethanol on the developing brain, little has been studied in terms of its effect on renal development. Gray et al. *(63)* examined the effects of multiple exposures to ethanol in the sheep model. They observed an 11% reduction in nephron number, though the overall kidney growth and the size of the fetus were not changed. Additionally there were no changes in gene expression so far as examined.

While some children with fetal alcohol syndrome have been reported to have kidney malformations—with small kidneys with malrotation and other anomalies—little is known about the relation between maternal alcohol intake during gestation and future cardiovascular health *(64–66)*.

Iron Deficiency

Iron deficiency during pregnancy in experimental models has been shown to result in offspring with hypertension. For example, Lewis et al. *(67)* found that restricting iron intake in the pregnant rat led to decreased birth weight in the pups and subsequent hypertension in adult life. Iron-restricted mothers were anemic at delivery, and their pups had lower hemoglobin levels as compared to normal offspring. At 3 months of age offspring remained anemic, and their systolic BP was elevated compared to BP in offspring of mothers that had not been iron restricted. Iron-restricted offspring had decreased fasting serum triglyceride levels, though fasting serum cholesterol and free fatty acid concentrations were similar in both groups. Insulin levels were not different between the groups. Thus, maternal iron restriction seemed to "program" offspring for future hypertension, with findings reminiscent of the maternal protein restriction model. Lisle et al. extended this work, with results suggesting a deficit in nephron number *(68)*. Subsequent work by Andersen et al. suggested that the adverse effects of maternal iron deficiency, studied with cultured rat embryos, could be rescued by restoration of iron in media *(69)*.

Iron deficiency is very common in pregnant women, even in industrialized nations *(70)*. Some studies have shown positive relationships between maternal hemoglobin and anemia *(71,72)*, while others have found no associations *(73,74)* and still others an inverse association *(75)*. Brion and colleagues *(76)* examined maternal anemia, iron intake during gestation, and blood pressure at age 7 in the Avon Longitudinal Study of Parents and Children. They found no effects, once data were adjusted for age, sex, and other confounders. If anything, blood pressure was lower in the offspring of anemic women.

PREMATURE BIRTH AND LATER BLOOD PRESSURE

Premature birth may occur prior to the completion of nephrogenesis *(77)*. Recently Gubhaju et al. *(78)* examined a primate model and found a high proportion of abnormal glomeruli in some but not all kidneys when animals were delivered at 125 days of gestation. There was no influence induced by providing glucocorticoids antenatally. The implications of their work to humans are not known at this time.

We do know that premature infants born early yet not surviving the neonatal period have hypertrophied glomeruli *(79)*. Further, premature infants of extremely low birth weight surviving into mid-childhood have been reported to have an increased amount of proteinuria *(80)*. Recently Hodgin et al. *(81)* reported that extremely low birth weight was a risk factor for secondary focal segmental glomerulosclerosis. Kistner et al. *(82)* examined blood pressures in women who had been born preterm and noted that there was a relative increase in systolic blood pressure as compared to those born at term.

POSSIBLE MECHANISMS OF PROGRAMMING

What are the mechanisms underlying the clinical and laboratory observations that perinatal events influence later cardiovascular and renal function? The coordinated developmental events involved in organogenesis are extremely complex *(3–6)*. It has been recognized for many years that toxic events that interrupt gestation can lead to such disordered development that a fetus does not survive *(3–6,83,84)*. For decades, toxicologic studies have constituted a major portion of new drug development, as well as a major medicolegal focus whenever a medication produces serious fetal abnormalities. In contrast to the effects of known toxins, the insults incurred by the fetus due to malnutrition do not generally produce clearly visible or identifiable abnormalities at birth.

To date, there have been several approaches to seek mechanisms responsible for perinatal programming. First, candidate genes and systems have been examined, most notably, to search for changes in steroid metabolism and feedback systems and to seek alterations in vasoactive systems such as the renin–angiotensin system, which are known to impact organogenesis and repair, and changes in biological systems that might lead to fibrogenesis.

Altered Steroid Metabolism

A number of observations support the idea that alterations in steroid metabolism can be caused by maternal diet and medication that can lead to changes in renal structure and function *(85)*. For example, protein restriction decreases the amount of placental 11β-hydroxysteroid dehydrogenase. Decreases in this enzyme, which inactivates maternal cortisol or corticosterone, lead to increased fetal exposure to glucocorticoids from the mother *(17)*. Such increased exposure may lead to steroid actions on nuclear receptors that might well influence the development of the kidney and vasculature. Infants with lower birth weight have been found to have placentas with relatively low 11β-hydroxysteroid dehydrogenase activity, supporting the concept that increased glucocorticoid exposure has been present *(51,85)*. This basic observation has led to the hypothesis that in conditions of low protein intake, placental 11βHSD is decreased, possibly leading to an increase in the amount of maternal steroids reaching the fetus with attendant changes in nephrogenesis. Indeed, dexamethasone administered to pregnant rats crosses the placenta yet is not metabolized by 11βHSD, leading to low birth weight pups with a propensity to become hypertensive as adults *(86,87)*. Carbenoxolone (an inhibitor of 11βHSD) also has resulted in low birth weight animals with a tendency toward hypertension in one study *(88)* but not in another *(89)*.

Alterations in Renal Tubular Transporter

Manning et al. *(90)* hypothesized that changes in the fetal kidney would program later inappropriate sodium retention in later life as one explanation for the hypertension observed. Thus, they examined the possible role of sodium transporters, speculating that at least one would demonstrate increased activity. Low-protein offspring showed evidence of upregulation of mRNA for two transporters, renal BSC1 and TSC at 4 weeks of age, prior to the development of hypertension.

Glomerular Hyperfiltration

Lucas *(91)* has reproduced the undernutrition model and examined in some detail what happens within hypertrophic glomeruli. In his model, dams subjected to 50% food restriction bore offspring with a decreased number of glomeruli that exhibited increased glomerular diameter, suggesting compensatory hypertrophy and hyperfiltration. He posited that glomerular hypertrophy would lead, ultimately, to renal damage and carried out morphologic, immunohistochemical, and functional studies in the offspring exposed to this energy restriction in utero. The offspring of restricted rats exhibited intense tubulointerstitial lesions and immunohistochemical alterations in the renal cortex—increased fibronectin and desmin expression in glomeruli and tubulointerstitium and increased vimentin and alpha-smooth muscle actin in the tubulointerstitial area from the renal cortex. Furthermore desmin was increased at the periphery of glomeruli, which implies likely podocyte injury. The investigators suggested that the aberrant glomerulogenesis in the offspring of the malnourished dams resulted in hyperfiltration and ensuing renal damage.

Alterations in the Renin–Angiotensin System

The intrarenal renin–angiotensin system (RAS) generally demonstrates altered expression in the offspring of mothers that have been subjected to protein restriction during gestation. The kidneys of rat pups born to protein-restricted mothers show dramatic decreases in renin mRNA protein immunostaining and angiotensin II levels *(20,21)*. The decrease in intrarenal angiotensin II is of particular interest, since that octapeptide is critical to normal growth and remodeling and thus important in nephrogenesis *(92)*. However, taken together, these data suggest that interruption of normal functions of the RAS could result in fewer nephrons, ultimately predisposing to hypertension in adult life *(93)*.

The two sexes are not similarly prone to experience perinatal programming given the same exposures. Thus, programming exhibits sexual dimorphism *(94)*. For example, Holemans et al. *(95)* showed that male offspring of mothers that had been administered low-protein diets in the latter half of pregnancy were far more susceptible to low birth weights than their female littermates. The female littermates then appeared to be resistant to elevated blood pressure as adults. Woods et al. have also noted that male pups were more susceptible to decreases of intrarenal renin and angiotensin II; males, but not females later became hypertensive *(94)*.

Endocrine Alterations

Vickers et al. *(96,97)* have induced maternal undernutrition throughout pregnancy, followed by postnatal hypercaloric nutrition in offspring to produce a rat model of metabolic syndrome. They observed the development of hyperphagia, obesity, hypertension, hyperinsulinemia, and hyperleptinemia in those offspring whose mothers had been subjected to undernutrition in pregnancy. This model has also been used to study the influence of IGF-I administration.

Growth Factors and Inflammation

Growth factors are important in nephrogenesis, and their alterations may lead to aberrant renal morphogenesis *(92,98)*. Rees et al. *(99)* have demonstrated that maternal protein deficiency leads to maternal decrease in circulating threonine and is associated with hepatic hypermethylation of DNA.

Other Mechanisms

The coordinated program necessary for the formation of the kidney requires several development and regression of the pronephros and mesonephros and the interaction of the mesonephros with the metanephros *(100)*. The changes wrought in perinatal programming would be more than likely reflected by subtle alterations in the process of nephrogenesis. The hypothesis and observation that adult hypertension is associated with fewer nephrons have been well articulated by Brenner and Mackenzie *(101)*. Fewer glomeruli have been reported in autopsies of human infants with intrauterine growth retardation, which is consistent with that theory *(79)*. The work of Kwong et al. *(102)* observed increased apoptosis in blastocysts of rats exposed to a low-protein diet in the preimplantation stage of gestation. Welham et al. *(103)* reported that protein restriction during gestation in the rat appears to be associated with increased apoptosis in mesenchymal cells. Welham et al. *(103)* noted that the metanephric mesenchyme, a subset of which is induced to form nephrons, is derived from the intermediate mesoderm. The intermediate mesoderm is also the source of the pronephros and mesonephros, which eventually become residual structures such as the Wolffian duct. Metanephric mesenchyme that is recruited via factors emanating from the ureteric bud to form the final kidney will undergo apoptosis unless rescued. Thus, increased apoptosis would presumably result in fewer generations of nephrons.

Oxidative stress and subsequent inflammation may be important in programming hypertension during gestation and the perinatal period. Work by Stewart et al. *(104)* in the rat model of maternal low-protein diet indicates that the offspring have evidence both of oxidative stress and of inflammation. Treatment of animals with mycophenolate and also the superoxide dismutase mimetic tempol lessened immune cell infiltration and increased renal nitrotyrosine levels.

Epigenetic Influences

Certain congenital anomalies of the kidney and urinary system are the result of monogenic mutations inherited via classic Mendelian genetics *(105–107)*. Changes in nephron number do occur in some of these disorders, which involve renal dysplasia, hypoplasia, and malformations (see Chapter 6 and *(106)*). However, more subtle alterations via epigenetic marking may be involved in perinatal programming *(106,108)*. Epigenetic alterations occur via DNA methylation and histone modification of chromatin or via proteins that associate with DNA. Such epigenetic changes can result in changes in both gene expression and stem cell lineage *(108–110)*. DNA-binding factors such as *Pax2* and *Pax8*, which are DNA-binding factors, are critical in renal development and have been proposed as means by which histone modification in the developing kidney might take place *(110)*.

Sodium resorption is important in the development of hypertension, and alterations in the expression of sodium transporters have been noted in offspring of dams subjected to protein restriction during gestation. Recently Zhang et al. reported that the collecting duct epithelial sodium channel is subjected to epigenetic control *(111)*. Kaneko et al. have published a recent review about the possible roles of epigenetics in organogenesis *(109)*.

What do all of these observations tell us? Basic studies provide substantial evidence that intrauterine events affect nephrogenesis, perhaps in subtle ways, the effects of which can only be observed later in life *(112)*. The propensity to develop hypertension, renal disease, and cardiovascular disease may well be initiated, at least in some persons, by intrauterine and perinatal events that impact organogenesis in subtle ways.

REFERENCES

1. Barker D, Bull A, Osmond C, Simmonds S. Fetal and placental size and risk of hypertension in adult life. BMJ. 1990;301:259–262.
2. Barker D, Godfrey K, Osmond C, Bull A. The relation of fetal length, ponderal index and head circumference to blood pressure and the risk of hypertension in adult life. Paediatr Perinat Epidemiol. 1992;6:35–44.
3. Baum M. Role of the kidney in the prenatal and early postnatal programming of hypertension. Am J Physiol Renal Physiol. 2010;298:F235–F247.
4. Nuyt AM, Alexander BT. Developmental programming and hypertension. Curr Opin Nephrol Hypertens. 2009;18:144–152.
5. Abitbol CL, Ingelfinger JR. Nephron mass and cardiovascular and renal disease risks. Semin Nephrol. 2009;29:445–454.
6. Dötsch J, Plank C, Amann K, Ingelfinger J. The implications of fetal programming of glomerular number and renal function. J Mol Med. 2009;87:841–848.
7. Brenner BM, Garcia DL, Anderson S. Glomeruli and blood pressure. Less of one, more the other? Am J Hypertens. 1988;1:335–347.
8. Keller G, Zimmer G, Mall G, Ritz E, Amann K. Nephron number in patients with primary hypertension. N Engl J Med. 2003;348:101–108.
9. Hoy WE, Bertram JF, Denton RD, Zimanyi M, Samuel T, Hughson MD. Nephron number, glomerular volume, renal disease and hypertension. Curr Opin Nephrol Hypertens. 2008;17:258–265.

10. Hughson MD, Gobe GC, Hoy WE, Manning RD Jr, Douglas-Denton R, Bertram JF. Associations of glomerular number and birth weight with clinicopathological features of African Americans and whites. Am J Kidney Dis. 2008;52:18–28.
11. Cass A, Cunningham J, Snelling P, Wang Z, Hoy W. End-stage renal disease in indigenous Australians: a disease of disadvantage. Ethn Dis. 2002;12:373–378.
12. Langley-Evans SC, Phillips GJ, Jackson AA. In utero exposure to maternal low protein diets induces hypertension in weanling rats, independently of maternal blood pressure changes. Clin Nutr. 1994;13:319–324.
13. Persson E, Jansson T. Low birth weight is associated with elevated adult blood pressure in the chronically catheterized guinea pig. Acta Physiol Scand. 1995;115:195.
14. Merlet-Benichou C, Gilbert T, Muffat-Joly M, Lelievre-Pegorier M, Leroy B. Intrauterine growth retardation leads to a permanent nephron deficit in the rat. Pediatr Nephrol. 1994;8:175–180.
15. Timofeeva NM, Egorova VV, Nikitina AA. Metabolic/food programming of enzyme systems in digestive and nondigestive organs of rats. Dokl Biol Sci. 2000;375:587–589.
16. Lelièvre-Pégorier M, Vilar J, Ferrier ML, Moreau E, Freund N, Gilbert T, Merlet-Bénichou C. Mild vitamin A deficiency leads to inborn nephron deficit in the rat. Kidney Int. 1998;54: 1455–1462.
17. Ortiz LA, Quan A, Weinberg A, Baum M. Effect of prenatal dexamethasone on rat renal development. Kidney Int. 2001;59:1663–1669.
18. Langley-Evans SC. Critical differences between two low protein diet protocols in the programming of hypertension in the rat. Int J Food Sci Nutr. 2000;51:11–17.
19. Langley-Evans SC, Welham SJM, Jackson AA. Fetal exposure to a maternal low protein diet impairs nephrogenesis and promotes hypertension in the rat. Life Sci. 1999;64:965–974.
20. Woods LL, Ingelfinger JR, Nyengaard JR, Rasch R. Maternal protein restriction suppresses the newborn renin-angiotensin system and programs adult hypertension in the rat. Pediatr Res. 2001;49:460–467.
21. Manning J, Vehaskari VM. Low birth weight-associated adult hypertension in the rat. Pediatr Nephrol. 2001;16:417–422.
22. Barker DJ, Osmond C, Golding J, Kuh D, Wadsworth ME. Growth in utero, blood pressure in childhood and adult life, and mortality from cardiovascular disease. BMJ. 1989;298:564–567.
23. Law CM, de Swiet M, Osmond C, Fayers PM, Barker DJ, Cruddas AM, Fall CH. Initiation of hypertension in utero and its amplification throughout life. BMJ. 1993;306:24–27.
24. Whincup PH, Cook DG, Shaper AG. Early influences on blood pressure: a study of children aged 5–7 years. BMJ. 1989;299:587–591.
25. Seidman D, Laor A, Gale R, Stevenson D, Mashiach S, Danon Y. Birth weight, current body weight and blood pressure in late adolescence. BMJ. 1991;302:1235–1237.
26. Whincup P, Cook D, Papacosta O, Walker M. Birth weight and blood pressure: cross sectional and longitudinal relations in childhood. BMJ. 1995;311:773–776.
27. Taylor SJ, Whincup PH, Cook DG, Papacosta O, Walker M. Size at birth and blood pressure: cross sectional study in 8–11 year old children. BMJ. 1997;314:475.
28. Hallan S, Euser AM, Irgens LM, Finken MJJ, Homen J, Dekker FW. Effect of intrauterine growth restriction on kidney function at young adult age: The Nord Trondelag Health (HUNT 2) study. Am J Kidney Dis. 2008;16:10–20.
29. Siewert-Delle A, Ljungman S. The impact of birth weight and gestational age on blood pressure in adult life: a population based study of 49-year old men. Am J Hypertens. 1998;11:946–953.
30. Huxley RR, Shiell AW, Law CM. The role of size at birth and postnatal catch-up growth in determining systolic blood pressure: a systematic review of the literature. J Hypertens. 2000;18:815–831.
31. Donker G, Labarthe DR, Harriat RB, Selwyn BJ, Wattigney W, Berenson GS. Low birth weight and blood pressure at age 7–11 years in a biracial sample. Am J Epidemiol. 1997;147:87–88.
32. Yiu V, Buka S, Zurakowski D, McCormick M, Brenner B, Jabs K. Relationship between birthweight and blood pressure in childhood. Am J Kid Dis. 1999;33:253–260.
33. Hales CN, Barker DJ. Type 2 (non-insulin-dependent) diabetes mellitus: the thrifty phenotype hypothesis. Diabetologia. 1992;35:595–601.
34. Barker DJP, Osmond C, Kajantie E, Eriksson JG. Growth and chronic disease: Findings in the Helsinki birth cohort. Ann Hum Biol. 2009;36:445–458.
35. Barker DJ, Bleker OP. Microalbuminuria in adults after prenatal exposure to the Dutch famine. J Am Soc Nephrol. 2005;16:189–194.
36. Painter RC, Roseboom TJ, van Montfrans GA, Bossuyt PMM, Krediet RT, Osmond C, Barker DJP, Bleker OP. Microalbuminuria in adults after prenatal exposure to the Dutch famine. J Am Soc Nephrol. 2005;16:189–194.

37. Yudkin JS, Phillips DI, Stanner S. Proteinuria and progressive renal disease: birth weight and microalbuminuria. Nephrol Dial Transplant. 1997;12(Suppl 2):10–13.

38. Wilson JG, Warkany J. Malformations in the genito-urinary tract induced by maternal vitamin A deficiency in the rat. Am J Anat. 1948;83:357–407.

39. Bhat PV, Manolescu DC. Role of vitamin A in determining nephron mass and possible relationship to hypertension. J Nutr. 2008;138:1407–1410.

40. Batourina E, Gim S, Bello N, Shy M, Clagett-Dame M, Srinivas S, Costantini F, Mendelsohn C. Vitamin A controls epithelial/mesenchymal interactions through Ret expression. Nat Genet. 2001;27:74–78.

41. Gilbert T, Merlet-Benichou C. Retinoids and nephron mass control. Pediatr Nephrol. 2000;14:1137–1144.

42. Merlet-Bénichou C, Vilar J, Lelièvre-Pégorier M, Gilbert T. Role of retinoids in renal development: pathophysiological implication. Curr Opin Nephrol Hypertens. 1999;8:39–43.

43. Mendelsohn C, Lohnes D, Décimo D, Lufkin T, LeMeur M, Chambon P, Mark M. Function of the retinoic acid receptors (RARs) during development. (II) Multiple abnormalities at various stages of organogenesis in RAR double mutants. Development. 1994;120:2749–2771.

44. Makrakis J, Zimanyi MA, Black MJ. Retinoic acid enhances nephron endowment in rats exposed to maternal protein restriction. Pediatr Nephrol. 2007;22:1861–1867.

45. Goodyer P, Kurpad A, Rekha S, Muthayya S, Dwarkanath P, Iyengar A, Philip B, Mhaskar A, Benjamin A, et al. Effects of maternal vitamin A status on kidney development: a pilot study. Pediatr Nephrol. 2007;22:209–214.

46. Darlow BA, Graham PJ. Vitamin A supplementation to prevent mortality and short and long-term morbidity in very low birthweight infants. Cochrane Database Syst Rev. 2007;4:CD000501.

47. Wintour EM, Moritz KM, Johnson K, Ricardo S, Samuel CS, Dodic M. Reduced nephron number in adult sheep, hypertensive as a result of prenatal glucocorticoid treatment. J Physiol. 2003;549:929–935.

48. Dodic M, Hantzis V, Duncan J, Rees S, Koukoulas I, Johnson K, Wintour M, Moritz K. Programming effects of short prenatal exposure to cortisol. FASEB J. 2002;16:1017–1026.

49. Dodic M, Peers A, Moritz K, Hantzis V, Wintour EM. No evidence for HPA reset in adult sheep with high blood pressure due to short prenatal exposure to dexamethasone. Am J Physiol Regul Integr Comp Physiol. 2002;282:R343–R350.

50. Dodic M, May CN, Wintour EM, Coghlan JP. An early prenatal exposure to excess glucocorticoid leads to hypertensive offspring in sheep. Clin Sci (Lond). 1998;94:149–155.

51. Seckl JR. Glucocorticoid programming of the fetus; adult phenotypes and molecular mechanisms. Mol Cell Endocrinol. 2001;185:61–71.

52. Doyle LW, Ford GW, Davis NM, et al. Antenatal corticosteroid therapy and blood pressure at 14 years of age in preterm children. Clin Sci (Lond). 2000;98:137–142.

53. Dessens AB, Haas HS, Koppe JG. Twenty-year follow-up of antenatal corticosteroid treatment. Pediatrics. 2000;105:E77.

54. Dalziel SR, Walker NK, Parag V, Mantell C, Rea HH, Rodgers A, Harding JE. Cardiovascular risk factors after antenatal exposure to betamethasone: 30-year follow-up of a randomized controlled trial. Lancet. 2005;365:1856–1862.

55. Finken MJJ, Keijzer-Veen MG, Dekker FW, Frolich M, Walther FJ, Romijn JA, Van der Heijden BJV, Wit JM, and on behalf of the Dutch POPS-19 Collaborative Study Group. Antenatal glucocorticoid treatment is not associated with long term metabolic risks in individuals born before 32 weeks of gestation. Arch Dis Child Fetal Neonatal Ed. 2008;93:F442–F447.

56. Contreras RJ, Wong DL, Henderson R, Curtis KS, Smith JC. High dietary NaCl early in development enhances mean arterial pressure of adult rats. Physiol Behav. 2000;71:173–181.

57. Alves da Silva A, Noronha IL, Oliveira IB, Malheiros DMC, Heimann JC. Renin–angiotensin system function and blood pressure in adult rats after perinatal salt overload. Nutr Metab Cardiovasc Dis. 2003;13:133–139.

58. Porter JP, King SH, Honeycutt AD. Prenatal high-salt diet in the Sprague-Dawley rat programs blood pressure and heart rate hyperresponsiveness to stress in adult female offspring. Am J Physiol Regul Integr Comp Physiol. 2007; 293:R334–R342.

59. Swenson SJ, Speth RC, Porter JP. Effect of a perinatal high-salt diet on blood pressure control mechanisms in young Sprague-Dawley rats. Am J Physiol Regul Integr Comp Physiol. 2004;286:R764–R770.

60. Vidonho AF Jr, da Silva AA, Catanozi S, Rocha JC, Beutel A, Carillo BA, Furukawa LN, Campos RR, de Toledo Bergamaschi CM, Carpinelli AR, Quintão EC, Dolnikoff MS, Heimann JC. Perinatal salt restriction: a new pathway to programming insulin resistance and dyslipidemia in adult Wistar rats. Pediatr Res. 2004;56:842–848.

61. Simonetti GD, Raio L, Surbek D, Nelle M, Frey FJ, Mohaupt MG. Salt sensitivity of children with low birth weight. Hypertension. 2008;52:625–630.

62. Thrift AG, Srikanth V, Fitzgerald SM, Kalyanram K, Kartik K, Hoppe CC, Walker KZ, Evans RG. The potential roles of high salt intake and maternal malnutrition in development of hypertension in disadvantaged populations. Clin Exp Pharmacol Physiol. 2010;37:e78–e90.

63. Gray SP, Kenna K, Bertram JF, Hoy WE, Yan EB, Bocking AD, Brien JF, Walker DW, Harding R, Moritz KM. Repeated ethanol exposure during late gestation decreases nephron endowment in fetal sheep. Am J Physiol Regul Integr Comp Physiol. 2008;295:R568–R574.

64. Taylor C, Jones KL, Jones MC, Kaplan GW. Incidence of renal anomalies in children prenatally exposed to ethanol. Pediatrics. 1994; 94:209–212.

65. Qazi Q, Masakawa A, Milman D, McGann B, Chua A, Haller J. Renal anomalies in fetal alcohol syndrome. Pediatrics. 1979;63:886–889.

66. Havers W, Majewski F, Olbing H, Eickenberg HU. Anomalies of the kidneys and genitourinary tract in alcoholic embryopathy. J Urol. 1980;124:108–110.

67. Lewis RM, Petry CJ, Ozanne SE, Hales CN. Effects of maternal iron restriction in the rat on blood pressure, glucose tolerance, and serum lipids in the 3-month-old offspring. Metabolism. 2001;50: 562–567.

68. Lisle SJ, Lewis RM, Petry CJ, Ozanne SE, Hales CN, Forhead AJ. Effect of maternal iron restriction during pregnancy on renal morphology in the adult rat offspring. Br J Nutr. 2003;90:33–39.

69. Andersen HS, Gambling L, Holtrop G, McArdle HJ. Maternal iron deficiency identifies critical windows for growth and cardiovascular development in the rat postimplantation embryo. J Nutr. 2006;136:1171–1177.

70. World Health Orgnization. Iron deficiency anaemia. Assessment, prevention and control. Geneva, Switzerland: World Health Organization, 2001. Available at http://www.who.int/nutrition/publications/en/ida_assessment_prevention_control.pdf [Last Accessed: February 1, 2010].

71. Godfrey KM, Forrester T, Barker DJ, et al. Maternal nutritional status in pregnancy and blood pressure in childhood. Br J Obstet Gynaecol. 1994;101:398–403.

72. Law CM, Barker DJ, Bull AR, Osmond C. Maternal and fetal influences on blood pressure. Arch Dis Child. 1991;66:1291–1295.

73. Belfort MB, Rifas-Shiman SL, Rich-Edwards JW, Kleinman KP, Oken E, Gillman MW. Maternal iron intake and iron status during pregnancy and child blood pressure at age 3 years. Int J Epidemiol. 2008;37:301–308.

74. Whincup P, Cook D, Papacosta O, Walker M, Perry I. Maternal factors and development of cardiovascular risk: evidence from a study of blood pressure in children. J Hum Hypertens. 1994;8:337–343.

75. Bergel E, Haelterman E, Belizan J, Villar J, Carroli G. Perinatal factors associated with blood pressure during childhood. Am J Epidemiol. 2000;151:594–601.

76. Brion MJ, Leary SJ, Smith GD, McArdle HJ, Ness AR. Maternal anemia, iron intake in pregnancy, and offspring blood pressure in the Avon Longitudinal Study of Parents and Children. Am J Clin Nutr. 2008;88:1126–1133.

77. Abitbol CL, Ingelfinger JR. Nephron mass and cardiovascular and renal disease risks. Semin Nephrol. 2009;29:445–454.

78. Gubhaju L, Sutherland MR, Yoder BA, Zulli A, Bertram JF, Black MJ. Is nephrogenesis affected by preterm birth? Studies in a non-human primate model. Am J Physiol Renal Physiol. 2009;297:1668–1677.

79. Rodriguez MM, Gomez A, Abitbol C, Chandar J, Montané B, Zilleruelo G. Comparative renal histomorphometry: a case study of oligonephropathy of prematurity. Pediatr Nephrol. 2005;20: 945–949.

80. Abitbol CL, Chandar J, Rodriguez MM, Berho M, Seeherunvong W, Freundlich M, Zilleruelo G. Obesity and preterm birth: additive risks in the progression of kidney disease in children. Pediatr Nephrol. 2009;24:1363–1370.

81. Hodgin JB, Rasoulpour M, Markowitz GS, D'Agati VD. Very low birth weight is a risk factor for secondary focal segmental glomerulosclerosis. Clin J Am Soc Nephrol. 2009;4:71–76.

82. Kistner A, Celsi G, Vanpee M, Jacobson SH. Increased systolic daily ambulatory blood pressure in adult women born preterm. Pediatr Nephrol. 2005;20:232–233.

83. Mantovani A, Calamandrei G. Delayed developmental effects following prenatal exposure to drugs. Curr Pharm Des. 2001;7:859–880.

84. Nagao T, Wada K, Marumo H, Yoshimura S, Ono H. Reproductive effects of nonylphenol in rats after gavage administration: a two-generation study. Reprod Toxicol. 2001;15:293–315.

85. Seckl JR, Benediktsson R, Lindsay RS, Brown RW. Placental 11 beta-hydroxysteroid dehydrogenase and the programming of hypertension. J Steroid Biochem Mol Biol. 1995;55:447–455.

86. Celsi G, Kistner A, Aizman R, Eklof AC, Ceccatelli S, de Santiago A, Jacobson SH. Prenatal dexamethasone causes oligonephronia, sodium retention and higher blood pressure in the offspring. Pediatr Res. 1998;44:317–322.

87. Benediktsson R, Lindsay RS, Noble J, Seckl JR, Edwards CRW. Glucocorticoid exposure in utero: a new model for adult hypertension. Lancet. 1993;341:339–341.
88. Langley-Evans SC. Maternal carbenoxolone treatment lowers birthweight and induces hypertension in the offspring of rats fed a protein-replete diet. Clin Sci (Lond). 1997;93:423–429.
89. Gomez-Sanchez, Elise P, Gomez-Sanchez CE. Maternal hypertension and progeny blood pressure: role of aldosterone and 11 beta-HSD. Hypertension. 1999;33:1369–1373.
90. Manning J, Beutler K, Knepper MA, Vehaskari VM. Upregulation of renal BSC1 and TSC and prenatally programmed hypertension. Am J Physiology Renal Physiol. 2002;283:F202–F206.
91. Lucas A. Programming by nutrition in man. In: Conning D, ed. Early Diet, Later Consequences: Proceedings of the Thirteenth British Nutrition Foundation Annual Conference. London: British Nutrition Federation; 1991:24.
92. Tufro-McReddie A, Romano LM, Harris JM, Ferber L, Gomez RA. Angiotensin II regulates nephrogenesis and renal vascular development. Am J Physiol. 1995;269:F110–F115.
93. Woods LL, Rasch R. Perinatal Ang II programs adult blood pressure, glomerular number, and renal function in rats. Am J Physiol. 1998;275:R1593–R1599.
94. Woods LL, Ingelfinger JR, Rasch R. Modest maternal protein restriction fails to program adult hypertension in female rats. Am J Physiol Regul Integr Comp Physiol. 2005;289:1131–1136.
95. Holemans K, Gerber R, Meurrens K, DeClerck F, Poston L, Van Assche F. Maternal food restriction in the second half of pregnancy affects vascular function but not blood pressure of rat female offspring. Br J Nutr. 1999;81:73–79.
96. Vickers MH, Ikenasio BA, Breier BH. IGF-I treatment reduces hyperphagia, obesity, and hypertension in metabolic disorders induced by fetal programming. Endocrinology. 2001;142:3964–3973.
97. Vickers MH, Reddy S, Ikenasio BA, Breier BH. Dysregulation of the adipoinsular axis—a mechanism for the pathogenesis of hyperleptinemia and adipogenic diabetes induced by fetal programming. J Endocrinol. 2001;170:323–332.
98. Muaku SM, Beauloye V, Thissen JP, Underwood LE, Fossion C, Gerard G, Ketelslegers JM, Maiter D. Long-term effects of gestational protein malnutrition on postnatal growth, insulin-like growth factor and IGF-binding proteins in rat progeny. Pediatr Res. 1996;39:649–655.
99. Rees WD, Hay SM, Buchan V, Antipatis C, Palmer RM. The effects of maternal protein restriction on the growth of the rat fetus and its amino acid supply. Br J Nutr. 1999;81:243–250.
100. Kuure S, Vuolteenaho R, Vainio S. Kidney morphogenesis: cellular and molecular regulation. Mech Dev. 2000;92:31–45.
101. Brenner BM, Mackenzie HS. Nephron mass as a risk factor for progression of renal disease. Kidney Int Suppl. 1997;63:S124–S127.
102. Kwong WY, Wild AE, Roberts P, Willis AC, Fleming TP. Maternal undernutrition during the preimplantation period of rat development causes blastocyst abnormalities and programming of postnatal hypertension. Dev Suppl. 2000;127:4195–4202.
103. Welham SJ, Wade A, Woolf AS. Protein restriction in pregnancy is associated with increased apoptosis of mesenchymal cells at the start of rat metanephrogenesis. Kidney Int. 2002;61:1231–1242.
104. Stewart T, Jung FF, Manning J, Vehaskari VM. Kidney immune cell infiltration and oxidative stress contribute to prenatally programmed hypertension. Kidney Int. 2005;68:2180–2188.
105. Sequeira Lopez ML, Gomez RA. The role of angiotensin II in kidney embryogenesis and kidney abnormalities. Curr Opin Nephrol Hypertens. 2004;13:117–122.
106. Schedl A. Renal abnormalities and their developmental origin. Nat Rev Genet. 2007;8:791–802.
107. Salomon R, Tellier AL, Attie-Bitach T, Amiel J, Vekemans M, Lyonnet S, et al. PAX2 mutations in oligomeganephronia. Kidney Int. 2001;59:457–462.
108. Barker DJ, Bagby SP, Hanson MA. Mechanisms of disease: in utero programming in the pathogenesis of hypertension. Nat Clin Pract Nephrol. 2006;2:700–707.
109. Kaneko K, Sato K, Michiue T, Okabayashi K, Ohnuma K, Danno H, et al. Developmental potential for morphogenesis in vivo and in vitro. J Exp Zool B Mol Dev Evol. 2008;310:492–503.
110. Waddington CH. Genetic assimilation of an acquired character. Evolution. 1953;7:118–126.
111. Zhang D, Yu Z-Y, Cruz P, Kong Q, Li S, Kone BC. Epigenetics and the control of epithelial sodium channel expression in collecting duct. Kidney Int. 2009;75:260–267.
112. Gluckman PD, Hanson MA, Cooper C, Thornburg KL. Effect of in utero and early-life conditions on adult health and disease. N Engl J Med.2008;359:61–73.

14 Familial Aggregation of Blood Pressure

Xiaoling Wang, MD, PhD
and Harold Snieder, PhD

CONTENTS

INTRODUCTION

In the first half of the last century, evidence for the familial aggregation of (elevated) blood pressure (BP) levels was largely anecdotal and based on case reports of clinicians until a number of large family studies in the 1960s showed familial resemblance of BP with correlations around 0.20 among first-degree relatives *(1,2)*. Relatively few observations were made in children in these early studies, which initiated a number of research projects in the 1970s investigating whether familial aggregation of BP could be detected in childhood. Zinner et al. *(3)*, for example, measured BP in 721 children between 2 and 14 years of age from 190 families. Sib–sib and mother–child correlations of 0.34 and 0.16, respectively, for systolic BP (SBP) and 0.32 and 0.17, respectively, for diastolic BP (DBP) were found. These results were largely confirmed in a follow-up of the same cohort 4 years later *(4)*. Findings were extended to even younger ages by two further studies that showed significant sibling BP aggregation with 1-month-old infants *(5)* and significant parent–offspring correlations between mothers and their newborn infants *(6)*.

Thus, these studies showed that a familial tendency to high (or low) BP is established early in life, but a number of questions remained unanswered. For example, it was unclear whether shared genes or shared environment caused the BP aggregation within families. Special study designs such as adoption or twin studies are necessary to effectively discriminate genetic from shared environmental influences, because these sources of familial resemblance are confounded within nuclear families. Furthermore, estimates

H. Snieder (✉)
Unit of Genetic Epidemiology & Bioinformatics, Department of Epidemiology, University Medical Center Groningen, University of Groningen, Groningen, The Netherlands
e-mail: h.snieder@epi.umcg.nl

From: *Clinical Hypertension and Vascular Diseases: Pediatric Hypertension*
Edited by: J. T. Flynn et al. DOI 10.1007/978-1-60327-824-9_14
© Springer Science+Business Media, LLC 2011

of the relative influence of genetic and environmental factors derived from, for example, cross-sectional twin studies are merely 'snapshots' of a specific point in time: they do not give information on underlying genetic and environmental sources of continuity and change in the development of cardiovascular disease or their intermediate traits such as BP or lipids *(7,8)*. Genetic (or environmental) influences on BP may thus be age dependent and can take two different forms *(9)*. First, the magnitude of these influences on BP can differ with age. Second, different genes or environmental factors may affect BP at different ages. For example, BP genes may switch on or off during certain periods in life, i.e., age-dependent gene expression.

Therefore, in this chapter we will review the available literature of twin and family studies to address two issues: the potential causes of familial aggregation of BP and the age dependency of genetic or environmental sources of BP variation (and covariation) within and between families.

CAUSES OF FAMILIAL AGGREGATION OF BP

Rationale Behind the Classic Twin Study

Two approaches that have been frequently used to study the contributions of genes and environment to variation in BP levels are family and twin studies. The first approach studies the resemblance in BP between parents and offspring or between siblings in nuclear families. The second approach examines the similarity in BP of monozygotic (MZ) and dizygotic (DZ) twin pairs. Resemblance between family members (including twins) can arise from a common environment shared by family members and from a (partially) shared genotype. These sources of familial resemblance are confounded within nuclear families, because there is no differential sharing of genotype among first-degree relatives. Both parent–offspring and sibling pairs share on average 50% of their genetic material. Therefore, special study designs are necessary to discriminate genetic from shared environmental influences. One possibility is the adoption design *(10)*, whose applicability is somewhat limited due to practical considerations. Far more popular are twin studies, which examine phenotypic (e.g., BP) similarity of MZ and DZ twin pairs. They offer a unique opportunity to distinguish between the influences of environment and heredity on resemblance between family members. In a twin design the separation of genetic and environmental variance is possible because MZ twins share 100% of their genetic makeup, whereas DZ twins only share on average 50% of their genes. If a trait is influenced by genetic factors, MZ twins should resemble each other to a greater extent than DZ twins. In the classic twin method, the difference between intraclass correlations for MZ twins and those for DZ twins is doubled to estimate heritability [$h^2 = 2(r_{MZ} - r_{DZ})$], which can be defined as the proportion of total phenotypic variance explained by genetic factors. Whenever the DZ correlation is larger than half the MZ correlation, this may indicate that part of the resemblance between twins is caused by shared environmental factors *(11)*. The twin method assumes that both types of twins share their environment to the same extent: the equal environment assumption. Although there has been some criticism on the equal environment assumption (e.g., *(12)*), most studies specifically carried out to test it have proved it to be valid. Even if shared environment differentially affects MZ and DZ twins, it is unlikely that this has a substantial effect on the trait under study *(11,13,14)*. Furthermore, BP levels in twins are representative of those in the general population *(15,16)*.

Use of quantitative genetic modeling to estimate these genetic and environmental variance components is now standard in twin research, and details of model fitting to twin data have been described elsewhere *(17,18)*. In short, the technique is based on the comparison of the variance–covariance matrices (or correlations) in MZ and DZ twin pairs and allows separation of the observed phenotypic variance, which can be decomposed into several contributing factors. Additive genetic variance (*A*) is the variance that results from the additive effects of alleles at each contributing locus. Dominance genetic variance (*D*) is the variance that results from the nonadditive effects of two alleles at the same locus summed over all loci that contribute to the variance of the trait. Shared (common) environmental variance (*C*) is the variance that results from environmental events shared by both members of a twin pair (e.g., rearing, school, neighborhood, diet). Specific (unique) environmental variance (*E*) is the variance that results from environmental effects that are not shared by members of a twin pair and also includes measurement error. Dividing each of these components by the total variance yields the different standardized components of variance, for example, the heritability which (in the absence of *D*) is the ratio of additive genetic variance to total phenotypic variance ($A/A + C + E$).

Heritability or Family Environment

Over the last 30 years a large number of twin studies have been conducted investigating the relative influence of genetic and environmental factors on BP variation, and Tables 1 and 2 summarize pediatric and adult studies, respectively. Only twin studies with a reasonably large sample size (>50 twin pairs total) were included. Although studies used different methods to estimate heritability, it is immediately obvious from these tables that the evidence for a sizeable contribution of genetic factors to BP is overwhelming, with most heritability estimates around 50–60%. The majority of these studies found no evidence for influence of shared family environment on BP. This was confirmed by the study of Evans et al. *(19)* in which heritabilities of BP were estimated in more than 4000 twin pairs from six different countries. Heritabilities of DBP were between 44 and 66% across samples. For SBP, the range of estimates were even narrower between 52 and 66%. Shared environmental factors did play an important role, except possibly in Finland. Given the huge number of twin pairs used in these analyses we may confidently assert that around 50% of the variance in BP is due to genetic factors. For adult twins no longer living in the same family household, this result might have been expected. However, for children it is more surprising that environmental factors shared within families, such as salt intake or physical exercise, apparently explain a negligible amount of variation in BP. Part of the explanation might be that even apparently environmental variables such as diet and exercise have a heritable component *(20–22)*. Another part of the story might be that many twin studies may lack the power to detect moderate size influences of common environment *(23,24)*. A few studies that either had large sample sizes *(25,26)* or used a more powerful multivariate approach *(27)* did find a small contribution of shared environment of around 10–20%. The conclusion seems nevertheless warranted that if not entirely, the familial aggregation of BP is still largely due to genes rather than environmental factors shared within the family.

Sex Effects on BP Heritability

The existence of sex differences in the influences of genetic and environmental factors on the phenotype can take several forms. Although autosomal genes are not expected to

Table 1
Pediatric Twin Studies Estimating Heritability (h^2) in Systolic (SBP) and Diastolic Blood Pressure (DBP), in Ascending Order According to Age

Study	Pairs of twins	Age Mean (SD)	Range	Race	Sex	h^2 SBP	DBP
Yu et al. (54)[a]	274 MZ, 65 DZ	? (?)	0.0–1.0	Chinese	m and f	0.29–0.55	0.27–0.45
Levine et al. (29)[b]	67 MZ, 99 DZ	? (?)	0.5–1.0	b and w	m and f	0.66	0.48
Havlik et al. (70)	72 MZ, 40 DZ			Black	m and f	0.46	0.51
	43 MZ, 42 DZ			White	m and f	0.11	0.71
	115 MZ, 82 DZ	7.0 (?)	?	All	m and f	0.23	0.53
Wang et al. (71)	75 MZ, 35 DZ	? (?)	7.0–12.0	Chinese	m and f	0.32	0.46
Schieken et al. (72)	71 MZM, 74 MZF, 23 DZM, 31 DZF, 52 DOS	11.1 (0.25)	?	White	Male	0.66	0.64
					Female	0.66	0.51
McIlhany et al. (30)	40 MZM, 47 MZF, 32 DZM, 36 DZF, 45 DOS	14.0 (6.5)	5.0–50.0	b and w	Male	0.41	0.56
					Female	0.78	0.61

Table 1
(continued)

Study	Pairs of twins	Age Mean (SD)	Range	Race	Sex	h² SBP	DBP
Snieder et al. (31)	75 MZM, 91 MZF 33 DZM, 31 DZF, 78 DOS	14.9 (3.0)	10.0–26.0	White	Male	0.57	0.45
					Female	0.57	0.45
	52 MZM, 58 MZF 24 DZM, 39 DZF, 50 DOS	14.6 (3.2)	10.0–26.0	Black	Male	0.57	0.58
					Female	0.57	0.58
Snieder et al. (7)	35 MZM, 33 MZF 31 DZM, 29 DZF, 28 DOS	16.8 (2.0)	13.0–22.0	White	Male	0.49	0.69
					Female	0.66	0.50

Abbreviations: MZF = monozygotic females, MZM = monozygotic males, DZF = dizygotic females, DZM = dizygotic males, DOS = dizygotic opposite sex, b and w = black and white combined, m and f = males and females combined, ? indicates that age is not reported in the original paper.

[a]Range of heritability estimates between 2 months and 1 year are given.

[b]Heritability estimates reported by Levine et al. (29) were doubled as outlined by Kramer (73).

Table 2

Adult Twin Studies Estimating Heritability (h^2) in Systolic (SBP) and Diastolic Blood Pressure (DBP), in Ascending Order According to Age

Study	Pairs of twins	Age Mean (SD)	Age Range	Race	Sex	H^2 SBP	H^2 DBP
Sims et al. (74)	40 MZM, 45 DZM	19.4 (3.0)	?	White	Male	0.68	0.76
Ditto (75)	20 MZM, 20 MZF, 20 DZM, 20 DZF, 20 DOS	20.0 (5.0)	12.0–44.0	White	Male Female	0.63 0.63	0.58 0.58
McCaffery et al. (76)	129 MZ, 66 DZ	21.3 (2.8)	18.0–30.0	94% White	m and f	0.48	0.51
Bielen et al. (77)	32 MZM 21 DZM	21.7 (3.7) 23.8 (3.9)	18.0–31.0	White	Male	0.69	0.32
Fagard et al. (35)	26 MZM 27 DZM	23.8 (4.2) 24.7 (4.8)	18.0–38.0	White	Male	0.64	0.73
Busjahn et al. (78)	100 MZ, 66 DZ	29.8 (12.0)	?	White	m and f	0.74	0.72
Slattery et al. (79)	77 MZM, 88 DZM	? (?)	22.0–66.0	White	Male	0.60	0.66
Vinck et al. (37)	150 MZ, 122 DZ	34.9 (?)	18.0–76.0	White	m and f	0.62	0.57
Jedrusik et al. (36)	39 MZ, 37 DZ	35.0 (8.0)	18.0–45.0	White	m and f	0.53	0.62
Williams et al. (80)	14 MZM, 44 MZF 9 DZM, 31 DZF, 11 DOS	36.4 (?)	17.0–65.0	White	Male Female	0.60 0.60	0.52 0.43

Table 2
(continued)

Study	Pairs of twins	Age Mean (SD)	Age Range	Race	Sex	H^2 SBP	H^2 DBP
Austin et al. (81)	233 MZF, 170 DZF	42.0 (?)	?	90% White	Female	0.35	0.26
Baird et al. (53)[a]	30 MZM, 28 MZF 35 DZM, 45 DZF, 60 DOS	43.7 (1.4)	40.5–46.5	White	Male Female	0.48 0.48	0.30 0.76
Snieder et al. (7)	43 MZM, 47 MZF 32 DZM, 39 DZF, 39 DOS	44.4 (6.7)	34.0–63.0	White	Male Female	0.40 0.63	0.42 0.61
Snieder et al. (26)	213 MZF, 556 DZF	45.4 (12.4)	18.0–73.0	White	Female	0.17	0.22
Feinleib et al. (82)	250 MZM, 264 DZM	? (?)	42.0–56.0	White	Male	0.60	0.61
Hong et al. (25)	41 MZM, 66 MZF 69 DZM, 111 DZF	63.0 (8.0)	>50.0	White	Male Female	0.56 0.56	0.32 0.32

For abbreviations see Table 1.
[a]DBP heritabilities were not reported in the original paper.

be different between males and females as a result of the random nature of chromosomal segregation during meiosis, it is possible that some genes (or environments) have greater impact in women than in men (or vice versa) or that some genes contributing to BP in women are distinct from genes contributing to BP in men *(28).* Sex differences in magnitude of genetic and environmental effects can be tested by comparing parameter estimates between males and females. If studies considered sex differences in heritabilities, estimates for males and females are listed separately in Tables 1 and 2. However, heritability estimates for males and females are remarkably similar. A number of studies even report the same heritabilities for the two sexes, indicating that estimates for males and females could be set equal as part of the model fitting process used in these studies. Lower correlations in DZ opposite-sex pairs compared to same-sex DZ pairs indicate that genetic or shared environmental influences may differ in kind between males and females, but this has never been reported for BP.

Ethnic Effects on BP Heritability

Genetic as well as environmental differences between different ethnic populations may result in different BP heritabilities. As shown in Tables 1 and 2 most twin studies were conducted in Caucasian populations and a few combined twins from different ethnic groups without reporting separate heritability estimates *(29,30).* To resolve the question whether the relative influence of genetic and environmental factors on BP in youth is different between black and white Americans we recently conducted a classic twin study including both ethnic groups living in the same area. In this first study to estimate and compare the relative influence of genetic and environmental factors on BP in a large sample of young black and white twins, heritability estimates of BP in black and white youth were not significantly different *(31).* Thus, concurrent with the few other twin studies of non-Caucasians as reported in Table 1, there seems to be no evidence for large differences in BP heritabilities between different ethnic groups. The fact that a similar amount of BP variation is explained by genetic factors within different ethnicities does not exclude the possibility; however, the actual genes responsible for this heritability differ between ethnic groups.

Twin Studies of Ambulatory BP

Conventional BP measures have shown their value in predicting adverse outcomes but provide only a snapshot of 24-h BP variability as seen in real life and might give an overestimation of real BP as a result of the white coat effect. The value of ambulatory BP (ABP) measurements is illustrated by studies showing that ABP is a better predictor of target organ damage and cardiovascular morbidity and mortality than BP measured in the clinic *(32).*

To circumvent disadvantages of conventional BP measures several twin studies have examined ABP, but the sample sizes of the initial studies have been small. Degaute et al. *(33)* evaluated 24-h ABP in a hospital research setting with 28 MZ and 16 DZ pairs of young adult males. The small sample size and the presentation of 33 different measures make interpretation of results difficult, but overall evidence suggested heritability on some characteristics of the 24-h profiles for DBP. Somes et al. *(34)* examined the heritability of ABP in 38 pairs of MZ twins, 17 pairs of same-sex DZ twins, and 11 pairs of opposite-sex DZ twins. Heritability estimates of 0.22 and 0.34 were observed for 24-h SBP and DBP, respectively. Fagard et al. *(35)* measured 24-h ABP in 26 MZ and 27 DZ male twin pairs aged 18–38 years. Using model fitting techniques, heritability ranged from 0.51 to 0.73 for 24-h, daytime, and nighttime SBP and DBP. The remaining variances were typically accounted for by unique environment (range = 0.27–0.40). Jedrusik et al. *(36)* measured 24-h ABP in 39 MZ and 37 DZ twin pairs aged 18–45 years and observed that heritabilities for 24-h, daytime, and nighttime SBP and DBP ranged between 0.37 and 0.79.

More recently, three twin studies with relatively large sample size using ABP monitoring have been conducted. Vinck et al. *(37)* measured conventional and ambulatory BP in 150 MZ and 122 DZ pairs. Heritabilities were similar (around 50%) for laboratory and ambulatory (daytime and nighttime) SBP and DBP irrespective of the chorionicity of the MZ twins *(38)*. Kupper et al. *(39)* evaluated daytime ABP in 230 MZ and 305 DZ twins and 257 singleton siblings with an average age of 31 years. A common genetic influence on morning, afternoon, and evening SBP and DBP was identified with the heritability ranging from 0.44 to 0.63. Importantly, by using the extended twin design (including singleton sibs), this study showed that results from twin studies on the genetics of ABP can be generalized to the singleton population. Finally, we measured 24-h ABP in 240 white American (105 pairs and 30 singletons) and 190 black American (82 pairs and 26 singletons) twins (mean ± SD age: 17.2 ± 3.4 years; range: 11.9–30.0 years) from the Georgia Cardiovascular Twin Study *(40)*. Inspired by evidence from prospective studies showing that nighttime BP is superior to daytime BP as a predictor of cardiac mortality *(41)*, we performed a bivariate analysis to test whether genetic influences on BP during nighttime are different from those during daytime. The model fitting showed no ethnic or gender differences for any of the measures, with heritabilities of 0.70 and 0.68 for SBP and 0.70 and 0.64 for DBP at daytime and nighttime, respectively. The bivariate analysis also indicated that about 56 and 33% of the heritabilities of nighttime SBP and DBP, respectively, could be attributed to genes that also influenced daytime levels. The specific heritabilities due to genetic effects only influencing nighttime values were 0.30 for SBP and 0.43 for DBP. Our findings suggest that the underlying genetic mechanisms for BP regulation change with the day–night shift.

Nocturnal BP fall is another interesting feature revealed by ABP. Studies have shown that individuals with a blunted nocturnal decline in BP (the so-called nondipping) display the highest risk because this pattern exposes these individuals to a greater cardiovascular load each day. Fava et al. *(42)* explored the genetic influence on nocturnal BP fall indexed by the night-to-day ratio and observed a heritability of 38% for systolic and 9% for diastolic dipping in 104 adult Swedish sibships. In our own study mentioned above, we used a liability threshold model to examine whether dipping as a categorical phenotype is heritable and observed a heritability of 59% for SBP dipping and 81% for DBP dipping *(40)*.

Heritability of BP Measured Under Challenged Conditions

In many studies, blood pressure is measured under certain standardized environmental challenges. For example, BP can be measured under mental or physical stress. In fact, such a challenged phenotype may be more heritable than its unchallenged counterpart, potentially offering important advantages for gene-finding studies.

This principle is illustrated by Gu et al. *(43)* who investigated the heritability of blood pressure responses to dietary sodium and potassium intake in 1906 individuals from 658 Chinese pedigrees. The intervention included a 7-day low-sodium diet followed by a 7-day high-sodium diet and a 7-day high-sodium plus potassium supplement diet. Baseline heritabilities under the natural diet of SBP and DBP were 0.31 and 0.32, respectively. These heritabilities increased significantly to a narrow range of values between 0.49 and 0.52 for both SBP and DBP in all three environmentally controlled dietary conditions. Interestingly, the authors showed that these increases in heritability estimates were caused not only by a decrease in unique environmental (or residual) variance, as might have been expected under environmentally controlled circumstances, but also by an equally large increase in additive genetic variance. Although Gu et al. *(43)* did not elaborate on this, such an increase in genetic variance may have been caused by (1) a larger effect during the dietary conditions of the same genes that also affect BP at rest, (2) an emergence of new genetic effects on BP specific to the dietary conditions, or (3) a combination of the two. Bivariate models that include both challenged and unchallenged conditions can distinguish between these possibilities and quantify genetic and environmental effects on levels of the challenged and unchallenged phenotypes. We recently used such an approach to investigate BP during a stress challenge and test for the existence of gene-by-stress interaction within the context of a classic twin study *(44)*. Cardiovascular reactivity to stress, measured as the averaged response to a choice reaction time and mental arithmetic test, was assessed for SBP and DBP in 160 adolescent and 212 middle-aged twin pairs. Genetic factors significantly contributed to individual differences in resting SBP and DBP in the adolescent and middle-aged cohorts (heritabilities between 0.49 and 0.59). The effect of these genetic factors was amplified by stress for both SBP and DBP in the adolescent cohort and for SBP in the middle-aged cohort. In addition, stress-specific genetic variation emerged for SBP in the adolescent cohort. Heritability of stress levels of SBP and DBP ranged from 0.67 to 0.72 in the adolescents and from 0.54 to 0.57 in the middle-aged cohort. On the basis of these results we concluded that exposure to stress may uncover new genetic variance and amplify the effect of genes that already influence the resting level *(44)*. This has clear implications for gene-finding studies. The genetic variation that emerges exclusively during stress can only be found in studies that have attempted to measure the stress levels of BP. Genetic variation that is amplified during stress can be detected using resting levels, but the genetic variance, and hence the power of the study, will be larger if stress levels are measured instead.

Influence of Obesity on Familial Aggregation of BP

In subjects of all ages, weight is probably the most important correlate of BP. The familial aggregation of BP may, therefore, to a certain extent be due to the familial aggregation of obesity. Schieken et al. *(45)* addressed this question in a pediatric population of 11-year-old twins. They observed highly significant correlations between SBP and weight ($r = 0.40$) as well as body mass index (BMI) ($r = 0.29$) that could largely be explained by common genes rather than common environmental effects influencing both SBP and weight (or BMI). The percentage of total SBP variance caused by genetic effects common to SBP and weight was 11.2%; for BMI this figure was 8%. No significant correlations between DBP and body size were found. Two further twin studies in adult males *(46)* and females *(47)* found evidence for a direct effect of BMI on BP rather than an effect of common genes (pleiotropy). Both mechanisms, however, imply that part of the genetic variation in BP can be explained by genes for obesity *(47)*.

Influence of Birth Weight on Familial Aggregation of BP

The association between low birth weight and increased BP, although modest, has been well established as shown by a meta-analysis of 34 studies: BP reduces 1–2 mmHg for every kilogram increase in birth weight for children and the effect increases to about 5 mmHg/kg in elderly people *(48)*. The fetal programming hypothesis states that this association is due to intrauterine malnutrition (reflected by low birth weight), which increases the risk of a number of chronic diseases in later life including hypertension. However, other factors such as socioeconomic status and genetic factors may also explain the inverse relation between birth weight and BP. By studying intrapair differences in twins (i.e., relate intrapair differences in birth weight with intrapair differences in outcome variables) the influence of confounding parental characteristics can be controlled. Furthermore, influence of genetic makeup can be eliminated in MZ twins and reduced in DZ twins. Using this intrapair twin design, Poulter et al. *(49)* found that BP tended to be lower among those twins of each pair that were heavier at birth, suggesting that the inverse association between birth weight and adult BP is independent of parental confounding variables. These results also point to the importance of environmental fetal nutrition factors that are different within twin pairs such as placental dysfunction rather than factors that are the same such as maternal nutrition. This was confirmed by a recent study *(50)* in Swedish twins in which a nested co-twin control analysis was performed in 594 DZ and 250 MZ twin pairs discordant for essential hypertension. The odds ratio for hypertension in relation to a 500-g decrease in birth weight was 1.34 (95% CI: 1.07–1.69) for DZ twins and 1.74 (95% CI: 1.13–2.70) for MZ twins, which suggests that the association between birth weight and the risk of hypertension is independent of both shared familial environment and genetic factors. On the other hand, there are also studies supporting the possibility that factors shared by twins confound the association between birth weight and blood pressure. For example, Christensen et al.'s study in 1311 pairs of adolescent twins found a decrease in SBP of 1.88 mmHg for every kilogram increase in birth weight in the overall sample, but a reduction of this effect was observed when intrapair analyses were used *(51)*. This was confirmed by a recent meta-analysis *(52)* in 3901 twin pairs in which the decrease in SBP for every kilogram increase in birth weight was –2.0 (95% CI: –3.2 to –0.8) mmHg in the unpaired analysis, but only –0.4 (95% CI: –1.5 to 0.7) mmHg in the paired analysis. Thus, the association between birth weight and SBP attenuated when familial factors were controlled for suggesting that they contribute to this association. However, neither study could convincingly show whether this familial confounding had a genetic or shared environmental origin. In summary, the relation between birth weight and BP is probably due to a combination of environmental and genetic factors, but the contribution to the familial aggregation of BP of genes influencing birth weight is likely to be small *(53)*.

AGE DEPENDENCY OF GENETIC EFFECTS ON BP

BP level changes as a function of age, but this trend is not a simple linear one. The age-specific increase in SBP and DBP suggests that different (genetic and environmental) mechanisms have their influence on BP in different periods of life. Not only the mean BP but also its population variance has been found to increase from adolescence to adulthood *(7)*. Such an increase in BP variance with age may be due to interindividual variation in the rise of BP over time and can only be explained by an increase in one or more of the underlying variance components, which can be genetic or environmental. Such changes in variance components may imply changes in heritabilities with age.

Cross-Sectional Studies

TWIN STUDIES

In both Table 1 (mean age <18 years) and Table 2 (mean age >18 years), studies are listed in ascending order according to age of the twin sample. Such a systematic overview of all studies may reveal any age-dependent trends in heritability, because each study yields heritability estimates representative of its specific age range. However, neither within the adult nor the pediatric age range can clear age trends in BP heritability be detected. Two studies in very young twins *(29,54)* confirm the conclusions from previously mentioned family studies that familial aggregation is established very early in life. These twin studies suggest that this can be ascribed to genetic factors. The above-mentioned study of Vinck et al. *(37)* specifically investigated stability of heritable and environmental influences on both conventional and ambulatory BP in three age groups: 18–29, 30–39, and ≥40 years. Their large sample of 150 MZ and 122 DZ twin pairs had considerable power but found no significant differences in genetic and environmental influences between age groups.

The conclusion seems, therefore, warranted that the relative influence of genetic factors on BP is stable across the life span.

FAMILY STUDIES

Parent–Offspring and Sibling Correlations. Another approach to investigating the age dependency of genetic and environmental effects is to compare parent–offspring data with data from siblings or twins. If there is an age-dependent genetic or environmental effect on the phenotype, one would expect the parent–offspring correlation to be lower than sibling or DZ twin correlations, as the latter are measured around the same age. This expectation was confirmed in a review by Iselius et al. *(55)*. They pooled the results from a large number of studies and arrived at a mean correlation for 14,553 parent–offspring pairs of 0.165 for SBP and 0.137 for DBP. Corresponding values for 11,839 sibling and DZ twin pairs were 0.235 (SBP) and 0.201 (DBP).

If, on the other hand, parents and their offspring are measured at the same age, a rise in parent–offspring correlations toward levels similar to sibling correlations is to be expected. This expectation was supported by data from Havlik et al. *(56)*, who measured SBP and DBP for 1141 parent pairs aged 48–51 years. After 20–30 years, blood pressures for 2497 of their offspring were measured. At this time, the offspring were of ages similar to those of their parents when they were measured. Parent–offspring correlations ranged between 0.13 and 0.25 for SBP and between 0.17 and 0.22 for DBP. These ranges were quite similar to the sibling-pair correlations, which were between 0.17 and 0.23 (SBP) and between 0.19 and 0.24 (DBP). An alternative explanation for the lower parent–offspring correlation compared to the sibling or DZ twin correlation could be the influence of genetic dominance *(25,57)*. However, an effect of dominance is hardly ever found for BP, and the similarity between correlations for parents and offspring (who do not share dominance variation) and siblings (who share 0.25 of their dominance variation) in the study of Havlik et al. *(56)* also suggests that dominance variation is not important.

Lower values for parent–offspring correlations are also likely to be the main reason for the peculiar finding that heritability estimates derived from family studies (which usually measure pairs of subjects at different ages) are generally lower than those derived from twin studies. Heritability estimates from family studies range from 0.17 to 0.45 for SBP and from 0.15 to 0.52 for DBP *(55,57,58)*, while estimates from twin studies are typically in the 0.40–0.70 range for both SBP and DBP *(19)* (see also Tables 1 and 2).

Age-Dependent Gene Expression. Two types of age-dependent effect could offer an explanation for the lower parent–offspring correlation compared to the sibling and DZ twin pair correlations. First, the influence of unique environmental factors may accumulate over a lifetime. Such an increase, however, would lead to lower heritabilities with age, which is not supported by the evidence presented in Tables 1 and 2. Second, different genes could influence BP in childhood and adulthood. This possibility is still compatible with the results of Tables 1 and 2, as heritability can remain stable across time even though different genes are influential at different times. The latter possibility is supported by data from Tambs et al. *(59)*. In a Norwegian sample with 43,751 parent–offspring pairs, 19,140 pairs of siblings, and 169 pairs of twins, correlations between relatives decreased as age differences between these relatives increased. A model specifying age-specific genetic additive effects and unique environmental effects fitted the data well. This model also estimated the extent to which genetic effects were age specific. As an example, the expected correlations for SBP and DBP in relatives with an age difference of 40 years were calculated. For SBP, 62% of the genetic variance at, for example, ages 20 and 60 is explained by genes that are common to both ages, and 38% is explained by age-specific genetic effects. The same values for DBP were 67 and 33%, respectively. The model used by Tambs et al. *(59)* assumes invariant heritabilities for BP throughout life. This assumption proved to be valid for SBP, whereas for DBP a very slight increase in heritability was detected. Using an extended twin-family design *(60)*, including in addition to younger twins and their parents, a group of middle-aged twins of the same age as the parents provided further support for age-specific genetic effects on BP that differ between childhood and adulthood *(7)*. Models allowing for these effects showed a slightly better fit for both SBP and DBP with genetic correlations across time equal to 0.76 for SBP and 0.72 for DBP. The slightly lower values found by Tambs et al. *(59)* (0.62 for SBP and 0.67 for DBP) might be explained by the larger age difference (40 years) in their example, compared to the age difference between parents and offspring in this study (30 years).

Longitudinal Studies

Although changes in phenotypic variance and their genetic and environmental components (i.e., heritability and environmentality) with age may be detected by comparing cross-sectional family and twin studies conducted in different age groups, only a longitudinal twin study, in which the same subjects are measured repeatedly, is informative about the stability of genetic and environmental factors. Such a study permits examination of two important questions. First, does the magnitude of genetic and environmental influences on the phenotypes of interest change over time? Second, do novel environmental and/or genetic influences on those phenotypes become apparent during the course of development?

To date four longitudinal twin studies have addressed the potential emergence of new genetic or environmental factors for BP in adult populations. Colletto et al. *(61)* analyzed resting SBP and DBP in 254 MZ and 260 dizygotic (DZ) male middle-aged twin pairs (average age 48 years) and again 9 later. Using a time series analysis of genetic and environmental components of variation, they found that shared family environmental effects were absent and that specific environmental influences were largely occasion specific. In contrast, genetic influences were in part the same across adulthood (60% of genetic variation at the later ages was already detected in middle age) and in part age specific (the remaining 40% of the genetic variation at later ages was unrelated to that expressed earlier). Despite these changing genetic influences, the estimated heritabilities remained relatively constant across ages at around 0.50. When the twins were measured again 6 years after the second measurement, the genetic influence had stabilized and no new genes were evident. A second study measured 298 same-sex elderly twin pairs at an average age of 65 years and again 6 years later and found that the same set of genes explained all genetic variance in BP across the 6-year follow-up *(62)*. That is, no evidence was found for new genes being switched on or off at different points in time. This was confirmed in two recent studies of Dutch and Australian twins *(63,64)* in which multivariate genetic analyses showed that BP tracking was entirely explained by the same genetic factors being expressed across time.

The above studies did not cover the important transition from childhood to adulthood. We recently conducted the first longitudinal twin study on BP *(65)* for the period between 14 and 18 years of age. Resting BP levels were measured twice in >500 pairs of white and black American twins, with an intervening period of 4.1 years. Structural equation modeling on BP showed the emergence of substantial new genetic variance in both ethnic groups. A possible explanation for this emergence of novel genetic effects between ages 14 and 18 years is that hormonal changes after puberty affect the activation and deactivation of genes influencing individual differences in BP regulation.

These results have important implications for gene-finding studies. In current gene-finding efforts for complex traits, large sample sizes are required to reach sufficient statistical power, especially when genome-wide association or linkage designs are used. It would be advantageous to be able to pool data from subjects at different ages on the assumption that the same set of genes underlies BP regulation across the life span. As we stated above, although most longitudinal studies in adults have confirmed this assumption and reported the presence of a single genetic factor explaining variance in BP over time, our study in youth showed that a significant part of the variance was explained by newly expressed genes between 14 and 18 years. This means that one should exercise caution pooling adolescent and adult subjects in large genome-wide linkage or association studies of BP. Further follow-up of our twin sample will enable us to determine at what age the genetic component stabilizes (i.e., at what age no further novel genetic effects are expressed).

SUMMARY AND CONCLUSIONS

This chapter has examined causes of familial aggregation of BP and whether and how underlying genetic or environmental influences, or both, are stable or change across the life span. Different types of genetically informative studies were discussed to shed some light on these questions.

Familial aggregation of BP is largely due to genes rather than familial environment, and heritability estimates are very similar across sex, ethnicity, and modes of measurement but appear higher under environmentally challenged conditions. Genes for obesity and possibly birth weight can explain part of the genetic variation in BP. In twin studies of BP level, no age trend in heritability could be detected. Findings in family studies of lower parent–offspring correlations compared to those for siblings and DZ twins indicate, however, that age may influence genetic or environmental effects on BP level. There are two possible explanations: the influence of unique environmental factors could increase with age or different genes could influence BP in different periods of life. The lack of an age trend in heritabilities of twin studies is inconsistent with the first explanation, because an increase of unique environmental variance in adulthood, without a commensurate increase in genetic variance, would lower the heritability estimate. On the other hand, the twin data are not inconsistent with the second hypothesis of genes switching on and off with age, because the overall influence of genes can remain stable even though different genes are responsible for the effect. A number of further studies, including longitudinal studies of both adolescent and middle-aged twins, offered additional support for the second hypothesis that partly different genes affect BP in different periods of life, such as childhood, middle age, and old age.

The study of the genetics of mechanisms involved in BP regulation in children might bring us closer to causal mechanisms. There is a considerable tracking of BP levels from childhood to adulthood (66), making BP at a young age an important predictor of adult levels (67). Longitudinal studies that follow children into adulthood can be used to study the influence of candidate genes for BP on the developmental trajectory of BP. Identification of these genes conferring susceptibility to development of essential hypertension in the general population will provide new avenues for treatment and prevention of this debilitating disease (68,69).

REFERENCES

1. Johnson BD, Epstein FH, Kjelsberg MO. Distributions and family studies of blood pressure and serum cholesterol levels in a total community—Tecumseh, Michigan. J Chron Dis. 1965;18:147–160.
2. Miall WE, Heneage P, Khosla T, Lovell HG, Moore F. Factors influencing the degree of resemblance in arterial pressure of close relatives. Clin Sci. 1967;33:271–283.
3. Zinner SH, Levy PS, Kass EH. Familial aggregation of blood pressure in childhood. N Eng J Med. 1971;284:401–404.
4. Zinner SH, Martin LF, Sacks F, Rosner B, Kass EH. A longitudinal study of blood pressure in childhood. Am J Epidemiol. 1974;100:437–442.
5. Hennekens CH, Jesse MJ, Klein BE, Gourley JE, Blumenthal S. Aggregation of blood pressure in infants and their siblings. Am J Epidemiol. 1976;103:457–463.
6. Lee YH, Rosner B, Gould JB, Lowe EW, Kass EH. Familial aggregation of blood pressures of newborn infants and their mother. Pediatrics. 1976;58:722–729.
7. Snieder H, vanDoornen LJP, Boomsma DI. Development of genetic trends in blood pressure levels and blood pressure reactivity to stress. In: Turner JR, Cardon LR, Hewitt JK, eds. Behavior Genetic Approaches in Behavioral Medicine. New York, NY: Plenum Press; 1995:105–130.
8. Snieder H, Boomsma DI, van Doornen LJP. Dissecting the genetic architecture of lipids, lipoproteins and apolipoproteins. Lessons from twin studies. Arterioscler Thromb Vasc Biol. 1999;19:2826–2834.
9. Snieder H. Path analysis of age-related disease traits. In: Spector TD, Snieder H, MacGregor AJ, eds. Advances in Twin and Sib-pair Analyses. London: Greenwich Medical Media; 2000:119–129.
10. Biron P, Mongeau JG, Bertrand D. Familial aggregation of blood pressure in 558 adopted children. Can Med Assoc J. 1976;115:773–774.
11. Plomin R, DeFries JC, McClearn GE. Behavioral Genetics. A Primer. New York, NY: W.H. Freeman; 1990.
12. Phillips DI. Twin studies in medical research: can they tell us whether diseases are genetically determined? Lancet. 1993;341:1008–1009.
13. Kendler KS, Neale MC, Kessler RC, Heath AC, Eaves LJ. A test of the equal-environment assumption in twin studies of psychiatric illness. Behav Genet. 1993;23:21–27.
14. Kyvik KO. Generalisability and assumptions of twin studies. In: Spector TD, Snieder H, MacGregor AJ, eds. Advances in Twin and Sib-Pair Analysis. London: Greenwich Medical Media; 2000:67–77.
15. Andrew T, Hart D, Snieder H, de Lange M, Spector TD, MacGregor AJ. Are twins and singletons comparable? A study of disease-related and lifestyle characteristics in adult women. Twin Res. 2001;4:464–477.
16. De Geus EJ, Posthuma D, Ijzerman RG, Boomsma DI. Comparing blood pressure of twins and their singleton siblings: Being a twin does not affect adult blood pressure. Twin Res. 2001;4:385–391.
17. Neale MC, Cardon LR. Methodologies for genetic studies of twins and families. Dordrecht: Kluwer, 1992.
18. Spector TD, Snieder H, MacGregor AJ. Advances in Twin and Sib-Pair Analysis. London: Greenwich Medical Media; 2000.
19. Evans A, Van Baal GC, McCarron P, DeLange M, Soerensen TI, De Geus EJ, Kyvik K, Pedersen NL, Spector TD, Andrew T, Patterson C, Whitfield JB, Zhu G, Martin NG, Kaprio J, Boomsma DI. The genetics of coronary heart disease: the contribution of twin studies. Twin Res. 2003;6:432–441.
20. de Castro JM. Heritability of diurnal changes in food intake in free-living humans. Nutrition. 2001;17:713–720.
21. Simonen SL, Perusse L, Rankinen T, Rice T, Rao DC, Bouchard C. Familial aggregation of physical activity levels in the Quebec family study. Med Sci Sports Exerc. 2002;34:1137–1142.

22. De Geus EJ, Boomsma DI, Snieder H. Genetic correlation of exercise with heart rate and respiratory sinus arrhythmia. Med Sci Sports Exerc. 2003;35:1287–1295.

23. Hopper JL. Why 'common' environmental effects' are so uncommon in the literature. In: Spector TD, Snieder H, MacGregor AJ, eds. Advances in Twin and Sib-pair Analysis. London: Greenwich Medical Media; 2000:151–165.

24. Middelberg RP, Spector TD, Swaminathan R, Snieder H. Genetic and environmental influences on lipids, lipoproteins, and apolipoproteins: effects of menopause. Arterioscler Thromb Vasc Biol. 2002;22: 1142–1147.

25. Hong Y, de Faire U, Heller DA, McClearn GE, Pedersen NL. Genetic and environmental influences on blood pressure in elderly twins. Hypertension. 1994;24:663–670.

26. Snieder H, Hayward CS, Perks U, Kelly RP, Kelly PJ, Spector TD. Heritability of central systolic pressure augmentation. A twin study. Hypertension. 2000;35:574–579.

27. Boomsma DI, Snieder H, de Geus EJ, van Doornen LJ. Heritability of blood pressure increases during mental stress. Twin Res. 1998;1:15–24.

28. Reynolds CA, Hewitt JK. Issues in the behavior genetic investigation of gender differences. In: Turner JR, Cardon LR, Hewitt JK, eds. Behavior Genetics Approaches in Behavioral Medicine. New York, NY: Plenum Press; 1995:189–199.

29. Levine RS, Hennekens CH, Perry A, Cassady J, Gelband H, Jesse MJ. Genetic variance of blood pressure levels in infant twins. Am J Epidemiol. 1982;116:759–764.

30. McIlhany ML, Shaffer JW, Hines EA. The heritability of blood pressure: an investigation of 200 pairs of twins using the cold pressor test. The Johns Hopkins Med J. 1974;136:57–64.

31. Snieder H, Harshfield GA, Dekkers JC, Treiber FA. Heritability of resting hemodynamics in African and European American youth. Hypertension. 2003;41:1196–1201.

32. Verdecchia P. Prognostic value of ambulatory blood pressure: current evidence and clinical implications. Hypertension. 2000;35:844–851.

33. Degaute JP, Van Cauter E, van de Borne P, Linkowski P. Twenty-four-hour blood pressure and heart rate profiles in humans. A twin study. Hypertension. 1994;23:244–253.

34. Somes GW, Harshfield GA, Alpert BS, Goble MM, Schieken RM. Genetic influences on ambulatory blood pressure patterns. The Medical College of Virginia Twin Study. Am J Hypertens. 1995;8:474–478.

35. Fagard R, Brguljan J, Staessen J, Thijs L, Derom C, Thomis M, Vlietinck R. Heritability of conventional and ambulatory blood pressures. A study in twins. Hypertension. 1995;26:919–924.

36. Jedrusik P, Januszewicz A, Busjahn A, Zawadzki B, Wocial B, Ignatowska-Switalska H, Berent H, Kuczynska K, Oniszczenko W, Strelau J, Luft FC, Januszewicz W. Genetic influence on blood pressure and lipid parameters in a sample of Polish twins. Blood Press. 2003;12:7–11.

37. Vinck WJ, Fagard RH, Loos R, Vlietinck R. The impact of genetic and environmental influences on blood pressure variance across age-groups. J Hypertens. 2001;19:1007–1013.

38. Fagard RH, Loos RJ, Beunen G, Derom C, Vlietinck R. Influence of chorionicity on the heritability estimates of blood pressure: a study in twins. J Hypertens. 2003;21:1313–1318.

39. Kupper N, Willemsen G, Riese H, Posthuma D, Boomsma DI, de Geus EJ. Heritability of daytime ambulatory blood pressure in an extended twin design. Hypertension. 2005;45:80–85.

40. Wang X, Ding X, Su S, Harshfield G, Treiber F, Snieder H. Genetic influences on daytime and nighttime blood pressure: similarities and differences. J Hypertens. 2009;27(12):2358–2364.

41. Fagard RH, Celis H, Thijs L, Staessen JA, Clement DL, De Buyzere ML, De Bacquer DA. Daytime and nighttime blood pressure as predictors of death and cause-specific cardiovascular events in hypertension. Hypertension. 2008;51:55–61.

42. Fava C, Burri P, Almgren P, Arcaro G, Groop L, Lennart Hulthen U, Melander O. Dipping and variability of blood pressure and heart rate at night are heritable traits. Am J Hypertens. 2005;18:1402–1407.

43. Gu D, Rice T, Wang S, Yang W, Gu C, Chen CS, Hixson JE, Jaquish CE, Yao ZJ, Liu DP, Rao DC, He J. Heritability of blood pressure responses to dietary sodium and potassium intake in a Chinese population. Hypertension. 2007;50:116–122.

44. De Geus EJ, Kupper N, Boomsma DI, Snieder H. Bivariate genetic modeling of cardiovascular stress reactivity: does stress uncover genetic variance? Psychosom Med. 2007;69:356–364.

45. Schieken RM, Mosteller M, Goble MM, Moskowitz WB, Hewitt JK, Eaves LJ, Nance WE. Multivariate genetic analysis of blood pressure and body size. The Medical College of Virginia Twin Study. Circulation. 1992;86:1780–1788.

46. Vinck WJ, Vlietinck R, Fagard RH. The contribution of genes, environment and of body mass to blood pressure variance in young adult males. J Hum Hypertens. 1999;13:191–197.

47. Allison DB, Heshka S, Neale MC, Tishler PV, Heymsfield SB. Genetic, environmental, and phenotypic links between Body Mass Index and blood pressure among women. Am J Med Genet. 1995;55: 335–341.

48. Law CM, Shiell AW. Is blood pressure inversely related to birth weight? The strength of evidence from a systematic review of the literature. J Hypertens. 1996;14:935–941.

49. Poulter NR, Chang CL, MacGregor AJ, Snieder H, Spector TD. Association between birth weight and adult blood pressure in twins: historical cohort study. Br Med J. 1999;319:1330–1333.

50. Bergvall N, Iliadou A, Johansson S, de Faire U, Kramer MS, Pawitan Y, Pedersen NL, Lichtenstein P, Cnattingius S. Genetic and shared environmental factors do not confound the association between birth weight and hypertension: a study among Swedish twins. Circulation. 2007;115:2931–2938.

51. Christensen K, Stovring H, McGue M. Do genetic factors contribute to the association between birth weight and blood pressure? J Epidemiol Community Health. 2001;55:583–587.

52. McNeill G, Tuya C, Smith WC. The role of genetic and environmental factors in the association between birthweight and blood pressure: evidence from meta-analysis of twin studies. Int J Epidemiol. 2004;33:995–1001.

53. Baird J, Osmond C, MacGregor A, Snieder H, Hales CN, Phillips DIW. Testing the fetal origins hypothesis in twins: the Birmingham twin study. Diabetologia. 2001;44:33–39.

54. Yu MW, Chen CJ, Wang CJ, Tong SL, Tien M, Lee TY, Lue HC, Huang FY, Lan CC, Yang KH. Chronological changes in genetic variance and heritability of systolic and diastolic blood pressure among Chinese twin neonates. Acta Genet Med Gemellol. 1990;39:99–108.

55. Iselius L, Morton NE, Rao DC. Family resemblance for blood pressure. Hum Hered. 1983;33:277–286.

56. Havlik RJ, Garrison RJ, Feinleib M, Kannel WB, Castelli WP, McNamara PM. Blood pressure aggregation in families. Am J Epidemiol. 1979;110:304–312.

57. Tambs K, Moum T, Holmen J, Eaves LJ, Neale MC, Lund-Larsen G, Naess S. Genetic and environmental effects on blood pressure in a Norwegian sample. Genet Epidemiol. 1992;9:11–26.

58. Hunt SC, Hasstedt SJ, Kuida H, Stults BM, Hopkins PN, Williams RR. Genetic heritability and common environmental components of resting and stressed blood pressures, lipids, and body mass index in Utah pedigrees and twins. Am J Epidemiol. 1989;129:625–638.

59. Tambs K, Eaves LJ, Moum T, Holmen J, Neale MC, Naess S, Lund-Larsen PG. Age-specific genetic effects for blood pressure. Hypertension. 1993;22:789–795.

60. Snieder H, van Doornen LJ, Boomsma DI. The age dependency of gene expression for plasma lipids, lipoproteins, and apolipoproteins. Am J Hum Genet. 1997;60:638–650.

61. Colletto GM, Cardon LR, Fulker DW. A genetic and environmental time series analysis of blood pressure in male twins. Genet Epidemiol. 1993;10:533–538.

62. Iliadou A, Lichtenstein P, Morgenstern R, Forsberg L, Svensson R, de Faire U, Martin NG, Pedersen NL. Repeated blood pressure measurements in a sample of Swedish twins: heritabilities and associations with polymorphisms in the renin-angiotensin-aldosterone system. J Hypertens. 2002;20: 1543–1550.

63. Hottenga JJ, Boomsma DI, Kupper N, Posthuma D, Snieder H, Willemsen G, de Geus EJ. Heritability and stability of resting blood pressure. Twin Res Hum Genet. 2005;8:499–508.

64. Hottenga JJ, Whitfield JB, de Geus EJ, Boomsma DI, Martin NG. Heritability and stability of resting blood pressure in Australian twins. Twin Res Hum Genet. 2006;9:205–209.

65. Kupper N, Ge D, Treiber FA, Snieder H. Emergence of novel genetic effects on blood pressure and hemodynamics in adolescence: the Georgia Cardiovascular Twin Study. Hypertension. 2006;47:948–954.

66. van Lenthe FJ, Kemper HCG, Twisk JWR. Tracking of blood pressure in children and youth. Am J Hum Biol. 1994;6:389–399.

67. Bao W, Threefoot SA, Srinivasan SR, Berenson GS. Essential hypertension predicted by tracking of elevated blood pressure from childhood to adulthood: The Bogalusa Heart Study. Am J Hypertens. 1995;8:657–665.

68. Snieder H, Harshfield GA, Barbeau P, Pollock DM, Pollock JS, Treiber FA. Dissecting the genetic architecture of the cardiovascular and renal stress response. Biol Psychol. 2002;61:73–95.

69. Imumorin IK, Dong Y, Zhu H, Poole JC, Harshfield GA, Treiber FA, Snieder H. A gene-environment interaction model of stress-induced hypertension. Cardiovasc Toxicol. 2005;5:109–132.

70. Havlik RJ, Garrison RJ, Katz SH, Ellison RC, Feinleib M, Myrianthopoulos NC. Detection of genetic variance in blood pressure of seven-year-old twins. Am J Epidemiol. 1978;109:512–516.

71. Wang Z, Ouyang Z, Wang D, Tang X. Heritability of blood pressure in 7- to 12-year-old Chinese twins, with special reference to body size effects. Genet Epidemiol. 1990;7:447–452.

72. Schieken RM, Eaves LJ, Hewitt JK, Mosteller M, Bodurtha JN, Moskowitz WB, Nance WE. Univariate genetic analysis of blood pressure in children (The Medical College of Virginia Twin Study). Am J Cardiol. 1989;64:1333–1337.

73. Kramer AA. Genetic variance of blood pressure levels in infant twins. Am J Epidemiol. 1984;119:651–652.

74. Sims J, Carroll D, Hewitt JK, Turner JR. A family study of developmental effects upon blood pressure variation. Acta Genet Med Gemellol. 1987;36:467–473.

75. Ditto B. Familial influences on heart rate, blood pressure, and self-report anxiety responses to stress: results from 100 twin pairs. Psychophysiology. 1993;30:635–645.

76. McCaffery JM, Pogue-Geile M, Debski T, Manuck SB. Genetic and environmental causes of covariation among blood pressure, body mass and serum lipids during young adulthood: a twin study. J Hypertens. 1999;17:1677–1685.

77. Bielen EC, Fagard R, Amery AK. Inheritance of blood pressure and haemodynamic phenotypes measured at rest and during supine dynamic exercise. J Hypertens. 1991;9:655–663.

78. Busjahn A, Li GH, Faulhaber HD, Rosenthal M, Becker A, Jeschke E, Schuster H, Timmermann B, Hoehe MR, Luft FC. β-2 adrenergic receptor gene variations, blood pressure, and heart size in normal twins. Hypertension. 2000;35:555–560.

79. Slattery ML, Bishop TD, French TK, Hunt SC, Meikle AW, Williams RR. Lifestyle and blood pressure levels in male twins in Utah. Genet Epidemiol. 1988;5:277–287.

80. Williams PD, Puddey IB, Martin NG, Beilin LJ. Platelet cytosolic free calcium concentration, total plasma calcium concentration and blood pressure in human twins: a genetic analysis. Clin Sci (Lond). 1992;82:493–504.

81. Austin MA, King MC, Bawol RD, Hulley SB, Friedman GD. Risk factors for coronary heart disease in adult female twins. Genetic heritability and shared environmental influences. Am J Epidemiol. 1987;125:308–318.

82. Feinleib M, Garrison RJ, Fabsitz R, Christian JC, Hrubec Z, Borhani NO, Kannel WB, Rosenman R, Schwartz JT, Wagner JO. The NHLBI twin study of cardiovascular disease risk factors: methodology and summary of results. Am J Epidemiol. 1977;106:284–295.

15

Influence of Dietary Electrolytes on Childhood Blood Pressure

Dawn K. Wilson, *PhD and* Sandra Coulon, BS

CONTENTS

Although the prevalence of hypertension (HTN) is relatively low during childhood and adolescence [1], an estimated 2.6–3.4% of children and adolescents have hypertensive blood pressure (BP) levels and 5.7–13.6% have prehypertensive BP levels [2,3]. BP patterns have been shown to track from childhood to the third and fourth decades of life [1,4], and elevated BP levels have been associated with increased risk of cardiovascular and renal diseases [5]. Hypertension and cardiovascular risk also increase with increasing rates of overweight and obesity, and prevention programs are needed to reduce these risks in youth [5–7]. Modifying intake of dietary electrolytes such as sodium and/or potassium has been shown to be an effective approach to BP reduction in adults [8–10], but there is less evidence for the benefit of this approach in children and adolescents [11]. Current recommendations for primary prevention of HTN, published by The National High Blood Pressure Education Program Coordinating Committee [12], involve a population approach and an intensive strategy for targeting individuals who are at increased risk for developing HTN in early adulthood. The Committee outlines a number of approaches that have proven effective for prevention of HTN. Two of these approaches include reducing sodium intake and maintaining an adequate intake of potassium. Evidence also suggests that addressing obesity-related hypertension through weight reduction and maintenance programs may be more efficacious when physical activity is incorporated into the intervention, and regular aerobic activity is strongly recommended for improving BP [13–15].

D.K. Wilson (✉)
Department of Psychology, Barnwell College, University of South Carolina, Columbia, SC, USA
e-mail: wilsondk@mailbox.sc.edu

From: *Clinical Hypertension and Vascular Diseases: Pediatric Hypertension*
Edited by: J. T. Flynn et al. DOI 10.1007/978-1-60327-824-9_15
© Springer Science+Business Media, LLC 2011

Identifying precursors or markers of HTN in youth is important for preventing the development of essential HTN. Two such markers include cardiovascular reactivity (CVR) and ambulatory BP profiles *(16–18)*. Cardiovascular reactivity is a measure of vasoconstriction in response to psychological or physical stressors. As a marker, hyperreactivity is conceptualized as a consequence of pre-existing cardiovascular damage or of heightened sympathetic tone that results in vasoconstriction and/or excessive cardiac output. As a mechanism, hyperreactive peaks are proposed to damage the intimal layer of arteries, contributing to the development of arteriosclerosis and subsequent HTN. Although there is controversy about the predictive value of CVR, prospective studies have shown that increased CVR to mental stress is predictive of later development of essential HTN *(17,19–23)*, although efforts to associate it with physiological correlates of HTN (i.e., left ventricular hypertrophy) have yielded mixed results *(16,24–27)*. Only a limited number of studies have been conducted examining the relationship between dietary electrolytes and CVR in youth, and the results of these studies have been inconsistent *(16)*.

Ambulatory BP profiles may be an important predictor or risk factor of future HTN in youth. Ambulatory BP (ABP) is a method for assessing an individual's daily fluctuations in BP and for identifying and evaluating factors associated with individual differences in BP responses in the natural environment. Previous research indicates that most people display lower BP values at nighttime during sleeping hours and higher BP values during waking hours *(18)*. In healthy individuals, average BP declines by 15% or more during sleeping hours, while for hypertensive patients the circadian rhythm is generally preserved. The 24-h BP profile, however, is shifted upward to a higher magnitude throughout the 24-h period *(28)*. A number of studies suggest that a blunted nocturnal decline in BP may be associated with greater cardiovascular risk *(18)*. For example, ambulatory BP nondipping status (defined as <10% decrease in BP from waking to sleeping) is a risk factor for the development of end-organ disease in essential HTN. Specifically, patients who are characterized as nondippers show a more frequent history of stroke and left ventricular hypertrophy (LVH) *(29–31)*. Studies from our laboratory indicate that even among healthy African-American adolescents, there is a 30% prevalence rate of nondipping status *(32,33)*. These findings have led us to investigate the dietary electrolyte factors that may influence the ABP pattern in youth.

Previous research indicates that dietary factors such as sodium and potassium significantly affect BP in adults, especially in industrialized countries *(34–37)*. At the cellular level, electrolytes are positively and negatively charged ions that moderate the conduction of electrical signals between cells and influence homeostasis within the body *(38)*. Electrolyte balance (i.e., balance of positively and negatively charged conductive ions) is essential for health and affects the regulation of hydration, blood pH, and motor functioning *(38)*. Although some controversy exists about the differential effects of electrolyte intake on BP in childhood, some studies indicate that the relation between environmental and genetic factors influences BP responses in children *(39–42)*. Specifically, some investigators have demonstrated that children as young as 0–3 years of age may be at higher risk for future cardiovascular complications because of differences in sodium handling and genetic phenotypes *(43)*, and that stress-induced excretion is a heritable phenotype which differentially affects African-Americans as compared to Caucasians *(39,44)*. Other investigators have demonstrated that positive changes in dietary sodium and potassium in the first two decades of life can reduce BP and cardiovascular risk *(35,36,45,46)*. Although the beneficial effects of decreasing sodium intake on BP have been more strongly supported than the effects of increasing potassium intake, few studies have been conducted that evaluate the influence of potassium on BP levels in youth *(47)*. The purpose of this chapter is to review the nutritional electrolyte-related determinants of BP in children and adolescents, especially focusing on the role of dietary sodium and potassium in regulating casual BP, BP reactivity, and circadian BP patterns in youth.

DIETARY SODIUM AND BLOOD PRESSURE IN YOUTH

Previous research suggests that casual BP is important in understanding the influence of genetic, environmental, and nutritional influences on the progression and development of HTN in children and young adults. In a recent national study of 1,658 youth (aged 4–18 years), He and MacGregor *(35)* showed a significant association between sodium intake and systolic BP after adjusting for age, sex, body mass index (BMI), and dietary potassium intake. The magnitude of the association was noted to be similar to that observed in a recent meta-analysis that evaluated the effects of sodium reduction on BP responses in youth *(35)*. In a comprehensive review, Simons-Morton and Obarzanck *(47)* critically evaluated 25 observational studies examining the association between sodium intake and casual BP in children and adolescents: 8 of the papers used self-report measures of dietary intake and 17 papers used urinary sodium excretion. Approximately 67% (two-thirds) of the urinary sodium studies that controlled for other factors (e.g., age, BMI, weight) in the analysis found a significant positive association with casual BP. One-third of the studies that had no control variables found a significant association with casual BP. Three of the four studies which relied on self-report measures of dietary intake and that controlled for other variables found significant positive associations between dietary sodium and casual systolic BP, diastolic BP, or both. Taken together, the studies reviewed above provide fairly consistent support for the role of sodium intake on BP regulation in children and adolescents. Intervention studies that aim to reduce the intake of sodium may be beneficial, although it is not clear whether youth can comply with long-term recommendations to reduce sodium intake.

Prior research shows that individuals who are at risk for cardiovascular complications such as African-Americans, hypertensive patients, and those with a positive family history of HTN are more likely to be salt sensitive *(48,49)* (i.e., show increased BP in response to high sodium intake). In a study examining the prevalence of salt sensitivity in normotensive African-American adolescents *(50)*, we demonstrated that 22% of healthy normotensive African-American adolescents were characterized as salt sensitive based on definitions established in the adult literature *(51)*. Falkner et al. *(49)* have also shown that salt-sensitive adolescents with positive family history of HTN had greater increases in BP with salt loading than did adolescents who were either salt resistant or had a negative family history of HTN. In a more recent study by Palacios et al. *(52)* African-American girls showed greater sodium retention in response to a low-sodium diet (57 mmol/day) than Caucasian girls, suggesting that sodium handling may contribute to underlying racial differences in susceptibility of developing HTN.

Several investigators have also examined the relationship between salt sensitivity and ambulatory BP profiles in children and adolescents. Wilson et al. examined the relationship between salt sensitivity and ambulatory BP dipping status *(53)*. A significantly greater percentage of salt-sensitive adolescents were classified as nondippers according to mean BP (<10% decrease in BP from awake to asleep) as compared to salt-resistant individuals. Harshfield et al. *(54)* also demonstrated that sodium intake is an important determinant of ambulatory BP profiles in African-American children and adolescents. These findings are consistent with de la Sierra et al. *(55)* who demonstrated higher awake BP values in normotensive salt-sensitive than in salt-resistant adults.

Rocchini et al. *(56)* conducted a series of studies examining BP sensitivity to sodium intake in obese adolescents. Obese adolescents showed greater decreases in casual BP after a shift from high to low sodium intake compared to nonobese adolescents. This BP sensitivity to the alteration of sodium intake was also positively correlated with plasma insulin concentration and hyperinsulinemia *(56)*. Consequently, sodium retention may be a mechanism underlying the higher concentrations of plasma insulin in obese adolescents. In another study by Lurbe et al. *(57)* 85 obese and 88 nonobese children (aged 3–19 years) participated in 24-h ambulatory BP monitoring and had their urinary sodium excretion rates determined. The interaction between sodium excretion and weight was negative, indicating a smaller rate of change in BP by sodium unit for obese than for nonobese participants. Obese participants also experienced higher ambulatory BP levels associated with the same levels of sodium excretion than nonobese participants. Taken together, these studies suggest that obesity may be associated with sodium regulation, in that obese youth are more likely to be sensitive to alterations in sodium intake than nonobese children.

Salt sensitivity has also been associated with nondipping status in adults *(30,31)*. The role of sodium intake in nocturnal BP has been studied by several investigators. Uzu et al. *(58)* found that nondipper nocturnal BP in salt-sensitive patients was normalized to a dipper pattern (drop from awake to asleep) with sodium restriction. Higashi et al. *(59)* also demonstrated that nocturnal decline in mean BP was significantly smaller in salt-sensitive patients with hypertension when compared to salt-resistant subjects with hypertension during a sodium-loading protocol.

The mechanism by which sodium sensitivity alters nighttime BP likely involves the sympathetic nervous system. Sympathetic nervous system arousal has been associated with differential handling of sodium following a behavioral challenge (video games) among individuals who are identified as retainers (those who show little excretion of sodium load in urine) *(60)*. In a biracial sample of normotensive children, Harshfield et al. *(54)* demonstrated a stronger relationship between sodium handling and casual BP in African-American versus caucasian adolescents. Harshfield et al. *(54)* also showed that African-American adolescents had a stronger association between 24-h urinary sodium excretion, casual BP, and BP during sleep, independent of the urinary potassium excretion, than Caucasian adolescents. For casual BP and nighttime ambulatory BP, the slope was positive and significant for African-Americans, but no relationship was shown for Caucasian adolescents. The findings reported by Harshfield and colleagues *(54,60)* and other investigators *(61)* suggest an interactive role for the sympathetic nervous system in sodium retention which may, in part, explain blunted nocturnal decline in ambulatory BP profiles observed in salt-sensitive individuals.

DIETARY POTASSIUM AND BLOOD PRESSURE IN YOUTH

The previously mentioned review by Simons-Morton and Obarzanck *(47)* included 12 observational studies examining the association of potassium intake and casual BP in children and adolescents. Nine of the observational studies used urinary measures of potassium excretion, and six of these studies controlled for other factors such as weight. Two of these studies showed a significant inverse relationship between potassium intake and casual BP, while three studies showed no relationship. One study showed an unexpected positive association between potassium intake and casual BP. Two studies that relied on self-report estimates of intake showed a significant inverse relationship between potassium intake and systolic or diastolic BP, while two additional studies showed no relationship. Taken together, these studies only provide partial support for the beneficial effect of high potassium on casual BP levels in youth. However, as Wilson et al. *(33)* have noted the effects of potassium may be most pronounced among salt-sensitive individuals, such as among African-Americans or those with a positive family history of HTN. These factors were not specifically addressed in Simons-Morton and Obarzanck's *(47)* extensive review of the literature.

Research examining the effects of potassium intake on CVR has been scarce. In general, these studies have been correlational and have shown beneficial effects in only a subgroup of individuals. For example, Berenson and colleagues *(62)* reported that African-American boys in the highest BP strata, who showed significant increases in BP reactivity, had lower urinary potassium excretion than Caucasians. Among adult populations, Morgan et al. *(63)* demonstrated in hypertensive patients that potassium supplementation (48 mmo1/24 h) prevented the rise in BP produced by postural changes.

Very few reports have characterized the relationship between plasma potassium and ambulatory BP in adults. Goto et al. *(64)* showed a significant negative association between daytime plasma potassium concentration and 24-h systolic and diastolic BP in patients with essential HTN. Plasma potassium was also inversely correlated with daytime and nighttime systolic and diastolic BP levels. Interpreting the relationship between a plasma electrolyte such as potassium and BP is difficult; however, because there are many factors known to influence plasma potassium values *(65,66)*. Although there are limitations of plasma potassium values, these results are consistent with prior epidemiological studies, which have shown negative associations between potassium intake, potassium excretion, and BP levels *(67)*.

NUTRITIONAL INTERVENTIONS AND BLOOD PRESSURE IN YOUTH

A number of studies to date have examined the prevalence of consumption of high-potassium/low-sodium foods (e.g., fruit and vegetable intake) among adolescent populations. In a report by Falkner and Michel *(68)*, average sodium intakes of urban children and adolescents in Philadelphia well exceeded their nutritional needs, determined by 24-h dietary recall assessments. These data are consistent with the Bogalusa Heart Study, a study that also assessed electrolyte intake among infants and children living in a rural biracial community *(69)*. In another study by Pomeranz et al. *(70)* increased BP levels were found among infants who received formula mixed with high-sodium tap water (196 mg/L) as compared to infants who received formula mixed with low-sodium minerals (32 mg/L) at 6 weeks of age. Among older youth, Cullen et al. *(71)* had 5,881 adolescents and young adults (aged 14–21 years) complete a survey on Youth Risk Behavior. Potassium intake related to fruit consumption declined for males and females during the high school years. Consistent with this finding, Neumark-Sztainer et al. *(72)* reported that among 30,000 adolescents who completed the Minnesota Health Survey, and who had inadequate potassium intake, 28% had inadequate fruit intake and 36% had inadequate vegetable intake. Several investigators, including Berenson et al. *(54,73,74)*, have also demonstrated that African-American children and adolescents show lower urinary potassium excretion rates than Caucasians of same age. Thus, targeting adolescents and minority adolescents for dietary interventions that emphasize high-potassium/low-sodium food choices may be particularly needed at this age of development, when emphasis on the importance of nutrition in youth seems to deteriorate.

Dietary electrolytes such as sodium, potassium, and the ratio of sodium/potassium are important in BP regulation. A number of studies have examined the influence of altering electrolyte intake on BP responses in children and adolescents (see Table 1). Table 1 provides a summary of the interventions in youth to date that have studied the effects of either reduced sodium intake, increased potassium intake, or the combination on BP responses. In general, the evidence is inconsistent but suggests that reducing sodium and increasing potassium seem to be effective strategies; however, further research is needed to determine the long-term compliance of such interventions in youth.

In a recent meta-analysis by He and MacGregor *(35)* ten trials were evaluated and it was shown that sodium reduction (ranging from 42 to 54%) in children demonstrated immediate decreases in BP. In a study by Miller et al. *(75)*, the effects of sodium restriction for 12 weeks (60 mEq/24 h) were evaluated on BP responses in Caucasian youth aged 3–30 years. They found a decrease in diastolic BP after adjusting for age, sex, height, and weight; however, the magnitude of change was minimal (–2 mmHg). Other investigators have also failed to demonstrate significant decreases in casual BP in Caucasian children during sodium restriction ranging from 4 weeks to 1 year of age *(76,77)*.

Researchers have demonstrated that subgroups of children and adolescents show greater decreases in BP responses to changes in sodium restriction. For example, Rocchini et al. *(78)* demonstrated that obese adolescents had significantly greater decreases in mean BP than nonobese adolescents when they went from a high-sodium diet to a low-sodium diet. Other researchers have also demonstrated greater reductions to alterations in sodium intake on casual BP responses in African-American children compared to Caucasian children *(79)*.

In their review, Simons-Morton and Obarzanek *(47)* also identified 11 relevant intervention studies, eight of which used a randomized controlled design that examined the effects of reducing sodium intake on casual BP in children and adolescents. The studies ranged in size from 10 to 191 participants (children and/or adolescents). Duration of the interventions ranged from 3 weeks to 3 years, with half lasting 3–4 weeks. Seven of the 11 studies reported reduced systolic BP, diastolic BP, or both. However, only four of these studies reported statistically significant effects. Effects were stronger for girls and for those with BMI less than 23. One study that evaluated the effects of increasing potassium was the Dietary Intervention Study in Children (DISC). Participants enrolled in this study had elevated low-density lipoprotein cholesterol. Assessments were done at baseline, 1 year, and 3 years. Longitudinal analyses revealed significant inverse associations between systolic BP and potassium, calcium, magnesium, protein, and fiber and significant inverse associations between diastolic BP and potassium, calcium, magnesium, protein, carbohydrates, and fiber. Direct associations were also found between fat intake and both systolic and diastolic BP. Multivariate models showed calcium, fiber, and fat to be the most important determinants of BP level in children with elevated low-density lipoprotein cholesterol.

Sinaiko et al. *(11)* tested the feasibility of a 3-year potassium supplementation or sodium reduction in preventing the rise in BP among adolescents. Adolescents who were in the upper 15th percentile of BP distribution were randomly assigned to potassium chloride supplementation (1 mmol/kg potassium chloride/day), a low-sodium diet (70 mmol sodium/day), or a placebo (normal diet plus placebo capsule). The results demonstrated that both the potassium supplementation and the sodium restriction interventions were effective in reducing the rise of casual BP in girls, but not in boys. The feasibility of long-term restriction of dietary sodium in boys may be limited.

Table 1
Effects of Dietary Sodium and Potassium Interventions on Blood Pressure in Youth

Authors	Intervention	Sample baseline demographics	Compliance	Findings
Sodium interventions				
Whitten et al. (United States) *(103)*	Two group RCT Duration=5 months/group with 8-year follow-up *Low-Sodium Infant Diet (LS; n=13)* Commercially available foods without sodium added (1.93 mmol/100 kcal) were provided to parents and fed to infants *Control Group (CTL; n=14)* Commercially available foods with sodium included (9.25 mmol/100 kcal) were provided to parents and fed to infants	$N = 27$ (F = 0 and M = 27) Healthy African-American male infants *Age (months)* = 3 *Race* = 100% African-American *Mean BP* = Not reported	*24-h UNa:* Samples were collected for 3 days via metabolic frames. Na concentration was 11.3 mmol/day in the LS group and 54.8 mmol/day in the CTL group *Food records:* Records showed a reduction in sodium intake consistent with UNa findings	The LS diet did not result in significant changes in BP in the LS group vs. the CTL, at 8-month (88/48 MBP vs. 90/49 MBP) or 8-year follow-up (103/75 MBP vs. 103/76 MBP). BP was significantly correlated with weight but not sodium intake, or sodium or potassium excretion at 8 months
Gillum et al. (United States) *(76)*	Two group RCT Duration=1 year *Family Education Program (FEP; n=41 [children + families])* Four biweekly 90-min lectures followed by 90-min maintenance sessions at bimonthly intervals. Educational materials covered physiological and dietary factors involved in BP. Parents were instructed to provide < 70 mmol Na/day to each family member	$N = 80$ children + their families (F = 61% FEP and F = 31% CTL) Children with SBP > 95th percentile for age and sex but SBP < 130 and DBP < 90 mmHg from the Minneapolis, MN public school system	*Food records (3 days):* The FEP group reported significantly lower sodium intake than the CTL group (~25 mmol decrease) *24-h UNa:* Overnight Na excretion did not differ between groups at baseline or 1 year. Poor parent compliance with urine collection method prevented the analyses of parental Na excretion	Based on 3-day food records sodium intake for the FEP group was ~ 25 mmol lower than the CTL group. FEP group participants who regularly attended sessions had sodium intake ~ 43 mmol lower those who did not attend sessions or who dropped out of the program.

Table 1
(continued)

Authors	Intervention	Sample baseline demographics	Compliance	Findings
	Control Group (CTL; n=39) No treatment	*Mean Age (year)* = 7.8 ± 0.7 (FEP); 8.0 ± 0.8 (CTL) *Race* = Not reported *Mean BP* = 111/65 (FEP); 115/69 (CTL)		Urinary sodium excretion did not differ between groups Blood pressure did not differ by group or change over time
Trevisan et al. (United States) *(104)*	Two group RCT Duration=10 weeks/group *Low-Sodium Diet (LS; n=12)* Diet included reduction of sodium intake by ~ 70% *Control Group (CTL; n=9)* Diet similar in composition to LS but without reduced sodium.	*N* = 21 Male and female students from a boarding high school *Age (years)* = 11–15 *Race* = Not reported *Mean SBP (mmHg)*= 108 (LS); 111 (CTL)	*24-h UNa:* There was a significant reduction in erythrocyte Na concentration in the LS group but no change in the CTL group. Random samples and duplicate meals were collected but results were not reported	Erythrocyte sodium concentration was reduced and a nonsignificant decline in SBP was observed in the LS group (−1.25±4.96 mmHg)

Table 1
(continued)

Authors	Intervention	Sample baseline demographics	Compliance	Findings
Hofman et al. (Netherlands) (105)	Two group RCT Duration=6 months *Low Sodium Infant Formula (LS; n=225)* Commercially available formula with 33% the concentration of sodium as the control formula. *Control Group (CTL; n=241)* Commercially available formula with sodium included (9.25 mmol/100 kcal) were provided to parents and fed to infants	N = 466 (F=49% and M=51%) Newborn infants born within 1 month of each other *Age (week)* = 1 *Race* = Not reported *Mean SBP (mmHg)* = 88 (LS); 87 (CTL)	*Spot UNa:*Na concentration was 22.7 mmol/L in the CTL group and 11.1 mmol/L in the LS group *Baby Food Delivered:* Mean Na consumed based on number of food deliveries was estimated to be 2.5 mol of Na in the CTL group and 0.89 mol of Na in the LS group	The LS formula group demonstrated a significant decrease in SBP at 25 weeks (−2.00 ±2.13 mmHg)
Cooper et al. (United States) (106)	Two group crossover RCT Duration=24-days/condition *Low-Sodium Diet (LS)* Diet included reduction of sodium intake by ~ 200–60 mmol/day via controlled cafeteria meals. Children were instructed not to add salt	N = 113 (F=66 and M=47) Adolescent students from a boarding high school without HTN or chronic illness *Mean Age (year)* = 16 *Race* = Not reported *Mean BP (mmHg)* = 109/61	*Overnight UNa:*Samples were collected in 42% (n= 48) of participants. Na concentration changed from 31 to 13 mmol/8 h. Duplicate meals were collected for 24-h period for three	Sodium intake was reduced by ~ 58% and SBP and DBP decreased nonsignificantly (−0.6±.70 mmHg; −1.40±1.0 mmHg) following the LS diet

Table 1
(continued)

Authors	Intervention	Sample baseline demographics	Compliance	Findings
	or condiments to meals and in-between meal snacks were provided. *Control Group (CTL)* Meals were same as LS group but without reduced sodium		random participants per group per week. Food samples were in close agreement with UNa	Participants with BMI below the median had significant decreases in SBP after the LS diet ($p<0.05$). Body size may influence BP response to sodium reduction
Calabrese and Tuthill (United States) (107)	Two group RCT Duration= 12-weeks/group *Low Sodium Water (LS; n=51)* Bottled water with low sodium (10 mg/L) was provided to children for drinking and family meal preparation and in school classrooms *Control (CTL; n=102)* Bottled water with high sodium (110 mg/L) was provided to children for drinking and family meal preparation and in school classrooms	$N = 153$ (F=75 and M=78) Fourth-grade school children in a community with high sodium in their water distribution system. Children were matched by sex, school, and baseline BP. *Mean Age (year)* = 9 *Race* = Not reported *Mean BP (mmHg)*= 99/58	*First-morning UNa:* Na concentration changed from 141 to 128 mmol/L in the LS group and from 121 to 124 mmol/L in the CTL group. No statistically significant differences were detected between boys and girls	BP levels among girls but not boys in the LS group demonstrated decreased BP over time when compared to the CTL group. Lack of effects for boys may have been due to undetected poorer compliance in boys or other explanations

Table 1
(continued)

Authors	Intervention	Sample baseline demographics	Compliance	Findings
Howe et al. (Australia) *(108)*	Two group crossover RCT Duration= 3-weeks/condition *Low Sodium Water (LS)* Parents and children were interviewed by a dietician who provided detailed instruction on adhering to a low-sodium diet *Control Group (CTL)* No treatment	$N = 21$ (F=48% and M=52%) Prehypertensive or hypertensive adolescents *Mean Age (year)* = 11–14 *Race* = Not reported *Mean BP (mmHg)* = 119/78	*Overnight UNa:* Na/creatinine ratio changed from 179.1 to 101.7 mmol/24 h. *Food Records:* Records showed a reduction in sodium intake consistent with UNa	Overnight UNa demonstrated a reduction in sodium intake of 43.3%. A slight decrease in DBP was demonstrated (−1.3±1.8 mmHg)
Tuthill and Calabrese (United States) *(109)*	Three group RCT Duration= 12-weeks/group *Morning Sodium Capsule (MS)* Participants took one capsule containing 2 g of sodium in the morning and one placebo capsule in the evening each day *Evening Sodium Capsule (ES)* Participants took one capsule containing 2 g of sodium in the evening and one placebo capsule in the morning each day *Placebo Control (CTL)* Participants took two placebo capsules each day	$N = 216$ (F=75 and M=78) Ninth through twelfth grade adolescent girls in a private boarding school. Children were matched by sex, school, and baseline BP. *Mean Age (year)* = 9 *Race* = Not reported *Mean BP* = 99/57 mmHg	*24-h UNa:* Urinalysis indicated that Na excretion was significantly higher in the MS and ES groups compared to the CTL group, and compliance was considered to be high	Though compliance was considered high and drop-out rates were low, between-group differences in BP were not detected in either SBP or DBP

Table 1
(continued)

Authors	Intervention	Sample baseline demographics	Compliance	Findings
Tochikubo et al. (Japan) (110)	Two group RCT Duration=10-weeks/group *Low Sodium Counseling and Self-Monitoring (LS+S; n=12)* Hypertension education and diet counseling including self-monitoring of urinary Cl excretion *Low Sodium Counseling (LS; n=9)* Hypertension education focusing on lowering sodium intake	N = 197 (F=17 and M=180) Borderline hypertensive (BHT) and normotensive (NT) students from six high schools in Japan *Age (year)* = 15–18 *Race* = Not reported *Mean SBP (mmHg)* = 150.3±9.8 (BHT); 117.7±12.2 (NT)	*24-h UNa and UK:* Mean BHT Na excretion was 211±94 and K excretion was 42.1±16.6. Mean NT Na excretion was 187±80 and K excretion was 39.5±23.6. Na concentration was significantly higher in the BHT group and K concentration was significantly lower	The LS group did not reduce blood pressure, but sodium excretion (−52 mEq/day), weight (−1.7 kg), and BP (−12/7 mmHg) decreased significantly in the LS+S group. Blood pressure of BHT adolescents may be decreased with dietary education and self-monitoring
Miller et al. (United States) (75)	One group CT Duration=12 weeks *Low-Sodium Diet (LS)* Families were instructed to reduce sodium intake to 60 mmol/day to ensure a reduction to 75 mmol/day. Families were instructed to otherwise maintain usual dietary practices	N = 149 (F=85 and M=64) Normotensive identical twin pairs, siblings, and parents recruited through a research twin panel and local schools *Mean Age (year)* = 9.7±.4 SEM (F); 10.6 ±.7 SEM (M) *Race* = 100% Caucasian *Mean BP (mmHg)* = 91/54 (F); 95/55 (M)	*Weekly UNa:* Na concentration decreased from baseline to 41.1±1.9 mmol/day (F) and 53.5±3.6 mmol/day (M) at the end of the LS diet	In both sexes there was a significant change in sodium excretion (p<0.001) without a change in potassium excretion. For boys there was no change in BP and for girls there was a small but significant decrease in DBP (p<0.05). Results suggest that compliance to modest sodium restriction may not consistently lower BP in normotensive children

Table 1
(continued)

Authors	Intervention	Sample baseline demographics	Compliance	Findings
Ellison et al. (United States) (111)	Two group crossover CT Duration=6 months/conditions *Low- Sodium Diet (LS; 309 students)* Diet included reduction of sodium intake by ~ 15–20% via controlled cafeteria meals and changes in food purchasing and preparation. *Control Group (CTL; 341 students)* Meals were same as LS group but without reduced sodium	N = 2 schools (F~51%, M~49%) Male and female students from two boarding high schools in the northeastern United States *Mean Age (year)* = 15 *Race*= ~77% Caucasian *Mean BP (mmHg)* = 107/64	*Food Records:* Each subject completed on average 4.5 food records during baseline and follow-up periods. Records showed that mean sodium intake was reduced by 15–20%	SBP significantly decreased during the LS diet (–1.7 mmHg, *p*<0.01) and DBP significantly decreased also (–1.5 mmHg, *p* < 0.01)
Myers (Australia) (112)	Two group crossover RCT Duration=2 weeks *Low-Sodium Diet (LS)* Participants were advised by a dietician to reduce sodium intake (77±37 mmol/day). Advice was based on previous diet history and 24-h UNa *High-Sodium Diet (HS)* Participants were advised to increase sodium intake (201±37 mmol/day). Advice was based on previous diet history and 24-h UNa	N=23 (F=100% and M=0%) Female sodium sensitive (SS) and insensitive (SI) children and adolescents whose parents were affiliated with a hospital in Newcastle, NSW. *Mean Age (year)* = 9 (SS); 12 (SI) *Race* = Not reported *Mean BP (mmHg)*= 108/67	*24-h UNa:* Na concentration changed from 158 to 66 mmol/24 h	Sodium intake was reduced by 58.2% based on UNa in the LS group. Both SBP and DBP decreased significantly in the LS group (–3.74±2 mmHg; –1.70±2 mmHg

Table 1
(continued)

Authors	Intervention	Sample baseline demographics	Compliance	Findings
Nader et al. (United States) (98)	Two group RCT Duration=1-year/group *Low-Sodium/Low-Fat diet (LS)* Three months of intensive educational group sessions promoting decreased sodium and fat intake and increased physical activity followed by 9 months of maintenance sessions *Control Group (CTL)* No treatment	*N* = 206 families (623 persons) Mexican-American and Caucasian families recruited through 15 matched elementary schools. Families were defined as one or more children in grades 5 or 6 and one or more adults in the same household *Mean Age (year)* = Not reported *Race* = 26% Caucasian families and 46% Mexican-American families *Mean BP (mmHg)* = Not reported	*Food Records, 24-h Recall, Food Frequency Questionnaire:* LS families reported improved eating habits	Significant differences between the LS and CTL groups ranged from 2.3 to 3.4 mmHg for SBP and DBP in both Mexican-American and Caucasian families Greater changes for dietary behaviors were observed than for physical activity in the LS group, and greater dietary change was reported by Caucasian than Mexican-American families
Rocchini et al. (United States) (78)	Two group crossover RCT Duration=2-weeks/condition *Low-Sodium Diet (LS)* Participants adhered to a four-day rotating meal plan with meals containing 20–30 mmol/day of sodium	*N* = 78 Obese (*n*=60) and nonobese (*n*=18) unmedicated adolescents recruited through pediatricians and school nurses	*Food Records:* Records analyzed for six randomly selected days during the low-sodium diet indicated that obese and nonobese participants had similar sodium intake (15.9±4.5 vs. 14.8±2.6 mmol/day)	Obese adolescents had a significantly greater decrease in mean BP when transitioning from a high-sodium diet to a low-sodium diet than nonobese adolescents (−12±1 mmHg vs. +1±2 mmHg; *p*<0.001)

Table 1
(continued)

Authors	Intervention	Sample baseline demographics	Compliance	Findings
	High-Sodium Diet (HS) Participants took five sodium chloride tablets in addition to their regular meals. The LS diet was formulated to be similar in calorie content as the HS diet	*Mean Age (year)* = 12.5±.5 SEM (obese); 12.5±.6 SEM (nonobese) *Race* = Not reported *Mean BP(mmHg)* = 125/74 (obese); 106/64 (nonobese)		BP in obese adolescents may be more sensitive to sodium intake
Howe et al. (Australia) *(113)*	Two group crossover RCT Duration=4 weeks/condition *Low-Sodium Diet (LS)* Weekly dietary counseling for both children and parents with low-sodium bread provided *Control Group (CTL)* Weekly dietary counseling for both children and parents with salt sachets provided	*N* = 100 (F=48% and M=52%) School children representing the top, middle, and bottom deciles of the blood pressure range *Age (years)* = 11–14 *Mean BP* = 115/60 mmHg	*First-morning UNa:* Na concentration decreased from 175.9 to 101.8 mmol/day in the LS condition. *Food Records:* A subset of participants completed records and showed a reduction in Na intake consistent with UNa findings	Sodium intake decreased by ~ 42% in the LS condition and both SBP and DBP declined (–.97±.68 mmHg; –.56±.71 mmHg) though not significantly
Gortmaker et al. (United States) *(100)*	Two group CT Duration=2 years *Eat Well and Keep Moving program (EWKM; n=6 schools)* Classroom teachers gave materials focused on decreasing high fat foods and television watching, and increasing fruit and vegetable intake and physical activity. The program provided links to school food services and families and wellness training programs to teachers	*N = 14 schools, 479 students* (F= 56% EWKM and F= 61% CTL) Children in grades 4 and 5 from public schools in Baltimore, MD.	Compliance not reported	Based on 24-h recall methods sodium intake did not differ between groups or change over time, though fruit and vegetable intake increased significantly more over time in the EWKM group than the CTL (*p*=0.01)

Table 1
(continued)

Authors	Intervention	Sample baseline demographics	Compliance	Findings
	Control Group (CTL; n=8 schools) No treatment	Mean Age (years) = 9.2 (EWKM); 9.1 (CTL) Race = 91% African-American Mean BP (mmHg) = 115/60		
Wilson and Ampey-Thornhill (United States) (97)	One group clinical trial Duration=5 days Low-Sodium Diet (LS) Children and families were given guidelines and several food items for maintaining a low-sodium diet	N = 184 (F=101 and M=83) Healthy normotensive, unmedicated African-American adolescents recruited from schools, churches, and local recreation centers in the southeastern United States Mean Age (year) = 14±1(F); 14±1 (M) Race = 100% African-American Mean BP (mmHg) = 101/56 (compliant F); 108/53 (compliant M)	24-h UNa: Compliance was defined as ≤ 50 mEq/24 h during the LS diet. Based on these criteria 77% of adolescents were compliant (n=114)	SBP trended toward decreasing in compliant participants but decreases were nonsignificant Compliant girls reported higher levels of familial dietary support, whereas compliant boys reported lower levels of familial dietary support. Higher dietary support may be associated with adherence in girls

Table 1
(continued)

Authors	Intervention	Sample baseline demographics	Compliance	Findings
Pomeranz et al. (Israel) (70)	Three group RCT Duration=8-weeks/group *Low Sodium Formula (LS; n=25)* Infant formula diluted with water with 1.4 mmol/L sodium concentration *High Sodium Formula (HS; n=33)* Infant formula diluted with water with 8.5 mmol/L sodium concentration *Control Group (CTL; n=15)* Infants were breastfed	N = 58 Newborn Jewish infants in a university-affiliated hospital. Infants from families with history of HTN excluded *Mean Age (week) =* 40±1.3 (LS); 40.2±1.1 (HS); 39.5±1.6 (CTL) *Race =* Not reported *Mean BP (mmHg) = Not reported*	*Spot UNa/creatinine:* Na content of the LS group was 57±1.9 mmol and 172±2 mmol for the high HS group. Days of noncompliance were eliminated from analyses	SBP, DBP, and creatinine ratios were significantly greater in the HS group than in the LS and CTL groups. Potassium concentrations were also decreased in the HS group At 24-week follow-up BP values in the LS group increased toward those of the HS group
Palacios et al. (United States) (52)	Two group crossover RCT Duration=2-months/condition *Low-Sodium Diet (LS)* 1 g/day, 43 mmol/day of sodium with fixed amounts of dietary potassium. *High-Sodium Diet (HS)* 4 g/day, 174 mmol/day of sodium with fixed amounts of dietary potassium. Packed foods were provided within a 4-day menu cycle and were of the same composition for both groups except for sodium variation	N = 36 (F= 100% and M= 0%) Matched African-American (n=22) and Caucasian (n=14) normotensive adolescent females *Mean Age (years) =* 12.4 (African-American); 13.2 (Caucasian) *Race =* 39% Caucasian and 61% African-American *Mean BP (mmHg) =* 113/59 (African-American); 113/55 (Caucasian)	*24-h UNa:* Na content of the LS group was 57±1.9 mmol and 172±2 mmol for the high HS group. Days of noncompliance were eliminated from analyses	Blood pressure significantly decreased (p<0.05) from baseline to the end of the study. African-American girls showed greater sodium retention in the HS condition than Caucasian girls, though blood pressure did not decrease despite increased sodium retention, nor did sodium excretion increase

Table 1
(continued)

Authors	Intervention	Sample baseline demographics	Compliance	Findings
Couch et al. (United States) (80)	Two group RCT Intervention=3 months/group *DASH Diet (DASH; n=29)* Initial counseling session with dietician to follow a modified DASH diet. Eight weekly and two biweekly phone calls with interventionists and biweekly mailings *Routine Care(RC; n=28)* Initial counseling session with dietician encouraging consumption of fruits, vegetables, grains, lean meats, and low-fat dairy	*N* = 57 (F=21 and M=36) Prehypertensive or hypertensive adolescents seeking treatment in a children's hypertension clinic *Mean Age (years)* = 14.3 ± 2.1 (DASH); 14.4 ± 2.1 (RC) *Race* = 40 Caucasian and 17 African-American *Mean BP (mmHg)* = 131/79 (DASH); 126/82 (RC)	Compliance not reported	The DASH group showed a greater decrease in SBP than the RC (−7.9% vs. −1.5%, *p* <0.01) There was an increase for DASH participants in fruit servings among DASH participants, with fruit servings increasing ~ 2/day and intake of high-sodium/ fat foods decreasing by ~ 0.8 servings/day. Intake of potassium and magnesium reportedly increased by 42 and 36%, respectively

Table 1
(continued)

Authors	Intervention	Sample baseline demographics	Compliance	Findings
Potassium interventions				
Wilson et al. (United States) (32)	Two group RCT Duration=4-weeks/group *High-Potassium Diet (HK; n=20)* 80 mmol/day of potassium with 4 weekly 1-h classes covering education, behavior skills, barriers, and strategies for increasing potassium consumption, and feedback on food record keeping and 24-h urine results. *Usual Diet Control (CTL; n=20)* Healthy diet program with weekly 1-h classes covering feedback on food record keeping and 24-h urine results	$N = 40$ (F=18 and M=22) Healthy normotensive African-American adolescents classified as dippers (>10% BP decrease from waking to sleeping; n=28) and nondippers ($\leq$10% BP decrease from waking to sleeping; n=12) *Mean Age (year)* = 14±1 (dippers); 14±1 (nondippers) *Race* = 100% African-American Mean BP *(mmHg)*= 109±63 mmHg (dippers); 112±61 mmHg (nondippers)	*24-h Urinary potassium:* Collections were obtained at weekly intervals. Urinary K levels increased in the HK group but not in the control group	Awake BP decreased for dippers in the HK group from baseline to post-treatment (119/67 to 114/64), but increased for nondippers (115/62 to 124/67)

Table 1
(continued)

Authors	Intervention	Sample baseline demographics	Compliance	Findings
Sorof et al. (United States) (84)	Three group crossover RCT; Duration=1-week/condition *Potassium Solution* 1.5 mmol/kg/day *Placebo Solution* Cherry syrup *CVR Stressors* Blood sampling, cold pressor, and video game	$N = 39$ (F=33 and M=17) Children aged 7–15 years recruited from schools and clinics with (n=22) and without (n=17) family history of essential HTN *Mean Age (year)* = 12 *Race*= 44% Caucasian and 56% African-American	*12-h Urinary potassium:* Significant increases in K excretion but overnight collections may not have captured compliance for entire week; children complained of unpleasant taste	CVR was not attenuated by the potassium solution compared to placebo. Potassium may need to be supplemented for > 1 week to produce positive effects Higher vegetable consumption in Caucasian children than in African- American children was associated with higher urinary potassium/creatinine ratio
Wilson et al. (United States) (33)	Two group RCT Duration=3-weeks/group *High-Potassium Diet (HK; n=26)* 80 mmol/day of K with 4 weekly 1-h classes covering education, behavior skills, barriers, and strategies for increasing K consumption, and feedback on food record keeping and 24-h urine results. *Usual Diet Control (CTL; n=32)* Normal diet program with weekly 1-h classes covering feedback on food record keeping and 24-h urine results	$N = 53$ (F=26 and M=27) Salt-sensitive (SS; n=16) and salt resistant (SR; n=37) African-American adolescents. Salt sensitivity was defined as an increase in MBP ≥ 5 mmHg in transitioning from a low- to high-sodium diet *Mean Age (year)* = 14±1 (SS); 14±1 (SR)	*24-h Urinary potassium:* Dietary K increased significantly over time in the HK group who had been nondippers achieved dipping status due to decreased nighttime DBP Participants in the CTL group did not show decreases in nighttime DBP. Increased potassium intake did not affect weight or sleep duration	At 3-week assessments all SS participants in the HK group who had been nondippers achieved dipping status due to decreased nighttime DBP (p<0.02) and K levels were significantly higher in the HK group vs. the CTL group

Table 1
(continued)

Authors	Intervention	Sample baseline demographics	Compliance	Findings
Mu et al. (China) *(114)*	Two group RCT Duration= 2-years/group *Potassium and Calcium Supplementation (KC; n=136)* Children were instructed to take a tablet consisting of 10 mmol potassium and 10 mmol calcium daily *Placebo Control (CTL; n=125)* Children were instructed to take a placebo tablet that was identical in appearance and taste to the potassium and calcium tablet All participants were instructed to maintain usual sodium intake	N = 261 (F=133 and M=128) School children in grades 3 and 4 with salt sensitivity (SS) and without salt sensitivity (NSS) from Hanzhong, China Mean Age (year) ~ 10.5 Race = 100% Asian Mean BP (mmHg) = 103/63 (SS/KC); 103/63 (NSS/KC); 103/63 (SS/CTL); 103/63 (NSS/CTL)	*Compliance not reported*	Blood pressure was lowered by 4.3–4.8 mmHg for SS children in the KC group, but not for NSS children. Decreases in night sodium excretion in SS children was significant (p<0.01) and was negatively correlated with increase in BP. Moderate increases in dietary calcium and potassium may promote urinary sodium excretion

Table 1
(continued)

Authors	Intervention	Sample baseline demographics	Compliance	Findings
Sodium and potassium interventions				
Sinaiko et al. (United States) *(11)*	Three group RCT Duration = 3-years/group *Low-Sodium Diet (LS; n= 70)* 70 mmol/day + nutrition counseling 7 times during months. 1–3 and then tri-monthly. Phone calls were made to reinforce instructions *Potassium Capsule (K; n= 71)* 1 mmol/kg/day, double blind *Placebo Capsule (CTL; n= 69)* Identical to potassium, double blind	$N = 210$ (F=105 and M=105) Minneapolis, MN public school students in grades 5–8 with SBP > 109 mmHg (boys) and 108 mmHg (girls) *Mean Age (year)* = 13.2 ± 0.1 *Race* = 86.5% Caucasian and 13.5% African-American *Mean BP (mmHg)* = 114/63 (LS); 114/67 (K); 114/65 (CTL)	*24-h UNa:* LS group did not achieve 70 mmol/day goal; No change in boys Na excretion (noncompliance); Reduced Na excretion in girls from baseline Percentage of expected capsule use: *Potassium capsule* 84.2%, range=77–93% *Placebo capsule* 91%, range=85–97%	No between-group differences were found for boys and BP increased over time For girls in sodium and potassium interventions BP increased less over time than for placebo groups but did not significantly decrease Differences between boys and girls may be due to poorer compliance in boys Poor compliance in the LS group challenges the feasibility of long-term sodium reduction in adolescents

Table 1
(continued)

Authors	Intervention	Sample baseline demographics	Compliance	Findings
Günther et al. (United States) (81)	Cross-sectional study *Type 1 diabetes (T1D; n= 2440)* *Type 2 diabetes (T2D; n= 390)* All participants' diets were analyzed and assessed for concurrence with eight food groups of the Dietary Approaches to Stop Hypertension (DASH) diet for increased fruit and vegetable intake	N = 2830 (F=54% and M=46%) Participants in the SEARCH for Diabetes in Youth trial aged 10–22 with type 1 or type 2 diabetes *Mean Age (year) =* 14.7–16.6 *Race T1D =* >71% Caucasian, >5% African-American, and >11% Hispanic *Race T2D =* >20% Caucasian, >30% African-American, >14% Hispanic, and >12% Native American *Mean BP (mmHg) =* 108/68	Participants' diets were analyzed using a self-report Food Frequency Questionnaire from which a DASH concurrence score was calculated	In youth with T1D adherence to DASH was inversely associated with HTN, where as in youth with T2D adherence to the DASH diet was not associated with reductions in the risk of HTN

BMI, body mass index; BP, blood pressure; CT, controlled trial; DBP, diastolic blood pressure; F, female; M, male; HTN, hypertension; RCT, randomized controlled trial; SBP, systolic blood pressure; UNa, urinary sodium.

In a study by Couch et al. *(80)*, the DASH diet was compared to routine care in a biracial sample of youth. Youth who were randomized to receive the DASH diet (rich in fruits and vegetables, potassium, and magnesium and low in total fat) showed a significantly greater decrease in systolic BP as compared to youth who were randomized to routine care. Those in the DASH diet also showed significant increases in fruit and vegetable intake, potassium, and magnesium and significant decreases in sodium intake and total fat as compared to the youth in the comparison group over the course of the 12-week intervention. In another recent study, Günther and colleagues *(81)* reported that youth with type 1 diabetes who demonstrated adherence to the DASH diet showed an inverse relationship with hypertension, independent of demographic, clinical, and behavioral characteristics. Note, however, that in the Günther et al. *(81)* study adherence to the DASH diet was not associated with such reductions in the risk of hypertension among youth with type 2 diabetes. Taken together, these studies suggest that the DASH diet may be a promising approach for improving cardiovascular risk factors such as elevated BP in some youth. Further research is needed to better determine the overall rate of compliance with the DASH diet relative to other approaches to reducing sodium intake and/or increasing potassium intake.

Some evidence indicates that dietary electrolyte intake plays an influential role in circulatory responses to stress. Falkner and colleagues *(82)* have conducted a number of investigations evaluating how altering dietary sodium affects CVR. One study evaluated 15 normotensive adolescent girls for 2 weeks, at rest and during mental arithmetic exercises, and before and after adding 10 g of sodium to their diet. The girls with a positive family history of essential HTN showed an increase in resting baseline and stress BP levels and the girls with a negative family history did not. These findings have been replicated in young adults *(83)*. However, for those with a positive family history of essential HTN, changes from baseline to stress were similar before and after salt loading.

Sorof et al. *(84)* examined whether CVR was inversely related to the dietary intake of potassium in 39 children. At baseline, the 24-h urinary potassium/creatinine ratio varied inversely with diastolic CVR in Caucasian children (who had a positive family history of HTN); however, CVR was not attenuated by potassium supplementation (1.5 mmol/kg/day of potassium citrate) compared to placebo. Urinary potassium/creatinine ratio was higher in Caucasian children than in African-American children and dietary potassium-modulated CVR in Caucasian children with a family history of HTN.

Consistent with this finding *(84)*, Wilson et al. *(33)* demonstrated no significant change in BP reactivity in African-American adolescents who complied with a 3-week high-potassium diet. Wilson et al. *(33)* also demonstrated, in a randomized control trial among adolescents, that increasing potassium was beneficial for reversing nondipping status and elevated nighttime BP in African-American adolescents. This study examined the effects of increasing dietary potassium on BP nondipping status in salt-sensitive and salt-resistant African-American adolescents. Urinary potassium excretion significantly increased in the treatment group (35 ± 7 to 57 ± 21 mmol/24 h). At baseline, a significantly greater percentage of salt-sensitive (44%) subjects were nondippers based on diastolic BP classifications ($p < 0.04$), compared to salt-resistant (7%) subjects. After the diet intervention, all of the salt-sensitive subjects in the high potassium group achieved a dipper BP status due to a drop in nocturnal diastolic BP (daytime 69 ± 5 vs. 67 ± 5; nighttime 69 ± 5 vs. 57 ± 6 mmHg). These results suggest that a positive relationship between dietary potassium intake and BP modulation exists, although daytime BP may be unchanged by a high-potassium diet. Our data are the first to indicate that increasing dietary potassium reversed nondipping status in salt-sensitive subjects, while having no effect on daytime BP. These findings in part corroborate other investigations that have shown beneficial effects of increasing potassium on BP responses in salt-sensitive populations. For example, Fujita and Ando *(85)* demonstrated that salt-sensitive hypertensives who were given a potassium supplement (96 mmol/24 h) while on a high-sodium diet showed significantly greater decreases in MBP after 3 days when compared to nonsupplemented hypertensive patients. Svetkey et al. *(86)* demonstrated a significant drop in both systolic and diastolic BP after 8 weeks of potassium supplementation (64 mmol/24 h vs. placebo) among mildly hypertensive patients.

A number of reviews on the influence of potassium on BP responses have also shown positive inverse associations between high potassium intake and BP responses in primarily adult populations *(12,67,87)*. The mechanisms underlying BP nondipping status are unknown. One potential mechanism by which potassium may alter nighttime BP may involve potassium-related natriuresis *(88,89)*. Restricting potassium intake leads to sodium retention; potassium supplementation results in a natriuresis. Some investigators suggest that the effect of potassium on urinary sodium excretion, plasma volume, and mean arterial pressure could be evidence of a potassium-mediated vasodilatory effect on BP *(67)*. If nondippers are characterized by elevated sympathetic nervous system activity and increased peripheral resistance during sleep, this potassium-mediated vasodilatory effect could explain the reversal of nondipping status in the Wilson et al. study *(33)*. Other studies that support this hypothesis show that intrabrachial arterial infusions of potassium chloride increase forearm blood flow and decrease forearm vascular resistance in healthy adults *(90,91)*. Potassium supplementation given in combination with a high-sodium diet also suppresses the increase in catecholamine responses typically seen in response to salt loading *(92)*. Previous studies have shown that total peripheral resistance and norepinephrine responses to stress are greater in offspring of hypertensives than in normotensives *(93)*. Several adult studies have also confirmed that sympathetic nervous system activation occurs in individuals with elevated nighttime BP *(94)*. Taken together, these data support the hypothesis that the sympathetic nervous system may have a controlling influence on nondipping BP status.

NUTRITION AND DIETARY COMPLIANCE IN YOUTH

Several lines of evidence suggest that targeting families may be important for promoting healthy dietary compliance in children and adolescents. Previous research has demonstrated moderate aggregation of dietary variables among adolescents and their parents *(95)*. Furthermore, because families share a genetic predisposition to health risk factors, family involvement may be important in motivating adolescents to improve their long-term eating habits. Parents and peers may serve as role models for adolescents by consuming foods that are healthy and by reinforcing dietary knowledge and behaviors learned in schools *(96)*.

Social support from family members may be one way that parental involvement may influence compliance with dietary interventions. Parents may encourage adolescents to adopt healthy dietary behaviors, which in turn may decrease the risk for cardiovascular disease and chronic illness. Wilson and Ampey-Thornhill *(97)* examined the relationship between gender, dietary social support (emotional), and compliance to a low-sodium diet. A total of 184 healthy African-American adolescents participated in an intensive 5-day low-sodium diet (50 mEq/2 h) as part of an HTN prevention program. Girls who were compliant (urinary sodium excretion [UnaV] <50 mEq/24 h) reported higher levels of dietary support from family members than boys who were compliant (UnaV <50 mEq/24 h).

In a study by Nader et al. *(98)*, Caucasian, African-American, and Mexican-American families were randomly assigned to a 3-month low-sodium, low-fat dietary program, or to a no-treatment group. The treatment group showed a greater increase in social support specific to diet than the no-treatment group. Taken together, these studies provide evidence that familial support may be important for increasing adolescents' compliance with healthy dietary programs that will ultimately decrease the risk of HTN and cardiovascular complications.

Another way that parents, teachers, and peers may influence adolescents' compliance with healthy eating habits is through role modeling. Cohen et al. *(99)* randomly assigned adolescents to peer-led or teacher-led promotions of a low-sodium, low-fat dietary intervention. At the end of the intervention, both groups showed equal effectiveness in changing nutritional habits. The peer-led group, however, was more effective in reducing BP.

Previous research also suggests that the incorporation of behavioral skills training and developmentally appropriate dietary interventions may be most effective in promoting long-term changes in sodium and/or potassium intake (e.g., increased fruit and vegetable intake). For example, in a study conducted by Gortmaker et al. *(100)* 1,295 sixth- and seventh-grade students from public schools in Massachusetts participated in a school-based intervention over 2 years to reduce the prevalence of obesity. The intervention was based on social cognitive theory (SCT) and behavioral choice theory. Treatment sessions were incorporated into the existing curricula, used classroom teachers, and targeted increasing their fruit and vegetable intake. Schools across four study sites were randomized to either the SCT treatment that focused on behavioral skills or a control condition. After 3 years, the intervention school children exhibited significant changes in improved knowledge, intentions, self-efficacy, dietary behavior, and perceived social reinforcement for healthy food choices.

Some studies have provided insight into the importance of targeting eating patterns for improving food choices related to high-potassium/low-sodium foods such as fruit and vegetable intake *(101)*. In 943 third to fifth graders, fruit juices accounted for 6.1% of the total food selections for boys and 6.6% for girls. Vegetables accounted for 15.7% of total selection for boys and 16.2% for girls. Fruit was more likely consumed for snacks than for meals and vegetables were eaten at the same rate for snacks, at lunch, and at supper. Consequently, targeting an increase in fruits in all meals may be one effective approach to improving electrolyte intake in children. Further research is needed, specifically more tests that systematically focus on the relevance of increasing fruit and vegetable intake throughout an entire day's eating episodes instead of sporadically.

Several studies have demonstrated sex differences in compliance to sodium restriction and dietary potassium supplementation. Sinaiko et al. *(11)* reported urinary electrolyte excretion data over the course of a 3-year intervention in fifth through eighth graders. Boys were less likely to comply with a sodium restriction of 70 mmol/day than girls. Subsequently, BP effects were only significant for girls. In a study by Wilson and Bayer *(102)*, boys were more likely than girls to comply with a 3-week dietary intervention of increasing potassium to 80 mmol/day intake. These studies suggest that boys, in particular, may be more likely to comply with high-potassium diets that emphasize adding foods to the diet, compared to low-sodium diets that focus on eliminating foods from the diet. Further research is needed to more fully explore the long-term effectiveness of dietary electrolyte interventions in boys vs. girls and among youth in general.

CONCLUSIONS AND IMPLICATIONS FOR FUTURE RESEARCH

In summary, the profile of elevated cardiovascular risk includes BP parameters such as high casual BP, elevated CVR, and nondipping ambulatory BP status. While much of the research to date has focused on adult populations, national efforts are continuing to move in the direction of prevention at the childhood level.

Reducing sodium and increasing potassium intake have been shown to be effective approaches for reducing the risk and development of HTN, yet much work remains to be done among children and adolescent populations. Research by our group suggests that compliance with high-potassium dietary interventions may be easier than with low-sodium diets. This chapter provides the basis for promoting effective nutritional-electrolyte-focused interventions. However, other important factors must be considered, including those related to obesity and sedentary lifestyles. Minority populations, including African-Americans, are at particularly high risk for developing HTN in early adulthood, and efforts should focus on preventing HTN in these and underserved communities. Continued efforts will be needed to assure prevention of obesity in underserved and minority youth. Abnormal sympathetic nervous system activity may be linked to the elevated BP parameters reviewed in this chapter. The role of dietary intake on BP markers suggests that further attention should be paid to promoting positive dietary lifestyle skills in youth. Promoting healthy diets that target decreasing sodium and increasing potassium may help to decrease sympathetic nervous system activation. The precise physiological mechanisms that underlie the observations reported in this chapter should be another focus of future investigations.

REFERENCES

1. Sinaiko AR, Gomez-Marin O, Prineas RJ. Prevalence of significant hypertension in junior high school-aged children. J Pediatr. 1989;114:664–669.
2. Muntner P, He J, Cutler J, Wildman RP, Whelton PK. Trends in blood pressure among children and adolescents. JAMA. 2004;291:2107–2113.
3. Ostchega Y, Carroll M, Prineas RJ, McDowell MA, Louis T, Tilert T. Trends of elevated blood pressure among children and adolescents: data from the National Health and Nutrition Examination Survey 1988–2006. Am J Hypertens. 2009;22:59–67.
4. Lauer RM, Clarke WR. Childhood risk factors for high adult blood pressure: the Muscatine study. Pediatrics. 1989;84:633–644.
5. Berenson GS, Srinivasan SR, Wattigney WA, Harsha DW. Obesity and cardiovascular risk in children. Ann N Y Acad Sci. 1993;699:93–103.
6. Chiolero A, Bovet P, Paradis G, Paccaud F. Has blood pressure increased in children in response to the obesity epidemic? Pediatrics. 2007;119:544–553.
7. Zhu H, Yan W, Ge D, et al. Relationships of cardiovascular phenotypes with healthy weight, at risk of overweight, and overweight in US youths. Pediatrics. 2008;121:115–122.
8. Carvalho JJ, Baruzzi FG, Howard PF, Poulter N, Alpers M, Stamler R. Blood pressure in four remote populations: INTERSALT study. Hypertension. 1989;14:238–246.
9. INTERSALT Cooperative Research Group. INTERSALT: An international study of electrolyte excretion and blood pressure. Results for 24-hour urinary sodium and potassium excretion. Br Med J. 1988;297:319–328.
10. Whelton PK, He J, Cutler JA, et al. Effects of oral potassium on blood pressure: meta-analysis of randomized controlled clinical trials. JAMA. 1997;277:1624–1632.
11. Sinaiko AR, Gomez-Marin O, Prineas R. Effect of a low sodium diet or potassium supplementation on adolescent blood pressure. Hypertension. 1993;21:989–994.
12. Whelton PK, He J, Appel LJ, et al. Primary prevention of hypertension: clinical and public health advisory from The National High Blood Pressure Education Program. National High Blood Pressure Education Program Coordinating Committee. JAMA. 2002;288:1882–1888.

13. Appel LJ, Brands MW, Daniels SR, Karanja N, Elmer PJ, Sacks FM, American Heart Association. Dietary approaches to prevent and treat hypertension: a scientific statement from the American Heart Association. Hypertension. 2006;47:296–308.
14. Falkner B, Daniels SR. Summary of the fourth report on the diagnosis, evaluation, and treatment of high blood pressure in children and adolescents. Hypertension. 2004;44:387–388.
15. National High Blood Pressure Education Program Working Group on High Blood Pressure in Children and Adolescents. The fourth report on the diagnosis, evaluation, and treatment of high blood pressure in children and adolescents. Pediatrics. 2004;114(Suppl):555–576.
16. Alpert BA, Wilson DK. Stress reactivity in childhood and adolescence. In: Turner JR, Sherwood A, Light K, eds. Individual Differences in Cardiovascular Response to Stress: Applications to Models of Cardiovascular Disease. New York, NY: Plenum; 1992:187–201.
17. Borghi C, Costa FV, Boschi S, Mussi A, Ambrosioni E. Predictors of stable hypertension in young borderline subjects: a five-year follow-up study. J Cardiovasc Pharmacol. 1986;8(Suppl): S138–S141.
18. Sica DA, Wilson DK. Sodium, potassium, the sympathetic nervous system, and the renin-angiotensis system: impact on the circadian variability in blood pressure. In: White WB, ed. Cardiovascular Chronobiology and Variability in Clinical Practice. Totowa, NJ: Humana; 2001:171–189.
19. Matthews KA, Katholi CR, McCreath H, et al. Blood pressure reactivity to psychological stress predicts hypertension in the CARDIA study. Circulation. 2004;110:74–78.
20. Masters KS, Hill RD, Kircher JC, Lensegrav Benson TL, Fallon JA. Religious orientation, aging, and blood pressure reactivity to interpersonal and cognitive stressors. Ann Behav Med. 2004;28: 171–178.
21. Roemmich JN, Smith JR, Epstein LH, Lambiase M. Stress reactivity and adiposity of youth. Obesity. 2007;15:2303–2310.
22. Barbeau P, Litaker MS, Harshfield GA. Impaired pressure natriuresis in obese youths. Obes Res. 2003;11:745–751.
23. Westmaas JL, Jamner LD. Paradoxical effects of social support on blood pressure reactivity among defensive individuals. Ann Behav Med. 2006;31:238–247.
24. Kaneda R, Kario K, Hoshide S, Umeda Y, Hoshide Y, Shimada K. Morning blood pressure hyper-reactivity is an independent predictor for hypertensive cardiac hypertrophy in a community-dwelling population. Am J Hypertens. 2005;18:1528–1533.
25. al'Absi M, Devereux RB, Rao DC, Kitzman D, Oberman A, Hopkins P, Arnett DK. Blood pressure stress reactivity and left ventricular mass in a random community sample of African-American and Caucasian men and women. Am J Cardiol. 2006;97:240–244.
26. Moseley JV, Linden W. Predicting blood pressure and heart rate change with cardiovascular reactivity and recovery: results from 3-year and 10-year follow up. Psychosom Med. 2006;68:833–843.
27. Stewart KJ, Ouyang P, Bacher AC, Lima S, Shapiro EP. Exercise effects on cardiac size and left ventricular diastolic function: relationships to changes in fitness, fatness, blood pressure and insulin resistance. Heart. 2006;92:893–898.
28. Verdecchia P, Schillaci G, Borgioni C, Ciucci A, Porcellati C. Prognostic significance of the white coat effect. Hypertension. 1997;29:1218–1224.
29. Kobrin I, Oigman W, Kumar A, et al. Diurnal variation of blood pressure in elderly patients with essential hypertension. J Am Geriatr Soc. 1984;32:896–899.
30. Verdecchia P, Schillaci G, Guerrieri M, et al. Circadian blood pressure changes and left ventricular hypertrophy in essential hypertension. Circulation. 1990;81:528–536.
31. Devereux RB, Pickering TG. Relationship between the level, pattern and variability of ambulatory blood pressure and target organ damage in hypertension. J Hypertens. 1991;9(Suppl):S34–S38.
32. Wilson DK, Sica DA, Devens M, Nicholson S. The influence of potassium intake on dipper and non-dipper blood pressure status in an African-American adolescent population. Blood Press Monit. 1996;1:447–455.
33. Wilson DK, Sica DA, Miller SB. Effects of potassium on blood pressure in salt-sensitive and salt-resistant adolescents. Hypertension. 1999;34:181–186.
34. Espeland MA, Kumanyika S, Yunis C, Zheng B, Brown WM, Jackson S, Wilson AC, Bahnson J. Electrolyte intake and nonpharmacologic blood pressure control. Ann Epidemiol. 2002;12: 587–595.
35. He FJ, MacGregor GA. Importance of salt in determining blood pressure in children: meta-analysis of controlled trials. Hypertension. 2006;48:861–869.
36. Savoca MR, Domel Baxter S, Ludwig DA, Evans CD, Mackey ML, Wilson ME, Hanevold C, Harshfield GA. A 4-day sodium-controlled diet reduces variability of overnight sodium excretion in free-living normotensive adolescents. J Am Diet Assoc. 2007;107:490–494.

37. Leong GM, Kainer G. Diet, salt, anthropological and hereditary factors in hypertension. Child Nephrol Urol. 1992;12:96–105.

38. Allison S. Fluid, electrolytes and nutrition. Clin Med. 2004;4:573–578.

39. Ge D, Su S, Zhu H, et al. Stress-induced sodium excretion: a new intermediate phenotype to study the early genetic etiology of hypertension? Hypertension. 2009;53:262–269.

40. Tobin MD, Timpson NJ, Wain LV, et al. Common variation in the WNK1 gene and blood pressure in childhood: the Avon Longitudinal Study of Parents and Children. Hypertension. 2008;52:974–979.

41. Kojima S, Inenaga T, Matsuoka H, et al. The association between salt sensitivity of blood pressure and some polymorphic factors. J Hypertens. 1994;12:797–801.

42. Weinberger MH, et al. Association of haptoglobin with sodium sensitivity and resistance of blood pressure. Hypertension. 1987;10:443–446.

43. Guerra A, Monteiro C, Breitenfeld L, et al. Genetic and environmental factors regulating blood pressure in childhood: prospective study from 0 to 3 years. J Hum Hypertens. 1997;11:233–238.

44. Hanevold CD, Pollock JS, Harshfield GA. Racial differences in microalbumin excretion in healthy adolescents. Hypertension. 2008;51:334–338.

45. Couch SC, Saelens BE, Levin L, Dart K, Falciglia G, Daniels SR. The efficacy of a clinic-based behavioral nutrition intervention emphasizing a DASH-type diet for adolescents with elevated blood pressure. J Pediatr. 2008;152:494–501.

46. Cook NR, Obarzanek E, Cutler JA, et al. Trials of Hypertension Prevention Collaborative Research Group. Joint effects of sodium and potassium intake on subsequent cardiovascular disease: the Trials of Hypertension Prevention follow-up study. Arch Intern Med. 2009;169:32–40.

47. Simons-Morton DG, Obarzanck E. Diet and blood pressure in children and adolescents. Pediatr Nephrol. 1997;11:244–249.

48. Weinberger MH, Miller JZ, Luft FC, et al. Definitions and characteristics of sodium sensitivity and blood pressure resistance. Hypertension. 1986;8:II127–II134.

49. Falkner B, Kushner H, Khalsa OK, et al. Sodium sensitivity, growth and family history of hypertension in young blacks. J Hypertens. 1986;4(Suppl):S381–S383.

50. Wilson DK, Bayer L, Krishnamoorthy JS, Ampey-Thornhill G, Nicholson SC, Sica DA. The prevalence of salt sensitivity in an African-American adolescent population. Ethn Dis. 1999;9:350–358.

51. Sullivan JM, Ratts TE. Sodium sensitivity in human subjects. Hemodynamic and hormonal correlates. Hypertension. 1988;11:717–723.

52. Palacios C, Wigertz K, Martin BR, Jackman L, Pratt JH, Peacock M, McCabe G, Weaver CM. Sodium retention in black and white female adolescents in response to salt intake. J Clin Endocrinol Metab. 2004;89:1858–1863.

53. Wilson DK, Sica DA, Miller SB. Ambulatory blood pressure and nondipping status in salt-sensitive versus salt-resistant black adolescents. Am J Hypertens. 1999;12:159–165.

54. Harshfield GA, Alpert BS, Pulliam DA, Willey ES, Somes GW, Stapleton FB. Sodium excretion and racial differences in ambulatory blood pressure patterns. Hypertension. 1991;18:813–818.

55. de la Sierra A, del Mar Lluch MM, Coca A, Aguilera MT, Sánchez M, Sierra C, Urbano-Márquez A. Assessment of salt sensitivity in essential hypertension by 24-h ambulatory blood pressure monitoring. Am J Hypertens. 1995;8:970–977.

56. Rocchini AP, Kolch V, Kveselis D, et al. Insulin and renal sodium retention in obese adolescents. Hypertension. 1989;14:367–374.

57. Lurbe E, Alvarez V, Liao Y, et al. Obesity modifies the relationship between ambulatory blood pressure and natriuresis in children. Blood Press Monit. 2000;5:275–280.

58. Uzu T, Ishikawa K, Fujita T, Nakamura S, Inenaga T, Kimura G. Sodium restriction shifts circadian rhythm of blood pressure from nondipper to dipper in essential hypertension. Circulation. 1997;96:1859–1862.

59. Higashi Y, Oshima T, Ozono R, Nakano Y, Matsuura H, Kambe M, Kajiyama G. Nocturnal decline in blood pressure is attenuated by NaCl loading in salt-sensitive patients with essential hypertension: noninvasive 24-hour ambulatory blood pressure monitoring. Hypertension. 1997;30:163–167.

60. Harshfield GA, Pulliam DA, Alpert BS. Patterns of sodium excretion during sympathetic nervous system arousal. Hypertension. 1991;17:1156–1160.

61. Light KC, Koepke JP, Obrist PA, Willis PW. Psychological stress induces sodium and fluid retention in men at high risk for hypertension. Science. 1983;220:429–431.

62. Berenson GS, Voors AW, Webber LS, Dalferes ER Jr, Harsha DW. Racial differences of parameters associated with blood pressure levels in children—the Bogalusa Heart Study. Metabolism. 1979;28:1218–1228.

63. Morgan T, Teow BH, Myers J. The role of potassium in control of blood pressure. Drugs. 1984;28(Suppl):I188–I195.

64. Goto A, Yamada K, Nagoshi H, et al. Relation of 24-h ambulatory blood pressure with plasma potassium in essential hypertension. J Hypertens. 1997;10:337–340.
65. Solomon R, Weinberg MS, Dubey A. The diurnal rhythm of plasma potassium: relationship to diuretic therapy. J Cardiovasc Pharmacol. 1991;17:854–859.
66. Struthers AD, Reid JL, Whitesmith R, Rodger JC. Effect of intravenous adrenaline on electrocardiogram, blood pressure, and serum potassium. Br Heart J. 1983;49:90–93.
67. Linas SL. The role of potassium in the pathogenesis and treatment of hypertension. Kidney Int. 1991;39:771–786.
68. Falkner B, Michel S. Blood pressure response to sodium in children and adolescents. Am J Clin Nutr. 1997;65(Suppl):618S–621S.
69. Frank GC, Webber LS, Nicklas TA, Berenson GS. Sodium, potassium, calcium, magnesium, and phosphorus intakes of infants and children: Bogalusa Heart Study. J Am Diet Assoc. Jul 1988;88:801–807.
70. Pomeranz A, Dolfin T, Korzets Z, Eliakim A, Wolach B. Increased sodium concentrations in drinking water increase blood pressure in neonates. J Hypertens. 2002;20:203–207.
71. Cullen KW, Koehly LM, Anderson C, et al. Gender differences in chronic disease risk behaviors through the transition out of high school. Am J Prev Med. 1999;17(1):1–7.
72. Neumark-Sztainer D, Story M, Resnick MD, Blum RW. Lessons learned about adolescent nutrition from the Minnesota Adolescent Health Survey. J Am Diet Assoc. 1998;98:1449–1456.
73. Berenson GS, Voors AW, Dalferes ER Jr, Webber LS, Shuler SE. Creatinine clearance, electrolytes, and plasma renin activity related to the blood pressure of white and black children—the Bogalusa Heart Study. J Lab Clin Med. 1979;93:535–548.
74. Pratt JH, Jones JJ, Miller JZ, Wagner MA, Fineberg NS. Racial differences in aldosterone excretion and plasma aldosterone concentrations in children. N Engl J Med. 1989;321:1152–1157.
75. Miller JZ, Weinberger MH, Daugherty SA, Fineberg NS, Christian JC, Grim CE. Blood pressure response to dietary sodium restriction in healthy normotensive children. Am J Clin Nutr. 1988;47:113–119.
76. Gillum RF, Elmer PJ, Prineas RJ. Changing sodium intake in children. The Minneapolis Children's Blood Pressure Study. Hypertension. 1981;3:698–703.
77. Watt GCM, Foy DJW, Hart JT, et al. Dietary sodium and arterial blood pressure: evidence against genetic susceptibility. Br Med J. 1985;291:1525–1528.
78. Rocchini AP, Key J, Bondie D, et al. The effect of weight loss on the sensitivity of blood pressure to sodium in obese adolescents. N Engl J Med. 1989;321:580–585.
79. Wilson DK, Becker JA, Alpert BS. Prevalence of sodium sensitivity in black versus white adolescents. Circulation. 1992;1(Suppl):13.
80. Couch SC, Saelens BE, Levin L, Dart K, Falciglia G, Daniels SR. The efficacy of a clinic-based behavioral nutrition intervention emphasizing a DASH-type diet for adolescents with elevated blood pressure. J Pediatr. 2008;152:494–501.
81. Günther AL, Liese AD, Bell RA, et al. Association between the dietary approaches to hypertension diet and hypertension in youth with diabetes mellitus. Hypertension. 2009;53:6–12.
82. Falkner B, Onesti G, Angelakos E. Effect of salt loading on the cardiovascular response to stress in adolescents. Hypertension. 1981;3(II):II195–II199.
83. Falkner B, Kushner H. Effect of chronic sodium loading on cardiovascular response in young blacks and whites. Hypertension. 1990;15:36–43.
84. Sorof JM, Forman A, Cole N, Jemerin JM, Morris RC. Potassium intake and cardiovascular reactivity in children with risk factors for essential hypertension. J Pediatr. 1997;131:87–94.
85. Fujita T, Ando K. Hemodynamic and endocrine changes associated with potassium supplementation in sodium-loaded hypertensives. Hypertension. 1984;6:184–192.
86. Svetkey LP, Yarger WE, Feussner JR, DeLong E, Klotman E. Double-blind, placebo-controlled trial of potassium chloride in the treatment of mild hypertension. Hypertension. 1987;9:444–450.
87. Cappuccio FP, MacGregor GA. Does potassium supplementation lower blood pressure? A meta-analysis of published trials. J Hypertens. 1991;9:465–473.
88. Krishna GG, Miller E, Kapoor S. Increased blood pressure during potassium depletion in normotensive men. N Engl J Med. 1989;320:1177–1182.
89. Weinberger MH, Luft FC, Bloch R, et al. The blood pressure-raising effects of high dietary sodium intake: racial differences and the role of potassium. J Am Coll Nutr. 1982;1:139–148.
90. Fujita T, Ito Y. Salt loads attenuate potassium-induced vasocilation of forearm vasculature in humans. Hypertension. 1993;21:772–778.
91. Phillips RJW, Robinson BF. The dilator response to K+ is reduced in the forearm resistance vessels of men with primary hypertension. Clin Sci. 1984;66:237–239.
92. Campese VM, Romoff MS, Levitan D, et al. Abnormal relationship between Na+ intake and sympathetic nervous activity in salt-sensitive patients with essential hypertension. Kidney Int. 1982;21:371–378.

93. Stamler R, Stamler J, Riedlinger WF, Algera G, Roberts RH. Family (parental) history and prevalence of hypertension. Results of a nationwide screening program. JAMA. 1979;241:43–46.
94. Kostic N, Secen S. Circadian rhythm of blood pressure and daily hormone variations. Med Pregl. 1997;50:37–40.
95. Patterson TL, Rupp JW, Sallis JF, Atkins CJ, Nader PR. Aggregation of dietary calories, fats, and sodium in Mexican-American and Anglo families. Am J Prev Med. 1988;4:75–82.
96. Perry CL, Luepker RV, Murray DM, Kurth C, Mullis R, Crockett S, Jacobs DR Jr. Parent involvement with children's health promotion: the Minnesota Home Team. Am J Public Health. 1988;78:1156–1160.
97. Wilson DK, Ampey-Thornhill G. The role of gender and family support on dietary compliance in an African American adolescent hypertension prevention study. Ann Behav Med. 2001;23:59–67.
98. Nader PR, Sallis JF, Patterson TL, et al. A family approach to cardiovascular risk reduction: results from the San Diego Family Health Project. Health Educ Q. 1989;16:229–244.
99. Cohen RY, Felix MR, Brownell KD. The role of parents and older peers in school-based cardiovascular prevention programs: implications for program development. Health Educ Q. 1989;16:245–253.
100. Gortmaker SL, Cheung LW, Peterson KE, et al. Impact of a school-based interdisciplinary intervention on diet and physical activity among urban primary school children: eat well and keep moving. Arch Pediatr Adolesc Med. 1999;153:975–983.
101. Simons-Morton BG, Baranowski T, Parcel GS, O'Hara NM, Matteson RC. Children's frequency of consumption of foods high in fat and sodium. Am J Prev Med. 1990;6:218–227.
102. Wilson DK, Bayer L. The role of diet in hypertension prevention among African-American adolescents. Ann Behav Med. 2002;24(Suppl):S198.
103. Whitten CF, Stewart RA. The effect of dietary sodium in infancy on blood pressure and related factors. Studies of infants fed salted and unsalted diets for five months at eight months and eight years of age. Acta Paediatr Scand. 1980;279(Suppl):1–17.
104. Trevisan M, Cooper R, Ostrow D, Miller W, Sparks S, Leonas Y, Allen A, Steinhauer M, Stamler J. Dietary sodium, erythrocyte sodium concentration, sodium-stimulated lithium efflux and blood pressure. Clin Sci (Lond). 1981;61:29s–32s.
105. Hofman A, Hazebroek A, Valkenburg HA. A randomized trial of sodium intake and blood pressure in newborn infants. JAMA. 1983;250:370–373.
106. Cooper R, Van Horn L, Liu K, Trevisan M, Nanas S, Ueshima H, Larbi E, Yu CS, Sempos C, LeGrady D, Stamler J. A randomized trial on the effect of decreased dietary sodium intake on blood pressure in adolescents. J Hypertens. 1984;2:361–366.
107. Calabrese EJ, Tuthill RW. The Massachusetts blood pressure study, part 3. Experimental reduction of sodium in drinking water: effect on blood pressure. Toxicol Ind Health. 1985;1:19–34.
108. Howe PRC, Jureidini KF, Smith RM. Sodium and blood pressure in children—a short-term dietary intervention study. Proc Nutr Soc Aust. 1985;10:121–124.
109. Tuthill RW, Calabrese EJ. The Massachusetts Blood Pressure Study, Part 4. Modest sodium supplementation and blood pressure change in boarding school girls. Toxicol Ind Health. 1985;1:35–43.
110. Tochikubo O, Sasaki O, Umemura S, Kaneko Y. Management of hypertension in high school students by using new salt titrator tape. Hypertension. 1986;8(12):1164–1171.
111. Ellison RC, Capper AL, Stephenson WP, Goldberg RJ, Hosmer DW Jr, Humphrey KF, Ockene JK, Gamble WJ, Witschi JC, Stare FJ. Effects on blood pressure of a decrease in sodium use in institutional food preparation: the Exeter-Andover Project. J Clin Epidemiol. 1989;42:201–208.
112. Myers JB. Reduced sodium chloride intake normalises blood pressure distribution. J Hum Hypertens. 1989;3:97–104.
113. Howe PRC, Cobiac L, Smith RM. Lack of effect of short-term changes in sodium intake on blood pressure in adolescent schoolchildren. J Hypertens. 1991;9:181–186.
114. Mu JJ, Liu ZQ, Liu WM, Liang YM, Yang DY, Zhu DJ, Wang ZX. Reduction of blood pressure with calcium and potassium supplementation in children with salt sensitivity: a 2-year double-blinded placebo-controlled trial. J Hum Hypertens. Jun 2005;19:479–483.

16 Ethnic Differences in Childhood Blood Pressure

Gregory A. Harshfield, PhD

CONTENTS

ETHNIC DIFFERENCES IN HYPERTENSION, MORBIDITY, AND MORTALITY

Ethnic differences in essential hypertension (EH) and blood pressure-related morbidity and mortality are well established. According to the 2009 report from the American Heart Association *(1)*, the prevalence of essential hypertension in blacks in the United States is among the highest in the world and continues to increase. From 1988–1994 to 1999–2002, the prevalence of EH in black adults increased by 5.6% (35.8–41.4%), and it was particularly high among black women at 44.0%. In contrast, the prevalence among white adults increased by only 1.8% (24.3–28.1%) *(2)*. Hypertension in blacks contributed to a 1.3 times greater rate of nonfatal stroke, a 1.8 times greater rate of fatal stroke, a 1.5 times greater rate of heart disease death, and a 4.2 times greater rate of end-stage kidney disease *(1)*.

G.A. Harshfield (✉)
Department of Pediatrics, Medical College of Georgia, The Georgia Prevention Institute, Augusta, GA, USA
e-mail: gharshfi@mail.mcg.edu

From: *Clinical Hypertension and Vascular Diseases: Pediatric Hypertension*
Edited by: J. T. Flynn et al. DOI 10.1007/978-1-60327-824-9_16
© Springer Science+Business Media, LLC 2011

DO ETHNIC DIFFERENCES IN BLOOD PRESSURE BEGIN IN YOUTH?

It is not clear when ethnic differences in blood pressure (BP) or EH become apparent. In the most recent edition of the *Hypertension Primer*, Morgenstern and Sinaiko *(3)* state "No significant differences have been found in blood pressure until adolescence." However, we identified in 56 studies that reported data for casual BP on black and white youth. Of these, 33 (62%) reported higher BPs for blacks, 10 (18%) reported higher BPs for whites, and 13 (23%) reported no differences. In 1993 Alpert and Fox *(4)* reviewed and performed a meta-analyses in which they observed that blacks had higher BP in 50% (19/38) of the comparisons for subjects 0–12 years, 66% (33/50) of the comparisons for subjects 13–18 years, 80% (4/5) of the comparisons for 19–24 years, and 100% (10/10) of the comparisons across the multiple age range. Overall, these data suggest that ethnic differences may not become apparent until an older age. Consistent with this hypothesis are the results of a study by Manatunga et al. *(5)* that examined ethnic differences in a prospective longitudinal assessment of BP in 345 white children and 164 black children. Each child had their BP measured every 6 months for 2–5.5 years. The mean BP and the mean rate of increase in BP over time were compared between gender-specific black and white groups. For both boys and girls, the mean systolic BP was 2 mmHg higher in black children than white children and the mean diastolic BP was 1.5 mmHg higher in black children than in white children. More importantly, the rate of increase in BP over time was significantly greater in blacks than whites. Voors et al. *(6)* reported on data from the Bogalusa Heart study. Black children had significantly higher BP than white children. This difference, starting before age 10, was largest in the children in the upper 5% of the BP ranks. Daniels et al. *(7)* evaluated ethnic differences in BP in girls aged 9–10 years in the National Heart, Lung, and Blood Institute Growth and Health Study (NGHS) and the extent to which these differences were explained by sexual maturation and body size. The NGHS enrolled 539 black and 616 white girls aged 9 years and 674 black and 550 white girls aged 10 years. The black girls compared to white girls had significantly higher systolic and diastolic BP (102/58 vs 100/56 mmHg). The stage of maturation was found to account for the difference. Daniels concluded that the effect of sexual maturation on BP appears to operate through height and body fat and that the effect of obesity may be more important for systolic BP than diastolic BP. Another study by Daniels et al. *(8)* assessed the longitudinal changes in BP in black and white adolescent girls and evaluated potential determinants of changes in BP, again including sexual maturation and body size. A total of 1213 black and 1166 white girls, aged 9 or 10 years at study entry, were followed up through age 14 with annual measurements of height, weight, skinfold thickness, stage of sexual maturation, BP, and other cardiovascular risk factors. Average BPs in black girls were generally 1–2 mmHg higher than in white girls of similar age over the course of the study. Age, race, stage of sexual maturation, height, and body mass index (kg/m^2) were all significant predictors of systolic BP and diastolic BP in longitudinal regression analyses. They observed that ethnic differences in BP were seen at all stages of maturation indicating additional factors are also important. Body mass index (BMI) had a lesser impact on BP in black girls; however, BMI increased at a greater rate with age in black girls which may have contributed to the ethnic differences in BP. Overall, in their study at higher BMIs there are no ethnic differences in BP; however, at lower BMIs black girls had higher BPs, which were not accounted for by maturation differences. Between ages 9 and 14, BMI increased with age at a greater rate in black girls, which helped account for the maintenance of ethnic differences in BP between ages 9 and 14. Liebman et al. *(9)* assessed BP levels, anthropometric parameters, and dietary intakes in 1981 and 1983 in a population of black ($n = 236$) and white ($n = 296$) adolescent girls aged 14 and 16 years in 1983. The 14-year-old black girls exhibited significantly higher mean SBP and DBPs than whites in both years. Body weight and Quetelet index were more strongly associated with BP than were height and triceps skinfold thickness. Rabinowitz et al. *(10)* assessed differences in the prevalence of BP ≥95th% (i.e., EH on an initial screening of 3349 students by race, sex, and age. The overall prevalence of EH in this urban adolescent population was 8.1%. Significant ethnic differences were present in females (blacks = 6.6% vs non-Hispanics = 2.9%, $p < 0.01$). Within the black females, EH occurred more frequently among the girls attending predominantly black public schools (7.7%) compared to an interracial parochial school (2.0%), $p < 0.001$. This difference could not be explained by weight, height, or the occurrence of obesity. However, the prevalence of obesity was higher in the adolescents with EH and among females with EH. Obesity was also present in a greater number of blacks than whites. The observed BP differences within black females, by school, may reflect a family–environment effect on cardiovascular risk.

In contrast to the studies cited above, other studies have not observed ethnic differences in BP. Rosner et al. *(11)* analyzed BPs from eight large epidemiologic studies published between 1978 and 1991 that included measurements of 47,196 children on 68,556 occasions for systolic BP and of 38,184 children on 52,053 occasions for diastolic BP. They conclude that "there are few substantive ethnic differences in either SBP or DBP during childhood and adolescence. The differences that were observed were small, inconsistent, and often explained by differences in body size." A longitudinal study by Baron et al. *(12)* did not find " substantial" ethnic differences in BPs between blacks, whites, and Mexican Americans prior to 20 years of age. Morrison et al. *(13)* also did not find ethnic differences in a biracial group of 682 schoolchildren, aged 6 through 19. Hohn et al. *(14)* assessed racial differences in BP levels in youth of Asian, black, Hispanic, and non-Hispanic white descent. They obtained BP measurements from 4577 ninth grade students during the spring of the years 1985–1989 (39% black, 30% Hispanic, 21% white, 10% Asian; 50% female) with a mean age of 15 years. They found no differences between black and white youth.

ETHNIC DIFFERENCES IN AMBULATORY BLOOD PRESSURE MONITORING

Ambulatory BP monitoring (ABPM) has become the standard for many physicians and scientists for the identification of individuals with EH and to assess the effectiveness of treatment *(12,15–21)*. ABPM has been proven to be superior to casual BP for the prediction of cardiovascular morbidity and mortality *(22–29)*. The use of ABPM is also recommended for use in children and adolescents *(30)* in whom it has been proven to be cost effective *(31)*.

In 1987, we presented data at the Interdisciplinary Conference On Hypertension in Blacks *(32)* from 35 black adults that showed a blunted nocturnal decline in BP, now referred to as non-dipping. Specifically, the subjects only showed about a 10% drop in BP from daytime to nighttime compared to a 15% drop which we had previously observed in white patients. This was the first report to our knowledge of this pattern in a healthy population. This ethnic difference has now been reported in a multitude of studies by many groups and is a well-established finding (for reviews, see *(33–35)*). Several studies demonstrated the clinical significance of the blunted nocturnal decline in BP in blacks. Fumo et al. *(36)* were the first to report that the pattern was associated with target organ changes to the heart, a finding confirmed by Mayet et al. *(37)* and Olutade et al. *(38)*. We demonstrated that the blunted nocturnal decline in black adolescents is associated with decreased renal function *(39)*. We also reported that the ethnic difference in ABPM is already apparent during adolescence *(40–43)*. Most recently, Wang et al. *(44)* of our group reported data for race differences in ABPM derived from a longitudinal study conducted at the GPI. Recordings were measured up to 12 times over 15 years for 312 black and 351 white subjects. We found significant ethnic differences in longitudinal trajectories. Black males had higher levels than white males and females, and black males and females showed a faster increase of BP with age, with greater differences in nighttime systolic BP than daytime BP.

Further studies identified factors related to the difference. Two of these factors, fitness *(45)* and body size *(46)*, are clearly related. Both decreased fitness level and increased body size had a greater effect on nighttime BP of African-Americans than Caucasians. The third factor was sodium intake *(47)*. We observed that sodium intake as determined by excretion was related to daytime and nighttime BP in African-Americans but not Caucasians. These findings are consistent with the well-known differences in the influence of sodium intake on casual BP (for recent reviews, see *(48–51)*). Further studies demonstrated that the differences in patterns are stable over time *(42,44)*.

ETHNIC DIFFERENCES IN BP-RELATED TARGET ORGAN DAMAGE IN YOUTH

Some studies suggest that black adolescents are characterized by greater BP-related target organ damage, although these findings are not universal. Burke et al. *(52)* using data from the Bogalusa Heart study did not observe ethnic differences for subjects aged 7–22. Daniels et al. *(53,54)* reported similar findings. Schieken et al. *(55)* reported data on twins aged 11–17 across 5 years. Blacks had greater left ventricular mass in visit that was not sustained across the visits. In contrast, we reported *(42)* greater LV mass in blacks with a mean age of 13 years which was associated with higher nighttime BP. Consistent with these results, Dekkers et al. *(56)* reported that ethnic differences in LV mass were expressed in early adolescence, and they persisted when controlling for socioeconomic status and anthropometric and hemodynamic variables. In another study, Kapuku et al. *(57)* reported data on a sample of 147 subjects aged 1–19 years tested on two occasions. Blacks compared to whites had greater relative wall thickness and left ventricular mass coupled with lower midwall fractional shortening ratio on both occasions.

We have also reported greater BP-related target organ damage to the kidney in black adolescents *(58)*. Specifically, in a sample of 317 adolescents, the blacks compared to whites had an approximately 10% greater rate of excretion of microalbumin. This pattern was in turn associated with impaired sodium regulation.

MECHANISMS UNDERLYING ETHIC DIFFERENCES IN BLOOD PRESSURE IN YOUTH

Many factors have been hypothesized to account for ethnic differences in BP and ABPM. These include genetic factors that control BP regulatory systems including the renin–angiotensin–aldosterone system, the sympathetic nervous system, the endothelial system, and inflammatory responses. We have been examining factors related to differences in BP regulation and the development of BP-related target organ damage within the Black pediatric population. Impaired sodium regulation is hypothesized to underlie the development and maintenance of EH in a significant percent of the hypertensive population. This is particularly true for high-risk populations that are characterized by a volume-dependent form of EH, including blacks and obese individuals (for recent reviews, see *(48–51)*). The hypothesis is based on the premise that BP is to maintain sodium homeostasis or sodium balance. This is accomplished by what is referred to as the renal-body fluid system *(59)*. The system operates as follows: a fall in BP such as would occur with severe hemorrhage increases the kidney's reabsorption of both water and sodium. This increases intracellular fluid volume, blood volume, and cardiac output to maintain BP and blood flow to the brain. Alternatively, an increase in BP increases the kidney's excretion of water (pressure diuresis) and sodium (pressure natriuresis), leading to a decrease in intracellular fluid volume and blood volume. This reduces cardiac output, which lowers BP. In normal individuals sodium homeostasis is maintained across a wide range of sodium intakes. In contrast, a higher level of BP is required to maintain sodium balance at high salt intake in individuals with a reduced ability to excrete sodium.

Blacks have a greater prevalence of stress-induced sodium retention. Light and Turner *(60)* examined 28 adults which included 14 blacks and 14 whites. The blacks had lower sodium excretion during a 1-h stress period, with a reduction in sodium excretion for 6 of the 14 black and 2 of the 14 white subjects. We *(61)* next reported race differences in stress-induced sodium retention using a protocol that examined concurrent changes in BP and sodium excretion across a series of tasks (playing video games, ice to forehead) in black and white youths with a positive family history of EH. The blacks had a greater increase in BP coupled with a smaller increase in sodium excretion averaged across the tasks. A second study *(62)* by our group tested 118 black youth. Of these, 38 (32%) retained sodium during stress. Sodium retention resulted in a cardiac output-related increase in BP across the stress period. This contrasted with the subjects that showed the expected increase in sodium during stress period was related to total peripheral resistance. Significantly, sodium retention resulted in a delay in the return of BP to pre-stress levels. This would be expected with the volume-mediated increase in BP which remains elevated until the volume expansion diminishes. As such, these individuals were exposed to a greater BP load than those individuals with the normal pressure natriuresis response. The third study by our group examined the interaction between race and sex on stress-induced sodium retention *(63)*. The 190 subjects included 94 boys (41 black, 53 white) and 96 girls (44 black, 52 white). Whites compared to blacks had a greater change in sodium excretion, as did boys compared to girls. The race by sex interaction was significant for the change in systolic BP, with white girls showing a smaller change than the other three race/sex groups.

Stress-induced sodium retention has also been demonstrated in animal models of EH. The initial report by Friedman and Iwai *(64)* was published in *Science* in 1976. They demonstrated that behavioral stress hastened the development of EH in Dahl salt-sensitive rats, a strain genetically predisposed to develop salt-sensitive EH. Koepke and his colleagues *(65,66)* performed a comprehensive series of studies on stress-induced sodium retention. They were among the first to describe stress-induced sodium retention in the spontaneously hypertensive rat model. They also demonstrated that high dietary sodium intake augmented the responses and that renal denervation corrected the impairment independent of sodium intake. Further studies localized two areas of the brain which contribute to this response pattern. Both of these areas are known to be involved in the perception of stress. Specifically, injection of a beta-2 receptor antagonist into the posterior hypothalamus or an alpha-2 receptor agonist into the amagdaloid nucleus abolished the renal responses. A subsequent study and more recent studies by others *(67–69)* suggest that the anti-natriuretic actions of stress-induced efferent renal sympathetic activity are the result of both direct actions on the kidney and resultant increases in angiotensin II. Lawler and Cox *(70)* developed an animal model of EH which they called the borderline hypertensive rat. The strain is normotensive unless it is exposed to either chronic stress or a high-sodium diet. Furthermore, stress-induced EH is associated with suppressed plasma renin activity, implicating impaired regulation of the renin–angiotensin–aldosterone system *(71)*. Of particular interest for the current study was the finding that this strain showed delayed recovery from an aversive conditioning task *(72)*. DiBona utilized the borderline hypertensive rat strain to examine the impact of stress on the development of EH. These studies confirmed previous results that demonstrated that the stress-induced sodium retention was the result of an increase in efferent renal sympathetic nerve activity *(73–77)*. A series of studies by Anderson et al. *(78–81)* examined the relationship between stress and sodium regulation in dogs. Their basic protocol was to expose two groups of dogs to avoidance conditioning training for 30 min a day for 15 days. One group was on a normal diet, and a second group received a constant rate of infusion of 185 mEq of sodium. The sodium-loaded dogs had a rapid development of EH. The EH was associated with immediate and sustained reductions in sodium excretion.

SUMMARY AND CONCLUSION

Overall, the studies suggest that black adolescents have higher levels of BP than their white counterparts. Furthermore, the differences are related to the premature development of BP-related target organ damage to the heart, vasculature, and kidneys. Of interest has been the research on the physiological mechanisms underlying differences within the black population. These data suggest significant heterogeneity in the mechanisms underlying BP regulation which is important for the treatment of hypertension in this population.

REFERENCES

1. Lloyd-Jones D, Adams R, Carnethon M, De Simone G, Ferguson TB, Flegal K, Ford E, Furie K, Go A, Greenlund K, Haase N, Hailpern S, Ho M, Howard V, Kissela B, Kittner S, Lackland D, Lisabeth L, Marelli A, McDermott M, Meigs J, Mozaffarian D, Nichol G, O'Donnell C, Roger V, Rosamond W, Sacco R, Sorlie P, Stafford R, Steinberger J, Thom T, Wasserthiel-Smoller S, Wong N, Wylie-Rosett J, Hong Y. Heart disease and stroke statistics—2009 update: a report from the American Heart Association Statistics Committee and Stroke Statistics Subcommittee. Circulation. Jan 27 2009;119(3):e21–e181.
2. Hertz RP, Unger AN, Cornell JA, Saunders E. Racial disparities in hypertension prevalence, awareness, and management. Arch Int Med. Oct 10 2005;165(18):2098–2104.
3. Morgenstern BZ, Sinaiko AR. Blood pressure in children. In: Izzo JL, Sica DA, Black HR, eds. Hypertension Primer, 4th ed. Philadelphia, PA: Lippencott, Williams & Wilkins; 2008:273–275.
4. Alpert BS, Fox ME. Racial aspects of blood pressure in children and adolescents. Pediatr Clin North Am. 1993;40:13–22.
5. Manatunga AK, Jones JJ, Pratt JH. Longitudinal assessment of blood pressure in black and white children. Hypertension. 1993;22:84–89.
6. Voors AW, Foster TA, Fredichs RR, Webber LS, Berenson GS. Studies of blood pressure in children, ages 5 to 14 years, in a total biracial community: the Bogalusa Heart Study. Circulation. 1976;54:319–327.
7. Daniels SR, Obarzanek E, Barton BA, Kimm SYS, Similo SL, Morrison JA. Sexual maturation and racial differences in blood pressure in girls: the National Heart, Lung, and Blood Institute Growth and Health Study. J Pediatr. 1996;129:208–213.
8. Daniels SR, McMahon RP, Obarzanek E, Waclawiw MA, Similo SL, Biro FM, Schreiber GB, Kimm SY, Morrison JA, Barton BA. Longitudinal correlates of change in blood pressure in adolescent girls. Hypertension. Jan 1998;31(1):97–103.

9. Liebman M, Chopin LF, Carter E, Clark AJ, Disney GW, Hegsted M, Kenney MA, Kirmani ZA, Koonce KL, Korslund MK, et al. Factors related to blood pressure in a biracial adolescent female population. Hypertension. Oct 1986;8(10):843–850.

10. Rabinowitz A, Kushner H, Falkner B. Racial differences in blood pressure among urban adolescents. J Adolesc Health. Jun 1993;14(4):314–318.

11. Rosner B, Prineas R, Daniels SR, Loggie J. Blood pressure differences between blacks and whites in relation to body size among US children and adolescents. Am J Epidemiol. May 15 2000;151(10): 1007–1019.

12. Baron AE, Freyer B, Fixler DE. Longitudinal blood pressures in blacks, whites, and Mexican Americans during adolescence and early adulthood. Am J Epidemiol. May 1986;123(5):809–817.

13. Morrison JA, Khoury P, Kelly K, Mellies MJ, Parrish E, Heiss G, Tyroler H, Glueck CJ. Studies of blood pressure in schoolchildren (ages 6–19) and their parents in an integrated suburban school district. Am J Epidemiol. Feb 1980;111(2):156–165.

14. Hohn AR, Dwyer KM, Dwyer JH. Blood pressure in youth from four ethnic groups: the Pasadena Prevention Project. J Pediatr. Sep 1994;125(3):368–373.

15. O'Brien E, Cox JP, O'Malley K. Ambulatory blood pressure measurement in the evaluation of blood pressure lowering drugs. J Hypertens. 1989;7:243–247.

16. Townsend RR, Ford V. Ambulatory blood pressure monitoring: coming of age in nephrology. J Am Soc Nephrol. Nov 1996;7(11):2279–2287.

17. White WB. Ambulatory blood-pressure monitoring in clinical practice. N Engl J Med. Jun 12 2003;348(24):2377–2378.

18. Pickering TG, Shimbo D, Haas D. Ambulatory blood-pressure monitoring. New Engl J Med. Jun 1 2006;354(22):2368–2374.

19. Conen D, Bamberg F. Noninvasive 24-h ambulatory blood pressure and cardiovascular disease: a systematic review and meta-analysis. J Hypertens. Jul 2008;26(7):1290–1299.

20. O'Brien E. Ambulatory blood pressure measurement: the case for implementation in primary care. Hypertension. Jun 2008;51(6):1435–1441.

21. Chavanu K, Merkel J, Quan AM. Role of ambulatory blood pressure monitoring in the management of hypertension. Am J Health Syst Pharm. Feb 1 2008;65(3):209–218.

22. Perloff D, Sokolow M, Cowan R. The prognostic value of ambulatory blood pressure. JAMA. 1983;249:2793–2798.

23. Pessina AC, Palatini P, DiMarco A, Mormino P, Fazio G, Libardoni M, Mos L, Casiglia E, DalPalu C. Continuous ambulatory blood pressure monitoring versus casual blood pressure in borderline hypertension. J Cardiovasc Pharm. 1986;8(Suppl 5):S93–S97.

24. Pickering TG, Devereux RB. Prediction of cardiovascular morbidity from ambulatory blood pressure monitoring. In: Meyer-Sabellek W, Anlauf M, Gotzen R, Steinfeld L, eds. Blood Pressure Measurements: New Techniques in Automatic and 24-hour Indirect Monitoring. Darmstadt: Steinkopff-Verlag; 1990:327–333.

25. Mancia G, Zanchetti A, Agabiti-Rosei E, Benemio G, De Cesaris R, Fogari R, Pessina A, Porcellati C, Rappelli A, Salvetti A, Trimarco B. Ambulatory blood pressure is superior to clinic blood pressure in predicting treatment-induced regression of left ventricular hypertrophy. SAMPLE Study Group. Study on Ambulatory Monitoring of Blood Pressure and Lisinopril Evaluation. Circulation. Mar 18 1997;95(6):1464–1470.

26. Devereux RB, Pickering TG, Harshfield GA, Kleinert HD, Denby L, Clark L, Pregibon D, Jason M, Kleiner B, Borer JS, Laragh JH. Left ventricular hypertrophy in patients with hypertension: importance of blood pressure response to regularly recurring stress. Circulation. Sep 1983;68(3):470–476.

27. Ohkubo T, Hozawa A, Nagai K, Kikuya M, Tsuji I, Ito S, Satoh H, Hisamichi S, Imai Y. Prediction of stroke by ambulatory blood pressure monitoring versus screening blood pressure measurements in a general population: the Ohasama study. J Hypertens. 2000;18(7):847–854.

28. Verdecchia P, Porcellati C, Schillaci G, Borgioni C, Ciucci A, Battistelli M, Guerrieri M, Gatteschi C, Zampi I, Santucci A, et al. Ambulatory blood pressure. An independent predictor of prognosis in essential hypertension. Hypertension. Dec 1994;24(6):793–801.

29. Kikuya M, Hansen TW, Thijs L, Bjorklund-Bodegard K, Kuznetsova T, Ohkubo T, Richart T, Torp-Pedersen C, Lind L, Ibsen H, Imai Y, Staessen JA. Diagnostic thresholds for ambulatory blood pressure monitoring based on 10-year cardiovascular risk. Circulation. Apr 24 2007;115(16):2145–2152.

30. Urbina E, Alpert B, Flynn J, Hayman L, Harshfield GA, Jacobson M, Mahoney L, McCrindle B, Mietus-Snyder M, Steinberger J, Daniels S. Ambulatory blood pressure monitoring in children and adolescents: recommendations for standard assessment: a scientific statement from the American Heart Association Atherosclerosis, Hypertension, and Obesity in Youth Committee of the council on cardiovascular disease in the young and the council for high blood pressure research. Hypertension. Sep 2008;52(3):433–451.

31. Swartz SJ, Srivaths PR, Croix B, Feig DI. Cost-effectiveness of ambulatory blood pressure monitoring in the initial evaluation of hypertension in children. Pediatrics. Dec 2008;122(6):1177–1181.

32. Harshfield GA, Hwang C, Edmundson J, Flores F, Grim CE. Circadian rhythm of blood pressure in blacks. Paper presented at International Conference on Hypertension in Blacks, Atlanta, 1987.
33. Harshfield GA, Treiber FA. Racial differences in ambulatory blood pressure monitoring-derived 24 h patterns of blood pressure in adolescents. Blood Press Monit. 1999;4(3):197–110.
34. Profant J, Dimsdale JE. Race and diurnal blood pressure patterns: a review and meta-analysis. Hypertension. 1999;33(5):1099–1104.
35. Harshfield GA, Wilson M. Ethnic differences in childhood blood pressure. In: Portman RJ, Sorof JM, Inglefinger J, eds. Pediatric Hypertension, Vol 1. Totowa, NJ: Humana Press; 2004:293–305.
36. Fumo M, Teeger S, Lang R, Bednarz J, Sareli P, Murphy M. Diurnal blood pressure variation and cardiac mass in American blacks and whites and South African blacks. Am J Hypertens. 1992;5:111–116.
37. Mayet J, Chapman N, Li CK, Shahi M, Poulter NR, Sever PS, Foale RA, Thom SA. Ethnic differences in the hypertensive heart and 24-hour blood pressure profile. Hypertension. 1998;31(5):1190–1194.
38. Olutade BO, Gbadebo TD, Porter VD, Wilkening B, Hall WD. Racial differences in ambulatory blood pressure and echocardiographic left ventricular geometry. Am J Med Sci. Feb 1998;315(2):101–109.
39. Harshfield G, Pulliam D, Alpert B. Ambulatory blood pressure and renal function in healthy children and adolescents. Am J Hypertens. 1994;7:282–285.
40. Harshfield GA, Alpert BS, Willey ES, Somes GW, Murphy JK, Dupaul LM. Race and gender influence ambulatory blood pressure patterns of adolescents. Hypertension. Dec 1989;14(6):598–603.
41. Harshfield GA, Pulliam DA, Alpert BS. Ambulatory blood pressure and renal function in healthy children and adolescents. Am J Hypertens. Mar 1994;7(3):282–285.
42. Harshfield GA, Treiber FA, Wilson ME, Kapuku GK, Davis HC. A longitudinal study of ethnic differences in ambulatory blood pressure patterns in youth. Am J Hypertens. Jun 2002;15(6):525–530.
43. Harshfield GA, Wilson ME, Treiber FA, Alpert BS. A comparison of ambulatory blood pressure patterns across populations. Blood Press Monit. Oct 2002;7(5):265–269.
44. Wang X, Poole JC, Treiber FA, Harshfield GA, Hanevold CD, Snieder H. Ethnic and gender differences in ambulatory blood pressure trajectories: results from a 15-year longitudinal study in youth and young adults. Circulation. Dec 19 2006;114(25):2780–2787.
45. Harshfield GA, Dupaul LM, Alpert BS, Christman JV, Willey ES, Murphy JK, Somes GW. Aerobic fitness and the diurnal rhythm of blood pressure in adolescents. Hypertension. 1990;15:810–814.
46. Harshfield GA, Barbeau P, Richey PA, Alpert BS. Racial differences in the influence of body size on ambulatory blood pressure in youths. Blood Press Monit. 2000;5(2):59–63.
47. Harshfield GA, Alpert BS, Pulliam DA, Willey ES, Somes GW, Stapelton FB. Sodium excretion and racial differences in ambulatory blood pressure patterns. Hypertension. Dec 1991;18(6):813–818.
48. Franco V, Oparil S. Salt sensitivity, a determinant of blood pressure, cardiovascular disease and survival. J Am Coll Nutr. Jun 2006;25(3 Suppl):247S–255S.
49. Weinberger MH. Pathogenesis of salt sensitivity of blood pressure. Curr Hypertens Rep. May 2006;8(2):166–170.
50. Orlov SN, Mongin AA. Salt-sensing mechanisms in blood pressure regulation and hypertension. Am J Physiol. Oct 2007;293(4):H2039–H2053.
51. Rodriguez-Iturbe B, Romero F, Johnson RJ. Pathophysiological mechanisms of salt-dependent hypertension. Am J Kidney Dis. Oct 2007;50(4):655–672.
52. Burke GL, Arcilla RA, Culpepper WS, Webber LS, Chiang YK, Berenson GS. Blood pressure and echocardiographic measures in children: the Bogalusa Heart Study. Circulation. Jan 1987;75(1):106–114.
53. Daniels SR, Meyer RA, Liang YC, Bove KE. Echocardiographically determined left ventricular mass index in normal children, adolescents and young adults. J Am Coll Cardiol. Sep 1988;12(3):703–708.
54. Daniels SR, Meyer RA, Strife CF, Lipman M, Loggie JM. Distribution of target-organ abnormalities by race and sex in children with essential hypertension. J Hum Hypertens. Apr 1990;4(2):103–104.
55. Schieken RM, Schwartz PF, Goble M. Tracking of left ventricular mass in children: race and sex comparisons: The MCVTwin Study. Circulation. 1998;97:1901–1906.
56. Dekkers C, Treiber FA, Kapuku G, Van Den Oord EJ, Snieder H. Growth of left ventricular mass in African American and European American youth. Hypertension. May 2002;39(5):943–951.
57. Kapuku GK, Treiber FA, Davis HC, Harshfield GA, Cook BB, Mensah GA. Hemodynamic function at rest, during acute stress, and in the field: predictors of cardiac structure and function 2 years later in youth. Hypertension. 1999;34(5):1026–1031.
58. Hanevold CD, Pollock JS, Harshfield GA. Racial differences in microalbumin excretion in healthy adolescents. Hypertension. Feb 2008;51(2):334–338.
59. Guyton AC. Textbook of Medical Physiology, 8th ed. Philadelphia, PA: W.B. Saunders Company; 1991.
60. Light KC, Turner JR. Stress-induced changes in the rate of sodium excretion in healthy black and white men. J Psychosom Res. 1992;36:497–508.

61. Harshfield GA, Treiber FA, Davis H, Kapuku GK. Impaired stress-induced pressure natriuresis is related to left ventricle structure in blacks. Hypertension. Apr 2002;39(4):844–847.
62. Harshfield G, Wilson M, Hanevold C, Kapuku G, Mackey L, Gillis D, Treiber F. Impaired stress-induced pressure natriuresis increases cardiovascular load in African American youths. Am J Hypertens. Oct 2002;15(10):903–906.
63. Harshfield GA, Hanevold C, Kapuku GK, Dong Y, Castles ME, Ludwig DA. The association of race and sex to the pressure natriuresis response to stress. Ethn Dis. 2007;17:498–302.
64. Friedman R, Iwai J. Genetic predisposition and stress-induced hypertension. Science. 1976;193:161–163.
65. Koepke JP, Copp UC, DiBona GF. The kidney in the pathogenesis of hypertension: role of the renal nerves. In: Kaplan N, Brenner B, Laragh J, eds. The Kidney in Hypertension, Vol 1. New York, NY: Raven Press; 1987:53–65.
66. Koepke JP. Effect of environmental stress on neural control of renal function. Miner Electrolyte Metab. 1989;15(1–2):83–87.
67. Veelken R, Hilgers KF, Stetter A, Siebert HG, Schmieder RE, Mann JF. Nerve-mediated antidiuresis and antinatriuresis after air-jet stress is modulated by angiotensin II. Hypertension. 1996;28(5):825–832.
68. Le Fevre ME, Guild SJ, Ramchandra R, Barrett CJ, Malpas SC. Role of angiotensin II in the neural control of renal function. Hypertension. Mar 2003;41(3):583–591.
69. Wagner C, Hinder M, Kramer BK, Kurtz A. Role of renal nerves in the stimulation of the renin system by reduced renal arterial pressure. Hypertension. 1999;34(5):1101–1105.
70. Lawler JE, Cox RH. The borderline hypertensive rat (BHR): a new model for the study of environmental factors in the development of hypertension. Pavlov J Biol Sci. 1985;20:101–115.
71. Lawler JE, Barker GF, Hubbard JW, Cox RH, Randall GW. Blood pressure and plasma renin activity response to chronic stress in the borderline hypertensive rat. Physiol Behav. 1984;32:101–105.
72. Sanders BJ, Cox RH, Lawler JE. Cardiovascular and renal responses to stress in borderline hypertensive rats. Am J Physiol. 1988;255:R431–R438.
73. DiBona GF. Stress and sodium intake in neural control of renal function in hypertension. Hypertension. 1991;17(Suppl III):III-2–III-6.
74. DiBona GF, Jones SY. Effect of acute NaCl depletion on NaCl-sensitive hypertension in borderline hypertensive rats. J Hypertens. 1992;10:125–129.
75. DiBona GF, Jones SY. Renal manifestations of NaCl sensitivity in borderline hypertensive rats. Hypertension. 1991;17:44–53.
76. DiBona GF, Sawin LL. Renal nerves in renal adaptation to dietary sodium restriction. Am J Physiol. 1983;245:F322–F328.
77. DiBona GF, Kopp UC. Neural control of renal function. Physiol Rev. 1977;77:75–197.
78. Anderson DE, Kearns WD, Belter WE. Progressive hypertension in dogs by avoidance conditioning and saline infusion. Hypertension. 1983;5:286–291.
79. Anderson DE, Dietz JR, Murphy P. Behavioral hypertension in sodium-loaded dogs is accompanied by sustained sodium retention. J Hypertens. 1986;5(1):101–105.
80. Anderson DE, Gomez-Sanchez C, Dietz JR. Suppression of renin and aldosterone in stress-salt hypertension in the dog. Am J Physiol. 1986;251:R181–R186.
81. Anderson DE, Gomez-Sanchez C, Dietz JR. Suppression of plasma renin and aldosterone in stress-salt hypertension in dogs. Am J Physiol. 1986;251(Regul Integr Comp Physiol 20):R181–R186.

17 Childhood Obesity and Blood Pressure Regulation

Albert P. Rocchini, MD

INTRODUCTION

Childhood obesity is the most common nutritional problem in children from both developed and non-developed countries. From the 1960s to 1990s, the prevalence of obesity in children grew from 5 to 11% *(1)*. In adults, obesity is recognized as an independent risk factor for the development of both hypertension and cardiovascular disease. In childhood there are data to demonstrate a strong relationship between childhood obesity and hypertension, type 2 diabetes mellitus, dyslipidemia, obstructive sleep apnea, left ventricular hypertrophy, and orthopedic problems. This chapter will summarize (1) the epidemiologic evidence that substantiates obesity as an independent risk factor for the development of hypertension in

A.P. Rocchini (✉)
Department of Pediatric Cardiology, C.S. Mott Children's Hospital, University of Michigan Medical School,
Ann Arbor, MI, USA
e-mail: rocchini@umich.edu

From: *Clinical Hypertension and Vascular Diseases: Pediatric Hypertension*
Edited by: J. T. Flynn et al. DOI 10.1007/978-1-60327-824-9_17
© Springer Science+Business Media, LLC 2011

both adults and children; (2) an explanation of how obesity may cause hypertension; (3) a brief summary of other cardiovascular abnormalities associated with obesity; and (4) a brief summary of how to manage the hypertensive obese child.

RELATIONSHIP BETWEEN OBESITY AND HIGH BLOOD PRESSURE

Epidemiological Studies Linking Obesity to Hypertension

The association between obesity and hypertension has been recognized since the early 1900s. Several large epidemiological studies documented the association between increasing body weight and an increase in blood pressure (2–13). For example, Symonds (4) analyzed 150,419 policyholders in the Mutual Life Insurance Corporation and documented that systolic and diastolic blood pressure increased with both age and weight. The Framingham study (5) documented that the prevalence of hypertension in obese individuals was twice that of those individuals who were normal weight. This relationship held up in all age groups of both women and men.

The association of obesity and hypertension in children has also been well documented. Rosner and co-workers (14) pooled data from eight large US epidemiological studies involving over 47,000 children. Irrespective of race, gender, and age, the risk of elevated blood pressure was significantly higher for children in the upper compared to the lower decile of body mass index. Freedman et al. (15) reported that overweight children were 4.5–2.4 times as likely to have elevated systolic and diastolic blood pressure. Similarly, Sorof et al. (16) reported a three times greater prevalence of hypertension in obese compared to non-obese adolescents in a school-based hypertension and obesity screening study. Thus, a large number of population-based studies have documented a strong association between obesity and hypertension in both sexes, in all age groups and for virtually every geographical and ethnic groups.

Relationship of Weight Gain to Blood Pressure Level

There have been no studies in humans that have investigated the effect of weight gain on blood pressure. However, in the dog, it has been shown that weight gain is directly related to an increase in blood pressure. Cash and Wood in 1938 (17) demonstrated that weight gain caused dogs with renal vascular hypertension to further increase their blood pressure. Rocchini et al. (18,19) and Hall et al. (20) found that normal mongrel dogs fed a high-fat diet gained weight and developed hypertension. In these dogs the hypertension was associated with sodium retention, hyperinsulinemia, and activation of the sympathetic nervous system.

Effect of Weight Loss on Blood Pressure Level

Weight loss is associated with a lowering of blood pressure. Haynes (21) reviewed the literature up to the mid-1980s on the relationship of weight loss to reductions in arterial pressure. He used strict criteria to examine only well-done studies and noted that there were only six studies available. Three of the six studies that meet Haynes criteria demonstrated a clear effect of weight loss on lowering arterial pressure. Many clinical trials published since the late 1970s have clearly documented the blood pressure lowering effect of weight loss (21–35). For example, the Hypertension Prevention Trial (23) documented that in individuals with borderline elevations in blood pressure a mean weight loss of 5 kg was associated with as much as a 5/3 mmHg decrease in blood pressure. Thus, based on numerous weight loss studies, calorie restriction and weight loss are associated with a reduction in blood pressure. In addition, it is clear that even modest weight loss (i.e., 10% loss of body weight) improves blood pressure, and many individuals achieve normal blood pressure levels without attaining their calculated ideal weight.

A limitation with the use of studies documenting that weight loss is associated with a reduction in blood pressure is that most studies do not address the long-term effect of weight change on blood pressure in subjects who are again placed on unrestricted diets. Dornfield and co-workers *(34)* reported that over a follow-up of 1–4 years after weight loss, changes in blood pressure still correlated with changes in body weight. However, recent data suggest that long-term weight loss may not reduce the incidence of hypertension. Sjöström et al. *(36)* compared the incidence of hypertension and diabetes in 346 patients undergoing gastric surgery with 346 obese control subjects who were matched on 18 variables. After 8 years, the surgical group had maintained a 16% weight loss, whereas the control subjects had a 1% weight gain. These investigators demonstrated that weight reduction in the surgical group had a dramatic effect on the 8-year incidence of diabetes, but had no effect on the 8-year incidence of hypertension. They *(37)* and others *(38)* previously documented that surgical weight loss positively affected blood pressure at 2 and 4 years of follow-up, but that this effect on blood pressure is lost after 8 years of follow-up. These authors have speculated "that remaining obesity in the surgically treated patients could have induced a reappearance of hypertension during the course of the study independent of ongoing weight maintenance." Therefore, Sjöström's study suggests that a relapse of hypertension after surgically induced weight loss does occur despite the maintenance of significant long-term weight loss and that the pathogenesis of recurrent hypertension is not well understood *(39)*.

Effect of Body Fat Distribution on Blood Pressure

The definition of obesity also contributes to the controversy regarding the independence of obesity as an etiological determinant of hypertension. Obesity is defined not just as an increase in body weight but rather as an increase in adipose tissue mass. Adipose tissue mass can be estimated by multiple techniques such as skinfold thickness, body mass index ([weight in kg]/[height in meters]^2), hydrostatic weighing, bioelectrical impedance, water dilution methods, computed tomography, and magnetic resonance imaging (MRI). In most clinical studies, body mass index is usually used as the index of adiposity. Obesity is generally defined as a body mass index of greater than 30 kg/m^2 in adults and >95th percentile for children and adolescents. In 1956, Jean Vague *(40)* reported that the cardiovascular and metabolic consequences of obesity were greatest in individuals whose fat distribution pattern favored the upper body segments. Since that observation, several population-based studies have demonstrated that upper body obesity is a more important cardiovascular risk factor than body mass index alone *(41–47)*. These studies suggest that increased visceral adipose tissue (VAT) as opposed to subcutaneous adipose tissue (SAT) relates better to the development of systemic hypertension. For example, the Normative Aging Study *(41)* has demonstrated that there is a significant relationship between abdominal circumference and diastolic blood pressure. In fact, the risk of developing hypertension was better predicted by upper body fat distribution than by either body weight or body mass index. Similarly, Fox et al. *(48)* demonstrated in 3001 participants from the Framingham Heart study that although both SAT and VAT are associated with the prevalence of hypertension, only VAT provides significant information above and beyond percent fat and waist circumference. In both children and young adults, Shear et al. *(42)* reported that blood pressure correlated strongly with upper body fat pattern, but not with measures of global obesity. Many investigators have demonstrated that the association of obesity to increased cardiovascular risk is primarily related to upper body adiposity *(49,50)*. There is limited information relating fat distribution to blood pressure in the pediatric population.

Finally, in dogs that develop hypertension by being fed a high-fat diet, they increase their abdominal circumference significantly more than their thoracic circumference *(51)*. MRI studies in fat-fed dogs also demonstrate a marked increase in omental and subcutaneous fat *(52)*. We also have preliminary data in dogs fed a high-fat diet that demonstrates a stronger relationship between the increase in blood pressure and the increase in abdominal circumference as compared to the increase in total body weight (Fig. 1).

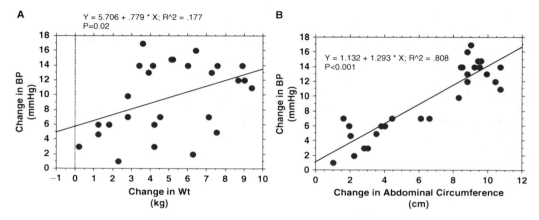

Fig. 1. The relationship between change in blood pressure and change in total body weight (panel A) or abdominal circumference (panel B) in seven dogs who received a high-fat diet for 5 weeks is depicted. Although blood pressure significantly correlates to the change in total body weight that the dogs experience when receiving the high-fat diet, the change in abdominal circumference is responsible significantly more of the variance in blood pressure.

Summary

We know that obesity is directly related to hypertension based on strong epidemiologic data, animal studies which demonstrate that weight gain causes hypertension, and many human studies which demonstrate that weight loss results in a reduction in blood pressure. In addition, it appears that it is abdominal adiposity, rather than general adiposity that is primarily related not only to the hypertension but also to the increased cardiovascular risk associated with being obese.

MECHANISM(S) WHEREBY OBESITY MIGHT CAUSE HYPERTENSION

The exact pathophysiologic mechanism whereby obesity causes hypertension is still unknown. Obesity hypertension is complex and multifactorial. It is clear that obesity hypertension directly relates to abnormal renal sodium handling and that this alteration in sodium handling is predominately mediated through activation of the sympathetic nervous system and to a lesser extent through activation of the renin–angiotensin–aldosterone system. However, what is less clear is how obesity initiates the activation of the sympathetic nervous system (Fig. 2).

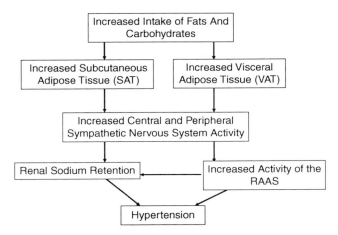

Fig. 2. A schematic representation for how the development of obesity might result in hypertension. SAT, subcutaneous adipose tissue; VAT, visceral adipose tissue; RAAS, rennin–angiotensin–aldosterone system.

Abnormal Renal Sodium Handling and Obesity Hypertension

Most investigators believe that fluid retention is the final common pathway that links obesity to hypertension. There is ample human and animal data linking obesity hypertension to fluid retention. Rocchini et al. *(33)* demonstrated that prior to weight loss, the blood pressure of a group of obese adolescents was very sensitive to dietary sodium intake; however, after weight loss, the obese adolescents lost their blood pressure sensitivity to sodium. These investigators demonstrated that when compared to non-obese adolescents, the obese adolescents have a renal-function relation (plot of urinary sodium excretion as a function of arterial pressure) that has a shallower slope. They demonstrated that the renal-function relationship is normalized by weight loss (Fig. 3).

There are also animal data that suggest that sodium retention is associated with obesity hypertension. In a dog model of obesity-induced hypertension, Rocchini et al. *(19)* demonstrated that during the first week of the high-fat diet, the increase in sodium retention appeared to best relate to an increase in plasma norepinephrine activity; whereas, during the latter weeks of the high-fat diet, an increase in plasma insulin appeared to be the best predictor of sodium retention. Rocchini also demonstrated that the hypertension associated with weight gain in the dog occurs only if adequate salt is present in the diet. Hall and co-workers *(53)* demonstrated that obesity-induced hypertension in the dog is associated with increased renal tubular sodium reabsorption since marked sodium retention occurred despite large increases in glomerular filtration and renal plasma flow. Granger et al. *(54)* demonstrated that dogs fed a high-fat diet develop an abnormal renal pressure–natriuresis relationship similar to that observed in obese adolescents.

The relationship between urinary sodium excretion and mean arterial pressure can be altered by intrinsic and extrinsic factors that are known to affect the ability of the kidney to excrete sodium (Table 1). Although both obese humans and animals can have compression of the kidney by the surrounding fat and that fat may penetrate the renal hilum into the sinuses surrounding the renal medulla *(55,56)*, it is unlikely that a fat-based structural change in the kidney is the major pathophysiological cause of the renal sodium retention associated with obesity. Based on both human and animal data, insulin resistance, activation

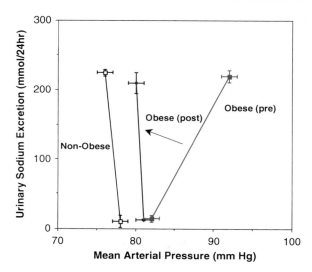

Fig. 3. Renal-function relations for 18 non-obese (X) and 60 obese adolescents before a weight loss program (*open square*) and the 36 obese adolescents who lost weight during a 20-week weight loss program (*closed square*). In comparison with the non-obese adolescents' renal-function relation, the obese adolescents' renal-function relation has a shallow slope (*p*<0.001). In those who lost weight, the slope increased (*arrow*). This increase was due to a decrease in the mean arterial pressure during the 2 weeks of the high-salt diet. From *(33)*.

Table 1
Factors That Produce Alterations in the Renal-Function Curves

  1. Constriction of the renal arteries and arterioles
  2. Changes in glomerular filtration coefficients
  3. Changes in the rate of tubular reabsorption
  4. Reduced renal mass
  5. Changing levels of renin–angiotensin activation
  6. Changing levels of aldosterone
  7. Changing levels of vasopressin
  8. Changing levels of insulin
  9. Changing levels of sympathetic nervous system activation
 10. Changing levels of atrial natriuretic hormone

of the renin–angiotensin–aldosterone system, and the sympathetic nervous system are the three most likely factors responsible for the altered renal-function curves observed in obesity.

Insulin Resistance

For years it has been recognized that hypertension is common in both obese and diabetic individuals. Glucose intolerance, independent of obesity, is also associated with hypertension *(57)*. In children, several studies have demonstrated a positive association between fasting insulin level and resting blood pressure *(58–62)*. Analysis of data from the San Antonio Heart Study has demonstrated an impressive pattern of overlap among hypertension, diabetes, and obesity. It has been estimated that by the fifth decade of life 85% of diabetic individuals are hypertensive and obese, 80% of obese subjects have abnormal glucose tolerance and are hypertensive, and 67% of hypertensive subjects are both diabetic and obese *(8,63)*. The relationship between insulin resistance and blood pressure has been observed in most populations *(64–67)*. Many investigators have suggested that insulin resistance may be the metabolic link that connects obesity to hypertension.

Factors known to improve insulin resistance are also associated with reductions in blood pressure. Weight loss has been documented to be associated with both a decrease in blood pressure and an improvement in insulin sensitivity *(68,69)*. The decline in blood pressure associated with exercise training programs seems to be limited to individuals who are initially hyperinsulinemic and have the greatest fall in plasma insulin level as a result of the training program *(69,70)*.

In addition to human data linking insulin and blood pressure, there are also animal data that suggest that insulin is an important regulator of blood pressure *(18,19,71–78)*.

Finally, there is evidence to suggest that in normal weight individuals, hyperinsulinemia and insulin resistance precede the development of hypertension. Young black males with borderline high blood pressure have higher insulin levels and more insulin resistance than normotensive black men *(64,65)*. In the Tecumseh Study *(79)*, individuals with borderline hypertension have higher plasma insulin levels and greater weight than normotensive individuals. Normotensive children with a family history of hypertension have higher insulin levels and more insulin resistance than children with no family history of hypertension *(80)*.

With respect to hypertension, one of the potentially important actions of insulin is the ability to induce renal sodium retention. Insulin resistance and/or hyperinsulinemia can result in chronic sodium retention. Insulin can enhance renal sodium retention both directly, through its effects on renal tubules *(81–83)*, and indirectly, through stimulation of the sympathetic nervous system and augmenting angiotensin II-mediated aldosterone secretion *(84,85)*. There are data to suggest that insulin resistance is directly related to sodium sensitivity in both obese and non-obese subjects. Rocchini et al. *(33)* demonstrated in obese adolescents that insulin resistance and sodium sensitivity of blood pressure are directly related. They demonstrated that the blood pressure of obese adolescents is more dependent on dietary sodium intake than the blood pressure of non-obese adolescents and that hyperinsulinemia and increased sympathetic nervous system activity appear to be responsible for the observed sodium sensitivity and hypertension. Finta et al. *(86)* showed that the endogenous hyperinsulinemia that occurs in obese subjects following a glucose meal can result in urinary sodium retention. In that study, the investigators also demonstrated that the obese adolescents who were the most sodium sensitive had significantly higher fasting insulin concentrations, higher glucose-stimulated insulin levels, and greater urine sodium retention in response to the oral glucose load. Finally in non-obese subjects with *(87)* or without *(83)* essential hypertension, there is a direct relationship between sodium sensitivity and insulin resistance.

There are also animal data that suggests that insulin resistance may be partly responsible for the sodium retention associated with obesity hypertension. In a dog model of obesity-induced hypertension, Rocchini et al. *(18,19)* demonstrated that during the first week of the high-fat diet, the increase in sodium retention appeared to best relate to an increase in plasma norepinephrine activity; whereas, during the latter weeks of the high-fat diet, an increase in plasma insulin appeared to be the best predictor of sodium retention.

In non-insulin-resistant subjects, both a concomitant decrease in proximal tubular sodium reabsorption and an increase in glomerular filtration oppose the direct effect of insulin to increase distal sodium retention. Hall and co-workers *(53)* demonstrated that obesity-induced hypertension in the dog is associated with increased renal tubular sodium reabsorption. Ter Maaten et al. *(88)* demonstrated that insulin-mediated glucose uptake was positively correlated with changes in glomerular filtration but not with changes in either proximal tubular sodium reabsorption or overall fractional sodium excretion. They speculated that insulin could only cause abnormal sodium retention if an additional antinatriuretic stimulus is present, such as through stimulation of the sympathetic activity, or augmenting angiotensin II-mediated aldosterone production.

In addition to sodium retention, selective insulin resistance may modulate the development of hypertension through changes in vascular structure and function, alterations in cation flux, activation of the renin–angiotensin–aldosterone system, and activation of the sympathetic nervous system.

However, in contrast to these and other reports *(8,64–69,89–92)* linking hyperinsulinemia to hypertension there have been other studies that have been unable to establish a relationship between hyperinsulinemia and high blood pressure. There is at least one study in obese hypertensive individuals *(93)*, which did not find a correlation between hyperinsulinemia and hypertension. In normal dogs, a chronic infusion of insulin, with or without an infusion of norepinephrine, failed to increase blood pressure *(25,94)*. In addition, even in those reports that have documented a relationship between insulin and blood pressure there is significant overlap in insulin resistance between those individuals who are hypertensive and those who are normotensive. No correlation has been found between blood pressure and plasma insulin or insulin sensitivity in Pima Indians *(95)*. Finally, we observed that when fat-fed dogs were treated with aspirin, an inhibitor of NF kappa B activation, insulin resistance did not develop as the dogs become obese, but the dogs still developed hypertension. Similarly, when fat-fed dogs were treated with alpha- and beta-blockade, using prazosin and atenolol, hypertension did not develop as the dogs become obese, but the dogs still developed insulin resistance *(96)*. Thus, from all of these studies it is clear that not all hypertensive subjects are insulin resistant and not all insulin-resistant subjects are hypertensive; therefore, hyperinsulinemia and/or insulin resistant is not either the major or sole mechanism responsible for the altered renal pressure–natriuresis relationship observed in obesity.

Renin–Angiotensin–Aldosterone System

The renin–angiotensin–aldosterone system is an important determinant of efferent glomerular arteriolar tone and tubular sodium reabsorption. Its activity is modulated by dietary salt ingestion, blood pressure, and the sympathetic nervous system. Therefore, alterations in the renin–angiotensin–aldosterone system could be expected to alter pressure–natriuresis. Enhanced activity of the renin–angiotensin–aldosterone system has been reported in obese humans and dogs *(32,85,97–102)*. Granger and co-workers *(102)* reported that plasma renin activity is 170% higher in obese dogs than in control dogs.

Aldosterone concentrations have been demonstrated to be abnormal in both human and animal obesity *(32,97–101)*. For example, Rocchini et al. *(97)* demonstrated that compared to non-obese adolescents, obese adolescents had significantly higher supine and 2-h upright aldosterone concentrations. Although plasma renin activity was not significantly different between the two groups of adolescents, they observed that a given increment in plasma renin activity produced a greater increment in aldosterone in the obese adolescents. Compared with an obese control group, weight loss resulted in both a significant decrease in plasma aldosterone and a significant decrease in the slope of the posture-induced relation between plasma renin activity and aldosterone. Goodfriend and Calhoun *(103)* suggested that increased plasma free fatty acids produced in obese individuals may stimulate aldosterone production independent of renin.

Insulin also has been shown to influence the renin–angiotensin–aldosterone system in both normal subjects *(84,104)* and in patients with diabetes *(105)*. For example, Rocchini et al. *(85)* measured the increase in plasma aldosterone after graded increases in intravenous angiotensin II before and after euglycemic hyperinsulinemia in seven chronically instrumented dogs. Euglycemic hyperinsulinemia resulted in a significantly greater (*p*<0.01) change in the angiotensin II-stimulated increments of plasma aldosterone than was observed when angiotensin II was administered alone. However, there was no dose dependence of insulin's effect on angiotensin II-stimulated aldosterone. In addition, although weight gain significantly increased angiotensin II-stimulated aldosterone. These authors speculated that increased plasma aldosterone concentration in some obese subjects maybe caused by increased adrenal sensitivity to angiotensin II.

Despite these results suggesting that obesity is associated with significant alterations in the renin–angiotensin–aldosterone system, Hall et al. *(53)* demonstrated that weight-related changes in blood pressure can occur in dogs independent of changes in angiotensin II, and de Paula et al. *(106)* demonstrated that the aldosterone antagonist, eplerenone, attenuated but did not prevent the sodium retention and hypertension associated with feeding dogs a high-fat diet. Thus, although the renin–angiotensin–aldosterone system may play an important role in the pathogenesis of obesity hypertension, it is not either the major or sole mechanism responsible for the altered renal pressure–natriuresis relationship observed in obesity.

Sympathetic Nervous System

For over 20 years it has been recognized that diet affects the sympathetic nervous system. Fasting suppresses sympathetic nervous system activity; whereas, overfeeding with either a high carbohydrate or high-fat diet simulates the sympathetic nervous system *(107–110)*. Insulin is believed to possibly be the signal that networks dietary intake and nutritional status to sympathetic activity. Glucose and insulin sensitive neurons in the ventromedial portion of the hypothalamus have been demonstrated to alter the activity of inhibitory pathways between the hypothalamus and the brain stem *(111)*. It has also been hypothesized that the physiological consequence of the link between dietary intake and sympathetic nervous system activity is to regulate energy expenditure in a hope to maintain weight homeostasis. Euglycemic hyperinsulinemia in both normal and obese humans and animals causes activation of the sympathetic nervous system as documented by increases in heart rate, blood pressure, and plasma norepinephrine *(30,85,112–115)*. Hyperinsulinemia is associated not only with an increase in circulating catecholamines but also with an increase in sympathetic nerve activity *(116)*. Landsberg and Krieger *(112)* suggested that in obese individuals the sympathetic nervous system is chronically activated in an attempt to prevent further weight gain, and that hypertension and other adverse cardiovascular effects of obesity are byproducts of the overactive sympathetic nervous system.

The Bogalusa Heart Study reported in a biracial group of children that resting heart rate was positively correlated with blood pressure and subscapular skinfold thickness *(117)*.

These investigators also demonstrated that a hyperdynamic cardiovascular state was associated with obesity *(118)*. Obese children are also reported to have increased heart rate variability and blood pressure variability as compared to non-obese children *(119)*. Microneurography, which directly measures sympathetic traffic to skeletal muscle, has consistently shown to be increased in obesity *(120)*.

Although many studies in obese individuals have demonstrated increased sympathetic nervous system activity, this has not been a universal finding *(121)*. Part of the controversy regarding the role of the sympathetic nervous system in obesity relates to relying on plasma levels of catecholamines as the index of sympathetic activity. Plasma norepinephrine levels provide an indirect assessment of systemic sympathetic activity, since they reflect the net balance between norepinephrine appearance and removal mechanisms and provide no information concerning what happens to norepinephrine after it is release from presynaptic sympathetic nerve terminals. Data from the Normative Aging Study *(41)* strongly suggest that obesity is associated with increased sympathetic nervous system activity. This study demonstrated that sympathetic activity, assessed by measuring 24-h urinary norepinephrine excretion, is directly related to abdominal girth, waist-to-hip ratio, and body mass index.

Previous studies in obese subjects have reported a positive association between sympathetic activity and increased blood pressure. In the fat-fed dog, Kassab et al. *(122)* demonstrated that renal denervation prevents both the sodium retention and the hypertension associated with weight gain but does not prevent insulin resistance. In addition, Eikelis et al. *(123)* using regional analysis of NE kinetics demonstrated increased renal NE spillover in obese subjects. In both animal and human studies, pharmacologic blockade of the sympathetic nervous system prevents the increase in blood pressure and sodium retention associated with obesity *(124,125)*. Finally, Lohmeier et al. *(126)* demonstrated that fat feeding of dogs causes a marked increase in the activity of the protein product of the immediate early gene *c-foss* in the baroreceptor sympathoexcitatory cells in the rostral ventrolateral medulla, a site known to be affected by both angiotensin II and leptin. Lohmeier's observations in obese dogs support the observations that sympathetic activity to the kidney and other vascular beds is increased in obesity hypertension *(122,123)*. Thus, activation of the sympathetic nervous systems appears to be one of the major factors responsible for both the altered renal-function relationship and hypertension observed in obesity. However, what is still unknown is what is the factor or factors responsible for activation of the sympathetic nervous system in obesity.

POSSIBLE MECHANISMS RESPONSIBLE FOR ACTIVATION OF THE SYMPATHETIC NERVOUS SYSTEM IN OBESITY

Since increased VAT appears to be the best predictor of hypertension *(3)*, it is likely that increased sympathetic activation is related to the metabolically active adipose tissue found in the visceral region. Visceral adipose tissue is known to secrete free fatty acids (FFAs), adipocytokines, and inflammatory cytokines into the portal circulation. Three possible mechanisms that may be responsible for the increase in sympathetic nervous system activity associated with obesity are increased FFA levels in the portal circulation, increased adipocytokines and inflammatory cytokine levels in the portal circulation, and/or central activation of the hypothalamic–sympathetic axis.

Increased Portal FFA and Increased Sympathetic Activation

Increased portal FFA may increase sympathetic activity through the development of insulin resistance and hyperinsulinemia. Arner *(127)* first suggested that the release into the portal vein of FFAs originating from the visceral fat might be responsible for the development of insulin resistance. There are a number of reports demonstrating that increasing FFAs by the infusion of a lipid emulsion leads, within hours, to substantial insulin resistance. Griffin et al. *(128)* demonstrated that FFAs interfere with insulin signaling at the level of a serine kinase cascade involving protein kinase C-θ, leading to defects in insulin signaling and glucose transport. Kabir et al. *(129)* demonstrated, in dogs fed a moderate-fat diet for 12 weeks, increased gene expression promoting lipid accumulation and lipolysis in visceral fat, as well as elevated rate-limiting gluconeogenic enzyme expression in the liver as evidence in favor of the portal FFA hypothesis.

Many investigators have documented that euglycemic hyperinsulinemia in both normal and obese humans and animals causes activation of the sympathetic nervous system as documented by increases in heart rate, blood pressure, and plasma norepinephrine *(85,112,116)*. However, it is unlikely that in obesity either hyperinsulinemia or insulin resistance is responsible for activation of the sympathetic nervous system or the subsequent development of hypertension since in the obese dog, Rocchini and co-workers *(96)* have demonstrated that insulin resistance and hypertension are dissociated from each other. Finally, in humans, long-term weight loss induced by bariatric surgery corrects the insulin resistance and hyperinsulinemia but does not prevent the hypertension *(39)*.

A second explanation for how increased portal FFAs could lead to activation of the sympathetic nervous system is that there is a known feedback mechanism relating FFA production and the sympathetic nervous system, whereby delivery of FFAs into the circulation results in sympathetic activation and conversely, sympathetic activity stimulates lipolysis. Grekin et al. *(130)* demonstrated that chronic portal venous infusion of an oleate solution and other long-chain fatty acids have a pressor effect that is mediated by the α-adrenergic component of the sympathetic nervous system. Thus, increased portal FFAs could be responsible for the initiation of both the hypertension and the insulin resistance associated with obesity.

Increased Inflammatory Cytokine Levels in the Portal Circulation Leading to Increased Sympathetic Activation

Visceral fat secretes substances like [TNF-α, IL-6, or decreased adiponectin] that may induce both insulin resistance and activation of the sympathetic nervous system. TNF-α and other proinflammatory cytokines elicit a broad spectrum of biological responses via their peripheral and central nervous system effects (Fig. 4). Because blood-borne cytokines are too large to readily cross the blood–brain barrier one possible route by which circulating cytokines might stimulate sympathetic activation is through activation of visceral sensory afferent nerves, particularly the abdominal vagus *(131)*.

Adipocytokines secreted from visceral fat may also play a role in the sympathetic activation associated with obesity. Both low levels of ghrelin and adiponectin have been reported to be associated with hypertension. Lin et al. *(132)* showed that ghrelin acts in the nucleus of the solitary tract to suppress renal sympathetic activity and to decrease arterial pressure.

In summary, the potential role of abdominally derived inflammatory cytokines and adipocytokines in obesity hypertension and activation of the sympathetic nervous system

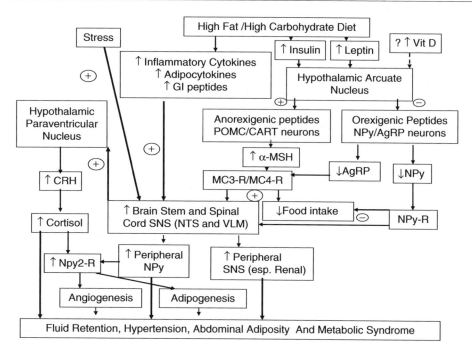

Fig. 4. A schematic representation of how ingestion of a diet high in fat and carbohydrates may be responsible for activation of the central and peripheral sympathetic nervous system (SNS) leading to the development of hypertension, abdominal adiposity, and the metabolic syndrome. The three locations in the central nervous system that are directly linking to central regulation of sympathetic activity are the hypothalamic arcuate nucleus, the hypothalamic paraventricular nucleus, and noradrenergic brain stem neurons in the nucleus tractus solitarii (NTS) and the ventrolateral medulla (VLM). A high-fat and carbohydrate diet through production of insulin and leptin can directly stimulate the arcuate nucleus to activate neurons expressing the anorexigenic peptides pro-opiomelanocortin (POMC) and cocaine-and amphetamine-regulated transcription (CART) and inhibition of neurons expressing the orexigenic peptides neuropeptide y (NPy) and agouti-related protein (AgRP). The resultant increase in production of alpha-melanocyte-stimulating hormone (α-MSH) and receptors (MC3-R/MC4-R) and the inhibition of production of AgRp and NYy and its receptors (NPy-R) results in both reduction in food intake and stimulation of the brain stem and spinal cord (SNS). Similarly, a diet high in fat and carbohydrates and /or stress can directly stimulate the NTS and VLM through production of inflammatory cytokines, adipocytokines, and gastrointestinal (GI) peptides. Once the NTS and VLM are activated, it can directly result in systemic activation of the SNS and the release of NPy leading to fluid retention and hypertension. The NTS and VLM through neural projections into the paraventricular nucleus of the hypothalamus result in release of corticotrophin-releasing hormone (CHR) and ultimately the production of cortisol from the adrenal gland that can both directly result in fluid retention, hypertension, and increased accumulation of abdominal fat or indirectly increasing the production NPy2-R that result in both increased angiogenesis and adipogenesis in abdominal fat.

remains controversial because of the limited amount of available data on the interaction between these substances and arterial pressure.

Activation of the Hypothalamic–Sympathetic Axis

The arcuate nucleus of the hypothalamus is a critical integrative center for the modulation of food intake and energy expenditure *(133)*. The arcuate nucleus contains at least two populations of neurons that have opposite influences on food intake and energy expenditure. One population expresses the anorexigenic precursor peptides pro-opiomelanocortin (POMC) and the cocaine- and amphetamine-regulated transcript (CART) peptides, whereas the other expresses the orexigenic peptides neuropeptide Y (NYP) and agouti-related protein (AgRP) (Fig. 4).

Leptin, a 167-amino acid hormone that is secreted exclusively by adipocytes, activates POMC-containing neurons to produce the anorexigenic peptide alpha-melanocyte-stimulating hormone (a-MSH) and reduces the release of orexigenic peptides NPY and AgRP *(134,135)*. Therefore, in the setting of excess food, the elevated leptin levels activate the anorexigenic and inhibit the orexigenic pathway. In addition, NPY/AgRP and POMC-containing neurons in the arcuate nucleus have direct projections to the paraventricular nucleus and to the lateral hypothalamus, both of which are implicated in autonomic nervous system regulation *(136,137)*.

Recent evidence from Eikelis and Esler *(138)* suggests that leptin may be the link between excess adiposity and increased cardiovascular sympathetic activity. Plasma leptin concentrations are known to correlate with the level of obesity. Eikelis et al. *(123)* using simultaneous arteriovenous blood sampling demonstrated that the increase in plasma leptin concentration in obese individuals is not from either the heart or from the portal circulation, but rather it is from peripheral adipose tissue and from the leptin produced in the brain and secreted into the systemic circulation.

Leptin and the sympathetic nervous system are intimately linked. There is a direct interaction between leptin and the sympathetic nervous system, leptin acting within the hypothalamus to cause activation of the central sympathetic outflow and stimulation of the adrenal medulla to release epinephrine. While leptin has been shown in animals to be associated with an increased sympathetic outflow to the kidney, adipose tissue, and skeletal muscle, Eikelis et al. *(123)* demonstrated in humans that of the measures of sympathoadrenal function tested, only total and renal norepinephrine spillover rates correlated with leptin secretion rate. These data and the report of Kassab et al. *(122)* that renal sympathetic denervation prevents the fluid retention and hypertension in the fat-fed dog are consistent with but does not prove the hypothesis that leptin may be a major factor responsible for the increase sympathetic activation observed in obesity. However, since leptin has been shown to be equally if not more correlated to SAT compared to VAT, leptin does not completely fit the observation of Fox et al. *(48)* that hypertension is more associated with VAT than SAT in obese individuals.

In addition to leptin, other central neuropeptides have been implicated in the development of obesity and hypertension. NPy is a peptide that is expressed in various regions of the nervous system including the hypothalamus, the amygdale, the hippocampus, the nucleus of the solitary tract, and peripheral sympathetic nerves. Npy plays an important role in several physiological functions including the regulation of feeding behavior through mediation of the actions of leptin and insulin, cardiovascular homoeostasis, regulation of the sympathetic nervous system, regulation of blood pressure, and control of the circadian rhythms. In addition to NPy being produced and released into the brain it is also produced and released into the systemic circulation from sympathetic nerves (Fig. 4). Systemically released NPy causes vasoconstriction, angiogenesis, and proliferation and differentiation of adipocytes and endothelial cells. Kuo et al. *(139)* demonstrated that stress, such as exposure to cold or aggression, causes the systemic release of NPy from sympathetic nerves, which in turn upregulates NPy and its receptors in a glucocorticoid-dependent manner in abdominal adipose tissue leading to diet-induced obesity and the development of hypertension and the metabolic syndrome. In addition, these investigators demonstrated that in stressed mice, fed a diet high in fat and sugar, blockade of NPy receptors with either using NPy receptor antagonists or using NPy fat-targeted knockout mice results in reduced abdominal fat and metabolic abnormalities. Thus, although centrally released NPy causes reduced central sympathetic activity and reduced blood pressure, when it is released peripherally through increased sympathetic nerve activity, NPy can cause vasoconstriction and hypertension. In addition, recent genetic association studies have demonstrated that the carriers of the T1128C polymorphism of the NPy gene have an increased prevalence of hypertension and cardiovascular disease *(140,141)*.

The precursor molecule POMC undergoes post-translational processing by prohormone convertases and generates the alpha-, beta-, and gamma-melanocyte-stimulating hormone (MSH) and adrenocorticotropin (ACTH). The importance of the melanocortin pathway in the regulation of food intake became evident after the characterization of the agouti obesity syndrome *(142)*. Alpha-MSH is the primary endogenous agonist for melanocortin receptors and plays an important role in the inhibition of food intake. Alpha-MSH has recently been shown to play a role in the regulation of blood pressure *(143,144)*.

Recently, vitamin D deficiency has been hypothesized as a cause of obesity and the metabolic syndrome *(145)*. Foss speculates that the metabolic and physiological changes observed as the metabolic syndrome, including hypertension and insulin resistance, could result from a "winter metabolism" which increases themogenic capacity. Foss speculates that the stimulus for the winter response is a fall in vitamin D due to reduced ultraviolet-B range sunlight exposure that occurs in mid-latitudes in autumn and winter. He proposes that a fall in circulating calcidiol is sensed in the hypothalamus and induces an increase in the body weight set point. A state of energy accrual ensues in which appetite is increased and energy expenditure reduced by activation of the AgRP/NPy neurons and inhibition of the POMC/CART neurons. The basis of this hypothesis is a body of evidence that demonstrates an inverse relationship between vitamin D status and both obesity and the metabolic syndrome *(146–149)*.

Finally, the similarities between Cushing's syndrome and the metabolic abnormalities associated with obesity hypertension have lead Bjorntrop and others to speculate that hypercortisolemia is involved in the pathogenesis of obesity hypertension *(150)*. There is evidence of increased secretion and turnover, resulting in normal or even lower than normal circulating concentration *(151)*. Measuring salivary cortisol, investigators have been able to demonstrate that normally regulated cortisol secretion is associated with "healthy" anthropometric, metabolic, and hemodynamic variables. However, upon perceived stress, cortisol secretion is increased and followed by insulin resistance, abdominal obesity, elevated blood pressure, and hyperlipidemia *(152,153)*. Rosmond and Bjorntrop *(154)* have demonstrated that diminished dexamethasone suppression is directly associated with obesity and elevation of leptin levels. Zahrezewska et al. *(155)* demonstrated in rats that glucocorticoids diminish leptin signals.

Bjorntorp and Rosmond *(150)* speculate that the two ways that elevated activity of the hypothalamic–pituitary adrenal axis could occur are either an elevated stimulation and/or a diminished feedback control. Elevated stimulation of the HPA axis can occur due to psychosocial and socioeconomic handicaps such as living alone, divorce, poor education, low social class, family member on unemployment, and problems at school, or even due to excess food intake *(156)*. With respect to causes of diminished feedback control of the HPA axis, Bjorntorp and others *(157–159)* demonstrated that a restriction fragment length polymorphism of the glucocorticoid receptor gene is associated with poorly controlled HPA axis function, as well as abdominal obesity, insulin resistance, and hypertension. Finally Kabir et al. *(129)* has demonstrated in mice that the combination of stress and a diet high in fat and sugar results in increased secretion of glucocorticoids which act as an upstream modulator of NPy activity. The increased activity of NPy and the NPy2 receptor is ultimately responsible for the development of obesity, hypertension, and the metabolic syndrome.

Therefore, Bjorntorp has suggested that many of the cardiovascular and physiologic consequences found in obese individuals could be due to "a discretely elevated cortisol secretion, discoverable during reactions to perceived stress in everyday life" *(160)*.

Summary

In summary, based on animal and human data, the best hypothesis for the mechanism of obesity hypertension is that ingestion of diet high in fat and sugar results in both increasing abdominal adiposity and activation of the hypothalamic–sympathetic axis. The combination of an increase in portal levels of FFA, increased secretion from visceral adipocytes of both adipocytokines (such as leptin) and inflammatory cytokines, stress and/or potentially even vitamin D deficiency is most likely responsible for the central activation of the hypothalamic–sympathetic axis. Activation of the hypothalamic–sympathetic axis produces increased renal sympathetic, activation of the renin–angiotensin–aldosterone system, fluid retention and ultimately in the development of systemic hypertension (Fig. 4).

OBESITY AS A CARDIOVASCULAR RISK FACTOR

The Framingham Heart Study *(5)* identified obesity and hypertension as independent risk factors for the development of cardiovascular disease. Obese normotensive and hypertensive men have a higher rate of coronary heart disease *(47)*. Manson et al. *(161)* has also reported that in women, the relative risk of fatal and nonfatal coronary heart disease increased from the lowest to the highest quartiles of obesity. Childhood obesity is associated with the development of early coronary artery pathology. The autopsies of 210 children aged 5–15 years who had suffered violent death were evaluated by Kotelainen *(162)*. Ponderal index was a significant predictor of heart weight and the presence of coronary artery intimal fatty streaks. In the Bogalusa Heart Study, Berenson et al. demonstrated that children and young adults who died of trauma showed an association between body mass index, systolic and diastolic blood pressure, and the presence of fatty streaks and fibrous plaques in the aorta and coronary arteries *(15,61)*. Recently Inge et al. *(163)* reported that following surgically induced weight loss adolescents experienced remission of type 2 diabetes and improved serum lipids and blood pressure.

Long-standing obesity is associated with preclinical and clinical left ventricular dilation *(164)* and impaired systolic function *(165,166)* with heart failure, frequently being the ultimate cause of death in markedly overweight individuals *(167)*.

A physiological change that may contribute to the association of obesity with left ventricular dilatation is sodium retention and a concomitant increase in blood volume and cardiac output. Many investigators *(168)* have reported that obesity is associated with an increased blood volume and cardiac output. However, the increment in cardiac output associated with obesity cannot be explained by an increase in adipose tissue perfusion alone; some have suggested that blood flow to the non-adipose mass must also be increased in obese subjects *(169,170)*. Thus, obesity is characterized by a relative volume expansion in the presence of restricted vascular capacity. The increase in volume in the presence of restricted vascular capacity may lead to left ventricular dilatation, increased left ventricular wall stress, and compensatory left ventricular hypertrophy *(165,169,170).* Hypertension increases afterload and as a consequence the left ventricle adapts with an increase in wall thickness. The combination of obesity and hypertension therefore creates a double burden on the heart, ultimately leading to the development of impaired ventricular function *(165–167,171,172).*

MacMahon et al. *(164)* reported that 50% of individuals who are more than 50% overweight have left ventricular hypertrophy. In children, adiposity is also one of the determinants of left ventricular mass. Urbina et al. reported that the major factors influencing left ventricular mass in childhood were linear growth, defined by height and measures of ponderosity *(173).* Daniels et al. reported that in children, lean body mass was the strongest determinant of left ventricular mass, but that fat mass and systolic blood pressure were also important predictors of left ventricular mass *(174,175).* As with blood pressure, weight loss can result in regression in the left ventricular hypertrophy *(164,176,177).* More recently, Ippisch et al. *(178)* demonstrated that surgically induced weight loss in morbidly obese adolescents resulted in a significant improvement in left ventricular mass and geometry, diastolic function, and cardiac workload.

Unlike the universal finding of left ventricular hypertrophy in obese individuals, not all studies have demonstrated impairment in left ventricular function. Schmeider and Messerli *(179)* reported that obese hypertensive individuals have normal global left ventricular systolic function as measured by left ventricular fractional shortening and velocity of circumferential fiber shorting. However, since both of these indices of left ventricular systolic function are dependent on ventricular preload and afterload, the results of Schmeider's study do not document that left ventricular contractility is normal. In fact, Blake and co-workers *(176)* demonstrated that despite a normal left ventricular ejection fraction at rest, obese individuals have an impaired left ventricular ejection fraction in response to dynamic exercise. Guillerno et al. *(171)* reported that the end-systolic wall stress to end-systolic volume index, a load-independent index of left ventricular function, is also abnormal in even mild or moderately obese individuals. These investigators also documented a significant inverse relationship between the index of end-systolic wall stress to end-systolic volume index and body mass index, diastolic diameter, and left ventricular mass index.

Abnormalities in left ventricular filling have also been reported to occur in obese individuals, i.e., decreased peak filling rate, duration of peak filling and left atrial emptying index *(176),* an increased isovolumic relaxation time, and an abnormal mitral valve Doppler filling pattern *(172).* Harada et al. *(180)* demonstrated that body mass index predicts left ventricular diastolic filling rate in asymptomatic obese children. Kanoupalis et al. *(181)* and Ippisch et al. *(178)* demonstrated that weight loss improves diastolic function.

The left ventricular hypertrophy, depressed myocardial contractility, and diastolic dysfunction can predispose individuals to excessive ventricular ectopy. Messerli et al. *(182)* reported that the prevalence of premature ventricular contractions was 30 times higher in obese individuals with eccentric left ventricular hypertrophy than in lean individuals.

Finally, as with hypertension, insulin resistance may be related to both the cardiac hypertrophy and abnormal cardiac function that is observed in many obese individuals. Nakajima et al. *(183)* reported that there is a direct relationship between intraabdominal fat accumulation and the cardiac abnormalities associated with obesity. Since increased upper body and intraabdominal fat accumulation relates to the presence of insulin resistance even without significant overall obesity, these investigators speculated that the cardiac dysfunction observed in obese individuals may be related to insulin resistance.

SUMMARY

Obesity is recognized as an independent risk factor for the development of cardiovascular disease. Obesity in both children and adults is associated with the development of cardiac dysfunction. Obese individuals have an increased risk for developing left ventricular dilatation, impaired systolic and diastolic dysfunction, and the development of left ventricular hypertrophy (Table 2).

Table 2
Cardiovascular Consequences of Obesity

1. Premature development of coronary atherosclerosis
2. Left ventricular hypertrophy
3. Left ventricular dilation
4. Left ventricular diastolic dysfunction
5. Left ventricular systolic dysfunction
6. Congestive heart failure

MANAGEMENT OF THE OBESE CHILD WITH HYPERTENSION

Weight loss is the cornerstone of hypertensive management in the obese individual. Weight loss in both adolescents and adults improves all of the cardiovascular abnormalities associated with obesity, including hypertension, dyslipemia, and sodium retention, structural abnormalities in resistant vessels, and left ventricular hypertrophy and dysfunction. It is also important to realize that the method by which weight loss is accomplished is important. Although weight loss in general results in a drop in resting systolic/diastolic blood pressure and heart rate, the greatest decrease in resting systolic blood pressure, peak exercise diastolic pressure, and heart rate can be achieved when the weight loss is incorporated with physical conditioning *(30)*. Similarly, a weight loss program that incorporates exercise along with caloric restriction produces the most favorable effects on insulin resistance *(30,70)*, dyslipidemia *(70,184)*, and vascular reactivity *(30,185)*. Endurance training in obese and non-obese individuals improves insulin resistance, in part, by increasing muscle oxidative capacity and increasing capillary density *(186,187)*. Most investigators believe that the additive effect of exercise to weight loss is related to the fact that exercise improves insulin resistance independent of weight loss.

In the morbidly obese adolescent, surgically induced weight loss also is accompanied by both an improvement in type 2 diabetes and a marked reduction of both blood pressure and other cardiovascular risk factors *(163,178)*.

Although weight loss and exercise are the cornerstones of blood pressure management in obese hypertensive individuals, most obese individuals are either unable or unwilling to lose weight or are unable to keep from regaining lost weight. Therefore, pharmacological therapy is frequently required in the hypertensive obese individual. The pharmacologic therapy of the obese hypertensive is divided into treatment of obesity and/or treatment of hypertension. The role of drug therapy in the treatment of childhood obesity is controversial. Many of the obesity drugs that have been tried in adults have resulted in complications, such as pulmonary hypertension and tricuspid regurgitation with fenfluramine/dexfenfluramine *(188)*. There have been few well-controlled studies to show that the available obesity drugs are well tolerated and effective for use in obese children. One medication that is currently approved for the treatment of obesity in adolescents is sibutramine, an inhibitor of reuptake of serotonin and norepinephrine. Although sibutramine is also associated with an increase in blood pressure in some patients, Daniels et al. *(189)* demonstrated that blood pressure decreased with sibutramine-induced weight loss in obese adolescents *(189)*. Orlistat is a gastrointestinal lipase inhibitor that is a safe and effective pharmacological treatment for childhood obesity *(190)*. Weight loss associated with Orlistat is associated with a decrease in blood pressure and other cardiovascular risk factors *(191)*.

In addition to the use of comprehensive, multidisciplinary weight loss programs and drugs, there also are new investigational strategies that can be used to treat obesity and it metabolic consequences. Wang et al. *(192)* recently reviewed the results of acupuncture in the treatment of obesity. These investigators demonstrated in a rat experimental model of obesity that electroacupuncture produced a significant reduction of both food intake and body weight as well as a reduction in lipids and other cardiovascular risk factors. They demonstrated that electroacupuncture stimulation produced an increased expression of the anorexigenic peptides α-MSH and CARR and a decreased expression of the orexigenic peptide NPy in the arcuate nucleus of the rat hypothalamus (Fig. 4). They also reported an open trial in 16 overweight humans which demonstrated that electrical acupoint stimulation produces a steady and significant decrease of body weight.

Experimental studies have shown that overactivation of the endocannabinoid (CB) system, a physiologic signaling system involved in regulating energy intake, fatty acid synthesis and storage, and glucose and lipid metabolism is associated with obesity, dyslipidemia, hypertension, and insulin resistance *(193)*. In clinical trials, rimonabant, the first selective CB1 receptor blocker, has resulted in substantial weight loss and significant improvement in lipid profiles and blood pressure *(194–196)*. The most commonly reported adverse events associated with rimonabant were nasopharyngitis, headache, back pain, nausea, influenza, and arthralgia. However, the most commonly associated reason for discontinuation of therapy was depressed mood disorders observed in 2.3–3.7% of patients. No trial of rimonabant has been reported in children and adolescents.

Finally, metformin is an older drug that has found new life in the treatment of obesity. For adolescents with morbid obesity and insulin resistance, including women with polycystic ovarian syndrome, the addition of metformin to a multidisciplinary weight loss program not only improved insulin resistance and lipid levels but also significantly reduced weight and body mass index *(197)*. Helvaci et al. *(198)* reported that the administration of metformin in 324 individuals with white-coat hypertension, only 279 who were overweight or obese, resulted in significant weight loss, improvement in there lipid profiles, and resolution of their white-coat hypertension. Thus, metformin appears to be an effective treatment not only of insulin resistance but also of white coat hypertension.

When choosing an antihypertensive agent for the obese child, it is important to remember that depending on the antihypertensive agents used, insulin resistance has been reported to improve, worsen, or remain unchanged. In general, thiazide diuretics *(92,199,200)* and β-blockers *(192,199)* are known to impair insulin sensitivity and glucose tolerance; calcium blockers do not seem to adversely affect carbohydrate metabolism *(201–203)*; indapamide and potassium-sparing diuretics do not influence glucose homeostasis *(204)*; and finally, angiotensin-converting enzyme inhibitors *(199)*, angiotensin II receptor blockers *(205)*, and α_1-blockers *(206,207)* may even improve glucose metabolism and insulin resistance. Recently, Rocchini et al. *(124)* demonstrated that clonidine, a centrally acting sympathetic agent, not only improved the hypertension associated with obesity but also improved the insulin resistance. Giugliano et al. *(208)* demonstrated that transdermal clonidine was effective in reducing blood pressure and improving insulin resistance in hypertensive individuals with non-insulin-dependent diabetes mellitus. Based on these two preliminary studies, it would appear that clonidine or other like drugs have a favorable profile for obese individuals with hypertension.

In addition to their unfavorable effect on insulin resistance, thiazide diuretics impair pancreatic insulin secretion *(209,210)* and increase LDL cholesterol and total cholesterol *(111,211)*. β-blockers are associated with a two- to threefold incidence of inducing diabetes mellitus *(212)* and are associated with a significant lowering of HDL cholesterol *(213,214)*. However, despite the different pharmacologic profiles of the antihypertensive drugs, there exists no clear recommendation for obese hypertensive individuals.

There is increasing data that confirm that angiotensin-converting enzyme inhibitors have specific benefit in individuals with diabetes, atherosclerosis, left ventricular dysfunction, and renal insufficiency *(215)*. In addition, one of the angiotensin receptor blockers, telmisartan has peroxisome proliferator-activated receptor-γ (PPAR-γ) activity. When compared to candesartan, telmisartan resulted in greater weight loss and more improvement in glucose tolerance in hypertensive patients with glucose intolerance. Telmisartan appears to have uniquely beneficial properties in individuals with obesity hypertension and the metabolic syndrome *(216)*.

Finally, there is one other class of agents, thiazolidinediones (pioglitazone, rosiglitazone, and troglitazone) that also appear to reverse insulin resistance, hypertension, and dyslipemia *(217,218)*. However, troglitazone recently has been associated with significant liver toxicity and fluid retention *(219)*. It is too early to know the role that these or similar agents will have in the treatment of childhood obesity hypertension.

SUMMARY

Although weight loss is the cornerstone of hypertensive management in the obese individual, many individuals will also require pharmacologic therapy. When choosing an antihypertensive medication, it is important to individualize the agent to the patient. Some agents such as thiazide diuretics and β-blockers can impair glucose tolerance and adversely alter plasma lipid levels. Whereas, angiotensin-converting enzyme inhibitors, angiotensin receptor blockers, and centrally acting sympathetic agents improve both the hypertension and the insulin resistance associated with obesity. Finally, angiotensin-converting enzyme inhibitors and angiotensin receptor blockers are also effective in reducing the development of congestive heart failure and reducing cardiovascular mortality.

FUTURE PERSPECTIVES

The prevalence and severity of obesity is increasing in children and adolescents. Based on this increased incidence of childhood obesity, we are currently facing an epidemic of childhood type II diabetes and hypertension *(220)*. In the past, most pediatricians have been taught that hypertension in children is a rare condition associates with renal disease. In reality, secondary hypertension in children has become far less common relative to primary (essential) hypertension. In a large pediatric hypertension practice, the typical hypertensive child is an otherwise healthy adolescent with obesity and some combination of cardiovascular risk factors associated with obesity. Obesity in childhood is a chronic medical condition and requires long-term treatment. It is hoped that with new discoveries more effective forms of treatment of childhood obesity will be developed.

REFERENCES

1. Ogden CL, Troiano RP, Briefel RR, Kuczmarski RJ, Flegal KM, Johnson CL. Prevalence of overweight among preschool children in the United States, 1971 through 1994. Pediatrics. 1997;99:E1.
2. Dublin LI. Report of the joint committee on mortality of the association of life insurance medical directors. The Actuarial Society of America; 1925.
3. Stamler R, Stamler J, Riedlinger WF, Algera G, Roberts R. Weight and blood pressure. Findings in hypertension screening of 1 million Americans. JAMA. 1978;240:1607–1609.
4. Symonds B. Blood pressure of healthy men and women. JAMA. 1923;8:232.
5. Hubert HB, Feinleib M, McNamara PM, Castelli WP. Obesity as an independent risk factor for cardiovascular disease: a 26-year follow-up of participants in the Framingham Heart Study. Circulation. 1983;67:968–977.
6. McMahon SW, Blacket RB, McDonald GJ, Hall W. Obesity, Alcohol consumption and blood pressure in Australian men and women: National Heart Foundation of Australia Risk Factor Prevalence Study. J Hypertens. 1984;2:85–91.
7. Bloom E, Swayne R, Yano K, MacLean C. Does obesity protect hypertensives against cardiovascular disease? JAMA. 1986;256:2972–2975.
8. Ferannini E, Haffner SM, Stern MP. Essential hypertension: an insulin-resistance state. J Cardiovasc Pharmacol. 1990;15(Suppl 5):S18–S25.
9. Manolio TA, Savage PJ, Burke GL, Liu KA, Wagenknecht LE, Sidney S, Jacobs DR Jr, Roseman JM, Donahue RP, Oberman A. Association of fasting insulin with blood pressure and lipids in young adults. The CARDIA Study. Atherosclerosis. 1990;10:430–436.
10. Larimore JW. A study of blood pressure in relation to type of bodily habitus. Arch Intern Med. 1923;31:567.
11. Levy RL, Troud WD, White PD. transient hypertension: its significance in terms of later development of sustained hypertension and cardiovascular-renal diseases. JAMA. 1944;126:82.
12. Hypertension Detection and Follow-Up Program Cooperative Group. Race, education and prevalence of hypertension. Am J Epidemiol. 1977;106:351–361.
13. Kannel W, Brand N, Skinner J, et al. The relation of adiposity to blood pressure and development of hypertension. The Framingham study. Ann Intern Med. 1967;67:48.
14. Rosner B, Prineas R, Daniels SR, Loggie J. Blood pressure differences between blacks and whites in relation to body size among US children and adolescents. Am J Epidemiol. 2000;151:1007–1019.
15. Freedman DS, Dietz WH, Srinivasan SR, Berenson GS. The relation of overweight to cardiovascular risk factors among children and adolescents: the Bogalusa Heart Study. Pediatrics. 199;103:1175–1182.
16. Sorof JM. Poffenbarger T, Franco K, Bernard L, Portman RJ. Isolated systolic hypertension, obesity, and hyperkinetic hemodynamic states in children. J Pediatr. 2002;140:660–666.
17. Cash JR, Wood Jr. Observations upon the blood pressure of dogs following changes in body weight. South Med J. 1938;31:270–282.
18. Rocchini AP, Moorehead C, Wentz E, Deremer S. Obesity-induced hypertension in the dog. Hypertension. 1987;9(Suppl III):III64–III68.
19. Rocchini AP, Moorehead CP, DeRemer S, Bondie D. Pathogenesis of weight-related changes in blood pressure in dogs. Hypertension. 1989;13;922–928.
20. Hall JE, Brands MW, Dixon WN, et al. Obesity-induced hypertension. Renal function and systemic hemodynamics. Hypertension. 1993;22:292–294.
21. Haynes R. Is weight loss an effective treatment for hypertension. Can J Physiol Pharmacol. 1985;64:825.
22. Langford H, Davis B, Blaufox D, et al. Effect of drug and diet treatment of mild hypertension on diastolic blood pressure. Hypertension. 1991;17:210.
23. Hypertension Prevention Treatment Group. The Hypertension Trial: Three-year effects of dietary changes on blood pressure. Arch Intern Med. 1990;150:153.
24. Davis BR, Blaufox D, Oberman A, Wassertheil-Smoller S, Zimbaldi N, Cutler JA, Kirchner K, Langford HG. Reduction in long-term antihypertensive medication requirements: effects of weight reduction by dietary intervention in overweight persons with mild hypertension. Arch Intern Med. 1993;153:1773–1782.
25. Fagerberg B, Andersson O, Isaksson B, et al. Blood pressure control during weight reduction in obese hypertensive men: separate effects of sodium and energy restriction. Br Med J. 1984;288:11.

26. Maxwell M, Kushiro T, Dornfeld L, et al. BP changes in obese hypertensive subjects during rapid weight loss. Comparison of restricted v unchanged salt intake. Arch Intern Med. 1984;144:1581.
27. Gillum R, Prineas R, Jeffrey R, et al. Nonpharmacological therapy of hypertension: the independent effects of weight reduction and sodium restriction in overweight borderline hypertensive patients. Am Heart J. 1983;105:128.
28. Reisen E. Weight reduction in the management of hypertension: epidemiologic and mechanistic evidence. Can J Physiol Pharmacol. 1985;64:818.
29. Reisen E, Abel R, Modan M, et al. Effect of weight loss without salt restriction on the reduction of blood pressure in overweight hypertensive patients. N Engl J Med. 1978;298:1.
30. Rocchini AP, Katch V, Anderson J, Hinderliter J, Becque D, Martin M, Marks C. Blood pressure and obese adolescents: effect of weight loss. Pediatrics. 1988;82;116–123.
31. Dahl LK, Silver L, Christie RW. The role of salt in the fall of blood pressure accompanying reduction in obesity. N Engl J Med. 1958;258:1186–1192.
32. Tuck MI, Sowers J, Dornfield L, Kledzik G, Maxwell M. The effect of weight reduction on blood pressure plasma renin activity and plasma aldosterone level in obese patients. N Engl J Med. 1981;304:930–933.
33. Rocchini AP, Key J, Bondie D, Chico R, Moorehead C, Katch V, Martin M. The effect of weight loss on the sensitivity of blood pressure to sodium in obese adolescents. N Engl J Med. 1989;321:580–585.
34. Dornfield TP, Maxwell MH, Waks AU, Schroth P, Tuck ML. Obesity and hypertension: long-term effects of weight reduction on blood pressure. Int J Obes. 1985;9:381–389.
35. Reisen E, Frohlich ED. Effects of weight reduction on arterial pressure. J Chronic Dis. 1982;33:887–891.
36. Sjöström CD, Peltonen M, Wedel H, Sjöström L. Differential long-term effects of intentional weight loss on diabetes and hypertension Hypertension. 2000;36:20–25.
37. Sjöström CD, Lissner L, Wedel H, Sjöström l. Reduction in incidence of diabetes, hypertension, and lipid disturbances after intentional weight loss induced by bariatric surgery: the SOS Intervention Study. Obes Res. 1999:7:477–484.
38. Carson JL Ruddy ME, Duff AE, Holems NJ, Cody RP, Brolin RE. The effect of gastric bypass surgery on hypertension in morbidly obese patients. Arch Intern Med. 1994;154:193–200.
39. Sjöström CD, Peltonen M, Sjöströml. Blood pressure and pulse pressure during long-term weight loss in the obese: the Swedish Obese Subjects (SOS) Intervention Study. Obes Res. 2001;9:188–195.
40. Vague J. The degree of masculine differentiation of obesities: a factor determining predisposition to diabetes, atherosclerosis, gout, and uric calculous disease. Am J Clin Nutr. 1956;4:20–34.
41. Landsberg L. Obesity and hypertension: experimental data. J Hypertens. 1992;10:S195–S201.
42. Shear CL, Freedman DS, Burke GL, Harsha DW, Berenson GS. Body fat patterning and blood pressure in children and young adults: the Bogalusa Heart Study. Hypertension. 1987;9:236–244.
43. Itallie V. Health implications of overweight and obesity in the United States. Ann Intern Med. 1985;103:983.
44. Kalkoff R, Hartz A, Rupley D, et al. Relationship of body fat distribution to blood pressure, carbohydrate tolerance, and plasma lipids in healthy obese women. J Lab Clin Med. 1983;102:621.
45. Kissebah A, Vydelingum N, Murray R, et al. Relation of body fat distribution to metabolic complications of obesity. J Clin Endocrinol Metab. 1982;54:254.
46. Peiris A, Sothmann M, Hoffmann R, et al. Adiposity, fat distribution, and cardiovascular risk. Ann Intern Med. 1989;110:867.
47. Donahue RP, Abbot RD, Bloom E, Reed DM, Yano K. Central obesity and coronary heart disease in men. Lancet. 1987;1:882–884.
48. Fox CS, Massaro JM, Hoffmann U, Pou KM, Maurovich-Horvat P, Liu CY, Masan RS, Murabito JM, Meigs JB, Cupples LA, D'Agostino RB Sr, O'Donnell CJ. Abdominal visceral and subcutaneous adipose tissue compartments: association with metabolic risk factors in the Framingham Heart Study. Circulation. 2007;116:39–48.
49. Lapidus L, Bengtsson C, Lissner L. Distribution of adipose tissue in relation to cardiovascular and total mortality as observed during 20 years in a prospective population study of women in Gothenburg, Sweden. Diabetes Res Clin Pract. 1990;10(Suppl 1):S185–S189.
50. Bjorntorp P. Portal adipose tissue as a generator of risk factors for cardiovascular disease and diabetes. Atherosclerosis. 1990;289:333–345.
51. Verwaerde P, Denard JM, Galinier M, Rouge P, Massabuau P, Galitsky J, Berlan M, Lafontan M, Montastruc JL. Changes in short-term variability of blood pressure and heart rate during the development of obesity-associated hypertension in high–fat fed dogs. J Hypertens. 1999;17:1135–1143.
52. Mitttelman SD, Van Citters GW, Kim SP, Davis DA, Dea MK, Hamilton-Wessler M, Bergman RN. Longitudinal compensation for fat-induced insulin resistance includes reduced insulin clearance and enhanced B-cell response. Diabetes. 2000;49:2116–2125.

53. Hall JE, Granger JP, Hester RL, Montani JP. Mechanisms of sodium balance in hypertension: role of pressure natriuresis. J Hypertens. 1986;4(Suppl 4):S57–S65.
54. Granger JP, West D, Scott J. Abnormal pressure natriuresis in the dog model of obesity-induced hypertension. Hypertension. 1994;23(Suppl I):I-8–I-11.
55. Hall JE, Brands MW, Henegar JR, Shek EW. Abnormal kidney function as a cause and a consequence of obesity hypertension. Clin Exp Pharmacol Physiol. 1998;25:58–64.
56. Hall JE. The kidney, hypertension and obesity. Hypertension. 2003;41:625–633.
57. Modan M, Halkin H, Almog S, et al. Hyperinsulinemia: a link between hypertension, obesity and glucose intolerance. J Clin Invest. 1985;75:809–817.
58. Voors AW, Radhakrishnamurthy B, Srinivasan SR, Webber LS, Berenson GS. Plasma glucose level related to blood pressure in 272 children, ages 7-15 years, sampled from a total biracial population. Am J Epidemiol. 1981;113:347–356.
59. Kanai H, Matsuzawa Y, Tokunaga K, Keno Y, Kobatake T, Fujiola S, Nakajima T, Tarui S. Hypertension in obese children: fasting serum insulin levels are closely correlated with blood pressure. Int J Obes. 1990;14:1047–1056.
60. Saito I, Nishino M, Kawabe H, Wainai H, Hasegawa C, Saruta T, Nagano S, Sekihhara T. Leisure time physical activity and insulin resistance in young obese students with hypertension. Am J Hypertens. 1992;5:915–918.
61. Chen W, Srinivasan SR, Elkasabany A, Berenson GS. Cardiovascular risk factors clustering features of insulin resistance syndrome (Syndrome X) in a biracial (Black-White) population of children, adolescents, and young adults: the Bogalusa Heart Study. Am J Epidemiol. 1999;150:667–674.
62. Young-Hyman D, Schlundt DG, Herman L, De Luca F, Counts D. Evaluation of the insulin resistance syndrome in a 5- to 10-year-old overweight/obese African-American children. Diabetes Care. 2001;24:1359–1364.
63. Haffner SM, Ferrannini E, Hazuda HP, et al. Clustering of cardiovascular risk factors in confirmed prehypertensive individuals: the San Antonio heart study. Diabetes. 1992;41:715–722.
64. Falkner B. Differences in blacks and whites with essential hypertension: biochemistry and endocrine. Hypertension. 1990;15:681–686.
65. Falkner B, Hulman S, Tannenbaum, et al. Insulin resistance and blood pressure in young black males. Hypertension. 1988;12:352–358.
66. Shen D-C, Shieh S-M, Fuh MM-T, et al. Resistance to insulin-stimulated-glucose uptake in patients with hypertension. J Clin Endocrinol Metab. 1988;66:580–583.
67. Darwin CH, Alpizar M, Buchanan TA, et al. Insulin resistance does not correlate with hypertension in Mexican American women. In 75th Annual Meeting Abstracts, Bethesda, MD, Endocrine Society Press, p. 233.
68. Pollare T, Lithell H, Berne C. Insulin resistance is a characteristic feature of primary hypertension independent of obesity. Metabolism. 1990;39:167–174.
69. Rocchini AP, Katch V, Schork A, Kelch RP. Insulin's role in blood pressure regulation during weight loss in obese adolescents. Hypertension. 1987;10:267–273.
70. Krotkorwski M, Mandroukas K, Sjostrom L, Sullivan L, Wetterquist H, Bjorntrop P. Effect of long-term physical training on body fat, metabolism and blood pressure in obesity. Metabolism. 1979;28:650–658.
71. Zavaroni I, Sander S, Scott S, Reaven GM. Effect of fructose feeding of insulin secretion and insulin action in the rat. Metabolism. 1980;29:970–973.
72. Hwang IS, Ho H, Hoffman BB, Reaven GM. Fructose-induced insulin and hypertension in rats. Hypertension. 1987;10:512–516.
73. Reaven GM, Ho H, Hoffman BB. Attenuation of fructose-induces hypertension in rats by exercise drainage. Hypertension. 1988;12:129–132.
74. Reaven GM, Ho H, Hoffamn BB. Somatostatin inhibition of fructose-induced hypertension. Hypertension. 1989;14:117–120.
75. Kurtz TW, Morris RC, Pershadsingh HA. The Zucker fatty rat as a genetic model of obesity and hypertension. Hypertension. 1989;13(6 Pt 2):896–901.
76. Mondon CE, Reaven GM. Evidence of abnormalities of insulin-stimulated glucose uptake in adipocytes isolates from spontaneously hypertensive rats with spontaneous hypertension. Metabolism. 1988;37:303–305.
77. Reaven GM, Chang H, Hoffman BB, Azhar S. Resistance to insulin-stimulated glucose uptake in adipocytes isolates from spontaneously hypertensive rats. Diabetes. 1989;38:1155–1160.
78. Finch D, Davis G, Bower J, Kirchner K. Effect of insulin on renal sodium handling in hypertensive rats. Hypertensive rats. Hypertension. 1990;15:514–518.
79. Julius S, Jamerson K, Media A, et al. The association of borderline hypertension with target organ changes and higher coronary risk. Tecumseh Blood Pressure Study. JAMA. 1990;264:354–358.

80. Ferrari P, Weidmann P, Shaw S, et al. Altered insulin sensitivity, hyperinsulinemia, and dyslipidemia in individuals with a hypertensive parent. Am J Med. 1991;91:589–596.

81. Rocchini AP, Katch V, Kveselis D, Moorehead C, Martin M, Lampman R, Gregory M. Insulin and renal sodium retention in obese adolescents. Hypertension. 1989;14:367–374.

82. DeFronzo RA, Cooke CR, Andres R, Fabona GR, Davis PJ. The effect of insulin on renal handling of sodium, potassium, calcium and phosphate in man. J Clin Invest. 1975;55:845–855.

83. Baum M. Insulin stimulates volume absorption in the proximal convoluted tubule. J Clin Invest. 1987;79:1104–1109.

84. Vierhapper H, Waldhausl W, Nowontny P. The effect of insulin on the rise in blood pressure and plasma aldosterone after angiotensin II in normal man. Clin Sci. 1983;64:383–386.

85. Rocchini AP, Moorehead C, DeRemer S, Goodfriend TL, Ball DL. Hyperinsulinemia and the aldosterone and pressor responses to angiotensin II. Hypertension. 1990;15:861–866.

86. Finta KM, Rocchini AP, Moorehead C, Key J, Katch V. Sodium retention in response to an oral glucose tolerance test in obese and nonobese adolescents. Pediatrics. 1992;90:442–446.

87. Rocchini AP. Insulin resistance, obesity, and hypertension. J Nutr. 1995;125(6 Suppl):1718S–1724S.

88. Ter Maaten JC, Bakker SJ, Serne EH, ter Wee PM, Donker AJ, Gans RO. Insulin's acute effects on glomerular filtration rate correlate with insulin sensitivity whereas insulin's acute effects on proximal tubular sodium reabsorption correlate with salt sensitivity in normal subjects. Nephrol Dial Transplant. 1999;14:2357–2363.

89. Ferrannini E, Buzzigoli G, Bonadonna R, et al. Insulin resistance in essential hypertension. N Engl J Med. 1987;317:350–357.

90. Lucas CP, Estigarribia JA, Daraga LL, Reaven GM. Insulin and blood pressure in obesity. Hypertension. 1985;7:702–706.

91. Sowers JR. Insulin resistance, hyperinsulinemia, dyslipidemia, hypertension, and accelerated atherosclerosis. J Clin Pharmacol. 1992;32:539–535.

92. Swislocki ALM, Hoffman BB, Reaven GM. Insulin resistance, glucose intolerance, and hyperinsulinemia in patients with hypertension. Am J Hypertens. 1989;2:419–423.

93. Grugni G, Ardizzi A, Dubini A, Guzzaloni G, Sartorio A, Morabito F. No correlation between insulin levels and high blood pressure in obese subjects. Horm Metab Res. 1990;22(2):124–125.

94. Hall JE, Brands MW, Kivlighn SD, Mizelle HL, Hidebrandt DA, Gaillard CA. Chronic hyperinsulinemia and blood pressure: interaction with catecholamines? Hypertension. 1990;15:519–527.

95. Brechtold P, Jorgens V, Finke C, et al. Epidemiology and hypertension. Int J Obes. 1981;5(Suppl 1):1–7.

96. Rocchini AP, Yang Q, Gokee A. Hypertension and insulin resistance are not directly related in obese dogs. Hypertension. 2004;43:1011–1016.

97. Rocchini AP, Katch VL, Grekin R, Moorehead C, Anderson J. Role for aldosterone in blood pressure regulation of obese adolescents. Am J Cardiol. 1986;57:613–618.

98. Hiramatsu K, Yamada T, Ichikawak T, Izumiyama T, Nagata H. Changes in endocrine activity to obesity in patients with essential hypertension. J Am Geriatr Soc. 1981;29:25–30.

99. Scavo D, Borgia C, Iacobelli A. Aspetti di funzione corticosurrenalica nell'obesita'. Nota VI. I1 comportamento della secrezione di aldosterone e della escrezione dei suoi metabolite nel corso di alcune prove dinamiche. Folia Endocrinol. 1968;21:591–602.

100. Scavo D, Iacobelli A, Borgia C. Aspetti fi funzione corticosurrenalica nell'obesita'. Nota V. La secrezonia giornlieia di aldosterone. Folia Endocrinol. 1968;21:577–590.

101. Spark RF, Arky RA, Boulter RP, Saudek CD, Obrian JT. Renin, aldosterone and glucagon in the natriureses of fasting. N Engl J Med. 1975;292:1335–1340.

102. Granger JP, West D, Scott J. Abnormal pressure natriuresis in the dog model of obesity-induced hypertension. Hypertension. 1994;23(Suppl I):I8–I11.

103. Goodfriend TL, Calhoun DA. Resistant hypertension, obesity, sleep apnea and aldosterone: theory and therapy. Hypertension. 2004;43:518–524.

104. Trovati M, Massucco P, Anfossi G, Caralot F, Mularoni E, Mattiello L, Rocca G, Emaneulli G. Insulin influences the renin-angiotensin-aldosterone system in humans. Metabolism. 1989;38:501–503.

105. Farfel Z, Iania A, Eliahou HE. Presence of insulin-renin-aldosterone-potassium interrelationship in normal subjects, disrupted in chronic hemodialysis patients. Clin Endrocrinol Metab. 1978;47:9–17.

106. de Paula RB, da Silva AA, Hall JE. Aldosterone antagonism attenuates obesity-induced hypertension and glomerular hyperfiltration. Hypertension. 2004;43:41–47.

107. Young JB, Landsberg L. Suppression of sympathetic nervous system during fasting. Science. 1977;196:1473–1475.

108. Young JB, Landsberg L. Stimulation of the sympathetic nervous system during sucrose feeding. Nature. 1977;269:615–617.

109. Landsberg L, Young JB. Fasting, feeding and regulation of the sympathetic nervous system. N Engl J Med. 1978;298:1295–1301.

110. Young JB, Saville ME, Rothwell NJ, Stock MJ, Landsberg L. Effect of diet and cold exposure on norepinephrine turnover in brown adipose tissue in the rat. J Clin Invest. 1982;69:1061–1071.

111. Landsberg L, Young JB. Insulin-mediated glucose metabolism in the relationship between dietary intake and sympathetic nervous system activity. Int J Obes. 1985;9:63–68.

112. Landsberg L, Krieger DR. Obesity, metabolism and the sympathetic nervous system. Am J Hypertens. 1989;2:125s–132s.

113. Young JB, Kaufman LN, Saville ME, Landsberg L. Increased sympathetic nervous system activity in rats fed a low protein diet: evidence against a role for dietary tyrosine. Am J Physiol. 1985;248:r627–r637.

114. Rowe JW, Young BY, Minaker KL, Stevens AL, Pallatta J, Landsberg L. Effect of insulin and glucose infusions on sympathetic nervous system activity in normal human man. Diabetes. 1981;30:219–225.

115. O'Hare JA, Minaker K, Young JB, Rowe JW, Pallotta JA, Landsberg L. Insulin increases plasma norepinephrine (NE) and lowers plasma potassium equally in lean and obese men [abstract]. Clin Res. 1985;33:441a.

116. Anderson EA, Hoffman RP, Balon TW, Sinkey CA, Mark AL. Hyperinsulinemia produces both sympathetic neural activation and vasodilation in normal humans. J Clin Invest. 1991;87:2246–2252.

117. Voors AW, Webber LS, Berenson GS. Resting heart rate and pressure-rate product of children in a total biracial community: the Bogalusa Heart Study. Am J Epidemiol. 1982;116:276–286.

118. Jiang X, Srinivasan SR, Urbina E, Berenson GS. Hyperdynamic circulation and cardiovascular risk in children and adolescents: the Bogalusa Heart Study. Circulation. 1995;91:1101–1106.

119. Riva P, Martini G, Rabbia F, Milan A, Paglieri C, Chiandussi L, Veglio F. Obesity and autonomic function in adolescents. Clin Exp Hypertens. 2001;23:57–67.

120. Alvarez GE, Beske SD, Ballard TP, et al. Sympathetic neural activation in visceral obesity. Circulation. 2002;106:2533–2536.

121. Young JB, Macdonald IA. Sympathoadrenal activity in human obesity: heterogeneity of findings since 1980. Int J Obes. 1992;16:959–967.

122. Kassab S, Kato T, Wilkins C, Chen R, Hall JE, Granger JP. Renal denervation attenuates the sodium retention and hypertension associated with obesity. Hypertension. 1995;25(part 2):893–897.

123. Eikelis N, Lambert G, Wiener G, Kaye D, Schlaich M, Morris M, Hastings J, Socratour F, Esler M. Extra-adipocyte release in humans obesity and its relation to sympathoadrenal function. Am J Physiol Endocrin Metab. 2004;286:E744–E752.

124. Rocchini AP, Mao HZ, Babu K, Marker P, Rocchini AJ. Clonidine prevents insulin resistance and hypertension in obese dogs. Hypertension. 1999;33:548–553.

125. Wofford MR, Anderson DC Jr, Brown CA, Jones DW, Miller ME, Hall HE. Antihypertensive effect of alpha- and beta-adrenergic blockade in obese and lean hypertensive subjects. Am J Hypertens. 2001;14:694–698.

126. Lohmeier TE, Warren S, Cunningham JT. Sustained activation of the central baroreceptor pathway in obesity hypertension. Hypertension. 2003;42:96–102.

127. Arner P. Not all fat is alike. Lancet. 1998;351:1301–1302.

128. Griffin ME, Marcucci MJ, Cline GW, Bell K, Barucci N, Lee D, Goodyear LJ, Kraegen EW, White MF, Shulman GI. Free fatty acid-induced insulin resistance is associated with activation of protein kinase C-θ and alteration in the insulin signaling cascade. Diabetes. 1999;48:1270–1274.

129. Kabir M, Catalano KJ, Ananthnarayan S, Kim SP, Van Citters GW, Dea MK, Bergman RN. Molecular evidence supporting the portal theory: a causative link between visceral adiposity and hepatic insulin resistance. Am J Physiol Endocrinol Metab. 2005;288:E454–E461.

130. Grekin RJ, Dumont CJ, Vollmer AP, Watts SW, Webb RC. Mechanisms in the pressor effects of hepatic portal venous fatty acid infusion. Am J Physiol. 1997;273:R324–R330.

131. Buller KM. Role of circumventricular organs in pro-inflammatory cytokine-induce activation of the hypothalamic-pituitary-adrenal axis. Clin Exp Pharmacol Physiol. 2001;28:581–589.

132. Lin Y, Matsumura K, Hukuhara M, Kafiyama S, Fujii K, Iida M. Ghrelin acts at the nucleus of the solitary tract to decrease arterial pressure in rats. Hypertension. 2004;43:977–982.

133. Cowley MA, Smart JL, Rubinstein M, et al. Leptin activates anoreigenic POMC neurons through a neural network in the arcuate nucleus. Nature. 2001;411:480–484.

134. Mizuno TM, Kleopoulos SP, Bergen HT, et al. Hypothalamic pro-opiomelanocortin mRNA is reduced by fasting and [corrected] in ob/ob and db/db mice , but is stimulated by leptin. Diabetes. 1998;47:294–297.

135. Korner J, Savontaus E, Chua SC, et al. Leptin regulation of Agrp and Npy mRNA in the rat hypothalamus. J Neuroendocrinol. 2001;13:959–966.

136. Elmquist JK. Hypothalamic pathways underlying the endocrine autonomic and behavioral effects of leptin. Physiol Behav. 2001;74:703–708.

137. Cone RD, Cowley MA, Butler AA, et al. The arcuate nucleus as a conduit for diverse signals relevant to energy homeostasis. Int J Obes Relat Metab Disord. 2001;25(Suppl 5):S63–S67.

138. Eikelis N, Esler M. The neurobiology of human obesity. Exp Physiol. 2005;90:673–682.
139. Kuo LE, Kitlinska JB, Tilan JU, Li L, Baker SB, Johnson MD, Lee EW, Burnett MS, Fricke ST, Kvetnansky R, Herzog H, Zukowska Z. Neuropeptide Y acts directly in the periphery on fat tissue and mediates stress-induced obesity and metabolic syndrome. Nat Med. 2007;13:803–811.
140. Karvonen MK, Valkonen VP, Lakka TA, et al. Leucine 7 to praline 7 polymorphism of the preroneuropeptide Y is associated with the progression of carotid atherosclerosis, blood pressure and serum lipids in Finnish men. Atherosclerosis. 2001;159:145–151.
141. Wallerstedt SM, Skritic S, Eriksson AL, Ohlsson C, Hedner T. Association analysis of polymorphism T1128C in the signal peptide of neuropeptide Y in a Swedish hypertensive population. J Hypertens. 2004;22:1277–1281.
142. Michaud EJ, Bultman SJ, Yang YK, et al. A molecular model for the genetic and phenotypic characteristics of the mouse lethal yell (a(Y)) mutation. Proc Natl Acad Sci USA. 1994;91:2562–2566.
143. Ni XP, Butler A, Cone RG, et al. Central receptors mediating the cardiovascular actions of melanocyte stimulating hormones. J Hypertens. 2006;24:2239–2246.
144. Matsumura K, Tsuchihashi T, Abe I, et al. Central a-melanocyte-stimulating hormone acts at melanocortin-4 receptor to activate sympathetic nervous system in conscious rabbits. Brain Res. 2002;948:145–148.
145. Foss YJ. Vitamin D deficiency is the cause of common obesity. Med Hypotheses. 2008;72:314–321.
146. Pittas AG, Lau J, Hu FB, Dawson-Hughes B. The role of vitamin D, calcium in type 2 diabetes. A systematic review and meta-analysis. J Clin Endocrinol Metab. 2007;92:2017–2029.
147. Ybarra J, Sanchez-Hernandez J, Perez A. Hypo-vitamin D and morbid obesity. Nurs Clin North Am. 2007;42:19–27.
148. Buffington C, Walker B, Cowan CSM Jr, Scruggs D. Vitamin D deficiency in the morbidly obese. Obes Surg. 1993;3:421–424.
149. Arunabh S, Pollack S, Yeh J, Aloia JF. Body fat content and 25-hydroxyvitamin P levels in healthy women. J Clin Endocrinol Metab. 2003;88:157–161.
150. Bjorntorp P, Rosmond R. Neuroendocrine abnormalities in visceral obesity. Int J Obes Relat Metab Disord. 2000;24(Suppl 2):S80–S85.
151. Strain GW, Zumoff B, Strain JL. Cortisol production in obesity. Metabolism. 1980;29:980–985.
152. Rosmond R, Dallman MF, Bjorntorp P. Stress-related cortisol secretion in men: relationships with abdominal obesity and endocrine, metabolic and hemodynamic abnormalities. J Clin Endocrinol Metab. 1998;83:1853–1859.
153. Kvist H, Chowdhury B, Grangard U, Tylen U, Sjostrom L. Total and visceral adipose tissue volumes derived from measurements with computed tomography in adult men and women. Predicative equations. Am J Clin Nutr. 1988;48:1351–1361.
154. Rosmond R, Bjorntorp P. The interactions between hypothalamic-pituitary-adrenal axis activity, testosterone, insulin-like growth factor I and abdominal obesity with metabolism and blood pressure in man. Int J Obes Relat Metab Disord. 1998;22:1184–1196.
155. Zahrezewska KE, Cusin J, Sainbury A, Pohner F, Jeanrenaud FR, Jeanrenaud B. Glucocorticoids are counterregulatory hormones to leptin. Towards an understanding of leptin resistance. Diabetes. 1997;46:717–719.
156. Rosmond R, Holm G, Bjorntorp P. Food-induced cortisol secretion relation to anthropometric, metabolic and hemodynamic variables in men Int J Obes Relat Metab Disord. 2000;24:95–105.
157. Rosmond R, Chagnon YC, Holm G, Changon M, Perusse L, Lindell K, Carlsson B, Bouchard C, Bjorntorp P. A glucocorticoid receptor gene marker is associated with abdominal obesity, leptin, and dysregulation of the hypothalamic-pituitary-adrenal axis. Obes Res. 2000;8:211–218.
158. Weaver J, Hitman GA, Kopelaman PG. An association between a Bc/I restriction fragment length polymorphism of the glucocorticoid receptor gene locus and hyperinsulinemia in obese women. J Mol Endocrinol. 1992;9:295–300.
159. Buemann B, Vohl MC, Chagnon M, Chagnon YC, Gagnon J, Perusse L, Dionne F, Despres JP, Tremblay A, Nadeau A, Bouchard C. Abdominal visceral fat is associated with a Bc/I restriction fragment length polymorphism at the glucocorticoid receptor gene locus. Obes Res. 1997;5:186–189.
160. Bjorntorp P, Rosmond R. Hypothalamic origin of the metabolic syndrome X. Ann N Y Acad Sci. 1999;892:308–311.
161. Manson JE, Colditz GA, Stampfer MJ, Willnet WC, Rosner B, Monson RR, Speizer FE, Hennekens CH. A prospective study of obesity and risk of coronary heart disease in women. N Engl J Med. 1990;322:882–889.
162. Kotelainen ML. Adiposity, cardiac size and precursors of coronary atherosclerosis in 5 to 15 year old children: a retrospective study of 210 violent deaths. Int J Obes. 1997;21:691–697.

163. Inge TH, Miyano G, Bean J, Melmrath M, Courcoulas A, Chen MK, Wilson K, Daniels SR, Garcia VF, Brandt ML, Dolan LM. Reversal of type 2 diabetes mellitus and improvements in cardiovascular risk factors after surgical weight loss in adolescents. Pediatrics. 2009;123:214–222.

164. MacMahon SW, Wicken DEL, MacDonald GJ. Effect of weight loss on left ventricular mass, a randomized controlled trial in young overweight hypertensive patients. N Engl J Med. 1985;314:334–339.

165. Alpert MA, Singh A, Terry BE, Kelly DL, Villarreal D, Mukerji V. Effect of exercise on left ventricular systolic function and reserve in morbid obesity. Am J Cardiol. 1989;63:1478–1482.

166. De Divittis O, Fazio S, Petitto M, Maddalena G, Contaldo F, Mancini M. Obesity and cardiac function. Circulation. 1981;64:477–482.

167. Alexander JK, Pettigrove JR. Obesity and congestive heart failure. Geriatrics. 1967;22:101–108.

168. Raison HJ, Achimastos A, Bouthier J, London G, Safar M. Intravascular volume, extracellular fluid volume, and total body water in obese and non-obese hypertensive patients. Am J Cardiol. 1983;51:165–170.

169. Reisin E, Frohlich ED, Messerli FH, Dreslinski GR, Dunn FG, Jones MM, Batson HM. Cardiovascular changes after weight reduction in obesity hypertension. Ann Int Med. 1983;98:315–319.

170. Lesser GT, Deutsch S. Measurement of adipose tissue blood flow and perfusion in man by uptake of 85-Kr. J Appl Physiol. 1967;23:621–631.

171. Guillerno E, Garavaglia E, Messerli FH, Nunez BD, Schmieder RE, Grossman E. Myocardial contractility and left ventricular function in obese patients with essential hypertension. Am J Cardiol. 1988;62: 594–597.

172. Stoddard MF, Tseuda K, Thomas M, Dillon S, Kupersmith J. The influence of obesity on left ventricular filing and systolic function. Am Heart J. 1992;124:694.

173. Urbina EM, Gidding SS, Bao W, Pickoff AS, Berdusis K, Berenson GS. Effect of body size, ponderosity, and blood pressure on left ventricular growth in children and young adults in the Bogalusa Heart Study. Circulation. 1995;91:2400–2406.

174. Daniels SR, Kimball TR, Morrison JA, Khoury P, Witt S, Meyer RA. Effect of lean body mass, fat mass, blood pressure, and sexual maturation on left ventricular mass in children and adolescents. Statistical, biological, and clinical significance. Circulation. 1995;92:3249–3254.

175. Daniels SR, Loggie JM, Khoury P, Kimball TR. Left ventricular geometry and severe left ventricular hypertrophy inchildren and adolescents with essential hypertension. Circulation. 1998;97: 1907–1911.

176. Blake J. Devereaux RB, Borer JS, Szulc M, Pappas TW, Laragh JH. Relation of obesity, high sodium intake, and eccentric left ventricular hypertrophy to left ventricular exercise dysfunction in essential hypertension. Am J Med. 1990;88:477–485.

177. Grossman E, Orren S, Messerli FH. Left ventricular filling in the systemic hypertension of obesity. Am J Cardiol. 1991;60:57–60.

178. Ippisch HM, Inge TH, Daniels SR, Wang B, Khoury PR, Witt SA, Glascock BJ, Garcia VF, Kimball TR. Reversibility of cardiac abnormalities in morbidly obese adolescents. J Am Coll Cardiol. 2009;8:1342–1348.

179. Schmeider RE, Messerli FH. Does obesity influence early target organ damage in hypertensive patients? Circulation. 1993;87:1482–1488.

180. Harada L, Orino T, Takada G. Body mass index can predict left ventricular diastolic filling in asymptomatic obese children. Pediatr Cardiol. 2001;22:273–278.

181. Kanoupalis E, Michaloudis D, Fraidakis O, Parthenakis F, Vardas P, Melissas J. Left ventricular function and cardiopulmonary performance following surgical treatment of morbid obesity. Obes Surg. 2001;11:552–558.

182. Messerli FH, Nunez BD, Ventura HO, Snyder DW. Overweight and sudden death: increased ventricular ectopy in cardiopathy in obesity. Arch Intern Med. 1987;147:1725–1728.

183. Nakajima T, Fugiola S, Tokunaga K, Matsuzawa Y, Tami S. Correlation of intraabdominal fat accumulation and left ventricular performance in obesity. Am J Cardiol. 1989;64:369–373.

184. Becque MD, Katch VL, Rocchini AP, Marks CR, Moorehead C. Coronary risk incidence of obese adolescents: reductions of exercise plus diet intervention. Pediatrics. 1988;81:605–612.

185. Rocchini AP, Moorehead C, Katch V, Key J, Finta KM. Forearm resistance vessel abnormalities and insulin resistance in obese adolescents. Hypertension. 1992;19:615–620.

186. Anderson P, Henriksson J. Capillary supply of the quadriceps femoris muscle of man: adaptive response to exercise. J Physiol. 1977;270:677–690.

187. Chi MMY, Hintz CS, Henriksson J. Chronic stimulation of mammalian muscle: enzyme changes in individual fibers. Am J Physiol. 1986;251:c633–c642.

188. Ryan DH, Bray GA, Helmcke F, Sander G, Volaufava J, Greenway F, Subramaniam P, Glancy DL. Serial echocardiographic and clinical evaluation of valvular regurgitation before, during, and after

treatment with fenfluramine or dexfenfluramine and mazindol or phentermine. Obes Res. 1999;7: 313–322.

189. Daniels SR, Long B, Crow S, Styne D, Sothern M, Vargas-Rodriguez I, Harris L, Walch J, Jasinsky O, Cwik K, Hewkin A, Blakesley V. Sibutramine. Adolescent study Group. Cardiovascular effects of sibutramine in the treatment of obese adolescents: results of a randomized, double-blind, placebo-controlled study. Pediatrics. 2007;120:e147–e157.

190. Ioannides-Demos LL, Proietto J, Tonkin AM, McNeil JJ. Safety of drug therapies used for weight loss and treatment of obesity. Drug Saf. 2006;29:277–302.

191. Ozkan B, Bereket A, Turan S, Keskin S. Addition of orlistat to conventional treatment in adolescents with severe obesity. Eur J Pediatr. 2004;163:738–741.

192. Wang F, Tian D, Han J. Electroacupuncture in the treatment of obesity. Neurochem Res. 2008;33:2023–2027.

193. Deedwania P. The endocannabinoid system and cardiometabolic risk: effect of CB1 receptor blockade on lipid metabolism. Int J Cardiol. 2008;131:305–312.

194. Van Gaal LF, Tissanen AM, Scheen AJ, Ziegler O, Rossner S. Effects of the cannabinoid-1 receptor blocker rimonabant on weight reduction and cardiovascular risk factors in overweight patients: 1-year experience from the RIO-Europe study. Lancet. 2005;365:1389–1397.

195. Despres JP, Golay A, Sjostrom L. Effects of rimonabant on metabolic risk factors in overweight patients with dyslipidemia. N Engl J Med. 2005;353:2121–2134.

196. Pi-Sunyer FX, Aronne LJ, Heshmati HM, Devin J, Rosenstock J. Effects of rimonabant, a canncbinoid-1 receptor blocker on weight and cardiometabolic factors in overweight or obese patients: RIO- North America: a randomized controlled trial. JAMA. 2006;295:761–775.

197. Glueck CJ, Aregawi D, Winiarska M, Agloria M, Kuo G, Sieve L. Metformin-diet ameliorates coronary heart disease risk factors and facilitates resumption of regular menses in adolescents with polycystic ovary syndrome. J Pediatr Endocrinol Metab. 2006;19:831–842.

198. Helvaci MR, Sevinc A, Camci C, Yalcin A. Treatment of white coat hypertension with metformin. Int Heart J. 2008;49:671–679.

199. Pollare T, Lithell H, Berne C. A comparison of the effects of hydrochlorothiazide and captopril on glucose and lipid metabolism in patients with hypertension. N Engl J Med. 1989;321:868–873.

200. Beardwood DM, Alden JS, Graham CA, et al. Evidence for a peripheral action of chlorothiazide in normal man. Metabolism. 1966;15:88–93.

201. Gill JS, Al-Hussary N, Anderson DC. Effect of nifedipine on glucose tolerance, serum insulin, and serum fructosamine in diabetic patients. Clin Ther. 1987;9:304–310.

202. Klauser R, Ptager R, Gaube S, et al. Metabolic effects on isradipine versus hydrochlorothiazide in diabetes mellitus. Hypertension. 1991;17:15–21.

203. Pollare T, Lithell H, Morlin C, et al. Metabolic effects of diltiazem and atenolol: results from a randomized, double blind study with parallel groups. J Hypertens. 1989;7:551–555.

204. Grunfeld CM, Chappell DA. Prevention of glucose intolerance of thiazide diuretics by maintenance of body potassium. Diabetes. 1983;32:106–111.

205. Trachtman H, Hainer JW, Sugg J, Teng R, Sorof JM, Radcliffe J. Candesartan in children with hypertension (CINCH) Investigators. Efficacy, safety, and pharmacokinetics of candesartan cilexetil in hypertension children aged 6 to 17 years. J Clin Hypertens. 2008;10:734–750.

206. Swislocki AL, Hoffman BB, Sheu WH, Chen YD, Reaven GM. Effect of prazosin treatment on carbohydrate and lipoprotein metabolism in patients with hypertension. Am J Med. 1989;86:14–18.

207. Pollare T, Lithell H, Selinus I, et al. Application of prazosin is associated with an increase of insulin sensitivity in obese patients with hypertension. Diabetologia. 1988;31:415–420.

208. Giugliano D, Acampora R, Marfella R, La Marca C, Marfella M, Nappo F, D'Onofrio F. Hemodynamic and metabolic effects of transdermal clonidine in patients with hypertension and non-insulin dependent diabetes mellitus. Am J Hypertens. 1998;11:184–189.

209. Fajans SS, Floyd JC, Knopf RF, et al. Benthiadiazine suppression of insulin release from normal and abnormal islet cell tissue of a man. J Clin Invest. 1966;45:481–493.

210. Amery A, Birkenhager W, Brixxo P. Glucose intolerance during diuretic therapy in elderly hypertensive patients. Med J. 1986;62:919–925.

211. Morgan TO. Metabolic effects of various antihypertensive agents. J Cardiovasc Pharmacol. 1990;15(Suppl 5):s39–s45.

212. Bergtsson C, Blhme T, Lapidus D. Do antihypertensive drugs precipitate diabetes? BMJ. 1984;289: 1495–1497.

213. Greenberg G, Brennan PJ, Miall WE. Effects of diuretic and β-Blocker therapy in the MRC trial. Am J Med. 1984;76:45–51.

214. Gemma G, Mantanari G, Suppe G, et al. Plasma lipid and lipoprotein changes in hypertensive patients treated with propranolol and prazosin. J Cardiovasc Pharmacol. 1982;4(Suppl 2):s233–s237.
215. Ferdinand KC. Update in pharmacologic treatment of hypertension. Cardiol Clin. 2001;19(2):279–294.
216. Makita S, Abiko A, Naganuma Y, Moriai Y, Nakmura M. Effects of telmisartan on adiponectin levels and body weight in hypertensive patients with glucose intolerance. Metab Clin Exp. 2008;57:1473–1478.
217. Kobayashi M, Iwanishi M, Egawa K, et al. Pioglitazone increases insulin sensitivity by activation insulin receptor kinase. Diabetes. 1992;41:476–483.
218. King AB. A comparison in a clinical setting of the efficacy and side effects of three thiazolidinediones. Diabetes Care. 2000;23:557–558.
219. Wagenaar LJ, Kuck EM, Hoekstra JB. Troglitazone is it all over? Netherlands J Med. 1999;55(1):4–12.
220. Rocchini AP. Childhood obesity and a diabetic epidemic. N Engl J Med. 2002;346(11):854–855.

18 Hypertension in Children with the Metabolic Syndrome or Type 2 Diabetes

Joseph T. Flynn, MD, MS

CONTENTS

INTRODUCTION

Of the many consequences of childhood obesity, the early development of type 2 diabetes (T2DM) is perhaps the most worrisome due to the long-term cardiovascular and renal sequelae of this condition. The metabolic syndrome (MS), a manifestation of insulin resistance that most commonly occurs in obese individuals, also has significant cardiovascular manifestations and commonly occurs in obese children and adolescents. This chapter reviews manifestations of hypertension in children with T2DM or the MS, with a significant focus on treatment considerations.

CLASSIFICATION OF BLOOD PRESSURE IN THE YOUNG

Traditional (hard) cardiovascular end points used to define levels of HTN in adults (myocardial infarction, stroke, etc.) do not occur in children and adolescents. Therefore, the definition of HTN in the young is a statistical one derived from analysis of a large database of BP obtained in healthy children and adolescents by screening projects such as

J.T. Flynn (✉)
Division of Nephrology, Seattle Children's Hospital, Seattle, WA, USA
e-mail: joesph.flynn@seattlechildrens.org

From: *Clinical Hypertension and Vascular Diseases: Pediatric Hypertension*
Edited by: J. T. Flynn et al. DOI 10.1007/978-1-60327-824-9_18
© Springer Science+Business Media, LLC 2011

Table 1
Classification of Hypertension in Children, Adolescents, and Adults

Blood pressure classification	Children and adolescents (≤ 17years of age)	Older adolescents (≥ 18 years of age) and adults
Normal	SBP and DBP <90th percentile	SBP <120 mmHg and DBP <80 mmHg
Prehypertension	SBP or DBP 90th–95th percentile; or if BP is >120/80 even if <90th percentile	SBP 120–139 mmHg or DBP 80–89 mmHg
Stage 1 hypertension	SBP or DBP ≥95th–99th percentile plus 5 mmHg	SBP 140–159 mmHg or DBP 90–99 mmHg
Stage 2 hypertension	SBP or DBP >99th percentile plus 5 mmHg	SBP ≥160 mmHg or DBP ≥100 mmHg

DBP, diastolic blood pressure; SBP, systolic blood pressure
Adapted from (1,2).

the NHANES. According to this approach, normal BP in children and adolescents is systolic and diastolic BP below the 90th percentile for age, gender, and height, while HTN is defined as systolic or diastolic BP persistently greater than the 95th percentile (1). Tables that list normative BP values for adolescents ≤17 years of age have been published; these are available elsewhere in this text. For older adolescents ≥18 years of age, the adult BP classification scheme issued by the Joint National Commission (2) should be followed. A comparison of the pediatric and adult BP classification schemes is presented in Table 1.

Common to both the pediatric and adult BP classification schemes is the concept of "prehypertension." This refers to BPs that would have been classified as "high-normal" in prior consensus recommendations. While the term prehypertension has proven to be controversial, it is meant to serve as a means of alerting patients and physicians alike of the potential for later development of HTN, and of the need to make lifestyle changes that might prevent this from occurring. This is particularly important for obese individuals. The same BP value of >120/80 is used in both adolescents and adults to designate prehypertension.

HYPERTENSION IN THE METABOLIC SYNDROME

The MS is a constellation of metabolic risk factors for developing atherosclerotic cardiovascular disease and diabetes mellitus, including dyslipidemia, insulin resistance, central obesity, and HTN. The prevalence of the metabolic syndrome in adults has been found to be 21.8% and it increases with increasing age: 6.7% for those 20–29 years old, 43.5% for 60–69 years old, and 42% for ≥70 years old (3). With 34% of the American adult population being overweight (body mass index [BMI] 25–29.9 kg/m^2), and 27% being obese (BMI ≥30 kg/m^2) (4), the MS is becoming increasingly prevalent.

While it is clear that components of the MS can also be identified in children and adolescents, a consensus definition for the MS has been difficult to reach for the pediatric population. A common approach has been to apply modified ATP III criteria, requiring three or more of the following: serum triglycerides (TGs) >95th percentile, HDL cholesterol <5th percentile, systolic or diastolic blood pressure (BP) >95th percentile, and impaired glucose tolerance *(5)*. Using these modified criteria, 39% of those who were moderately obese and 50% of those who were severely obese had the MS. The prevalence increased with increasing degrees of insulin resistance when adjusting for race and degree of obesity. Using more stringent criteria, the prevalence of MS in the NHANES III was 29% in obese subjects (BMI ≥95th percentile), 6.8% in overweight subjects (BMI 85th–95th percentiles), and 0.1% in normal weight subjects (BMI <85th percentile) *(6)*.

Recently, the International Diabetes Federation (IDF) Task Force on Epidemiology and Prevention of Diabetes has proposed a new consensus definition for the MS in childhood that utilizes different criteria for different age groups (Table 2) *(7)*. Central to this definition is the use of waist circumference to define risk. Waist circumference has recently been shown to be an independent predictor of insulin resistance, lipid levels, and blood pressure *(8)*; use of waist circumference percentiles in the proposed IDF definition is felt to account for changes associated with growth. It is unclear, however, why the IDF chose an absolute BP level instead of a BP percentile to denote elevated BP in the 6–16-year-old group. As has been pointed out in a recent review, this definition of the pediatric MS will require validation in large-scale studies before it can be widely adopted *(9)*.

Given that elevated BP is one of the criteria for diagnosis of the MS, it follows that the majority of individuals with the MS will exhibit some degree of BP elevation. The MS has been identified as a strong independent predictor of cardiovascular events in hypertensive individuals, amplifying the cardiovascular risk associated with HTN *(10)*. Recent studies indicate that the process of atherosclerosis starts at an early age and is already linked to obesity and other components of the MS in childhood *(11)*. This makes accurate identification and appropriate treatment of children and adolescents with the MS an important priority for our healthcare system.

Table 2
Proposed IDF Definition of MS in Children and Adolescents

Age 6 to <10 years
- Obesity ≥90th percentile as assessed by waist circumference
- Metabolic syndrome cannot be diagnosed, but further measurements should be made if family history of metabolic syndrome, type 2 diabetes mellitus, dyslipidemia, cardiovascular disease, hypertension, or obesity

Age 10 to <16 years
- Obesity ≥90th percentile (or adult cutoff if lower) as assessed by waist circumference
- Triglycerides ≥1.7 mmol/l
- HDL cholesterol <1.03 mmol/l
- Blood pressure ≥130 mmHg systolic or ≥85 mmHg diastolic
- Glucose ≥5.6 mmol/l (oral glucose tolerance test recommended) or known type 2 diabetes mellitus

Age >16 years
- Use existing IDF criteria for adults

HDL, High-density lipoprotein; IDF, International Diabetes Federation

HYPERTENSION IN TYPE 2 DIABETES

In adults with type 2 diabetes (T2DM), hypertension is common. Recent data from the NHANES 1999–2004 survey indicate that overall over 70% of prevalent adults with T2DM have coexisting hypertension, and that the prevalence has been increasing over the past decade *(12)*. Indeed, a significant proportion of adults with newly diagnosed T2DM are already hypertensive at the time of diagnosis *(13)*. Hypertension in adults with T2DM is often poorly controlled, with only about 30% of patients achieving the recommended target BP of <130/80 *(12)*. Consequently, there is a high rate of stroke and other severe cardiovascular disease in adults with T2DM, and premature death from cardiovascular causes is common *(14)*.

Not surprisingly, fewer data are available on the prevalence of hypertension in children and adolescents with T2DM. In a recent analysis of data from the SEARCH for diabetes in youth study, among approximately 2,100 children aged 3–19 years old with diabetes, the prevalence of BP above the 90th percentile or treatment with antihypertensive medications was 22% among those with T1DM vs. 73% among those with T2DM—however, there were fewer than 100 subjects with T2DM in the study sample *(15)*. Other reported prevalences of hypertension in youth with T2DM range from 8 to 36% *(16)*, which is certainly lower than in adults, but still greater than in unselected pediatric populations, even given the effects of the childhood obesity epidemic *(17)*. Some of these studies are characterized by use of nonstandard definitions of hypertension, or reliance on single measurements of BP, which limits the conclusions that can be made regarding prevalence.

In a study of obese minority adolescents with and without T2DM that incorporated ambulatory blood pressure monitoring (ABPM) *(18)*, we found ambulatory hypertension in 39% of those with T2DM, compared to only 8% of those without T2DM. Nearly all ABPM variables, including mean awake and sleep BP and awake and sleep BP loads *(19)*, were significantly higher in the T2DM subjects. Blunted nocturnal dipping, however, was common in both groups, affecting 58% of those with T2DM and 42% of those without T2DM, suggesting that blunted dipping may be an early manifestation of elevated cardiovascular risk in obese youth whether or not T2DM has developed. Of note, abnormal ambulatory BP profiles in youth with T2DM were accompanied by a high incidence of microalbuminuria *(18)*, suggesting that as in adults, there is early development of renal damage in pediatric patients with T2DM.

Clearly, better data are needed regarding the prevalence of hypertension and other cardiovascular risk factors in youth with T2DM. It is likely that given the increasing prevalence of T2DM in children and adolescents, particularly among specific minority groups *(20,21)*, large-scale studies can be conducted to prospectively study this important risk factor. Incorporation of ambulatory BP monitoring and consensus definitions of hypertension into such studies will be needed to produce the most accurate assessment of early cardiovascular disease in T2DM.

PATHOPHYSIOLOGY

A detailed discussion of the mechanisms underlying the development of hypertension in patients with the MS or T2DM is beyond the scope of this chapter, but a few key points deserve emphasis. Since there is considerable overlap with obesity-related hypertension, the interested reader should see Chapter 17. Additionally, discussions of this form of hypertension in adults *(14,22)* would also be pertinent to adolescents with either the MS or T2DM.

Insulin resistance is clearly the major pathophysiologic mechanism involved in the development of hypertension in both the MS and T2DM. Landsberg has noted that "...insulin resistance in the obese is a mechanism evolved for limiting further weight gain. Like any compensatory mechanism, however, there is a price to pay. In this situation, that price is the hyperinsulinemia and sympathetic activation which, via effects on the blood vessels, the heart and the kidneys, exerts a prohypertensive effect that, in susceptible individuals, causes hypertension" (23). There are several lines of evidence linking hyperinsulinemia with increased sympathetic nervous system (SNS) activation and hypertension, including the finding of elevated levels of plasma catecholamines, and abrogration of hypertension after adrenergic blockade (24,25). While there are likely multiple mechanisms involved in activation of the SNS in the MS and T2DM (26), hyperinsulinemia is one of the most important.

There are many other mechanisms by which hyperinsulinemia may contribute to the development of hypertension. First and foremost among these is altered renal handling of sodium, leading to hypertension through an expansion of plasma volume. Insulin increases renal sodium reabsorption, possibly in the distal nephron, although this is not completely certain (27). It is likely that increased activity of renal sympathetic nerves is responsible at least in part for this effect (28). Elevated circulating levels of aldosterone, which have been demonstrated in salt-sensitive obese adolescents, may also be involved (29). Importantly, these effects of hyperinsulinemia on renal sodium handling can be reversed with weight loss (29).

Another mechanism by which hyperinsulinemia may elevate blood pressure is through effects on vascular structure and function. Although insulin when infused directly into local vascular beds acts as a vasodilator (30), in hypertensive subjects this effect is probably offset by vasoconstriction mediated by increased sympathetic nervous activity (30,31). In addition, impaired vasodilatation in response to insulin infusion has been demonstrated in obese individuals (32). Alternatively, insulin may act to stimulate vascular smooth muscle proliferation in resistance vessels via activation of the local renin–angiotensin system (33), thereby leading to increased peripheral vascular resistance due to vascular medial hypertrophy. In this way, hyperinsulinemia would lead to hypertension by increasing systemic vascular resistance. This mechanism is supported by recent studies demonstrating altered vascular structure and function in obese youth with and without T2DM (34).

THERAPY

Since elevated BP is one of the defining criteria of the MS, and since many patients, including adolescents, may already be hypertensive at the time of diagnosis of T2DM, treatment of elevated BP will be required in many, if not most, children and adolescents diagnosed with either the MS or T2DM. Given the common pathophysiology of hypertension in both the MS and T2DM, treatment of both conditions will be discussed collectively in the remaining sections of this chapter.

Role of Nonpharmacologic Therapy

(Also see Chapter 30.)

While the effects on BP may be modest in magnitude, weight loss, aerobic exercise, and dietary modifications have all been shown to successfully reduce BP in children and adolescents, and are therefore considered primary treatment in children with obesity-related

HTN *(1)*. Studies in obese adolescents have demonstrated that modest weight loss not only decreases BP but, importantly for those with the MS or T2DM, also improves other cardiovascular risk factors such as dyslipidemia and insulin resistance *(35–37)*. In studies where a reduction in body mass index of about 10% was achieved, short-term reductions in BP were in the range of 8–12 mmHg. Unfortunately, weight loss is difficult and frequently unsuccessful. Additionally, even intensive efforts at weight loss in childhood may be followed by recidivism and an increased prevalence of adverse consequences of obesity in adulthood *(38)*. However, identifying a medical complication of obesity such as the MS or T2DM can perhaps provide the necessary motivation for patients and families to make the appropriate lifestyle changes.

Similarly, exercise training over 3–6 months has been shown to result in a reduction of 6–12 mmHg for systolic BP and 3–5 mmHg for diastolic BP *(39)*. However, cessation of regular exercise is generally promptly followed by a rise in BP to preexercise levels. Aerobic exercise activities such as running, walking, or cycling are usually preferred to static forms of exercise in the management of HTN. Many children may already be participating in one or more appropriate activities and may only need to increase the frequency and/or intensity of these activities to produce a reduction in their BP. At the very least, the amount of time spent in sedentary activities such as television viewing should be restricted to <2 h/day *(40)*. Increasing physical activity may not only reduce BP, but can help with weight loss and/or maintenance, and has been proven to be effective in preventing the development of T2DM *(41)*.

For best results in terms of BP reduction and weight control, exercise should probably be combined with dietary changes such as those discussed below. Such an approach has been shown to improve markers of insulin resistance in obese adolescents *(41,42)*. The combination of dietary changes and exercise training may also improve vascular function in addition to reducing BP *(43)*.

Dietary modification in the management of HTN in children and adolescents has received a great deal of attention. Nutrients that have been examined include the obvious, such as sodium, potassium, and calcium, as well as folate, caffeine, and other substances. Manipulation of sodium intake has received extensive study *(44)*. Many authors have noted that the typical dietary sodium intakes of children and adolescents, at least in the United States, far exceed any nutritional requirements for sodium. Trials of dietary sodium restriction in hypertensive children and adolescents have had mixed results, with some studies showing no benefit, and others showing a modest reduction in BP in obese adolescents but not in lean adolescents *(29)*. This suggests that dietary sodium restriction may have a role in treatment of children and adolescents with the MS or T2DM, a substantial proportion of whom are likely to be salt sensitive.

Other nutrients that have been examined in hypertensive children and adolescents include potassium and calcium, both of which have been shown to have antihypertensive effects. A recent 2-year trial of potassium and calcium supplementation in hypertensive, salt-sensitive Chinese children demonstrated that this combination significantly reduced systolic BP *(45)*. Therefore, a diet that is low in sodium and enriched with potassium and calcium may be more effective in reducing BP than a diet that restricts sodium only.

An example of such a diet is the so-called "DASH" diet, which has been shown to have an antihypertensive effect in adults with HTN, even in those receiving antihypertensive medication *(46,47)*. The basic elements of the DASH eating plan are logical to apply the treatment of hypertensive children, especially if accompanied by counseling from a pediatric dietitian. A recent study in a population of mostly obese adolescents with either prehypertension or Stage 1 HTN confirmed that a DASH-type eating plan is effective in reducing BP in the young *(48)*. The DASH diet also incorporates higher intake of such micronutrients as folate, which may have an antihypertensive effect, as well as measures designed to reduce dietary fat intake, an important strategy given the frequent presence of both HTN and dyslipidemia in children and adolescents with the MS or T2DM.

Cardiovascular Effects of Oral Hypoglycemic Agents

It has become apparent over recent years that many of the agents used to improve insulin sensitivity in individuals with the MS or T2DM have important cardiovascular effects as well. Although treatment with these agents will not obviate the need for antihypertensive medications in most affected individuals, their potential impact on BP deserves consideration.

Metformin, which is widely used in patients with T2DM, is a biguanide antihyperglycemic drug that lowers hepatic glucose production, lowers plasma free fatty acid levels, and improves insulin sensitivity, primarily by increasing peripheral glucose uptake in skeletal muscle and adipose tissue *(48–50)*. Studies in rats with streptozotocin-induced diabetes have demonstrated that metformin reduces BP and restores aortic endothelial function *(51)*. Human studies, however, have not uniformly demonstrated a significant effect of metformin on BP.

Manzella et al. randomized 128 subjects with T2DM to either metformin or placebo in order to examine the effect of metformin on BP and the SNS. While metformin treatment resulted in a significant improvement in cardiac sympathovagal balance as assessed by heart rate variability, no changes were noted in mean arterial BP *(52)*. In another study, metformin was given for 12 weeks to obese subjects with T2DM managed with either dietary therapy alone or sulfonylurea monotherapy. Although metformin, either as monotherapy or in combination with a sulfonylurea, improved glycemic control, there was no significant effect on BP *(53)*. Finally, Stakos et al. randomized subjects with insulin resistance and normal glucose tolerance to receive glipizide 5 mg/day, metformin 500 mg/day, or placebo for 2 years. Patients in the metformin and placebo groups had a mild but significant decrease in systolic and diastolic BP, while the glipizide group had a mild but nonsignificant decrease in BP *(54)*. Clearly, metformin alone will be insufficient treatment for hypertension in the MS or T2DM, but it may have some beneficial cardiovascular effects.

Rosiglitazone, a thiazolidinedione, binds to the peroxisome proliferator-activated receptor-gamma (PPAR-γ), a transcription factor that regulates the expression of genes that involved in glucose production, transport, and utilization in the liver, adipose tissue, and muscle *(50)*. Rosiglitazone has been shown to improve vascular function and ameliorate BP in hypertensive transgenic mice *(55)*. Negro et al. compared the effects of rosiglitazone and metformin vs. metformin alone on BP and metabolic parameters of diabetic patients *(56)*. After 1 year of treatment with both rosiglitazone and metformin, a significant reduction of systolic and diastolic BP was demonstrated by ambulatory BP monitoring. In a similar study, rosiglitazone treatment produced a significant reduction in ambulatory BP that was correlated with improvements in insulin sensitivity *(57)*. Rosiglitazone has also been studied in combination with metformin with or without the addition of glimepiride, a second-generation sulfonylurea, in hypertensive type 2 diabetic patients *(58)*. Subjects were randomized to treatment with either metformin + glimepiride or metformin + rosiglitazone. Mean BP was not significantly improved at any time in the group that received glimepiride + metformin; however, BP significantly improved at 12 months in those who received rosiglitazone + metformin. The antihypertensive effect of rosiglitazone appeared to be mainly related to decreased insulin resistance and improvement in endothelial function *(58)*.

Pioglitazone, another thiazolidinedione, was studied in patients with T2DM who had abnormal nocturnal BP on ambulatory BP monitoring. Subjects were randomized to either metformin + placebo or metformin + pioglitazone. After 8 weeks of treatment, the metformin + pioglitazone group had reduced nocturnal BP values which were independent of changes in metabolic parameters *(59)*.

Acarbose is a glucose oxidase inhibitor which delays the absorption of glucose, resulting in a reduction of postprandial blood glucose levels. The STOP-NIDDM (Study to Prevent Non-Insulin-Dependent Diabetes Mellitus) trial examined the effect of acarbose on the progression of patients with impaired glucose tolerance (IGT) to diabetes, HTN, and cardiovascular disease *(60)*. After a mean follow-up of 3.3 years, treatment with acarbose resulted in a 25% relative risk reduction in the development of T2DM, a 34% risk reduction in the development of new cases of HTN, and a 49% risk reduction in the development of cardiovascular events. Another study by Rachmani et al. examined the effect of 24 weeks of acarbose treatment on insulin resistance in obese hypertensive subjects with normal glucose tolerance *(61)*. Insulin resistance improved in the acarbose group; however, BP declined equally in the two groups.

Although mostly limited to studies conducted in adults, these data suggest that many of the agents used to improve insulin sensitivity in patients with the MS and/or T2DM may have additional benefits in lowering BP. Further studies conducted in the young might provide a clearer picture of the effects of these agents on cardiovascular risk. At any rate, since the data are not consistent, it is unlikely that treatment with these agents alone would be sufficient to control HTN, making combination treatment with antihypertensive drugs necessary in many affected children and adolescents.

Antihypertensive Drug Therapy

INDICATIONS FOR ANTIHYPERTENSIVE DRUG THERAPY

Even with successful weight loss, exercise, dietary changes, and use of the oral hypoglycemic agents discussed above, antihypertensive medications will be needed in many patients with the MS or T2DM in order to achieve the desired BP. Despite the potential theoretical benefits of initiation of drug therapy early in life, it is important to recognize that the long-term consequences of untreated HTN in a child or adolescent remain unknown. Similarly, there is a lack of data on the benefits of therapy in the pediatric age group, as well as on the long-term effects of antihypertensive medications on growth and development, which add further uncertainty to the decision to initiate drug treatment. However, since accelerated cardiovascular disease occurs commonly in adult patients with the MS or T2DM, there is added impetus for starting drug therapy in the young.

As recommended by the National High Blood Pressure Education Program *(1)*, definite indications for initiating pharmacologic therapy in a child or adolescent include the following:

- Stage 2 hypertension (see Table 1)
- Symptomatic hypertension
- Secondary hypertension

- Hypertensive target-organ damage
- Diabetes (types 1 and 2)
- Persistent hypertension despite nonpharmacologic measures.

Thus far, although it might seem reasonable to add the presumptive diagnosis of the MS as an additional indication for initiating drug therapy, no consensus organization has yet endorsed this, probably because of the difficulties defining the MS in pediatrics as discussed earlier. At the very least, children and adolescents with the MS and BP above the prehypertensive range who do not comply with or respond to a reasonable (6–12-month) trial of nonpharmacologic measures should probably be prescribed antihypertensive medications due to the likely risk of progression of the MS to frank diabetes, and because of the increased risk of development of atherosclerosis in these patients.

CHOICE OF ANTIHYPERTENSIVE MEDICATION

The general topic of drug therapy in childhood hypertension is covered in detail in Chapter 31, so the following discussion will be limited to specific aspects pertinent to the MS and T2DM. One of the general principles of treatment of hypertension that is important to highlight here is consideration of comorbidities that may preferentially favor one class of drug over another. The best example of this principle can be found in the JNC-7 report *(2)*, which highlighted a list of "compelling indications" that, based upon the results of large-scale clinical trials, necessitate the use of specific drug classes. Included in the list of compelling indications is diabetes, and drug classes listed as indicated included ACE inhibitors, angiotensin receptor antagonists, diuretics, beta-blockers, and calcium channel blockers. Choosing between these in a patient with T2DM might depend upon the presence or absence of microalbuminuria, in which case an agent affecting the renin–angiotensin system would be favored *(62)*. Unfortunately, a similar evidence base is lacking for pediatric patients, as studies including subjects with comorbid conditions have not been conducted in the young.

Probably, the most important issue to consider in the selection of an antihypertensive agent in the pediatric patient with the MS or T2DM is the drug's effect on insulin sensitivity. Alpha-adrenergic blockers, for example, are well known to improve insulin sensitivity and have been advocated for use in treatment of HTN in individuals with impaired glucose tolerance and/or frank diabetes *(63,64)*. Alpha-blockers lower triglyceride and free fatty acid levels, and have no effect on total, high-density, or low-density cholesterol *(64)*, important considerations given the common finding of dyslipidemia in the MS and T2DM. The benefits of alpha-blockade have also been demonstrated in a study of the combined alpha- and beta-blocker carvedilol, which effectively reduced BP without worsening selected metabolic parameters in adults with the MS *(65)*.

Calcium channel blockers have also been demonstrated to have beneficial effects on insulin sensitivity in patients with essential HTN *(66,67)*, so by extension would be appropriate for use in individuals with the MS. Even more encouraging is blockade of the renin–angiotensin system with angiotensin-converting enzyme (ACE) inhibitors or angiotensin receptor blockers (ARBs). These agents have been shown to have either neutral or beneficial effects on glucose metabolism, and have the potential to prevent the development of diabetes in individuals with the MS *(68,69)*. Some of the newer ARBs appear to activate PPAR-γ, producing the beneficial effects of the thiazolidinediones without the weight gain and other adverse effects sometimes seen with those agents *(70)*. Therefore, many authors recommend ACE inhibitors and ARBs as the first-line agents for treatment of

HTN in patients with the MS *(71)*. The well-known activation of the renin–angiotensin system in obesity *(72)* would provide additional rationale for use of ACE inhibitors in children and adolescents with the MS or T2DM.

In contrast to the above, diuretics and beta-adrenergic blockers are usually thought to have "diabetogenic" potential *(73)* and might therefore be avoided as initial agents in treating HTN in patients with coexisting MS *(74)*. This position is supported by recent analysis of data from the ALLHAT study *(75)* that demonstrated a greater incidence of new-onset diabetes in the group treated with chlorthalidone compared to those treated with amlodipine or lisinopril *(76)*. However, this may have been the result of use of chlorthalidone in combination with the beta-blocker atenolol, which was the most commonly prescribed second-line agent in ALLHAT. The combination of a thiazide diuretic and beta-blocker is thought to be particularly diabetogenic *(77)*. However, other authors have argued that the adverse effects of diuretics and beta-blockers have been overstated, and that these classes of agents can be used judiciously in such patients, particularly as second-line agents, given the imperative to control BP and prevent the development of more significant cardiovascular disease *(71)*.

Finally, adherence to prescribed therapy is another important issue that should be considered in the treatment of HTN because most patients have so few symptoms. In adolescents, this is particularly difficult because they often do not like to remember to take their medications and do not like to be perceived as different from their peers. If BP control can be achieved with a single drug that is taken once a day, this will improve the likelihood of compliance with taking the medication and should be taken into consideration when the initial agent is chosen. Adverse effects of the chosen agent should also be considered. Some classes of antihypertensive agents, particularly newer ones such as ACEIs and ARBs, have a lower incidence of adverse effects *(78)* and may be preferable when compliance is a concern. There are also combination preparations available that can improve compliance when more than one agent is needed to achieve the desired goal BP *(79)*. Early institution of combination therapy in treating hypertensive patients with T2DM has been advocated and appears to be supported by several recent clinical trials in adults *(80)*.

GOALS OF THERAPY

In adults with complicated HTN such as that seen in T2DM, a lower treatment goal (130/80) is recommended than in those with uncomplicated HTN (140/90) *(2)*. This recommendation is gain based upon the results of large-scale clinical trials involving thousands of patients. Lacking large-scale trials in pediatric hypertension, the NHBPEP has developed a similar recommendation for children based upon expert opinion: For children with uncomplicated primary HTN and no hypertensive target organ damage, goal BP should be <95th percentile for age, gender, and height, whereas for children with secondary HTN, diabetes, or hypertensive target organ damage, goal BP should be <90th percentile for age, gender, and height *(1)*. By extension, the 90th percentile should probably be the target BP for children and young adolescents with the MS. In older hypertensive adolescents aged ≥18 years with the MS or T2DM, JNC-7 guidelines should be followed.

SUMMARY

The increasing prevalence of obesity in children and adolescents is unfortunately being accompanied by numerous complications, including the MS and T2DM. Although there is still some uncertainty regarding the optimal definition of the MS in the young, signs of insulin resistance are common and its consequences, most notably HTN, are readily detectable. HTN in obese children with or without T2DM is characterized by abnormalities on ambulatory BP monitoring and may be diagnosed earlier using this technique. Therapy of such children should begin with lifestyle modifications, as these measures have been proven effective in reducing BP and also in preventing progression to full-blown T2DM. Some oral hypoglycemic agents appear to have BP-lowering effects in adults, but pediatric data are lacking. When antihypertensive drugs are necessary, consideration should be given to the agent's effect on insulin sensitivity. In addition to better studies of drug therapies, there is clearly a need for increased efforts to prevent childhood obesity so that these complications can be avoided altogether.

REFERENCES

1. National High Blood Pressure Education Program Working Group on High Blood Pressure in Children and Adolescents. The fourth report on the diagnosis, evaluation, and treatment of high blood pressure in children and adolescents. Bethesda, Maryland. National Institute of Health, NIH publication 05:5267, 2005.
2. Chobanian AV, Bakris GL, Black HR, et al. The seventh report of the Joint National Committee on Prevention, Detection, Evaluation, and Treatment of High Blood Pressure: the JNC 7 report. JAMA. 2003;289:2560–2572.
3. Ford ES, Giles WH, Dietz WH. Prevalence of the metabolic syndrome among US adults. Findings from the Third National Health and Nutrition Examination Survey. JAMA. 2002;287:356–359.
4. National Center for Health Statistics, Prevalence of Overweight and Obesity Among Adults: United States, 1999–2002. http://www.cdc.gov/nchs/products/pubs/pubd/hestats/obese/obse99.htm [Accessed June 23, 2009].
5. Weiss R, Dziura J, Burgert TS, et al. Obesity and the metabolic syndrome in children and adolescents. N Engl J Med. 2004;350:2362–2374.
6. Cook S, Weitzman M, Auinger P, et al. Prevalence of a metabolic syndrome phenotype in adolescents: findings from the third National Health and Nutrition Examination Survey 1998–1994. Arch Pediatr Adolesc Med. 2003;157:821–827.
7. Zimmet P, Alberti G, Kaufman F, et al. The metabolic syndrome in children and adolescents. Lancet. 2007;369:2059–2061.
8. Lee S, Bacha F, Arslanian SA. Waist circumference, blood pressure, and lipid components of the metabolic syndrome. J Pediatr. 2006;149:809–816.
9. Steinberger J, Daniels SR, Eckel RH, et al. Progress and challenges in metabolic syndrome in children and adolescents: a scientific statement from the American Heart Association Atherosclerosis, Hypertension, and Obesity in the Young Committee of the Council on Cardiovascular Disease in the Young; Council on Cardiovascular Nursing; and Council on Nutrition, Physical Activity, and Metabolism. Circulation. 2009;119:628–647.
10. Schillaci G, Pirro M, Vaudo G, et al. Prognostic value of the metabolic syndrome in essential hypertension. J Am Coll Cardiol. 2004;43:1817–1822.
11. Berenson GS, Srinivasan SR, Bao W, et al. Association between multiple cardiovascular risk factors and atherosclerosis in children and young adults. N Engl J Med. 1998;338:1650–1656.
12. Suh DC, Kim CM, Choi IS, et al. Trends in blood pressure control and treatment among type 2 diabetes with comorbid hypertension in the United States: 1988–2004. J Hypertens. 2009;27:1908–1916.
13. Hypertension in Diabetes Study (HDS): I. Prevalence of hypertension in newly presenting type 2 diabetic patients and the association with risk factors for cardiovascular and diabetic complications. J Hypertens. 1993;11:309.
14. Mugo MN, Link D, Stump CS, Sowers JR. Insulin resistance and diabetes in hypertension. In: Lip GYH, Hall JE, eds. Comprehensive Hypertension. Philadelphia, PA: Mosby; 2007:681–692.
15. Rodriguez BL, Fujimoto WY, Mayer-Davis EJ, et al. Prevalence of cardiovascular disease risk factors in U.S. children and adolescents with diabetes: the SEARCH for diabetes in youth study. Diabetes Care. 2006;29:1891–1896.
16. Dean HJ, Sellers EAC. Comorbidities and microvascular complications of type 2 diabetes in children and adolescents. Pediatr Diabetes. 2007;8(Suppl 9):35–41.
17. Flynn JT. Hypertension in the young: epidemiology, sequelae, therapy. Nephrol Dial Transplant. 2009;24:370–375.

18. Ettinger LM, Freeman K, DiMartino-Nardi JR, Flynn JT. Microalbuminuria and abnormal ambulatory blood pressure in adolescents with type 2 diabetes mellitus. J Pediatr. 2005;147: 67–73.
19. Urbina EM, Alpert B, Flynn J, et al. Ambulatory blood pressure monitoring in children and adolescents: recommendations for standard assessment. Hypertension. 2008;52:433–451.
20. Dabelea D, Bell RA, D'Agostino RB Jr, et al. Incidence of diabetes in youth in the United States. JAMA. 2007;297:2716–2724.
21. Shaw J. Epidemiology of childhood type 2 diabetes and obesity. Pediatr Diabetes. 2007;8 (Suppl. 9):7–15.
22. Redon J, Cifkova R, Laurent S, et al. Mechanisms of hypertension in the cardiometabolic syndrome. J Hypertens. 2009;27:441–451.
23. Landsberg L. Insulin-mediated sympathetic stimulation: role in the pathogenesis of obesity-related hypertension (or, how insulin affects blood pressure, and why). J Hypertens. 2001;19:523–528.
24. Rocchini AP. Obesity hypertension. Am J Hypertens. 2002;15:50S–52S.
25. Tentolouris N, Liatis S, Katsilambros N. Sympathetic system activity in obesity and metabolic syndrome. Ann N Y Acad Sci. 2006;1083:129–152.
26. Straznicky NE, Eikelis N, Lambert EA, Esler MD. Mediators of sympathetic activation in metabolic syndrome obesity. Curr Hypertens Rep. 2008;10:440–447.
27. Gupta AK, Clark RV, Kirchner KA. Effects of insulin on renal sodium excretion. Hypertension. 1992;19:I78–I82.
28. Esler M, Rumantir M, Wiesner G, et al. Sympathetic nervous system and insulin resistance: from obesity to diabetes. Am J Hypertens. 2001;14:304S–309S.
29. Rocchini AP, Key J, Bondie D, et al. The effect of weight loss on the sensitivity of blood pressure to sodium in obese adolescents. N Engl J Med. 1989;321:580–585.
30. Anderson EA, Hoffman RP, Balon TW, et al. Hyperinsulinemia produces both sympathetic neural activation and vasodilation in normal humans. J Clin Invest. 1991;87:2246–2252.
31. Reaven GM, Lithell H, Landsberg L. Hypertension and associated metabolic abnormalities—the role of insulin resistance and the sympathoadrenal system. N Engl J Med. 1996;334:374–381.
32. Laakso M, Edelman SV, Brechtel G, Baron AD. Decreased effect of insulin to stimulate skeletal muscle blood flow in obese man. A novel mechanism for insulin resistance. J Clin Invest. 1990;85: 1844–1852.
33. Kamide K, Hori MT, Zhu JH, et al. Insulin and insulin-like growth factor-I promotes angiotensinogen production and growth in vascular smooth muscle cells. J Hypertens. 2000; 18:1051–1056.
34. Urbina EM, Kimball TR, McCoy CE, et al. Youth with obesity and obesity-related type 2 diabetes mellitus demonstrate abnormalities in carotid structure and function. Circulation. 2009;119:2913–2919.
35. Rocchini AP, Katch V, Anderson J, et al. Blood pressure in obese adolescents: Effect of weight loss. Pediatrics. 1988;82:16–23.
36. Williams CL, Hayman LL, Daniels SR, et al. Cardiovascular health in childhood: a statement for health professionals from the Committee on Atherosclerosis, Hypertension, and Obesity in the Young (AHOY) of the Council on Cardiovascular Disease in the Young, American Heart Association. Circulation. 2002;106: 143–160.
37. Reinehr T, Andler W. Changes in the atherogenic risk factor profile according to degree of weight loss. Arch Dis Child. 2004;89:419–422.
38. Togashi K, Masuda H, Rankinen T, et al. A 12-year follow-up study of treated obese children in Japan. Int J Obes Relat Metab Disord. 2002;26:770–777.
39. Alpert BS. Exercise as a therapy to control hypertension in children. Int J Sports Med. 2000;21(Suppl 2):S94–S96.
40. Daniels SR, Arnett DK, Eckel RH, et al. Overweight in children and adolescents: pathophysiology, consequences, prevention, and treatment. Circulation. 2005;111:1999–2012.
41. Diabetes Prevention Program Research Group. Reduction in the incidence of type 2 diabetes with lifestyle modification or metformin. N Engl J Med. 2002;346:393–403.
42. Ben Ounis O, Elloumi M, Ben Chiekh I, et al. Effects of two-month physical-endurance and diet-restriction programmes on lipid profiles and insulin resistance in obese adolescent boys. Diabetes Metab. 2008;34:595–600.
43. Ribeiro MM, Silva AG, Santos NS, et al. Diet and exercise training restore blood pressure and vasodilatory responses during physiological maneuvers in obese children. Circulation. 2005;111:1915–1923.
44. Falkner B, Michel S. Blood pressure response to sodium in children and adolescents. Am J Clin Nutr. 1997;65(2 Suppl):618S–621S.
45. Mu JJ, Liu ZQ, Liu WM, et al. Reduction of blood pressure with calcium and potassium supplementation in children with salt sensitivity: a 2-year double-blinded placebo-controlled trial. J Hum Hypertens. 2005;19:479–483.

46. Appel LJ, Moore TJ, Obarzanek E, et al. A clinical trial of the effects of dietary patterns on blood pressure. N Engl J Med. 1997;336:1117–1124.
47. Appel L, Brands, M, Daniels SR, et al. Dietary approaches to prevent and treat hypertension: a scientific statement from the American Heart Association. Hypertension. 2006;47:296–308.
48. Couch SC, Saelens BE, Levin L, et al. The efficacy of a clinic-based behavioral nutrition intervention emphasizing a DASH-type diet for adolescents with elevated blood pressure. J Pediatr. 2008;152: 494–501.
49. Vague P. Is metformin more than an oral hypoglycaemic agent? Diabetes Metab. 2003;29(4 Pt 2):6S5–6S7.
50. Wellington K. Rosiglitazone/metformin. Drugs. 2005;65:1581–1592.
51. Majithiya JB, Balaraman R. Metformin reduces blood pressure and restores endothelial function in aorta of streptozotocin-induced diabetic rats. Life Sci. 2006;78:2615–2624.
52. Manzella D, Grella R, Esposito K, et al. Blood pressure and cardiac autonomic nervous system in obese type 2 diabetic patients: effect of metformin administration. Am J Hypertens. 2004;17:223–227.
53. Abbasi F, Chu JW, McLaughlin T, et al. Effect of metformin treatment on multiple cardiovascular disease risk factors in patients with type 2 diabetes mellitus. Metabolism. 2004;53:159–164.
54. Stakos DA, Schuster DP, Sparks EA, et al. Long term cardiovascular effects of oral antidiabetic agents in non-diabetic patients with insulin resistance: double blind, prospective, randomised study. Heart. 2005;91:589–594.
55. Ryan MJ, Didion SP, Mathur S, et al. PPAR(gamma) agonist rosiglitazone improves vascular function and lowers blood pressure in hypertensive transgenic mice. Hypertension. 2004;43:661–666.
56. Negro R, Mangieri T, Dazzi D, et al. Rosiglitazone effects on blood pressure and metabolic parameters in nondipper diabetic patients. Diabetes Res Clin Pract. 2005;70:20–25.
57. Sarafidis PA, Lasaridis AN, Nilsson PM, et al. Ambulatory blood pressure reduction after rosiglitazone treatment in patients with type 2 diabetes and hypertension correlates with insulin sensitivity increase. J Hypertens. 2004;22:1769–1777.
58. Derosa G, Cicero AF, Gaddi AV, et al. Long-term effects of glimepiride or rosiglitazone in combination with metformin on blood pressure control in type 2 diabetic patients affected by the metabolic syndrome: a 12-month double-blind, randomized clinical trial. Clin Ther. 2005;27:1383–1391.
59. Negro R, Dazzi D, Hassan H, Pezzarossa A. Pioglitazone reduces blood pressure in non-dipping diabetic patients. Minerva Endocrinol. 2004;29:11–17.
60. Chiasson JL. Acarbose for the prevention of diabetes, hypertension, and cardiovascular disease in subjects with impaired glucose tolerance: the Study to Prevent Non-Insulin-Dependent Diabetes Mellitus (STOP-NIDDM) Trial. Endocr Pract. 2006;12(Suppl 1):25–30.
61. Rachmani R, Bar-Dayan Y, Ronen Z, et al. The effect of acarbose on insulin resistance in obese hypertensive subjects with normal glucose tolerance: a randomized controlled study. Diabetes Obes Metab. 2004;6:63–68.
62. Ritz E, Dikow R. Hypertension and antihypertensive treatment of diabetic nephropathy. Nat Clin Pract Nephrol. 2006;2:562–567.
63. Giorda C, Appendino M, Mason MG, et al. Alpha 1-blocker doxazosin improves peripheral insulin sensitivity in diabetic hypertensive patients. Metabolism. 1995;44:673–676.
64. Inukai T, Inukai Y, Matsutomo R, et al. Clinical usefulness of doxazosin in patients with type 2 diabetes complicated by hypertension: effects on glucose and lipid metabolism. J Int Med Res. 2004;32: 206–213.
65. Uzunlulu M, Oguz A, Yorulmaz E. The effect of carvedilol on metabolic parameters in patients with metabolic syndrome. Int Heart J. 2006;47:421–430.
66. Harano Y, Kageyama A, Hirose J, et al. Improvement of insulin sensitivity for glucose metabolism with the long-acting Ca-channel blocker amlodipine in essential hypertensive subjects. Metabolism. 1995;44: 315–319.
67. Koyama Y, Kodama K, Suzuki M, Harano Y. Improvement of insulin sensitivity by a long-acting nifedipine preparation (nifedipine-CR) in patients with essential hypertension. Am J Hypertens. 2002;15:927–931.
68. Scheen AJ. Renin-angiotensin system inhibition prevents type 2 diabetes mellitus. Part 2. Overview of physiological and biochemical mechanisms. Diabetes Metab. 2004;30:498–505.
69. Gillespie EL, White CM, Kardas M, et al. The impact of ACE inhibitors or angiotensin II type I receptor blockers on the development of new-onset type 2 diabetes. Diabetes Care. 2005;28:2261–2266.
70. Pershadsingh HA. Treating the metabolic syndrome using angiotensin receptor antagonists that selectively modulate peroxisome proliferator-activated receptor-gamma. Int J Biochem Cell Biol. 2006;38:766–781.
71. Asfaha S, Padwal R. Antihypertensive drugs and incidence of type 2 diabetes: evidence and implications for clinical practice. Curr Hypertens Rep. 2005;7:314–322.
72. Hall JE. The kidney, hypertension, and obesity. Hypertension. 2003;41:625–633.

73. Izzedine H, Launay-Vacher V, Deybach C, et al. Drug-induced diabetes mellitus. Expert Opin Drug Saf. 2005;4:1097–1099.
74. Verdecchia P, Angeli F, Reboldi GP, Gattobigio R. New-onset diabetes in treated hypertensive patients. Curr Hypertens Rep. 2005;7:174–179.
75. ALLHAT Officers and Coordinators for the ALLHAT Collaborative Research Group. Major outcomes in high-risk hypertensive patients randomized to angiotensin-converting enzyme inhibitor or calcium channel blocker vs. diuretic: the Antihypertensive and Lipid-Lowering Treatment to Prevent Heart Attack Trial (ALLHAT). J Am Med Assoc. 2002;288:2981–2997.
76. Punzi HA, Punzi CF. Metabolic issues in the Antihypertensive and Lipid-Lowering Heart Attack Trial study. Curr Hypertens Rep. 2004;6:106–110.
77. Manson JM, Dickinson HO, Nicholson DJ, et al. The diabetogenic potential of thiazide-type diuretic and beta-blocker combinations in patients with hypertension. J Hypertens. 2005;23:1777–1781.
78. Anonymous. After the diagnosis: adherence and persistence with hypertension therapy. Am J Manag Care. 2005;11(13 Suppl):S395–S399.
79. Wells T, Stowe C. An approach to the use of antihypertensive drugs in children and adolescents. Curr Ther Res Clin Exp. 2001;62:329.
80. Reboldi G, Gentile G, Angeli F, Verdecchia P. Choice of ACE inhibitor combinations in hypertensive patients with type 2 diabetes: update after recent clinical trials. Vasc Health Risk Manage. 2009;5: 411–427.

19 Primary Hypertension

Gaurav Kapur, MD
and Tej K. Mattoo, MD, DCH, FRCP (UK), FAAP

CONTENTS

INTRODUCTION

Pickering stated, "The relationship between arterial pressure and mortality is quantitative, the higher the pressure the worse the prognosis" *(1)*. Primary hypertension (HTN), which affects almost 20% of adults and is a major public health issue, is believed to have its antecedents during childhood. Therefore, it is important that those providing care to children approach the issue of HTN both as a societal challenge and as a disease affecting discrete individuals.

DEFINITIONS AND TECHNIQUES

HTN in children, unlike in adults, does not affect a large percentage of the pediatric population. Due to this, most of the data on HTN in children are from tertiary centers reporting a preponderance of secondary HTN. As reviewed by Flynn *(2)*, examination of this data shows shift toward higher reported prevalence (up to 50%) of primary HTN in children. Criteria for making a diagnosis of primary HTN are summarized in Table 1. As per the current recommendations, BP readings of more than 95th percentile for sex, age, and height on three separate occasions are required for diagnosing HTN. The most widely used

G. Kapur (✉)
Department of Pediatric Nephrology, Children's Hospital of Michigan, Wayne State University School of Medicine, Detroit, MI, USA
e-mail: gkapur@med.wayne.edu

From: *Clinical Hypertension and Vascular Diseases: Pediatric Hypertension*
Edited by: J. T. Flynn et al. DOI 10.1007/978-1-60327-824-9_19
© Springer Science+Business Media, LLC 2011

Table 1
Criteria to Use in Diagnosing Primary HTN in Children

Primary criteria

➢ An average of 2–3 readings of systolic BP and/or diastolic BP exceeding the 95th
  percentile for age, gender, and height repeated three times over a 2–3-month period

or

➢ Ambulatory blood pressure measurements over a 24-h period that exceed the 95th
  percentile for age-matched controls (lack of diastolic HTN and normal dipping on
  ABPM are more consistent with primary HTN)

and

➢ Unable to identify a known secondary cause of HTN

Supportive criteria

➢ Stage 1 HTN on presentation
➢ Children obese on presentation (BMI>95th percentile)
➢ Family history of HTN
➢ Idiopathic HTN associated with high, normal, or low PRA
➢ Abnormal response to mental stress
➢ Evidence of end-organ effect; fundoscopic changes, cardiac enlargement by
  electrocardiogram and/or echocardiogram (suggestive of long standing HTN)

nomograms for BP in children are those reported by the Fourth Task Force Report on Blood
Pressure in Children and Adolescents *(3)*. According to the recommendations of the Fourth
Task Force Report, pediatric HTN is now categorized into pre-HTN (SBP or DBP between
90th and 95th percentile or greater than 120/80), stage 1 HTN (SBP or DBP ≤ 95th–99th
percentile plus 5 mmHg), and stage 2 HTN (SBP>99th percentile plus 5 mmHg). Based on
these recommendations, primary HTN in children is usually mild or stage 1 HTN and is
often associated with a family history of HTN or cardiovascular disease. Other comorbid
conditions associated with primary HTN in children, which increase the risk for cardiovascular disease, include abnormal lipid profile, glucose intolerance, and sleep abnormalities. HTN definition is an arbitrary division in the continuum of BP, concurrent with an
increased risk of recognizable morbidity and mortality that becomes increasingly prevalent
as BP increases. A pragmatic definition of HTN would be the level of systolic BP and/or
diastolic BP above which recognizable morbidity occurs. As of this writing, there are no
data that adequately define this in children. Not everyone agrees with the current definition because only the first BP reading was used to define normal values for the 83,000
children included in the BP nomograms for children and adolescents *(3,4)*. It is noteworthy that a comparison of normal BP readings reported by 10 different investigators reveals
that the highest and lowest (50th and 95th) percentile values for boys differ by 20 mmHg
(5). Other confounding factors in BP measurement in children include the cuff size, number of measurements, type of instruments used, patient position (supine or sitting), and the
choice of sound (Korotkoff (K) 4 versus K 5) used for defining diastolic BP *(3)*. Ambulatory blood pressure monitoring (ABPM) has been used increasingly in the past decade
to diagnose HTN, define diurnal BP variability in normal and hypertensive populations
(including children) *(6)*, and evaluate therapy. ABPM is essential for diagnosing white-coat

HTN and may sometimes help to distinguish primary versus secondary HTN in children. Nocturnal dipping during ABPM is believed to reflect decreased sympathetic nervous system activity. BP load and non-dipping have been associated with end-organ changes and possibly higher risk for secondary HTN *(7)*. Masked HTN is a condition in which subjects classified as normotensive by conventional office measurement are hypertensive with ABPM or self-measurement. Lurbe et al. have estimated the prevalence of masked HTN at 9% in children/adolescents with persistence in 50% of these patients *(8)*. Lurbe et al. *(8)* and Stabouli et al. *(9)* have reported progression to sustained hypertension and hypertensive end-organ damage (increased left ventricular mass index) in patients with masked hypertension. These findings make a case for treatment of patients with masked HTN to prevent cardiovascular complications of hypertension.

PATHOGENESIS OF HTN *(10–12)*

An overview of the steps involved in the generation and a persistent phase of HTN (Tables 2 and 3) serves as a basis upon which risk factors, clinical evaluation, and treatment of primary HTN in children are better understood. HTN occurs when the sum of cardiac output (CO) and total peripheral resistance (TPR) increases. Each parameter is influenced by other factors, which may increase or decrease the relative contribution of volume and/or vasoconstrictor components of the BP formula. The factors involved in increasing BP during the generation and maintenance phases of primary HTN are often different. In one form, the increase in CO during its early stages has been attributed to a hyperkinetic circulation characterized by increased heart rate (HR), cardiac index, and forearm blood flow secondary to increased sympathetic tone and cardiac contractility *(13)*. Fixed persistent primary HTN is characterized by an increase in TPR and a return to a normal CO. In the second form, early HTN is characterized by increased left ventricular (LV) mass, as also reported in normotensive offspring of hypertensive parents. These observations raise the possibility that repeated neural stimulation and upregulation of cardiac receptors may be the primary event in the onset of primary HTN *(14)*. The observed changes, from that of an increased to normal CO, and an increased TPR over time, enable a constant blood flow to organs in experimental animals and humans. The proposed mechanisms for these changes include (1) auto-regulation, an intrinsic feature of vasculature characterized by increased flow-induced vasoconstriction, and (2) vascular structural changes including hypertrophy and eventually fibrosis. According to Folkow hypothesis *(15)*, peripheral resistance increase

Table 2
The Basic Blood Pressure Formula and Its Physiologic Transformation to HTN

1. Pressure equals flow times resistance
2. BP = volume times resistance
3. BP = CO times total peripheral resistance
4. BP = flow (preload + contractility) × resistance (arteriolar functional contraction + vessel anatomical changes), e.g., BP = Flow × Resistance
5. HTN = a net increase in CO and/or increased peripheral resistance

Table 3
Factors Involved in the Generation and/or Persistence of HTN

Cardiac output

Preload

Increased fluid volume

➢ Renal sodium retention: genetic factors, decreased glomerular filtration surface, and renin aldosterone effect

➢ Excess sodium intake

Volume redistribution

➢ Sympathetic nervous system overactivity: genetic factors, stress (personal and environmental), and renin angiotensin excess

Contractility

➢ Sympathetic nervous system overactivity and genetic factors

Total peripheral resistance

Functional vasoconstriction

➢ Renin angiotensin excess, sympathetic nervous system overactivity, genetic influence on cell membrane function, and endothelins

Structural constriction

➢ Folkow hypothesis, renin–angiotensin excess, sympathetic nervous system overactivity, endothelins, and hyperinsulinemia

in hypertension of any etiology is most likely related to increased vascular mass. This amplifies the extent of contraction resulting from vasoactive stimuli and, thus, markedly increases resistance to blood flow and systemic blood pressure in the vessels of hypertensive patients. There is controversy over the primary mechanisms involved, as they may operate independently or collectively. The presence of functional versus irreversible structural changes explains response to therapy and the potential reversibility of the hypertensive process aggravated by obesity, stress, and/or excessive salt intake.

Electrolytes

In chronically hypertensive individuals it is hypothesized that the normal relationship between BP and natriuresis is reset at a higher level, which may be genetically determined. Abundant evidence exists to support a major role of sodium in the etiology of essential hypertension (Table 4). Salt-sensitive individuals are estimated at 25–50% of the adult population and in them BP changes correlate with an increase or decrease in salt intake. Genetic renal defects linked with abnormal sodium homeostasis in primary HTN include increased efferent arteriolar tone leading to increased sodium reabsorption, congenital reduction in the number of nephrons and filtering surface *(16)*, nephron heterogeneity *(17)*, and non-modulation that involves abnormal adrenal and renal responses to angiotensin (ANG) II infusions *(18)*. Intake of other ions like calcium and potassium also influences BP. Increased potassium intake by Dutch children over a 7-year period was associated with a mean yearly increase in systolic BP of 1.4 mmHg, while children ingesting a low potassium intake experienced a systolic BP raise of 2.4 mmHg per year *(19)*. Low calcium intake or its

Table 4
Role of Sodium in Primary HTN

Experimental evidence

➤ High salt intake increases renal vascular vasoconstriction, catecholamine release, and NaK ATPase inhibitor ouabain, which in turn leads to increase in intracellular calcium and sodium

➤ In salt-sensitive patients with essential HTN, BP varies directly with changes in sodium intake

➤ Decreases in salt intake in people with borderline high BP may prevent the onset of HTN

➤ The time and the quantity of sodium administration to rats genetically predisposed to HTN determine the onset and the level of BP

➤ Similar mother and offspring BP response to sodium restriction supports a genetic predisposition to salt sensitivity

Epidemiologic evidence

➤ Significant correlations between salt intake and BP have been demonstrated in large population studies

➤ Primitive isolated societies with naturally ingesting low-sodium diets do not develop HTN, nor does BP rise with age

➤ Primitive isolated societies increase their BP after being exposed to environments where excess sodium is ingested

---

increased excretion can lead to hyperparathyroidism, which presumably causes hypertension by altering contractility in vascular smooth muscle *(20)*.

Hormones (10,11)

RAAS (Renin–Angiotensin–Aldosterone System): The renin–angiotensin–*aldosterone* system (RAAS) influences both elements of the BP formula. ANG II binding to AT1 receptors in vascular smooth muscle increases contractility as well as sensitivity to catecholamines. Binding within the adrenal gland leads to increased aldosterone production, sodium retention by the kidney, and volume expansion. The AT2 receptor, which is not involved in the vascular/smooth muscle contraction, is known to play a role in cell differentiation and hypertrophy. Studies have shown that aldosterone receptor antagonist improves endothelial dysfunction, increases NO, and prevents nephrosclerosis.

Catecholamines: Sympathetic nervous system (SNS) activity can function as an initiator and as a secondary contributing factor. Stress and/or a primary catecholamine regulation defect in the brain may directly cause vascular vasoconstriction. SNS stimuli from the vasomotor center activate efferent pathways causing norepinephrine release at peripheral nerve endings, which in turn stimulate adrenergic receptors. Circulating epinephrine derived from the adrenal medulla can stimulate norepinephrine release through the stimulation of presynaptic β2 receptors. Excessive circulating catecholamines increase the BP response to a sodium load. Baroreceptor reflex arc dysfunction occurs in some patients with primary HTN. Usually, elevated BP leads to reflex lowering of the BP by reducing sympathetic outflow from vasomotor centers and increasing vagal tone. The responsiveness of this system resets itself to a higher level with BP elevations and plays a role in the persistence of HTN. Although *Dopamine* is a modulator of systemic BP, with additional actions on fluid and sodium intake, no mutations have linked patients' primary HTN or genetic HTN in rats to the D1 receptor. One D1 and D2 receptor polymorphism has been associated with HTN; however, the mechanism is unclear. The systemic affects of the *natriuretic peptides (A, B, and C)* result in reduction of both preload and afterload, especially in conditions with intravascular volume expansion. Mutations in ANP genes have been described in hypertensive patients and other cardiovascular disease.

Endothelial-Derived Hormones: Endothelin (ET-1) signals through ET-A and ET-B receptor subtypes. The balance between the vasoconstrictor effects of ET-A and vasodilator effects of ET-B determines the overall effects of ET-1. Nitrous oxide (NO), synthesized by the endothelium form L-arginine, is predominantly a vasodilator. The balance between NO and endothelium-derived vasodilators and the SNS maintains the vascular tone. Neuronal NO has also been shown to influence the autonomic regulation of BP. Other hormones linked to blood pressure regulation include adenosine (endothelium derived), triiodothyronine, and adrenomedullin peptide.

Genetic Influences

The theory of impaired genetic homeostasis postulates *(21)* that the mismatch between genes involved in the regulation of BP and the acculturated changes in our society accounts for the recent increase in documented HTN. Low birth weight, increased placental weight, and HTN *(22)* result in a phenotype that is insulin resistant and hypertensive and possibly associated with abnormalities in 11β-hydroxysteroid dehydrogenase activity *(23)*. Synchronicity, a process by which growth spurts are associated with increases in BP, may be accelerated in genetically prone hypertensive individuals *(24)*. Allometric dysfunction, a process by which somatic and renal growth fail to match each other, might lead to HTN if environmental factors enable excessive non-genetically determined growth to occur *(25)*. The failure of renal vascular remodeling to occur during fetal and postnatal life might alter the expected decreases in the activity of RAS and/or sodium regulatory mechanisms. Premature telomere shortening, a process associated with normal aging, may lead to HTN *(26)*. Finally, perturbation in neural development of the sympathetic nervous system and/or cardiac β1 receptors may predispose newborns to develop a hyperkinetic circulation and therefore HTN *(27)*.

PREDICTORS OF PRIMARY HTN

Tracking (12) refers to the pattern of repeated BP measurements over a period of time. The clinical importance of tracking in children with annual BP over the age of 3 years is related to the ability to predict BP status later in childhood and adulthood. Children who are hypertensive are more likely to remain hypertensive throughout childhood and as adults, particularly in the presence of a family history of HTN, increased body weight, or increased left ventricular mass *(28,29)*. The Muscatine study *(30)* has demonstrated that in children with two or more systolic or diastolic BP readings above the 90th percentile or any SBP reading above the 90th percentile, 24–25% of adult readings were above the 90th percentile while in children with three BP readings less than the 90th percentile, 6–7% of adult readings were above the 90th percentile. A recent meta-analysis of published studies on BP tracking confirms the presence of childhood BP tracking into adulthood across diverse populations, with stronger association seen with older ages *(31)*.

RISK FACTORS INVOLVED IN CHILDHOOD PRIMARY HTN *(10–12)*

Age and Gender

Children have lower BP levels in comparison to adults, but the levels progressively increase as the child ages, with a linear rise from 1 to 13 years. This increase is related more to body size than age. Primary HTN is the most common cause of HTN in older children especially in the post-pubertal group. The prevalence of HTN and pre-HTN is greater in boys than in girls *(32)*. Also, in girls BP rises rapidly between 6 and 11 years of age, than it does from 12 to 17 years, while the opposite is seen in boys *(10)*.

Race and Ethnicity

The prevalence of primary HTN is clearly influenced by race and ethnicity *(33)*. Native Americans have the same or higher rate of primary HTN as Hispanics who have the same or lower BP than Caucasians. The prevalence of HTN in blacks is twice that of whites, has an earlier onset, and is associated with more end-organ damage. Muntner et al. *(34)* and Din-Dzietham et al. *(35)* have also reported on the prevalence of higher BP levels in minority youth. These differences are most likely quantitative *(36)* for the characteristics of the hypertensive process are similar in blacks and whites when corrected for age, cardiovascular and renal damage, and level of BP *(37)*. Blacks have higher sleep and less dipping in their nighttime ABPM values than age-matched whites *(38)*. Blacks experience a greater degree of renal global, segmental, and interstitial sclerosis than whites at an earlier age, despite having similar BP and degrees of proteinuria *(39)*. Possible factors include increased salt sensitivity, activity of the RAAS (genetic polymorphism), and transforming growth factor β. Several studies have reported that blacks have a poorer response to both angiotensin-converting enzyme (ACE) inhibitors and calcium channel blockers. The addition of a diuretic to these agents improves the response.

Renin Profiling

Laragh et al. have proposed that patients with primary HTN can be divided into three groups: normo, hyper, and hypo reninemic based on renin profiling, e.g., the comparison of plasma renin activity (PRA) to sodium excretion *(40)*. This group concluded that high-renin primary HTN patients are at greater risk for vasoocclusive events such as stroke, infarction, and renal failure, while those with low-renin primary HTN are volume over-expanded and less likely to experience the aforementioned end-organ damage. Moreover, they suggest that drug therapy should be targeted at the underlying primary pathophysiology and renin inhibitors and diuretics be, respectively, used to treat patients with high- and low-renin primary HTN. Limited studies in children have included renin profiling, and the incidence of low-renin HTN is estimated at 19% *(41)*. There are currently no long-term data on the outcome of hypertensive children, who were renin profiled at diagnosis. Studies have also shown that PRA is higher in those with high uric acid levels and inversely related to fractional excretion of uric acid in hypertensive patients *(42)*. This suggests the presence of altered glomerulotubular balance in hypertensive patients. Feig et al. have recently reported that hyperuricemia (uric acid>5.5 mg/dl) is more commonly associated with primary HTN compared to secondary or white-coat HTN *(43)*. Flynn et al. have reported that high PRA is associated with higher BP load and correlates positively with diastolic BP, but not with systolic BP *(44)*.

White-Coat HTN (WCH)

WCH or isolated office HTN is defined as office BP readings ≥95th percentile but with normal values outside the clinical setting. The estimated prevalence of WCH is around 35% in children being evaluated for persistently elevated casual BP and 44% in children with a family history of primary HTN *(45)*. The prevalence of white-coat HTN is higher when the office values reveal borderline or mild HTN and much lower with moderate or severe HTN *(46)*. Similar to adults, a retrospective study in children has shown that WCH is possibly a prehypertensive condition with increased left ventricular mass and progression to sustained HTN *(47)*. Increased urinary excretion of cortisol and endothelin in adolescents with WCH identifies a group with distinct metabolic abnormalities *(48)*. Since urinary endothelin is derived from the kidney, these findings support a dysregulation of renal function. It is possible that WCH in children represents two populations: one that is destined to develop primary HTN (prehypertensive) *(49)* and one that remains normotensive outside the clinical setting.

Fetal Development

Baker first proposed that HTN in adult life is associated with retarded fetal growth and this relationship becomes stronger as the patient ages *(22)*. Postulated mechanisms include insulin resistance, exposure of a malnourished fetus to maternal glucocorticoids that alter subsequent steroid sensitivity, as well as the metabolism of placenta cortisol *(50)*, and the presence of a reduced number of glomeruli. The net result is a reduced number of glomeruli (as much as 25% in experimental animals), a decreased glomerular surface area, and a reduction in glomerular filtration rate (GFR) per nephron *(51)*. The impaired nephron function eventually leads to HTN.

Obesity

Obesity, which is found in 35–50% of hypertensive adolescents, is one of the most important factors involved in both the generation and persistence of childhood primary HTN. Prevalence studies, including tracking studies of weight change and BP in young adults *(52)*, have reported an increase in childhood obesity and HTN in obese subjects. The relationship between elevated BP and weight begins in early childhood and has been reported to occur as early as 5 years *(53)*. The Muscatine Study showed that changes in ponderosity over 11 years correlated directly with BP changes *(30)*. Obesity is associated with "metabolic syndrome," which is characterized by insulin resistance, an atherogenic dyslipidemia, activation of the sympathetic nervous system, and an increased tendency for thrombosis—suggest using a reference for metabolic syndrome. Other suggested mechanisms of obesity-related HTN include hyperinsulinemia, hyperproinsulinemia, renal sodium retention, increased sympathetic activity, increased plasma volume, increased levels of dehydroepiandrosterone *(54)*, and increased CO (for further discussion, see Chapter 17).

Increased plasma aldosterone activity in obese adolescents correlates with increases in their mean BP; the BP level falls when weight loss occurs *(55)*.

Salt Intake (Table 4)

The average sodium intake in American diet has increased almost fivefold to approximately 3400 mg/day, a level sufficiently high enough to enable high-BP expression in salt-sensitive individuals *(56)*. Also, epidemiologic studies have shown that BP levels are higher in societies with high salt intake *(10)*. Experimental studies have shown that the amount and time of introduction of sodium in the diet of newborn rats influences the onset and persistence of HTN. In human neonates, the ingestion of lower sodium (4 mEq/L) containing formula after birth was associated with a 2.1 mmHg lower BP after 6 months *(57)*. Even though this difference did not persist a few years later, it is still possible that a lifelong effect may be seen. The findings of the Intersalt study *(58)* and PREMIER study *(59)* challenge the recommendations regarding the DASH (dietary approaches to stop HTN) diet as central component of combined lifestyle modification for HTN treatment. Furthermore, the DASH study recommendations are limited due to a follow-up of only 30 days, and the association between sodium intake and risk from adverse events has not been demonstrated in non-obese subjects. In children, this issue is further complicated as sodium is essential for normal growth and development.

Exercise

Exercise (aerobic and static) transiently increases BP. Exercise provides a number of benefits: increased caloric expenditure, appetite suppression, and improved exercise tolerance. Serum cholesterol and triglyceride levels inversely relate to the level of exercise. The BP response of hypertensive adolescents to exercise is similar to that of normotensive adolescents, but starts and finishes at higher levels *(60)*. In adolescents, peak SBP >210 mmHg, and a rise in DBP with dynamic exercise, is occasionally used to determine the need for antihypertensive drug therapy *(61)*.

Lipids and Cigarette Smoking

Chronic smoking itself does not increase BP; it is associated with increased cholesterol levels and lower levels of high-density lipoprotein (HDL), which increase the risk of atherogenesis *(62)*. Prolonged elevation of cholesterol is strongly associated with an increased risk of coronary artery disease. Evaluations of the coronary arteries and aorta of 35 children and young adults dying from non-coronary artery disease events revealed fatty aortic streaks in 61%, coronary artery fibrous streaks and/or plaques in 85%, and raised plaques in 25% *(62)*. The extent of involvement correlated directly with total cholesterol and low-density lipoprotein (LDL) and, inversely, with the ratio of HDL to LDL cholesterol. Obesity is the most common cause of hypertriglyceridemia, often associated with a low HDL in adolescents. It is well known that inherited disorders of lipid metabolism increase the risk of early cardiovascular disease.

Genetics

Approximately 60–70% of HTN in families can be attributed to genetic factors and the remainder to environmental factors *(63)*. Comparison of dizygotic with monozygotic twins supports a hereditary estimate of 0.72 and 0.28 for DBP and SBP, respectively *(64)* (for further discussion, see Chapter 14). The observations that dizygotic correlations are higher than other first-degree relatives support a role for shared environmental cause *(65)*. Attempts to identify specific candidate genes involved in primary HTN have yielded inconsistent results. Such differences may reflect environmental factors, the influence of other genes, evolutionary diversion (race and ethnicity), and study design and/or technical issues. At least 25–30 genes have been suggested as contributors to the hypertensive process (Table 5 *(66)*). ACE/ID polymorphisms are believed to play a major role in both the onset of primary HTN and its treatment. Individuals homozygotic for the D allele have higher levels of ACE. The DD genotype has been associated in some, but not all, studies with a reduced antiproteinuric effect to ACE inhibitor antihypertensive agents. In such patients, AT1 receptor blockades may improve BP response and retard progression of renal disease *(67)*. The genes controlling plasma angiotensinogen (AGT) clearly influence BP while those involved in ACE production do not *(68)*. The Gly460Trp variant of the α-adducin gene has been associated with HTN more in blacks *(69)* than in whites. A number of renal transplantation experiments, between genetic strains of primary HTN and normotensive rats, as well as

Table 5
Partial Listing of Chromosomes, Genes, and Flanking Markers Involved in HTN

Chromosome 5q31-q34 (marker bordering region D5S2093), ADRB2 allele Arg16Gly

* β-adrenoceptor-G-protein system: chromosome 20q13.2, gene GNAS1 exon 5, allele Fok1.chromosome 12p13, gene GNB3, exon 10. Allele C825T

α-adducin

* Chromosome 4p, gene alpha adducin. Allele Gly460Trp
* Catecholamine synthetic enzymes: (a) dopamine-β-hydroxylase gene, (b) phenylethanolamine *N*-methyltransferase gene, and (c) tyrosine hydroxylase gene
* Chromosome 18q *(74)*
* Genomic array identified genes: (a) 2p22.1-2p21, 5p33.3-5q34, 6q23.1-6q24.1, 15q23.1-15q26.1; (b) chromosome 11q, marker D11S934; and (c) chromosome 15q, marker D158203
* Lipoprotein metabolism

Chromosome 8p22, gene lipoprotein lipase

* Chromosome 2p24, gene apolipoprotein, and allele β 3′ promoter hypervariable region
* Miscellaneous genes: (a) glucagon receptor, (b) glucocorticoid receptor, (c) prostacyclin synthase, and (d) transforming growth factor β (TGF-β) 1 gene
* Renal kallikrein-kinin system: (a) chromosome 19q13 and (b) gene tissue kallikrein (KLK1) 5′ proximal promoter
* Renin–angiotensin–aldosterone system: (a) angiotensinogen gene alleles M235T, A-6G, and A-20C and (b) ACE locus deletion/insertion (D/I) polymorphism intron 16
* Aldosterone synthase (CYP11B2 on chromosome 8p21) alleles –344T
* Epithelial sodium channel (ENaC): subunit β T594M mutation (nearby β gene 16p12.3) *(75)*

Adapted unless otherwise stated from *(66)*.

human transplantation *(70)*, support the concept that the genetic composition of the kidney plays a role in determining HTN.

Stress

Stress of all types can increase BP. Poverty, socio-cultural factors, racial issues, and migrations are also known to increase BP. Both SBP and DBP can be correlated with chronic hostility, nervousness, and the demanding perception of environment in adolescents *(71)*. Type A behavior is associated with increases in SBP, but not in DBP *(72)*. Three models of psychosocial stress that might explain the genesis of primary HTN are the Defense Defeat Model, Demand Control, and Lifestyle Incongruity Index *(73)*. These models deal with issues such as fight flight, control, aggression, depression, subordination, the relationship between psychologic demand factored by the available latitude of decision-making, and differences between occupational and social class and achievement versus accomplishment.

CONCLUSION

The increasing diagnosis of primary hypertension in children represents an important shift in our understanding of pediatric hypertension. Primary hypertension in children is a diagnosis of exclusion and children need to be evaluated for any underlying secondary causes. An understanding of the pathophysiology, genetic mechanisms underlying primary HTN in children, holds the promise of modification of behavioral traits, designer drug therapy, and improved interpretation of gene expression (thereby likely gene therapy in future). This will help in addressing both the public health issues and individual needs of hypertensive children and adults.

REFERENCES

1. Pickering G. Mechanisms, methods, management in hypertension: definitions, natural histories and consequences. In: Laragh J, ed. Hypertension Manual. New York, NY: York Medical books; 1973:3–10.
2. Flynn JT. What's new in pediatric hypertension? Curr Hypertens Rep. 2001;3:503–510.
3. National High Blood Pressure Education Program Working Group on High Blood Pressure in Children and Adolescents. The fourth report on the diagnosis, evaluation, and treatment of high blood pressure in children and adolescents. Pediatrics. 2004;114:555–576.
4. Task Force on Blood Pressure Control in Children. National Heart, Lung, and Blood Institute, Bethesda, Maryland. Report of the Second Task Force on Blood Pressure Control in Children—1987. Pediatrics. 1987;79:1–25.
5. Park M, Troxler, RG. Systemic hypertension. In: Park M, Troxler RG, eds. Pediatric Cardiology for Practitioners, 4th ed. St. Louis, MO: Mosby; 2002:408–416.
6. Sorof JM, Portman RJ. Ambulatory blood pressure monitoring in the pediatric patient. J Pediatr. 2000;136:578–586.
7. Belsha CW, Wells TG, McNiece KL, Seib PM, Plummer JK, Berry PL. Influence of diurnal blood pressure variations on target organ abnormalities in adolescents with mild essential hypertension. Am J Hypertens. 1998;11:410–417.
8. Lurbe E, Torro I, Alvarez V, et al. Prevalence, persistence, and clinical significance of masked hypertension in youth. Hypertension. 2005;45:493–498.
9. Stabouli S, Kotsis V, Toumanidis S, Papamichael C, Constantopoulos A, Zakopoulos N. White-coat and masked hypertension in children: association with target-organ damage. Pediatr Nephrol. 2005;20: 1151–1155.

10. Bender J, Bonilla-Felix MA, Portman RJ. Epidemiology of hypertension. In: Avner EA, Harmon WE, Niaudet P, eds. Pediatric Nephrology, 5th ed. Philadelphia, PA: Lippincott Williams and Wilkins; 2004:1125–1152.

11. Blumenfeld J, Laragh JH. Essential hypertension. In: Brenner BM, ed. The Kidney, 7th ed. Philadelphia, PA: Saunders; 2004:2023–2064.

12. Matoo TK. Epidemiology, risk factors, and etiology of hypertension in children and adolescents. In: UpToDate, Basow DS, ed. UpToDate, Waltham, MA, 2009. http://www.uptodate.com/online/content/topic.do?topicKey=pedineph/19132. [Accessed February 14, 2009].

13. Julius S, Krause L, Schork NJ, et al. Hyperkinetic borderline hypertension in Tecumseh, Michigan. J Hypertens. 1991;9:77–84.

14. Korner PI, Bobik A, Angus JJ. Are cardiac and vascular "amplifiers" both necessary for the development of hypertension? Kidney Int Suppl. 1992;37:S38–S44.

15. Folkow B. Physiological aspects of primary hypertension. Physiol Rev. 1982;62:347–504.

16. Brenner BM, Garcia DL, Anderson S. Glomeruli and blood pressure. Less of one, more the other? Am J Hypertens. 1988;1:335–347.

17. Sealey JE, Blumenfeld JD, Bell GM, Pecker MS, Sommers SC, Laragh JH. On the renal basis for essential hypertension: nephron heterogeneity with discordant renin secretion and sodium excretion causing a hypertensive vasoconstriction-volume relationship. J Hypertens. 1988;6:763–777.

18. Hollenberg NK, Adams DF, Solomon H, et al. Renal vascular tone in essential and secondary hypertension: hemodynamic and angiographic responses to vasodilators. Medicine (Baltimore). 1975;54:29–44.

19. Geleijnse JM, Grobbee DE, Hofman A. Sodium and potassium intake and blood pressure change in childhood. BMJ. 1990;300:899–902.

20. Staessen J, Sartor F, Roels H, et al. The association between blood pressure, calcium and other divalent cations: a population study. J Hum Hypertens. 1991;5:485–494.

21. Neel JV, Weder AB, Julius S. Type II diabetes, essential hypertension, and obesity as "syndromes of impaired genetic homeostasis": the "thrifty genotype" hypothesis enters the 21st century. Perspect Biol Med. 1998;42:44–74.

22. Baker D. Fetal and Infant Origins of Adult Disease. London: BMJ; 1993.

23. Seckl JR. Glucocorticoids, feto-placental 11 beta-hydroxysteroid dehydrogenase type 2, and the early life origins of adult disease. Steroids. 1997;62:89–94.

24. Akahoshi M, Soda M, Carter RL, et al. Correlation between systolic blood pressure and physical development in adolescence. Am J Epidemiol. 1996;144:51–58.

25. Weder AB, Schork NJ. Adaptation, allometry, and hypertension. Hypertension. 1994;24:145–156.

26. Aviv A, Aviv H. Reflections on telomeres, growth, aging, and essential hypertension. Hypertension. 1997;29:1067–1072.

27. Julius S, Quadir H, Gajendragadhkar S. Hyperkinetic state: a precursor of hypertension? A longitudinal study of borderline hypertension. In: Gross F, Strasser T, eds. Mild Hypertension: Natural History and Management. London: Pittman; 1979:116–126.

28. Katz SH, Hediger ML, Schall JI, et al. Blood pressure, growth and maturation from childhood through adolescence. Mixed longitudinal analyses of the Philadelphia Blood Pressure Project. Hypertension. 1980;2:55–69.

29. Shear CL, Burke GL, Freedman DS, Berenson GS. Value of childhood blood pressure measurements and family history in predicting future blood pressure status: results from 8 years of follow-up in the Bogalusa Heart study. Pediatrics. 1986;77:862–869.

30. Lauer RM, Clarke WR. Childhood risk factors for high adult blood pressure: the Muscatine study. Pediatrics. 1989;84:633–641.

31. Chen X, Wang Y. Tracking of blood pressure from childhood to adulthood: a systematic review and meta-regression analysis. Circulation. 2008;117:3171–3180.

32. Dasgupta K, O'Loughlin J, Chen S, et al. Emergence of sex differences in prevalence of high systolic blood pressure: analysis of a longitudinal adolescent cohort. Circulation. 2006;114:2663–2670.

33. Cornoni-Huntley J, LaCroix AZ, Havlik RJ. Race and sex differentials in the impact of hypertension in the United States. The National Health and Nutrition Examination Survey I Epidemiologic Follow-up Study. Arch Intern Med. 1989;149:780–788.

34. Muntner P, He J, Cutler JA, Wildman RP, Whelton PK. Trends in blood pressure among children and adolescents. JAMA. 2004;291:2107–2113.

35. Din-Dzietham R, Liu Y, Bielo MV, Shamsa F. High blood pressure trends in children and adolescents in national surveys, 1963 to 2002. Circulation. 2007;116:1488–1496.

36. Flack JM, Peters R, Mehra VC, Nasser SA. Hypertension in special populations. Cardiol Clin. 2002;20:303–319, vii.

37. Flack JM, Gardin JM, Yunis C, Liu K. Static and pulsatile blood pressure correlates of left ventricular structure and function in black and white young adults: the CARDIA study. Am Heart J. 1999;138: 856–864.

38. Harshfield GA, Alpert BS, Pulliam DA, Somes GW, Wilson DK. Ambulatory blood pressure recordings in children and adolescents. Pediatrics. 1994;94:180–184.

39. Marcantoni C, Ma LJ, Federspiel C, Fogo AB. Hypertensive nephrosclerosis in African Americans versus Caucasians. Kidney Int. 2002;62:172–180.

40. Brunner HR, Laragh JH, Baer L, et al. Essential hypertension: renin and aldosterone, heart attack and stroke. N Engl J Med. 1972;286:441–449.

41. Kilcoyne MM. Adolescent hypertension. II. Characteristics and response to treatment. Circulation. 1974;50:1014–1019.

42. Prebis JW, Gruskin AB, Polinsky MS, Baluarte HJ. Uric acid in childhood essential hypertension. J Pediatr. 1981;98:702–707.

43. Feig DI, Johnson RJ. Hyperuricemia in childhood primary hypertension. Hypertension. 2003;42:247–252.

44. Flynn JT, Alderman MH. Characteristics of children with primary hypertension seen at a referral center. Pediatr Nephrol. 2005;20:961–966.

45. Hornsby JL, Mongan PF, Taylor AT, Treiber FA. 'White coat' hypertension in children. J Fam Pract. 1991;33:617–623.

46. Sorof JM, Poffenbarger T, Franco K, Portman R. Evaluation of white coat hypertension in children: importance of the definitions of normal ambulatory blood pressure and the severity of casual hypertension. Am J Hypertens. 2001;14:855–860.

47. Kavey RE, Kveselis DA, Atallah N, Smith FC. White coat hypertension in childhood: evidence for end-organ effect. J Pediatr. 2007;150:491–497.

48. Vaindirlis I, Peppa-Patrikiou M, Dracopoulou M, Manoli I, Voutetakis A, Dacou-Voutetakis C. "White coat hypertension" in adolescents: increased values of urinary cortisol and endothelin. J Pediatr. 2000;136: 359–364.

49. Matthews KA, Woodall KL, Allen MT. Cardiovascular reactivity to stress predicts future blood pressure status. Hypertension. 1993;22:479–485.

50. Benediktsson R, Lindsay RS, Noble J, Seckl JR, Edwards CR. Glucocorticoid exposure in utero: new model for adult hypertension. Lancet. 1993;341:339–341.

51. Woods LL. Fetal origins of adult hypertension: a renal mechanism? Curr Opin Nephrol Hypertens. 2000;9:419–425.

52. Khoury P, Morrison JA, Mellies MJ, Glueck CJ. Weight change since age 18 years in 30- to 55-year-old whites and blacks. Associations with lipid values, lipoprotein levels, and blood pressure. JAMA. 1983;250:3179–3187.

53. Gutin B, Basch C, Shea S, et al. Blood pressure, fitness, and fatness in 5- and 6-year-old children. JAMA. 1990;264:1123–1127.

54. Katz SH, Hediger ML, Zemel BS, Parks JS. Blood pressure, body fat, and dehydroepiandrosterone sulfate variation in adolescence. Hypertension. 1986;8:277–284.

55. Rocchini AP, Katch VL, Grekin R, Moorehead C, Anderson J. Role for aldosterone in blood pressure regulation of obese adolescents. Am J Cardiol. 1986;57:613–618.

56. Eaton SB, Konner M, Shostak M. Stone agers in the fast lane: chronic degenerative diseases in evolutionary perspective. Am J Med. 1988;84:739–749.

57. Hofman A, Hazebroek A, Valkenburg HA. A randomized trial of sodium intake and blood pressure in newborn infants. JAMA. 1983;250:370–373.

58. Intersalt Cooperative Research Group. Intersalt: an international study of electrolyte excretion and blood pressure. Results for 24 hour urinary sodium and potassium excretion. BMJ. 1988;297:319–328.

59. Appel LJ, Champagne CM, Harsha DW, et al. Effects of comprehensive lifestyle modification on blood pressure control: main results of the PREMIER clinical trial. JAMA. 2003;289:2083–2093.

60. Wilson SL, Gaffney FA, Laird WP, Fixler DE. Body size, composition, and fitness in adolescents with elevated blood pressures. Hypertension. 1985;7:417–422.

61. Jung FF, Ingelfinger JR. Hypertension in childhood and adolescence. Pediatr Rev. 1993;14:169–179.

62. Berenson GS, Mcmann CA, Voors, AW, et al. Cardiovascular Risk Factors in Children: The Early Natural History of Atherosclerosis and Essential Hypertension. New York, NY: Oxford University Press; 1990.

63. Ward R. Familial aggregation and genetic epidemiology of blood pressure. In: Laragh J, Brenner B, ed. Hypertension-Pathophysiology, Diagnosis and Management. New York, NY: Raven; 1990:81–100.

64. Christian JC. Twin studies of blood pressure. In: Filer LJ, Laver RM, eds. Children's blood pressure. Report of the 88th Ross conference on Pediatric Research. Ross Laboratories, Columbus; 1985:51–55.

65. Feinleib M, Garrison R, Borhani N. Studies of hypertension in twins. In: Paul O, ed. Epidemiology and Control of Hypertension. New York, NY: Stratton Intercontinental Medical Book Corp; 1975:3–20.
66. Timberlake DS, O'Connor DT, Parmer RJ. Molecular genetics of essential hypertension: recent results and emerging strategies. Curr Opin Nephrol Hypertens. 2001;10:71–79.
67. Van Essen GG, Rensma PL, de Zeeuw D, et al. Association between angiotensin-converting-enzyme gene polymorphism and failure of renoprotective therapy. Lancet. 1996;347:94–95.
68. Smithies O, Kim HS, Takahashi N, Edgell MH. Importance of quantitative genetic variations in the etiology of hypertension. Kidney Int. 2000;58:2265–2280.
69. Barlassina C, Norton GR, Samani NJ, et al. Alpha-adducin polymorphism in hypertensives of South African ancestry. Am J Hypertens. 2000;13:719–723.
70. Curtis JJ, Luke RG, Dustan HP, et al. Remission of essential hypertension after renal transplantation. N Engl J Med. 1983;309:1009–1015.
71. Southard DR, Coates TJ, Kolodner K, Parker FC, Padgett NE, Kennedy HL. Relationship between mood and blood pressure in the natural environment: an adolescent population. Health Psychol. 1986;5:469–480.
72. Siegel JM, Matthews KA, Leitch CJ. Blood pressure variability and the type A behavior pattern in adolescence. J Psychosom Res. 1983;27:265–272.
73. Pickering T. Psychosocial stress and hypertension: clinical and experimental evidence. In: Swales J, ed. Textbook of Hypertension. Oxford: Blackwell Scientific; 1994:640–654.
74. Kristjansson K, Manolescu A, Kristinsson A. Linkage of essential hypertension to chromosome 18q. Hypertension. 2002;39:1044–1049.
75. Hyndman ME, Parson HG, Verma S, et al. Mutation in endothelial nitric oxide synthase is associated with hypertension. Hypertension. 2002;39:919–922.

20 Secondary Forms of Hypertension

Kjell Tullus, MD, PhD, FRCPCH

INTRODUCTION

In most studies, hypertension in children has been secondary to an identifiable cause in a large majority of those studied [1,2]. This has changed during the relatively recent epidemic of childhood obesity, where primary hypertension in many centers now is the most common cause form of hypertension [3]. In adults primary hypertension is the dominating diagnosis. This chapter will discuss those cases where a cause for the hypertension has been possible to identify. It is quite possible that in the future some children that presently are diagnosed with primary or essential hypertension will be found to have an underlying diagnosis.

The causes of secondary hypertension vary considerably with the age of the child. They can be defined as acute forms of hypertension related to an acute episode of a disease or its treatment, or chronic secondary hypertension. The blood pressure in the former children often normalizes when the acute disease is resolved while in latter often the problem persists for many years, even indefinitely. Of course, some children with acute hypertension will develop a more sustained or chronic disease.

K. Tullus (✉)
Department of Nephrology, Great Ormond Street Hospital for Children, London, UK
e-mail: tulluk@gosh.nhs.uk

From: *Clinical Hypertension and Vascular Diseases: Pediatric Hypertension*
Edited by: J. T. Flynn et al. DOI 10.1007/978-1-60327-824-9_20
© Springer Science+Business Media, LLC 2011

ACUTE SECONDARY HYPERTENSION

There are numerous causes for acute transiently increased BP (Table 1), the most common being acute renal failure or acute glomerulonephritis (GN). Two common diagnoses in children are hemolytic uremic syndrome (HUS) and post-streptococcal GN. Salt and water retention is a prime mechanism behind this hypertension. Many cases of GN and in particular diagnoses causing impaired blood flow by narrowing of blood vessels, as in vasculitides or HUS, may also have a renin-mediated process. Salt and water overload of other causes (e.g., iatrogenic) can also cause hypertension.

Paradoxical hypertension can be seen in children with intravascular volume depletion as such as in the acute phase of nephrotic syndrome *(4)*. This form of hypertension is caused

Table 1
Causes of Acute Transient Hypertension

Renal parenchymal disease
   Acute glomerulonephritis
   Acute tubulointerstitial nephritis
   Hemolytic uremic syndrome
Acute renal failure of any cause
Acute urinary tract obstruction
Salt and water overload
   With acute renal failure
   Iatrogenic—giving too much salt and water
   Iatrogenic—salt retaining hormone treatments
Vascular
   Renal vein and renal artery thrombosis
   Embolic disease
   Vasculitis
   Renal compression—tumor, post-trauma, or surgery
Neurological
   Raised intracranial pressure
   Guillain–Barré
   Poliomyelitis
   Dysautonomia
Drug mediated
   Oral contraceptives
   Sympathomimetic drugs
   Erythropoietin
   Drugs for hyperactivity in ADHD
   Illicit drugs e.g. cocaine and amphetamine
Diet mediated
   Alcohol
   Licorice

by renin release to produce vasoconstriction, and normalizes after volume repletion. Several neurological conditions can cause hypertension, in particular increased intracranial pressure but also conditions such as Guillain–Barré syndrome and poliomyelitis *(5,6)*.

Many drugs, including not only illicit drugs such as cocaine, but also prescribed agents such as corticosteroids, can cause severe hypertension (Table 1) *(7)*.

CHRONIC SECONDARY HYPERTENSION

The causes of chronic secondary hypertension are quite different in different age groups. In neonates the most common are malformations in the kidney or coarctation of the aorta (CoA) (Table 2) *(8)*. Problems related to prematurity and its treatment, including chronic lung disease and thrombotic events of the renal arteries or veins, are also important. A more thorough discussion of neonatal hypertension is found in Chapter 21. In older infants renal malformations and renovascular disease (RVD) become the predominant diagnoses (Table 3).

Table 2
Common Causes of Hypertension in Neonates

Renal artery or vein thrombosis due to umbilical catheter
Renal venous thrombosis
Congenital renal malformations
Coarctation
Chronic lung disease
Post-ECMO
Midaortic syndrome and/or renal artery stenosis

Table 3
Common Causes of Hypertension in Infants

Renal parenchymal disease
Renovascular disease
Medication
Chronic lung disease

An overview of the most common causes of hypertension seen at Great Ormond Street Hospital for Children is given in Table 4. Such a list will, however, vary from hospital to hospital and also from time period to time period but gives a general impression of the most common diagnoses. I will here discuss the most important causes of secondary hypertension in more detail (Table 5).

Table 4
Causes of Sustained Hypertension at Great Ormond
Street Hospital for Children

Renal scarring	36%
Glomerulonephritis	23%
Renovascular hypertension	10%
Coarctation	9%
Polycystic kidneys	6%
Post-HUS	4%
Idiopathic	3.5%
Catecholamine excess	3%
Wilms' tumors	2.5%
Miscellaneous	4.5%

Table 5
Causes of Chronic Hypertension

Parenchymal renal disease
  CAKUT
  Chronic glomerulonephritis
  Polycystic kidney diseases
  Other parenchymal kidney diseases
  After an acute kidney disease such as HUS
Renovascular disease
  Fibromuscular dysplasia
  Sometimes with midaortic syndrome
Chronic renal failure
  Often worsening with worsening renal function
Tumors
Coarctation of aorta
Pulmonary
  Chronic lung disease of the newborn
Endocrine
  Catecholamine excess
    Pheochromocytoma
    Paraganglioma
    Neuroblastoma
  Corticosteroid excess
    Iatrogenic
    Cushing's disease
    Conn's syndrome
Monogenic disorders
  See Chapter 6

RENAL PARENCHYMAL DISEASES

Twenty-five percent of children with chronic kidney disease are either hypertensive or prehypertensive *(9)*. Several parenchymal kidney diseases in particular have hypertension as an important symptom. These include CAKUT (congenital abnormalities of the kidneys and the urinary tract), chronic glomerulonephritides and polycystic kidney diseases. Volume expansion due to reduced sodium excretion and increased activity in the renin–angiotensin axis are two important mechanisms for this hypertension. Others are reduced production of vasodilators and activation of the adrenergic system *(10)*.

CAKUT

CAKUT represents a heterogeneous group of children with congenital damage to the renal parenchyma. This diagnosis is the most common in children with renal impairment. Many different diagnostic terms are used for similar conditions emphasizing different diagnostic or etiological aspects. Some stem from a proposed etiology such as reflux nephropathy or obstructive nephropathy, others are based on a pathological diagnosis such as hypoplastic or dysplastic kidneys and "chronic pyelonephritis" while others are based on the radiological appearance, for example, multicystic dysplastic kidneys. A further commonly used term is scarred kidneys, implying secondary kidney damage due to a process such as acute pyelonephritis. These diagnostic labels are often neither in clinical practice nor in most scientific studies used with a clear distinction between them. It is often difficult to separate congenital dysplastic kidneys from kidneys harmed from acute infections and no consensus on how to best define these diagnoses exists.

These diagnostic difficulties most likely explain the great variation in the reported frequency of high blood pressure in different studies in these children. A population-based study of all children with renal scarring detected during a 10 year period and followed for a mean of 17 years found similar 24-h blood pressure in the children with renal scars compared to those without *(11)*. This contrasts markedly to other studies in more selected populations, such as that from Great Ormond Street Hospital for Children, where renal scarring was the most common cause (36%) for hypertension and up to 20% all children with a renal scar were estimated to get high blood pressure *(12)*. A study from eastern Europe showed that children with more extensive kidney scars on their DMSA scan had higher BP than children with no scars or less extensive scars *(13)*.

Many children with congenital malformations have tubular dysfunction, with impaired reabsorption of sodium, and inability to concentrate their urine. They do therefore often loose both salt and water, which explains why a majority of these children have normal or low blood pressure. Please also see Chapter 22.

Chronic Glomerulonephritides

Children with long-standing ongoing inflammation in their kidneys frequently have high blood pressure as one major symptom. The cause of this high blood pressure is multifactorial, with water retention, vascular constriction, and renin release as important components. Children with chronic GN resulting in chronic renal impairment frequently have persistent proteinuria, which has been associated with a greater likelihood of having hypertension compared to children without proteinuric renal disease *(9)*.

Autosomal Recessive Polycystic Kidney Disease and Autosomal Dominant Polycystic Kidney Disease

Children with polycystic kidneys often have high blood pressure as an important symptom even before they develop impaired kidney function. In autosomal recessive polycystic kidney disease (ARPKD), the high blood pressure is often evident already during the first month of life. Also children with autosomal dominant polycystic kidney disease (ADPKD) do often display hypertension long before any signs of impairment of kidney function *(14,15)* (Fig. 1). The mechanisms behind the hypertension are debated, with activation of the renin–angiotensin system still most likely being of major importance *(16)*.

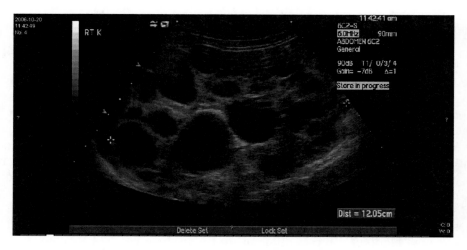

Fig. 1. Renal ultrasound of the right kidney of a 1-month-old boy with ADPKD and severe hypertension.

Aggressive treatment of the blood pressure, in particular with agents blocking the RAS, is hoped to be able to slow down the progression of renal failure, but no clear evidence exists to support that notion *(17)*.

Hypertension After Severe Acute Renal Diseases

Children with acute kidney diseases such as HUS often suffer from very difficult-to-treat high blood pressure during the acute phase of the disease. In some of these children, in particular those with atypical HUS, the high blood pressure persists also after the acute episode, and management of the blood pressure remains a very important issue *(18)*. This is particularly true as the pressure stress on the endothelium caused by the hypertension might trigger further relapses of the HUS. Ambulatory blood pressure recordings have shown that also a high proportion of children who have recovered from severe HUS caused by Shiga toxin-producing *Escherichia coli* have persistent hypertension *(19)*.

Hypertension Associated with Severe Renal Failure

Children in end-stage renal failure, children on dialysis, or children who had a kidney transplant are frequently hypertensive. For a thorough discussion of hypertension in these conditions, please see Chapter 23.

RENOVASCULAR DISEASE

RVD causes some 10% of hypertension in children, and has been extensively reviewed elsewhere *(20)*. It is important to diagnose as it is potentially curable with interventional treatment. The extent of RVD ranges from the with narrowing of only one renal artery to the large group of children with extensive involvements of their vascular tree *(21)*. In 53–78% of cases there is involvement of both renal arteries and in a third there is also intrarenal small artery disease *(22,23)*. A large group (20–48%) of these children have associated midaortic syndrome (MAS) (Fig. 2) *(24,25)*, that is, narrowing of the abdominal aorta. Involvement of the celiac axis and the superior and inferior mesenteric arteries occurs in 53% of cases and cerebral artery disease is also found in a large proportion.

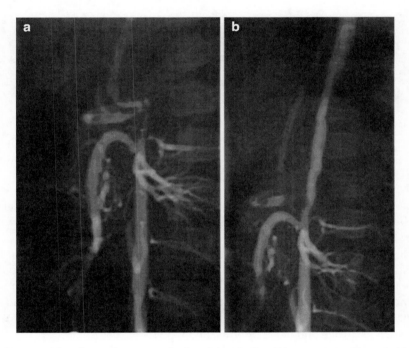

Fig. 2. Severe midaortic syndrome seen before (**a**) and after (**b**) treatment with angioplasty.

There are many causes of RVD in children and they are quite different than those in adults where atherosclerotic disease is the predominant diagnosis. In children a developmental abnormality of the vessel wall is the most common diagnosis *(26,27)*. This is often called fibromuscular dysplasia, but it is uncommon to have pathological confirmation of the diagnosis. The typical pattern with so-called beading on angiography is also often not present (Fig. 3a). Certain syndromes, in particular neurofibromatosis type 1 and William syndrome, are overrepresented among children with RVD even if most children with these syndromes do not have RVD *(28–30)*. Children with vasculitis can also develop clinically significant narrowing of their renal arteries. In some reports, Takayasu's disease is an important cause while we at Great Ormond Street Hospital in London see very few of those cases *(31,32)*. Tumors, radiation, and trauma can also cause significant RVD.

RVD is in a large proportion of children progressive. The number of blood vessels, renal and extra renal, that are involved can increase and the severity of the lesion is often seen to worsen over time. There are no known ways to predict the further course in a single child.

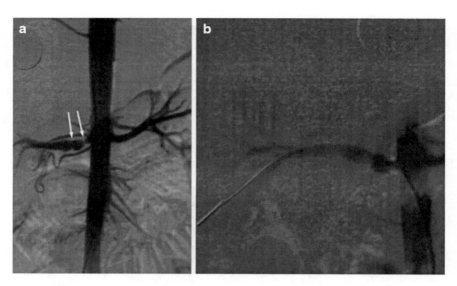

Fig. 3. (**a**) Typical beaded appearance of a renal artery with severe stenosis. (**b**) After treatment with angioplasty.

The hypertension in RVD is caused by a combination of renin-mediated mechanisms and sodium-related volume expansion. Increased sympathetic nervous system activity can also play a role.

Children with RVH do often present with very high BP; it is not uncommon for patients to have systolic blood pressure well above 200 mmHg, with maximum blood pressure even reaching 300 mmHg in some cases. The clinical presentation of these children is very variable. Many children (26–70%) are completely asymptomatic, and are diagnosed as a chance finding, but some can present with severe, potentially life-threatening cerebral or cardiac symptoms such as stroke and heart failure *(23,33–35)*.

The most reliable way to diagnose RVD is with digital subtraction angiography (DSA), which is the only method that can reliably define the extent of the RVD *(21,36)*. Angiography is, however, invasive and general anesthesia is needed in most cases. Other less invasive investigations are therefore used to help to define the group of children that need to undergo DSA. These investigations include those commonly used for all children with high BP, including routine laboratory studies. For example, elevated plasma renin activity or aldosterone, or low to low normal serum potassium can often be seen in children with RVD, but are not always present. Thus, a high index of suspicion needs to be maintained when investigating children with otherwise unexplained severe hypertension.

Renal Doppler ultrasound may in some cases be very helpful in detecting RVD but is in a many cases unable to detect the renal artery stenosis *(37–39)*. The resistance index has been used to measure blood flow in kidneys but the sensitivity is too low for it to rule a need for angiography *(40)*. Pre- and post-captopril renal scintigraphy has been widely used to screen for RVD, based on the concept of reduced blood flow to the kidney or part of the kidney after administration of the angiotensin-converting enzyme inhibitor (ACEi) *(41)* can be seen as reduced relative function of one kidney or as a new uptake defect in on or both kidneys. The sensitivity (50–73%) of this investigation has, however, not been shown to be good enough to make the use of this procedure useful in clinical practice *(38,42–46)*.

Newer imaging modalities such as computed tomography angiography (CTA) and magnetic resonance angiography (MRA) can be helpful in detecting and monitoring vascular lesions. No studies on MRA or CTA exist in children with suspected RVD. The sensitivity and specificity in adult patients is between 64–93% and 64–94%, respectively *(20,38,47,48)*. Both these methods have problems with smaller blood vessels with a sensitivity of 85% in detecting clinically significant stenosis of the coronary arteries in adult patients *(49)*. As children have smaller blood vessels, this might be a bigger problem in the younger population. In our own experience, we have seen that CTA and MRA can both over- and underdiagnose RVD in children.

Measurement of renal vein renins is in many cases helpful in deciding how to treat a child with RVD *(50–52)*. It is performed at the same time as the angiography where the femoral vein is catheterized and blood is sampled from the inferior vena cava and from the main renal veins and their main branches in both kidneys. This information can be used in the defining which part of the kidney(s) that seems to produce increased levels of renin and thus to decide which of often several artery stenosis that should be given priority in the treatment.

The treatment of children with RVD should be managed by a multidisciplinary team and should be based on a combination of antihypertensive drugs, angioplasty, and surgery. Medicines are useful in most children with RVH and are often needed as adjunctive therapy in children who have successfully undergone surgery or angioplasty. It is important not to use an ACEi in these children as this very often can cause a major deterioration in the function of the affected kidney(s) *(53)*. This can in cases with unilateral renal artery stenosis only be monitored with renal scintigraphy as serum creatinine is not sensitive enough to detect deterioration of the function in one kidney.

With modern technology, angioplasty can cure or improve the blood pressure in at least 50% of children *(35,54,55)* (Fig. 3). The angioplastied artery has in many children a tendency to undergo restenosis. In some cases, a stent can be placed to keep the artery open *(35,56–58)* (Fig. 4). The lumen of some stents will with time narrow down. This can be due to intimal hyperplasia within the stent or due to thrombosis of the stent. In adult coronary arteries, stents coated with an anti-proliferative agent such as sirolimus have been used to reduce the occurrence of intimal hyperplasia. This does however seem to increase the risk of early thrombosis of the stents and no clear scientific opinion on which stent is preferred exists at the present time *(59)*.

Some children not amenable to angioplasty can be treated with ethanol ablation of a part of a kidney *(52,60)*. This is particularly useful in polar arteries supplying only a small part of one kidney. Surgery should only be used in children where angioplasty has not achieved good enough blood pressure control. There are many different surgical options including nephrectomy of a kidney with very little function and different revascularization procedures. Nephrectomy is often very successful at curing the blood pressure in particular if there is unilateral disease *(61,62)*. We have occasionally seen kidneys that on a pretreatment DMSA scans demonstrated <10% function that after successful angioplasty or revascularization surgery have recovered up to 50% relative function (Tse personal communication). These kidneys may survive on collateral circulation that in ordinary circumstances does not result in meaningful kidney function, but the function can sometimes be recovered. We use the size of the affected kidney on ultrasound to decide when to try to recover function or to go directly to nephrectomy.

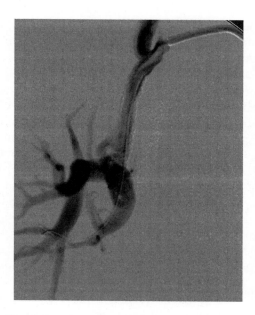

Fig. 4. Renal artery stented after angioplasty.

Revascularization surgery can be performed in several different ways: surgery on the renal arteries with autologous or synthetic grafts inserted or aortic reconstruction with or without a synthetic graft *(62–64)*. The autologous grafts can be the splenic or the gastroduodenal artery that is pulled to the kidney, part of the saphenous vein or internal iliac artery. Dacron is often used for the synthetic grafts (Fig. 5). The surgery on the renal arteries can sometimes be so complicated and time consuming that it needs to be done outside of the

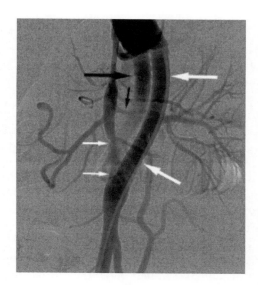

Fig. 5. A so-called trouser graft from upper aorta linking on to lower aorta (*big white arrow*) and left renal artery (*big black arrow*).

child with an ensuing autotransplantation. With complicated pathology such as bilateral stenosis and MAS, a so-called trouser graft can be used that goes from the aorta above the MAS down to the aorta below the MAS and one or both renal arteries.

With increasing use of angioplasty the children needing surgery have become more and more complicated. Despite this, the results of revascularization surgery are generally very good. We and other authors achieve cure or improvement in 90% of the children undergoing surgery *(61,65)*.

RENAL TUMORS

Different tumors can cause hypertension through two primary mechanisms: direct pressure on the renal blood vessels or aorta, or through hormones secreted from the tumor (see below). Wilms' tumors cause hypertension in a majority of cases, but also other more uncommon renal tumors such as reninomas and occasionally hamartomas can also cause HT *(66–68)*.

COARCTATION OF THE AORTA

CoA accounts for a few percent of children with high blood pressure. It is amenable to potentially curable surgical treatment and is therefore important to diagnose early *(69,70)*. CoA is mostly diagnosed in newborn children or infants but may be detected at later ages. The classical lesion is narrowing of the aorta just below the origin of the left subclavian artery. CoA is not normally associated with narrowing of other blood vessels. The cause of hypertension presurgery is renal hypoperfusion with increased renin–angiotensin activity. When hypertension persists postsurgery, it is most likely caused by both renin and sympathetic nervous system activities *(71–73)*.

The presenting symptoms are mostly detection of a murmur or raised blood pressure on measurement. The diagnosis is normally suspected clinically from the combination of higher blood pressures in the arms compared to the legs, the sometimes absent femoral pulses and the systolic ejection murmur that sometimes is heard better in the back. The diagnosis is confirmed with echocardiography. Angiography is still the method that best can both define anatomy and give hemodynamic data, but MRA and CTA are increasingly used *(69)*.

The optimal treatment for coarctation has with time become controversial *(74)*. The treatment of choice used to be surgical, with excision of the narrowed part of the aorta and end-to-end anastomosis. This seems to still be the preferred method in neonates and infants. In older children and in adults, balloon angioplasty is used more and more sometimes also with stenting *(75)*. This is, however, particularly in smaller children quite controversial *(70)*.

Narrowing can occur also in other parts of the aorta. Typical is narrowing of the abdominal aorta. This was previously called abdominal coarctation but the modern preferred term is MAS. MAS is in most cases related to other vascular pathology and seems in children to fall into the same spectrum as RVD (see above).

The BP in children with CoA does mostly normalize postsurgery. However a significant proportion of children will still need some antihypertensive treatment also after the surgery. This risk seems to increase over several decades and is higher in children treated at an age of more than 1 year compared to children who were treated during their infancy *(72,76)*. This can be caused by reoccurrence of the stenosis but is in most cases not fully understood.

PULMONARY CAUSES

There is a well-known relation between chronic lung disease of prematurity and high blood pressure in neonates *(77,78)*. For details please see Chapter 21. The mechanisms behind this blood pressure are not fully understood but treatment with steroids can play a role. Chronic hypoxia has also been thought to be of importance.

ENDOCRINE

Endocrine causes of high blood pressure can mainly be divided into those that are caused by excess catecholamines or excess corticosteroids.

Catecholamine Excess

Catecholamine excess is a very important but rare cause of hypertension in childhood as it is amenable to curative surgery *(79,80)*. It is regarded to cause 1% or less of all childhood high blood pressure. The lesions can mostly be divided into pheochromocytoma (80%) and paraganglioma; and occasionally a neuroblastoma can produce catecholamines that cause high blood pressure *(81,82)*. Pheochromocytomas are tumors that arise from chromaffin cells in the adrenal medulla while paragangliomas arise from the sympathetic or the parasympathetic paraganglia. The parasympathetic paragangliomas are normally nonfunctioning.

Pheochromocytomas and paragangliomas are often familial and in some studies more than 50% related to a mutation in one of the *VHL* (von Hippel–Lindau type 2), *SDH* (succinate dehydrogenase; paraganglioma syndrome) B and D, *MEN2* (multiple endocrine neoplasia type 2), or *NF1* (neurofibromatosis type 1) genes *(79,83)*. All these are inherited in an autosomal dominant manner. The mechanism might be via impaired apoptosis of sympathetic neuronal precursor cells. A majority of these tumors are benign but a significant proportion are malignant. Histopathological evaluation after surgery is very important to confirm the diagnosis and to attempt to quantify the risk of malignancy and recurrence *(84)*. Certain mutations, in particular the SDHD, have a higher risk of malignancy *(85)*.

Children with pheochromocytomas can present in very different ways, most with some degree of hypertension that can be sustained (60–90%) or variable *(86,87)*. Other classical symptoms are those related to very high blood pressure or to the increased catecholamine levels such as headache, sweating, flushing, palpitation, syncope, blurred vision, tremor, panic attacks, and weight loss. In some reports, only 60% of children with pheochromocytoma had high blood pressure *(88)*.

The diagnosis is based on increased urinary levels of adrenalin and noradrenalin often measure as 24-h excretions *(89,90)*. Fractionated plasma metanephrines show the highest sensitivity, 97%, and can be test of choice in high risk children. VMA (vanillylmandelic acid) and HVA (homovanillic acid) have a too low sensitivity to rule out pheochromocytoma *(91)*. Imaging includes ultrasound, CT, or abdominal MRI depending on local facilities. All these methods can in most cases define the tumor, but MRI seems to be the method of choice *(92)*. Whole-body metaiodobenzylguanidine (MIBG) [123]I scan has an important role in helping with the diagnosis and to evaluate the extent of the disease, including defining multiple occurrences and relapsing lesions. Its sensitivity seems, however, not to be better than 80–90% but the specificity approaches 100% *(93,94)*. Labeled somatostatin is an alternative method that has been used in cases with negative MIBG. A biopsy before surgery should normally be avoided as handling of the tumor can lead to release of cate-cholamines with severe peaks of high blood pressure leading to stroke or arrhythmias.

The blood pressure is best controlled by the combination of an α- and β-sympathetic blockade often using phenoxybenzamine and a short-acting β-blocking agent as propranolol *(82,95)*. The α-adrenoceptor blockade opposes the vasoconstriction that is induced by the catecholamine excess while the β-blockade opposes reflex tachycardia that can occur from the vasodilatation. β-Blockade on its own should not be used as it can result in worsening blood pressure from not blocking the α-receptors.

Induction of anesthesia and manipulation of the tumor can cause unpredictable release of catecholamines that can cause hypertensive crisis with stroke and arrhythmias. It is impor-tant that the above-mentioned pharmacological blockade is in place before the surgery. Liberal salt intake and keeping the child well hydrated is important to reduce surgical risks *(96)*. Metyrosine that competitively inhibits catecholamine biosynthesis can also have a role in minimizing intra-operative risks *(97)*. A very gentle anesthetic procedure keeping the patient very calm is also very important. Acute rises of the blood pressure during surgery might need to be controlled with intravenous antihypertensives. Hypotension can also occur when the venous drainage of the tumor is blocked and the tumor is removed. Treatment with pressor agents such as dopamine or catecholamines might be needed in that situation. Post-operative hypoglycemia should be monitored for *(96)*. Recently, laparoscopic surgery of abdominal and thoracic tumors has become more common *(88,96,98,99)*.

The histopathology of the tumor is important to confirm the diagnosis but cannot accu-rately predict the further behavior of the tumors. There are attempts to try to quantify the risk of malignancy with a combination of pathological criteria and expression of certain markers that can be helpful in understanding the long-term prognosis *(84)*. Long-term follow-up is needed throughout life to detect tumor relapses and development of tumors at other sites. Screening is done by regular blood pressure measurements and regular mon-itoring of urinary or plasma catecholamines. This is particularly important in children with defined genetic mutations *(85)*.

Corticosteroid Excess

The most common cause for hypertension from corticosteroid excess is treatment with glucocorticoids. In these children the high blood pressure can be a problem necessitating treatment with multiple antihypertensive medications. The pathophysiology is uncertain but activation of the renin–angiotensin system and sodium retention due to mineralocorticoid effects of the steroid are most often thought to be involved. This form of hypertension will resolve when it is possible to reduce doses or discontinue the medication completely.

Cushing's syndrome caused by excessive production of ACTH or glucocorticoids is far less common in children *(100,101)*. This can be caused by an ACTH-secreting hypotha-lamic tumor, by ACTH production elsewhere, or by corticosteroid-producing tumors or adrenal hyperplasia. The diagnosis can in these unusual cases mostly be suspected from the classical clinical habitus; round face, truncal obesity, acne, and abdominal striae. These children do also display delayed growth and sometimes virilization and pseudoprecocious puberty *(102)*. In infants McCune–Albright syndrome is a major cause of Cushing's syn-drome *(103)*.

The diagnosis is confirmed by urine and blood testing of cortisol and ACTH levels *(104)*. Surgical resection is usually curative but can be very challenging. The hypothalamic lesions should be treated with a transsphenoidal approach *(105)*.

Raised levels of aldosterone from adrenal tumors (Conn's syndrome) are extremely rare conditions in children *(106)*. The mineralocorticoid excess leads to salt and water retention. The condition should be suspected in cases with low to low normal serum potassium and metabolic alkalosis. Surgical treatment should be curative.

Congenital adrenal hyperplasia, in particular the 11β-hydroxylase deficiency and the much less common 17α-hydroxylase deficiency, can cause hypertension *(107,108)* (see also Chapter 6). The 11β-hydroxylase defect leads to decreased secretion of cortisone and cortisol and excess production androgens. This stimulates secretion of pituitary ACTH and excess adrenal production of DOC (11-deoxycorticosterone) that has mineralocorticoid effects in high concentrations. These children also exhibit symptoms of virilization and ambiguous genitalia.

Children with 17α-hydroxylase deficiency lack both cortisol and androgens and are thus not virilized and often not diagnosed before they develop their hypertension, hypokalemia, and hypogonadism in adolescence *(109)*.

Other very uncommon causes of real or apparent mineralocorticoid excess (AME) are Liddle's syndrome, glucocorticoid-remediable aldosteronism (GRA), and Gordon's syndrome. These syndromes that have taught us a lot on molecular mechanisms and tubular function are described in more detail in Chapter 6.

REFERENCES

1. Gill DG, Mendes de CB, Cameron JS, Joseph MC, Ogg CS, Chantler C. Analysis of 100 children with severe and persistent hypertension. Arch Dis Child. Dec 1976;51(12):951–956.
2. Wyszynska T, Cichocka E, Wieteska-Klimczak A, Jobs K, Januszewicz P. A single pediatric center experience with 1025 children with hypertension. Acta Paediatr. Mar 1992;81(3):244–246.
3. Sorof J, Daniels S. Obesity hypertension in children: a problem of epidemic proportions. Hypertension. Oct 2002;40(4):441–447.
4. Bissler JJ, Welch TR, Loggie JM. Paradoxical hypertension in hypovolemic children. Pediatr Emerg Care. Dec 1991;7(6):350–352.
5. Cooper WO, Daniels SR, Loggie JM. Prevalence and correlates of blood pressure elevation in children with Guillain-Barre syndrome. Clin Pediatr (Phila). Oct 1998;37(10):621–624.
6. Perlstein MA, Ndelman MB, Rosner DC, Wehrle P. Incidence of hypertension in poliomyelitis. Pediatrics. June 1953;11(6):628–633.
7. Ferdinand KC. Substance abuse and hypertension. J Clin Hypertens (Greenwich). Jan 2000;2(1):37–40.
8. Flynn JT. Neonatal hypertension: diagnosis and management. Pediatr Nephrol. Apr 2000;14(4):332–341.
9. Flynn JT, Mitsnefes M, Pierce C, et al. Blood pressure in children with chronic kidney disease: a report from the Chronic Kidney Disease in Children study. Hypertension. Oct 2008;52(4):631–637.
10. Martinez-Maldonado M. Hypertension in end-stage renal disease. Kidney Int Suppl. Dec 1998;68: S67–S72.
11. Wennerstrom M, Hansson S, Hedner T, Himmelmann A, Jodal U. Ambulatory blood pressure 16-26 years after the first urinary tract infection in childhood. J Hypertens. Apr 2000;18(4):485–491.
12. Goonasekera CD, Shah V, Wade AM, Barratt TM, Dillon MJ. 15-Year follow-up of renin and blood pressure in reflux nephropathy. Lancet. Mar 1996 9;347(9002):640–643.
13. Patzer L, Seeman T, Luck C, Wuhl E, Janda J, Misselwitz J. Day- and night-time blood pressure elevation in children with higher grades of renal scarring. J Pediatr. Feb 2003;142(2):117–122.
14. Avner ED. Childhood ADPKD: answers and more questions. Kidney Int. May 2001;59(5):1979–1980.
15. Sedman A, Bell P, Manco-Johnson M, et al. Autosomal dominant polycystic kidney disease in childhood: a longitudinal study. Kidney Int. Apr 1987;31(4):1000–1005.
16. Chapman AB, Schrier RW. Pathogenesis of hypertension in autosomal dominant polycystic kidney disease. Semin Nephrol. Nov 1991;11(6):653–660.
17. Davis ID, MacRae DK, Sweeney WE, Avner ED. Can progression of autosomal dominant or autosomal recessive polycystic kidney disease be prevented? Semin Nephrol. Sept 2001;21(5):430–440.
18. Taylor CM. Hemolytic-uremic syndrome and complement factor H deficiency: clinical aspects. Semin Thromb Hemost. June 2001;27(3):185–190.

19. Krmar RT, Ferraris JR, Ramirez JA, et al. Ambulatory blood pressure monitoring after recovery from hemolytic uremic syndrome. Pediatr Nephrol. Oct 2001;16(10):812–816.

20. Tullus K, Brennan E, Hamilton G, et al. Renovascular hypertension in children. Lancet. Apr 2008;371(9622):1453–1463.

21. Vo NJ, Hammelman BD, Racadio JM, Strife CF, Johnson ND, Racadio JM. Anatomic distribution of renal artery stenosis in children: implications for imaging. Pediatr Radiol. Oct 2006;36(10):1032–1036.

22. Daniels SR, Loggie JM, McEnery PT, Towbin RB. Clinical spectrum of intrinsic renovascular hypertension in children. Pediatrics. Nov 1987;80(5):698–704.

23. Deal JE, Snell MF, Barratt TM, Dillon MJ. Renovascular disease in childhood. J Pediatr. Sept 1992;121(3):378–384.

24. Panayiotopoulos YP, Tyrrell MR, Koffman G, Reidy JF, Haycock GB, Taylor PR. Mid-aortic syndrome presenting in childhood. Br J Surg. Feb 1996;83(2):235–240.

25. Sethna CB, Kaplan BS, Cahill AM, Velazquez OC, Meyers KE. Idiopathic mid-aortic syndrome in children. Pediatr Nephrol. Jul 2008;23(7):1135–1142.

26. Sandmann W, Schulte KM. Multivisceral fibromuscular dysplasia in childhood: case report and review of the literature. Ann Vasc Surg. Sept 2000;14(5):496–502.

27. Slovut DP, Olin JW. Fibromuscular dysplasia. N Engl J Med. Apr 2004 ;350(18):1862–1871.

28. Criado E, Izquierdo L, Lujan S, Puras E, del Mar EM. Abdominal aortic coarctation, renovascular, hypertension, and neurofibromatosis. Ann Vasc Surg. May 2002;16(3):363–367.

29. Kurien A, John PR, Milford DV. Hypertension secondary to progressive vascular neurofibromatosis. Arch Dis Child. May 1997;76(5):454–455.

30. Daniels SR, Loggie JM, Schwartz DC, Strife JL, Kaplan S. Systemic hypertension secondary to peripheral vascular anomalies in patients with Williams syndrome. J Pediatr. Feb 1985;106(2):249–251.

31. Hari P, Bagga A, Srivastava RN. Sustained hypertension in children. Indian Pediatr. Mar 2000;37(3):268–274.

32. McCulloch M, Andronikou S, Goddard E, et al. Angiographic features of 26 children with Takayasu's arteritis. Pediatr Radiol. Apr 2003;33(4):230–235.

33. Estepa R, Gallego N, Orte L, Puras E, Aracil E, Ortuno J. Renovascular hypertension in children. Scand J Urol Nephrol. Oct 2001;35(5):388–392.

34. McTaggart SJ, Gulati S, Walker RG, Powell HR, Jones CL. Evaluation and long-term outcome of pediatric renovascular hypertension. Pediatr Nephrol. Sept 2000;14(10–11):1022–1029.

35. Shroff R, Roebuck DJ, Gordon I, et al. Angioplasty for renovascular hypertension in children: 20-year experience. Pediatrics. Jul 2006;118(1):268–275.

36. Shahdadpuri J, Frank R, Gauthier BG, Siegel DN, Trachtman H. Yield of renal arteriography in the evaluation of pediatric hypertension. Pediatr Nephrol. Aug 2000;14(8–9):816–819.

37. Brun P, Kchouk H, Mouchet B, et al. Value of Doppler ultrasound for the diagnosis of renal artery stenosis in children. Pediatr Nephrol. Feb 1997;11(1):27–30.

38. Eklof H, Ahlstrom H, Magnusson A, et al. A prospective comparison of duplex ultrasonography, captopril renography, MRA, and CTA in assessing renal artery stenosis. Acta Radiol. Oct 2006;47(8):764–774.

39. Garel L, Dubois J, Robitaille P, et al. Renovascular hypertension in children: curability predicted with negative intrarenal Doppler US results. Radiology. May 1995;195(2):401–405.

40. Li JC, Wang L, Jiang YX, et al. Evaluation of renal artery stenosis with velocity parameters of Doppler sonography. J Ultrasound Med. Jun 2006;25(6):735–742.

41. Dondi M. Captopril renal scintigraphy with 99mTc-mercaptoacetyltriglycine (99mTc-MAG3) for detecting renal artery stenosis. Am J Hypertens. Dec 1991;4(12 Pt 2):737S–740S.

42. Arora P, Kher V, Singhal MK, et al. Renal artery stenosis in aortoarteritis: spectrum of disease in children and adults. Kidney Blood Press Res. 1997;20(5):285–289.

43. Fommei E, Ghione S, Hilson AJ, et al. Captopril radionuclide test in renovascular hypertension: a European multicentre study. European Multicentre Study Group. Eur J Nucl Med. Jul 1993;20(7):617–623.

44. Minty I, Lythgoe MF, Gordon I. Hypertension in paediatrics: can pre- and post-captopril technetium-99m dimercaptosuccinic acid renal scans exclude renovascular disease? Eur J Nucl Med. Aug 1993;20(8):699–702.

45. Ng CS, de Bruyn R, Gordon I. The investigation of renovascular hypertension in children: the accuracy of radio-isotopes in detecting renovascular disease. Nucl Med Commun. Nov 1997;18(11):1017–1028.

46. Abdulsamea S, Anderson P, Biassoni L, Brennan E, McLaren CA, Marks SD, Roebuck DJ, Selim S, Tullus K. Pre- and post-captopril renal scintigraphy as a screening test for renovascular hypertension in children. Pediatr Nephrol. 2010;25:317–322.

47. Hacklander T, Mertens H, Stattaus J, et al. Evaluation of renovascular hypertension: comparison of functional MRI and contrast-enhanced MRA with a routinely performed renal scintigraphy and DSA. J Comput Assist Tomogr. Nov 2004;28(6):823–831.

48. Vasbinder GB, Nelemans PJ, Kessels AG, et al. Accuracy of computed tomographic angiography and magnetic resonance angiography for diagnosing renal artery stenosis. Ann Intern Med. Nov 2004;141(9):674–682.
49. Miller JM, Rochitte CE, Dewey M, et al. Diagnostic performance of coronary angiography by 64-row CT. N Engl J Med. Nov 2008;359(22):2324–2336.
50. Dillon MJ, Ryness JM. Plasma renin activity and aldosterone concentration in children. Br Med J. Nov 1975;4(5992):316–319.
51. Goonasekera CD, Shah V, Wade AM, Dillon MJ. The usefulness of renal vein renin studies in hypertensive children: a 25-year experience. Pediatr Nephrol. Nov 2002;17(11):943–949.
52. Teigen CL, Mitchell SE, Venbrux AC, Christenson MJ, McLean RH. Segmental renal artery embolization for treatment of pediatric renovascular hypertension. J Vasc Interv Radiol. Feb 1992;3(1):111–117.
53. Wong H, Hadi M, Khoury T, Geary D, Rubin B, Filler G. Management of severe hypertension in a child with tuberous sclerosis-related major vascular abnormalities. J Hypertens. Mar 2006;24(3):597–599.
54. Konig K, Gellermann J, Querfeld U, Schneider MB. Treatment of severe renal artery stenosis by percutaneous transluminal renal angioplasty and stent implantation: review of the pediatric experience: apropos of two cases. Pediatr Nephrol. May 2006;21(5):663–671.
55. McLaren CA, Roebuck DJ. Interventional radiology for renovascular hypertension in children. Tech Vasc Interv Radiol. Dec 2003;6(4):150–157.
56. Imamura H, Isobe M, Takenaka H, Kinoshita O, Sekiguchi M, Ohta M. Successful stenting of bilateral renal artery stenosis due to fibromuscular dysplasia assessed by use of pressure guidewire technique: a case report. Angiology. Jan 1998;49(1):69–74.
57. Ing FF, Goldberg B, Siegel DH, Trachtman H, Bierman FZ. Arterial stents in the management of neurofibromatosis and renovascular hypertension in a pediatric patient: case report of a new treatment modality. Cardiovasc Intervent Radiol. Nov 1995;18(6):414–418.
58. Liang CD, Wu CJ, Fang CY, Ko SF. Endovascular stent placement for management of total renal artery occlusion in a child. J Invasive Cardiol. Jan 2002;14(1):32–35.
59. Lange RA, Hillis LD. Coronary revascularization in context. N Engl J Med. Mar 2009;360(10): 1024–1026.
60. Ishijima H, Ishizaka H, Sakurai M, Ito K, Endo K. Partial renal embolization for pediatric renovascular hypertension secondary to fibromuscular dysplasia. Cardiovasc Intervent Radiol. Sept 1997;20(5): 383–386.
61. Hegde S, Coulthard MG. Follow-up of early unilateral nephrectomy for hypertension. Arch Dis Child Fetal Neonatal Ed. Jul 2007;92(4):F305–F306.
62. Stanley JC, Criado E, Upchurch GR Jr, et al. Pediatric renovascular hypertension: 132 primary and 30 secondary operations in 97 children. J Vasc Surg. Dec 2006;44(6):1219–1228.
63. O'Neill JA Jr, Berkowitz H, Fellows KJ, Harmon CM. Midaortic syndrome and hypertension in childhood. J Pediatr Surg. Feb 1995;30(2):164–171.
64. Stanley JC, Zelenock GB, Messina LM, Wakefield TW. Pediatric renovascular hypertension: a thirty-year experience of operative treatment. J Vasc Surg. Feb 1995;21(2):212–226.
65. Staderman MB, Montinin G, Hamilton G, Roebuck DJ, McLaren CA, Dillon MJ, Marks SD, Tullus K. Nephrology Dialysis Transplantation. 2010;25:807–813.
66. Haab F, Duclos JM, Guyenne T, Plouin PF, Corvol P. Renin secreting tumors: diagnosis, conservative surgical approach and long-term results. J Urol. Jun 1995;153(6):1781–1784.
67. Steinbrecher HA, Malone PS. Wilms' tumour and hypertension: incidence and outcome. Br J Urol. Aug 1995;76(2):241–243.
68. Warshaw BL, Anand SK, Olson DL, Grushkin CM, Heuser ET, Lieberman E. Hypertension secondary to a renin-producing juxtaglomerular cell tumor. J Pediatr. Feb 1979;94(2):247–250.
69. McCrindle BW. Coarctation of the aorta. Curr Opin Cardiol. Sept 1999;14(5):448–452.
70. Walhout RJ, Plokker HW, Meijboom EJ, Doevendans PA. Advances in the management and surveillance of patients with aortic coarctation. Acta Cardiol. Dec 2008;63(6):771–782.
71. Bagby SP. Acute responses to arterial pressure and plasma renin activity to converting enzyme inhibition (SQ 20,881) in serially studied dogs with neonatally-induced coarctation hypertension. Hypertension. Jan 1982;4(1):146–154.
72. Roegel JC, Heinrich E, De JW, et al. Vascular and neuroendocrine components in altered blood pressure regulation after surgical repair of coarctation of the aorta. J Hum Hypertens. Aug 1998;12(8):517–525.
73. Yagi S, Kramsch DM, Madoff IM, Hollander W. Plasma renin activity in hypertension associated with coarctation of the aorta. Am J Physiol. Sept 1968;215(3):605–610.
74. Hamilton JR. Surgical controversies: coarctation. Cardiol Young. Jan 1998;8(1):50–53.
75. Wong D, Benson LN, Van Arsdell GS, Karamlou T, McCrindle BW. Balloon angioplasty is preferred to surgery for aortic coarctation. Cardiol Young. Feb 2008;18(1):79–88.

76. Seirafi PA, Warner KG, Geggel RL, Payne DD, Cleveland RJ. Repair of coarctation of the aorta during infancy minimizes the risk of late hypertension. Ann Thorac Surg. Oct 1998;66(4):1378–1382.

77. Abman SH. Monitoring cardiovascular function in infants with chronic lung disease of prematurity. Arch Dis Child Fetal Neonatal Ed. Jul 2002;87(1):F15–F18.

78. Emery EF, Greenough A. Neonatal blood pressure levels of preterm infants who did and did not develop chronic lung disease. Early Hum Dev. Dec 1992;31(2):149–156.

79. Armstrong R, Sridhar M, Greenhalgh KL, et al. Phaeochromocytoma in children. Arch Dis Child. Oct 2008;93(10):899–904.

80. Havekes B, Romijn JA, Eisenhofer G, Adams K, Pacak K. Update on pediatric pheochromocytoma. Pediatr Nephrol. May 2009;24(5):943–950.

81. Lenders JW, Eisenhofer G, Mannelli M, Pacak K. Phaeochromocytoma. Lancet. Aug 2005;366(9486):665–675.

82. Pacak K, Eisenhofer G, Ahlman H, et al. Pheochromocytoma: recommendations for clinical practice from the First International Symposium. October 2005. Nat Clin Pract Endocrinol Metab. Feb 2007;3(2):92–102.

83. de Krijger RR, Petri BJ, van Nederveen FH, et al. Frequent genetic changes in childhood pheochromocytomas. Ann N Y Acad Sci. Aug 2006;1073:166–176.

84. Tischler AS, Kimura N, McNicol AM. Pathology of pheochromocytoma and extra-adrenal paraganglioma. Ann N Y Acad Sci. Aug 2006;1073:557–570.

85. Neumann HP, Pawlu C, Peczkowska M, et al. Distinct clinical features of paraganglioma syndromes associated with SDHB and SDHD gene mutations. JAMA. Aug 25 2004;292(8):943–951.

86. Barontini M, Levin G, Sanso G. Characteristics of pheochromocytoma in a 4- to 20-year-old population. Ann N Y Acad Sci. Aug 2006;1073:30–37.

87. Pham TH, Moir C, Thompson GB, et al. Pheochromocytoma and paraganglioma in children: a review of medical and surgical management at a tertiary care center. Pediatrics. Sept 2006;118(3):1109–1117.

88. Ludwig AD, Feig DI, Brandt ML, Hicks MJ, Fitch ME, Cass DL. Recent advances in the diagnosis and treatment of pheochromocytoma in children. Am J Surg. Dec 2007;194(6):792–796.

89. Sawka AM, Jaeschke R, Singh RJ, Young WF Jr. A comparison of biochemical tests for pheochromocytoma: measurement of fractionated plasma metanephrines compared with the combination of 24-hour urinary metanephrines and catecholamines. J Clin Endocrinol Metab. Feb 2003;88(2):553–558.

90. Weise M, Merke DP, Pacak K, Walther MM, Eisenhofer G. Utility of plasma free metanephrines for detecting childhood pheochromocytoma. J Clin Endocrinol Metab. May 2002;87(5):1955–1960.

91. Bockenhauer D, Rees L, Neumann H, Foo Y. A sporadic case of paraganglioma undetected by urine metabolite screening. Pediatr Nephrol. Oct 2008;23(10):1889–1891.

92. Erickson D, Kudva YC, Ebersold MJ, et al. Benign paragangliomas: clinical presentation and treatment outcomes in 236 patients. J Clin Endocrinol Metab. 2001;86(11):5210–5216.

93. Nielsen JT, Nielsen BV, Rehling M. Location of adrenal medullary pheochromocytoma by I-123 metaiodobenzylguanidine SPECT. Clin Nucl Med. Sept 1996;21(9):695–699.

94. van der HE, de Herder WW, Bruining HA, et al. [(123)I]metaiodobenzylguanidine and [(111)In]octreotide uptake in benign and malignant pheochromocytomas. J Clin Endocrinol Metab. Feb 2001;86(2):685–693.

95. Goldstein RE, O'Neill JA Jr, Holcomb GW III, et al. Clinical experience over 48 years with pheochromocytoma. Ann Surg. Jun 1999;229(6):755–764.

96. Hack HA. The perioperative management of children with phaeochromocytoma. Paediatr Anaesth. 2000;10(5):463–476.

97. Pacak K. Preoperative management of the pheochromocytoma patient. J Clin Endocrinol Metab. Nov 2007;92(11):4069–4079.

98. Brunt LM, Lairmore TC, Doherty GM, Quasebarth MA, DeBenedetti M, Moley JF. Adrenalectomy for familial pheochromocytoma in the laparoscopic era. Ann Surg. May 2002;235(5):713–720.

99. Kravarusic D, Pinto-Rojas A, Al-Assiri A, Sigalet D. Laparoscopic resection of extra-adrenal pheochromocytoma—case report and review of the literature in pediatric patients. J Pediatr Surg. Oct 2007;42(10):1780–1784.

100. Nieman LK, Ilias I. Evaluation and treatment of Cushing's syndrome. Am J Med. Dec 2005;118(12):1340–1346.

101. Savage MO, Chan LF, Grossman AB, Storr HL. Work-up and management of paediatric Cushing's syndrome. Curr Opin Endocrinol Diabetes Obes. Aug 2008;15(4):346–351.

102. Peters CJ, Ahmed ML, Storr HL, et al. Factors influencing skeletal maturation at diagnosis of paediatric Cushing's disease. Horm Res. 2007;68(5):231–235.

103. Kirk JM, Brain CE, Carson DJ, Hyde JC, Grant DB. Cushing's syndrome caused by nodular adrenal hyperplasia in children with McCune-Albright syndrome. J Pediatr. Jun 1999;134(6):789–792.
104. Batista DL, Riar J, Keil M, Stratakis CA. Diagnostic tests for children who are referred for the investigation of Cushing syndrome. Pediatrics. Sept 2007;120(3):e575–e586.
105. Joshi SM, Hewitt RJ, Storr HL, et al. Cushing's disease in children and adolescents: 20 years of experience in a single neurosurgical center. Neurosurgery. Aug 2005;57(2):281–285.
106. Abasiyanik A, Oran B, Kaymakci A, Yasar C, Caliskan U, Erkul I. Conn syndrome in a child, caused by adrenal adenoma. J Pediatr Surg. Mar 1996;31(3):430–432.
107. Ferrari P, Bianchetti M, Frey FJ. Juvenile hypertension, the role of genetically altered steroid metabolism. Horm Res. 2001;55(5):213–223.
108. Migeon CJ. Over 50 years of progress in the treatment of the hypertensive form of congenital adrenal hyperplasia due to steroid 11-beta-hydroxylase deficiency. Commentary on Simm PJ and Zacharin MR: successful pregnancy in a patient with severe 11-beta-hydroxylase deficiency and novel mutations in CYP11B1 gene (Horm Res. 2007;68:294–297). Horm Res. 2007;68(6):298–299.
109. Biglieri EG, Kater CE. 17 Alpha-hydroxylation deficiency. Endocrinol Metab Clin North Am. Jun 1991;20(2):257–268.

21 Neonatal Hypertension

Joseph T. Flynn, MD, MS

Contents

INTRODUCTION

Hypertension as a clinical problem in newborn infants was first recognized in the 1970s *(1)*. However, recent advances in our ability to identify, evaluate, and care for premature infants have lead to an increased awareness of neonatal hypertension, not only in the neonatal intensive care unit (NICU) but also in the neonatal follow-up clinic. This chapter will focus on the differential diagnosis of hypertension in the neonate, the optimal diagnostic evaluation, and both acute and chronic antihypertensive therapy.

INCIDENCE/EPIDEMIOLOGY

It is difficult to ascertain the actual incidence of hypertension in neonates because there is no generally accepted definition of hypertension for this age group *(2,3)*. One study of preterm infants admitted to six NICUs in New England demonstrated that 28% of infants with birth weights <1500 g had at least one blood pressure that was considered "hypertensive" *(2)*. Clearly, few of these infants had sustained hypertension. At the other extreme, hypertension is considered so unusual in otherwise healthy term infants that routine blood pressure determination is not recommended for this group by consensus organizations *(4)*.

J.T. Flynn (✉)
Division of Nephrology, Seattle Children's Hospital, Seattle, WA, USA
e-mail: joseph.flynn@seattlechildrens.org

From: *Clinical Hypertension and Vascular Diseases: Pediatric Hypertension*
Edited by: J. T. Flynn et al. DOI 10.1007/978-1-60327-824-9_21
© Springer Science+Business Media, LLC 2011

Despite these issues, most authors agree that the actual incidence of hypertension in neonates is quite low, ranging from 0.2 to 3% in most reports *(5–9)*. The incidence may be somewhat higher in premature and otherwise high-risk newborns. In a review of over 3000 infants admitted to a Chicago NICU, the overall incidence of hypertension was found to be 0.81% *(8)*. Hypertension was considerably more common in infants with bronchopulmonary dysplasia, patent ductus arteriosus, intraventricular hemorrhage or that had indwelling umbilical arterial catheters. In this latter group, approximately 9% of the infants with these conditions developed hypertension. Similar risk factors for hypertension were identified in a recent study of approximately 2600 infants admitted to a tertiary NICU in Canberra, Australia *(9)*. Aside from prematurity, umbilical artery catheterization, chronic lung disease, and antenatal steroid administration were the most significant risk factors for the development of hypertension *(9)*.

These high-risk infants are also at risk for the development of hypertension long after discharge from the NICU. In a retrospective review of over 650 infants seen in follow-up after discharge from a teaching hospital NICU, Friedman and Hustead found an incidence of hypertension (defined as a systolic blood pressure >113 mmHg on three consecutive visits over 6 weeks) of 2.6% *(10)*. Hypertension in this study was detected at a mean age of approximately 2 months post-term when corrected for prematurity. The hypertensive infants tended to have lower initial Apgar scores and slightly longer NICU stays than infants who remained normotensive, indicating a somewhat greater likelihood of developing hypertension in sicker babies, a finding similar to that of Singh et al. *(8)*.

In yet another study of NICU "graduates," risk factors for higher blood pressure were found to include difficult delivery, prolonged ventilatory support, and hypertension in the nursery *(11)*. Nephrocalcinosis has also been described as a risk factor for future hypertension in infancy *(12)*. Even with the increasing rates of survival of premature infants, however, hypertension remains a relatively infrequent clinical problem that is primarily confined to the NICU or neonatal follow-up clinic.

DIFFERENTIAL DIAGNOSIS

As in older infants and children, the causes of hypertension in neonates are numerous (Table 1), with the two largest categories being renovascular and other renal parenchymal diseases. More specifically, umbilical artery catheter-associated thromboembolism affecting either the aorta or the renal arteries probably accounts for the majority of cases of hypertension seen in the typical NICU. A clear association between use of umbilical arterial catheters and development of arterial thrombi was first demonstrated in the early 1970s by Neal and colleagues *(13)*. They performed aortography at the time of umbilical artery removal in 19 infants, demonstrating thrombus formation in 18 of the 19 infants, as well as several instances of clot fragmentation and embolization. Thrombosis was also seen at autopsy in 7 of 12 additional infants who had died, for an overall incidence of 25 out of 31 infants, or approximately 81% of infants studied.

Following Neal's report, the association between umbilical arterial catheter-associated thrombi and the development of neonatal hypertension was confirmed by several other investigators *(14–19)*. Hypertension was demonstrated in infants who had undergone umbilical arterial catheterization even when thrombi were unable to be demonstrated in the renal arteries. Reported rates of thrombus formation have generally been much lower than in Neal's study, typically about 25% *(14,20,21)*. Although there have been several studies that have examined the duration of line placement and line position ("low" vs. "high") as

Table 1
Causes of Neonatal Hypertension

Renovascular	Medications/intoxications
Thromboembolism	Infant
Renal artery stenosis	Adrenergic agents
Mid-aortic coarctation	Caffeine
Renal venous thrombosis	Dexamethasone
Compression of renal artery	Erythropoietin
Abdominal aortic aneurysm	Pancuronium
Idiopathic arterial calcification	Phenylephrine
Congenital rubella syndrome	Theophylline
Renal parenchymal disease	Vitamin D intoxication
Congenital	Maternal
Polycystic kidney disease	Cocaine
Multicystic-dysplastic kidney	Heroin
disease	Neoplasia
Tuberous sclerosis	Wilms tumor
Ureteropelvic junction obstruction	Mesoblastic nephroma
Unilateral renal hypoplasia	Neuroblastoma
Primary megaureter	Pheochromocytoma
Congenital nephrotic syndrome	Neurologic
Renal tubular dysgenesis	Pain
Acquired	Intracranial hypertension
Acute tubular necrosis	Seizures
Cortical necrosis	Familial dysautonomia
Interstitial nephritis	Subdural hematoma
Hemolytic-uremic syndrome	Miscellaneous
Obstruction (stones, tumors)	Total parenteral nutrition (TPN)
Pulmonary	Closure of abdominal wall defect
Bronchopulmonary dysplasia	Adrenal hemorrhage
Pneumothorax	Hypercalcemia
Cardiac	Traction
Thoracic aortic coarctation	ECMO
Endocrine	Birth asphyxia
Congenital adrenal hyperplasia	
Hyperaldosteronism	
Hyperthyroidism	
Pseudohypoaldosteronism type II	
(Gordon syndrome)	

factors involved in thrombus formation, these data have not been conclusive *(20,21)*. Thus, the assumption has been made that the cause of hypertension in such cases is related to thrombus formation at the time of line placement, probably related to disruption of the vascular endothelium of the umbilical artery. Such thrombi may then embolize to the kidneys, causing areas of infarction and increased renin release. A similar phenomenon has been reported in infants with dilatation of the ductus arteriosus *(22)*.

The Cochrane Group has regularly examined the controversy regarding umbilical artery catheter placement and complications *(23)*. They analyzed five randomized clinical trials and one study using alternate assignments to compare the incidence of complications such as thrombus formation. The placement of a catheter tip was defined as high when located in the descending aorta above the diaphragm and low when located in the descending aorta above the bifurcation but below the renal arteries. The reviewers concluded that high catheter position causes fewer clinically obvious ischemic complications and possibly decreases the frequency of aortic thrombosis. As far as hypertension was concerned, however, it was concluded that it seems to appear with equal frequency among infants with high and low umbilical artery catheter placements.

Other renovascular problems may also lead to neonatal hypertension. Renal venous thrombosis (Fig. 1) classically presents with the triad of hypertension, gross hematuria, and an abdominal mass. Hypertension may be quite severe in such cases and may persist beyond the neonatal period *(24–26)*. Fibromuscular dysplasia leading to renal arterial stenosis is another important cause of renovascular hypertension in the neonate. Many of these infants may have main renal arteries that appear normal on angiography but demonstrate significant branch vessel disease that can cause severe hypertension *(27–29)*. In addition, renal arterial stenosis may also be accompanied by mid-aortic coarctation and cerebral vascular stenoses *(27,30)*. Other vascular abnormalities may also lead to hypertension in the neonate, including idiopathic arterial calcification *(31,32)* and renal artery stenosis secondary to congenital rubella infection *(33)*. Congenital aortic aneurysm is a rare condition producing renovascular hypertension that may be fatal because of intractable congestive heart failure *(34)*. Finally, mechanical compression of one or both renal arteries by tumors, obstructed/hydronephrotic kidneys, or other abdominal masses may also lead to hypertension.

The next largest group of infants with hypertension are those who have congenital renal parenchymal abnormalities. It is well known that both autosomal dominant and autosomal recessive polycystic kidney disease (PKD) may present in the newborn period with severe nephromegaly and hypertension *(35–37)*. With recessive PKD (Fig. 2), the majority of affected infants will be discovered to be hypertensive during the first year of life, and presentation in the first month of life is common *(35,36)*. The most severely affected infants with recessive PKD are at risk for development of congestive heart failure due to severe, malignant hypertension. Although much less common than in PKD, hypertension has also

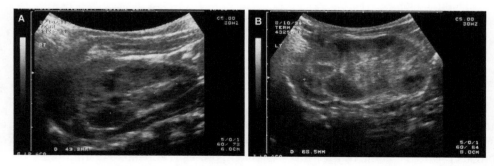

Fig. 1. Renal venous thrombosis. (**a**) Renal ultrasound demonstrating normal right kidney. (**b**) Renal ultrasound demonstrating affected left kidney. The kidney is enlarged and swollen, with loss of normal corticomedullary differentiation.

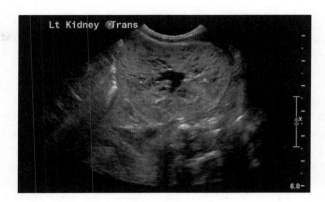

Fig. 2. Transverse ultrasound image demonstrating increased echogenicity, loss of corticomedullary differentiation, and medullary microcyst formation classic of autosomal recessive polycystic kidney disease.

been reported in infants with unilateral multicystic-dysplastic kidneys *(6,38–40)*. This is somewhat paradoxical, as such kidneys are usually thought to be non-functioning. In fact, the case has been made that hypertension in such patients is the result of another coexisting urologic abnormality such as parenchymal scarring *(41)*. Another recently described cause of severe neonatal hypertension related to dysplasia is unilateral tubular dysgenesis *(42)*.

Renal obstruction may be accompanied by hypertension, even in the absence of renal arterial compression. This has been seen, for example, in infants with congenital uretero-pelvic junction obstruction *(6,8,9,43)* and sometimes may persist following surgical correction of the obstruction *(44)*. Hypertension has also been described in babies with congenital primary megaureter *(45)*. Ureteral obstruction by other intra-abdominal masses may also be accompanied by hypertension. The mechanism of hypertension in such instances is unclear, although the renin–angiotensin system has been implicated *(46,47)*. Finally, unilateral renal hypoplasia may also present with hypertension *(48)*, although this is uncommon. The importance of congenital urologic malformations as a cause of neonatal hypertension was recently highlighted in a referral series from Brazil *(43)*. In that series, 13/15 infants with hypertension had urologic causes. Median age at diagnosis of hypertension was 20 days (range 5–70 days), emphasizing the need for regular BP measurement in infants with urologic malformations in order to detect hypertension *(49)*.

Hypertension due to acquired renal parenchymal disease is less common than that due to congenital renal abnormalities. However, severe ATN, interstitial nephritis, or cortical necrosis may be accompanied by significant hypertension *(6,8)* usually on the basis of volume overload or presumed activation of the renin–angiotensin system. Hemolytic uremic syndrome, which has been described in both term and preterm infants *(50)*, is usually also accompanied by hypertension. Such hypertension may be extremely difficult to control, requiring treatment with multiple agents.

Hypertension as a consequence of bronchopulmonary dysplasia (BPD) was first described in the mid-1980s by Abman and colleagues *(51)*. In a study of 65 infants discharged from a neonatal intensive care unit, the instance of hypertension in infants with BPD was 43% vs. an incidence of 4.5% in infants without BPD. Investigators were unable to identify a clear cause of hypertension, but postulated that hypoxemia might be involved. Over half of the infants with BPD who developed hypertension did not display it until after discharge from the NICU, highlighting the need for measurement of blood pressure in NICU "graduates," whether or not they have lung disease *(9,49)*.

Abman's findings have been reproduced by other investigators, most recently in 1998 by Alagappan *(52)*, who found that hypertension was twice as common in very low birth weight infants with BPD compared to the incidence in all very low birth weight infants. Since all of the hypertensive infants required supplemental oxygen and aminophylline, development of hypertension appeared to be correlated with the severity of pulmonary disease. Anderson and colleagues have demonstrated that the more severe the bronchopulmonary dysplasia, the higher the likelihood of the development of increased blood pressure *(53)*. Severity was defined as a greater need for diuretics (91% of the hypertensive group vs. 55% of the normotensive group, $p<0.05$) and bronchodilators (91% of the hypertensive group vs. 37% of the normotensive group, $p<0.001$).

Although updated studies are needed, these observations reinforce the impression that infants with severe BPD are clearly at increased risk and need close monitoring for the development of hypertension. This is especially true in infants who require ongoing treatment with theophylline preparations and/or corticosteroids.

Hypertension may also be seen in disorders of several other organ systems. Coarctation of the thoracic aorta is easily detected in the newborn period and has been reported in numerous case series of neonatal hypertension. Hypertension may persist in these infants even after surgical repair of the coarctation. Repair early in infancy seems to lead to an improved long-term outcome compared to delayed repair *(54)*. Endocrine disorders, particularly congenital adrenal hyperplasia, hyperaldosteronism, and hyperthyroidism, constitute easily recognizable clinical entities that have been reported to cause hypertension in neonates *(55–58)*. Similarly, pseudohypoaldosteronism type II (Gordon syndrome) should be suspected in the hypertensive infant with hyperkalemia and metabolic acidosis. The interested reader should consult Chapter 6 for a full discussion of Gordon syndrome and other monogenic forms of hypertension, some of which may present in infancy.

Iatrogenic causes of hypertension comprise another important category of diagnoses. Medications commonly administered to infants for the treatment of pulmonary disease such as dexamethasone and aminophylline have clearly been shown to elevate blood pressure *(59–61)*. The risks of dexamethasone-induced hypertension have been clearly illustrated in a multicenter study conducted by the Neonatal Research Network *(61)*. In this study of 220 very low birth weight infants (birth weight 501–1000 g) randomized to receive either dexamethasone or placebo because of the need for mechanical ventilation, the incidence of systolic BP >90 mmHg was significantly higher in the dexamethasone group ($p=0.01$ compared to placebo), as was the likelihood of being treated for hypertension ($p=0.04$).

In addition, high doses of adrenergic agents, prolonged use of pancuronium, or administration of phenylephrine ophthalmic drops *(62)* may raise blood pressure. Erythropoietin therapy has also been implicated in the development of neonatal hypertension *(63)*. Hypertension in these infants typically resolves when the offending agent is discontinued or its dose reduced. For infants receiving prolonged parenteral nutrition (TPN), hypertension may result from salt and water overload, or from hypercalcemia, caused either directly by excessive calcium intake or indirectly by vitamin A or D intoxication.

Substances ingested during pregnancy may also lead to significant problems with hypertension in the neonate. In particular, maternal cocaine use may have a number of undesirable effects on the developing kidney that may lead to hypertension *(64)*. Hypertension has also been reported to occur in infants of drug-addicted mothers withdrawing from heroin.

Tumors, including neuroblastoma, Wilms tumor, and mesoblastic nephroma, may all present in the neonatal period and may produce hypertension, either because of compression of the renal vessels or ureters or because of production of vasoactive substances such as renin or catecholamines (9,65–69). Neurologic problems such as seizures, intracranial hypertension, and pain constitute fairly common causes of episodic hypertension. In the typical modern NICU, postoperative pain must not be overlooked as a cause of hypertension. Provision of adequate analgesia may constitute the only required "antihypertensive medication" in such infants.

There are numerous other miscellaneous causes of hypertension in neonates (Table 1). Of these, hypertension associated with extracorporeal membrane oxygenation (ECMO) deserves comment. This may be seen in up to 50–90% of infants requiring ECMO (70–72) and may result in serious complications, including intracranial hemorrhage (73) and increased mortality (71). Multiple antihypertensive medications may be needed to achieve blood pressure control (72). Despite extensive investigation, the exact pathogenesis of this form of hypertension remains poorly understood. Fluid overload, altered handling of sodium and water, activation of the renin–angiotensin system, and derangements in atrial baroreceptor function have all been proposed as causative factors (72). Given the widespread and increasing use of ECMO both in neonates and in older children, further investigation of this problem is clearly needed.

DEFINITION OF HYPERTENSION

Establishing a definition for hypertension in neonates is difficult due to the rapid changes in blood pressure in the immediate postnatal period and is even more difficult in preterm neonates due to similar issues. Just as blood pressure in older children has been demonstrated to increase with increasing age and body size, studies in both term and preterm infants have demonstrated that blood pressure in neonates increases with both gestational and postconceptual age, as well as with birth weight (73–79). Additionally, blood pressure increases over the first few days of life (80,81), gradually stabilizing by about 5 days of age. Updated normative data for blood pressure in term infants over the first few days of life have recently been published (81).

Extremely useful data describing the various influences on neonatal blood pressure have been published by Zubrow and associates (78), who prospectively obtained serial blood pressure measurements from 695 infants admitted to several NICUs in a large metropolitan area over a period of 3 months. They then defined the mean blood pressures and upper and lower 95% confidence limits for the infants studied. Their data clearly demonstrated that blood pressure increases with increasing gestational age, birthweight, and postconceptual age (Figs. 3, 4, and 5). Since the diagnosis of hypertension in older children is based upon identifying those with blood pressures at the upper end of the distribution (i.e., above the 95th percentile), an approach to identifying hypertension in neonates would be to consider an infant's blood pressure to be elevated if it consistently was above the upper 95% confidence interval for infants of similar gestational or postconceptual age.

For older infants (1–12 months of age) found to be hypertensive following discharge from the NICU or for ongoing follow-up of persistently hypertensive neonates, the percentile curves published in the Second Task Force report (Fig. 6) (82) remain the only available reference data. Based on serial blood pressure measurements obtained from nearly 13,000 infants, these curves allow blood pressure to be characterized as normal or elevated not only by age and gender but also by size, albeit to a somewhat limited extent.

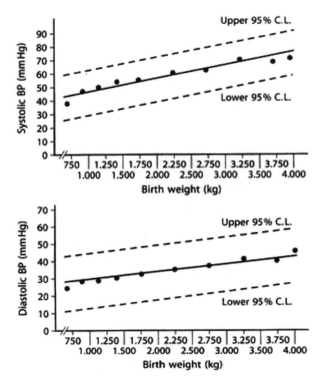

Fig. 3. Linear regression of mean systolic (**a**) and diastolic (**b**) blood pressures by birth weight on day 1 of life, with 95% confidence limits (*upper* and *lower dashed lines*). Reprinted with permission from Macmillan Publishers *(78)*, copyright 1995.

Hypertension in this age group would be defined as blood pressure elevation above the 95th percentile for infants of similar age, size, and gender. Updated normative blood pressure data for this age group are urgently needed and may perhaps be generated by the National Children's Study currently underway in the United States.

BLOOD PRESSURE MEASUREMENT

As in older children, it is crucial that blood pressure is being measured accurately so that hypertensive infants will be correctly identified. Fortunately, in most acutely ill neonates, blood pressure is usually monitored directly via an indwelling arterial catheter either in the radial or in the umbilical artery. This method provides the most accurate BP readings and is clearly preferable to other methods *(83)*. In addition to accurately measuring blood pressures, such catheters are also crucial in careful management of hypertension, particularly in infants with extremely severe blood pressure elevation. This will be discussed in more detail later in the chapter.

Automated, oscillometric devices are the most common alternative method of blood pressure measurement in most NICUs. Although accurate, readings obtained by such devices may differ significantly from intra-arterial readings. When comparing blood pressures obtained from 31 newborns with these two techniques, Low et al. *(84)* reported that the average oscillometric pressures were significantly lower than the intra-arterial

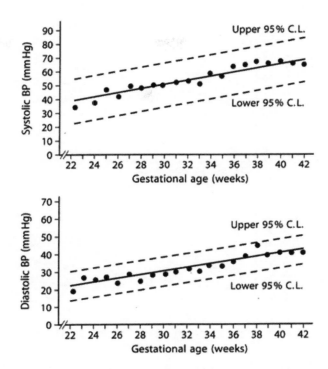

Fig. 4. Linear regression of mean systolic (**a**) and diastolic (**b**) blood pressures by gestational age on day 1 of life, with 95% confidence limits (*upper* and *lower dashed lines*). Reprinted with permission from Macmillan Publishers *(78)*, copyright 1995.

pressures. The systolic was lower by 1 mmHg, the mean by 5.3 mmHg, and the diastolic by 4.6 mmHg. These differences may need to be taken into account when determining whether an infant's blood pressure is normal or elevated.

Despite the fact that blood pressure readings obtained by oscillometric devices may differ slightly from intra-arterial BP measurements, they are easy to use and provide the ability to follow blood pressure trends over time. They are especially useful for infants who require BP monitoring after discharge from the NICU *(85)*. When using such devices, however, attention should be paid to using a properly sized cuff and also to the extremity used. Most normative blood pressure data, not only in infants but also in older children, have been collected using blood pressures obtained in the right arm *(82)*. Since blood pressures obtained in the leg may be higher than those obtained in the arm *(6–87)*, the use of other extremities for routine blood pressure determination may complicate the evaluation of hypertension. Nursing staff should document the extremity used for blood pressure determinations and try to use the same extremity for subsequent determinations if possible. Finally, the infant's state of activity may also affect the accuracy of BP readings. Increased activity, including oral feeding, increases blood pressure *(88)*. It may therefore be important to obtain BP readings while infants are sleeping in order to obtain the most accurate readings.

These issues have been highlighted in a study by Nwanko et al. of blood pressure in low birth weight term and preterm infants *(89)*. It was demonstrated that blood pressure was significantly lower in the prone than supine position and that the first reading was significantly higher than the third. Nwanko et al. concluded that a standardized protocol

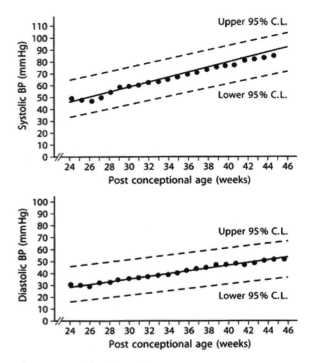

Fig. 5. Linear regression of mean systolic (**a**) and diastolic (**b**) blood pressures by postconceptual age in weeks, with 95% confidence limits (*upper* and *lower dashed lines*). Reprinted with permission from Macmillan Publishers *(78)*, copyright 1995.

is necessary in order to accurately measure BP in neonates. They recommended checking blood pressures 1.5 h after the last feeding or intervention, applying an appropriately sized cuff (two-thirds the length of the limb segment and 75% of the limb circumference), waiting 15 more minutes for stillness, then obtaining three successive readings at 2-min intervals. Using proper technique, it should be possible to correctly identify infants with hypertension requiring further evaluation.

DIAGNOSTIC EVALUATION

Diagnosing the etiology of hypertension is a straightforward task in most hypertensive neonates. A relatively focused history should be obtained, paying attention to determining whether there were any pertinent prenatal exposures, as well as to the particulars of the infant's nursery course and any concurrent conditions. The procedures that the infant has undergone (e.g., umbilical catheter placement) should be reviewed, and the current medication list should be scrutinized.

The physical examination, likewise, should be focused on obtaining pertinent information to assist in narrowing the differential diagnosis. Blood pressure readings should be obtained in all four extremities in order to rule out coarctation of the thoracic aorta. The general appearance of the infant should be assessed, with particular attention paid to the presence of dysmorphic features that may indicate an obvious diagnosis such as congenital adrenal hyperplasia. Careful cardiac and abdominal examination should be performed. The

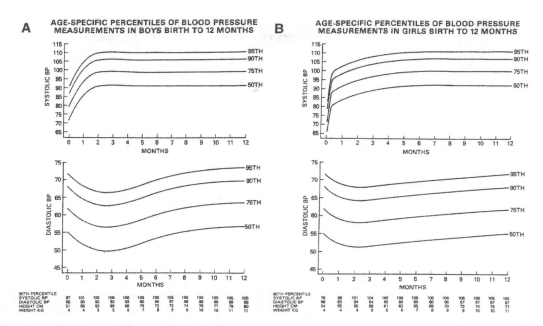

Fig. 6. Age-specific percentiles for blood pressure in boys (**a**) and girls (**b**) from birth to 12 months of age. Reprinted from Task Force on Blood Pressure Control in Children *(82)*, National Heart, Lung and Blood Institutes, National Institutes of Health, Bethesda, MD.

presence of a flank mass or of an epigastric bruit may point the clinician toward diagnosis of either ureteropelvic junction obstruction or renal artery stenosis, respectively.

In most instances, few laboratory data are needed in the evaluation of neonatal hypertension, as the correct diagnosis is usually suggested by the history and physical examination. It is important to assess renal function, as well as to examine a specimen of the urine in order to ascertain the presence of renal parenchymal disease. Chest X-ray may be useful as an adjunctive test in infants with congestive heart failure or in those with a murmur on physical examination. Other diagnostic studies, such as cortisol, aldosterone, or thyroxine levels, should be obtained when there is history suggesting endocrine hypertension (Table 2).

Determination of plasma renin activity is frequently recommended in the assessment of neonates with hypertension, although there are few data on what constitutes normal values for infants, particularly for premature infants. Available data indicate that renin values are typically quite high in infancy, at least in term newborns *(90,91)*. Although renal artery stenosis and thromboembolic phenomenon are typically considered high-renin forms of hypertension, a peripheral renin level may not be elevated in such infants despite the presence of significant underlying pathology. Conversely, plasma renin may be falsely elevated by medications that are commonly used in the NICU, such as aminophylline *(92)*. At the other end of the spectrum, plasma renin activity will be profoundly suppressed in some genetic forms of hypertension (see Chapter 6). With proper interpretation, assessment of plasma renin activity may be helpful in the evaluation of some infants and is therefore usually included as part of the initial laboratory evaluation.

The role of various imaging modalities in the evaluation of neonatal hypertension has been reviewed in detail elsewhere *(93)*, so only a few comments will be made here.

Table 2
Diagnostic Testing in Neonatal Hypertension

Generally useful	Useful in selected infants
Urinalysis (and/or culture)	Thyroid studies
CBC and platelet count	Urine VMA/HVA
Electrolytes	Aldosterone
BUN, creatinine	Cortisol
Calcium	Echocardiogram
Plasma renin	Abdominal/pelvic
Chest X-ray	ultrasound
Renal ultrasound with Doppler	VCUG
	Aortography and/or renal
	arteriography
	Nuclear scan
	(DTPA/Mag-3)

Ultrasound imaging of the genitourinary tract is a relatively inexpensive, noninvasive, and quick study that should be obtained in all hypertensive infants. An accurate renal ultrasound can help uncover potentially correctable causes of hypertension such as renal venous thrombosis *(24)*, may detect aortic and/or renal arterial thrombi *(14)*, and can identify anatomic renal abnormalities or other congenital renal diseases. Doppler evaluation should be added, especially in acutely hypertensive infants, primarily to identify absent venous flow, which is diagnostic of renal venous thrombosis. For these reasons, ultrasound has largely replaced intravenous pyelography, which has little if any use in the routine assessment of neonatal hypertension.

For infants with extremely severe blood pressure elevation, angiography may be necessary. A formal angiogram utilizing the traditional femoral venous approach offers the most accurate method of diagnosing renal arterial stenosis, particularly given the high incidence of intrarenal branch vessel disease in children with fibromuscular dysplasia *(27,28)*. Even though there have been significant advances in both computed tomographic and magnetic resonance angiography, these techniques still cannot provide detailed images of branch vessels in infants and young children *(28,29)*. In extremely small infants, or where appropriate facilities are not available, it may be necessary to defer angiography, managing the hypertension medically until the baby is large enough for an angiogram to be performed safely.

Although nuclear scanning has been shown in some studies to demonstrate abnormalities of renal perfusion caused by thromboembolic phenomenon, in our practice it has had little role in the assessment of infants with hypertension, primarily due to the difficulties in obtaining accurate, interpretable results in this age group. In proper hands, it may be useful as an adjunctive study in the evaluation of infants with suspected renovascular hypertension *(93)*. Other imaging studies, including echocardiograms and voiding cystourethrograms, should be obtained as clinically indicated.

TREATMENT

With a few exceptions (for example, congestive heart failure) generally accepted indications for treatment of hypertensive neonates have not been established. It is therefore up to the individual clinician to decide which infants should receive antihypertensive medications. Although long-term follow-up data of untreated hypertensive infants are not available, it is reasonable to assume that as in older children, long-standing hypertension in the neonate may cause left ventricular hypertrophy or other target organ damage. Therefore, consideration should be given to treatment of any infant with sustained hypertension (as defined above).

Although today's clinician has available an ever-expanding list of agents that can be used for treatment of neonatal hypertension (Table 3), practically none of these medications have been systematically studied in neonates, and there are no antihypertensive medications with FDA-approved indications for use in hypertensive infants. It is unfortunate that infants remain excluded from the clinical trials of antihypertensive agents that have been conducted in children under the auspices of the 1997 Food and Drug Administration Modernization Act *(94)*. Physicians who care for hypertensive neonates must therefore rely upon case series data, older clinical trials, and personal experience for guidance in selecting the appropriate agent for a particular neonate.

Prior to initiating antihypertensive drug therapy, however, the infant's clinical status should be assessed and any easily correctable iatrogenic causes of hypertension addressed. These may include infusions of inotropic agents or administration of other medications known to elevate blood pressure, volume overload, or pain. Following this, an antihypertensive agent should be chosen that is not only appropriate for the specific clinical situation but also directed to the pathophysiology of the infant's hypertension whenever possible.

For the majority of acutely ill infants, particularly those with severe hypertension, continuous intravenous infusions are the most appropriate approach. The advantage of intravenous infusions are numerous, most importantly including the ability to quickly increase or decrease the rate of infusion to achieve the desired level of blood pressure control. Infusions may also allow the infant's blood pressure to be kept within a relatively narrow range. This stands in stark contrast to the wide fluctuations in blood pressure frequently seen when intermittently administered intravenous agents are utilized. As in patients of any age with malignant hypertension, care should be taken to avoid too rapid a reduction in blood pressure *(95)* in order to avoid cerebral ischemia and hemorrhage, a problem that premature infants in particular are already at increased risk for due to the immaturity of their periventricular circulation. Here again, continuous infusions of intravenous antihypertensives offer a distinct advantage over intermittently administered agents.

Although comprised of single-center, retrospective studies, a growing body of literature suggests that the intravenous calcium channel antagonist nicardipine is appropriate for use as a first-line agent in severely hypertensive infants *(96–98)*. This drug offers the advantage of quick onset of action, which allows the patient's blood pressure to be easily titrated to and maintained at the desired level *(99)*. It may also be continued for prolonged periods of time without apparent decrease in antihypertensive efficacy *(98)*. Other intravenous antihypertensives that have been successfully used in neonates include esmolol *(100)*, labetalol, and nitroprusside *(101)*. Whatever agent is used, blood pressure should be monitored continuously via an indwelling arterial catheter or else by frequently repeated (Q10–15 min) cuff readings so that the dose can be titrated to achieve the desired degree of blood pressure control.

For some infants, intermittently administered intravenous agents do have a role in therapy. Hydralazine and labetalol in particular may be useful in infants with mild-to-moderate hypertension that are not yet candidates for oral therapy because of gastrointestinal dysfunction. Enalaprilat, the intravenous angiotensin-converting enzyme

Table 3
Recommended Doses for Selected Antihypertensive Agents for Treatment of Hypertensive Infants

Class	Drug	Route	Dose	Interval	Comments
ACE inhibitors	Captopril	Oral	<3months: 0.01–0.5 mg/kg/dose Max 2 mg/kg/day >3months: 0.15–0.3 mg/kg/dose Max 6 mg/kg/day	TID	1. First dose may cause rapid drop in BP, especially if receiving diuretics 2. Monitor serum creatinine and K^+ 3. Intravenous enalaprilat *not* recommended—see text
	Enalapril	Oral	0.08–0.6 mg/kg/day	QD–BID	
	Lisinopril	Oral	0.07–0.6 mg/kg/day	QD	
α- and β-antagonists	Labetalol	Oral	0.5–1.0 mg/kg/dose Max 10 mg/kg/day	BID–TID	Heart failure, BPD relative contraindications
		IV	0.20–1.0 mg/kg/dose 0.25–3.0 mg/kg/h	Q4–6 h Infusion	
	Carvedilol	Oral	0.1 mg/kg/dose up to 0.5 mg/kg/dose	BID	May be useful in heart failure
β-Antagonists	Esmolol	IV	100–500 mcg/kg/min	Infusion	Very short-acting—constant infusion necessary
	Propranolol	Oral	0.5–1.0 mg/kg/dose Max 8–10 mg/kg/day	TID	Monitor heart rate; avoid in BPD
Calcium channel blockers	Amlodipine	Oral	0.05–0.3 mg/kg/dose Max 0.6 mg/kg/day	QD	All may cause mild reflex tachycardia
	Isradipine	Oral	0.05–0.15 mg/kg/dose Max 0.8 mg/kg/day	QID	
	Nicardipine	IV	1–4 mcg/kg/min	Infusion	

Table 3
(continued)

Class	Drug	Route	Dose	Interval	Comments
Central α-agonist	Clonidine	Oral	5–10 mcg/kg/day Max 25 mcg/kg/day	TID	May cause mild sedation
Diuretics	Chlorothiazide	Oral	5–15 mg/kg/dose	BID	Monitor electrolytes
	Hydrochlorothiazide	Oral	1–3 mg/kg/dose	QD	
	Spironolactone	Oral	0.5–1.5 mg/kg/dose	BID	
Vasodilators	Hydralazine	Oral	0.25–1.0 mg/kg/dose Max 7.5 mg/kg/day	TID–QID	Tachycardia and fluid retention are common side effects
		IV	0.15– 0.6 mg/kg/dose	Q4h	
	Minoxidil	Oral	0.1–0.2 mg/kg/dose	BID–TID	Tachycardia and fluid retention common side effects; prolonged use causes hypertrichosis
	Sodium nitroprusside	IV	0.5–10 mcg/kg/min	Infusion	Thiocyanate toxicity can occur with prolonged (>72 h) use or in renal failure

Abbreviations: BID, twice daily; BPD, bronchopulmonary dysplasia; IV, intravenous; QD, once daily; QID, four times daily; TID, three times daily.

inhibitor, has also been reported to be useful in the treatment of neonatal renovascular hypertension *(102,103)*, despite the lack of an established safe and effective pediatric (let alone neonatal) dose. However, in our experience, this agent should be used with extreme caution, if at all. Even doses at the lower end of published ranges may lead to significant, prolonged hypotension and oliguric acute renal failure in neonates.

Oral antihypertensive agents (Table 3) are best reserved for infants with less severe hypertension or infants whose acute hypertension has been controlled with intravenous infusions and are ready to be transitioned to chronic therapy. Again, no guidelines exist to help choose what agents are appropriate for use in neonates. At least one recent report indicates that ACE inhibitors and calcium channel blockers are common choices in infants requiring oral antihypertensive therapy *(43)*. A recent analysis of a large administrative database of NICU encounters from 36 children's hospitals in the United States indicated that hypertensive neonates are exposed to multiple antihypertensive agents, with direct vasodilators, ACE inhibitors, and calcium channel blockers among the most commonly used classes of agents (D. Blowey MD, Pediatric Academic Societies meeting, Washington, DC, May 14, 2005).

Captopril in particular is a useful agent for many causes of neonatal hypertension *(104,105)* and is commonly used in many NICUs despite the concerns of some pediatric nephrologists about the long-term effects of ACE inhibitors on renal maturation in premature infants. Based on this concern, at our center, captopril is typically avoided until the preterm infant has reached a corrected postconceptual age of 44 weeks. If captopril is chosen, the starting dose should be extremely low, especially in premature infants, as they may have an exaggerated fall in blood pressure following captopril administration. Adverse neurologic effects have been described in infants following captopril-related hypotension *(105)*, highlighting the need for close blood pressure monitoring after administration of this agent. Other ACE inhibitors (enalapril, lisinopril, etc.) have no doubt been used in neonates, but there are no published data on safe and effective doses.

When a vasodilator is indicated, the second-generation calcium channel blocker isradipine may be superior to the older agents hydralazine and minoxidil since it can be compounded into a stable suspension *(106)* that can be dosed with accuracy, even in tiny infants *(107)*. Use of short-acting nifedipine is no longer recommended because of the difficulty in administering small doses and because of the rapid, profound, and short-lived blood pressure reduction typically produced by this agent *(108)*. The third-generation calcium channel blocker amlodipine may also be useful for long-term management of neonatal hypertension. Like isradipine, it may be compounded into a stable suspension and can therefore be dosed accurately, even in small infants *(99)*.

If either an ACE inhibitor such as captopril or a vasodilator is chosen as the initial agent and if the infant's blood pressure is unable to be controlled by that agent alone, the addition of a diuretic will frequently result in the desired degree of blood pressure control. Beta-blockers may need to be avoided in chronic therapy of neonatal hypertension, particularly in infants with chronic lung disease. In such infants, diuretics may have a beneficial effect not only in controlling blood pressure but also in improving pulmonary function *(109)*. Interestingly, we have observed numerous infants with chronic lung disease over the years who "suddenly" became hypertensive after the withdrawal of chronic diuretic therapy. Although this observation is based on anecdotal experience, one could speculate that these infants had chronic lung disease-associated hypertension all along that was being "masked" by the diuretics being prescribed for their lung disease.

Surgery is indicated for treatment of neonatal hypertension in a limited set of circumstances *(110)*. In particular, hypertension caused by ureteral obstruction or aortic coarctation is best approached surgically. For infants with renal arterial stenosis, it may be necessary to manage the infant medically until it has grown sufficiently to undergo definitive repair of the vascular abnormalities *(111)*. However, unilateral nephrectomy may be needed in rare cases *(112)*. Infants with hypertension secondary to Wilms tumor or neuroblastoma will require surgical tumor removal, possibly following chemotherapy. A case has also been made by some authors for removal of multicystic-dysplastic kidneys because of the risk of development of hypertension *(38–40)*, although this is controversial *(41)*. Infants with malignant hypertension secondary to polycystic kidney disease may require bilateral nephrectomy. Fortunately, such severely affected infants are quite rare.

LONG-TERM OUTCOME

Few studies examining the long-term outcome of neonatal hypertension have been published. Fortunately, some data are available for the largest category of hypertensive infants, namely those with hypertension related to an umbilical arterial catheter *(113,114)*. Although better data are needed, available information and personal experience suggest that in such babies, hypertension will usually resolve over time. Some of these infants may require increases in their antihypertensive medications in the first several months following discharge from the nursery as they undergo rapid growth. Following this, it is usually possible to "wean" their antihypertensives by making no further dose increases as the infant continues to grow, followed by later discontinuation of treatment. Home blood pressure monitoring by the parents is a crucially important component of this process. Home blood pressure equipment, usually an oscillometric device, should be arranged for all infants discharged from the NICU on antihypertensive medications, and home blood pressure data should be used in guiding continuation or discontinuation of antihypertensive medications.

Some forms of neonatal hypertension may persist beyond infancy. In particular, PKD and other forms of renal parenchymal disease may continue to cause hypertension throughout childhood *(35–37,115)*. Infants with renal venous thrombosis may also remain hypertensive, and some of these children will ultimately benefit from removal of the affected kidney *(24,25)*. Persistent or late/"recurrent" hypertension may also be seen in children who have undergone repair of renal artery stenosis or thoracic aortic coarctation. Reappearance of hypertension in these situations should prompt a search for restenosis by the appropriate imaging studies.

What are sorely needed at this point are true long-term outcome studies of infants with neonatal hypertension. Since many of these infants are delivered prior to the completion of nephron development, it is possible that they may not develop the full complement of glomeruli normally seen in term infants. Reduced nephron mass has been hypothesized to be a risk factor for the development of hypertension in adulthood *(116,117)*. Thus, it may be possible that hypertensive neonates (and possibly also normotensive premature neonates) are at increased risk compared to term infants for the development of hypertension in late adolescence or early adulthood. Since we are now entering the era in which the first significantly premature NICU "graduates" are reaching their second and third decades of life, it is possible that appropriate studies can be conducted to address this question.

CONCLUSIONS

Blood pressure in neonates depends on a variety of factors, including gestational age, postnatal age, and birth weight. Hypertension can be seen in a variety of situations in the modern NICU and is especially common in infants who have undergone umbilical arterial catheterization or who have chronic lung disease. A careful diagnostic evaluation should lead to determination of the underlying cause of hypertension in most infants. Treatment decisions should be tailored to the severity of the hypertension and may include intravenous and/or oral therapy. Hypertension will resolve in most infants over time, although a small number may have persistent blood pressure elevation throughout childhood. Further study is needed to obtain better normative data on blood pressure in infancy and to define the long-term outcome of hypertensive neonates.

REFERENCES

1. Adelman RD. Neonatal hypertension. Pediatr Clin North Am. 1978;25:99–110.
2. Al-Aweel I, Pursley DM, Rubin LP, Shah B, Weisberger S, Richardson DK. Variations in prevalence of hypotension, hypertension and vasopressor use in NICUs. J Perinatol. 2001;12:272–278.
3. Watkinson M. Hypertension in the newborn baby. Arch Dis Child Fetal Neonatal Ed. 2002;86:F78–F81.
4. American Academy of Pediatrics Committee on Fetus and Newborn. Routine evaluation of blood pressure, hematocrit and glucose in newborns. Pediatrics. 1993;92:474–476.
5. Inglefinger JR. Hypertension in the first year of life. In: Inglefinger JR, ed. Pediatric Hypertension. Philadelphia, PA: W.B. Saunders; 1982:229–240.
6. Buchi KF, Siegler RL. Hypertension in the first month of life. J Hypertens. 1986;4:525–528.
7. Skalina MEL, Kliegman RM, Fanaroff AA. Epidemiology and management of severe symptomatic neonatal hypertension. Am J Perinatol. 1986;3:235–239.
8. Singh HP, Hurley RM, Myers TF. Neonatal hypertension: incidence and risk factors. Am J Hypertens. 1992;5:51–55.
9. Seliem WA, Falk MC, Shadbolt B, Kent AL. Antenatal and postnatal risk factors for neonatal hypertension and infant follow-up. Pediatr Nephrol. 2007;22:2081–2087.
10. Friedman AL, Hustead VA. Hypertension in babies following discharge from a neonatal intensive care unit. Pediatr Nephrol. 1987;1:30–34.
11. Dgani J, Arad I. Measurement of systolic blood pressure in the follow-up of low birth weight infants. J Perinat Med. 1992;20:365–370.
12. Schell-Feith EA, Kist-van Holthe JE, van Zwieten PH, Zonderland HM, Holscher HC, Swinkels DW, Brand R, Berger HM, van der Heijden BJ. Preterm neonates with nephrocalcinosis: natural course and renal function. Pediatr Nephrol. 2003;18:1102–1108.
13. Neal WA, Reynolds JW, Jarvis CW, Williams HJ. Umbilical artery catheterization: demonstration of arterial thrombosis by aortography. Pediatrics. 1972;50:6–13.
14. Seibert JJ, Taylor BJ, Williamson SL, Williams BJ, Szabo JS, Corbitt SL. Sonographic detection of neonatal umbilical-artery thrombosis: clinical correlation. Am J Roentgenol. 1987;148:965–968.
15. Ford KT, Teplick SK, Clark RE. Renal artery embolism causing neonatal hypertension. Radiology. 1974;113:169–170.
16. Bauer SB, Feldman SM, Gellis SS, Retik AB. Neonatal hypertension: a complication of umbilical-artery catheterization. N Engl J Med. 1975;293:1032–1033.
17. Plumer LB, Kaplan GW, Mendoza SA. Hypertension in infants—a complication of umbilical arterial catheterization. J Pediatr. 1976;89:802–805.
18. Merten DF, Vogel JM, Adelman RD, Goetzman, BW, Bogren HG. Renovascular hypertension as a complication of umbilical arterial catheterization. Radiology. 1978;126:751–757.
19. Brooks WG, Weibley RE. Emergency department presentation of severe hypertension secondary to complications of umbilical artery catheterization. Pediatr Emerg Care. 1987;3:104–106.
20. Goetzman BW, Stadalnik RC, Bogren HG, Balnkenship WJ, Ikeda RM, Thayer J. Thrombotic complications of umbilical artery catheters: a clinical and radiographic study. Pediatrics. 1975;56:374–379.
21. Wesström G, Finnström O, Stenport G. Umbilical artery catheterization in newborns. I. Thrombosis in relation to catheter type and position. Acta Paediatr Scand. 1979;68:575–581.

22. Durante D, Jones D, Spitzer R. Neonatal arterial embolism syndrome. J Pediatr. 1976;89:978–981.

23. Barrington KJ. Umbilical artery catheters in the newborn: effects of position of the catheter tip (review). Cochrane Database Syst Rev. 1999;1:CD000505. DOI: 10.1002/14651858.CD000505.

24. Evans DJ, Silverman M, Bowley NB. Congenital hypertension due to unilateral renal vein thrombosis. Arch Dis Child. 1981;56:306–308.

25. Mocan H, Beattie TJ, Murphy AV. Renal venous thrombosis in infancy: long-term follow-up. Pediatr Nephrol. 1991;5:45–49.

26. Kiessling SG, Wadhwa N, Kriss VM, Iocono J, Desai NS. An unusual case of severe therapy-resistant hypertension in a newborn. Pediatrics. 2007;119(1):e301–e304.

27. Deal JE, Snell MF, Barratt TM, Dillon MJ. Renovascular disease in childhood. J Pediatr. 1992;121: 378–384.

28. Vo NJ, Hammelman BD, Racadio JM, Strife CF, Johnson ND, Racadio JM. Anatomic distribution of renal artery stenosis in children: implications for imaging. Pediatr Radiol. 2006;36:1032–1036.

29. Tullus K, Brennan E, Hamilton G, Lord R, McLaren CA, Marks SD, Roebuck DJ. Renovascular hypertension in children. Lancet. 2008;371:1453–1463.

30. Sethna CB, Kaplan BS, Cahill AM, Velazquez OC, Meyers KE. Idiopathic mid-aortic syndrome in children. Pediatr Nephrol. 2008;23:1135–1142.

31. Milner LS, Heitner R, Thomson PD, Levin SE, Rothberg AD, Beale P, Ninin DT. Hypertension as the major problem of idiopathic arterial calcification of infancy. J Pediatr. 1984;105: 934–938.

32. Ciana G, Colonna F, Forleo V, Brizzi F, Benettoni A, de Vonderweid U. Idiopathic arterial calcification of infancy: effectiveness of prostaglandin infusion for treatment of secondary hypertension refractory to conventional therapy: case report. Pediatr Cardiol. 1997;18:67–71.

33. Dorman DC, Reye RDK, Reid RR. Renal-artery stenosis in the rubella syndrome. Lancet. 1966;1: 790–792.

34. Kim ES, Caitai JM, Tu J, Nowygrod R, Stolar CJ. Congenital abdominal aortic aneurysm causing renovascular hypertension, cardiomyopathy and death in a 19-day-old neonate. J Pediatr Surg. 2001;36: 1445–1449.

35. Zerres K, Rudnik-Schöneborn S, Deget F, Holtkamp U, Brodehl J, Geisert J, Schärer K. The Arbeitsgemeinschaft für Pädiatrische Nephrologie. Autosomal recessive polycystic kidney disease in 115 children: clinical presentation, course and influence of gender. Acta Paediatr. 1996;85:437–445.

36. Guay-Woodford LM, Desmond RA. Autosomal recessive polycystic kidney disease: the clinical experience in North America. Pediatrics. 2003;111:1072–1080.

37. Fick GM, Johnson AM, Strain JD, Kimberling WJ, Kumar S, Manco-Johnson ML, Duley IT, Gabow PA. Characteristics of very early onset autosomal dominant polycystic kidney disease. J Am Soc Nephrol. 1993;3:1863–1870.

38. Susskind MR, Kim KS, King LR. Hypertension and multicystic kidney. Urology. 1989;34:362–366.

39. Angermeier KW, Kay R, Levin H. Hypertension as a complication of multicystic dysplastic kidney. Urology. 1992;39:55–58.

40. Webb NJA, Lewis MA, Bruce J, Gough DCS, Ladusans EJ, Thomson APJ, Postlethwaite RJ. Unilateral multicystic dysplastic kidney: the case for nephrectomy. Arch Dis Child. 1997;76:31–34.

41. Husmann DA. Renal dysplasia: the risks and consequences of leaving dysplastic tissue in situ. Urology. 1998;52:533–536.

42. Delaney D, Kennedy SE, Tobias VH, Farnsworth RH. Congenital unilateral renal tubular dysgenesis and severe neonatal hypertension. Pediatr Nephrol. 2009;24:863–867.

43. Lanzarini VV, Furusawa EA, Sadeck L, Leone CR, Vaz FAC, Koch VH. Neonatal arterial hypertension in nephrourological malformations in a tertiary care hospital. J Hum Hypertens. 2006;20: 679–683.

44. Gilboa N, Urizar RE. Severe hypertension in newborn after pyeloplasty of hydronephrotic kidney. Urology. 1983;22:179–182.

45. Oliveira EA, Diniz JS, Rabelo EA, Silva JM, Pereira AK, Filgueiras MT, Soares FM, Sansoni RF. Primary megaureter detected by prenatal ultrasonography: conservative management and prolonged follow-up. Urol Nephrol. 2000;32:13–18.

46. Cadnapaphornchai P, Aisenbrey G, McDonald KM, Burke TJ, Schrier RW. Prostaglandin-mediated hyperemia and renin-mediated hypertension during acute ureteral obstruction. Prostaglandins. 1978;16: 965–971.

47. Riehle RA Jr, Vaughan ED Jr. Renin participation in hypertension associated with unilateral hydronephrosis. J Urol. 1981;126:243–246.

48. Tokunaka S, Osanai H, Hashimoto H, Takamura T, Yachiku S, Mori Y. Severe hypertension in infant with unilateral hypoplastic kidney. Urology. 1987;29:618–620.

49. National High Blood Pressure Education Program Working Group on High Blood Pressure in Children and Adolescents. The fourth report on the diagnosis, evaluation, and treatment of high blood pressure in children and adolescents. Pediatrics. 2004;114:555–576.

50. Wilson BJ, Flynn JT. Familial, atypical hemolytic uremic syndrome in a premature infant. Pediatr Nephrol. 1998;12:782–784.

51. Abman SH, Warady BA, Lum GM, Koops BL. Systemic hypertension in infants with bronchopulmonary dysplasia. J Pediatr. 1984;104:929–931.

52. Alagappan A. Malloy MH. Systemic hypertension in very low-birth weight infants with bronchopulmonary dysplasia: incidence and risk factors. Am J Perinatol. 1998;15:3–8.

53. Anderson AH, Warady BA, Daily DK, Johnson JA, Thomas MK. Systemic hypertension in infants with severe bronchopulmonary dysplasia: associated clinical factors. Am J Perinatol. 1993;10: 190–193.

54. Beekman RH. Coarctation of the aorta. In: Emmanouilides GC, Riemenschneider TA, Allen HD, Gutgesell HP, eds. Moss and Adams' Heart Disease in Infants, Children and Adolescents: Including the Fetus and Young Adult, 5th ed. Baltimore, MD: Williams and Wilkins; 1995:1111–1133.

55. Mimouni M, Kaufman H, Roitman A, Moraq C, Sadan N. Hypertension in a neonate with 11 beta-hydroxylase deficiency. Eur J Pediatr. 1985;143:231–233.

56. White PC. Inherited forms of mineralocorticoid hypertension. Hypertension. 1996;28:927–936.

57. Pozzan GB, Armanini D, Cecchetto G, Opocher G, Rigon F, Fassina A, Zacchello F. Hypertensive cardiomegaly caused by an aldosterone-secreting adenoma in a newborn. J Endocrinol Invest. 1997;20: 86–89.

58. Schonwetter BS, Libber SM, Jones D Jr, Park KJ, Plotnick LP. Hypertension in neonatal hyperthyroidism. Am J Dis Child. 1983;137:954–955.

59. Greenough A, Emery EF, Gamsu HR. Dexamethasone and hypertension in preterm infants. Eur J Pediatr. 1992;151:134–135.

60. Smets K, Vanhaesebrouck P. Dexamethasone associated systemic hypertension in low birth weight babies with chronic lung disease. Eur J Pediatr. 1996;155:573–575.

61. Stark AR, Carlo WA, Tyson JE, Papile L-A, Wright LL, Shankaran S, Donovan EF, Oh W, Bauer CR, Saha S, Poole WK, Stoll BJ. Adverse effects of early dexamethasone treatment in extremely-low-birth-weight infants. N Engl J Med. 2001;344:95–101.

62. Greher M, Hartmann T, Winkler M, Zimpfer M, Crabnor CM. Hypertension and pulmonary edema associated with subconjunctival phenylephrine in a 2-month old child during cataract extraction. Anesthesiology. 1998;88:1394–1396.

63. Chen JM, Jeng MJ, Chiu SY, Lee YS, Soong WJ, Hwang B, Tang RB. Conditions associated with hypertension in a high-risk premature infant. J Chin Med Assoc. 2008;71:485–490.

64. Horn PT. Persistent hypertension after prenatal cocaine exposure. J Pediatr. 1992;121:288–291.

65. Weinblatt ME, Heisel MA, Siegel SE. Hypertension in children with neurogenic tumors. Pediatrics. 1983;71:947–951.

66. Malone PS, Duffy PG, Ransley PG, Risdon RA, Cook T, Taylor M. Congenital mesoblastic nephroma, renin production, and hypertension. J Pediatr Surg. 1989;24:599–600.

67. Steinmetz JC. Neonatal hypertension and cardiomegaly associated with a congenital neuroblastoma. Pediatr Pathol. 1989;9:577–582.

68. Haberkern CM, Coles PG, Morray JP, Kennard SC, Sawin RS. Intraoperative hypertension during surgical excision of neuroblastoma: case report and review of 20 years' experience. Anesth Analg. 1992;75: 854–858.

69. Madre C, Orbach D, Baudouin V, Brisse H, Bessa F, Schleiermacher G, Pacquement H, Doz F, Michon J. Hypertension in childhood cancer: a frequent complication of certain tumor sites. J Pediatr Hematol Oncol. 2006;28:659–664.

70. Boedy RF, Goldberg AK, Howell CG Jr, Hulse E, Edwards EG, Kanto WP. Incidence of hypertension in infants on extracorporeal membrane oxygenation. J Pediatr Surg. 1990;25:258–261.

71. Becker JA, Short BL, Martin GR. Cardiovascular complications adversely affect survival during extracorporeal membrane oxygenation. Crit Care Med. 1998;26:1582–1586.

72. Heggen JA, Fortenberry JD, Tanner AJ, Reid CA, Mizzell DW, Pettignano R. Systemic hypertension associated with venovenous extracorporeal membrane oxygenation for pediatric respiratory failure. J Pediatr Surg. 2004;39:1626–1631.

73. Sell LL, Cullen ML, Lerner GR, Whittlesey GC, Shanley CJ, Klein MD. Hypertension during extracorporeal membrane oxygenation: cause, effect and management. Surgery. 1987;102: 724–730.

74. de Swiet M, Fayers P, Shinebourne EA. Systolic blood pressure in a population of infants in the first year of life: the Brompton study. Pediatrics. 1980;65:1028–1035.

75. Versmold HT, Kitterman JA, Phibbs RH, Gregory GA, Tooley WH. Aortic blood pressure during the first 12 hours of life in infants with birth weight 610 to 4220 grams. Pediatrics. 1981;67:607–613.

76. Tan KL. Blood pressure in very low birth weight infants in the first 70 days of life. J Pediatr. 1988;112:266–270.

77. McGarvey ST, Zinner SH. Blood pressure in infancy. Semin Nephrol. 1989;9:260–266.

78. Zubrow AB, Hulman S, Kushner H, Falkner B. Determinants of blood pressure in infants admitted to neonatal intensive care units: a prospective multicenter study. J Perinatol. 1995;15:470–479.

79. Georgieff MK, Mills MM, Gomez-Marin O, Sinaiko AR. Rate of change of blood pressure in premature and full term infants from birth to 4 months. Pediatr Nephrol. 1996;10:152–155.

80. Hegyi T, Anwar M, Carbone MT, Ostfeld B, Hiatt M, Koons A, Pinto-Martin J, Paneth N. Blood pressure ranges in premature infants: II. The first week of life. Pediatrics. 1996;97:336–342.

81. Kent AL, Kecskses Z, Shadbolt B, Falk MC. Normative blood pressure data in the early neonatal period. Pediatr Nephrol. 2007;22:1335–1341.

82. Task force on blood pressure control in children. Report of the second task force on blood pressure control in children. Pediatrics. 1987;79:1–25.

83. Elliot SJ, Hansen TN. Neonatal hypertension. In: Long WA, ed. Fetal and Neonatal Cardiology. Philadelphia, PA: W.B. Saunders; 1990:492–498.

84. Low JA, Panagiotopoulos C, Smith JT, Tang W, Derrick EJ. Validity of newborn oscillometric blood pressure. Clin Invest Med. 1995;18:163–167.

85. Park MK, Menard SM. Normative oscillometric blood pressure values in the first 5 years of life in an office setting. Am J Dis Child. 1989;143:860–864.

86. DeSwiet M, Peto J, Shinebourne EA. Difference between upper and lower limb blood pressure in neonates using Doppler technique. Arch Dis Child. 1974;49:734–735.

87. Crapanzano MS, Strong WB, Newman IR, Hixon RL, Casal D, Linder CW. Calf blood pressure: clinical implications and correlations with arm blood pressure in infants and young children. Pediatrics. 1996;97:220–224.

88. Park MK, Lee D. Normative arm and calf blood pressure values in the newborn. Pediatrics. 1989;83:240–243.

89. Nwankwo MU, Lorenz JM, Gardiner JC. A standard protocol for blood pressure measurement in the newborn. Pediatrics. 1997;99:E10.

90. Tannenbaum J, Hulman S, Falkner B. Relationship between plasma renin concentration and atrial natriuretic peptide in the human newborn. Am J Perinatol. 1990;7:174–177.

91. Krüger C, Rauh M, Dörr HG. Immunoreactive renin concentration in healthy children from birth to adolescence. Clin Chim Acta. 1998;274:15–27.

92. Cannon ME, Twu BM, Yang CS, Hsu CH. The effect of theophylline and cyclic adenosine 3', 5'-monophosphate on renin release by afferent arterioles. J Hypertens. 1989;7:569–576.

93. Roth CG, Spottswood SE, Chan JC, Roth KS. Evaluation of the hypertensive infant: a rational approach to diagnosis. Radiol Clin North Am. 2003;41:931–944.

94. Flynn JT. Successes and shortcomings of the Food and Drug Modernization Act. Am J Hypertens. 2003;16:889–891.

95. Flynn JT, Tullus K. Severe hypertension in children and adolescents: pathophysiology and treatment. Pediatr Nephrol. 2009;24:1101–1112.

96. Gouyon JB, Geneste B, Semama DS, Francoise M, Germain JF. Intravenous nicardipine in hypertensive preterm infants. Arch Dis Child Fetal Neonatal Ed. 1997;76:F126–F127.

97. Milou C, Debuche-Benouachkou V, Semama DS, Germain JF, Gouyon JB. Intravenous nicardipine as a first-line antihypertensive drug in neonates. Intensive Care Med. 2000;26:956–958.

98. Flynn, JT, Mottes TA, Brophy PB, Kershaw DB, Smoyer WE, Bunchman TE. Intravenous nicardipine for treatment of severe hypertension in children. J Pediatr. 2001;139:38–43.

99. Flynn JT, Pasko DA. Calcium channel blockers: pharmacology and place in therapy of pediatric hypertension. Pediatr Nephrol. 2000;15:302–316.

100. Wiest DB, Garner SS, Uber WE, Sade RM. Esmolol for the management of pediatric hypertension after cardiac operations. J Thorac Cardiovasc Surg. 1998;115:890–897.

101. Deal JE, Barratt TM, Dillon MJ. Management of hypertensive emergencies. Arch Dis Child. 1992;67:1089–1092.

102. Wells TG, Bunchman TE, Kearns GL. Treatment of neonatal hypertension with enalaprilat. J Pediatr. 1990;117:664–667.

103. Mason T, Polak MJ, Pyles L, Mullett M, Swanke C. Treatment of neonatal renovascular hypertension with intravenous enalapril. Am J Perinatol. 1992;9:254–257.

104. Sinaiko AR, Kashtan CE, Mirkin BL. Antihypertensive drug therapy with captopril in children and adolescents. Clin Exp Hypertens. 1986;A8:829–839.

105. Perlman JM, Volpe JJ. Neurologic complications of captopril treatment of neonatal hypertension. Pediatrics. 1989;83:47–52.
106. MacDonald JL, Johnson CE Jacobson P. Stability of isradipine in an extemporaneously compounded oral liquid. Am J Hosp Pharm. 1994;51:2409–2411.
107. Flynn JT, Warnick SJ. Isradipine treatment of hypertension in children: a single-center experience. Pediatr Nephrol. 2002;17:748–753.
108. Flynn JT. Safety of short-acting nifedipine in children with severe hypertension. Exp Opin Drug Safety. 2003,2:133–139.
109. Englehardt B, Elliott S, Hazinski TA. Short- and long-term effects of furosemide on lung function in infants with bronchopulmonary dysplasia. J Pediatr. 1986;109:1034–1039.
110. Hendren WH, Kim SH, Herrin JT, Crawford JD. Surgically correctable hypertension of renal origin in childhood. Am J Surg. 1982;143:432–442.
111. Bendel-Stenzel M, Najarian JS, Sinaiko AR. Renal artery stenosis: long-term medical management before surgery. Pediatr Nephrol. 1995;10:147–151.
112. Kiessling SG, Wadhwa N, Kriss VM, Iocono J, Desai NS. An unusual case of severe therapy-resistant hypertension in a newborn. Pediatrics. 2007;119:e301–e304.
113. Adelman RD. Long-term follow-up of neonatal renovascular hypertension. Pediatr Nephrol. 1987;1: 35–141.
114. Caplan MS, Cohn RA, Langman CB, Conway JA, Ahkolnik A, Brouillette RT. Favorable outcome of neonatal aortic thrombosis and renovascular hypertension. J Pediatr. 1989;115:291–295.
115. Roy S, Dillon MJ, Trompeter RS, Barratt TM. Autosomal recessive polycystic kidney disease: long-term outcome of neonatal survivors. Pediatr Nephrol. 1997;11:302–306.
116. Mackenzie HS, Lawler EV, Brenner BM. Congenital olionephropathy. The fetal flaw in essential hypertension? Kidney Int. 1996;55:S30–S34.
117. Keller G, Zimmer G, Mall G, Ritz E, Amann K. Nephron number in patients with primary hypertension. N Engl J Med. 2003;348:101–108.

22 Hypertension in Chronic Kidney Disease

Franz Schaefer, MD

Contents

Kidney disease is the most common identifiable cause of secondary hypertension in childhood. In this chapter, the prevalence, pathophysiology, and treatment of renal hypertension will be reviewed, with an emphasis on recent clinical trial results demonstrating the benefits of aggressive treatment of hypertension on the rate of progression of chronic kidney disease.

PREVALENCE OF RENAL HYPERTENSION IN CHILDHOOD

Numerous recent clinical trials have established that hypertension is one of the earliest and most prevalent complications of pediatric chronic kidney disease (CKD). Among 366 children with CKD followed at a single center, the prevalence of hypertension according to office blood pressure was 70%, increasing from 63% in CKD stage 1 to >80% in stages 3–5 [1]. The fraction of patients with uncontrolled hypertension despite antihypertensive treatment increased from 9% in CKD stage 1 to 20% in stage 5. Similarly, in the chronic kidney disease in children (CKiD) study in North America, the prevalence of elevated blood pressure among 432 children with moderate CKD (>90th percentile; based upon auscultatory office BP) was 25% for systolic BP and 23% for DBP [2]. A significant proportion of these children were not receiving antihypertensive medications, implying that hypertension in pediatric CKD is frequently missed. Finally, in a cross-sectional multicenter survey of 24-h blood pressure performed by the ESCAPE trial group in 508 children with stages 2–4 CKD,

F. Schaefer (✉)
Division of Paediatric Nephrology, Center for Paediatric and Adolescent Medicine, University of Heidelberg,
Im Neuenheimer Feld 151, 69120 Heidelberg, Germany
e-mail: franz_schaefer@med.uni-heidelberg.de

From: *Clinical Hypertension and Vascular Diseases: Pediatric Hypertension*
Edited by: J. T. Flynn et al. DOI 10.1007/978-1-60327-824-9_22
© Springer Science+Business Media, LLC 2011

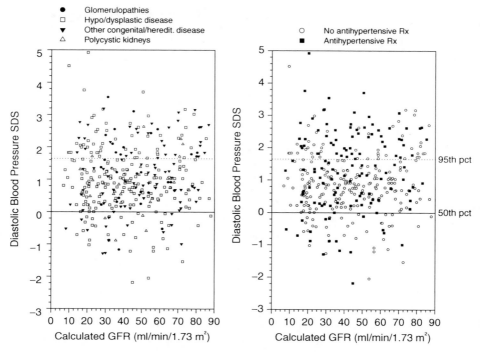

Fig. 1. Blood pressure in 508 children with chronic kidney disease. Distribution of diastolic blood pressure SDS is depicted according to underlying disease (*left panel*) and by prevalent antihypertensive medication (*right panel*). Data were obtained as part of a trial screening procedure in 33 European pediatric nephrology units (ESCAPE Network). Diastolic blood pressure values were converted to SDS using the European pediatric reference values for casual blood pressure of de Man et al. *(139)*.

the prevalence of controlled or uncontrolled (diastolic) hypertension was 46% (Fig. 1) *(3)*. Among the patients receiving antihypertensive treatment, 30% had elevated blood pressure. Blood pressure was largely independent of the current glomerular filtration rate.

UNDERLYING DISORDERS

Renovascular Disease

Renovascular hypertension is defined as hypertension resulting from lesions that impair blood flow to a part, or all, of one or both kidneys *(4,5)*. It accounts for about 10% of pediatric patients (20% of infants) presenting with persistent hypertension. Renal artery stenosis by fibromuscular dysplasia is the most frequent underlying disorder (70%), affecting the main renal artery and/or, more commonly, intrarenal vessels *(6)*. Fibromuscular dysplasia occurs in familial traits in the majority of cases *(7)*; the genetics are consistent with an autosomal dominant inheritance with variable and often no clinical effect. Neurofibromatosis, von Recklinghausen's disease, constitutes a major subgroup among children with fibromuscular dysplasia, accounting for at least 15% of all pediatric cases of renal artery stenosis *(4,8)*. Another frequent genetic cause of renal artery stenosis is Williams–Beuren syndrome *(9)*. In these and other hereditary syndromes, renal artery stenosis is usually combined with anomalies of extrarenal arteries. The combination with aortic coarctation is known as the middle aortic syndrome *(10)*. Apart from vascular malformation complexes, it is frequently caused by Takayasu disease, an unspecific aorto-arteriitis of autoimmune origin common in non-white populations *(11)*. Renovascular hypertension may also be due to other systemic vasculitic disorders, such as panarteriitis nodosa or scleroderma.

Renoparenchymal Disease

Hypertension is very common in various forms of glomerulonephritis. Whereas acute, e.g., post-streptococcal, glomerulonephritis usually induces a reversible rise in blood pressure, chronic glomerular disease is commonly associated with persistent hypertension. The most common underlying histopathological entities associated with hypertension even in the absence of renal failure are focal segmental glomerulosclerosis, membranoproliferative glomerulonephritis, and crescentic glomerulonephritis. Persistent hypertension is also common in patients who have recovered from hemolytic uremic syndrome. Moreover, a high prevalence of secondary hypertension is observed in glomerulonephritis secondary to systemic vasculitis, such as lupus erythematosus. Renoparenchymal hypertension is not limited to glomerular disease, but is also observed in tubulointerstitial disorders leading to renal scarring. Recurrent pyelonephritis, reflux nephropathy, obstructive uropathies, and polycystic kidney disease all lead to tubulointerstitial fibrosis and tubular atrophy. Scarring processes induce local renin and angiotensin synthesis, although peripheral renin activity usually remains normal.

The underlying disease seems to be a more important determinant of hypertension than the actual degree of renal dysfunction. At any given level of GFR, children with acquired glomerulopathies or polycystic kidney disease tend to have higher blood pressure than patients with renal hypoplasia and/or uropathies. In the survey of the ESCAPE trial group, the prevalence of hypertension was 88% in patients with acquired glomerulopathies, 38% in children with hypo/dysplastic kidney disorders, and 57% in other congenital or hereditary renal diseases (Fig. 1).

PATHOMECHANISMS OF HYPERTENSION IN CHRONIC KIDNEY DISEASE

Blood pressure can be elevated by an increase in cardiac output and/or of total peripheral resistance. Both mechanisms can be affected by a plethora of different mechanisms in CKD *(12)*. Figure 2 gives an overview of the most important pathways involved.

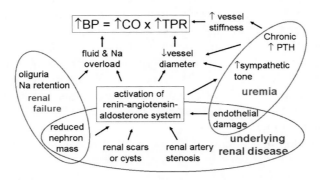

Fig. 2. Physiopathological mechanisms of hypertension in chronic kidney disease. From *(12)*, with permission.

Sodium and Water Retention

Sodium retention and consequent *fluid overload* have long been recognized as a critical cause of hypertension in CKD. In a seminal study, Coleman and Guyton showed that infusion of normal saline in anephric dogs leads to hypertension characterized by an initial increase in plasma volume and cardiac output followed by an increased peripheral vascular resistance *(13)*. Extracellular fluid expansion is most consistently found in hypertensive ESRD patients.

Hypertensive children on dialysis have lower residual urine output than their normotensive peers *(14)*. Strict enforcement of dry weight and normalization of sodium by reduced salt intake and slow long hemodialysis or additional ultrafiltration sessions have been shown to normalize blood pressure without the need for antihypertensives in adults and children *(15,16)* (also see Chapter 23). Plasma volume is elevated and correlated with blood pressure in renal disease, but not in essential hypertension.

On the other hand, the correlation between interdialytic weight gain and blood pressure is weak, suggesting that additional volume-independent mechanisms must affect blood pressure in CKD *(17–22)*. Also, the high prevalence of arterial hypertension in early CKD, when plasma and extracellular fluid volumes tend to be normal *(23)*, supports a role of fluid-independent mechanisms. This is particularly remarkable in children with renal hypo/dysplasia, who tend to lose considerable amounts of sodium and water and yet are commonly hypertensive. The blood pressure lowering efficacy of diuretics in early CKD is no proof for a leading role of salt and water retention in the pathogenesis of hypertension, since loop diuretics interfere with the vascular actions of angiotensin II independent of their saluretic effect *(24,25)*.

The most compelling evidence for volume-independent mechanisms of hypertension in CKD comes from patients undergoing bilateral nephrectomy. In dialyzed children, nephrectomy lowers mean blood pressure despite causing anuria *(26)*. The removal of the native kidneys markedly reduces blood pressure and total peripheral vascular resistance, suggesting an excessive vasopressor effect of failing kidneys. Of interest, previously hypertensive, but not previously normotensive, patients respond to salt and water loading by an increase in blood pressure. Hence, the vascular tone must be affected by kidney-related as well as by kidney-unrelated mechanisms.

Renin–Angiotensin–Aldosterone System

Activation of the renin–angiotensin–aldosterone system plays a pivotal role in renal hypertension. While plasma renin activity is typically found to be markedly elevated only in patients with renal artery stenosis, many patients with CKD have 'inappropriately normal' renin levels (i.e., lower levels would be expected considering their degree of hypertension and fluid overload *(27,28)*). The infusion of normal saline fails to suppress plasma renin activity in patients with CKD stage 5 *(28)*. Hyperreninemia occurs probably due to renin secretion in poorly perfused areas, such as cysts, scars or after microangiopathic damage, or tubulointerstitial inflammation *(29,30)*, and leads to angiotensin II-mediated vasoconstriction as well as aldosterone-mediated salt retention, thus increasing both total peripheral resistance and blood volume.

In addition to mediating systemic vasoconstriction and fluid retention, angiotensin is synthesized locally and regulates growth and differentiation in many tissues including the kidneys. The local angiotensin tone in the diseased kidney is affected by multiple mechanisms, independently of plasma renin activity. Locally formed angiotensin II increases transglomerular pressure and stimulates mesangial cell proliferation, glomerular hypertrophy, and tubulointerstitial fibrosis both directly and via regulation of growth factors and cytokines such as endothelin-1 and TGF-β. Moreover, in CKD renal angiotensin II upregulates afferent neuronal activity originating from the kidney, contributing to sympathetic overstimulation. Additional delayed effects of a high local angiotensin II tone include microinflammation, cardiac hypertrophy, and endothelial cell damage *(31)*; these conditions further aggravate hypertension and end-organ damage.

Sympathetic Hyperactivation

Clinical and experimental evidence suggests that sympathetic overactivity may play a key role in the pathogenesis of hypertension in CKD. Sympathetic nerve activity is markedly increased in CKD and dialyzed patients *(32,33)* and persists even after renal transplantation as long as the native kidneys are in place. After bilateral nephrectomy, sympathetic nerve activity normalizes, concomitantly with a reduction in blood pressure *(32)*. Treatment with ACE inhibitors, but not calcium channel blockers, normalizes sympathetic activity, suggesting an effect of the renal angiotensin tone on afferent neural signaling *(33)* (Fig. 2). The mechanisms underlying this phenomenon are as yet unclear and may include afferent signals from the failing kidney.

In rodent models of acute and chronic renal disease, intrarenal afferent sensory neural pathways are activated which connect with the hypothalamic vasomotor control center, resulting in a rise in blood pressure sustained by noradrenergic mechanisms *(34)*. Renal denervation improves both hypertension and increased sympathetic activity *(35)*. In addition, abnormalities in dopaminergic neurotransmission and the accumulation of leptin have been postulated to be involved in CKD-associated sympathetic hyperactivation *(36,37)*. Overactivation of the sympathetic drive is also observed in renovascular and polycystic kidney disease-related hypertension *(38)*, where renal afferent nervous input is probably triggered by renal ischemia.

Recent research has suggested an important role of renalase, an amine oxidase mainly expressed by the kidneys, in the regulation of blood pressure and cardiac function *(39)*. Renalase expression and enzymatic activity are rapidly turned on by modest increases in blood pressure and by brief surges in plasma catecholamines. The active enzyme degrades circulating catecholamines, causing a fall in blood pressure. The renalase knockout mouse (KO) is hypertensive and exquisitely sensitive to cardiac ischemia. Renalase expression is markedly deficient in animal models of CKD. Blood renalase levels are inversely correlated with glomerular filtration rate and are markedly reduced in patients with end-stage kidney disease. Renalase deficiency may thus contribute to the sympathetic overactivation, hypertension, and cardiac disease associated with CKD.

Endothelial Factors

The vascular endothelium exerts important endocrine and paracrine functions, including active control of the vascular tone. Endothelium-dependent vasodilation is impaired in CKD *(40,41)*.

The key vasodilatory factor secreted by the endothelium is nitric oxide (NO), the absence of which causes severe hypertension *(42)*. NO production is decreased in CKD *(43,44)* as a result of impaired biosynthesis and bioavailability of L-arginine, reduced NO synthase (NOS) expression, and increased circulating endogenous NOS inhibitors *(45)*. Asymmetric dimethylarginine (ADMA), a potent NOS inhibitor, accumulates in CKD due to impaired renal excretion and enzymatic degradation. In hemodialysis patients circulating ADMA concentrations are increased five- to tenfold (43,46,47). ADMA independently predicts overall mortality and cardiovascular events in patients with ESRD as well as progression of CKD (48,49), but these findings do not appear to be related to clinical differences in blood pressure (50). A recent study in children with mild to moderate CKD showed no relationship of ADMA levels with 24-h blood pressure load (51). Moreover, the specificity of ADMA accumulation in uremia has been questioned, since ADMA is also elevated in patients with atherosclerotic disease and normal kidney function (47).

Endothelin-I (ET-1), a peptide secreted mainly by vascular endothelial cells, is the most potent vasoconstrictor known to date. In addition, ET-1 affects salt and water homeostasis via interaction with the renin–angiotensin–aldosterone system, vasopressin, and atrial natriuretic peptide and stimulates the sympathetic nervous system (52). ET-1 overexpression renders mice susceptible to salt-induced hypertension and renal damage (53). In the rat remnant kidney model of CKD as well as in ESRD patients, ET-1 plasma levels are increased in correlation with blood pressure (54). Hence, circulating and possibly renal ET-1 may contribute to hypertension in CKD. Notably, ACE inhibitors reduce ET-1 expression and attenuate ET-I-induced hypertension by inhibiting the catabolism of vasodilatory kinins (55,56).

Calcium and Parathyroid Hormone

Secondary hyperparathyroidism starts early in the course of CKD. PTH has multiple effects on the cardiovascular system. When infused acutely, PTH lowers blood pressure in a dose-dependent fashion via its well-established vasodilatory effect (57). In contrast, a consistent positive correlation between blood pressure and serum PTH levels is observed in patients with chronic hyperparathyroidism (58). Chronically elevated PTH leads to intracellular calcium accumulation in vascular smooth muscle cells, enhancing their sensitivity to calcium and norepinephrine (59,60). This effect can be blocked by calcium channel antagonists (60).

The enhancement of pressor responses by PTH and dysregulation of cytosolic calcium may be mediated in part via suppression of eNOS expression. In the remnant kidney rat model of CKD, reduced aortic eNOS protein abundance was observed, which could be reversed by parathyroidectomy and calcium channel blockade (61) (Fig. 3).

Apart from PTH, cytosolic calcium is regulated by (Na,K)-ATPase. The activity of this transmembranous carrier protein is reduced in CKD by accumulation of circulating digitalis-like substances, which may contribute to the proposed cytosolic calcium-mediated hyperresponsiveness of vascular smooth muscle cells to endogenous vasoconstrictors.

Intrauterine Programming

Environmental influences in intrauterine life may predispose individuals to hypertension, dyslipidemia, and cardiovascular disease in later life. Barker and coworkers first proposed that intrauterine malnutrition, indicated by low birth weight, is associated with type II diabetes mellitus, hypertension, dyslipidemia, and cardiovascular disease in adult life (62). Furthermore, intrauterine malnutrition appears to be associated with reduced nephronogenesis. Maternal protein intake appears to be critical for fetal nephron endowment. Similarly, exposure to excess glucocorticoids leads to a decrease in nephron number by 30–40% in rodents and sheep (63), associated with marked hypertension in post-adolescent life.

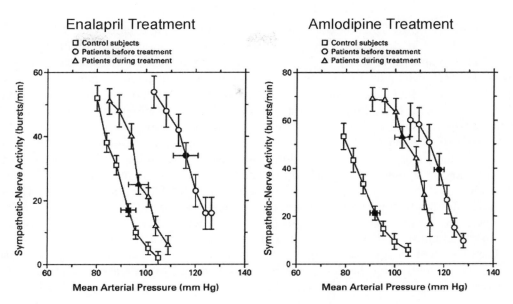

Fig. 3. Baroreflex response of sympathetic nerve activity to changes in mean arterial pressure in patients with CKD before and after 4 weeks of treatment with enalapril ($n=14$, *left panel*) or amlodipine ($n=10$, *right panel*) and in control subjects. Both drugs lowered baseline blood pressure to the same degree. Enalapril, which lowered resting sympathetic nerve activity and heart rate, shifted baroreflex curves downward and nearly normalized sympathetic nerve activity. By contrast, amlodipine increased resting muscle sympathetic nerve activity and the baroreflex response curve was shifted upward, implying that sympathetic activity remained elevated over a range of blood pressure levels. Adapted from *(33)*, with permission.

A disproportionate reduction in kidney size suggesting reduced nephron mass is evident by ultrasound in children with intrauterine growth retardation antenatally and at birth *(64,65)*. A possible link between reduced nephron endowment and the development of hypertension has been suggested by an autopsy study in subjects with essential hypertension and matched non-hypertensive controls, which disclosed a reduction in total kidney nephron number by almost 50% in the hypertensive subjects, which was compensated by a twofold increase in glomerular size *(66)*. While this observation appears compatible with the concept of Brenner implying that a congenital reduction in nephron endowment predisposes to hypertension as a long-term consequence of glomerular hyperfiltration and glomerulosclerosis *(67)*, glomerulosclerosis was very mild in the hypertensive oligonephronic humans and absent in the sheep model *(63,66)*. Also, unilateral nephrectomy leads to hypertension only when performed during the period of active nephrogenesis in rats and sheep *(68,69)*, and children with unilateral renal agenesis have higher 24-h blood pressure than children losing one kidney shortly after birth *(70)*.

Additional mechanisms of prenatal blood pressure imprinting have been suggested such as persistent upregulation of renal angiotensinogen and angiotensin receptors and increased sodium channel expression *(71,72)*, which may operate independently of nephron endowment. Hence, reduced renal mass and CKD may not be causally linked, but both be secondary to intrauterine malnutrition. Finally, it is possible that abnormalities in genes controlling nephron development could also affect the predisposition for hypertension *(73)*.

Pharmacological Hypertension

A number of drugs commonly administered in CKD can cause 'iatrogenic' hypertension. For example, a blood pressure elevation is commonly seen upon institution of *erythropoietin* (EPO) treatment, possibly due to arterial wall remodeling causing increased vascular resistance *(74)*. EPO may act directly on voltage-independent calcium channels on smooth muscle cells, leading to a decreased sensitivity to the vasodilatory action of nitric oxide *(75)*. Calcium channel antagonist therapy as a mechanistically logical approach for EPO-induced hypertension has been successfully tested in the rat model *(76)*.

Glucocorticoids lead to fluid retention by their mineralocorticoid effect. *Calcineurin inhibitors* cause vasoconstriction of glomerular afferent arterioles and hyperplasia of the juxtaglomerular apparatus with subsequent increased release of renin and angiotensin II *(77)*. Increased circulating catecholamines and endothelin-1 precursors and an increased renal sodium absorption via the Na-K-2Cl co-transporter in the loop of Henle *(78)* have also been demonstrated after cyclosporine A treatment, especially when cyclosporine is administered intravenously. Tacrolimus appears to be somewhat less hypertensiogenic than cyclosporine A at bioequivalent doses *(79)*. Treatment with *growth hormone* leads to water and sodium retention by the distal nephron *(80)* mediated by increased intrarenal IGF-1. However, GH does not appear to increase blood pressure in children with CKD *(81)*.

HYPERTENSION AND PROGRESSION OF CHRONIC RENAL FAILURE

A large body of evidence from epidemiological studies and clinical trials indicates that hypertension is an important risk factor for progressive renal disease. In the multiple risk factor intervention trial (MRFIT) which followed more than 330,000 men over up to 16 years the initial blood pressure quantitatively predicted the risk of developing end-stage renal disease; even the high-normal blood pressure range was associated with a twofold renal risk *(82)*. Numerous interventional trials have demonstrated that lowering blood pressure preserves kidney function in hypertensive patients at risk for progressive renal disease (Table 1) *(83–94,95)*.

Besides hypertension, proteinuria is a major risk factor for renal failure progression. Although hypertension aggravates proteinuria and the two risk factors are strongly interrelated in patients with CKD *(2)*, they independently impact on renal survival. Two prospective pediatric trials have demonstrated that hypertension and proteinuria are major independent risk factors for progressive renal failure also in children with CKD *(95,96)* (Fig. 4). In the following we will discuss the pathologic mechanisms by which hypertension and proteinuria contribute to renal disease progression, and the resulting concepts of pharmacologic renoprotection in children with CKD.

Mechanisms of CKD Progression

The current concepts of the mechanisms leading to progressive renal failure are summarized in Fig. 5. Healthy kidneys protect their glomerular tufts from the effects of systemic blood pressure variations by judicious adaptation of the afferent arteriolar tone, leading to a stable filtration pressure over a wide range of systemic BP. This autoregulation is thought

Table 1
Randomized Clinical Trials Demonstrating Renoprotective Effect of Antihypertensive
Treatment in Adult Patients. See Text for Details

Source	Patient population	Renal outcome	ACEI/ARB comparison vs. other AHT	ACEI/ARB superior
Parving et al. (132)	Type 1 DM	Slowed decline in GFR	No	...
Peterson et al. (83)	Nondiabetic	Slowed decline in GFR	No	...
Lewis et al. (86)	Type 1 DM	Decreased risk for ESRD, doubling SCr, and death	Yes, ACEI	Yes
Bakris et al. (92)	Type 2 DM	Slowed decline in GFR	Yes, ACEI	Yes
UK Prospective Diabetes Study group (94)	Type 2 DM	Decreased risk of proteinuria	Yes, ACEI	No
Zucchelli et al. (89)	Nondiabetic renal disease	Slowed decline in GFR	Yes, ACEI	No
Hannedouche et al. (90)	Nondiabetic renal disease	Slowed decline in GFR	Yes, ACEI	No
Kamper et al. (87)	Nondiabetic renal disease	Slowed decline in GFR	Yes, ACEI	Yes
Toto et al. (84)	Hypertensive nephrosclerosis	Slowed decline in GFR	Yes, ACEI	No
Ihle et al. (91)	Nondiabetic renal disease	Slowed decline in GFR	Yes, ACEI	Yes
Maschio et al. (85)	Nondiabetic renal disease	Decreased risk for ESRD	Yes, ACEI	Yes
GISEN group (93)	Glomerulonephritis	Decreased risk for ESRD	Yes, ACEI	Yes
AASK group (109)	Nondiabetic renal disease	Decreased risk for ESRD, 50% GFR loss, and death	Yes, ACEI	Yes
Parving et al. (136)	Type 2 DM	Decreased risk of proteinuria	Yes, ARB	Yes
Lewis et al. (137)	Type 2 DM	Decreased risk for ESRD, doubling Scr	Yes, ARB	Yes

Table 1
(continued)

Source	Patient population	Renal outcome	ACEI/ARB comparison vs. other AHT	ACEI/ARB superior
RENAAL group (138)	Type 2 DM	Decreased risk for ESRD, doubling Scr	Yes, ARB	Yes
Wühl et al. (95)	Children with CKD	Decreased risk for ESRD, 50% GFR loss	Fixed dose ACEI in all patients; intensified BP control by non-RAS agents	–

ACEI indicates angiotensin-converting enzyme inhibitor; ARB, angiotensin type I receptor blocker; AHT, antihypertensive agents; DM, diabetes mellitus; GFR, glomerular filtration rate; ESRD, end-stage renal disease; SCr, serum creatinine; Nondiabetic renal disease includes patients with hypertensive nephrosclerosis, glomerular disease, tubulointerstitial diseases, and autosomal dominant polycystic disease.
Adapted from Toto (135).

to be defective in CKD (97), resulting in unrestrained transmission of systemic blood pressure to the glomeruli. Hypertension and preexisting renal damage converge on the level of glomerular transcapillary pressure. According to the Brenner hypothesis, any critical reduction in functional renal mass leads to hyperfiltration and intraglomerular hypertension in the remaining nephrons (67). The increased filtration pressure causes, or aggravates pre-existing, proteinuria. The exposure of tubular and mesangial structures to macromolecular proteins elicits a marked and persistent tissue response. This is characterized by the release of vasoactive peptides and growth factors such as angiotensin II (Ang II), endothelin-1, and others (98), which further increase intraglomerular hypertension by preferentially constricting the efferent arterioles and/or by inducing glomerular hypertrophy. Independently of its glomerular hemodynamic effects, Ang II interferes with tubulointerstitial tissue homeostasis. Ang II stimulates the synthesis and release of TGF-β which, via its downstream mediator connective tissue growth factor (CTGF), stimulates collagen and matrix protein synthesis. In addition, angiotensin and aldosterone induce the local release of inhibitors of tissue proteases such as TIMP-1, TIMP-2, and PAI-1. Increased production and diminished degradation of matrix proteins result in excessive deposition of fibrous filaments. Moreover, proteinuria and enhanced Ang II formation stimulate the synthesis and release of several pro-inflammatory cytokines and chemokines such as RANTES and MCP-1 and of the transcription factor NFkB (99,100). These mediators enhance macrophage infiltration, matrix deposition, interstitial fibrosis, and tubular cell apoptosis. In addition, proteinuria induces complement activation and oxidative stress to the tubular epithelial cells (101–103).

Another possible mechanism of progressive renal damage has been identified in animal models of hypertensive glomerulopathy (104). Once glomerulosclerosis is established, synechial glomerular capillaries may continue to produce ultrafiltrate which is misdirected into the paraglomerular and peritubular space, resulting in a local inflammatory and fibrotic tissue response and atrophy of the nephron.

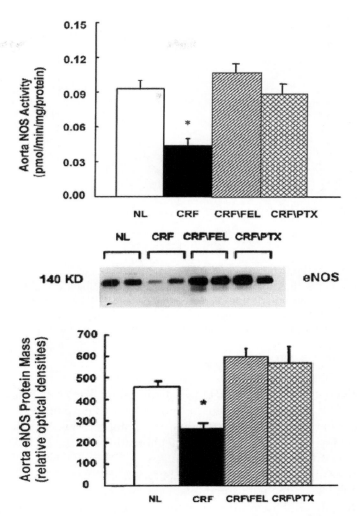

Fig. 4. Reduced NOS activity (*upper panel*) and eNOS protein expression in thoracic aorta of 5/6 nephrectomized uremic rats: NOS protein abundance and activity are restored both by calcium channel blockade (FEL, felodipine treatment) and by parathyroidectomy (PTX). From *(61)* with permission.

Antihypertensive and Nephroprotective Treatment Strategies in CKD

The epidemiological evidence and pathophysiological insights described above have stimulated the search for rational management strategies of CKD-associated hypertension. These relate to both blood pressure targets and preferred antihypertensive choices.

BP TARGET

For adult patients with CKD due to diabetic or nondiabetic nephropathies, meta-analyses of antihypertensive trials showed an almost linear relationship between achieved blood pressure and the rate of GFR loss *(105)*.

Consequently, the Seventh Report of the Joint National Committee on Prevention, Detection, Evaluation, and Treatment of High Blood Pressure (JNC7) has recommended

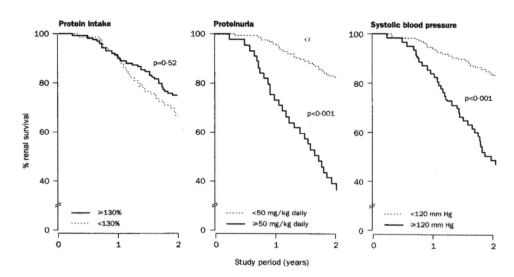

Fig. 5. Lacking effect of restricted protein intake on renal survival (defined as less than 10 ml/min/1.73 m² GFR loss during 2 years of observation) in 200 children with CKD (left panel). Secondary analysis revealed markedly poorer renal survival in children with proteinuria >50 mg/kg per day (middle panel) and systolic blood pressure greater than 120 mmHg. From *(96)*, with permission.

a blood pressure goal of <130/80 mmHg in patients with CKD or diabetes, as compared to <140/90 mmHg in hypertension of other origin. This was despite the fact that controlled randomized trials have not unanimously confirmed renoprotective superiority of very strict blood pressure control in patients with adult nephropathies. In the MDRD trial, proteinuric patients randomized for a low blood pressure goal (<120/75) showed improved long-term renal survival over up to 10 years *(106,107)*, but may have been biased by the preferential use of ACE inhibitors in the intensified treatment arm. In the REIN-2 trial, additional BP lowering targeting to <130/80 mmHg by addition of felodipine to ramipril did not improve renal survival *(108)*. In the AASK trial, forced blood pressure lowering to 92 mmHg mean arterial pressure in African-Americans with hypertensive nephrosclerosis did not affect the rate of GFR loss *(109)*. In the ABCD trial, a lower blood pressure target did not improve renal survival in hypertensive diabetic patients, whereas normotensive patients benefited from lowering blood pressure to the low normal range *(106–110)*.

In children with CKD, available consensus recommendations state that for children with CKD, the resting/office blood pressure target should be the 90th percentile for age, gender, and height. More recently, the Efficacy of Strict Blood Pressure Control and ACE inhibition in Renal Failure Progression in Pediatric Patients (ESCAPE) trial has provided evidence for a renoprotective effect of intensified blood pressure control based upon ambulatory BP monitoring *(95)*. Children randomized to a target 24-h mean arterial pressure below the 50th percentile for age were 35% less likely to lose 50% GFR or progress to end-stage renal disease within 5 years than children with 24-h mean arterial blood pressure between the 50th and 95th percentiles (Fig. 6). The renoprotective effect of low normal BP was independent of RAS inhibition since all subjects received the same dose of the ACE inhibitor ramipril.

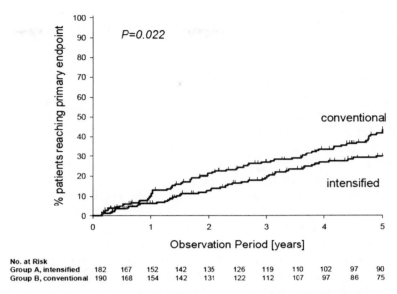

Fig. 6. Improved renal survival by intensified blood pressure control, targeting at 24-h mean arterial pressure below 50th percentile for age, sex, and height, in children with CKD (ESCAPE trial). From *(95)*, with permission.

While the benefit was most pronounced in children with glomerular disorders, it was also significant in children with renal hypodysplasia, the most common cause of CKD in children. Survival analysis stratified by the achieved 24-h blood pressure throughout the 5-year observation period suggested that any 24-h blood pressure exceeding the 50th percentile was associated with a compromised renal outcome (Table 2). Proteinuria was an important modifier of the renoprotective efficacy of intensified BP control. The improvement of renal survival by intensified BP control was mainly related to patients with significant proteinuria.

Apart from the renoprotective effect of intensified BP control, preliminary evidence from the ESCAPE trial suggests that BP reduction to the low normal range is associated with regression of left ventricular hypertrophy in children with CKD, although no

Table 2

Likelihood of Losing >50% GFR or Progressing to End-Stage Renal Disease by Achieved 24-H MAP in Children with CKD. Renal Survival Benefit Was Statistically Significant for Any Arbitrary Cutoff Blood Pressure Criterion Down to the 50th Percentile *(95)*

Achieved BP	Below	Above	p
25th percentile	66.3	66.8	0.63
50th percentile	73.6	57.3	0.005
75th percentile	70.1	49.9	0.001
90th percentile	70.7	29.2	<0.001
95th percentile	71.1	16.4	<0.001

linear relationship between BP reduction and LVH regression was observed *(111,112)*. Altogether, the results of the ESCAPE trial provide a rationale for targeting the 50th 24-h BP percentile in proteinuric, and at least the 75th percentile in non-proteinuric children with mild to moderate CKD.

CHOICE OF ANTIHYPERTENSIVE DRUGS

The multiple mechanisms by which Ang II is involved in renal failure progression provide a rationale for the hypothesis that renin–angiotensin system (RAS) antagonists might confer specific nephroprotection beyond their antihypertensive properties. RAS antagonists lower transglomerular pressure and proteinuria and suppress local growth factor, cytokine, and chemokine release, with subsequent reduction of glomerular hypertrophy and sclerosis, as well as tubulointerstitial inflammation and fibrosis *(95)* (Fig. 7). To date, most albeit not all randomized clinical trials disclosed a superior renoprotective efficacy of RAS antagonists (ACE inhibitors and angiotensin type I receptor blockers (ARBs) alike) in adults with diabetic and nondiabetic CKD. Several meta-analyses have confirmed the specific nephroprotective benefit of RAS antagonists, although the effect size is somewhat controversial *(113,114)*. One analysis suggested that the renoprotection conferred by ACE inhibitors may in part be independent of their antihyper and even of their anti-action *(113)*. RAS antagonists are therefore considered the pharmacological option of first choice in hypertensive CKD patients and are even indicated in non-hypertensive patients with proteinuric, progressive CKD.

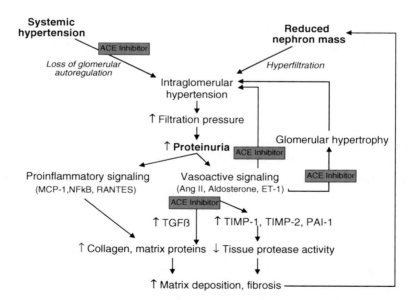

Fig. 7. Mechanisms of disease progression in CKD and sites of action of ACE inhibitors. See text for details.

Published information regarding the use of RAS antagonists for BP control and nephroprotection in children with CKD includes small uncontrolled studies showing stable renal function in post-HUS children during long-term ACE inhibition *(115)*, stable GFR during losartan treatment in children with proteinuric CKD *(116)*, and attenuated histologic progression in children with IgA nephropathy receiving combined RAS blockade

(117). Furthermore, the ESCAPE trial demonstrated efficient BP and short-term proteinuria reduction by the ACE inhibitor ramipril in 400 children with stages 2–4 CKD *(118)*. The drug was very well tolerated throughout 5 years of follow-up, with only 6% of patients requiring discontinuation due to acute increases in serum creatinine ($n=12$), hyperkalemia ($n=9$), or hypotensive episodes ($n=2$) *(95)*. However, it was not possible to assess the effect of ACE inhibition on long-term GFR preservation in this trial since all subjects received ramipril at the same fixed dose. Hence, the nephroprotective efficacy of RAS blockade in children has not been demonstrated by the ESCAPE trial.

The adult study populations in which the concept has been established mainly comprised patients with acquired glomerulopathies. In children, hypo/dysplastic renal malformations and other congenital or hereditary disorders are preponderant. It could be argued that hyperfiltering nephrons in renal hypoplasia should be susceptible to the specific renal effects of RAS inhibition. Hyper- and proteinuria clearly predict CKD progression also in children *(96)*, and extensive tubulointerstitial fibrosis is commonly found in progressive pediatric nephropathies such as obstructive and refluxive nephropathies, nephronophthisis. These arguments provide a rationale for pharmacological renoprotection by RAS inhibition in children with CKD. However, individual subsets of pediatric kidney disease may remain unresponsive to RAS inhibition. Of note, polycystic kidney disease is the only disease entity identified to date in which ACE inhibition has not proven renoprotective *(119)*.

There is some evidence suggesting that the RAS is incompletely suppressed by ACE inhibition alone, and the possibility of partial secondary resistance due to compensatory upregulation of ACE-independent angiotensin II production has been suggested ('aldosterone escape') *(120–122)*. In the pediatric ESCAPE trial proteinuria was initially reduced by ACE inhibition by about 50% *(118)*. However, proteinuria subsequently gradually rebounded to pre-treatment levels within 3 years despite ongoing ramipril therapy, continued suppression of circulating ACE activity, and persistently excellent blood pressure control *(95)*. Since residual protein excretion on treatment was predictive of renal survival, breakthrough proteinuria may limit the long-term therapeutic benefit of ACE inhibition in CKD.

In theory, breakthrough proteinuria should not occur with drug classes blocking the RAS further downstream such as ARBs or aldosterone receptor blockers. Recent research suggests that the doses required to achieve the maximal antiproteinuric effect of ARBs may be much higher than the maximally active antihypertensive doses. Significant additional proteinuria lowering was achieved without increased side effects in adults by 64 and even 128 mg of candesartan, which has no additional blood pressure lowering effect beyond daily doses of 16–32 mg *(123)*. Hence, ARBs and potentially selective aldosterone receptor blockers such as eplerenone, dose titrated to maximal antiproteinuric action, may become the first-line pharmacological approach in proteinuric CKD.

Proteinuria can also be minimized by combined use of ACEIs and ARBs *(124–126)*. Whereas an earlier randomized trial had suggested improved renal survival with ACEI–ARB combination therapy *(124)*, a recent mega-trial in 28,000 patients showed no better patient or renal survival and slightly increased incidences of hyperkalemia and acute renal failure in patients on combined high-dose ramipril and telmisartan as compared to monotherapies *(127,128)*. Hyperkalemia is also the limiting factor for combinations of ACEIs with mineralocorticoid receptor blockers *(129)*.

In the ESCAPE trial, BP control (24 h MAP <95th percentile) was achieved with ACE inhibitor monotherapy in only 57% of children. Intensified BP control was achieved in two-third of patients in the intervention arm; this was accomplished by ramipril alone in 52% and by combination therapy (1.5 additional drugs on average) in 47% of patients. Hence, a significant number of pediatric CKD patients require multidrug antihypertensive therapy. The choice of additional antihypertensive drugs in children with CKD is largely arbitrary. Dihydropyridine calcium channel blockers have no antiproteinuric effect and may actually promote proteinuria and more rapid CKD progression *(130)*. However, their combination with ARBs provides very powerful blood pressure lowering and even conferred a patient survival advantage as compared to the combination of ARB with thiazide diuretics (*(131)* and unpublished results of ACCOMPLISH Trial).

Non-dihydropyridine calcium channel blockers (diltiazem and verapamil) are antiproteinuric and therefore potentially renoprotective, but have a weaker effect on blood pressure *(130)*. The use of β-receptor blockers appears rational in view of the sympathetic overactivation in CKD. Metoprolol and atenolol were the first antihypertensive drugs used to demonstrate nephroprotective effects of good blood pressure control *(132)*. Newer β-blockers, e.g., carvedilol, exert a significantly greater antiproteinuric effect than atenolol at comparable blood pressure reduction *(133,134)*.

ACKNOWLEDGMENTS

This work was supported by a grant from the KfH Foundation for Preventive Medicine.

REFERENCES

1. Wong H, Mylera K, Feber J, Drukker A, Filler G. Prevalence of complications in children with chronic kidney disease according to KDOQI. Kidney Int. 2006;70:585–590.
2. Flynn JT, Mitsnefes M, Pierce C, Cole SR, Parekh RS, Furth SL, Warady BA. Blood pressure in children with chronic kidney disease: a report from the Chronic Kidney Disease in Children study. Hypertension. 2008;52:631–637.
3. Wühl E, Schaefer F, Mehls O. Prevalence and current treatment policies of hypertension and proteinuria in children with chronic renal failure in Europe. In: Timio M, Wizemann V, Venanzi S, eds. Cardionephrology. Cosenza, Editoriale Bios; 1999:85–88.
4. Brun P. Hypertension artérielle rénovasculaire. In: Loirat C, Niaudet P, eds. Néphrologie pédiatrique. Paris, Doin; 1993:203–211.
5. Hiner L, Falkner B. Renovascular hypertension in children. Pediatr Clin North Am. 1993;40:123–140.
6. Deal JE, Snell MF, Barratt TM, Dillon MJ. Renovascular disease in childhood. J Pediatr. 1992;121: 378–384.
7. Rushton AR. The genetics of fibromuscular dysplasia. Arch Intern Med. 1980;140:233–236.
8. Pilmore HL, Na Nagara MP, Walker RI. Neurofibromatosis and renovascular hypertension in early pregnancy. Nephrol Dial Transplant. 1997;12:187–189.
9. Pober BR, Lacro RV, Rice C, Mandell V, Teele RL. Renal findings in 40 individuals with Williams syndrome. Am J Med Genet. 1993;46:271–274.
10. Sumboonananda A, Robinson BL, Gedroye WMW, Saxton HM, Reidy JF, Haycock GB. Middle aortic syndrome. Arch Dis Child. 1992;67:501–505.
11. Wiggelinkhuizen J, Cremin BJ. Takayasu arteritis and renovascular hypertention in childhood. Pediatrics. 1978;62:209–217.
12. Hadtstein C, Schaefer F. Hypertension in children with chronic kidney disease: pathophysiology and management. Pediatr Nephrol. 2008;23:363–371.
13. Coleman TG, Guyton AM. Hypertension caused by salt loading in the dog. 3. Onset transients of cardiac output and other circulatory variables. Circ Res. 1969;25:153–160.
14. Tkaczyk M, Nowicki M, Balasz-Chmielewska I, Boguszewska-Baczkowska H, Drozdz D, Kollataj B, Jarmolinski T, Jobs K, Killis-Pstrusinska K, Leszczynska B, Makulska I, Runowski D, Stankiewicz R, Szczepanska M, Wiercinski R, Grenda R, Kanik A, Pietrzyk JA, Roszkowska-Blaim M, Szprynger K, Zachwieja J, Zajaczkowska MM, Zoch-Zwierz W, Zwolinska D, Zurowska A. Hypertension in dialysed children: the prevalence and therapeutic approach in Poland—a nationwide survey. Nephrol Dial Transplant. 2006;21:736–742.

15. Charra B, Calemard E, Ruffet M, Chazot C, Terrat JC, Vanel T, Laurent G. Survival as an index of adequacy of dialysis. Kidney Int. 1992;41:1286–1291.
16. Ozkahya M, Toz H, Unsal A, Ozerkan F, Asci G, Gurgun C, Akcicek F, Mees FJ. Treatment of hypertension in dialysis patients by ultrafiltration: role of cardiac dilatation and time factor. Am J Kidney Dis. 1999;34:218–222.
17. Sorof JM, Brewer ED, Portmann RJ. Ambulatory blood pressure monitoring and interdialytic weight gain in children receiving chronic hemodialysis. Am J Kidney Dis. 1999;33:667–674.
18. Rahman M, Fu P, Sehgal AR, Smith MC. Interdialytic weight gain, compliance with dialysis regime, and age are independent predictors of blood pressure in hemodialysis patients. Am J Kidney Dis. 2000;35:257–265.
19. Rahman M, Dixit A, Donley V, Gupta S, Hanslik T, Lacson E, Ogundipe A, Weigel K, Smith MC. Factors associated with inadequate blood pressure control in hypertensive hemodialysis patients. Am J Kidney Dis. 1999;33:498–506.
20. Lingens N, Soergel M, Loirat C, Busch C, Lemmer B, Schärer K. Ambulatory blood pressure monitoring in paediatric patients treated by regular hemodialysis and peritoneal dialysis. Pediatr Nephrol. 1995;9:167–172.
21. Chazot C, Charra B, Laurent G, Didier C, Vo Van C, Terrat JC, Calenard E, Vanel T, Ruffet M. Interdialysis blood pressure control by long hemodialysis sessions. Nephrol Dial Transplant. 1995;10: 831–837.
22. Savage T, Fabbian F, Giles M, Tomson CRV, Raine AEG. Interdialytic weight gain and 48-hr blood pressure in haemodialysis patients. Nephrol Dial Transplant. 1997;12:2308–2311.
23. Blumberg A, Nelp WB, Hegström RM, Scribner BH. Extracellular volume in patients with chronic renal disease treated for hypertension by sodium restriction. Lancet. 1967;2:69–73.
24. Muniz P, Fortuno A, Zalba G, Fortuno MA, Diez J. Effects of loop diuretics on angiotensin II-stimulated vascular smooth muscle cells growth. Nephrol Dial Transplant. 2001;16:14–17.
25. Fortuno A, Muniz P, Zalba G, Fortuno MA, Diez J. The loop diuretic torasemide interferes with endothelin-1 actions in the aorta of hypertensive rats. Nephrol Dial Transplant. 2001;16:18–21.
26. Klein IH, Ligtenberg G, Oey PL, Koomans HA, Blankestijn PJ. Sympathetic activity is increased in polycystic kidney disease and is associated with hypertension. J Am Soc Nephrol. 2001;12: 2427–2433.
27. Brass H, Ochs HG, Armbruster H, Heintz R. Plasma renin activity (PRA) and aldosterone (PA) in patients with chronic glomerulonephritis (GN) and hypertension. Clin Nephrol. 1976;5:57–60.
28. Warren DJ, Ferris TF. Renin secretion in renal hypertension. Lancet. 1970;1(7639):159–162.
29. Ibrahim HN, Hostetter TH. The renin-aldosterone axis in two models of reduced renal mass in the rat. J Am Soc Nephrol. 1998;9:72–76.
30. Loghman-Adham M, Soto CE, Inagami T, Cassis L. The intrarenal renin-angiotensin system in autosomal dominant polycystic kidney disease. Am J Physiol Renal Physiol. 2004;287(4):F775–F788.
31. Wolf G, Butzmann U, Wenzel UO. The renin-angiotensin system and progression of renal disease: from hemodynamics to cell biology. Nephron Physiol. 2003;93:P3–P13.
32. Converse RLJ, Jacobsen TN, Toto RD, Jost CM, Cosentino F, Fouad-Tarazi F, Victor RG. Sympathetic overactivity in patients with chronic renal failure. N Engl J Med. 1992;327:1912–1918.
33. Ligtenberg G, Blankenstijn PJ, Oey PL, Klein IH, Dijkhorst-Oei LT, Boomsma F, Wieneke GH, van Huffelen AC, Koomans HA. Reduction of sympathetic hyperactivity by enalapril in patients with chronic renal failure. N Engl J Med. 1999;340:1321–1328.
34. Campese VM. The kidney and the neurogenic control of blood pressure in renal disease. J Nephrol. 2003;13:221–224.
35. Ye S, Ozgur B, Campese VM. Renal afferent impulses, the posterior hypothalamus, and hypertension in rats with chronic renal failure. Kidney Int. 1997;51:722–727.
36. Kuchel OG, Shigetomi S. Dopaminergic abnormalities in hypertension associated with moderate renal insufficiency. Hypertension. 1994;23:I240–I245.
37. Wolf G, Chen S, Han DC, Ziyadeh FN. Leptin and renal disease. Am J Kidney Dis. 2002;39:1–11.
38. Miyajima E, Yamada Y, Yoshida Y, Matsukawa T, Shionoiri H, Tochikubo O, Ishii M. Muscle sympathetic nerve activity in renovascular hypertension and primary aldosteronism. Hypertension. 1991;17: 1057–1062.
39. Xu J, Li G, Wang P, Velazquez H, Yao X, Li Y, Wu Y, Peixoto A, Crowley S, Desir GV. Renalase is a novel, soluble monoamine oxidase that regulates cardiac function and blood pressure. J Clin Invest. 2005;115:1275–1280.
40. Thambyrajah J, Landray MJ, McGlynn FJ, Jones HJ, Wheeler DC, Townend JN. Abnormalities of endothelial function in patients with predialysis renal failure. Heart. 2000;83:205–209.

41. Hussein G, Bughdady Y, Kandil ME, Bazaraa HM, Taher H. Doppler assessment of brachial artery flow as a measure of endothelial dysfunction in pediatric chronic renal failure. Pediatr Nephrol. 2008;23: 2025–2030.
42. Baylis C, Vallance P. Effects of NO deficiency. Curr Opin Nephrol Hypertens. 1996;5:80–88.
43. Schmidt RJ, Domico J, Samsell LS, Yokota S, Tracy C, Sorkin MI, Engels K, Baylis C. Indices of activity of the nitric oxide system in hemodialysis patients. Am J Kidney Dis. 1999;34:228–234.
44. Schmitt RJ, Yokota S, Tracy C, Sorkin M, I, Baylis C. Nitric oxide production is low in end-stage renal disease patients on peritoneal dialysis. Am J Physiol. 1999;276:794–797.
45. Baylis C: Nitric oxide deficiency in chronic kidney disease. Am J Physiol Renal Physiol. 2008;294: F1–F9.
46. Vallance P, Leone A, Collier J, Moncada S. Accumulation of an endogenous inhibitor of nitric oxide synthesis in chronic renal failure. Lancet 1992;339:572–575.
47. Kielstein JT, Böger RH, Bode-Böger SM, Schäffer J, Barbey M, Koch KM, Fröhlich JC. Asymmetric dimethylarginine plasma concentrations differ in patients with end-stage renal disease: Relationship to treatment method and atherosclerotic disease. J Am Soc Nephrol. 1999;10:594–600.
48. Zoccali C, Bode-Böger S, Mallamaci F, Benedetto F, Tripepi G, Malatino L, Cataliotto A, Bellanuova I, Fermo I, Frölich J, Böger R. Plasma concentration of asymmetrical dimethylarginine and mortality in patients with end-stage renal disease: a prospective study. Lancet. 2001;358:2113–2117.
49. Fliser D, Kronenberg F, Kielstein JT, Morath C, Bode-Böger SM, Haller H, Ritz E. Asymmetric dimethy-larginine and progression of chronic kidney disease: the mild to moderate kidney disease study. J Am Soc Nephrol. 2005;16:2254–2256.
50. Anderstam B, Katzarski K, Bergström J. Serum levels of NO, NG-dimethyl-L-Arginine, a potential endogenous nitric oxide inhibitor in dialysis patients. J Am Soc Nephrol. 1997;8:1437–1442.
51. Brooks ER, Langman CB, Wang S, Price HE, Hodges AL, Darling L, Yang AZ, Smith FA. Methy-lated arginine derivatives in children and adolescents with chronic kidney disease. Pediatr Nephrol. 2009;24:129–134.
52. Agapitov AV, Haynes WG. Role of endothelin in cardiovascular disease. J Renin Angiotensin Aldosterone Syst. 2002;3:1–15.
53. Shindo T, Kurihara H, Maemura K, Kurihara Y, Ueda O, Suzuki H, Kuwaki T, Ju KH, Wang Y, Ebi-hara A, Nishimatsu H, Moriyama N, Fukuda M, Akimoto Y, Hirano H, Morita H, Kumada M, Yazaki YNR, Kimura K. Renal damage and salt-dependent hypertension in aged transgenic mice overexpressing endothelin-1. J Mol Med. 2002;80:69–70.
54. Lariviere R, Lebel M. Endothelin-1 in chronic renal failure and hypertension. Can J Physiol Pharmacol. 2003;81:607–621.
55. Largo R, Gomez Garre D, Liu XH, Alonso J, Blanco J, Plaza JJ, Egido J. Endothelin-1 upregulation in the kidney of uninephrectomized spontaneously hypertensive rats and its modification by the angiotensin-converting enzyme inhibitor quinapril. Hypertension. 1997;29:1178–1185.
56. Elmarakby AA, Morsing P, Pollock DM. Enalapril attenuates endothelin-1-induced hypertension via increased kinin survival. Am J Physiol Heart Circ Physiol. 2003;284:1899–1903.
57. McCarron DA, Ellison DH, Anderson S. Vasodilatation mediated by human PTH 1.34 in the sponta-neously hypertensive rats. Am J Physiol. 1984;246:96–100.
58. Raine AE, Bedford L, Simpson AW, Ashley CC, Brown R, Woodhead JS, Ledingham JG. Hyper-parathyroidism, platelet intracellular free calcium and hypertension in chronic renal failure. Kidney Int. 1993;43:700–705.
59. Iseki K, Massry SG, Campese VM. Effects of hypercalcemia and parathyroid hormone on blood pressure in normal and renal failure rats. Am J Physiol. 1986;250:924–929.
60. Schiffl H, Fricke H, Sitter T. Hypertension secondary to early-stage kidney disease: The pathogenetic role of altered cytosolic calcium (Ca2+) homeostasis of vascular smooth muscle cells. Am J Kidney Dis. 1993;21:51–57.
61. Vaziri ND, Ni X, Wang Q, Oveisi F, Zhou XJ. Downregulation of nitric oxide synthase in chronic renal insufficiency: role of excess PTH. Am J Physiol Renal Physiol. 1998;274:F642–F649.
62. Barker DJ, Eriksson JG, Forsen T, Osmond C. Fetal origins of adult disease: strength of effects and biological basis. Int J Epidemiol. 2002;31:1235–1239.
63. Baum M, Ortiz L, Quan A. Fetal origins of cardiovascular disease. Curr Opin Pediatr. 2003;12:166–170.
64. Silver LE, Decamps PJ, Kost LM, Platt LD, Castro LC. Intrauterine growth restriction is accompanied by decreased renal volume in the human fetus. Am J Obstet Gynecol. 2003;188:1320–1325.
65. Manalich R, Reyes L, Herera M, Melendi C, Fundora I. Relationship between weight at birth and the number and size of renal glomeruli in humans: a histomorphometric study. Kidney Int. 2000;58:770–773.
66. Keller G, Zimmer G, Mall G, Ritz E, Amann K: Nephron number in patients with primary hypertension. N Engl J Med. 2003;348:101–108.

67. Brenner BM. Nephron adaptation to renal injury or ablation. Am J Physiol. 1985;249:F324–F327.
68. Woods LL. Fetal origins of adult hypertension; a renal mechanism? Curr Opin Nephrol Hypertens. 2000;9:419–425.
69. Moritz KM, Wintour EM, Dodic M. Fetal uninephrectomy leads to postnatal hypertension and compromised renal function. Hypertension. 2002;39:1071–1076.
70. Mei-Zahav M, Korzets Z, Cohen I, Kessler O, Rathaus V, Wolach B, Pomeranz A. Ambulatory blood pressure monitoring in children with a solitary kidney – a comparison between unilateral renal agenesis and uninephrectomy. Blood Press Monit. 2001;6:263–267.
71. Moritz KM, Johnson K, Douglas-Denton R, Wintour EM, Dodic M. Maternal glucocorticoid treatment programs alterations in the renin-angiotensin system of the ovine fetal kidney. Endocrinology. 2002;143:4455–4463.
72. Manning J, Beutler K, Knepper MA, Vehaskari VM. Upregulation of renal BSC1 and TSC in prenatally programmed hypertension. Am J Physiol Renal Physiol. 2002;283:F202–F206.
73. Ingelfinger JR. Is microanatomy destiny? N Engl J Med. 2003;348:99–100.
74. Carlini RG, Reyes AA, Rothstein M. Recombinant human erythropoietin stimulates angiogenesis in vitro. Kidney Int. 1995;47:740–745.
75. Vaziri ND. Mechanism of erythropoietin-induced hypertension. Am J Kidney Dis. 1999;33:821–828.
76. Ni Z, Wang XQ, Vaziri ND. Nitric oxide metabolism in erythropoietin-induced hypertension: effect of calcium channel blockade. Hypertension. 1988;32:724–729.
77. Busauschina A, Schnuelle P, van der Woude FJ. Cyclosporine nephrotoxicity. Transplant Proc. 2004;36:229S–233S.
78. Esteva-Font C, Ars E, Guillen-Gomez E, Campistol JM, Sanz L, Jiménez W, Knepper MA, Torres F, Torra R, Ballarin JA, Fernández-Llama P. Cyclosporine-induced hypertension is associated with increased sodium transporter of the loop of Henle (NKCC2). Nephrol Dial Transplant. 2007;22:2810–2816.
79. Neu AM, Ho PL, Fine RN, Furth SL, Fivush BA. Tacrolimus vs. cyclosporine A as primary immunosuppression in pediatric renal transplantation: a NAPRTCS study. Pediatr Transplant. 2003;7:217–222.
80. Johannson G, Sverrisdóttir YB, Ellegard L, Lundberg PA, Herlitz H. GH increases extracellular volume by stimulating sodium reabsorbtion in the distal nephron and preventing pressure natriuresis. J Clin Endocrinol Metab. 2002;87:1743–1749.
81. Vimalachandra D, Hodson EM, Willis NS, Craig JC, Cowell C, Knight JF. Growth hormone for children with chronic kidney disease. Cochrane Database Syst Rev. 2006;3:CD003264.
82. Klag MJ, Whelton PK, Randall BL, Neaton JD, Brancati FL, Ford CE, Shulman NB, Stamler J. Blood pressure and end-stage renal disease in men. Hypertension. 1996;13:180–193.
83. Peterson JC, Adler S, Burkart JM, Greene T, Hebert LA, Hunsicker LG, King AJ, Klahr S, Massry SG, Seifter LJ. Blood pressure control, proteinuria, and the progression of renal disease: the modification of diet in renal disease study. Ann Intern Med. 1995;123:754–762.
84. Toto RD, Mitchell HC, Smith RD, Lee HC, McIntire D, Pettinger WA. "Strict" blood pressure control and progression of renal disease in hypertensive nephrosclerosis. Kidney Int. 1995;48:851–859.
85. Maschio G, Alberti D, Janin G, Locatelli F, Mann JF, Motolese M, Ponticelli C, Ritz E, Zucchelli P. Effect of angiotensin-converting-enzyme inhibitor benazepril on the progression of chronic renal insufficiency. N Engl J Med. 1996;334:939–945.
86. Lewis EJ, Hunsicker LG, Raymond PB, Rohde RD, for the Collaborative Study Group. The effect of Angiotensin-Converting-Enzyme inhibition on diabetic nephropathy. N Engl J Med. 1993;329:1456–1462.
87. Kamper AL, Strandgaard S, Leyssac P. Effect of enalapril on the progression of chronic renal failure: a randomized controlled trial. Am J Hypertens. 1992;5:423–430.
88. Bantis C, Ivens K, Kreusser W, Koch M, Klein-Vehne N, Grabensee B, Heering P. Influence of genetic polymorphisms of the renin-angiotensin system on IgA nephropathy. Am J Nephrol. 2004;24:258–267.
89. Zucchelli P, Zuccalà A, Borghi M, Fusaroli M, Sasdelli M, Stallone C, Sanna G, Gaggi R. Long-term comparison between captopril and nifedipine in the progression of renal insufficiency. Kidney Int. 1992;42:452–458.
90. Hannedouche T, Landais P, Goldfarb B, el Esper N, Fournier A, Godin M, Durand D, Chanard J, Mihnin F, Suo JM. Randomised controlled trial of enalapril and beta blockers in non-diabetic chronic renal failure. BMJ. 1994;309:833–837.
91. Ihle BU, Whitworth JA, Shahinfar S, Cnaan A, Kincaid-Smith PS, Becker GJ. Angiotensin-converting-enzyme inhibition in non-diabetic progressive renal insufficiency: a controlled double-blind trial. Am J Kidney Dis. 1996;27:489–495.
92. Bakris GL, Copley JB, Vicknair N, Sadler R, Leurgans S. Calcium channel blockers vs. other antihypertensive therapies on progression of NIDDM associated nephropathy. Kidney Int. 1996;50:1641–1650.

93. The GISEN Group (Gruppo Italiano di Studi Epidemiologici in Nefrologia). Randomised placebo-controlled trial of effect of ramipril on decline in glomerular filtration rate and risk of terminal renal failure in proteinuric, non-diabetic nephropathy. Lancet. 1997;349:1857–1863.

94. UK Prospective Diabetes Study Group. Efficacy of atenolol and captopril in reducing risk of macrovascular and microvascular complications in type-II diabetes. BMJ. 1998;317:713–720.

95. Wühl E, Trivelli A, Picca S, Litwin M, Peco-Antic A, Zurowska A, Testa S, Jankauskiene A, Emre S, Caldas-Afonso A, Anarat A, Niaudet P, Mir S, Bakkaloglu A, Enke B, Montini G, Wingen A-M, Sallay P, Jeck N, Berg U, Caliskan S, Wygoda S, Hohbach-Hohenfellner K, Dusek J, Urasinski T, Arbeiter K, Neuhaus T, Gellermann J, Drozdz D, Fischbach M, Möller K, Wigger M, Peruzzi L, Mehls O. Strict blood pressure control and renal failure progression in children. N Engl J Med. 2009;361:1639–1650.

96. Wingen AM, Fabian Bach C, Schaefer F, Mehls O. European Study Group for Nutritional Treatment of Chronic Renal Failure in Childhood. Randomised multicentre study of a low-protein diet on the progression of chronic renal failure in children. Lancet. 1997;349:1117–1123.

97. Christensen PK, Hommel EE, Clausen P, Feldt-Rasmussen B, Parving HH. Impaired autoregulation of the glomerular filtration rate in patients with nondiabetic nephropathies. Kidney Int. 1999;56:1517–1521.

98. Largo R, Gomez-Garre D, Soto K, Marron B, Blanco J, Gazapo RM, Plaza JJ, Egido J. Angiotensin-converting enzyme is upregulated in the proximal tubules of rats with intense proteinuria. Hypertension. 1999;33:732–739.

99. Benigni A, Remuzzi G. How renal cytokines and growth factors contribute to renal disease progression. Am J Kidney Dis. 2001;37:21–24.

100. Gomez-Garre D, Largo R, Tejera N, Fortes J, Manzabeitia F, Egidio J. Activation of NF-Kappa B in tubular epithelial cells of rats with intense proteinuria: role of angiotensin II and endothelin-1. Hypertension. 2001;37:1171–1178.

101. Nangaku M, Pippin J, Couser W. Complement membrane attack complex (C5b-9) mediates interstitial disease in experimental nephrotic syndrome. J Am Soc Nephrol. 1999;10:2323–2331.

102. Nangaku M, Pippin J, Couser W. C6 mediates chronic progression of tubulointerstitial damage in rat with remnant kidneys. J Am Soc Nephrol. 2002;13:928–936.

103. Chen L, Zhang BH, Harris DC. Evidence suggesting that nitric oxide mediates iron-induced toxicity in cultured proximal tubule cells. Am J Physiol. 1998;274:18–25.

104. Kriz W, Hartmann I, Hosser H, Hähnel B, Kränzlin B, Provoost A, Gretz N. Tracer studies in the rat demonstrate misdirected filtration and pertubular filtrate spreading in nephrons with segmental glomerulosclerosis. J Am Soc Nephrol. 2001;12:496–506.

105. Bakris GL, Williams M, Dworkin L, Elliot WJ, Epstein M, Toto R, Tuttle K, Douglas J, Hsueh W, Sowers J. Preserving renal function in adults with hypertension and diabetes: a consensus approach. National Kidney Foundation Hypertension and Diabetes Executive Committees Working Group. Am J Kidney Dis. 2000;36:646–661.

106. Klahr S, Levy AD, Beck GJ. The effects of dietary protein restriction and blood-pressure control on the progression of chronic renal disease. N Engl J Med. 1994;330:877–884.

107. Sarnak MJ, Greene T, Wang X, Beck G, Kusek JW, Collins AJ, Levey AS. The effect of a lower target blood pressure on the progression of kidney disease: long-term follow-up of the modification of diet in renal disease study. Ann Intern Med. 2005;142:342–351.

108. Ruggenenti P, Perna A, Loriga G, Ganeva M, Ene-Iordache B, Turturro M, Lesti M, Perticucci E, Chakarski IN, Leonardis D, Garini G, Sessa A, Basile C, Alpa M, Scanziani R, Sorba G, Zoccali C, Remuzzi G, REIN-2 Study Group. Blood pressure control for renoprotection in patients with non-diabetic chronic renal disease (REIN-2): multicenter, randomized controlled trial. Lancet. 2005;365:939–946.

109. Wright JTJ, Bakris G, Greene T, Agodoa LY, Appel LJ, Charleston J, Cheek DA, Douglas-Baltimore JG, Gassman J, Glassock R, Hebert L, Jamerson K, Lewis J, Phillips RA, Toto RD, Middleton JP, Rostand SG. Effect of blood pressure lowering and antihypertensive drug class on progression of hypertensive kidney disease. JAMA. 2002;288:2421–2431.

110. Schrier RW, Estacio RO, Mehler PS, Hiatt WR. Appropriate blood pressure control in hypertensive and normotensive type 2 diabetes mellitus: a summary of the ABCD trial. Nat Clin Pract Nephrol. 2008;3:428–438.

111. Matteucci MC, Picca S, Chinali M, Mastrostefano A, de Simone G, Mehls O, Wühl E, Schaefer F, and the ESCAPE Group. Regression of left ventricular hypertrophy and normalization of myocardial contractility by ACE inhibition in children with CKD. Pediatr Nephrol. 2007;22:Abstract 278 (FC).

112. Wühl E, Schaefer F. Therapeutic strategies to slow chronic kidney disease progression. Pediatr Nephrol. 2008;23:705–716.

113. Jafar TH, Schmid CH, Landa M, Giatras J, Toto R, Remuzzi G, Maschio G, Brenner BM, Kamper A, Zucchelli P, Becker G, Himmelmann A, Bannister K, Landais P, Shahinfar S, DeJong P, DeZeeuw D, Lau

J, Levey AS, for the ACE Inhibition in Progressive Renal Disease Study Group. Angiotensin-converting enzyme inhibitors and progression of nondiabetic renal disease. A meta-analysis of patient-level data. Ann Intern Med. 2001;135:73–87.

114. Casas JP, Weiliang C, Loukogeorgakis S, Vallance P, Smeeth L, Hingorani AD, MacAllister RJ: Effect of inhibitors of the renin-angiotensin system and other antihypertensive drugs on renal outcomes: systematic review and meta-analysis. Lancet. 2005;366:2026–2033.

115. Van Dyck M, Proesmans W. Renoprotection by ACE inhibitors after severe hemolytic uremic syndrome. Pediatr Nephrol. 2004;19:688–690.

116. Ellis D, Vats A, Moritz ML, Reitz S, Grosso MJ, Janosky JE. Long-term antiproteinuric and renoprotective efficacy and safety of losartan in children with proteinuria. J Pediatr. 2003;143:89–97.

117. Tanaka H, Suzuki K, Nakahata T, Tsugawa K, Konno Y, Tsuruga K, Ito E, Waga S. Combined therapy of enalapril and losartan attenuates histologic progression in immunoglobulin A nephropathy. Pediatr Int. 2004;46:576–579.

118. Wühl E, Mehls O, Schaefer F, ESCAPE trial group. Antihypertensive and antiproteinuric efficacy of ramipril in children with chronic renal failure. Kidney Int. 2004;66:768–776.

119. Ruggenenti P, Perna A, Gherardi G, Benigni A, Remuzzi G. Chronic proteinuric nephropathies: outcomes and response to treatment in a prospective cohort of 352 patients with different patterns of renal injury. Am J Kidney Dis. 2000;35:1155–1165.

120. Mooser V, Nussberger J, Juillerat L, Burnier M, Waeber B, Bidiville J, Pauly N, Brunner HR. Reactive hyperreninemia is a major determinant of plasma angiotensin II during ACE inhibition. J Cardiovasc Pharmacol. 1990;15:276–282.

121. van den Meiracker AH, Man in't Veld AJ, Admiraal PJ, Ritsema van Eck HJ, Boomsma F, Derkx FH, Schalenkamp MA. Partial escape of angiotensin converting enzyme (ACE) inhibition during prolonged ACE inhibitor treatment: does it exist and does it affect the antihypertensive response? J Hypertens. 1992;10:803–812.

122. Shiigai T, Shichiri M. Late escape from the antiproteinuric effect of ACE inhibitors in nondiabetic renal disease. Am J Kidney Dis. 2001;37:477–483.

123. Schmieder RE, Klingbeil AU, Fleischmann EH, Veelken R, Delles C. Additional antiproteinuric effect of ultrahigh dose candesartan: a double-blind, randomized, prospective study. J Am Soc Nephrol. 2005;16:3038–3045.

124. Nakao N, Yoshimura A, Morita H, Takada M, Kayano T, Ideura T. Combination treatment of angiotensin-II receptor blocker and angiotensin-converting-enzyme inhibitor in non-diabetic renal disease (COOPER-ATE): a randomised controlled trial. Lancet. 2003;361:117–124.

125. Campbell R, Sangalli F, Perticucci E, Aros C, Viscarra C, Perna A, Remuzzi A, Bertocchi F, Fagiani L, Remuzzi G, Ruggenenti P. Effects of combined ACE inhibitor and angiotensin II antagonist treatment in human chronic nephropathies. Kidney Int. 2003;63:1094–1103.

126. MacKinnon M, Shurraw S, Akbari A, Knoll GA, Jaffey J, Clark HD. Combination therapy with an angiotensin receptor blocker and an ACE inhibitor in proteinuric renal disease: a systematic review of the efficacy and safety data. Am J Kidney Dis. 2006;48:8–20.

127. ONTARGET Investigators, Yusuf S, Teo KK, Pogue J, Dyal L, Copland I, Schumacher H, Dagenais G, Sleigth P, Anderson C. Telmisartan, ramipril, or both in patients at high risk for vascular events. N Engl J Med. 2008;358:1547–1559.

128. Mann JF, Schmieder RF, McQueen M, Dyal L, Schumacher H, Pogue J, Wang X, Maggioni A, Budaj A, Chaithiraphan S, Dickstein K, Keltai M, Metsärinne K, Oto A, Parkhomenko A, Piegas LS, Svedsen TL, Teo KK, Yusuf S, ONTARGET Investigators. Renal outcomes with telmisartan, ramipril, or both, in people at high vascular risk (the ONTARGET study): a multicentre, randomised, double-blind, controlled trial. Lancet. 2008;372:547–553.

129. Epstein M, Buckalew V, Altamirano J, Roniker B, Krause S, Kleimann J. Eplerenone reduces proteinuria in type II diabetes mellitus: implications for aldosterone involvement in the pathogenesis of renal dysfunction. J Am Coll Cardiol. 2002;39(Suppl. 1):249.

130. Remuzzi G, Ruggenenti P, Benigni A. Understanding the nature of renal disease progression. Kidney Int. 1997;51:2–15.

131. Flack JM, Hilkert R. Single-pill combination of amlodipine and valsartan in the management of hypertension. Expert Opin Pharmacother. 2009;10:1979–1994.

132. Parving HH, Andersen AR, Smidt UM, Svendsen PA. Early aggressive antihypertensive treatment reduces rate of decline in kidney function in diabetic nephropathy. Lancet. 1983;1:1175–1179.

133. Marchi F, Ciriello G. Efficacy of carvedilol in mild to moderate essential hypertension and effects on microalbuminuria: a multicenter, randomized. open-label, controlled study versus atenolol. Adv Ther. 1995;12:212–221.

134. Fassbinder W, Quarder O, Waltz A. Treatment with carvedilol is associated with a significant reduction in microalbuminuria: a multicenter randomized study. Int J Clin Pract. 1999;53:519–522.

135. Toto R. Angiotensin II subtype 1 receptor blockers and renal function. Arch Intern Med. 2001;161: 1492–1499.

136. Parving H, Lehnert H, Brochner-Mortensen J, Gomis R, Andersen S, Arner P, Irbesartan in patients with type 2 diabetes and microalbuminuria Study Group. The effect of irbesartan on the development of diabetic nephropathy in patients with type 2 diabetes. N Engl J Med. 2001;345:870–878.

137. Lewis EJ, Hunsicker LG, Clarke WL, Berl T, Pohl MA, Lewis JB, Ritz E, Atkins RC, Rohde R, Raz I, Collaborative Study Group. Renoprotective effect of the angiotensin-receptor antagonist irbesartan in patients with nephropathy due to type 2 diabetes. N Engl J Med. 2001;345:851–860.

138. Brenner BM, Cooper ME, DeZeeuw D, Keane WF, Mitch WE, Parving HH, Remuzzi G, Sanpinn SM, Zhan Z, Shahinfar S, RENAAL Study Investigators. Effects of losartan on renal and cardiovascular outcomes in patients with type 2 diabetes and nephropathy. N Engl J Med. 2001;345:861–869.

139. de Man SA, André JL, Bachmann HJ, Grobbee DE, Ibsen KK, Laaser U, Lippert P, Hofmann A. Blood pressure in childhood: pooled findings of six European studies. J Hypertens. 1991;9:109–114.

23 Hypertension in End-Stage Renal Disease

Tomáš Seeman, MD, PhD

INTRODUCTION

Hypertension is a frequent finding in children with end-stage renal disease (ESRD), occurring more often than in children with chronic kidney disease. The origin comes from the chronically diseased kidney (see preceding chapter), but additional risk factors appear in dialyzed and transplanted children, such as fluid overload, immunosuppressive drugs, or obesity. Hypertension is one of the most important risk factors for cardiovascular morbidity and mortality in children with ESRD. Furthermore, cardiovascular events are the most common cause of death in these patients. Therefore, the treatment of hypertension is one of the most important strategies in dialyzed and transplanted children to improve their survival.

HYPERTENSION IN CHILDREN ON DIALYSIS

Measurement of Blood Pressure in Dialyzed Children

CASUAL BLOOD PRESSURE

The same guidelines for measuring blood pressure (BP) used for normal children (see Chapter 7) apply to children on peritoneal dialysis (PD). However, in measuring BP in children on hemodialysis (HD), the general rule to use the right upper extremity must often be disregarded if a right arm arteriovenous fistula is present because compression of the fistula may contribute to access failure. In order to avoid difficulties in measuring BP in the upper extremities with arteriovenous fistulas, some authors proposed to use the legs to measure BP. However, systolic BP readings from the dorsalis pedis artery have yielded

T. Seeman (✉)
Department of Pediatrics, University Hospital Motol, Charles University Prague, 2nd Faculty of Medicine, Prague, Czech Republic
e-mail: tomas.seeman@lfmotol.cuni.cz

From: *Clinical Hypertension and Vascular Diseases: Pediatric Hypertension*
Edited by: J. T. Flynn et al. DOI 10.1007/978-1-60327-824-9_23
© Springer Science+Business Media, LLC 2011

values 15 mmHg higher than arm pressures *(1)* and therefore are not comparable. Blood pressure measurement obtained in the thigh gives also higher BP values than in the arm *(2)*. Automated oscillometric BP monitors are increasingly used also in dialyzed children; however, they should be used and obtained values interpreted with caution because they give significantly higher BP values than auscultatory devices in adults as well as in children *(3,4)*.

Controversies still exist surrounding the timing of BP measurement in HD patients. Casual readings are usually taken immediately after the start of HD session, but this so-called predialytic BP overestimates the mean systolic interdialytic systolic BP by 10 mmHg, whereas the postdialytic BP may underestimate it by 7 mmHg in adult patients *(5)*. Some authors believe that postdialytic readings better reflect the interdialytic BP *(6)*, whereas others prefer predialytic BP as a guide for treatment *(7)*. A variety of influences account for these differences before, during, and after HD; changes in volume, neural signaling, local and systemic hormonal release, and vascular tone. A composite of BP measurements over a period of several weeks rather than isolated readings during one HD session (predialytic or postdialytic BP) should be used for guidance *(8)*. Volume-related differences might be present also between morning and evening BP in patients undergoing automated overnight PD with significant ultrafiltration.

AMBULATORY BLOOD PRESSURE

Ambulatory BP monitoring (ABPM) improves the evaluation of the BP status in HD as well as in PD patients. The many advantages of ABPM (see Chapter 29) are particularly evident in ESRD patients. The white coat hypertension and white coat effect play a more minor role than in other patient groups in adults *(9)*. Conflicting data on white coat hypertension exist in dialyzed children, Koch et al. showed no white coat hypertension, whereas Lingens et al. showed 31% of dialyzed children to be reclassified as normotensive whose casual BP values were in the normotensive range *(10,11)*. Studies in adult HD patients have shown that ABPM is relatively reproducible and less variable than casual pre- or postdialytic BP; however, the reproducibility of the BP decrease during sleep (nocturnal dip) is poor, because up to 43% of patients change their nocturnal dip category after repeated measurements *(12)*. This reflects many influences that affect circadian BP patterns in dialyzed patients and that change with time (especially changes in body volume and sodium that affect nocturnal BP dip). The issue of reproducibility of nocturnal dip has not yet been studied in children. Interdialytic weight gain has been shown to correlate with ambulatory BP in children *(13)*; however, other study failed to demonstrate any correlation between interdialytic weight gain and BP *(11)*. Therefore, this issue deserves further investigation. The main advantage of ABPM, the possibility to evaluate circadian changes of BP, is particularly important in ESRD patients, in view of the prognostic significance of nocturnal dipping *(14)*. Furthermore, the results of ABPM correlate also in dialyzed adults and children better with markers of target-organ damage, such as left ventricular hypertrophy, than of casual BP *(15,16)*.

In dialyzed children, casual BP measurement and ABPM results are poorly correlated. A third of children appearing normotensive by casual readings have to be reclassified to hypertensive when examined by ABPM or the converse *(11)*. Sorof et al. *(13)* found a wide range of error for casual BP relative to ABPM, confirming the unreliable character of casual readings. Interdialytic BP monitoring with an ABPM monitor is therefore the most reproducible method and is thought to best represent BP in dialysis patients *(8)*.

HOME BLOOD PRESSURE

Home BP performed regularly by the patients or by their parents has been shown to give lower values than clinic BP in most children *(17)*. It is an important method for control of hypertension in dialyzed children and a valuable supplement to ABPM that can also increase the compliance of patients with antihypertensive therapy.

Definition and Prevalence of Hypertension in Dialyzed Children

Since children with ESRD are often growth retarded, problems with the definition of HTN may occur, because no normative data for casual BP are available for children with heights below the 5th height percentile *(18)* and since available normative data for pediatric ABPM, while indexed to height in centimeters, do not exist for children with heights <120 cm *(19)*. It has been suggested that looking at norms for the age at which the child's height would fall in the 50th percentile should suffice. However, this maneuver may result in an underestimate of the normal BP range for such children. Therefore, normative data for casual BP should be taken for the 5th–95th height percentile *(18)* and normative data for ABPM for the patient's height regardless of the patient's age *(19)*.

In general, casual BP readings in dialyzed patients are subject to sampling errors, mainly because of the great influence of the rapidly changing volume status (as previously noted). Even repeated casual measurements are not able to reflect circadian changes. It appears that in all ESRD patients, HTN can be better defined by applying ABPM than by casual recordings.

The prevalence of HTN in dialyzed children ranges significantly, mainly depending on the method of BP measurement and the time of the measurement. In the first weeks or months after the start of dialysis therapy, BP tends to decrease and often allows reduction in antihypertensive medication *(20)*. However, HTN persists in a high proportion in chronically dialyzed children. This observation was confirmed in large pediatric dialysis populations followed in registry studies. In Europe, 55% of patients under 15 years of age on maintenance dialysis received antihypertensive drugs and despite receiving antihypertensive therapy, 45% of HD patients and 31% of PD patients maintained BP levels of 10 mmHg or more above the 95th percentile *(21)*. An American multicenter study reported that 53% of HD and 40% of PD patients (including adolescents) received antihypertensive drugs 2 years after dialysis initiation *(22)*. Recently, the American Midwest Pediatric Nephrology Consortium Study found HTN, defined as mean casual BP ≥95th percentile, in 59% of HD children *(23)*. Similar observations were reported by the Mid-European Pediatric Peritoneal Dialysis Study Group, by the North American Pediatric Renal Transplant Cooperative Study, or by the nationwide survey in Poland *(24–26)*. These multicenter studies were based on casual BP measurements.

Using ABPM, which provides a more detailed analysis, Lingens et al. *(11)* found that 33% of children and adolescents on long-term HD and 70% on PD were hypertensive, as defined by standard reference data obtained from casual readings. The predialysis plasma levels of atrial natriuretic peptide (ANP), as an indicator of the volume status, correlated highly with daytime BP in both HD and PD patients. This is in agreement with the finding of Sorof et al. who found a correlation of the ambulatory BP and interdialytic weight gain *(13)*, but in discordance with the finding of Lingens et al. who found no correlation between these parameters *(11)*.

An attenuated nocturnal dip in BP has been observed in many adult patients receiving dialysis treatment. This reduced nocturnal dipping may lead to nocturnal HTN, which presents an unfavorable prognostic sign associated with higher cardiovascular mortality *(27,28)*. In the study by Lingens et al. *(11)*, the median nocturnal decline of mean systolic and diastolic BP was 4 and 7% in children on HD and 9 and 12% in PD children, respectively, which is lower than in healthy children. In the Finnish investigation, a decreased nocturnal decline (non-dipping, defined as nighttime BP decrease <10%) was noted in 40% of children on PD *(29)*.

Etiology and Pathogenesis of Hypertension in Dialyzed Children

The two main pathogenic mechanisms contributing to HTN, before and after initiation of dialysis therapy, are hypervolemia and increased vasoconstriction. Volume overload seems to be the major pathogenic factor, first outlined by Guyton et al. *(30)*. Diminished glomerular filtration rate and sodium excretory capacity result in water and sodium retention in the body, thereby increasing venous return and cardiac output. In order to prevent hyperperfusion of tissues, vasoconstriction ensues via autoregulation. This mechanism operates, however, only after some time lag. For example, it may take several weeks until volume changes in dialyzed adult patients are translated into changes in BP *(31)*. After the disappearance of edema, HTN may persist until strict control of hypervolemia, e.g., by extension of the dialysis time, and may finally reduce BP *(32)*. However, hypervolemia may also occur in the absence of HTN.

Increased peripheral vascular resistance caused by humoral factors inappropriate to the volume state is another explanation of HTN in dialyzed patients *(33)*. Activation of the renin–angiotensin–aldosterone system (RAAS) was demonstrated by high plasma renin activity *(34)* in adult patients on HD treatment *(35)*. In addition, the local RAAS in the vessel walls appears to be activated in renal failure.

Furthermore, increased sympathetic activity, correlating highly with systemic BP, was documented in dialyzed adults *(36)*. In children, a two- to fourfold increase in plasma noradrenalin and adrenalin levels was noted during an HD session *(34)*. Sympathetic overactivity appears to be mediated by an afferent signal arising in the failing kidney and HD patients who had undergone bilateral nephrectomy display normalization of the sympathetic activity *(37)*. The finding of structural abnormalities of coronary and great arteries in experimental CRF and dialyzed patients further supports the role of elevated peripheral vascular resistance and impaired elasticity of great vessels in the pathogenesis of HTN in ESRD *(38)*.

Another concept used to explain HTN in ESRD relates to the abnormal endothelial release of hemodynamically active compounds. Elevated plasma levels of the vasoconstrictor endothelin-1 have been reported in HD patients *(39)*. Endothelium-dependent vasodilatation has been reported to be impaired in uremia, reflected by reduced release or action of nitric oxide (NO) *(40)*, possibly related to the accumulation of circulating inhibitors of NO synthetase (e.g., asymmetric dimethyl-L-arginine, ADMA) in the plasma of adult ESRD patients as well as of children with CKD *(41,42)*.

Finally, HTN in ESRD is related to the duration of HTN in the predialysis period and, therefore, to the original renal disease and chronic vascular changes (i.e., the Folkow hypothesis) as well as to declining residual renal function during dialysis *(43)*. This suggests that HTN in ESRD patients is a progressive disease related also to falling glomerular filtration rate and diuresis, the preservation of which might improve BP control and possibly also modify cardiovascular risk. Potential risk factors responsible for the development of HTN in dialyzed children are summarized in Table 1.

Table 1
Causes of Hypertension in Dialysed Children

Extracellular volume overload and sodium retention

Inappropriate high renin–angiotensin system in relationship to high volume and sodium body content leading to increased vasoconstriction

Sympathetic overactivity

Impaired endothelium-dependent vasodilatation with reduced synthesis of NO and increased levels of vasoconstrictors (e.g., endothelin-1)

Hypertension derived from the failing kidney (e.g., residual renal function, increased renin secretion, and sympathetic activity)

Genetic factors

Iatrogenic factors (e.g., rh-EPO, steroids for primary disease)

Secondary hyperparathyroidism

High dialysate sodium concentration

Inadequate dialysis regimen

Complications of Hypertension in Dialyzed Children

Complications from HTN are mainly produced by vascular damage and may concern different organs. Before efficient antihypertensive therapy became available, involvement of the central nervous system was one of the most frightening manifestations of severe HTN in children with ESRD *(44)*. The kidneys may be damaged further by elevated BP—residual renal function may be compromised by HTN during dialysis therapy.

In the long run, functional and structural abnormalities of the heart are the most important consequences of chronic HTN in pediatric ESRD patients. Echocardiography usually reveals normal systolic left ventricular (LV) function in the absence of severe HTN, anemia, or cardiac failure *(45)* and normal LV contractility *(46)*. However, LV diastolic dysfunction occurs in about half of the adult dialysis patients and has also been demonstrated in children *(47)*.

Four main structural abnormalities of the heart have been described in adult patients with CRF and ESRD with or without HTN *(38)*: (1) LV hypertrophy (LVH); (2) expansion of the nonvascular cardiac interstitium leading to intracardial fibrosis; (3) changes of the vascular architecture (thickening of intramyocardial arterioles and reduction of capillary length density); and (4) myocardial calcification. LVH is most relevant cardiac abnormality in children with ESRD.

LVH is a strong and independent predictor of death and cardiac failure in adult dialysis patients *(48)*. Risk main factors for the development of LVH are systolic HTN, anemia, hyperparathyroidism, coronary artery disease, hypervolemia, and prolonged dialysis therapy. Two forms of LVH may be distinguished *(49)*: concentric (or symmetric) LVH caused by the pressure overload, leading to disproportionate overgrowth of cardiomyocytes with thickening of both interventricular septum and left ventricular posterior wall (i.e., increased left ventricular mass LVM), but normal cavity dimension (i.e., normal relative wall thickness RWT) and eccentric (or asymmetric) LVH caused mainly by volume overload, resulting primarily in dilatation of the LV chamber (increased RWT) and increased wall thickness sufficient to counterbalance the dilatation with predominant thickening of the interventricular septum and a low LV to volume ratio. In ESRD, both forms of LVH may be present and have also been described in dialyzed children in 70–80% of cases *(50,51)*. On the contrary, the third abnormal finding of the cardiac geometry found on the echocardiography, namely concentric remodeling (i.e., increased RWT but normal LVM), is only rarely seen in pediatric ESRD patients *(51)*.

Although LVH is an adaptive response to chronic pressure and volume overload (allowing maintenance of systolic function), its persistence may become detrimental because it impairs diastolic compliance and reduces coronary perfusion reserve *(48)*. Reduced diastolic filling is closely associated with LVH and increased stiffness of the LV chamber owing to collagen accumulation.

Many reports have described LVH in children with ESRD *(45)*. Echocardiographic examination provides reliable data but requires large experience of the investigator and cooperative patients. In addition, there is still some controversy surrounding the optimal expression of LV mass data in children with renal disease. The currently most often used expression of LV mass is the left ventricular mass index (LVMI) corrected to body size (height raised to a power of 2.7, i.e., $g/m^{2.7}$) and definition of LVH as a LVMI greater than the 95th percentile for normal children and adolescents *(52)*.

In the largest echocardiographic study reported in children with ESRD (aged <15 years), 51% of patients on HD and 29% on PD exhibited LVH. However, no methodological details were collected in this European ERA/EDTA pediatric registry *(21)*. Since then, several single centers have published detailed data on LV mass in children and adolescents with ESRD. In the study by Mitsnefes et al. *(50)*, LV mass was increased by the start of dialysis therapy and did not change after a mean follow-up of 10 months. Risk factors for LVH were lower hemoglobin level (anemia), longer duration of renal disease prior to start of dialysis, and higher systolic BP. The degree of LVH indexed to body size (e.g., $g/m^{2.7}$) seems to be similar in pediatric and adult patients, although small children were rarely assessed.

There are discrepant data on whether LVH is more prevalent in children on PD or HD. An American study has shown that children on HD have more often LVH (85%) than children on PD (68%, *(53)*). Similarly, the Finnish study has demonstrated only 45% of PD children to have LVH that highly correlated with the severity of HTN (pressure overload) and ANP level, a marker of hypervolemia *(29)*. On the contrary, the results from a German study showed similar LV mass index with both modes of treatment *(45)*. It is therefore likely that the prevalence of LVH is dependent more on the overall control of BP and volume status than on dialysis modality.

In adults on long-term HD, LVH may regress; this has been attributed to improved control of HTN, hypervolemia, or anemia *(54)*. Such regression of LV mass is associated with better survival *(55)*. In adults, LV mass may also decrease after conversion from conventional to daily nighttime HD, associated with a drop of BP *(56)*. In children, only very few studies have investigated LV mass longitudinally during long-term dialysis. In the Midwest Pediatric Nephrology Consortium study, no normalization of LV geometry was observed during 2 years of HD *(51)*. On the contrary, in a French study, a significant reduction of LVH in HD children has been reached during a median follow-up of 18 months *(57)*. The reduction of LVH was associated with the reduction of BP, extracellular volume (represented by increased plasma protein), and improvement of anemia.

Left ventricular hypertrophy in ESRD is frequently associated with vascular lesions in the heart and great vessels, which have been extensively investigated in adult patients *(38)*. Two recent studies, which used new noninvasive imaging techniques (electron-beam computed tomography and high-resolution Doppler ultrasonography), revealed a high prevalence of coronary calcifications and wall thickening of the carotid arteries (coronary intima media thickness, cIMT) in former pediatric patients evaluated as young adults after long-standing dialysis and transplantation *(58,59)*. Histologic examination study of the internal iliac arteries at the time of transplantation (i.e., after long-term dialysis) confirmed these clinical investigations that used noninvasive markers of vascular lesions such as cIMT. The most recent study by Civilibal et al. on patients in the pediatric age group has demonstrated increased cIMT also in dialyzed pediatric patients, with no differences seen between children on HD and PD *(60)*. Diastolic BP was the only independent significant predictor of cIMT in this pediatric study showing the early evolution of cardiovascular morbidity in pediatric ESRD patients and clearly demonstrating that better management of hypertension may be the priority for preventing or improving cardiovascular damage in these patients.

It is well established that the high mortality of adult patients with ESRD is related to long-standing HTN. The mortality risk is increased by a large interdialytic weight gain, a high nocturnal BP, and an increased pulse pressure (difference of systolic BP and diastolic BP) *(61,62)*. Long-term studies have demonstrated that adequate BP control improves the survival of adult ESRD patients *(63)*.

Since the start of the dialysis era, there has been a remarkable decrease in early cardiovascular mortality in children and adolescents with ESRD *(64,65)*. The late cardiovascular mortality has been studied only rarely in pediatric patients. According to the US Renal Data System, 1.1 and 2.0 cardiac death per 100 patient years were recorded in dialyzed pediatric ESRD patients at the age of 0–15 years in white and black subjects, respectively (normal about 0.1 in healthy children, i.e., 1000 times less than in ESRD children), rising to 2.3 for all patients reaching the age of 20–30 years *(66)*. According to this study, cardiovascular mortality corresponds to approximately 20–30% of all deaths encountered in dialyzed children and young adults up to 30 years.

It should be stressed that late fatal cardiovascular events, such as myocardial infarction and cerebrovascular accidents, are the result of both specific (uremic) and unspecific (traditional atherosclerotic) risk factors. However, because the cardiovascular mortality in children with ESRD is up to 1000 times higher than in healthy children, mainly the disease-specific—uremic—risk factors are responsible for such a tremendous increased mortality in ESRD children.

A more detailed study from the Netherland Dutch Cohort Study analyzed the data from patients who required the initiation of renal replacement therapy from birth to 15 years of age between 1972 and 1992. Such children had an overall mortality of 1.6 per 100 patient years, a 31-fold increase in death rate compared to normal population of same-aged children *(65)*. Patients who had spent more time on dialysis than with a functioning renal allograft had a seven times higher mortality rate. Altogether, 41% of deaths in children on both treatments were attributed to cardiovascular causes. An interesting and clinically important finding was that patients with long-standing HTN had a threefold higher risk of death than normotensive patients. Cerebrovascular accidents on dialysis treatment were by far the most frequent cardiovascular cause encountered in this study.

Therefore, the very high cardiovascular mortality risk in dialyzed children can be decreased mainly by decreasing the time spending on dialysis (i.e., early transplantation, seven times lower risk of death in transplanted than in dialyzed children) and rigorous treatment of hypertension (threefold increased risk of death in hypertensive children).

Evaluation of Hypertensive Children on Dialysis

Every pediatric patient with ESRD should be regarded as potentially hypertensive (due to the very high prevalence of hypertension including nighttime HTN) and should undergo a systematic evaluation.

Casual BP recordings obtained by oscillometric devices should be regularly checked by auscultatory methods and, preferably, by ABPM as well (see "Measurement of BP" and "Definition of HTN in ESRD"). ABPM is especially helpful in HD patients, because it allows a better recognition of intra- and postdialytic (particular nocturnal) BP changes when continued over 24 or 48 h *(14)*. It is also a useful method for evaluation of BP rhythms in children on PD. Furthermore, ABPM allows better monitoring of antihypertensive treatment and improves patient compliance in children on all forms of renal replacement therapy (RRT). ABPM should therefore be performed regularly in all dialyzed children, at least every 6–12 months, regardless of values of casual BP.

Given the known prognostic significance of cardiovascular lesions and hypertensive end-organ damage (especially LVH) in pediatric ESRD patients, early and regularly repeated monitoring, especially of cardiac function and geometry, is required, even in the absence of any clinical signs of cardiovascular disease *(45)*. There is no doubt that the collaboration of the nephrologist with and experienced pediatric cardiologist and/or radiologist considerably facilitates the cardiovascular care of children with ESRD.

The traditional markers of cardiovascular morbidity and mortality should also be checked in dialyzed children *(60)*. They include mainly dyslipidemia, obesity, and diabetes. Early treatment of these risk factors may improve the overall unfavorable long-term cardiovascular morbidity and mortality in pediatric ESRD patients.

Volume changes should regularly and carefully be checked in hypertensive patients undergoing HD or PD. The absence of clinical signs of edema and normal pre- and postdialytic BP values are not reliable signs of normovolemia. Therefore, additional methods to recognize increased intravascular volume should be applied in children with severe HTN or marked lability of BP. These methods include bioimpedance *(67)*, sonography of the inferior vena cava diameter *(68)*, and determination of the ANP in plasma *(29)*. Although these methods are not sufficiently validated in large series of children with ESRD, their use may help in determining the individual "dry weight" at which child must carefully be maintained. It should be noted that intravascular volume is reconstituted only a few hours after the end of an HD session *(6)*. A new technique that can help in assessment of child's dry weight is noninvasive monitoring of the hematocrit in HD patients. This method has recently been studied also in pediatric HD patients *(69)*.

Treatment of Hypertensive Children on Dialysis

Control of volume status is the primary goal in the treatment of hypertensive children undergoing long-term HD or PD *(33)* as the most important cause of HTN is intravascular volume overload. Use of multiple antihypertensive drugs in the setting of fluid overload is inappropriate and very often ineffective *(70)*. Therefore, the appropriate initial management of HTN in a dialyzed child is gradual fluid extraction to control BP and achieve an ideal "dry weight," i.e., the weight at which most of the excess fluid has been extracted *(71)*. In the clinical practice, in every hypertensive patient newly admitted to dialysis therapy, one should try to gradually withdraw any antihypertensive medication within 1–2 months in concert with a tolerable dietary salt and fluid restriction (which also help to decrease thirst). During this period the true "dry weight" should become evident (see "Evaluation"). Non-invasive monitoring of hematocrit, if available, may facilitate accurate establishment of dry weight *(69)*. In some patients (especially without severe HTN before initiation of dialysis), normal normalization of HTN by these measures may be obtained without antihypertensive drugs. The therapeutic results should be checked regularly by ABPM, with the aim to obtain normal daytime, as well as nighttime, BP values. The target "dry weight" should be periodically reassessed and adjusted according to the child's growth and changes in muscle or fat mass.

Since compliance with the strict procedures necessitated by ESRD and dialysis is often difficult, the dialysis prescription often has to be modified to better control BP, e.g., switching to longer, more frequent (e.g., daily) or nocturnal HD sessions or by minimizing the sodium content of food and dialysate fluid. In a randomized crossover study performed in adult patients, daily HD sessions (six times 2 h/week over 6 months) were able to reduce extracellular water, mean 24-h BP, and LV mass significantly, compared with conventional HD (three times 4 h/week), and antihypertensive medication was able to be stopped or lowered in most subjects *(72)*. Most recently, similar study has been performed also in children in which after a 16-week study with frequent HD (six times/week) the patients exhibited progressive reduction in casual predialysis BP, discontinuation of antihypertensive medication, and decreased BP load by ABPM *(73)*. Similar results were obtained in adult patients switched from conventional to nocturnal dialysis *(56)*. In other studies, reduction of predialysis BP was obtained by gradually lowering the dialysate sodium content during HD sessions *(74)*. However, fluid removal is sometimes limited by hypotensive episodes occurring during the HD procedure, related either to exaggerated ultrafiltration or to concurrent use of high doses of diuretics or antihypertensive drugs. Therefore, antihypertensive drugs should be, whenever possible, withdrawn before attempts at reaching adequate fluid removal during HD procedure to minimize hypotensive episode and to be able to reach the true dry weight. Another measure how to improve BP control in dialyzed children and to reduce dialysis-associated events is a standard noninvasive monitoring (NIMV) of hematocrit algorithm. In a recent 6-month study using NIVM of hematocrit on 20 pediatric HD patients, there was a decrease in postdialytic casual BP, daytime ambulatory BP, number of antihypertensive medications prescribed, and rate of intradialytic events related to ultrafiltration *(69)*.

Whether conversion from HD to PD has any persistent favorable effect on the BP status is controversial. On the other hand, prolonged conservation of residual urine volume during HD or PD treatment generally allows for dialysis with a less stringent dialytic volume control. From this point of view, HD leads to faster loss of residual diuresis than PD and can therefore be potentially associated with increased risk of HTN during long-term HD treatment when residual urine output is decreasing *(75)*. Above all, application of all criteria for adequate dialysis is important in both hypertensive and normotensive pediatric dialysis patients.

Another important issue in the treatment of HTN in dialyzed patients is sodium restriction. It can be obtained by dietary, dialysis, or pharmacological measures. Salt-restricted diet (<6 g/day) has been shown to reduce peripheral vascular resistance and BP in adult patients *(76)*. However, the compliance with the sodium-restricted diet is low, especially if it has to be combined with fluid restrictions. No pediatric data are available on the effect of salt-restricted diet on BP in ESRD patients. Dialysis regimen with low-sodium dialysate fluid concentration (135–136 mmol/l) can reduce BP in adult patients *(77)*. Similar effect is expected also in pediatric patients; however, no studies have been performed in children. The use of diuretics can decrease the sodium content in the body and reduce BP in dialysis patients; however, it is not possible to use them in anuric or severely oliguric patients.

It is generally agreed that antihypertensive drugs should be used in dialyzed children only if BP remains elevated, despite seemingly adequate volume and sodium control—i.e., after reaching dry weight. Since no controlled studies have been performed in this group of patients, the optimal drug therapy remains empiric, based on the investigations performed in other hypertensive populations. Angiotensin-converting enzyme (ACE) inhibitors and calcium channel blockers (CCBs) appear to be the most frequently used antihypertensive agents used in dialyzed children. In the EDTA study, they were given to 62 and 56% of children on HD and PD, respectively, followed by beta-blockers (35 and 44%, respectively), alone or in combination with other drugs *(21)*. In the recent nationwide survey in Poland, ACE inhibitors and CCBs were given to 50 and 46% of dialyzed children, respectively *(26)*. The antihypertensive drugs mentioned are usually well tolerated, but the prescribing physician must note their multiple side effects, contraindications, and dose modifications in renal failure most carefully (see Chapter 31).

There are emerging data that suggest that ACE inhibitors and angiotensin receptor blockers may have a greater effect on decreasing cardiovascular morbidity and mortality in dialyzed patients than other groups of antihypertensive drugs *(78)*. However, some trials showed important BP differences between investigated groups of patients and are therefore partly inconclusive whether ACE inhibitors and ARBs have cardioprotective effects beyond their BP-lowering effects. CCBs have also been shown to reduce LV mass and may be used even in the presence of volume overload. The less frequent application of beta-blocking agents in children with ESRD may be related to their side effects (bradycardia, hyperlipidemia, etc.), but according to a recent study in adults, they contribute to improved survival *(62)*. In many cases, the hypotensive agents, as well as diuretics, have to be combined in order to obtain adequate BP control. In the Polish nationwide survey, 66% of treated children received two or more antihypertensive drugs *(26)*. Despite all these efforts, the control of HTN in dialyzed children is still rather poor. Tkaczyk et al. showed that the effectiveness of antihypertensive treatment in pediatric patients on HD and PD was only 58% *(26)*. Drug-resistant HTN is rare and usually the result of inadequate ultrafiltration (fluid overload), but may also be due to a paradoxical (heightened) response of the RAAS to ultrafiltration.

HYPERTENSION IN CHILDREN AFTER RENAL TRANSPLANTATION

Introduction

Hypertension is a common and serious complication in patients after renal transplantation *(79,80)*. It is an important risk factor for cardiovascular morbidity and mortality in transplanted patients *(81)*. Furthermore, it is a strong risk factor for impaired graft survival in adult and pediatric patients *(82–84)*.

Measurement of BP in Transplanted Children

Casual blood pressure should be measured during every outpatient transplant follow-up visit. However, casual BP has its limitations, mainly in that it can neither distinguish between true and white coat hypertension nor measure BP during sleep. It has been shown in several studies that ambulatory blood pressure monitoring (ABPM) is a better method for BP evaluation than CBP measurement in children after renal transplantation *(83)*. The main reasons are the ability of ABPM to reveal white coat hypertension and to measure BP during nighttime. Furthermore, ABPM is superior to casual BP in regard to better correlation with target-organ damage such as left ventricular hypertrophy *(85)* and the ability to diagnose masked hypertension (i.e., normal casual BP but increased ambulatory daytime BP) in children with ESRD and after transplantation. Finally, the results of ABPM are more closely related to renal function in transplanted patients than the results of casual BP *(86)*. Therefore, regular use of ABPM is recommended in all patients after renal transplantation regardless of the values of casual BP. How frequently ABPM should be used in transplanted children is not clear; however, it is evident from the superiority of ABPM over CBP that ABPM should be performed at least once a year in every transplanted child and at least 6 months after every change in antihypertensive therapy.

An interesting finding of several studies *(87,88)* is the predominance of nighttime hypertension in these patients. This finding further stresses the importance of ABPM with its monitoring of BP values during the night that are usually elevated in hypertensive transplanted children.

Reduced physiological decrease of BP during the night (nocturnal dip) has been revealed in 30–72% of transplanted children *(87,88)*. Adult transplant patients who are non-dippers have greater left ventricular mass than dippers *(89)*. However, in a pediatric study no significant difference in the left ventricular mass index between children with normal and attenuated nocturnal BP dip was found *(88)*.

Home BP self-measurement is also an important method for measurement of BP. It is increasingly used as a valuable supplement to casual BP and also ABPM in children with chronic renal failure or on renal replacement therapy *(17)*. It is especially recommended in children receiving antihypertensive medication.

Definition and Prevalence of Hypertension in Transplanted Children

The same definition is used for transplanted children as for healthy children or children on dialysis. The prevalence of hypertension in children after renal transplantation ranges considerably between 58 and 89% *(79,80,87,88)*. The reason for the wide range in the prevalence of hypertension is based mainly on the different methods of BP measurement and different definitions of hypertension in various trials. Studies using casual BP measurements always report lower prevalence of hypertension than studies that used ABPM. This phenomenon clearly underlines the importance of ABPM since it also measures BP during the night when BP is often increased in transplanted patients *(90)*. Moreover, children should be defined as hypertensive on the basis of two criteria—use of antihypertensive drugs and current BP level, and control of hypertension should also be assessed according to these criteria. Children on antihypertensive drugs with normal current BP level should be regarded as having *controlled* hypertension and children on antihypertensive drugs with elevated current BP level should be regarded as having *uncontrolled* hypertension. The main reason for this differentiation is the fact that it has been shown in several trials that transplanted patients with controlled hypertension have the same graft survival as spontaneous normotensive patients (i.e., normal BP without antihypertensive drugs). In contrast, patients with uncontrolled hypertension have significantly worse graft survival *(84,91)*. Therefore, using only one category of hypertension (regardless of the therapeutic control of hypertension) or antihypertensive drugs as the only criterion for definition of hypertension without knowing the current level of BP would lead to misinterpretation of the importance of the influence of BP on the overall prognosis of transplanted patients.

Etiology and Pathogenesis of Hypertension in Transplanted Children

The etiology of post-transplant hypertension is multifactorial *(79,80,92)*. The main causes are summarized in Table 2. Hypertension prior to transplantation caused mainly by the diseased native kidney is believed to be a significant risk factor for the presence of hypertension after successful renal transplantation *(99,92)*.

Table 2
Causes of Hypertension in Transplanted Children

Recipient's native kidney

Immunosuppresive drugs (steroids, cyclosporine A, tacrolimus)

Graft dysfunction (acute rejection, chronic allograft nephropathy—dysfunction)

Kidney from cadaveric, borderline, or hypertensive donor

Renal graft artery stenosis

Overweight/excessive post-transplant weight gain

Genetic factors (primary hypertension, genes of RAAS)

Recurrent or de novo renal disease

Others (e.g., polycythemia, pyelonephritis, ureteric obstruction, lymphocele)

Children receiving kidneys from deceased donors are more frequently hypertensive than children receiving grafts from living donors *(80,92)*. The lower prevalence of hypertension among children after living donor transplantation could be one of the reasons for better graft survival of the living donor grafts in comparison with cadaver. This hypothesis is supported by the results of a single center study which shows that post-transplant hypertension is, together with episodes of acute rejection, the only independent determinant of graft survival in children after living donor transplantation *(93)*.

Steroids are well-known risk factor for post-transplant hypertension. Several factors, such as sodium retention or increase in cardiac output and renal vascular resistance, induce steroid-related hypertension. Elimination of steroids in stable patients showed reduction of BP in adult as well as in pediatric patients *(94,95)*, and children with steroid avoidance immunosuppressive protocol showed improvement in hypertension *(96)*. In a cross-sectional study the patients on alternate dose steroid treatment showed significantly lower prevalence of hypertension than children on daily steroid medication *(88)* and other studies showed that conversion from daily to alternate dose steroid therapy significantly reduces BP *(97)*. Therefore, adoption of steroid-sparing or steroid-free immunosuppression regimens can be considered as a treatment strategy for improving control of BP in transplanted children.

With the introduction of the calcineurin inhibitor cyclosporine, there has been a dramatic increase in the prevalence of post-transplant hypertension *(92)*. Hypertension induced by cyclosporine is caused by several mechanisms *(98)*. Gordjani et al. *(92)* showed in their large single center study on 102 children that high trough levels of cyclosporine (>400 ng/ml) were associated with a significantly higher incidence of hypertension in comparison to children with levels <400 ng/ml (91 vs. 57%). The newer calcineurin inhibitor tacrolimus also has hypertensinogenic effects similar to cyclosporine. In the only randomized controlled trial comparing cyclosporine and tacrolimus-based immunosuppression in pediatric renal transplanted patients, there were no significant differences in the prevalence of hypertension between children treated with cyclosporine and those with tacrolimus *(99)*. New immunosuppressive agents such as mycophenolate mofetil, sirolimus, or everolimus do not have BP increasing effects, and therefore their use is a further option to improve the control of hypertension in transplanted children *(98)*.

Renal graft dysfunction is another risk factor for post-transplant hypertension; however, there is a dual relationship between BP and graft dysfunction. On the one hand, graft dysfunction elevates BP while on the other hand, elevated BP accelerates decline of graft function. In adults, impaired graft function is associated with elevated BP and increased risk of hypertension *(86,91,100)*. In a single center study, Mitsnefes et al. did not find any difference in mean calculated glomerular filtration rate or acute rejection episodes between normotensive and hypertensive children *(84)*. However, hypertensive children had poor allograft function (glomerular filtration rate GFR <50 ml/min/1.73 m^2) more frequently than normotensive patients, whereas children with normal BP more frequently had normal graft function (GFR >75 ml/min/1.73 m^2).

Current body weight or change of body weight is a well-known and potent determinant of BP level in adults and children *(101)* and most children gain weight after renal transplantation *(102)*. Therefore, control of body weight should be recommended in all children after renal transplantation to improve BP control.

Stenosis of the graft artery has become a rare cause of hypertension with current surgical technique using aortic patches *(103)*. Doppler ultrasonography, magnetic resonance angiography, and spiral CT angiography are noninvasive techniques that can be used to identify this; however, in some cases, a traditional arteriogram may need to be performed. The treatment of choice is percutaneous transluminal angioplasty; surgery should be reserved for cases of angioplasty failure.

The development of recurrent or de novo glomerulonephritis may be associated with the occurrence of hypertension, although these conditions are not common causes of significant post-transplant hypertension.

Complications of Hypertension in Transplanted Children

Hypertension is a strong predictor of graft loss. The most robust evidence comes from the results of the large multicenter Collaborative Transplant Study (CTS) published by Opelz et al. *(82)* which showed that there is a linear negative relationship between casual BP and renal graft survival. This is true not only for adults but also for children <18 years. This relationship between BP and graft survival has been later confirmed by many other studies in adult and pediatric patients *(81,84)*. The results from the NAPRTCS registry showed that the use of antihypertensive medication, a definition for hypertension in this retrospective analysis, is associated with higher graft failure *(80)*. Increased BP is therefore clearly associated with decreased graft survival. Despite these clear findings, it is still a matter of debate whether post-transplant hypertension is a real cause of chronic allograft dysfunction or only the result of renal dysfunction or both. Several findings from retrospective studies such as from the study done by Mitsnefes et al. *(84)* showing that hypertension is associated with allograft failure in children with normal graft function but not in children with severely impaired graft function suggest that hypertension is not only a marker of graft dysfunction but also a direct cause of renal graft damage (Fig. 1).

Similar to the general population, hypertension is associated with increased cardiovascular morbidity also in the population of transplanted patients. Left ventricular hypertrophy (LVH) is a frequent type of cardiac end-organ damage in hypertensive children after renal transplantation occurring in 50–82% children *(87,88)*. Matteucci et al. *(104)* found a correlation between left ventricular mass index (LVMI) and mean 24-h systolic BP; however, another study done by Morgan et al. *(87)* could not find any relationship between LVMI and ambulatory BP data. However, in a recent study, Kitzmueller et al. found a correlation between LVMI and ABPM data at repeated measurement but not at baseline suggesting that control of BP, i.e., change of BP level during longitudinal follow-up, is important for the maintenance of the myocardial architecture *(105)*.

Hypertension is also a risk factor for increased cardiovascular mortality seen in transplanted adult patients *(106)*. Similar studies in children are rare. The Dutch Cohort Study has demonstrated that hypertension is one of the most powerful risk factor for cardiovascular morbidity and mortality also in children after renal transplantation *(65)*. In this study cardiovascular events were the most common cause of death and hypertensive children had a three times higher risk of overall mortality than normotensive children.

Evaluation of Hypertensive Children After Renal Transplantation

Casual BP should be measured during every outpatient visit and regular use of ABPM is recommended in all patients after renal transplantation regardless of the values of casual BP (at least once a year). The diagnostic evaluation of hypertension in transplanted children should consider the multiple etiologies of post-transplant HTN (Table 2). Echocardiography should be assessed at least once a year to determine the presence or absence of hypertensive target-organ damage on the heart.

Treatment of Hypertensive Children After Renal Transplantation

There is clear evidence from the observational studies on the correlation between BP and cardiovascular morbidity, mortality, and graft function that post-transplant hypertension must be treated at least as it is in the general pediatric population or in children with chronic kidney disease. If an identified treatable cause of hypertension is detected (such as renal graft artery stenosis, recurrence of primary disease, ureteric stenosis), the primary disease leading to BP elevation should be treated.

Many other issues on the treatment of hypertension in children after renal hypertension are less clear or even controversial. There are no studies comparing different classes of antihypertensive drugs in children after renal transplantation; therefore, it is not known whether one class of drugs is better than another in transplanted patients. Historically, calcium channel blockers (CCBs) have been considered the drugs of choice for post-transplant hypertension because they counteract the afferent arteriolar vasoconstriction caused by calcineurin inhibitors and reduce their nephrotoxicity *(107)*.

There has been some concern that angiotensin-converting enzyme inhibitors (ACE inhibitors) or angiotensin receptor blockers (ARBs) may deteriorate graft function in case of undiagnosed graft artery stenosis or due to the preferential efferent arteriolar vasodilation and reduction of intraglomerular pressure. However, it has been demonstrated that ACE inhibitors are safe and effective drugs in adult as well as pediatric transplant patients *(108,109)*. Furthermore, ACE inhibitors and ARBs can slow the progression of chronic native kidney diseases in adults mainly by long-term reduction of intraglomerular pressure. The data on the renoprotective ability of ACE inhibitors in children are still lacking. The

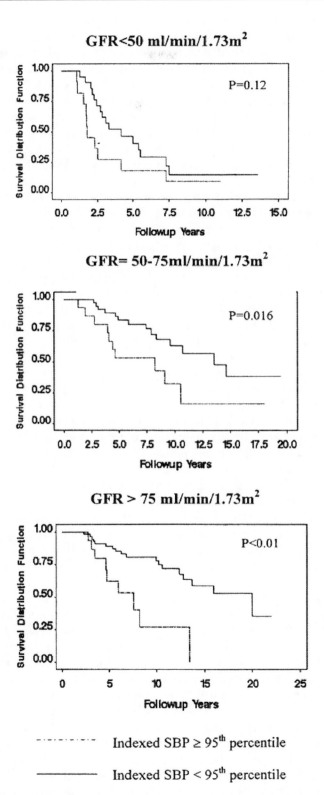

Fig. 1. Renal allograft survival by 1-year indexed systolic BP and 1-year graft function (reprinted from Mitsnefes et al. *(84)*, figure 2).

ability of ACE inhibitors to slow the progression of chronic allograft nephropathy (CAN), which is the most common cause of late graft loss, has never been proven in a prospective interventional trial on adult or pediatric patients. Some retrospective studies have shown promising results such as stabilization or even an improvement in patient survival and graft function in patients with CAN *(109,110)*. However, the results from CTS published recently did not show any improvement of patient or graft survival in patients treated with ACE inhibitors *(111)*. Therefore, this issue is still controversial and needs prospective interventional trials to resolve this controversy. At present, there are no data on the use of angiotensin receptor blockers (ARBs) in children after renal transplantation. However, in adults, there are several small single center studies showing that ARB can also be used in transplanted patients *(112)*.

Beta-blockers are also effective drugs in transplanted patients *(113)*. However, beta-blockers are not able to reduce proteinuria as ACE inhibitors do. A further disadvantage of beta-blockers is their negative metabolic effects (increased lipid levels or impaired glucose tolerance), which may further contribute to the increased risk of cardiovascular disease in these patients.

Sodium retention is often present after renal transplantation, and therefore diuretics are important antihypertensive drugs in these patients as well. Thiazide diuretics should be preferred in patients with normal graft function, whereas loop diuretics should be given in patients with impaired graft function. Diuretics may also have detrimental metabolic effects such as hyperlipidemia, hyperuricemia, or hyperglycemia. Potassium-sparing diuretics are used rarely due to their risk of hyperkalemia.

All four major classes of antihypertensive drugs can therefore be used in transplanted patients. Post-transplant hypertension has a multifactorial etiology and is often severe; therefore, combination therapy is usually needed to control it. Which drug should be used as a first-line treatment remains the individual decision of the physician because it has not been consistently shown that one class is better than other in renal transplant recipients *(107)*. In most pediatric renal transplantation centers, the most commonly used antihypertensive drugs are CCB, which are given to 38–65% of transplanted children *(87,88,90)*. The second most commonly prescribed drugs are ACE inhibitors and beta-blockers. Diuretics are given less frequently to transplanted children.

Non-pharmacological lifestyle measures (reduction of increased body weight, reduction of salt intake, and physical activity) should be encouraged even during antihypertensive drug therapy as they target the risk factors not only for hypertension but also for cardiovascular morbidity and mortality of the patients (obesity, increased salt intake, and physical inactivity).

It is still a matter of debate what should be the target BP for patients after renal transplantation. The National Kidney Foundation Task Force on Cardiovascular Disease recommends a target BP level <130/85 for adult renal allograft recipients and <125/75 for proteinuric patients similar to guidelines for the management of hypertension in patients with diabetic nephropathy *(114)*. However, there are no prospective interventional trials showing that target BP lower than the conventional cutoff of 140/90 will improve graft function and long-term graft survival. The same is true also for pediatric renal transplant recipients. The results of a most recent large European multicenter study (ESCAPE trial) showed that reduction of ambulatory 24-h BP <50th percentile leads to significantly slower progression of chronic renal insufficiency in children comparing to children with BP between 50th and 95th percentile *(115)*. However, it is not known whether these results can be extrapolated to transplanted children. The current recommendation of the Fourth report of the National High BP Education Program Working Group on High BP in Children recommends target BP <90th percentile for children with chronic kidney diseases *(18)*.

While no such recommendation has yet been made for the management of hypertension after renal transplantation, adoption of this target would seem logical *(116)*.

The control of hypertension in children after transplantation is still not adequate. Only a minority of children treated for hypertension after kidney transplantation has BP at least below the target BP level recommended for the healthy population, i.e., <95th percentile *(88)*. The prevalence of persistent hypertension despite antihypertensive treatment (i.e., prevalence of uncontrolled hypertension) ranged between 45 and 82% in the recent pediatric studies using ABPM *(87,88)*. This means that only 18–55% of children after renal transplantation had hypertension controlled by drugs with BP at least <95th percentile. These data suggest that there is a high potential for improvement of antihypertensive therapy in children after renal transplantation.

The reasons for the insufficient antihypertensive therapy in transplanted patients have not been thoroughly investigated. Many factors, such as chronic allograft dysfunction, need for lifelong use of blood pressure elevating immunosuppressive drugs (steroids, cyclosporine, and tacrolimus), obesity, salt retention, renin secretion from diseased native kidneys, and the fear of ACE inhibitors in transplanted patients are discussed as the major reasons for inadequate BP control in transplanted patients. Last, noncompliance can play an important role in the control of hypertension, particularly in adolescent patients. Therefore, adherence to the recommended antihypertensive drugs should be checked during every outpatient visit.

An important issue is whether the poor control of hypertension can be improved and whether improved control of hypertension can stabilize or even improve graft function or cardiac complications. Results from CTS group showed in adults that improved control of BP is associated with improved long-term graft and patient survival *(117)*. Two recent studies have demonstrated promising result on this issue also in children. In a prospective interventional trial on intensified treatment of hypertension, it was shown that the ambulatory BP could be significantly reduced after 2 years by increasing the number of antihypertensive drugs, especially ACE inhibitors and diuretics and that children who remained hypertensive during a 2-year interventional trial on BP control lost significant graft function compared to children in whom BP was lowered to normotensive range despite similar graft function at the beginning of the trial (Fig. 2) *(118)*. In the second most recent study, left ventricular

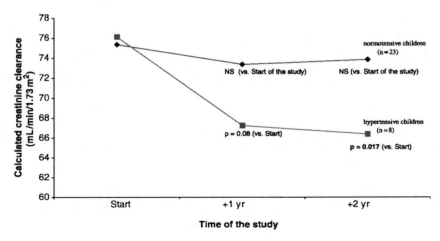

Fig. 2. Graft function in children being normotensive and hypertensive at 2 years during 2-year interventional study (reprinted from Seeman et al. *(118)*, figure 3).

mass index improved and the prevalence of LVH decreased from 54 to 8% in transplanted children in comparison to the same children being on dialysis, and these positive changes of cardiac structure were associated with decrease of systolic and diastolic BP index *(119)*.

Acknowledgments

Supported by the Ministry of Education of the Czech Republic VZ MŠMT No 0021620819 and Ministry of Health VZ MZ No 0006420301, MZOFNM2005.

REFERENCES

1. Frauman AC, Lansing LM, Fennell RS. Indirect blood pressure measurement in undergoing hemodialysis: a comparison of brachial and dorsalis pedis auscultatory sites. AANNT J. 1984;11:19–21.
2. Park MK, Lee DH, Johnson GA. Oscillometric blood pressures in the arm, thigh, and calf in healthy children and those with aortic coarctation. Pediatrics. 1993;91:761–765.
3. Rahman M, Griffin V, Kumar A, Manzoor F, Wright FJ Jr, Smith MC. A comparison of standardized versus "usual" blood pressure measurements in hemodialysis patients. Am J Kidney Dis. 2002;39: 1226–1230.
4. Menard SW, Park MK, Yuan CH. The San Antonio Biethnic Children's Blood Pressure Study: auscultatory findings. J Pediatr Health Care. 1999;13:237–244.
5. Coomer RW, Schulman G, Breyer JA, Shyr Y. Ambulatory blood pressure monitoring in dialysis patients and estimation of mean interdialytic blood pressure. Am J Kidney Dis. 1997;29:678–684.
6. Luik AJ, Kooman P, Leuwissen KML. Hypertension in haemodialysis patients: is it only hypervolemia? Nephrol Dial Transplant. 1997;12:1557–1560.
7. Conion PJ, Walshe JJ, Heinle S. Predialysis systolic blood pressure correlates strongly with mean 24-hour systolic blood pressure and left ventricular mass in stable hemodialysis patients. J Am Soc Nephrol. 1996;7:2658–2663.
8. Sankaranarayaan N, Santos SF, Peixoto AJ. Blood pressure measurement in dialysis patients. Adv Chron Kidney Dis. 2004;11:134–142.
9. Ritz E, Schwenger V, Zeier M, Rychlik I. Ambulatory blood pressure monitoring: fancy gadgetry or clinically useful exercise? Nephrol Dial Transplant. 2001;16:1550–1554.
10. Koch VH, Furusawa EA, Ignes E, Okay Y, Mion Junior D. Ambulatory blood pressure monitoring in chronically dialyzed pediatric patients. Blood Press Monit. 1999;4:213–216.
11. Lingens N, Soergel M, Loirat C, Busch D, Lemmer B, Schärer K. Ambulatory blood pressure monitoring in pediatric patients treated by regular haemodialysis and peritoneal dialysis. Pediatr Nephrol. 1995;9:167–172.
12. Peixoto AJ, Santos SF, Mendes RB, Crowley ST, Maldonado R, Orias M, Mansoor GA, White WB. Am J Kidney Dis. 2000;36:983–990.
13. Sorof JM, Brewer ED, Portman RJ. Ambulatory blood pressure monitoring and interdialytic weight gain in children receiving chronic hemodialysis. Am J Kidney Dis. 1999;33:667–674.
14. Covic A, Goldsmith D. Ambulatory blood pressure monitoring: an essential tool for blood pressure assessment in uraemic patients. Nephrol Dial Transplant. 2002;17:1737–1741.
15. Peixoto AJ, White WB. Ambulatory blood pressure monitoring in chronic renal disease: technical aspects and clinical relevance. Curr Opin Nephrol Hypertens. 2002;11:507–516.
16. Sorof JM. Ambulatory blood pressure monitoring in pediatric end-stage renal disease: chronic dialysis and transplantation. Blood Press Monit. 1999;4:171–174.
17. Bald M, Böhm W, Feldhoff C, Bonzel KE. Home blood pressure self-measurement in children and adolescents with renal replacement therapy. Klin Padiatr. 2001;213:21–25.
18. National High Blood Pressure Education Program Working Group on High Blood Pressure in Children and Adolescents. The fourth report on the diagnosis, evaluation, and treatment of high blood pressure in children and adolescents. Pediatrics. 2004;114:555–557.
19. Soergel M, Kirschstein M, Busch C, Danne T, Gellermann J, Holl R, Krull F, Reichert H, Reusz GS, Rascher W. Oscillometric twenty-four-hour ambulatory blood pressure values in healthy children and adolescents: a multicenter trial including 1141 subjects. J Pediatr. 1997;130:178–184.
20. Schärer K, Rauh W, Ulmer HE. The management of hypertension in children with chronic renal failure. In: Giovannelli G, New MI, Gorini S, eds. Hypertension in Children and Adolescents. New York, NY: Raven; 1981:239–250.

21. Loirat C, Ehrich JH, Geerlings W, Jones EH, Landais P, Loirat C, Mallick NP, Margreiter R, Raine AE, Salmela K. Report on management of renal failure in Europe XXII, 1992. Nephrol Dial Transplant. 1994;9(Suppl 1):26–40.

22. Lerner GR, Warady BA, Sullivan EK, Alexander SR. Chronic dialysis in children and adolescents. The 1996 report of the North American Pediatric Renal Transplant Cooperative Study. Pediatr Nephrol. 1999;13:404–417.

23. VanDeVoorde RG, Barletta GM, Chand DH, Dresner IG, Lane J, Leiser J, Lin JJ, Pan CG, Patel H, Valentini RP, Mitsnefes MM. Blood pressure control in pediatric hemodialysis: the Midwest pediatric nephrology consortium Study. Pediatr Nephrol. 2007;22:547–553.

24. Schaefer F, Klaus G, Müller-Wiefel D, Mehls O. Mid-European Pediatric Peritoneal Dialysis Study Group. Current practice of peritoneal dialysis in children: results of a longitudinal survey. Perit Dial Int. 1999;19:S445–S449.

25. Mitsnefes MM, Stablein D. Hypertension in pediatric patients on long-term dialysis: a report of the North American Pediatric Renal Transplant Cooperative Study (NAPRTCS). Am J Kidney Dis. 2005;45: 309–315.

26. Tkaczyk M, Nowicki M, Balasz-Chmielewska I, et al. Hypertension in dialysed children: the prevalence and therapeutic approach in Poland—a nationwide survey. Nephrol Dial Transplant. 2006;21: 736–742.

27. Amar J, Vernier I, Rossignol E, Bongard V, Arnaud C, Conte JJ, Salvador M, Chamontin B. Nocturnal blood pressure and 24-hour pulse pressure are potent indicators of mortality in hemodialysis patients. Kidney Int. 2000;57:2485–2491.

28. Liu M, Takahashi H, Morita Y, Maruyama S, Mizumo M, Yuzawa Y, Watanabe M, Toriyama T, Kawahara H, Matsuo S. Non-dipping is a potent predictor of cardiovascular mortality and is associated with autonomic dysfunction in haemodialysis patients. Nephrol Dial Transplant. 2003;18:563–569.

29. Holttä T, Happonen JM, Rönnholm K, Fyhrquist F, Holmberg C. Hypertension, cardiac state, and the role of volume overload during peritoneal dialysis. Pediatr Nephrol. 2001;16:324–331.

30. Guyton AC, Granger HJ, Coleman TG. Autoregulation of the total systemic circulation and its relation to control of cardiac output and arterial pressure. Circ Res. 1971;28(Suppl 1):93–97.

31. Charra B, Bergstrom J, Scribner BH. Blood pressure control in dialysis patients: importance of the lag phenomenon. Am J Kidney Dis. 1998;32:720–724.

32. Katzarski KS, Charra B, Luik AJ, Nisell J, Divino Filho JC, Leypoldt JK, Leunissen KM, Laurent G, Bergström J. Fluid state and blood pressure control in patients treated with long and short hemodialysis. Nephrol Dial Transplant. 1999;14:369–375.

33. Hörl MP, Hörl WH. Hemodialysis-associated hypertension: pathophysiology and therapy. Am J Kidney Dis. 2002;39:227–244.

34. Rauh W, Hund E, Sohl G, Rascher W, Mehls O, Schärer K. Vasoactive hormones in children with chronic renal failure. Kidney Int. 1983;24(Suppl 15):16–21.

35. Mailloux LU. Hypertension in chronic renal failure and ESRD: prevalence, pathophysiology, and outcomes. Semin Nephrol. 2001;21:146–156.

36. Orth SR, Amann K, Strojek K, Ritz E. Sympathetic overactivity and arterial hypertension in renal failure. Nephrol Dial Transplant. 2001;16(Suppl 1):67–69.

37. Converse RL Jr, Jacobsen TN, Toto RD, Jost CM, Cosentino F, Fouad-Tarazi F, Victor RG. Sympathetic overactivity in patients with chronic renal failure. N Engl J Med. 1992;327:1912–1928.

38. Ritz E, Amann K, Törnig J, Schwartz U, Stein G. Some cardiac abnormalities in renal failure. Adv Nephrol. 1997;27:85–103.

39. Erkan E, Devarajan P, Kaskel F. Role of nitric oxide, endothelin-1, and inflammatory cytokines in blood pressure regulation in hemodialysis patients. Am J Kidney Dis. 2002;40:76–81.

40. Passauer J, Bussemaker E, Range U, Plug M, Gross P. Evidence in vivo showing increase of nitric oxide generation and impairment of endothelium dependent vasodilatation in normotensive patients on chronic hemodialysis. J Am Soc Nephrol. 2000;11:1726–1734.

41. Xiao S, Wagner L, Schmidt RJ, Baylis C. Circulating endothelial nitric oxide synthase inhibitory factor in some patients with chronic renal disease. Kidney Int. 2001;59:1466–1472.

42. Wang S, Vicente FB, Miller A, Brooks ER, Price HE, Smith FA. Measurement of arginine derivates in pediatric patients with chronic kidney disease using high-performance liquid chromatography-tandem mass spectrometry. Clin Chem Lab Med. 2007;45:1305–1312.

43. Menon MK, Naimark DM, Bargman JM, Vas SI, Oreopoulos DG. Long-term blood pressure control in a cohort of peritoneal dialysis patients and its association with residual renal function. Nephrol Dial Transplant. 2001;16:2207–2213.

44. Schärer K, Benninger C, Heimann A, Rascher W. Involvement of the central nervous system in renal hypertension. Eur J Pediatr. 1993;152:59–63.

45. Schärer K, Schmidt KG, Soergel M. Cardiac function and structure in patients with chronic renal failure. Pediatr Nephrol. 1999;13:951–965.

46. Colan SD, Sanders SP, Ingelfinger JR, Harmon W. Left ventricular mechanics and contractile state in children and young adults with end-stage renal disease: effect of dialysis and transplantation. J Am Coll Cardiol. 1987;10:1085–1094.

47. Goren A, Glaser I, Drukker A. Diastolic function in children and adolescents on dialysis and after kidney transplantation: an echocardiographic assessment. Pediatr Nephrol. 1993;7:725–728.

48. Middleton RJ, Parfrey PS, Foley RN. Left ventricular hypertrophy in the renal patient. J Am Soc Nephrol. 2001;12:1079–1084.

49. London GM. The concept of ventricular vascular coupling: functional and structural alterations of the hearth and arterial vessels of the heart go in parallel. Nephrol Dial Transplant. 1998;13:250–253.

50. Mitsnefes MM, Daniels SR, Schwartz SM, Khoury P, Strife CF. Changes in left ventricular mass in children and adolescents during chronic dialysis. Pediatr Nephrol. 2001;16:318–325.

51. Mitsnefes MM, Barletta GM, Dresner IG, Chand DH, Geary D, Lin JJ, Patel H. Severe cardiac hypertrophy and long-term dialysis: the Midwest Pediatric Nephrology Consortium study. Pediatr Nephrol. 2006;21:1167–1170.

52. De Simone G, Devereux RB, Daniels SR, Koren MJ, Meyer RA, Laragh JH. Effect of growth on variability of left ventricular mass: assessment of allometric signals in adults and children and their capacity to predict cardiovascular risk. J Am Coll Cardiol. 1995;25:1056–1062.

53. Mitsnefes MM, Daniels SR, Schwartz SM, Meyer RA, Khoury P, Strife CF. Severe left ventricular hypertrophy in pediatric dialysis: prevalence and predictors. Pediatr Nephrol. 2000;14:898–902.

54. Washio M, Okuda S, Mizou CT, Mizoue T, Kiyama S, Ando T, Sanai T, Hirakata H, Nanishi F, Kiyohara C, Ogimoto I, Fujishima M. Risk factors for left ventricular hypertrophy in chronic hemodialysis patients. Clin Nephrol. 1997;47:362–366.

55. London GM, Pannier B, Guerin AP, Blacher J, Marchais SJ, Darne B, Metivier F, Adda H, Safar ME. Alterations of left ventricular hypertrophy and survival of patients receiving hemodialysis: follow-up of an interventional study. J Am Soc Nephrol. 2001;12:2759–2767.

56. Chan CF, Floras JS, Miller JA, Richardson RM, Pierratos A. Regression of left ventricular hypertrophy after conversion to nocturnal hemodialysis. Kidney Int. 2002;61:2235–2239.

57. Ulinski T, Genty J, Viau C, Tillous-Borde I, Deschenes G. Reduction of left ventricular hypertrophy in children undergoing hemodialysis. Pediatr Nephrol. 2006;21:1171–1178.

58. Goodman WG, Goldin J, Kuizon BD, Yoon C, Gales B, Sider D, Wang Y, Chung J, Emerick A, Greaser L, Elashoff RM, Salusky IB. Coronary artery calcification in young adults with end-stage renal disease who are undergoing dialysis. N Engl J Med. 2000;342:1478–1483.

59. Oh J, Wunsch R, Turzer M, Bahner M, Raqqi P, Querfeld U, Mehls O, Schaefer F. Advanced coronary and carotid arteriopathy in young adults with childhood-onset chronic renal failure. Circulation. 2002;106:100–105.

60. Civilibal M, Caliskan S, Oflaz H, Sever L, Candan C, Canpolat N, Kasapcopur O, Bugra Z, Arisoy N. Traditional and "new" cardiovascular risk markers and factors in pediatric dialysis patients. Pediatr Nephrol. 2007;22:1021–1029.

61. Amar J, Vernier I, Rossignol E. Nocturnal blood pressure and 24-hour pulse pressure are potent indicators of mortality in hemodialysis patients. Kidney Int. 2000;57:2485–2491.

62. Foley RN, Herzog CA, Collins AJ. Blood pressure and long-term mortality in United States hemodialysis patients: USRDS waves 3 and 4 study. Kidney Int. 2002;62:1784–1790.

63. Mailloux LU, Haley WE. Hypertension in the ESRD patient: pathophysiology, therapy, outcomes, and future directions. Am J Kidney Dis. 1998;32:705–719.

64. Reiss U, Wingen AM, Schärer K. Mortality trends in pediatric patients with chronic renal failure. Pediatr Nephrol. 1996;10:602–605.

65. Groothoff JW, Gruppen MP, Offringa M, Hutten J, Lilien MR, Van De Kar NJ, Wolff ED, Davin JC, Heymans HS. Mortality and causes of death of end-stage renal disease in children: a Dutch cohort study. Kidney Int. 2002;61:621–629.

66. Parekh RS, Carroll CE, Wolfe RA, Port FK. Cardiovascular mortality in children and young adults with end-stage kidney disease. J Pediatr. 2002;141:191–197.

67. Wühl E, Frisch C, Schärer K, Mehls O. Assessment of total body water in pediatric patients on dialysis. Nephrol Dial Transplant. 1996;11:75–80.

68. Dietel T, Filler G, Grenda R, Wolfish N. Bioimpedance and inferior vena cave diameter for assessment of dialysis dry weight. Pediatr Nephrol. 2000;14:903–907.

69. Patel HP, Goldstein SL, Mahan JD, Smith B, Fried CB, Currier H, Flynn JT. A standard, noninvasive monitoring of hematocrit algorithm improves blood pressure control in pediatric hemodialysis patients. Clin J Am Soc Nephrol. 2007;2:252–257.

70. Cheigh JS, Milite C, Sullivan JF, Rubin AL, Stenzel KH. Hypertension is not adequately controlled in hemodialysis patients. Am J Kidney Dis. 1992;19:453–459.

71. Ifudu O. The concept of "dry weight" in maintenance hemodialysis: flaws in clinical application. Int J Artif. Organs. 1996;7:384–386.

72. Fagugli RM, Reboldi G, Quintalini G, Pasini P, Ciao G, Cicconi B, Pasticci F, Kaufman JM, Buoncristiani U. Short daily hemodialysis: blood pressure control and left ventricular mass reduction in hypertensive hemodialysis patients. Am J Kidney Dis. 2001;38:371–376.

73. Goldstein SL, Silverstein DM, Leung JC, Feig DI, Soletsky B, Knight C, Warady BA. Frequent hemodialysis with NxStage system in pediatric patients receiving maintenance hemodialysis. Pediatr Nephrol. 2008;23:129–135.

74. Krautzig S, Janssen U, Koch KM, Granolleeras S, Shaldon S. Dietary salt restriction and reduction of dialysate sodium to control hypertension in maintenance hemodialysis patients. Nephrol Dial Transplant. 1998;13:552–553.

75. Feber J, Schärer K, Schaefer F, Míková M, Janda J. Residual renal function in children on haemodialyis and peritoneal dialysis therapy. Pediatr Nephrol. 1994;8:579–583.

76. Özkahya M, Ok E, Cirit M, Aydin S, Akcicek F, Basci A, Dorhout Mees EJ. Regression of left ventricular hypertrophy in hemodialysis patients by ultrafiltration and reduced salt intake without antihypertensive drugs. Nephrol Dial Transplant. 1998;13:1489–1493.

77. Flanigan MJ, Khairullah QT, Lim VS. Dialysate sodium delivery can alter chronic blood pressure management. Am J Kidney Dis. 1997;29:383–391.

78. Kjeldsen SE. Julius S. Hypertension mega-trials with cardiovascular end points: effect of angiotensin-converting enzyme inhibitors and angiotensin receptor blockers. Am Heart J. 2004;148:747–754.

79. Baluarte HJ, Gruskin AB, Ingelfinger JR, Tejani A. Analysis of hypertension in children post renal transplantation—a report of the North American Pediatric Renal Transplant Cooperative Study (NAPRTCS). Pediatr Nephrol. 1994;8:570–573.

80. Sorof JM, Sullivan EK, Tejani A, Portman RJ. Antihypertensive medication and renal allograft failure: A North American Pediatric Renal Transplant Cooperative Study report. J Am Soc Nephrol. 1999;10: 1324–1330.

81. Tutone VK, Mark PB, Stewart GA, Tan CC, Rodger RSC, Geddes CC, Jardine AG. Hypertension, antihypertensive agents and outcomes following renal transplantation. Clin Transplant. 2005;19:181–192.

82. Opelz G, Wujciak T, Ritz E for the Collaborative Transplant Study. Association of chronic kidney graft failure with recipient blood pressure. Kidney Int. 1998;53:217–222.

83. Mitsnefes MM, Omoloja A, McEnery PT. Short-term pediatric renal transplant survival: blood pressure and allograft function. Pediatr Transpl. 2001;5:160–165.

84. Mitsnefes MM, Khoury PR, McEnery PT. Early posttransplantation hypertension and poor long-term renal allograft survival in pediatric patients. J Pediatr. 2003;143:98–103.

85. Mitsnefes MM, Portman RJ. Ambulatory blood pressure monitoring in pediatric renal transplantation. Pediatr Transplant. 2003;7:86–92.

86. Jacobi J, Rockstroh J, John S, Schreiber M, Schlaich MP, Neumayer HH, Schmieder RE. Prospective analysis of the value of 24-hour ambulatory blood pressure on renal function after kidney transplantation. Transplantation. 2000;70:819–827.

87. Morgan H, Khan I, Hashmi A, Hebert D, Balfe JW. Ambulatory blood pressure monitoring after renal transplantation in children. Pediatr Nephrol. 2001;16:843–847.

88. Seeman T, Šimková E, Kreisinger J, Vondrák K, Dušek J, Gilík J, Feber J, Dvořák P, Janda J. Control of hypertension in children after renal transplantation. Pediatr Transplant. 2006;10:316–322.

89. Lipkin GW, Tucker B, Giles M, Raine AE. Ambulatory blood pressure and left ventricular mass in cyclosporin- and non-cyclosporin-treated renal transplant recipients. J Hypertens. 1993;11:439–442.

90. McGlothan KR, Wyatt RJ, Ault BH, Hastings MC, Rogers T, DiSessa T, Jones DP. Predominance of nocturnal hypertension in pediatric renal allograft recipients. Pediatr Transplant. 2006;10: 558–564.

91. Vianello A, Mastrosimone S, Calconi G, Gatti PL, Calzavara P, Maresca MC. The role of hypertension as damaging factor for kidney grafts under cyclosporine therapy. Am J Kidney Dis. 1993;21(Suppl 1): 79–83.

92. Gordjani A, Offner G, Hoyer PF, Brodehl J. Hypertension after renal transplantation in patients treated with cyclosporine and azathioprine. Arch Dis Child. 1990;65:275–279.

93. El-Husseini AA, Foda MA, Shokeir AA, Shebab El-Din AB, Sobh MA, Ghoneim MA. Determinants of graft survival in pediatric and adolescent live donor kidney transplant recipients: a single center experience. Pediatr Transplant. 2005;9:763–760.

94. Kasiske BL, Ballantyne CM. Cardiovascular risk associated with immunosuppression in renal transplantation. Transplant Rev. 2002;16:1–21.

95. Hocker B, John U, Plank C, Wuhl E, Weber LT, Misselwitz J, Rascher W, Mehls O, Tonshoff B. Successful withdrawal of steroids in pediatrics renal transplant recipients receiving cyclosporine A and mycopheno-late mofetil treatment: results after four years. Transplantation. 2004;78:228–234.

96. Sarwal MM, Vidhun JR, Alexander SR, Satterwhite T, Millan M, Salvatierra O Jr. Continued superior out-come with modification and lengthened follow-up of a steroid-avoidance pilot with extended daclizumab induction in pediatric renal transplantation. Transplantation. 2003;76:1331–1339.

97. Curtis JJ, Galla JH, Kotchen TA, Lucas B, McRoberts JW, Luke RG. Prevalence of hypertension in a renal transplant population on alternate-day steroid therapy. Clin Nephrol. 1976;5:123–127.

98. Büscher R, Vester U, Wingen AM, Hoyer PF. Pathomechanisms and the diagnosis of arterial hypertension in pediatric renal allograft recipients. Pediatr Nephrol. 2004;19:1202–1211.

99. Trompeter R, Filler G, Webb NJ, Watson AR, Milford DV, Tyden G, Grenda R, Janda J, Hughes D, Ehrich JH, Klare B, Zacchello G, Bjorn Brekke I, McGraw M, Perner F, Ghio L, Balzar E, Friman S, Gusmano R, Stolpe J. Randomized trial of tacrolimus versus cyclosporin microemulsion in renal transplantation. Pediatr Nephrol. 2002;17:141–149.

100. Cheigh JS, Haschemeyer RH, Wang JCL, Riggio RR, Tapia L, Stenzel KH, Rubin AL. Hypertension in kidney transplant recipients. Effect on long-term renal allograft survival. Am J Hypertens. 1989;2: 341–348.

101. Lurbe E, Alvarez V, Liao Y, Tacons J, Cooper R, Cremades B, Torro I, Redon J. The impact of obesity and body fat distribution on ambulatory blood pressure in children and adolescents. Am J Hypertens. 1998;11:418–424.

102. Hanevold CD, Ho PL, Talley L, Mitsnefes MM. Obesity and renal transplant outcome: a report of the North American Pediatric Renal Transplant Cooperative Study. Pediatrics. 2005;115:352–356.

103. Fung LC, McLorie GA, Khoury AR. Donor aortic cuff reduces the rate of anastomotic arterial stenosis in pediatric renal transplantation. J Urol. 1995;154:909–913.

104. Matteucci MC, Giordano U, Calzolari A, Turchetta A, Santilli A, Rizzoni G. Left ventricular hypertro-phy, treadmill tests, and 24-hour blood pressure in pediatric transplant patients. Kidney Int. 1999;56: 1566–1570.

105. Kitzmueller E, Vécsei A, Pichler J, Bohm M, Muller T, Vargha R, Csaicsich D, Aufricht C. Changes of blood pressure and left ventricular mass in pediatric renal transplantation. Pediatr Nephrol. 2004;19: 1385–1389.

106. Kasiske BL, Guijarro C, Massy ZA, Wiederkehr MR, Ma JZ. Cardiovascular disease after renal trans-plantation. J Am Soc Nephrol. 1996;7:158–165.

107. Curtis JJ. Treatment of hypertension in renal allograft patients: Does drug selection make a difference. Kidney Int. 1997;52(Suppl 63):S75–S77.

108. Stigant CE, Cohen J, Vivera M, Zaltzman JS. ACE inhibitors and angiotensin II antagonists in renal transplantation: an analysis of safety and efficacy. Am J Kidney Dis. 2000;35:58–63.

109. Arbeiter K, Pichler A, Stemberger R, Mueller T, Ruffingshofer D, Vargha R, Balzar E, Aufricht C. ACE inhibition in the treatment of children after renal transplantation. Pediatr Nephrol. 2004;19: 222–226.

110. Heinze G, Mitterbauer C, Regele H, Kramar R, Winkelmayer WC, Curhan GC, Oberbauer R. Angiotensin-converting enzyme inhibitor or angiotensin II type 1 receptor antagonist therapy is associated with prolonged patient and graft survival after renal transplantation. J Am Soc Nephrol. 2006;17:889–899.

111. Opelz G, Zeier M, Laux G, Morath C, Dohler B. No improvement of patient or graft survival in trans-plant recipients treated with angiotensin-converting enzyme inhibitors or angiotensin II type 1 receptor blockers: a collaborative transplant study report. J Am Soc Nephrol. 2006;17:3257–3262.

112. Calvino J, Lens XM, Romero R, Sánchez-Guisande D. Long-term anti-proteinuric effect of losartan in renal transplant recipients treated for hypertension. Nephrol Dial Transplant. 2000;15:82–86.

113. Hausberg M, Barenbrock M, Hohage H, Müller S, Heidenreich S, Rahn KH. ACE inhibitor ver-sus β-blocker for the treatment of hypertension in renal allograft recipients. Hypertension. 1999;33: 862–868.

114. Task force on cardiovascular disease. Special report from the National Kidney Foundation. Am J Kidney Dis. 1998;32(Suppl 3):1–121.

115. Schaefer F. Intensified blood pressure control in pediatric chronic kidney disease: results of the ESCAPE trial. Pediatr Nephrol. 2007;22:1415.

116. Flynn JT. Hypertension and future cardiovascular disease in pediatric renal transplant recipients. Pediatr Transplant. 2006;10:276–278.

117. Opelz G, Dohler B. Collaborative Transplant Study. Improved long-term outcomes after renal transplan-tation associated with blood pressure control. Am J Transplant. 2005;5:2725–2731.

118. Seeman T, Šimková E, Kreisinger J, Vondrák K, Dušek J, Gilík J, Dvořák P, Janda J. Improved control of hypertension in children after renal transplantation: Results of a two-yr interventional trial. Pediatr Transplant. 2007;11:491–497.
119. Becker-Cohen R, Nir A, Ben-Shalom E, Rinat C, Feinstein S, Farber B, Frishberg Y. Improved left ventricular mass index in children after renal transplantation. Pediatr Nephrol. 2008;23:1545–1550.

24 Sequelae of Hypertension in Children and Adolescents

Donald J. Weaver, Jr, MD, PhD
and Mark M. Mitsnefes, MD, MS

CONTENTS

INTRODUCTION
SEQUELAE OF CHRONIC HYPERTENSION
SEQUELAE OF ACUTE HYPERTENSIVE CRISIS
CONCLUSIONS
REFERENCES

INTRODUCTION

Hypertension is a significant public health challenge because of its high prevalence as well as its associated complications including cerebrovascular disease, renal failure, and heart failure *(1)*. In fact, hypertension is the second leading cause of end-stage renal disease (ESRD) among adults in the USA *(2)*. Moreover, hypertension is the leading risk factor for cardiovascular mortality and ranked third as a cause of disability-adjusted life years in adults *(1,3)*. A recent study examining the economic burden of chronic cardiovascular disease suggested that medical expenditures attributable to hypertension account for 8% of annual US healthcare costs at more than 20 billion dollars *(3)*. There is also increasing evidence that the pathogenesis of hypertension begins in childhood, and hypertension in children is a risk factor for development of adult cardiovascular disease *(4,5)*. However, hypertension in children is often underdiagnosed, and the alterations in end-organ structure and function noted in adult hypertensive patients begin in childhood *(6,7)*. Since treatment of hypertension has been shown to improve cardiovascular outcomes and to reduce the risk for development of these complications in the adult population, prompt recognition of these alterations in children and adolescents may prevent future morbidity and mortality in these patients *(8)*.

D.J. Weaver (✉)
Division of Nephrology and Hypertension, Department of Pediatrics, Levine Children's Hospital at Carolinas Medical Center, Charlotte, NC, USA
e-mail: jack.weaver@carolinashealthcare.org

From: *Clinical Hypertension and Vascular Diseases: Pediatric Hypertension*
Edited by: J. T. Flynn et al. DOI 10.1007/978-1-60327-824-9_24
© Springer Science+Business Media, LLC 2011

SEQUELAE OF CHRONIC HYPERTENSION

Primary hypertension in children and adolescents is generally thought to be an asymptomatic disease not associated with emergent adverse events. However, even in the early stages of hypertension, children and adolescents experience nonspecific symptoms that can impact lifestyle. Croix and Feig *(9)* recently reported that hypertensive children at initial evaluation are more likely to experience sleep disturbances and daytime fatigue than normotensive children. Moreover, 64% of hypertensive children are more likely to complain of nonspecific symptoms including headache, chest pain, and shortness of breath than normotensive children at initial evaluation *(9)*. More strikingly, treatment of hypertension significantly reduced the prevalence of these complaints 6 months following initiation of therapy highlighting the importance of screening and recognition of early hypertension *(9)*. In addition to the symptoms described above that affect quality of life and school performance, childhood hypertension leads to abnormalities in several organ systems with the potential for significant long-term morbidity as outlined below (Table 1).

Table 1
End-Organ Alterations in Pediatric Patients with
Chronic Hypertension

Cardiac structure
     Increased left atrial size
     Left ventricular hypertrophy
Cardiac function
     Diastolic dysfunction
Vascular structure
     Increased cIMT
     Arterial stiffening
     Atheromatous changes
Renal function
     Microalbuminuria
Retinal vasculature
     Arteriolar narrowing
     Tortuosity
     AV nicking
Cognition
     Short-term memory
     Attention/concentration

Cardiac Structure and Function

Hypertension is a major risk factor for development of congestive heart failure, and randomized controlled trials have demonstrated a consistent decrease in risk for development of congestive heart failure upon lowering of elevated blood pressure in adults *(10,11)*. In the classical paradigm for the pathogenesis of hypertensive heart disease, development of LV failure is preceded by alterations in both left atrial and ventricular geometry *(12)*. The changes in ventricular geometry occur in two different patterns *(12)*. In concentric

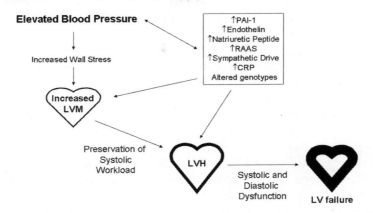

Fig. 1. Pathogenesis of left ventricular hypertrophy in pediatric patients with chronic hypertension. Renin–angiotensin–aldosterone axis (RAAS), left ventricular mass (LVM), left ventricular hypertrophy (LVH), C-reactive protein (CRP), plasminogen activator inhibitor-1 (PAI-1).

LV hypertrophy, parallel addition of sarcomeres causes an increase in the cross-sectional area and diameter of the cardiac myocytes *(13)*. These alterations lead to a significant increase in LV wall thickness out of proportion to an increase in size of the LV cavity *(13)*. In contrast, a symmetric increase in wall thickness as well as LV cavity size results in eccentric LVH as a result of sarcomere addition in series. Hypertension is generally associated with development of concentric hypertrophy as increased blood pressure and pulse pressure oppose LV ejection inducing increased LV wall stress (Fig. 1) *(14)*. In addition to left ventricular stress, numerous nonhemodynamic factors are thought to influence the development of altered left ventricular geometry including neurohormonal activation, biomarkers of inflammation, and hemostatic factors (Fig. 1) *(15–19)*. Recently, a central role for the renin–angiotensin–aldosterone axis (RAAS) was proposed based on a cross-sectional study examining the contribution of several biomarkers including C-reactive protein, plasminogen activator inhibitor-1, B-type natriuretic peptide, renin, and aldosterone *(20)*. The investigators found that the aldosterone–renin ratio alone was significantly associated with development of both concentric and eccentric remodeling *(20)*. Regardless of the mechanism, these alterations are thought to provide for normalization of afterload and preservation of systolic performance early in the development of hypertension (Fig. 1) *(15)*. However, as myocardial oxygen demand increases due to increased cardiac mass and persistently elevated wall stress, a decrease in coronary artery oxygen reserve is noted leading to increased apoptosis and cardiac cell death (Fig. 1) *(15)*. Furthermore, abnormalities in myocardial electrical conduction in the hypertrophied muscle also trigger the development of arrhythmias.

In terms of atrial structure, left atrial enlargement is associated with duration of elevated blood pressure, the levels of sustained systolic blood pressure, and pulse pressure in the general adult population *(21)*. However, only age, race, and obesity were significant predictors of left atrial size in hypertensive adults *(22)*. Although not consistently associated with hypertension, the presence of left atrial enlargement is significant because it is associated with development of cardiac arrhythmias, cerebrovascular events, and death in hypertensive adults *(23)*. Although data are limited in the pediatric population, Daniels et al. *(24)* studied a cohort of 112 pediatric patients with hypertension and found that 51% of patients had left atrial dimensions above the 95% upper confidence limit. In statistical analysis, height, body mass index, and systolic blood pressure were independent predictors for left atrial enlargement *(24)*. Interestingly, left ventricular geometry was also an independent predictor of left atrial size, and children with eccentric left ventricular hypertrophy demonstrated increased left atrial size compared to patients with other forms of left ventricular geometry *(24)*. Although the cross-sectional nature of this study prevented elucidation of cause and effect, the authors speculated that the hypertrophied left ventricle may demonstrate impaired diastolic filling necessitating increased left atrial mass *(24)*. The prognostic value of these findings in pediatric patients remains to be determined.

Left ventricular hypertrophy is a frequent finding in adults with hypertension. Data from several studies have suggested that the prevalence of left ventricular hypertrophy in hypertensive adults ranges from 33 to 81% *(25,26)*. More importantly, LVH has been noted to be a risk factor for cardiovascular disease, cardiovascular morbidity, ventricular arrhythmias, and cardiovascular death *(27,28)*. Abnormalities in left ventricular structure are also present in 40% of children and adolescents with hypertension *(29,30)*. A recent retrospective analysis demonstrated that the prevalence of LVH increased with severity of hypertension. Specifically, patients with normal blood pressures were noted to have a prevalence of LVH of 5.7%, whereas patients with stage 1 hypertension had a prevalence of 18% compared to 32% in patients with stage 2 hypertension *(31)*. A separate study of 184 children who were referred for evaluation of hypertension at three centers demonstrated a prevalence of LVH of 41% at initial presentation *(32)*. In this study, children with LVH were more likely to have a higher BMI and to be non-white compared to those without LVH. Surprisingly, after controlling for age, sex, and height, no associations between blood pressure parameters at the initial visit and LVH were detected *(32)*. In contrast, Richey et al. *(33)* detected associations between development of LVH and systolic blood pressure as well as 24-h systolic blood pressure load. In addition, LVM has correlated with serum uric acid and homocysteine levels *(30)*.

In addition to LV structure, diastolic dysfunction is a well-recognized complication of hypertension in adults affecting up to 45% of patients even in the absence of LV hypertrophy *(34)*. Similar findings have been reported in pediatric patients with hypertension *(35,36)*. Recently, Border et al. *(37)* compared the ventricular function of 50 pediatric patients with essential hypertension to 53 normotensive, healthy controls. In agreement with other reports, the authors did not detect any differences in markers of systolic function including shortening fraction, ejection fraction, or midwall shortening between the two groups *(37)*. However, when indices of both ventricular relaxation and compliance were measured using both M-mode and tissue Doppler echocardiography, significant differences between the two groups were observed *(37)*. When compared to the controls, 39% of hypertensive patients demonstrated abnormal left ventricular compliance similar to adult studies *(37)*. Regression analysis revealed that LV mass was the only significant predictor of LV compliance, whereas BMI predicted LV relaxation providing further evidence that compensatory changes in LV geometry could lead to maladaptive alterations in LV function *(37)*.

Vascular Structure

In parallel with cardiac abnormalities, hypertension induces alterations in the structure and function of the arterial tree *(38)*. The mechanisms underlying these changes are multifactorial and incompletely understood (Fig. 2) *(39,40)*. Increased pulse pressure in

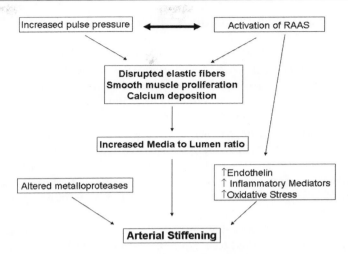

Fig. 2. Vascular adaptation in pediatric patients with chronic hypertension. Renin–angiotensin–aldosterone axis (RAAS).

hypertension alters the orderly arrangement of elastic fibers within the media of the artery leading to fragmentation and an associated increase in both collagen and calcium deposition within the vascular wall (Fig. 2) *(39)*. Because elastin influences smooth muscle proliferation and migration, this redistribution of elastin fibers leads to dedifferentiation of smooth muscle cells and arterial wall hypertrophy (Fig. 2) *(40)*. Mechanical stress also alters the activity of matrix metalloproteinases which are essential for maintenance of the extracellular matrix of the arterial wall (Fig. 2) *(39)*. Continued wall stress enhances production of endothelin, a potent vasoconstrictor which when combined with other inflammatory mediators contributes to significant endothelial dysfunction (Fig. 2). Ultimately, these changes lead to structural reduction of the arterial lumen diameter and increased arterial stiffness (Fig. 2) *(39)*.

To evaluate these alterations, vascular ultrasound has emerged as a noninvasive means to assess changes in vascular structure and risk of future cardiovascular events *(41)*. Specifically, altered carotid artery intimal–medial thickness (cIMT) has been demonstrated to be a surrogate marker for the presence and degree of atherosclerosis as well as for occurrence of future coronary events in adults *(41)*. In a study of 32 patients referred to a pediatric hypertension clinic, 28% of patients demonstrated increased cIMT *(42)*. Although associations with blood pressure parameters were not detected in their analysis, the presence of increased cIMT was significantly associated with the presence of LVH suggesting a common pathway of cardiovascular adaptation to increased pressure and wall stress *(42)*. Similarly, in the Bogalusa Heart Study, office-based systolic and diastolic blood pressures in childhood did not predict cIMT in adulthood *(43)*. Lande et al. *(44)* compared the cIMT results of 28 patients with newly diagnosed hypertension to 28 BMI-matched controls in an effort to control for the confounding effects of obesity on cIMT. These results demonstrated that cIMT was increased in hypertensive children relative to controls independent of BMI *(44)*. Furthermore, a strong correlation was observed between cIMT and several ABPM-based measurements including daytime systolic blood pressure load and daytime systolic blood pressure index *(44)*. In contrast, associations between office-based blood pressure measurements and cIMT were not detected *(44)*. These findings validated previous reports that alterations in the vascular tree occur in childhood and correlate with blood pressure load as assessed by ABPM.

In addition to cIMT, pulse wave velocity is a widely used noninvasive method to assess arterial stiffness *(45)*. In principle, a central pressure wave is generated upon left ventricular contraction during systole. The magnitude and speed of the pressure wave are influenced by multiple factors including left ventricular contraction, blood viscosity, and properties of the arterial tree. The wave advances until it encounters a branch point or other alterations in vascular structure. At that time, the wave is reflected back toward its origin. Physiologically, the reflected wave is important because early in diastole it augments coronary blood flow *(45)*. However, in the presence of noncompliant arteries, the reflected wave returns to central circulation during late systole increasing cardiac workload and decreasing the pressure support for coronary artery blood flow. Using this technology, elevations in childhood blood pressure consistently predicted arterial stiffening in adulthood in the Bogalusa Heart Study *(46)*. A recent report demonstrated that pulse wave velocity is increased in hypertensive adolescents compared to normotensive controls *(47)*. In a separate report, elevated mean blood pressure independently predicted elevated pulse wave velocity in a larger cross-sectional study of over 200 adolescents *(48)*. Together, these studies suggest that arterial compliance and elasticity are impaired early in hypertension.

These findings are also supported by autopsy studies. The Pathobiological Determinants of Atherosclerosis in Youth (PDAY) study examined the role of various risk factors for development of atherosclerosis in 3000 accident victims aged 15–34 years who underwent autopsy *(49)*. In their analysis, hypertension significantly augmented the risk for development of atherosclerosis in the cerebral arteries *(49)*. In a separate follow-up study, hypertension also enhanced formation of raised lesions from fatty streaks in the abdominal aortas *(50)*. Interestingly, this association was only observed in African-American subjects and not in white subjects *(49,50)*. However, the PDAY study used the intimal thickness of the renal arteries as a surrogate marker for blood pressure which may confound the association *(51)*. In contrast, the Bogalusa Heart Study found that systolic and diastolic blood pressures in addition to several other traditional risk factors for cardiovascular disease were associated with development of fatty streaks and fibrous plaques in both the aorta and the coronary arteries *(52,53)*. Together, these studies suggest that elevated blood pressure contributes to both initiation and progression of atherosclerosis.

The Kidneys

Hypertension is the second leading cause of end-stage kidney disease in the USA. However, despite its prevalence, the pathologic mechanisms through which mild, chronic elevations in blood pressure induce alterations in renal function are not completely understood, and histological examinations suggest that multiple molecular pathways may be involved in nephron loss *(54)*. Loss of renal autoregulation as a result of arterial stiffening, low-grade chronic inflammation, oxidative stress, and altered renin–angiotensin activity are all thought to contribute to renal dysfunction in the context of hypertension *(54)*.

Although common in adults, children with elevated blood pressures typically do not demonstrate clinically apparent alterations in renal function. However, subtle alterations in renal function may be present. For example, the presence of microalbuminuria is thought to be an early marker for hypertensive renal disease *(55)*. More importantly, microalbuminuria is associated with increased risk of cardiovascular as well as all-cause mortality in adult patients with primary hypertension *(56)*. As part of the Bogalusa Heart Study,

Hoq et al. *(57)* demonstrated that elevated childhood blood pressure was associated with the development of microalbuminuria in young African-Americans. Although not observed in white subjects, these observations suggest that even early hemodynamic alterations exert subtle alterations in renal function in the context of other specific genetic and environmental factors. In agreement with these findings, Lubrano et al. *(58)* assessed GFR and proteinuria in 146 children with prehypertension as well as 104 normotensive children. Relative to controls, a significant reduction in GFR was detected in patients with prehypertension (90 vs. 110 ml/min/1.73 m^2). Moreover, proteinuria was increased in patients with prehypertension (145 vs. 66 mg/m^2/24 h) *(58)*. Although the GFR and degree of proteinuria reported by the authors did not exceed values accepted as normal, these results suggested that mild elevations in blood pressure may induce subtle impairment in renal function *(58)*.

Studies have also linked the development of changes in renal function to development of cardiovascular complications in hypertensive pediatric patients. Specifically, Assadi *(59)* examined the relationship between left ventricular hypertrophy, microalbuminuria, and C-reactive protein (CRP). In this study, estimated GFR, blood pressure, and left ventricular mass (LVM) were determined in 64 patients referred to pediatric nephrology clinic. The results demonstrated a correlation between blood pressure, LVH, and presence of microalbuminuria *(59)*. In regression analysis, CRP, microalbuminuria, and systolic blood pressure were independent predictors of LVH *(59)*. The author speculates that inflammation and microalbuminuria portend increased cardiovascular risk in pediatric patients with hypertension *(59)*. As a result, pharmacologic regimens that target these parameters may improve cardiovascular outcomes in this patient population *(59)*.

The Retina

In a recent study of 800 hypertensive adult patients, the prevalence of early retinal vascular changes was 78% using direct ophthalmoscopy *(60)*. Several studies have also detected associations between development of hypertensive-induced retinal changes and other macrovascular complications of hypertension such as development of left ventricular hypertrophy and carotid artery stiffness *(61)*. Several population-based studies have also suggested that individuals with retinal microvascular changes have increased cardiovascular morbidity and mortality *(62)*. However, there have been few studies examining retinal alterations in pediatric patients with elevated blood pressures. A small case series of 21 infants with hypertension demonstrated that almost 50% of these patients had retinal microvascular alterations similar to those found in adults *(63)*. In a second study of 97 children with essential hypertension, the prevalence of arteriolar narrowing was 41%, tortuosity was 14%, and arteriovenous nicking was 8% *(64)*. In a separate study, Daniels et al. *(65)* examined the predictors of retinal vascular abnormalities in 50 pediatric patients with essential hypertension. In their analysis, diastolic blood pressure and a smaller rise in systolic blood pressure during exercise were independently associated with vascular anomalies *(65)*. In agreement with these findings, the Singapore Malay Eye Study reported strong associations between retinal arteriolar narrowing and blood pressure in young adults with hypertension *(66)*.

Cognition

In adults, hypertension increases the risk of cerebrovascular disease and stroke. It is also associated with the development of subcortical and periventricular white matter lesions *(67)*. Although the etiology of these lesions is unclear, several studies have suggested that elevated blood pressure impairs cognitive functioning in adults *(67)*. Recently, the

Maine–Syracuse Study examined the cognitive functioning of approximately 1500 patients using multiple domains on the Wechsler Adults Intelligence Scale *(68)*. Significant inverse associations between blood pressure parameters and cognitive functioning were observed including measures of psychomotor speed, concept formation, and abstract reasoning abilities *(68)*. Although limited by its cross-sectional design, these results indicated that hypertension is associated with poor performance in several aspects of cognition *(68)*. In agreement with this, Lande et al. *(69)* recently studied the relationship of elevated blood pressure and cognition in school-age children and adolescents. Of the 5077 children studied, 3.4% and 1.6% had systolic and diastolic blood pressures above the 90th percentile, respectively *(69)*. Children with elevated systolic blood pressures but not with diastolic blood pressures demonstrated lower scores on assessments of short-term memory, attention, and concentration *(69)*. Although limited, these data highlight the need for further assessment of cognitive impairment in children with hypertension as well as the need for vigilant screening for hypertension in children to prevent further deterioration of cognitive functioning.

SEQUELAE OF ACUTE HYPERTENSIVE CRISIS

Central Nervous System

Central nervous system abnormalities are typically the most prevalent of end-organ complications in hypertensive crises in children *(70,71)*. Cerebral autoregulation is responsible for maintaining constant cerebral blood flow despite alterations in blood pressure *(72)*. However, as mean arterial pressure increases, disruption of the vascular endothelium and blood–brain barrier leads to fibrinoid deposition within the vascular lumen *(72)*. The cerebral vasculature will dilate in an effort to improve perfusion, but these changes ultimately lead to edema and microhemorrhages primarily affecting the white matter in the parietal–occipital regions of the brain *(73)*. As an imbalance between oxygen supply and demand develops, cerebral infarction can develop *(73)*. In one case series of pediatric patients, visual symptoms were noted in 9% of children, seizures in 25%, encephalopathy in 25%, facial palsy in 12%, and hemiplegia in 8% *(74)*. Although reversible with appropriate blood pressure control, prompt recognition is required to prevent long-term complications, especially the visual outcome of these patients as there have been reports of permanent decline in visual acuity following treatment of hypertensive crisis *(75–78)*. Browning et al. *(77)* described four cases with vision impairment during an episode of malignant hypertension. Of the cases, two patients demonstrated normalization of visual acuity, whereas two patients with prolonged blood pressures of 220/180 had permanent impairment of visual acuity *(77)*. In contrast, Logan et al. *(78)* reported three cases with permanent reductions in visual acuity despite normal-appearing optic discs. In terms of neurocognitive outcomes, Trompeter et al. *(79)* found that outcomes were not significantly different when compared to a control group that consisted of children with chronic renal disease.

Cardiovascular System

Cardiovascular complications are also common in severe hypertension *(71)*. Activation of the RAAS axis leads to an increase in systemic vascular resistance and increased myocardial oxygen demand as a result of increased left ventricular (LV) wall tension *(80)*. In an attempt to compensate for increased LV tension, myocytes become hypertrophic *(81)*. In addition, enhanced deposition of extracellular matrix within the ventricle occurs further increasing the oxygen demand of the heart. Continued activation of the renin–angiotensin axis results in enhanced sodium absorption and increased total body water further worsening ventricular load *(80)*. Because of increased metabolic demands, focal ischemia can develop impairing both left ventricular contraction and relaxation *(81)*. Ultimately, the left ventricle is unable to overcome the abrupt increase in systemic vascular resistance causing left ventricular failure and congestive heart failure *(82)*. In one case series involving adult and pediatric patients, heart failure was seen in 36% of patients, acute myocardial infarction was seen in 12% of patients, and aortic dissection was noted in 2% of patients *(74)*. It is important to emphasize that clinical findings of congestive heart failure are especially common in neonates with severe hypertension *(83)*.

The Kidneys

Acute renal insufficiency due to altered renal autoregulation and subsequent renal ischemia is also a complication of severe hypertension *(71)*. Similar to the central nervous system, renal autoregulation provides for constant renal blood flow and glomerular filtration between mean arterial pressures of 80 and 160 mmHg. However, at extremes of arterial pressure, intraglomerular pressure will fluctuate directly with systemic pressure and the afferent and efferent arterioles are unable to prevent alterations in glomerular filtration leading to ischemia and renal failure. Histologic examination of renal biopsy specimens from patients with renal insufficiency secondary to malignant hypertension demonstrates an obliterative vasculopathy with fibrinoid necrosis and occasional thrombosis of interlobular arteries *(84)*. The presence of thrombosis and microangiopathic hemolysis is thought to portend a poor prognosis *(84)*. In a study of 51 adult patients with malignant hypertension, 46 patients demonstrated renal insufficiency with 67% of patients presenting with a serum creatinine greater than 2.3 mg/dl *(85)*. More importantly, 30% of patients in the study remained on chronic hemodialysis *(85)*. In a study by Gudbrandsson, 50% of patients in hypertensive crisis presented with renal failure *(86)*. In contrast to adults, data examining the prevalence of renal failure in pediatric patients with hypertensive crisis are limited. Several early case studies have suggested a prevalence of 50% with up to one-third of patients requiring renal replacement therapy *(87–90)*. Development of significant hematuria and proteinuria was also detected in these patients *(87,89)*.

CONCLUSIONS

As illustrated above, significant alterations in end-organ structure and function develop in pediatric patients with hypertension. These data reinforce the importance of prompt recognition and treatment of hypertension in the pediatric population. However, additional studies are required to demonstrate the long-term significance of these alterations and the effect of pharmacologic intervention on altering the progression of end-organ damage in the pediatric population. Improved treatment strategies as well as a better understanding of appropriate blood pressure targets should lead to enhanced long-term outcomes in these patients.

REFERENCES

1. Kearney PM, Whelton M, Muntner P, et al. Global burden of hypertension: analysis of worldwide data. Lancet. 2005;365:217–223.
2. United States Renal Data System (USRDS) 2008. Annual Report www.usrds.org.

3. Trogdon JG, Nwaise IA, Tangka FK, et al. The economic burden of chronic cardiovascular disease for major insurers. Health Promot Pract. 2007;8:234–242.
4. Elksabany AM, Urbina EM, Daniels SR, et al. Prediction of adult hypertension by K4 and K5 diastolic blood pressure in children: the Bogalusa Heart Study. J Pediatr. 1998;132:687–692.
5. Chen X, Wang Y. Tracking of blood pressure for childhood to adulthood: a systematic review and meta-regression analysis. Circulation. 2008;117:3171–3180.
6. Hansen ML, Gunn PW, Kaelber DC. Underdiagnosis of hypertension in children and adolescents. JAMA. 2007;298:874–879.
7. Mitsnefes MM. Hypertension in children and adolescents. Pediatr Clin North Am. 2006;53: 493–512.
8. Neaton JD, Grimm RH Jr, Prineas RJ, et al. Treatment of mild hypertension study. Final results. JAMA. 1993;270:713–724.
9. Croix B, Feig DI. Childhood hypertension is not a silent disease. Pediatr Nephrol. 2006;21: 527–532.
10. Haider AW, Larson MG, Franklin SS, et al. Systolic blood pressure, diastolic blood pressure, and pulse pressure as predictors of risk for congestive heart failure in the Framingham Heart Study. Ann Intern Med. 2003;138:10–16.
11. Kostis JB, Davis BR, Cutler J, et al., for the SHEP cooperative Research Group. Prevention of heart failure by antihypertensive drug treatment in older persons with isolated systolic hypertension. JAMA. 1997;278:212–216.
12. Kenchaiah S, Pfeffer MA. Cardiac remodeling in systemic hypertension. Med Clin North Am. 2004;88:115–130.
13. Lorell BH, Carabello BA. Left ventricular hypertrophy: pathogenesis, detection, and prognosis. Circulation. 2000;102:470–479.
14. Opie LH, Commerford PJ, Gersh BJ, et al. Controversies in ventricular remodeling. Lancet. 2006;367: 356–367.
15. Cohn JN, Ferrari R, Sharpe N, on behalf of an International Forum on Cardiac remodeling. Cardiac remodeling-concepts and clinical implications: a consensus paper from an international forum on cardiac remodeling. J Am Coll Cardiol. 2000;35:569–582.
16. Drazner MH. The transition from hypertrophy to failure: How certain are we? Circulation. 2005;112: 936–938.
17. Bowman JC, Steinberg SF, Jiang T, et al. Expression of protein kinase C beta in the heart causes hypertrophy in adult mice and sudden death in neonates. J Clin Invest. 1997;100:2189–2195.
18. Brull D, Dhamrait S, Myerson S, et al. Bradykinin B2BKR receptor polymorphism and left ventricular growth response. Lancet. 2001;358:1155–1156.
19. Muscholl MW, Schunkert H, Muders F, et al. Neurohormonal activity and left ventricular geometry in patients with essential arterial hypertension. Am Heart J. 1998;135:58–66.
20. Velagaleti RS, Gona P, Levy D, et al. Relations of biomarkers representing distinct biological pathways to left ventricular geometry. Circulation. 2008;118:2252–2258.
21. Benjamin EJ, D'Agostino RB, Belanger AJ, et al. Left atrial size and the risk of stroke and death: The Framingham Heart Study. Circulation. 1995;92:835–841.
22. Gottdiener JS, Reda DJ, Williams DW, et al. Left atrial size in hypertensive men: influence of obesity, race, and age. J Am Coll Cardiol. 1997;29:651–658.
23. Vaziri S, Lauer M, Benjamin E, et al. Influence of blood pressure on left atrial size. Hypertension. 1995;25:1155–1160.
24. Daniels SR, Witt SA, Glascock B, et al. Left atrial size in children with hypertension: the influence of obesity, blood pressure, and left ventricular mass. J Pediatr. 2002;141:186–190.
25. Kannel WB, Gordon T, Castelli, et al. Electrocardiographic left ventricular hypertrophy and risk of coronary heart disease: the Framingham study. Ann Intern Med. 1970;72:813–822.
26. Pewsner D, Juni P, Egger M, et al. Accuracy of electrocardiography in diagnosis of left ventricular hypertrophy in arterial hypertension: systematic review. BMJ. 2008;335:711.
27. Levy, D, Garrison RJ, Savage DD, et al. Prognostic implications of echocardiographically determined left ventricular mass in the Framingham Heart Study. N Engl J Med. 1990;322:1561–1566.
28. Verdecchia P, Carini G, Circo A, et al. Left ventricular mass and cardiovascular morbidity in essential hypertension: the MAVI study. J Am Coll Cardiol. 2001;38:1829–1835.
29. Sorof JM, Turner J, Martin DS, et al. Cardiovascular risk factors and sequelae in hypertensive children identified by referral versus school-based screening. Hypertension. 2004;43:214–218.
30. Litwin M, Niemirska A, Sladowska J, et al. Left ventricular hypertrophy and arterial wall thickening in children with essential hypertension. Pediatr Nephrol. 2006;21:811–819.

31. McNiece KL, Gupta-Malhotra M, Samuels J, et al. Left ventricular hypertrophy in hypertensive adolescents: Analysis of risk by 2004 National High Blood Pressure Education Program Working Group staging criteria. Hypertension. 2007;50:392–395.

32. Brady TM, Fivush B, Flynn JT, et al. Ability of blood pressure to predict left ventricular hypertrophy in children with primary hypertension. J Pediatr. 2008;152:73–78.

33. Richey PA, DiSessa TG, Hastings MC, et al. Ambulatory blood pressure and increased left ventricular mass in children at risk for hypertension. J Pediatr. 2008;152:343–348.

34. Fagard R, Pardaens K. Left ventricular diastolic function predicts outcome in uncomplicated hypertension. Am J Hypertens. 2001;14:504–508.

35. Snider AR, Gidding SS, Rocchini AP, et al. Doppler evaluation of left ventricular diastolic filling in children with systemic hypertension. Am J Cardiol. 1985;56:921–926.

36. Johnson MC, Bergerse LJ, Beck A, et al. Diastolic function and tachycardia in hypertensive children. Am J Hypertens. 1999;12:1009–1114.

37. Border WL, Kimball TR, Witt SA, et al. Diastolic filling abnormalities in children with essential hypertension. J Pediatr. 2007;150:503–509.

38. Laurent S, Boutouyrie P. Recent advances in arterial stiffness and wave reflection in human hypertension. Hypertension. 2007;49:1202–1206.

39. Humphrey JD. Mechanisms of arterial remodeling in hypertension. Coupled roles of wall shear and intramural stress. Hypertension. 2008;52:195–200.

40. Duprez DA. Role of the renin-angiotensin-aldosterone system in vascular remodeling and inflammation: a clinical review. J Hypertens. 2006;24:983–991.

41. Hodis HN, Mack WJ, LaBree L, et al. The role of carotid arterial intima-media thickness in predicting clinical coronary events. Ann Intern Med. 1998;128:262–269.

42. Sorof JM, Alexandrov AV, Cardwell G, et al. Carotid artery intimal-medial thickness and left ventricular hypertrophy in children with elevated blood pressure. Pediatrics. 2003;111:61–66.

43. Li S, Chen W, Srinivasan SR, et al. Childhood cardiovascular risk factors and carotid vascular changes in adulthood: the Bogalusa Heart Study. JAMA. 2003;290:2271–2276.

44. Lande MB, Carson NL, Roy J, et al. Effects of childhood primary hypertension on carotid intima media thickness: a matched controlled study. Hypertension. 2006;48:40–44.

45. Lim HS, Lip GYH. Arterial stiffness: beyond pulse wave velocity and its measurement. J Hum Hypertens. 2008;22:656–658.

46. Li, S, Chen W, Srinivasan SR. Childhood blood pressure as a predictor of arterial stiffness in young adults. Hypertension. 2004;43:541–546.

47. Niboshi A, Hamaoka K, Sakata K, et al. Characteristics of brachial-ankle pulse wave velocity in Japanese children. Eur J Pediatr. 2006;165;625–629.

48. Im JA, Lee JW, Shim JY, et al. Association between brachial-ankle pulse wave velocity and cardiovascular risk factors in healthy adolescents. J Pediatr. 2007;150:247:251.

49. McGill HC Jr, Strong JP, Tracy RE, et al. Pathobiological Determinants of Atherosclerosis in Youth (PDAY) Research Group. Relation of a postmortem renal index of hypertension to atherosclerosis in youth. Arterioscler Thromb Vasc Biol. 1995:15:2222–2228.

50. McGill HC, McMahan A, Herderick EE, et al. Effects of coronary heart disease risk factors on atherosclerosis of selected regions of the aorta and right coronary artery. Arterioscler Thromb Vasc Biol. 2000;20: 836–845.

51. McMahan CA, Gidding SS, Malcom GT, et al. Comparison of coronary heart disease risk factors in autopsied young adults from the PDAY study with living young adults from the CARDIA study. Cardiovasc Pathol. 2007;16:151–158.

52. Newman WP III, Freedman DS, Voors AW, et al. Relation of serum lipoprotein levels and systolic blood pressure to early atherosclerosis: the Bogalusa Heart Study. N Engl J Med. 1986;314:138–144.

53. Berenson GS, Srinivasan SR, Bao W, et al. Association between multiple cardiovascular risk factors and atherosclerosis in children and young adults. The Bogalusa Heart Study. N Engl J Med. 1998;335: 1650–1656.

54. Hill GS. Hypertensive nephrosclerosis. Curr Opin Nephrol Hypertens. 2008;17:266–270.

55. Cirillo M, Stellato D, Laurenzi M, et al. Pulse pressure and isolated systolic hypertension: association with microalbuminuria. The GUBBIO Study Collaborative Research Group. Kidney Int. 2000;58:1211–1218.

56. Hillege HL, Fidler V, Diercks GF, et al. Urinary albumin excretion predicts cardiovascular and noncardiovascular mortality in the general population. Circulation. 2002;106:1777–1782.

57. Hoq S, Chen W, Srinivasan SR, et al. Childhood blood pressure predicts adult microalbuminuria in African Americans, but not in whites: The Bogalusa Heart Study. Am J Hypertens. 2002;15:1036–1041.

58. Lubrano R, Travasso E, Raggi C, et al. Blood pressure load, proteinuria, and renal function in pre-hypertensive children. Pediatr Nephrol. 2009;24:823–831.

59. Assadi F. Relation of left ventricular hypertrophy to microalbuminuria and c-reactive protein in children and adolescents with essential hypertension. Pediatr Cardiol. 2008;29:580–584.
60. Cuspidi C, Salerno M, Salerno DE, et al. High prevalence of retinal vascular changes in never-treated essential hypertensives: an inter- and intra-observer reproducibility study with non-mydriatic retinography. Blood Press. 2004;13:25–30.
61. Porta M, Grosso A, Vegio F. Hypertensive retinopathy: there's more than meets the eye. J Hypertens. 2005;23:683–696.
62. Liao D, Cooper L, Cai J, et al. The prevalence and severity of white matter lesions, their relationship with age, ethnicity, gender, and cardiovascular disease risk factors: the ARIC study. Neuroepidemiology. 1997;16:149–162.
63. Skalina MEL, Annable WL, Kleigman RM, et al. Hypertensive retinopathy in the newborn infant. J Pediatr. 1983;103:781–786.
64. Daniels SR, Lipman MJ, Burke MJ, et al. The prevalence of retinal vascular abnormalities in children and adolescents with essential hypertension. Am J Ophthalmol. 1991;111:205–208.
65. Daniels SR, Lipman MJ, Burke MJ, et al. Determinants of retinal vascular abnormalities in children and adolescents with essential hypertension. J Hum Hypertens. 1993;7:223–228.
66. Sun C, Liew G, Wang JJ, et al. Retinal vascular caliber, blood pressure, and cardiovascular risk factors in an Asian population: the Singapore Malay Eye Study. Invest Ophthalmol Vis Sci. 2008;49:1784–1790.
67. Van Boxtel MPJ, Henskens LHG, Kroon AA, et al. Ambulatory blood pressure, asymptomatic cerebrovascular damage and cognitive function in essential hypertension. J Hum Hypertens. 2006;20:5–13.
68. Robbins MA, Elias MF, Elias PK, et al. Blood pressure and cognitive function in an African-American and a Caucasian-American sample: the Maine-Syracuse Study. Psychosom Med. 2005;67:707–714.
69. Lande MB, Kaczorowski JM, Auinger P, et al. Elevated blood pressure and decreased cognitive function among school-age children and adolescents in the United States. J Pediatr. 2003;143:720–724.
70. Adelman RD, Coppo R, Dillon MJ. The emergency management of severe hypertension. Pediatr Nephrol. 2000;14:422–427.
71. Flynn JT. Tullus K. Severe hypertension in children and adolescents: pathophysiology and treatment. Pediatr Nephrol. 2009;24:1101–1112.
72. Van Lieshout JJ, Wieling W, Karemaker JM et al. Syncope, cerebral perfusion, and oxygenation. J Appl Physiol. 2003;94:833–848.
73. Immick RV, van den Born BJ, van Montfrans GA, et al. Impaired cerebral autoregulation in patients with malignant hypertension. Circulation. 2004;110:2241–2245.
74. Zampaglione B, Pascale C, Marchiso M, et al. Hypertensive urgencies and emergencies: prevalence and clinical presentation. Hypertension. 1996;27:144–147.
75. Lee VH, Wijdicks E FM, Manno EM, et al. Clinical spectrum of reversible posterior leukoencephalopathy syndrome. Arch Neurol. 2008;65:205–210.
76. Hulse JA, Taylor DS, Dillon MJ. Blindness and paraplegia in severe childhood hypertension. Lancet. 1979;2:553–556.
77. Browning AC, Mengher LS, Gregson RM, et al. Visual outcome of malignant hypertension in young people. Arch Dis Child. 2001;85:401–403.
78. Logan P, Eustace P, Robinson R. Hypertensive retinopathy: a cause of decreased visual acuity in children. J Pediatr Opthamol Strabismus. 1992;29:287–289.
79. Trompeter RS, Smith RL, Hoare RD, et al. Neurological complication of arterial hypertension. Arch Dis Child. 1982;57:913–917.
80. Aggarwal M, Khan IA. Hypertensive crisis: hypertensive emergencies and urgencies. Cardiol Clin. 2006;24:135–146.
81. Nadar S, Beevers DG, Lip GY. Echocardiographic changes in patients with malignant phase hypertension: the West Birmingham Malignant Hypertension Registry. J Hum Hypertens. 2005;19:69–75.
82. Frohlich ED. Target organ involvement in hypertension: a realistic promise of prevention and reversal. Med Clin North Am. 2004;88:1–9.
83. Deal JE, Barratt TM, Dillon MJ. Management of hypertensive emergencies. Arch Dis Child. 1992;67:1089–1092.
84. Van den Born BJH, Honnebier UPF, Koopmans RP, et al. Microangiopathic hemolysis and renal failure in malignant hypertension. Hypertension. 2005;45:246–251.
85. Guerin C, Gonthier R, Berthoux FC. Long-term prognosis in malignant and accelerated hypertension. Nephrol Dial Transplant. 1988;3:33–37.
86. Gudbrandsson T, Hansson L, Herlitz H, et al. Malignant hypertension. Improving prognosis in a rare disease. Acta Med Scand. 1979;206:495–499.
87. Gill DG, Mehdes da Costa B, Cameron JS, et al. Analysis of 100 children with severe and persistent hypertension. Arch Dis Child. 1976;51:951–956.

88. Kumar P, Aurora P, Khmer V, et al. Malignant hypertension in children in India. Nephrol Dial Transplant. 1996;11:1261–1266.
89. Tanaka H, Tatiana T, Suzuki K, et al. Acute renal failure due to hypertension: malignant hypertension in an adolescent. Pediatr Int. 2003;45:342–344.
90. Adelman RD, Russo J. Malignant hypertension: recovery of renal function after treatment with antihypertensive medications and hemodialysis. J Pediatr. 1981;98:766–768.

25 Sleep Apnea and Hypertension

Alisa A. Acosta, MD, MPH

Contents

INTRODUCTION

Sleep disordered breathing (SDB) encompasses all forms of respiratory disorders specific to sleep *(1)*. There is a spectrum of SDB ranging from mild to severe with the most severe form being obstructive sleep apnea (OSA) *(2)*. In adults, OSA has been linked to cardiovascular disease, specifically hypertension (HTN) *(3)*. The association between systemic HTN and OSA is well documented in both cross-sectional and prospective population studies *(4–6)*. These studies not only demonstrate an association between the two conditions, but one study also documented OSA preceding the development of HTN *(6)*. Additionally, OSA has been associated with drug-resistant HTN in adults *(7,8)* which may be partially mediated by aldosterone *(9,10)*. The relationship between OSA and HTN is so well defined in adults that OSA is now recognized as an identifiable cause of HTN and should be considered during the evaluation for elevated blood pressure (BP) *(11)*. The National High Blood Pressure Education Working Group for Children and Adolescents made a similar recommendation to evaluate for OSA as a comorbid condition in children with HTN *(12)*. However, the relationship between SDB and HTN is not as clear in children. Regardless, there is evidence to suggest an association between these two conditions, but the causal relationship is still unknown.

A.A. Acosta (✉)
Pediatric Nephrology, Children's Hospital at Scott and White, Texas A&M College of Medicine, 2401 South 31st
Street, Temple, TX, USA
e-mail: aacosta@swmail.sw.org

From: *Clinical Hypertension and Vascular Diseases: Pediatric Hypertension*
Edited by: J. T. Flynn et al. DOI 10.1007/978-1-60327-824-9_25
© Springer Science+Business Media, LLC 2011

DEFINITIONS AND EPIDEMIOLOGY OF SDB

OSA in children as defined by the American Thoracic Society is a sleep-related breathing disorder "characterized by prolonged partial upper airway obstruction and/or intermittent complete obstruction (obstructive apnea) that disrupts normal ventilation during sleep and normal sleep patterns" *(13)*. Specifically, an obstructive apnea is a cessation in ventilation despite effort for 10 s or 2 breath cycles in older children, or despite effort for 6 s or 1.5–2 breath cycles in infants *(14)*. An obstructive hypopnea is a decrease in airflow by at least 50% despite effort occurring at the same time or during breath cycles associated with a desaturation or arousal *(13)*. Both of these events contribute to the apnea/hypopnea index (AHI) defined as the total number of apneas and hypopneas per hour of sleep (also referred to as the respiratory disturbance index, RDI) *(14)*. AHI can only be measured by polysomnography (PSG), the gold standard for diagnosing SDB. An AHI > 1 is considered abnormal in children *(15)* contrary to adult guidelines that specify an AHI > 5 as the cutoff for the diagnosis of OSA *(16)*. When partial upper airway obstruction results in hypercapnia, these episodes are referred to as obstructive hypoventilation. Obstructive hypoventilation requires measurement of end-tidal CO_2 ($ETCO_2$) and is defined by an $ETCO_2$ > 45 mmHg for more than 60% of total sleep time or any $ETCO_2$ > 53 mmHg *(15)*.

Another form of SDB is the upper airway resistance syndrome (UARS) characterized by partial obstruction of the upper airway leading to arousals and sleep fragmentation without gas exchange abnormalities *(17)*. UARS was first described in children in 1982, but the actual term was first used in reference to adults *(18,19)*. Despite the lack of abnormal ventilation or oxygenation, excessive daytime somnolence is a common symptom among adults and children with UARS *(18–21)*. Children can also present with hyperactivity *(18)*. For the diagnosis of UARS, certain techniques and measurements are required during PSG. A nasal cannula/pressure transducer and an esophageal catheter can measure the esophageal pressure allowing for the detection of more subtle changes in breathing patterns during sleep *(21)*. If an esophageal catheter is not available, UARS can be diagnosed by the presence of asynchronous movements of the chest and abdomen followed by arousal, but this paradoxical breathing can be a normal feature during sleep in children less than 3 years old *(20)*. In contrast to patients with OSA, these patients are less likely to be obese, have more orthostatic symptoms, and have low or normal BP *(21)*.

Finally, snoring without obstructive apneas, frequent arousals, or gas exchange abnormalities define primary snoring *(22)*. Inherent in the definition, primary snoring is a diagnosis of exclusion requiring evaluation for other forms of SDB *(14)*. Historically, primary snoring was thought to be a benign condition, but studies do not always distinguish primary snoring from other forms of SDB *(22)*. One study made this distinction and excluded children with abnormalities on PSG other than snoring *(23)*. In this study, there were significant differences in neurobehavioral testing between children with primary snoring and those without snoring or SDB. Overall, both groups scored in the average range, but those with primary snoring scored significantly less than the normal controls. This study suggests primary snoring may not be benign and should be considered separately from other forms of SDB and normal controls. Table 1 summarizes the terms and definitions for SDB. Together, primary snoring, UARS, obstructive hypoventilation, and OSA represent the spectrum of SDB from mild to severe *(20)*.

The prevalence of SDB in children is difficult to determine because of the heterogeneity in the studies assessing prevalence. Despite the availability of definitions and normative values for SDB, there is still no universal consensus on the criteria required for the diagnosis

Table 1
Sleep Disordered Breathing Terms and Definitions

SDB term	Definition
Obstructive apnea	Complete or partial upper airway obstruction with cessation in ventilation despite respiratory effort
Obstructive hypopnea	Decrease in airflow by at least 50% despite effort
Apnea hypopnea index (respiratory disturbance index)	Total number of apneas and hypopneas per hour of sleep
Primary snoring	Snoring without abnormalities on PSG
Upper airway resistance syndrome	Partial upper airway obstruction causing arousals without gas exchange abnormalities
Obstructive hypoventilation	Partial upper airway obstruction resulting in hypercapnia
Obstructive sleep apnea	Obstructive apneas disrupting normal sleep patterns and normal ventilation during sleep

(14,17). In addition, most prevalence studies were based primarily on a variety of question-naires with few studies performing diagnostic testing for confirmation. Recently, Lumeng and Chervin *(24)* performed a systematic review of epidemiologic studies on SDB and when applicable, performed a meta-analysis to adjust for the heterogeneity of results from the different studies. They found the prevalence of snoring as reported by parents ranged from 1.5 to 14.8%, and the meta-analysis of relevant studies revealed a prevalence of almost 7.5% (95% confidence interval, 5.75–9.61). Parent-reported SDB ranged from around 4 to 11%, and this range extended even further in both directions to 0.1–13% when SDB was diagnosed by PSG and other diagnostic testing. However, a majority of the studies that used diagnostic testing reported a prevalence of around 1–4%.

CLINICAL PRESENTATION AND DIAGNOSIS

Snoring is the most common presenting symptom of SDB in children *(18)*, but there is no correlation between the loudness or intensity of snoring and the severity of SDB *(22)*. Parents may also report the child having difficulty breathing while asleep or even witness apneas described as pauses in breathing usually followed by gasping, choking, or arousal *(1)*. Arousals may occur frequently without apneic spells manifesting as nighttime restlessness *(25)*. Parents may also observe paradoxical breathing movements representing continued attempts at respiration during upper airway obstruction. Other clinical features during sleep include sweating and posturing with a hyperextended neck to promote airway patency *(20,25)*. Enuresis has also been reported to occur in higher proportions in children with SDB *(26)*. Additionally, studies have shown symptoms of enuresis improve after adenotonsillectomy *(27,28)*. Daytime symptoms may include morning headache, chronic mouth breathing, or behavior and attention problems resembling attention deficit hyperactivity disorder (ADHD) *(14,18)*. Older children may also present with an ADHD-type picture, but they will more likely complain of daytime somnolence and fatigue especially if obesity is also present *(25)*. Obesity is another risk factor for SDB in addition to craniofacial disorders and retro/micrognathia. However, the most common feature seen on physical exam is adenotonsillar hypertrophy, a finding more common in younger children because of the progressive increase in lymphoid tissue till about 12 years of age *(1)*. The degree of hypertrophy has been shown to correlate with the duration of obstructive apneas but not with the number of obstructive apneas *(29)*. Adenotonsillar hypertrophy may be less important in obese children. In a retrospective review of over 400 children with a mean age of 6.5 years and OSA, adenotonsillar size correlated with the AHI for non-obese children but not for obese children *(30)*. The obese group had a significantly higher Mallampati score than the non-obese group. The Mallampati score is based on how much the visual site of the soft palate, fauces, uvula, and tonsillar pillars is obscured with tongue protrusion. The higher the score, the more obscured the view, which suggests crowding of the upper airway even in the absence of adenotonsillar hypertrophy. The presence of any of these symptoms (Table 2) on history or physical exam should prompt further evaluation for SDB.

Table 2
Clinical Signs and Symptoms of Sleep Disordered Breathing

Snoring

Difficulty breathing while sleeping

Witnessed apneas

Paradoxical breathing movements

Arousals/restlessness

Sweating during sleep

Posturing to promote airway patency

Enuresis

Chronic mouth breathing

Morning headache

Behavior or attention problems

Daytime somnolence

Obesity

Adenotonsillary hypertrophy

Further evaluation for SDB typically includes referral to a sleep medicine clinic and/or a PSG. There have been many alternative diagnostic methods studied to confirm the presence of SDB without having to endure the burden and cost of a full overnight PSG in a sleep laboratory. Questionnaires are a good screening tool but cannot distinguish between primary snoring and OSA *(25)*. Audiotaping and/or videotaping may again screen for OSA and perhaps even detect apneas, but other abnormalities such as hypoventilation and hypopneas cannot accurately be detected without additional monitoring. Other techniques include continuous pulse oximetry recording and electrocardiography, but both techniques are limited because of technical application or lack of larger validation studies. Home monitoring studies have been used with some success proving to be both reproducible and valid in the context of a research protocol *(31)*. Regardless, no substitute has proven to be as sensitive and specific in diagnosing SDB as the gold standard, an overnight PSG in a sleep laboratory *(22)*. Initially, the respiratory indices and values used to diagnose OSA in adults were applied to children. However, because children have different physiology and respiratory rates than adults, guidelines for defining the various respiratory events were developed specifically for pediatrics *(13)*. Subsequently, normal values were published to aid in the interpretation of PSG in children *(15)*, but the correlation of these values to adverse outcomes is not established *(22)*. Therefore, the diagnostic criteria and the classification for the severity of SDB is not consistent in the pediatric literature making it difficult to compare multiple studies.

PATHOPHYSIOLOGY

The pathophysiology of SDB in children is complex and not entirely understood, but the two main factors of the upper airway underlying the pathology in children appear to be structural and functional. Structurally, when measured endoscopically, or noninvasively by pharyngometry or MRI, children with SDB have smaller cross-sectional areas and/or volumes of the upper airway than children without SDB *(32–34)*. On MRI, affected children were also found to have larger adenoids, tonsils, and soft palates *(32)*. Functionally, upper airway patency is maintained during sleep by neuromuscular responses to ventilation, oxygenation, and airway pressure *(17,35)*. On a cross-sectional analysis of children and adults, this response to pressure decreased with age and body mass index (BMI) *(36)*. Additionally, children with OSA were found to have a decreased response to hypercapnia and intermittent acute negative pressure during sleep when compared to controls *(37)*. Not only is the response affected, but Gozal and Burnside *(38)* demonstrated more upper airway collapsibility during wakefulness in children with an AHI $\geq$ 5. The combination of narrower airways and increased susceptibility to upper airway collapse during sleep are two major contributing factors for the development of SDB in children.

The mechanism underlying the relation between SDB and HTN is complex and multifactorial, and most of the information comes from adult data. The autonomic nervous system plays a major role, but other factors have been identified including vasoactive substances, endothelial dysfunction, and intrathoracic changes. Normally, heart rate, BP, and sympathetic activity decline during sleep, but intermittent hypoxemia, hypercapnia, and arousals activate the sympathetic nervous system *(39,40)*. These surges in sympathetic activity during sleep result in increased BP and heart rate that can persist into wakefulness *(41)*. The vasoactive substances found to correlate with OSA in adults include endothelin *(42)* and aldosterone, but increased aldosterone has been limited to adults with resistant HTN *(9,10)*. Other vasoactive substances are believed to contribute to endothelial dysfunction in adults. In response to nocturnal hypoxemia, an altered production of these substances by the endothelial cells, (decreased nitric oxide and increased endothelin-1), results in vasoconstriction *(43)*. There is evidence of endothelial dysfunction in children with OSA that improved after adenotonsillectomy *(38)*. Finally, changes in intrathoracic pressure may contribute to the autonomic responses during sleep in patients with OSA leading to activation of the sympathetic nervous system and ultimately raising BP *(40)*. In addition to raising BP, intrathoracic pressure may also have an effect on ventricular remodeling because of the transmural gradients created across the atria, ventricles, and aorta. Left ventricular transmembrane pressure is a reflection of the afterload on the left ventricle, and elevated left ventricular transmembrane pressures were detected during the ventilatory period following an obstructive apnea in adults with congestive heart failure *(44)*. This increase in cardiac afterload following obstructive apneas may explain the presence of left ventricular hypertrophy (LVH) in patients with OSA independent of BP *(45)*.

SDB AND HYPERTENSION

Similar to the epidemiologic studies of SDB in children, studies evaluating the association of BP with SDB are heterogeneous and differ by the methods and criteria used to diagnose SDB and to measure BP. Some studies measured casual BP either with oscillometric devices *(46,47)*, calibrated sphygmomanometers *(48)*, or mercury manometers *(49)*. The remaining studies measured ambulatory blood pressure (ABP) during wake and sleep *(50–53)* or only in relation to the PSG *(54,55)*. Most of the studies analyzed raw BP values, but some studies indexed BP to the 95th percentile according to various reference values in order to assess HTN status. In regards to SDB, participants were divided into two or three groups depending on AHI or snoring. Among the studies analyzing the association between BP and SDB (Table 3), there is no clear consensus on how the two conditions relate. One of the earliest reports in children was a case series by Guilleminault et al. *(56)* where five of the eight children with sleep apnea had HTN. A later study assessing BP during PSG found significantly higher wake and sleep diastolic BP in children with OSA than those with primary snoring *(55)*. There was no difference in systolic BP between the two groups. However, when the groups were combined, both systolic and diastolic BP significantly correlated with the AHI.

Subsequent studies reported similar findings but also detected a difference in systolic BP *(48,52,54)*. One study divided the participants into high AHI (AHI $\geq$ 10) and low AHI (AHI < 10) groups and used a BP index defined as the difference between mean BP and cutoff values for age *(54)*. Those with high AHI had a significantly increased systolic and diastolic BP index, but only the diastolic BP index correlated with the AHI. A more recent study defined three SDB groups by AHI but excluded primary snorers (AHI < 1 and snoring > 3 times per week): (1) AHI < 1, (2) AHI between 1 and 5, and (3) AHI > 5 *(52)*. Mean BP was converted to a z-score according to the LMS method described by Wuhl et al. *(57)* There was no difference in the BP z-score between groups 1 and 2, but group 3 had a significantly higher wake and sleep systolic, diastolic, and mean arterial BP z-score than groups 1 and 2. Furthermore, group 3 had a significant association with wake systolic BP that was no longer significant after controlling for BMI. A different study evaluating BP as a component of the metabolic syndrome in adolescents also demonstrated patients with SDB (AHI $\geq$ 5) had significantly higher systolic and diastolic BP even after adjusting for age and BMI percentile *(48)*.

Other studies were less consistent with the differences in diastolic BP *(46,50,51,53)*. Leung et al. *(53)* compared a high AHI (AHI $\geq$ 5) and a low AHI (AHI < 5) group by 24-h ABP variables with a BP index defined as the measured BP divided by the 95th percentile for ABP *(53)*. This study also detected greater systolic and diastolic BP indices in the high AHI group, but the difference in diastolic BP was isolated to sleep measurements. Another study with the largest study population to complete PSG did not find a difference in diastolic BP among the three SDB groups: (1) no SDB, AHI < 1; (2) mild SDB, AHI 1 to < 5; and (3) moderate SDB, AHI $\geq$ 5) *(46)*. However, there was a significant increasing trend in the systolic and mean arterial BP across the groups. Furthermore, to delineate a threshold in AHI, the authors compared BP across SDB groups with incremental increases in AHI (i.e.,

Table 3
Comparison of Blood Pressure Studies and Sleep Disordered Breathing in Children

Source	SDB classification	Method of BP measurement	Method of BP analysis	Systolic BP results	Diastolic BP results	Mean arterial BP results	Nocturnal dip
Guilleminault et al. (56)	Case series of patients with OSA	NR	Presence or absence of HTN	NR	NR	NR	N/A
Marcus et al. (55)	OSA vs primary snoring	Oscillometric during PSG	BP index	No difference	Elevated wake and sleep	NR	No difference
Kohyama et al. (54)	Low vs high AHI	Oscillometric during PSG	BP index	Elevated wake and REMS	Elevated wake and REMS	NR	No difference
Li et al. (52)	Controls, mild, moderate SDB by AHI	ABPM	z-score	Elevated wake and sleep	Elevated wake and sleep	Elevated wake and sleep	No difference
Redline et al. (48)	SDB vs no SDB	Aneroid manometer	Raw values	Elevated	Elevated	NR	N/A
Leung et al. (53)	Low vs high AHI	ABPM	BP index	Elevated wake and sleep	Elevated sleep	NR	No difference
Bixler et al. (46)	Controls, mild, moderate SDB by AHI	Oscillometric	Raw values	Elevated	No difference	Elevated	N/A
Kaditis et al. (47)	Snorers vs non-snorers by questionnaire	Oscillometric	Raw values	No difference	No difference	NR	N/A
Amin et al. (50)	Controls, mild, moderate SDB by AHI	ABPM	BP index and BP variability	No difference	Lower during wake	No difference	Linear trend across SDB groups

Table 3
(continued)

Source	SDB classification	Method of BP measurement	Method of BP analysis	Systolic BP results	Diastolic BP results	Mean arterial BP results	Nocturnal dip
Amin et al. (51)	Controls, mild, moderate SDB by AHI	ABPM	Raw values	Elevated wake	Elevated wake and sleep	Elevated wake and sleep	NR
Enright et al. (49)	RDI	Mercury manometer	HTN vs normal	HTN associated with RDI	HTN associated with RDI	NR	N/A
Reade et al. (65)	OSA vs non-OSA	Manual BP	BP score	Elevated	Elevated	NR	N/A

SDB, sleep disordered breathing; BP, blood pressure; NR, not reported; HTN, hypertension; N/A, not applicable; PSG, polysomnography; AHI, apnea hypopnea index; REMS, rapid eye movement sleep; ABPM, ambulatory blood pressure monitor; RDI, respirator disturbance index.

AHI $\geq$ 1, AHI $\geq$ 2, etc.), the strongest association was between systolic BP and the group with an AHI $\geq$ 5. For this study, BP was not indexed to reference levels to account for the differences in age, gender, and height, and sleep BP was not measured.

Only one study failed to detect any difference in BP between SDB groups, but these groups were defined by questionnaire alone into habitual and non-habitual snorers (47). One study actually detected a lower diastolic BP in the group with the highest AHI (50). This study defined three groups by AHI: (1) primary snorers, no evidence of nocturnal hypoventilation and an AHI <1; (2) Group 2, AHI from 1 to 5; and (3) Group 3, AHI > 5. For this study, 24-h ABP was measured and BP index ((measured BP – 95th percentile)/95th percentile × 100) was compared across the three groups. The authors also analyzed BP variability defined as the average standard deviation of awake and sleep systolic, diastolic, and mean arterial BP. Of all the BP variables including average wake and sleep systolic, diastolic, and mean arterial BP, only wake diastolic BP was significantly different among the three SDB groups with the lowest level in Group 3. On the contrary, there was a dose-dependent increase in wake systolic BP variability across the three groups. A similar trend was demonstrated for wake mean arterial BP and for all sleep BP. The authors propose the variability in BP during both sleep and wakefulness suggests autonomic instability in children with SDB resulting in BP dysregulation. The same group later performed a separate but similar, more rigorous study and did detect significantly elevated BPs (except for sleep systolic BP) in those with an AHI > 5 compared to controls with an AHI <1 (51). Furthermore, the relative predictive contributions of AHI and BMI were similar for all measures of BP except sleep diastolic BP where AHI had a significantly greater effect. In this study, an additional BP variable was evaluated, the morning surge, defined as the slope of BP from the beginning of the last hour of sleep to the end of the first hour of awakening. In adults, the morning surge has been associated with cardiovascular events such as myocardial infarction and stroke (59–61). The children in this study with severe SDB had a morning BP surge significantly higher for systolic, diastolic, and mean arterial BP than the controls. This was the first study evaluating the association of the morning surge with SDB in children, and its implication in children is currently unknown. Although echocardiographic measures of the left ventricle were assessed in this study, there was no report of their relationship to the morning surge.

Despite significant BP differences among a variety of SDB groups, none of the groups had mean BPs consistent with HTN defined by a BP $\geq$ 95th percentile according to reference values for casual measurement (12) or for ambulatory measurements (57,62). Enright et al. (49) evaluated BP in terms of HTN and dichotomized BP into HTN or normal (49). In their study, the RDI was a significant predictor for systolic and/or diastolic HTN, but HTN was defined as a BP $\geq$ 90th percentile for age, gender, and height (58). One of the previously mentioned studies by Leung et al. (53) also estimated HTN prevalence defined as a mean wake, sleep, and/or total ABP $\geq$ 95th percentile for ABP reference values (62). They found the prevalence of HTN was significantly greater in the high-AHI group. However, when the participants were combined regardless of AHI group, AHI was not a significant predictor of HTN except among those with obesity.

Obesity must be considered when analyzing the relationship between SDB and HTN since obesity is associated with both conditions (63,64). In the previous study by Li et al. (52), BMI was found to be a confounding factor for wake systolic BP, that is, the association was no longer significant when controlled for BMI. However, the other previously mentioned studies that used PSG to determine SDB status found both BMI and SDB variables (i.e., AHI) to have an independent effect on BP (46,49–55). In one of the studies, SDB remained a significant predictor of BP when controlled for BMI, but the effect of BMI on BP was not reported *(48)*. There was one study, not yet mentioned, specifically designed to address the interaction between SDB, BP, and obesity *(65)*. The specific aim was to assess if OSA was associated with an increased risk of HTN in obese children on a retrospective analysis of children who had undergone PSG, BP, and anthropometric measurement. OSA was defined by an apnea index > 1 or the lowest oxygen saturation associated with an obstructive apnea < 90%. A BP score was defined as the ratio of the measured BP to the 95th percentile for age, gender, and height *(58)*, and BMI score was the ratio of measured BMI to the 95th percentile. Participants were classified and analyzed in three separate manners: (1) OSA versus non-OSA, (2) obese versus non-obese, and (3) obese hypertensives versus obese normotensives. For the three separate analyses, there was a significantly higher prevalence of HTN and obesity in the OSA group; a higher prevalence of HTN and OSA in the obese group; and a higher prevalence of OSA in the obese hypertensives. Furthermore, on multiple regression analysis, the hypopnea index and BMI score were significant predictors for systolic and diastolic BP score for the OSA and the obese groups. For obese hypertensives, only BMI was significant for systolic BP score. The interaction between OSA, HTN, and obesity is significant, and all of these studies suggest there is an independent effect of BP and BMI on SDB. An interaction between BMI and SDB on BP also exists, but the causal relationship of this interaction and the effect on BP is yet to be elucidated.

NOCTURNAL DIPPING

BP has a normal physiologic decline during sleep commonly referred to as the nocturnal dip *(66)*. The normal mean nocturnal dip is typically 10–20% less than the mean daytime BP *(67)*. Abnormal nocturnal BP patterns can vary from a minimal decline in nocturnal BP (<10% dip) to a rise in nocturnal BP above normal daytime values *(68)*. The prevalence of nondipping in adults with OSA is 48–84% *(8,69,70)*. When compared to controls in one study, only patients with OSA were nondippers even though one of the controls had HTN. After controlling for several variables including age and BMI, only the RDI was a significant predictor of nondipping status *(70)*. In children, the relationship between nocturnal dipping status and SDB has not been consistent *(50,52–55)*. From the previously mentioned studies evaluating BP during sleep and wake, most do not show a statistically significant difference in the proportion of nondippers among children with SDB compared to those without SDB *(52–55)*. Two of the studies demonstrated a higher proportion of nondippers in the SDB group compared to the group without SDB (29 vs 19% and 12 vs 4%, respectively), but the difference was not statistically significant *(54,55)*. Rather than comparing the proportion of nondippers, two studies examined the mean nocturnal dip per group defined by AHI (AHI < 1, AHI 1–5, and AHI > 5) *(50,52)*. In the first study, the average nocturnal dip per group significantly decreased for systolic, diastolic, and mean arterial BP across the three groups *(50)*. The proportion of nondippers per group was not reported, but the mean nocturnal dip was blunted (< 10%) for systolic BP in both groups with an AHI > 1. In the second study, there was no difference in the mean nocturnal dip nor the proportion of nondippers per group *(52)*. The inability to consistently demonstrate significant differences in the nocturnal dip among SDB groups is likely another result of the heterogeneity among studies. Regardless, a child or adolescent undergoing evaluation for elevated BP with an abnormal nocturnal dip on ABP monitoring warrants further screening and/or evaluation for SDB, especially in the presence of other risk factors.

LEFT VENTRICULAR GEOMETRY

LVH is the most commonly recognized surrogate marker of end-organ damage in children and adolescents with systemic HTN (12). In adults with OSA, the intermittent obstructive apneas lead to an increase in afterload (44) possibly contributing to the development of LVH. Therefore, patients with both HTN and OSA may have an even greater risk of LVH. Adult data suggest that LVH is independently associated with OSA (45,71). One of the first studies addressing left ventricular geometry and SDB in children reported patients with OSA had a significantly increased left ventricular mass index (LVMI) without a difference in right ventricular dimensions when compared to primary snorers (72). Furthermore, on stepwise multiple regression analysis, AHI was the only significant predictor of LVMI even when age, gender, and BMI were forced into the model. Participants with an AHI > 10 were about 11 times more likely to have LVH independent of age, gender, and BMI. Resting BP was not a significant predictor and, therefore, not included in the final model. This dose-dependent effect of the severity of SDB on LVMI was consistent in a later report from the same group with additional participants (73). A separate study from the same group with different participants measured ABP in addition to resting BP and divided the study population into three SDB groups according to AHI: (1) controls, AHI < 1 and no history of obstructive breathing during sleep; (2) moderate, AHI 1 to < 5; (3) severe, AHI ≥ 5 (51). They found a progressive, but insignificant, increase in LVMI across the three groups with worsening AHI. There was a difference in left ventricular relative wall thickness between controls and the severe SDB group, and all BP parameters (wake and sleep systolic, diastolic, and mean arterial BP) were significant predictors for this relationship. One additional study evaluated echocardiographic parameters in adolescents with SDB compared to controls and found a correlation between the RDI and left ventricular posterior wall thickness, but LVMI was similar in the two groups (74). Although evidence suggests LVMI increases with worsening AHI, there has not been a clear, independent association demonstrated between LVH and SDB in children and adolescents.

TREATMENT

Adenotonsillectomy is generally the first-line treatment for OSA in children (22). Other surgical treatment options include uvulopalatoplasty, nasal surgery, maxillofacial surgery, or even in extreme cases tracheotomy, but these are rarely necessary (17). For those who are not surgical candidates or fail to have a response to surgery, continuous positive airway pressure (CPAP) is a nonsurgical alternative (22). CPAP is fairly well tolerated in children, but for effectiveness, compliance is crucial and can be poor secondary to minor side effects such as rhinorrhea, nasal congestion, or dryness (1). Studies have demonstrated significant improvement in the AHI and in behavioral and cognitive symptoms after treatment of SDB (75,76), and some studies have even shown an improvement in left ventricular geometry and/or function (73,77). For example, one of the previously mentioned studies by Amin et al. (73) compared pretreatment and posttreatment left ventricular diastolic function by mitral inflow velocity. Treatment for SDB either consisted of adenotonsillectomy ± uvulopalatoplasty or CPAP. Pretreatment, there was a progressive decline in diastolic function across the SDB groups correlating with increasing severity. Posttreatment, regardless of therapy, the SDB groups had an improvement in diastolic function to a level similar to controls (primary snorers). Another study reported significant baseline differences between the SDB and control groups in regards to left ventricular measures and compliance, but after adenotonsillectomy, measurements in the SDB group were no longer different from controls *(77)*. Few studies have reported the treatment effect of SDB on BP in children. In the aforementioned case series by Guilleminault et al. *(56)* five of the eight patients with OSA had HTN at presentation. Those who underwent adenotonsillectomy and demonstrated improvement of symptoms on follow-up PSG were no longer hypertensive on follow-up. Two patients with HTN had extreme cases of OSA and required tracheotomy. Both cases also showed significant improvement in SDB symptoms and resolution of HTN after surgery. One study specifically evaluated the effect of adenotonsillectomy on BP in children *(78)*. Children with complete resolution of SDB after surgery (AHI < 1) had a significant decrease in diastolic BP but not in systolic BP. Although the association between drug-resistant HTN and OSA has been described in adults *(7,8)*, there are currently no reports in children. However, in a child with risk factors for SDB and difficult to control HTN the presence of SDB should be considered.

CONCLUSION

Despite the heterogeneity, the studies in children and adolescents suggest that a relationship exists between elevated BP/BP variability and SDB. This relationship is significant independent of obesity, but obesity also has an independent association with SDB and with HTN *(63,64)*. How the three conditions interact and whether there is a causal relationship among the conditions is unknown and requires further investigation. In adults, both HTN and SDB are independently associated with significant cardiovascular events. Fortunately, the same cardiovascular events do not occur in children, but the changes in left ventricular structure and function have been shown to occur. Similar to obesity, these left ventricular changes are associated with both HTN and SDB and after treatment of SDB alone, the changes improve. Therefore, the evaluation of a child with HTN should identify clinical signs and symptoms of SDB during the history and physical exam. Snoring and adenotonsillar hypertrophy are the two most common risk factors for SDB in children, and the presence of either sign in a child with HTN warrants further evaluation for SDB, especially if obesity is also present.

REFERENCES

1. Marcus CL. Sleep-disordered breathing in children. Curr Opin Pediatr. 2000;12:208–212.
2. Benninger M, Walner D. Obstructive sleep-disordered breathing in children. Clin Cornerstone. 2007;9(Suppl 1):S6–S12.
3. Somers VK, White DP, Amin R, et al. Sleep apnea and cardiovascular disease: An American Heart Association/American College of Cardiology Foundation Scientific Statement from the American Heart Association Council for High Blood Pressure Research Professional Education Committee, Council on Clinical Cardiology, Stroke Council, and Council on Cardiovascular Nursing. In Collaboration with the National Heart, Lung, and Blood Institute National Center on Sleep Disorders Research (National Institutes of Health). Circulation. 2008;118:1080–1111.
4. Lavie P, Herer P, Hoffstein V. Obstructive sleep apnoea syndrome as a risk factor for hypertension: population study. BMJ. 2000;320:479–482.
5. Nieto FJ, Young TB, Lind BK, et al. Association of sleep-disordered breathing, sleep apnea, and hypertension in a large community-based study. Sleep Heart Health Study. JAMA. 2000;283:1829–1836.
6. Peppard PE, Young T, Palta M, Skatrud J. Prospective study of the association between sleep-disordered breathing and hypertension. N Engl J Med. 2000;342:1378–1384.
7. Grote L, Hedner J, Peter JH. Sleep-related breathing disorder is an independent risk factor for uncontrolled hypertension. J Hypertens. 2000;18:679–685.

8. Logan AG, Perlikowski SM, Mente A, et al. High prevalence of unrecognized sleep apnoea in drug-resistant hypertension. J Hypertens. 2001;19:2271–2277.
9. Calhoun DA, Nishizaka MK, Zaman MA, Harding SM. Aldosterone excretion among subjects with resistant hypertension and symptoms of sleep apnea. Chest. 2004;125:112–117.
10. Pratt-Ubunama MN, Nishizaka MK, Boedefeld RL, Cofield SS, Harding SM, Calhoun DA. Plasma aldosterone is related to severity of obstructive sleep apnea in subjects with resistant hypertension. Chest. 2007;131:453–459.
11. Chobanian AV, Bakris GL, Black HR, et al. Seventh report of the joint national committee on prevention, detection, evaluation, and treatment of high blood pressure. Hypertension. 2003;42:1206–1252.
12. National High Blood Pressure Education Program Working Group on High Blood Pressure in Children and Adolescents. The fourth report on the diagnosis, evaluation, and treatment of high blood pressure in children and adolescents. Pediatrics. 2004;114:555–576.
13. Standards and indications for cardiopulmonary sleep studies in children. American Thoracic Society. Am J Respir Crit Care Med. 1996;153:866–878.
14. Sargi Z, Younis RT. Pediatric obstructive sleep apnea: current management. ORL J Otorhinolaryngol Relat Spec. 2007;69:340–344.
15. Marcus CL, Omlin KJ, Basinki DJ, et al. Normal polysomnographic values for children and adolescents. Am Rev Respir Dis. 1992;146:1235–1239.
16. Sleep-related breathing disorders in adults: recommendations for syndrome definition and measurement techniques in clinical research. The report of an American academy of sleep medicine task force. Sleep. 1999;22:667–689.
17. Ray RM, Bower CM. Pediatric obstructive sleep apnea: the year in review. Curr Opin Otolaryngol Head Neck Surg. 2005;13:360–365.
18. Guilleminault C, Winkle R, Korobkin R, Simmons B. Children and nocturnal snoring: Evaluation of the effects of sleep related respiratory resistive load and daytime functioning. Eur J Pediatr. 1982;139:165–171.
19. Guilleminault C, Stoohs R, Clerk A, Cetel M, Maistros P. A cause of excessive daytime sleepiness. the upper airway resistance syndrome. Chest. 1993;104:781–787.
20. Ng DK, Chow PY, Chan CH, Kwok KL, Cheung JM, Kong FY. An update on childhood snoring. Acta Paediatr. 2006;95:1029–1035.
21. Bao G, Guilleminault C. Upper airway resistance syndrome – one decade later. Curr Opin Pulm Med. 2004;10:461–467.
22. Section on Pediatric Pulmonology, Subcommittee on Obstructive Sleep Apnea Syndrome. American Academy of Pediatrics. Clinical practice guideline: diagnosis and management of childhood obstructive sleep apnea syndrome. Pediatrics. 2002;109:704–712.
23. O'Brien LM, Mervis CB, Holbrook CR, et al. Neurobehavioral implications of habitual snoring in children. Pediatrics. 2004;114:44–49.
24. Lumeng JC, Chervin RD. Epidemiology of pediatric obstructive sleep apnea. Proc Am Thorac Soc. 2008;5:242–252.
25. Muzumdar H, Arens R. Diagnostic issues in pediatric obstructive sleep apnea. Proc Am Thorac Soc. 2008;5:263–273.
26. Brooks LJ, Topol HI. Enuresis in children with sleep apnea. J Pediatr. 2003;142:515–518.
27. Firoozi F, Batniji R, Aslan AR, Longhurst PA, Kogan BA. Resolution of diurnal incontinence and nocturnal enuresis after adenotonsillectomy in children. J Urol. 2006;175:1885–1888; discussion 1888.
28. Weissbach A, Leiberman A, Tarasiuk A, Goldbart A, Tal A. Adenotonsilectomy improves enuresis in children with obstructive sleep apnea syndrome. Int J Pediatr Otorhinolaryngol. 2006;70:1351–1356.
29. Brooks LJ, Stephens BM, Bacevice AM. Adenoid size is related to severity but not the number of episodes of obstructive apnea in children. J Pediatr. 1998;132:682–686.
30. Dayyat E, Kheirandish-Gozal L, Sans Capdevila O, Maarafeya MM, Gozal D. Obstructive sleep apnea in children: relative contributions of body mass index and adenotonsillar hypertrophy. Chest. 2009;136:137–144.
31. Goodwin JL, Enright PL, Kaemingk KL, et al. Feasibility of using unattended polysomnography in children for research – report of the tucson children's assessment of sleep apnea study (TuCASA). Sleep. 2001;24:937–944.
32. Arens R, McDonough JM, Costarino AT, et al. Magnetic resonance imaging of the upper airway structure of children with obstructive sleep apnea syndrome. Am J Respir Crit Care Med. 2001;164:698–703.
33. Isono S, Shimada A, Utsugi M, Konno A, Nishino T. Comparison of static mechanical properties of the passive pharynx between normal children and children with sleep-disordered breathing. Am J Respir Crit Care Med. 1998;157:1204–1212.
34. Monahan KJ, Larkin EK, Rosen CL, Graham G, Redline S. Utility of noninvasive pharyngometry in epidemiologic studies of childhood sleep-disordered breathing. Am J Respir Crit Care Med. 2002;165:1499–1503.

35. Katz ES, D'Ambrosio CM. Pathophysiology of pediatric obstructive sleep apnea. Proc Am Thorac Soc. 2008;5:253–262.

36. Marcus CL, Lutz J, Hamer A, Smith PL, Schwartz A. Developmental changes in response to subatmospheric pressure loading of the upper airway. J Appl Physiol. 1999;87:626–633.

37. Marcus CL, Katz ES, Lutz J, Black CA, Galster P, Carson KA. Upper airway dynamic responses in children with the obstructive sleep apnea syndrome. Pediatr Res. 2005;57:99–107.

38. Gozal D, Burnside MM. Increased upper airway collapsibility in children with obstructive sleep apnea during wakefulness. Am J Respir Crit Care Med. 2004;169:163–167.

39. Somers VK, Dyken ME, Mark AL, Abboud FM. Sympathetic-nerve activity during sleep in normal subjects. N Engl J Med. 1993;328:303–307.

40. Malhotra A, Loscalzo J. Sleep and cardiovascular disease: an overview. Prog Cardiovasc Dis. 2009;51:279–284.

41. Somers VK, Dyken ME, Clary MP, Abboud FM. Sympathetic neural mechanisms in obstructive sleep apnea. J Clin Invest. 1995;96:1897–1904.

42. Gjorup PH, Sadauskiene L, Wessels J, Nyvad O, Strunge B, Pedersen EB. Abnormally increased endothelin-1 in plasma during the night in obstructive sleep apnea: relation to blood pressure and severity of disease. Am J Hypertens. 2007;20:44–52.

43. Phillips BG, Narkiewicz K, Pesek CA, Haynes WG, Dyken ME, Somers VK. Effects of obstructive sleep apnea on endothelin-1 and blood pressure. J Hypertens. 1999;17:61–66.

44. Tkacova R, Rankin F, Fitzgerald FS, Floras JS, Bradley TD. Effects of continuous positive airway pressure on obstructive sleep apnea and left ventricular afterload in patients with heart failure. Circulation. 1998;98:2269–2275.

45. Hedner J, Ejnell H, Caidahl K. Left ventricular hypertrophy independent of hypertension in patients with obstructive sleep apnoea. J Hypertens. 1990;8:941–946.

46. Bixler EO, Vgontzas AN, Lin HM, et al. Blood pressure associated with sleep-disordered breathing in a population sample of children. Hypertension. 2008;52:841–846.

47. Kaditis AG, Alexopoulos EI, Kostadima E, et al. Comparison of blood pressure measurements in children with and without habitual snoring. Pediatr Pulmonol. 2005;39:408–414.

48. Redline S, Storfer-Isser A, Rosen CL, et al. Association between metabolic syndrome and sleep-disordered breathing in adolescents. Am J Respir Crit Care Med. 2007;176:401–408.

49. Enright PL, Goodwin JL, Sherrill DL, Quan JR, Quan SF, Tucson Children's Assessment of Sleep Apnea study. Blood pressure elevation associated with sleep-related breathing disorder in a community sample of white and hispanic children: the Tucson children's assessment of sleep apnea study. Arch Pediatr Adolesc Med. 2003;157:901–904.

50. Amin RS, Carroll JL, Jeffries JL, et al. Twenty-four-hour ambulatory blood pressure in children with sleep-disordered breathing. Am J Respir Crit Care Med. 2004;169:950–956.

51. Amin R, Somers VK, McConnell K, et al. Activity-adjusted 24-hour ambulatory blood pressure and cardiac remodeling in children with sleep disordered breathing. Hypertension. 2008;51:84–91.

52. Li AM, Au CT, Sung RY, et al. Ambulatory blood pressure in children with obstructive sleep Apnoea: a community based study. Thorax. 2008;63:803–809.

53. Leung LC, Ng DK, Lau MW, et al. Twenty-four-hour ambulatory BP in snoring children with obstructive sleep apnea syndrome. Chest. 2006;130:1009–1017.

54. Kohyama J, Ohinata JS, Hasegawa T. Blood pressure in sleep disordered breathing. Arch Dis Child. 2003;88:139–142.

55. Marcus CL, Greene MG, Carroll JL. Blood pressure in children with obstructive sleep apnea. Am J Respir Crit Care Med. 1998;157:1098–1103.

56. Guilleminault C, Eldridge FL, Simmons FB, Dement WC. Sleep apnea in eight children. Pediatrics. 1976;58:23–30.

57. Wuhl E, Witte K, Soergel M, Mehls O, Schaefer F, German Working Group on Pediatric Hypertension. Distribution of 24-h ambulatory blood pressure in children: Normalized reference values and role of body dimensions. J Hypertens. 2002;20:1995–2007.

58. Rosner B, Prineas RJ, Loggie JM, Daniels SR. Blood pressure nomograms for children and adolescents, by height, sex, and age, in the United States. J Pediatr. 1993;123:871–886.

59. Amici A, Cicconetti P, Sagrafoli C, et al. Exaggerated morning blood pressure surge and cardiovascular events. A 5-year longitudinal study in normotensive and well-controlled hypertensive elderly. Arch Gerontol Geriatr. 2008.

60. Kario K, Pickering TG, Hoshide S, et al. Morning blood pressure surge and hypertensive cerebrovascular disease: role of the alpha adrenergic sympathetic nervous system. Am J Hypertens. 2004;17:668–675.

61. Kario K, Pickering TG, Umeda Y, et al. Morning surge in blood pressure as a predictor of silent and clinical cerebrovascular disease in elderly hypertensives: a prospective study. Circulation. 2003;107:1401–1406.

62. Soergel M, Kirschstein M, Busch C, et al. Oscillometric twenty-four-hour ambulatory blood pressure values in healthy children and adolescents: a multicenter trial including 1141 subjects. J Pediatr. 1997;130:178–184.

63. Sorof J, Daniels S. Obesity hypertension in children: a problem of epidemic proportions. Hypertension. 2002;40:441–447.

64. Redline S, Tishler PV, Schluchter M, Aylor J, Clark K, Graham G. Risk factors for sleep-disordered breathing in children. Associations with obesity, race, and respiratory problems. Am J Respir Crit Care Med. 1999;159:1527–1532.

65. Reade EP, Whaley C, Lin JJ, McKenney DW, Lee D, Perkin R. Hypopnea in pediatric patients with obesity hypertension. Pediatr Nephrol. 2004;19:1014–1020.

66. Urbina E, Alpert B, Flynn J, et al. Ambulatory blood pressure monitoring in children and adolescents: recommendations for standard assessment. A Scientific Statement from the American Heart Association Atherosclerosis, Hypertension, and Obesity in Youth Committee of the Council on Cardiovascular Disease in the Young and the Council for High Blood Pressure Research. Hypertension. 2008;52:433–451.

67. Pickering TG. Should we be evaluating blood pressure dipping status in clinical practice? J Clin Hypertens (Greenwich). 2005;7:178–182.

68. Flynn JT. What's new in pediatric hypertension? Curr Hypertens Rep. 2001;3:503–510.

69. Loredo JS, Ancoli-Israel S, Dimsdale JE. Sleep quality and blood pressure dipping in obstructive sleep apnea. Am J Hypertens. 2001;14:887–892.

70. Suzuki M, Guilleminault C, Otsuka K, Shiomi T. Blood pressure "dipping" and "non-dipping" in obstructive sleep apnea syndrome patients. Sleep. 1996;19:382–387.

71. Sukhija R, Aronow WS, Sandhu R, et al. Prevalence of left ventricular hypertrophy in persons with and without obstructive sleep apnea. Cardiol Rev. 2006;14:170–172.

72. Amin RS, Kimball TR, Bean JA, et al. Left ventricular hypertrophy and abnormal ventricular geometry in children and adolescents with obstructive sleep apnea. Am J Respir Crit Care Med. 2002;165:1395–1399.

73. Amin RS, Kimball TR, Kalra M, et al. Left ventricular function in children with sleep-disordered breathing. Am J Cardiol. 2005;95:801–804.

74. Sanchez-Armengol A, Rodriguez-Puras MJ, Fuentes-Pradera MA, et al. Echocardiographic parameters in adolescents with sleep-related breathing disorders. Pediatr Pulmonol. 2003;36:27–33.

75. Shine NP, Lannigan FJ, Coates HL, Wilson A. Adenotonsillectomy for obstructive sleep apnea in obese children: effects on respiratory parameters and clinical outcome. Arch Otolaryngol Head Neck Surg. 2006;132:1123–1127.

76. Suen JS, Arnold JE, Brooks LJ. Adenotonsillectomy for treatment of obstructive sleep apnea in children. Arch Otolaryngol Head Neck Surg. 1995;121:525–530.

77. Gorur K, Doven O, Unal M, Akkus N, Ozcan C. Preoperative and postoperative cardiac and clinical findings of patients with adenotonsillar hypertrophy. Int J Pediatr Otorhinolaryngol. 2001;59:41–46.

78. Apostolidou MT, Alexopoulos EI, Damani E, et al. Absence of blood pressure, metabolic, and inflammatory marker changes after adenotonsillectomy for sleep apnea in Greek children. Pediatr Pulmonol. 2008;43:550–560.

26 Hypertension and Exercise

Rae-Ellen W. Kavey, MD, MPH

NORMAL BP RESPONSE TO EXERCISE

In normal children, the physiologic blood pressure response to exercise is complex, involving increases in stroke volume and heart rate, changes in peripheral resistance, and a response to sympathetic output. With dynamic exercise, the increase in cardiac output is accompanied by a continuous steep rise in heart rate and systolic blood pressure, a small decrease in diastolic blood pressure, and a significant decrease in systemic vascular resistance *(1–5)*. The rise in systolic BP is higher in boys than in girls and it increases in both sexes with increasing age and body size *(2)*. Both lean body mass and fat mass are important hemodynamic determinants of blood pressure *(6)*. Consistent racial differences in the BP response to exercise have not been reported *(7)*. With treadmill exercise testing, systolic BPs as high as 250 mmHg have been recorded in healthy normotensive adolescent males.

With static or isometric exercise, there is an abrupt increase in both systolic and diastolic BPs, a modest increase in heart rate, stable or limited decline in stroke volume, a small increase in cardiac output, and no change in systemic vascular resistance *(4,8–10)*. The increase in systolic and diastolic BPs can be marked. In young adult male weight lifters, extremely high blood pressures, exceeding 400/300 mmHg, have been reported from direct intra-arterial recordings *(11)*.

R.-E.W. Kavey (✉)
Division of Pediatric Cardiology, University of Rochester Medical Center, Rochester, NY, USA
e-mail: rae-ellen_kavey@urmc.rochester.edu

From: *Clinical Hypertension and Vascular Diseases: Pediatric Hypertension*
Edited by: J. T. Flynn et al. DOI 10.1007/978-1-60327-824-9_26
© Springer Science+Business Media, LLC 2011

BP MEASUREMENT WITH EXERCISE TESTING

The role of exercise testing in the evaluation of children and adolescents with defined cardiac problems and in those with potentially cardiac symptoms continues to increase. Current guidelines from the American Heart Association published in 2006 review the equipment requirements, exercise protocols, and required measurements for safe and effective assessment of exercise performance in the pediatric age group *(12)*. Blood pressure responses to exercise testing have been reported for both bicycle ergometer and treadmill exercise testing in a variety of populations *(2–5,7,13–26)*, with exercise blood pressures monitored manually or with automated instruments *(12,27)*. The use of varying protocols makes direct comparison of these results difficult.

There is agreement that regardless of the protocol or equipment, systolic BP rises continuously with dynamic exercise, with the difference from baseline to peak exertion increasing as age and body surface area increase. By contrast, diastolic blood pressure is stable or decreases slightly during exercise. Upper versus lower extremity blood pressure gradients with exercise testing have been evaluated in normal children and adolescents and are very small: mean arm–leg gradient at rest was –5 mmHg, increasing to 4, 2, and 1 mmHg at 1, 3, and 4 min postexercise *(28)*. In adults, a maximum normal systolic BP response to exercise testing has been defined as 220 mmHg. However, measurement of BP response with radial artery catheterization in adults during exercise testing reveals that direct systolic BP was significantly greater than cuff systolic BP by a mean of 29 mmHg with maximal exercise systolic BP exceeding 240 mmHg in 20% of subjects *(29)*. Defining the normal maximum BP response to exercise in adolescents has been challenging with cuff systolic BPs as high as 250 mmHg being recorded in studies of normotensive postpubertal male athletes *(2,30)*. The AHA guidelines state that ". . . there is no evidence of danger when the systolic blood pressure reaches the 250-mmHg range during exercise in an asymptomatic child or adolescent" *(12)*.

BP RESPONSE TO EXERCISE IN PEDIATRIC SUBPOPULATIONS

Children and Adolescents with Hypertension

The BP response to exercise correlates best with resting BP and this is true across the BP distribution in normal children and in those with hypertension *(4)*. For children with hypertension, the change in SBP and DBP with dynamic and isometric exercise is similar to that seen in nonhypertensive subjects but BPs are higher, paralleling those of normotensive children at a higher level *(30–35)*. With effective treatment, exercise BP decreases in parallel with changes in office and ambulatory BP. The 2005 Bethesda Conference recommendations on competitive exercise in individuals with cardiovascular disease address systemic hypertension without distinguishing children and adolescents from adults *(36)*. The BP-lowering effects of repetitive exercise are reviewed and regular dynamic activity is recommended. Intensive resistive training is not recommended. Athletic participation is limited only "until BP is controlled by appropriate treatment". Other expert commentaries have also recommended routine dynamic exercise and no exercise limitation in hypertensive children and adolescents on therapy *(30,37–39)*.

Children at Increased Risk for Future Hypertension and/or Cardiovascular Disease

In normotensive adults, an exaggerated BP response to exercise testing has been shown to predict future hypertension and increased cardiovascular risk *(40–42)*. In children, the predictive value of exercise BP has been also been evaluated. From 3.4 years of follow-up in the Muscatine study, subsequent systolic BP was best predicted from initial resting blood pressure, maximal exercise systolic BP, and left ventricular mass. Only exercise blood pressure effectively predicted subsequent LV mass *(43)*. In normotensive adolescents, systolic BP response to exercise was significantly higher in those with a family history of hypertension than in controls with a negative family history *(44)*. In 7- to 10-year-old boys with a family history of premature myocardial infarction, a significantly greater systolic blood pressure and total peripheral resistance was demonstrated in response to bicycle ergometer testing *(45)*. In a larger group from the same laboratory, 1-year stability was demonstrated for dynamic pressor responses in children from hypertensive families *(46)*. Evaluation of the pressor response to treadmill exercise in 6- to 7-year-old black and white children showed that stress responses are predictive of resting cardiovascular function at 2.5 year follow-up *(47)*. In a study of Dutch adolescents and young adults, exercise responses to isometric exercise and bicycle ergometry were compared in those with two hypertensive parents and those with normotensive parents. By contrast with other reports, the offspring of hypertensive parents were found to have increased total peripheral resistance during isometric exercise and an attenuated increase in stroke volume with dynamic exercise but no increase in blood pressure *(48)*. In a small series of boys with severe hypercholesterolemia, exercise systolic and diastolic blood pressures were found to be significantly higher than those of normolipidemic controls, suggesting altered control of arterial vascular tone in this setting *(49)*. Among children and adolescents with white coat hypertension defined by elevated office blood pressures with normal ambulatory BP recordings, 38% had an exaggerated BP response to treadmill exercise, compared with 63% of those with sustained hypertension. This was felt to suggest that white coat hypertension in childhood may represent a true prehypertensive state *(35)*. In summary, the BP response to exercise appears to be exaggerated in children who are at increased risk for early atherosclerotic disease.

Congenital Heart Disease

There are three congenital cardiac diagnoses in which the blood pressure response to exercise has been extensively evaluated: postoperative coarctation of the aorta, aortic stenosis, and hypertrophic cardiomyopathy. The characteristic exercise BP responses are summarized below.

Coarctation of the Aorta

After repair of coarctation of the aorta, long-term follow-up studies document persistent hypertension, significant cardiovascular morbidity, and premature mortality despite elimination of resting arm–leg pressure gradient *(50–52)*. An upper body hypertensive response to exercise and development of a significant arm–leg gradient have been well described in these patients, even when resting blood pressures are normal *(53–56)*. This has been attributed to a variety of mechanisms, including histologic and physiologic abnormalities of the aortic wall *(57)*, altered baroreceptor function *(58)*, increased vascular resistance and abnormal vasodilator function in the upper body *(59)*, increased norepinephrine response to exercise with increased plasma renin levels *(60)*, altered flow around the surgically altered aortic arch *(61)*, and altered mechanics at the repair site *(62,63)*. The significance of isolated exercise hypertension in postcoarctectomy patients and its relation to clinical outcome is not known and some have suggested that exercise testing results in this context are not meaningful *(64)*. However, exercise-induced hypertension has been shown to correlate with increased carotid intima–media thickness, a subclinical measure of atherosclerosis, suggesting that it may contribute to the ultimate development of clinical cardiovascular disease *(65)*. In the context of known increased risk, the presence of exercise-induced hypertension, especially if associated with increased LV mass, may identify a group of postcoarctectomy patients who warrant antihypertensive treatment. Cardioselective beta-blockade has been shown to be effective in this setting *(66)*.

Aortic Stenosis

As might be anticipated with obstruction to left ventricular outflow, the exercise response of patients with aortic stenosis is often abnormal. In adult series, the increase in cardiac output with exercise is reduced, approximately 50–60% of normal *(67,68)*. With exercise testing, this is associated with a blunted blood pressure rise, the development of anginal or presyncopal symptoms, and the onset of significant ST depression in one-third to two-thirds of asymptomatic adult patients, with abnormal results correlating best with resting gradient *(69)*. Several recent prospective series have shown that in asymptomatic patients, an abnormal exercise test is strongly predictive of an adverse outcome (the onset of clinical symptoms in daily life, aortic valve surgery or sudden death) over relatively short-term (12–36 months) follow-up *(70–73)*. In Europe, exercise testing has been recommended to aid in clinical decision-making in asymptomatic patients with moderate gradients every year and with severe gradients every 6 months *(74)*. In the 2008 ACC/AHA guidelines for management of aortic valvular disease, exercise testing is recommended in asymptomatic adults with moderate Doppler gradients above 50 mmHg *(75)*.

In children with aortic valve stenosis, results have been less consistent. Beginning in the 1960s, characteristic ischemic ECG changes of ST segment depression with exercise have been reported in children with aortic valve stenosis; the presence and severity of the ischemic response correlated with the magnitude of the aortic valve gradient *(76–78)*. In the 1970s, a series of investigators reported lower systolic BP rise with exercise in children with aortic stenosis compared with normal children and suggested that the exercise BP response, combined with analysis of electrocardiographic changes, could be used to quantify the severity of stenosis *(79–81)*. However, in one of the largest series, 70 children with isolated AS, maximal exercise responses for work load, heart rate, and peak working capacity were reduced compared with normal controls, but neither maximal blood pressure response nor ECG abnormalities correlated with the severity of the outflow gradient *(82)*. Unfortunately, there was no physiologic measure of exercise effort to validate comparison among the patients with aortic stenosis and controls. A later report of exercise testing during cardiac catheterization demonstrated that aortic stenosis patients with exercise-induced ST-segment depression had significantly higher exercise LV pressure, higher LVOT gradient, and lower aortic systolic BP with a correspondingly higher LV-O2 supply–demand ratio, supporting the conception of myocardial ischemia as the etiology of ischemic electrocardiographic findings *(83)*. Two more relatively recent studies have demonstrated a greater increase in QT interval with exercise in patients with AS compared with controls and this has been suggested as a potential mechanism for rare cases of serious ventricular arrhythmias and sudden death in this population *(84,85)*. Finally, a recent survey-based review of current practice among academic pediatric cardiology programs in managing patients with aortic stenosis reported that 28% of programs use exercise testing as part of the routine evaluation and follow-up of children with moderate and severe aortic stenosis *(86)*. The most recent Bethesda Conference guidelines on competitive athletics in children with heart disease require exercise testing results in patients with moderate aortic stenosis to determine exercise recommendations *(87)*.

Hypertrophic Cardiomyopathy

Sudden death is a dreaded and relatively common occurrence in patients with hypertrophic cardiomyopathy (HCM)and the risk of sudden death is greatest in children and young adults *(88–90)*. Exercise hypotension has been well documented in this setting, occurring in approximately a third of patients, and is strongly associated with young age and a family history of sudden death *(91)*. Invasive studies have shown that the failure to increase blood pressure appropriately during exercise is a consequence of an inappropriate vasodilator response in non-exercising vascular beds leading to an exaggerated fall in systemic vascular resistance, impaired diastolic filling capacity, and a blunted increase in stroke volume *(92,93)*. Left ventricular outflow tract gradient has been shown to increase markedly when measured immediately after exercise; independent predictors of an increase in outflow gradient with exercise included a history of syncope or presyncope *(94,95)*. An abnormal exercise blood pressure response has also been related to subendocardial ischemia in patients with HCM *(96)*. Finally, a recent study using ambulatory radionuclide monitoring demonstrated that an abnormal blood pressure response was associated with exercise-induced left ventricular systolic dysfunction and impairment in oxygen consumption *(97)*. In prospective studies from both tertiary referral centers and community-based populations, an abnormal BP response to exercise was observed in 11–37% of patients. On subsequent follow-up, an abnormal BP response to exercise was shown to be associated with increased risk of sudden cardiac death with high-negative but low-positive predictive accuracy *(98–100)*. In addition to the abnormal hemodynamic response, exercise testing and ambulatory ECG monitoring demonstrate a high prevalence of atrial and ventricular arrhythmias *(101)*.

While most of the studies reported above have included children and adolescents, there have been some that have exclusively evaluated children with hypertrophic cardiomyopathy. In a small series from Japan, exercise BP response was reduced in all ten patients with HCM and two had a hypotensive response to exercise *(102)*. A series of 23 patients with HCM, aged 6–23 years, with previous history of cardiac arrest, syncope, or a family history of sudden cardiac death underwent exercise thallium scintigraphy, electrophysiologic study, and ambulatory ECG monitoring *(103)*. In this highly selected patient group, all patients with a history of syncope or cardiac arrest had inducible ischemia on thallium scintigraphy and a majority had LV cavity dilation. BP response to exercise is not reported. In a continuous series of 99 pediatric patients with HCM, all less than 18 years of age, treadmill exercise results were reported in 43 *(104)*. All patients survived testing but 19% developed chest pain with significant ST depression and 42% had a hypotensive response to exercise. Mean exercise duration was reduced for the group. Unfortunately, exercise results were only available for 1 of the subset of 12 patients from the whole group who went on to sudden death; in that child, there was a BP drop with exercise. Finally, a consecutive series of children with HCM were evaluated by echocardiography, ambulatory ECG monitoring, and exercise testing *(105)*. Of the 38 children who underwent exercise testing, 16 were symptomatic and 50% of these had a blunted BP response to exercise, compared with 10% of asymptomatic children. Maximum oxygen consumption (VO2max) was significantly lower in the symptomatic patients and by linear regression analysis, there was a significant inverse relationship between NYHA class and VO2max. Children with HCM had significantly decreased early diastolic tissue Doppler velocities for ventricular inflow compared with controls and in regression analysis, early transmitral left ventricular filling velocity predicted death, cardiac arrest, or ventricular tachycardia. Maximum oxygen consumption with exercise was most predictive of subsequent symptomatology.

The 2005 Bethesda Conference recommendations on competitive athletics in children and adults with cardiovascular disease recommend limitation from all competitive sports in individuals with a probable or unequivocal clinical diagnosis of HCM, regardless of age or prior treatment *(106)*. However, in genotype positive–phenotype negative individuals, regular exercise stress testing is recommended. If blood pressure response and exercise tolerance remain normal and there are no exercise-related ventricular arrhythmias, no restriction from competitive athletics is recommended.

EXERCISE AS NONPHARMACOLOGIC TREATMENT OF ESSENTIAL HYPERTENSION

When essential hypertension begins in childhood, a nonpharmacologic approach to lowering BP is preferable when possible since initiation of drug treatment has known significant side effects. In other parts of this book, the BP-lowering effects of weight loss and diet change are presented. Here, the BP-lowering effect of exercise is reviewed.

Many epidemiologic studies have shown a strong relationship between higher levels of regular physical activity and lower blood pressure. The DISC study was a randomized clinical trial of a reduced saturated fat and cholesterol diet in 8- to 10-year-old children with moderate baseline cholesterol elevation. Over a 3-year period, self-reported levels of physical activity were significantly correlated with blood pressure: for every 100 estimated-metabolic-equivalent hours of physical activity, there was a decrease of 1.15 mmHg in systolic BP *(107)*. In the Muscatine study, a subset of the cohort underwent assessment of physical fitness. Increased fitness and strength correlated inversely with BP over a 5-year interval *(108)*. In the Northern Ireland Young Hearts project, a random cohort of 12- to 15-year-old adolescents underwent cardiovascular risk assessment. Over a 3-year interval, there was a significant relationship between increased self-reported physical activity and lower blood pressure *(109)*. Finally, in the Young-HUNT study from Norway, activity levels, weight measures, and BPs were evaluated in more than 8000 adolescents. In this population, low levels of physical activity were significantly associated with higher mean diastolic BP and increased odds of overweight and obesity *(110)*.

The effects of specific activity interventions on blood pressure in children and adolescents have been evaluated in a series of randomized controlled trials. These have been systematically reviewed in a recent meta-analysis *(111)*. The review included 12 trials representing 16 outcomes in 1266 subjects. Sample size ranged from 16 to over 500 subjects and age ranged from 7 to 19 years. The training period varied from 8 to 36 weeks with frequency ranging from two to five times a week and duration from 10 to 75 min per session. Ten trials used primarily aerobic training and two used resistance training. Collectively, the studies showed a 1% reduction in systolic BP and a 3% reduction in diastolic BP. Two subsequent trials confirm significant blood pressure-lowering effects of exercise in children *(112,113)*. Although the magnitude of change in blood pressure in these studies is not large, it occurs at a time when blood pressure is normally increasing. Both the longitudinal studies and the intervention studies indicate that the age-related rise in blood pressure may be blunted by frequent, regular activity. Combining this with knowledge of the strong association between hypertension and obesity and the established benefits of exercise in weight control, regular dynamic physical activity should be a standard part of the management of essential hypertension in children and adolescents.

EXERCISE RECOMMENDATIONS IN HYPERTENSIVE ATHLETES

Activity recommendations for specific BP-related subgroups of children have been included throughout this chapter. As noted in the section describing the exercise response in hypertensive children and adolescents, the 2005 Bethesda Conference recommendations on competitive exercise in individuals with cardiovascular disease address systemic hypertension without distinguishing children and adolescents from adults (36). The BP-lowering effects of repetitive exercise are reviewed and regular dynamic activity is recommended. Intensive resistive training is not recommended. Participation in competitive athletics is limited only "until BP is controlled by appropriate treatment". The American Academy of Pediatrics Committee on Sports Medicine and Fitness recommends restriction from weight- and powerlifting, body building, and strength training in children with hypertension; participation in competitive sports is given a "qualified yes" (114). In previous guidelines from the AAP that focused specifically on children with hypertension, children with severe hypertension are limited from competitive sports until BP is adequately controlled (115). Many other expert commentaries have also recommended regular dynamic exercise and no exercise limitation in hypertensive children and adolescents on effective therapy (30,37–39).

Overall, the consensus appears to be no dynamic exercise limitations in children and adolescents once BP has been treated. There are some reservations about static exercise in hypertensive patients. However, beyond the potential for extreme pressure elevation with resistance training that has been documented in normotensive subjects, the basis for this is limited, especially in light of studies documenting a fall in blood pressure with a sustained resistance training program (11,111).

REFERENCES

1. Braden DS, Strong WB. Cardiovascular responses to exercise in childhood. Am J Dis Child. 1990;144:1255–1260.
2. Wanne OPS, Haapoja E. Blood pressure during exercise in healthy children. Eur J Appl Physiol. 1988;58:62–67.
3. Riopel DA, Taylor AB, Hohn AR. Blood pressure, heart rate, pressure-rate product and electrocardiographic changes in healthy children during treadmill exercise. Am J Cardiol. 1979;44:697–704.
4. Schieken RM, Clarke WR, Lauer RM. The cardiovascular responses to exercise in children across the blood pressure distribution: the Muscatine Study. Hypertension. 1983;5:71–78.
5. Ahmad F, Kavey REW, Kveselis DA, Gaum WE. Responses of non-obese white children to treadmill exercise. J Pediatr. 2001;139:284–290.
6. Daniels SR, Kimball TR, Khoury P, Witt S, Morrison JA. Correlates of the hemodynamic determinants of blood pressure. Hypertension. 1996;28:37–41.
7. Pate RR, Matthews C, Alpert BS, Strong WB, DuRant RH. Systolic blood pressure response to exercise in black and white preadolescent and early adolescent boys. Arch Pediatr Adolesc Med. 1994;148:1027–1031.
8. Laird WP, Fixler DE, Huffines FD. Cardiovascular response to isometric exercise in normal adolescents. Circulation. 1979;59:651–654.
9. Rowland T, Heffernan K, Jae SY, Echols G, Fernhall B. Cardiovascular responses to static exercise in boys: insights from tissue Doppler imaging. Eur J Appl Physiol. 2006;97:637–642.
10. Ferrara LA, Mainenti G, Fasano ML, Maroyya T, Borrelli R, Mancini M. Cardiovascular response to mental stress and to handgrip in children. Jpn Heart J. 1991;32:645–654.
11. MacDougall JD, Tuxen D, Sale DG, Moroz JR, Sutton JR. Arterial blood pressure response to heavy resistance exercise. J Appl Physiol. 1985;58:785–790.
12. Paridon SM, Alpert BS, Boas SR, Cabrera ME, Caldarera LL, Daniels SR, Kimball TR, Knilans TK, Nixon PA, Rhodes J, Yetman AT. Clinical stress testing in the pediatric age group. A statement from the American Heart Association Council on Cardiovascular Disease in the Young, Committee on Atherosclerosis, Hypertension and Obesity in Youth. Circulation. 2006;113:1905–1920.

13. Adams FH, Linde LM, Miyake H. The physical working capacity of normal school children: I. California. Pediatrics. 1961;28:55–64.

14. Adams FH, Bengtsson E, Bervan H, Wegelium C. The physical working capacity of normal school children: II. Swedish city and country. Pediatrics. 1961;30:243.

15. Godfrey S, Davis CTM, Wozniak E, Bawles CA. Cardiorespiratory response to exercise in normal children. Clin Sci. 1971;40:419–442.

16. Strong WB, Spencer D, Miller MD, Salehbhai M. The physical working capacity of healthy black children. Am J Dis Child. 1978;132:244.

17. Thapar MK, Strong WB, Miller MD, Leatherbury L, Salehbhai M. Exercise electro-cardiography of healthy black children. Am J Dis Child. 1978;132:592.

18. Lock JE, Einzig S, Moller JH. Hemodynamic responses to exercise in normal children. Am J Cardiol. 1978;41:1278.

19. Cumming GR, Everatt D, Hastmen L. Bruce treadmill test in children: normal values in a clinic population. Am J Cardiol. 1978;40:69–75.

20. James FW, Kaplan S, Glueck CJ, Tsay J-V, Knight MJS, Sarwar CJ. Responses of normal children and young adults to controlled bicycle exercise. Circulation. 1980;61:902–912.

21. Alpert BS, Dover EV, Booker DL, Martin AM, Strong WB. Blood pressure response to dynamic exercise in healthy children—black vs white. J Pediatr. 1981;99:556–560.

22. Alpert BS, Flood NL, Strong WB, Dover EV, DuRant RH, Martin AM, Booker DL. Responses to ergometer exercise in a healthy biracial population of children. J Pediatr. 1982;101:538–545.

23. Washington RL, van Gundy JC, Cohen C, Sondheimer HM, Wolfe RR. Normal aerobic and anaerobic exercise data for North American school-age children. J Pediatr. 1988;112:223–233.

24. Maffulli N, Greco L, Greco L, D'Alterio D. Treadmill exercise in Neopolitan children and adolescents. Acta Pediatr. 1994;83:106–112.

25. Lenk MK, Alehan D, Celiker A, Alpay F, Sarici U. Bruce treadmill test in healthy Turkish children: endurance time, heart rate, blood pressure and electrocardiographic changes. Turk J Pediatr. 1998;40: 167–175.

26. Becker M deM C, Barbosa e Silva O, Goncalves IE, Victor EG. Arterial blood pressure in adolescents during exercise stress testing. Arq Bras Cardiol. 2007;88:297–300.

27. Alpert BS, Flood NL, Balfour IC, Strong WB. Automated blood pressure measurement during ergometer exercise in children. Cathet Cardiovasc Diagn. 1982;8:525–533.

28. Knecht SK, Mays WA, Gerdes YM, Claytor RP, Knilans TK. Exercise evaluation of upper- versus lower-extremity blood pressure gradients in pediatric and young adult participants. Pediatr Exerc Sci. 2007;18:344–348.

29. Rasmussen PH, Staats BA, Driscoll DJ, Beck KC, Bonekat HW, Wilcox WD. Direct and indirect blood pressure during exercise. Chest. 1985;87:743–748.

30. Dlin R. Blood pressure response to dynamic exercise in healthy and hypertensive youths. Pediatrician. 1986;13:34–43.

31. Nudel DB, Gootman N, Brunson SC, Stenzler A, Shenker IR, Gauthier BG. Exercise performance of hypertensive adolescents. Pediatrics. 1980;65:1073–1078.

32. Fixler DE, Laird WP, Browne R, Fitzgerald V, Wilson S, Vance R. Response of hypertensive adolescents to dynamic and isometric exercise stress. Pediatrics. 1979;64:579–583.

33. Wilson SL, Gaffney A, Laird WP, Fixler DE. Body size, composition and fitness in adolescents with elevated blood pressures. Hypertension. 1985;7:417–422.

34. Klein AA, McCrory WW, Engle MA, Rosenthal R, Ehlers KH. Sympathetic nervous system and exercise tolerance in normotensive and hypertensive adolescents. J Am Coll Cardiol. 1984;3:381–386.

35. Kavey REW, Kveselis DA, Atallah N, Smith FC. White coat hypertension in childhood: evidence for end-organ effect. J Pediatr. 2007;150:491–197.

36. Kaplan NM, Gidding SS, Pickering TG, Wright JT. 36th Bethesda Conference: eligibility recommendations for competitive athletes with cardiovascular abnormalities. Task Force 5: systemic hypertension. J Am Coll Cardiol. 2005;45:1326–1333.

37. Kaminer SJ, Hixon RL, Strong WB. Evaluation and recommendations for participation in athletics for children with heart disease. Curr Opin Pediatr. 1995;7:595–600.

38. Alpert BS. Exercise in hypertensive children and adolescents: any harm done? Pediatr Cardiol. 1999;20:66–69.

39. Strong WB, Malina RM, Blimkie CJR, Daniels SR, Dishman RK, Gutin B, Hergenroeder AC, Must A, Nixon PA, Pivarnik JM, Rowland T, Trost S, Trudeau F. Evidence based physical activity for school-age youth. J Pediatr. 2005;146:732–737.

40. Dlin RA, Hanne N, Silverberg DS, Bar-Or O. Follow-up of normotensive men with exaggerated blood pressure response to exercise. Am Heart J. 1983;106:316–320.

41. Manolio TA, Burke GL, Savage PJ, Gardin JM, Oberman A. Exercise blood pressure response and 5-year risk of elevated blood pressure in a cohort of young adults: the CARDIA study. Am J Hypertens. 1994;7:234–241.

42. Lewis GD, Gona P, Larson MG, Plehn JF, Benjamin EJ, O'Donnell CJ, Levy D, Vasan RS, Wang TJ. Exercise blood pressure and the risk of incident cardiovascular disease (from the Framingham heart study). Am J Cardiol. 2008;101:1614–1620.

43. Mahoney LT, Schieken RM, Clarke WR, Lauer RM. Left ventricular mass and exercise responses predict future blood pressure: the Muscatine Study. Hypertension. 1988;12:206–213.

44. Molineux D, Steptoe A. Exaggerated blood pressure responses to submaximal exercise in normotensive adolescents with a family history of hypertension. J Hypertens. 1988;6:361–365.

45. Treiber FA, Strong WB, Arensman FW, Forrest T, Davis H, Musante L. Family history of myocardial infarction and hemodynamic responses to exercise in young black boys. Am J Dis Child. 1991;145: 1029–1033.

46. Treiber FA, Murphy JK, Davis H, Raunikar RA, Pflieger K, Strong WB. Pressor reactivity, ethnicity, and 24-hour ambulatory monitoring in children from hypertensive families. Behav Med. 1994;20: 133–142.

47. Treiber FA, Turner JR, Davis H, Thompson W, Levy M, Strong WB. Young children's cardiovascular stress responses predict resting cardiovascular functioning $2\frac{1}{2}$ years later. J Cardiovasc Risk. 1996;3: 95–100.

48. de Visser DC, van Hooft IMS, van Doornen LJP, Orlebeke JF, Grobbee DE. Cardiovascular response to physical stress in offspring of hypertensive parents: Dutch Hypertension and Offspring Study. J Hum Hypertens. 1996;10:781–788.

49. Kavey R-EW, Kveselis DA, Gaum WE. Exaggerated blood pressure response to exercise in children with increased low-density lipoprotein cholesterol. Am Heart J. 1997;133:162–168.

50. Maron BJ, Humphries JO, Rowe RD, Mellitis EG. Prognosis of surgically corrected coarctation of the aorta: a 20 year postoperative appraisal. Circulation. 1973;47:119–126.

51. Cohen M, Fuster V, Steele PM, Driscoll D, McGoon DC. Coarctation of the aorta: long-term follow-up and prediction of outcome after surgical correction. Circulation. 1989;80:840–845.

52. Toro-Salazar OH, Steinberger J, Thomas W, Rocchini AP, Carpenter B, Moller JH. Long-term follow-up of patients after coarctation of the aorta repair. Am J Cardiol. 2002;89:541–547.

53. Markham LW, Knecht SK, Daniels SR, Mays WA, Khoury PR, Knilans TK. Development of exercise-induced arm-leg gradient and abnormal arterial compliance in patients with repaired coarctation of the aorta. Am J Cardiol. 2004;94:1200–1202.

54. Freed MD, Rocchini A, Rosenthal A, Nadas AS, Castaneda AR. Exercise-induced hypertension after surgical repair of coarctation of the aorta. Am J Cardiol. 1979;43:253–258.

55. Sigurdardottir LY, Helgason H. Exercise-induced hypertension after corrective surgery for coarctation of the aorta. Pediatr Cardiol. 1996;17:301–307.

56. Ruttenberg HD. Pre- and post-operative exercise testing of the child with coarctation of the aorta. Pediatr Cardiol. 1999;20:33–37.

57. Sehested J, Baandrup U, Mikkelsen E. Different reactivity and structure of the prestenotic and poststenotic aorta in human coarctation. Implications for baroreceptor function. Circulation. 1982;65:1060–1066.

58. Beekman RH, Katz BP, Moorehead-Steffens C, Rocchini AP. Altered baroreceptor function in children with systolic hypertension after coarctation repair. Am J Cardiol. 1983;52:112–117.

59. Gidding SS, Rocchini AP, Moorehead C, Schork MA, Rosenthal A. Increased foream vascular reactivity in patients with hypertension after repair of coarctation. Circulation. 1985;71:495–499.

60. Ross RD, Clapp SK, Gunther S, Paridon SM, Humes RA, Farooki ZQ, Pinsky WW. Augmented norepinephrine and renin output in response to maximal exercise in hypertensive coarctectomy patients. Am Heart J. 1992;123:1293–1299.

61. Ou P, Bonnet D, Auriacombe L, Pedroni E, Balleux F, Sidi D, Mousseaux E. Late systemic hypertension and aortic arch geometry after successful repair of coarctation of the aorta. Eur Heart J. 2004;25: 1853–1859.

62. Ong CM, Canter CE, Gutierrez RF, Sekarski DR, Goldring DR. Increased stiffness and persistent narrowing of the aorta after successful repair of coarctation of the aorta: relationship to left ventricular mass and blood pressure at rest and with exercise. Am Heart J. 1992;123:1594–1600.

63. Kimball TR, Reynolds JM, Mays WA, Khoury P, Claytor RP, Daniels SR. Persistent hyperdynamic cardiovascular state at rest and during exercise in children after successful repair of coarctation of the aorta. J Am Coll Cardiol. 1994;24:194–200.

64. Swan L, Goyal S, Hsia C, Webb G, Gatzoulis MA. Exercise systolic blood pressures are of questionable value in the assessment of the adult with a previous coarctation repair. Heart. 2003;89:189–192.

65. Vriend JWJ, de Groot E, Bouma BJ, Hrudova J, Kastelein JJP, Tijssen JGP, Mulder BJM. Carotid intima-media thickness in post-coarctectoy patients with exercise-induced hypertension. Heart. 2005;91: 962–963.
66. Kavey RE, Cotton JL, Blackman MS. Atenolol therapy for exercise-induced hypertension after aortic coarctation repair. Am J Cardiol. 1990;66:1233–1236.
67. Richardson JW, Anderson FL, Tsagaris TJ. Rest and exercise hemodynamic studies in patients with isolated aortic valve stenosis. Cardiology. 1979;64:1–11.
68. Clyne CA, Arrighi JA, Maron BJ, Dilsizian V, Bonow RO, Cannon RO III. Systemic and left ventricular responses to exercise stress in asymptomatic patients with valvular aortic stenosis. Am J Cardiol. 1991;68:1469–1476.
69. Iung B, Baron G, Butchart EG. A prospective survey of patients with valvular heart disease in Europe: the Euro heart survey on valvular heart disease. Eur Heart J. 2003;24:1231–1243.
70. Otto CM, Burwash IG, Legget ME, Munt BI, Fujioka M, Healy NL, Kraft CD, Miyake-Hull CY, Schwaegler RG. Prospective study of asymptomatic valvular aortic stenosis. Circulation. 1997;95:2262–2270.
71. Amato MCM, Moffa PJ, Werner KE, Ramires JAF. Treatment decision in asymptomatic aortic valve stenosis: role of exercise testing. Heart. 2001;86:381–386.
72. Das P, Rimington H, Chambers J. Exercise testing to stratify risk in aortic stenosis. Eur Heart J. 2005;26:1309–1313.
73. Peidro R, Brion G, Angelino A. Exercise testing in asymptomatic aortic stenosis. Cardiology. 2007;108:258–264.
74. Pierard LA, Lancellotti P. Stress testing in valve disease. Heart. 2007;93:766–772.
75. Bonow RO, Carabello BA, Chatterjee K, de Leon AC Jr, Faxon DP, Freed MD, Gaasch WH, Lytle BW, Nishimura RA, O'Gara PT, O'Rourke RA, Otto CM, Shah PM, Shanewise JS. 2008 Focused Update Incorporated Into the ACC/AHA 2006 Guidelines for the Management of Patients with Valvular Heart Disease: a Report of the American College of Cardiology/American Heart Association Task Force on Practice Guidelines. Circulation. 2008;118:e523–e661.
76. Huggenholz PE, Lees MM, Nadas AS. The scalar electrocardiogram, vectorcardiogram and exercise electrocardiogram in the assessment of congenital aortic stenosis. Circulation. 1962;26:79–91.
77. Halloran KH. The telemetered exercise electrocardiogram in congenital aortic stenosis. Pediatrics. 1971;47:31–39.
78. Chandramouli B, Ehmke DA, Lauer RM. Exercise-induced electrocardiographic changes in children with congenital aortic stenosis. J Pediatr. 1975;87:725–730.
79. Alpert BS, Kartodihardjo W, Harp R, Izukawa T, Strong WB. Exercise blood pressure response—a predictor of severity of aortic stenosis in children. J Pediatr. 1981;98:763–765.
80. Whitmer JT, James FW, Kaplan S, Schwartz DC, Sandker Knight MJ. Exercise testing in children before and after surgical treatment of aortic stenosis. Circulation. 1981;63:254–263.
81. James FW, Schwartz DB, Kaplan S, Spilkin SP. Exercise electrocardiogram, blood pressure and working capacity in young patients with valvular or subvalvular aortic stenosis. Am J Cardiol. 1982;50:769–775.
82. Alpert BS, Moes DM, Durant RH, Strong WB, Flood NL. Hemodynamic responses to ergometer exercise in children and young adults with left ventricular pressure or volume overload. Am J Cardiol. 1983;52:563–567.
83. Kveselis DA, Rocchini AP, Rosenthal A, Crowley DC, MacDonald D, Snider AR, Moorehead C. Hemodynamic determinants of exercise-induced ST-segment depression in children with valvar aortic stenosis. Am J Cardiol. 1985;55:1133–1139.
84. Bastianon V, Del Bolgia F, Boscioni M, Gobbi V, Marzano MC, Colloridi V. Altered cardiac repolarization during exercise in congenital aortic stenosis. Pediatr Cardiol. 1993;14:23–27.
85. Yilmaz G, Ozme S, Ozme, Ozer S, Tokel K, Celiker A. Estimation by exercise testing of children with mild and moderate aortic stenosis. Pediatr Int. 2000;42: 48–52.
86. Khalid O, Luzenberg DM, Sable C; Benavidez O, Geva T, Hann B, Abdulla R. Aortic stenosis: the spectrum of practice. Pediatr Cardiol. 2006;27:661–669.
87. Graham TP, Driscoll DJ, Gersony WM, Newburger JW, Rocchini A, Towbin JA. 36th Bethesda Conference: eligibility recommendations for competitive athletes with cardiovascular abnormalities. Task Force 2: congenital heart disease. J Am Coll Cardiol. 2005;45:1326–1333.
88. McKenna WJ, Deanfield J, Faruqui A, England D, Oakley CM, Goodwin JF. Prognosis in hypertrophic cardiomyopathy. Am J Cardiol. 1981;47:532–538.
89. Fiddler GI, Tajik AJ, Weidman WH, McGoon DC, Ritter DG, Giuliana ER. Idiopathic hypertrophic subaortic stenosis in the young. Am J Cardiol. 1978;42:793–799.
90. Maron BJ, Tajik AJ, Ruttenberg HD, Graham TP, Atwood VBE, Lie JT, Roberts WC. Hypertrophic cardiomyopathy in infants: clinical features and natural history. Circulation. 1982;65:7–17.

91. Frenneaux MP, Counihan PJ, Chikamori T, Caforio ALP, McKenna WJ. Abnormal blood pressure response in hypertrophic cardiomyopathy. Circulation. 1990;82:1995–2002.
92. Ciampi Q, Betocchi S, Volante A, et al. Haemodynamic determinants of exercise induced hypotension in hypertrophic cardiomyopathy. J Am Coll Cardiol. 2002;40:278–284.
93. Lele SS, Thomson HL, Seo H, et al. Exercise capacity in hypertrophic cardiomyopathy: role of stroke volume limitation, heart rate and diastolic filling characteristics. Circulation. 1995;92: 2886–2894.
94. Klues HG, Leuner C, Kuhn H. Left ventricular outflow tract obstruction in patients with hypertrophic cardiomyopathy: increase in gradient after exercise. J Am Coll Cardiol. 1992;19:527–533.
95. Shah JS, Esteban MTT, Thaman R, Sharma R, Mist B, Pantazis A, Ward D, Kohli SK, Demetrescu C, Sevdalis E, Keren A, Pellerin D, McKenna WJ, Elliott PM. Prevalence of exercise-induced left ventricular outflow obstruction in symptomatic patients with non-obstructive hypertrophic cardiomyopathy. Heart. 2008;94:1288–1294.
96. Yoshida N, Ikeda H, Wada T, et al. Exercise-induced abnormal blood pressure responses are related to subendocardial ischemia in hypertrophic cardiomyopathy. J Am Coll Cardiol. 1998;32: 1938–1942.
97. Ciampi Q, Betocchi S, Losi MAL, Ferro A, Cuocolo A, Lombardi R, Villari B, Chiarello M. Abnormal blood pressure response to exercise and oxygen consumption in patients with hypertrophic cardiomyopathy. J Nucl Cardiol. 2007;14:869–875.
98. Sadoul N, Prasad K, Elliot PM, et al. Prospective prognostic assessment of blood pressure response during prospective prognostic assessment of blood pressure response during exercise in patients with hypertrophic cardiomyopathy. Circulation. 1997;96:2987–2991.
99. Olivotto I, Maron BJ, Montereggi A, et al. Prognostic value of systemic blood pressure response during exercise in a community-based population with hypertrophic cardiomyopathy. J Am Coll Cardiol. 1999;33:2044–2051.
100. Maki S, Ikeda H, Muro A, et al. Predictors of sudden cardiac death in hypertrophic cardiomyopathy. Am J Cardiol. 1998;82:774–778.
101. Savage DD, Seides SF, Maron BJ, Myers DJ, Epstein SE. Prevalence of arrhythmias during 24-hour electrocadiographic monitoring and exercise testing in patients with obstructive and nonobstructive hypertrophic cardiomyopathy. Circulation. 1979;59:866–875.
102. Sumitomo N, Ito S, Harada K, Kobayashi H, Okuni M. Treadmill exercise test in children with cardiomyopathy and postmyocarditic hypertrophy. Heart Vessels. 1986;1:47–50.
103. Dilsizian V, Bonow RO, Epstein SE, Fananapazir L. Myocardial ischemia detected by thallium scintigraphy is frequently related to cardiac arrest and syncope in young patients with hypertrophic cardiomyopathy. J Am Coll Cardiol. 1993;22:796–804.
104. Yetman AT, Hamilton RM, Benson LN, McCrindle BW. Long-term outcome and prognostic determinants in children with hypertrophic cardiomyopathy. J Am Coll Cardiol. 1998;32:1943–1950.
105. McMahon CJ, Nagueh SF, Pignatelli RH, Denfield SW, Dreyer WJ, Price JF, Clunie S, Bezold LI, Hays AL, Towbin JA, Eidem BW. Characterization of left ventricular diastolic function by tissue Doppler imaging and clinical status in children with hypertrophic cardiomyopathy. Circulation. 2004;109: 1756–1762.
106. Maron BJ, Ackerman MJ, Nishimura RA, Pyeritz RE, Towbin JA, Udelson JE. 36th Bethesda Conference: eligibility recommendations for competitive athletes with cardiovascular abnormalities. Task Force 4: HCM and other cardiomyopathies, mitral valve prolapse, myocarditis, and Marfan Syndrome. J Am Coll Cardiol. 2005;45:1340–1345.
107. Gidding SS, Barton BA, Dorgan JA, Kimm SYS, Kwiterovich PO, Lasser NL, Robson AM, Stevens VJ, Van Horn L, Simons-Morton DG. Higher self-reported physical activity is associated with lower systolic blood pressure: the Dietary Intervention Study in Childhood (DISC). Pediatrics. 2006;118: 2388–2393.
108. Janz KF, Dawson JD, Mahoney LT. Increases in physical fitness during childhood improve cardiovascular health during adolescence: the Muscatine Study. Int J Sports Med. 2002;23(Suppl 1):S15–S21.
109. Boreham C, Twisk J, van Mechelen W, Savage M, Strain J, Cran G. Relationships between the development of biological risk factors for coronary heart disease and lifestyle parameters during adolescence: the Northern Ireland Young Hearts Project. Public Health. 1999;113:7–12.
110. Fasting MH. Nilsen TIL, Holmen TL, Vik T. Lifestyle related blood pressure and body weight in adolescence: cross sectional data from the Young-HUNT study, Norway. BMC Public Health. 2008;8: 111–121.
111. Kelley GA, Kelley KS, Tran ZV. The effects of exercise on resting blood pressure in children and adolescents: a meta-analysis of randomized controlled trials. Prev Cardiol. 2003;6:8–16.

112. Obert P, Mandigouts S, Nottin S, Vinet A, N'Guyen LD, Lecoq AM. Cardiovascular responses to endurance training in children: effect of gender. Eur J Clin Invest. 2003;33:199–208.
113. Ribeiro MM, Silva AG, Santos NS, Guazzelle I, Matos LNJ, Trombetta IC, Halpern A, Negrao CE, Villares SMF. Diet and exercise training restore blood pressure and vasodilatory responses during physiological maneuvers in obese children. Circulation. 2005;111:1915–1923.
114. American Academy of Pediatrics Committee on Sports Medicine and Fitness: Medical conditions affecting sports participation. Pediatrics. 2001;107:1205–1209.
115. American Academy of Pediatrics Committee on Sports Medicine and Fitness. Athletic participation by children and adolescents who have systemic hypertension. Pediatrics. 1997;99:885–888.

27 Hypertension in the Developing World

Vera H. Koch, MD

THE EPIDEMIOLOGICAL TRANSITION OF THE DEVELOPING WORLD

In the past, the diseases that have occurred among people in developed and developing countries have largely been attributed to the socioeconomic status of each country (*1*). In developed countries, the health problems have largely been associated with increased wealth providing the opportunity to spend extra resources on poor health habits such as sedentary lifestyle and increased fat intake. In contrast, the diseases that have occurred among people in developing countries have been largely attributed to poverty, poor infrastructure, and limited access to care. These factors lead to famine, the spread of infectious disease, and reduced life spans.

The present picture of health problems around the world, however, now reflects a different reality. In 2002, the two most common causes of death in the world were ischemic heart disease (accounting for more than 7 million deaths) and cerebrovascular disease (approximately 5.5 million deaths) (*1*); these comprised 12.6 and 9.6%, respectively, of all deaths worldwide (*2*). One may presume that the majority of these deaths occurred in developed countries, but when countries are grouped according to their state of economic and demographic development and their mortality patterns, it is possible to realize that the number of deaths from cerebrovascular disease in developed countries comprised less than one-third of deaths from this disease worldwide. Similar distribution patterns

V.H. Koch (✉)
Department of Pediatrics, Instituto da Criança, Hospital das Clínicas da Faculdade de Medicina, Universidade de São Paulo (USP), São Paulo, SP, Brazil
e-mail: vkoch@terra.com.br

From: *Clinical Hypertension and Vascular Diseases: Pediatric Hypertension*
Edited by: J. T. Flynn et al. DOI 10.1007/978-1-60327-824-9_27
© Springer Science+Business Media, LLC 2011

emerge for ischemic heart disease *(3)*. Thus, despite the fact that the burden of disease in developed countries still largely reflects the problems associated with wealth, there is an enormous burden of chronic non-communicable diseases among populations in developing countries *(4)*.

The emergence of chronic diseases in developing countries is thought to be due to changes in the demographic structure of the population, as well as to epidemiological transitions *(1)*. These changes have traditionally occurred with economic development, have evolved over hundreds to thousands of years, and have involved an evolution from times of high mortality and low population growth to periods of increased life spans and receding pandemics. The final progression is then on to degenerative and man-made diseases, such as cardiovascular disease, resulting from major social and economic changes *(1)*. In modern times, however, the transition is happening at a faster pace due to urbanization, free trade and economic globalization, foreign investment, and promotional marketing *(5)*. Presently, although developing countries are experiencing a decline in the prevalence of infectious diseases, this is far outweighed high rates of both infectious and chronic diseases.

The risk factors underlying the emergence of non-communicable disease in these developing countries follow the same patterns as those identified previously in the current established market economies. These include increased levels of alcohol consumption, tobacco smoking, obesity, physical inactivity, and low fruit and vegetable intake. In parallel with this, there is also increased evidence of high cholesterol levels and, in particular, high blood pressure *(6)*.

The emergence of the cardiovascular disease (CVD) epidemic in the developing countries during the past two to three decades has attracted little public health response, even within these countries. In a recent literature search of the MEDLINE database *(7)*, conducted in search of published studies, which reported the prevalence of hypertension in representative population samples, the reported prevalence of hypertension varied around the world, with the lowest prevalence in rural India (3.4% in men and 6.8% in women) and the highest prevalence in Poland (68.9% in men and 72.5% in women). Awareness of hypertension was reported for 46% of the studies and varied from 25.2% in Korea to 75% in Barbados, treatment varied from 10.7% in Mexico to 66% in Barbados, and control (blood pressure <140/90 mmHg while on antihypertensive medication) varied from 5.4% in Korea to 58% in Barbados. The authors concluded that although hypertension is an important public health challenge in both economically developing and developed countries, significant numbers of individuals with hypertension are unaware of their condition and, among those with diagnosed hypertension, treatment is frequently inadequate.

The present high burden of CVD deaths is in itself an adequate reason for attention; however, another important cause for concern is the early age of CVD deaths in the developing countries compared with the developed countries. In 1990, the proportion of CVD deaths occurring below the age of 70 years was 26.5% in the developed countries compared with 46.7% in the developing countries *(8)*. The contrast between the truly developed countries (22.8% of CVD deaths at <70 years) and a large developing country like India (52.2%) was even sharper *(8)*. Therefore, the contribution of the developing countries to the global burden of CVD, in terms of disability adjusted years of life lost, was 2.8 times higher than that of the developed countries.

As a consequence of the epidemiological transition, life expectancy in developing countries has risen, due to a decline in deaths occurring in infancy, childhood, and adolescence, and was related to more effective public health responses to perinatal, infectious, and nutritional deficiency disorders and to improved economic indicators such as per capita income and social indicators such as female literacy in some areas. The increasing longevity provides longer periods of exposure to the risk factors of CVD *(9)*, resulting in a greater probability of clinically manifest CVD events *(10)* and leading to a projected rise in both proportional and absolute CVD mortality rates in the developing countries *(1)*. Hypertension is projected to be one of the major risk factors underlying the global burden of disease in 2020 *(4)*.

THE FETAL ORIGINS HYPOTHESIS AND DOHAD—DEVELOPMENTAL ORIGIN OF HEALTH AND ADULT DISEASE

The "early" or "fetal" origins of adult disease hypothesis was originally put forward and further developed by David Barker and colleagues in Southampton in the United Kingdom which stated that environmental factors, particularly nutrition, act in early life to program the risks for the early onset of cardiovascular and metabolic disease in adult life and premature death *(11–22)*. Before the fetal origins hypothesis was articulated, an association between early-life events and later cardiovascular disease had been proposed on more than one occasion *(23–25)*. In 1992, Hales and Barker *(26)* coined the term the "thrifty phenotype" hypothesis, derived from the prior "thrifty genotype" hypothesis *(27)* proposed by Neel, to suggest that "thrifty" genes were selected during evolution at a time when food resources were scarce and that they resulted in a "fast insulin trigger" and thus an enhanced capacity to store fat, which placed the individual at risk of insulin resistance and type 2 diabetes. The thrifty phenotype hypothesis, however, suggested that when the fetal environment is poor, there is an adaptive response, which optimizes the growth of key body organs to the detriment of others and leads to an altered postnatal metabolism, which is designed to enhance postnatal survival under conditions of intermittent or poor nutrition. It was proposed that these adaptations only became detrimental when nutrition was more abundant in the postnatal environment, than it had been in the prenatal environment *(26,28)*. This concept is consistent with the definition of "programming" by Lucas in 1991 *(29)* as either the induction, deletion, or impaired development of a permanent somatic structure or the "setting" of a physiological system by an early stimulus or insult operating at a "sensitive" period, resulting in long-term consequences for function. One of the crucial elements of this definition is the concept of a sensitive or "critical" period during which specific nutritional perturbations may operate to cause long-term changes in development and adverse outcomes in later life *(30,31)*. Germ cell maturation, fertilization, blastocyst formation, differentiation, organogenesis, fetal growth and development, postnatal growth and development, puberty, and pregnancy are considered critical windows of developmental plasticity; each stage can be affected by programming mechanisms of adult disease *(32–34)*. As in other species, developmental plasticity attempts to "tune" gene expression to produce a phenotype best suited to the predicted later environment *(35)*. When the resulting phenotype is matched to its environment, the organism will remain healthy. When there is a mismatch, the individual's ability to respond to environmental challenges may be inadequate and risk of disease increases. Thus, the degree of the mismatch determines the individual's susceptibility to chronic disease *(36)*.

The processes of phenotypic induction through developmental plasticity produce integrated changes in a range of organs via epigenetic processes. They establish a life-course strategy for meeting the demands of the predicted later environment *(36,37)*, producing a range of effects in cardiovascular and metabolic homeostasis, growth and body composition, cognitive and behavioral development, reproductive function, repair processes, and longevity—some of which are associated with increased risk of cardiovascular and metabolic disease, "precocious" puberty, osteoporosis, and some forms of cancer. Understanding the underlying epigenetic processes thus holds the key to understanding the underlying pathophysiology and to developing approaches to early diagnosis, prevention, and treatment of these diseases.

The term "epigenetic" was created by Waddington *(38)* to refer developmental environment influences on the mature phenotype. It is now used to refer to structural changes to genes that do not alter the nucleotide sequence. Of particular relevance is methylation of specific CpG dinucleotides (cytosine and guanine adjacent to each other in the genome, linked by a phosphodiester bond) in gene promoters and alterations in DNA packaging arising from chemical modifications of the chromatin histone core around which DNA wraps. The modifications include acetylation, methylation, ubiquitination, and phosphorylation *(39)*.

The degree of mismatch can by definition be increased by either poorer environmental conditions during development or richer conditions later or both *(36)*. Such changes are of considerable importance in developing societies going through rapid socioeconomic transitions and represents an important risk factor for CVD in the populations of developing countries as vast numbers of poorly nourished infants have been born in the past several decades and have been benefitting from a steady improvement in child survival, which will lead to a higher proportion of such infants surviving to adult life.

Evidence of Epigenetic Mechanisms in Animals and Its Importance as a Cause of Adult Nephropathy and Arterial Hypertension

Birth weight is a crude surrogate for the broad spectrum of specific adverse events that may impair fetal growth in humans; therefore, experimental models have been developed to probe postnatal outcomes after specific interventions that are relevant to human pregnancy, including nutrient deficits and placental insufficiency *(40)*. Attention continues to focus primarily on fetal growth. Impaired growth during this critical period of organ development may have an impact on disease risk by permanently reducing the number of functional units, including nephrons *(41)*. In the years since, investigators have induced such developmental programming of adverse health outcomes in many animal species with the use of different interventions, ranging from the modification of the maternal or grandmaternal diet to the prenatal administration of glucocorticoid hormones, ligation of the uterine artery, experimentally produced anemia, and alteration of postnatal growth *(32)*. These perturbations can result in the adverse development of organs or organ systems directly or in adaptive responses that may be beneficial in the short term but deleterious in the long run. Because such experiments in animals involve environmental changes, they do not address purely genetic influences, but epigenetic processes may play a key role in the mechanisms underlying these phenomena *(32)*.

Several animal studies were devised to evaluate the effect of perinatal interventions on renal organogenesis and postnatal renal function. Table 1 depicts some of these studies and the main results in the offspring.

Table 1
A Selection of Intervention Studies Performed in Pregnant Rats to Evaluate Renal Organogenesis and Postnatal Renal Function in the Offspring

Author	Intervention	Outcome
Gilbert et al. *(42)*	Late gestational exposition to gentamycin	• Oligonephronia • Early nephron compensatory adaptation • Progressive glomerular sclerosis
Celsi et al. *(43)*	Gestational exposition to dexamethasone	• Oligonephronia • Early nephron compensatory adaptation • Arterial hypertension • ⇓ GFR • Albuminuria • ⇓ Urinary sodium excretion rate and fractional sodium excretion • ⇑ Sodium tissue content was higher
Lelièvre-Pégorier et al. *(44)*	Gestational exposition to mild vitamin A deficiency	• Oligonephronia
Vehaskari et al. *(45)*	Gestational exposition to low-protein diets	• Oligonephronia • Apoptosis • ⇓ PRA • ⇑ Aldosterone • Arterial hypertension
Woods et al. *(46)*	Gestational exposition to low-protein diets	• Oligonephronia • Glomerular enlargement • ⇓ Renal renin mRNA • Arterial hypertension
Pham et al. *(47)*	Uteroplacental insufficiency	• Oligonephronia • Apoptosis • Arterial hypertension

Evidence of Epigenetic Mechanisms in Animals and Its Importance as a Cause of Adult Nephropathy and Arterial Hypertension

Human studies have provided evidence suggesting nongenomic inheritance across generations. Patterns of smoking, diet, and exercise can affect risk across more than one generation *(48)*. During the 1944/1945 famine in the Netherlands, previously adequately nourished women were subjected to low caloric intake and associated environmental stress. Pregnant women exposed to famine in late pregnancy gave birth to smaller babies *(49)*. Famine exposure at different stages of gestation was variously associated with an increased risk of obesity, coronary heart disease, elevated albuminuria, later insulin resistance, and

Table 2
List of Selected Epidemiological Studies Investigating the Association of Birth Weight and/or Prematurity with Different Clinical Outcomes Along the Human Life Cycle in Developing Countries and Underprivileged Populations

Author	Country	Population	Outcome	Aggravating influence
Levitt et al. (64)	South Africa	5-year-old children	Inverse relation between BW and SBP	–
Law et al. (65)	China, Guatemala, Chile, Sweden	3- to 6-year-old children Term pregnancy BW > 2.5 kg	Inverse relation between BW and BP	Current WT
Bavdekar et al. (66)	India	8-year-old children	Inverse relation between BW and – SBP – Fasting plasma insulin – Plasma total and LDL cholesterol concentrations	Catch-up growth in previously growth-restricted children
Walker et al. (67)	Jamaica	11- to 12-year-old children	Inverse relation between SBP and BW	Postnatal growth retardation Current WT
Barros and Victora (68)	Brazil	14- to 15-year-olds	No association between BW and BP	Arterial hypertension More frequently diagnosed in adolescents born SGA
Adair and Cole (69)	Philippines	14- to 16-year-olds	Higher prevalence of elevated BP in low BW males	Weight gain from late childhood into adolescence in males with low BW
Nelson et al. (70)	PIMA Indians (USA)	Adults Type 2 diabetes	Association of ↑ albuminuria with BW <2.5 kg BW >4.5 kg	
Hoy et al. (71)	Australian Aborigines	Adults	Inverse relation between BW and albuminuria	

BP, blood pressure; SBP, systolic blood pressure; BW, birth weight.

dyslipidemia *(50)*. Second-born infants of females exposed in the first trimester in utero did not have the expected increase in birth weight with increasing birth order *(49)*.

Barker and colleagues' observations extended the range of diseases associated with low birth weight: to include atherosclerosis, coronary heart disease, type 2 diabetes mellitus, metabolic syndrome, stroke, and chronic bronchitis *(11–22)*. These observations have been corroborated and extended by other epidemiologic studies and studies in twins *(50–61)*.

The interest in this field has grown rapidly over the past decade. However, the most critical questions in this field remain unanswered. First, which of the children who have biochemical markers of metabolic disease will go on and develop overt metabolic disease in adult life? Second, what are the initiating events that trigger persistent metabolic programming? Third, what are the mechanisms that lead to adverse programmed metabolic changes *(62)*? The low birth weight group includes those born small for gestational age (SGA), premature, or following in vitro fertilization (IVF), which is often associated with both SGA and prematurity. These three common childhood groups are likely to have been exposed to an adverse environment during different phases of early development and might endure future morbid consequences of this exposure. However, it is important to emphasize that associations of birth weight with adult disease outcomes have been found in studies which included term pregnancies and birth weight >2500 g *(63)*.

A list of selected epidemiological studies investigating the association of birth weight with different clinical outcomes along the human life cycle in developing countries and underprivileged populations is shown in Table 2.

THE FUTURE OF CARDIOVASCULAR DISEASE IN THE DEVELOPING WORLD

As we have discussed there is a high burden of CVD morbidity and mortality in the developing countries, affecting individuals at a younger age than observed in developed countries *(8)*. As a consequence of the epidemiological transition, life expectancy in developing countries has risen; the increasing longevity provides longer periods of exposure to the risk factors of CVD, resulting in a greater probability of clinically manifest CVD events *(10)*.

The survivors of an economic transition period are more likely to present the phenotype of lower birth weight coupled with either stunting or a higher body mass index in childhood or adulthood which appears to be associated with the highest risks of morbid cardiovascular, renal, and metabolic outcomes into adulthood.

According to the World Health Organization *(72)*, 30 million low birth weight babies are born annually (23.8% of all births). Although the global prevalence of such births is slowly dropping, it is as high as 30% in many developing countries, frequently as a consequence of poor nutritional status and inadequate nutritional intake for women during pregnancy. Besides its negative impact on birth weight and early development, low birth weight results in substantial costs to the health sector and imposes a significant burden on society as a whole. Table 3 shows the WHO data on percentage and number of low birth weight infants (LBW) according to the world region and WHO development classification in 2000. The high prevalence of short stature in children of developing countries is depicted in Fig. 1, showing high rates in important areas of the world, including India.

An enormous task awaits developing countries, as national strategies to control the CVD epidemic must be developed and effectively implemented by individual countries. In par-

Table 3
Percentage and Number of Low Birth Weight Infants (LBW) According to the World Region and World Health Organization Region Development Classification, 2000

	% LBW	No LBW/1000	No live births/1000
World	15.5	20,629	132,882
Developed	7.0	916	13,100
Less developed	16.5	19,713	119,721
África	14.3	4320	30,305
Ásia	18.3	14,195	77,490
Europe	6.4	460	7185
Latin America and Caribbean	10.0	1171	11,671
North America	7.7	348	4479
Oceania	10.5	27	255

Modified from *(73)*.

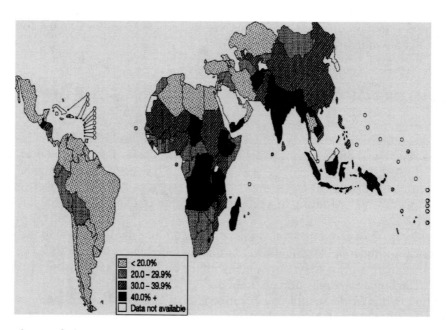

Fig. 1. Prevalence of short stature in children younger than 5 years of age in developing countries (from *(74)*).

allel, individual national efforts could be definitely strengthened by regional and global initiatives by international agencies concerned with health-care program facilitation, policy development and research funding. It is of utmost importance that, along with vigorous efforts to optimize childhood growth, researchers and policymakers identify, quantify, and evaluate strategies to modify prenatal and perinatal determinants of adverse adult health outcomes. Valuable initiatives can be found in WHO's "Working with individuals, families and communities to improve maternal and newborn health 2003" *(75)* and the "Making pregnancy safer" program *(76)*, which emphasize the need for professional assistance during pregnancy in addition to provision of a balanced diet, a safe environment, and avoidance of tobacco use. These programs also emphasize the importance of breast-feeding during at least the first 6 months to ensure child health and survival. Breast-feeding is also important for provision of sufficient caloric intake for growth, without incurring in the dangers of overfeeding and higher weight gain in early childhood, which are associated with the use of nutrient-enriched formula, and may predispose to hypertension and metabolic syndrome in later life *(77,78)*.

Schoolchildren and adolescents cannot be forgotten as it is mandatory to ensure their access to a properly balanced nutrition and lifestyle orientation, which includes alcohol and tobacco avoidance, daily exercise, and weight control *(79)*. These principles should be also ensured for the general population with age and gender adaptations.

Other essential components of a CVD control program would be the following: (1) establishment of efficient systems for estimation of CVD-related burden of disease and its secular trends; (2) estimation of the levels of established CVD risk factors (e.g., smoking, elevated cholesterol, or blood pressure) in representative population samples to help identify risk factors that require immediate intervention; (3) evaluation of emerging risk factors (e.g., glucose, abdominal obesity, fibrinolytic status, homocysteine) that may be of special relevance to the populations concerned; (4) identification of the determinants of health behavior that influence the levels of both traditional and emerging risk factors in the specific context of each society; and (5) development of a health policy that will integrate population-based measures for CVD risk modification and cost-effective case management strategies for individuals who have clinically manifested CVD or are detected to be at a high risk of developing it.

All of these require a strengthening of policy-relevant research that can support and evaluate CVD control programs in the developing countries. The challenge of CVD control is especially complex in settings in which epidemiological data related to the incidence of fatal and nonfatal CVD events as well as population-attributable risk of various risk factors of CVD are not readily or reliably available at present *(80)*.

REFERENCES

1. Omran A. The epidemiologic transition. A theory of the epidemiology of population change. Milbank Q. 1971;49:509–538.
2. World Health Organization. The World Heath Report 2002: reducing risks, promoting healthy life. World Health Organization, Geneva. Available at http://www.who.int/whr/2002/en/. [Last Accessed on February 28, 2009].
3. World Health Organization. The World Heath Report 2003: shaping the future. Annex 2. World Health Organization, Geneva. Available at http://www.who.int/whr/2003/en/Annex2-en.pdf. [Last Accessed on February 23, 2009].
4. Reid CM, Thrift AG. Hypertension 2020: confronting tomorrow's problem today. Clin Exp Pharmacol Physiol. 2005;32:374–376.
5. Yach D. The global burden of chronic disease: overcoming impediments to prevention and control. JAMA. 2004;291:2616–2622.
6. Guidelines Subcommittee. WHO–ISH hypertension guidelines for the management of hypertension. J Hypertens. 1999;17:151–183.
7. Kearney PM, Whelton M, Reynolds K, Whelton PK, He J. Worldwide prevalence of hypertension: a systematic review. J Hypertens. 2004;22:11–19.
8. Murray CJL, Lopez AD. Global Comparative Assessments in the Health Sector. Geneva, Switzerland: World Health Organization; 1994.

9. Barker DJ, Osmond C. Infant mortality, childhood nutrition, and ischaemic heart disease in England and Wales. Lancet. 1986;1:1077–1081.
10. Reddy KS. Cardiovascular disease in India. World Health Stat Q. 1993;46:101–107.
11. Barker DJ, Osmond C, Golding J, Kuh D, Wadsworth ME. Growth in utero, blood pressure in childhood and adult life, and mortality from cardiovascular disease. Bone Miner J. 1989;298:564–567.
12. Barker DJ, Osmond C, Law CM. The intrauterine and early postnatal origins of cardiovascular disease and chronic bronchitis. J Epidemiol Community Health. 1989;43:237–240.
13. Barker DJ, Winter PD, Osmond C, Margetts B, Simmonds SJ. Weight in infancy and death from ischaemic heart disease. Lancet. 1989;2:577–580.
14. Barker DJP, Osmond C, Winter PD, Margetts BM, Simmonds SJ. Weight in infancy and death from ischaemic heart disease. Lancet 1989;2:577–580.
15. Barker DJ. The fetal and infant origins of adult disease. BMJ. 1990;301:1111.
16. Barker DJ, Bull AR, Osmond C, Simmonds SJ. Fetal and placental size and risk of hypertension in adult life. Bone Miner J. 1990;301:259–262.
17. Barker DJP, Hales CN, Fall CHD, Osmond C, Phipps K, Clark PMS. Type 2 (non-insulin-dependent) diabetes mellitus, hypertension and hyperlipidemia (syndrome X): relation to reduced fetal growth. Diabetologia. 1993;36:62–67.
18. Barker DJP, Martyn CN, Osmond C, Haleb CN, Fall CHD. Growth in utero and serum cholesterol concentrations in adult life. BMJ. 1993;307:1524–1527.
19. Martyn CN, Barker DJP, Jespersen S, Greenwald S, Osmond C, Berry C. Growth in utero, adult blood pressure and arterial compliance. Br Heart J. 1995;73:116–121.
20. Barker DJP. Fetal origins of coronary heart disease. BMJ. 1995;311:171–174.
21. Barker DJ, Eriksson JG, Forsen T, Osmond C. Fetal origins of adult disease: strength of effects and biological basis. Int J Epidemiol. 2002;31:1235–1239.
22. Barker DJP. Developmental origins of adult health and disease. J Epidemiol Community Health. 2004;58:114–115.
23. Kermack WO, McKendrick AG, McKinlay PL. Death-rates in Great Britain and Sweden. Some general regularities and their significance. Lancet. 1934;i:698–703.
24. Forsdahl A. Are poor living conditions in childhood and adolescence an important risk factor for arteriosclerotic heart disease? Br J Prev Soc Med. 1977;31:91–95.
25. Wadsworth ME, Cripps HA, Midwinter RE, Colley JR. Blood pressure in a national birth cohort at the age of 36 related to social and familial factors, smoking, and body mass. Br Med J. 1985;291:1534–1538.
26. Hales CN, Barker DJ. Type 2 (non-insulin-dependent) diabetes mellitus: the thrifty phenotype hypothesis. Diabetologia. 1992;35:595–601.
27. Neel JV. Diabetes mellitus: a "thrifty" genotype rendered detrimental by "progress"? Am J Hum Genet. 1962;14:353–362.
28. Hales CN, BarkerDJ. The thrifty phenotype hypothesis. Br Med Bull. 2001;60:5–20.
29. Lucas A. Programming by early nutrition in man. Ciba Found Symp. 1991;156:38–50.
30. Thoman EB, Levine S. Hormonal and behavioral changes in the rat mother as a function of early experience treatments of the offspring. Physiol Behav. 1970;5:1417–1421.
31. Wiesel TN, Hubel DH. Comparison of the effects of unilateral and bilateral eye closure on cortical unit responses in kittens. J Neurophysiol. 1965;28:1029–1040.
32. Mcmillen C; Robinson JS. Developmental origins of the metabolic syndrome: prediction, plasticity, and programming. Physiol Rev. 2005;85:571–633.
33. West-Eberhard MJ. Developmental Plasticity and Evolution. Oxford University Press, New York, NY; 2003.
34. Bateson P, Barker D, Clutton-Brock T, Deb D, Foley RA, Gluckman P, Godfrey K, Kirkwood T, Mirazón Lahr M, Macnamara J, Metcalfe NB, Monaghan P, Spencer HG, Sultan SE. Developmental plasticity and human health. Nature. 2004;430:419–421.
35. Gluckman PD, Hanson MA. Living with the past: evolution, development and patterns of disease. Science. 2004;305:1733–1736.
36. Gluckman PD, Hanson MA. Mismatch: How Our World No Longer Fits Our Bodies. Oxford University Press, Oxford; 2006.
37. Gluckman PD, Hanson MA, Beedle AS. Early life events and their consequences for later disease; a life history and evolutionary perspective. Am J Hum Biol. 2007;19:1–19.
38. Waddington CH. The Strategy of the Genes: A Discussion of Some Aspects of Theoretical Biology. Macmillan, New York, NY; 1957.
39. Godfrey KM, Lillycrop KA, Burdge GC, Gluckman PD, Hanson MA. Epigenetic mechanisms and the mismatch concept of the developmental origins of health and disease. Pediatr Res. 2007;61(5 Part 2) Supplement:5R–10R.

40. Armitage JA, Khan IY, Taylor PD, Nathanielsz PW, Poston L. Developmental programming of the metabolic syndrome by maternal nutritional imbalance: how strong is the evidence from experimental models in mammals? J Physiol. 2004;561:355–377.

41. Bagby SP. Maternal nutrition, low nephron number, and hypertension in later life: pathways of nutritional programming. J Nutr. 2007;137:1066–1072.

42. Gilbert T, Lelievre-Pegorier M, Merlet-Benichou C. Long-term effects of mild oligonephronia induced in utero by gentamicin in the rat. Pediatr Res. 1991;30(5):450–456.

43. Celsi G, Kistner A, Aizman R, Eklöf AC, Ceccatelli S, de Santiago A, Jacobson SH. Prenatal dexamethasone causes oligonephronia, sodium retention, and higher blood pressure in the offspring. Pediatr Res. 1998;44:317–322.

44. Lelièvre-Pégorier M, Vilar J, Ferrier ML, Moreau E, Freund N, Gilbert T, Merlet-Bénichou C. Mild vitamin A deficiency leads to inborn nephron deficit in the rat. Kidney Int. 1998;54:1455–1462.

45. Vehaskari VM, Aviles DH, Manning J. Prenatal programming of adult hypertension in the rat. Kidney Int. 2001;59:238–245.

46. Woods LL, Ingelfinger JR, Nyengaard JR, Rasch R. Maternal protein restriction suppresses the newborn renin-angiotensin system and programs adult hypertension in rats. Pediatr Res. 2001;49:460–467.

47. Pham TD, MacLennan NK, Chiu CT, Laksana GS, Hsu JL, Lane RH. Uteroplacental insufficiency increases apoptosis and alters p53 gene methylation in the full-term IUGR rat kidney. Am J Physiol Regul Integr Comp Physiol. 2003;285:R962–R970.

48. Brook JS, Whiteman M, Brook DW. Transmission of risk factors across three generations. Psychol Rep. 1999;85:227–241.

49. Lumey LH, Stein AD. Offspring birth weights after maternal intrauterine undernutrition: a comparison within sibships. Am J Epidemiol. 1997;146:810–819.

50. Painter RC, Roseboom TJ, Bleker OP. Prenatal exposure to the Dutch famine and disease in later life: an overview. Reprod Toxicol. 2005;20:345–352.

51. Curhan GC, Willett WC, Rimm EB, Spiegelman D, Ascherio AL, Stampfer MJ. Birth weight and adult hypertension, diabetes mellitus, and obesity in US men. Circulation. 1996;94:3246–3250.

52. Boyko EJ. Proportion of type 2 diabetes cases resulting from impaired fetal growth. Diabetes Care. 2000;23:1260–1264.

53. Eriksson JG, Osmond C, Barker DJ. Pathways of infant and childhood growth that lead to type 2 diabetes. Diabetes Care. 2003;26:3006–3010.

54. Law CM, de Swiet M, Osmond C, Fayers PM, Barker DJ, Cruddas AM, Fall CH. Initiation of hypertension in utero and its amplification throughout life. BMJ. 1993;306:24–27.

55. Whincup P, Cook D, Papacosta O, Walker M. Birth weight and blood pressure: cross sectional and longitudinal relations in childhood. BMJ. 1995;311(7008):773–776.

56. Uiterwaal CS, Anthony S, Launer LJ, Witteman JC, Trouwborst AM, Hofman A, Grobbee DE. Birth weight, growth, and blood pressure: an annual follow-up study of children aged 5 through 21 years. Hypertension. 1997;(2 Pt 1):267–271.

57. Barker DJ, Osmond C, Forsén TJ, Kajantie E, Eriksson JG. Trajectories of growth among children who have coronary events as adults. N Engl J Med. 2005;353(17):1802–1809.

58. Kajantie E, Osmond C, Barker DJ, Forsén T, Phillips DI, Eriksson JG. Size at birth as a predictor of mortality in adulthood: a follow-up of 350 000 person-years. Int J Epidemiol. 2005;34:655–663.

59. Lackland DT, Bendall HE, Osmond C, Egan BM, Barker DJ. Low birth weights contribute to high rates of early-onset chronic renal failure in the Southeastern United States. Arch Intern Med. 2000;160(10):1472–1476.

60. Keijzer-Veen MG, Schrevel M, Finken MJ, Dekker FW, Nauta J, Hille ET, Frölich M, van der Heijden BJ. Dutch POPS-19 Collaborative Study Group. Microalbuminuria and lower glomerular filtration rate at young adult age in subjects born very premature and after intrauterine growth retardation. J Am Soc Nephrol. 2005;16:2762–2768.

61. Bergvall N, Iliadou A, Johansson S, de Faire U, Kramer MS, Pawitan Y, Pedersen NL, Lichtenstein P, Cnattingius S. Genetic and shared environmental factors do not confound the association between birth weight and hypertension: a study among Swedish twins. Circulation. 2007;115:2931–2938.

62. Cutfield WS, Hofman PL, Mitchell M, Morison IM. Could epigenetics play a role in the developmental origins of health and disease. Pediatr Res. 2007;61(5 Part 2) Supplement:68R–75R.

63. Lurbe E, Torro I, Rodríguez C, Alvarez V, Redón J. Birth weight influences blood pressure values and variability in children and adolescents. Hypertension. 2001;38(3):389–393.

64. Levitt NS, Steyn K, De Wet T, Morrell C, Edwards R, Ellison GT, Cameron N. An inverse relation between blood pressure and birth weight among 5 year old children from Soweto, South Africa. J Epidemiol Community Health. 1999;53(5):264–268.

65. Law CM, Egger P, Dada O, Delgado H, Kylberg E, Lavin P, Tang GH, von Hertzen H, Shiell AW, Barker DJ. Body size at birth and blood pressure among children in developing countries. Int J Epidemiol. 2001;30(1):52–57.

66. Bavdekar A, Yajnik CS, Fall CHD, et al. Insulin resistance syndrome in 8-year-old Indian children: small at birth, big at 8 years, or both? Diabetes. 1999;48:2422–2429.

67. Walker SP, Gaskin P, Powell CA, Bennett FI, Forrester TE, Grantham-McGregor S. The effects of birth weight and postnatal linear growth retardation on blood pressure at age 11–12 years. J Epidemiol Community Health. 2001;55(6):394–398.

68. Barros FC, Victora CG. Increased blood pressure in adolescents who were small for gestational age at birth: a cohort study in Brazil. Int J Epidemiol. 1999;28:676–681.

69. Adair LS, Cole TJ. Rapid child growth raises blood pressure in adolescent boys who were thin at birth. Hypertension. 2003;41:451–456.

70. Nelson RG, Morgenstern H, Bennett PH. Birth weight and renal disease in Pima Indians with type 2 diabetes mellitus. Am J Epidemiol. 1998;148:650–656.

71. Hoy WE, Rees M, Kile E, Mathews JD, Wang Z. A new dimension to the Barker hypothesis: low birth-weight and susceptibility to renal disease. Kidney Int. 1999;56:1072–1077.

72. World Health Organization. Feto-maternal nutrition and low birth weight. World health Organization, Geneva. Available at: http://www.who.int/nutrition/topics/feto_maternal/en. [Last Accessed on February 23, 2009].

73. http://www.who.int/reproductive-health/publications/low_birthweight/low_birthweight_estimates.pdf. [Last Accessed on February 23, 2009].

74. de Onis M, Blössner M. The World Health Organization Global Database on Child Growth and Malnutrition: methodology and applications. Int J Epidemiol. 2003;32(4):518–526.

75. http://www.who.int/reproductive-health/publications/ifc/ifc.pdf. [Last Accessed on February 23, 2009].

76. http://www.who.int/making_pregnancy_safer/en/. [Last Accessed on February 23, 2009].

77. Singhal A, Cole TJ, Lucas A. Early nutrition in preterm infants and later blood pressure: two cohorts after randomised trials. Lancet. 2001;357(9254):413–419.

78. Singhal A, Fewtrell M, Cole TJ, Lucas A. Low nutrient intake and early growth for later insulin resistance in adolescents born preterm. Lancet. 2003;361(9363):1089–1097.

79. http://www.who.int/cardiovascular_diseases/guidelines/Fulltext.pdf. [Last Accessed on February 23, 2009].

80. Reddy KS, Yusuf S. Emerging epidemic of cardiovascular disease in developing countries. Circulation. 1998;97:596–601.

IV EVALUATION AND MANAGEMENT OF PEDIATRIC HYPERTENSION

28 Evaluation of the Hypertensive Pediatric Patient

Rita D. Swinford, MD
and Ronald J. Portman, MD

CONTENTS

INTRODUCTION

A clinical challenge to the successful treatment of children with hypertension is in the identification and then thorough evaluation of children with elevated blood pressure (BP) *(1)*. In this light, consideration must be given to the causative spectrum of hypertension in pediatric patients as it is broad and changes with age. Most infants, toddlers, and school-aged children must be presumed to have secondary hypertension, with primary hypertension most prevalent in adolescence. For children with severe hypertension, those above the 99th percentile, careful, comprehensive, and immediate evaluation is required. A rule of thumb for the identification of children with secondary hypertension is when the hypertension is severe and the child is young, with the highest sensitivity found in the youngest and most severely hypertensive. However, this may not always be the case, and therefore evaluation is important as the cause may be remediable and benefit from pharmacologic therapy. Recommendations for pharmacologic treatment are based on the presence of symptomatic hypertension, evidence of end-organ damage and/or stage 2 hypertension, or stage 1 hypertension unresponsive to lifestyle modification *(2)*. Not to be discounted are children in high-risk diagnostic groups, e.g., diabetes mellitus and chronic kidney disease (CKD), whose onset of premature atherosclerosis leads to early cardiovascular disease. Recent recommendations for treatment based on risk stratification by disease process are now available *(3)*.

R.D. Swinford (✉)

Division of Pediatric Nephrology and Hypertension, Department of Pediatrics, University of Texas at Houston, Houston, TX, USA

e-mail: rita.d.swinford@uth.tmc.edu

From: *Clinical Hypertension and Vascular Diseases: Pediatric Hypertension*
Edited by: J. T. Flynn et al. DOI 10.1007/978-1-60327-824-9_28
© Springer Science+Business Media, LLC 2011

Unlike in adults, the diagnosis of pediatric hypertension predominantly is founded on epidemiologic and expert opinion data rather than being driven by evidence-based outcomes *(2)*. Recently, however, a 5-year randomized trial has been published showing the benefit of renoprotective therapy on retarding the progression of renal disease in children *(4)*; hopefully, this will lead to development of evidence-based treatment recommendations. The necessity for further studies and revised guidelines has become increasingly clear as mounting evidence shows that even mild hypertension in children and adolescents is much more common than previously described *(5,6)*. A shift in BP distribution to higher levels is now seen in children and adolescents very likely secondary to the global obesity epidemic. We now understand that children with elevated BPs mature into adults with hypertension, and this underscores the importance of control *(7)*.

Technologic advances have seen the widespread introduction of oscillometric devices for BP measurement which have the advantage of ease of use and little interobserver variability. These devices determine BP indirectly by determining the mean arterial pressure from the point of maximum oscillations and then by calculating the SBP and DBP using proprietary and unpublished algorithms. Unfortunately, short oscillatory cycles, as is sometimes seen in children, can lead to errors in measurement. Validation of the oscillometric method is recommended, but few devices have been validated successfully; those that have been can be found at the web site www.dableducation.org. Studies that compare oscillometric devices to auscultatory sphygmomanometry show poor correlation, highlighting the need for confirmation by auscultatory methods. As BP is a continuous variable, assuming a single clinic BP (CBP) measurement representative of the patient's true BP pattern may not be reasonable; ambulatory BP monitoring (ABPM), on the other hand, is considered to be superior to CBP for the prediction of cardiovascular events. With this in mind, ABPM is now increasingly recognized as being indispensable for the diagnosis and management of hypertension *(8–11)*. Urbina et al., in a 2008 American Heart Association scientific statement, reported that the 24-h ABPM had utility in the assessment of hypertension in children and adolescents *(10)*. In children, not dissimilar to adults, ABPM is found to correlate with left ventricular mass in both hypertensive and normotensive patients. In children, however, a relationship is seen with LVM and nocturnal systolic BP and BP load *(12,13)*. McNiece et al. in 2007 linked the severity of hypertension to the odds of having left ventricular hypertrophy *(14)*. Others have shown thicker carotid arteries with higher ABPM levels *(15,16)*.

The use of home BP measurement in children and adolescents has limited evidence, but can be a technique for BP monitoring, suggest the diagnosis of white coat hypertension (WCH), and monitor antihypertensive therapy. Wuhl et al. in 2004 compared ABPM with self-measurement of BP and clinic BPs in children with chronic kidney disease. They were able to show that while SMBP did improve clinic BP's sensitivity to detect hypertension, 20% of hypertensive children were missed, proving that ABPM remained superior in the evaluation of hypertension *(17)*. Home monitoring of BP in children and adolescents can be used as a supplement in the assessment of hypertension in clinical practice, particularly for the detection of white coat and masked hypertension. Home BP monitoring advantages include lower cost and user acceptance *(18)*.

That said, the traditional pattern of a higher prevalence of secondary hypertension compared to primary hypertension in adolescence is changing, with primary hypertension becoming increasingly evident during early adolescence and even late childhood. Indeed, with the exception of childhood asthma, hypertension may now be the most common chronic disease of childhood. The causal factor responsible for the apparent dramatic increase in prevalence of primary hypertension is *obesity*, now considered a global phenomenon associated with an increased risk for the development of cardiovascular and renal disease *(19)*. Approximately 60% of overweight (BMI > 95th percentile) youths have at least one risk factor for future cardiovascular disease, including elevation of BP, abnormal lipids, and insulin resistance *(20)*. ABPM may facilitate the differentiation of

Table 1
Phases of Hypertension Evaluation

Phase 1: Is the Patient Truly Hypertensive in the Non-medical Setting?
   Ambulatory blood pressure monitoring
   Self-measured blood pressure
   School-based blood pressure measurements

Phase 2: Screening
   CBC
   Urinalysis
   Urine culture
   Serum chemistries
      Electrolytes (potassium, sodium, chloride, bicarbonate, glucose)
      Creatinine, BUN
   Lipoprotein profiling (serum total cholesterol, with high-density lipoprotein, low-density lipoprotein, and triglycerides)
   Renal ultrasound with Doppler
   Echocardiogram/EKG

Phase 3: Definition of Abnormalities
   Renal imaging
      • Renal ultrasound with Doppler plus/minus radionuclide scan
      • VCUG
   Renovascular imaging (noninvasive), CT or MRI angiography
   Captopril challenge
   Renin profiling
   Aldosterone, catecholamine profiling
   Abdominal imaging; CT or ultrasound

Phase 3a: Identification of End-Organ Damage
   Echocardiography
   Retinal examination
   Urine protein quantification

Phase 4: Determination of Significance and Remediability of Abnormalities
   Arteriography (conventional or digital subtraction angiography)
   Renal vein renin collection
   Renal biopsy
   MIBG scans (pheochromocytoma)

primary from secondary hypertension as adolescents with secondary hypertension have been shown to have greater nocturnal systolic BP loads and daytime and nocturnal diastolic BP loads than similarly aged children with primary hypertension *(21)*.

Once it has been determined that a child has an elevated BP and that this BP elevation is persistent, the following guide is anticipated to aid in the diagnostic evaluation (Tables 1 and 2). We use the term 'phase' of evaluation in an attempt to lessen confusion with 'stages' of hypertension used in Table 3.

Phase 1: Is the Patient Truly Hypertensive in the Non-medical Setting? (Confirmation of Hypertension with ABPM or Objective SMBP)
Phase 2: Screening for Hypertension
A. Why does the patient have hypertension? (Etiology)
B. What has hypertension done to the patient's body already? (End-organ damage)

Table 2
Questions to be Addressed in Phase 2 Evaluation After the Hypertension Has Been Confirmed

Test	Design
What has hypertension done to the patient?	
Examination of history	
Measurement of growth	
Urinalysis	Renal disease (microalbuminuria, proteinuria, hematuria)
Echocardiogram	Left ventricular hypertrophy
Poor growth	Chronic kidney disease
Fundoscopic examination	Chronic hypertension
Hemoglobin/hematocrit	Renal dysfunction/anemia of CRF
Serum electrolytes, Ca, and phosphate	Renal dysfunction
What other risk factors for cardiovascular/kidney disease are present?	
Fasting blood sugar	Diabetes
Elevated HgA1c	Diabetes
Glucosuria	Diabetes
Weight	Obesity
Lipoprotein analysis	Hypercholesterolemia; hypertriglyceridemia
Family history	Cardiovascular, obesity
Personal history	Medications, smoking, inactivity
Why does the patient have hypertension?	
Serum electrolytes	1° or 2° aldosteronism
BUN and S_{cr}	Renal dysfunction
Uric acid	Primary HTN marker (?)
Renal ultrasound	Anatomic or pathologic etiology
Urinalysis	Hematuria/proteinuria (nephritis, renal masses)
Weight	Obesity

Table 3
Classification of Hypertension in Children and Adolescents

Normal blood pressure	SBP and DBP <90th percentile
Prehypertension	SBP or DBP ≥90th percentile but <95th percentile
Hypertension	SBP or DBP ≥95th percentile
Stage 1 hypertension	SBP or DBP from 95th percentile to 99th percentile plus 5 mmHg
Stage 2 hypertension	SBP or DBP >99th percentile plus 5 mmHg

SBP = systolic blood pressure; DBP = diastolic blood pressure.
Percentiles are for sex, age, and height for blood pressure measured on at least three separate occasions.
Characterized by higher percentile if SBP or DBP percentiles are different.
Adapted from *(2)*.

C. What other risk factor for cardiovascular/kidney disease does the patient have? (Comorbidities)

Phase 3: Definition of Abnormalities
Phase 4: Determination of Significance and Remediability of Abnormality

EVALUATION

Phase 1: Is the Patient Truly Hypertensive in the Non-medical Setting?

When a child is found to have an elevated BP this should elicit, *before* a thorough evaluation is performed, further validation of the possible hypertension. Preferably three measurements should be taken in an upper extremity at least 2 min apart and the average of these compared to the Fourth Report nomograms at each measurement session *(2)*. Accurate measurement of BP is dependent on a number of factors including use of the appropriate sized cuff. For example, increasing body weight is associated with an increase in arm circumference which accentuates the importance of recognizing the relationship between arm circumference and BP cuff size and its impact on accurate BP measurement. If a BP cuff is used with an inappropriate small cuff, BP may be falsely overestimated.

Confirmation of BP elevation should be repeated on at least three separate occasions unless it is severe (greater than or equal to stage 2 hypertension) or the child is symptomatic. In the latter case, one should make immediate referral to a specialist in pediatric hypertension or admission to a hospital or emergency room. SMBP can also be performed preferably with a recording monitor and with the caveats previously mentioned. School nurses can be useful in collecting additional measurements which can then be faxed to complete the record. However, school BP equipment may not be regularly calibrated and the training of school nurses may vary widely; therefore, proper training of the nurses and validation of equipment used at local schools is time well spent. Ideally ABPM should be used to confirm the diagnosis of hypertension and to exclude the diagnosis of WCH *(22)*. One must also note that a small percentage of patients similar to those reported by Lurbe and colleagues *(23)* who have normal casual BP measurements have elevated ambulatory BP measurement, i.e., masked hypertension. With regard to the association of ABPM with end-organ damage for adults and children, those with WCH have a prevalence of end-organ damage not different from normotensive subjects. Conversely, those with masked hypertension have end-organ damage prevalence not dissimilar from children with true hypertension *(24)*. An algorithm for the evaluation of hypertension using different BP measurement techniques can be found in Fig. 1. In the case where ABPM is unavailable multiple CBP or self-measured BP can be used.

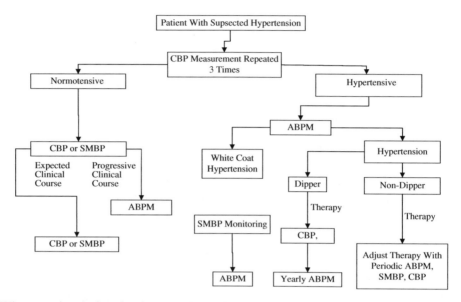

Fig. 1. When a patient is found to have an elevated BP on initial evaluation or screening, BP should be repeated at least twice. If the patient is determined to be normotensive after repeated measures, follow-up BP measurements should be taken every 6 months to a year. One must be mindful that the patient may still have a non-dipping pattern placing them in a higher risk category or masked hypertension. One should follow the patient's clinical course and if proceeds as expected, CBP or SMBP can be used to follow the patient. However, if features are unexplained such as proteinuria or symptoms are present with elevation of BP an ABPM should be performed. If the patient has hypertension by casual measurement, ABPM may be performed to diagnose WCH as well as determine altered BP patterns. If WCH is found, SMBP can be effective in monitoring the WCH and ABPM can be repeated if clinical course varies from expected. If ABPM confirms the hypertension, the patient can then be categorized by dipping status. A patient with a dipping pattern may be followed with CBP or SMBP with occasional ABPM monitoring as needed. However, a patient with a non-dipping pattern can only be practically monitored by ABPM which should be used along with CBP and SMBP as needed to maintain and assure adequate circadian BP control. The significance and chronicity of BP abnormalities should also be confirmed by assessment of end-organ damage.

Phase 2: Screening for Hypertension

WHY DOES THE PATIENT HAVE HYPERTENSION?

The etiology of hypertension by age group is listed in Table 4. The exact percentages at each age group are unknown; however, the younger the patient and the more severe the hypertension, the more likely that the hypertension is secondary. Many adolescents have primary hypertension; however, the percentage of secondary causes in this age group remains higher than that in adults, and thus all pediatric patients must be screened for secondary causes. Renal or renovascular causes of hypertension account for ~90% of

Table 4
Most Common Causes of Secondary Hypertension: By Age

Age group	Etiology
Newborn	Renal artery or venous thrombosis
	Renal artery stenosis
	Congenital renal abnormalities
	Coarctation of the aorta
	Bronchopulmonary dysplasia
First year	Renovascular disease
	Renal parenchymal disease
	Coarctation of the aorta
	Iatrogenic (medication, volume)
	Tumor
Infancy to 6 years	Renal parenchymal disease
	Renovascular disease
	Coarctation of the aorta
	Tumor
	Endocrine causes[a]
	Iatrogenic
	Essential hypertension
Age 6–10 years	Renal parenchymal disease
	Essential hypertension
	Renovascular disease
	Coarctation of the aorta
	Endocrine causes
	Tumor
	Iatrogenic
Adolescence, age 12–18 years	Essential hypertension
	Iatrogenic
	Renal parenchymal disease
	Endocrine causes
	Coarctation of the aorta

[a]Shaded areas are uncommon for category.

secondary causes with 2% contributed from abnormalities of the aorta and 0.5% from pheochromocytoma *(25,26)*. The National High Blood Pressure Education Program Working Group on High Blood Pressure in Children and Adolescents (NHBPEP) has published a useful algorithm for childhood hypertension evaluation and management *(2)*.

The personal and family history of hypertension and/or cardiovascular disease (Table 5) is a key starting point for the assessment of childhood hypertension; other important risk factors include metabolic syndrome and sleep-disordered breathing (either from obstructive sleep apnea or from snoring). Symptoms related to hypertension may be caused by the disease, related to the cause of the hypertension, nonspecific or absent. The newborn may

Table 5
Relevant Questions for the Hypertensive History

Family history

Essential hypertension
   ? medications/diet control
   ? salt sensitive
   ? obesity
Systemic disease
? endocrine
     hyperthyroidism, diabetes
   ? obesity
   ? cardiovascular disease
     early myocardial infarction/stroke
   ? hyperlipoproteinemia
   ? kidney disease
     kidney failure, dialysis, or transplantation

Medications
  Anti-inflammatory agents: steroidal and nonsteroidal
  Decongestants (pseudoephedrine)
  Stimulants: caffeine, ritalin, adderall
  Antidepressants: tricyclics

  Calcineurin inhibitors: cyclosporine, tacrolimus
Weight change
  Weight loss or gain?
  Time frame for interval change in weight

    Weight loss as with pheochromocytoma
    Weight gain as with exo- or endogenous steroids
Neonatal history: umbilical arterial catheter; neonatal asphyxia, bronchopulmonary dysplasia

Trauma

Systemic disease
  Systemic lupus erythematosus
  olyarteritis
  Flushing, sweating, headaches, palpitations as in pheochromocytoma or neuroblastoma
  Neurofibromatosis
  Scleroderma
  Urinary tract infections or history of unexplained or explained fevers

Substance abuse
  Amphetamines
  Other

appear to have sepsis, feeding disorders, or neurologic abnormalities, while older patients frequently are asymptomatic but may complain of nonspecific symptoms such as abdominal pain, epistaxis, chest pain, or headache. Children can have subtle abnormalities that are difficult to attribute to hypertension such as personality changes, irritability, or changes in school performance. The hypertension-oriented history should be directed at eliciting evidence of systemic diseases, use of medications including those which elevate BP (oral contraceptives, bronchodilators, cyclosporin, corticosteroids, decongestants, performance-enhancing substances, tobacco, and illicit drugs), congenital disorders, symptoms related to hypertension (headache, irritability), neonatal history (use of umbilical catheters, neonatal asphyxia), growth pattern, present and past history of kidney or urologic disorders including urinary tract infections, symptoms suggestive of an endocrine etiology (change in weight, sweating, flushing, fevers, palpitations, muscle cramps), and family history of hypertension or other cardiovascular morbid or mortal events.

The physical examination should address direct attention to detecting causes of secondary hypertension (Table 6). In the majority of children with hypertension, however, the physical examination will be normal. For a child in the first year of life, secondary causes of hypertension are the rule, and even when no etiology is detected secondary hypertension should still be suspected (Table 4). In older children, by contrast, secondary hypertension has a different spectrum (Table 4). The physical examination should focus on symptoms and signs of hypertension (Table 7). For all age groups with hypertension, kidney disease is a common etiology where approximately 60–90% is secondary to renal parenchymal or renovascular disease *(25,26)*. Physical examination may reveal cranial (infants), neck, back, or abdominal bruits, where stenotic lesions cause turbulent blood flow or asymmetric lower versus upper extremity pulses signifying a possible aortic coarctation. Evidence for secondary hypertension can also be supported by the finding on physical examination of hypertensive retinopathy, neurofibromas, café-au-lait spots, lesions of tuberous sclerosis, or thyromegaly. Initial evaluation should also assess four extremity BP measurements to screen for coarctation of the aorta. Physical examination should include calculation of the body mass index (BMI) because of the strong association between obesity and hypertension.

The child with confirmed hypertension should be screened with laboratory testing and imaging to find identifiable causes, comorbid conditions, and ascertainment of end-organ damage. A serum creatinine and estimation (Schwartz formula) *(27)* of glomerular filtration rate (GFR) or actual GFR measurement either by 24-h urine collection for creatinine or obtaining a formal clearance study with a marker such as iothalamate are also fundamental *(28)*. The importance of a complete urinalysis with urinary protein or microalbumin and sterilely collected urine for culture cannot be overemphasized. Proteinuria or hematuria may be revealed and indicates possible glomerular disease or other non-glomerular conditions such as pyelonephritis, obstructive uropathy, and interstitial nephritis. Additional testing can be chosen by examining the individual and family history. A young child with stage 2 hypertension or in those with systemic symptoms should have extensive evaluation, whereas the older or obese child with a significant family history of say diabetes or other cardiovascular risks will have a more streamlined approach for the metabolic abnormality.

A renal ultrasound is a simple and informative noninvasive test and appropriate for the initial screening. The prevalence of abnormalities revealed by a renal ultrasound may be low; however, the importance of findings and noninvasive nature make it a valued screening test. The information provided can reveal asymmetrically sized kidneys, which would suggest vesicoureteral reflux, obstruction, unilateral infection, or possible kidney

Table 6
Physical Examination: Clues to the Etiology of Hypertension

Body habitus	*Thinness*—pheochromocytoma, hyperthyroidism, renal disease (growth failure)
	Obesity—Cushing's disease
	Virilized—congenital adrenal hyperplasia
	Rickets—chronic renal disease
Skin	*Neurofibromas*—neurofibromatosis
	Café-au-lait spots—pheochromocytoma
	Tubers, ash-leaf spots—tuberous sclerosis
	Bruising—Cushing's disease, trauma
	Rashes: vasculitis—collagen vascular disease or nephritic
	Impetigo—acute nephritis
	striae—Cushing's disease
	Needle tracks—iatrogenic hypertension
Head and face	*Unusual shape*—mass lesion
	Round facies (moon)—Cushing's syndrome
	Elfin facies—William's syndrome
	Seventh nerve palsy—severe hypertension
Eyes	*EOM palsy*—nonspecific
	Fundal changes—nonspecific
	Proptosis—hyperthyroidism
Neck	*Goiter*—hyperthyroidism
	Bruit—carotid or vertebral stenosis; suggestive of fibromuscular dysplasia
Lungs	*Rales, rhonchi*—nonspecific? cardiac decompensation
Heart	*Failure*—same as for enlarged heart
	Rub—? chronic renal disease with hypertension
	Enlargement
Abdomen	*Masses*—Wilm's tumor, neuroblastoma, hydronephrosis, polycystic kidney disease
	Hepatomegaly—heart failure
	Hepatosplenomegaly—infantile polycystic disease
	Scars—GU surgery
	Bruit—renovascular disease
	Edema—renal/renovascular disease
Back/flank	*Bruit*—renovascular disease
	Flank tenderness—pyelonephritis, obstruction, acute nephritis
	Scoliosis—? hypertension secondary to renal compression
Pelvis	*Mass*—obstructive, neuroblastoma
Genitalia	*Ambiguous, virilized*—congenital adrenal hyperplasia
Extremities	*Disparity in BP, pulse, delayed refill*—coarctation
	Edema
Neurologic	*Bell's palsy*—nonspecific
	Encephalopathy—nonspecific
	Personality changes—nonspecific
	Changes in school performance–nonspecific

Table 7
Physical Signs or Symptoms Suggestive of Secondary Hypertension

Sign or symptom	Comment
CNS	
Hypertensive crisis	Severe hypertension with underlying encephalopathy
Bell's palsy	Often associated with severe hypertension
Hypertensive retinopathy	In children, rarely found in essential hypertension but good staging unavailable
Skin	
Neurofibromas	Pheochromocytoma/renovascular lesions
Café-au-lait spots	Pheochromocytoma/renovascular lesions
Lesions of tuberous sclerosis	Renal cysts, vascular lesions
Rash	
of systemic lupus erythematosus	Lupus nephritis
or Henoch–Schonlein purpura	Henoch–Schonlein nephritis/vasculitis
Needle tracks	Drug abuse, iatrogenic hypertension
Neck	
Goiter	Hyperthyroidism
Lungs	
Picture of bronchopulmonary dysplasia	Associated hypertension
Pulmonary edema	Volume overload associated hypertension: acute glomerulonephritis or chronic renal insufficiency
Heart	
Failure	Volume overload associated hypertension: acute glomerulonephritis or chronic renal insufficiency
Endocrine/genetic	
Multiple endocrinopathy	Pheochromocytoma
Turner's syndrome	Coarctation of the aorta
Williams syndrome	Renovascular hypertension
Van Hippel–Lindau	Pheochromocytoma
Abdominal	
Bruits	Renovascular hypertension
Enlarged kidneys	Polycystic disease, obstructive uropathy, renal inflammatory disorders (pyelonephritis, nephritis)

dysplasia, and symmetrically enlarged kidneys indicating potential infective (pyelonephritis) or glomerular disease. Additionally the renal ultrasound easily documents renal calculi, nephrocalcinosis, renal parenchymal cysts, polycystic kidney disease, or multicystic dysplastic kidney. Doppler waveform analysis of the renal hilum can also provide information as to the patency of the vessels; however, its sensitivity for diagnosis of renal artery stenosis is limited, particularly in infants and children and in the detection of intrarenal lesions and incomplete stenoses in older children or adolescents *(29,30)*.

Serum electrolytes most commonly will be normal; however, alterations of potassium concentrations can indicate primary or secondary hyperaldosteronism, particularly when the potassium is low and there is a concomitant metabolic alkalosis. Liddle's syndrome, the syndrome of apparent mineralocorticoid excess, Gordon's syndrome, and glucocorticoid remediable aldosteronism and other forms of monogenic hypertension are often associated with this electrolyte pattern and altered renin and aldosterone levels (Fig. 2) *(31)*. By contrast, elevated potassium in conjunction with a metabolic acidosis may suggest kidney disease. Indeed, this diagnosis may be supported by an elevation in serum creatinine or one may find nephrocalcinosis on renal ultrasound indicating a renal tubular defect. Importantly, values of serum creatinine for pediatric patients differ with increasing age and often can be misinterpreted as 'normal' when in fact a significant loss of kidney mass/function has occurred despite the use of Schwartz formula *(32)*.

Syndrome	K$^+$	pH	Renin	Aldo	Specific Treatment	Gene Loci	Gene
GRA	↓	↑	↓	↑	Spironolactone (Amiloride, triamterene)	8q	Chimeric gene (CYP11B1/ CYP11B2)
Liddle's syndrome	↓	↑	↓	↓	Amiloride, triamterene	16p	β and γ subunit of ENaC
AME	↓	↑	↓	↓	Spironolactone (Amiloride, triamterene)	16q	11-β-HSD
MR	↓	↑	↓	↓	None, multiple drug therapy	4q	MR
Gordon's syndrome	↑	↓	↓	↓	Hydrochlorothiazide	1q 12p13 17p	WNK1 WNK4
HBS	N	N	N (↓)	N	None, multiple drug therapy	12p11	Unknown

NOTE. Contrary to the rest, the HBS is not salt sensitive and features normal values for the shown parameters. Abbreviations: K$^+$, potassium; Aldo, aldosterone.
GRA: glucocorticoid-remediable aldosteronism
AME: Apparent mineralocorticord excess
MR: Mineralocorticoid receptor mutation
HBS: Hypertension brachydactyly syndrome

Fig. 2. Monogenic forms of hypertension. GRA: glucocorticoid-remediable aldosteronism; AME: apparent mineralocorticoid excess; MR: mineralocorticoid receptor mutation; HBS: hypertension brachydactyly syndrome.

WHAT ARE THE CONSEQUENCES OF HYPERTENSION: END-ORGAN DAMAGE?

The relationship of hypertension to end-organ damage is critical to the true definition of hypertension and discussed in detail by Sorof et al. *(33)*. The evaluation of hypertension is not solely to determine where the measured level of BP exceeds some epidemiologically derived number, but rather to ascertain the level of this endothelial disease marker associated with end-organ damage. The evaluation of end-organ damage should include a complete assessment of the cardiovascular system (including blood vessels), kidneys, and nervous system. This assessment can assist in determining the chronicity and the severity of the hypertension. Fundoscopy, typically reserved for patients with severe hypertension, rarely discloses hemorrhages or exudates but may reveal arteriolar narrowing and arteriovenous nicking. As few studies of retinal abnormalities have been conducted in hypertensive children, there has been no development of a standardized grading system for hypertensive retinopathy in children. Daniels et al. using direct ophthalmoscopy showed that 51% of children with primary hypertension had retinal abnormalities *(34)*. More recently, Mitchell et al. examined children aged 6–8 years, where for every 10 mmHg increase in systolic blood pressure, a narrowing of 1.93–2.08 μm was seen in the retinal arterioles *(35)*.

LVH is a clear and independent risk factor for cardiovascular morbidity and mortality in adult patients, but its significance is less clear for children unless it is severe or found to compromise cardiac function. The echocardiogram is more sensitive than the electrocardiogram for the determination of left ventricular hypertrophy/index *(36)*. ABPM has been shown to have a significant correlation to left ventricular mass index where casual BP measurements do not. Specifically the best predictors include the 24 h wake or sleep mean BP, BP load, or BP index *(33)*. Additionally, further evidence for hypertension's role in causing end-organ damage in pediatrics emanates from the correlation of the carotid intimal–medial thickness and left ventricular mass index with hypertension and obesity *(37)*. There is a growing body of evidence which demonstrates an association with non-dipping status (failure of BP to decline with sleep) and an increased risk of adverse events *(10–12,15,16,38,39)*. Additional markers of end-organ damage include elevated microalbumin excretion, which is especially important in, patients with CKD, and the obese as a marker of hypertensive end-organ damage. The presence of end-organ damage in a child is an absolute indication for pharmacologic treatment of hypertension *(2)*.

WHAT OTHER RISK FACTORS FOR CARDIOVASCULAR DISEASE MAY BE PRESENT?

The major modifiable cardiovascular risk factors are hypertension, diabetes, smoking, hyperlipidemia, and proteinuria (chronic kidney disease) and should be evaluated during the initial screening process. A reasonable list of tests for cardiovascular risk assessment includes a fasting lipoprotein analysis including cholesterol, triglycerides, HDL, LDL, VLDL, a fasting glucose and insulin for assessment of insulin resistance, microalbumin excretion, echocardiography, and kidney function. However, not all of these studies have been endorsed by consensus organizations for routine screening *(2)*.

Phase 3: What Is the Definition of Abnormality?

Phase 3 evaluation is designed to further clarify and define abnormalities identified during phase 1 in any of the three categories of etiology, risk factors, and end-organ damage determination. Concerning etiology, performance of stage 3 evaluation should be done for the very young hypertensive patient or for those with severe hypertension even if phase 1 is unremarkable (Table 3). At this point, we aim to find the abnormality, but specifically limit the diagnostic tests to match the patient. For instance, if the patient by history and physical examination has stigmata of hyperthyroidism, e.g., weight loss, enlargement of thyroid, proptosis, we might perform a thyroid panel, but not for everyone. Individual consideration should be given to measurement of plasma levels of various endocrine or vasoactive hormones as well as 24-h excretion rates of various hormones based on prior findings. Imaging studies provide information on the condition of the renal parenchyma and renovascular dysfunction. Renal ultrasound with Doppler flow analysis in conjunction with other studies can reveal the etiology for diagnosis of certain kidney lesions. Radionuclide renal scanning can be very helpful as it can assess renal function, perfusion, obstruction, and presence of renal scarring. Radionuclide scintigraphy to assess scarring may use either ^{99m}Tc dimercaptosuccinic acid (DMSA), ^{99m}Tc glucoheptonate (DTPA), or ^{99m}Tc mercaptoacetyltriglycine (Mag3) and can be done with diuretics to help assess for the presence of obstructive hydronephrosis. In children with a history of urinary tract infections and the diagnosis of vesicoureteral reflux or bladder abnormalities is entertained, voiding cystourethrography should also be performed. Detection of proteinuria requires either quantitation of protein excretion with the first morning urine using a urinary protein to creatinine ratio or a 24-h urine collection for protein and creatinine (split into supine and upright fractions to assess for orthostatic proteinuria).

Abnormalities of the mesenteric, splenic, and hepatic vessels often accompany renovascular disease in children. A certain percentage of these children may have neurofibromatosis type 1 (NF-1) *(40,41)* or abdominal coarctation *(42–44)* or intracranial disease *(45)*. In our experience, Doppler ultrasound is a very specific but insensitive test for renovascular hypertension. Screening for renal artery stenosis in children with captopril scans has also been unrewarding. Magnetic resonance angiography may become a valuable tool for detection of renal artery stenosis in children, but no large studies have yet validated the technology. It may be used as a screening test, but if there is a high index of suspicion, arteriography, the gold standard, should still be performed.

If other risk factors are identified, testing and/or appropriate referral should be performed. For example, glucose intolerance should be further evaluated with assessment of glycosylated hemoglobin (HgA1c), glucose tolerance testing, and referral to endocrinology as appropriate. Elevated serum lipoproteins in the obese could suggest dietary causes or rarely hypothyroidism. Familial forms of hyperlipidemia such as abnormalities in number or function of LDL receptors should also be assessed.

Phase 4: Determination of Significance and Remediability of Abnormality

At this point, having found an abnormality we now look for a test or series of tests that will provide information regarding the medical or surgical correctability of the problem.

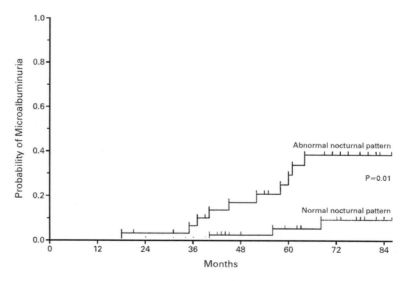

Fig. 3. Kaplan–Meier curves showing the probability of microalbuminuria according to the pattern of daytime and nighttime systolic pressure. The probability of microalbuminuria differed significantly between the two groups ($p = 0.01$ by the log-rank test; chi-square $= 6.217$ with 1 df). The risk of microalbuminuria was 70% lower in the subjects with a normal nocturnal pattern than in those with an abnormal nocturnal pattern *(46)*.

If a renal artery stenosis is detected by renovascular imaging, renal vein renins may provide further evidence for surgical correction. If an elevated serum metanephrine or urinary catecholamines are found suggesting a pheochromocytoma, then an octreotide or metaiodobenzylguanidine (MIBG) scan would aid in localization for surgical correction. A finding of significant proteinuria or hematuria with RBC casts would suggest a renal biopsy be performed. This information is also helpful in determining the type of antihypertensive therapy to be used. If abnormalities in serum renin or aldosterone consistent with the genetic syndromes outlined in Fig. 3 are found, specific therapies such as amiloride or spironolactone are suggested *(47,48)*. Finding of CKD or diabetes can suggest the use of drugs affecting the renin–angiotensin system such as ACE inhibitors or angiotensin receptor blockade.

SUMMARY

While cardiovascular end points or the presence of hypertensive end-organ damage should be the basis for the definition of pediatric hypertension, this is not currently the case. Primary hypertension, as defined by BP measurements exceeding the 95th percentile for height with no underlying cause, is increasing in prevalence, particularly in older children and adolescents with hypertension risk factors, e.g., obesity. We recommend the evaluation of the pediatric hypertensive patient be performed in phases beginning with the confirmation of hypertension beyond the office measurement (phase 1). This confirmation should be followed by the screening phase which further defines (a) the etiology of the hypertension knowing that younger patients are more likely to have a secondary etiology and older patients primary hypertension, (b) other risk factors for cardiovascular/kidney disease, and (c) hypertensive end-organ damage. Phase 3 defines the abnormalities in either (a), (b), or (c), and the fourth and final phase is the determination of the significance of observed findings.

We recommend pharmacologic treatment of all children and adolescents with persistent hypertension due to the believed risk of end-organ damage and the lack of long-term efficacy of non-pharmacologic therapy as a sole therapy. Evidence-based definitions of pediatric hypertension and the indication for treatment are currently evolving as well as the introduction of new information for areas of pre- and postnatal causes of hypertension; genetics of hypertension; the relationship of obesity, diabetes, and CKD to hypertension; the use of ABPM in the evaluation of childhood hypertension; and the introduction of new pharmacologic therapy. Clearly, the information presented in this text has improved our understanding of the pathogenesis, diagnosis, and treatment of childhood hypertension; however, significant advances remain to be made. The most efficient tests and evaluation pathways for determining which children have secondary forms of hypertension or who are at risk for end-organ damage have also yet to be determined.

REFERENCES

1. Falkner, BE. Treatment of hypertensive children and adolescents. In: Isso JL, Black HR, eds. Hypertension Primer, 3rd ed. Philadelphia, PA: Lippincott Williams & Wilkins; 2003:494–497.
2. US Department of Health and Human Services. National Institutes of Health. National Heart, Lung, Blood Institute. The fourth report on the diagnosis, evaluation and treatment of high blood pressure in children and adolescents. NIH Publication No. 05-5267 May 2005;1–42.
3. Lande MB, Flynn JT. Treatment of hypertension in children and adolescents. Pediatr Nephrol. 2009;24:1939–1949.

4. The ESCAPE Trial Group. Strict blood-pressure control and progression of renal failure in children. N Engl J Med. 361;17:1639–1650.
5. Kavey RE, Allada V, Daniels SR, Hayman LL, McCrindle BW, et al. Cardiovascular risk reduction in high-risk pediatric patients: a scientific statement from the American Heart Association Expert Panel on Population and Prevention Science. Circulation. 2006;114:2710–2738.
6. Falkner B. Hypertension in children and adolescents: epidemiology and natural history. Pediatr Nephrol. 2010;25:1219–1224.
7. Julius S, Nesbitt SD, Egan BM, Weber MA, Michelson EL, Kaciroti N, et al. Feasibility of treating pre-hypertension with an angiotensin-receptor blocker for the Trial of Preventing Hypertension (TROPHY) Study Investigators. N Engl J Med. 2006;354:1685–1697.
8. Swartz SJ, Srivaths PR, Croix B, Feig DI. Cost-effectiveness of ambulatory blood pressure monitoring in the initial evaluation of hypertension in children. Pediatrics. 2008;122:1177–1181.
9. Lurbe E, Cifkova R, Cruickshank JK, Dillon MJ, Ferreira I, Invitti C, et al. Management of high blood pressure in children and adolescents: recommendations of the European Society of Hypertension. J Hypertens. 2009;1719–1742.
10. Urbina E, Alpert B, Flynn J, Hayman L, Gregory A, et al. Ambulatory blood pressure monitoring in children and adolescents: recommendations for standard assessment. A scientific statement from the American Heart Association Atherosclerosis, Hypertension, and Obesity in Youth Committee of the Council on Cardiovascular Disease in the Young and the Council for High Blood Pressure Research. Hypertension. 2009;52:433–451.
11. Clement DL, De Buyzere ML, De Bacquer DA, Fagard RH, Gheeraert PJ, Missault LH, Braun JJ, Six RO, Van Der Niepen P, O'Brien E. For the Office versus Ambulatory Pressure Study investigators. Prognostic value of ambulatory blood-pressure recordings in patients with treated hypertension. New Engl J Med. 2002;348:2407–2415.
12. Amin R, Somers VK, McConnell, K, Willging P, Myer C, Sherman M, et al. Activity-adjusted 24-hour ambulatory blood pressure and cardiac remodeling in children with sleep disordered breathing. Hypertension. 2008;51:84–91.
13. Karavanaki K, Kazianis G, Konstantopoulos I, Tsouvalas E, Karayianni C. Early signs of left ventricular dysfunction in adolescents with type 1 diabetes mellitus: the importance of impaired circadian modulation of blood pressure and heart rate. J Endocrinol Invest. 2008;31:289–296.
14. McNiece KL, Gupta-Malhotra M, Samuels J, Bell C, Garcia K, Poffengbarger T, et al. Left ventricular hypertrophy in hypertensive adolescents: analysis of risk by 2004 National High Blood Pressure Education Program Working Group Staging Criteria. Hypertension. 2007;50:392–395.
15. Covic A, Goldsmith DJA, Georgescu GC, Ackrill P. Relationships between blood pressure variability and left ventricular parameters in hemodialysis and renal transplant patients. Nephrology. 1998;4:87–94.
16. Appel LJ, Robinson KA, Guallar E, Erlinger T, Masood SO, Jehn M, Fleisher LA, Bass EB. Utility of blood pressure monitoring outside of the clinic setting. Evidence/Technology Assessment, No 63, U.S. Department of Health and Human Service, Agency for Healthcare Research and Quality, 2002. Available at http://www.ahrq.gov/downloads/pub/evidence/pdf/utbp/utbp.pdf. [Last accessed February 4, 2010].
17. Wuhl E, Hadtstein C, Mehls O, Schaefer F. ESCAPE Trial Group home, clinic, and ambulatory blood pressure monitoring in children with chronic renal failure. Pediatr Res. 2004;55:492–497.
18. Stergious GS, Karpettas N, Kapoyiannis A, Stefandidi CJ, Vazeou A. Home blood pressure monitoring in children and adolescents: a systematic review. J Hypertens. 2009;27:1941–1947.
19. Lurbe E, Alvarez V, Redon J. Obesity, body fat distribution, and ambulatory blood pressure in children and adolescents. J Clin Hypertens. 2001;3:362–367.
20. Barlow SE, Dietz WH, Klish WJ, Trowbridge FL. Medical evaluation of overweight children and adolescents: reports from pediatricians, pediatric nurse practitioners, and registered dietitians. Pediatrics. 2002;110:222–228.
21. Flynn JT. Differentiation between primary and secondary hypertension in children using ambulatory blood pressure monitoring. Pediatrics. 2002;110:89–93.
22. Gimpel C, Wuhl E, Arbeiter K, Drozdz D, Trivelli A, Charbit M, et al. Superior consistency of ambulatory blood pressure monitoring in children: implications for clinical trials. J Hypertens. 2009;27(8):1568–1574.
23. Lurbe E, Toor I, Paya R, Alvarez V, Redon J. Masked hypertension in adolescents. Am J Hypertens. 2003;16:237A.
24. Stabouli S, Kotsis V, Zakopoulos N. Ambulatory blood pressure monitoring and target organ damage in pediatrics. J Hypertens. 2007;25:1979–1986.
25. Londe S. Causes of hypertension in the young. Pediatr Clin North Am. 1978;25(1):55–65.
26. Luma GB, Spiotta RT. Hypertension in children and adolescents. Am Fam Physician. 2006;73:1558–1568.
27. Schwartz GJ, Brion LP, Spitzer A. The use of plasma creatinine concentration for estimating glomerular filtration rate in infants, children, and adolescents. Pediatr Clin North Am. 1987;34(3):571–590.

28. Hall PM, Rolin H. Iothalmate clearance and its use in large-scale clinical trials. Curr Opin Nephrol Hypertens. 1995;3:510–513.

29. Olin JW, Piedmonte MA, Young JR. The utility of duplex ultrasound scanning of the renal arteries for diagnosing significant renal artery stenosis. Ann Intern Med. 1995;122:833–838.

30. Brun P, Kchouk H, Mouchet B. Value of Doppler ultrasound for the diagnosis of renal artery stenosis in children. Pediatr Nephrol. 1997;11:27–30.

31. Toka HR, Luft FC. Monogenic forms of human hypertension. Semin Nephrol. 2002;22:81–88.

32. Lemly KV. Estimating GFR in children: Schwartz redux. Nat Rev Nephrol. 2009;5:310–311.

33. Sorof JM, Poffenbarger T, Franco K, Portman R. Evaluation of white coat hypertension in children: importance of the definitions of normal ambulatory blood pressure and the severity of casual hypertension. Am J Hypertens. 2001;14:855–860.

34. Daniels SR, Lipman MU, Berke JM. The prevalence of retinal vascular abnormalities in children and adolescents with essential hypertension. Am J Ophthalmol. 1991;111:205–208.

35. Mitchell P, Cheung N, Dettuseth K, Taylor B, Rochitchira E, Wang JJ, et al. Blood pressure and retinal arteriolar narrowing in children. Hypertension. 2007;49:1156–1162.

36. Daniels SR, Loggie JM, Khoury P, Kimball TR. Left ventricular geometry and severe left ventricular hypertrophy in children and adolescents with essential hypertension. Circulation. 1998;97:1907–1911.

37. Sorof JM, Alexandrov AV, Cardwell G, Portman RJ. Carotid artery intimal-medial thickness and left ventricular hypertrophy in children with elevated blood pressure. Pediatrics. 2003;111:61–66.

38. McConnell K, Somers VKL, Kimball T, Daniels S, VanDyke R, Fenchel M, et al. Baroreflex gain in children with obstructive sleep apnea. Am J Respir Crit Care Med. 2009;180:42–48.

39. McGlothan KR, Wyatt RJ, Ault BH, Hastings MC, Rogers T, DiSessa T, et al. Predominance of nocturnal hypertension in pediatric renal allograft recipients. Pediatr Transplant. 2006;10:558–564.

40. Loughridge LW. Renal abnormalities in the Marfan syndrome. Q J Med. 1959;28:531–544.

41. Glushien AS, Mansuy MM, Littman DS. Pheochromocytoma: its relationship to neurocutaneous syndromes. Am J Med. 1953;14:318–327.

42. Alpert BS, Bain HH, Balfe JW. Role of the renin-angiotensin-aldosterone system in hypertensive children with coarctation of the aorta. Am J Cardiol. 1979;43:828–831.

43. Becker AE, Becker MJ, Edward JE. Anomalies associated with coarctation of aorta. Circulation. 1979;41:1067–1069.

44. Morriss M, McNamara D. Coarctation of the aorta. In: Garson A, Bricker J, McNamara D, eds. Science and Practice of Pediatric Cardiology. Philadelphia, PA: Lea&Febiger; 1990:1353–1365.

45. Wiggelinkhuizen J, Cremin BJ. Takayasu arteritis and renovascular hypertension in childhood. Pediatrics. 1978;62:209–217.

46. Lurbe E, Redon J, Kesani A, et al. Increase in nocturnal blood pressure and progression to microalbuminuria in type I diabetes. N Engl J Med. 2002;347:797–805.

47. Vehaskari, M. Heritable forms of hypertension. Pediatr Nephrol. 2009;24:1929–1937.

48. Martinez-Aguayo A, Fardell C. Genetics of hypertensive syndrome. Horm Res. 2009;71:253–259.

29

The Role of Ambulatory Blood Pressure Monitoring in Diagnosis of Hypertension and Evaluation of Target Organ Damage

Empar Lurbe, MD, PhD *and Josep Redon,* MD, PhD, FAHA

CONTENTS

INTRODUCTION

The goal of blood pressure (BP) measurement in children and adolescents is to provide strategies for promoting cardiovascular health which should be integrated into a comprehensive pediatric health-care program. Blood pressure, however, is a parameter that changes on a beat-to-beat basis in response to a variety of physiological and environmental stimuli. Nevertheless, casual BP measurement has provided the basis for present knowledge of the potential risk associated with hypertension *(1)* and has guided patient management for many years *(2)*. A few BP measurements obtained in the office, on the contrary, may not necessarily reflect the true BP of an individual. Subsequently, a better characterization of BP level and variability could lead to a better stratification of risk. This line of reasoning has led consequently to the development of methods that permit the acquisition of a large number of measurements under normal living conditions *(3)*. The possibility of carrying out repeated ambulatory BP measurements using automatic or semiautomatic devices allows for the gathering of more representative values of BP and for observing the behavior of BP

E. Lurbe (✉)
Pediatric Nephrology Department, Department of Pediatrics, Consorcio Hospital General Universitario de Valencia, University of Valencia, Spain; CIBERobn, Instituto de Salud Carlos III, Spain
e-mail: empar.lurbe@uv.es

From: *Clinical Hypertension and Vascular Diseases: Pediatric Hypertension*
Edited by: J. T. Flynn et al. DOI 10.1007/978-1-60327-824-9_29
© Springer Science+Business Media, LLC 2011

during both moments of activity and rest *(4)*. Indeed, over the last few years ambulatory BP monitoring has been introduced in pediatric populations, contributing to a significant increase in the bulk of knowledge of crucial clinically relevant issues *(5)*.

Ambulatory BP measurement is now increasingly recognized as being indispensable to the diagnosis and management of hypertension *(6)*, and it has contributed significantly to our understanding of hypertension by revealing or "unmasking" blood pressure phenomena that were not readily apparent using traditional techniques of measurement in clinical practice. These have included the dipping and non-dipping patterns of nocturnal BP *(7)* and white-coat hypertension *(8)* to which now must be added masked hypertension *(9)*, a condition in which subjects classified as normotensive by conventional office or clinic measurement are hypertensive with ambulatory BP monitoring. Likewise, the better relationship of ambulatory BP measurements with the presence of organ damage and the prognosis to develop it have provided additional support to ambulatory BP as a clinical valuable tool in the research, evaluation, and management of high BP in children and adolescents *(5)*.

The use of ambulatory BP monitoring is now recommended in several situations by the Fourth Report on the Diagnosis, Evaluation and Treatment in Children and Adolescents *(10)*, the American Heart Association Atherosclerosis, Hypertension, and Obesity in Youth Committee *(11)*, and the Recommendations of the European Society of Hypertension *(12)* (Table 1). These documents have established the currently known conditions where ambulatory BP monitoring is useful and where it will provide additional information in children and adolescents.

Table 1
Recommendations for 24-H Ambulatory BP
Monitoring *(12)*

During the process of diagnosis
Confirm hypertension before starting antihypertensive
   drug treatment
Type 1 diabetes
Chronic kidney disease
Renal, liver, or heart transplant

During antihypertensive drug treatment
Evaluation of refractory hypertension
Assessment of BP control in children with organ damage
Symptoms of hypotension

Clinical trials

Other clinical conditions
Autonomic dysfunction
Suspicion of catecholamine-secreting tumors

Aside from the assessment of refractory hypertension or drug-induced hypotension, ambulatory BP monitoring is useful in the evaluation of white-coat hypertension and in target organ injury risk. Furthermore, ambulatory BP monitoring gives additional BP information in chronic renal failure, diabetes, and autonomic neuropathy. In these diseases, in which abnormal circadian variability is frequent and worsens the prognosis, ambulatory BP monitoring is the only method capable of assessing the absence of circadian rhythm.

AMBULATORY BLOOD PRESSURE MONITORING IN THE DIAGNOSIS

Since pediatricians agree on operational thresholds ambulatory BP monitoring has become an established instrument for the diagnosis of hypertension in children and adolescents *(13,14)*. By using not only office but also ambulatory BP, four possible situations arise. Two of these have values in agreement for normotension or hypertension. Two have values that are discrepant. The latter two are known as white-coat and masked hypertension. In sustained normotension or hypertension, both office and daytime ambulatory BP were normal and elevated, respectively. White-coat hypertension is the transient elevation of a patient's BP in response to the observer measuring the BP *(15,16)*. It has been characterized by a normal daytime ambulatory BP yet with elevated office BP. The opposite phenomenon, masked hypertension, consists of elevated daytime or awake ambulatory BP with normal office BP *(17)*.

Besides the fact that there was higher mean ambulatory BP than office BP in the individual patient, the discrepancies have clinical relevance. How common and important the intraindividual differences are within clinical and ambulatory BP is the keystone to the use of ambulatory BP monitoring as a diagnostic tool. The prevalence and significance of the two discrepant conditions, white-coat hypertension and masked hypertension, are not well understood and differ according to the characteristics of the subjects analyzed. The main studies in the prevalence and significance of white-coat and masked hypertension are shown in Table 2.

Table 2
Studies on White-Coat and Masked Hypertension in Children and Adolescents

Author	Population characteristics	Prevalence white coat (%)	Prevalence masked	Association TOD
Sorof et al. *(16)*	71 referred subjects	31	–	–
Matsuoka et al. *(19)*	202 normo-hypertension	47	–	–
Matsuoka and Awazu *(24)*	138 normo-hypertension	–	11	–
Lurbe et al. *(17)*	592 population study	1.7	7.6	LVH in masked
Stabouli et al. *(18)*	85 referred subjects	12.9	9.4	LVH in masked
McNiece et al. *(20)*	163 referred subjects	Stage 1—34 Stage 2—15	20	LVH in masked
Kavey et al. *(21)*	119 referred subjects	52	–	LVH in white coat
Lande et al. *(22)*	217 referred subjects	31	–	–
Stergiou et al. *(23)*	102 referred subjects	18	11	–

White Coat

The prevalence of white-coat hypertension, the first of the two discrepant conditions to be recognized, differs largely among the studies published, ranging from very low values to very high values as much as 44% *(16)*, since it depends not only on the threshold selected to define hypertension by using ambulatory BP values but also on the population included and the procedure of office BP measurements.

The elevated figures for the white-coat phenomenon are dependent at least in part on the defining threshold for the upper limit of normality for ambulatory BP. The higher the ambulatory BP threshold, the greater the white-coat phenomenon. Sometimes the thresholds used are the same for both ambulatory and office BP. If not, they have been selected comparing age- and height-based reference values for office BP with height-based values for ambulatory BP. Another factor is the kind of population included. Sorof et al. *(16)* and Stabouli et al. *(18)* in two studies, which included children referred to a hypertension clinic, reported that white-coat hypertension was present in 44 and 12.9% of the subjects, respectively. Other studies also performed in referred subjects had figures within the previously mentioned *(19–23)*. In contrast, one study which included healthy children and adolescents diagnosed only 1% to have white-coat hypertension *(17)*. This very low prevalence was not only dependent on the kind of population studied but also on the method used to assess the office BP values, since BP status was qualified using the average of three measurements and office BP was measured by nurses which reduce the potential for alarm reaction.

Concerning the significance of white-coat hypertension, children with white-coat hypertension tended to have a higher left ventricular mass index than confirmed normotensives did, although no significant differences were observed between the groups *(16,18,20)*. Furthermore, there are currently no data on the long-term follow-up of children found to have white-coat hypertension upon initial assessment, and questions concerning reproducibility of the phenomenon and whether the white-coat phenomenon in adolescents is an innocuous phenomenon or a prelude to future permanent adult hypertension need to be clarified. Thus, there is presently insufficient evidence in children to assert that normal ambulatory BP in conjunction with a persistently elevated casual BP is necessarily reassuring.

Masked

The opposite phenomenon, the so-called masked hypertension, occurred in approximately 10% of children and adolescents in studies which have explored this condition *(17,18,23)*, although higher prevalence has been reported in other, 22% *(20)*. Key issues such as the persistence and the significance of the phenomenon were analyzed in a prospective study *(17)*. Follow-up of 234 adolescents demonstrated that the abnormal elevation of the daytime ambulatory BP persisted in nearly 40%. Furthermore, 1 out of 10 subjects with masked hypertension is predisposed to the development of sustained hypertension and has a higher left ventricular mass index with a prevalence of left ventricular hypertrophy of 22% *(20)* and 10% *(24)*.

Adolescents with persistent masked hypertension were more than twice as likely to have a parental history of hypertension. Other characteristics observed in those with masked hypertension were that they had a higher ambulatory pulse rate and body mass index than did normotensive subjects. These three characteristics, alone or in combination, predispose subjects to the development of hypertension and an increase in cardiovascular risk later in life *(17)*. Parental history of hypertension, tachycardia, and high body mass index are usually accompanied by stimulation of the sympathetic nervous system, which together with the elevated daytime BP and obesity might underlie the development of left ventricular hypertrophy in youth with masked hypertension even before its preceding to sustained hypertension *(25,26)*.

Because both hypertension and left ventricular hypertrophy are harbingers of adverse cardiovascular outcomes later in life *(27,28)*, masked hypertension in childhood should be regarded as a condition that requires further follow-up and intervention in whom this disorder persists. From a therapeutic point of view, masked hypertension in pediatric patients is an indicator for further follow-up and the institution of lifestyle measures, which promote cardiovascular health and have the potential to decrease BP or delay the development of hypertension. Once persistent for 1 year, masked hypertension may be an indication for BP-lowering treatment, especially in children and adolescents with a positive family history of hypertension. Whether or not pharmacological treatment should be initiated in such cases must await supporting evidence.

As for the existence of white-coat or masked hypertension in children, its importance as a clinical entity will depend on whether it carries risk for future cardiovascular outcome. Despite the scarce information available, recent research has added essential information that can help in the better design of future studies to answer practical questions and delineate clinical recommendations. The superiority of ambulatory over office BP underlines the diagnostic complementarity of ambulatory monitoring to conventional BP measurement at the office. Furthermore, a paper from Mancia and coworkers *(29)* established that each BP elevation (office, home, or ambulatory) carries an increase in risk mortality that adds to that of the other BP elevations. If the three, office, home, or ambulatory, show normal BP values, the risk is lower compared to subjects that have at least one of the three BPs elevated. If the elevation exists in two, the risk is even higher. Furthermore, if the three BPs are elevated, the risk is the highest.

Masked hypertension in children presents pediatricians with the serious problem of identifying subjects with the condition. This gives rise to a very pertinent question. Which children need ambulatory BP monitoring? Although the question has yet to be resolved, ambulatory BP monitoring is useful not only for stratifying risk in individual subjects but also for providing data which will add to our knowledge of this issue. Clearly, it is not practical to perform ambulatory BP monitoring in all subjects with normotension in the office or clinic to unmask those with ambulatory hypertension, but we have to face the reality that children with masked hypertension may be seriously disadvantaged if ambulatory BP monitoring is not performed. Once masked hypertension is detected, repeated office BP measurements should be encouraged to detect the potential progressive rise in BP values.

Clinical Significance of Discrepant Phenomenon

The occurrence of white-coat hypertension and the reverse phenomenon of masked hypertension in at least 10% of children and adolescents introduce the potential for misdiagnosing subjects who present themselves to doctors for BP measurement. This estimate, which is conservative, must surely make ambulatory BP monitoring an indispensable research tool for the diagnosis and management of hypertension in children and adolescents *(30)*, mainly in those at higher risk. The finding that masked and white-coat hypertension occur in at least 10 and 21% of the moderate and severely obese, respectively, emphasizes the likelihood of misdiagnosing clinically relevant BP problems in obese youths *(31)*.

When to Use Ambulatory Blood Pressure Monitoring in the Diagnosis

Considering the current information above updated, ambulatory BP monitoring in children and adolescents should be performed during the process of diagnoses of hypertension in the following conditions: Confirm hypertension before starting antihypertensive drug treatment; type 1 diabetes; chronic kidney disease; and renal, liver, or heart transplant *(12)* (see Table 1).

AMBULATORY BLOOD PRESSURE MONITORING AND HYPERTENSION-INDUCED ORGAN DAMAGE

Once hypertension is confirmed, organ damage evaluation should include heart, great vessels, and kidney due to the importance of subclinical organ damage as an intermediate stage in the continuum of vascular disease. Cardiovascular damage develops in parallel to renal damage, although the cardiovascular sequelae of childhood-onset hypertension, such as left ventricular hypertrophy and dysfunction and atherosclerosis, may not become clinically relevant before adulthood. Subsequently, evaluation of organ damage is also useful as an intermediate end point for monitoring treatment-induced protection.

Ambulatory BP monitoring has provided knowledge about the role of the BP components on the development of hypertension-induced organ damage. Hypertension in children as defined by casual BP values, however, is not well correlated to any particular form of hypertensive target organ damage. Ambulatory BP monitoring may overcome these limitations; therefore, ambulatory BP monitoring became an established instrument for the evaluation and prognosis *(5)* due to the ability to obtain more accurate and reproducible BP values *(31)* and the estimation of circadian variability *(32)*, a parameter that had demonstrated additional value in the evaluation of hypertension and its impact in organ damage.

Renal Diseases

Renal disease in children is frequently associated with high BP. An increase in BP as a consequence of kidney disease contributes to the progression of renal damage. A rapid progression of renal damage may result in end-stage renal insufficiency during childhood. Cardiovascular damage develops in parallel to this, although the cardiovascular sequelae of childhood-onset HTN, such as left ventricular hypertrophy and dysfunction and atherosclerosis, may not become clinically relevant before adulthood. With the decline in the number of functional nephrons, a further increase in BP occurs, creating a vicious cycle which progresses to end-stage renal disease. Furthermore, progressive vascular disease compromises renal blood supply and contributes still further to the vicious cycle by increasing renal damage.

Evidence of the importance of ambulatory BP values in the progression of renal disease has come from several clinical studies in children with or without established renal insufficiency. Besides the GFR reduction, an increase in urinary albumin excretion is a marker of hypertension-induced renal damage. Proteinuria is a marker of glomerular damage in primary and secondary glomerulopathies that can increase as a consequence of elevated BP values, so it should be targeted by lowering BP. Even small amounts of urinary albumin excretion (UAE) and microalbuminuria are correlated with the progression of nephropathy and to a higher cardiovascular risk. Initially, information came from cross-sectional studies which demonstrated a clustering of cardiovascular risk factors and organ damage associated with a subtle increase in UAE. The role of microalbuminuria assessment in pediatrics, however, is limited to diabetics.

The regular use of ambulatory BP monitoring in patients with renal disease not only permits a better assessment of BP control but also frequently uncovers circadian variability abnormalities. A blunted nocturnal BP fall, the non-dipper pattern, is characteristic for renal failure, whichever the etiology. The role of the pattern as either a marker or a pathogenic factor for kidney damage has been stressed in many studies *(33)*.

Patients with a decrease in glomerular filtration rate (GFR) are likely to show less of a nocturnal dip in BP and frequently show an increase in nocturnal versus daytime BP levels when these are compared with the BP profiles from normotensives or hypertensives with a normal GFR *(34–36)*. The prevalence of non-dipping rises, however, with worsening renal function, reaching statistical significance once plasma creatinine is elevated to levels greater than 400 μmol/l *(34)*. When GFR decreases to extremely low levels of <10 ml/min, and creatinine reaches values greater than 600 μmol/l, more than 70% of these end-stage renal disease subjects show the non-dipper pattern. This figure is practically the same as that seen in patients during renal replacement therapy.

After renal transplantation, an abnormal BP decline in nighttime occurs almost universally in adults as well as in children *(37–42)*. Some of these patients may experience reverse dipping, with nighttime BP exceeding daytime BP. In a study by Sorof et al. *(40)*, 72% of the patients have an attenuated decline in nocturnal systolic BP, with 24% having greater nighttime BP than daytime BP.

Even in the absence of renal insufficiency, the prevalence of the non-dipper pattern is high in such diseases as autosomic dominant polycystic kidney disease *(43)*, reflux nephropathy *(44,45)*, and type 1 diabetes *(46)*. It is from the last disease where the greatest of amount information has been obtained.

The spectrum of abnormalities of circadian BP variability through all the nephropathy stages of type 1 diabetes shows that about 58% of the microalbuminuric and 80% of the proteinuric subjects have a persistently blunted BP fall during night. The reduction in the BP nocturnal fall is independent of the disease duration *(47)*. In type 1 diabetes, the presence of persistent microalbuminuria represents an early BP dysregulation during sleep even in the absence of hypertension. When overt nephropathy is established, hypertension is present and abnormalities in the circadian BP profile are more conspicuous. A pathogenic role of nocturnal systolic BP has been related to the development of microalbuminuria in normotensive type 1 diabetics *(48)*. An increase in BP during sleep precedes the development of microalbuminuria, whereas in those whose BP decreased normally during sleep the progression to microalbuminuria was less frequent.

Mechanisms underlying the circadian variation abnormality are not well understood. The potential role of sympathetic overdrive has been ruled out in a study comparing plasma norepinephrine values in dipper and non-dipper end-stage renal disease subjects *(49)*. Some authors affirm that the presence of the non-dipper pattern in subjects with end-stage renal disease depends rather on the presence of autonomic neuropathy or corticosteroid treatment than on the end-stage renal disease itself *(50)*, although when GFR decreases, the prevalence of non-dipper pattern increases.

Whether or not the abnormal circadian variability may contribute to further kidney damage is a matter of debate. Some evidence supports the potential role of systemic BP transmission as a mechanism of inducing renal damage, whereas other evidence supports the non-dipping pattern as a consequence of the renal damage itself. Neither the cause nor the consequence interpretations of these data are mutually exclusive. In some cases, higher BP values during nighttime may contribute to the progression toward renal insufficiency, while in other cases the values are but a consequence of the altered renal function itself. In the latter, higher BP may also participate in accelerating the loss of renal function, contributing in turn to more severe hypertension.

There is practical utility associated with the assessment of circadian variability. First it can be used in the prognosis of disease. Second, it can aid in the identification of patients with suboptimal BP control.

The presence of nocturnal hypertension can contribute not only to a faster decline in renal function over time but also to the development of more severe hypertensive cardiovascular disease. Assessing nocturnal BP as a target for protecting against kidney damage seems to be important in the treatment of renal disease, although the optimal nocturnal BP goal needs to be defined in prospective studies.

Until now BP values which are consistently above the 95th percentile for age, sex, and height have determined the need to initiate antihypertensive treatment in children and adolescents *(10)*. Nevertheless, the presence of a non-dipping pattern, when BP values are below the 95th percentile, has not been deemed sufficient cause to start treatment. Future studies need to be conducted to address this specific point.

Heart

The abnormal increase of left ventricular mass and/or geometry has been recognized as one of the most important markers of risk for hypertension-induced cardiovascular morbidity and mortality in adults. In children and adolescents, the relationship between hypertension and left ventricular mass is more difficult to recognize because children and adolescents grow rapidly and their BP increases with age.

Cross-sectional studies have shown that the major determinants of left ventricular growth are body size and sex, with a smaller contribution made by BP *(51,52)*. The important contribution of the somatic growth and the recognition that lean body mass contributes somewhat more to cardiac growth than fat mass were nicely demonstrated in the Bogalusa Heart Study *(53)*. In a longitudinal study, left ventricular mass tracks from early to late adolescence to about the same degree as other important risk factors, such as BP and cholesterol *(54)*. Recently, the potential role of adiposity in the increment of left ventricular mass has been highlighted. Adiposity and left ventricular mass are related in childhood, and this association tracks and becomes stronger in young adulthood. Moreover, the increase in left ventricular mass from the child to the young adult is related to the degree of increase in body mass index *(55)*.

Studies of normal and hypertensive children have found that systolic BP and left ventricular mass index are positively associated across a wide range of BP values, with no clear threshold to predict pathologically increased left ventricular mass index. Sensitivity and response to hemodynamic load seems to vary with age, sex, and ethnicity, which explains some of the differences among published results.

Although epidemiological studies do not help to establish the difference between appropriate and excessive increases in left ventricular mass, operational thresholds have been established. Both the allometric definition of excessive mass (>51 g/m^2) and the percentile distribution of mass and geometry have been recommended. Using these operational thresholds, a few studies have analyzed the prevalence of left ventricular hypertrophy in not only healthy but also hypertensive children and adolescents. In hypertensive children, the prevalence of left ventricular hypertrophy ranges from 24 to 40% in different pediatric studies (56–59).

The relationship between left ventricular mass index and systolic BP is more evident when BP is measured using 24-h ambulatory BP monitoring (60–62). Consequently, hemodynamic load seems to play a more important role in the growth of left ventricular mass than previously recognized by using office BP. According to this, left ventricular mass tends to be greater in those groups with a higher ambulatory BP. In one cross-sectional study, both subjects with sustained hypertension and masked hypertensives had significantly higher left ventricular mass index than confirmed normotensive (20). Moreover, in a group with adolescents who had sustained masked hypertension, left ventricular mass index was significantly higher than that observed in normotensive adolescents (17).

Vessels

Hypertension-induced abnormalities in arterial structure and function are important because they underlie many adverse effects. Assessment of vascular damage, however, received little attention prior to the advent of the advanced ultrasound technology which permits noninvasive study of vascular walls and lumen. Intima-media thickness measurement at the carotid artery is the most common of the methods to assess structural abnormalities. Since age and sex influence the values of intima-media thickness (63), measured values should be related to percentiles or expressed as standard deviation scores.

In the few pediatric studies available, hypertensive children and adolescents tend to have an increase of intima-media thickness compared to those of normotensive controls (57,64,65), although one study did not observe differences among normotensives and white-coat, masked, or sustained hypertensives (18). Moreover, a relationship between intima-media thickness and endothelial function has been established in the Cardiovascular Risk in Young Finns Study (66). The impact of other cardiovascular risk factors besides hypertension, such as cholesterol levels or smoking, needs to be considered in the interpretation of intima-media thickness levels, since these have been associated with intima-media thickness as well (67). Moreover, measurement is not trivial and subject to some observer bias. Hence, despite the increasing evidence for its predictive value in cardiovascular disease, carotid intima-media thickness assessments have not yet been recommended universally for routine clinical use (10,12). Up to now, the information about the relationship between carotid wall thickness and ambulatory BP came from only two studies in obese children. While in one of them (68) no relationship between carotid wall thickness and ambulatory BP was observed, the other provided strong evidence that carotid intima-media thickness is increased in childhood primary hypertension independent of the effect of obesity (69).

REFERENCES

1. MacMahon S, Peto R, Cutler J, Collins R, Sorlie P, Neaton J, Abbot R, Godwin J, Dyer A, Stamler J. Blood pressure, stroke and coronary heart disease. Part I, prolonged differences in blood pressure: prospective observational studies corrected for the regression dilution bias. Lancet. 1990;335:765–774.

2. Chobanian AV, Alderman MH, DeQuattro V, Frohlich ED, Gifford RW, Hill MN, Kaplan NM, Langford HG, Moore MA, Nickey WA, Porush JG, Thomson GE, Winston MC, Dustan HP, Krishan I, Moser M, Cutler JA, Horan MJ, Payne GH, Roccella EJ, Weiss SM. The 1988 report of the joint national committee on detection, evaluation, and treatment of high blood pressure. Arch Intern Med. 1988;148: 1023–1038.

3. Littler WA, Honour AH, Pugsley DJ, Sleight P. Continuous recording of direct arterial pressure in unrestricted patients: its role in the diagnosis and management of high blood pressure. Circulation. 1975;51:1101–1106.

4. Mancia G, Parati G, Pomidossi G, Di Rienzo M. Validity and usefulness of non-invasive ambulatory blood pressure monitoring. J Hypertens. 1985;3(Suppl 2):S5–S11.

5. Lurbe E, Sorof JM, Daniels SR. Clinical and research aspects of ambulatory blood pressure monitoring in children. J Pediatr. 2004;144:7–16.

6. O'Brien E. Ambulatory blood pressure measurement is indispensable to good clinical practice. J Hypertens. 2003;21(Suppl 2):S11–S18.

7. O'Brien E, Sheridan J, O'Malley K. Dippers and non-dippers. Lancet. 1988;2:397.

8. Pickering TG, James GD, Boddie C, Harshfield GA, Blank S, Laragh JH. How common is white-coat hypertension? JAMA. 1988;259:225–228.

9. Pickering TG, Davidson K, Gerin W, Schwartz JE. Masked hypertension. Hypertension. 2002;40: 795–796.

10. National High Blood Pressure Education Program Working Group on High Blood Pressure in Children and Adolescents. The fourth report on the diagnosis, evaluation and treatment of high blood pressure in children and adolescents. Pediatrics. 2004;114:555–576.

11. Urbina E, Alpert B, Flynn J, Hayman L, Harshfield GA, Jacobson M, Mahoney L, McCrindle B, Mietus-Snyder M, Steinberger J, Daniels S. American Heart Association Atherosclerosis, Hypertension, and Obesity in Youth Committee. Ambulatory blood pressure monitoring in children and adolescents: recommendations for standard assessment: a scientific statement from the American Heart Association Atherosclerosis, Hypertension, and Obesity in Youth Committee of the council on cardiovascular disease in the young and the council for high blood pressure research. Hypertension. 2008;52:433–451.

12. Lurbe E, CifkovaR, Cruickshank JK, Dillon MJ, Ferreira I, Invitti C, Kuznetsova T, Laurent S, Mancia G, Morales-Olivas F, Rascher W, Redon J, Schaefer F, Seeman T, Stergiou G, Wühl E, Zanchetti A. Management of high blood pressure in children and adolescents: recommendations of the European Society of Hypertension. J Hypertens. 2009;27:1719–1742.

13. Lurbe E, Redon J, Liao Y, Tacons J, Cooper RS, Alvarez V. Ambulatory blood pressure monitoring in normotensive children. J Hypertens. 1994;12:1417–1423.

14. Wuhl E, Witte K, Soergel M, Mehls O, Schaefer F. German Working Group on Pediatric Hypertension. Distribution of 24-h ambulatory blood pressure in children: normalized reference values and role of body dimensions. J Hypertens. 2002;20:1995–2007.

15. Hornsby JL, Mongan PF, Taylor AT, Treiber FA. 'White coat' hypertension in children. J Fam Pract. 1991;33:617–623.

16. Sorof JM, Poffenbarger T, Franco K, Portman R. Evaluation of white-coat hypertension in children: importance of the definitions of normal ambulatory blood pressure and the severity of casual hypertension. Am J Hypertens. 2001;14:855–860.

17. Lurbe E, Torro I, Alvarez V, Nawrot T, Paya R, Redon J, Staessen JA. Prevalence, persistence, and clinical significance of masked hypertension in youth. Hypertension. 2005;45:493–498.

18. Stabouli S, Kotsis V, Toumanidis S, Papamichael C, Constantopoulos A, Zakopoulos N. White-coat and masked hypertension in children: association with target organ damage. Pediatr Nephrol. 2005;20: 1151–1155.

19. Matsuoka S, Kawamura K, Honda M, Awazu M. White coat effect and white coat hypertension in pediatric patients. Pediatr Nephrol. 2002;17:950–953.

20. McNiece KL, Gupta-Malhotra M, Samuels J, Bell C, Garcia K, Poffenbarger T, Sorof JM, Portman RJ, National High Blood Pressure Education Program Working Group. Left ventricular hypertrophy in hypertensive adolescents: analysis of risk by 2004 National High Blood Pressure Education Program Working Group staging criteria. Hypertension. 2007;50:392–395.

21. Kavey RE, Kveselis DA, Atallah N, Smith FC. White coat hypertension in childhood: evidence for endorgan effect. J Pediatr. 2007;150:491–497.

22. Lande MB, Meagher CC, Fisher SG, Belani P, Wang H, Rashid M. Left ventricular mass index in children with white coat hypertension. J Pediatr. 2008;153:50–54.

23. Stergiou GS, Nasothimiou E, Giovas P, Kapoyiannis A, Vazeou A. Diagnosis of hypertension in children and adolescents based on home versus ambulatory blood pressure monitoring. J Hypertens. 2008;26:1556–1562.

24. Matsuoka S, Awazu M. Masked hypertension in children and young adults. Pediatr Nephrol. 2004;19: 651–654.

25. Palatini P, Julius S. Heart rate and the cardiovascular risk. J Hypertens. 1997;15:3–17.

26. Julius S, Valentini M, Palatini P. Overweight and hypertension: a 2 way street? Hypertension. 2000;35: 807–813.

27. Bobrie G, Chatellier G, Genes N, Clerson P, Vaur L, Vaisse B, Menard J, Mallion JM. Cardiovascular prognosis of "masked hypertension" detected by blood pressure self-measurement in elderly treated hypertensive patients. JAMA. 2004;291:1342–1349.

28. Bjorklund K, Lind L, Zethelius B, Andrén B, Lithell H. Isolated ambulatory hypertension predicts cardiovascular morbidity in elderly men. Circulation. 2003;107:1297–1302.

29. Mancia G, Facchetti R, Bombelli M, Grassi G, Sega R. Long-term risk of mortality associated with selective and combined elevation in office, home and ambulatory blood pressure. Hypertension. 2006;47: 846–853.

30. O'Brien E. Unmasking hypertension. Hypertension. 2005;45:481–482.

31. Lurbe E, Invitti C, Torro I, Maronati A, Aguilar F, Sartorio G, Redon J, Parati G. The impact of the degree of obesity on the discrepancies between office and ambulatory blood pressure values in youth. J Hypertens. 2006;24:1557–1564.

32. Lurbe E, Thijs L, Redón J, Alvarez V, Tacons J, Staessen J. Diurnal blood pressure curve in children and adolescents. J Hypertens. 1996;14:41–46.

33. Lurbe E, Redon J. Assessing ambulatory blood pressure in renal diseases: Facts and concerns. Nephrol Dial Transplant. 1999;14:2564–2568.

34. Portaluppi F, Montanari L, Massari M, Di Chiara V, Capanna M. Loss of nocturnal decline of blood pressure in hypertension due to chronic renal failure. Am J Hypertens. 1991;4:20–26.

35. Luik AJ, Struijk DG, Gladziwa U, von Olden RW, von Hooff JP, de Leeuw PW, Leunissen KM. Diurnal blood pressure variations in haemodialysis and CAPD patients. Nephrol Dial Transplant. 1994;9: 1616–1621.

36. Farmer CK, Goldsmith DJ, Cox J, Dallyn P, Kingswood JC, Sharpstone P. An investigation of the effect of advancing uraemia, renal replacement therapy and renal transplantation on blood pressure diurnal variability. Nephrol Dial Transplant. 1997;12:2301–2307.

37. Faria Mdo S, Nunes JP, Ferraz JM, Fernandes J, Praca A, Pestana M, Oliveira G, Guerra L, Polónia JJ. 24 hour blood pressure profile early after renal transplantation. Rev Port Cardiol. 1995;14: 227–231.

38. Lingens N, Dobos E, Lemmer B, Scharer K. Nocturnal blood pressure elevation in transplanted pediatric patients. Kidney Int Suppl. 1996;55:S175–S176.

39. Mistnefes M, Portman R. Ambulatory blood pressure monitoring in pediatric renal transplantation. Pediatr Transplant. 2003;7:86–92.

40. Sorof JM, Poffenbarger T, Portman R. Abnormal 24-hour blood pressure patterns in children after renal transplantation. Am J Kidney Dis. 2000;35:681–686.

41. Calzolari A, Giordano U, Matteucci M, Pastore E, Turchetta A, Rizzoni G, Alpert B. Hypertension in young patients after renal transplantation: ambulatory blood pressure monitoring versus casual blood pressure. Am J Hypertens. 1998;11:497–501.

42. Morgan H, Khan I, Hashmi A, Hebert D, McCrindle B, Balfe JW. Ambulatory blood pressure monitoring after renal transplantation in children. Pediatr Nephrol. 2001;16:843–847.

43. Li Kam Wa TC, Macnicol AM, Watson ML. Ambulatory blood pressure in hypertensive patients with autosomal dominant polycystic kidney disease. Nephrol Dial Transplant. 1997;12:2075–2080.

44. Lama G, Tedesco MA, Graziano L, Calabrese E, Grassia C, Natale F, Pacileo G, Rambaldi PF, Esposito-Salsano M. Reflux nephropathy and hypertension: correlation with the progression of renal damage. Pediatr Nephrol. 2003;18:241–245.

45. Patzer L, Seeman T, Luck C, Wühl E, Janda J, Misselwitz J. Day and night time blood pressure elevation in children with higher grades of renal scarring. J Pediatr. 2003;142:117–122.

46. Lurbe A, Redón J, Pascual JM, Tacons J, Alvarez V, Batlle D. Altered blood pressure during sleep in normotensive subjects with type I diabetes. Hypertension. 1993;21:227–235.

47. Lurbe E, Redon J, Pascual JM, Tacons J, Alvarez V. The spectrum of circadian blood pressure changes in type 1 diabetic patients. J Hypertens. 2001;19:1421–1428.

48. Lurbe E, Redon J, Kesani A, Pascual JM, Tacons J, Alvarez V, Batlle D. Increase in nocturnal blood pressure and progression to microalbuminuria in Type 1 diabetes. N Engl J Med. 2002;347:797–805.

49. van de Borne P, Tielemans C, Collart F, Vanherweghem JL, Degaute JP. Twenty-four-hour blood pressure and heart rate patterns in chronic hemodialysis patients. Am J Kidney Dis. 1993;22:419–425.

50. Redon J, Lurbe E. Ambulatory blood pressure and the kidney: implications for renal dysfunction. In: Epstein M, ed. Calcium Antagonists in Clinical Medicine. Philadelphia, PA: Hanley & Belfus; 2002: 665–679.

51. Malcolm DD, Burns TL, Mahoney LT, Lauer RM. Factors affecting left ventricular mass in childhood: the Muscatine study. Pediatrics. 1993;92:703–709.
52. de Simone G, Devereux RB, Daniels SR, Koren MJ, Meyer RA, Laragh JH. Effect of growth on variability of left ventricular mass: assessment of allometric signals in adults and children and their capacity to predict cardiovascular risk. J Am Coll Cardiol. 1995;25:1056–1062.
53. Urbina EM, Gidding SS, Bao W, Pickoff AS, Berdusis K, Berenson GS. Effect of body size, ponderosity, and blood pressure on left ventricular growth in children and young adults in the Bogalusa Heart Study. Circulation. 1995;91:2400–2406.
54. Schieken RM, Schwartz PF, Goble MM. Tracking of left ventricular mass in children: race and sex comparisons: the MCV Twin Study. Medical College of Virginia. Circulation. 1998;97:1901–1906.
55. Sivanandam S, Sinaiko AR, Jacobs DR Jr, Steffen L, Moran A, Steinberger J. Relation of increase in adiposity to increase in left ventricular mass from childhood to young adulthood. Am J Cardiol. 2006;98: 411–415.
56. Flynn JT, Alderman MH. Characteristics of children with primary hypertension seen at a referral center. Pediatr Nephrol. 2005;20:961–966.
57. Litwin M, Niemirska A, Sladowska J, Antoniewicz J, Daszkowska J, Wierzbicka A, Wawer ZT, Grenda R. Left ventricular hypertrophy and arterial wall thickening in children with essential hypertension. Pediatr Nephrol. 2006;21:811–819.
58. Daniels SR, Loggie JM, Khoury P, Kimball TR. Left ventricular geometry and severe left ventricular hypertrophy in children and adolescents with essential hypertension. Circulation. 1998;97:1907–1911.
59. Sorof JM, Cardwell G, Franco K, Portman RJ. Ambulatory blood pressure and left ventricular mass index in hypertensive children. Hypertension. 2002;39:903–908.
60. Richey PA, Disessa TG, Hastings MC, Somes GW, Alpert BS, Jones DP. Ambulatory blood pressure and increased left ventricular mass in children at risk for hypertension. J Pediatr. 2008;152:343–348.
61. Maggio AB, Aggoun Y, Marchand LM, Martin XE, Herrmann F, Beghetti M, Farpour-Lambert NJ. Associations among obesity, blood pressure, and left ventricular mass. J Pediatr. 2008;152:489–493.
62. Stabouli S, Kotsis V, Rizos Z, Toumanidis S, Karagianni C, Constantopoulos A, Zakopoulos N. Left ventricular mass in normotensive, prehypertensive and hypertensive children and adolescents. Pediatr Nephrol. 2009;24:1545–1551.
63. Jourdan C, Wühl E, Litwin M, Fahr K, Trelewicz J, Jobs K, Schenk JP, Grenda R, Mehls O, Troger J, Schaefer F. Normative values for intima-media thickness and distensibility of large arteries in healthy adolescents. J Hypertens. 2005;23:1707–1715.
64. Sass C, Herbeth B, Chapet O, Siest G, Visvikis S, Zannad F. Intima-media thickness and diameter of carotid and femoral arteries in children, adolescents and adults from the Stanislas cohort: effect of age, sex, anthropometry and blood pressure. J Hypertens. 1998;16:1593–1602.
65. Sorof JM, Alexandrov AV, Cardwell G, Portman RJ. Carotid artery intimal-medial thickness and left ventricular hypertrophy in children with elevated blood pressure. Pediatrics. 2003;111:61–66.
66. Juonala M, Viikari JS, Laitinen T, Marniemi J, Helenius H, Rönnemaa T, Raitakari OT. Interrelations between brachial endothelial function and carotid intima-media thickness in young adults. The Cardiovascular Risk in Young Finns Study. Circulation. 2004;110:2918–2923.
67. Davis PH, Dawson JD, Riley WA, Lauer RM. Carotid intimal-medial thickness is related to cardiovascular risk factors measured from childhood through middle age: the Muscatine study. Circulation. 2001;104:2815–2819.
68. Aggoun Y, Farpour-Lambert NJ, Marchand LM, Golay E, Maggio AB, Beghetti M. Impaired endothelial and smooth muscle functions and arterial stiffness appear before puberty in obese children and are associated with elevated ambulatory blood pressure. Eur Heart J. 2008;29:792–799.
69. Lande MB, Carson NL, Roy J, Meagher CC. Effects of childhood primary hypertension on carotid intima media thickness: a matched controlled study. Hypertension. 2006;48:40–44.

30 Nonpharmacologic Treatment of Pediatric Hypertension

R. Thomas Collins, II, MD
and Bruce S. Alpert, MD

Contents

INTRODUCTION

During childhood, elevated systolic and/or diastolic blood pressure (BP) is commonly secondary to diseases of the kidneys, endocrine system, and/or cardiovascular system. When diagnostic evaluation does not reveal a cause for the elevation in BP, the condition is referred to as essential, or idiopathic, hypertension (HTN). Over 90% of HTN in adults is essential HTN; there are well over 60 million Americans with essential HTN. Much has been written about research to control essential HTN in adults; relatively less work has been done concerning children. Many pharmacologic approaches, such as β (beta)-blockade, angiotensin-converting enzyme (ACE) inhibition, afterload reduction, and α (alpha)-blockade, have been successful in lowering BP. When essential HTN occurs in childhood, a nonpharmacologic approach to lowering BP is preferable so that the patient may not require lifelong medication. Long-term use of medications may be associated with significant side effects and produce associated morbidity and/or mortality.

Several nonpharmacologic approaches have been successful in lowering BP in adults and children. These include weight loss, exercise, stress reduction, and alterations in electrolyte intake, in particular Na^+, K^+, and Cl^-. Chapter 15, by Dr. Wilson, discusses the effects of dietary electrolytes on BP. Chapter 17, by Dr. Rocchini, provides evidence that weight loss may control essential HTN. These findings will not be repeated in this chapter. The

R.T. Collins (✉)
University of Arkansas for Medical Sciences, College of Medicine, Division of Cardiology, Arkansas Children's Hospital, Little Rock, AR, USA
e-mail: rtcollins@uams.edu

From: *Clinical Hypertension and Vascular Diseases: Pediatric Hypertension*
Edited by: J. T. Flynn et al. DOI 10.1007/978-1-60327-824-9_30
© Springer Science+Business Media, LLC 2011

specific areas covered herein are exercise and stress reduction. More research is needed in both areas.

EXERCISE

Several years ago, Alpert and Wilmore *(1)* published a review of data relating to the effects of activity/exercise on BP in healthy children and adolescents, as well as in those with elevated BP. If BP was normal prior to the exercise intervention, there was no measurable change in systolic (S) BP or diastolic (D) BP after the program. At the time of that review, there were seven studies that reported data relating to changes in BP in children and adolescents with essential HTN in response to an exercise/activity intervention. An extensive literature review by one author failed to find additional, recent studies addressing this issue.

The first documented research concerning exercise was an abstract in 1979 by Laird et al. *(2)*. They studied seven boys, aged 15–16 years. The intervention was a 2-month program of weight lifting, presumably both an aerobic and an isometric activity. They measured SBP, DBP, and left ventricular (LV) mass. The change in SBP was small, from a mean of 134 to 131 mmHg. The inclusion criteria of essential HTN identified in these subjects, whose SBP prior to the intervention was only 134 mmHg, weaken the value of the study somewhat. The DBP change from pre- to postexercise was from a mean of 78 to 80 mmHg. A similar, insignificant change in LV mass occurred, from 198 to 202 g. The important conclusion from this abstract was that resistance training did not lead to an increase in BP, which had been thought of as a possibility. The authors concluded that "hypertensive" youth did not need to be restricted from resistance training.

Shortly thereafter, Frank and coworkers *(3)* reported data from the Bogalusa Heart Study on 48 children (gender unspecified) from 8 to 18 years of age whose BPs were in the top decile of a group of 1604 youth followed in that study. The subjects were receiving antihypertensive medications. The intervention included both dietary and exercise components; the exercise component was not rigorously described. The intervention was successful, lowering both SBP and DBP by 9 mmHg each. Because the patients had dietary, exercise, and pharmacologic treatments simultaneously, no conclusions may be drawn as to the effectiveness of exercise alone in this group of Caucasians and African-Americans.

In 1983 and 1984, Hagberg and colleagues *(4,5)* published two articles from studies in 25 children, 19 of whom were boys. The mean age was 15.6 years, and all attended public schools. There were 6 African-Americans and 19 Caucasians. A control group was included, rendering these findings statistically more robust. The subjects underwent a 3-day/week, 30–40-min/day aerobic program supervised by school physical education faculty. The subjects were identified as hypertensive through carefully performed screenings. The variables measured prior to the 6-month training period and after 9 months of detraining included SBP, DBP, and VO_2 max. The study results are summarized in Table 1. The effects of the program were more pronounced in boys compared to girls; the mixed-gender control group experienced no training-induced changes. There were no racial differences. The positive changes were all reversed with detraining. This small controlled trial supports the hypothesis that aerobic exercise lowers BP in adolescents with essential HTN. The expected drops in BP should be approximately 8 mmHg for SBP and 5 mmHg for DBP.

The Hagberg team *(6)* expanded their studies by utilizing an aerobic program followed by weight training. There were 6 children in the treatment group and 17 controls. The aerobic program consisted of 5 months of endurance training (running) at 60–75% of VO_2

Table 1
Hagberg et al. *(4,5)* Study Results

Condition	Systolic BP (mmHg)	Diastolic BP (mmHg)	VO₂ max (mL/kg/min)
Pretraining	137	80	43
End of training	129*	75*	48
Detraining	139	78	43

*$p < 0.01$.

max. Each session lasted 30–50 min and occurred 3 days/week. After the aerobic training phase, the youths switched to a weight training program consisting of 12–15 repetitions of 14 exercises. That phase also lasted 5 months. The subjects then detrained for 12 months. The SBP fell from 143 to 130 mmHg following the aerobic sessions and to 126 mmHg at the end of the endurance training. After detraining it rose to 142 mmHg. The changes with exercise were of statistical significance. The parallel changes of DBP were from 80 to 77, 73, and 74 mmHg, none of which were statistically significant. There were decreases in measured systemic vascular resistance in response to both endurance and weight training. These studies continue to support the concept that both endurance and weight training have beneficial effects on SBP and, to a lesser degree, DBP in youth with essential HTN. The group of six children was too small to draw conclusions with respect to either gender or ethnicity.

More recently, Danforth et al. *(7)* used a simple cycle ergometer or jogging/walking program in a group of 12 African-American children (mean age 11.5 years) of low socioeconomic status. The sessions were 30 min/day, 3 days/week for 12 weeks. The target intensity was 60–80% of maximal heart rate (HR). The results are shown in Table 2. The intervention led to a 9 mmHg reduction in SBP and a 9 mmHg decrease in DBP, both of which were statistically significant. The DBP returned to baseline after detraining; however, there was a lasting effect of the reduction after detraining for SBP. The compliance (attendance) was an outstanding 96%. The decrease in BP was not related to a change in weight. This study shows that inexpensive programs may yield results similar to those involving more expensive equipment or which last more than 3 months.

The final study on which we comment comes from a very productive research team in Denmark *(8)*. The Odense Schoolchild Study has produced numerous significant results. In this particular publication, results from 137 children (68 normotensives and 69 hypertensives) were reported. The children were 9–11 years of age. The 8-month intervention involved three additional 50-min sessions of school physical education per week. The

Table 2
Danforth et al. *(7)* Study Results

Condition	Systolic BP (mmHg)	Diastolic BP (mmHg)
Initial	130	84
Posttraining	121*	75*
Detraining	123*	85

*$p < 0.01$ vs initial.

variables reported were SBP, DBP, and VO$_2$ max. The SBP in the "hypertensive" boys decreased from 113 to 107 mmHg ($p < 0.05$). No significant change occurred in the DBP values. There was a slight but significant increase in VO$_2$ max, 52–54 mL/min/kg. No statistically significant changes in SBP or DBP occurred in the hypertensive girls. During the 8-month study, data were collected at 3 months to assess interval changes; none occurred. The significant results all occurred at the end of the 8-month period. This is the largest series published to date and concludes that boys appear to benefit more than girls from an intensive exercise intervention.

In summary, endurance (aerobic) exercise led to reductions of SBP and DBP, but seldom to completely normal levels. The "hypertensives" generally did not have BP elevations much greater than the normotensive/hypertensive cutoffs. The one study that used only resistance training (2) did not show a reduction in BP, but when resistance training was performed following an aerobic program, the reductions in BP were maintained. There has been a concern that children with essential HTN should not participate in resistance training. No study showed a deleterious effect. Accordingly, we do not believe that children with essential HTN who do not show evidence of end-organ damage such as stroke, renal failure, or increased LV mass need to be excluded from resistance training.

From available data, it is not possible to state what is the minimal frequency, intensity, or duration of exercise that will lead to reductions of SBP or DBP. From a public health standpoint, exercise should be lifelong in duration. Recent recommendations (1) have been for three or more sessions per week, 30 or more minutes per day, and at least at 60% VO$_2$ max.

Future studies should enroll children with more severe elevations of BP. Children of all ethnicities should be included. The reason for the apparently better results in male, compared to female, children needs to be investigated. For optimal efficiency these studies should be multicenter. An organization such as the North American Society for Pediatric Exercise Medicine could be a valuable resource for such a study. We hope that the readers of this chapter will appreciate the paucity of rigorous data and will seek to provide future studies to define the much needed data.

STRESS REDUCTION

The relevance of stress reduction for the treatment of essential HTN dates back to early theories regarding the pathogenesis of the disorder. Clinical and empirical data implicate stress as an important factor for the development and maintenance of HTN in certain persons and provide a rationale for the use of stress management techniques in at-risk persons. With respect to children and adolescents, such nonpharmacologic approaches are especially important, since elevated BP in childhood often relates to essential HTN in early adulthood, and clinical trials have not conclusively determined the long-term risk–benefit ratio of antihypertensive drug therapy for youth (9). Consequently, current guidelines for treating childhood HTN are conservative; when essential HTN is the likely diagnosis in the context of mild BP elevations, interventions that emphasize lifestyle or health-promoting behavioral changes are recommended.

In general, nonpharmacologic therapies for essential HTN encompass strategies aimed at weight reduction, dietary modification, and physical activity. Considerably less attention has been devoted to stress reduction, per se; this disparity is even more apparent for pediatric HTN patients. This is surprising given the effectiveness of stress reduction techniques such as biofeedback and relaxation training for a variety of medical conditions affecting children, including fecal *(10)* and urinary *(11–13)* incontinence, headache *(12,13)*, and asthma *(14)*. One possible explanation for the lack of carryover may be the relatively recent incorporation of BP measurement in the routine pediatric examination *(9)*. Reluctance on the part of some physicians to inquire about recreational behaviors (e.g., drinking, smoking) that may have negative overall effects on young patients *(15)* also may contribute to a lack of perceived need for more formal treatment recommendations that emphasize stress reduction in children and adolescents with essential HTN.

Research has demonstrated that stress elicits significant increases in BP and other hemodynamic parameters in children. Furthermore, a number of studies have shown that these BP responses to stress predict future elevations in resting BP in children and adolescents over periods of several months to years *(16–22)*. Consequently, the utilization of techniques to reduce reactivity to stress during childhood may prevent the development of essential HTN across the life span.

Two studies provide some support for the use of stress reduction in children at risk for developing essential HTN *(23,24)*. Utilizing nonsomatic therapies, these studies reported substantial changes in BP, or behaviors associated with elevated BP, in disparate samples of children. Although the lasting effects of these interventions are not known, these studies underscore the importance of stress and stress reduction in childhood HTN.

The first investigation examined the effects of Medical Resonance Therapy Music (MRT-Music) in a sample of children with transient HTN following the nuclear accident in Chernobyl *(23)*. Sixty children with varying degrees of BP elevation were exposed to twice-daily MRT-Music treatments for 3 weeks while in the hospital. Treatment sessions lasted 20–30 min and occurred under conditions designed to maximize relaxation. Pre- and post-treatment comparisons of basic hemodynamic parameters revealed a strong treatment effect for both SBP and DBP, with a normalization of overall BP to age-appropriate levels. This effect was particularly pronounced for those children with higher, compared to lower, levels of HTN at the onset of treatment.

The second study examined the relationship between religion and various parameters of cardiovascular (CV) health in a sample of 137 immigrants between 18 and 71 years of age *(24)*. Regression analyses indicated strong associations among demographic, social support, and physical health measures for this group of individuals deemed to be at risk for BP elevations secondary to immigration-related stress. After ruling out a number of competing explanations for the observed relationships, the author concluded that religious commitment had a beneficial effect on CV health, as indicated by significantly lower rates of HTN, as well as significantly lower SBP and DBP levels among those high on both quantitative and qualitative indices of religious commitment. This association was particularly strong for younger persons in the sample. The author discussed this relationship in terms of social support and noted that religious participation appeared to remove a source of stress among immigrants by facilitating feelings of social cohesion and a sense of belonging. Although over one-third of the sample was classified as hypertensive, it is unclear how many participants were adolescents, as opposed to adults. Nevertheless, the study provided support for the positive effects of church attendance and religious commitment on CV health in general and BP elevations in particular, among both youthful and older immigrants.

Four studies of nonpharmacologic stress reduction treatments for normotensive children have implications for the management of childhood HTN. One study evaluated the effects of gender and family support on dietary compliance and BP in a sample of 184 African-American adolescents who participated in a 5-day low-Na+ diet as part of a HTN prevention program *(25)*. Compliance was defined as urine Na+ excretion ≤50 mEq/24 h at the completion of the dietary intervention. A trend toward lower SBP was observed among compliant participants, but the effect diminished after controlling for body mass index. Moreover, dietary compliance was moderated by social support and gender. These findings suggest that social support may play a role in improving dietary compliance and, subsequently, BP control among adolescents at risk for developing essential HTN.

Another study evaluated the impact of transcendental meditation (TM) at rest and during acute psychological stress in high school students *(26)*. Adolescents with high-normal BP were randomly assigned to either a TM or a health education control group. Pre- and postintervention comparisons revealed significant group differences, with TM participants exhibiting greater decreases in resting SBP and greater declines in SBP during a car driving simulation task compared to control group peers.

In contrast, generally unfavorable results have been reported for the use of progressive muscle relaxation (PMR) in the treatment of adolescents with high BP *(27,28)*. Compared to wait-list controls, significant declines in SBP were observed in teenagers upon completion of a 3-month school-based PMR program. At follow-up 4 months later, however, group differences in BP were no longer significant *(27)*. Similarly, 4 months of relaxation training, combined with increased physical activity, failed to yield BP differences in comparisons of community boys with nontreated peers *(28)*.

SUMMARY

Given the link between elevated BP during childhood and the development of adult HTN, the need for interventions aimed at reducing disease development in at-risk youth is apparent. Stress has been identified as an important contributor to the progression and maintenance of HTN in certain individuals. Nonpharmacologic techniques that minimize stress to achieve and maintain normal BP are particularly relevant for children because clinical trials have not conclusively determined the long-term risk–benefit ratio of antihypertensive drug therapy for young patients. When essential HTN is the likely diagnosis in the context of mild BP elevations in children and adolescents, interventions that emphasize lifestyle or health-promoting behavioral changes are recommended *(9)*. Stress reduction is an example of such an approach. In addition to using stress reduction techniques to treat children with essential HTN, these methods may be useful for children with high-normal BP and may provide adjunctive benefit to more intensive therapies for young patients with severe disease.

REFERENCES

1. Alpert B, Wilmore J. Physical activity and blood pressure in adolescents. Pediatr Exerc Sci. 1994;6:361–380.
2. Laird WP, Fixler DE, Swanborn CD. Cardiovascular effects of weight training in hypertensive adolescents. Med Sci Sports Exerc. 1979;11:78 (abstract).
3. Frank GC, Farris RP, Ditmarsen P, Voors AW, Berenson GS. An approach to primary preventive treatment for children with high blood pressure in a total community. J Am Coll Nutr. 1982;1:357–374.
4. Hagberg JM, Goldring D, Ehsani AA, Heath GW, Hernandez A, Schechtman K, Holloszy JO. Effect of exercise training on the blood pressure and hemodynamic features of hypertensive adolescents. Am J Cardiol. 1983;52:763–768.
5. Hagberg JM, Goldring D, Heath GW, Ehsani AA, Hernandez A, Holloszy JO. Effect of exercise training on plasma catecholamines and haemodynamics of adolescent hypertensives during rest, submaximal exercise and orthostatic stress. Clin Physiol. 1984;4:117–124.

6. Hagberg JM, Ehsani AA, Goldring D, Hernandez A, Sinacore DR, Holloszy JO. Effect of weight training on blood pressure and hemodynamics in hypertensive adolescents. J Pediatr. 1984;104:147–151.
7. Danforth JS, Allen KD, Fitterling JM, Danforth JA, Farrar D, Brown M, Drabman RS. Exercise as a treatment for hypertension in low-socioeconomic-status black children. J Consult Clin Psychol. 1990;58:237–239.
8. Hansen HS, Froberg K, Hyldebrandt N, Nielsen JR. A controlled study of eight months of physical training and reduction of blood pressure in children: the Odense schoolchild study. BMJ. 1991;303:682–685.
9. Report of the Second Task Force on Blood Pressure Control in Children—1987. Task force on blood pressure control in children. National Heart, Lung, and Blood Institute, Bethesda, Maryland. Pediatrics. 1987;79:1–25.
10. Borowitz SM, Cox DJ, Sutphen JL, Kovatchev B. Treatment of childhood encopresis: a randomized trial comparing three treatment protocols. J Pediatr Gastroenterol Nutr. 2002;34:378–384.
11. Rhodes C. Effective management of daytime wetting. Paediatr Nurs. 2000;12:14–17.
12. Arndorfer RE, Allen KD. Extending the efficacy of a thermal biofeedback treatment package to the management of tension-type headaches in children. Headache. 2001;41:183–192.
13. Grazzi L, Andrasik F, D'Amico D, Leone M, Moschiano F, Bussone G. Electromyographic biofeedback-assisted relaxation training in juvenile episodic tension-type headache: clinical outcome at three-year follow-up. Cephalalgia. 2001;21:798–803.
14. Malhi P. Psychosocial issues in the management and treatment of children and adolescents with asthma. Indian J Pediatr. 2001;68(Suppl 4):S48–S52.
15. Ellen JM, Franzgrote M, Irwin CE Jr, Millstein SG. Primary care physicians' screening of adolescent patients: a survey of California physicians. J Adolesc Health. 1998;22:433–438.
16. Murphy JK, Alpert BS, Walker SS, Willey ES. Children's cardiovascular reactivity: stability of racial differences and relation to subsequent blood pressure over a one-year period. Psychophysiology. 1991;28:447–457.
17. Murphy JK, Alpert BS, Walker SS. Ethnicity, pressor reactivity, and children's blood pressure. Five years of observations. Hypertension. 1992;20:327–332.
18. Malpass D, Treiber FA, Turner JR, Davis H, Thompson W, Levy M, Strong WB. Relationships between children's cardiovascular stress responses and resting cardiovascular functioning 1 year later. Int J Psychophysiol. 1997;25:139–144.
19. Treiber FA, Turner JR, Davis H, Thompson W, Levy M, Strong WB. Young children's cardiovascular stress responses predict resting cardiovascular functioning 2 1/2 years later. J Cardiovasc Risk. 1996;3:95–100.
20. Kelsey RM, Barnard M, Alpert BS. Race, SES, and cardiovascular reactivity to cold stress as longitudinal predictors of blood pressure in adolescents. Am J Hypertension. 2001;14:250A (abstract).
21. Borghi C, Costa FV, Boschi S, Mussi A, Ambrosioni E. Predictors of stable hypertension in young borderline subjects: a five-year follow-up study. J Cardiovasc Pharmacol. 1986;8(Suppl 5):S138–S141.
22. Falkner B, Kushner H, Onesti G, Angelakos ET. Cardiovascular characteristics in adolescents who develop essential hypertension. Hypertension. 1981;3:521–527.
23. Sidorenko VN. Effects of the medical resonance therapy music on haemodynamic parameter in children with autonomic nervous system disturbances. Integr Physiol Behav Sci. 2000;35:208–211.
24. Walsh A. Religion and hypertension: testing alternative explanations among immigrants. Behav Med. 1998;24:122–130.
25. Wilson DK, Ampey-Thornhill G. The role of gender and family support on dietary compliance in an African American adolescent hypertension prevention study. Ann Behav Med. 2001;23:59–67.
26. Barnes VA, Treiber FA, Davis H. Impact of Transcendental Meditation on cardiovascular function at rest and during acute stress in adolescents with high normal blood pressure. J Psychosom Res. 2001;51:597–605.
27. Ewart CK, Harris WL, Iwata MM, Coates TJ, Bullock R, Simon B. Feasibility and effectiveness of school-based relaxation in lowering blood pressure. Health Psychol. 1987;6:399–416.
28. Rauhala E, Alho H, Hanninen O, Helin P. Relaxation training combined with increased physical activity lowers the psychophysiological activation in community-home boys. Int J Psychophysiol. 1990;10:63–68.

31 Pharmacotherapy of Pediatric Hypertension

Douglas L. Blowey, MD

CONTENTS

Hypertension is the primary cause of cardiovascular disease in humans. In adults, hypertension is clearly linked to an increased risk of stroke, ischemic heart disease, congestive heart failure, and kidney disease *(1)*. Fortunately, the devastating cardiovascular health outcomes seen in the adult population are infrequently seen in children, but the seemingly benign nature of hypertension in children may be more a result of the duration of exposure rather than any disease, developmental, or physiologic factor. Emerging evidence suggests that the pathophysiology of cardiovascular disease and resultant adverse health outcomes begins during childhood and, if left unattended, will likely culminate in the clinical presentation of cardiovascular disease as an adult. The evidence pointing to a pediatric onset of adult cardiovascular disease includes the finding of left ventricular hypertrophy (LVH) and increased carotid intimal–medial thickness (cIMT) in many children with hypertension *(2–6)*, as well as epidemiologic studies finding an association between cardiovascular disease as an adult and high blood pressure readings as a youth *(7–10)*.

Compared to adults where normal blood pressure is defined based on the risk of adverse health outcomes, hypertension in children and adolescents is based on the normative

D.L. Blowey (✉)
Department of Pediatrics, Children's Mercy Hospital and Clinics, University of Missouri-Kansas City School of Medicine, Kansas City, MO, USA
e-mail: dblowey@cmh.edu

From: *Clinical Hypertension and Vascular Diseases: Pediatric Hypertension*
Edited by: J. T. Flynn et al. DOI 10.1007/978-1-60327-824-9_31
© Springer Science+Business Media, LLC 2011

distribution of BP in healthy children and adolescents and is defined as average systolic blood pressure (SBP) and/or diastolic blood pressure (DBP) that exceeds the 95th percentile for gender, age, and height on repeated occasions (11). Those children not meeting the criterion for hypertension but potentially at risk for developing hypertension or hypertensive-related cardiovascular disease (e.g., "pre-hypertension") are defined as children and adolescents with average SBP and/or DBP between the 90th and 95th percentile for gender, age, and height or BP levels greater than 120/80 mmHg. In the general population the prevalence of hypertension in children and adolescence is approximately 1–4% (12). The prevalence of "pre-hypertension" has not been clearly delineated but is likely substantial. The prevalence of hypertension in children with chronic kidney disease, solid organ transplantation, and obesity is greatly increased and at times may occur in up to 70% of the at-risk population (13).

Adequate control of blood pressure in adults, irrespective of the means by which the blood pressure is lowered, reduces the rate of cardiovascular mortality, stroke, and congestive heart failure events (1). While there can be concomitant conditions associated with HTN that are compelling indications for the use of a particular antihypertensive agent, such as the desire to prescribe an angiotensin-converting enzyme (ACE) inhibitor or angiotensin II receptor antagonist (ARB) in a patient with proteinuric chronic kidney disease (CKD) or diabetes mellitus (DM) due to the additional renoprotective effect independent of the reduction in blood pressure (14–16), there appears to be similar protection against cardiovascular disease among the different classes of antihypertensive agents when adequately titrated to achieve desired BP goal. With this in mind, the current emphasis in the treatment of hypertension is not focused on which of the numerous and often redundant antihypertensive drugs should be selected, but rather on using a sufficient amount of drug or drugs to control BP. In response to the 1997 Food and Drug Administration Act and the 2002 Best Pharmaceuticals in Children Act that provided patent extensions in return for pediatric studies, a number of antihypertensive agents have been evaluated in children providing some limited information on the safety and effectiveness of antihypertensive agents in children with hypertension. While the recent influx of information is encouraging, there continues to be gaps between the extent of pediatric-specific information that is available and what is needed to make rationale therapeutic decisions about the pharmacologic treatment of the hypertensive child. Specifically, there is a great need for individual and comparative studies evaluating the effect of antihypertensive agents on long-term health outcomes or biological markers of cardiovascular disease (e.g., LVH, cIMT) in children with hypertension.

In the absence of objective information on the long-term health risks of hypertension in children and adolescents and on the impact of lifestyle or pharmacologic interventions on clinically significant outcome measures, the decision to begin pharmacologic therapy in children with high blood pressure is arbitrary. Most experts seem to agree that pharmacologic therapy should be strongly considered in children with symptomatic hypertension, concomitant chronic kidney disease, or diabetes mellitus and in those children demonstrating hypertensive target-organ damage (e.g., LVH, cIMT, retinopathy). Less clear is when to initiate pharmacologic therapy for the asymptomatic child with persistent hypertension that has not responded to a trial of lifestyle modifications or the asymptomatic child that has other cardiovascular risk factors such as obesity, sleep apnea, or lipid abnormalities. In the absence of evidence, a common approach is to consider adding a pharmacologic agent to the treatment regimen after a 6–12-month trial of lifestyle modification.

PRINCIPLES OF ANTIHYPERTENSIVE THERAPY

Any child that consistently has blood pressure measurements exceeding 90% for age, gender, and height when measured with the appropriate techniques *(11)* warrants some form of intervention, and therapeutic lifestyle changes are an important component of treatment in all children and adolescents with elevated BP irrespective of the plan to initiate pharmacologic therapy. In some children blood pressure may be adequately controlled by a combination of weight reduction (in overweight children), regular physical activity, and the ingestion of a diet rich in fruits and vegetables and low in salt (i.e., the Dietary Approaches to Stop Hypertension or DASH diet) *(17)*. The potential for normalization of blood pressure with time in children with presumed hypertension was noted in a pediatric study where 17% of hypertensive children enrolled in an antihypertensive drug trial had normalization of their blood pressure during the 2-week placebo screening period and 34% of children randomized to placebo had normalization of blood pressure during the 12-week study *(18)*. Although therapeutic lifestyle changes may not result in adequate control of BP, the principles should continue to be emphasized upon the introduction of antihypertensive drugs as continuance of therapeutic lifestyle changes may facilitate the pharmacologic control of blood pressure. In addition, the successful and continued implementation of therapeutic lifestyle changes may have an ongoing and progressive effect on blood pressure (e.g., continued weight loss or improved physical conditioning) that may permit the withdrawal of the pharmacologic support with time.

Antihypertensive drugs lower BP by altering one of the physiologic components responsible for arterial pressure, namely cardiac output and peripheral vascular resistance. At its core, the therapeutic actions of BP lowering for all antihypertensive drugs result from their ability to either lower peripheral vascular resistance, reduce cardiac output, or both. Peripheral vascular resistance can be reduced through direct relaxation of the smooth muscle in the resistance vessels or indirectly by interfering with the effector signals of one of the many systems, such as the sympathetic nervous system or renin–angiotensin–aldosterone system, that cause constriction of resistance vessels. A reduction in cardiac output may be achieved by a decrease in myocardial contractility or a decrease in the ventricular filling pressure that may accompany a change in venous pressure or blood volume. A classification of antihypertensive drugs by the primary mechanism of action is shown in Table 1. As BP is maintained by a complex, coordinated, and often overlapping set of regulatory systems, drug-induced lowering of blood pressure that occurs by interference with one component of the regulatory system (e.g., vasodilation) often results in a reactive change in another component of the regulatory system (e.g., tachycardia, enhanced salt, and water reabsorption) that counteracts or blunts the blood pressure-lowering effect. For this reason, the use of more than one drug with a different mechanism of action is often required to effectively lower blood pressure. While there may be formulation and dosage concerns when applied to children, the pharmaceutical industry has long recognized the blood pressure-lowering benefits of combining treatment with different classes of antihypertensive agents and has marketed several combination products (Table 4).

To date, the antihypertensive drug trials that have been completed in children and adolescents have shown that a variety of antihypertensive agents are capable of lowering blood pressure in children with hypertension. While helpful, the information from these studies is limited by the small number of patients treated during the clinical trials, the short duration of therapy, and lack of meaningful health outcome end points. Likewise, comparative studies of antihypertensive agents in children have not been completed.

Table 1
Classification of Antihypertensive Drugs and Mechanism of Action

Drug classification	Primary mechanism of action
Angiotensin-converting enzyme inhibitors	Decreases angiotensin II-induced constriction of resistance vessels
Angiotensin II receptor antagonist	Blocks angiotensin II-induced constriction of resistance vessels
Calcium channel blockers	Decreases constriction of resistance vessels

Diuretics
  1. Thiazide and thiazide-like agents
  2. Loop diuretics
  3. Potassium sparing
	Reduces ventricular filling pressure by volume reduction. Long-term use results in decreased vascular resistance

Renin inhibitors	Decreases angiotensin II-induced constriction of resistance vessels

Sympatholytic drugs
  1. α-Adrenergic antagonist
  2. β-Adrenergic antagonist
  3. Mixed adrenergic antagonist
  4. Centrally acting agents
  5. Adrenergic neuron-blocking agent
	Reduces cardiac contractility and/or decreases constriction of resistance vessels

Vasodilators	Decreases constriction of resistance vessels

Due to the heterogeneous nature of childhood hypertension with a high rate of secondary causes, especially in the young child, most practitioners have abandoned the indiscriminant stepped-care approach for an individualized approach to antihypertensive drug therapy *(19)*. With an individualized approach, the initial antihypertensive drug is chosen based on the presumed mechanism and severity of hypertension; concomitant diseases and therapies; availability of appropriate formulations (e.g., suspension and dosage choices); and, when available, pediatric safety, pharmacokinetics, and efficacy data. In general, individualized therapy begins with a low dose of the initial drug (Table 5) and is slowly titrated upward, based on the blood pressure response or side effects. Unless clinically warranted, dose titration should proceed slowly, especially with antihypertensive drugs that have a long biological half-life (e.g., amlodipine), so that the blood pressure response at each dose level can be fully evaluated. An alternative antihypertensive agent can be substituted if no response or significant side effects are observed (Table 2). A second drug is added to the current regimen if the response to the first drug is inadequate but well-tolerated and correctable causes of an inadequate response are addressed (Table 3). When a second agent is needed for blood pressure control, diuretics appear to be the most useful as they have been shown to have an additive blood pressure-lowering effect when added to other classes of antihypertensive agents. If blood pressure is controlled with a second drug, a fixed combination preparation can be substituted if the appropriate dosing formulation is available (Table 4). Once blood pressure is controlled for 6–12 months and target-organ damage has regressed or resolved, an effort to decrease the dosage or number of antihypertensive medications should be considered. Lifestyle modifications are maintained during step-down therapy and

Table 2
Clinical Problems with Antihypertensive Drugs

ACE inhibitors/AT II receptor antagonist
    Use with caution in patients with bilateral renal artery stenosis or
      renal artery stenosis in a solitary kidney
    Use during pregnancy associated with fetal and neonatal toxicity
    Cough, hypotension, angioedema, renal failure, hyperkalemia,
      neutropenia
Renin inhibitors
    Angioedema, hyperkalemia, diarrhea (high dose)
Calcium channel blockers
    Profound and unexpected drops in BP seen with short-acting
      nifedipine
    Flushing, headache, fatigue, palpitations, edema
Vasodilators
    Fluid retention, edema, palpitations
    Minoxidil—hypertrichosis
    Hydralazine—lupus-like syndrome (greater in slow acetlylators)
β-Adrenergic antagonists
    Use with caution in patients with bronchial asthma, heart failure,
      diabetes mellitus
    Fatigue, cold extremities, sedation, bradycardia, abnormalities of
      lipid and glucose metabolism
Peripheral α-adrenergic antagonist
    Orthostatic hypotension with "first-dose effect"
Centrally acting α-adrenergic agonist
    Rebound hypertension with abrupt withdrawal
    Sedation, dry mouth, headache
Diuretics
    Potassium loss, volume depletion
    Hearing loss (loop diuretics), hyperkalemia (potassium-sparing
      diuretics)

Table 3
Causes of Inadequate Response to Antihypertensive Therapy

Inappropriate measurement technique
Damaged/improperly calibrated equipment
Noncompliance with prescribed therapy
  Medication noncompliance
  Dietary noncompliance (e.g., low salt, fluid restriction)
  Lifestyle modification noncompliance (failure to lose weight, exercise, . . .)

Table 3
(continued)

Progression of underlying disease
  Worsening renal failure
  Arteritis/vasculitis
Inappropriate drug for underlying mechanism of HTN
Dose of antihypertensive medications too low
Drug interactions
  Sympathomimetics, illicit drugs
  Caffeine
  Oral contraceptives, corticosteroids, cyclosporine, tacrolimus
  NSAIDs
Drug metabolism
  Rapid inactivation (e.g., rapid acetylator with hydralazine)
  Slow bioactivation of prodrug (e.g., losartan, irbesartan)
  Other undefined pharmacogenetic variant (e.g., sodium channel mutation)

Table 4
Antihypertensive Fixed-Drug Combinations (Products Available in USA)

Drug	Formulation	Cost/day
ACE inhibitors (+) diuretics		
Benazepril (+) HCTZ	5 mg/6.25 mg; 10/12.5; 20/12.5; 20/25	$1.05
Captopril (+) HCTZ	25 mg/15 mg; 50/15; 25/25; 50/25	$0.72
Enalapril (+) HCTZ	5 mg/12.5 mg; 10/25	$1.19
Lisinopril (+) HCTZ	10 mg/12.5 mg; 20/12.5; 20/25	$1.34
Moexipril (+) HCTZ	7.5 mg/12.5 mg; 15/12.5; 15/25	$1.38
Quinapril (+) HCTZ	10 mg/12.5 mg; 20/12.5; 20/25	$1.22
ACE inhibitors (+) CCBs		
Benazepril (+) amlodipine	10 mg/2.5 mg; 10/5; 20/5	$3.56
Trandolapril (+) verapamil ER	1 mg/240 mg; 2/180; 2/240; 4/240	$3.27
AT II receptor antagonists (+) diuretics		
Candesartan (+) HCTZ	16 mg/12.5 mg; 32/12.5	$3.16
Eprosartan (+) HCTZ	600 mg/12.5 mg	$3.44
Irbesartan (+) HCTZ	150 mg/12.5 mg; 300/12.5; 300/25	$3.13
Losartan (+) HCTZ	50 mg/12.5 mg; 100/12.5; 100/25	$2.60

Table 4
(continued)

Drug	Formulation	Cost/day
Olmesartan (+) HCTZ	20 mg/12.5 mg; 40/12.5; 40/25	$3.06
Telmisartan (+) HCTZ	40 mg/12.5 mg; 80/12.5; 80/25	$2.57
Valsartan (+) HCTZ	80 mg/12.5 mg; 160/12.5; 160/25; 320/12.5; 320/25	$2.80
AT II receptor antagonist (+) CCBs		
Olmesartan (+) amlodipine	20 mg/5 mg; 20/10; 40/5; 40/10	$3.06
Valsartan (+) amlodipine	160 mg/5 mg; 160/10; 320/5; 320/10	$3.53
AT II receptor antagonist (+) CCBs (+) diuretic		
Valsartan (+) amlodipine (+) HCTZ	160 mg/5 mg/12.5 mg; 160/5/25 160/10/12.5; 160/10/25; 320/10/25	$3.13
Renin inhibitor (+) diuretic		
Aliskiren (+) HCTZ	150 mg/12.5 mg; 150/25; 300/12.5; 300/25	$2.82
β-Adrenergic antagonist (+) diuretics		
Atenolol (+) chlorthalidone	50 mg/25 mg; 100/25	$0.90
Bisoprolol (+) HCTZ	2.5 mg/6.25 mg; 5/6.25; 10/6.25	$1.14
Propranolol (+) HCTZ	40 mg/25 mg; 80/25	$0.53
Metoprolol (+) HCTZ	50 mg/25 mg; 100/25; 100/50	$1.80
Vasodilators (+) diuretics		
Hydralazine (+) HCTZ	25 mg/25 mg; 50/50;	$1.56
Sympatholytics (+) diuretics		
Clonidine (+) chlorthalidone	0.1 mg/15 mg; 0.2/15; 0.3/15 1 mg/0.5 mg; 2/0.5; 5/0.5	$1.22
Diuretics (+) potassium-sparing diuretics		
HCTZ (+) spironolactone	25 mg/25 mg; 50/50	$0.50
HCTZ (+) triamterene	25 mg/37.5 mg; 25/50; 50/75	$0.35
HCTZ (+) amiloride	50 mg/5 mg	$0.42

HCTZ: hydrochlorothiazide.
Cost/day: based on average AWP and initial adult dosing recommendations.

drug reductions should be made methodically and slowly in order to fully assess the blood pressure response with each change.

There are clinical situations where a specific class of drug has proven more effective or beneficial for reasons independent of blood pressure lowering *(20,21)*. In the child with diabetes mellitus and microabluminuria or proteinuria, an ACE inhibitor is recommended as ACE inhibitors have been shown to slow the loss of renal function in adults with diabetic proteinuric renal disease *(14)*. Although outcome studies have not been performed with angiotensin II (AT II) receptor antagonists, these agents may also be beneficial for patients in whom ACE inhibitors are indicated, but the patients are unable to tolerate ACE inhibitors. ACE inhibitors are also recommended for children with proteinuric kidney disease or chronic kidney disease. The loss of kidney function in adults with proteinuric kidney disease is slowed in those receiving ACE inhibitors *(15,22,23)*.

In the absence of an absolute indication for a specific antihypertensive drug, the trend in the treatment of hypertension in children has been the use of ACE inhibitors, long-acting dihydropyridine calcium channel blockers (CCBs), and AT II receptor antagonists. These agents have gained favor due to the low side-effect profile, long duration of action requiring once- or twice-daily dosing, and the availability of formulations that allow for pediatric dosing. However, the use of agents that interfere with the angiotensin system in girls of childbearing potential is tempered by the potential fetal and neonatal adverse effects. For many of the newer antihypertensive drugs, pharmacokinetic and efficacy studies have been completed providing for the rational use of these agents in children. Although many of the traditional agents are still available for use in children with hypertension, it is unlikely that efficacy and pharmacokinetic studies will be performed and the pediatric dosing information will continue to be based on the reported experience in a few patients. Other antihypertensive agents that may be reasonably used as first-line agents include thiazide-type diuretics, β-adrenergic antagonists, and peripheral α–adrenergic antagonists. The α-adrenergic antagonists such a doxazosin, prazosin, and terazosin may be useful in the obese adolescent with "insulin-resistant syndrome" due to the minimal effect of the drug on lipid and carbohydrate metabolism and the reported enhanced sympathetic activity in such patients *(24,25)*. Vasodilators (e.g., hydralazine, minoxidil) and central α-adrenergic agonists (e.g., clonidine, guanfacine) are to be considered second-line agents. The role of the newest class of antihypertensive medications, renin inhibitors, in the treatment of pediatric hypertension is yet to be determined. See Table 5 for dosing recommendations.

Angiotensin-Converting Enzyme (ACE) Inhibitors

Angiotensin-converting enzyme catalyzes the conversion of angiotensin I to angiotensin II, which in turn influences blood pressure by direct vasoconstriction of the arterial vasculature, increased sympathetic nervous system activity, direct cardiovascular inotropic effect, and aldosterone-enhanced salt and water retention. ACE inhibitors, such as benazepril, captopril, enalapril, fosinopril, lisinopril, moexipril, perindopril, quinapril, ramipril, and trandolapril, reversibly inhibit the enzyme and block the formation of angiotensin II and the degradation of the vasodilatory peptide bradykinin.

Because renal and renovascular diseases are frequent causes of childhood hypertension, ACE inhibitors are commonly prescribed. ACE inhibitors are well tolerated by children and lower blood pressure in hypertensive children in a dose-dependent manner *(26–34)*. Neonates appear to be extremely sensitive to the blood pressure-lowering effects of ACE

Table 5

Suggested Dosing of Antihypertensive Medication in Children and Adolescents

Drug	Pediatric dosing	Adult dosing	Formulation	Cost/day
ACE inhibitors				
Benazepril[R]	Initial: 0.2 mg/kg QD Max: 0.6 mg/kg/day [40 mg/day]	Initial: 10 mg/day Max: 80 mg/day	T: 5 mg/10/20/40 Extemp: 2 mg/ml	$1.05
Captopril[R]	Initial: 0.2–0.5 mg/kg Q 6–12 h or 12.5–25 mg/dose BID/TID Max: 6 mg/kg/day	Initial: 25 mg BID/TID Max: 450 mg/day	T: 12.5 mg/25/50/100 Extemp: 1 mg/ml	$1.50–2.25
Enalapril[R]	Initial: 0.08 mg/kg QD Max: 0.6 mg/kg/day [40 mg/day]	Initial: 2.5–5 mg QD Max: 40 mg/day	T: 2.5 mg/5/10/20 Extemp: 1 mg/ml	$1.02
Fosinopril[R]	Initial: 0.1 mg/kg QD Max: Not established	Initial: 10 mg QD Max: 80 mg/day	T: 10 mg/20/40	$1.19
Lisinopril[R]	Initial: 0.07 mg/kg QD [5 mg/day] Max: 0.6 mg/kg/day [40 mg/day]	Initial: 10 mg QD Max: 80 mg/day	T: 2.5 mg/5/10/20/30/40 Extemp: 1 mg/ml; 2 mg/ml	$0.99
Moexipril[R]	No data	Initial: 7.5 mg QD Max: 60 mg/day	T: 7.5 mg/15	$1.38
Perindopril[R]	No data	Initial: 4 mg QD Max: 16 mg/day	T: 2 mg/4/8	$2.56
Quinapril[R]	Initial: 0.1–0.2 mg/kg QD [5–10 mg QD] Max: No information	Initial: 10 mg QD Max: 80 mg/day	T: 5 mg/10/20/40	$1.22
Ramipril[R]	No data	Initial: 2.5 mg QD Max: 20 mg/day	C/T: 1.25 mg/2.5/5/10	$2.00

Table 5
(continued)

Drug	Pediatric dosing	Adult dosing	Formulation	Cost/day
Trandolapril[R]	No data	Initial: 1 mg QD Max: 8 mg/day	T: 1 mg/2/4	$1.20
AT II receptor antagonists				
Candesartan	Initial: 0.13 mg/kg QD Max: 16 mg QD	Initial: 16 mg QD Max: 32 mg/day	T: 4 mg/8/16/32	$2.30
Eprosartan	No data	Initial: 600 mg QD Max: 800 mg/day	T: 400 mg/600	$3.24
Irbesartan	Initial: >6 y/o 75 mg QD Max: 150 mg/day	Initial: 150 mg QD Max: 300 mg/day	T: 75 mg/150/300	$2.36
Losartan	Initial: >6 y/o 0.7 mg/kg QD [>20 kg: 25 mg; >50 kg: 50 mg] Max: [>20 kg: 50 mg; >50 kg: 100 mg]	Initial: 50 mg QD Max: 100 mg/day	T: 25 mg/50/100	$2.37
Olmesartan	No data	Initial: 20 mg QD Max:: 40 mg QD	T: 5 mg/20/40	$2.38
Telmisartan	No data	Initial: 40 mg QD Max: 80 mg/day	T: 20 mg/40/80	$2.40
Valsartan	Initial: 1–2 mg/kg QD [40 mg/day] Max: 3.4 mg/kg [160 mg/day]	Initial: 80 mg QD Max: 320 mg/day	T: 40 mg/80/160/320 Extemp: 4 mg/ml	$2.60
Renin inhibitors				
Aliskiren	No data	Initial: 150 mg QD Max: 300 mg/day	T: 150 mg/300	$2.82

Table 5
(continued)

Drug	Pediatric dosing	Adult dosing	Formulation	Cost/day
Calcium channel blockers				
Amlodipine	Initial: 0.1–0.2 mg/kg QD [2.5–5 mg] Max: 0.6 mg/kg [10 mg]	Initial: 5 mg QD Max: 10 mg/day	T: 2.5 mg/5/10 Extemp: 1 mg/ml	$1.72
Diltiazem	*There are numerous formulations and dosing recommendations, please consult reference text*			
Felodipine	Initial: 2.5 mg QD Max: 10 mg/day	Initial: 5 mg QD Max: 10 mg/day	T(ER): 2.5 mg/5/10	$1.51
Isradipine	Initial: 0.15–0.2 mg/kg/day *Regular:* ÷BID/TID *CR:* ÷QD/BID	Initial: *Regular:* 2.5 mg BID *CR:* 5 mg QD Max: 20 mg/day	C: 2.5 mg/5 CR: 5 mg/10 Extemp: 1 mg/ml	*Regular:* $2.60 *CR:* $2.86
Nifedipine	0.25 mg/kg/dose Q 4–6 h	Not recommended in adults	C: 10 mg/20	
Nifedipine ER	Initial: 0.25 mg/kg ÷ QD/BID Max: Not established	Initial: 30 mg QD Max: 180 mg/day	T: 30 mg/60/90	$1.36
Nisoldipine	No data	Initial: 20 mg QD Max: 60 mg/day	T: 10 mg/20/30/40 [original formulation]	$2.55
Verapamil	*There are numerous formulations and dosing recommendations, please consult reference text*			

Table 5
(continued)

Drug	Pediatric dosing	Adult dosing	Formulation	Cost/day
Diuretics				
Amiloride[R]	Initial: 0.4–0.625 mg/kg QD Max: 20 mg	Initial: 5–10 mg QD Max: 20 mg	T: 5 mg	$1.25
Chlorothiazide[R]	Initial: 10–20 mg/kg ÷ QD/BID Max: <2 y/o 375 mg/day >2 y/o 1 g/day	Initial: 125–500 mg QD/BID Max: 2 g/day	T: 250 mg/500 Susp: 250 mg/5 ml	$0.25–0.50
Chlorthalidone[R]	Initial: 0.3 mg/kg QD/QOD Max: 2 mg/kg/day [50 mg/day]	Initial: 15 mg QD Max: 50 mg QD	T: 15 mg/ 25/50/100	$0.23
Hydrochlorothiazide	Initial: 1–2 mg/kg ÷ QD/BID Max: <2 y/o 37.5 mg/day >2 y/o 50 mg/day	Initial: 25 mg QD/BID Max: 100 mg/day	C: 12.5 mg T: 25 mg/50 Soln: 50 mg/5 ml	$0.09–0.18
Spironolactone[R]	Initial: 1 mg/kg ÷ QD/BID Max: 3 mg/kg/day—may need higher doses with mineralocorticoid excess	Initial: 25 mg QD/BID Max: 200 mg/day	T: 25 mg/50/100 Extemp: 5 mg/ml; 1 mg/ml	$0.46–0.92
Triamterene[R]	Initial: 1–2 mg/kg/day ÷ BID Max: 3–4 mg/kg/day [300 mg]	Initial: 50–100 mg QD/BID Max: 300 mg/day	C: 50 mg/100	$1.29–2.58
Vasodilators				
Hydralazine[R]	Initial: 0.7–1 mg/kg ÷ BID/QID Max: 7.5 mg/kg/day [100 mg]	Initial: 10 mg QID Max: 300 mg/day	T: 10 mg/25/50/100 Extemp: 20 mg/5 ml	$1.64

Table 5
(continued)

Drug	Pediatric dosing	Adult dosing	Formulation	Cost/day
Minoxidil[R]	Initial: 0.1–0.2 mg/kg ÷ QD/BID [5 mg] Max: 50 mg/day	Initial: 2.5–5 mg QD Max: 100 mg/day	T: 2.5 mg/10 Extemp: 2 mg/ml	$0.85
β-Adrenergic antagonists				
Acebutolol[R] (ISA)	No data	Initial: 400–800 mg QD Max: 1200 mg/day	C: 200 mg/400	$1.34
Atenolol[R] (B1-selective)	Initial: 0.5–1 mg/kg QD Max: 2 mg/kg/day [100]	Initial: 25–50 mg QD Max: 100 mg/day	T: 25 mg/50/100 Extemp: 2 mg/ml	$0.85
Bisoprolol[R] (B1-selective)	No data	Initial: 5 mg QD Max: 20 mg/day	T: 5 mg/10	$1.23
Metoprolol ER	Initial: 1 mg/kg QD [50 mg] Max: 2 mg/kg [100 mg]	Initial: 50–100 mg QD Max: 400 mg/day	T(ER): 25 mg/50/100/200 Extemp: 10 mg/ml	$0.90
Nadolol[R]	No data	Initial: 40–80 mg QD Max: 640 mg/day	T: 20 mg/40/80/120/160	$1.05
Propranolol	Initial: 0.5–1 mg/kg ÷ BID/TID Max: 16 mg/kg/day	Initial: 40 mg BID LA: 80 mg QD Max: 640 mg/day	T: 10 mg/20/40/60/80 LA: 60 mg/80/120/160 Extemp: 1 mg/ml	$1.38 CR: $2.40
Timolol	No data	Initial: 10 mg BID Max: 60 mg/day	T: 5 mg/10/20	$1.00
Labetalol (α- and β-)	Initial: 1–3 mg/kg/day ÷ BID Max: 10–20 mg/kg [1200 mg]	Initial: 100 mg BID Max: 2.4 g/day	T: 100 mg/200/300 Extemp: 10 mg/ml	$1.00
Carvedilol (α- and β-)	No data	Initial: 6.25 mg BID Max: 50 mg/day	T: 3.125 mg/6.25/12.5/25 C(ER): 10 mg/20/40/80	$4.20 ER: $4.54

Table 5
(continued)

Drug	Pediatric dosing	Adult dosing	Formulation	Cost/day
Central α-adrenergic agonists				
Clonidine	Initial: <12 y/o: 5–10 mcg/kg ÷ BID/TID >12 y/o: 0.2 mg/kg ÷ BID/TID Max: Not established	Initial: 0.1 mg BID Max: 2.4 mg/day	T: 0.1 mg/0.2/0.3 Transdermal: 0.1 mg/0.2/0.3	$0.50 TD:$4.26
Guanfacine[R]	Max: 0.9 mg/day No data	Initial: 1 mg QD Max: 2 mg/day	T: 1 mg/2	$0.71
α-adrenergic antagonists				
Doxazosin	Initial: 1 mg QD Max: 4 mg/day	Initial: 1 mg QD Max: 16 mg/day	T: 1 mg/2/4/8	0.92
Prazosin	Initial: 0.05–0.1 mg/kg ÷ BID/TID Max: 0.5 mg/kg/day	Initial: 1 mg BID/TID Max: 20 mg/day	C: 1 mg/2/5	$0.64–0.96
Terazosin	No data	Initial: 1 mg QD Max: 20 mg/day	C: 1 mg/2/5/10	$1.60

R: dosing adjustments/concerns with renal dysfunction.
Cost/day: based on average AWP using initial adult dosing recommendations.

inhibitors, and the dosage should be significantly lower than the dosage recommended for older children *(35,36)* (see Chapter 21).

Captopril has a beneficial blood pressure-lowering effect in children with renal parenchymal and renovascular disease *(26,28–31)*; however, the increased incidence of cough and need for more frequent dosing have led to greater use of the newer, longer acting ACE inhibitors (e.g., enalapril, lisinopril). Once-daily dosing with enalapril or lisinopril lowers trough blood pressure in a dose-dependent manner in children with hypertension *(32,33)*. In these prospective studies, the lowest dosage group (0.02 mg/kg) did not have a consistent blood pressure-lowering response, and the initial recommended dosage for both agents is 0.08 mg/kg given once daily. In a fairly large study from a pediatric perspective, the effectiveness, safety, and dose–response relationship of fosinopril were studied in 253 children with high or high-normal blood pressure *(37)*. Treatment with fosinopril significantly lowered systolic and diastolic blood pressure during the 4-week study. Because there was no apparent dose–response relationship the initial recommended dose for children is 0.1 mg/kg given once daily; however, a post hoc analysis suggested that black children may require higher doses to produce similar blood pressure-lowering effects *(38)*. If a child is receiving a moderate dose of an ACE inhibitor and the blood pressure-lowering effect diminishes toward the end of the dosing interval (e.g., trough BP) twice-daily dosing should be considered prior to adding a second antihypertensive drug. The pharmacokinetic parameters of enalapril and quinapril in hypertensive children are similar to those reported for adults *(39,40)*.

The most common adverse effects reported in children receiving ACE inhibitors include cough, hypotension, and deterioration of renal function *(41,42)*. The decline in renal function and hypotension is noted most in neonates or children with preexisting renal disease or volume depletion and is uncommon in the well-hydrated child with normal renal function. Less common adverse effects include angioedema, hyperkalemia, rash, anemia, and leukopenia *(43)*.

The use of ACE inhibitors during pregnancy has been associated with fetal and neonatal toxicity. ACE inhibitor fetopathy is typically associated with ACE inhibitor exposure during the second and third trimesters of pregnancy and characterized by fetal hypotension, anuria-oliogohydramnios, growth restriction, pulmonary hypoplasia, renal tubular dysplasia, and hypocalvaria *(44)*. More recently, ACE inhibitor exposure during the first trimester has been associated with an increased risk of birth defects, namely cardiovascular abnormalities *(45)*. Because of the potential adverse fetal and neonatal effects, ACE inhibitors should probably not be used as the initial treatment for hypertension in this population unless the expected benefit clearly exceeds the potential risk such as might be the situation in adolescent girls with CKD, DM, or difficult to control/resistant hypertension. Adolescents of childbearing potential that are prescribed ACE inhibitors are to be informed of the potential risks of ACE inhibitors on the developing fetus and counseled on proper birth control measures. ACE inhibitors are contraindicated in children with a history of angioedema and should be used with great caution in children with bilateral renal artery stenosis or renal artery stenosis in a solitary kidney.

ANGIOTENSIN II (AT II) RECEPTOR ANTAGONISTS

AT II receptor antagonists block the binding of angiotensin II to the angiotensin receptor (type 1) located in vascular smooth muscle and the adrenal gland. AT II receptor antagonists prevent the pressor effect of angiotensin II and inhibit angiotensin II-stimulated aldosterone secretion from the adrenal gland.

Similar to ACE inhibitors, AT II receptor antagonists appear to be well tolerated and effectively lower blood pressure in hypertensive children as monotherapy or delivered with other antihypertensive agents *(46–50)*. The pharmacokinetic profile of valsartan and irbesartan in children is similar to that observed in adult patients with hypertension. Once-daily candesartan effectively reduced clinic and 24-h ambulatory blood pressure in 11 children studied by Franks et al. *(46)*. Similarly, valsartan effectively lowered blood pressure in a group of 88 children less than 5 years of age with untreated or inadequately treated hypertension *(50)*. As would be expected, the majority of these young children had an underlying urologic or kidney disease associated with hypertension. Finally, although primarily a pharmacokinetic study, Sakarcan et al. *(47)* detected a BP-lowering effect in a group of children receiving irbesartan.

There are relatively few reports of adverse effect of AT II receptor antagonist in the pediatric studies with an adverse effect profile similar to placebo. The most commonly reported adverse events in the pediatric studies were concurrent infectious illnesses which are common in this population. Other reported events include hyperkalemia, headache, and rare events of pruritus, malaise, hepatitis, decreased appetite, and blurred vision. Due to the fetal and neonatal toxicity noted with drugs that act on the renin–angiotensin system *(44,45)*, AT II receptor antagonist should not be given during pregnancy, and their use in adolescents of childbearing potential should be undertaken with caution as described in the preceding section on ACE inhibitors. If prescribed, adolescents of childbearing potential are to be informed of the potential risks and counseled on proper birth control measures.

RENIN INHIBITORS

Renin inhibitors block the circulating enzyme renin that catalyzes the conversion of the substrate angiotensinogen to the inactive peptide angiotensin I. Angiotensin I is converted to the active peptide angiotensin II, which in turn influences blood pressure by direct vasoconstriction of the arterial vasculature, increased sympathetic nervous system activity, direct cardiovascular inotropic effect, and aldosterone-enhanced salt and water retention.

Studies of direct renin inhibitors in children are currently in progress, and no data are presently available on their effectiveness or safety in the pediatric population. Aliskiren, the only direct renin inhibitor currently available, effectively lowers systolic and diastolic BP in adults *(51)*. The most common adverse effect associated with higher does of aliskiren was diarrhea.

CALCIUM CHANNEL BLOCKERS (CCBS)

The contraction of cardiac and vascular smooth muscle and peripheral vascular resistance are dependent on the inward flux of calcium. Dihydropyridine calcium channel blockers (CCBs) such as amlodipine, felodipine, isradipine, nicardipine, nifedipine, and nisoldipine inhibit the inward movement of calcium and cause relaxation of the arterial vasculature and decreased peripheral vascular resistance. In contrast to non-dihydropyridine CCBs such as verapamil and diltiazem, dihydropyridine CCBs have a negligible effect on cardiac conduction and contractility.

CCBs effectively lower blood pressure in hypertensive children and are well tolerated *(52,53)*. Amlodipine lowered the systolic and diastolic blood pressure of hypertensive children in a dose-dependent manner when administered once daily *(54)*. Amlodipine is ideally suited for the treatment of childhood hypertension because the prolonged elimination half-life (e.g., >30 h) permits once-daily dosing and the physicochemical properties allow the drug to be compounded as a liquid suspension (extemporaneous formulation) that permits treatment of children unable to swallow tablets/capsules and allows dose titration in small increments. In children able to swallow a tablet or capsule formulation, sustained release of nifedipine appears to be well tolerated.

The most common adverse effects reported in children receiving CCBs include flushing, headache, peripheral edema, and fatigue *(55–57)*. Other reported adverse effects include gingival hyperplasia, chest pain, and nausea and vomiting *(43)*.

The use of short-acting nifedipine or other short-acting CCBs in children with hypertension is not recommended for long-term therapy, and their use to control acute elevations of blood pressure is controversial *(58–61)*. Short-acting nifedipine in adult patients is associated with an increased risk of adverse cardiac and neurologic events *(21,62)*. In general, short-acting nifedipine appears to be effective in children with acute blood pressure elevation *(58)*; however, profound and unpredictable drops in blood pressure have been observed in children receiving short-acting nifedipine, occasionally resulting in catastrophic CNS events *(63)*. When used, the initial nifedipine dosage should be 0.1–0.25 mg/kg and should be avoided in children with an underlying acute CNS injury *(58,64)*.

DIURETICS

Thiazide diuretics are the most common and effective diuretics prescribed for hypertension. Loop diuretics are not useful as long-term antihypertensive agents due to the adaptive processes that limit their effectiveness *(65)* but may be effective as adjuvant therapy in volume-overloaded patients that are resistant to the effects of thiazide diuretics, such as patients with chronic renal failure. The potassium-sparing diuretics (e.g., spironolactone and amiloride) are specifically indicated for hypertension due to mineralocorticoid excess and to diminish thiazide and loop diuretic-induced hypokalemia.

The initial blood pressure-lowering effect of thiazide diuretics results from an increased urinary loss of sodium and extracellular fluid volume contraction. With chronic dosing, sodium balance and extracellular fluid volume return toward normal; however, the lower blood pressure is maintained by a decline in peripheral vascular resistance. The mechanism(s) responsible for the changes in vascular resistance are unclear. The antihypertensive response to thiazide diuretics is dependent on sodium intake, and a high-sodium intake will attenuate the antihypertensive effect and is a common cause of apparent resistance to therapy (Table 5).

Thiazide diuretics, alone or in combination with β-adrenergic antagonists, lower blood pressure in children with hypertension *(18,66)*. In a placebo-controlled trial examining the blood pressure-lowering effect of the combination drug bisoprolol/hydrochlorothiazide, systolic and diastolic blood pressures were significantly reduced as compared to a group of children randomized to placebo *(18)*.

The thiazide dose–antihypertensive response relationship in adults is relatively flat, such that there is little further blood pressure lowering but increased incidence of adverse effects with larger doses. Common adverse effects with diuretics are hypokalemia, hyponatremia, alkalosis, and extracellular fluid volume depletion. Caution is suggested when adding an ACE inhibitor to a child receiving diuretics as the diuretic-induced volume depletion may increase the risk of hypotension and renal dysfunction. Ototoxicity is a reported side effect of loop diuretics, and the risk increases with high doses, kidney failure, and concomitant use of other ototoxic drugs such as aminoglycosides.

β-ADRENERGIC RECEPTOR ANTAGONISTS

β-Adrenergic receptor antagonists decrease blood pressure through several mechanisms including decreased cardiac output, decreased secretion of renin and aldosterone, altered central nervous system sympathetic activity, and potentiation of natriuretic peptides.

Cardioselective β-adrenergic receptor antagonists such as acebutolol, atenolol, bisoprolol, and metoprolol have a greater affinity for the beta$_1$-adrenergic receptor, whereas nonselective drugs such as carvedilol, labetalol, nadolol, propranolol, and timolol interact with both beta$_1$- and beta$_2$-adrenergic receptors. The preferential effect of cardioselective drugs for beta$_1$-adrenergic receptors is relative, and at higher doses, cardioselective drugs will inhibit the beta$_2$-adrenergic receptors that are located in bronchial musculature. The clinical importance of intrinsic sympathetic activity is not well defined. Carvedilol and labetalol are nonselective beta-adrenergic receptor antagonists that also have peripheral alpha$_1$-adrenergic blocking activity.

Beta-adrenergic receptor antagonists lower blood pressure in hypertensive children when used alone or in combination with other antihypertensive agents *(18,66–68)*. Great interindividual variation exists in the amount of propranolol needed to lower blood pressure as propranolol is metabolized by the liver prior to entering the systemic circulation (e.g., first-pass effect). This results in unpredictable plasma concentrations following oral administration and a wide range of effective dosages. The combination drug bisoprolol and hydrochlorothiazide lowered systolic and diastolic blood pressure in children with hypertension *(18)*. Metoprolol, a cardioselective agent, effectively lowered blood pressure in a group of hypertensive adolescents *(69)*.

The most common adverse effects from beta-adrenergic receptor antagonists are related to the central nervous system and include dizziness, light-headedness, fatigue, depression, and hallucinations. Other adverse effects are bradycardia, postural hypotension, cold extremities, and nausea. Beta-adrenergic receptor antagonists can mask the premonitory signs associated with hypoglycemia in diabetic patients and should not be used in patients with bronchospastic disease.

CENTRALLY ACTING SYMPATHOLYTIC AGENTS

Stimulation of the alpha$_2$-adrenergic receptors in the central nervous system decreases sympathetic outflow. Centrally acting agents such as clonidine and guanabenz are commonly reserved for hypertension recalcitrant to multiple antihypertensive drugs. Clonidine may be the preferred antihypertensive agent in children receiving pharmacologic treatment of a hyperactivity disorder. The reported experience with centrally acting agents is limited to adolescents with essential hypertension *(70–72)*.

Side effects are common with the use of centrally acting agents. Dry mouth, sedation, fatigue, dizziness, weakness, and constipation are typically dose related and tend to decrease with continued dosing. Discontinuation of centrally acting agents should be gradual as abrupt withdrawal can result in symptoms such as agitation, headache, tremor, and hypertension.

PERIPHERAL ADRENERGIC ANTAGONIST

Alpha$_1$-adrenergic receptor antagonist such as doxazosin, prazosin, and terazosin blocks the pressor effect of adrenergic stimulation on the vasculature resulting in reduced arteriolar resistance and venous capacitance. Alpha$_1$-adrenergic receptor antagonists are usually reserved for severe or drug-resistant hypertension and are infrequently prescribed in children. The alpha$_1$-adrenergic receptor antagonists can be considered for initial therapy in children with the insulin-resistant syndrome, a syndrome characterized by obesity, insulin resistance, lipid abnormalities, and hypertension, as the syndrome is associated with sympathetic overactivity *(73)*, and alpha$_1$-adrenergic receptor antagonists have positive effect on the lipid profile.

The first-dose phenomenon, a marked postural hypotensive response that occurs shortly after the initial dose or with a dosage increase, is common and more likely to occur in patients receiving diuretics or beta-adrenergic receptor antagonists. The most common adverse effects associated with alpha$_1$-adrenergic receptor antagonists are dizziness, headache, fatigue, palpitations, and nausea.

VASODILATORS

Vasodilators such as hydralazine and minoxidil produce arteriolar vasodilation through a direct action on vascular smooth muscle. Minoxidil successfully lowers blood pressure in children *(74,75)* but is best reserved for severe and drug-resistant forms of hypertension.

The predominant side effects of vasodilators are fluid and salt retention and cardiac stimulation. Cardiac output is increased by enhanced venous return and sympathetic activity. Patients with poorly compliant ventricles, such as patients with severe left ventricular hypertrophy and diastolic dysfunction, may develop heart failure when prescribed vasodilators. Concomitant treatment with diuretics or beta-adrenergic receptor antagonist may modify the fluid retention and cardiac stimulation. Flushing, headache, palpitations, hypotension, and palpitation are commonly observed with vasodilators. Growth of hair on the face, back, arms, and legs occurs in all patients receiving minoxidil and can be very distressing for young girls. Hydralazine can cause a drug-induced lupus syndrome.

REFERENCES

1. National Institutes of Health, National Heart, Lung, and Blood Institute, National High Blood Pressure Program. The seventh report of the joint national committee on prevention, detection, evaluation, and treatment of high blood pressure. Report No. 04-5230. 2004.
2. Sorof JM, Alexandrov AV, Cardwell G, Portman RJ. Carotid artery intimal-medial thickness and left ventricular hypertrophy in children with elevated blood pressure. Pediatrics. 2003;111:61–66.
3. Litwin M, Trelewicz J, Wawer Z, Antoniewicz J, Wierzbicka A, Rajszys P, Grenda R. Intima-media thickness and arterial elasticity in hypertensive children: controlled study. Pediatr Nephrol. 2004;19:767–774.
4. Lande MB, Carson NL, Roy J, Meagher CC. Effects of childhood primary hypertension on carotid intima-media thickness: a matched controlled study. Hypertension. 2006;48:40–44.
5. Sorof JM, Cardwell G, Franco K, Portman RJ. Ambulatory blood pressure and left ventricular mass index in hypertensive children. Hypertension. 2002;39(4):903–908.
6. Sorof J, Hanevold C, Portman R, Daniels S. Left ventricular hypertrophy in hypertensive children: A report from the international pediatric hypertension association. Am J Hypertens. 2002;15[4 (part 2 of 2)]:31A (Abstract).
7. Tracy RE, Newman WP III, Wattigney WA, Berenson GS. Risk factors and atherosclerosis in youth autopsy findings of the Bogalusa Heart Study. Am J Med Sci. 1995;310(Suppl 1):S37–S41.

8. Knoflach M, Kiechl S, Kind M, Said M, Sief R, Gisinger M, van der Zee R, Gaston H, Jarosch E, Willeit J, Wick G. Cardiovascular Risk Factors and Atherosclerosis in Young Males: ARMY Study (Atherosclerosis Risk-Factors in Male Youngsters) Circulation. 2003;108:1064–1069.

9. Li S, Chen W, Srinivasan SR, Bond MG, Tang R, Urbina EM, Berenson GS. Childhood cardiovascular risk factors and carotid vascular changes in adulthood: the Bogalusa Heart Study. JAMA. 2003;290(17):2271–2276. Erratum in: JAMA. 2003;290(22):2943.

10. Lauer RM, Clarke WR. Childhood risk factors for high adult blood pressure: The Muscatine study. Pediatrics. 1984;84:633–641.

11. National High Blood Pressure Education Program Working Group on High Blood Pressure in Children and Adolescents. The fourth report on the diagnosis, evaluation, and treatment of high blood pressure in children and adolescents. Pediatrics. 2004;114(2 Suppl 4th Report):555–576.

12. Sinaiko AR, Gomez-Marin O, Prineas RJ. Prevalence of "significant" hypertension in junior high school-aged children: the children and adolescent blood pressure program. J Pediatr. 1989;114:664–669.

13. Wong H, Mylrea K, Feber J, Drukker A, Filler G. Prevalence of complications in children with chronic kidney disease according to KDOQI. Kidney Int. 2006;70:585–590.

14. Lewis EJ, Hunsicker LG, Bain RP, Rohde RD. The effect of angiotensin-converting-enzyme inhibition on diabetic nephropathy. The Collaborative Study Group. N Engl J Med. 1993;329(20):1456–1462.

15. Coppo R, Peruzzi L, Amore A, Piccoli A, Cochar P, Stone R, Kirschstein M, Linne T. IgACE: a placebo-controlled, randomized trial of angiotensin-converting enzyme inhibitors in children and young people with IgA nephropathy and moderate proteinuria. J Am Soc Nephrol. 2007;18:1880–1888.

16. Pfeffer MA, Braunwald E, Moye LA, Basta L, Brown EJ Jr, Cuddy TE, et al. Effect of captopril on mortality and morbidity in patients with left ventricular dysfunction after myocardial infarction. Results of the survival and ventricular enlargement trial. The SAVE Investigators. N Engl J Med. 1992;327(10):669–677.

17. United States Department of Health and Human Services, National Institutes of Health, National Heart Lung, and Blood Institute. Your Guide to Lowering Your Blood Pressure With DASH. http://www.nhlbi.nih.gov/health/public/heart/hbp/dash/ [Accessed October 5, 2010].

18. Sorof JM, Cargo P, Graepel J, Humphrey D, King E, Rolf C, et al. Beta-Blocker/thiazide combination for treatment of hypertensive children: a randomized double-blind, placebo-controlled trial. Pediatr Nephrol. 2002;17(5):345–350.

19. Wells T, Stowe C. An approach to the use of antihypertensive drugs in children and adolescents. Curr Ther Res Clin Exp. 2001;62(4):329–350.

20. Agodoa LY, Appel L, Bakris GL, Beck G, Bourgoignie J, Briggs JP, et al. Effect of ramipril vs amlodipine on renal outcomes in hypertensive nephrosclerosis: a randomized controlled trial. JAMA. 2001;285(21):2719–2728.

21. Pahor M, Psaty BM, Alderman MH, Applegate WB, Williamson JD, Cavazzini C, et al. Health outcomes associated with calcium antagonists compared with other first-line antihypertensive therapies: a meta-analysis of randomized controlled trials. Lancet. 2000;356(9246):1949–1954.

22. Ruggenenti P, Perna A, Gherardi G, Benini R, Remuzzi G. Chronic proteinuric nephropathies: outcomes and response to treatment in a prospective cohort of 352 patients with different patterns of renal injury. Am J Kidney Dis. 2000;35(6):1155–1165.

23. Gansevoort RT, de Zeeuw D, de Jong PE. Long-term benefits of the antiproteinuric effect of angiotensin-converting enzyme inhibition in nondiabetic renal disease. Am J Kidney Dis. 1993;22(1):202–206.

24. Sorof JM, Poffenbarger T, Franco K, Bernard L, Portman RJ. Isolated systolic hypertension, obesity, and hyperkinetic hemodynamic states in children. J Pediatr. 2002;140(6):660–666.

25. Rocchini AP. Adolescent obesity and hypertension. Pediatr Clin North Am. 1993;40(1):81–92.

26. Leckman JF, Detlor J, Harcherik DF, Young G, Anderson GM, Shaywitz BA, et al. Acute and chronic clonidine treatment in Tourette's syndrome: a preliminary report on clinical response and effect on plasma and urinary catecholamine metabolites, growth hormone, and blood pressure. J Child Psychiatry. 1983;22(5):433–440.

27. Miller K, Atkin B, Rodel Jr PV, Walker JF. Enalapril: A well-tolerated and efficacious agent for the pediatric hypertensive patient. J Cardiovasc Pharmacol. 1987;10(Suppl 7):S154–S156.

28. Morsi MR, Madina EH, Anglo AA, Soliman AT. Evaluation of captopril versus reserpine and furosemide in treating hypertensive children with acute post-streptococcal glomerulonephritis. Acta Paediatr. 1992;81:145–149.

29. Bendig L, Temesvari A. Indications and effects of captopril therapy in childhood. Acta Physiologica Hungarica. 1988;72:121–129.

30. Sagat T, Sasinka M, Furkova K, Milovsky V, Riedel R, Tordova E. Treatment of renal hypertension in children by captopril. Clin Exp Hypertens A. 1986;8(4–5):853–857.

31. Callis L, Vila A, Catala J, Gras X. Long-term treatment with captopril in pediatric patients with severe hypertension and chronic renal failure. Clin Exp Hypertens A. 1986;8(4–5):847–851.

32. Soffer BA, Shahinfar S, Shaw WC, Zhang Z, Herrera P, Frame V, et al. Effects of the Ace inhibitor, enalapril, in children age 6–16 years with hypertension. Pediatr Res. 2000;47(4): (Abstract).

33. Herrera P, Soffer B, Zhang Z, Miller K, Cano F, Hernandez O, et al. Effects of the ACE inhibitor, lisinopril (L), in children age 6-16 years with hypertension. Am J Hypertens. 2002;14(4 part 2):32A (Abstract).

34. Seeman T, Dusek J, Feber J, Vondrak K, Janda J. Treatment of hypertension with ramipril in children with renal diseases. Am J Hypertens. 2002;15(4 part 2):204A–205A (Abstract).

35. Tack ED, Perlman JN. Renal failure in sick hypertensive premature infants receiving captopril therapy. J Pediatr. 1988;112:805–810.

36. Sinaiko AR, Mirkin BL, Hendrick DA, Green TP, O'Dea RF. Antihypertensive effect and elimination kinetics of captopril in hypertensive children with renal disease. J Pediatr. 1983;103:799–805.

37. Li JS, Berezny K, Kilaru R, Hazan L, Portman R, Hogg R, Jenkins RD, Kanani P, Cottrill CM, Mattoo TK, Zharkova L, Kozlova L, Weisman I, Deitchman D, Califf RM. Is the extrapolated adult dose of fosinopril safe and effective in treating hypertensive children? Hypertension. Sept 2004;44(3):289–293.

38. Menon S, Berezny KY, Kilaru R, Benjamin DK Jr, Kay JD, Hazan L, Portman R, Hogg R, Deitchman D, Califf RM, Li JS. Racial differences are seen in blood pressure response to fosinopril in hypertensive children. Am Heart J. Aug 2006;152(2):394–399.

39. Wells T, Rippley R, Hogg R, Sakarcan A, Blowey D, Walson P, et al. The pharmacokinetics of enalapril in children and infants with hypertension. J Clin Pharmacol. 2001;41:1064–1074.

40. Blumer JL, Daniels SR, Dreyer WJ, Batisky D, Walson PD, Roman D, Ouellet D. Pharmacokinetics of quinapril in children: assessment during substitution for chronic angiotensin-converting enzyme inhibitor treatment. J Clin Pharmacol. Feb 2003;43(2):128–132.

41. von Vigier RO, Mozzettini S, Truttmann AC, Meregalli P, Ramelli GP, Bianchetti MG. Cough is common in children prescribed converting enzyme inhibitors. Nephron. 2000;84:98.

42. Bianchetti MG, Caflisch M, Oetliker OH. Cough and converting enzyme inhibitors. Eur J Pediatr. 1992;151:225–226.

43. Blowey DL. Safety of the newer antihypertensive agents in children. Expert Opin Drug Saf. 2002;1(1):39–43.

44. Sedman AB, Kershaw DB, Bunchman TE. Recognition and management of angiotensin converting enzyme inhibitor fetopathy. Pediatr Nephrol. 1995;9:382–385.

45. Cooper WO, Hernandez-Diaz S, Arbogast PG, Dudley JA, Dyer S, Gideon PS, Hall K, Ray WA. Major congenital malformations after first-trimester exposure to ACE inhibitors. N Engl J Med. 2006;354(23):2443–2451.

46. Franks AM, O'Brien CE, Stowe CD, Wells TG, Gardner SF: Candesartan cilexetil effectively reduces blood pressure in hypertensive children. Ann Pharmacother. Oct 2008;42(10):1388–1395.

47. Sakarcan A, Tenney F, Wilson JT, Stewart JJ, Adcock KG, Wells TG, Vachharajani NN, Hadjilambris OW, Slugg P, Ford NF, Marino MR. The pharmacokinetics of Irbesartan in hypertensive children and adolescents. J Clin Pharmacol. Jul 2001;41(7):742–749.

48. Shahinfar S, Cano F, Soffer BA, Ahmed T, Santoro EP, Zhang Z, Gleim G, Miller K, Vogt B, Blumer J, Briazgounov I. A double-blind, dose-response study of losartan in hypertensive children. Am J Hypertens. Feb 2005;18(2 Pt 1):183–190.

49. Blumer J, Batisky DL, Wells T, Shi V, Solar-yohay S, Sunkara G. Pharmacokinetics of valsartan in pediatric and adolescent subjects with hypertension. J Clin Pharmacol. 2009;49:235–241.

50. Flynn JT, Meyers KEC, Neto JP, Meneses RdeP, Zurowska A, Bagga A, Mattheyse L, Shi V, Gupte J, Solar-Yohay S, Han G. Efficacy and safety of the angiotensin receptor blocker valsartan in children with hypertension aged 1 to 5 years. Hypertension. 2008;52:222–228.

51. Gradman AH, Schmieder RE, Lins RL, Nussberger J, Chiang Y, Bedigian MP. Aliskiren, a novel orally effective renin inhibitor, provides dose-dependent antihypertensive efficacy and placebo-like tolerability in hypertensive patients. Circulation. Mar 1 2005;111(8):1012–1018.

52. Flynn JT, Pasko D. Calcium channel blockers: pharmacology and place in therapy of pediatric hypertension. Pediatr Nephrol. 2000;15:302–316.

53. Sinaiko AR. Clinical pharmacology of converting enzyme inhibitors, calcium channel blockers and diuretics. J Hum Hypertens. 1994;8:389–394.

54. Flynn JT, Hogg RJ, Portman RJ, Saul JP, Miller K, Sanders SP, et al. A randomized, placebo-controlled trial of amlodipine in the treatment of children with hypertension. Am J Hypertens. 2002;15(4 part 2):31A–32A (Abstract).

55. Flynn JT, Smoyer WE, Bunchman TE. Treatment of hypertensive children with amlodipine. Am J Hypertens. 2000;13(10):1061–1066.

56. Silverstein DM, Palmer J, Baluarte HJ, Brass C, Conley SB, Polinsky MS. Use of calcium-channel blockers in pediatric renal transplant recipients. Pediatr Transplant. 1999;3(4):288–292.

57. Tallian KB, Nahata MC, Turman MA, Mahan JD, Hayes JR, Mentser MI. Efficacy of amlodipine in pediatric patients with hypertension. Pediatr Nephrol. 1999;13:304–310.

58. Egger DW, Deming DD, Hamada N, Perkin RM, Sahney S. Evaluation of the safety of short-acting nifedipine in children with hypertension. Pediatr Nephrol. 2002;17:35–40.

59. Truttmann AC, Zehnder-Schlapbach S, Bianchetti MG. A moratorium should be placed on the use of short acting nifedipine for hypertensive crises (letter). Pediatr Nephrol. 1998;12:259–261.

60. Sinaiko AR, Daniels S. The use of short-acting nifedipine in children with hypertension: another example of the need for comprehensive drug testing in children. J Pediatr. 2001;139:7–9.

61. Flynn JT. Nifedipine in the treatment of hypertension in children. J Pediatr. 2002;140(6):787–788.

62. Psaty BM, Heckbert SR, Koepsell TD, Siscovick DS, Raghunathan TE, Weiss NS, et al. The risk of myocardial infarction associated with antihypertensive drug therapies. JAMA. 1995;274:620–625.

63. Gauthier B, Trachtman H. Short-acting nifedipine (letter). Pediatr Nephrol. 1997;11:786–787.

64. Levene MI, Gibson NA, Fenton AC, Papathoma E, Barnett D. The use of a calcium-channel blocker, nicardipine, for severely asphyxiated newborn infants. Dev Med Child Neurol. 1990;32:567–574.

65. Ellison D. Adaptation to diuretic drugs. In: Seldin D, Giebisch G, eds. Diuretic Agents: Clinical Physiology and Pharmacology. San Diego, CA, Academic; 1997:209–232.

66. Bachmann H. Propranolol versus chlorthalidone—a prospective therapeutic trial in children with chronic hypertension. Helv Paediatr Acta. 1984;39:55–61.

67. Potter DE, Schambelan M, Salvatierra O Jr, Orloff S, Holliday MA. Treatment of high-renin hypertension with propranolol in children after renal transplantation. J Pediatr. 1977;90(2):307–311.

68. Griswold WR, McNeal R, Mendoza SA, Sellers BB, Higgins S. Propranolol as an antihypertensive agent in children. Arch Dis Child. 1978;53(7):594–596.

69. Falkner B, Lowenthal DT, Affrime MB. The pharmacodynamic effectiveness of metoprolol in adolescent hypertension. Pediatr Pharmacol. 1982;2(1):49–55.

70. Falkner B, Onesti G, Lowenthal DT, Affrime MB. Effectiveness of centrally acting drugs and diuretics in adolescent hypertension. Clin Pharmacol Ther. 1982;32(5):577–583.

71. Walson PD, Rath A, Kilbourne K, Deitch MW. Guanabenz for adolescent hypertension. Pediatr Pharmacol. 1984;4:1–6.

72. Falkner B, Lowenthal DT, Onesti G. Dynamic exercise response in hypertensive adolescent on clonidine therapy: Clonidine therapy in adolescent hypertension. Pediatr Pharmacol. 1980;1:121–128.

73. Sorof JM. Systolic hypertension in children: benign or beware? Pediatr Nephrol. 2001;16(6):517–525.

74. Sinaiko AR, Mirkin BL. Management of severe childhood hypertension with minoxidil: a controlled clinical study. J Pediatr. 1977;91(1):138–142.

75. Pennisi AJ, Takahashi M, Bernstein BH, Singsen BH, Uittenbogaart C, Ettenger RB, et al. Minoxidil therapy in children with severe hypertension. J Pediatr. 1977;90(5):813–819.

32 Management of Hypertensive Emergencies

Craig W. Belsha, MD

CONTENTS

INTRODUCTION

Severe, symptomatic hypertension occurs infrequently in childhood but when present often signifies a life-threatening emergency. The clinician needs to approach this situation with a sense of urgency to reduce blood pressure (BP) and limit end-organ damage while avoiding overly aggressive therapy which may also lead to ischemia and further injury. This chapter discusses the causes, pathophysiology, evaluation, and treatment of severe hypertension.

DEFINITIONS OF HYPERTENSIVE CRISES, EMERGENCIES, AND URGENCIES

Hypertension in childhood is classified by The Fourth Report on the Diagnosis, Evaluation, and Treatment of High Blood Pressure in Children and Adolescents into two

C.W. Belsha (✉)
Department of Pediatrics, SSM Cardinal Glennon Children's Medical Center, Saint Louis University, St. Louis, MO, USA
e-mail: belshacw@slu.edu

From: *Clinical Hypertension and Vascular Diseases: Pediatric Hypertension*
Edited by: J. T. Flynn et al. DOI 10.1007/978-1-60327-824-9_32
© Springer Science+Business Media, LLC 2011

Table 1
Hypertension Stages

Stage	Pediatric criteria	Adult criteria
1	SBP or DBP > 95th to 99th percentile plus 5 mmHg	140–159/90–99 mmHg
2	SBP or DBP > 99th percentile plus 5 mmHg	≥160/100 mmHg

SBP, systolic blood pressure, DBP, diastolic blood pressure.
Adapted from *(1,4)*.

stages *(1)*. Stage 1 hypertension is designated for blood pressure levels from the 95th percentile to 5 mmHg above the 99th percentile for age, gender, and height while Stage 2 hypertension is designated for levels above the 99th percentile plus 5 mmHg. The purpose of this staging system is to help distinguish mild hypertension from more severe hypertension where more immediate and extensive evaluation is indicated (Table 1) *(1)*. School-based screenings report an incidence of Stage 1 hypertension in 2.6% and Stage 2 hypertension in 0.6% in adolescent students when blood pressure was measured on three separate occasions *(2)*. While the width of the blood pressure range in Stage 1 hypertension is 12–15 mmHg, individuals with Stage 2 hypertension may have a blood pressure level just a few or many mmHg above the Stage 2 limit. Patients with Stage 1 or 2 hypertension may be asymptomatic or have a range of clinical signs or symptoms *(3)*.

The terminology used to further categorize severe hypertension as a hypertensive crisis, emergency, or urgency has not been rigorously defined in childhood. The most recent report of the Joint National Committee on Detection, Evaluation and Treatment of Hypertension, JNC 7, considers blood pressure values above 180/120 mmHg in adults to constitute a "hypertensive crisis" *(4,5)*. This is a value 20 mmHg above the lower limit for Stage 2 hypertension in adults. While there is no absolute level of blood pressure that constitutes a hypertensive crisis in childhood or adolescence, values would be expected, as with adults, to usually exceed the Stage 2 limit.

Hypertensive emergencies and hypertensive urgencies are considered to be two forms of a hypertensive crisis. Severe hypertension with the presence of life-threatening symptoms or target-organ injury defines a hypertensive emergency. In a hypertensive urgency, the blood pressure could be similarly elevated, but less significant symptoms would be present and no acute target-organ injury *(5,6)*. For example, a hypertensive child presenting with encephalopathy or heart failure would be considered as experiencing a hypertensive emergency while a hypertensive teenager with a headache and vomiting would be classified as experiencing a hypertensive urgency. Perioperative hypertension is also considered to be a hypertensive urgency *(5,6)*.

Other terms have also been used to describe severe hypertension. "Accelerated hypertension" is used to describe a recent significant rise over baseline blood pressure that is associated with target-organ damage. "Malignant hypertension" describes the association of elevated BP in association with encephalopathy or nephropathy. This term, however, has been removed from National and International Blood Pressure Control guidelines and is best referred to as a hypertensive emergency *(5,6)*. In the International Classification of Diseases (ICD 9) coding system, "malignant hypertension" refers to any situation with severe high arterial blood pressure and not just to elevated BP associated with encephalopathy or nephropathy *(7)*. This term is no longer a coding modifier in the proposed ICD 10 system. Confusion regarding the definitions and use of these terms has led some authors to avoid the distinction between hypertensive emergencies or urgencies and consider a classification scheme of severe hypertension with or without severe symptoms or end-organ injury *(8,9)*.

ORGAN SYSTEMS SUSCEPTIBLE TO HYPERTENSIVE INJURY

Damage to organs in a hypertensive emergency may involve the brain (seizures, focal deficits, hemorrhage), eye (papilledema, hemorrhages, exudates), kidneys (renal insufficiency), and heart (congestive heart failure). Reports dating back to the 1960s have demonstrated an association between severely elevated blood pressure and hypertensive target-organ damage in children. In 1963, Still and Cottom reviewed their experience with 55 children with severely elevated blood pressure (diastolic BP > 120 mmHg) and evidence of cardiomegaly on clinical exam or left ventricular hypertrophy on electrocardiogram (ECG) *(10)*. Neurologic complications (facial palsy, convulsions, cerebrovascular lesions) were present in one-third of these patients and papilledema in 36%. Unfortunately, due to the lack of effective therapy, 31 of 55 (56%) died as a result of complications from hypertension. In a 1992 report by Deal, 82 of 110 children (75%) requiring "emergent" treatment for an average blood pressure of 180/127 mmHg had evidence of injury to at least one organ system (Table 2). Fortunately, long-term outcome was improved with only 4% experiencing sustained neurologic damage *(11)*. Another report from 1987 on 27 children and adolescents with renovascular hypertension with mean BP at presentation of 172/114 mmHg (age 5 months to 20 years) found that 85% had evidence of target-organ abnormalities *(12)*. Eighteen of 27 (66%) had left ventricular hypertrophy by ECG, 16 of 27 (60%) had retinal vascular lesions, and 3 of 27 (11%) had renal failure.

Table 2
Signs and Symptoms of Hypertensive Emergencies

Hypertensive retinopathy	27%
Hypertensive encephalopathy	25%
Convulsions	25%
Left ventricular hypertrophy	13%
Facial palsy	12%
Visual symptoms	9%
Hemiplegia	8%
Cranial bruits	5%
BP > 99th% without organ damage	24%

BP, blood pressure.
Adapted from *(11)*.

ETIOLOGIES OF SEVERE HYPERTENSION

In contrast to adults where uncontrolled primary hypertension is the most common etiology of hypertensive emergencies, severe hypertension in children is generally considered to be secondary to disorders of the kidney, heart, or endocrine systems *(13,14)*. Older case series have reported renal problems as the cause of hypertensive emergencies or urgencies in children in over 80% of patients *(11)*. A more recent series of children treated with an intravenous antihypertensive agent reported that 55% had associated renal disease *(15)*.

With the increasing presence of primary hypertension in adolescence, this may become a more frequent etiology of severe hypertension in the future.

The etiologies of severe hypertension in children may vary with age and parallel the underlying causes of hypertension in each age group *(16)*. In neonates, renovascular disease secondary to an aortic or renal thrombus related to an umbilical artery catheter is a common cause of a hypertensive emergency as well as congenital renal anomalies and coarctation of the aorta. Outside of the newborn period, children may have renal parenchymal disease such as glomerulonephritis or reflux nephropathy or renovascular disease or endocrine disease. In adolescents, renal parenchymal diseases may also be seen, but additional causes of severe hypertension may include pre-eclampsia and drug intoxication (cocaine, amphetamines). While most adults presenting to the emergency department with severe hypertension have a known diagnosis of hypertension (80%) *(17)*, this would appear to be less common in childhood. Among adults with known hypertension, common reasons for severe BP elevation may include running out of medication (16%) and noncompliance (12%). These circumstances may also occur in childhood. Fluid overload in dialysis patients may be another cause for severe symptomatic hypertension *(18,19)*. Abrupt withdrawal of either a beta-blocker or clonidine may result in "rebound" hypertension that may require urgent intervention *(20)*.

PATHOPHYSIOLOGY

One of the key homeostatic mechanisms to prevent organ injury is autoregulation. While present in many tissues, autoregulation of cerebral blood flow is the most well studied *(21,22)*. This mechanism attempts to maintain a constant cerebral blood flow in the presence of a broad range of perfusion pressures. This constancy occurs due to cerebral arteriolar vasoconstriction with increasing perfusion pressure and vasodilatation with decreasing perfusion pressure. Other factors influencing cerebral blood flow include cerebral metabolic demand and blood oxygen and carbon dioxide content *(23)*. In adults, autoregulation appears to be present over the mean arterial pressure range from 60 to 150 mmHg *(24)*. Autoregulation appears early in development and is present in later fetal and neonatal lambs and neonatal dogs and humans *(25,26)*. While the autoregulation limits in the human preterm and full-term newborn have not been established with certainty, the approximate range appears to be from 25 to 50 mmHg mean arterial pressure *(25)*. The autoregulatory plateau appears to be more narrow in the newborn and increases with maturation. Autoregulation is rendered inoperative by factors leading to pronounced cerebral vasodilatation (hypercarbia, hypoxia, hypoglycemia, postasphyxial state). In these situations, cerebral blood flow becomes pressure-passive, increasing susceptibility to hyperperfusion with increased cerebral perfusion pressure and ischemia with lower perfusion pressure *(25)*.

In adults with uncontrolled chronic hypertension, there is a shift in the autoregulatory curve, providing constant cerebral blood flow at higher mean arterial pressures *(24)*. This shift may develop as a result of structural changes in the cerebral vasculature. While protecting against hyperperfusion at severely elevated blood pressure, this shift in the limits of autoregulation may lead to cerebral ischemia if blood pressure is rapidly lowered to a normotensive level. In acute hypertension, this shift in the autoregulatory curve has not occurred, making individuals more susceptible to hyperperfusion states at high pressures, but less susceptible to ischemia when BP is rapidly reduced to the normal range. While differences exist in cerebral autoregulation between healthy boys and girls and adolescents and adults *(27–29)*, the effects of chronic hypertension on developmental differences in cerebral autoregulation during childhood and adolescence remain unknown.

When blood pressure exceeds the upper limits of the autoregulatory range, the compensatory response of vasoconstriction is inadequate and cerebral blood flow increases proportionately with the mean arterial pressure. This leads to forced vasodilatation, endothelial dysfunction, and edema formation as fluid is forced through the capillary walls of the blood–brain barrier resulting in the development of hypertensive encephalopathy *(30)*. This impairment in autoregulation has been demonstrated in severely hypertensive adults *(31)*, and studies have demonstrated differential effects of antihypertensive agents on cerebral blood flow during blood pressure reduction *(32)*. Recent studies have demonstrated a role for the delta protein kinase C (δ(delta)PKC) signaling pathway on alterations in endothelial cell tight junctions in the blood–brain barrier (BBB) in hypertensive encephalopathy *(33,34)*. Inhibition of δ(delta)PKC led to stability of the BBB in a hypertensive rat model, suggesting this may be a therapeutic target for prevention of BBB disruption in this condition.

The mechanisms of hypertension leading to development of hypertensive emergencies often involve the renin–angiotensin–aldosterone system *(9,35–37)*. These have been reviewed in detail elsewhere *(38)*. High renin and aldosterone are often found in renovascular and other renal causes of hypertension. Activation of this system leads to vasoconstriction via angiotensin II production and sodium retention through the effects of aldosterone on the kidneys. Angiotensin II may also promote endothelial dysfunction and increased expression of proinflammatory cytokines such as NF-Kβ(beta). Other mechanisms leading to severe blood pressure elevation may include fluid overload, as may occur in acute kidney injury or chronic kidney disease, activation of the sympathetic nervous system by secretion of vasoactive substances as in a pheochromocytoma and medications *(39)*.

CLINICAL PRESENTATION

Children with severe hypertension may present with major symptoms or be asymptomatic *(3)*. After confirming that blood pressure has been measured with the proper size cuff and technique, the initial history and physical exam should focus on symptoms and signs of end-organ damage *(40,41)*. These may include central nervous system findings such as a change in behavior, seizures, vision changes, headache, altered mental status, confusion, focal weakness, or other neurologic signs. Orthopnea, shortness of breath, and edema may suggest congestive heart failure and hematuria, flank pain, "cola-colored" urine, and oliguria suggest renal disease.

Signs of end-organ damage may include those of hypertensive encephalopathy including lethargy, confusion, and coma *(42,43)*. Facial nerve palsy has also been a CNS finding in children with a hypertensive emergency *(44–47)*. Hemorrhages or exudates and papilledema are frequently reported on fundoscopic exam *(48–50)*. Tachypnea, pulmonary edema, a gallop rhythm, or a new heart murmur may suggest congestive heart failure. Additional signs may include peripheral edema suggesting fluid overload in renal disease or an abdominal bruit suggesting renovascular hypertension. Exopthalmos may be associated with hyperthyroidism and an abdominal mass may be seen with Wilm's tumor, polycystic kidney disease, neuroblastoma, or congenital renal anomalies *(51,52)*. Skin lesions such as café-au-lait spots and axillary freckling may suggest neurofibromatosis which may be associated with renovascular hypertension or pheochromocytoma *(53)*. Diminished femoral pulses or reduced blood pressure in the legs suggest coarctation of the aorta *(40)*. It is also important to look for signs of child abuse or other CNS trauma which may lead to hypertension through the development of increased intracranial pressure as these situations require therapy directed to preserve the cerebral perfusion pressure and should not be managed with antihypertensive medications *(35)*.

EVALUATION OF CHILDREN WITH HYPERTENSIVE CRISES

The evaluation of children with a hypertensive emergency should include a urinalysis to look for hematuria and proteinuria as evidence of underlying renal disease. Electrolytes, blood urea nitrogen, and creatinine should be measured to evaluate renal function. A complete blood count should be obtained to look for evidence of a microangiopathic hemolytic anemia *(54)*. Adolescent girls should have a pregnancy test as pre-eclampsia may present with severely elevated blood pressure *(55)*. A chest radiograph can screen for cardiac hypertrophy and vascular congestion. An echocardiogram is also helpful if heart failure is suspected or to look for left ventricular hypertrophy, but should not delay the institution of therapy. A urine toxicology screen may be considered in some clinical settings as well as a renal ultrasound to evaluate for renal causes of hypertension *(56,57)*. If signs of encephalopathy are present, a computed tomography study of the head should be obtained to evaluate cerebral edema, intracranial hemorrhage, and stroke and to differentiate hypertensive encephalopathy from intracranial injury or mass lesion. More complex studies such as brain magnetic resonance imaging can be performed at a later date to evaluate for edema of white matter in the parieto-occipital regions as seen in posterior reversible leukoencephalopathy syndrome (PRES) *(58–63)*. If renovascular hypertension is suspected, other imaging modalities such as computed tomography angiography, magnetic resonance angiography, or direct renal angiography may be considered after blood pressure is stabilized *(57,64,65)*.

TREATMENT OF SEVERE HYPERTENSION

The patient with a hypertensive emergency ideally should be managed in the intensive care unit where careful monitoring of blood pressure and neurologic status is possible. Blood pressure should be measured frequently, preferably by continuous intra-arterial monitoring. Initiation of treatment should not be delayed, however, for arterial cannulation. Frequent automated oscillometric or manual auscultatory readings may be adequate methods of blood pressure measurement initially. Noninvasive blood pressure measurements would be adequate as well for most patients with a hypertensive urgency. The airway, breathing, and circulation status of the patient should be frequently assessed and endotracheal intubation performed if mental status is depressed or in the presence of respiratory failure. Seizures should be stopped with anticonvulsants such as lorazepam. Two intravenous access lines should be present to prevent sudden loss of access for antihypertensive medications *(35)*.

A number of antihypertensive medications are available with established efficacy *(66)*. Unfortunately, few have undergone rigorous testing in children and less than half of current IV antihypertensive agents marketed in the USA have pediatric labeling *(9)*. There have been no randomized clinical trials of management of pediatric hypertensive emergencies to evaluate the optimal medication and rate or degree of blood pressure reduction. Meta-analysis of adult studies also fails to prove beneficial effects of treatment on morbidity and mortality *(67)*. Most of these trials, however, involved small numbers of patients with differing definitions for enrollment and outcome, treatment regimens, and length of follow-up

(68). Optimal treatment will remain more opinion- than evidenced based until additional studies have been completed.

Adult and pediatric guidelines recommend that blood pressure be reduced in a controlled manner in hypertensive emergencies with continuous intravenous medications *(1,4).* Evidence supporting this view includes a report by Deal et al. comparing treatment complications in 53 children receiving intravenous labetalol and/or sodium nitroprusside infusion as compared with an earlier time period in 57 children of intravenous bolus injection of diazoxide and/or hydralazine. About 23% of patients treated with bolus therapy versus 4% of those treated with infusions experienced complications. All seven children with permanent neurologic injury were treated with bolus therapy *(11).*

The goal for antihypertensive treatment in children is to reduce blood pressure to <95th percentile, unless concurrent conditions such as cardiac or renal disease or diabetes are present when BP should be lowered to <90th percentile *(1).* As noted above, children with chronic uncontrolled hypertension may be at much greater risk than those with acute hypertension to have decreased cerebral blood flow and ischemia with rapid normalization of blood pressure. The Fourth Report on the Diagnosis, Evaluation, and Treatment of High Blood Pressure in Children and Adolescents recommends lowering blood pressure by ≤25% in the first 8 h after presentation and then gradually normalizing the blood pressure over 26–48 h to prevent complications of treatment *(1).* In a hypertensive urgency, evaluation should occur immediately and treatment begun to lower BP over a course of hours to days with either intravenous or oral antihypertensives depending on the child's symptomatology.

Intravenous antihypertensives which have proven most useful in treating severe hypertension include nicardipine, labetolol, sodium nitroprusside, and hydralazine. Additional intravenous agents which may be occasionally useful include esmolol, fenoldopam, and possibly enalaprilat. Oral medications recommended for acute hypertensive urgencies include clonidine, isradipine, and minoxidil. Each of these will be reviewed below. Suggested doses for these agents can be found in Table 3.

Diazoxide, an intravenous direct vasodilator used frequently in the past by bolus injection *(69–71),* is no longer recommended as a first-line antihypertensive agent for hypertensive emergencies *(1)* due to a long half-life and unpredictable duration of action *(9,72).* Use of short-acting nifedipine has been abandoned in adults *(73)* due to significant adverse events, but continues to be used by some pediatric centers. While single and multicenter retrospective reviews have suggested this medication is safe and effective with in-hospital use *(74–76),* others have pointed to difficulties in accurately dosing this medication, availability of other medications, and reports of adverse neurologic events as evidence against its continued use *(77–82).* Short-acting nifedipine is not included in the Fourth Report on the Diagnosis, Evaluation, and Treatment of High Blood Pressure in Children and Adolescents for treatment of hypertension *(1).*

Sodium nitroprusside, a direct vasodilator of arteriolar and venous smooth muscle cells, has been used for treatment of severe hypertension in childhood since the 1970s *(83,84).* The recommended dosage by continuous infusion is 0.53–10 µg/kg/min *(1).* Nitroprusside acts by releasing nitric oxide which dilates arterioles and venules and reduces total peripheral resistance. This decreases preload and afterload, allowing use of this agent for severe congestive heart failure as well as in severe hypertension. Use may result in modest tachycardia. Nitroprusside has a rapid onset of action within 30 s which results in rapid lowering of blood pressure. The antihypertensive effect disappears within a few minutes of stopping the medication *(85).* Toxicity occurs as a result of the metabolism of nitroprusside

Table 3
Antihypertensive Drugs for Treatment of Severe Hypertension

Drug	Class	Dose	Route	Comments
Emergencies (severe hypertension with life-threatening symptoms)				
Esmolol	β(beta)-blocker	100–500 µg/kg/min	IV infusion	Very short-acting; constant infusion. May cause bradycardia
Hydralazine[a]	Vasodilator	0.2–0.6 mg/kg/dose	IV bolus or IM	Causes reflex tachycardia, headaches, fluid retention
Labetolol	α(alpha)- and β(beta)-blocker	Bolus: 0.2–1 mg/kg/dose up to 40 mg/dose Infusion: 0.25–3 mg/kg/h	IV infusion or bolus	Use with caution in asthma, heart failure. Preferred in neurologic emergency
Nicardipine	Calcium channel blocker	1–2 µg/kg/min	IV infusion	May cause reflex tachycardia. Preferred in neurologic emergency
Sodium nitroprusside	Vasodilator	0.53–10 µg/kg/min	IV infusion	Associated with cyanide, thiocyanate toxicity. Monitor levels with (>48 h) use or in hepatic or renal dysfunction
Urgencies (severe hypertension with less significant symptoms)				
Clonidine[b]	Central α(alpha)-agonist	0.05–0.1 mg/kg/dose may be repeated up to 0.8 mg total dose	po	Side effects include sedation, dry mouth
Enalaprilat	ACE inhibitor	0.05–0.1 mg/kg/dose up to 1.25 mg/dose	IV bolus	May cause prolonged hypotension, oliguria, and hyperkalemia
Fenoldopam	Dopamine receptor agonist	0.2–0.8 µg/kg/min	IV infusion	Produced modest reduction in BP in a pediatric clinical trial up to age 12 years
Isradipine	Calcium channel blocker	0.05–0.1 mg/kg/dose	po	Stable suspension can be compounded
Minoxidil	Vasodilator	0.1–0.2 mg/kg/dose	po	Most potent oral vasodilator, long-acting

IV, indicated intravenous; IM, intramuscular; po, oral; ACE, angiotensin-converting enzyme; HTN, hypertension.

[a]May be used in initial treatment of hypertensive emergency at 0.1 mg/kg dose.

[b]Limited reported pediatric experience, smaller doses may be needed in younger children.

Adapted from (1).

to cyanide and thiocyanate. Toxic accumulation of cyanide leads to development of metabolic acidosis with elevated lactate levels, tachycardia, altered consciousness, dilated pupils, and methemoglobinemia. Cyanide levels (toxic > 2 μg/mL) should be monitored in the setting of hepatic dysfunction *(86)*. Thiocyanate toxicity is suggested by symptoms of altered mental status, nausea, seizures, skin rash, psychosis, anorexia, or coma *(72)*. Thiocyanate levels should be monitored daily if used for >48 h, with dosages above 4 μg/kg/min or with renal dysfunction. Levels should be less than 50 mg/L. The nitroprusside infusion should be discontinued if signs and symptoms of cyanide or thiocyanate toxicity are present. Thiosulfate administration may facilitate the conversion of cyanide to thiocyanate by donating a sulfur group *(72)*, which may lessen the risk of toxicity. Most authorities recommend limiting nitroprusside use to situations where no other suitable agents are available or to brief periods of time *(6,9)*.

Labetolol is a combined α(alpha)$_1$ and β(beta)-adrenergic blocking agent. When given intravenously, rather than orally, it may allow for controlled reduction in blood pressure *(87)*. The α(alpha)$_1$ blocking effect leads to vasodilatation and reduced peripheral vascular resistance with little effect on cardiac output. Due to its β(beta)-blocking effects, heart rate is usually maintained or slightly reduced. Hypotensive effects of a single dose appear within 2–5 min, peak at 5–15 min, and last up to 2–4 h *(87)*. The medication is metabolized by the liver and elimination is not altered by renal dysfunction. Labetolol is 3–7 times more potent as a β-blocker than α(alpha)-blocker *(87)*. The beta effects may lead to bronchospasm and bradycardia and use of labetolol is contraindicated in acute left ventricular failure. It should be used with caution in diabetic patients as it may prevent the signs and symptoms of hypoglycemia. It is recommended for hypertension management in neurologic emergencies such as hypertensive encephalopathy as it does not increase intracranial pressure *(88,89)*. As compared with sodium nitroprusside, systemic and cerebral vascular resistance are decreased proportionally, maintaining cerebral blood flow to a greater extent with labetolol *(32)*. Case series in children have demonstrated its usefulness in the pediatric population *(11,90)*. Labetalol may be given as a bolus of 0.2–1 mg/kg/dose up to a 40 mg maximum dose or as a continuous infusion of 0.25–3 mg/kg/h with a maximum 24 h dose of 300 mg *(1,6)*.

Nicardipine, a second-generation dihydropyridine calcium channel blocker, has greater selectivity for vascular smooth muscle than cardiac myocytes. It has strong cerebral and coronary vasodilatory activity and minimal inotropic cardiac effects leading to favorable effects on myocardial oxygen balance *(91)*. Efficacy in reducing blood pressure was similar to IV sodium nitroprusside in adults. Modest tachycardia may be seen with the use of this agent. Onset of action with this medication is rapid within 1–2 min and duration of action of a single dose is 3 h. Nicardipine undergoes liver metabolism and the dosage is unaffected by renal dysfunction. Like labetolol, it is recommended for hypertension management in neurologic emergencies such as hypertensive encephalopathy as it does not increase intracranial pressure *(88,89)*.

The effectiveness of nicardipine in childhood has been shown in a number of pediatric series involving children as young as age 9 days to age 18 years *(92–98)*. It has proven to be safe and is generally well tolerated. The recommended pediatric dosage is 1–3 μg/kg/min *(1)*. Like most other agents, it has not been evaluated by clinical trials in the pediatric population. A multicenter trial was recently terminated when the drug was sold by the sponsor of the trial. Reported adverse effects include headache, hypotension, nausea, and vomiting. The manufacturer recommends that IV nicardipine be administered by continuous infusion at a concentration of 0.1 mg/mL. Studies have shown stability when mixed at concentrations of 0.5 mg/mL thus enabling critically ill patients to be administered smaller volumes of the drug *(99).* Phlebitis has been reported at the site of administration with higher dosage concentrations *(95),* suggesting the medication should in this situation be given through a central line.

Hydralazine is a direct vasodilator of arteriolar smooth muscle. The mechanism of action is unclear, although it may involve alterations in intracellular calcium metabolism *(85).* Hydralazine-induced vasodilatation leads to stimulation of the sympathetic nervous system resulting in tachycardia, increased renin release, and fluid retention. The onset of action is within 5–30 min after intravenous administration *(72).* Average maximum decrease in blood pressure occurs 10–80 min after intravenous administration *(9).* This medication can be given intramuscularly. The recommended dosage for pediatric patients is 0.1–0.6 mg/kg/dose given intravenously every 4–6 h *(1,86).* Given as a bolus rather than continuous intravenous medication, hydralazine may be more useful in an individual with a hypertensive urgency that is unable to tolerate oral medications than in a hypertensive emergency. An intravenous dosage of 0.1 mg/kg could be used as an initial step for blood pressure reduction in an emergency situation until a medication such as labetolol or nicardipine has been prepared by the hospital pharmacy.

Esmolol is an ultrashort-acting cardioselective β(beta)-blocking agent. Onset of action with this medication is within 60 s with offset of action in 10–20 min. Metabolism of this agent is by rapid hydrolysis of ester linkages by RBC esterases and is not dependent on hepatic or renal function. Pharmacokinetics of this agent in children did not differ from adults *(100,101).* A trial in children with coarctation of the aorta included 116 patients less than age 6 years who received esmolol at low (125 µg/kg), medium (250 µg/kg), or high dose (500 µg/kg). Systolic blood pressure decreased significantly from baseline on averaged by 6–12.2 mmHg by group, but failed to show a dose–response relationship. Heart rate reduction ranged 7.4–13.2 beats/min by group and no serious adverse events occurred *(101).* Pediatric studies with this agent in noncardiac conditions have not been reported.

Fenoldopam is a dopamine D_1 receptor agonist that does not act at D_2 receptors. This leads to vasodilatation of renal, coronary, and cerebral arteries as well as peripheral vasodilatation. Onset of action is within 5 min with 50% of the maximal blood pressuring lowering effect occurring within 15 min and maximal effect by 1 h. The duration of action after stopping the medication is 30–60 min. This medication has been effective in reducing blood pressure in adults with hypertensive emergencies where it has proven to be as effective as nitroprusside *(6,102).* It has also been used as a renal protective drug in critically ill adult and pediatric patients *(102,103).* One pediatric trial conducted in 77 children aged 1 month to 12 years undergoing controlled hypotension during surgery compared response to one of the four doses of fenoldopam (0.05, 0.2, 0.8, or 3.2 µg/kg/min) *(104).* Dosages of 0.8 and 3.2 µg/kg/min significantly decreased blood pressure but resulted in increases in heart rate of 9–17 beats/min. The effective dose range appeared to be higher (0.8–1.2 µg/kg/min) than as labeled for adults (0.05–0.3 µg/kg/min). Only a single case report of use of this agent for a hypertensive emergency in childhood has been reported *(105).*

Enalaprilat, an intravenous angiotensin-converting enzyme (ACE) inhibitor, produces vasodilatation and decreases peripheral vascular resistance. Onset of action is 30–60 min and duration of action is 4–6 h. Elimination is primarily renal, and dosage adjustment is needed if the patient has renal impairment. Blood pressure reduction is variable, and hypotension may occur more often in high renin states *(6).* One pediatric case series in ten premature neonates receiving doses of 7.4–22.9 µg/kg per 24 h demonstrated a reduction in mean arterial pressure within 30 min of enalaprilate administration that persisted generally for a median of 12 h *(106)*. Side effects included hypotension, oliguria, elevated serum creatinine, and transient hyperkalemia in some infants. Given the higher baseline plasma renin activity, and incidence of renovascular hypertension in childhood, this medication is infrequently used in the pediatric age group.

Clevidipine is a new, third-generation calcium channel blocking agent recently approved for use in adults with severe hypertension. This medication inhibits L-type calcium channels, thus relaxing vascular smooth muscle in small arteries resulting in a reduction of peripheral vascular resistance. Onset of action is 2–4 min with offset of effect in 5–15 min. Like esmolol, this medication is rapidly metabolized by RBC esterases and not affected by hepatic or renal function *(107)*. Clevidipine by continuous infusion effectively reduced BP in adult cardiac surgery patients and was more effective at maintaining systolic BP within preset target limits than intravenous nitroglycerin or nitroprusside in preoperative patients. It was as effective as nicardipine in the postoperative setting. In adults with acute severe hypertension, clevidipine lowered blood pressure in most patients (88.9%) to the prescribed target within 30 min of initiation of treatment *(108)*. Pediatric studies with this agent are expected in the near future.

Clonidine is a centrally acting α(alpha)$_2$-adrenergic agonist which decreases cerebral sympathetic outflow. Its onset of action is 30–60 min after administration and duration is 6–8 h. It should be avoided in patients with altered mental status because of its common side effect of drowsiness. Other complications of this therapy may include dry mouth, occasional dizziness, and the development of hypertensive crisis upon abrupt discontinuation of therapy *(20)*. Oral clonidine loading in adults utilizes an initial dosage of 0.1–0.2 mg followed by hourly dosages of 0.05–0.1 mg until goal BP is achieved or a total of 0.7 mg has been given. This approach to treatment of severe hypertension is reported to be successful at reaching target BP in 93% of adult patients *(109)*. Hypotension occurred more often in volume-depleted patients. Average total dose requirements have ranged in studies from 0.26 to 0.45 mg. While published reports of clonidine treatment in childhood is limited to chronic oral or transdermal therapy in adolescents *(110,111)*, suggested dosages for severe hypertension in children have been given *(1)*.

Isradipine is a second-generation dihydropyridine calcium channel blocker which acts selectively on L-type channels on vascular smooth muscle, but not myocardial cells. Because it does not affect myocardial contractility, it can be used in patients with decreased myocardial function *(112)*. Onset of action is by 1 h with peak effect at 2–3 h when administered orally *(113)*. Medication half-life is 3–8 h. A stable extemporaneous suspension of isradipine may be compounded for use in small children *(114)*. Several pediatric series of the use of this medication for management of hypertension have been reported *(115–117)*. Isradipine given sublingually to 27 adults with severe hypertension demonstrated a reduction of mean arterial pressure of 22% by 2 h *(118)*. A recent report in 218 children with acute hypertension receiving isradipine at a mean dosage of 0.08 mg/kg (0.02–0.22 mg/kg) demonstrated a median decrease in systolic BP of 15.7% and diastolic BP of 23.4%. The greatest decrease in BP was observed in children below age 2 years. Higher dosages were associated with more frequent drop in mean arterial pressure >25%. The most common adverse events included vomiting, nausea, and headache *(119)*.

Minoxidil, an oral antihypertensive, is metabolized to minoxidil sulfate which opens K^+ channels in vascular smooth muscle cells permitting K^+ efflux, hyperpolarization, and relaxation of smooth muscle. This produces arteriolar vasodilatation and a reduction in BP and peripheral vascular resistance. Peak concentrations of minoxidil occur 1 h after oral administration, though the peak antihypertensive effect is later, possibly due to delayed formation of the active metabolite. Duration of action may be up to 24 h. Tachycardia may develop with minoxidil use as well as salt and water retention *(85)*. Reported use in childhood includes severe chronic hypertension refractory to other medications and for acute BP elevations in children with chronic hypertension *(120,121)*.

CONCLUSION

Severe, symptomatic hypertension requires immediate evaluation and rapid institution of antihypertensive therapy. Use of continuous infusions is recommended to allow BP reduction in a controlled manner, avoiding overly aggressive therapy that may also lead to ischemia and further injury. A number of medications are available, although much remains to be learned about optimal treatment of this condition in childhood.

REFERENCES

1. National High Blood Pressure Education Program Working Group on High Blood Pressure in Children and Adolescents. The fourth report on the diagnosis, evaluation, and treatment of high blood pressure in children and adolescents. National Institute or Health publication 05:5267. Bethesda, MD: National Heart, Lung, and Blood Institute; 2005.
2. McNiece KL, Poffenbarger TS, Turner JL, et al. Prevalence of hypertension and pre-hypertension among adolescents. J Pediatr. 2007;150(6):640–644, 644.e1.
3. Croix B, Feig DI. Childhood hypertension is not a silent disease. Pediatr Nephrol. 2006;21(4):527–532.
4. Chobanian AV, Bakris GL, Black HR, et al. Seventh report of the joint national committee on prevention, detection, evaluation, and treatment of high blood pressure. Hypertension. 2003;42(6):1206–1252.
5. Varon J. Treatment of acute severe hypertension: current and newer agents. Drugs. 2008;68(3):283–297.
6. Marik PE, Varon J. Hypertensive crises: challenges and management. Chest. 2007;131(6):1949–1962.
7. I C D-9-C M Guidelines, Conversions & Tabular, 6th edn. 2008. Available at http://www.cdc.gov/nchs/datawh/ftpserv/ftpicd9/ftpicd9.htm [Accessed March 5, 2009].
8. Adelman RD, Coppo R, Dillon MJ. The emergency management of severe hypertension. Pediatr Nephrol. 2000;14(5):422–427.
9. Flynn J, Tullus K. Severe hypertension in children and adolescents: pathophysiology and treatment. Pediatr Nephrol. 2009;24(6):1101–1112.
10. Still JL, Cottom D. Severe hypertension in childhood. Arch Dis Child. 1967;42(221):34–39.
11. Deal JE, Barratt TM, Dillon MJ. Management of hypertensive emergencies. Arch Dis Child. 1992;67(9):1089–1092.
12. Daniels SR, Loggie JM, McEnery PT, Towbin RB. Clinical spectrum of intrinsic renovascular hypertension in children. Pediatrics. 1987;80(5):698–704.
13. Groshong T. Hypertensive crisis in children. Pediatr Ann. 1996;25(7):368–371, 375–376.
14. Fivush B, Neu A, Furth S. Acute hypertensive crises in children: emergencies and urgencies. Curr Opin Pediatr. 1997;9(3):233–236.
15. Flynn JT, Mottes TA, Brophy PD, et al. Intravenous nicardipine for treatment of severe hypertension in children. J Pediatr. 2001;139(1):38–43.
16. Constantine E, Linakis J. The assessment and management of hypertensive emergencies and urgencies in children. Pediatr Emerg Care. 2005;21(6):391–396; quiz 397.
17. Bender SR, Fong MW, Heitz S, Bisognano JD. Characteristics and management of patients presenting to the emergency department with hypertensive urgency. J Clin Hypertens (Greenwich). 2006;8(1):12–18.
18. Sorof JM, Brewer ED, Portman RJ. Ambulatory blood pressure monitoring and interdialytic weight gain in children receiving chronic hemodialysis. Am J Kidney Dis. 1999;33(4):667–674.
19. Mitsnefes M, Stablein D. Hypertension in pediatric patients on long-term dialysis: a report of the North American Pediatric Renal Transplant Cooperative Study (NAPRTCS). Am J Kidney Dis. 2005;45(2):309–315.
20. Geyskes GG, Boer P, Dorhout Mees EJ. Clonidine withdrawal. Mechanism and frequency of rebound hypertension. Br J Clin Pharmacol. 1979;7(1):55–62.
21. Strandgaard S, Olesen J, Skinhoj E, Lassen NA. Autoregulation of brain circulation in severe arterial hypertension. Br Med J. 1973;1(5852):507–510.

22. Strandgaard S, Paulson OB. Cerebral autoregulation. Stroke. 1984;15(3):413–416.
23. Vavilala MS, Lee LA, Lam AM. Cerebral blood flow and vascular physiology. Anesthesiol Clin North Am. 2002;20(2):247–264, v.
24. Paulson OB, Waldemar G, Schmidt JF, Strandgaard S. Cerebral circulation under normal and pathologic conditions. Am J Cardiol. 1989;63(6):2C–5C.
25. Volpe JJ. Hypoxic-ischemic encephalopathy: biochemical and physiological aspects. In: Neurology of the Newborn, 5th ed. Philadelphia, PA: Saunders Elsevier; 2008:291–324.
26. Pryds O, Edwards AD. Cerebral blood flow in the newborn infant. Arch Dis Child Fetal Neonatal Ed. 1996;74(1):F63–F69.
27. Vavilala MS, Newell DW, Junger E, et al. Dynamic cerebral autoregulation in healthy adolescents. Acta Anaesthesiol Scand. 2002;46(4):393–397.
28. Vavilala MS, Kincaid MS, Muangman SL, et al. Gender differences in cerebral blood flow velocity and autoregulation between the anterior and posterior circulations in healthy children. Pediatr Res. 2005;58(3):574–578.
29. Tontisirin N, Muangman SL, Suz P, et al. Early childhood gender differences in anterior and posterior cerebral blood flow velocity and autoregulation. Pediatrics. 2007;119(3):e610–e615.
30. Gardner CJ, Lee K. Hyperperfusion syndromes: insight into the pathophysiology and treatment of hypertensive encephalopathy. CNS Spectr. 2007;12(1):35–42.
31. Immink RV, van den Born BH, van Montfrans GA, et al. Impaired cerebral autoregulation in patients with malignant hypertension. Circulation. 2004;110(15):2241–2245.
32. Immink RV, van den Born BH, van Montfrans GA, et al. Cerebral hemodynamics during treatment with sodium nitroprusside versus labetalol in malignant hypertension. Hypertension. 2008;52(2):236–240.
33. Qi X, Inagaki K, Sobel RA, Mochly-Rosen D. Sustained pharmacological inhibition of deltaPKC protects against hypertensive encephalopathy through prevention of blood-brain barrier breakdown in rats. J Clin Invest. 2008;118(1):173–182.
34. Chou W, Messing RO. Hypertensive encephalopathy and the blood-brain barrier: is deltaPKC a gatekeeper? J Clin Invest. 2008;118(1):17–20.
35. Flynn J. Management of Hypertensive Emergencies and Urgencies in Children. UpToDate. Available at http://www.utdol.com/online/content/topic.do?topicKey=ped_symp/9567&selectedTitle=2~128&source=search_result#1 [Accessed April 20, 2009].
36. Patel HP, Mitsnefes M. Advances in the pathogenesis and management of hypertensive crisis. Curr Opin Pediatr. 2005;17(2):210–214.
37. Blumenfeld JD, Laragh JH. Management of hypertensive crises: the scientific basis for treatment decisions. Am J Hypertens. 2001;14(11 Pt 1):1154–1167.
38. Flynn JT, Woroniecki RP. Pathophysiology of hypertension. In: Avner ED, Harmon WE, Niaudet P, eds. Pediatric Nephrology, 5th ed. Philadelphia, PA: Lippincott Williams & Wilkins; 2004:1153–1177.
39. Grossman E, Messerli FH. Secondary hypertension: interfering substances. J Clin Hypertens (Greenwich). 2008;10(7):556–566.
40. Farine M, Arbus GS. Management of hypertensive emergencies in children. Pediatr Emerg Care. 1989;5(1):51–55.
41. Suresh S, Mahajan P, Kamat D. Emergency management of pediatric hypertension. Clin Pediatr (Phila). 44(9):739–745.
42. Wright RR, Mathews KD. Hypertensive encephalopathy in childhood. J Child Neurol. 1996;11(3):193–196.
43. Hu M, Wang H, Lin K, et al. Clinical experience of childhood hypertensive encephalopathy over an eight year period. Chang Gung Med J. 31(2):153–158.
44. Trompeter RS, Smith RL, Hoare RD, Neville BG, Chantler C. Neurological complications of arterial hypertension. Arch Dis Child. 1982;57(12):913–917.
45. Harms MM, Rotteveel JJ, Kar NC, Gabreëls FJ. Recurrent alternating facial paralysis and malignant hypertension. Neuropediatrics. 2000;31(6):318–320.
46. Lewis VE, Peat DS, Tizard EJ. Hypertension and facial palsy in middle aortic syndrome. Arch Dis Child. 2001;85(3):240–241.
47. Tirodker UH, Dabbagh S. Facial paralysis in childhood hypertension. J Paediatr Child Health. 2001;37(2):193–194.
48. Skalina ME, Annable WL, Kliegman RM, Fanaroff AA. Hypertensive retinopathy in the newborn infant. J Pediatr. 1983;103(5):781–786.
49. Browning AC, Mengher LS, Gregson RM, Amoaku WM. Visual outcome of malignant hypertension in young people. Arch Dis Child. 2001;85(5):401–403.
50. Shroff R, Roebuck DJ, Gordon I, et al. Angioplasty for renovascular hypertension in children: 20-year experience. Pediatrics. 2006;118(1):268–275.

51. Madre C, Orbach D, Baudouin V, et al. Hypertension in childhood cancer: a frequent complication of certain tumor sites. J Pediatr Hematol Oncol. 2006;28(10):659–664.
52. Grinsell M, Norwood V. At the bottom of the differential diagnosis list: unusual causes of pediatric hypertension. Pediatr Nephrol. 2008. 24(11):2137–2146.
53. Fossali E, Signorini E, Intermite RC, et al. Renovascular disease and hypertension in children with neurofibromatosis. Pediatr Nephrol. 2000;14(8–9):806–810.
54. Belsha CW. Pediatric hypertension in the emergency department. Ann Emerg Med. 2008;51(3 Suppl):S21–S23.
55. Barton JR. Hypertension in pregnancy. Ann Emerg Med. 2008;51(3 Suppl):S16–S17.
56. Roth CG, Spottswood SE, Chan JCM, Roth KS. Evaluation of the hypertensive infant: a rational approach to diagnosis. Radiol Clin North Am. 2003;41(5):931–944.
57. Tullus K, Brennan E, Hamilton G, et al. Renovascular hypertension in children. Lancet. 2008;371(9622):1453–1463.
58. Pavlakis SG, Frank Y, Chusid R. Hypertensive encephalopathy, reversible occipitoparietal encephalopathy, or reversible posterior leukoencephalopathy: three names for an old syndrome. J Child Neurol. 1999;14(5):277–281.
59. Kwon S, Koo J, Lee S. Clinical spectrum of reversible posterior leukoencephalopathy syndrome. Pediatr Neurol. 2001;24(5):361–364.
60. Ishikura K, Ikeda M, Hamasaki Y, et al. Posterior reversible encephalopathy syndrome in children: its high prevalence and more extensive imaging findings. Am J Kidney Dis. 2006;48(2):231–238.
61. Prasad N, Gulati S, Gupta RK, et al. Spectrum of radiological changes in hypertensive children with reversible posterior leucoencephalopathy. Br J Radiol. 2007;80(954):422–429.
62. Onder AM, Lopez R, Teomete U, et al. Posterior reversible encephalopathy syndrome in the pediatric renal population. Pediatr Nephrol. 2007;22(11):1921–1929.
63. Sanjay KM, Partha PC. The posterior reversible encephalopathy syndrome. Indian J Pediatr. 2008;75(9):953–955.
64. Shahdadpuri J, Frank R, Gauthier BG, Siegel DN, Trachtman H. Yield of renal arteriography in the evaluation of pediatric hypertension. Pediatr Nephrol. 2000;14(8–9):816–819.
65. Vade A, Agrawal R, Lim-Dunham J, Hartoin D. Utility of computed tomographic renal angiogram in the management of childhood hypertension. Pediatr Nephrol. 2002;17(9):741–747.
66. Cherney D, Straus S. Management of patients with hypertensive urgencies and emergencies: a systematic review of the literature. J Gen Intern Med. 2002;17(12):937–945.
67. Perez MI, Musini VM. Pharmacological interventions for hypertensive emergencies: a Cochrane systematic review. J Hum Hypertens. 2008;22(9):596–607.
68. Messerli FH, Eslava DJ. Treatment of hypertensive emergencies: blood pressure cosmetics or outcome evidence? J Hum Hypertens. 2008;22(9):585–586.
69. Kohaut EC, Wilson CJ, Hill LL. Intravenous diazoxide in acute poststreptococcal glomerulonephritis. J Pediatr. 1975;87(5):795–798.
70. McLaine PN, Drummond KN. Intravenous diazoxide for severe hypertension in childhood. J Pediatr. 1971;79(5):829–832.
71. McCrory WW, Kohaut EC, Lewy JE, Lieberman E, Travis LB. Safety of intravenous diazoxide in children with severe hypertension. Clin Pediatr (Phila). 1979;18(11):661–663, 666–667, 671.
72. Porto I. Hypertensive emergencies in children. J Pediatr Health Care. 14(6):312–317.
73. Grossman E, Messerli FH, Grodzicki T, Kowey P. Should a moratorium be placed on sublingual nifedipine capsules given for hypertensive emergencies and pseudoemergencies? JAMA. 276(16):1328–1331.
74. Blaszak RT, Savage JA, Ellis EN. The use of short-acting nifedipine in pediatric patients with hypertension. J Pediatr. 2001;139(1):34–37.
75. Egger DW, Deming DD, Hamada N, Perkin RM, Sahney S. Evaluation of the safety of short-acting nifedipine in children with hypertension. Pediatr Nephrol. 2002;17(1):35–40.
76. Yiu V, Orrbine E, Rosychuk RJ, et al. The safety and use of short-acting nifedipine in hospitalized hypertensive children. Pediatr Nephrol. 2004;19(6):644–650.
77. Flynn JT. Safety of short-acting nifedipine in children with severe hypertension. Expert Opin Drug Saf. 2003;2(2):133–139.
78. Calvetta A, Martino S, von Vigier RO, et al. "What goes up must immediately come down!" Which indication for short-acting nifedipine in children with arterial hypertension? Pediatr Nephrol. 2003;18(1):1–2.
79. Leonard MB, Kasner SE, Feldman HI, Schulman SL. Adverse neurologic events associated with rebound hypertension after using short-acting nifedipine in childhood hypertension. Pediatr Emerg Care. 2001;17(6):435–437.
80. Castaneda MP, Walsh CA, Woroniecki RP, Del Rio M, Flynn JT. Ventricular arrhythmia following short-acting nifedipine administration. Pediatr Nephrol. 2005;20(7):1000–1002.

81. Truttmann AC, Zehnder-Schlapbach S, Bianchetti MG. A moratorium should be placed on the use of short-acting nifedipine for hypertensive crises. Pediatr Nephrol. 1998;12(3):259.

82. Sasaki R, Hirota K, Masuda A. Nifedipine-induced transient cerebral ischemia in a child with Cockayne syndrome. Anaesthesia. 1997;52(12):1236.

83. Gordillo-Paniagua G, Velásquez-Jones L, Martini R, Valdez-Bolaños E. Sodium nitroprusside treatment of severe arterial hypertension in children. J Pediatr. 1975;87(5):799–802.

84. Luderer JR, Hayes AH, Dubnsky O, Berlin CM. Long-term administration of sodium nitroprusside in childhood. J Pediatr. 1977;91(3):490–491.

85. Hoffman B. Therapy of hypertension. In: Laurence L Brunton, Lazo JS, Parker KL, eds. Goodman & Gillman's the Pharmacological Basis of Therapeutics, 11th ed. New York, NY: McGraw Hill; 2006: 845–868.

86. Robertson J, Shilkofski N, eds. The Harriet Lane Handbook, 17th ed. Philadelphia, PA: Elsevier Mosby; 2005:899.

87. Goa KL, Benfield P, Sorkin EM. Labetalol. A reappraisal of its pharmacology, pharmacokinetics and therapeutic use in hypertension and ischaemic heart disease. Drugs. 1989;37(5):583–627.

88. Rose JC, Mayer SA. Optimizing blood pressure in neurological emergencies. Neurocrit Care. 2004;1(3):287–299.

89. Pancioli AM. Hypertension management in neurological emergencies. Ann Emerg Med. 2008;51(Suppl 3):S24–S27.

90. Bunchman TE, Lynch RE, Wood EG. Intravenously administered labetalol for treatment of hypertension in children. J Pediatr. 1992;120(1):140–144.

91. Curran MP, Robinson DM, Keating GM. Intravenous nicardipine: its use in the short-term treatment of hypertension and various other indications. Drugs. 2006;66(13):1755–1782.

92. Treluyer JM, Hubert P, Jouvet P, Couderc S, Cloup M. Intravenous nicardipine in hypertensive children. Eur J Pediatr. 1993;152(9):712–714.

93. Gouyon JB, Geneste B, Semama DS, Françoise M, Germain JF. Intravenous nicardipine in hypertensive preterm infants. Arch Dis Child Fetal Neonatal Ed. 1997;76(2):F126–F127.

94. Michael J, Groshong T, Tobias JD. Nicardipine for hypertensive emergencies in children with renal disease. Pediatr Nephrol. 1998;12(1):40–42.

95. Tenney F, Sakarcan A. Nicardipine is a safe and effective agent in pediatric hypertensive emergencies. Am J Kidney Dis. 2000;35(5):E20.

96. Milou C, Debuche-Benouachkou V, Semama DS, Germain JF, Gouyon JB. Intravenous nicardipine as a first-line antihypertensive drug in neonates. Intensive Care Med. 2000;26(7):956–958.

97. McBride BF, White CM, Campbell M, Frey BM. Nicardipine to control neonatal hypertension during extracorporeal membrane oxygen support. Ann Pharmacother. 2003;37(5):667–670.

98. Nakagawa TA, Sartori SC, Morris A, Schneider DS. Intravenous nicardipine for treatment of postcoarctectomy hypertension in children. Pediatr Cardiol. 25(1):26–30.

99. Baaske DM, DeMay JF, Latona CA, Mirmira S, Sigvardson KW. Stability of nicardipine hydrochloride in intravenous solutions. Am J Health Syst Pharm. 1996;53(14):1701–1705.

100. Adamson PC, Rhodes LA, Saul JP, et al. The pharmacokinetics of esmolol in pediatric subjects with supraventricular arrhythmias. Pediatr Cardiol. 2006;27(4):420–427.

101. Tabbutt S, Nicolson SC, Adamson PC, et al. The safety, efficacy, and pharmacokinetics of esmolol for blood pressure control immediately after repair of coarctation of the aorta in infants and children: a multicenter, double-blind, randomized trial. J Thorac Cardiovasc Surg. 2008;136(2): 321–328.

102. Murphy MB, Murray C, Shorten GD. Fenoldopam: a selective peripheral dopamine-receptor agonist for the treatment of severe hypertension. N Engl J Med. 2001;345(21):1548–1557.

103. Moffett BS, Mott AR, Nelson DP, Goldstein SL, Jefferies JL. Renal effects of fenoldopam in critically ill pediatric patients: a retrospective review. Pediatr Crit Care Med. 2008;9(4):403–406.

104. Hammer GB, Verghese ST, Drover DR, Yaster M, Tobin JR. Pharmacokinetics and pharmacodynamics of fenoldopam mesylate for blood pressure control in pediatric patients. BMC Anesthesiol. 2008;8:6.

105. Lechner BL, Pascual JF, Roscelli JD. Failure of fenoldopam to control severe hypertension secondary to renal graft rejection in a pediatric patient. Mil Med. 2005;170(2):130–132.

106. Wells TG, Bunchman TE, Kearns GL. Treatment of neonatal hypertension with enalaprilat. J Pediatr. 1990;117(4):664–667.

107. Deeks ED, Keating GM, Keam SJ. Clevidipine: a review of its use in the management of acute hypertension. Am J Cardiovasc Drugs. 2009;9(2):117–134.

108. Pollack CV, Varon J, Garrison NA, et al. Clevidipine, an intravenous dihydropyridine calcium channel blocker, is safe and effective for the treatment of patients with acute severe hypertension. Ann Emerg Med. 2009;53(3):329–338.

109. Houston MC. Treatment of hypertensive emergencies and urgencies with oral clonidine loading and titration. A review. Arch Intern Med. 1986;146(3):586–589.
110. Falkner B, Onesti G, Lowenthal DT, Affrime MB. The use of clonidine monotherapy in adolescent hypertension. Chest. 1983;83(2 Suppl):425–427.
111. Falkner B, Thanki B, Lowenthal DT. Transdermal clonidine in the treatment of adolescent hypertension. J Hypertens Suppl. 1985;3(4):S61–S63.
112. Sahney S. A review of calcium channel antagonists in the treatment of pediatric hypertension. Paediatr Drugs. 2006;8(6):357–373.
113. Flynn JT, Pasko DA. Calcium channel blockers: pharmacology and place in therapy of pediatric hypertension. Pediatr Nephrol. 2000;15(3–4):302–316.
114. MacDonald JL, Johnson CE, Jacobson P. Stability of isradipine in an extemporaneously compounded oral liquid. Am J Hosp Pharm. 1994;51(19):2409–2411.
115. Johnson CE, Jacobson PA, Song MH. Isradipine therapy in hypertensive pediatric patients. Ann Pharmacother. 1997;31(6):704–707.
116. Strauser LM, Groshong T, Tobias JD. Initial experience with isradipine for the treatment of hypertension in children. South Med J. 2000;93(3):287–293.
117. Flynn JT, Warnick SJ. Isradipine treatment of hypertension in children: a single-center experience. Pediatr Nephrol. 2002;17(9):748–753.
118. Saragoça MA, Portela JE, Plavnik F, et al. Isradipine in the treatment of hypertensive crisis in ambulatory patients. J Cardiovasc Pharmacol. 1992;19(Suppl 3):S76–S78.
119. Miyashita Y, Peterson D, Flynn J. Isradipine Effectively Lowers Blood Pressure in Hospitalized Children with Acute Hypertension. Available at http://www.abstracts2view.com/pas/ search.php?search=do&intMaxHits=10&where%5B%5D=&andornot%5B%5D=&query=hypertension [Accessed April 22, 2009] 2009.
120. Pennisi AJ, Takahashi M, Bernstein BH, et al. Minoxidil therapy in children with severe hypertension. J Pediatr. 1977;90(5):813–819.
121. Strife CF, Quinlan M, Waldo FB, et al. Minoxidil for control of acute blood pressure elevation in chronically hypertensive children. Pediatrics. 1986;78(5):861–865.

33 Pediatric Antihypertensive Clinical Trials

Jennifer S. Li, MD, MHS, Daniel K. Benjamin Jr., MD, PhD, MPH, Thomas Severin, MD, and Ronald J. Portman, MD

CONTENTS

INTRODUCTION
PEDIATRIC ANTIHYPERTENSIVE CLINICAL TRIAL DESIGN
CLINICAL EFFICACY STUDIES
CONCLUSION
REFERENCES

INTRODUCTION

Historically, systemic hypertension was felt to occur in 1–4% of children *(1–5)*; however, the prevalence is now increasing because of the influence of childhood obesity *(6,7)*. Over the past three decades, childhood obesity has increased dramatically and has been deemed an epidemic by the Centers for Disease Control and Prevention *(8)*. The 2002 National Health and Nutrition Examination Survey reported that the prevalence of overweight and obese children aged 6–19 years was 31%, a 45% increase from the previous survey *(9)*. Not only is the prevalence of pediatric hypertension increasing, but also the condition is frequently underdiagnosed *(10,11)*. In younger children, hypertension is often secondary to an underlying disorder while primary (or essential) hypertension accounts for up to 95% of cases in adolescents *(12,13)*. Hypertension in this age group is linked to obesity and risk factors associated with metabolic syndrome that can lead to cardiovascular disease in later life, including lipid abnormalities and insulin resistance. Obesity has been linked to comorbid conditions in children, including type 2 diabetes mellitus, hypertension, and hyperlipidemia *(14,15)*.

There is major concern that the increasing prevalence of these cardiovascular risk factors in children will lead to a dramatic rise in adult cardiovascular disease and neurologic

J.S. Li (✉)
Department of Pediatrics, Duke University Medical Center, Durham, NC, USA
e-mail: jennifer.li@duke.edu

From: *Clinical Hypertension and Vascular Diseases: Pediatric Hypertension*
Edited by: J. T. Flynn et al. DOI 10.1007/978-1-60327-824-9_33
© Springer Science+Business Media, LLC 2011

events. The presence of obesity, type 2 diabetes, hyperlipidemia, and hypertension in childhood has been linked to elevated left ventricular mass and carotid intima-media thickness, as well as peripheral endothelial dysfunction (15–18). The presence and severity of coronary atherosclerotic plaque in asymptomatic young adults are related to the number of risk factors present, including higher body mass index, hypertension, and hyperlipidemia (19). A Danish study of 275,835 adults found that childhood body mass index was significantly associated with coronary artery events in adulthood (20).

Given these trends, the number of children prescribed antihypertensive medications is likely to increase in coming years. Therapy for this condition is hampered, however, by uncertainty over the efficacy and safety of antihypertensive medicines in children. Agents that have been extensively tested and that have a long history of use in adults are often not supported by adequate data obtained in children; drug treatment of hypertension therefore presents a challenge for the pediatrician.

In response to the small number of clinical drug trials in children, the US Congress passed the Food and Drug Administration Modernization Act (FDAMA) in 1997 providing for an additional 6-month period of marketing exclusivity to a pharmaceutical company that responds to a Food and Drug Administration (FDA)—issued written request for studies of their drug in pediatric patients (21,22). The program was extended in January 2002 when Congress passed the Best Pharmaceuticals for Children Act and was subsequently renewed in September 2007. This program has been very successful in stimulating drug studies in children, and, as a result of the program, >200 drug labeling changes have been enacted for children (22–24). The European Medicines Agency (EMEA) has recently started to require drug studies in children and has begun to receive pediatric investigation plans (PIPS) for new molecular entities, including antihypertensive products. Also, under the European Union Pediatric Regulation for already authorized and patented medicinal products, a PIP is required if a sponsor wants to apply for a variation of an existing marketing authorization (e.g., to add a new indication [including pediatric], a new pharmaceutical form, or a new route of administration). For off-patent medicines developed specifically for pediatric use and with an appropriate formulation, a new marketing authorization—the pediatric-use marketing authorization (PUMA)—can be obtained.

Approximately half of the products studied for US pediatric exclusivity have been found to have substantive differences in dosing, safety, or efficacy in children when compared with adult populations (25). Twenty-nine of 131 drugs examined were found to be ineffective when studied in children. Several products that did not demonstrate efficacy (or for which a statistically significant dose response was not observed) were oral antihypertensive agents known to be effective in adults.

This chapter will present an overview of the pediatric antihypertensive studies done to date and will focus on the clinical trial design and factors associated with success or failure of the clinical trials.

PEDIATRIC ANTIHYPERTENSIVE CLINICAL TRIAL DESIGN

The FDA allows for several types of trial designs in the written request for an antihypertensive agent. The written request, issued by FDA before initiation of pediatric exclusivity studies, contains the required elements of the requested studies, including indication, number of studies, age ranges, trial design, sample sizes, and need for a pediatric formulation (25). In the written requests for antihypertensive drugs, the FDA allows for four efficacy trial designs (Fig. 1) (26). Of note, it is not necessary for the dose-ranging study to show that a certain drug is effective in treating pediatric hypertension in order for

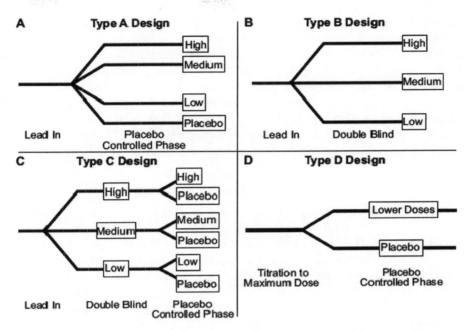

Fig. 1. During the double-blind phase, all of the patients received drug. A, Type A trial design; B, Type B trial design; C, Type C trial design; D, Type D trial design.

its manufacturer to be eligible for exclusivity. However, trial data must be "interpretable," in accordance with the guidelines in order for the drug manufacturer to be eligible for patent extension. In other words, the study should show that the drug is either effective or ineffective. Thus, a trial not eligible for exclusivity is one that does not show a clear result; not one that shows a medication to be ineffective. Conducting these trials is further complicated by ethical and methodological issues unique to pediatric research *(27,28)*, in addition to compliance with the formal guidelines.

Trial Design A

In trial design A, patients are randomized to placebo or one of a few different dosages of the test medication (Fig. 1). It is recommended that the dosages be chosen to provide exposure in a range from slightly less than those achieved by the lowest approved adult dosage to slightly more than those achieved by the highest approved adult dosage. After a few weeks of treatment, the trial is analyzed by examining the slope of the placebo-corrected change in blood pressure from baseline as a function of dosage. A negative slope (i.e., the reduction in blood pressure increases as treatment dosage increases) indicates that the trial was successful, or that the test drug was effective. If the slope were not different from zero, the drug is considered ineffective. The major advantage of this trial type is its straightforward design and analysis. Both successful and unsuccessful trials are considered to be interpretable and therefore responsive to the written request.

However, the placebo-controlled design can lead to slow recruitment because parents are often uncomfortable with the possibility that their child may be placed on placebo. These trials can employ a 3:1 randomization scheme (thereby 3 times as many children receive active product) but some parents still have significant concerns about their child's participation, especially if the trial drug is available off-label. The knowledge that one could use a 3:1 randomization scheme was not evident in the early days of pediatric antihypertensive trials and thus this option was not frequently chosen by companies. In addition, some institutional review boards (IRBs) question the ethics of conducting placebo-controlled trials in children in general, in part due to the potential risk of adverse events while not on active therapy *(27,28)*. We have recently evaluated adverse events in subjects while on placebo in ten antihypertensive trials and observed no differences in the rates of adverse events reported between the patients who received placebo and those who received active drug. Therefore, despite the theoretic concerns over use of placebo *(27)*, short-term exposure to placebo in pediatric trials of antihypertensive medications appears to be safe *(29)*.

Trial Design B

To avoid the issues associated with a placebo-controlled trial, trial design B involves randomization to one of three dosages of the test medication as in trial A, but without a placebo arm (Fig. 1). If analysis of trial design B reveals a negative slope of the dose–response curve, the trial is considered successful and responsive to the written request. However, if the slope were zero, it would not be possible to determine whether this was due to the absence of an effect, or if all doses were too low or too high. Therefore, the trial would be considered uninterpretable. Thus, a negative trial would be unresponsive to the written request. This trial has the simplest design of the four and avoids the aforementioned ethical and patient recruitment issues associated with placebo-controlled trials in children. However, it involves significant risk for manufacturers compared with the other trials, in that only a positive outcome is considered responsive to the written request. More importantly, the ethics of enrolling pediatric patients in a trial in which the outcome may not be interpretable are questionable. Finally, the lack of controls does not allow adequate assessment of safety.

Trial Design C

Trial design C employs a more complex design in order to avoid use of a true placebo arm as in trial design B, while adding the ability to obtain interpretable results regardless of the outcome of the trial, as in trial A (Fig. 1). Trial design C begins like trial design B with randomization to one of a few dosages of the study drug. In addition, it includes a randomized withdrawal phase. At the end of the treatment period, patients are rerandomized to continue on their assigned treatments or to be withdrawn to placebo, with close followup and withdrawal to open-label treatment. The analysis of the treatment phase is similar to that of trial design B. If the slope of the dose–response curve is negative, the trial is considered successful and responsive to the written request. However, if the slope is zero during the treatment phase, the addition of the withdrawal phase allows further analysis and interpretation of the trial. For example, if the treatment phase dose–response curve slope was zero, but the withdrawal phase demonstrated a rise in blood pressure with withdrawal to placebo, this indicates that the dosages used during the treatment phase were too high. If blood pressure did not change significantly with withdrawal to placebo, this suggests that all dosages were too low, or that the drug was ineffective. Thus, as in trial design A, the trial would be considered interpretable regardless of the outcome, and therefore, responsive to the written request. Having two chances to meet eligibility for exclusivity is a major advantage of this trial design. In addition, minimizing the use of an explicit placebo arm likely makes this type of trial more appealing when presented to parents and IRBs.

Trial Design D

In trial design D, the entire trial is built around randomized drug withdrawal (Fig. 1). In this trial, patients are force-titrated to maximal tolerated dosages of the drug, and then randomly withdrawn to lower dosages, including placebo, with close follow-up, and discretionary withdrawal to open-label therapy. The analysis of this type of trial is similar to that of trial design C. Much like trial design C, trial design D minimizes the use of a placebo arm. However, the close follow-up and risk of adverse events that come with titration to maximal dosages are considerable disadvantages, and can result in recruitment problems. Further, since all patients begin the placebo withdrawal period at the highest dose of study drug, a very effective or long-acting drug may still be effective even after the short 2–3 week withdrawal period and be interpreted as a negative study as the BP in the placebo group would not rise, such as was seen in the first pediatric ramipril study (R Portman, personal communication).

CLINICAL EFFICACY STUDIES

The passage of the Food and Drug Administration Modernization Act in 1997 has been the single greatest stimulus for the recent proliferation of industry-sponsored trials of antihypertensive agents in children *(30)*. Figure 2 lists the various studies completed to date. The results of many, but not all, of the clinical trials of antihypertensive agents in children

Drug	Trial Design	Sample size	Dose response	Label change
Amlodipine	C	268	No	Yes
Benazepril	D	107	No	Yes
Bisoprolol	A	94	Yes	No
Candesartan	A	240	No	Pending
Enalapril	C	110	Yes	Yes
Eplerenone	C	304	No	Yes (negative)
Felodipine	D	133	No	No
Fosinopril	C	253	No	Yes
Irbesartan	C	318	No	Yes (negative)
Lisinopril	C	115	Yes	Yes
Losartan	C	175	Yes	Yes
Metoprolol	A	140	No	Yes
Quinapril	A	112	No	No
Ramipril	D	219	No	No
Valsartan	C	351	No age 1-5/Yes age 6-16	Yes

Fig. 2. Clinical trials in pediatric hypertension. The list includes drug, trial design, sample size, dose response (yes/no), and label change (yes/no).

have resulted in publications in scientific journals *(31–43)*. Furthermore, the Best Pharmaceuticals for Children Act now requires the FDA to publish the results of its internal analyses of the trial results submitted by sponsors on the Internet *(24)*. A recent review summarizes the advances in our knowledge about the use of antihypertensive agents in children and provides updated recommendations on the optimal use of antihypertensive agents in children and adolescents who require pharmacologic treatment *(30)*. Of note, however, most of these studies failed to show a dose response. As this pattern emerged, we sought to determine why these trials failed to show dose response in children and hypothesized that difficulties in dosing might be the cause of trial failure *(44)*. Using meta-analytic techniques applied to the clinical trial data as submitted to the FDA, we determined that several factors are important which were predictive of trial success. These factors are discussed below.

Development and Use of a Liquid Formulation

Several of the trials of orally administered antihypertensive agents (particularly those used in the trials that failed to show a dose response) did not develop a pediatric (e.g., liquid) formulation and, thus, exhibited a wide range in exposure within each weight stratum. This is because precise dosing is not feasible using a limited number of tablets; liquid formulations allow for more precise dosing per kilogram. An ideal oral drug for children should be effective, be well tolerated, have good stability, and have good palatability with acceptable taste, aftertaste, and smell. Modern medications are complex mixtures containing many other components besides the active ingredient. These are called "inert ingredients," or excipients and consist of bulk materials, flavorings, sweeteners, and coloring agents. These excipients increase the bulk, add desirable color, mask the unpleasant taste and smell, and facilitate a uniform mixture of the active ingredient in the final marketed preparation. Unlike the active ingredients, excipients are not well regulated in most countries. Although mostly well tolerated, some adverse events and idiosyncratic reactions are well known for a variety of excipients. These components play a critical role, especially in liquid and chewable preparations that are mostly consumed by infants and children *(45)*. Development of a liquid formulation is often challenging because bioavailability can be unreliable, and dissolving the agent in liquid can require high concentrations of alcohol. In addition, stability and bioequivalence testing of liquid formulations also require additional time and expense. Moreover, it is important that the liquid formulation be palatable and often crushed tablets suspended in an aqueous medium are bitter which ultimately will affect drug compliance. Despite these issues, pediatric formulations should be requested in the Pediatric Drug Development Programs whenever possible. Development of these formulations is now more economically feasible because of benefits provided to companies for successfully completing trials requested by FDA as part of this program.

Primary Endpoint

Many successful trials used change in diastolic blood pressure (DBP) as the primary endpoint. Several unsuccessful studies (e.g., trials of amlodipine, irbesartan, and fosinopril) used change in sitting systolic blood pressure (SBP) as the primary outcome. We evaluated the reduction in SBP and DBP related to several agents and found that a reduction in DBP was more closely related to the dosage of agent administered. For example, in the enalapril trial where DBP elevation was the entry criteria, the dosage was more closely related to a reduction in DBP than SBP (coefficient 0.19 [$P=0.001$] versus coefficient 0.12 [$P=0.08$]).

We also observed a closer relationship between DBP reduction and dosage in the lisinopril trial (coefficient 0.12 [$P=0.001$] versus coefficient 0.08 [$P=0.09$]).

The reason for this closer relationship between DBP reduction and dosage may be related to the fact that there is less variability associated with measurement of DBP compared to SBP. DBP may have less physiological variability but also the change in DBP may be more difficult to detect by BP measurement. This reduction in variability may contribute to the success of DBP as the primary endpoint. Perhaps more likely is the fact that inclusion of DBP as a primary entry criteria tends to select children with secondary forms of hypertension. These patients are more likely to respond to drugs affecting the renin–angiotensin–aldosterone system, as seen with the lisinopril, enalapril, and losartan studies.

Systolic hypertension is however threefold more common in children and adolescents than diastolic hypertension, and the motivation to use SBP as the primary endpoint therefore likely derives from feasibility, a common problem in conducting pediatric drug trials. However, another important consideration is that SBP is a surrogate measurement that has been long accepted in adult patients because of its close relationship with hard endpoints of stroke, congestive heart failure, and myocardial infarction. These events are rare in children but the best BP correlate to any form of end-organ damage in children, i.e., left ventricular hypertrophy, is SBP. Thus, it seems that there would be definite benefit to the patient to test an antihypertensive medication for reduction in SBP. A primary study endpoint of mean arterial blood pressure that incorporates both SBP and DBP values might prove advantageous, and this possibility should be explored in future trials. Perhaps, even more beneficial would be the use of ambulatory BP monitoring in pediatric clinical trials for antihypertensive medications. One study has shown that the standard deviations of office casual blood pressure responses were up to 39% larger than those of ambulatory BP monitoring. Depending on the magnitude of the expected antihypertensive effect and trial design, the utilization of ABPM in antihypertensive drug efficacy studies may allow reduction of sample sizes by 57–75% *(46)*.

Dose Range

The dose range received by children randomly assigned to low- and high-dosage groups is extremely variable between trials. For example, in the amlodipine trial which did not show a dose response, there was only a twofold difference between the high- and low-dosage groups. Children in the high-dosage group received 5 mg and children in the low-dosage group received 2.5 mg. In the fosinopril, valsartan, and irbesartan trials, a similar pattern of lack of dose response was also seen with small dosing ranges at six-, eight-, and ninefold, respectively. The enalapril, lisinopril, and losartan trials (which were successful in demonstrating a dose response) had considerably higher dosing ranges, at 32-fold, 32-fold, and 20-fold, respectively. The successful trials thus incorporated a wide range of doses. The lowest clinical trial dose should be lower than the lowest approved dose in adults, and the highest clinical trial dose should at least be twofold higher than the highest approved dose in adults, unless contraindicated for safety concerns. In some of these situations, there had been a conflict between FDA, investigators, and IRBs in this regard. The FDA has requested higher doses than approved in adults, leaving investigators and IRBs in a difficult situation of using a dose higher than its approval in adults. With the knowledge from these early trials, hopefully this issue will not arise in future trials.

None of the failed trials investigated dose ranges higher than the corresponding adult doses. For example, the highest irbesartan dosage was 4.5 mg/kg, whereas adult data indicate that most adults need dosages up to 150–300 mg (~2–4 mg/kg for a 75-kg child) for better blood pressure control. Data obtained from irbesartan use in adults showed that effects on blood pressure increase at dosages ≥600 mg (~8 mg/kg for a 75-kg child), and the maximum irbesartan dosage studied in adults was 900 mg. These doses, however, were not included in the drug's label, making IRB approval of this high dose in a pediatric clinical trial problematic at the time.

In contrast, successful trials provided large differences across low-, medium-, and high-dosage strata. Successful trials used dosages much lower (nearly placebo) than the dosages approved in adults. For example, the recommended initial lisinopril dose in adults is 10 mg, and the usual dose range is 20–40 mg. The lowest dosage used in the pediatric clinical trial was 0.625 mg, thus providing a wider range for exploring dose response.

The selection of wide dosage ranges has important pharmacokinetic/pharmacodynamic implications because closely spaced dosages will likely yield overlapping exposures among dose groups. If overlap is substantial, the dose response could appear flat and, thus, fail to demonstrate a significant dose–response relationship.

Another important aspect of early antihypertensive trials in children was that pharmacokinetic studies were often performed simultaneously with safety and efficacy trials and thus the information was not available for use in determining dosing. Under current pediatric drug development programs, these studies are performed before embarking on subsequent phase 3 trials in children.

Dose by Weight

Weight-based dosing strategies were inconsistent in the trials. The amlodipine trial did not incorporate individual subject weight in dosing but rather gave all children in the low-dosage arm 2.5 mg of product and all children in the high-dosage arm 5 mg of product. This dosing strategy resulted in the following paradox: a 100-kg subject randomly assigned to "high" dosage received 0.05 mg/kg, and a 20-kg subject randomly assigned to "low" dosage received 0.125 mg/kg. In the low-dosage group, one fourth of subjects received >0.06 mg/kg, and one fourth of the high-dosage group received <0.06 mg/kg. Although blood pressure did not show a dose response to amlodipine as randomized, increased dosage on a milligram per kilogram basis was associated with a decrease in blood pressure.

The fosinopril trial also failed to demonstrate a dose response, although it incorporated individual subject weight into the dosing. However, the weight-based strategy of dosing in this trial was limited in that no child received a dosage >40 mg. Thus, children randomly assigned to medium dosage who weighed <30 kg received more fosinopril (in milligrams per kilogram) than the heaviest subjects randomly assigned to high dosage. Similar to the amlodipine trial, blood pressure dose response was not associated with product as randomized, but increased dosing on a milligram per kilogram basis was associated with blood pressure reduction.

CONCLUSION

As a result of legislative incentives, much has been learned about the treatment of hypertension in children and adolescents in the last decade. This expansion of our knowledge base allows for improved understanding of efficacy and safety of these agents. Understanding clinical trial design in pediatric studies is paramount: lack of liquid formulation development, poor dose selection, and failure to fully incorporate weight and pediatric pharmacology into trial design likely led to the difficulties observed in several antihypertensive pediatric exclusivity trials. The BP measurement to use as the primary endpoint of these trials remains controversial.

These data may be applicable to efforts to improve pediatric clinical trial design by government agencies, clinicians, and pharmaceutical sponsors in both North America and Europe. In the future, we recommend that pediatric antihypertensive trials do the following:

- develop an exposure–response model using adult data and published pediatric data and use this model to perform clinical trial simulations of pediatric studies and to explore competing trial designs and analysis options,
- work with FDA/EU Paediatric Committee to design global pediatric trials by leveraging previous quantitative knowledge,
- routinely collect blood samples at informative time points to assess the pharmacokinetics in each subject to ascertain exposure–response analysis and perform these pharmacokinetic and pharmacodynamic trials before the initiation of safety and efficacy trials, and
- consider the use of ambulatory blood pressure monitoring to assess efficacy as part of the clinical trial design.

In addition, studies of the comparative effectiveness, long-term safety, and effects of antihypertensive agents on growth, maturation, and neurocognitive development are needed. Additional studies might also explore effects on vascular reactivity and the impact of pharmacologic treatment on long-term outcomes such as development of cardiovascular morbidity and mortality.

REFERENCES

1. Rames LK, Clarke WR, Connor WE, Reiter MA, Lauer RM. Normal blood pressure and the evaluation of sustained blood pressure elevation in childhood: the Muscatine study. Pediatrics. 1978;61:2245–2251.
2. Reichman LN, Cooper BM, Blumenthal S, Block G, O'Hare D, Chaves AD, Alderman MH, Deming QB, Farber SJ, Thomson GE. Hypertension testing among high school students: I. Surveillance procedures and results. J Chron Dis. 1975;28:161–171.
3. Kilcoyne MM, Richter RW, Alsup PA. Adolescent hypertension: I. Detection and prevalence. Circulation. 1974;50:758–764.
4. Fixler DE, Laird WP. Validity of mass blood pressure screening in children. Pediatrics. 1983;72:459–463.
5. Sinaiko AR, Gomex-Marin O, Prineas RJ. "Significant" diastolic hypertension in pre-high school black and white children: the children and adolescent blood pressure program. Am J Hypertens. 1988;1:178–180.
6. Sorof J, Daniels S. Obesity hypertension in children: a problem of epidemic proportions. Hypertension. 2002;40:441–447.
7. Ogden CL, Flegal KM, Carroll MC, John CL. Prevalence and trends in overweight among US children and adolescents, 1999–2000. JAMA. 2002;288:1728–1732.
8. Strauss RS, Pollack HA. Epidemic increase in childhood overweight, 1986–1998. JAMA. 2001;286: 2845–2848.
9. Hedley AA, Ogden CL, Johnson CL, Carroll MD, Curtin LR, Flegal KM. Prevalence of overweight and obesity among US children, adolescents, and adults, 1999–2002. JAMA. 2004;291:2847–2850.
10. Sorof JM, Lai D, Turner J, Poffenbarger T, Portman RJ. Overweight, ethnicity, and the prevalence of hypertension in school-aged children. Pediatrics. 2004;113(3 Pt 1):475–482.
11. Hansen ML, Gunn PW, Kaelber DC. Underdiagnosis of hypertension in children and adolescents. JAMA. 2007;298(8):874–879.
12. Luma GB, Spiotta RT. Hypertension in children and adolescents. Am Fam Physician. 2006;73(9): 1558–1568.
13. Flynn JT. Evaluation and management of hypertension in childhood. Prog Pediatr Cardiol. 2001;12(2): 177–188.
14. Berenson GS, Pickoff AS. Preventive cardiology and its potential influence on the early natural history of adult heart diseases: the Bogalusa Heart Study and the Heart Smart Program. Am J Med Sci. 1995;310(Suppl 1):S133–S138.

15. Chinali M, de Simone G, Roman MJ, Lee ET, Best LG, Howard BV, Devereux RB. Impact of obesity on cardiac geometry and function in a population of adolescents: the strong heart study. J Am Coll Cardiol. 2006;47:2267–2273.

16. Woo KS, Chook P, Yu CW, Sung RY, Qiao M, Leung SS, Lam CW, Metreweli C, Celermajer DS. Overweight in children is associated with arterial endothelial dysfunction and intima-media thickening. Int J Obes Relat Metab Disord. 2004;28:852–857.

17. Davis PH, Dawson JD, Riley WA, Lauer RM. Carotid intimal-medial thickness is related to cardiovascular risk factors measured from childhood through middle age: the Muscatine study. Circulation. 2001;104:2815–2819.

18. Raitakari OT, Juonala M, Kahonen M, Taittonen L, Laitinen T, Maki-Torkko N, Jarvisalo MJ, Uhari M, Rokinen E, Ronnemaa T, Akerblom HK, Viikari JS. Cardiovascular risk factors in childhood and carotid intima-media thickness in adulthood: the Cardiovascular Risk in Young Finns Study. JAMA. 2003;290:2277–2283.

19. Berenson GS, Srinivasan SR, Bao W, Newman WP III, Tracy RE, Wattigney WA. Association between multiple cardiovascular risk factors and atherosclerosis in children and young adults. N Engl J Med. 1998;338:1650–1656.

20. Baker JL, Olsen LW, Sorensen TIA. Childhood body-mass index and the risk of coronary heart disease in adulthood. N Engl J Med. 2007;357:2329–2337.

21. Public Law 105-115: Food and Drug Administration Modernization Act of 1997. Adopted November 21, 1997. Available at http://www.fda.gov/oc/fdama/default.htm. [Last Accessed October 4, 2010].

22. Benjamin DK Jr, Smith PB, Murphy MD, Roberts R, Mathis L, Avant D, Califf RM, Li JS. Peer-reviewed publication of clinical trials completed for pediatric exclusivity. JAMA. 2006;296:1266–1273.

23. Li JS, Eisenstein EL, Grabowski HG, Reid ED, Mangum B, Schulman KA, Goldsmith JV, Murphy MD, Califf RM, Benjamin DK Jr. Economic return of clinical trials performed under the pediatric exclusivity program. JAMA. 2007;297:480–488.

24. United States Food and Drug Administration. Pediatric Exclusivity Labeling Changes. Available at http://www.fda.gov/downloads/ScienceResearch/SpecialTopics/PediatricTherapeuticsResearch/UCM 163159.pdf. [Last Accessed October 4, 2010].

25. Rodriguez W, Selen A, Avant D, Chaurasia C, Crescenzi T, Gieser G, Di Giacinto J, Huang SM, Lee P, Mathis L, Murphy D, Murphy S, Roberts R, Sachs HS, Suarez S, Tandon V, Uppoor RS. Improving pediatric dosing through pediatric initiatives: what we have learned. Pediatrics. 2008;121(3):530–539.

26. Pasquali SK, Sanders SP, Li JS. Oral antihypertensive trial design and analysis under the pediatric exclusivity provision. Am Heart J. 2002;144:608–614.

27. Flynn JT. Ethics of placebo use in pediatric clinical trials: the case of antihypertensive drug studies. Hypertension. 2003;42:865–869.

28. Committee on Drugs, American Academy of Pediatrics. Guidelines for the ethical conduct of studies to evaluate drugs in pediatric populations. Pediatrics. 1995;95:286–294.

29. Smith PB, Li JS, Murphy MD, Califf RM, Benjamin DK Jr. Safety of placebo controls in pediatric hypertension trials. Hypertension. 2008;51:1–5.

30. Flynn JT, Daniels SR. Pharmacologic treatment of hypertension in children and adolescents. J Pediatr. 2006;149:746–754.

31. Flynn JT, Newburger JW, Daniels SR, Sanders SP, Portman RJ, Hogg RJ. A randomized, placebo-controlled trial of amlodipine in children with hypertension. J Pediatr. 2004;145:353–359.

32. Sorof JM, Cargo P, Graepel J, Humphrey D, King E, Rolf C, et al. Beta-blocker/thiazide combination for treatment of hypertensive children: a randomized double-blind, placebo-controlled trial. Pediatr Nephrol. 2002;17:345–350.

33. Trachtman H, Hainer JW, Sugg J, Teng R, Sorof JM, Radcliffe J. Candesartan in Children with Hypertension (CINCH) investigators. Efficacy, safety, and pharmacokinetics of candesartan cilexetil in hypertensive children aged 6 to 17 years. J Clin Hypertens (Greenwich). 2008;10: 743–750.

34. Wells T, Frame V, Soffer B, Shaw W, Zhang Z, Herrera P, et al. A double-blind, placebo-controlled, dose-response study of the effectiveness and safety of enalapril for children with hypertension. J Clin Pharmacol. 2002;42:870–880.

35. Li J, Flynn JT, Davis I, Portman R, Ogawa M, Pressler M. Randomized, double-blind trial of the aldosterone receptor antagonist eplerenone in hypertensive children [abstract]. J Clin Hypertens (Greenwich). 2008;9(10 Suppl A):A152–A153.

36. Trachtman H, Frank R, Mahan JD, Portman R, Restaino I, Matoo TK, et al. Clinical trial of extended-release felodipine in pediatric essential hypertension. Pediatr Nephrol. 2003;18:548–553.

37. Li JS, Berezny K, Kilaru R, Hazan L, Portman R, Hogg R, et al. Is the extrapolated adult dose of fosinopril safe and effective in treating hypertensive children? Hypertension. 2004;44:289–293.
38. Sakarcan A, Tenney F, Wilson JT, Stewart JJ, Adcock KG, Wells TG, et al. The pharmacokinetics of irbesartan in hypertensive children and adolescents. J Clin Pharmacol. 2001;41:742–749.
39. Soffer B, Zhang Z, Miller K, Vogt BA, Shahinfar S. A double-blind, placebo-controlled, dose-response study of the effectiveness and safety of lisinopril for children with hypertension. Am J Hypertens. 2003;16:795–800.
40. Shahinfar S, Cano F, Soffer BA, Ahmed T, Santoro EP, Zhang Z, et al. A double-blind, dose–response study of losartan in hypertensive children. Am J Hypertens. 2005;18:183–190.
41. Batisky DL, Sorof JM, Sugg J, Llewellyn M, Klibaner M, Hainer JW, Portman RJ, Falkner B, Toprol-XL Pediatric Hypertension Investigators. Efficacy and safety of extended release metoprolol succinate in hypertensive children 6 to 16 years of age: a clinical trial experience. J Pediatr. 2007;150(2):134–139, 139.e1.
42. Blumer JL, Daniels SR, Dreyer WJ, Batisky D, Walson PD, Roman D, et al. Pharmacokinetics of quinapril in children: assessment during substitution for chronic angiotensin-converting enzyme inhibitor treatment. J Clin Pharmacol. 2003;43:128–132.
43. Flynn JT, Meyers KEC, Neto JP, Meneses R, Zurowska A, Bagga A, Mattheyse L, Shi V, Gupte J, Solar-Yohay S, Han G, for the Pediatric Valsartan Study Group. Efficacy and safety of the angiotensin receptor blocker valsartan in children with hypertension aged 1 to 5 years. Hypertension. 2008;52: 222–228.
44. Benjamin DK Jr, Smith PB, Jadhav P, Gobburu JV, Murphy MD, Hasselblad V, Baker-Smith C, Califf RM, Li JS. Pediatric antihypertensive trial failures: analysis of endpoints and dose range. Hypertension. 2008; 51:834–840.
45. Pawar S, Kumar A. Issues in the formulation of drugs for oral use in children: role of excipients. Paediatr Drugs. 2002;4:371–379.
46. Gimpel C, Wühl E, Arbeiter K, et al. Superior consistency of ambulatory blood pressure monitoring in children: implications for clinical trials. J Hypertens. 2009;27:1568–1574.

Subject Index

Note: The letters 'f' and 't' following locators refer to figures and tables respectively.

A

ABPM, *see* Ambulatory blood pressure monitoring (ABPM)
ABPM and hypertension-induced organ damage
  casual BP values, 522
  heart, 524–525
    body size and sex, 524
    LVMI and SBP, 525
  renal diseases
    abnormalities of circadian BP variability, 523
    glomerular filtration rate (GFR), 523
    microalbuminuria, role of, 523
    nocturnal hypertension, 524
    non-dipper pattern, prevalence of, 523
    proteinuria, 523
    urinary albumin excretion (UAE), 523
  vessels, 525
    abnormalities in arterial structure and function, 525
ABPM in diagnosis, role of
  clinical significance, 521–522
  24-H ambulatory BP monitoring, 518t
  and hypertension-induced organ damage, *see* ABPM and hypertension-induced organ damage
  white-coat and masked hypertension, 520–521
    studies on, 519t
ABPM monitors, 162–169
  blood pressure rhythmicity (ultradian rhythms), 168
  in child with SBP/DBP, 169f
  equipment, 162

frequency for ABPM measurements, 168
guidelines for diagnosis/treatment of high BP, 162
for healthy Caucasian children, 163t–168t
measurement technology
  AAMI, 162
  British protocols (BHS), 162
  Korotkoff sound (K4 *vs.* K5), 162
national hypertension leagues, 162
physical activity, 169
recording, ABPM, 168
  daytime and nighttime, 169
software equipment, 162
  nocturnal BP dipping, 162
standard cuff sizes, 162
Accelerated hypertension, 560
Acute hypertensive crisis
  cardiovascular system, 450–451
    focal ischemia, 451
    heart failure, 451
    increased myocardial oxygen demand, 450
  central nervous system, 450
    cerebral infarction, 450
    hypertensive crisis, 450
    visual symptoms, 450
  kidneys, 451
    acute renal insufficiency, 451
    chronic hemodialysis, 451
    hematuria and proteinuria, 451
    renal replacement therapy, 451
    thrombosis and microangiopathic hemolysis, 451

From: *Clinical Hypertension and Vascular Diseases: Pediatric Hypertension*
Edited by: J. T. Flynn et al. DOI 10.1007/978-1-60327-824-9
© Springer Science+Business Media, LLC 2011

ESSENTIAL
CELL BIOLOGY

FIFTH EDITION

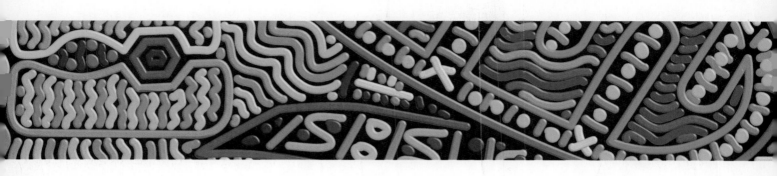

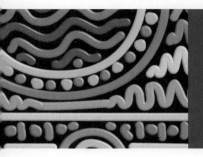

FIFTH
EDITION

ESSENTIAL
CELL BIOLOGY

Bruce Alberts
UNIVERSITY OF CALIFORNIA, SAN FRANCISCO

Karen Hopkin
SCIENCE WRITER

Alexander Johnson
UNIVERSITY OF CALIFORNIA, SAN FRANCISCO

David Morgan
UNIVERSITY OF CALIFORNIA, SAN FRANCISCO

Martin Raff
UNIVERSITY COLLEGE LONDON (EMERITUS)

Keith Roberts
UNIVERSITY OF EAST ANGLIA (EMERITUS)

Peter Walter
UNIVERSITY OF CALIFORNIA, SAN FRANCISCO

W. W. NORTON & COMPANY
NEW YORK • LONDON

W. W. Norton & Company has been independent since its founding in 1923, when William Warder Norton and Mary D. Herter Norton first published lectures delivered at the People's Institute, the adult education division of New York City's Cooper Union. The firm soon expanded its program beyond the Institute, publishing books by celebrated academics from America and abroad. By midcentury, the two major pillars of Norton's publishing program—trade books and college texts—were firmly established. In the 1950s, the Norton family transferred control of the company to its employees, and today—with a staff of four hundred and a comparable number of trade, college, and professional titles published each year—W. W. Norton & Company stands as the largest and oldest publishing house owned wholly by its employees.

Editors: Betsy Twitchell and Michael Morales
Associate Editor: Katie Callahan
Editorial Consultant: Denise Schanck
Senior Associate Managing Editor, College: Carla L. Talmadge
Editorial Assistants: Taylere Peterson and Danny Vargo
Director of Production, College: Jane Searle
Managing Editor, College: Marian Johnson
Managing Editor, College Digital Media: Kim Yi
Media Editor: Kate Brayton
Associate Media Editor: Gina Forsythe
Media Project Editor: Jesse Newkirk
Media Editorial Assistant: Katie Daloia
Ebook Production Manager: Michael Hicks
Content Development Specialist: Todd Pearson
Marketing Manager, Biology: Stacy Loyal
Director of College Permissions: Megan Schindel
Permissions Clearer: Sheri Gilbert
Composition: Emma Jeffcock of EJ Publishing Services
Illustrations: Nigel Orme
Design Director: Hope Miller Goodell
Designer: Matthew McClements, Blink Studio, Ltd.
Indexer: Bill Johncocks
Manufacturing: Transcontinental Interglobe—Beauceville, Quebec

Permission to use copyrighted material is included alongside the appropriate content.

Library of Congress Cataloging-in-Publication Data

Names: Alberts, Bruce, author.
Title: Essential cell biology / Bruce Alberts, Karen Hopkin, Alexander
  Johnson, David Morgan, Martin Raff, Keith Roberts, Peter Walter.
Description: Fifth edition. | New York : W.W. Norton & Company, [2019] |
  Includes index.
Identifiers: LCCN 2018036121 | **ISBN 9780393679533 (hardcover)**
Subjects: LCSH: Cytology. | Molecular biology. | Biochemistry.
Classification: LCC QH581.2 .E78 2019 | DDC 571.6—dc23 LC record available at
https://lccn.loc.gov/2018036121

W. W. Norton & Company, Inc., 500 Fifth Avenue, New York, NY 10110
wwnorton.com
W. W. Norton & Company Ltd., 15 Carlisle Street, London W1D 3BS

3 4 5 6 7 8 9 0

PREFACE

Nobel Prize–winning physicist Richard Feynman once noted that nature has a far, far better imagination than our own. Few things in the universe illustrate this observation better than the cell. A tiny sac of molecules capable of self-replication, this marvelous structure constitutes the fundamental building block of life. We are made of cells. Cells provide all the nutrients we consume. And the continuous activity of cells makes our planet habitable. To understand ourselves—and the world of which we are a part—we need to know something of the life of cells. Armed with such knowledge, we—as citizens and stewards of the global community—will be better equipped to make well-informed decisions about increasingly sophisticated issues, from climate change and food security to biomedical technologies and emerging epidemics.

In *Essential Cell Biology* we introduce readers to the fundamentals of cell biology. The Fifth Edition introduces powerful new techniques that allow us to examine cells and their components with unprecedented precision—such as super-resolution fluorescence microsocopy and cryoelectron microscopy—as well as the latest methods for DNA sequencing and gene editing. We discuss new thinking about how cells organize and encourage the chemical reactions that make life possible, and we review recent insights into human origins and genetics.

With each edition of *Essential Cell Biology*, its authors re-experience the joy of learning something new and surprising about cells. We are also reminded of how much we still don't know. Many of the most fascinating questions in cell biology remain unanswered. How did cells arise on the early Earth, multiplying and diversifying through billions of years of evolution to fill every possible niche—from steaming vents on the ocean floor to frozen mountaintops—and, in doing so, transform our planet's entire environment? How is it possible for billions of cells to seamlessly cooperate and form large, multicellular organisms like ourselves? These are among the many challenges that remain for the next generation of cell biologists, some of whom will begin a wonderful, lifelong journey with this textbook.

Readers interested in learning how scientific inquisitiveness can fuel breakthroughs in our understanding of cell biology will enjoy the stories of discovery presented in each chapter's "How We Know" feature. Packed with experimental data and design, these narratives illustrate how biologists tackle important questions and how experimental results shape future ideas. In this edition, a new "How We Know" recounts the discoveries that first revealed how cells transform the energy locked in food molecules into the forms used to power the metabolic reactions on which life depends.

As in previous editions, the questions in the margins and at the end of each chapter not only test comprehension but also encourage careful thought and the application of newly acquired information to a broader biological context. Some of these questions have more than one valid answer and others invite speculation. Answers to all of the questions are included at the back of the book, and many provide additional information or an alternative perspective on material presented in the main text.

More than 160 video clips, animations, atomic structures, and high-resolution micrographs complement the book and are available online. The movies are correlated with each chapter and callouts are highlighted in color. This supplemental material, created to clarify complex and critical concepts, highlights the intrinsic beauty of living cells.

For those who wish to probe even more deeply, *Molecular Biology of the Cell*, now in its sixth edition, offers a detailed account of the life of the cell. In addition, *Molecular Biology of the Cell, Sixth Edition: A Problems Approach*, by John Wilson and Tim Hunt, provides a gold mine of thought-provoking questions at all levels of difficulty. We have drawn upon this tour-de-force of experimental reasoning for some of the questions in *Essential Cell Biology*, and we are very grateful to its authors.

Every chapter of *Essential Cell Biology* is the product of a communal effort: both text and figures were revised and refined as drafts circulated from one author to another—many times over and back again! The numerous other individuals who have helped bring this project to fruition are credited in the Acknowledgments that follow. Despite our best efforts, it is inevitable that errors will have crept into the book, and we encourage eagle-eyed readers who find mistakes to let us know, so that we can correct them in the next printing.

Acknowledgments

The authors acknowledge the many contributions of professors and students from around the world in the creation of this Fifth Edition. In particular, we received detailed reviews from the following instructors who had used the fourth edition, and we would like to thank them for their important contributions to our revision:

Delbert Abi Abdallah, Thiel College, Pennsylvania
Ann Aguanno, Marymount Manhattan College
David W. Barnes, Georgia Gwinnett College
Manfred Beilharz, The University of Western Australia
Christopher Brandl, Western University, Ontario
Marion Brodhagen, Western Washington University
David Casso, San Francisco State University
Shazia S. Chaudhry, The University of Manchester, United Kingdom
Ron Dubreuil, The University of Illinois at Chicago
Heidi Engelhardt, University of Waterloo, Canada
Sarah Ennis, University of Southampton, United Kingdom
David Featherstone, The University of Illinois at Chicago
Yen Kang France, Georgia College
Barbara Frank, Idaho State University
Daniel E. Frigo, University of Houston
Marcos Garcia-Ojeda, University of California, Merced
David L. Gard, The University of Utah
Adam Gromley, Lincoln Memorial University, Tennessee
Elly Holthuizen, University Medical Center Utrecht, The Netherlands
Harold Hoops, The State University of New York, Geneseo
Bruce Jensen, University of Jamestown, North Dakota
Andor Kiss, Miami University, Ohio
Annette Koenders, Edith Cowan University, Australia
Arthur W. Lambert, Whitehead Institute for Biomedical Research
Denis Larochelle, Clark University, Massachusetts
David Leaf, Western Washington University
Esther Leise, The University of North Carolina at Greensboro
Bernhard Lieb, University of Mainz, Germany

Julie Lively, Louisiana State University
Caroline Mackintosh, University of Saint Mary, Kansas
John Mason, The University of Edinburgh, Scotland
Craig Milgrim, Grossmont College, California
Arkadeep Mitra, City College, Kolkata, India
Niels Erik Møllegaard, University of Copenhagen
Javier Naval, University of Zaragoza, Spain
Marianna Patrauchan, Oklahoma State University
Amanda Polson-Zeigler, University of South Carolina
George Risinger, Oklahoma City Community College
Laura Romberg, Oberlin College, Ohio
Sandra Schulze, Western Washington University
Isaac Skromne, University of Richmond, Virginia
Anna Slusarz, Stephens College, Missouri
Richard Smith, University of Tennessee Health Science Center
Alison Snape, King's College London
Shannon Stevenson, University of Minnesota Duluth
Marla Tipping, Providence College, Rhode Island
Jim Tokuhisa, Virginia Polytechnic Institute and State University
Guillaume van Eys, Maastricht University, The Netherlands
Barbara Vertel, Rosalind Franklin University of Medicine and Science, Illinois
Jennifer Waby, University of Bradford, United Kingdom
Dianne Watters, Griffith University, Australia
Allison Wiedemeier, University of Louisiana at Monroe
Elizabeth Wurdak, St. John's University, Minnesota
Kwok-Ming Yao, The University of Hong Kong
Foong May Yeong, National University of Singapore

We are also grateful to those readers who alerted us to errors that they found in the previous edition.

Working on this book has been a pleasure, in part due to the many people who contributed to its creation. Nigel Orme again worked closely with author Keith Roberts to generate the entire illustration program with his usual skill and care. He also produced all of the artwork for both cover and chapter openers as a respectful digital tribute to the "squeeze-bottle" paintings of the American artist Alden Mason (1919–2013). As in previous editions, Emma Jeffcock did a brilliant job in laying out the whole book and meticulously incorporated our endless corrections. We owe a special debt to Michael Morales, our editor at Garland Science, who coordinated the whole enterprise. He oversaw the initial reviewing, worked closely with the authors on their chapters, took great care of us at numerous writing meetings, and kept us organized and on schedule. He also orchestrated the wealth of online materials, including all video clips and animations. Our copyeditor, Jo Clayton, ensured that the text was stylistically consistent and error-free. At Garland, we also thank Jasmine Ribeaux, Georgina Lucas, and Adam Sendroff.

For welcoming our book to W. W. Norton and bringing this edition to print, we thank our editor Betsy Twitchell, as well as Roby Harrington, Drake McFeely, Julia Reidhead, and Ann Shin for their support. Taylere Peterson and Danny Vargo deserve thanks for their assistance as the book moved from Garland to Norton and through production. We are grateful to media editor Kate Brayton and content development specialist Todd Pearson, associate editors Gina Forsythe and Katie Callahan, and media editorial assistant Katie Daloia whose coordination of electronic media development has resulted in an unmatched suite of resources for cell biology students and instructors alike. We are grateful for marketing manager Stacy Loyal's tireless enthusiasm and advocacy for our book. Megan Schindel, Ted Szczepanski, and Stacey Stambaugh are all owed thanks for navigating the permissions for this edition. And Jane Searle's able management of production, Carla Talmadge's incredible attention to detail, and their shared knack for troubleshooting made the book you hold in your hands a reality.

Denise Schanck deserves extra special thanks for providing continuity as she helped shepherd this edition from Garland to Norton. As always, she attended all of our writing retreats and displayed great wisdom in orchestrating everything she touched.

Last but not least, we are grateful, yet again, to our colleagues and our families for their unflagging tolerance and support. We give our thanks to everyone in this long list.

Resources for Instructors and Students

INSTRUCTOR RESOURCES

wwnorton.com/instructors

Smartwork5

Smartwork5 is an easy-to-use online assessment tool that helps students become better problem solvers through a variety of interactive question types and extensive answer-specific feedback. All Smartwork5 questions are written specifically for the book, are tagged to Bloom's levels and learning objectives, and many include art and animations. Get started quickly with our premade assignments or take advantage of Smartwork5's flexibility by customizing questions and adding your own content. Integration with your campus LMS saves you time by allowing Smartwork5 grades to report right to your LMS gradebook, while individual and class-wide performance reports help you see students' progress.

Interactive Instructor's Guide

An all-in-one resource for instructors who want to integrate active learning into their course. Searchable by chapter, phrase, topic, or learning objective, the Interactive Instructor's Guide compiles the many valuable teaching resources available with *Essential Cell Biology*. This website includes activities, discussion questions, animations and videos, lecture outlines, learning objectives, primary literature suggestions, medical topics guide, and more.

Coursepacks

Easily add high-quality Norton digital media to your online, hybrid, or lecture course. Norton Coursepacks work within your existing learning management system. Content is customizable and includes chapter-based, multiple-choice reading quizzes, text-based learning objectives, access to the full suite of animations, flashcards, and a glossary.

Test Bank

Written by Linda Huang, University of Massachusetts Boston, and Cheryl D. Vaughan, Harvard University Division of Continuing Education, the revised and expanded Test Bank for *Essential Cell Biology* includes 65–80 questions per chapter. Questions are available in multiple-choice, matching, fill-in-the-blank, and short-answer formats, with many using art from the textbook. All questions are tagged to Bloom's taxonomy level, learning objective, book section, and difficulty level, allowing instructors to easily create meaningful exams. The Test Bank is available as downloadable PDFs or Word files from wwnorton.com/instructors.

Animations and Videos

Streaming links give access to more than 130 videos and animations, bringing the concepts of cell biology to life. The movies are correlated with each chapter and callouts are highlighted in color.

Figure-integrated Lecture Outlines

All of the figures are integrated in PowerPoint, along with the section and concept headings from the text, to give instructors a head start creating lectures for their course.

Image Files

Every figure and photograph in the book is available for download in PowerPoint and JPG formats from wwnorton.com/instructors.

STUDENT RESOURCES

digital.wwnorton.com/ecb5

Animations and Videos

Streaming links give access to more than 130 videos and animations, bringing the concepts of cell biology to life. Animations can also be accessed via the ebook and in select Smartwork5 questions. The movies are correlated with each chapter and callouts are highlighted in color.

Student Site

Resources for self-study are available on the student site, including multiple-choice quizzes, cell explorer slides, challenge and concept questions, flashcards, and a glossary.

ABOUT THE AUTHORS

BRUCE ALBERTS received his PhD from Harvard University and is a professor in the Department of Biochemistry and Biophysics at the University of California, San Francisco. He was the editor in chief of *Science* from 2008 to 2013 and served as president of the U.S. National Academy of Sciences from 1993 to 2005.

KAREN HOPKIN received her PhD from the Albert Einstein College of Medicine and is a science writer. Her work has appeared in various scientific publications, including *Science*, *Proceedings of the National Academy of Sciences*, and *The Scientist*, and she is a regular contributor to *Scientific American*'s daily podcast, "60-Second Science."

ALEXANDER JOHNSON received his PhD from Harvard University and is a professor in the Department of Microbiology and Immunology at the University of California, San Francisco.

DAVID MORGAN received his PhD from the University of California, San Francisco, where he is a professor in the Department of Physiology and vice dean for research in the School of Medicine.

MARTIN RAFF received his MD from McGill University and is emeritus professor of biology at the Medical Research Council Laboratory for Molecular Cell Biology at University College London.

KEITH ROBERTS received his PhD from the University of Cambridge and was deputy director of the John Innes Centre. He is emeritus professor at the University of East Anglia.

PETER WALTER received his PhD from The Rockefeller University in New York and is a professor in the Department of Biochemistry and Biophysics at the University of California, San Francisco, and an investigator of the Howard Hughes Medical Institute.

LIST OF CHAPTERS and SPECIAL FEATURES

CONTENTS

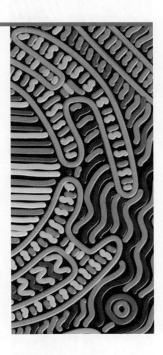

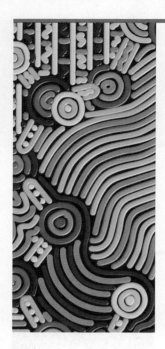

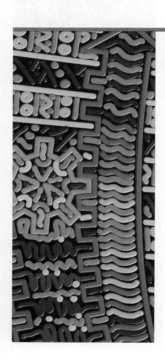

CHAPTER 4

Protein Structure and Function   117

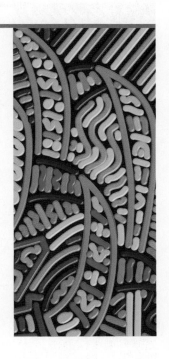

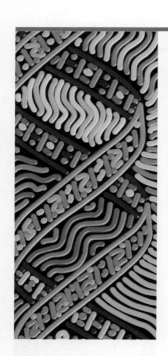

CHAPTER 5

DNA and Chromosomes   173

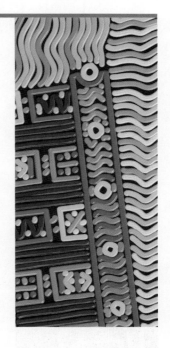

CHAPTER 6

DNA Replication and Repair   199

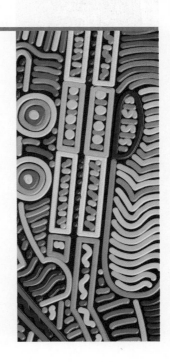

CHAPTER 7

From DNA to Protein: How Cells Read the Genome   227

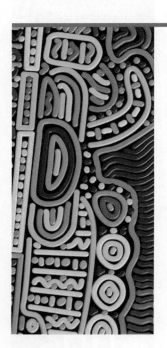

CHAPTER 8

Control of Gene Expression   267

CHAPTER 9

How Genes and Genomes Evolve   297

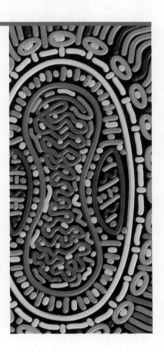

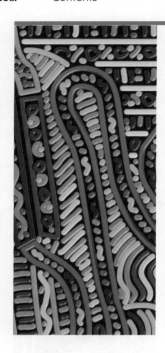

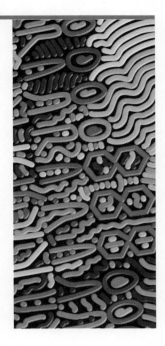

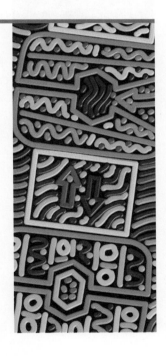

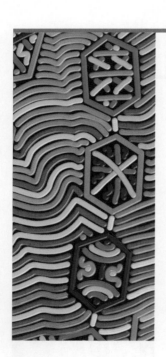

CHAPTER 13

How Cells Obtain Energy from Food   427

CHAPTER 14

Energy Generation in Mitochondria and Chloroplasts 455

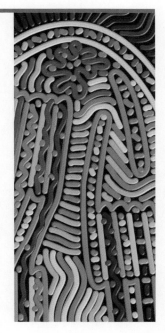

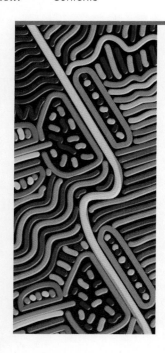

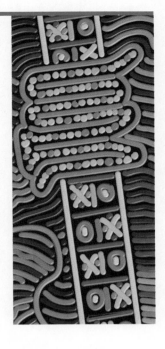

CHAPTER 16

Cell Signaling 533

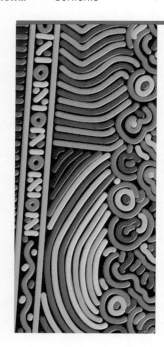

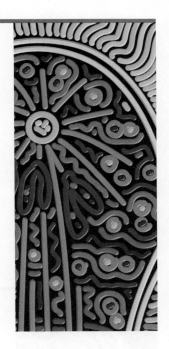

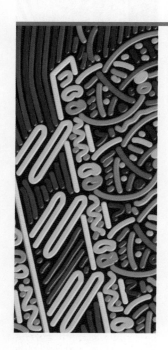

CHAPTER 19

Sexual Reproduction and Genetics 651

CHAPTER 20

Cell Communities: Tissues, Stem Cells, and Cancer   691

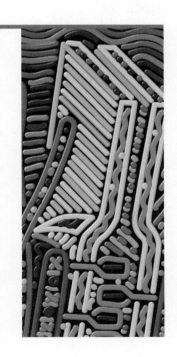

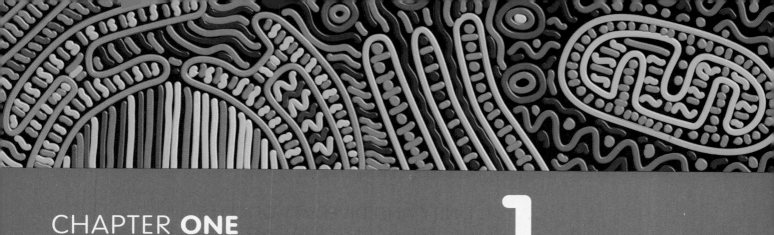

CHAPTER ONE

1

Cells: The Fundamental Units of Life

What does it mean to be living? Petunias, people, and pond scum are all alive; stones, sand, and summer breezes are not. But what are the fundamental properties that characterize living things and distinguish them from nonliving matter?

The answer hinges on a basic fact that is taken for granted now but marked a revolution in thinking when first established more than 175 years ago. All living things (or *organisms*) are built from **cells**: small, membrane-enclosed units filled with a concentrated aqueous solution of chemicals and endowed with the extraordinary ability to create copies of themselves by growing and then dividing in two. The simplest forms of life are solitary cells. Higher organisms, including ourselves, are communities of cells derived by growth and division from a single founder cell. Every animal or plant is a vast colony of individual cells, each of which performs a specialized function that is integrated by intricate systems of cell-to-cell communication.

Cells, therefore, are the fundamental units of life. Thus it is to *cell biology*—the study of cells and their structure, function, and behavior—that we look for an answer to the question of what life is and how it works. With a deeper understanding of cells, we can begin to tackle the grand historical problems of life on Earth: its mysterious origins, its stunning diversity produced by billions of years of evolution, and its invasion of every conceivable habitat on the planet. At the same time, cell biology can provide us with answers to the questions we have about ourselves: Where did we come from? How do we develop from a single fertilized egg cell? How is each of us similar to—yet different from—everyone else on Earth? Why do we get sick, grow old, and die?

UNITY AND DIVERSITY OF CELLS

CELLS UNDER THE MICROSCOPE

THE PROKARYOTIC CELL

THE EUKARYOTIC CELL

MODEL ORGANISMS

In this chapter, we introduce the concept of cells: what they are, where they come from, and how we have learned so much about them. We begin by looking at the great variety of forms that cells can adopt, and we take a preliminary glimpse at the chemical machinery that all cells have in common. We then consider how cells are made visible under the microscope and what we see when we peer inside them. Finally, we discuss how we can exploit the similarities of living things to achieve a coherent understanding of all forms of life on Earth—from the tiniest bacterium to the mightiest oak.

UNITY AND DIVERSITY OF CELLS

Biologists estimate that there may be up to 100 million distinct species of living things on our planet—organisms as different as a dolphin and a rose or a bacterium and a butterfly. Cells, too, differ vastly in form and function. Animal cells differ from those in a plant, and even cells within a single multicellular organism can differ wildly in appearance and activity. Yet despite these differences, all cells share a fundamental chemistry and other common features.

In this section, we take stock of some of the similarities and differences among cells, and we discuss how all present-day cells appear to have evolved from a common ancestor.

Cells Vary Enormously in Appearance and Function

When comparing one cell and another, one of the most obvious places to start is with size. A bacterial cell—say a *Lactobacillus* in a piece of cheese—is a few **micrometers**, or µm, in length. That's about 25 times smaller than the width of a human hair. At the other extreme, a frog egg—which is also a single cell—has a diameter of about 1 millimeter (mm). If we scaled them up to make the *Lactobacillus* the size of a person, the frog egg would be half a mile high.

Cells vary just as widely in their shape (**Figure 1–1**). A typical nerve cell in your brain, for example, is enormously extended: it sends out its electrical signals along a single, fine protrusion (an axon) that is 10,000 times longer than it is thick, and the cell receives signals from other nerve cells through a collection of shorter extensions that sprout from its body like the branches of a tree (see Figure 1–1A). A pond-dwelling *Paramecium*, on the other hand, is shaped like a submarine and is covered with thousands of *cilia*—hairlike projections whose sinuous, coordinated beating sweeps the cell forward, rotating as it goes (Figure 1–1B). A cell in the surface layer of a plant is squat and immobile, surrounded by a rigid box of cellulose with an outer waterproof coating of wax (Figure 1–1C). A macrophage in the body of an animal, by contrast, crawls through tissues, constantly pouring itself into new shapes, as it searches for and engulfs debris, foreign microorganisms, and dead or dying cells (Figure 1–1D). A fission yeast is shaped like a rod (Figure 1–1E), whereas a budding yeast is delightfully spherical (see Figure 1–14). And so on.

Cells are also enormously diverse in their chemical requirements. Some require oxygen to live; for others the gas is deadly. Some cells consume little more than carbon dioxide (CO_2), sunlight, and water as their raw materials; others need a complex mixture of molecules produced by other cells.

These differences in size, shape, and chemical requirements often reflect differences in cell function. Some cells are specialized factories for the production of particular substances, such as hormones, starch, fat, latex, or pigments. Others, like muscle cells, are engines that burn fuel to do mechanical work. Still others are electricity generators, like the modified muscle cells in the electric eel.

Some modifications specialize a cell so much that the cell ceases to proliferate, thus producing no descendants. Such specialization would be senseless for a cell that lived a solitary life. In a multicellular organism, however, there is a division of labor among cells, allowing some cells to become specialized to an extreme degree for particular tasks and leaving them dependent on their fellow cells for many basic requirements. Even the most basic need of all, that of passing on the genetic instructions of the organism to the next generation, is delegated to specialists—the egg and the sperm.

Living Cells All Have a Similar Basic Chemistry

Despite the extraordinary diversity of plants and animals, people have recognized from time immemorial that these organisms have something in common, something that entitles them all to be called living things. But while it seemed easy enough to recognize life, it was remarkably difficult to say in what sense all living things were alike. Textbooks had to settle for defining life in abstract general terms related to growth, reproduction, and an ability to actively alter their behavior in response to the environment.

The discoveries of biochemists and molecular biologists have provided an elegant solution to this awkward situation. Although the cells of all living things are enormously varied when viewed from the outside, they are fundamentally similar inside. We now know that cells resemble one another to an astonishing degree in the details of their chemistry. They are composed of the same sorts of molecules, which participate in the same types of chemical reactions (discussed in Chapter 2). In all organisms, genetic information—in the form of *genes*—is carried in DNA molecules. This information is written in the same chemical code, constructed out of the same chemical building blocks, interpreted by essentially the same chemical machinery, and replicated in the same way when a cell or

---

QUESTION 1–1

"Life" is easy to recognize but difficult to define. According to one popular biology text, living things:
1. Are highly organized compared to natural inanimate objects.
2. Display homeostasis, maintaining a relatively constant internal environment.
3. Reproduce themselves.
4. Grow and develop from simple beginnings.
5. Take energy and matter from the environment and transform it.
6. Respond to stimuli.
7. Show adaptation to their environment.
Score a person, a vacuum cleaner, and a potato with respect to these characteristics.

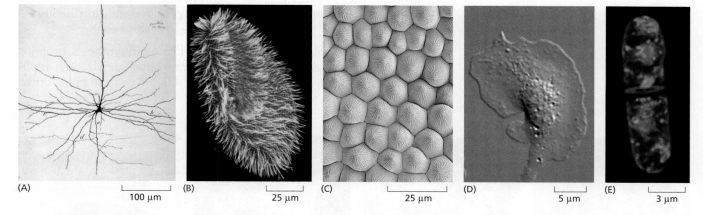

(A) ⊢ 100 μm ⊣ (B) ⊢ 25 μm ⊣ (C) ⊢ 25 μm ⊣ (D) ⊢ 5 μm ⊣ (E) ⊢ 3 μm ⊣

Figure 1–1 Cells come in a variety of shapes and sizes. Note the very different scales of these micrographs. (A) Drawing of a single nerve cell from a mammalian brain. This cell has a single, unbranched extension (axon), projecting toward the top of the image, through which it sends electrical signals to other nerve cells, and it possesses a huge branching tree of projections (dendrites) through which it receives signals from as many as 100,000 other nerve cells. (B) *Paramecium*. This protozoan—a single giant cell—swims by means of the beating cilia that cover its surface. (C) The surface of a snapdragon flower petal displays an orderly array of tightly packed cells. (D) A macrophage spreads itself out as it patrols animal tissues in search of invading microorganisms. (E) A fission yeast is caught in the act of dividing in two. The medial septum (stained *red* with a fluorescent dye) is forming a wall between the two nuclei (also stained *red*) that have been separated into the two daughter cells; in this image, the cells' membranes are stained with a *green* fluorescent dye. (A, Herederos de Santiago Ramón y Cajal, 1899; B, courtesy of Anne Aubusson Fleury, Michel Laurent, and André Adoutte; C, courtesy of Kim Findlay; D, from P.J. Hanley et al., *Proc. Natl Acad. Sci. USA* 107:12145–12150, 2010. With permission from National Academy of Sciences; E, courtesy of Janos Demeter and Shelley Sazer.)

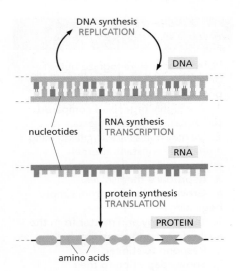

Figure 1–2 In all living cells, genetic information flows from DNA to RNA (transcription) and from RNA to protein (translation)—an arrangement known as the central dogma. The sequence of nucleotides in a particular segment of DNA (a gene) is transcribed into an RNA molecule, which can then be translated into the linear sequence of amino acids of a protein. Only a small part of the gene, RNA, and protein is shown.

organism reproduces. Thus, in every cell, long polymer chains of **DNA** are made from the same set of four monomers, called *nucleotides*, strung together in different sequences like the letters of an alphabet. The information encoded in these DNA molecules is read out, or *transcribed*, into a related set of polynucleotides called **RNA**. Although some of these RNA molecules have their own regulatory, structural, or chemical activities, most are *translated* into a different type of polymer called a **protein**. This flow of information—from DNA to RNA to protein—is so fundamental to life that it is referred to as the *central dogma* (**Figure 1–2**).

The appearance and behavior of a cell are dictated largely by its protein molecules, which serve as structural supports, chemical catalysts, molecular motors, and much more. Proteins are built from *amino acids*, and all organisms use the same set of 20 amino acids to make their proteins. But the amino acids are linked in different sequences, giving each type of protein molecule a different three-dimensional shape, or *conformation*, just as different sequences of letters spell different words. In this way, the same basic biochemical machinery has served to generate the whole gamut of life on Earth (**Figure 1–3**).

Living Cells Are Self-Replicating Collections of Catalysts

One of the most commonly cited properties of living things is their ability to reproduce. For cells, the process involves duplicating their genetic material and other components and then dividing in two—producing a pair of daughter cells that are themselves capable of undergoing the same cycle of replication.

It is the special relationship between DNA, RNA, and proteins—as outlined in the central dogma (see Figure 1–2)—that makes this self-replication possible. DNA encodes information that ultimately directs the assembly of proteins: the sequence of nucleotides in a molecule of DNA dictates the sequence of amino acids in a protein. Proteins, in turn, catalyze the replication of DNA and the transcription of RNA, and they participate in the translation of RNA into proteins. This feedback loop between proteins and polynucleotides underlies the self-reproducing behavior of living things (**Figure 1–4**). We discuss this complex interdependence between DNA, RNA, and proteins in detail in Chapters 5 through 8.

In addition to their roles in polynucleotide and protein synthesis, proteins also catalyze the many other chemical reactions that keep the self-replicating system shown in Figure 1–4 running. A living cell can break down

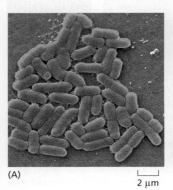
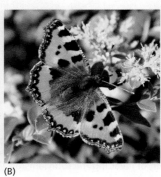
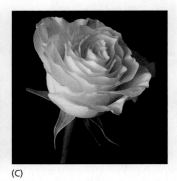
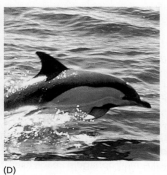

(A) 2 μm (B) (C) (D)

Figure 1–3 All living organisms are constructed from cells. (A) A colony of bacteria, (B) a butterfly, (C) a rose, and (D) a dolphin are all made of cells that have a fundamentally similar chemistry and operate according to the same basic principles. (A, courtesy of Janice Carr; D, courtesy of Jonathan Gordon, IFAW.)

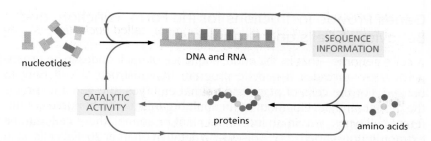

Figure 1–4 Life is an autocatalytic process. DNA and RNA provide the sequence information (*green* arrows) that is used to produce proteins and to copy themselves. Proteins, in turn, provide the catalytic activity (*red* arrows) needed to synthesize DNA, RNA, and themselves. Together, these feedback loops create the self-replicating system that endows living cells with their ability to reproduce.

nutrients and use the products to both make the building blocks needed to produce polynucleotides, proteins, and other cell constituents and to generate the energy needed to power these biosynthetic processes. We discuss these vital metabolic reactions in detail in Chapters 3 and 13.

Only living cells can perform these astonishing feats of self-replication. Viruses also contain information in the form of DNA or RNA, but they do not have the ability to reproduce by their own efforts. Instead, they parasitize the reproductive machinery of the cells that they invade to make copies of themselves. Thus, viruses are not truly considered living. They are merely chemical zombies: inert and inactive outside their host cells but able to exert a malign control once they gain entry. We review the life cycle of viruses in Chapter 9.

All Living Cells Have Apparently Evolved from the Same Ancestral Cell

When a cell replicates its DNA in preparation for cell division, the copying is not always perfect. On occasion, the instructions are corrupted by *mutations* that change the sequence of nucleotides in the DNA. For this reason, daughter cells are not necessarily exact replicas of their parent.

Mutations can create offspring that are changed for the worse (in that they are less able to survive and reproduce), changed for the better (in that they are better able to survive and reproduce), or changed in a neutral way (in that they are genetically different but equally viable). The struggle for survival eliminates the first, favors the second, and tolerates the third. The genes of the next generation will be the genes of the survivors.

For many organisms, the pattern of heredity may be complicated by sexual reproduction, in which two cells of the same species fuse, pooling their DNA. The genetic cards are then shuffled, re-dealt, and distributed in new combinations to the next generation, to be tested again for their ability to promote survival and reproduction.

These simple principles of genetic change and selection, applied repeatedly over billions of cell generations, are the basis of **evolution**—the process by which living species become gradually modified and adapted to their environment in more and more sophisticated ways. Evolution offers a startling but compelling explanation of why present-day cells are so similar in their fundamentals: they have all inherited their genetic instructions from the same common ancestral cell. It is estimated that this cell existed between 3.5 and 3.8 billion years ago, and we must suppose that it contained a prototype of the universal machinery of all life on Earth today. Through a very long process of mutation and natural selection, the descendants of this ancestral cell have gradually diverged to fill every habitat on Earth with organisms that exploit the potential of the machinery in a seemingly endless variety of ways.

QUESTION 1–2

Mutations are mistakes in the DNA that change the genetic plan from that of the previous generation. Imagine a shoe factory. Would you expect mistakes (i.e., unintentional changes) in copying the shoe design to lead to improvements in the shoes produced? Explain your answer.

Genes Provide Instructions for the Form, Function, and Behavior of Cells and Organisms

A cell's **genome**—that is, the entire sequence of nucleotides in an organism's DNA—provides a genetic program that instructs a cell how to behave. For the cells of plant and animal embryos, the genome directs the growth and development of an adult organism with hundreds of different cell types. Within an individual plant or animal, these cells can be extraordinarily varied, as we discuss in detail in Chapter 20. Fat cells, skin cells, bone cells, and nerve cells seem as dissimilar as any cells could be. Yet all these *differentiated cell types* are generated during embryonic development from a single fertilized egg cell, and they contain identical copies of the DNA of the species. Their varied characters stem from the way that individual cells use their genetic instructions. Different cells *express* different genes: that is, they use their genes to produce some RNAs and proteins and not others, depending on their internal state and on cues that they and their ancestor cells have received from their surroundings—mainly signals from other cells in the organism.

The DNA, therefore, is not just a shopping list specifying the molecules that every cell must make, and a cell is not just an assembly of all the items on the list. Each cell is capable of carrying out a variety of biological tasks, depending on its environment and its history, and it selectively uses the information encoded in its DNA to guide its activities. Later in this book, we will see in detail how DNA defines both the parts list of the cell and the rules that decide when and where these parts are to be made.

CELLS UNDER THE MICROSCOPE

Today, we have access to many powerful technologies for deciphering the principles that govern the structure and activity of the cell. But cell biology started without these modern tools. The earliest cell biologists began by simply looking at tissues and cells, and later breaking them open or slicing them up, attempting to view their contents. What they saw was to them profoundly baffling—a collection of tiny objects whose relationship to the properties of living matter seemed an impenetrable mystery. Nevertheless, this type of visual investigation was the first step toward understanding tissues and cells, and it remains essential today in the study of cell biology.

Cells were not made visible until the seventeenth century, when the **microscope** was invented. For hundreds of years afterward, all that was known about cells was discovered using this instrument. *Light microscopes* use visible light to illuminate specimens, and they allowed biologists to see for the first time the intricate structure that underpins all living things.

Although these instruments now incorporate many sophisticated improvements, the properties of light—specifically its wavelength—limit the fineness of detail these microscopes reveal. *Electron microscopes*, invented in the 1930s, go beyond this limit by using beams of electrons instead of beams of light as the source of illumination; because electrons have a much shorter wavelength, these instruments greatly extend our ability to see the fine details of cells and even render some of the larger molecules visible individually.

In this section, we describe various forms of light and electron microscopy. These vital tools in the modern cell biology laboratory continue to improve, revealing new and sometimes surprising details about how cells are built and how they operate.

The Invention of the Light Microscope Led to the Discovery of Cells

By the seventeenth century, glass lenses were powerful enough to permit the detection of structures invisible to the naked eye. Using an instrument equipped with such a lens, Robert Hooke examined a piece of cork and in 1665 reported to the Royal Society of London that the cork was composed of a mass of minute chambers. He called these chambers "cells," based on their resemblance to the simple rooms occupied by monks in a monastery. The name stuck, even though the structures Hooke described were actually the cell walls that remained after the plant cells living inside them had died. Later, Hooke and his Dutch contemporary Antoni van Leeuwenhoek were able to observe living cells, seeing for the first time a world teeming with motile microscopic organisms.

For almost 200 years, such instruments—the first light microscopes—remained exotic devices, available only to a few wealthy individuals. It was not until the nineteenth century that microscopes began to be widely used to look at cells. The emergence of cell biology as a distinct science was a gradual process to which many individuals contributed, but its official birth is generally said to have been signaled by two publications: one by the botanist Matthias Schleiden in 1838 and the other by the zoologist Theodor Schwann in 1839. In these papers, Schleiden and Schwann documented the results of a systematic investigation of plant and animal tissues with the light microscope, showing that cells were the universal building blocks of all living tissues. Their work, and that of other nineteenth-century microscopists, slowly led to the realization that all living cells are formed by the growth and division of existing cells—a principle sometimes referred to as the *cell theory* (**Figure 1–5**). The implication that living organisms do not arise spontaneously but can be generated only from existing organisms was hotly contested, but it was finally confirmed

Figure 1–5 New cells form by growth and division of existing cells. (A) In 1880, Eduard Strasburger drew a living plant cell (a hair cell from a *Tradescantia* flower), which he observed dividing in two over a period of 2.5 hours. Inside the cell, DNA (*black*) can be seen condensing into chromosomes, which are then segregated into the two daughter cells. (B) A comparable living plant cell photographed through a modern light microscope. (B, from P.K. Hepler, *J. Cell Biol.* 100:1363–1368, 1985. With permission from Rockefeller University Press.)

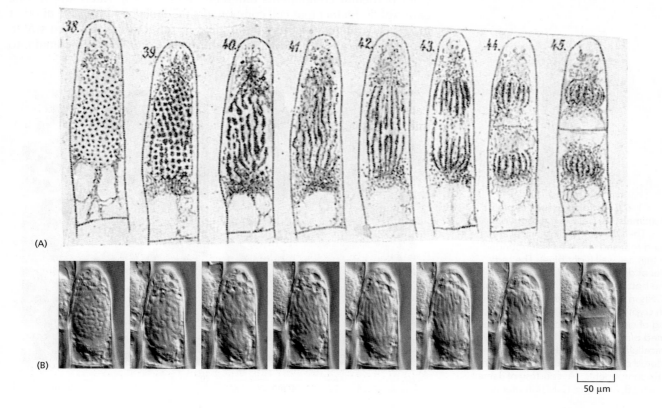

(A)

(B)

50 μm

QUESTION 1–3

You have embarked on an ambitious research project: to create life in a test tube. You boil up a rich mixture of yeast extract and amino acids in a flask, along with a sprinkling of the inorganic salts known to be essential for life. You seal the flask and allow it to cool. After several months, the liquid is as clear as ever, and there are no signs of life. A friend suggests that excluding the air was a mistake, since most life as we know it requires oxygen. You repeat the experiment, but this time you leave the flask open to the atmosphere. To your great delight, the liquid becomes cloudy after a few days, and, under the microscope, you see beautiful small cells that are clearly growing and dividing. Does this experiment prove that you managed to generate a novel life-form? How might you redesign your experiment to allow air into the flask, yet eliminate the possibility that contamination by airborne microorganisms is the explanation for the results? (For a ready-made answer, look up the classic experiments of Louis Pasteur.)

in the 1860s by an elegant set of experiments performed by Louis Pasteur (see Question 1–3).

The principle that cells are generated only from preexisting cells and inherit their characteristics from them underlies all of biology and gives the subject a unique flavor: in biology, questions about the present are inescapably linked to conditions in the past. To understand why present-day cells and organisms behave as they do, we need to understand their history, all the way back to the misty origins of the first cells on Earth. Charles Darwin provided the key insight that makes this history comprehensible. His theory of evolution, published in 1859, explains how random variation and natural selection gave rise to diversity among organisms that share a common ancestry. When combined with the cell theory, the theory of evolution leads us to view all life, from its beginnings to the present day, as one vast family tree of individual cells. Although this book is primarily about how cells work today, we will encounter the theme of evolution again and again.

Light Microscopes Reveal Some of a Cell's Components

If a very thin slice is cut from a suitable plant or animal tissue and viewed using a light microscope, it is immediately apparent that the tissue is divided into thousands of small cells. In some cases, the cells are closely packed; in others, they are separated from one another by an *extracellular matrix*—a dense material often made of protein fibers embedded in a gel of long sugar chains. Each cell is typically about 5–20 μm in diameter. If care has been taken to keep the specimen alive, particles will be seen moving around inside its individual cells. On occasion, a cell may even be seen slowly changing shape and dividing into two (see Figure 1–5 and Movie 1.1).

Distinguishing the internal structure of a cell is difficult, not only because the parts are small, but also because they are transparent and mostly colorless. One way around the problem is to stain cells with dyes that color particular components differently (Figure 1–6). Alternatively, one can exploit the fact that cell components differ slightly from one another in refractive index, just as glass differs in refractive index from water, causing light rays to be deflected as they pass from the one medium into

Figure 1–6 Cells form tissues in plants and animals. (A) Cells in the root tip of a fern. The DNA-containing nuclei are stained *red*, and each cell is surrounded by a thin cell wall (*light blue*). The *red* nuclei of densely packed cells are seen at the bottom corners of the preparation. (B) Cells in the crypts of the small intestine. Each crypt appears in this cross section as a ring of closely packed cells (with nuclei stained *blue*). The ring is surrounded by extracellular matrix, which contains the scattered cells that produced most of the matrix components. (A, courtesy of James Mauseth; B, Jose Luis Calvo/Shutterstock.)

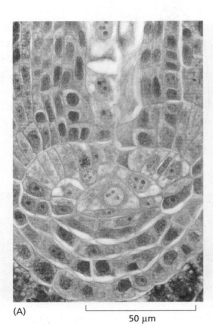

(A)   50 μm

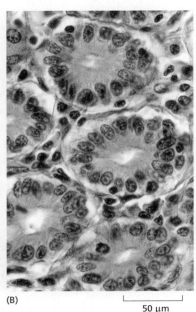

(B)   50 μm

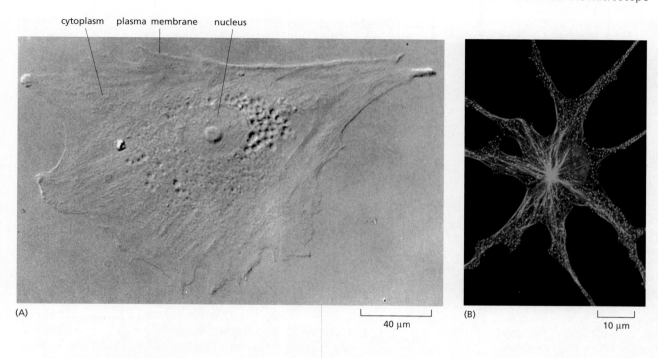

cytoplasm plasma membrane nucleus

(A) 40 μm

(B) 10 μm

the other. The small differences in refractive index can be made visible by specialized optical techniques, and the resulting images can be enhanced further by electronic processing (**Figure 1–7A**).

As shown in Figures 1–6B and 1–7A, typical animal cells visualized in these ways have a distinct anatomy. They have a sharply defined boundary, indicating the presence of an enclosing membrane, the **plasma membrane**. A large, round structure, the *nucleus*, is prominent near the middle of the cell. Around the nucleus and filling the cell's interior is the **cytoplasm**, a transparent substance crammed with what seems at first to be a jumble of miscellaneous objects. With a good light microscope, one can begin to distinguish and classify some of the specific components in the cytoplasm, but structures smaller than about 0.2 μm—about half the wavelength of visible light—cannot normally be resolved; points closer than this are not distinguishable and appear as a single blur.

In recent years, however, new types of light microscope called **fluorescence microscopes** have been developed that use sophisticated methods of illumination and electronic image processing to see fluorescently labeled cell components in much finer detail (**Figure 1–7B**). The most recent super-resolution fluorescence microscopes, for example, can push the limits of resolution down even further, to about 20 nanometers (nm). That is the size of a single **ribosome**, a large macromolecular complex in which RNAs are translated into proteins. These super-resolution techniques are described further in Panel 1–1 (pp. 12–13).

The Fine Structure of a Cell Is Revealed by Electron Microscopy

For the highest magnification and best resolution, one must turn to an **electron microscope**, which can reveal details down to a few nanometers. Preparing cell samples for the electron microscope is a painstaking process. Even for light microscopy, a tissue often has to be *fixed* (that is, preserved by pickling in a reactive chemical solution), supported by *embedding* in a solid wax or resin, cut, or *sectioned,* into thin slices, and *stained* before it is viewed. (The tissues in Figure 1–6 were prepared in

Figure 1–7 Some of the internal structures of a cell can be seen with a light microscope. (A) A cell taken from human skin and grown in culture was photographed through a light microscope using interference-contrast optics (described in Panel 1–1, pp. 12–13). The nucleus is especially prominent, as is the small, round nucleolus within it (discussed in Chapter 5 and see Panel 1–2, p. 25). (B) A pigment cell from a frog, stained with fluorescent dyes and viewed with a confocal fluorescence microscope (discussed in Panel 1–1). The nucleus is shown in *purple,* the pigment granules in *red,* and the microtubules—a class of protein filaments in the cytoplasm—in *green.* (A, courtesy of Casey Cunningham; B, courtesy of Stephen Rogers and the Imaging Technology Group of the Beckman Institute, University of Illinois, Urbana.)

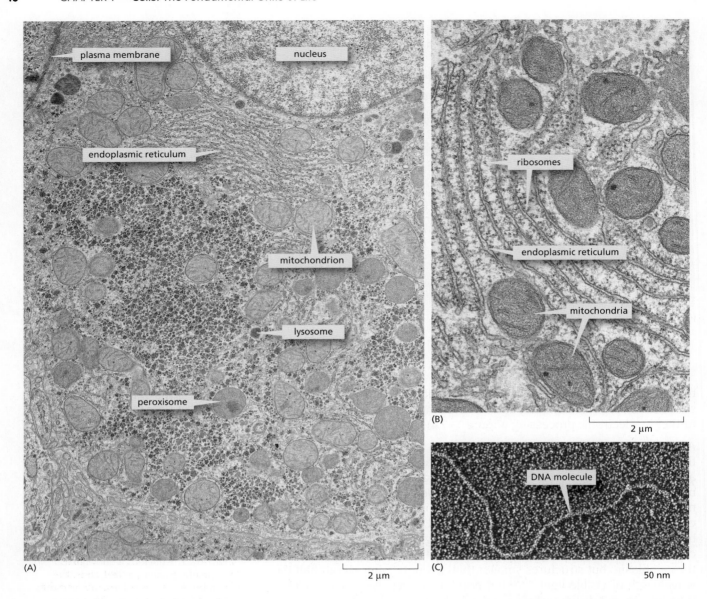

(A)   2 μm

(B)   2 μm

(C)   50 nm

Figure 1–8 The fine structure of a cell can be seen in a transmission electron microscope. (A) Thin section of a liver cell showing the enormous amount of detail that is visible. Some of the components to be discussed later in the chapter are labeled; they are identifiable by their size, location, and shape. (B) A small region of the cytoplasm at higher magnification. The smallest structures that are clearly visible are the ribosomes, each of which is made of 80–90 or so individual protein and RNA molecules; some of the ribosomes are free in the cytoplasm, while others are bound to a membrane-enclosed organelle—the endoplasmic reticulum—discussed later (see Figure 1–22). (C) Portion of a long, threadlike DNA molecule isolated from a cell and viewed by electron microscopy. (A and B, by permission of E.L. Bearer and Daniel S. Friend; C, courtesy of Mei Lie Wong.)

this way.) For electron microscopy, similar procedures are required, but the sections have to be much thinner and there is no possibility of looking at living cells.

When thin sections are cut, stained with electron-dense heavy metals, and placed in the electron microscope, much of the jumble of cell components becomes sharply resolved into distinct **organelles**—separate, recognizable substructures with specialized functions that are often only hazily defined with a conventional light microscope. A delicate membrane, only about 5 nm thick, is visible enclosing the cell, and similar membranes form the boundary of many of the organelles inside (**Figure 1–8A and B**). The plasma membrane separates the interior of the cell from its external environment, while *internal membranes* surround most organelles. All of these membranes are only two molecules thick (as discussed in Chapter 11). With an electron microscope, even individual large molecules can be seen (**Figure 1–8C**).

The type of electron microscope used to look at thin sections of tissue is known as a *transmission electron microscope*. This instrument is, in principle, similar to a light microscope, except that it transmits a beam of

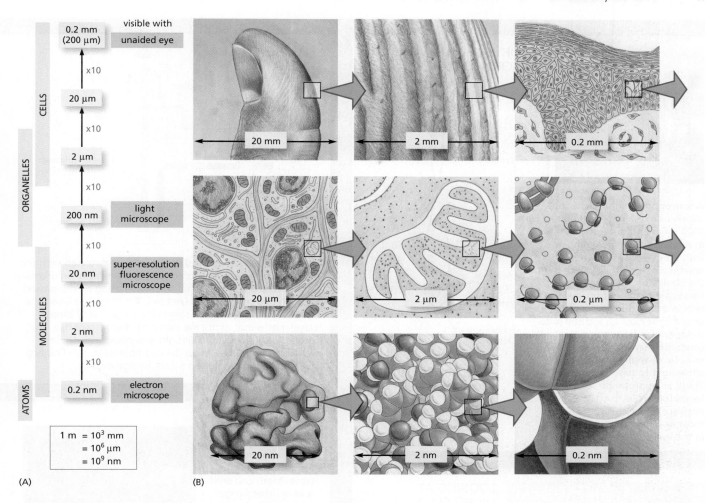

(A)

(B)

electrons rather than a beam of light through the sample. Another type of electron microscope—the *scanning electron microscope*—scatters electrons off the surface of the sample and so is used to look at the surface detail of cells and other structures. These techniques, along with the different forms of light microscopy, are reviewed in **Panel 1–1** (pp. 12–13).

Even the most powerful electron microscopes, however, cannot visualize the individual atoms that make up biological molecules (**Figure 1–9**). To study the cell's key components in atomic detail, biologists have developed even more sophisticated tools. Techniques such as x-ray crystallography or cryoelectron microscopy, for example, can be used to determine the precise positioning of atoms within the three-dimensional structure of protein molecules and complexes (discussed in Chapter 4).

THE PROKARYOTIC CELL

Of all the types of cells that have been examined microscopically, *bacteria* have the simplest structure and come closest to showing us life stripped down to its essentials. Indeed, a bacterium contains no organelles other than ribosomes—not even a nucleus to hold its DNA. This property—the presence or absence of a nucleus—is used as the basis for a simple but fundamental classification of all living things. Organisms whose cells have a nucleus are called **eukaryotes** (from the Greek words *eu*, meaning "well" or "truly," and *karyon*, a "kernel" or "nucleus"). Organisms whose cells do not have a nucleus are called **prokaryotes** (from *pro*, meaning "before").

Figure 1–9 How big are cells and their components? (A) This chart lists sizes of cells and their component parts, the units in which they are measured, and the instruments needed to visualize them. (B) Drawings convey a sense of scale between living cells and atoms. Each panel shows an image that is magnified by a factor of 10 compared to its predecessor—producing an imaginary progression from a thumb, to skin, to skin cells, to a mitochondrion, to a ribosome, and ultimately to a cluster of atoms forming part of one of the many protein molecules in our bodies. Note that ribosomes are present inside mitochondria (as shown here), as well as in the cytoplasm. Details of molecular structure, as shown in the last two bottom panels, are beyond the power of the electron microscope.

CONVENTIONAL LIGHT MICROSCOPY

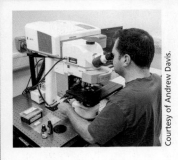

Courtesy of Andrew Davis.

A conventional light microscope allows us to magnify cells up to 1000 times and to resolve details as small as 0.2 μm (200 nm), a limitation imposed by the wavelike nature of light, not by the quality of the lenses. Three things are required for viewing cells in a light microscope. First, a bright light must be focused onto the specimen by lenses in the condenser. Second, the specimen must be carefully prepared to allow light to pass through it. Third, an appropriate set of lenses (objective, tube, and eyepiece) must be arranged to focus an image of the specimen in the eye.

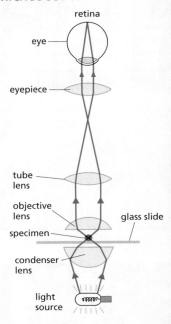

retina

eye

eyepiece

tube lens

objective lens

specimen

glass slide

condenser lens

light source

the light path in a light microscope

LOOKING AT LIVING CELLS

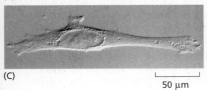

(A)

(B)

(C)

50 μm

The same unstained, living animal cell (fibroblast) in culture viewed with
(A) the simplest, bright-field optics;
(B) phase-contrast optics;
(C) interference-contrast optics.
The two latter systems exploit differences in the way light travels through regions of the cell with differing refractive indices. All three images can be obtained on the same microscope simply by interchanging optical components.

FIXED SAMPLES

Most tissues are neither small enough nor transparent enough to examine directly in the microscope. Typically, therefore, they are chemically fixed and cut into thin slices, or *sections*, that can be mounted on a glass microscope slide and subsequently stained to reveal different components of the cells. A stained section of a plant root tip is shown here (D).

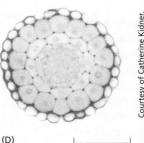

(D)

50 μm

Courtesy of Catherine Kidner.

FLUORESCENCE MICROSCOPY

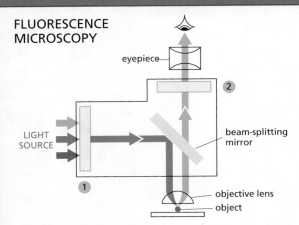

eyepiece

2

beam-splitting mirror

LIGHT SOURCE

objective lens

object

1

Fluorescent dyes used for staining cells are detected with the aid of a *fluorescence microscope*. This is similar to an ordinary light microscope, except that the illuminating light is passed through two sets of filters (*yellow*). The first (1) filters the light before it reaches the specimen, passing only those wavelengths that excite the particular fluorescent dye. The second (2) blocks out this light and passes only those wavelengths emitted when the dye fluoresces. Dyed objects show up in bright color on a dark background.

FLUORESCENT PROBES

Fluorescent molecules absorb light at one wavelength and emit it at another, longer wavelength. Some fluorescent dyes bind specifically to particular molecules in cells and can reveal their location when the cells are examined with a fluorescence microscope.

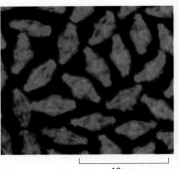

10 μm

Courtesy of William Sullivan.

In these dividing nuclei in a fly embryo, the stain for DNA fluoresces *blue*. Other dyes can be coupled to antibody molecules, which then serve as highly specific staining reagents that bind selectively to particular molecules, showing their distribution in the cell. Because fluorescent dyes emit light, they allow objects even smaller than 0.2 μm to be seen. Here, a microtubule protein in the mitotic spindle (see Figure 1–28) is stained *green* with a fluorescent antibody.

CONFOCAL FLUORESCENCE MICROSCOPY

A confocal microscope is a specialized type of fluorescence microscope that builds up an image by scanning the specimen with a laser beam. The beam is focused onto a single point at a specific depth in the specimen, and a pinhole aperture in the detector allows only fluorescence emitted from this same point to be included in the image.

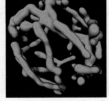

2 μm

Courtesy of Stefan Hell.

Scanning the beam across the specimen generates a sharp image of the plane of focus—an *optical* section. A series of optical sections at different depths allows a three-dimensional image to be constructed, such as this highly branched mitochondrion in a living yeast cell.

SUPER-RESOLUTION FLUORESCENCE MICROSCOPY

Several recent and ingenious techniques have allowed fluorescence microscopes to break the usual resolution limit of 200 nm. One such technique uses a sample that is labeled with molecules whose fluorescence can be reversibly switched on and off by different colored lasers. The specimen is scanned by a nested set of two laser beams, in which the central beam excites fluorescence in a very small spot of the sample, while a second beam—wrapped around the first—switches off fluorescence in the surrounding area. A related approach allows the positions of individual fluorescent molecules to be accurately mapped while others nearby are switched off. Both approaches slowly build up an image with a resolution as low as 20 nm. These new super-resolution methods are being extended into 3-D imaging and real-time live cell imaging.

Courtesy of Carl Zeiss Microscopy, LLC.

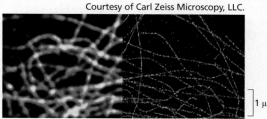

1 µm

Microtubules viewed with conventional fluorescence microscope (*left*) and with super-resolution optics (*right*). In the super-resolution image, the microtubule can be clearly seen at the actual size, which is only 25 nm in diameter.

TRANSMISSION ELECTRON MICROSCOPY

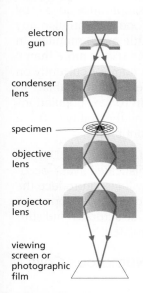

electron gun

condenser lens

specimen

objective lens

projector lens

viewing screen or photographic film

Courtesy of Andrew Davis.

The electron micrograph below shows a small region of a cell in a thin section of testis. The tissue has been chemically fixed, embedded in plastic, and cut into very thin sections that have then been stained with salts of uranium and lead.

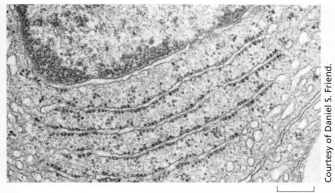

Courtesy of Daniel S. Friend.

0.5 µm

The transmission electron microscope (TEM) is in principle similar to a light microscope, but it uses a beam of electrons, whose wavelength is very short, instead of a beam of light, and magnetic coils to focus the beam instead of glass lenses. Because of the very small wavelength of electrons, the specimen must be very thin. Contrast is usually introduced by staining the specimen with electron-dense heavy metals. The specimen is then placed in a vacuum in the microscope. The TEM has a useful magnification of up to a million-fold and can resolve details as small as about 1 nm in biological specimens.

SCANNING ELECTRON MICROSCOPY

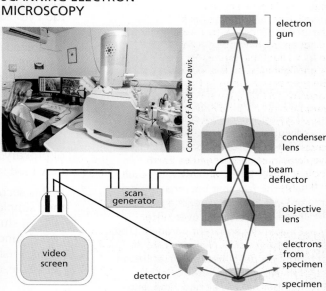

Courtesy of Andrew Davis.

electron gun

condenser lens

beam deflector

scan generator

objective lens

video screen

detector

electrons from specimen

specimen

In the scanning electron microscope (SEM), the specimen, which has been coated with a very thin film of a heavy metal, is scanned by a beam of electrons brought to a focus on the specimen by magnetic coils that act as lenses. The quantity of electrons scattered or emitted as the beam bombards each successive point on the surface of the specimen is measured by the detector, and is used to control the intensity of successive points in an image built up on a video screen. The microscope creates striking images of three-dimensional objects with great depth of focus and can resolve details down to somewhere between 3 nm and 20 nm, depending on the instrument.

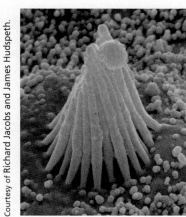

Courtesy of Richard Jacobs and James Hudspeth.

1 µm

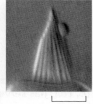

5 µm

Scanning electron micrograph of stereocilia projecting from a hair cell in the inner ear (*left*). For comparison, the same structure is shown by light microscopy, at the limit of its resolution (*above*).

Figure 1–10 Bacteria come in different shapes and sizes. Typical spherical, rodlike, and spiral-shaped bacteria are drawn to scale. The spiral cells shown are the organisms that cause syphilis.

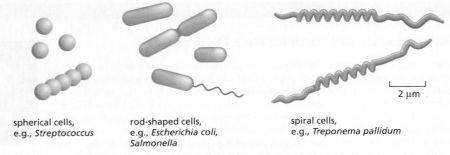

spherical cells,
e.g., *Streptococcus*

rod-shaped cells,
e.g., *Escherichia coli*,
Salmonella

spiral cells,
e.g., *Treponema pallidum*

2 µm

Prokaryotes are typically spherical, rodlike, or corkscrew-shaped (**Figure 1–10**). They are also small—generally just a few micrometers long, although some giant species are as much as 100 times longer than this. Prokaryotes often have a tough protective coat, or cell wall, surrounding the plasma membrane, which encloses a single compartment containing the cytoplasm and the DNA. In the electron microscope, the cell interior typically appears as a matrix of varying texture, without any obvious organized internal structure (**Figure 1–11**). The cells reproduce quickly by dividing in two. Under optimum conditions, when food is plentiful, many prokaryotic cells can duplicate themselves in as little as 20 minutes. In only 11 hours, a single prokaryote can therefore give rise to more than 8 billion progeny (which exceeds the total number of humans currently on Earth). Thanks to their large numbers, rapid proliferation, and ability to exchange bits of genetic material by a process akin to sex, populations of prokaryotic cells can evolve fast, rapidly acquiring the ability to use a new food source or to resist being killed by a new antibiotic.

In this section, we offer an overview of the world of prokaryotes. Despite their simple appearance, these organisms lead sophisticated lives—occupying a stunning variety of ecological niches. We will also introduce the two distinct classes into which prokaryotes are divided: bacteria and *archaea* (singular, archaeon). Although they are structurally indistinguishable, archaea and bacteria are only distantly related.

Prokaryotes Are the Most Diverse and Numerous Cells on Earth

Most prokaryotes live as single-celled organisms, although some join together to form chains, clusters, or other organized, multicellular structures. In shape and structure, prokaryotes may seem simple and limited, but in terms of chemistry, they are the most diverse class of cells on the planet. Members of this class exploit an enormous range of habitats, from hot puddles of volcanic mud to the interiors of other living cells, and they vastly outnumber all eukaryotic organisms on Earth. Some are aerobic, using oxygen to oxidize food molecules; some are strictly anaerobic and are killed by the slightest exposure to oxygen. As we discuss later in this chapter, *mitochondria*—the organelles that generate energy in eukaryotic cells—are thought to have evolved from aerobic bacteria that took

QUESTION 1–4

A bacterium weighs about 10^{-12} g and can divide every 20 minutes. If a single bacterial cell carried on dividing at this rate, how long would it take before the mass of bacteria would equal that of the Earth $(6 \times 10^{24}$ kg)? Contrast your result with the fact that bacteria originated at least 3.5 billion years ago and have been dividing ever since. Explain the apparent paradox. (The number of cells N in a culture at time t is described by the equation $N = N_0 \times 2^{t/G}$, where N_0 is the number of cells at zero time, and G is the population doubling time.)

Figure 1–11 The bacterium *Escherichia coli* (*E. coli*) has served as an important model organism. An electron micrograph of a longitudinal section is shown here; the cell's DNA is concentrated in the lightly stained region. Note that *E. coli* has an outer membrane and an inner (plasma) membrane, with a thin cell wall in between. The many flagella distributed over its surface are not visible in this micrograph. (Courtesy of E. Kellenberger.)

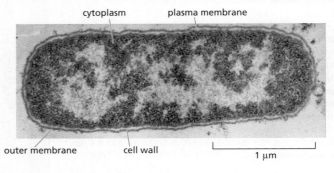

cytoplasm   plasma membrane

outer membrane   cell wall   1 µm

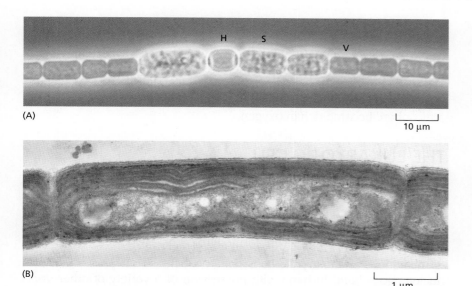

(A)

10 µm

(B)

1 µm

Figure 1–12 Some bacteria are photosynthetic. (A) *Anabaena cylindrica* forms long, multicellular chains. This light micrograph shows specialized cells that either fix nitrogen (that is, capture N_2 from the atmosphere and incorporate it into organic compounds; labeled H), fix CO_2 through photosynthesis (labeled V), or become resistant spores (labeled S) that can survive under unfavorable conditions. (B) An electron micrograph of a related species, *Phormidium laminosum*, shows the intracellular membranes where photosynthesis occurs. As shown in these micrographs, some prokaryotes can have intracellular membranes and form simple multicellular organisms. (A, courtesy of David Adams; B, courtesy of D.P. Hill and C.J. Howe.)

to living inside the anaerobic ancestors of today's eukaryotic cells. Thus our own oxygen-based metabolism can be regarded as a product of the activities of bacterial cells.

Virtually any organic, carbon-containing material—from wood to petroleum—can be used as food by one sort of bacterium or another. Even more remarkably, some prokaryotes can live entirely on inorganic substances: they can get their carbon from CO_2 in the atmosphere, their nitrogen from atmospheric N_2, and their oxygen, hydrogen, sulfur, and phosphorus from air, water, and inorganic minerals. Some of these prokaryotic cells, like plant cells, perform *photosynthesis*, using energy from sunlight to produce organic molecules from CO_2 (**Figure 1–12**); others derive energy from the chemical reactivity of inorganic substances in the environment (**Figure 1–13**). In either case, such prokaryotes play a unique and fundamental part in the economy of life on Earth, as other living organisms depend on the organic compounds that these cells generate from inorganic materials.

Plants, too, can capture energy from sunlight and carbon from atmospheric CO_2. But plants unaided by bacteria cannot capture N_2 from the atmosphere. In a sense, plants even depend on bacteria for photosynthesis: as we discuss later, it is almost certain that the organelles in the plant cell that perform photosynthesis—the *chloroplasts*—have evolved from photosynthetic bacteria that long ago found a home inside the cytoplasm of a plant-cell ancestor.

The World of Prokaryotes Is Divided into Two Domains: Bacteria and Archaea

Traditionally, all prokaryotes have been classified together in one large group. But molecular studies have determined that there is a gulf within the class of prokaryotes, dividing it into two distinct *domains*—the **bacteria** and the **archaea**—which are thought to have diverged from a common prokaryotic ancestor approximately 3.5 billion years ago. Remarkably, DNA sequencing reveals that, at a molecular level, the members of these two domains differ as much from one another as either does from the eukaryotes. Most of the prokaryotes familiar from everyday life—the species that live in the soil or make us ill—are bacteria. Archaea are found not only in these habitats but also in environments that are too hostile for most other cells: concentrated brine, the hot acid of volcanic springs,

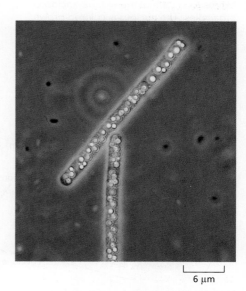

6 µm

Figure 1–13 A sulfur bacterium gets its energy from H_2S. *Beggiatoa*, a prokaryote that lives in sulfurous environments, oxidizes H_2S to produce sulfur and can fix carbon even in the dark. In this light micrograph, yellow deposits of sulfur can be seen inside two of these bacterial cells. (Courtesy of Ralph S. Wolfe.)

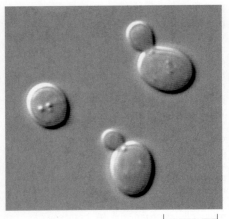

Figure 1–14 Yeasts are simple, free-living eukaryotes. The cells shown in this micrograph belong to the species of yeast, *Saccharomyces cerevisiae*, used to make dough rise and turn malted barley juice into beer. As can be seen in this image, the cells reproduce by growing a bud and then dividing asymmetrically into a large mother cell and a small daughter cell; for this reason, they are called budding yeast.

the airless depths of marine sediments, the sludge of sewage treatment plants, pools beneath the frozen surface of Antarctica, as well as in the acidic, oxygen-free environment of a cow's stomach, where they break down ingested cellulose and generate methane gas. Many of these extreme environments resemble the harsh conditions that must have existed on the primitive Earth, where living things first evolved before the atmosphere became rich in oxygen.

THE EUKARYOTIC CELL

Eukaryotic cells, in general, are bigger and more elaborate than bacteria and archaea. Some live independent lives as single-celled organisms, such as amoebae and yeasts (**Figure 1–14**); others live in multicellular assemblies. All of the more complex multicellular organisms—including plants, animals, and fungi—are formed from eukaryotic cells.

By definition, all eukaryotic cells have a nucleus. But possession of a nucleus goes hand-in-hand with possession of a variety of other organelles, most of which are membrane-enclosed and common to all eukaryotic organisms. In this section, we take a look at the main organelles found in eukaryotic cells from the point of view of their functions, and we consider how they came to serve the roles they have in the life of the eukaryotic cell.

The Nucleus Is the Information Store of the Cell

The **nucleus** is usually the most prominent organelle in a eukaryotic cell (**Figure 1–15**). It is enclosed within two concentric membranes that form

Figure 1–15 The nucleus contains most of the DNA in a eukaryotic cell. (A) This drawing of a typical animal cell shows its extensive system of membrane-enclosed organelles. The nucleus is colored *brown*, the nuclear envelope is *green*, and the cytoplasm (the interior of the cell outside the nucleus) is *white*. (B) An electron micrograph of the nucleus in a mammalian cell. Individual chromosomes are not visible because at this stage of the cell-division cycle the DNA molecules are dispersed as fine threads throughout the nucleus. (B, by permission of E.L. Bearer and Daniel S. Friend.)

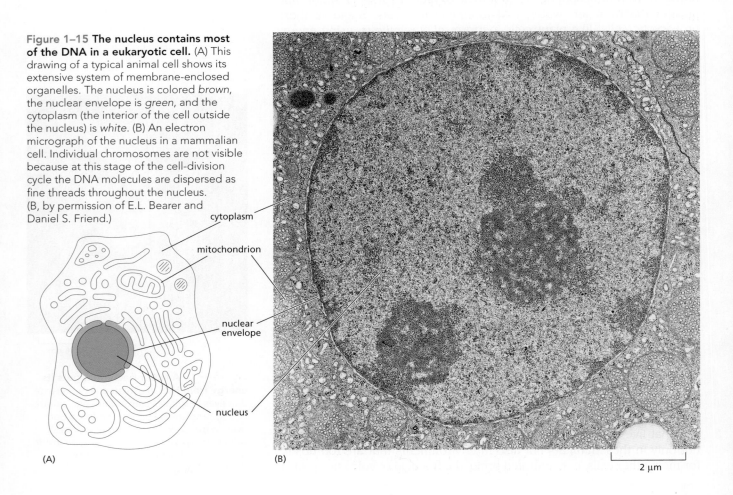

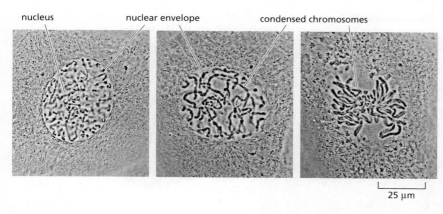

nucleus   nuclear envelope   condensed chromosomes

25 µm

Figure 1–16 **Chromosomes become visible when a cell is about to divide.** As a eukaryotic cell prepares to divide, its DNA molecules become progressively more compacted (condensed), forming wormlike chromosomes that can be distinguished in the light microscope (see also Figure 1–5). The photographs here show three successive steps in this chromosome condensation process in a cultured cell from a newt's lung; note that in the last micrograph on the right, the nuclear envelope has broken down. (Courtesy of Conly L. Rieder, Albany, New York.)

the *nuclear envelope*, and it contains molecules of DNA—extremely long polymers that encode the genetic information of the organism. In the light microscope, these giant DNA molecules become visible as individual **chromosomes** when they become more compact before a cell divides into two daughter cells (**Figure 1–16**). DNA also carries the genetic information in prokaryotic cells; these cells lack a distinct nucleus not because they lack DNA, but because they do not keep their DNA inside a nuclear envelope, segregated from the rest of the cell contents.

Mitochondria Generate Usable Energy from Food Molecules

Mitochondria are present in essentially all eukaryotic cells, and they are among the most conspicuous organelles in the cytoplasm (see Figure 1–8B). In a fluorescence microscope, they appear as worm-shaped structures that often form branching networks (**Figure 1–17**). When seen with an electron microscope, individual mitochondria are found to be enclosed in two separate membranes, with the inner membrane formed into folds that project into the interior of the organelle (**Figure 1–18**).

Microscopic examination by itself, however, gives little indication of what mitochondria do. Their function was discovered by breaking open cells and then spinning the soup of cell fragments in a centrifuge; this treatment separates the organelles according to their size and density. Purified mitochondria were then tested to see what chemical processes they could perform. This revealed that mitochondria are generators of chemical energy for the cell. They harness the energy from the oxidation of food molecules, such as sugars, to produce *adenosine triphosphate*, or *ATP*—the basic chemical fuel that powers most of the cell's activities. Because the mitochondrion consumes oxygen and releases CO_2 in the course of this activity, the entire process is called *cell respiration*—essentially, breathing at the level of a cell. Without mitochondria, animals, fungi, and plants would be unable to use oxygen to extract the energy they need from the food molecules that nourish them. The process of cell respiration is considered in detail in Chapter 14.

Mitochondria contain their own DNA and reproduce by dividing. Because they resemble bacteria in so many ways, they are thought to derive from bacteria that were engulfed by some ancestor of present-day eukaryotic

Figure 1–17 **Mitochondria can vary in shape and size.** This budding yeast cell, which contains a green fluorescent protein in its mitochondria, was viewed in a super-resolution confocal fluorescence microscope. In this three-dimensional image, the mitochondria are seen to form complex branched networks. (From A. Egner, S. Jakobs, and S.W. Hell, *Proc. Natl. Acad. Sci. U.S.A* 99:3370–3375, 2002. With permission from National Academy of Sciences.)

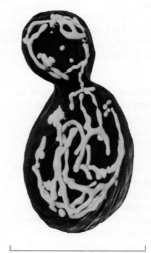

10 µm

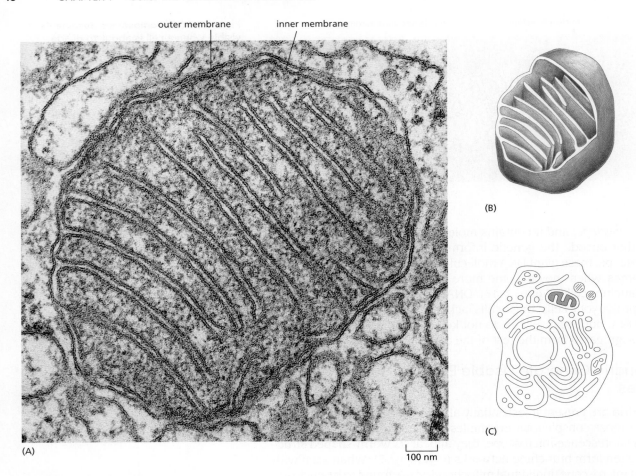

outer membrane   inner membrane

(B)

(C)

(A)

100 nm

Figure 1–18 Mitochondria have a distinctive internal structure. (A) An electron micrograph of a cross section of a mitochondrion reveals the extensive infolding of the inner membrane. (B) This three-dimensional representation of the arrangement of the mitochondrial membranes shows the smooth outer membrane (*gray*) and the highly convoluted inner membrane (*red*). The inner membrane contains most of the proteins responsible for energy production in eukaryotic cells; it is highly folded to provide a large surface area for this activity. (C) In this schematic cell, the innermost compartment of the mitochondrion is colored *orange*. (A, courtesy of Daniel S. Friend, by permission of E.L. Bearer.)

Figure 1–19 Mitochondria are thought to have evolved from engulfed bacteria. It is virtually certain that mitochondria evolved from aerobic bacteria that were engulfed by an archaea-derived, early anaerobic eukaryotic cell and survived inside it, living in symbiosis with their host. As shown in this model, the double membrane of present-day mitochondria is thought to have been derived from the plasma membrane and outer membrane of the engulfed bacterium; the membrane derived from the plasma membrane of the engulfing ancestral cell was ultimately lost.

cells (**Figure 1–19**). This evidently created a *symbiotic* relationship in which the host eukaryote and the engulfed bacterium helped each other to survive and reproduce.

Chloroplasts Capture Energy from Sunlight

Chloroplasts are large, green organelles that are found in the cells of plants and algae, but not in the cells of animals or fungi. These organelles have an even more complex structure than mitochondria: in addition to their two surrounding membranes, they possess internal stacks of membranes containing the green pigment *chlorophyll* (**Figure 1–20**).

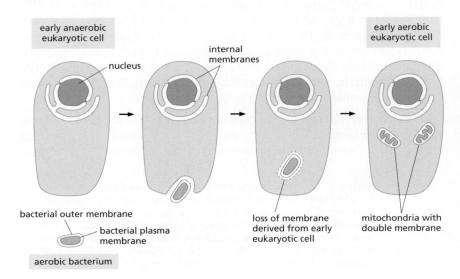

early anaerobic eukaryotic cell

early aerobic eukaryotic cell

internal membranes

nucleus

bacterial outer membrane

bacterial plasma membrane

aerobic bacterium

loss of membrane derived from early eukaryotic cell

mitochondria with double membrane

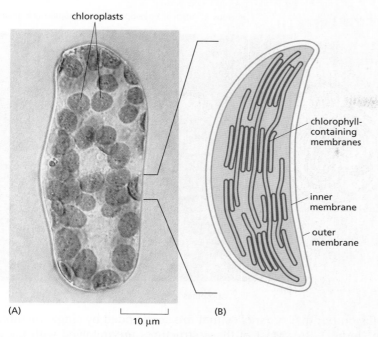

(A)

10 µm

(B)

Figure 1–20 Chloroplasts in plant cells capture the energy of sunlight. (A) A single cell isolated from a leaf of a flowering plant, seen in the light microscope, showing many green chloroplasts. (B) A drawing of one of the chloroplasts, showing the inner and outer membranes, as well as the highly folded system of internal membranes containing the green chlorophyll molecules that absorb light energy. (A, courtesy of Preeti Dahiya.)

Chloroplasts carry out **photosynthesis**—trapping the energy of sunlight in their chlorophyll molecules and using this energy to drive the manufacture of energy-rich sugar molecules. In the process, they release oxygen as a molecular by-product. Plant cells can then extract this stored chemical energy when they need it, in the same way that animal cells do: by oxidizing these sugars and their breakdown products, mainly in the mitochondria. Chloroplasts thus enable plants to get their energy directly from sunlight. They also allow plants to produce the food molecules—and the oxygen—that mitochondria use to generate chemical energy in the form of ATP. How these organelles work together is discussed in Chapter 14.

Like mitochondria, chloroplasts contain their own DNA, reproduce by dividing in two, and are thought to have evolved from bacteria—in this case, from photosynthetic bacteria that were engulfed by an early aerobic eukaryotic cell (**Figure 1–21**).

Internal Membranes Create Intracellular Compartments with Different Functions

Nuclei, mitochondria, and chloroplasts are not the only membrane-enclosed organelles inside eukaryotic cells. The cytoplasm contains a

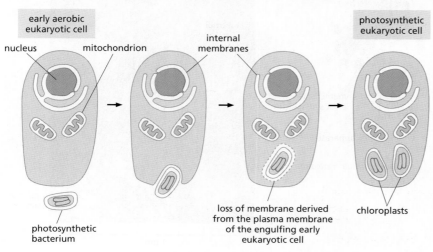

Figure 1–21 Chloroplasts almost certainly evolved from engulfed photosynthetic bacteria. The bacteria are thought to have been taken up by early eukaryotic cells that already contained mitochondria.

Figure 1–22 The endoplasmic reticulum produces many of the components of a eukaryotic cell. (A) Schematic diagram of an animal cell shows the endoplasmic reticulum (ER) in *green*. (B) Electron micrograph of a thin section of a mammalian pancreatic cell shows a small part of the ER, of which there are vast amounts in this cell type, which is specialized for protein secretion. Note that the ER is continuous with the membranes of the nuclear envelope. The black particles studding the region of the ER (and nuclear envelope) shown here are ribosomes, structures that translate RNAs into proteins. Because of its appearance, ribosome-coated ER is often called "rough ER" to distinguish it from the "smooth ER," which does not have ribosomes bound to it. (B, courtesy of Lelio Orci.)

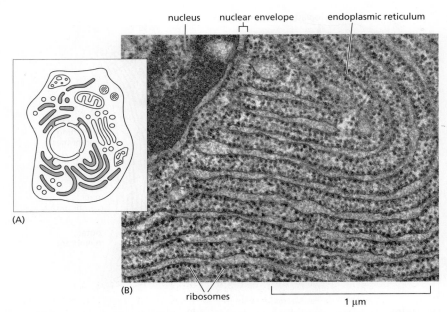

profusion of other organelles that are surrounded by single membranes (see Figure 1–8A). Most of these structures are involved with the cell's ability to import raw materials and to export both useful substances and waste products that are produced by the cell (a topic we discuss in detail in Chapter 12).

The **endoplasmic reticulum** (**ER**) is an irregular maze of interconnected spaces enclosed by a membrane (**Figure 1–22**). It is the site where most cell-membrane components, as well as materials destined for export from the cell, are made. This organelle is enormously enlarged in cells that are specialized for the secretion of proteins. Stacks of flattened, membrane-enclosed sacs constitute the **Golgi apparatus** (**Figure 1–23**),

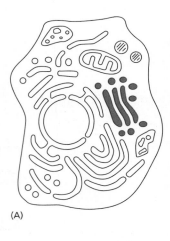

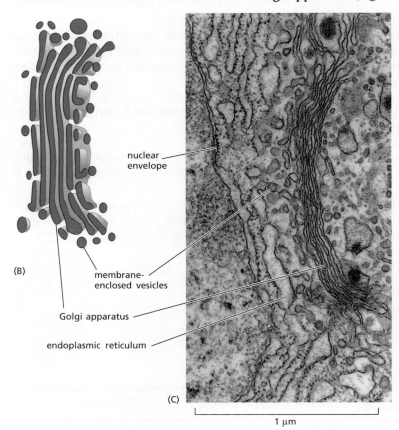

Figure 1–23 The Golgi apparatus is composed of a stack of flattened, membrane-enclosed discs. (A) Schematic diagram of an animal cell with the Golgi apparatus colored *red*. (B) More realistic drawing of the Golgi apparatus. Some of the vesicles seen nearby have pinched off from the Golgi stack; others are destined to fuse with it. Only one stack is shown here, but several can be present in a cell. (C) Electron micrograph that shows the Golgi apparatus from a typical animal cell. (C, courtesy of Brij L. Gupta.)

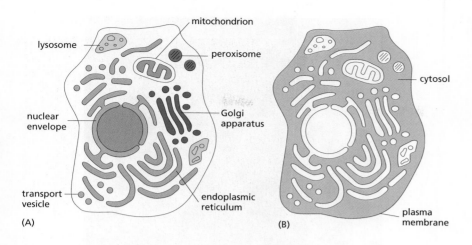

Figure 1–24 Membrane-enclosed organelles are distributed throughout the eukaryotic cell cytoplasm. (A) The various types of membrane-enclosed organelles, shown in different colors, are each specialized to perform a different function. (B) The cytoplasm that fills the space outside of these organelles is called the cytosol (colored *blue*).

which modifies and packages molecules made in the ER that are destined to be either secreted from the cell or transported to another cell compartment. *Lysosomes* are small, irregularly shaped organelles in which intracellular digestion occurs, releasing nutrients from ingested food particles into the cytosol and breaking down unwanted molecules for either recycling within the cell or excretion from the cell. Indeed, many of the large and small molecules within the cell are constantly being broken down and remade. *Peroxisomes* are small, membrane-enclosed vesicles that provide a sequestered environment for a variety of reactions in which hydrogen peroxide is used to inactivate toxic molecules. Membranes also form many types of small *transport vesicles* that ferry materials between one membrane-enclosed organelle and another. All of these membrane-enclosed organelles are highlighted in **Figure 1–24A**.

A continual exchange of materials takes place between the endoplasmic reticulum, the Golgi apparatus, the lysosomes, the plasma membrane, and the outside of the cell. The exchange is mediated by transport vesicles that pinch off from the membrane of one organelle and fuse with another, like tiny soap bubbles that bud from and combine with other bubbles. At the surface of the cell, for example, portions of the plasma membrane tuck inward and pinch off to form vesicles that carry material captured from the external medium into the cell—a process called *endocytosis* (**Figure 1–25**). Animal cells can engulf very large particles, or even entire foreign cells, by endocytosis. In the reverse process, called *exocytosis*, vesicles from inside the cell fuse with the plasma membrane and release their contents into the external medium (see Figure 1–25); most of the hormones and signal molecules that allow cells to communicate with one another are secreted from cells by exocytosis. How membrane-enclosed organelles move proteins and other molecules from place to place inside the eukaryotic cell is discussed in detail in Chapter 15.

The Cytosol Is a Concentrated Aqueous Gel of Large and Small Molecules

If we were to strip the plasma membrane from a eukaryotic cell and remove all of its membrane-enclosed organelles—including the nucleus, endoplasmic reticulum, Golgi apparatus, mitochondria, chloroplasts, and so on—we would be left with the **cytosol** (**Figure 1–24B**). In other words, the cytosol is the part of the cytoplasm that is not contained within intracellular membranes. In most cells, the cytosol is the largest single compartment. It contains a host of large and small molecules, crowded together so closely that it behaves more like a water-based gel than a

IMPORT BY ENDOCYTOSIS

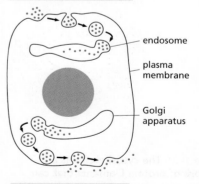

endosome

plasma membrane

Golgi apparatus

EXPORT BY EXOCYTOSIS

Figure 1–25 Eukaryotic cells engage in continual endocytosis and exocytosis across their plasma membrane. They import extracellular materials by endocytosis and secrete intracellular materials by exocytosis. Endocytosed material is first delivered to membrane-enclosed organelles called endosomes (discussed in Chapter 15).

Figure 1–26 The cytosol is extremely crowded. This atomically detailed model of the cytosol of *E. coli* is based on the sizes and concentrations of 50 of the most abundant large molecules present in the bacterium. RNAs, proteins, and ribosomes are shown in different colors (Movie 1.2). (From S.R. McGuffee and A.H. Elcock, *PLoS Comput. Biol.* 6:e1000694, 2010.)

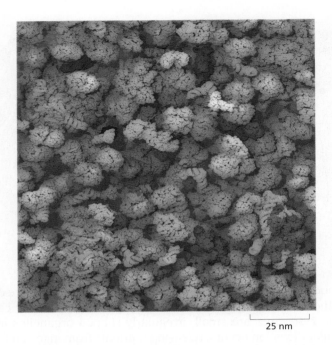

25 nm

QUESTION 1–5

Suggest a reason why it would be advantageous for eukaryotic cells to evolve elaborate internal membrane systems that allow them to import substances from the outside, as shown in Figure 1–25.

liquid solution (**Figure 1–26**). The cytosol is the site of many chemical reactions that are fundamental to the cell's existence. The early steps in the breakdown of nutrient molecules take place in the cytosol, for example, and it is here that most proteins are made by ribosomes.

The Cytoskeleton Is Responsible for Directed Cell Movements

The cytosol is not just a structureless soup of chemicals and organelles. Using an electron microscope, one can see that in eukaryotic cells the cytosol is criss-crossed by long, fine filaments. Frequently, the filaments are seen to be anchored at one end to the plasma membrane or to radiate out from a central site adjacent to the nucleus. This system of protein filaments, called the **cytoskeleton**, is composed of three major filament types (**Figure 1–27**). The thinnest of these filaments are the *actin filaments*; they are abundant in all eukaryotic cells but occur in especially large numbers inside muscle cells, where they serve as a central part of the machinery responsible for muscle contraction. The thickest filaments in the cytosol are called *microtubules* (see Figure 1–7B), because they have the form of minute hollow tubes; in dividing cells, they become reorganized into a spectacular array that helps pull the duplicated chromosomes

Figure 1–27 The cytoskeleton is a network of protein filaments that can be seen criss-crossing the cytoplasm of eukaryotic cells. The three major types of filaments can be detected using different fluorescent stains. Shown here are (A) actin filaments, (B) microtubules, and (C) intermediate filaments. Intermediate filaments are not found in the cytoplasm of cells with cell walls, such as plant cells. (A, Molecular Expressions at Florida State University; B, courtesy of Nancy Kedersha; C, courtesy of Clive Lloyd.)

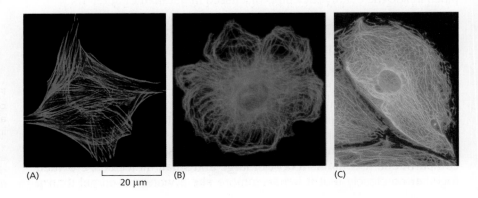

(A) 20 μm (B) (C)

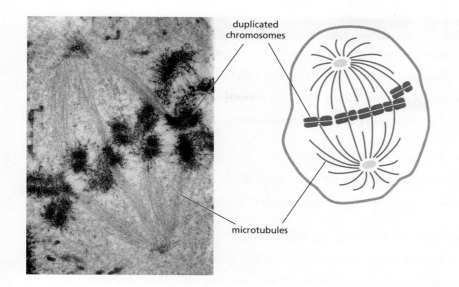

duplicated
chromosomes

microtubules

Figure 1–28 Microtubules help segregate the chromosomes in a dividing animal cell. A transmission electron micrograph and schematic drawing show duplicated chromosomes attached to the microtubules of a mitotic spindle (discussed in Chapter 18). When a cell divides, its nuclear envelope breaks down and its DNA condenses into visible chromosomes, each of which has duplicated to form a pair of conjoined chromosomes that will ultimately be pulled apart into separate daughter cells by the spindle microtubules. See also Panel 1–1, pp. 12–13. (Photomicrograph courtesy of Conly L. Rieder, Albany, New York.)

apart and distribute them equally to the two daughter cells (**Figure 1–28**). Intermediate in thickness between actin filaments and microtubules are the *intermediate filaments*, which serve to strengthen most animal cells. These three types of filaments, together with other proteins that attach to them, form a system of girders, ropes, and motors that gives the cell its mechanical strength, controls its shape, and drives and guides its movements (Movie 1.3 and Movie 1.4).

Because the cytoskeleton governs the internal organization of the cell as well as its external features, it is as necessary to a plant cell—boxed in by a tough cell wall—as it is to an animal cell that freely bends, stretches, swims, or crawls. In a plant cell, for example, organelles such as mitochondria are driven in a constant stream around the cell interior along cytoskeletal tracks (Movie 1.5). And animal cells and plant cells alike depend on the cytoskeleton to separate their internal components into two daughter cells during cell division (see Figure 1–28).

The cytoskeleton's role in cell division may be its most ancient function. Even bacteria contain proteins that are distantly related to those that form the cytoskeletal elements involved in eukaryotic cell division; in bacteria, these proteins also form filaments that play a part in cell division. We examine the cytoskeleton in detail in Chapter 17, discuss its role in cell division in Chapter 18, and review how it responds to signals from outside the cell in Chapter 16.

The Cytosol Is Far from Static

The cell interior is in constant motion. The cytoskeleton is a dynamic jungle of protein ropes that are continually being strung together and taken apart; its filaments can assemble and then disappear in a matter of minutes. *Motor proteins* use the energy stored in molecules of ATP to trundle along these tracks and cables, carrying organelles and proteins throughout the cytoplasm, and racing across the width of the cell in seconds. In addition, the large and small molecules that fill every free space in the cell are knocked to and fro by random thermal motion, constantly colliding with one another and with other structures in the cell's crowded cytosol.

Of course, neither the bustling nature of the cell's interior nor the details of cell structure were appreciated when scientists first peered at cells in a microscope; our knowledge of cell structure accumulated slowly.

TABLE 1–1 HISTORICAL LANDMARKS IN DETERMINING CELL STRUCTURE

1665	Hooke uses a primitive microscope to describe small chambers in sections of cork that he calls "cells"
1674	Leeuwenhoek reports his discovery of protozoa. Nine years later, he sees bacteria for the first time
1833	Brown publishes his microscopic observations of orchids, clearly describing the cell nucleus
1839	Schleiden and Schwann propose the cell theory, stating that the nucleated cell is the universal building block of plant and animal tissues
1857	Kölliker describes mitochondria in muscle cells
1879	Flemming describes with great clarity chromosome behavior during mitosis in animal cells
1881	Cajal and other histologists develop staining methods that reveal the structure of nerve cells and the organization of neural tissue
1898	Golgi first sees and describes the Golgi apparatus by staining cells with silver nitrate
1902	Boveri links chromosomes and heredity by observing chromosome behavior during sexual reproduction
1952	Palade, Porter, and Sjöstrand develop methods of electron microscopy that enable many intracellular structures to be seen for the first time. In one of the first applications of these techniques, Huxley shows that muscle contains arrays of protein filaments—the first evidence of a cytoskeleton
1957	Robertson describes the bilayer structure of the cell membrane, seen for the first time in the electron microscope
1960	Kendrew describes the first detailed protein structure (sperm whale myoglobin) to a resolution of 0.2 nm using x-ray crystallography. Perutz proposes a lower-resolution structure for hemoglobin
1965	de Duve and his colleagues use a cell-fractionation technique to separate peroxisomes, mitochondria, and lysosomes from a preparation of rat liver
1968	Petran and collaborators make the first confocal microscope
1970	Frye and Edidin use fluorescent antibodies to show that plasma membrane molecules can diffuse in the plane of the membrane, indicating that cell membranes are fluid
1974	Lazarides and Weber use fluorescent antibodies to stain the cytoskeleton
1994	Chalfie and collaborators introduce green fluorescent protein (GFP) as a marker to follow the behavior of proteins in living cells
1990s–2000s	Betzig, Hell, and Moerner develop techniques for super-resolution fluorescence microscopy that allow observation of biological molecules too small to be resolved by conventional light or fluorescence microscopy

A few of the key discoveries are listed in **Table 1–1**. In addition, **Panel 1–2** (p. 25) summarizes the main differences between animal, plant, and bacterial cells.

Eukaryotic Cells May Have Originated as Predators

Eukaryotic cells are typically 10 times the length and 1000 times the volume of prokaryotic cells, although there is huge size variation within each category. They also possess a whole collection of features—a nucleus, a versatile cytoskeleton, mitochondria, and other organelles—that set them apart from bacteria and archaea.

When and how eukaryotes evolved these systems remains something of a mystery. Although eukaryotes, bacteria, and archaea must have diverged from one another very early in the history of life on Earth (discussed in Chapter 14), the eukaryotes did not acquire all of their distinctive features at the same time (**Figure 1–29**). According to one theory, the ancestral eukaryotic cell was a predator that fed by capturing other cells. Such a way of life requires a large size, a flexible membrane, and a cytoskeleton to help the cell move and eat. The nuclear compartment may have evolved to keep the DNA segregated from this physical and chemical

QUESTION 1–6

Discuss the relative advantages and disadvantages of light and electron microscopy. How could you best visualize a living skin cell, a yeast mitochondrion, a bacterium, and a microtubule?

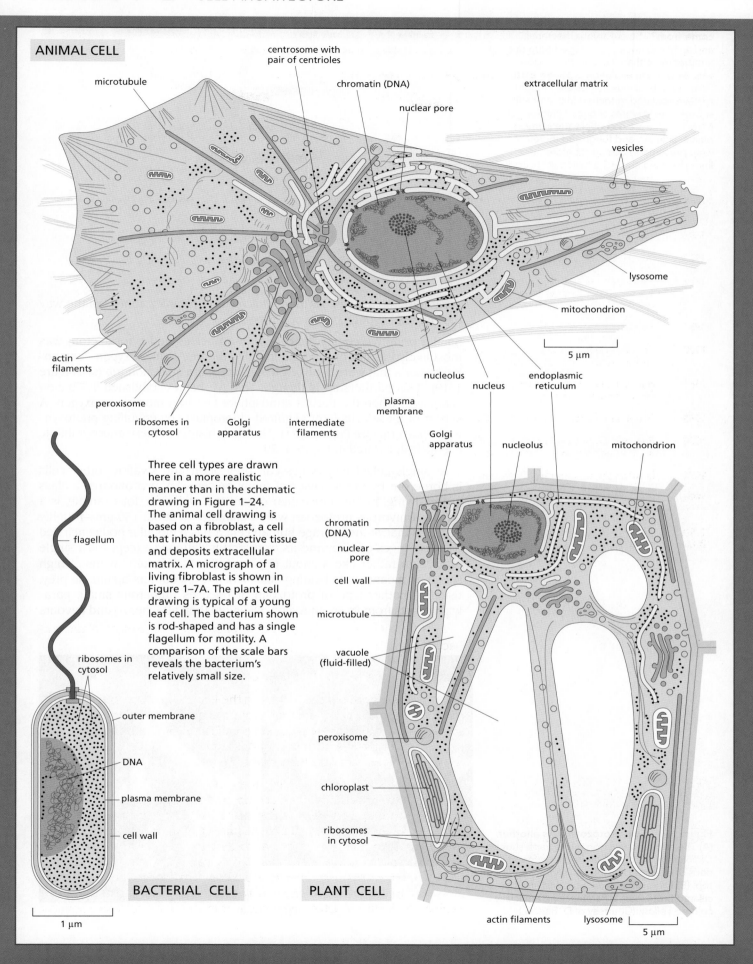

ANIMAL CELL

microtubule

centrosome with pair of centrioles

chromatin (DNA)

nuclear pore

extracellular matrix

vesicles

lysosome

mitochondrion

5 μm

actin filaments

peroxisome

ribosomes in cytosol

Golgi apparatus

intermediate filaments

plasma membrane

nucleolus

nucleus

endoplasmic reticulum

Three cell types are drawn here in a more realistic manner than in the schematic drawing in Figure 1–24. The animal cell drawing is based on a fibroblast, a cell that inhabits connective tissue and deposits extracellular matrix. A micrograph of a living fibroblast is shown in Figure 1–7A. The plant cell drawing is typical of a young leaf cell. The bacterium shown is rod-shaped and has a single flagellum for motility. A comparison of the scale bars reveals the bacterium's relatively small size.

flagellum

ribosomes in cytosol

outer membrane

DNA

plasma membrane

cell wall

Golgi apparatus

nucleolus

mitochondrion

chromatin (DNA)

nuclear pore

cell wall

microtubule

vacuole (fluid-filled)

peroxisome

chloroplast

ribosomes in cytosol

BACTERIAL CELL

PLANT CELL

actin filaments

lysosome

1 μm

5 μm

Figure 1–29 Where did eukaryotes come from? The eukaryotic, bacterial, and archaean lineages diverged from one another more than 3 billion years ago—very early in the evolution of life on Earth. Some time later, eukaryotes are thought to have acquired mitochondria; later still, a subset of eukaryotes acquired chloroplasts. Mitochondria are essentially the same in plants, animals, and fungi, and therefore were presumably acquired before these lines diverged about 1.5 billion years ago.

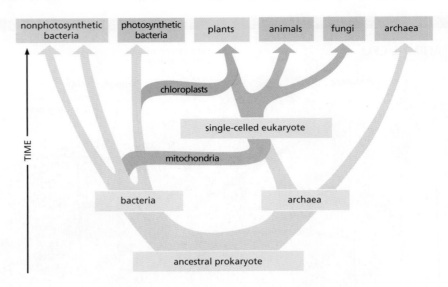

hurly-burly, so as to allow more delicate and complex control of the way the cell reads out its genetic information.

Such a primitive eukaryotic cell, with a nucleus and cytoskeleton, was most likely the sort of cell that engulfed the free-living, oxygen-consuming bacteria that were the likely ancestors of the mitochondria (see Figure 1–19). This partnership is thought to have been established 1.5 billion years ago, when the Earth's atmosphere first became rich in oxygen. A subset of these cells later acquired chloroplasts by engulfing photosynthetic bacteria (see Figure 1–21). The likely history of these endosymbiotic events is illustrated in Figure 1–29.

That single-celled eukaryotes can prey upon and swallow other cells is borne out by the behavior of many present-day **protozoans**: a class of free-living, motile, unicellular organisms. *Didinium*, for example, is a large, carnivorous protozoan with a diameter of about 150 μm—roughly 10 times that of the average human cell. It has a globular body encircled by two fringes of cilia, and its front end is flattened except for a single protrusion rather like a snout (**Figure 1–30A**). *Didinium* swims at high speed by means of its beating cilia. When it encounters a suitable prey, usually another type of protozoan, it releases numerous small, paralyzing darts from its snout region. *Didinium* then attaches to and devours

Figure 1–30 One protozoan eats another. (A) The scanning electron micrograph shows *Didinium* on its own, with its circumferential rings of beating cilia and its "snout" at the top. (B) *Didinium* is seen ingesting another ciliated protozoan, a *Paramecium*, artificially colored *yellow*. (Courtesy of D. Barlow.)

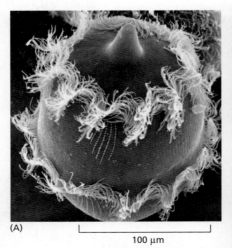

(A)

100 μm

(B)

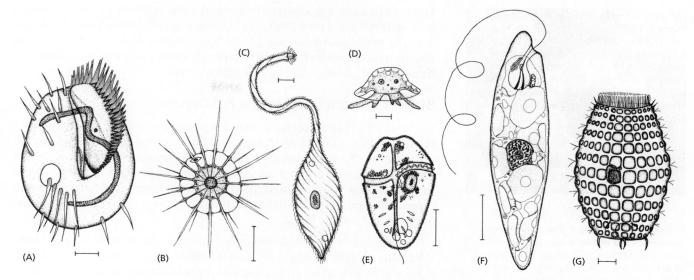

the other cell, inverting like a hollow ball to engulf its victim, which can be almost as large as itself (**Figure 1–30B**).

Not all protozoans are predators. They can be photosynthetic or carnivorous, motile or sedentary. Their anatomy is often elaborate and includes such structures as sensory bristles, photoreceptors, beating cilia, stalklike appendages, mouthparts, stinging darts, and musclelike contractile bundles. Although they are single cells, protozoans can be as intricate and versatile as many multicellular organisms (**Figure 1–31**). Much remains to be learned about fundamental cell biology from studies of these fascinating life-forms.

MODEL ORGANISMS

All cells are thought to be descended from a common ancestor, whose fundamental properties have been conserved through evolution. Thus, knowledge gained from the study of one organism contributes to our understanding of others, including ourselves. But certain organisms are easier than others to study in the laboratory. Some reproduce rapidly and are convenient for genetic manipulations; others are multicellular but transparent, so the development of all their internal tissues and organs can be viewed directly in the live animal. For reasons such as these, biologists have become dedicated to studying a few chosen species, pooling their knowledge to gain a deeper understanding than could be achieved if their efforts were spread over many different species. Although the roster of these representative organisms is continually expanding, a few stand out in terms of the breadth and depth of information that has been accumulated about them over the years—knowledge that contributes to our understanding of how all cells work. In this section, we examine some of these **model organisms** and review the benefits that each offers to the study of cell biology and, in many cases, to the promotion of human health.

Molecular Biologists Have Focused on *E. coli*

In molecular terms, we understand the workings of the bacterium *Escherichia coli*—*E. coli* for short—more thoroughly than those of any other living organism (see Figure 1–11). This small, rod-shaped cell normally lives in the gut of humans and other vertebrates, but it also grows happily and reproduces rapidly in a simple nutrient broth in a culture bottle.

Figure 1–31 An assortment of protozoans illustrates the enormous variety within this class of single-celled eukaryotes. These drawings are done to different scales, but in each case the scale bar represents 10 μm. The organisms in (A), (C), and (G) are ciliates; (B) is a heliozoan; (D) is an amoeba; (E) is a dinoflagellate; and (F) is a euglenoid. To see the latter in action, watch Movie 1.6. Because these organisms can only be seen with the aid of a microscope, they are also referred to as microorganisms. (From M.A. Sleigh, The Biology of Protozoa. London: Edward Arnold, 1973. With permission from Edward Arnold.)

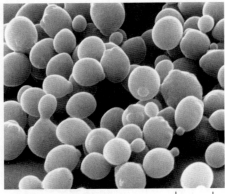

Figure 1–32 **The yeast *Saccharomyces cerevisiae* is a model eukaryote.** In this scanning electron micrograph, a number of the cells are captured in the process of dividing, which they do by budding. Another micrograph of the same species is shown in Figure 1–14. (Courtesy of Ira Herskowitz and Eric Schabtach.)

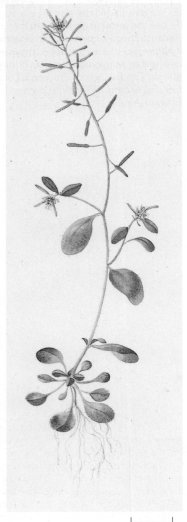

Figure 1–33 ***Arabidopsis thaliana*, the common wall cress, is a model plant.** This small weed has become the favorite organism of plant molecular and developmental biologists. (Courtesy of Toni Hayden and the John Innes Centre.)

Most of our knowledge of the fundamental mechanisms of life—including how cells replicate their DNA and how they decode these genetic instructions to make proteins—has come from studies of *E. coli*. Subsequent research has confirmed that these basic processes occur in essentially the same way in our own cells as they do in *E. coli*.

Brewer's Yeast Is a Simple Eukaryote

We tend to be preoccupied with eukaryotes because we are eukaryotes ourselves. But humans are complicated and reproduce slowly. So to get a handle on the fundamental biology of eukaryotes, we study a simpler representative—one that is easier and cheaper to keep and reproduces more rapidly. A popular choice has been the budding yeast *Saccharomyces cerevisiae* (**Figure 1–32**)—the same microorganism that is used for brewing beer and baking bread.

S. cerevisiae is a small, single-celled fungus that is at least as closely related to animals as it is to plants. Like other fungi, it has a rigid cell wall, is relatively immobile, and possesses mitochondria but not chloroplasts. When nutrients are plentiful, *S. cerevisiae* reproduces almost as rapidly as a bacterium. Yet it carries out all the basic tasks that every eukaryotic cell must perform. Genetic and biochemical studies in yeast have been crucial to understanding many basic mechanisms in eukaryotic cells, including the cell-division cycle—the chain of events by which the nucleus and all the other components of a cell are duplicated and parceled out to create two daughter cells. The machinery that governs cell division has been so well conserved over the course of evolution that many of its components can function interchangeably in yeast and human cells (**How We Know**, pp. 30–31). Darwin himself would no doubt have been stunned by this dramatic example of evolutionary conservation.

Arabidopsis Has Been Chosen as a Model Plant

The large, multicellular organisms that we see around us—both plants and animals—seem fantastically varied, but they are much closer to one another, in their evolutionary origins and their basic cell biology, than they are to the great host of microscopic single-celled organisms. Whereas bacteria, archaea, and eukaryotes separated from each other more than 3 billion years ago, plants, animals, and fungi diverged only about 1.5 billion years ago, and the different species of flowering plants less than 200 million years ago (see Figure 1–29).

The close evolutionary relationship among all flowering plants means that we can gain insight into their cell and molecular biology by focusing on just a few convenient species for detailed analysis. Out of the several hundred thousand species of flowering plants on Earth today, molecular biologists have focused their efforts on a small weed, the common wall cress *Arabidopsis thaliana* (**Figure 1–33**), which can be grown indoors in large numbers: one plant can produce thousands of offspring within 8–10 weeks. Because genes found in *Arabidopsis* have counterparts in agricultural species, studying this simple weed provides insights into the development and physiology of the crop plants upon which our lives depend, as well as into the evolution of all the other plant species that dominate nearly every ecosystem on the planet.

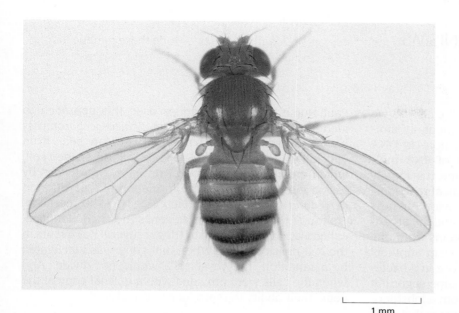

Figure 1–34 *Drosophila melanogaster* is a favorite among developmental biologists and geneticists. Molecular genetic studies on this small fly have provided a key to the understanding of how all animals develop. (Edward B. Lewis. Courtesy of the Archives, California Institute of Technology.)

1 mm

Model Animals Include Flies, Worms, Fish, and Mice

Multicellular animals account for the majority of all named species of living organisms, and the majority of animal species are insects. It is fitting, therefore, that an insect, the small fruit fly *Drosophila melanogaster* (**Figure 1–34**), should occupy a central place in biological research. The foundations of classical genetics (which we discuss in Chapter 19) were built to a large extent on studies of this insect. More than 80 years ago, genetic analysis of the fruit fly provided definitive proof that genes—the units of heredity—are carried on chromosomes. In more recent times, *Drosophila*, more than any other organism, has shown us how the genetic instructions encoded in DNA molecules direct the development of a fertilized egg cell (or *zygote*) into an adult multicellular organism containing vast numbers of different cell types organized in a precise and predictable way. *Drosophila* mutants with body parts strangely misplaced or oddly patterned have provided the key to identifying and characterizing the genes that are needed to make a properly structured adult body, with gut, wings, legs, eyes, and all the other bits and pieces—all in their correct places. These genes—which are copied and passed on to every cell in the body—define how each cell will behave in its social interactions with its sisters and cousins, thus controlling the structures that the cells can create, a regulatory feat we return to in Chapter 8. More importantly, the genes responsible for the development of *Drosophila* have turned out to be amazingly similar to those of humans—far more similar than one would suspect from the outward appearances of the two species. Thus the fly serves as a valuable model for studying human development as well as the genetic basis of many human diseases.

Another widely studied animal is the nematode worm *Caenorhabditis elegans* (**Figure 1–35**), a harmless relative of the eelworms that attack the

QUESTION 1–7

Your next-door neighbor has donated $100 in support of cancer research and is horrified to learn that her money is being spent on studying brewer's yeast. How could you put her mind at ease?

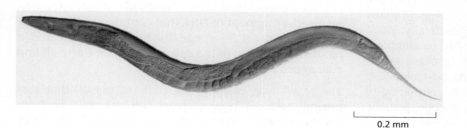

Figure 1–35 *Caenorhabditis elegans* is a small nematode worm that normally lives in the soil. Most individuals are hermaphrodites, producing both sperm and eggs (the latter of which can be seen just beneath the skin along the underside of the animal). *C. elegans* was the first multicellular organism to have its complete genome sequenced. (Courtesy of Maria Gallegos.)

0.2 mm

LIFE'S COMMON MECHANISMS

All living things are made of cells, and all cells—as we have discussed in this chapter—are fundamentally similar inside: they store their genetic instructions in DNA molecules, which direct the production of RNA molecules that direct the production of proteins. It is largely the proteins that carry out the cell's chemical reactions, give the cell its shape, and control its behavior. But how deep do these similarities between cells—and the organisms they comprise—really run? Are proteins from one organism interchangeable with proteins from another? Would an enzyme that breaks down glucose in a bacterium, for example, be able to digest the same sugar if it were placed inside a yeast cell or a cell from a lobster or a human? What about the molecular machines that copy and interpret genetic information? Are they functionally equivalent from one organism to another? Insights have come from many sources, but the most stunning and dramatic answer came from experiments performed on humble yeast cells. These studies, which shocked the biological community, focused on one of the most fundamental processes of life—cell division.

Division and discovery

All cells come from other cells, and the only way to make a new cell is through division of a preexisting one. To reproduce, a parent cell must execute an orderly sequence of reactions, through which it duplicates its contents and divides in two. This critical process of duplication and division—known as the *cell-division cycle*, or *cell cycle* for short—is complex and carefully controlled. Defects in any of the proteins involved can be devastating to the cell.

Fortunately for biologists, this acute reliance on crucial proteins makes them easy to identify and study. If a protein is essential for a given process, a mutation that results in an abnormal protein—or in no protein at all—can prevent the cell from carrying out the process. By isolating organisms that are defective in their cell-division cycle, scientists have worked backward to discover the proteins that control progress through the cycle.

The study of cell-cycle mutants has been particularly successful in yeasts. Yeasts are unicellular fungi and are popular organisms for such genetic studies. They are eukaryotes, like us, but they are small, simple, rapidly reproducing, and easy to manipulate genetically. Yeast mutants that are defective in their ability to complete cell division have led to the discovery of many genes that control the cell-division cycle—the so-called *Cdc* genes—and have provided a detailed understanding of how these genes, and the proteins they encode, actually work.

Paul Nurse and his colleagues used this approach to identify *Cdc* genes in the yeast *Schizosaccharomyces pombe*, which is named after the African beer from which it was first isolated. *S. pombe* is a rod-shaped cell, which grows by elongation at its ends and divides by fission into two, through the formation of a partition in the center of the rod (see Figure 1–1E). The researchers found that one of the *Cdc* genes they had identified, called *Cdc2*, was required to trigger several key events in the cell-division cycle. When that gene was inactivated by a mutation, the yeast cells would not divide. And when the cells were provided with a normal copy of the gene, their ability to reproduce was restored.

It's obvious that replacing a faulty *Cdc2* gene in *S. pombe* with a functioning *Cdc2* gene from the same yeast should repair the damage and enable the cell to divide normally. But what about using a similar cell-division gene from a different organism? That's the question the Nurse team tackled next.

Next of kin

Saccharomyces cerevisiae is another kind of yeast and is one of a handful of model organisms biologists have chosen to study to expand their understanding of how eukaryotic cells work. Also used to brew beer, *S. cerevisiae* divides by forming a small bud that grows steadily until it separates from the mother cell (see Figures 1–14 and 1–32). Although *S. cerevisiae* and *S. pombe* differ in their style of division, both rely on a complex network of interacting proteins to get the job done. But could the proteins from one type of yeast substitute for those of the other?

To find out, Nurse and his colleagues prepared DNA from healthy *S. cerevisiae*, and they introduced this DNA into *S. pombe* cells that contained a temperature-sensitive mutation in the *Cdc2* gene that kept the cells from dividing when the heat was turned up. And they found that some of the mutant *S. pombe* cells regained the ability to proliferate at the elevated temperature. If spread onto a culture plate containing a growth medium, the rescued cells could divide again and again to form visible colonies, each containing millions of individual yeast cells (**Figure 1–36**). Upon closer examination, the researchers discovered that these "rescued" yeast cells had received a fragment of DNA that contained the *S. cerevisiae* version of *Cdc2*—a gene that had been discovered in pioneering studies of the cell cycle by Lee Hartwell and colleagues.

The result was exciting, but perhaps not all that surprising. After all, how different can one yeast be from another? A more demanding test would be to use DNA

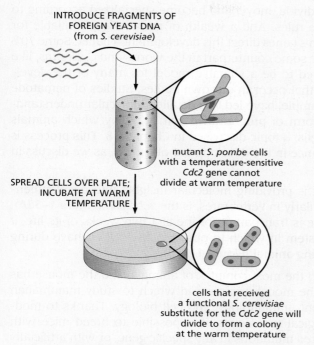

INTRODUCE FRAGMENTS OF
FOREIGN YEAST DNA
(from *S. cerevisiae*)

mutant *S. pombe* cells
with a temperature-sensitive
Cdc2 gene cannot
divide at warm temperature

SPREAD CELLS OVER PLATE;
INCUBATE AT WARM
TEMPERATURE

cells that received
a functional *S. cerevisiae*
substitute for the *Cdc2* gene will
divide to form a colony
at the warm temperature

Figure 1–36 *S. pombe* mutants defective in a cell-cycle gene can be rescued by the equivalent gene from *S. cerevisiae.* DNA is collected from *S. cerevisiae* and broken into large fragments, which are introduced into a culture of mutant *S. pombe* cells dividing at room temperature. We discuss how DNA can be manipulated and transferred into different cell types in Chapter 10. These yeast cells are then spread onto a plate containing a suitable growth medium and are incubated at a warm temperature, at which the mutant Cdc2 protein is inactive. The rare cells that survive and proliferate on these plates have been rescued by incorporation of foreign DNA fragments containing the *Cdc2* gene, allowing them to divide normally at the higher temperature.

from a more distant relative. So Nurse's team repeated the experiment, this time using human DNA. And the results were the same. The human equivalent of the *S. pombe Cdc2* gene could rescue the mutant yeast cells, allowing them to divide normally.

Gene reading

This result was much more surprising—even to Nurse. The ancestors of yeast and humans diverged some

1.5 billion years ago. So it was hard to believe that these two organisms would orchestrate cell division in such a similar way. But the results clearly showed that the human and yeast proteins are functionally equivalent. Indeed, Nurse and colleagues demonstrated that the proteins are almost exactly the same size and consist of amino acids strung together in a very similar order; the human Cdc2 protein is identical to the *S. pombe* Cdc2 protein in 63% of its amino acids and is identical to the equivalent protein from *S. cerevisiae* in 58% of its amino acids (**Figure 1–37**). Together with Tim Hunt, who discovered a different cell-cycle protein called cyclin, Nurse and Hartwell shared a 2001 Nobel Prize for their studies of key regulators of the cell cycle.

The Nurse experiments showed that proteins from very different eukaryotes can be functionally interchangeable and suggested that the cell cycle is controlled in a similar fashion in every eukaryotic organism alive today. Apparently, the proteins that orchestrate the cycle in eukaryotes are so fundamentally important that they have been conserved almost unchanged over more than a billion years of eukaryotic evolution.

The same experiment also highlights another, even more basic point. The mutant yeast cells were rescued, not by direct injection of the human protein, but by introduction of a piece of human DNA. Thus the yeast cells could read and use this information correctly, indicating that, in eukaryotes, the molecular machinery for reading the information encoded in DNA is also similar from cell to cell and from organism to organism. A yeast cell has all the equipment it needs to interpret the instructions encoded in a human gene and to use that information to direct the production of a fully functional human protein.

The story of Cdc2 is just one of thousands of examples of how research in yeast cells has provided critical insights into human biology. Although it may sound paradoxical, the shortest, most efficient path to improving human health will often begin with detailed studies of the biology of simple organisms such as brewer's or baker's yeast.

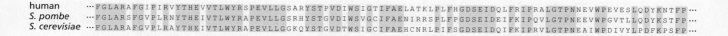

human ···FGLARAFGIPIRVYTHEVVTLWYRSPEVLLGSARYSTPVDIWSIGTIFAELATKLPLFHGDSEIDQLFRIPRALGTPNNEVWPEVESLQDYKNTFP···
S. pombe ···FGLARSFGVPLRNYTHEIVTLWYRAPEVLLGSRHYSTGVDIWSVGCIFAENIRRSPLFPGDSEIDEIFKIPQVLGTPNEEVWPGVTLLQDYKSTFP···
S. cerevisiae ···FGLARAFGVPLRAYTHEIVTLWYRAPEVLLGGKQYSTGVDTWSIGCIFAEHCNRLPIFSGDSEIDQIFKIPRVLGTPNEAIWPDIVYLPDFKPSFP···

Figure 1–37 The cell-division-cycle proteins from yeasts and human are very similar in their amino acid sequences. Identities between the amino acid sequences of a region of the human Cdc2 protein and a similar region of the equivalent proteins in *S. pombe* and *S. cerevisiae* are indicated by *green* shading. Each amino acid is represented by a single letter.

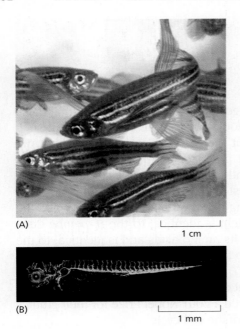

(A)

|_____| 1 cm

(B)

|_____| 1 mm

Figure 1–38 Zebrafish are popular models for studies of vertebrate development. (A) These small, hardy, tropical fish—a staple in many home aquaria—are easy and cheap to breed and maintain. (B) They are also ideal for developmental studies, as their transparent embryos develop outside the mother, making it easy to observe cells moving and changing their characters in the living organism as it develops. In this image of a two-day-old embryo, taken with a confocal microscope, a green fluorescent protein marks the developing lymphatic vessels and a red fluorescent protein marks developing blood vessels; regions where the two fluorescent markers coincide appear *yellow*. (A, courtesy of Steve Baskauf; B, from H.M. Jung et al., *Development* 144:2070–2081, 2017.)

roots of crops. Smaller and simpler than *Drosophila*, this creature develops with clockwork precision from a fertilized egg cell into an adult that has exactly 959 body cells (plus a variable number of egg and sperm cells)—an unusual degree of regularity for an animal. We now have a minutely detailed description of the sequence of events by which this occurs—as the cells divide, move, and become specialized according to strict and predictable rules. And a wealth of mutants are available for testing how the worm's genes direct this developmental ballet. Some 70% of human genes have some counterpart in the worm, and *C. elegans*, like *Drosophila*, has proved to be a valuable model for many of the developmental processes that occur in our own bodies. Studies of nematode development, for example, have led to a detailed molecular understanding of *apoptosis*, a form of programmed cell death by which animals dispose of surplus cells, a topic discussed in Chapter 18. This process is also of great importance in the development of cancer, as we discuss in Chapter 20.

Another animal that is providing molecular insights into developmental processes, particularly in vertebrates, is the *zebrafish* (**Figure 1–38A**). Because this creature is transparent for the first two weeks of its life, it provides an ideal system in which to observe how cells behave during development in a living animal (**Figure 1–38B**).

Mammals are among the most complex of animals, and the mouse has long been used as the model organism in which to study mammalian genetics, development, immunology, and cell biology. Thanks to modern molecular biological techniques, it is possible to breed mice with deliberately engineered mutations in any specific gene, or with artificially constructed genes introduced into them (as we discuss in Chapter 10). In this way, one can test what a given gene is required for and how it functions. Almost every human gene has a counterpart in the mouse, with a similar DNA sequence and function. Thus, this animal has proven an excellent model for studying genes that are important in both human health and disease.

Biologists Also Directly Study Humans and Their Cells

Humans are not mice—or fish or flies or worms or yeast—and so many scientists also study human beings themselves. Like bacteria or yeast, our individual cells can be harvested and grown in culture, where investigators can study their biology and more closely examine the genes that govern their functions. Given the appropriate surroundings, many human cell types—indeed, many cell types of animals or plants—will survive, proliferate, and even express specialized properties in a culture dish. Experiments using such cultured cells are sometimes said to be carried out *in vitro* (literally, "in glass") to contrast them with experiments on intact organisms, which are said to be carried out *in vivo* (literally, "in the living").

Although not true for all cell types, many cells—including those harvested from humans—continue to display the differentiated properties appropriate to their origin when they are grown in culture: fibroblasts, a major cell type in connective tissue, continue to secrete proteins that form the extracellular matrix; embryonic heart muscle cells contract spontaneously in the culture dish; nerve cells extend axons and make functional connections with other nerve cells; and epithelial cells join together to form continuous sheets, as they do inside the body (**Figure 1–39** and Movie 1.7). Because cultured cells are maintained in a controlled environment, they are accessible to study in ways that are often not possible *in vivo*. For example, cultured cells can be exposed to hormones or growth factors,

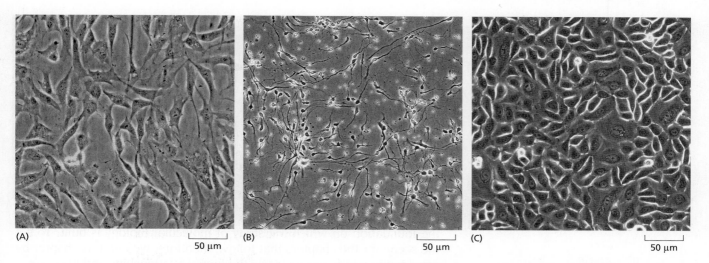

(A)   50 µm   (B)   50 µm   (C)   50 µm

Figure 1–39 Cells in culture often display properties that reflect their origin. These phase-contrast micrographs show a variety of cell types in culture. (A) Fibroblasts from human skin. (B) Human neurons make connections with one another in culture. (C) Epithelial cells from human cervix form a cell sheet in culture. (Micrographs courtesy of ScienCell Research Laboratories, Inc.)

and the effects that these signal molecules have on the shape or behavior of the cells can be easily explored. Remarkably, certain human embryo cells can be coaxed into differentiating into multiple cell types, which can self-assemble into organlike structures that closely resemble a normal organ such as an eye or brain. Such *organoids* can be used to study developmental processes—and how they are derailed in certain human genetic diseases (discussed in Chapter 20).

In addition to studying our cells in culture, humans are also examined directly in clinics. Much of the research on human biology has been driven by medical interests, and the medical database on the human species is enormous. Although naturally occurring, disease-causing mutations in any given human gene are rare, the consequences are well documented. This is because humans are unique among animals in that they report and record their own genetic defects: in no other species are billions of individuals so intensively examined, described, and investigated.

Nevertheless, the extent of our ignorance is still daunting. The mammalian body is enormously complex, being formed from thousands of billions of cells, and one might despair of ever understanding how the DNA in a fertilized mouse egg cell directs the generation of a mouse rather than a fish, or how the DNA in a human egg cell directs the development of a human rather than a mouse. Yet the revelations of molecular biology have made the task seem eminently approachable. As much as anything, this new optimism has come from the realization that the genes of one type of animal have close counterparts in most other types of animals, apparently serving similar functions (Figure 1–40). We all have a common evolutionary origin, and under the surface it seems that we share the same molecular mechanisms. Flies, worms, fish, mice, and humans thus provide a key to understanding how animals in general are made and how their cells work.

Comparing Genome Sequences Reveals Life's Common Heritage

At a molecular level, evolutionary change has been remarkably slow. We can see in present-day organisms many features that have been preserved through more than 3 billion years of life on Earth—about one-fifth of the age of the universe. This evolutionary conservatism provides

Figure 1–40 Different species share similar genes. The human baby and the mouse shown here have remarkably similar white patches on their foreheads because they both have defects in the same gene (called *Kit*), which is required for the normal development, migration, and maintenance of some skin pigment cells. (Courtesy of R.A. Fleischman, *Proc. Natl. Acad. Sci. U.S.A.* 88:10885–10889, 1991.)

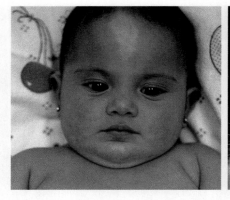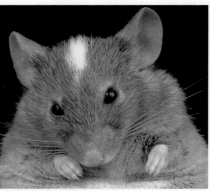

the foundation on which the study of molecular biology is built. To set the scene for the chapters that follow, therefore, we end this chapter by considering a little more closely the family relationships and basic similarities among all living things. This topic has been dramatically clarified by technological advances that have allowed us to determine the complete genome sequences of thousands of organisms, including our own species (as discussed in more detail in Chapter 9).

The first thing we note when we look at an organism's genome is its overall size and how many genes it packs into that length of DNA. Prokaryotes carry very little superfluous genetic baggage and, nucleotide-for-nucleotide, they squeeze a lot of information into their relatively small genomes. *E. coli*, for example, carries its genetic instructions in a single, circular, double-stranded molecule of DNA that contains 4.6 million nucleotide pairs and 4300 protein-coding genes. (We focus on the genes that code for proteins because they are the best characterized, and their numbers are the most certain. We review how genes are counted in Chapter 9.) The simplest known bacterium contains only about 500 protein-coding genes, but most prokaryotes have genomes that contain at least 1 million nucleotide pairs and 1000–8000 protein-coding genes. With these few thousand genes, prokaryotes are able to thrive in even the most hostile environments on Earth.

The compact genomes of typical bacteria are dwarfed by the genomes of typical eukaryotes. The human genome, for example, contains about 700 times more DNA than the *E. coli* genome, and the genome of an amoeba contains about 100 times more than ours (**Figure 1–41**). The rest of the

Figure 1–41 Organisms vary enormously in the size of their genomes. Genome size is measured in nucleotide pairs of DNA per haploid genome; that is, per single copy of the genome. (The body cells of sexually reproducing organisms such as ourselves are generally diploid: they contain two copies of the genome, one inherited from the mother, the other from the father.) Closely related organisms can vary widely in the quantity of DNA in their genomes (as indicated by the length of the *green* bars), even though they contain similar numbers of functionally distinct genes; this is because most of the DNA in large genomes does not code for protein, as discussed shortly. (Data from T.R. Gregory, 2008, Animal Genome Size Database: www.genomesize.com.)

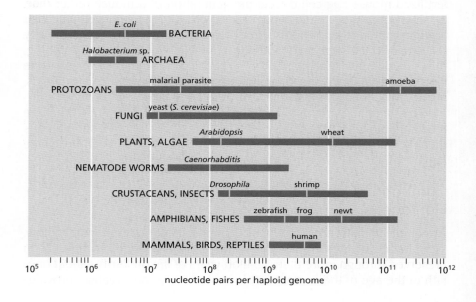

TABLE 1–2 SOME MODEL ORGANISMS AND THEIR GENOMES		
Organism	Genome Size* (Nucleotide Pairs)	Approximate Number of Protein-coding Genes
Homo sapiens (human)	3200×10^6	19,000
Mus musculus (mouse)	2800×10^6	22,000
Drosophila melanogaster (fruit fly)	180×10^6	14,000
Arabidopsis thaliana (plant)	103×10^6	28,000
Caenorhabditis elegans (roundworm)	100×10^6	22,000
Saccharomyces cerevisiae (yeast)	12.5×10^6	6600
Escherichia coli (bacterium)	4.6×10^6	4300

*Genome size includes an estimate for the amount of highly repeated, noncoding DNA sequence, which does not appear in genome databases.

model organisms we have described have genomes that fall somewhere between *E. coli* and human in terms of size. *S. cerevisiae* contains about 2.5 times as much DNA as *E. coli*; *D. melanogaster* has about 10 times more DNA than *S. cerevisiae*; and *M. musculus* has about 20 times more DNA than *D. melanogaster* (Table 1–2).

In terms of gene numbers, however, the differences are not so great. We have only about five times as many protein-coding genes as *E. coli*, for example. Moreover, many of our genes—and the proteins they encode— fall into closely related family groups, such as the family of hemoglobins, which has nine closely related members in humans. Thus the number of fundamentally different proteins in a human is not very many times more than in the bacterium, and the number of human genes that have identifiable counterparts in the bacterium is a significant fraction of the total.

This high degree of "family resemblance" is striking when we compare the genome sequences of different organisms. When genes from different organisms have very similar nucleotide sequences, it is highly probable that they descended from a common ancestral gene. Such genes (and their protein products) are said to be **homologous**. Now that we have the complete genome sequences of many different organisms from all three domains of life—archaea, bacteria, and eukaryotes—we can search systematically for homologies that span this enormous evolutionary divide. By taking stock of the common inheritance of all living things, scientists are attempting to trace life's origins back to the earliest ancestral cells. We return to this topic in Chapter 9.

Genomes Contain More Than Just Genes

Although our view of genome sequences tends to be "gene-centric," our genomes contain much more than just genes. The vast bulk of our DNA does not code for proteins or for functional RNA molecules. Instead, it includes a mixture of sequences that help regulate gene activity, plus sequences that seem to be dispensable. The large quantity of regulatory DNA contained in the genomes of eukaryotic multicellular organisms allows for enormous complexity and sophistication in the way different genes are brought into action at different times and places. Yet, in the end, the basic list of parts—the set of proteins that the cells can make, as specified by the DNA—is not much longer than the parts list of an automobile, and many of those parts are common not only to all animals, but also to the entire living world.

That DNA can program the growth, development, and reproduction of living cells and complex organisms is truly amazing. In the rest of this book, we will try to explain what is known about how cells work—by examining their component parts, how these parts work together, and how the genome of each cell directs the manufacture of the parts the cell needs to function and to reproduce.

ESSENTIAL CONCEPTS

- Cells are the fundamental units of life. All present-day cells are believed to have evolved from an ancestral cell that existed more than 3 billion years ago.

- All cells are enclosed by a plasma membrane, which separates the inside of the cell from its environment.

- All cells contain DNA as a store of genetic information and use it to guide the synthesis of RNA molecules and proteins. This molecular relationship underlies cells' ability to self-replicate.

- Cells in a multicellular organism, though they all contain the same DNA, can be very different because they turn on different sets of genes according to their developmental history and to signals they receive from their environment.

- Animal and plant cells are typically 5–20 μm in diameter and can be seen with a light microscope, which also reveals some of their internal components, including the larger organelles.

- The electron microscope reveals even the smallest organelles, but specimens require elaborate preparation and cannot be viewed while alive.

- Specific large molecules can be located in fixed or living cells by fluorescence microscopy.

- The simplest of present-day living cells are prokaryotes—bacteria and archaea: although they contain DNA, they lack a nucleus and most other organelles and probably resemble most closely the original ancestral cell.

- Different species of prokaryotes are diverse in their chemical capabilities and inhabit an amazingly wide range of habitats.

- Eukaryotic cells possess a nucleus and other organelles not found in prokaryotes. They probably evolved in a series of stages, including the acquisition of mitochondria by engulfment of aerobic bacteria and (for cells that carry out photosynthesis) the acquisition of chloroplasts by engulfment of photosynthetic bacteria.

- The nucleus contains the main genetic information of the eukaryotic organism, stored in very long DNA molecules.

- The cytoplasm of eukaryotic cells includes all of the cell's contents outside the nucleus and contains a variety of membrane-enclosed organelles with specialized functions: mitochondria carry out the final oxidation of food molecules and produce ATP; the endoplasmic reticulum and the Golgi apparatus synthesize complex molecules for export from the cell and for insertion in cell membranes; lysosomes digest large molecules; in plant cells and other photosynthetic eukaryotes, chloroplasts perform photosynthesis.

- Outside the membrane-enclosed organelles in the cytoplasm is the cytosol, a highly concentrated mixture of large and small molecules that carry out many essential biochemical processes.

- The cytoskeleton is composed of protein filaments that extend throughout the cytoplasm and are responsible for cell shape and movement and for the transport of organelles and large molecular complexes from one intracellular location to another.

- Free-living, single-celled eukaryotic microorganisms are complex cells that, in some cases, can swim, mate, hunt, and devour other microorganisms.

- Animals, plants, and some fungi are multicellular organisms that consist of diverse eukaryotic cell types, all derived from a single fertilized egg cell; the number of such cells cooperating to form a large, multicellular organism such as a human runs into thousands of billions.

- Biologists have chosen a small number of model organisms to study intensely, including the bacterium *E. coli*, brewer's yeast, a nematode worm, a fly, a small plant, a fish, mice, and humans themselves.

- The human genome has about 19,000 protein-coding genes, which is about five times as many as *E. coli* and about 5000 more than the fly.

KEY TERMS

archaeon	endoplasmic reticulum	model organism
bacterium	eukaryote	nucleus
cell	evolution	organelle
chloroplast	fluorescence microscope	photosynthesis
chromosome	genome	plasma membrane
cytoplasm	Golgi apparatus	prokaryote
cytoskeleton	homologous	protein
cytosol	micrometer	protozoan
DNA	microscope	ribosome
electron microscope	mitochondrion	RNA

QUESTIONS

QUESTION 1–8

By now you should be familiar with the following cell components. Briefly define what they are and what function they provide for cells.

A. cytosol

B. cytoplasm

C. mitochondria

D. nucleus

E. chloroplasts

F. lysosomes

G. chromosomes

H. Golgi apparatus

I. peroxisomes

J. plasma membrane

K. endoplasmic reticulum

L. cytoskeleton

M. ribosome

QUESTION 1–9

Which of the following statements are correct? Explain your answers.

A. The hereditary information of a cell is passed on by its proteins.

B. Bacterial DNA is found in the cytoplasm.

C. Plants are composed of prokaryotic cells.

D. With the exception of egg and sperm cells, all of the nucleated cells within a single multicellular organism have the same number of chromosomes.

E. The cytosol includes membrane-enclosed organelles such as lysosomes.

F. The nucleus and a mitochondrion are each surrounded by a double membrane.

G. Protozoans are complex organisms with a set of specialized cells that form tissues such as flagella, mouthparts, stinging darts, and leglike appendages.

H. Lysosomes and peroxisomes are the sites of degradation of unwanted materials.

QUESTION 1–10

Identify the different organelles indicated with letters in the electron micrograph of a plant cell shown below. Estimate the length of the scale bar in the figure.

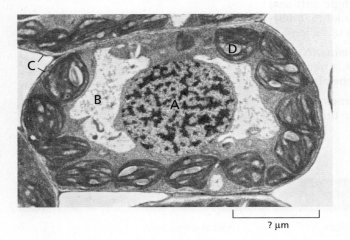

? μm

QUESTION 1–11

There are three major classes of protein filaments that make up the cytoskeleton of a typical animal cell. What are they, and what are the differences in their functions? Which cytoskeletal filaments would be most plentiful in a muscle cell or in an epidermal cell making up the outer layer of the skin? Explain your answers.

QUESTION 1–12

Natural selection is such a powerful force in evolution because organisms or cells with even a small reproductive advantage will eventually outnumber their competitors. To illustrate how quickly this process can occur, consider a cell culture that contains 1 million bacterial cells that double every 20 minutes. A single cell in this culture acquires a mutation that allows it to divide faster, with a generation time of only 15 minutes. Assuming that there is an unlimited food supply and no cell death, how long would it take before the progeny of the mutated cell became predominant in the culture? (Before you go through the calculation, make a guess: do you think it would take about a day, a week, a month, or a year?) How many cells of either type are present in the culture at this time? (The number of cells N in the culture at time t is described by the equation $N = N_0 \times 2^{t/G}$, where N_0 is the number of cells at zero time and G is the generation time.)

QUESTION 1–13

When bacteria are cultured under adverse conditions—for example, in the presence of a poison such as an antibiotic—most cells grow and divide slowly. But it is not uncommon to find that the rate of proliferation is restored to normal after a few days. Suggest why this may be the case.

QUESTION 1–14

Apply the principle of exponential growth of a population of cells in a culture (as described in Question 1–12) to the cells in a multicellular organism, such as yourself. There are about 10^{13} cells in your body. Assume that one cell has acquired mutations that allow it to divide in an uncontrolled manner to become a cancer cell. Some cancer cells can proliferate with a generation time of about 24 hours. If none of the cancer cells died, how long would it take before 10^{13} cells in your body would be cancer cells? (Use the equation $N = N_0 \times 2^{t/G}$, with t the time and G the generation time. Hint: $10^{13} \approx 2^{43}$.)

QUESTION 1–15

"The structure and function of a living cell are dictated by the laws of chemistry, physics, and thermodynamics." Provide examples that support (or refute) this claim.

QUESTION 1–16

What, if any, are the advantages in being multicellular?

QUESTION 1–17

Draw to scale the outline of two spherical cells, one a bacterium with a diameter of 1 μm, the other an animal cell with a diameter of 15 μm. Calculate the volume, surface area, and surface-to-volume ratio for each cell. How would the latter ratio change if you included the internal membranes of the animal cell in the calculation of surface area (assume internal membranes have 15 times the area of the plasma membrane)? (The volume of a sphere is given by $4\pi r^3/3$ and its surface by $4\pi r^2$, where r is its radius.) Discuss the following hypothesis: "Internal membranes allowed bigger cells to evolve."

QUESTION 1–18

What are the arguments that all living cells evolved from a common ancestor cell? Imagine the very "early days" of evolution of life on Earth. Would you assume that the primordial ancestor cell was the first and only cell to form?

QUESTION 1–19

Looking at some pond water with a light microscope, you notice an unfamiliar rod-shaped cell about 200 μm long. Knowing that some exceptional bacteria can be as big as this or even bigger, you wonder whether your cell is a bacterium or a eukaryote. How will you decide? If it is not a eukaryote, how will you discover whether it is a bacterium or an archaeon?

Chemical Components of Cells

At first sight, it is difficult to comprehend that living creatures are merely chemical systems. Their incredible diversity of form, their seemingly purposeful behavior, and their ability to grow and reproduce all seem to set them apart from the world of solids, liquids, and gases that chemistry normally describes. Indeed, until the late nineteenth century, it was widely believed that all living things contained a vital force—an "animus"—that was responsible for their distinctive properties.

We now know that there is nothing in a living organism that disobeys chemical or physical laws. However, the chemistry of life is indeed a special kind. First, it is based overwhelmingly on carbon compounds, the study of which is known as *organic chemistry*. Second, it depends almost exclusively on chemical reactions that take place in a watery, or *aqueous*, environment and in the relatively narrow range of temperatures experienced on Earth. Third, it is enormously complex: even the simplest cell is vastly more complicated in its chemistry than any other chemical system known. Fourth, it is dominated and coordinated by collections of large **polymers**—molecules made of many chemical **subunits** linked end-to-end—whose unique properties enable cells and organisms to grow and reproduce and to do all the other things that are characteristic of life. Finally, the chemistry of life is tightly regulated: cells deploy a wide variety of mechanisms to make sure that each of their chemical reactions occurs at the proper rate, time, and place.

Because chemistry lies at the heart of all biology, in this chapter, we briefly survey the chemistry of the living cell. We will meet the molecules from which cells are made and examine their structures, shapes, and chemical properties. These molecules determine the size, structure, and functions

CHEMICAL BONDS

SMALL MOLECULES IN CELLS

MACROMOLECULES IN CELLS

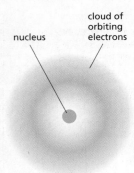

Figure 2–1 An atom consists of a nucleus surrounded by an electron cloud. The dense, positively charged nucleus contains nearly all of the atom's mass. The much lighter and negatively charged electrons occupy space around the nucleus, as governed by the laws of quantum mechanics. The electrons are depicted as a continuous cloud, because there is no way of predicting exactly where an electron is at any given instant. The density of shading of the cloud is an indication of the probability that electrons will be found there.

The diameter of the electron cloud ranges from about 0.1 nm (for hydrogen) to about 0.4 nm (for atoms of high atomic number). The nucleus is very much smaller: about 5×10^{-6} nm for carbon, for example. If this diagram were drawn to scale, the nucleus would not be visible.

of living cells. By understanding how they interact, we can begin to see how cells exploit the laws of chemistry and physics to survive, thrive, and reproduce.

CHEMICAL BONDS

Matter is made of combinations of *elements*—substances such as hydrogen or carbon that cannot be broken down or interconverted by chemical means. The smallest particle of an element that still retains its distinctive chemical properties is an *atom*. The characteristics of substances other than pure elements—including the materials from which living cells are made—depend on which atoms they contain and the way that these atoms are linked together in groups to form *molecules*. To understand living organisms, therefore, it is crucial to know how the chemical bonds that hold atoms together in molecules are formed.

Cells Are Made of Relatively Few Types of Atoms

Each **atom** has at its center a dense, positively charged nucleus, which is surrounded at some distance by a cloud of negatively charged **electrons**, held in orbit by electrostatic attraction to the nucleus (**Figure 2–1**). The nucleus consists of two kinds of subatomic particles: **protons**, which are positively charged, and *neutrons*, which are electrically neutral. The *atomic number* of an element is determined by the number of protons present in its atom's nucleus. An atom of hydrogen has a nucleus composed of a single proton; so hydrogen, with an atomic number of 1, is the lightest element. An atom of carbon has six protons in its nucleus and an atomic number of 6 (**Figure 2–2**).

The electric charge carried by each proton is exactly equal and opposite to the charge carried by a single electron. Because the whole atom is electrically neutral, the number of negatively charged electrons surrounding the nucleus is therefore equal to the number of positively charged protons that the nucleus contains; thus the number of electrons in an atom also equals the atomic number. All atoms of a given element have the same atomic number, and we will see shortly that it is this number that dictates each element's chemical behavior.

Neutrons have essentially the same mass as protons. They contribute to the structural stability of the nucleus: if there are too many or too few, the nucleus may disintegrate by radioactive decay. However, neutrons do not alter the chemical properties of the atom. Thus an element can exist in several physically distinguishable but chemically identical forms, called *isotopes*, each having a different number of neutrons but the same

Figure 2–2 The number of protons in an atom determines its atomic number. Schematic representations of an atom of carbon and an atom of hydrogen are shown. The nucleus of every atom except hydrogen consists of both positively charged protons and electrically neutral neutrons; the atomic weight equals the number of protons plus neutrons. The number of electrons in an atom is equal to the number of protons, so that the atom has no net charge.

In contrast to Figure 2–1, the electrons are shown here as individual particles. The concentric *black* circles represent in a highly schematic form the "orbits" (that is, the different distributions) of the electrons. The neutrons, protons, and electrons are in reality minuscule in relation to the atom as a whole; their size is greatly exaggerated here.

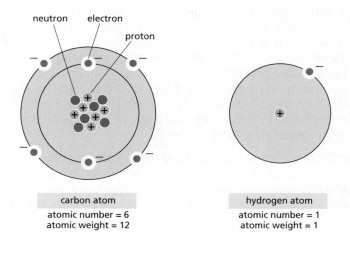

carbon atom
atomic number = 6
atomic weight = 12

hydrogen atom
atomic number = 1
atomic weight = 1

number of protons. Multiple isotopes of almost all the elements occur naturally, including some that are unstable—and thus radioactive. For example, while most carbon on Earth exists as carbon 12, a stable isotope with six protons and six neutrons, also present are small amounts of an unstable isotope, carbon 14, which has six protons and eight neutrons. Carbon 14 undergoes radioactive decay at a slow but steady rate, a property that allows archaeologists to estimate the age of organic material.

The **atomic weight** of an atom, or the **molecular weight** of a molecule, is its mass relative to the mass of a hydrogen atom. This value is equal to the number of protons plus the number of neutrons that the atom or molecule contains; because electrons are so light, they contribute almost nothing to the total mass. Thus the major isotope of carbon has an atomic weight of 12 and is written as ^{12}C. The unstable carbon isotope just mentioned has an atomic weight of 14 and is written as ^{14}C. The mass of an atom or a molecule is generally specified in *daltons*, one dalton being an atomic mass unit essentially equal to the mass of a hydrogen atom.

Atoms are so small that it is hard to imagine their size. An individual carbon atom is roughly 0.2 nm in diameter, so it would take about 5 million of them, laid out in a straight line, to span a millimeter. One proton or neutron weighs approximately $1/(6 \times 10^{23})$ gram. As hydrogen has only one proton—thus an atomic weight of 1—1 gram of hydrogen contains 6×10^{23} atoms. For carbon—which has six protons and six neutrons, and an atomic weight of 12—12 grams contain 6×10^{23} atoms. This huge number, called **Avogadro's number**, allows us to relate everyday quantities of chemicals to numbers of individual atoms or molecules. If a substance has a molecular weight of X, X grams of the substance will contain 6×10^{23} molecules. This quantity is called one *mole* of the substance (**Figure 2–3**). The concept of mole is used widely in chemistry as a way to represent the number of molecules that are available to participate in chemical reactions.

There are about 90 naturally occurring elements, each differing from the others in the number of protons and electrons in its atoms. Living things, however, are made of only a small selection of these elements, four of which—carbon (C), hydrogen (H), nitrogen (N), and oxygen (O)—constitute 96% of any organism's weight. This composition differs markedly from that of the nonliving, inorganic environment on Earth (**Figure 2–4**) and is evidence that a distinctive type of chemistry operates in biological systems.

The Outermost Electrons Determine How Atoms Interact

To understand how atoms come together to form the molecules that make up living organisms, we have to pay special attention to each atom's electrons. Protons and neutrons are welded tightly to one another in an atom's nucleus, and they change partners only under extreme conditions—during radioactive decay, for example, or in the interior of the sun or a nuclear reactor. In living tissues, only the electrons of an atom undergo rearrangements. They form the accessible part of the atom and specify the chemical rules by which atoms combine to form molecules.

Electrons are in continuous motion around the nucleus, but motions on this submicroscopic scale obey different laws from those we are familiar with in everyday life. These laws dictate that electrons in an atom can exist only in certain discrete regions of movement—very roughly speaking, in distinct orbits. Moreover, there is a strict limit to the number of electrons that can be accommodated in an orbit of a given type, a so-called *electron shell*. The electrons closest on average to the positively charged nucleus are attracted most strongly to it and occupy the inner,

A **mole** is X grams of a substance, where X is the molecular weight of the substance. A mole will contain 6×10^{23} molecules of the substance.

1 mole of carbon weighs 12 g
1 mole of glucose weighs 180 g
1 mole of sodium chloride weighs 58 g

A **one molar solution** has a concentration of 1 mole of the substance in 1 liter of solution. A 1 M solution of glucose, for example, contains 180 g/L, and a one millimolar (1 mM) solution contains 180 mg/L.

The standard abbreviation for gram is g; the abbreviation for liter is L.

Figure 2–3 What's a mole? Some simple examples of moles and molar solutions.

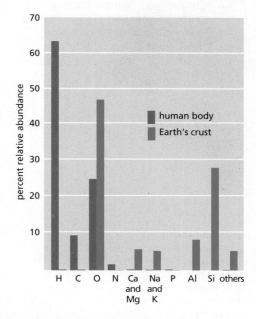

Figure 2–4 The distribution of elements in the Earth's crust differs radically from that in the human body. The abundance of each element is expressed here as a percentage of the total number of atoms present in a biological or geological sample (water included). Thus, for example, more than 60% of the atoms in the human body are hydrogen atoms, and nearly 30% of the atoms in the Earth's crust are silicon atoms (Si). The relative abundance of elements is similar in all living things.

Figure 2–5 An element's chemical reactivity depends on the degree to which its outermost electron shell is filled. All of the elements commonly found in living organisms have outermost shells that are not completely filled. The electrons in these incomplete shells (here shown in *red*) can participate in chemical reactions with other atoms. Inert gases (*yellow*), in contrast, have completely filled outermost shells (*gray*) and are thus chemically unreactive.

atomic number

	element	electron shell			
		I	II	III	IV
1	Hydrogen (H)	●			
2	Helium (He)	●●			
6	Carbon (C)	●●	●●●●		
7	Nitrogen (N)	●●	●●●●●		
8	Oxygen (O)	●●	●●●●●●		
10	Neon (Ne)	●●	●●●●●●●●		
11	Sodium (Na)	●●	●●●●●●●●	●	
12	Magnesium (Mg)	●●	●●●●●●●●	●●	
15	Phosphorus (P)	●●	●●●●●●●●	●●●●●	
16	Sulfur (S)	●●	●●●●●●●●	●●●●●●	
17	Chlorine (Cl)	●●	●●●●●●●●	●●●●●●●	
18	Argon (Ar)	●●	●●●●●●●●	●●●●●●●●	
19	Potassium (K)	●●	●●●●●●●●	●●●●●●●●	●
20	Calcium (Ca)	●●	●●●●●●●●	●●●●●●●●	●●

QUESTION 2–1

A cup containing exactly 18 g, or 1 mole, of water was emptied into the Aegean Sea 3000 years ago. What are the chances that the same quantity of water, scooped today from the Pacific Ocean, would include at least one of these ancient water molecules? Assume perfect mixing and an approximate volume for the world's oceans of 1.5 billion cubic kilometers (1.5×10^9 km^3).

most tightly bound shell. This innermost shell can hold a maximum of two electrons. The second shell is farther away from the nucleus, and can hold up to eight electrons. The third shell can also hold up to eight electrons, which are even less tightly bound. The fourth and fifth shells can hold 18 electrons each. Atoms with more than four shells are very rare in biological molecules.

The arrangement of electrons in an atom is most stable when all the electrons are in the most tightly bound states that are possible for them—that is, when they occupy the innermost shells, closest to the nucleus. Therefore, with certain exceptions in the larger atoms, the electrons of an atom fill the shells in order—the first before the second, the second before the third, and so on. An atom whose outermost shell is entirely filled with electrons is especially stable and therefore chemically unreactive. Examples are helium with 2 electrons (atomic number 2), neon with 2 + 8 electrons (atomic number 10), and argon with 2 + 8 + 8 electrons (atomic number 18); these are all inert gases. Hydrogen, by contrast, has only one electron, which leaves its outermost shell half-filled, so it is highly reactive. The atoms found in living organisms all have outermost shells that are incompletely filled, and they are therefore able to react with one another to form molecules (Figure 2–5).

Because an incompletely filled electron shell is less stable than one that is completely filled, atoms with incomplete outer shells have a strong tendency to interact with other atoms so as to either gain or lose enough electrons to fill the outermost shell. This electron exchange can be achieved either by transferring electrons from one atom to another or by sharing electrons between two atoms. These two strategies generate the two types of **chemical bonds** that can bind atoms strongly to one another: an *ionic bond* is formed when electrons are donated by one atom to another, whereas a *covalent bond* is formed when two atoms share a pair of electrons (Figure 2–6).

An H atom, which needs only one more electron to fill its only shell, generally acquires this electron by sharing—forming one covalent bond with another atom. The other most common elements in living cells—C, N, and O, which have an incomplete second shell, and P and S, which have an incomplete third shell (see Figure 2–5)—also tend to share electrons; these elements thus fill their outer shells by forming several covalent bonds. The number of electrons an atom must acquire or lose (either by sharing or by transfer) to attain a filled outer shell determines the number of bonds that the atom can make.

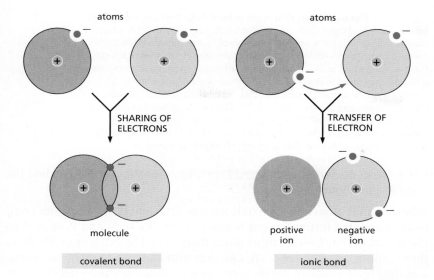

atoms   atoms

SHARING OF ELECTRONS   TRANSFER OF ELECTRON

molecule   positive ion   negative ion

covalent bond   ionic bond

Figure 2–6 Atoms can attain a more stable arrangement of electrons in their outermost shell by interacting with one another. A covalent bond is formed when electrons are shared between atoms. An ionic bond is formed when electrons are transferred from one atom to the other. The two cases shown represent extremes; often, covalent bonds form with a partial transfer (unequal sharing of electrons), resulting in a polar covalent bond, as we discuss shortly.

Because the state of the outer electron shell determines the chemical properties of an element, when the elements are listed in order of their atomic number we see a periodic recurrence of elements that have similar properties. For example, an element with an incomplete second shell containing one electron will behave in a similar way as an element that has filled its second shell and has an incomplete third shell containing one electron. The metals, for example, have incomplete outer shells with just one or a few electrons, whereas, as we have just seen, the inert gases have full outer shells. This arrangement gives rise to the *periodic table* of the elements, outlined in **Figure 2–7**, in which the elements found in living organisms are highlighted in color.

Covalent Bonds Form by the Sharing of Electrons

All of the characteristics of a cell depend on the molecules it contains. A **molecule** is a cluster of atoms held together by **covalent bonds**, in which electrons are shared rather than transferred between atoms. The shared electrons complete the outer shells of the interacting atoms. In the simplest possible molecule—a molecule of hydrogen (H_2)—two H atoms, each with a single electron, share their electrons, thus filling their outermost shells. The shared electrons form a cloud of negative charge that is densest between the two positively charged nuclei. This electron density helps to hold the nuclei together by opposing the mutual repulsion between the positive charges of the nuclei, which would otherwise force them apart. The attractive and repulsive forces are precisely in balance

QUESTION 2–2

A carbon atom contains six protons and six neutrons.
A. What are its atomic number and atomic weight?
B. How many electrons does it have?
C. How many additional electrons must it add to fill its outermost shell? How does this affect carbon's chemical behavior?
D. Carbon with an atomic weight of 14 is radioactive. How does it differ in structure from nonradioactive carbon? How does this difference affect its chemical behavior?

Figure 2–7 When ordered by their atomic number into the periodic table, the elements fall into vertical columns in which the atoms have similar properties. This is because the atoms in the same vertical column must gain or lose the same number of electrons to attain a filled outer shell, and they therefore behave similarly when forming bonds with other atoms. Thus, for example, both magnesium (Mg) and calcium (Ca) tend to give away the two electrons in their outer shells to form ionic bonds with atoms such as chlorine (Cl), which need extra electrons to complete their outer shells.

The chemistry of life is dominated by lighter elements. The four elements highlighted in *red* constitute 99% of the total number of atoms present in the human body and about 96% of our total weight. An additional seven elements, highlighted in *blue*, together represent about 0.9% of our total number of atoms. Other elements, shown in *green*, are required in trace amounts by humans. It remains unclear whether those elements shown in *yellow* are essential in humans or not.

The atomic weights shown here are those of the most common isotope of each element. The vertical *red* line represents a break in the periodic table where a group of large atoms with similar chemical properties has been removed.

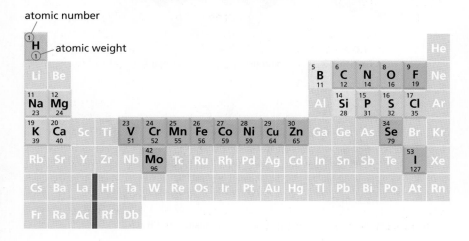

atomic number

atomic weight

two hydrogen atoms

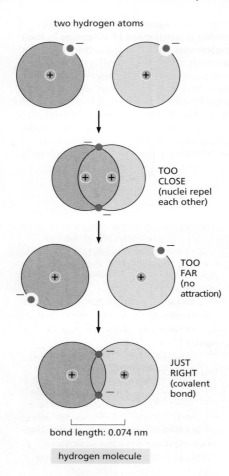

TOO CLOSE (nuclei repel each other)

TOO FAR (no attraction)

JUST RIGHT (covalent bond)

bond length: 0.074 nm

hydrogen molecule

Figure 2–8 The hydrogen molecule is held together by a covalent bond. Each hydrogen atom in isolation has a single electron, which means that its first (and only) electron shell is incompletely filled. By coming together to form a hydrogen molecule (H_2, or hydrogen gas), the two atoms are able to share their electrons, so that each obtains a completely filled first shell, with the shared electrons adopting modified orbits around the two nuclei. The covalent bond between the two atoms has a defined length—0.074 nm, which is the distance between the two nuclei. If the atoms were closer together, the positively charged nuclei would repel each other; if they were farther apart, they would not be able to share electrons as effectively.

when these nuclei are separated by a characteristic distance, called the *bond length* (**Figure 2–8**).

Whereas an H atom can form only a single covalent bond, the other common atoms that form covalent bonds in cells—O, N, S, and P, as well as the all-important C—can form more than one. The outermost shells of these atoms, as we have seen, can accommodate up to eight electrons, and they form covalent bonds with as many other atoms as necessary to reach this number. Oxygen, with six electrons in its outer shell, is most stable when it acquires two extra electrons by sharing with other atoms, and it therefore forms up to two covalent bonds. Nitrogen, with five outer electrons, forms a maximum of three covalent bonds, while carbon, with four outer electrons, forms up to four covalent bonds—thus sharing four pairs of electrons (see Figure 2–5).

When one atom forms covalent bonds with several others, these multiple bonds have definite orientations in space relative to one another, reflecting the orientations of the orbits of the shared electrons. Covalent bonds between multiple atoms are therefore characterized by specific bond angles, as well as by specific bond lengths and bond energies (**Figure 2–9**). The four covalent bonds that can form around a carbon atom, for example, are arranged as if pointing to the four corners of a regular tetrahedron. The precise orientation of the covalent bonds around carbon dictates the three-dimensional geometry of all organic molecules.

Some Covalent Bonds Involve More Than One Electron Pair

Most covalent bonds involve the sharing of two electrons, one donated by each participating atom; these are called *single bonds*. Some covalent bonds, however, involve the sharing of more than one pair of electrons.

Figure 2–9 Covalent bonds are characterized by particular geometries. (A) The spatial arrangement of the covalent bonds that can be formed by oxygen, nitrogen, and carbon. (B) Molecules formed from these atoms therefore have precise three-dimensional structures defined by the bond angles and bond lengths for each covalent linkage. A water molecule, for example, forms a "V" shape with an angle close to 109°.

In these ball-and-stick models, the different colored balls represent different atoms, and the sticks represent the covalent bonds. The colors traditionally used to represent the different atoms—*black* (or *dark gray*) for carbon, *white* for hydrogen, *blue* for nitrogen, and *red* for oxygen—were established by the chemist August Wilhelm Hofmann in 1865, when he used a set of colored croquet balls to build molecular models for a public lecture on "the combining power of atoms."

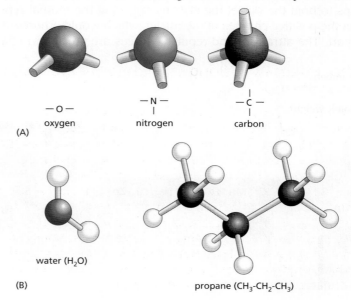

—O—
oxygen

—N—
 |
nitrogen

 |
—C—
 |
carbon

(A)

water (H_2O)

propane (CH_3-CH_2-CH_3)

(B)

Four electrons can be shared, for example, two coming from each participating atom; such a bond is called a *double bond*. Double bonds are shorter and stronger than single bonds and have a characteristic effect on the geometry of molecules containing them. A single covalent bond between two atoms generally allows the rotation of one part of a molecule relative to the other around the bond axis. A double bond prevents such rotation, producing a more rigid and less flexible arrangement of atoms (**Figure 2–10**). This restriction has a major influence on the three-dimensional shape of many macromolecules.

Some molecules contain atoms that share electrons in a way that produces bonds that are intermediate in character between single and double bonds. The highly stable benzene molecule, for example, is made up of a ring of six carbon atoms in which the bonding electrons are evenly distributed, although the arrangement is sometimes depicted as an alternating sequence of single and double bonds. **Panel 2–1** (pp. 66–67) reviews the covalent bonds commonly encountered in biological molecules.

Electrons in Covalent Bonds Are Often Shared Unequally

When the atoms joined by a single covalent bond belong to different elements, the two atoms usually attract the shared electrons to different degrees. Covalent bonds in which the electrons are shared unequally in this way are known as *polar covalent bonds*. A **polar** structure (in the electrical sense) is one in which the positive charge is concentrated toward one atom in the molecule (the positive pole) and the negative charge is concentrated toward another atom (the negative pole). The tendency of an atom to attract electrons is called its **electronegativity**, a property that was first described by the chemist Linus Pauling.

Knowing the electronegativity of atoms allows one to predict the nature of the bonds that will form between them. For example, when atoms with different electronegativities are covalently linked, their bonds will be polarized. Among the atoms typically found in biological molecules, oxygen and nitrogen (with electronegativities of 3.4 and 3.0, respectively) attract electrons relatively strongly, whereas an H atom (with an electronegativity of 2.1) attracts electrons relatively weakly. Thus the covalent bonds between O and H (O–H) and between N and H (N–H) are polar (**Figure 2–11**). An atom of C and an atom of H, by contrast, have similar electronegativities (carbon is 2.6, hydrogen 2.1) and attract electrons more equally. Thus the bond between carbon and hydrogen, C–H, is relatively nonpolar.

Covalent Bonds Are Strong Enough to Survive the Conditions Inside Cells

We have already seen that the covalent bond between two atoms has a characteristic length that depends on the atoms involved (see Figure 2–10). A further crucial property of any chemical bond is its strength. *Bond strength* is measured by the amount of energy that must be supplied to break the bond, usually expressed in units of either kilocalories per mole (kcal/mole) or kilojoules per mole (kJ/mole). A kilocalorie is the amount of energy needed to raise the temperature of 1 liter of water by 1°C. Thus, if 1 kilocalorie of energy must be supplied to break 6×10^{23} bonds of a specific type (that is, 1 mole of these bonds), then the strength of that bond is 1 kcal/mole. One kilocalorie is equal to about 4.2 kJ, which is the unit of energy universally employed by physical scientists and, increasingly, by cell biologists as well.

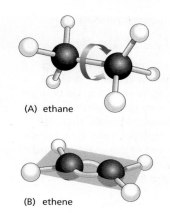

(A) ethane

(B) ethene

Figure 2–10 Carbon–carbon double bonds are shorter and more rigid than carbon–carbon single bonds. (A) The ethane molecule, with a single covalent bond between the two carbon atoms, shows the tetrahedral arrangement of the three single covalent bonds between each carbon atom and its three attached H atoms. The CH_3 groups, joined by a covalent C–C bond, can rotate relative to one another around the bond axis. (B) The double bond between the two carbon atoms in a molecule of ethene (ethylene) alters the bond geometry of the carbon atoms and brings all the atoms into the same plane; the double bond prevents the rotation of one CH_2 group relative to the other.

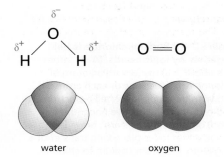

water   oxygen

Figure 2–11 In polar covalent bonds, the electrons are shared unequally. Comparison of electron distributions in the polar covalent bonds in a molecule of water (H_2O) and the nonpolar covalent bonds in a molecule of oxygen (O_2). In H_2O, electrons are more strongly attracted to the oxygen nucleus than to the H nucleus, as indicated by the distributions of the partial negative (δ^-) and partial positive (δ^+) charges.

To get an idea of what bond strengths mean, it is helpful to compare them with the average energies of the impacts that molecules continually undergo owing to collisions with other molecules in their environment—their thermal, or heat, energy. Typical covalent bonds are stronger than these thermal energies by a factor of 100, so they are resistant to being pulled apart by thermal motions. In living organisms, covalent bonds are normally broken only during specific chemical reactions that are carefully controlled by highly specialized protein catalysts called *enzymes*.

Ionic Bonds Form by the Gain and Loss of Electrons

In some substances, the participating atoms are so different in electronegativity that their electrons are not shared at all—they are transferred completely to the more electronegative partner. The resulting bonds, called **ionic bonds**, are usually formed between atoms that can attain a completely filled outer shell most easily by donating electrons to—or accepting electrons from—another atom, rather than by sharing them. For example, returning to Figure 2–5, we see that a sodium (Na) atom can achieve a filled outer shell by giving up the single electron in its third shell. By contrast, a chlorine (Cl) atom can complete its outer shell by gaining just one electron. Consequently, if a Na atom encounters a Cl atom, an electron can jump from the Na to the Cl, leaving both atoms with filled outer shells. The offspring of this marriage between sodium, a soft and intensely reactive metal, and chlorine, a toxic green gas, is table salt (NaCl).

When an electron jumps from Na to Cl, both atoms become electrically charged **ions**. The Na atom that lost an electron now has one less electron than it has protons in its nucleus; it therefore has a net single positive charge (Na^+). The Cl atom that gained an electron now has one more electron than it has protons and has a net single negative charge (Cl^-). Because of their opposite charges, the Na^+ and Cl^- ions are attracted to each other and are thereby held together by an ionic bond (**Figure 2–12A**). Ions held together solely by ionic bonds are generally called *salts* rather than molecules. A NaCl crystal contains astronomical numbers of Na^+ and Cl^- ions packed together in a precise, three-dimensional array with their opposite charges exactly balanced: a crystal only 1 mm across contains about 2×10^{19} ions of each type (**Figure 2–12B and C**).

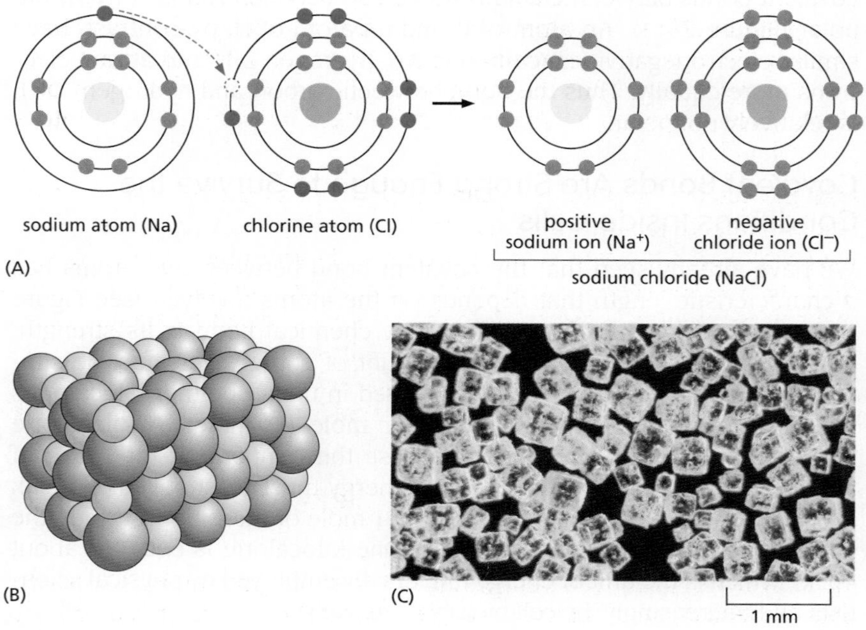

sodium atom (Na)   chlorine atom (Cl)   positive sodium ion (Na^+)   negative chloride ion (Cl^-)

(A)   sodium chloride (NaCl)

Figure 2–12 **Sodium chloride is held together by ionic bonds.** (A) An atom of sodium (Na) reacts with an atom of chlorine (Cl). Electrons of each atom are shown in their different shells; electrons in the chemically reactive (incompletely filled) outermost shells are shown in *red*. The reaction takes place with transfer of a single electron from sodium to chlorine, forming two electrically charged atoms, or ions, each with complete sets of electrons in their outermost shells. The two ions have opposite charge and are held together by electrostatic attraction. (B) The product of the reaction between sodium and chlorine, crystalline sodium chloride, contains sodium and chloride ions packed closely together in a regular array in which the charges are exactly balanced. (C) Color photograph of crystals of sodium chloride.

(B)   (C)   1 mm

Because of the favorable interaction between ions and water molecules (which are polar), many salts (including NaCl) are highly soluble in water. They dissociate into individual ions (such as Na⁺ and Cl⁻), each surrounded by a group of water molecules. Positive ions are called *cations* and negative ions are called *anions*. Small inorganic ions such as Na⁺, Cl⁻, K⁺, and Ca²⁺ play important parts in many biological processes, including the electrical activity of nerve cells, as we discuss in Chapter 12.

In aqueous solution, ionic bonds are 10–100 times weaker than the covalent bonds that hold atoms together in molecules. But, as we will see, such weak interactions nevertheless play an important role in the chemistry of living things.

Hydrogen Bonds Are Important Noncovalent Bonds for Many Biological Molecules

Water accounts for about 70% of a cell's weight, and most intracellular reactions occur in an aqueous environment. Thus the properties of water have put a permanent stamp on the chemistry of living things. In each molecule of water (H_2O), the two covalent H–O bonds are highly polar because the O is strongly attractive for electrons whereas the H is only weakly attractive. Consequently, in each water molecule, there is a preponderance of positive charge on the two H atoms and negative charge on the O. When a positively charged region of one water molecule (that is, one of its H atoms) comes close to a negatively charged region (that is, the O) of a second water molecule, the electrical attraction between them can establish a weak bond called a **hydrogen bond** (Figure 2–13A).

These bonds are much weaker than covalent bonds and are easily broken by random thermal motions. Thus each bond lasts only an exceedingly short time. But the combined effect of many weak bonds is far from trivial. Each water molecule can form hydrogen bonds through its two H atoms to two other water molecules, producing a network in which hydrogen bonds are being continually broken and formed (see Panel 2–3, pp. 70–71). It is because of these interlocking hydrogen bonds that water at room temperature is a liquid—with a high boiling point and high surface tension—and not a gas. Without hydrogen bonds, life as we know it could not exist.

Hydrogen bonds are not limited to water. In general, a hydrogen bond can form whenever a positively charged H atom held in one molecule by a polar covalent linkage comes close to a negatively charged atom—typically an oxygen or a nitrogen—belonging to another molecule (Figure 2–13B). Hydrogen bonds can also occur between different parts of a single large molecule, where they often help the molecule fold into a particular shape.

Like molecules (or salts) that carry positive or negative charges, substances that contain polar bonds and can form hydrogen bonds also mix well with water. Such substances are termed **hydrophilic**, meaning that they are "water-loving." A large proportion of the molecules in the aqueous environment of a cell fall into this category, including sugars, DNA, RNA, and a majority of proteins. **Hydrophobic** ("water-fearing") molecules, by contrast, are uncharged and form few or no hydrogen bonds, and they do not dissolve in water. These and other properties of water are reviewed in Panel 2–2 (pp. 68–69).

Four Types of Weak Interactions Help Bring Molecules Together in Cells

Much of biology depends on specific but transient interactions between one molecule and another. These associations are mediated by

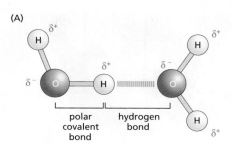

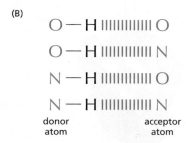

Figure 2–13 Noncovalent hydrogen bonds form between water molecules and between many other polar molecules.
(A) A hydrogen bond forms between two water molecules. The slight positive charge associated with the hydrogen atom is electrically attracted to the slight negative charge of the oxygen atom. (B) In cells, hydrogen bonds commonly form between molecules that contain an oxygen or nitrogen. The atom bearing the hydrogen is considered the H-bond donor and the atom that interacts with the hydrogen is the H-bond acceptor.

QUESTION 2–4

True or false? "When NaCl is dissolved in water, the water molecules closest to the ions will tend to preferentially orient themselves so that their oxygen atoms face the sodium ions and face away from the chloride ions." Explain your answer.

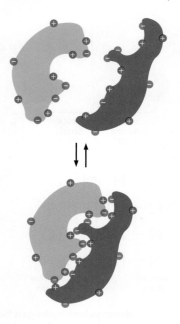

Figure 2–14 A large molecule, such as a protein, can bind to another protein through noncovalent interactions on the surface of each molecule. In the aqueous environment of a cell, many individual weak interactions could cause the two proteins to recognize each other specifically and form a tight complex. Shown here is a set of electrostatic attractions between complementary positive and negative charges.

noncovalent bonds, such as the hydrogen bonds just discussed. Although these noncovalent bonds are individually quite weak, their energies can sum to create an effective force between two molecules.

The ionic bonds that hold together the Na$^+$ and Cl$^-$ ions in a salt crystal (see Figure 2–12) represent a second form of noncovalent bond called an **electrostatic attraction**. Electrostatic attractions are strongest when the atoms involved are fully charged, as are Na$^+$ and Cl$^-$ ions. But a weaker electrostatic attraction can occur between molecules that contain polar covalent bonds (see Figure 2–11). Like hydrogen bonds, electrostatic attractions are extremely important in biology. For example, any large molecule with many polar groups will have a pattern of partial positive and negative charges on its surface. When such a molecule encounters a second molecule with a complementary set of charges, the two will be drawn to each other by electrostatic attraction. Even though water greatly reduces the strength of these attractions in most biological settings, the large number of weak noncovalent bonds that form on the surfaces of large molecules can nevertheless promote strong and specific binding (**Figure 2–14**).

A third type of noncovalent bond, called a **van der Waals attraction**, comes into play when any two atoms approach each other closely. These nonspecific interactions spring from fluctuations in the distribution of electrons in every atom, which can generate a transient attraction when the atoms are in very close proximity. These weak attractions occur in all types of molecules, even those that are nonpolar and cannot form ionic or hydrogen bonds. The relative lengths and strengths of these three types of noncovalent bonds are compared to the length and strength of covalent bonds in **Table 2–1**.

The fourth effect that often brings molecules together is not, strictly speaking, a bond at all. In an aqueous environment, a **hydrophobic force** is generated by a pushing of nonpolar surfaces out of the hydrogen-bonded water network, where they would otherwise physically interfere with the highly favorable interactions between water molecules. Hydrophobic forces play an important part in promoting molecular interactions—in particular, in building cell membranes, which are constructed largely from *lipid molecules* with long hydrocarbon tails. In these molecules, the H atoms are covalently linked to C atoms by nonpolar bonds (see Panel 2–1, pp. 66–67). Because the H atoms have almost no net positive charge, they cannot form effective hydrogen bonds to other molecules, including water. As a result, lipids can form the thin membrane barriers that keep the aqueous interior of the cell separate from the surrounding aqueous environment.

All four types of weak chemical interactions important in biology are reviewed in **Panel 2–3** (pp. 70–71).

TABLE 2–1 LENGTH AND STRENGTH OF SOME CHEMICAL BONDS			
Bond Type	Length* (nm)	Strength (kJ/mole)	
		In Vacuum	In Water
Covalent	0.10	377 [90]**	377 [90]
Noncovalent: ionic bond	0.25	335 [80]	12.6 [3]
Noncovalent: hydrogen bond	0.17	16.7 [4]	4.2 [1]
Noncovalent: van der Waals attraction (per atom)	0.35	0.4 [0.1]	0.4 [0.1]

*The bond lengths and strengths listed are approximate, because the exact values will depend on the atoms involved.
**Values in brackets are kcal/mole. 1 kJ = 0.239 kcal and 1 kcal = 4.184 kJ.

Some Polar Molecules Form Acids and Bases in Water

One of the simplest kinds of chemical reaction, and one that has profound significance for cells, takes place when a molecule with a highly polar covalent bond between a hydrogen and another atom dissolves in water. The hydrogen atom in such a bond has given up its electron almost entirely to the companion atom, so it exists as an almost naked positively charged hydrogen nucleus—in other words, a *proton* (H^+). When the polar molecule becomes surrounded by water molecules, the proton will be attracted to the partial negative charge on the oxygen atom of an adjacent water molecule (see Figure 2–11); this proton can thus dissociate from its original partner and associate instead with the oxygen atom of the water molecule, generating a **hydronium ion** (H_3O^+) (**Figure 2–15A**). The reverse reaction—in which a hydronium ion releases a proton—also takes place very readily, so in an aqueous solution, billions of protons are constantly flitting to and fro between one molecule and another.

Substances that release protons when they dissolve in water, thus forming H_3O^+, are termed **acids**. The higher the concentration of H_3O^+, the more acidic the solution. Even in pure water, H_3O^+ is present at a concentration of 10^{-7} M, as a result of the movement of protons from one water molecule to another (**Figure 2–15B**). By tradition, the H_3O^+ concentration is usually referred to as the H^+ concentration, even though most protons in an aqueous solution are present as H_3O^+. To avoid the use of unwieldy numbers, the concentration of H^+ is expressed using a logarithmic scale called the **pH scale**. Pure water has a pH of 7.0 and is thus neutral—that is, neither acidic (pH <7) nor basic (pH >7).

Acids are characterized as being strong or weak, depending on how readily they give up their protons to water. Strong acids, such as hydrochloric acid (HCl), lose their protons easily. Acetic acid, on the other hand, is a weak acid because it holds on to its proton fairly tightly when dissolved in water. Many of the acids important in the cell—such as molecules containing a carboxyl (COOH) group—are weak acids (see Panel 2–2, pp. 68–69). Their tendency to give up a proton with some reluctance is exploited in a variety of cellular reactions.

Because protons can be passed readily to many types of molecules in cells, thus altering the molecules' characters, the H^+ concentration inside a cell—its pH—must be closely controlled. Acids will give up their protons more readily if the H^+ concentration is low (and the pH is high) and will hold onto their protons (or accept them back) when the H^+ concentration is high (and the pH is low).

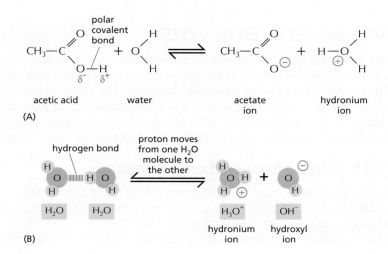

Figure 2–15 **Protons move continuously from one molecule to another in aqueous solutions.** (A) The reaction that takes place when a molecule of acetic acid dissolves in water. At pH 7, nearly all of the acetic acid molecules are present as acetate ions. (B) Water molecules are continually exchanging protons with each other to form hydronium and hydroxyl ions. These ions in turn rapidly recombine to form water molecules.

Figure 2–16 **In aqueous solutions, the concentration of hydroxyl (OH⁻) ions increases as the concentration of H₃O⁺ (or H⁺) ions decreases.** The product of the two values, [OH⁻] x [H⁺], is always 10^{-14} (moles/liter)². At neutral pH, [OH⁻] = [H⁺], and both ions are present at 10^{-7} M. Also shown are examples of common solutions along with their approximate pH values.

	$[H^+]$ moles/liter	pH	$[OH^-]$ moles/liter	some solutions and their pH values
ACIDIC	1	0	10^{-14}	battery acid (0.5)
	10^{-1}	1	10^{-13}	stomach acid (1.5)
	10^{-2}	2	10^{-12}	lemon juice (2.3), cola (2.5)
	10^{-3}	3	10^{-11}	orange juice (3.5)
	10^{-4}	4	10^{-10}	beer (4.5)
	10^{-5}	5	10^{-9}	black coffee (5.0), acid rain (5.6)
	10^{-6}	6	10^{-8}	urine (6.0), milk (6.5)
NEUTRAL	10^{-7}	7	10^{-7}	pure water (7.0)
BASIC	10^{-8}	8	10^{-6}	sea water (8.0)
	10^{-9}	9	10^{-5}	hand soap (9.5)
	10^{-10}	10	10^{-4}	milk of magnesia (10.5)
	10^{-11}	11	10^{-3}	household ammonia (11.9)
	10^{-12}	12	10^{-2}	non-phosphate detergent (12.0)
	10^{-13}	13	10^{-1}	bleach (12.5)
	10^{-14}	14	1	caustic soda (13.5)

QUESTION 2–5

A. Are there H₃O⁺ ions present in pure water at neutral pH (i.e., at pH = 7.0)? If so, how are they formed?
B. If they exist, what is the ratio of H₃O⁺ ions to H₂O molecules at neutral pH? (Hint: the molecular weight of water is 18, and 1 liter of water weighs 1 kg.)

Molecules that accept protons when dissolved in water are called **bases**. Just as the defining property of an acid is that it raises the concentration of H₃O⁺ ions by donating a proton to a water molecule, so the defining property of a base is that it raises the concentration of hydroxyl (OH⁻) ions by removing a proton from a water molecule. Sodium hydroxide (NaOH) is basic (the term *alkaline* is also used). NaOH is considered a strong base because it readily dissociates in aqueous solution to form Na⁺ ions and OH⁻ ions. Weak bases—which have a weak tendency to accept a proton from water—however, are more important in cells. Many biologically important weak bases contain an amino (NH₂) group, which can generate OH⁻ by taking a proton from water: $-NH_2 + H_2O \rightarrow -NH_3^+ + OH^-$ (see Panel 2–2, pp. 68–69).

Because an OH⁻ ion combines with a proton to form a water molecule, an increase in the OH⁻ concentration forces a decrease in the H⁺ concentration, and vice versa (**Figure 2–16**). A pure solution of water contains an equal concentration (10^{-7} M) of both ions, rendering it neutral (pH 7). The interior of a cell is kept close to neutral by the presence of **buffers**: mixtures of weak acids and bases that will adjust proton concentrations around pH 7 by releasing protons (acids) or taking them up (bases) whenever the pH changes. This give-and-take keeps the pH of the cell relatively constant under a variety of conditions.

SMALL MOLECULES IN CELLS

Having looked at the ways atoms combine to form small molecules and how these molecules behave in an aqueous environment, we now examine the main classes of small molecules found in cells and their biological roles. Amazingly, we will see that a few basic categories of molecules, formed from just a handful of different elements, give rise to all the extraordinary richness of form and behavior displayed by living things.

A Cell Is Formed from Carbon Compounds

If we disregard water, nearly all the molecules in a cell are based on carbon. Carbon is outstanding among all the elements in its ability to form large molecules. Because a carbon atom is small and has four electrons and four vacancies in its outer shell, it readily forms four covalent bonds with other atoms (see Figure 2–9). Most importantly, one carbon atom can link to other carbon atoms through highly stable covalent C–C bonds, producing rings and chains that can form the backbone of complex molecules with no obvious upper limit to their size. These carbon-containing compounds are called **organic molecules**. By contrast, all other molecules, including water, are said to be **inorganic**.

In addition to containing carbon, the organic molecules produced by cells frequently contain specific combinations of atoms, such as the methyl ($-CH_3$), hydroxyl ($-OH$), carboxyl ($-COOH$), carbonyl ($-C=O$), phosphoryl ($-PO_3^{2-}$), and amino ($-NH_2$) groups. Each of these **chemical groups** has distinct chemical and physical properties that influence the behavior of the molecule in which the group occurs, including whether the molecule tends to gain or lose protons when dissolved in water and with which other molecules it will interact. Knowing these groups and their chemical properties greatly simplifies understanding the chemistry of life. The most common chemical groups and some of their properties are summarized in Panel 2–1 (pp. 66–67).

Cells Contain Four Major Families of Small Organic Molecules

The small organic molecules of the cell are carbon compounds with molecular weights in the range 100–1000 that contain up to 30 or so carbon atoms. They are usually found free in solution in the cytosol and have many different roles. Some are used as *monomer* subunits to construct the cell's polymeric *macromolecules*—its proteins, nucleic acids, and large polysaccharides. Others serve as energy sources, being broken down and transformed into other small molecules in a maze of intracellular metabolic pathways. Many have more than one role in the cell—acting, for example, as both a potential subunit for a macromolecule and as an energy source. The small organic molecules are much less abundant than the organic macromolecules, accounting for only about one-tenth of the total mass of organic matter in a cell. But small organic molecules adopt a huge variety of chemical forms. Nearly 4000 different kinds of small organic molecules have been detected in the well-studied bacterium *Escherichia coli*.

All organic molecules are synthesized from—and are broken down into—the same set of simple compounds. Both their synthesis and their breakdown occur through sequences of simple chemical changes that are limited in variety and follow step-by-step rules. As a consequence, the compounds in a cell are chemically related, and most can be classified into a small number of distinct families. Broadly speaking, cells contain four major families of small organic molecules: the *sugars*, the *fatty acids*, the *amino acids*, and the *nucleotides* (**Figure 2–17**). Although many compounds present in cells do not fit into these categories, these four families of small organic molecules—together with the macromolecules made by linking them into long chains—account for a large fraction of a cell's mass (**Table 2–2**).

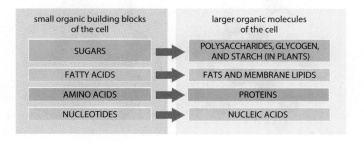

Figure 2–17 **Sugars, fatty acids, amino acids, and nucleotides are the four main families of small organic molecules in cells.** They form the monomeric building blocks, or subunits, for larger organic molecules, including most of the macromolecules and other molecular assemblies of the cell. Some, like the sugars and the fatty acids, are also energy sources.

TABLE 2–2 THE CHEMICAL COMPOSITION OF A BACTERIAL CELL		
Substance	Percent of Total Cell Weight	Approximate Number of Types in Each Class
Water	70	1
Inorganic ions	1	20
Sugars and precursors	1	250
Amino acids and precursors	0.4	100
Nucleotides and precursors	0.4	100
Fatty acids and precursors	1	50
Other small molecules	0.2	3000
Phospholipids	2	4*
Macromolecules (nucleic acids, proteins, and polysaccharides)	24	3000

*There are four classes of phospholipids, each of which exists in many varieties (discussed in Chapter 4).

Sugars Are both Energy Sources and Subunits of Polysaccharides

The simplest **sugars**—the monosaccharides—are compounds with the general formula $(CH_2O)_n$, where n is usually 3, 4, 5, or 6. Glucose, for example, has the formula $C_6H_{12}O_6$ (**Figure 2–18**). Because of this simple formula, sugars, and the larger molecules made from them, are called *carbohydrates*. The formula, however, does not adequately define the molecule: the same set of carbons, hydrogens, and oxygens can be joined together by covalent bonds in a variety of ways, creating structures with different shapes. Thus glucose can be converted into a different sugar—mannose or galactose—simply by switching the orientations of specific –OH groups relative to the rest of the molecule (**Panel 2–4**, pp. 72–73). In addition, each of these sugars can exist in either of two forms, called the D-form and the L-form, which are mirror images of each other. Sets of molecules with the same chemical formula but different structures are called *isomers*, and mirror-image pairs of such molecules are called

Figure 2–18 **The structure of glucose, a monosaccharide, can be represented in several ways.** (A) A structural formula in which the atoms are shown as chemical symbols, linked together by solid lines representing the covalent bonds. The thickened lines are used to indicate the plane of the sugar ring and to show that the –H and –OH groups are not in the same plane as the ring. (B) Another kind of structural formula that shows the three-dimensional structure of glucose in a so-called "chair configuration." (C) A ball-and-stick model in which the three-dimensional arrangement of the atoms in space is indicated. (D) A space-filling model, which, as well as depicting the three-dimensional arrangement of the atoms, also shows the relative sizes and surface contours of the molecule (**Movie 2.1**). The atoms in (C) and (D) are colored as in Figure 2–9: C, *black*; H, *white*; O, *red*. This is the conventional color-coding for these atoms and will be used throughout this book.

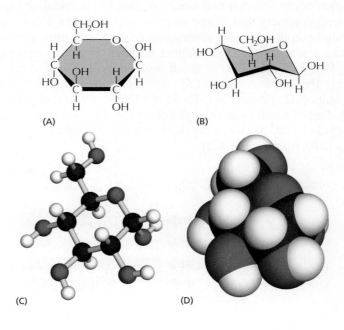

optical isomers. Isomers are widespread among organic molecules in general, and they play a major part in generating the enormous variety of sugars. A more complete outline of sugar structures and chemistry is presented in Panel 2–4.

Monosaccharides can be linked by covalent bonds—called glycosidic bonds—to form larger carbohydrates. Two monosaccharides linked together make a disaccharide, such as sucrose, which is composed of a glucose and a fructose unit. Larger sugar polymers range from the *oligosaccharides* (trisaccharides, tetrasaccharides, and so on) up to giant *polysaccharides*, which can contain thousands of monosaccharide subunits (*monomers*). In most cases, the prefix *oligo-* is used to refer to molecules made of a small number of monomers, typically 2 to 10 in the case of oligosaccharides. Polymers, in contrast, can contain hundreds or thousands of subunits.

The way sugars are linked together illustrates some common features of biochemical bond formation. A bond is formed between an –OH group on one sugar and an –OH group on another by a **condensation reaction**, in which a molecule of water is expelled as the bond is formed (**Figure 2–19**). The subunits in other biological polymers, including nucleic acids and proteins, are also linked by condensation reactions in which water is expelled. The bonds created by all of these condensation reactions can be broken by the reverse process of **hydrolysis**, in which a molecule of water is consumed. Generally speaking, condensation reactions, which synthesize larger molecules from smaller subunits, are energetically unfavorable; hydrolysis reactions, which break down larger molecules into smaller subunits, are energetically favorable (**Figure 2–20**).

Because each monosaccharide has several free hydroxyl groups that can form a link to another monosaccharide (or to some other compound), sugar polymers can be branched, and the number of possible polysaccharide structures is extremely large. For this reason, it is much more difficult to determine the arrangement of sugars in a complex polysaccharide than it is to determine the nucleotide sequence of a DNA molecule or the amino acid sequence of a protein, in which each unit is joined to the next in exactly the same way.

The monosaccharide *glucose* has a central role as an energy source for cells, as we explain in Chapter 13. It is broken down to smaller molecules in a series of reactions, releasing energy that the cell can harness to do useful work. Cells use simple polysaccharides composed only of glucose units—principally *glycogen* in animals and *starch* in plants—as long-term stores of glucose, held in reserve for energy production.

Sugars do not function exclusively in the production and storage of energy. They are also used, for example, to make mechanical supports. The most abundant organic molecule on Earth—the *cellulose* that forms plant cell walls—is a polysaccharide of glucose. Another extraordinarily abundant organic substance, the *chitin* of insect exoskeletons and fungal cell walls, is also a polysaccharide—in this case, a linear polymer of a sugar derivative called *N*-acetylglucosamine (see Panel 2–4, pp. 72–73). Other polysaccharides, which tend to be slippery when wet, are the main components of slime, mucus, and gristle.

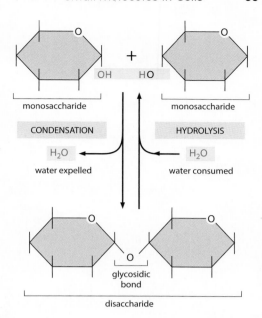

Figure 2–19 Two monosaccharides can be linked by a covalent glycosidic bond to form a disaccharide. This reaction belongs to a general category of reactions termed *condensation reactions*, in which two molecules join together as a result of the loss of a water molecule. The reverse reaction (in which water is added) is termed *hydrolysis*.

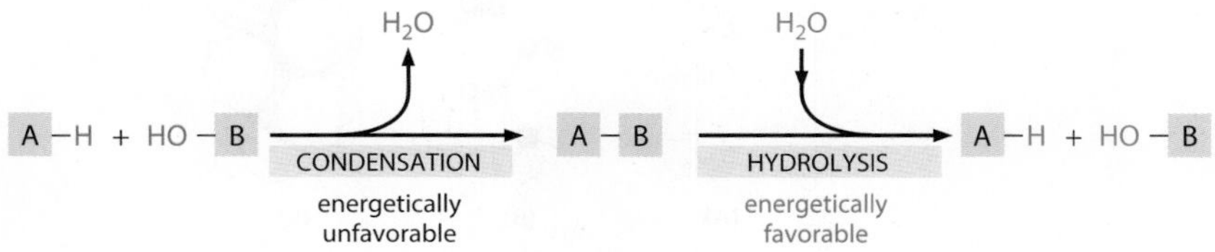

Figure 2–20 Condensation and hydrolysis are reverse reactions. The large polymeric macromolecules of the cell are formed from subunits (or monomers) by condensation reactions, and they are broken down by hydrolysis. Condensation reactions are energetically unfavorable; thus macromolecule formation requires an input of energy, as we discuss in Chapter 3.

Smaller oligosaccharides can be covalently linked to proteins to form *glycoproteins*, or to lipids to form glycolipids (**Panel 2–5**, pp. 74–75), which are both found in cell membranes. The sugar side chains attached to glycoproteins and glycolipids in the plasma membrane are thought to help protect the cell surface and often help cells adhere to one another. Differences in the types of cell-surface sugars form the molecular basis for the human blood groups, information that dictates which blood types can be used during transfusions.

Fatty Acid Chains Are Components of Cell Membranes

A **fatty acid** molecule, such as *palmitic acid*, has two chemically distinct regions. One is a long hydrocarbon chain, which is hydrophobic and not very reactive chemically. The other is a carboxyl (–COOH) group, which behaves as an acid (carboxylic acid): in an aqueous solution, it is ionized (–COO⁻), extremely hydrophilic, and chemically reactive (**Figure 2–21**). Molecules—such as fatty acids—that possess both hydrophobic and hydrophilic regions are termed *amphipathic*. Almost all the fatty acid molecules in a cell are covalently linked to other molecules by their carboxylic acid group (see Panel 2–5, pp. 74–75).

The hydrocarbon tail of palmitic acid is *saturated*: it has no double bonds between its carbon atoms and contains the maximum possible number of hydrogens. Some other fatty acids, such as oleic acid, have *unsaturated* tails, with one or more double bonds along their length. The double bonds create kinks in the hydrocarbon tails, interfering with their ability to pack together. Fatty acid tails are found in cell membranes, where the tightness of their packing affects the fluidity of the membrane. The many different fatty acids found in cells differ only in the length of their hydrocarbon chains and in the number and position of the carbon–carbon double bonds (see Panel 2–5).

Fatty acids serve as a concentrated food reserve in cells: they can be broken down to produce about six times as much usable energy, gram for gram, as glucose. Fatty acids are stored in the cytoplasm of many cells in the form of fat droplets composed of *triacylglycerol* molecules—compounds made of three fatty acid chains covalently joined to a glycerol molecule (**Figure 2–22** and see Panel 2–5). Triacylglycerols are the animal fats found in meat, butter, and cream, and the plant oils such as corn oil and olive oil. When a cell needs energy, the fatty acid chains

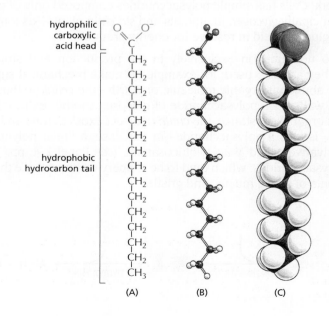

Figure 2–21 Fatty acids have both hydrophobic and hydrophilic components. The hydrophobic hydrocarbon chain is attached to a hydrophilic carboxylic acid group. Different fatty acids have different hydrocarbon tails. Palmitic acid is shown here. (A) Structural formula, showing the carboxylic acid head group in its ionized form, as it exists in water at pH 7. (B) Ball-and-stick model. (C) Space-filling model (**Movie 2.2**).

can be released from triacylglycerols and broken down into two-carbon units. These two-carbon units are identical to those derived from the breakdown of glucose, and they enter the same energy-yielding reaction pathways, as described in Chapter 13.

Fatty acids and their derivatives, including triacylglycerols, are examples of **lipids**. Lipids are loosely defined as molecules that are insoluble in water but soluble in fat and organic solvents such as benzene. They typically contain long hydrocarbon chains, as in the fatty acids, or multiple linked aromatic rings, as in the *steroids* (see Panel 2–5).

The most unique function of fatty acids is in the establishment of the **lipid bilayer**, the structure that forms the basis for all cell membranes. These thin sheets, which enclose all cells and surround their internal organelles, are composed largely of *phospholipids* (**Figure 2–23**).

Like triacylglycerols, most phospholipids are constructed mainly from fatty acids and glycerol. In these phospholipids, however, the glycerol is joined to two fatty acid chains, rather than to three as in triacylglycerols. The remaining –OH group on the glycerol is linked to a hydrophilic phosphate group, which in turn is attached to a small hydrophilic compound such as choline (see Panel 2–5, pp. 74–75). With their two hydrophobic fatty acid tails and a hydrophilic, phosphate-containing head, phospholipids are strongly amphipathic. This characteristic amphipathic composition and shape gives them very different physical and chemical properties from triacylglycerols, which are predominantly hydrophobic. In addition to phospholipids, cell membranes contain differing amounts of other lipids, including *glycolipids*, which are structurally similar to phospholipids but contain one or more sugars instead of a phosphate group.

Thanks to their amphipathic nature, pure phospholipids readily form membranes in water. These lipids can spread over the surface of water to form a monolayer, with their hydrophobic tails facing the air and their hydrophilic heads in contact with the water. Alternatively, two of these phospholipid layers can readily combine tail-to-tail in water to form the phospholipid sandwich that is the lipid bilayer (see Chapter 11).

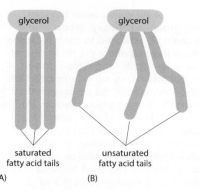

Figure 2–22 The properties of fats depend on the length and saturation of the fatty acid chains they carry. Fatty acids are stored in the cytosol of many cells in the form of droplets of *triacylglycerol* molecules made of three fatty acid chains joined to a glycerol molecule. (A) Saturated fats are found in meat and dairy products. (B) Plant oils, such as corn oil, contain unsaturated fatty acids, which may be monounsaturated (containing one double bond) or polyunsaturated (containing multiple double bonds). The presence of these double bonds causes plant oils to be liquid at room temperature. Although fats are essential in the diet, saturated fats raise the concentration of cholesterol in the blood, which tends to clog the arteries, increasing the risk of heart attacks and strokes.

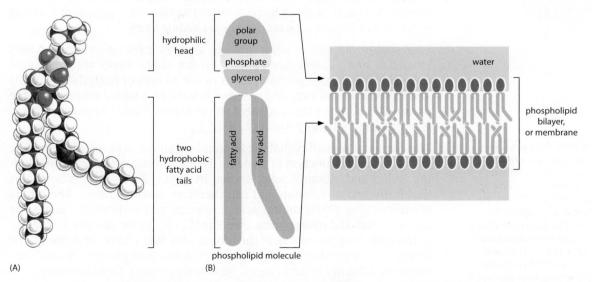

Figure 2–23 Phospholipids can aggregate to form cell membranes. Phospholipids contain two hydrophobic fatty acid tails and a hydrophilic head. (A) Phosphatidylcholine is the most common phospholipid in cell membranes. (B) Diagram showing how, in an aqueous environment, the hydrophobic tails of phospholipids pack together to form a lipid bilayer. In the lipid bilayer, the hydrophilic heads of the phospholipid molecules are on the outside, facing the aqueous environment, and the hydrophobic tails are on the inside, where water is excluded.

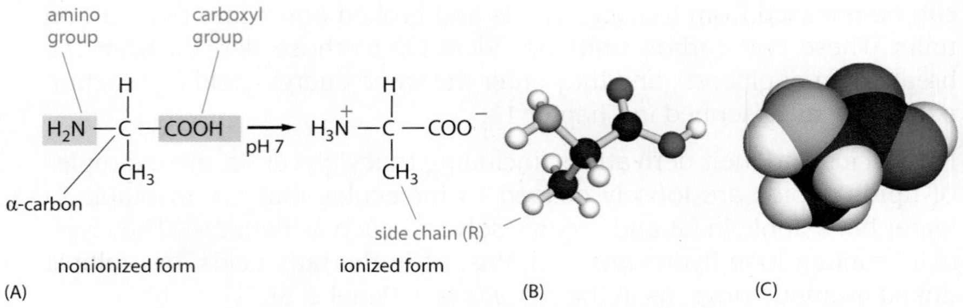

Figure 2–24 All amino acids have an amino group, a carboxyl group, and a side chain (R) attached to their α-carbon atom. In the cell, where the pH is close to 7, free amino acids exist in their ionized form; but, when they are incorporated into a polypeptide chain, the charges on their amino and carboxyl groups are lost. (A) The amino acid shown is alanine, one of the simplest amino acids, which has a methyl group (CH₃) as its side chain. Its amino group is highlighted in *blue* and its carboxyl group in *red*. (B) A ball-and-stick model and (C) a space-filling model of alanine. In (B) and (C), the N atom is *blue* and the O atom is *red*.

Figure 2–24 All amino acids have an amino group, a carboxyl group, and a side chain (R) attached to their α-carbon atom. In the cell, where the pH is close to 7, free amino acids exist in their ionized form; but, when they are incorporated into a polypeptide chain, the charges on their amino and carboxyl groups are lost. (A) The amino acid shown is alanine, one of the simplest amino acids, which has a methyl group (CH₃) as its side chain. Its amino group is highlighted in *blue* and its carboxyl group in *red*. (B) A ball-and-stick model and (C) a space-filling model of alanine. In (B) and (C), the N atom is *blue* and the O atom is *red*.

QUESTION 2–6

Why do you suppose only L-amino acids and not a random mixture of the L- and D-forms of each amino acid are used to make proteins?

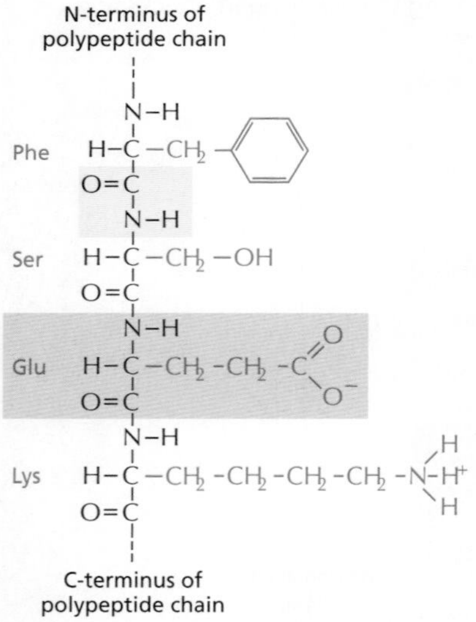

Figure 2–25 Amino acids in a protein are held together by peptide bonds. The four amino acids shown are linked together by three peptide bonds, one of which is highlighted in *yellow*. One of the amino acids, glutamic acid, is shaded in *gray*. The amino acid side chains are shown in *red*. The N-terminus of the polypeptide chain is capped by an amino group, and the C-terminus ends in a carboxyl group. The sequence of amino acids in a protein is abbreviated using either a three-letter or a one-letter code, and the sequence is always read starting from the N-terminus (see Panel 2–6, pp. 76–77). In the example given, the sequence is Phe-Ser-Glu-Lys (or FSEK).

Amino Acids Are the Subunits of Proteins

Amino acids are small organic molecules with one defining property: they all possess a carboxylic acid group and an amino group, both attached to a central α-carbon atom (**Figure 2–24**). This α-carbon also carries a specific side chain, the identity of which distinguishes one amino acid from another.

Cells use amino acids to build **proteins**—polymers made of amino acids, which are joined head-to-tail in a long chain that folds up into a three-dimensional structure that is unique to each type of protein. The covalent bond between two adjacent amino acids in a protein chain is called a *peptide bond*, and the resulting chain of amino acids is therefore also known as a *polypeptide*. Peptide bonds are formed by condensation reactions that link one amino acid to the next. Regardless of the specific amino acids from which it is made, the polypeptide always has an amino (NH₂) group at one end—its *N-terminus*—and a carboxyl (COOH) group at its other end—its *C-terminus* (**Figure 2–25**). This difference in the two ends gives a polypeptide a definite directionality—a structural (as opposed to electrical) polarity.

Twenty types of amino acids are commonly found in proteins, each with a different side chain attached to its α-carbon atom (**Panel 2–6**, pp. 76–77). How this precise set of 20 amino acids came to be chosen is one of the mysteries surrounding the evolution of life; there is no obvious chemical reason why other amino acids could not have served just as well. But once the selection had been locked into place, it could not be changed, as too much chemistry had evolved to exploit it. Switching the types of amino acids used by cells—whether bacterial, plant, or animal—would require the organism to retool its entire metabolism to cope with the new building blocks.

Like sugars, all amino acids (except glycine) exist as optical isomers termed D- and L-forms (see Panel 2–6). But only L-forms are ever found in proteins (although D-amino acids occur as part of bacterial cell walls and in some antibiotics, and D-serine is used as a signal molecule in the brain). The origin of this exclusive use of L-amino acids to make proteins is another evolutionary mystery.

The chemical versatility that the 20 standard amino acids provide is vitally important to the function of proteins. Five of the 20 amino acids—including lysine and glutamic acid, shown in Figure 2–25—have side chains that form ions in solution and can therefore carry a charge. The others are uncharged. Some amino acids are polar and hydrophilic, and some are nonpolar and hydrophobic (see Panel 2–6). As we discuss in Chapter 4, the collective properties of the amino acid side chains underlie all the diverse and sophisticated functions of proteins. And proteins, which constitute half the dry mass of a cell, lie at the center of life's chemistry.

Nucleotides Are the Subunits of DNA and RNA

DNA and RNA are built from subunits called **nucleotides**. Nucleotides consist of a nitrogen-containing ring compound linked to a five-carbon

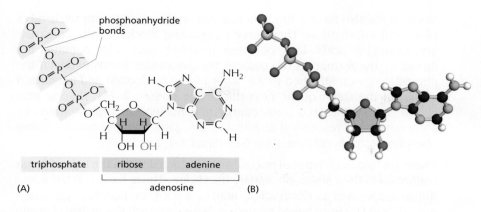

Figure 2–26 Adenosine triphosphate (ATP) is a crucially important energy carrier in cells. (A) Structural formula, in which the three phosphate groups are shaded in *yellow*. The presence of the OH group on the second carbon of the sugar ring (*red*) distinguishes this sugar as ribose. (B) Ball-and-stick model (Movie 2.3). In (B), the P atoms are *yellow*.

sugar that has one or more phosphate groups attached to it (**Panel 2–7**, pp. 78–79). The sugar can be either ribose or deoxyribose. Nucleotides containing ribose are known as *ribonucleotides*, and those containing deoxyribose are known as *deoxyribonucleotides*.

The nitrogen-containing rings of all these molecules are generally referred to as *bases* for historical reasons: under acidic conditions, they can each bind an H⁺ (proton) and thereby increase the concentration of OH⁻ ions in aqueous solution. There is a strong family resemblance between the different nucleotide bases. *Cytosine* (C), *thymine* (T), and *uracil* (U) are called *pyrimidines*, because they all derive from a six-membered pyrimidine ring; *guanine* (G) and *adenine* (A) are purines, which bear a second, five-membered ring fused to the six-membered ring. Each nucleotide is named after the base it contains (see Panel 2–7, pp. 78–79). A base plus its sugar (without any phosphate group attached) is called a *nucleoside*.

Nucleoside di- and triphosphates can act as short-term carriers of chemical energy. Above all others, the ribonucleoside triphosphate known as **adenosine triphosphate**, or **ATP** (**Figure 2–26**), participates in the transfer of energy in hundreds of metabolic reactions. ATP is formed through reactions that are driven by the energy released from the breakdown of foodstuffs. Its three phosphates are linked in series by two *phosphoanhydride* bonds (see Panel 2–7). Rupture of these phosphate bonds by hydrolysis releases large amounts of useful energy, also known as *free energy* (see Panel 3–1, pp. 94–95). Most often, it is the terminal phosphate group that is split off—or transferred to another molecule—to release energy that can be used to drive biosynthetic reactions (**Figure 2–27**). Other nucleotide derivatives serve as carriers for other chemical groups. All of this is described in Chapter 3.

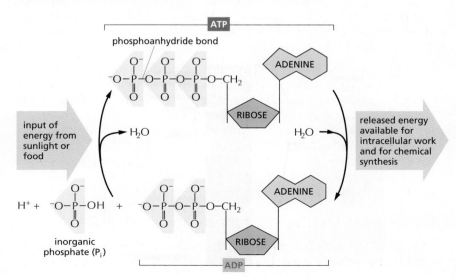

Figure 2–27 ATP is synthesized from ADP and inorganic phosphate, and it releases energy when it is hydrolyzed back to ADP and inorganic phosphate. The energy required for ATP synthesis is derived from either the energy-yielding oxidation of foodstuffs (in animal cells, fungi, and some bacteria) or the capture of light (in plant cells and some bacteria). The hydrolysis of ATP releases energy that is used to drive many processes inside cells. Together, the two reactions shown form the ATP cycle.

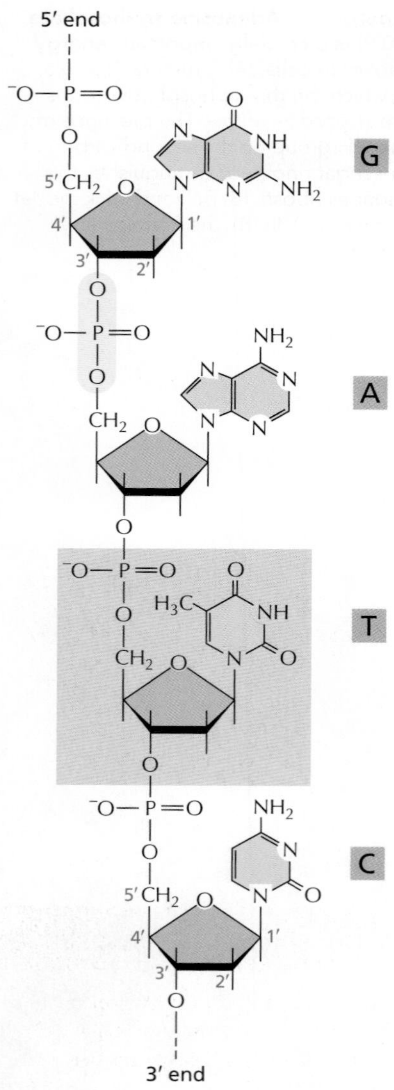

5' end

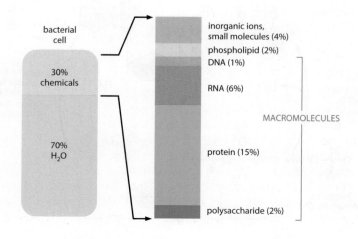

Figure 2–28 A short length of one chain of a deoxyribonucleic acid (DNA) molecule shows the covalent phosphodiester bonds linking four consecutive nucleotides. Because the bonds link specific carbon atoms in the sugar ring—known as the 5' and 3' carbon atoms—one end of a polynucleotide chain, the 5' end, has a free phosphate group and the other, the 3' end, has a free hydroxyl group. One of the nucleotides, T, is shaded in *gray*, and one phosphodiester bond is highlighted in *yellow*. The linear sequence of nucleotides in a polynucleotide chain is commonly abbreviated using a one-letter code, and the sequence is always read from the 5' end. In the example illustrated, the sequence is GATC.

Figure 2–29 Macromolecules are abundant in cells. The approximate composition (by mass) of a bacterial cell is shown. The composition of an animal cell is similar.

Nucleotides also have a fundamental role in the storage and retrieval of biological information. They serve as building blocks for the construction of *nucleic acids*—long polymers in which nucleotide subunits are linked by the formation of covalent *phosphodiester bonds* between the phosphate group attached to the sugar of one nucleotide and a hydroxyl group on the sugar of the next nucleotide (**Figure 2–28**). Nucleic acid chains are synthesized from energy-rich nucleoside triphosphates by a condensation reaction that releases inorganic pyrophosphate during phosphodiester bond formation (see Panel 2–7, pp. 78–79).

There are two main types of nucleic acids, which differ in the type of sugar contained in their sugar–phosphate backbone. Those based on the sugar ribose are known as **ribonucleic acids**, or **RNA**, and contain the bases A, G, C, and U. Those based on deoxyribose (in which the hydroxyl group at the 2' position of the ribose carbon ring is replaced by a hydrogen) are known as **deoxyribonucleic acids**, or **DNA**, and contain the bases A, G, C, and T (T is chemically similar to the U in RNA; see Panel 2–7). RNA usually occurs in cells in the form of a single-stranded polynucleotide chain, but DNA is virtually always in the form of a double-stranded molecule: the DNA double helix is composed of two polynucleotide chains that run in opposite directions and are held together by hydrogen bonds between the bases of the two chains (see Panel 2–3, pp. 70–71).

The linear sequence of nucleotides in a DNA or an RNA molecule encodes genetic information. The two nucleic acids, however, have different roles in the cell. DNA, with its more stable, hydrogen-bonded helix, acts as a long-term repository for hereditary information, while single-stranded RNA is usually a more transient carrier of molecular instructions. The ability of the bases in different nucleic acid molecules to recognize and pair with each other by hydrogen-bonding (called *base-pairing*)—G with C, and A with either T or U—underlies all of heredity and evolution, as explained in Chapter 5.

MACROMOLECULES IN CELLS

On the basis of mass, macromolecules are by far the most abundant of the organic molecules in a living cell (**Figure 2–29**). They are the principal building blocks from which a cell is constructed and also the components that confer the most distinctive properties on living things. Intermediate in size and complexity between small organic molecules and organelles, **macromolecules** are constructed simply by covalently linking small

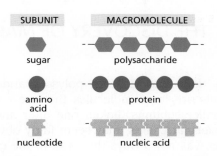

Figure 2–30 **Polysaccharides, proteins, and nucleic acids are made from monomeric subunits.** Each macromolecule is a polymer formed from small molecules (called monomers or subunits) that are linked together by covalent bonds.

organic **monomers**, or subunits, into long chains, or polymers (**Figure 2–30** and **How We Know**, pp. 60–61). Yet they have many unexpected properties that could not have been predicted from their simple constituents. For example, it took a long time to determine that the nucleic acids, DNA and RNA, store and transmit hereditary information (see How We Know, Chapter 5, pp. 193–195).

Proteins are especially versatile and perform thousands of distinct functions. Many proteins act as highly specific *enzymes* that catalyze the chemical reactions that take place in cells. For example, one enzyme in plants, called ribulose bisphosphate carboxylase, converts CO_2 to sugars, thereby creating most of the organic matter used by the rest of the living world. Other proteins are used to build structural components: tubulin, for example, self-assembles to make the cell's long, stiff microtubules (see Figure 1–27B), and histone proteins assemble into disc-like structures that help wrap up the cell's DNA in chromosomes. Yet other proteins, such as myosin, act as molecular motors to produce force and movement. We examine the molecular basis for many of these wide-ranging functions in later chapters. Here, we consider some of the general principles of macromolecular chemistry that make all of these activities possible.

Each Macromolecule Contains a Specific Sequence of Subunits

Although the chemical reactions for adding subunits to each polymer are different in detail for proteins, nucleic acids, and polysaccharides, they share important features. Each polymer grows by the addition of a monomer onto one end of the polymer chain via a condensation reaction, in which a molecule of water is lost for each subunit that is added (**Figure 2–31**). In all cases, the reactions are catalyzed by specific enzymes, which ensure that only the appropriate monomer is incorporated.

The stepwise polymerization of monomers into a long chain is a simple way to manufacture a large, complex molecule, because the subunits are added by the same reaction performed over and over again by the same set of enzymes. In a sense, the process resembles the repetitive operation of a machine in a factory—with some important differences. First, apart from some of the polysaccharides, most macromolecules are made from a set of monomers that are slightly different from one another; for example, proteins are constructed from 20 different amino acids (see Panel 2–6, pp. 76–77). Second, and most important, the polymer chain is not assembled at random from these subunits; instead, the subunits are added in a particular order, or **sequence**.

The biological functions of proteins, nucleic acids, and many polysaccharides are absolutely dependent on the particular sequence of subunits in the linear chains. By varying the sequence of subunits, the cell could in principle make an enormous diversity of the polymeric molecules. Thus, for a protein chain 200 amino acids long, there are 20^{200} possible combinations ($20 \times 20 \times 20 \times 20...$ multiplied 200 times), while for a DNA molecule 10,000 nucleotides long (small by DNA standards), with its four different nucleotides, there are $4^{10,000}$ different possibilities—an unimaginably large number. Thus the machinery of polymerization must

QUESTION 2–7

What is meant by "polarity" of a polypeptide chain and by "polarity" of a chemical bond? How do the meanings differ?

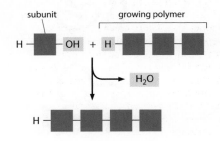

Figure 2–31 **Macromolecules are formed by adding subunits to one end of a chain.** In a condensation reaction, a molecule of water is lost with the addition of each monomer to one end of the growing chain. The reverse reaction—the breakdown of the polymer—occurs by the addition of water (hydrolysis). See also Figure 2–19.

HOW WE KNOW

THE DISCOVERY OF MACROMOLECULES

The idea that proteins, polysaccharides, and nucleic acids are large molecules that are constructed from smaller subunits, linked one after another into long molecular chains, may seem fairly obvious today. But this was not always the case. In the early part of the twentieth century, few scientists believed in the existence of such biological polymers built from repeating units held together by covalent bonds. The notion that such "frighteningly large" macromolecules could be assembled from simple building blocks was considered "downright shocking" by chemists of the day. Instead, they thought that proteins and other seemingly large organic molecules were simply heterogeneous aggregates of small organic molecules held together by weak "association forces" (Figure 2–32).

The first hint that proteins and other organic polymers are large molecules came from observing their behavior in solution. At the time, scientists were working with various proteins and carbohydrates derived from foodstuffs and other organic materials—albumin from egg whites, casein from milk, collagen from gelatin, and cellulose from wood. Their chemical compositions seemed simple enough: like other organic molecules, they contained carbon, hydrogen, oxygen, and, in the case of proteins, nitrogen. But they behaved oddly in solution, showing, for example, an inability to pass through a fine filter.

Why these molecules misbehaved in solution was a puzzle. Were they really giant molecules, composed of an unusually large number of covalently linked atoms? Or were they more like a colloidal suspension of particles—a big, sticky hodgepodge of small organic molecules that associate only loosely?

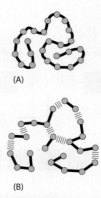

(A)

(B)

Figure 2–32 What might an organic macromolecule look like? Chemists in the early part of the twentieth century debated whether proteins, polysaccharides, and other apparently large organic molecules were (A) discrete particles made of an unusually large number of covalently linked atoms or (B) a loose aggregation of heterogeneous small organic molecules held together by weak forces.

One way to distinguish between the two possibilities was to determine the actual size of one of these molecules. If a protein such as albumin were made of molecules all identical in size, that would support the existence of true macromolecules. Conversely, if albumin were instead a miscellaneous conglomeration of small organic molecules, these should show a whole range of molecular sizes in solution.

Unfortunately, the techniques available to scientists in the early 1900s were not ideal for measuring the sizes of such large molecules. Some chemists estimated a protein's size by determining how much it would lower a solution's freezing point; others measured the osmotic pressure of protein solutions. These methods were susceptible to experimental error and gave variable results. Different techniques, for example, suggested that cellulose was anywhere from 6000 to 103,000 daltons in mass (where 1 dalton is approximately equal to the mass of a hydrogen atom). Such results helped to fuel the hypothesis that carbohydrates and proteins were loose aggregates of small molecules rather than true macromolecules.

Many scientists simply had trouble believing that molecules heavier than about 4000 daltons—the largest compound that had been synthesized by organic chemists—could exist at all. Take hemoglobin, the oxygen-carrying protein in red blood cells. Researchers tried to estimate its size by breaking it down into its chemical components. In addition to carbon, hydrogen, nitrogen, and oxygen, hemoglobin contains a small amount of iron. Working out the percentages, it appeared that hemoglobin had one atom of iron for every 712 atoms of carbon—and a minimum weight of 16,700 daltons. Could a molecule with hundreds of carbon atoms in one long chain remain intact in a cell and perform specific functions? Emil Fischer, the organic chemist who determined that the amino acids in proteins are linked by peptide bonds, thought that a polypeptide chain could grow no longer than about 30 or 40 amino acids. As for hemoglobin, with its purported 700 carbon atoms, the existence of molecular chains of such "truly fantastic lengths" was deemed "very improbable" by leading chemists.

Definitive resolution of the debate had to await the development of new techniques. Convincing evidence that proteins are macromolecules came from studies using the ultracentrifuge—a device that uses centrifugal force to separate molecules according to their size (see Panel 4–3, pp. 164–165). Theodor Svedberg, who designed the machine in 1925, performed the first studies. If a protein were really an aggregate of smaller molecules, he reasoned, it would appear as a smear of molecules of different sizes when sedimented in an ultracentrifuge. Using hemoglobin as his test protein, Svedberg found that the centrifuged sample revealed a single, sharp band with a molecular weight of 68,000 daltons. The finding strongly supported the theory that proteins are true macromolecules (**Figure 2–33**).

Additional evidence continued to accumulate throughout the 1930s, when other researchers were able to obtain crystals of pure protein that could be studied by x-ray diffraction. Only molecules with a uniform size and shape can form highly ordered crystals and diffract x-rays in such a way that their three-dimensional structure can be determined, as we discuss in Chapter 4. A heterogeneous suspension could not be studied in this way.

We now take it for granted that large macromolecules carry out many of the most important activities in living cells. But chemists once viewed the existence of such polymers with the same sort of skepticism that a zoologist might show on being told that "In Africa, there are elephants that are 100 meters long and 20 meters tall." It took decades for researchers to master the techniques required to convince everyone that molecules ten times larger than anything they had ever encountered were a cornerstone of biology. As we shall see throughout this book, such a labored pathway to discovery is not unusual, and progress in science—as in the discovery of macromolecules—is often driven by advances in technology.

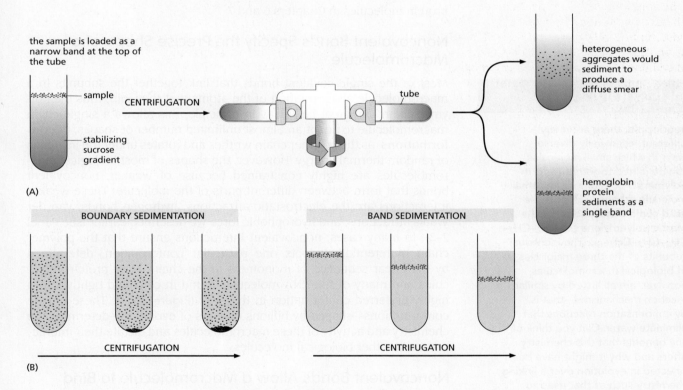

Figure 2–33 The ultracentrifuge helped to settle the debate about the nature of macromolecules. In the ultracentrifuge, centrifugal forces exceeding 500,000 times the force of gravity can be used to separate proteins or other large molecules. (A) In a modern ultracentrifuge, samples are loaded in a thin layer on top of a gradient of sucrose solution formed in a tube. The tube is placed in a metal rotor that is rotated at high speed in a vacuum. Molecules of different sizes sediment at different rates, and these molecules will therefore move as distinct bands in the sample tube. If hemoglobin were a loose aggregate of heterogeneous peptides, it would show a broad smear of sizes after centrifugation (top tube). Instead, it appears as a sharp band with a molecular weight of 68,000 daltons (bottom tube). Although the ultracentrifuge is now a standard, almost mundane, fixture in most biochemistry laboratories, its construction was a huge technological challenge. The centrifuge rotor must be capable of spinning centrifuge tubes at high speeds for many hours at constant temperature and with high stability to avoid disrupting the gradient and ruining the samples. In 1926, Svedberg won the Nobel Prize in Chemistry for his ultracentrifuge design and its application to chemistry. (B) In his actual experiment, Svedberg filled a special tube in the centrifuge with a homogeneous solution of hemoglobin; by shining light through the tube, he then carefully monitored the moving boundary between the sedimenting protein molecules and the clear aqueous solution left behind (so-called boundary sedimentation). The more recently developed method shown in (A) is a form of band sedimentation.

Figure 2–34 Most proteins and many RNA molecules fold into a particularly stable three-dimensional shape, or conformation. This shape is directed mostly by a multitude of weak, noncovalent, intramolecular bonds. If the folded macromolecules are subjected to conditions that disrupt noncovalent bonds, the molecule becomes a flexible chain that loses both its conformation and its biological activity.

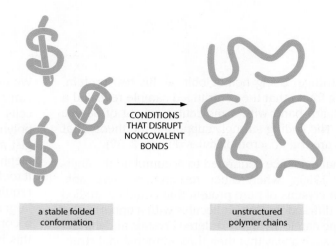

CONDITIONS THAT DISRUPT NONCOVALENT BONDS

a stable folded conformation

unstructured polymer chains

---

be subject to a sensitive control that allows it to specify exactly which subunit should be added next to the growing polymer end. We discuss the mechanisms that specify the sequence of subunits in DNA, RNA, and protein molecules in Chapters 6 and 7.

Noncovalent Bonds Specify the Precise Shape of a Macromolecule

Most of the single covalent bonds that link together the subunits in a macromolecule allow rotation of the atoms that they join; thus the polymer chain has great flexibility. In principle, this allows a single-chain macromolecule to adopt an almost unlimited number of shapes, or **conformations**, as the polymer chain writhes and rotates under the influence of random thermal energy. However, the shapes of most biological macromolecules are highly constrained because of weaker, noncovalent bonds that form between different parts of the molecule. These weaker interactions are the electrostatic attractions, hydrogen bonds, van der Waals attractions, and hydrophobic force we described earlier (see Panel 2–3). In many cases, noncovalent interactions ensure that the polymer chain preferentially adopts one particular conformation, determined by the linear sequence of monomers in the chain. Most protein molecules and many of the RNA molecules found in cells fold tightly into a highly preferred conformation in this way (**Figure 2–34**). These unique conformations—shaped by billions of years of evolution—determine the chemistry and activity of these macromolecules and dictate their interactions with other biological molecules.

Noncovalent Bonds Allow a Macromolecule to Bind Other Selected Molecules

As we discussed earlier, although noncovalent bonds are individually weak, they can add up to create a strong attraction between two molecules when these molecules fit together very closely, like a hand in a glove, so that many noncovalent bonds can occur between them (see Panel 2–3). This form of molecular interaction provides for great specificity in the binding of a macromolecule to other small and large molecules, because the multipoint contacts required for strong binding make it possible for a macromolecule to select just one of the many thousands of different molecules present inside a cell. Moreover, because the strength of the binding depends on the number of noncovalent bonds that are

QUESTION 2–8

In principle, there are many different, chemically diverse ways in which small molecules can be joined together to form polymers. For example, the small molecule ethene ($CH_2=CH_2$) is used commercially to make the plastic polyethylene (...–CH_2–CH_2–CH_2–CH_2–CH_2–...). The individual subunits of the three major classes of biological macromolecules, however, are all linked by similar reaction mechanisms—that is, by condensation reactions that eliminate water. Can you think of any benefits that this chemistry offers and why it might have been selected in evolution over a linking chemistry such as that used to produce polyethylene?

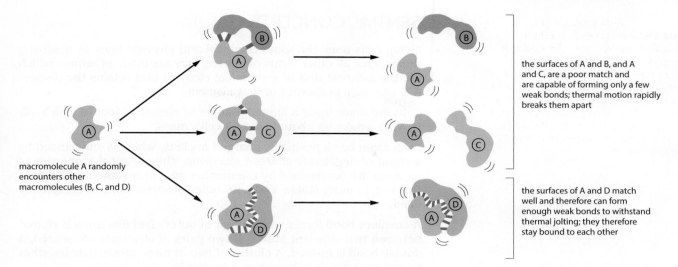

the surfaces of A and B, and A and C, are a poor match and are capable of forming only a few weak bonds; thermal motion rapidly breaks them apart

the surfaces of A and D match well and therefore can form enough weak bonds to withstand thermal jolting; they therefore stay bound to each other

macromolecule A randomly encounters other macromolecules (B, C, and D)

Figure 2–35 Noncovalent bonds mediate interactions between macromolecules. They can also mediate interactions between a macromolecule and small molecules (see **Movie 2.4**).

formed, associations of almost any strength are possible. As one example, binding of this type makes it possible for proteins to function as enzymes. Enzymes recognize their substrates via noncovalent interactions, and an enzyme that acts on a positively charged substrate will often use a negatively charged amino acid side chain to guide the substrate to its proper position. We discuss such interactions in greater detail in Chapter 4.

Noncovalent bonds can also stabilize associations between any two macromolecules, as long as their surfaces match closely (**Figure 2–35**). Such associations allow macromolecules to be used as building blocks for the formation of much larger structures. For example, proteins often bind together into multiprotein complexes that function as intricate machines with multiple moving parts, carrying out such complex tasks as DNA replication and protein synthesis (**Figure 2–36**). In fact, noncovalent bonds account for a great deal of the complex chemistry that makes life possible.

QUESTION 2–9

Why could covalent bonds not be used in place of noncovalent bonds to mediate most of the interactions of macromolecules?

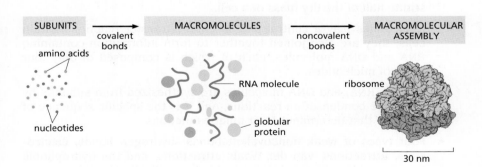

Figure 2–36 Both covalent bonds and noncovalent bonds are needed to form a macromolecular assembly such as a ribosome. Covalent bonds allow small organic molecules to join together to form macromolecules, which can assemble into large macromolecular complexes via noncovalent bonds. Ribosomes are large macromolecular machines that synthesize proteins inside cells. Each ribosome is composed of about 90 macromolecules (proteins and RNA molecules), and it is large enough to see in the electron microscope (see Figure 7–34). The subunits, macromolecules, and ribosome shown here are drawn roughly to scale.

ESSENTIAL CONCEPTS

- Living cells obey the same chemical and physical laws as nonliving things. Like all other forms of matter, they are made of atoms, which are the smallest unit of a chemical element that retains the distinctive chemical properties of that element.

- Cells are made up of a limited number of elements, four of which—C, H, N, O—make up about 96% of a cell's mass.

- Each atom has a positively charged nucleus, which is surrounded by a cloud of negatively charged electrons. The chemical properties of an atom are determined by the number and arrangement of its electrons: it is most stable when its outer electron shell is completely filled.

- A covalent bond forms when a pair of outer-shell electrons is shared between two adjacent atoms; if two pairs of electrons are shared, a double bond is formed. A cluster of two or more atoms held together by covalent bonds is known as a molecule.

- When an electron jumps from one atom to another, two ions of opposite charge are generated; these ions are held together by mutual attraction, forming a noncovalent ionic bond.

- Cells are 70% water by weight; the chemistry of life therefore takes place in an aqueous environment.

- Living organisms contain a distinctive and restricted set of small, carbon-based (organic) molecules, which are essentially the same for every living species. The main categories are sugars, fatty acids, amino acids, and nucleotides.

- Sugars are a primary source of chemical energy for cells and can also be joined together to form polysaccharides or shorter oligosaccharides.

- Fatty acids are an even richer energy source than sugars, but their most essential function is to form lipid molecules that assemble into sheet-like cell membranes.

- The vast majority of the dry mass of a cell consists of macromolecules—mainly polysaccharides, proteins, and nucleic acids (DNA and RNA); these macromolecules are formed as polymers of sugars, amino acids, or nucleotides, respectively.

- The most diverse and versatile class of macromolecules are proteins, which are formed from 20 types of amino acids that are covalently linked by peptide bonds into long polypeptide chains. Proteins constitute half of the dry mass of a cell.

- Nucleotides play a central part in energy-transfer reactions within cells; they are also joined together to form information-containing RNA and DNA molecules, each of which is composed of only four types of nucleotides.

- Protein, RNA, and DNA molecules are synthesized from subunits by repetitive condensation reactions, and it is the specific sequence of subunits that determines their unique functions.

- Four types of weak noncovalent bonds—hydrogen bonds, electrostatic attractions, van der Waals attractions, and the hydrophobic force—enable macromolecules to bind specifically to other macromolecules or to selected small molecules.

- Noncovalent bonds between different regions of a polypeptide or RNA chain allow these chains to fold into unique shapes (conformations).

KEY TERMS

acid	electrostatic attraction	molecule
amino acid	fatty acid	monomer
atom	hydrogen bond	noncovalent bond
atomic weight	hydrolysis	nucleotide
ATP	hydronium ion	organic molecule
Avogadro's number	hydrophilic	pH scale
base	hydrophobic	polar
buffer	hydrophobic force	polymer
chemical bond	inorganic	protein
chemical group	ion	proton
condensation reaction	ionic bond	RNA
conformation	lipid	sequence
covalent bond	lipid bilayer	subunit
DNA	macromolecule	sugar
electron	molecular weight	van der Waals attraction
electronegativity		

QUESTIONS

QUESTION 2–10

Which of the following statements are correct? Explain your answers.

A. An atomic nucleus contains protons and neutrons.

B. An atom has more electrons than protons.

C. The nucleus is surrounded by a double membrane.

D. All atoms of the same element have the same number of neutrons.

E. The number of neutrons determines whether the nucleus of an atom is stable or radioactive.

F. Both fatty acids and polysaccharides can be important energy stores in the cell.

G. Hydrogen bonds are weak and can be broken by thermal energy, yet they contribute significantly to the specificity of interactions between macromolecules.

QUESTION 2–11

To gain a better feeling for atomic dimensions, assume that the page on which this question is printed is made entirely of the polysaccharide cellulose, whose molecules are described by the formula $(C_nH_{2n}O_n)$, where n can be a quite large number and is variable from one molecule to another. The atomic weights of carbon, hydrogen, and oxygen are 12, 1, and 16, respectively, and this page weighs 5 g.

A. How many carbon atoms are there in this page?

B. In cellulose, how many carbon atoms would be stacked on top of each other to span the thickness of this page (the size of the page is 21.2 cm × 27.6 cm, and it is 0.07 mm thick)?

C. Now consider the problem from a different angle. Assume that the page is composed only of carbon atoms. A carbon atom has a diameter of 2×10^{-10} m (0.2 nm); how many carbon atoms of 0.2 nm diameter would it take to span the thickness of the page?

D. Compare your answers from parts B and C and explain any differences.

QUESTION 2–12

A. How many electrons can be accommodated in the first, second, and third electron shells of an atom?

B. How many electrons would atoms of the elements listed below have to gain or lose to obtain a completely filled outer shell?

helium	gain __	lose __
oxygen	gain __	lose __
carbon	gain __	lose __
sodium	gain __	lose __
chlorine	gain __	lose __

C. What do the answers tell you about the reactivity of helium and the bonds that can form between sodium and chlorine?

QUESTION 2–13

The elements oxygen and sulfur have similar chemical properties because they both have six electrons in their outermost electron shells. Indeed, both elements form molecules with two hydrogen atoms, water (H_2O) and hydrogen sulfide (H_2S). Surprisingly, at room temperature, water is a liquid, yet H_2S is a gas, despite sulfur being much larger and heavier than oxygen. Explain why this might be the case.

QUESTION 2–14

Write the chemical formula for a condensation reaction of two amino acids to form a peptide bond. Write the formula for its hydrolysis.

CARBON SKELETONS

Carbon has a unique role in the cell because of its ability to form strong covalent bonds with other carbon atoms. Thus carbon atoms can join to form:

chains

branched trees

rings

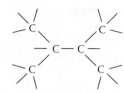

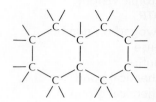

also written as

also written as

also written as

COVALENT BONDS

A covalent bond forms when two atoms come very close together and share one or more of their outer-shell electrons. Each atom forms a fixed number of covalent bonds in a defined spatial arrangement.

SINGLE BONDS: two electrons shared per bond

DOUBLE BONDS: four electrons shared per bond

The precise spatial arrangement of covalent bonds influences the three-dimensional structure and chemistry of molecules. In this review panel, we see how covalent bonds are used in a variety of biological molecules.

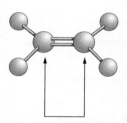

Atoms joined by two or more covalent bonds cannot rotate freely around the bond axis. This restriction has a major influence on the three-dimensional shape of many macromolecules.

C–H COMPOUNDS

Carbon and hydrogen together make stable compounds (or groups) called hydrocarbons. These are nonpolar, do not form hydrogen bonds, and are generally insoluble in water.

$$H-\overset{\overset{\displaystyle H}{|}}{\underset{\underset{\displaystyle H}{|}}{C}}-H$$

$$H-\overset{\overset{\displaystyle H}{|}}{\underset{\underset{\displaystyle H}{|}}{C}}-H$$

methane   methyl **group**

part of the hydrocarbon "tail" of a fatty acid molecule

ALTERNATING DOUBLE BONDS

A carbon chain can include double bonds. If these are on alternate carbon atoms, the bonding electrons move within the molecule, stabilizing the structure by a phenomenon called *resonance*.

Alternating double bonds in a ring can generate a very stable structure.

the truth is somewhere between these two structures

benzene

often written as

C–O COMPOUNDS

Many biological compounds contain a carbon covalently bonded to an oxygen. For example,

alcohol

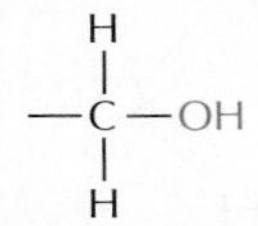

The –OH is called a hydroxyl group.

aldehyde

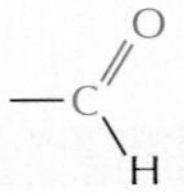

ketone

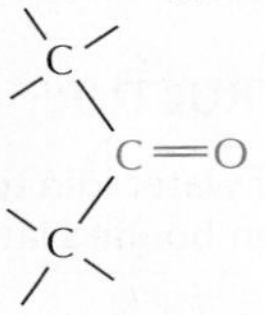

The C=O is called a carbonyl group.

carboxylic acid

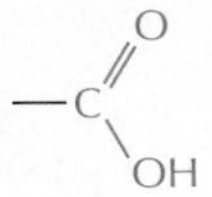

The –COOH is called a carboxyl group. In water, this loses an H^+ ion to become $-COO^-$.

esters

Esters are formed by combining an acid and an alcohol.

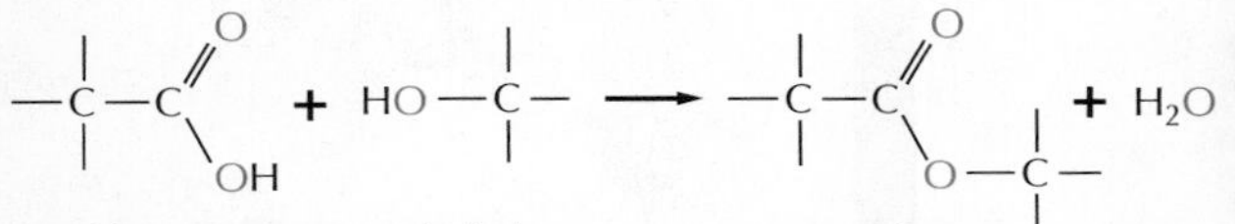

acid + alcohol → ester + H_2O

C–N COMPOUNDS

Amines and amides are two important examples of compounds containing a carbon linked to a nitrogen.

Amines in water combine with an H^+ ion to become positively charged.

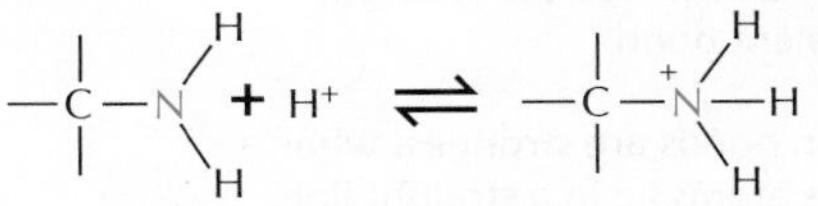

Amides are formed by combining an acid and an amine. Unlike amines, amides are uncharged in water. An example is the peptide bond that joins amino acids in a protein.

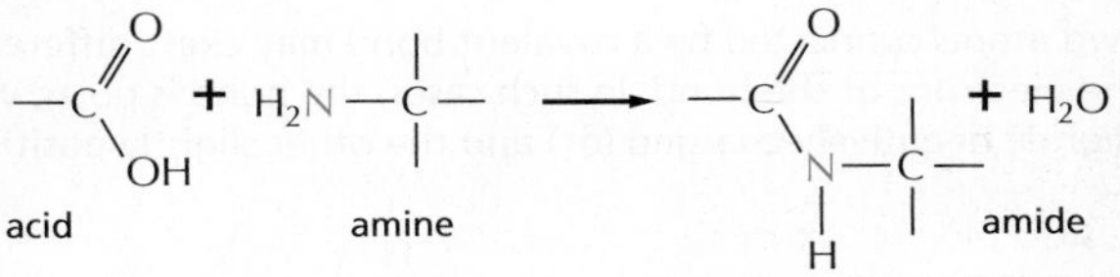

acid + amine → amide + H_2O

Nitrogen also occurs in several ring compounds, including important constituents of nucleic acids: purines and pyrimidines.

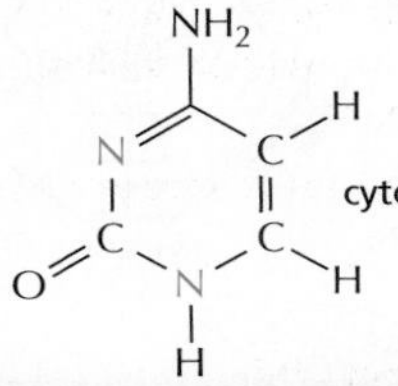

cytosine (a pyrimidine)

SULFHYDRYL GROUP

The $-\overset{|}{\underset{|}{C}}-SH$ is called a sulfhydryl group. In the amino acid cysteine, the sulfhydryl group may exist in the reduced form, $-\overset{|}{\underset{|}{C}}-SH$ or more rarely in an oxidized, cross-bridging form, $-\overset{|}{\underset{|}{C}}-S-S-\overset{|}{\underset{|}{C}}-$

PHOSPHATES

Inorganic phosphate is a stable ion formed from phosphoric acid, H_3PO_4. It is also written as P_i.

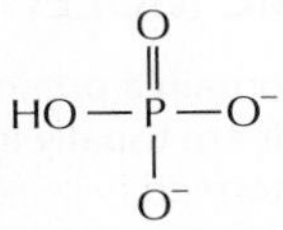

Phosphate esters can form between a phosphate and a free hydroxyl group. Phosphate groups are often covalently attached to proteins in this way.

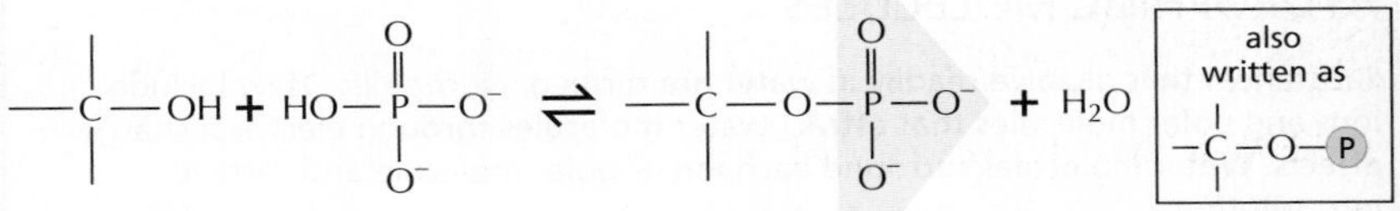

also written as

The combination of a phosphate and a carboxyl group, or two or more phosphate groups, produces an acid anhydride. Because compounds of this type release a large amount of free energy when the bond is broken by hydrolysis in the cell, they are often said to contain a "high-energy" bond.

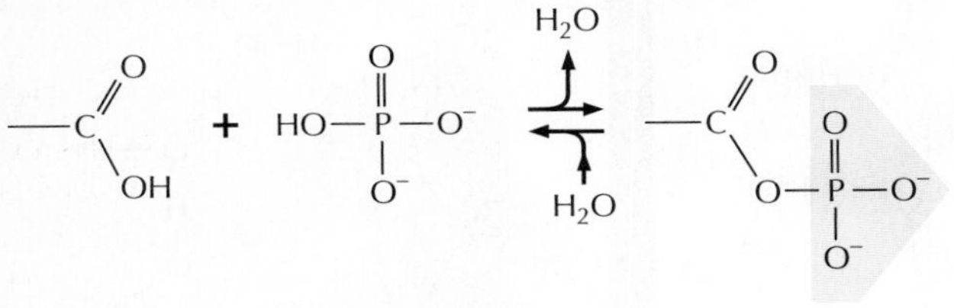

"high-energy" acyl phosphate bond (carboxylic–phosphoric acid anhydride) found in some metabolites

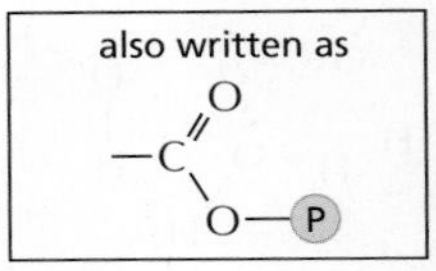

also written as

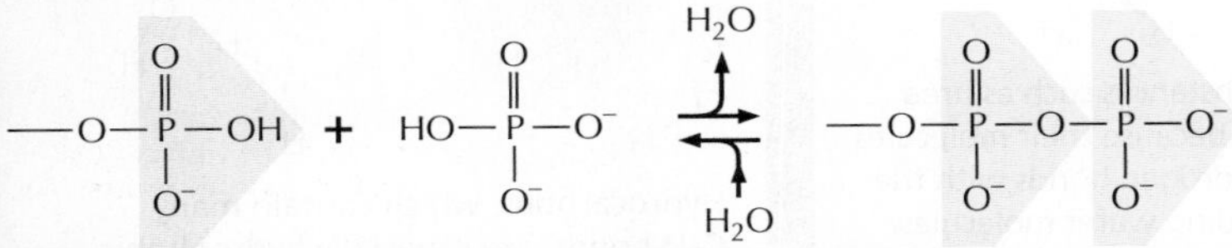

"high-energy" phosphoanhydride bond found in molecules such as ATP

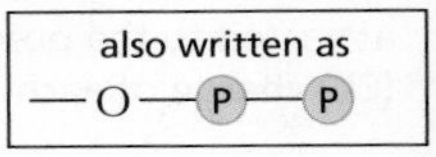

also written as

HYDROGEN BONDS

Because they are polarized, two adjacent H_2O molecules can form a noncovalent linkage known as a hydrogen bond. Hydrogen bonds have only about 1/20 the strength of a covalent bond.

Hydrogen bonds are strongest when the three atoms lie in a straight line.

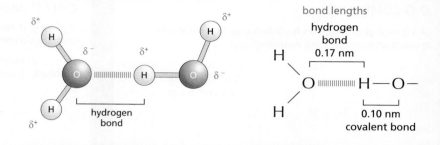

bond lengths

hydrogen
bond
0.17 nm

0.10 nm
covalent bond

WATER

Two atoms connected by a covalent bond may exert different attractions for the electrons of the bond. In such cases, the bond is polar, with one end slightly negatively charged (δ^-) and the other slightly positively charged (δ^+).

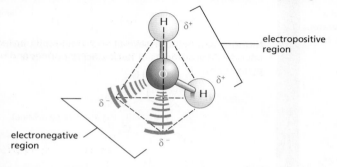

electropositive region

electronegative region

Although a water molecule has an overall neutral charge (having the same number of electrons and protons), the electrons are asymmetrically distributed, making the molecule polar. The oxygen nucleus draws electrons away from the hydrogen nuclei, leaving the hydrogen nuclei with a small net positive charge. The excess of electron density on the oxygen atom creates weakly negative regions at the other two corners of an imaginary tetrahedron. On these pages, we review the chemical properties of water and see how water influences the behavior of biological molecules.

WATER STRUCTURE

Molecules of water join together transiently in a hydrogen-bonded lattice.

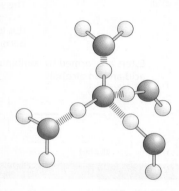

The cohesive nature of water is responsible for many of its unusual properties, such as high surface tension, high specific heat capacity, and high heat of vaporization.

HYDROPHILIC MOLECULES

Substances that dissolve readily in water are termed hydrophilic. They include ions and polar molecules that attract water molecules through electrical charge effects. Water molecules surround each ion or polar molecule and carry it into solution.

Ionic substances such as sodium chloride dissolve because water molecules are attracted to the positive (Na$^+$) or negative (Cl$^-$) charge of each ion.

Polar substances such as urea dissolve because their molecules form hydrogen bonds with the surrounding water molecules.

HYDROPHOBIC MOLECULES

Substances that contain a preponderance of nonpolar bonds are usually insoluble in water and are termed hydrophobic. Water molecules are not attracted to such hydrophobic molecules and so have little tendency to surround them and bring them into solution.

Hydrocarbons, which contain many C–H bonds, are especially hydrophobic.

WATER AS A SOLVENT

Many substances, such as household sugar (sucrose), dissolve in water. That is, their molecules separate from each other, each becoming surrounded by water molecules.

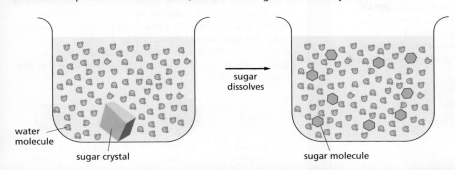

sugar dissolves

water molecule

sugar crystal

sugar molecule

When a substance dissolves in a liquid, the mixture is termed a solution. The dissolved substance (in this case sugar) is the solute, and the liquid that does the dissolving (in this case water) is the solvent. Water is an excellent solvent for hydrophilic substances because of its polar bonds.

ACIDS

Substances that release hydrogen ions (protons) into solution are called acids.

$$HCl \longrightarrow H^+ + Cl^-$$

hydrochloric acid   hydrogen ion   chloride ion
(strong acid)

Many of the acids important in the cell are not completely dissociated, and they are therefore weak acids—for example, the carboxyl group (–COOH), which dissociates to give a hydrogen ion in solution.

carboxyl group
(weak acid)

Note that this is a reversible reaction.

HYDROGEN ION EXCHANGE

Positively charged hydrogen ions (H^+) can spontaneously move from one water molecule to another, thereby creating two ionic species.

hydronium ion   hydroxyl ion

often written as: $H_2O \rightleftharpoons H^+ + OH^-$

hydrogen ion   hydroxyl ion

Because the process is rapidly reversible, hydrogen ions are continually shuttling between water molecules. Pure water contains equal concentrations of hydronium ions and hydroxyl ions (both 10^{-7} M).

pH

The acidity of a solution is defined by the concentration (conc.) of hydronium ions (H_3O^+) it possesses, generally abbreviated as H^+. For convenience, we use the pH scale, where

$$pH = -\log_{10}[H^+]$$

For pure water

$$[H^+] = 10^{-7} \text{ moles/liter}$$

$$pH = 7.0$$

H^+ conc. moles/liter		pH
1		0
10^{-1}		1
10^{-2}		2
10^{-3}	ACIDIC	3
10^{-4}		4
10^{-5}		5
10^{-6}		6
10^{-7}		7
10^{-8}		8
10^{-9}		9
10^{-10}		10
10^{-11}	BASIC	11
10^{-12}		12
10^{-13}		13
10^{-14}		14

BASES

Substances that reduce the number of hydrogen ions in solution are called bases. Some bases, such as ammonia, combine directly with hydrogen ions.

$$NH_3 + H^+ \longrightarrow NH_4^+$$

ammonia   hydrogen ion   ammonium ion

Other bases, such as sodium hydroxide, reduce the number of H^+ ions indirectly, by producing OH^- ions that then combine directly with H^+ ions to make H_2O.

$$NaOH \longrightarrow Na^+ + OH^-$$

sodium hydroxide   sodium ion   hydroxyl ion
(strong base)

Many bases found in cells are partially associated with H^+ ions and are termed weak bases. This is true of compounds that contain an amino group (–NH₂), which has a weak tendency to reversibly accept an H^+ ion from water, thereby increasing the concentration of free OH^- ions.

$$-NH_2 + H^+ \rightleftharpoons -NH_3^+$$

WEAK NONCOVALENT CHEMICAL BONDS

Organic molecules can interact with other molecules through three types of short-range attractive forces known as *noncovalent bonds*: van der Waals attractions, electrostatic attractions, and hydrogen bonds. The repulsion of hydrophobic groups from water is also important for these interactions and for the folding of biological macromolecules.

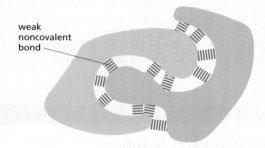

weak noncovalent bond

Weak noncovalent bonds have less than 1/20 the strength of a strong covalent bond. They are strong enough to provide tight binding only when many of them are formed simultaneously.

HYDROGEN BONDS

As already described for water (see Panel 2–2, pp. 68–69), hydrogen bonds form when a hydrogen atom is "sandwiched" between two electron-attracting atoms (usually oxygen or nitrogen).

Hydrogen bonds are strongest when the three atoms are in a straight line:

$$\text{O—H} \|\|\|\|\|\|\|\| \text{O} \qquad \text{N—H} \|\|\|\|\|\|\|\| \text{O}$$

Examples in macromolecules:

Amino acids in a polypeptide chain can be hydrogen-bonded together in a folded protein.

Two bases, G and C, are hydrogen-bonded in a DNA double helix.

VAN DER WAALS ATTRACTIONS

If two atoms are too close together, they repel each other very strongly. For this reason, an atom can often be treated as a sphere with a fixed radius. The characteristic "size" for each atom is specified by a unique van der Waals radius. The contact distance between any two noncovalently bonded atoms is the sum of their van der Waals radii.

H	C	N	O
0.12 nm radius	0.2 nm radius	0.15 nm radius	0.14 nm radius

At very short distances, any two atoms show a weak bonding interaction due to their fluctuating electrical charges. The two atoms will be attracted to each other in this way until the distance between their nuclei is approximately equal to the sum of their van der Waals radii. Although they are individually very weak, such van der Waals attractions can become important when two macromolecular surfaces fit together very closely, because many atoms are involved.

Note that when two atoms form a covalent bond, the centers of the two atoms (the two atomic nuclei) are much closer together than the sum of the two van der Waals radii. Thus,

0.4 nm	0.15 nm	0.13 nm
two non-bonded carbon atoms	two carbon atoms held by a single covalent bond	two carbon atoms held by a double covalent bond

HYDROGEN BONDS IN WATER

Any two atoms that can form hydrogen bonds to each other can alternatively form hydrogen bonds to water molecules. Because of this competition with water molecules, the hydrogen bonds formed in water between two peptide bonds, for example, are relatively weak.

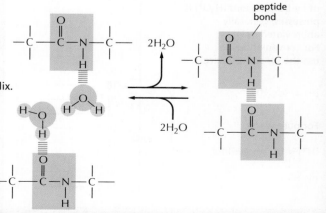

peptide bond

$2H_2O$

ELECTROSTATIC ATTRACTIONS

Electrostatic attractions occur both between fully charged groups (ionic bond) and between partially charged groups on polar molecules.

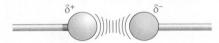

The force of attraction between the two partial charges, δ^+ and δ^-, falls off rapidly as the distance between the charges increases.

In the absence of water, ionic bonds are very strong. They are responsible for the strength of such minerals as marble and agate, and for crystal formation in common table salt, NaCl.

Cl$^-$

Na$^+$

a crystal of NaCl

ELECTROSTATIC ATTRACTIONS IN WATER

Charged groups are shielded by their interactions with water molecules. Electrostatic attractions are therefore quite weak in water.

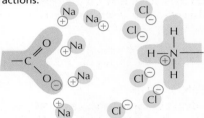

Inorganic ions in solution can also cluster around charged groups and further weaken these electrostatic attractions.

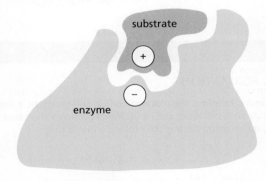

Despite being weakened by water and inorganic ions, electrostatic attractions are very important in biological systems. For example, an enzyme that binds a positively charged substrate will often have a negatively charged amino acid side chain at the appropriate place.

substrate

+

−

enzyme

HYDROPHOBIC FORCES

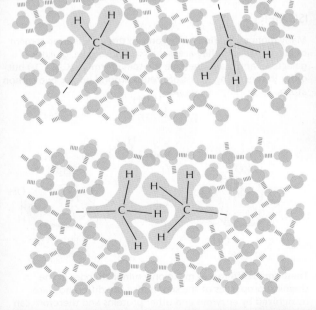

Water forces hydrophobic groups together in order to minimize their disruptive effects on the water network formed by the hydrogen bonds between water molecules. Hydrophobic groups held together in this way are sometimes said to be held together by "hydrophobic bonds," even though the attraction is actually caused by a repulsion from water.

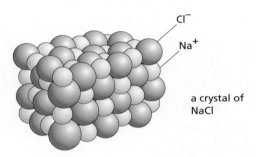

PANEL 2–4 AN OUTLINE OF SOME OF THE TYPES OF SUGARS

MONOSACCHARIDES

Monosaccharides usually have the general formula $(CH_2O)_n$, where n can be 3, 4, 5, or 6, and have two or more hydroxyl groups. They either contain an aldehyde group ($-C\overset{O}{\underset{H}{\diagdown}}$) and are called aldoses, or a ketone group ($\diagup C=O$) and are called ketoses.

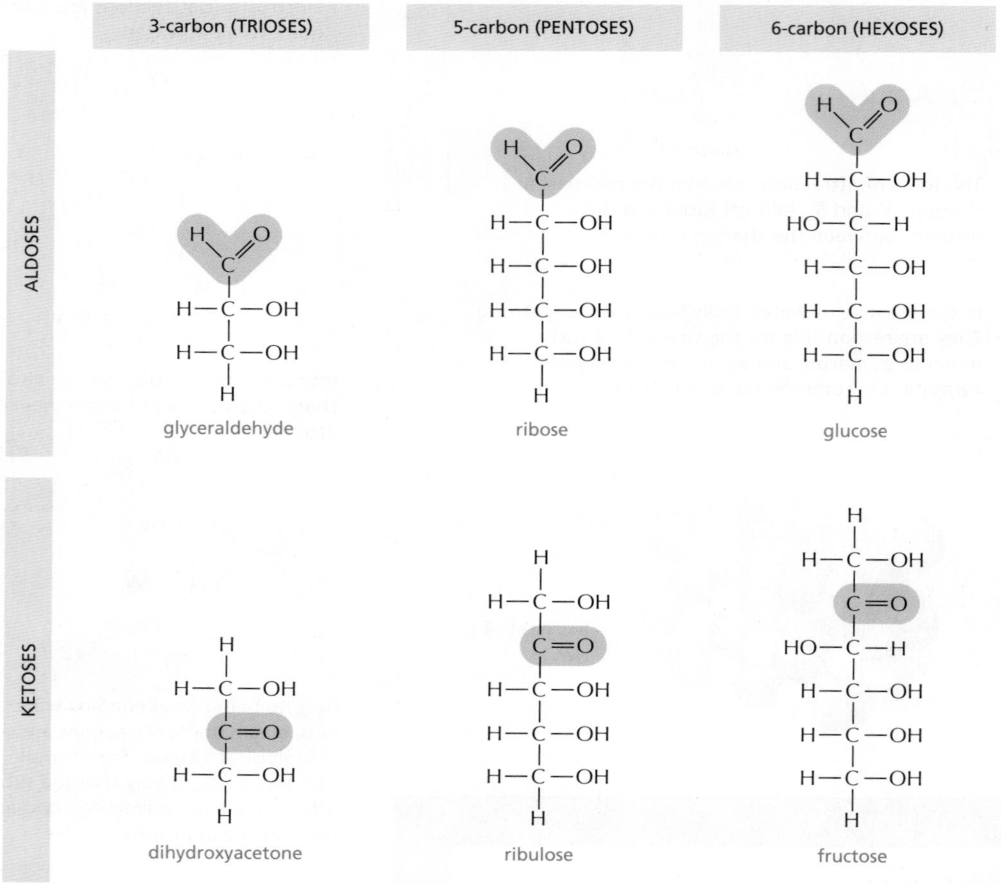

	3-carbon (TRIOSES)	5-carbon (PENTOSES)	6-carbon (HEXOSES)
ALDOSES	glyceraldehyde	ribose	glucose
KETOSES	dihydroxyacetone	ribulose	fructose

RING FORMATION

In aqueous solution, the aldehyde or ketone group of a sugar molecule tends to react with a hydroxyl group of the same molecule, thereby closing the molecule into a ring.

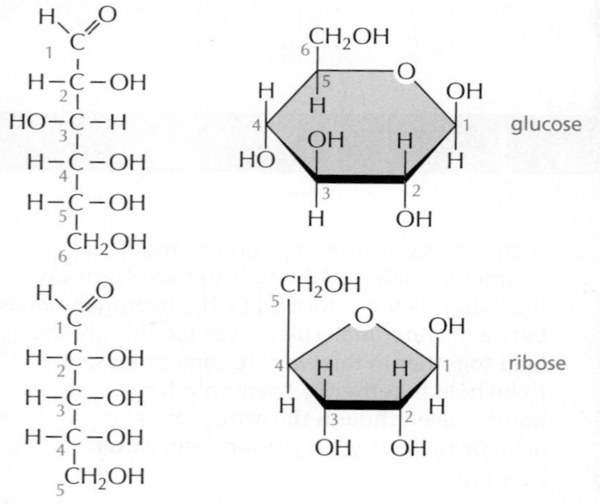

glucose

ribose

Note that each carbon atom has a number.

ISOMERS

Many monosaccharides differ only in the spatial arrangement of atoms—that is, they are isomers. For example, glucose, galactose, and mannose have the same formula ($C_6H_{12}O_6$) but differ in the arrangement of groups around one or two carbon atoms.

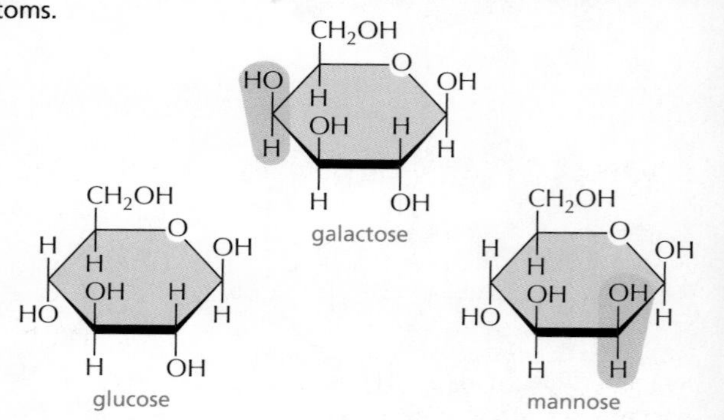

galactose

glucose

mannose

These small differences make only minor changes in the chemical properties of the sugars. But the differences are recognized by enzymes and other proteins and therefore can have major biological effects.

α AND β LINKS

The hydroxyl group on the carbon that carries the aldehyde or ketone can rapidly change from one position to the other. These two positions are called α and β.

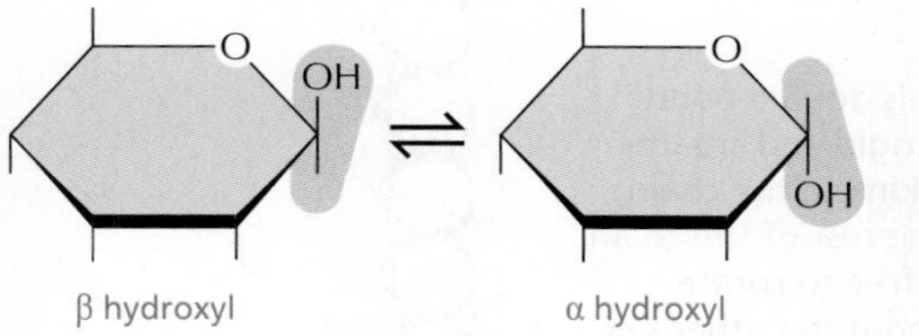

β hydroxyl   α hydroxyl

As soon as one sugar is linked to another, the α or β form is frozen.

SUGAR DERIVATIVES

The hydroxyl groups of a simple monosaccharide, such as glucose, can be replaced by other groups.

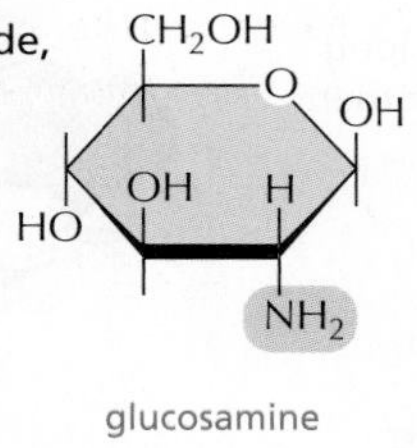

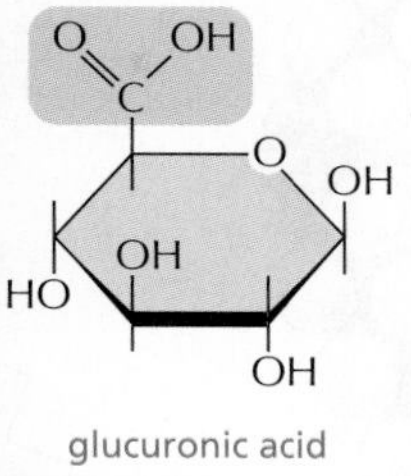

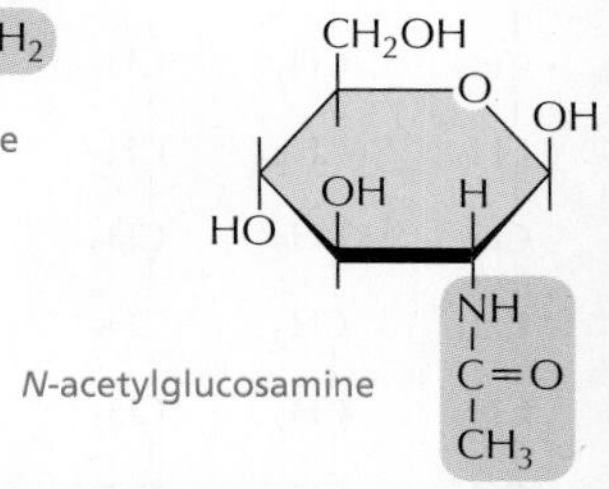

glucuronic acid

glucosamine

N-acetylglucosamine

DISACCHARIDES

The carbon that carries the aldehyde or the ketone can react with any hydroxyl group on a second sugar molecule to form a disaccharide. Three common disaccharides are

maltose (glucose + glucose)
lactose (galactose + glucose)
sucrose (glucose + fructose)

The reaction forming sucrose is shown here.

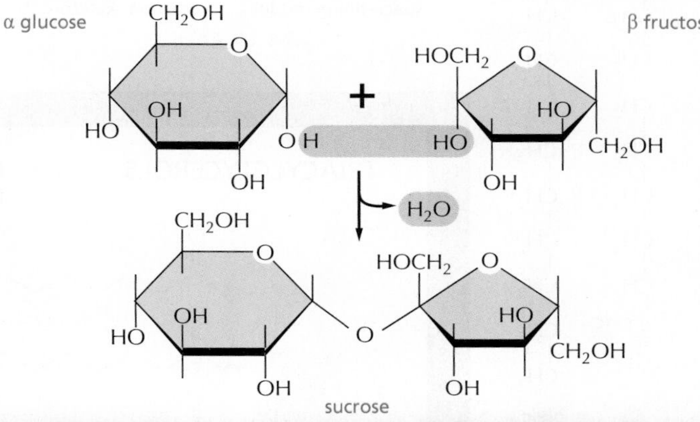

α glucose   β fructose

H_2O

sucrose

OLIGOSACCHARIDES AND POLYSACCHARIDES

Large linear and branched molecules can be made from simple repeating sugar subunits. Short chains are called oligosaccharides, and long chains are called polysaccharides. Glycogen, for example, is a polysaccharide made entirely of glucose subunits joined together.

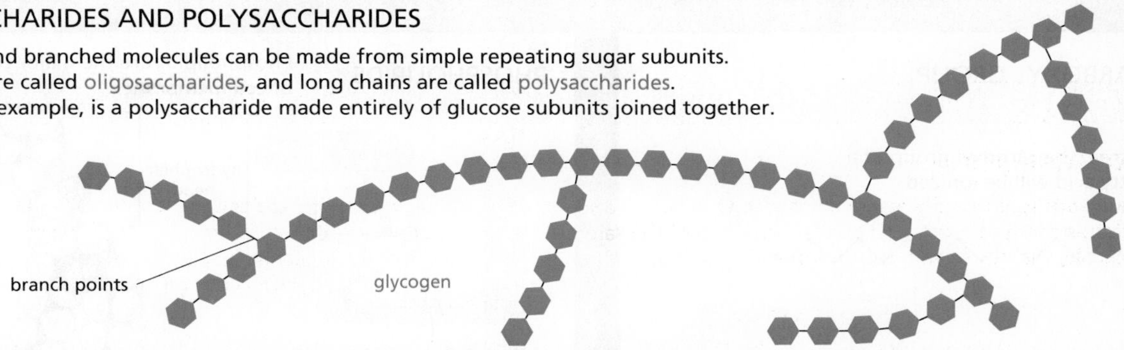

branch points   glycogen

COMPLEX OLIGOSACCHARIDES

In many cases, a sugar sequence is nonrepetitive. Many different molecules are possible. Such complex oligosaccharides are usually linked to proteins or to lipids, as is this oligosaccharide, which is part of a cell-surface molecule that defines a particular blood group.

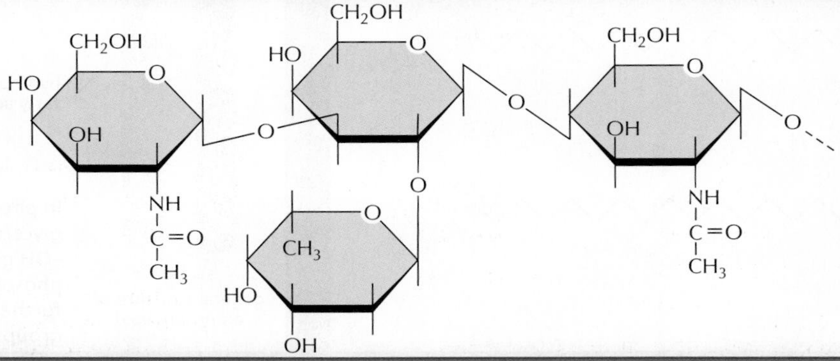

FATTY ACIDS

All fatty acids have a carboxyl group at one end and a long hydrocarbon tail at the other.

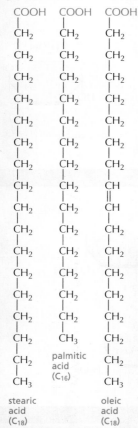

COOH   COOH   COOH
CH₂   CH₂   CH₂

stearic acid (C₁₈)

palmitic acid (C₁₆)

oleic acid (C₁₈)

Hundreds of different kinds of fatty acids exist. Some have one or more double bonds in their hydrocarbon tail and are said to be unsaturated. Fatty acids with no double bonds are saturated.

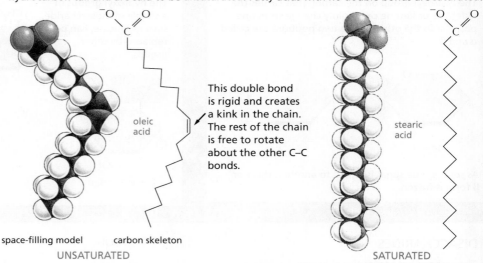

oleic acid

space-filling model   carbon skeleton

UNSATURATED

This double bond is rigid and creates a kink in the chain. The rest of the chain is free to rotate about the other C–C bonds.

stearic acid

SATURATED

TRIACYLGLYCEROLS

Fatty acids are stored in cells as an energy reserve (fats and oils) through an ester linkage to glycerol to form triacylglycerols.

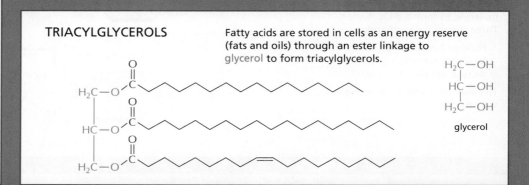

glycerol

CARBOXYL GROUP

If free, the carboxyl group of a fatty acid will be ionized.

But more often it is linked to other groups to form either esters

or amides.

PHOSPHOLIPIDS

Phospholipids are the major constituents of cell membranes.

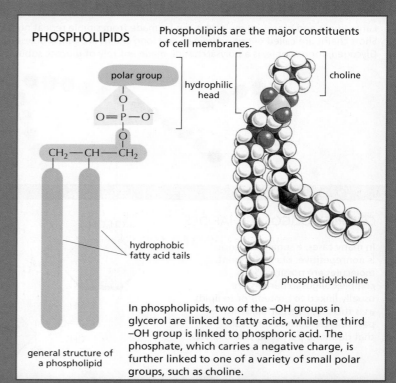

polar group

hydrophilic head

$O=P-O^-$

$CH_2-CH-CH_2$

hydrophobic fatty acid tails

general structure of a phospholipid

choline

phosphatidylcholine

In phospholipids, two of the –OH groups in glycerol are linked to fatty acids, while the third –OH group is linked to phosphoric acid. The phosphate, which carries a negative charge, is further linked to one of a variety of small polar groups, such as choline.

LIPID AGGREGATES

Fatty acids have a hydrophilic head and a hydrophobic tail.

In water, they can form either a surface film or small, spherical micelles.

surface film

micelle

Their derivatives can form larger aggregates held together by hydrophobic forces:

Triacylglycerols form large, spherical fat droplets in the cell cytoplasm.

Phospholipids and glycolipids form self-sealing *lipid bilayers*, which are the basis for all cell membranes.

200 nm or more

◄—— 4 nm ——►

OTHER LIPIDS

Lipids are defined as water-insoluble molecules that are soluble in organic solvents. Two other common types of lipids are steroids and polyisoprenoids. Both are made from isoprene units.

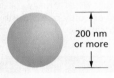

$$CH_3$$
$$C{-}CH{=}CH_2$$
$$CH_2$$ isoprene

STEROIDS

Steroids have a common multiple-ring structure.

OH

HO

cholesterol—found in many cell membranes

O

testosterone—male sex hormone

GLYCOLIPIDS

Like phospholipids, these compounds are composed of a hydrophobic region, containing two long hydrocarbon tails, and a polar region, which contains one or more sugars. Unlike phospholipids, there is no phosphate.

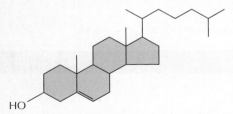

galactose

sugar

H   OH   H   O
C   C   C   CH₂
C   H   C
H
NH
C
O

a simple glycolipid

POLYISOPRENOIDS

Long-chain polymers of isoprene

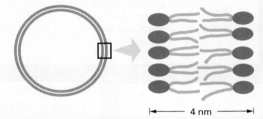

O⁻
O=P—O⁻
O

dolichol phosphate—used to carry activated sugars in the membrane-associated synthesis of glycoproteins and some polysaccharides

FAMILIES OF AMINO ACIDS

The common amino acids are grouped according to whether their side chains are

    acidic
    basic
    uncharged polar
    nonpolar

These 20 amino acids are given both three-letter and one-letter abbreviations.

Thus: alanine = Ala = A

BASIC SIDE CHAINS

lysine
(Lys, or K)

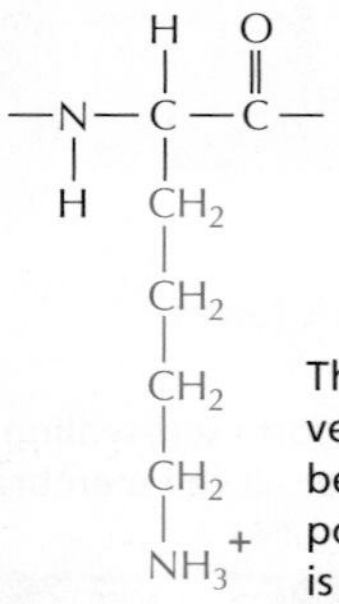

This group is very basic because its positive charge is stabilized by resonance (see Panel 2–1).

arginine
(Arg, or R)

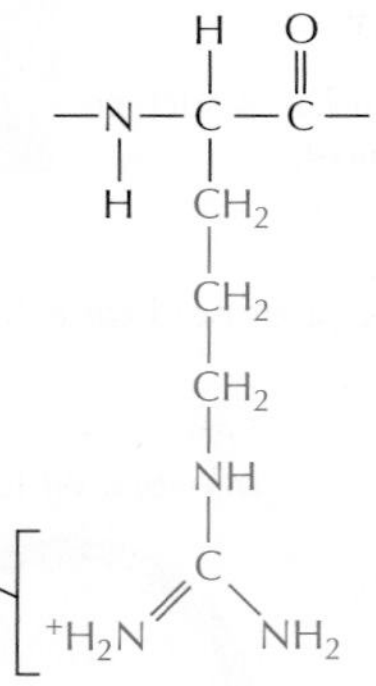

histidine
(His, or H)

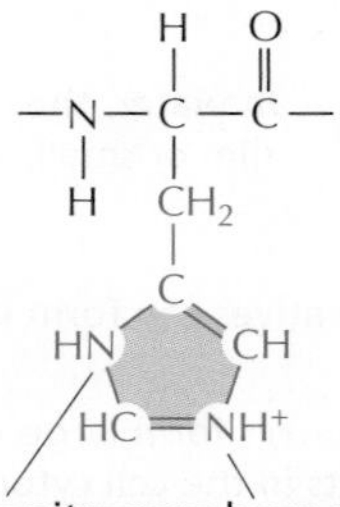

These nitrogens have a relatively weak affinity for an H^+ and are only partly positive at neutral pH.

THE AMINO ACID

The general formula of an amino acid is

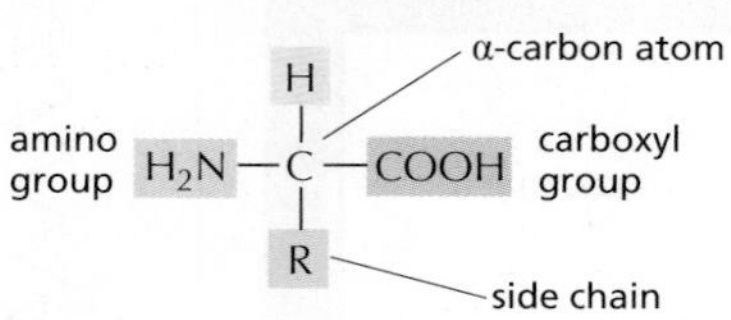

amino group H_2N — α-carbon atom — carboxyl group COOH

side chain R

R is commonly one of 20 different side chains. At pH 7, both the amino and carboxyl groups are ionized.

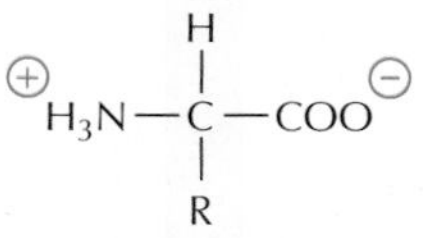

$$\overset{\oplus}{H_3N} - \underset{R}{\overset{H}{C}} - COO^{\ominus}$$

OPTICAL ISOMERS

The α-carbon atom is asymmetric, allowing for two mirror-image (or stereo-) isomers, L and D.

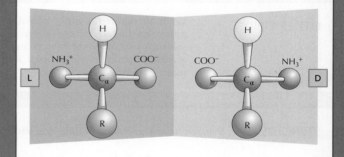

Proteins contain exclusively L-amino acids.

PEPTIDE BONDS

In proteins, amino acids are joined together by an amide linkage, called a peptide bond.

The four atoms involved in each peptide bond form a rigid planar unit (*red* box). There is no rotation around the C–N bond.

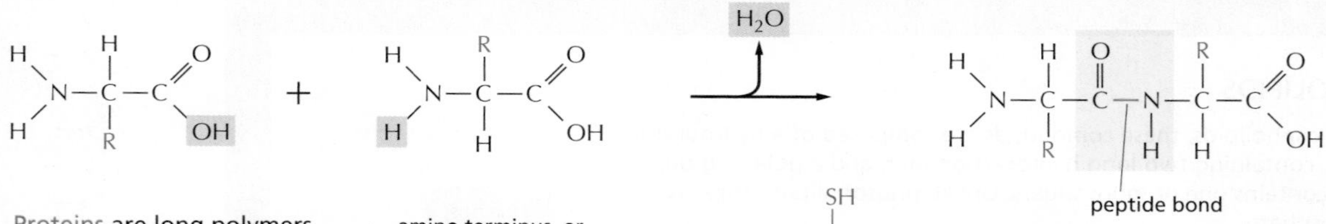

H_2O

peptide bond

Proteins are long polymers of amino acids linked by peptide bonds, and they are always written with the N-terminus toward the left. Peptides are shorter, usually fewer than 50 amino acids long. The sequence of this tripeptide is histidine-cysteine-valine.

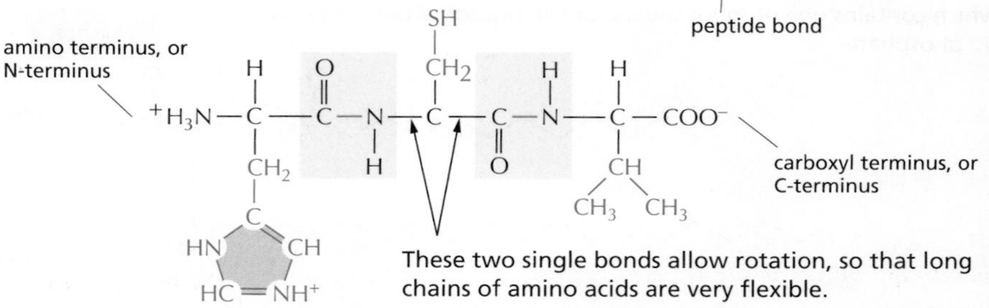

amino terminus, or N-terminus

carboxyl terminus, or C-terminus

These two single bonds allow rotation, so that long chains of amino acids are very flexible.

ACIDIC SIDE CHAINS

aspartic acid

(Asp, or D)

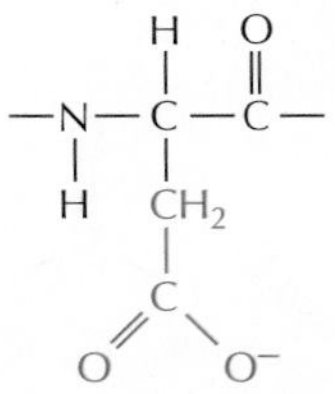

glutamic acid

(Glu, or E)

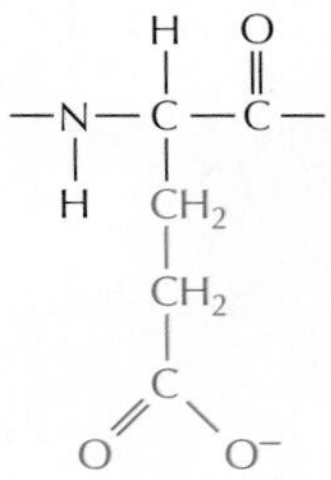

UNCHARGED POLAR SIDE CHAINS

asparagine

(Asn, or N)

glutamine

(Gln, or Q)

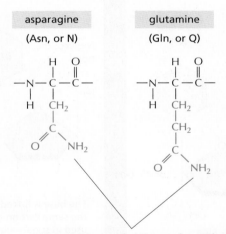

Although the amide N is not charged at neutral pH, it is polar.

serine

(Ser, or S)

threonine

(Thr, or T)

tyrosine

(Tyr, or Y)

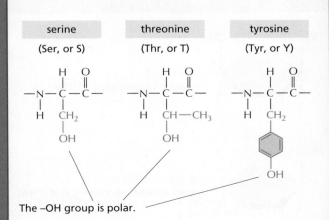

The –OH group is polar.

NONPOLAR SIDE CHAINS

alanine

(Ala, or A)

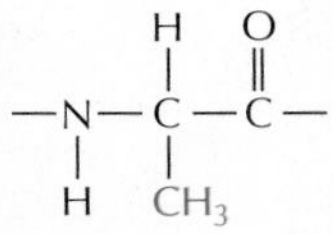

valine

(Val, or V)

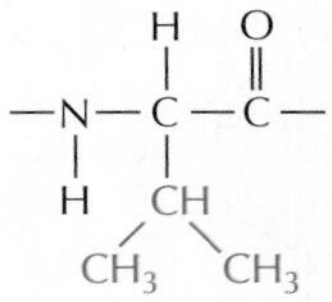

leucine

(Leu, or L)

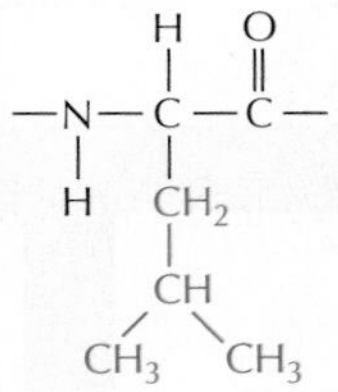

isoleucine

(Ile, or I)

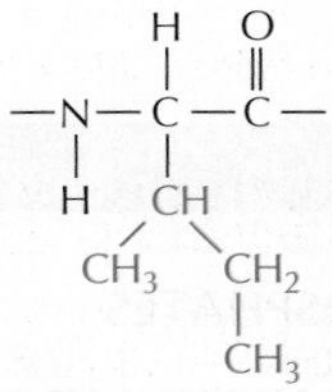

proline

(Pro, or P)

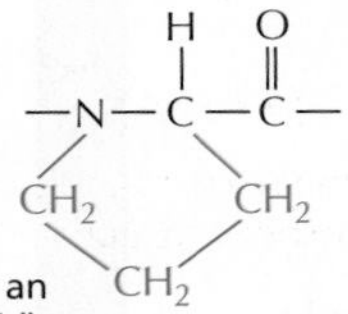

(actually an imino acid)

phenylalanine

(Phe, or F)

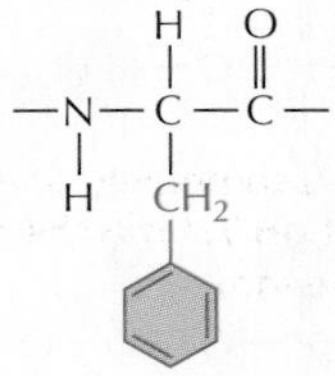

methionine

(Met, or M)

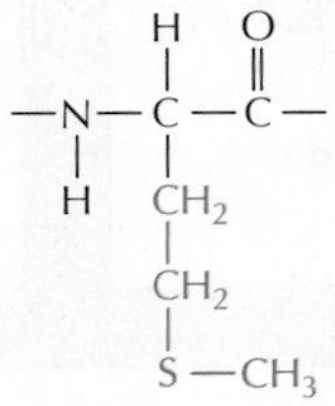

tryptophan

(Trp, or W)

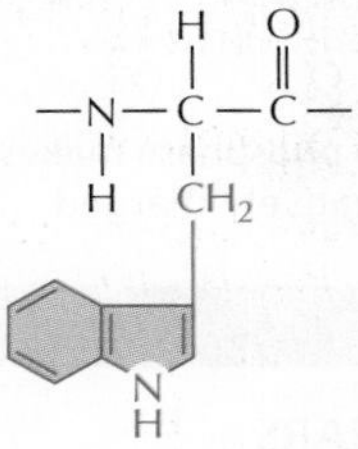

glycine

(Gly, or G)

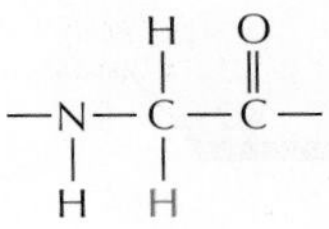

cysteine

(Cys, or C)

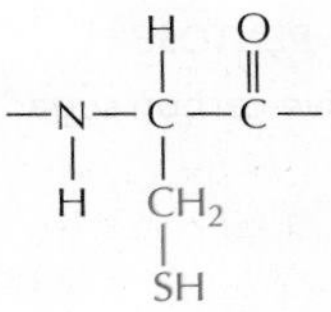

A disulfide bond (red) can form between two cysteine side chains in proteins.

$$--CH_2-S-S-CH_2--$$

PANEL 2–7 A SURVEY OF THE NUCLEOTIDES

BASES

The bases are nitrogen-containing ring compounds, either pyrimidines or purines.

uracil

cytosine

thymine

adenine

guanine

PYRIMIDINE

PURINE

PHOSPHATES

The phosphates are normally joined to the C5 hydroxyl of the ribose or deoxyribose sugar (designated 5'). Mono-, di-, and triphosphates are common.

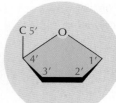

as in AMP

as in ADP

as in ATP

The phosphate makes a nucleotide negatively charged.

NUCLEOTIDES

A nucleotide consists of a nitrogen-containing base, a five-carbon sugar, and one or more phosphate groups.

BASE

PHOSPHATE

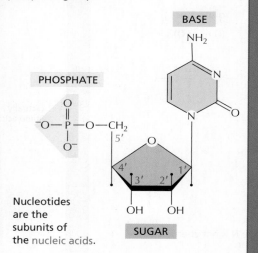

5'

4'   1'

3'   2'

Nucleotides are the subunits of the nucleic acids.

SUGAR

BASE–SUGAR LINKAGE

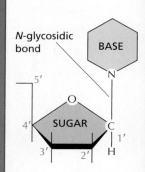

N-glycosidic bond

BASE

5'

4'   SUGAR

3'   2'   1'

H

The base is linked to the same carbon (C1) used in sugar–sugar bonds.

SUGARS

PENTOSE

a five-carbon sugar

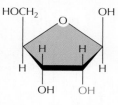

two kinds of pentoses are used

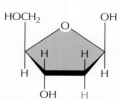

β-D-ribose
used in ribonucleic acid (RNA)

β-D-2-deoxyribose
used in deoxyribonucleic acid (DNA)

Each numbered carbon on the sugar of a nucleotide is followed by a prime mark; therefore, one speaks of the "5-prime carbon," etc.

NOMENCLATURE

The names can be confusing, but the abbreviations are clear.

BASE	NUCLEOSIDE	ABBR.
adenine	adenosine	A
guanine	guanosine	G
cytosine	cytidine	C
uracil	uridine	U
thymine	thymidine	T

Nucleotides and their derivatives can be abbreviated to three capital letters. Some examples follow:

AMP = adenosine monophosphate
dAMP = deoxyadenosine monophosphate
UDP = uridine diphosphate
ATP = adenosine triphosphate

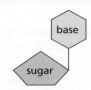

BASE + SUGAR = NUCLEOSIDE

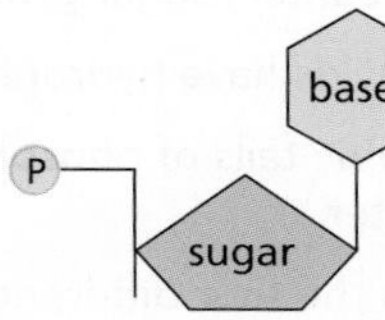

BASE + SUGAR + PHOSPHATE = NUCLEOTIDE

NUCLEIC ACIDS

To form nucleic acid polymers, nucleotides are joined together by phosphodiester bonds between the 5′ and 3′ carbon atoms of adjacent sugar rings. The linear sequence of nucleotides in a nucleic acid chain is abbreviated using a one-letter code, such as AGCTT, starting with the 5′ end of the chain.

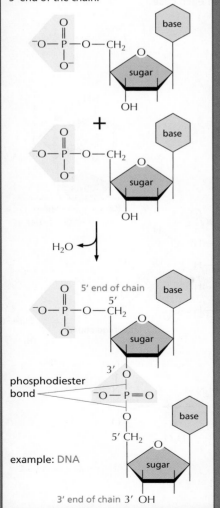

example: DNA

NUCLEOTIDES AND THEIR DERIVATIVES HAVE MANY OTHER FUNCTIONS

1. As nucleoside di- and triphosphates, they carry chemical energy in their easily hydrolyzed phosphoanhydride bonds.

phosphoanhydride bonds

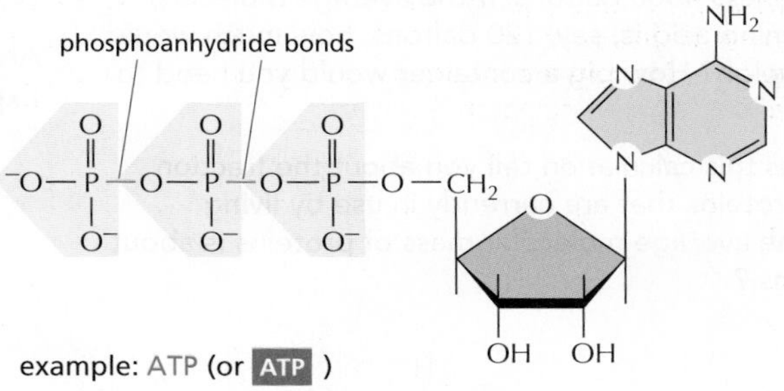

example: ATP (or ATP)

2. They combine with other groups to form coenzymes.

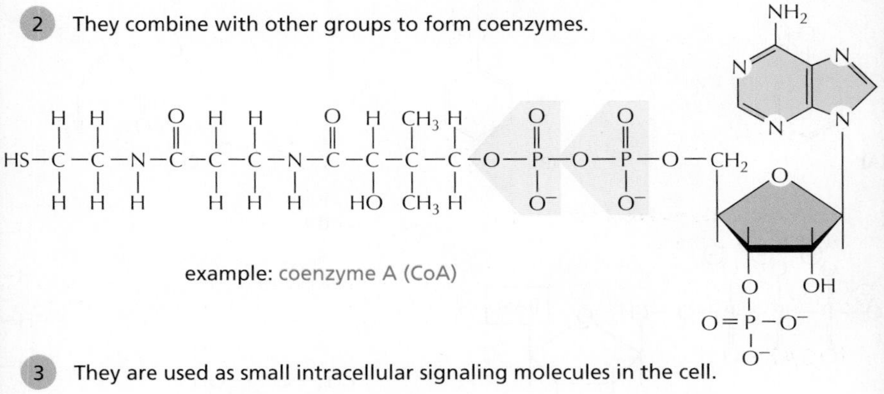

example: coenzyme A (CoA)

3. They are used as small intracellular signaling molecules in the cell.

example: cyclic AMP

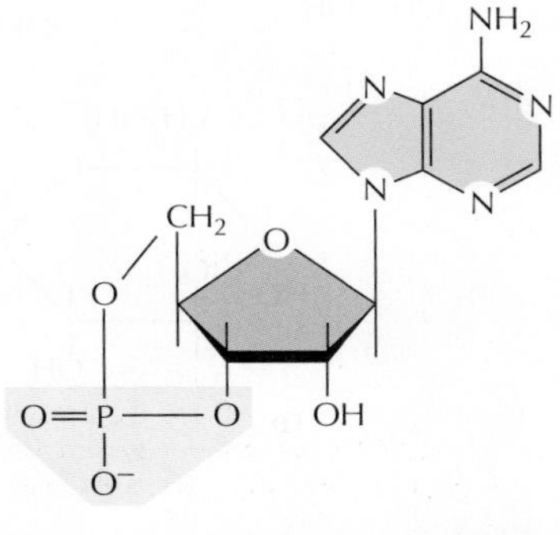

QUESTION 2–15

Which of the following statements are correct? Explain your answers.

A. Proteins are so remarkably diverse because each is made from a unique mixture of amino acids that are linked in random order.

B. Lipid bilayers are macromolecules that are made up mostly of phospholipid subunits.

C. Nucleic acids contain sugar groups.

D. Many amino acids have hydrophobic side chains.

E. The hydrophobic tails of phospholipid molecules are repelled from water.

F. DNA contains the four different bases A, G, U, and C.

QUESTION 2–16

A. How many different molecules composed of (a) two, (b) three, and (c) four amino acids, linked together by peptide bonds, can be made from the set of 20 naturally occurring amino acids?

B. Assume you were given a mixture consisting of one molecule each of all possible sequences of a smallish protein of molecular mass 4800 daltons. If the average molecular mass of an amino acid is, say, 120 daltons, how much would the sample weigh? How big a container would you need to hold it?

C. What does this calculation tell you about the fraction of possible proteins that are currently in use by living organisms (the average molecular mass of proteins is about 30,000 daltons)?

QUESTION 2–17

This is a biology textbook. Explain why the chemical principles that are described in this chapter are important in the context of modern cell biology.

QUESTION 2–18

A. Describe the similarities and differences between van der Waals attractions and hydrogen bonds.

B. Which of the two bonds would form (a) between two hydrogens bound to carbon atoms, (b) between a nitrogen atom and a hydrogen bound to a carbon atom, and (c) between a nitrogen atom and a hydrogen bound to an oxygen atom?

QUESTION 2–19

What are the forces that determine the folding of a macromolecule into a unique shape?

QUESTION 2–20

Fatty acids are said to be "amphipathic." What is meant by this term, and how does an amphipathic molecule behave in water? Draw a diagram to illustrate your answer.

QUESTION 2–21

Are the formulas in Figure Q2–21 correct or incorrect? Explain your answer in each case.

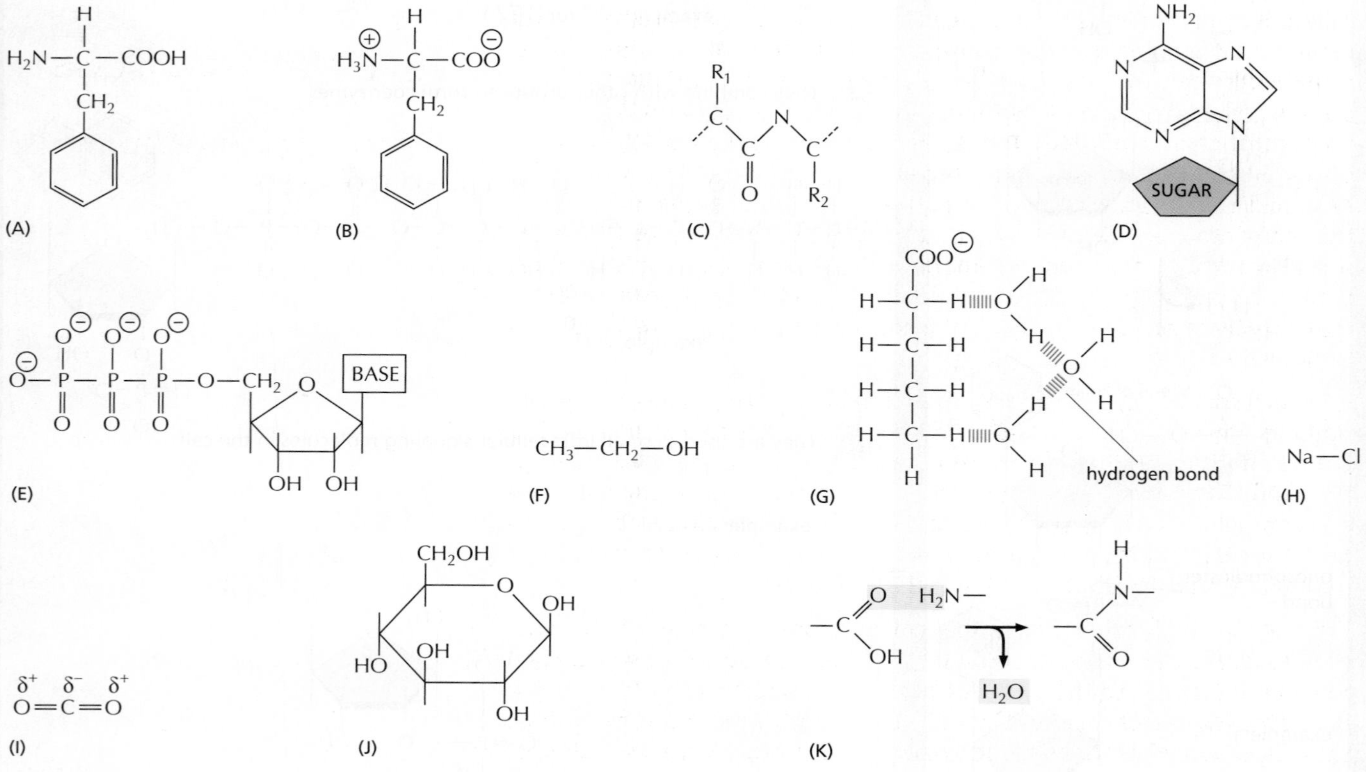

Figure Q2–21

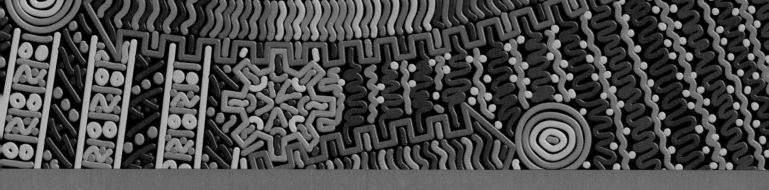

Energy, Catalysis, and Biosynthesis

One property above all makes living things seem almost miraculously different from nonliving matter: they create and maintain order in a universe that is tending always toward greater disorder. To accomplish this remarkable feat, the cells in a living organism must continuously carry out a never-ending stream of chemical reactions to maintain their structure, meet their metabolic needs, and stave off unrelenting chemical decay. In these reactions, small organic molecules—amino acids, sugars, nucleotides, and lipids—can be taken apart or modified to supply the many other small molecules that the cell requires. These molecules are also used to construct an enormously diverse range of large molecules, including the proteins, nucleic acids, and other macromolecules that constitute most of the mass of living systems and endow them with their distinctive properties.

Each cell can be viewed as a tiny chemical factory, performing many millions of reactions every second. This incessant activity requires both a source of atoms in the form of food molecules and a source of energy. Both the atoms and the energy must come, ultimately, from the nonliving environment. In this chapter, we discuss why cells require energy, and how they use energy and atoms from their environment to create and maintain the molecular order that makes life possible.

Most of the chemical reactions that cells perform would normally occur only at temperatures that are much higher than those inside a cell. Each reaction therefore requires a major boost in chemical reactivity to enable it to proceed rapidly within the cell. This boost is provided by a large set of specialized proteins called *enzymes*, each of which accelerates, or *catalyzes*, just one of the many possible reactions that a particular

THE USE OF ENERGY BY CELLS

FREE ENERGY AND CATALYSIS

ACTIVATED CARRIERS AND BIOSYNTHESIS

Figure 3–1 A series of enzyme-catalyzed reactions forms a linked pathway. Each chemical reaction is catalyzed by a distinct enzyme. Together, this set of enzymes, acting in series, converts molecule A to molecule F.

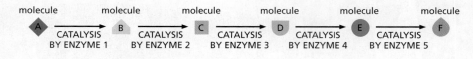

molecule could in principle undergo. These enzyme-catalyzed reactions are usually connected in series, so that the product of one reaction becomes the starting material for the next (**Figure 3–1**). The long, linear reaction pathways that result are in turn linked to one another, forming a complex web of interconnected reactions.

Rather than being an inconvenience, the necessity for *catalysis* is a benefit, as it allows the cell to precisely control its **metabolism**—the sum total of all the chemical reactions it needs to carry out to survive, grow, and reproduce. This control is central to the chemistry of life.

Two opposing streams of chemical reactions occur in cells: the *catabolic* pathways and the *anabolic* pathways. The catabolic pathways (**catabolism**) break down foodstuffs into smaller molecules, thereby generating both a useful form of energy for the cell and some of the small molecules that the cell needs as building blocks. The anabolic, or *biosynthetic*, pathways (**anabolism**) use the energy harnessed by catabolism to drive the synthesis of the many molecules that form the cell. Together, these two sets of reactions constitute the metabolism of the cell (**Figure 3–2**).

The details of the reactions that comprise cell metabolism are part of the subject matter of *biochemistry*, and they need not concern us here. But the general principles by which cells obtain energy from their environment and use it to create order are central to cell biology. We therefore begin this chapter by explaining why a constant input of energy is needed to sustain living organisms. We then discuss how enzymes catalyze the reactions that produce biological order. Finally, we describe the molecules inside cells that carry the energy that makes life possible.

THE USE OF ENERGY BY CELLS

Left to themselves, nonliving things eventually become disordered: buildings crumble and dead organisms decay. Living cells, by contrast, not only maintain but actually generate order at every level, from the large-scale structure of a butterfly or a flower down to the organization of the molecules that make up such organisms (**Figure 3–3**). This property of life is made possible by elaborate molecular mechanisms that extract energy from the environment and convert it into the energy stored in chemical bonds. Biological structures are therefore able to maintain their form, even though the materials that form them are continually being broken down, replaced, and recycled. Your body has the same basic structure it had 10 years ago, even though you now contain atoms that, for the most part, were not part of your body then.

Figure 3–2 Catabolic and anabolic pathways together constitute the cell's metabolism. During catabolism, a major portion of the energy stored in the chemical bonds of food molecules is dissipated as heat. But some of this energy is converted to the useful forms of energy needed to drive the synthesis of new molecules in anabolic pathways, as indicated.

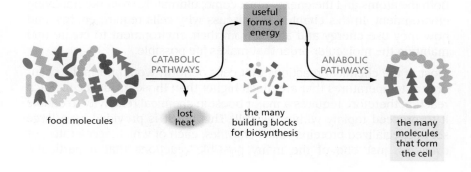

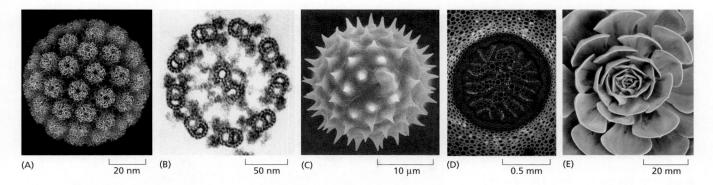

(A) ⊢——⊣ 20 nm   (B) ⊢——⊣ 50 nm   (C) ⊢——⊣ 10 μm   (D) ⊢——⊣ 0.5 mm   (E) ⊢——⊣ 20 mm

Biological Order Is Made Possible by the Release of Heat Energy from Cells

The universal tendency of things to become disordered is expressed in a fundamental law of physics called the *second law of thermodynamics.* This law states that in the universe as a whole, or in any isolated system (a collection of matter that is completely cut off from the rest of the universe), the degree of disorder can only increase. The second law of thermodynamics has such profound implications for living things that it is worth restating in several ways.

We can express the second law in terms of probability by stating that *systems will change spontaneously toward those arrangements that have the greatest probability.* Consider a box in which 100 coins are all lying heads up. A series of events that disturbs the box—for example, someone jiggling it a bit—will tend to move the arrangement toward a mixture of 50 heads and 50 tails. The reason is simple: there is a huge number of possible arrangements of the individual coins that can achieve the 50–50 result, but only one possible arrangement that keeps them all oriented heads up. Because the 50–50 mixture accommodates a greater number of possibilities and places fewer constraints on the orientation of each individual coin, we say that it is more "disordered." For the same reason, one's living space will become increasingly disordered without an intentional effort to keep it organized. Movement toward disorder is a spontaneous process, and requires a periodic input of energy to reverse it (Figure 3–4).

Figure 3–3 Biological structures are highly ordered. Well-defined, ornate, and beautiful spatial patterns can be found at every level of organization in living organisms. Shown are: (A) protein molecules in the coat of a virus (a parasite that, although not technically alive, contains the same types of molecules as those found in living cells); (B) the regular array of microtubules seen in a cross section of a sperm tail; (C) surface contours of a pollen grain; (D) cross section of a fern stem, showing the patterned arrangement of cells; and (E) a spiral array of leaves, each made of millions of cells. (A, courtesy of Robert Grant, Stéphane Crainic, and James M. Hogle; B, courtesy of Lewis Tilney; C, courtesy of Colin MacFarlane and Chris Jeffree; D, courtesy of Jim Haseloff.)

"SPONTANEOUS" REACTION
as time elapses →

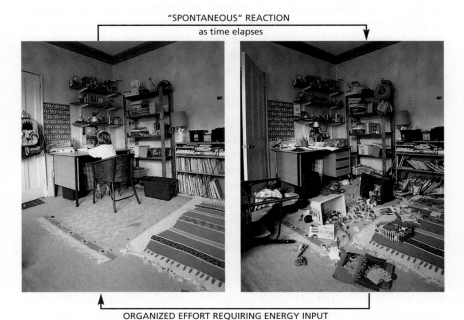

ORGANIZED EFFORT REQUIRING ENERGY INPUT

Figure 3–4 The spontaneous tendency toward disorder is an everyday experience. Reversing this natural tendency toward disorder requires an intentional effort and an input of energy. In fact, from the second law of thermodynamics, we can be certain that the human intervention required will release enough heat to the environment to more than compensate for the reestablishment of order in this room.

Figure 3–5 Living cells do not defy the second law of thermodynamics. In the diagram on the left, the molecules of both the cell and the rest of the universe (the environment) are depicted in a relatively disordered state. In addition, *red* arrows suggest the relative amount of thermal motion of the molecules both inside and outside the cell. In the diagram on the right, the cell has taken in energy from food molecules, carried out a reaction that gives order to the molecules that the cell contains, and released heat (*yellow* arrows) into the environment. The released heat increases the disorder in the cell's surroundings—as depicted here by the increase in thermal motion of the molecules in the environment and the distortion of those molecules due to enhanced vibration and rotation. The second law of thermodynamics is thereby satisfied, even as the cell grows and constructs larger molecules.

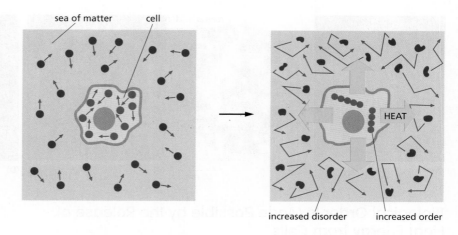

The measure of a system's disorder is called the **entropy** of the system, and the greater the disorder, the greater the entropy. Thus another way to express the second law of thermodynamics is to say that systems will change spontaneously toward arrangements with greater entropy. Living cells—by surviving, growing, and forming complex communities and even whole organisms—generate order and thus might appear to defy the second law of thermodynamics. This is not the case, however, because a cell is not an isolated system. Rather, a cell takes in energy from its environment—in the form of food, inorganic molecules, or photons of light from the sun—and uses this energy to generate order within itself, forging new chemical bonds and building large macromolecules. In the course of performing the chemical reactions that generate order, some energy is inevitably lost in the form of heat (see Figure 3–2). Heat is energy in its most disordered form—the random jostling of molecules (analogous to the random jostling of the coins in the box). Because the cell is not an isolated system, the heat energy produced by metabolic reactions is quickly dispersed into the cell's surroundings. There, the heat increases the intensity of the thermal motions of nearby molecules, thereby increasing the entropy of the cell's environment (**Figure 3–5**).

To satisfy the second law of thermodynamics, the amount of heat released by a cell must be great enough that the increased order generated inside the cell is more than compensated for by the increased disorder generated in the environment. In other words, the chemical reactions inside a cell must increase the total entropy of the entire system: that of the cell plus its environment. Thanks to the cell's activity, the universe thereby becomes more disordered—and the second law of thermodynamics is obeyed.

Cells Can Convert Energy from One Form to Another

Where does the heat released by cells as they generate order come from? To understand that, we need to consider another important physical law. According to the *first law of thermodynamics*, energy cannot be created or destroyed—but it can be converted from one form to another (**Figure 3–6**). Cells take advantage of this law of thermodynamics, for example, when they convert the energy from sunlight into the energy in the chemical bonds of sugars and other small organic molecules during photosynthesis. Although the chemical reactions that power such energy conversions can change how much energy is present in one form or another, the first law tells us that the total amount of energy in the universe must always be the same.

Heat, too, is a product of energy conversion. When an animal cell breaks down foodstuffs, some of the energy in the chemical bonds in the food

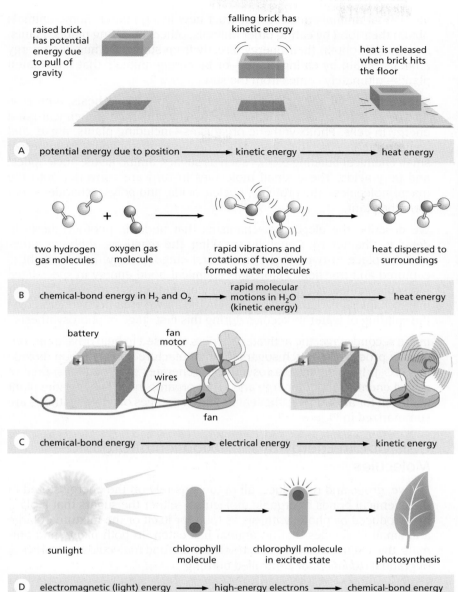

Figure 3–6 Different forms of energy are interconvertible, but the total amount of energy must be conserved. (A) We can use the height and weight of the brick to predict exactly how much heat will be released when it hits the floor. (B) The large amount of chemical-bond energy released when water (H_2O) is formed from H_2 and O_2 is initially converted to very rapid thermal motions in the two new H_2O molecules; however, collisions with other H_2O molecules almost instantaneously spread this kinetic energy evenly throughout the surroundings (heat transfer), making the new H_2O molecules indistinguishable from all the rest. (C) Cells can convert chemical-bond energy into kinetic energy to drive, for example, molecular motor proteins; however, this occurs without the intermediate conversion of chemical energy to electrical energy that a man-made appliance such as this fan requires. (D) Some cells can also harvest the energy from sunlight to form chemical bonds via photosynthesis.

molecules (chemical-bond energy) is converted into the thermal motion of molecules (heat energy). This conversion of chemical energy into heat energy causes the universe as a whole to become more disordered—as required by the second law of thermodynamics. But a cell cannot derive any benefit from the heat energy it produces unless the heat-generating reactions are directly linked to processes that maintain molecular order inside the cell. It is the tight coupling of heat production to an increase in order that distinguishes the metabolism of a cell from the wasteful burning of fuel in a fire. Later in this chapter, we illustrate how this coupling occurs. For the moment, it is sufficient to recognize that—by directly linking the "burning" of food molecules to the generation of biological order—cells are able to create and maintain an island of order in a universe tending toward chaos.

Photosynthetic Organisms Use Sunlight to Synthesize Organic Molecules

All animals live on energy stored in the chemical bonds of organic molecules, which they take in as food. These food molecules also provide the

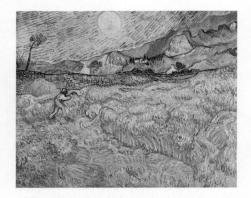

Figure 3–7 With few exceptions, the radiant energy of sunlight sustains all life. Trapped by plants and some microorganisms through photosynthesis, light from the sun is the ultimate source of all energy for humans and other animals. (*Wheat Field Behind Saint-Paul Hospital with a Reaper* by Vincent van Gogh. Courtesy of Museum Folkwang, Essen.)

QUESTION 3–1

Consider the equation
light energy + CO_2 + H_2O →
sugars + O_2 + heat energy
Would you expect this reaction to occur in a single step? Why must heat be generated in the reaction? Explain your answers.

atoms that animals need to construct new living matter. Some animals obtain their food by eating other animals, others by eating plants. Plants, by contrast, obtain their energy directly from sunlight. Thus, the energy animals obtain by eating plants—or by eating animals that have eaten plants—ultimately comes from the sun (**Figure 3–7**).

Solar energy enters the living world through **photosynthesis**, a process that converts the electromagnetic energy in sunlight into chemical-bond energy in cells. Photosynthetic organisms—including plants, algae, and some bacteria—use the energy they derive from sunlight to synthesize small chemical building blocks such as sugars, amino acids, nucleotides, and fatty acids. These small molecules in turn are converted into the macromolecules—the proteins, nucleic acids, and polysaccharides—that form the plant.

We describe the elegant mechanisms that underlie photosynthesis in detail in Chapter 14. Generally speaking, the reactions of photosynthesis take place in two stages. In the first stage, energy from sunlight is captured and transiently stored as chemical-bond energy in specialized molecules called *activated carriers*, which we discuss in more detail later in the chapter. All of the oxygen (O_2) in the air we breathe is generated by the splitting of water molecules during this first stage of photosynthesis.

In the second stage, the activated carriers are used to help drive a *carbon-fixation* process, in which sugars are manufactured from carbon dioxide gas (CO_2). In this way, photosynthesis generates an essential source of stored chemical-bond energy and other organic materials—for the plant itself and for any animals that eat it. The two stages of photosynthesis are summarized in **Figure 3–8**.

Cells Obtain Energy by the Oxidation of Organic Molecules

To live, grow, and reproduce, all organisms rely on the energy stored in the chemical bonds of organic molecules—either the sugars that a plant has produced by photosynthesis as food for itself or the mixture of large and small molecules that an animal has eaten. In both plants and animals, this chemical energy is extracted from food molecules by a process of gradual *oxidation*, or controlled burning.

Earth's atmosphere is about 21% oxygen. In the presence of oxygen, the most energetically stable form of carbon is CO_2 and that of hydrogen is H_2O; the oxidation of carbon-containing molecules is therefore energetically very favorable. A cell is able to obtain energy from sugars or other organic molecules by allowing the carbon and hydrogen atoms in these molecules to combine with oxygen—that is, become *oxidized*—to produce CO_2 and H_2O, respectively. This complex step-wise process by which food molecules are broken down to produce energy is known as **cell respiration**.

Photosynthesis and cell respiration are complementary processes (**Figure 3–9**). Plants, animals, and microorganisms have existed together on this

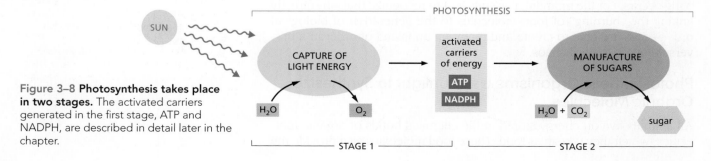

Figure 3–8 Photosynthesis takes place in two stages. The activated carriers generated in the first stage, ATP and NADPH, are described in detail later in the chapter.

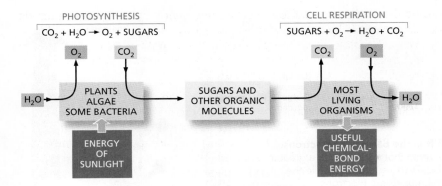

Figure 3–9 Photosynthesis and cell respiration are complementary processes in the living world. The left side of the diagram shows how photosynthesis—carried out by plants and photosynthetic microorganisms—uses the energy of sunlight to produce sugars and other organic molecules from the carbon atoms in CO_2 in the atmosphere. In turn, these molecules serve as food for other organisms. The right side of the diagram shows how cell respiration in most organisms—including plants and other photosynthetic organisms—uses O_2 to oxidize food molecules, releasing the same carbon atoms in the form of CO_2 back to the atmosphere. In the process, the organisms obtain the useful chemical-bond energy that they need to survive.

The first cells on Earth are thought to have been capable of neither photosynthesis nor cell respiration (discussed in Chapter 14). However, photosynthesis must have preceded cell respiration on the Earth, because there is strong evidence that billions of years of photosynthesis were required to release enough O_2 to create an atmosphere that could support respiration.

planet for so long that they have become an essential part of each other's environments. The oxygen released by photosynthesis is consumed by nearly all organisms for the oxidative breakdown of organic molecules. And some of the CO_2 molecules that today are incorporated into organic molecules by photosynthesis in a green leaf were released yesterday into the atmosphere by the respiration of an animal, a fungus, or the plant itself—or by the burning of fossil fuels. Carbon atoms therefore pass through a huge cycle that involves the entire *biosphere*—the collection of living things on Earth—as they move between individual organisms (**Figure 3–10**).

Oxidation and Reduction Involve Electron Transfers

The cell does not oxidize organic molecules in one step, as occurs when organic material is burned in a fire. Through the use of enzyme catalysts, metabolism directs the molecules through a series of chemical reactions, few of which actually involve the direct addition of oxygen. Before we consider these reactions, we need to explain what is meant by oxidation.

Although the term **oxidation** literally means the addition of oxygen atoms to a molecule, oxidation is said to occur in any reaction in which electrons are transferred between atoms. Oxidation, in this sense, involves the removal of electrons from an atom. Thus, Fe^{2+} is oxidized when it loses an electron to become Fe^{3+}. The converse reaction, called **reduction**, involves the addition of electrons to an atom. Fe^{3+} is reduced when it gains an electron to become Fe^{2+}, and a chlorine atom is reduced when it gains an electron to become Cl^-.

Because the number of electrons is conserved in a chemical reaction (there is no net loss or gain), oxidation and reduction always occur simultaneously: that is, if one molecule gains an electron in a reaction (reduction), a second molecule must lose the electron (oxidation).

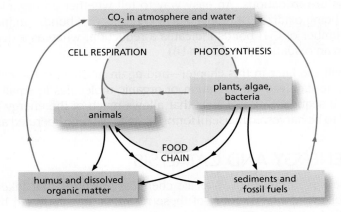

Figure 3–10 Carbon atoms cycle continuously through the biosphere. Individual carbon atoms are incorporated into organic molecules of the living world by the photosynthetic activity of plants, algae, and bacteria. They then pass to animals and microorganisms—as well as into organic material in soil and oceans—and are ultimately restored to the atmosphere in the form of CO_2 when organic molecules are oxidized by cells during respiration or burned by humans as fossil fuels. In this diagram, the *green* arrow denotes an uptake of CO_2, whereas the *red* arrows indicate CO_2 release.

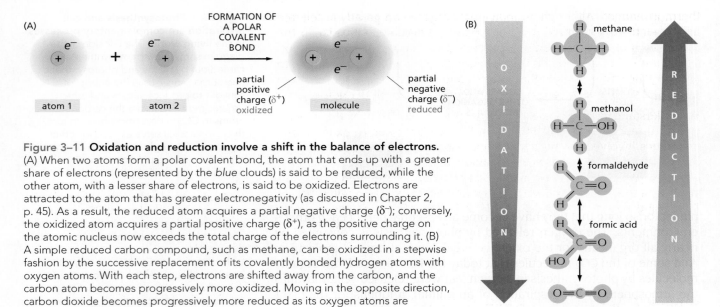

Figure 3–11 Oxidation and reduction involve a shift in the balance of electrons. (A) When two atoms form a polar covalent bond, the atom that ends up with a greater share of electrons (represented by the *blue* clouds) is said to be reduced, while the other atom, with a lesser share of electrons, is said to be oxidized. Electrons are attracted to the atom that has greater electronegativity (as discussed in Chapter 2, p. 45). As a result, the reduced atom acquires a partial negative charge (δ^-); conversely, the oxidized atom acquires a partial positive charge (δ^+), as the positive charge on the atomic nucleus now exceeds the total charge of the electrons surrounding it. (B) A simple reduced carbon compound, such as methane, can be oxidized in a stepwise fashion by the successive replacement of its covalently bonded hydrogen atoms with oxygen atoms. With each step, electrons are shifted away from the carbon, and the carbon atom becomes progressively more oxidized. Moving in the opposite direction, carbon dioxide becomes progressively more reduced as its oxygen atoms are replaced by hydrogens to yield methane.

Why is a "gain" of electrons referred to as a "reduction"? The term arose before anything was known about the movement of electrons. Originally, reduction reactions involved a liberation of oxygen—for example, when metals are extracted from ores by heating—which caused the samples to become lighter; in other words, "reduced" in mass.

It is important to recognize that the terms oxidation and reduction apply even when there is only a partial shift of electrons between atoms. When a carbon atom becomes covalently bonded to an atom with a strong affinity for electrons—oxygen, chlorine, or sulfur, for example—it gives up more than its equal share of electrons to form a *polar covalent bond*. The positive charge of the carbon nucleus now slightly exceeds the negative charge of its electrons, so that the carbon atom acquires a partial positive charge (δ^+) and is said to be oxidized. Conversely, the carbon atom in a C–H bond has somewhat more than its share of electrons; it acquires a partial negative charge (δ^-) and so is said to be reduced (**Figure 3–11A**).

In such oxidation–reduction reactions, electrons generally do not travel alone. When a molecule in a cell picks up an electron (e^-), it often picks up a proton (H^+) at the same time (protons being freely available in water). The net effect in this case is to add a hydrogen atom to the molecule:

$$A + e^- + H^+ \rightarrow AH$$

Even though a proton is involved (in addition to the electron), such *hydrogenation* reactions are reductions, and the reverse *dehydrogenation* reactions are oxidations. An easy way to tell whether an organic molecule is being oxidized or reduced is to count its C–H bonds: an increase in the number of C–H bonds indicates a reduction, whereas a decrease indicates an oxidation (**Figure 3–11B**).

As we will see later in this chapter—and again in Chapter 13—cells use enzymes to catalyze the oxidation of organic molecules in small steps, through a sequence of reactions that allows much of the energy that is released to be harvested in useful forms, instead of being liberated as heat.

FREE ENERGY AND CATALYSIS

Life depends on the highly specific chemical reactions that take place inside cells. The vast majority of these reactions are catalyzed by proteins called **enzymes**. Enzymes, like cells, must obey the second law of thermodynamics. Although an individual enzyme can greatly accelerate an energetically favorable reaction—one that produces disorder in the universe—it cannot force an energetically unfavorable reaction to occur. Cells, however, must do just that in order to grow and divide—or just to survive. They must build highly ordered and energy-rich molecules from small and simple ones—a process that requires an input of energy.

To understand how enzymes promote the acceleration of the specific chemical reactions needed to sustain life, we first need to examine the energetics involved. In this section, we consider how the free energy of molecules contributes to their chemistry, and we see how free-energy changes—which reflect how much total disorder is generated in the universe by a reaction—influence whether and how a reaction will proceed. Examining these energetic concepts will reveal how enzymes working together can exploit the free-energy changes of different reactions to drive the energetically unfavorable reactions that produce biological order. This type of enzyme-assisted catalysis is crucial for cells: without it, life could not exist.

Chemical Reactions Proceed in the Direction That Causes a Loss of Free Energy

Paper burns readily, releasing into the atmosphere water and carbon dioxide as gases, while simultaneously releasing energy as heat:

$$\text{paper} + O_2 \rightarrow \text{smoke} + \text{ashes} + \text{heat} + CO_2 + H_2O$$

This reaction occurs in only one direction: smoke and ashes never spontaneously gather carbon dioxide and water from the heated atmosphere and reconstitute themselves into paper. When paper burns, most of its chemical energy is dissipated as heat. This heat is not lost from the universe, since energy can never be created or destroyed; instead, it is irretrievably dispersed in the chaotic random thermal motions of molecules. In the language of thermodynamics, there has been a release of *free energy*—that is, energy that can be harnessed to do work or drive chemical reactions. This release reflects a loss of orderliness in the way the energy and molecules had been stored in the paper; the greater the free-energy change, the greater the amount of disorder created in the universe when the reaction occurs.

We will discuss free energy in more detail shortly, but a general principle can be summarized as follows: chemical reactions proceed only in the direction that leads to a loss of free energy. In other words, the spontaneous direction for any reaction is the direction that goes "downhill." A "downhill" reaction in this sense is said to be energetically favorable.

Enzymes Reduce the Energy Needed to Initiate Spontaneous Reactions

Although the most energetically favorable form of carbon under ordinary conditions is CO_2, and that of hydrogen is H_2O, a living organism will not disappear in a puff of smoke, and the book in your hands will not burst spontaneously into flames. This is because the molecules in both the living organism and the book are in a relatively stable state, and they cannot be changed to lower-energy states without an initial input of energy. In other words, a molecule requires a boost over an energy barrier before it can undergo a chemical reaction that moves it to a lower-energy (more stable) state. This boost is known as the **activation energy** (**Figure 3–12A**). In the case of a burning book, the activation energy is provided by the heat of a lighted match. But cells can't raise their temperature to drive biological reactions. Inside cells, the push over the energy barrier is aided by enzymes.

QUESTION 3–2

In which of the following reactions does the *red* atom undergo an oxidation?
A. $Na \rightarrow Na^+$ (Na atom → Na⁺ ion)
B. $Cl \rightarrow Cl^-$ (Cl atom → Cl⁻ ion)
C. $CH_3CH_2OH \rightarrow CH_3CHO$
        (ethanol → acetaldehyde)
D. $CH_3CHO \rightarrow CH_3COO^-$
        (acetaldehyde → acetic acid)
E. $CH_2=CH_2 \rightarrow CH_3CH_3$
        (ethene → ethane)

Figure 3–12 Even energetically favorable reactions require activation energy to get them started. (A) Compound Y (a reactant) is in a relatively stable state; thus energy is required to convert it to compound X (a product), even though X is at a lower overall energy level than Y. This conversion will not take place, therefore, unless compound Y can acquire enough *activation energy* (energy *a* minus energy *b*) from its surroundings to undergo the reaction that converts it into compound X. This energy may be provided by means of an unusually energetic collision with other molecules. For the reverse reaction, X ⟶ Y, the activation energy required will be much larger (energy *a* minus energy *c*); this reaction will therefore occur much more rarely. The total energy change for the energetically favorable reaction Y ⟶ X is energy *c* minus energy *b*, a negative number, which corresponds to a loss of free energy. (B) Energy barriers for specific reactions can be lowered by catalysts, as indicated by the line marked *d*. Enzymes are particularly effective catalysts because they greatly reduce the activation energy for the reactions they catalyze. Note that activation energies are always positive.

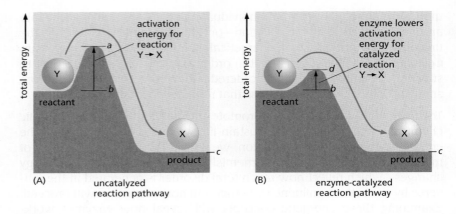

(A) uncatalyzed reaction pathway

(B) enzyme-catalyzed reaction pathway

Each enzyme binds tightly to one or two molecules, called **substrates**, and holds them in a way that greatly reduces the activation energy needed to facilitate a specific chemical interaction between them (**Figure 3–12B**). A substance that can lower the activation energy of a reaction is termed a **catalyst**; catalysts increase the rate of chemical reactions because they allow a much larger proportion of the random collisions with surrounding molecules to kick the substrates over the energy barrier, as illustrated in **Figure 3–13** and **Figure 3–14A**. Enzymes are among the most effective catalysts known. They can speed up reactions by a factor of as much as 10^{14}—that is, trillions of times faster than the same reactions would proceed without an enzyme catalyst. Enzymes therefore allow reactions that would not otherwise occur to proceed rapidly at the normal temperature inside cells.

Unlike the effects of temperature, enzymes are highly selective. Each enzyme usually speeds up—or *catalyzes*—only one particular reaction out of the several possible reactions that its substrate molecules could undergo. In this way, enzymes direct each of the many different molecules in a cell along specific reaction pathways (**Figure 3–14B** and **C**), thereby producing the compounds that the cell actually needs.

Like all catalysts, enzyme molecules themselves remain unchanged after participating in a reaction and can therefore act over and over again (**Figure 3–15**). In Chapter 4, we will discuss further how enzymes work, after we have looked in detail at the molecular structure of proteins.

The Free-Energy Change for a Reaction Determines Whether It Can Occur

According to the second law of thermodynamics, a chemical reaction can proceed only if it results in a net (overall) increase in the disorder of

Figure 3–13 Lowering the activation energy greatly increases the probability that a reaction will occur. At any given instant, a population of identical substrate molecules will have a range of energies, distributed as shown on the graph. The varying energies come from collisions with surrounding molecules, which make the substrate molecules jiggle, vibrate, and spin. For a molecule to undergo a chemical reaction, the energy of the molecule must exceed the activation-energy barrier for that reaction (*dashed* lines); for most biological reactions, this almost never happens without enzyme catalysis. Even with enzyme catalysis, only a small fraction of substrate molecules (*red* shaded area) will experience the highly energetic collisions needed to reach an energy state high enough for them to undergo a reaction.

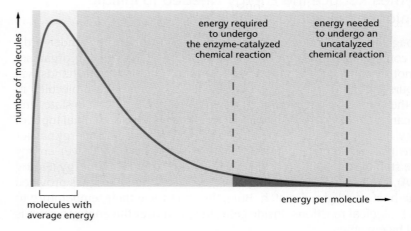

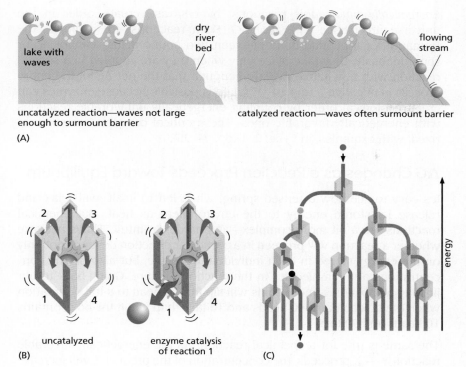

Figure 3–14 Enzymes catalyze reactions by lowering the activation-energy barrier. (A) The dam represents the activation energy, which is lowered by enzyme catalysis. Each *green* ball represents a potential substrate molecule that is bouncing up and down in energy level owing to constant encounters with waves, an analogy for the thermal bombardment of substrate molecules by surrounding water molecules. When the barrier—the activation energy—is lowered significantly, the balls (substrate molecules) with sufficient energy can roll downhill, an energetically favorable movement. (B) The four walls of the box represent the activation-energy barriers for four different chemical reactions that are all energetically favorable because the products are at lower energy levels than the substrates. In the left-hand box, none of these reactions occurs because even the largest waves are not large enough to surmount any of the energy barriers. In the right-hand box, enzyme catalysis lowers the activation energy for reaction number 1 only; now the jostling of the waves allows the substrate molecule to pass over this energy barrier, allowing reaction 1 to proceed (Movie 3.1). (C) A branching set of reactions with a selected set of enzymes (*yellow* boxes) serves to illustrate how a series of enzyme-catalyzed reactions—by controlling which reaction will take place at each junction—determines the exact reaction pathway followed by each molecule inside the cell.

the universe (see Figure 3–5). Disorder increases when useful energy that could be harnessed to do work is dissipated as heat. The useful energy in a system is known as its **free energy**, or **G**. And because chemical reactions involve a transition from one molecular state to another, the term that is of most interest to chemists and cell biologists is the **free-energy change**, denoted **ΔG** ("Delta G").

Let's consider a collection of molecules. ΔG measures the amount of disorder created in the universe when a reaction involving these molecules takes place. *Energetically favorable* reactions, by definition, are those that create disorder in the universe by decreasing the free energy of the system to which they belong; in other words, they have a *negative ΔG* (**Figure 3–16**).

A reaction can occur spontaneously only if ΔG is negative. On a macroscopic scale, an energetically favorable reaction with a negative ΔG is the relaxation of a compressed spring into an expanded state, which releases its stored elastic energy as heat to its surroundings. On a microscopic scale, an energetically favorable reaction—one with a negative ΔG—occurs when salt (NaCl) dissolves in water. Note that just because a reaction can occur spontaneously does not mean it will occur quickly. The decay of diamonds into graphite is a spontaneous process—but it takes millions of years.

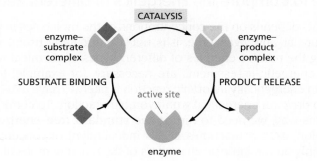

Figure 3–15 Enzymes convert substrates to products while remaining unchanged themselves. Catalysis takes place in a cycle in which a substrate molecule (*red*) binds to an enzyme and undergoes a reaction to form a product molecule (*yellow*), which then gets released. Although the enzyme participates in the reaction, it remains unchanged.

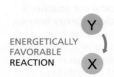

ENERGETICALLY
FAVORABLE
REACTION

The free energy of Y
is greater than the free
energy of X. Therefore
ΔG is negative (< 0), and
the disorder of the
universe increases when
Y is converted to X.

this reaction can occur spontaneously

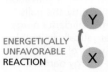

ENERGETICALLY
UNFAVORABLE
REACTION

If the reaction X→ Y
occurred, ΔG would
be positive (> 0), and
the universe would
become more
ordered.

this reaction can occur only if
it is driven by being coupled to a second,
energetically favorable reaction

Figure 3–16 Energetically favorable reactions have a negative ΔG, whereas energetically unfavorable reactions have a positive ΔG. Imagine, for example, that molecule Y has a free energy (G) of 10 kilojoules (kJ) per mole, whereas X has a free energy of 4 kJ/mole. The reaction Y → X therefore has a ΔG of –6 kJ/mole, making it energetically favorable.

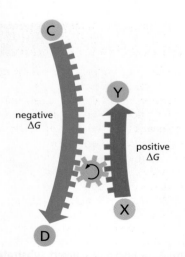

negative
ΔG

positive
ΔG

Figure 3–17 Reaction coupling can drive an energetically unfavorable reaction. The energetically unfavorable (ΔG > 0) reaction X → Y cannot occur unless it is coupled to an energetically favorable (ΔG < 0) reaction C → D, such that the net free-energy change for the pair of reactions is negative (less than 0).

Energetically unfavorable reactions, by contrast, create order in the universe; they have a *positive* ΔG. Such reactions—for example, the formation of a peptide bond between two amino acids—cannot occur spontaneously; they take place only when they are coupled to a second reaction with a negative ΔG large enough that the net ΔG of the entire process is negative (**Figure 3–17**). Life is possible because enzymes can create biological order by coupling energetically unfavorable reactions with energetically favorable ones. These critical concepts are summarized, with examples, in **Panel 3–1** (pp. 94–95).

ΔG Changes as a Reaction Proceeds Toward Equilibrium

It's easy to see how a tensed spring, when left to itself, will relax and release its stored energy to the environment as heat. But chemical reactions are a bit more complex—and harder to intuit. That's because whether a reaction will proceed in a particular direction depends not only on the energy stored in each individual molecule, but also on the concentrations of the molecules in the reaction mixture. Going back to our jiggling box of coins, more coins will flip from a head to a tail orientation when the box contains 90 heads and 10 tails than when the box contains 10 heads and 90 tails.

The same is true for a chemical reaction. As the energetically favorable reaction Y → X proceeds, the concentration of the product X will increase and the concentration of the substrate Y will decrease. This change in relative concentrations of substrate and product will cause the ratio of Y to X to shrink, making the initially favorable ΔG less and less negative. Unless more Y is added, the reaction will slow and eventually stop.

Because ΔG changes as products accumulate and substrates are depleted, chemical reactions will generally proceed until they reach a state of **equilibrium**. At that point, the rates of the forward and reverse reactions are equal, and there is no further net change in the concentrations of substrate or product (**Figure 3–18**). For reactions at chemical equilibrium, ΔG = 0, so the reaction will not proceed forward or backward, and no work can be done.

Such a state of chemical inactivity would be incompatible with life, inevitably allowing chemical decay to overcome the cell. Living cells work hard to avoid reaching a state of complete chemical equilibrium. They are constantly exchanging materials with their environment: replenishing nutrients and eliminating waste products. In addition, many of the individual reactions in the cell's complex metabolic network also exist in disequilibrium because the products of one reaction are continually being siphoned off to become the substrates in a subsequent reaction. Rarely do products and substrates reach concentrations at which the forward and reverse reaction rates are equal.

The Standard Free-Energy Change, ΔG°, Makes It Possible to Compare the Energetics of Different Reactions

Because ΔG depends on the concentrations of the molecules in the reaction mixture at any given time, it is not a particularly useful value for comparing the relative energies of different types of chemical reactions. But such energetic assessments are necessary, for example, to predict whether an energetically favorable reaction is likely to have a ΔG negative enough to drive an energetically unfavorable reaction. To compare reactions in this way, we need to turn to the **standard free-energy change** of a reaction, **ΔG°**. A reaction's ΔG° is independent of concentration; it depends only on the intrinsic characters of the reacting molecules, based

FOR THE ENERGETICALLY FAVORABLE REACTION Y → X,

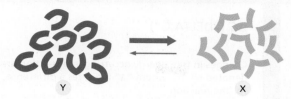

Y   X

when X and Y are at equal concentrations, [Y] = [X], the formation of X is energetically favored. In other words, the ΔG of Y → X is negative and the ΔG of X → Y is positive. Nevertheless because of thermal bombardments, there will always be some X converting to Y.

THUS, FOR EACH INDIVIDUAL MOLECULE,

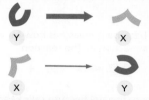

Y   X

conversion of Y to X will occur often.

X   Y

Conversion of X to Y will occur less often than the transition Y → X, because it requires a more energetic collision.

Therefore, if one starts with an equal mixture, the ratio of X to Y molecules will increase

EVENTUALLY, there will be a large enough excess of X over Y to just compensate for the slow rate of X → Y, such that the number of X molecules being converted to Y molecules each second is exactly equal to the number of Y molecules being converted to X molecules each second. At this point, the reaction will be at equilibrium.

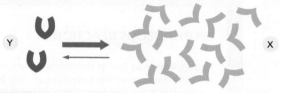

Y   X

AT EQUILIBRIUM, there is no net change in the ratio of Y to X, and the ΔG for both forward and backward reactions is zero.

Figure 3–18 **Reactions will eventually reach a chemical equilibrium.** At that point, the forward and the backward fluxes of reacting molecules are equal and opposite. The widths of the arrows indicate the relative rates at which an *individual molecule* converts.

on their behavior under ideal conditions where the concentrations of all the reactants are set to the same fixed value of 1 mole/liter in aqueous solution.

A large body of thermodynamic data has been collected from which $\Delta G°$ can be calculated for most metabolic reactions. Some common reactions are compared in terms of their $\Delta G°$ in Panel 3–1 (pp. 94–95).

The ΔG of a reaction can be calculated from $\Delta G°$ if the concentrations of the reactants and products are known. For the simple reaction Y → X, their relationship follows this equation:

$$\Delta G = \Delta G° + RT \ln \frac{[X]}{[Y]}$$

where $\Delta G°$ is in kilojoules per mole, [Y] and [X] denote the concentrations of Y and X in moles/liter (a mole is 6×10^{23} molecules of a substance), ln is the natural logarithm, and RT is the product of the gas constant, R, and the absolute temperature, T. At 37°C, $RT = 2.58$.

From this equation, we can see that when the concentrations of reactants and products are equal—in other words, [X]/[Y] = 1—the value of ΔG equals the value of $\Delta G°$ (because ln 1 = 0). Thus when the reactants and products are present in equal concentrations, the direction of the reaction depends entirely on the intrinsic properties of the molecules.

QUESTION 3–3

Consider the analogy of the jiggling box containing coins that was described on page 83. The reaction, the flipping of coins that either face heads up (H) or tails up (T), is described by the equation H ↔ T, where the rate of the forward reaction equals the rate of the reverse reaction.
A. What are ΔG and $\Delta G°$ in this analogy?
B. What corresponds to the temperature at which the reaction proceeds? What corresponds to the activation energy of the reaction? Assume you have an "enzyme," called jigglase, which catalyzes this reaction. What would the effect of jigglase be and what, mechanically, might jigglase do in this analogy?

FREE ENERGY

This panel reviews the concept of free energy and offers examples showing how changes in free energy determine whether—and how—biological reactions occur.

The molecules of a living cell possess energy because of their vibrations, rotations, and movement through space, and because of the energy that is stored in the bonds between individual atoms.

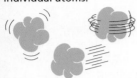

The free energy, G (in kJ/mole), measures the energy of a molecule that could in principle be used to do useful work at constant temperature, as in a living cell. Energy can also be expressed in calories (1 joule = 0.24 calories).

REACTIONS CAUSE DISORDER

Think of a chemical reaction occurring in a cell that has a constant temperature and volume. This reaction can produce disorder in two ways.

1 Changes of bond energy of the reacting molecules can cause heat to be released, which disorders the environment around the cell.

2 The reaction can decrease the amount of order in the cell—for example, by breaking apart a long chain of molecules, or by disrupting an interaction that prevents bond rotations.

PREDICTING REACTIONS

To predict the outcome of a reaction (Will it proceed to the right or to the left? At what point will it stop?), we must determine its standard free-energy change ($\Delta G°$).
This quantity represents the gain or loss of free energy as one mole of reactant is converted to one mole of product under "standard conditions" (all molecules present in aqueous solution at a concentration of 1 M and pH 7.0).

 driving force

$\Delta G°$ for some reactions

glucose 1-P ⟶ glucose 6-P	–7.3 kJ/mole
sucrose ⟶ glucose + fructose	–23 kJ/mole
ATP ⟶ ADP + P	–30.5 kJ/mole
glucose + $6O_2$ ⟶ $6CO_2$ + $6H_2O$	–2867 kJ/mole

ΔG ("DELTA G")

Changes in free energy occurring in a reaction are denoted by ΔG, where "Δ" indicates a difference. Thus, for the reaction

$$A + B \longrightarrow C + D$$

ΔG = free energy (C + D) minus free energy (A + B)

ΔG measures the amount of disorder caused by a reaction: the change in order inside the cell, plus the change in order of the surroundings caused by the heat released.

ΔG is useful because it measures how far away from equilibrium a reaction is. The reaction

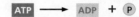

has a large negative ΔG because cells keep the reaction a long way from equilibrium by continually making fresh ATP. However, if the cell dies, then most of its ATP will be hydrolyzed until equilibrium is reached; at equilibrium, the forward and backward reactions occur at equal rates and $\Delta G = 0$.

SPONTANEOUS REACTIONS

From the second law of thermodynamics, we know that the disorder of the universe can only increase. ΔG is *negative* if the disorder of the universe (reaction plus surroundings) *increases*.

In other words, a chemical reaction that occurs spontaneously must have a negative ΔG:

$$G_{products} - G_{reactants} = \Delta G < 0$$

EXAMPLE: The difference in free energy of 100 mL of 10 mM sucrose (common sugar) and 100 mL of 10 mM glucose plus 10 mM fructose is about –23 joules. Therefore, the hydrolysis reaction that produces two monosaccharides from a disaccharide (sucrose → glucose + fructose) can proceed spontaneously.

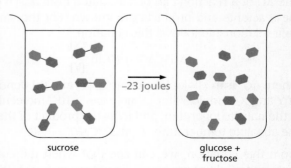

sucrose   glucose + fructose

In contrast, the reverse reaction (glucose + fructose → sucrose), which has a ΔG of +23 joules, could not occur without an input of energy from a coupled reaction.

REACTION RATES

A spontaneous reaction is not necessarily a rapid reaction: a reaction with a negative free-energy change (ΔG) will not necessarily occur rapidly by itself. Consider, for example, the combustion of glucose in oxygen:

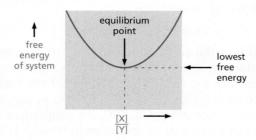

$$\Delta G° = -2867 \text{ kJ/mole}$$

Even this highly favorable reaction may not occur for centuries unless enzymes are present to speed up the process. Enzymes are able to catalyze reactions and speed up their rate, but they cannot change the $\Delta G°$ of a reaction.

CHEMICAL EQUILIBRIA

A fixed relationship exists between the standard free-energy change of a reaction, $\Delta G°$, and its equilibrium constant K. For example, the reversible reaction

$$Y \rightleftharpoons X$$

will proceed until the ratio of concentrations [X]/[Y] is equal to K (note: square brackets [ ] indicate concentration). At this point, the free energy of the system will have its lowest value.

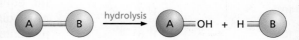

At 37°C, $\quad \Delta G° = -5.94 \log_{10} K \quad$ (see text, p. 96)

$$K = 10^{-\Delta G°/5.94}$$

For example, the reaction

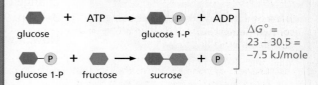

glucose 1-P $\qquad$ glucose 6-P

has $\Delta G° = -7.3$ kJ/mole. Therefore, its equilibrium constant

$$K = 10^{(7.3/5.94)} = 10^{(1.23)} = 17$$

So the reaction will reach steady state when

$$[\text{glucose 6-P}]/[\text{glucose 1-P}] = 17$$

COUPLED REACTIONS

Reactions can be "coupled" together if they share one or more intermediates. In this case, the overall free-energy change is simply the sum of the individual $\Delta G°$ values. A reaction that is unfavorable (has a positive $\Delta G°$) can for this reason be driven by a second, highly favorable reaction.

SINGLE REACTION

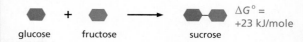

glucose $\qquad$ fructose $\qquad$ sucrose $\qquad$ $\Delta G° = +23$ kJ/mole

NET RESULT: reaction will not occur

ATP $\longrightarrow$ ADP + Ⓟ $\quad \Delta G° = -30.5$ kJ/mole

NET RESULT: reaction is highly favorable

COUPLED REACTIONS

glucose + ATP $\longrightarrow$ glucose 1-P + ADP

glucose 1-P + fructose $\longrightarrow$ sucrose + Ⓟ

$\Delta G° = 23 - 30.5 = -7.5$ kJ/mole

NET RESULT: sucrose is made in a reaction driven by the hydrolysis of ATP

HIGH-ENERGY BONDS

One of the most common reactions in the cell is hydrolysis, in which a covalent bond is split by adding water.

A—B $\xrightarrow{\text{hydrolysis}}$ A—OH + H—B

The $\Delta G°$ for this reaction is sometimes loosely termed the "bond energy." Compounds such as acetyl phosphate and ATP, which have a large negative $\Delta G°$ of hydrolysis in an aqueous solution, are said to have "high-energy" bonds.

	$\Delta G°$ (kJ/mole)
acetyl–Ⓟ $\longrightarrow$ acetate + Ⓟ	–43.1
ATP $\longrightarrow$ ADP + Ⓟ	–30.5
glucose 6-P $\longrightarrow$ glucose + Ⓟ	–13.8

(Note that, for simplicity, H_2O is omitted from the above equations.)

TABLE 3–1 RELATIONSHIP BETWEEN THE STANDARD FREE-ENERGY CHANGE, $\Delta G°$, AND THE EQUILIBRIUM CONSTANT

Equilibrium Constant [X]/[Y]	Standard Free-Energy Change ($\Delta G°$) for Reaction Y → X (kJ/mole)
10^5	–29.7
10^4	–23.8
10^3	–17.8
10^2	–11.9
10	–5.9
1	0
10^{-1}	5.9
10^{-2}	11.9
10^{-3}	17.8
10^{-4}	23.8
10^{-5}	29.7

Values of the equilibrium constant were calculated for the simple chemical reaction Y → X, using the equation given in the text.

The $\Delta G°$ values given here are in kilojoules per mole at 37°C. As explained in the text, $\Delta G°$ represents the free-energy difference under standard conditions (where all components are present at a concentration of 1 mole/liter).

From this table, we see that if there is a favorable free-energy change of –17.8 kJ/mole for the transition Y → X, there will be 1000 times more molecules of X than of Y at equilibrium ($K = 1000$).

The Equilibrium Constant Is Directly Proportional to $\Delta G°$

As mentioned earlier, all chemical reactions tend to proceed toward equilibrium. Knowing where that equilibrium lies for any given reaction will reveal which way the reaction will proceed—and how far it will go. For example, if a reaction is at equilibrium when the concentration of the product is ten times the concentration of the substrate, and we begin with a surplus of substrate and little or no product, the reaction will continue to proceed forward. The ratio of substrate to product at this equilibrium point is called the reaction's **equilibrium constant**, K. For the simple reaction Y → X,

$$K = \frac{[X]}{[Y]}$$

where [X] is the concentration of the product and [Y] is the concentration of the substrate at equilibrium. In the example we just described, $K = 10$.

The equilibrium constant depends on the intrinsic properties of the molecules involved, as expressed by $\Delta G°$. In fact, the equilibrium constant is directly proportional to $\Delta G°$. Let's see why.

At equilibrium, the rate of the forward reaction is exactly balanced by the rate of the reverse reaction. At that point, $\Delta G = 0$, and there is no net change of free energy to drive the reaction in either direction (see Panel 3–1, pp. 94–95).

Now, if we return to the equation presented on page 93,

$$\Delta G = \Delta G° + RT \ln \frac{[X]}{[Y]}$$

we can see that, at equilibrium at 37°C, where $\Delta G = 0$ and the constant $RT = 2.58$, this equation becomes:

$$\Delta G° = -2.58 \ln \frac{[X]}{[Y]}$$

In other words, $\Delta G°$ is directly proportional to the equilibrium constant, K:

$$\Delta G° = -2.58 \ln K$$

If we convert this equation from natural log (ln) to the more commonly used base-10 logarithm (log), we get

$$\Delta G° = -5.94 \log K$$

This equation reveals how the equilibrium ratio of Y to X, expressed as the equilibrium constant K, depends on the intrinsic character of the molecules, as expressed in the value of $\Delta G°$. Thus, for the reaction we presented, Y → X, where $K = 10$, $\Delta G° = -5.94$ kJ/mole. In fact, for every 5.94 kJ/mole difference in free energy at 37°C, the equilibrium constant for a reaction changes by a factor of 10, as shown in Table 3–1. Thus, the more energetically favorable the reaction, the more product will accumulate when the reaction proceeds to equilibrium. For a reaction with a $\Delta G°$ of –17.8 kJ/mole, K will equal 1000, which means that at equilibrium, there will be 1000 molecules of product for every molecule of substrate present.

In Complex Reactions, the Equilibrium Constant Includes the Concentrations of All Reactants and Products

We have so far discussed the simplest of reactions, Y → X, in which a single substrate is converted into a single product. But inside cells, it is more common for two reactants to combine to form a single product: A + B → AB. How can we predict how this reaction will proceed?

The same principles apply, except that in this case the equilibrium constant K includes the concentrations of both of the reactants, in addition to the concentration of the product:

$$K = [AB]/[A][B]$$

The concentrations of both reactants are multiplied in the denominator because the formation of product AB depends on the collision of A and B, and these encounters occur at a rate that is proportional to $[A] \times [B]$ (**Figure 3–19**). As with single-substrate reactions, $\Delta G° = -5.94 \log K$ at 37°C. Thus, the relationship between K and $\Delta G°$ is the same as that shown in Table 3–1.

The Equilibrium Constant Also Indicates the Strength of Noncovalent Binding Interactions

The concept of free-energy change does not apply only to chemical reactions where covalent bonds are being broken and formed. It is also used to quantitate the strength of interactions in which one molecule binds to another by means of noncovalent interactions (discussed in Chapter 2, p. 48). Two molecules will bind to each other if the free-energy change for the interaction is negative; that is, the free energy of the resulting complex is lower than the sum of the free energies of the two partners when unbound. Noncovalent interactions are immensely important to cells. They include the binding of substrates to enzymes, the binding of transcription regulators to DNA, and the binding of one protein to another to make the many different structural and functional protein complexes that operate in a living cell.

The equilibrium constant, K, used to describe reactions in which covalent bonds are formed and broken, also reflects the binding strength of a noncovalent interaction between two molecules. This binding strength is a very useful quantity because it indicates how specific the interaction is between the two molecules. When molecule A binds to molecule B to form the complex AB, the reaction proceeds until it reaches equilibrium. At which point the number of association events precisely equals the number of dissociation events; at this point, the concentrations of reactants A and B, and of the complex AB, can be used to determine the equilibrium constant K (see Figure 3–19).

K becomes larger as the *binding energy*—that is, the energy released in the binding interaction—increases. In other words, the larger K is, the greater is the drop in free energy between the dissociated and associated states, and the more tightly the two molecules will bind. Even a

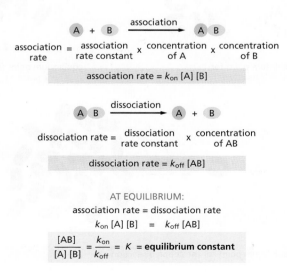

Figure 3–19 **The equilibrium constant, K, for the reaction A + B → AB depends on the concentrations of A, B, and AB.** Molecules A and B must collide in order to interact, and the association rate is therefore proportional to the product of their individual concentrations $[A] \times [B]$. As shown, the ratio of the rate constants k_{on} and k_{off} for the association (bond formation) and the dissociation (bond breakage) reactions, respectively, is equal to the equilibrium constant, K.

Consider 1000 molecules of A and 1000 molecules of B in the cytosol of a eukaryotic cell. The concentration of both will be about 10^{-9} M.

If the equilibrium constant (K) for A + B → AB is 10^{10} liters/mole, then at equilibrium there will be

270	270	730
A molecules	B molecules	AB complexes

If the equilibrium constant is a little weaker, say 10^8 liters/mole—a value that represents a loss of 11.9 kJ/mole of binding energy from the example above, or 2–3 fewer hydrogen bonds—then there will be

915	915	85
A molecules	B molecules	AB complexes

Figure 3–20 Small changes in the number of weak bonds can have drastic effects on a binding interaction. This example illustrates the dramatic effect of the presence or absence of a few weak noncovalent bonds in the interaction between two cytosolic proteins.

change of a few noncovalent bonds can have a striking effect on a binding interaction, as illustrated in **Figure 3–20**. In this example, a loss of 11.9 kJ/mole of binding energy, equivalent to eliminating a few hydrogen bonds from a binding interaction, can be seen to cause a dramatic decrease in the amount of complex that exists at equilibrium.

For Sequential Reactions, the Changes in Free Energy Are Additive

Now we return to our original concern regarding how cells can generate and maintain order. And more specifically: how can enzymes catalyze reactions that are energetically unfavorable?

One way they do so is by directly coupling energetically unfavorable reactions with energetically favorable ones. Consider, for example, two sequential reactions,

$$X \rightarrow Y \text{ and } Y \rightarrow Z$$

where the $\Delta G°$ values are +21 and –54 kJ/mole, respectively. (Recall that a mole is 6×10^{23} molecules of a substance.) The unfavorable reaction, $X \rightarrow Y$, will not occur spontaneously. However, it can be driven by the favorable reaction $Y \rightarrow Z$, provided that the second reaction follows the first. That's because the overall free-energy change for the coupled reaction is equal to the sum of the free-energy changes for each individual reaction. In this case, the $\Delta G°$ for the coupled reaction, $X \rightarrow Y \rightarrow Z$, will be –33 kJ/mole, making the overall pathway energetically favorable.

Cells can therefore cause the energetically unfavorable transition, $X \rightarrow Y$, to occur if an enzyme catalyzing the $X \rightarrow Y$ reaction is supplemented by a second enzyme that catalyzes the energetically favorable reaction, $Y \rightarrow Z$. In effect, the reaction $Y \rightarrow Z$ acts as a "siphon," pulling the conversion of all of molecule X to molecule Y, and then to molecule Z (**Figure 3–21**). Several of the reactions in the long pathway that converts sugars into CO_2 and H_2O are energetically unfavorable. This pathway nevertheless

Figure 3–21 An energetically unfavorable reaction can be driven by an energetically favorable follow-on reaction that acts as a chemical siphon. (A) At equilibrium, there are twice as many X molecules as Y molecules. (B) At equilibrium, there are 25 times more Z molecules than Y molecules. (C) If the reactions in (A) and (B) are coupled, nearly all of the X molecules will be converted to Z molecules, as shown. In terms of energetics, the $\Delta G°$ of the $Y \rightarrow Z$ reaction is so negative that, when coupled to the $X \rightarrow Y$ reaction, it lowers the ΔG of $X \rightarrow Y$. This is because the ΔG of $X \rightarrow Y$ decreases as the ratio of Y to X declines (see Figure 3–18).

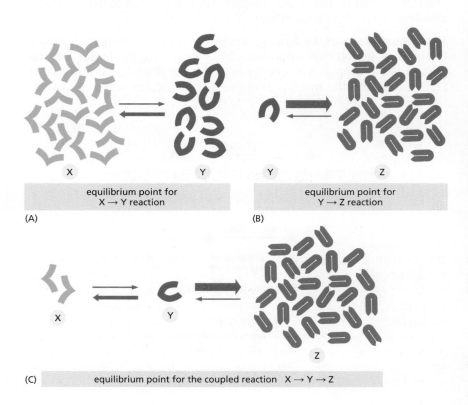

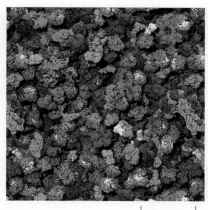

Figure 3–22 The cytosol is crowded with various molecules. Only the macromolecules, which are drawn to scale and displayed in different colors, are shown. Enzymes and other macromolecules diffuse relatively slowly in the cytosol, in part because they interact with so many other macromolecules. Small molecules, by contrast, can diffuse nearly as rapidly as they do in water (see Movie 1.2). (From S.R. McGuffee and A.H. Elcock, *PLoS Comput. Biol.* 6(3): e1000694, 2010.)

25 nm

proceeds rapidly to completion because the total $\Delta G°$ for the series of sequential reactions has a large negative value.

Forming a sequential pathway, however, is not the answer for many other metabolic needs. Often the desired reaction is simply $X \rightarrow Y$, without further conversion of Y to some other product. Fortunately, there are other, more general ways of using enzymes to couple reactions together, involving the production of activated carriers that can shuttle energy from one reaction site to another, as we discuss shortly.

Enzyme-catalyzed Reactions Depend on Rapid Molecular Collisions

Thus far we have talked about chemical reactions as if they take place in isolation. But the cytosol of a cell is densely packed with molecules of various shapes and sizes (**Figure 3–22**). So how do enzymes and their substrates, which are present in relatively small amounts in the cytosol of a cell, manage to find each other? And how do they do it so quickly? Observations indicate that a typical enzyme can capture and process about a thousand substrate molecules every second.

Rapid binding is possible because molecular motions are enormously fast—very much faster than the human mind can easily imagine. Because of heat energy, molecules are in constant motion and consequently will explore the cytosolic space very efficiently by wandering randomly through it—a process called **diffusion**. In this way, every molecule in the cytosol collides with a huge number of other molecules each second. As these molecules in solution collide and bounce off one another, an individual molecule moves first one way and then another, its path constituting a *random walk* (**Figure 3–23**).

Although the cytosol of a cell is densely packed with molecules of various shapes and sizes, experiments in which fluorescent dyes and other labeled molecules are injected into the cell cytosol show that small organic molecules diffuse through this aqueous gel nearly as rapidly as they do through water. A small organic molecule, such as a substrate, takes only about one-fifth of a second on average to diffuse a distance of 10 µm. Diffusion is therefore an efficient way for small molecules to move limited distances in the cell.

Because proteins diffuse through the cytosol much more slowly than do small molecules, the rate at which an enzyme will encounter its substrate depends on the concentration of the substrate. The most abundant substrates are present in the cell at a concentration of about 0.5 mM. Because pure water is 55 M, there is only about one such substrate molecule in the cell for every 10^5 water molecules. Nevertheless, the site on an enzyme that binds this substrate will be bombarded by about 500,000 random collisions with the substrate every second! For a substrate concentration tenfold lower (0.05 mM), the number of collisions drops to 50,000 per second, and so on. These incredibly numerous collisions play a critical role in life's chemistry.

QUESTION 3–4

For the reactions shown in Figure 3–21, sketch an energy diagram similar to that in Figure 3–12 for the two reactions alone and for the combined reactions. Indicate the standard free-energy changes for the reactions $X \rightarrow Y$, $Y \rightarrow Z$, and $X \rightarrow Z$ in the graph. Indicate how enzymes that catalyze these reactions would change the energy diagram.

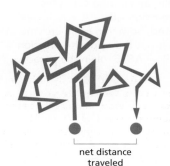

net distance
traveled

Figure 3–23 A molecule traverses the cytosol by taking a random walk. Molecules in solution move in a random fashion due to the continual buffeting they receive in collisions with other molecules. This movement allows small molecules to diffuse rapidly throughout the cell cytosol (Movie 3.2).

Noncovalent Interactions Allow Enzymes to Bind Specific Molecules

The first step in any enzyme-catalyzed chemical reaction is the binding of the substrate. Once this step has taken place, the substrate must remain bound to the enzyme long enough for the chemistry to occur. The association of enzyme and substrate is stabilized by the formation of multiple, weak bonds between the participating molecules. These weak interactions—which can include hydrogen bonds, van der Waals attractions, and electrostatic attractions (discussed in Chapter 2)—persist until random thermal motion causes the molecules to dissociate again.

When two colliding molecules have poorly matching surfaces, few noncovalent bonds are formed, and their total energy is negligible compared with that of thermal motion. In this case, the two molecules dissociate as rapidly as they come together (see Figure 2–35). As we saw in Figure 3–20, even small changes in the number of noncovalent bonds made between two interacting molecules can have a dramatic effect on their ability to form a complex. Poor noncovalent bond formation is what prevents unwanted associations from forming between mismatched molecules, such as those between an enzyme and the wrong substrate. Only when the enzyme and substrate are well matched do they form many weak interactions. It is these numerous noncovalent bonds that keep them together long enough for a covalent bond in the substrate molecule to be formed or broken, converting substrate to product.

Enzymes are remarkable catalysts, capturing substrates and releasing products in mere milliseconds. But though an enzyme can lower the activation energy for a reaction, such as $Y \rightarrow X$ (see Figure 3–12), it is important to note that the same enzyme will also lower the activation energy for the reverse reaction $X \rightarrow Y$ to exactly the same degree. That's because the same noncovalent bonds are formed with the enzyme whether the reaction goes forward or backward. The forward and backward reactions will therefore be accelerated by the same factor by an enzyme, and the equilibrium point for the reaction—and thus its $\Delta G°$—remains unchanged (**Figure 3–24**).

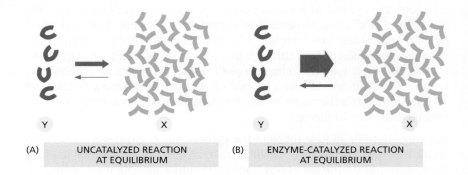

(A) UNCATALYZED REACTION AT EQUILIBRIUM

(B) ENZYME-CATALYZED REACTION AT EQUILIBRIUM

Figure 3–24 Enzymes cannot change the equilibrium point for reactions. Enzymes, like all catalysts, speed up the forward and reverse rates of a reaction by the same amount. Therefore, for both the (A) uncatalyzed and (B) catalyzed reactions shown here, the number of molecules undergoing the transition $Y \rightarrow X$ is equal to the number of molecules undergoing the transition $X \rightarrow Y$ when the ratio of X molecules to Y molecules is 7 to 1, as illustrated. In other words, both the catalyzed and uncatalyzed reactions will eventually reach the same equilibrium point, although the catalyzed reaction will reach equilibrium much faster.

ACTIVATED CARRIERS AND BIOSYNTHESIS

Much of the energy released by an energetically favorable reaction such as the oxidation of a food molecule must be stored temporarily before it can be used by cells to fuel energetically unfavorable reactions, such as the synthesis of all the other molecules needed by the cell. In most cases, the energy is stored as chemical-bond energy in a set of **activated carriers**, small organic molecules that contain one or more energy-rich covalent bonds. These molecules diffuse rapidly and carry their bond energy from the sites of energy generation to the sites where energy is used either for **biosynthesis** or for the many other energy-requiring activities that a cell must perform (Figure 3–25). In a sense, cells use activated carriers like money to pay for the energetically unfavorable reactions that otherwise would not take place.

Activated carriers store energy in an easily exchangeable form, either as a readily transferable chemical group or as readily transferable ("high-energy") electrons. They can serve a dual role as a source of both energy and chemical groups for biosynthetic reactions. As we shall discuss shortly, the most important activated carriers are *ATP* and two molecules that are close chemical cousins, *NADH* and *NADPH*.

An understanding of how cells transform the energy locked in food molecules into a form that can be used to do work required the dedicated effort of the world's finest chemists (How We Know, pp. 102–103). Their discoveries, amassed over the first half of the twentieth century, marked the dawn of the study of biochemistry.

The Formation of an Activated Carrier Is Coupled to an Energetically Favorable Reaction

When a fuel molecule such as glucose is oxidized inside a cell, enzyme-catalyzed reactions ensure that a large part of the free energy released is captured in a chemically useful form, rather than being released wastefully as heat. When your cells oxidize the sugar from a chocolate bar, that energy allows you to power metabolic reactions; burning that same chocolate bar in the street will get you nowhere, warming the environment while producing no metabolically useful energy.

In cells, energy capture is achieved by means of a special form of **coupled reaction**, in which an energetically favorable reaction is used to drive an energetically unfavorable one, so that an activated carrier or some other useful molecule is produced. Such coupling requires enzyme catalysis, which is fundamental to all of the energy transactions in the cell.

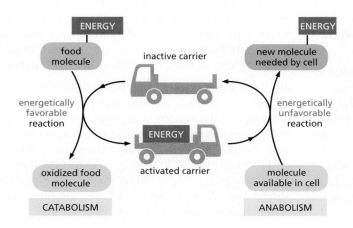

Figure 3–25 **Activated carriers can store and transfer energy in a form that cells can use.** By serving as intracellular energy shuttles, activated carriers perform their function as go-betweens that link the release of energy from the breakdown of food molecules (catabolism) to the energy-requiring biosynthesis of small and large organic molecules (anabolism).

HOW WE KNOW

"HIGH-ENERGY" PHOSPHATE BONDS POWER CELL PROCESSES

Cells require a continuous stream of energy to generate and maintain order, while acquiring the materials they need to survive, grow, and reproduce. But even as late as 1921, very little was known about how energy—which for animal cells is derived from the breakdown of nutrients—is biochemically transformed, stored, and released for work in the cell. It would take the efforts of a handful of biochemists, many of whom worked with Otto Meyerhof—a pioneer in the field of cell metabolism—to get a handle on this fundamental problem.

Muscling in

Meyerhof was trained as a physician in Heidelberg, Germany, and he had a strong interest in physiological chemistry; in particular, he wondered how energy is transformed during chemical reactions in cells. He recognized that between its initial entry in the form of food and its final dissipation as heat, a large amount of energy must be made available by a series of intermediate chemical steps that allow the cell or organism to maintain itself in a state of dynamic equilibrium.

To explore how these mysterious chemical transformations power the work done by cells, Meyerhof focused his attention on muscle. Muscle tissue could be isolated from an animal, such as a frog, and stimulated to contract with a pulse of electricity. And contraction provided a dramatic demonstration of the conversion of energy to a usable, mechanical form.

When Meyerhof got started, all that was known about the chemistry of contraction is that, in active muscle tissue, lactic acid is generated by a process of fermentation. As Meyerhof's first order of business, he demonstrated that this lactic acid comes from the breakdown of glycogen—a branched polymer made of glucose units that serves as an energy store in animal cells, particularly in muscle (see Panel 2–4, p. 73).

While Meyerhof focused on the chemistry, English physiologist Archibald "A.V." Hill determined that working muscles give off heat, both as they contract and as they recover; further, he found that the amount of heat correlates with how hard the muscle is working.

Hill and Meyerhof then showed that the heat produced during muscle relaxation was linked to the resynthesis of glycogen. A portion of the lactic acid made by the muscle would be completely oxidized to CO_2 and water, and the energy from this oxidative breakdown would be used to convert the remaining lactic acid back to glycogen. This conversion of glycogen to lactic acid—and back again—provided the first evidence of cyclical energy transformation in cells (**Figure 3–26**). And in 1922, it earned Meyerhof and Hill a Nobel Prize.

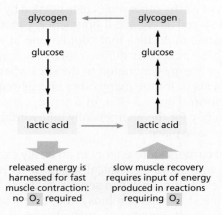

Figure 3–26 A "lactic acid cycle" was thought to supply the energy needed to power muscle contraction. Preparations of frog muscle were stimulated to contract while being held at constant length (isometric contraction). As shown, contraction was accompanied by the breakdown of glycogen and the formation of lactic acid. The energy released by this oxidation was thought to somehow power muscle contraction. Lactic acid is converted back to glycogen as the muscle recovers.

In the mail

But did the conversion of glycogen into lactic acid directly power the mechanical work of muscle contraction? Meyerhof had thought so—until 1927, when a letter arrived from Danish physiologist Einar Lundsgaard. In it, Lundsgaard told Meyerhof of the surprising results of some experiments he had performed both on isolated muscles and in living rabbits and frogs. Lundsgaard had injected muscles with iodoacetate, a compound that inhibits an enzyme involved in the breakdown of sugars (as we discuss in Chapter 13). In these iodoacetate-treated muscles, fermentation was blocked and no lactic acid could be made.

What Lundsgaard discovered was that the poisoned muscles continued to contract. Indeed, animals injected with the compound at first "behaved quite normally," wrote Fritz Lipmann, a biochemist who was working in Meyerhof's laboratory. But after a few minutes, they suddenly keeled over, their muscles frozen in rigor.

But if the formation of lactic acid was not providing fuel for muscle contraction, what was? Lundsgaard went on to show that the source of energy for muscle contraction in poisoned muscles appeared to be a recently discovered molecule called creatine phosphate. When lactic acid formation was blocked by iodoacetate, muscle contraction was accompanied by the hydrolysis of creatine phosphate. When the supply of creatine phosphate was exhausted, muscles seized up permanently.

"The turmoil that this news created in Meyerhof's laboratory is difficult to realize today," wrote Lipmann. The finding contradicted Meyerhof's theory that lactic acid formation powered muscle contraction. And it pointed toward not just an alternative molecule, but a whole new idea: that certain phosphate bonds, when hydrolyzed, could provide energy. "Lundsgaard had discovered that the muscle machine can be driven by phosphate-bond energy, and he shrewdly realized that this type of energy was 'nearer,' as he expressed it, to the conversion of metabolic energy into mechanical energy than lactic acid," wrote Lipmann.

But rather than being upset, Meyerhof welcomed Lundsgaard to his lab in Heidelberg, where he was serving as director of the Kaiser Wilhelm Physiology Institute. There, Lundsgaard made very careful measurements showing that the breakdown of creatine phosphate—and the heat it generated—closely tracked the amount of tension generated by intact muscle.

The most direct conclusion that could be drawn from these observations is that the hydrolysis of creatine phosphate supplied the energy that powers muscle contraction. But in one of his papers published in 1930, Lundsgaard was careful to note that there was another possibility: that in normal muscle, both lactic acid formation and creatine phosphate hydrolysis transferred energy to a third, yet-to-be identified system. This is where ATP comes in.

Squiggle P

Even before Lundsgaard's eye-opening observations, Meyerhof had an interest in the amount of energy contained in various metabolic compounds, particularly those that contained phosphate. He thought that metabolic energy sources might be identified by finding naturally occurring molecules that release unusually large amounts of heat when hydrolyzed. Creatine phosphate was one of those compounds. Another was ATP, which had been discovered in 1929—by Meyerhof's assistant, chemist Karl Lohmann, and, at the same time, by biochemists Cyrus Fiske and Yellapragada Subbarow working in America.

By 1935, Lohmann had demonstrated that the hydrolytic breakdown of creatine phosphate occurs through the transfer of its phosphate group to ADP to form ATP. It is the hydrolysis of ATP that serves as the direct source of energy for muscle contraction; creatine phosphate provides a reservoir of "high-energy" phosphate groups that replenish depleted ATP and maintain the needed ratio of ATP to ADP (**Figure 3–27**).

In 1941, Lipmann published a 63-page review in the inaugural issue of *Advances in Enzymology*. Entitled "The metabolic generation and utilization of phosphate bond

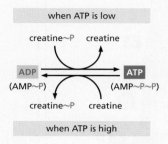

Figure 3–27 Creatine phosphate serves as an intermediate energy store. An enzyme called creatine kinase transfers a phosphate group from creatine phosphate to ADP when ATP concentrations are low; the same enzyme can catalyze the reverse reaction to generate a pool of creatine phosphate when ATP concentrations are high. Here, the "high-energy" phosphate bonds are symbolized by ~P. AMP is adenosine monophosphate (see Figure 3–41).

energy," this article introduced the symbol ~P (or "squiggle P") to denote an energy-rich phosphate bond—one whose hydrolysis yields enough energy to drive energetically unfavorable reactions and processes (**Figure 3–28**).

Although several molecules contain such high-energy phosphate bonds (see Panel 3–1, p. 95), it is the hydrolysis of ATP that provides the driving force for most of the energy-requiring reactions in living systems, including the contraction of muscles, the transport of substances across membranes, and the synthesis of macromolecules including proteins, nucleic acids, and carbohydrates. Indeed, in a memorial written after the death of Meyerhof in 1951, Lipmann—who would shortly win his own Nobel Prize for work on a different activated carrier—wrote: "The discovery of ATP thus was the key that opened the gates to the understanding of the conversion mechanisms of metabolic energy."

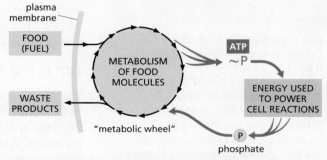

Figure 3–28 High-energy phosphate bonds generate an energy current (*red*) that powers cell reactions. This diagram, modeled on a figure published in Lipmann's 1941 article in *Advances in Enzymology*, shows how energy released by the metabolism of food molecules (represented by the "metabolic wheel") is captured in the form of high-energy phosphate bonds (~P) of ATP, which are used to power all other cell reactions. After the high-energy bonds are hydrolyzed, the inorganic phosphate released is recycled and reused, as indicated.

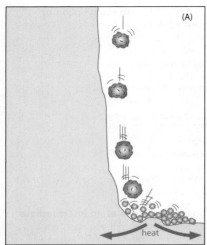

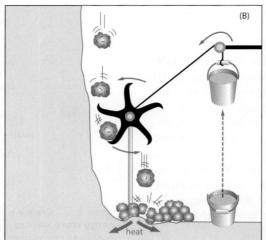

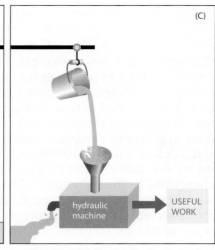

kinetic energy of falling rocks is transformed into heat energy only

part of the kinetic energy is used to lift a bucket of water, and a correspondingly smaller amount is transformed into heat

the potential energy stored in the raised bucket of water can be used to drive hydraulic machines that carry out a variety of useful tasks

Figure 3–29 A mechanical model illustrates the principle of coupled chemical reactions. (A) The spontaneous reaction shown could serve as an analogy for the direct oxidation of glucose to CO_2 and H_2O, which produces only heat. (B) The same reaction is coupled to a second reaction, which could serve as an analogy for the synthesis of activated carriers. (C) The energy produced in (B) is in a more useful form than in (A) and can be used to drive a variety of otherwise energetically unfavorable reactions.

To provide an everyday representation of how coupled reactions work, let's consider a mechanical analogy in which an energetically favorable chemical reaction is represented by rocks falling from a cliff. The kinetic energy of falling rocks would normally be entirely wasted in the form of heat generated by friction when the rocks hit the ground (**Figure 3–29A**). By careful design, however, part of this energy could be used to drive a paddle wheel that lifts a bucket of water (**Figure 3–29B**). Because the rocks can now reach the ground only after moving the paddle wheel, we say that the energetically favorable reaction of rocks falling has been directly coupled to the energetically unfavorable reaction of lifting the bucket of water. Because part of the energy is used to do work in (B), the rocks hit the ground with less velocity than in (A), and correspondingly less energy is wasted as heat. The energy saved in the elevated bucket of water can then be used to do useful work (**Figure 3–29C**).

Analogous processes occur in cells, where enzymes play the role of the paddle wheel in Figure 3–29B. By mechanisms that we discuss in Chapter 13, enzymes couple an energetically favorable reaction, such as the oxidation of food molecules, to an energetically unfavorable reaction, such as the generation of activated carriers. As a result, the amount of heat released by the oxidation reaction is reduced by exactly the amount of energy that is stored in the energy-rich covalent bonds of the activated carrier. That saved energy can then be used to power a chemical reaction elsewhere in the cell.

ATP Is the Most Widely Used Activated Carrier

The most important and versatile of the activated carriers in cells is **ATP** (adenosine 5′-triphosphate). Just as the energy stored in the raised bucket of water in Figure 3–29B can be used to drive a wide variety of hydraulic machines, ATP serves as a convenient and versatile store, or currency, of energy that can be used to drive a variety of chemical reactions in cells. As shown in **Figure 3–30**, ATP is synthesized in an energetically unfavorable *phosphorylation* reaction, in which a phosphate group is added to **ADP** (adenosine 5′-diphosphate). When required, ATP gives up this energy packet in an energetically favorable hydrolysis to ADP and inorganic phosphate (P_i). The regenerated ADP is then available to be used for another round of the phosphorylation reaction that forms ATP, creating an ATP cycle in the cell.

QUESTION 3–7

Use Figure 3–29B to illustrate the following reaction driven by the hydrolysis of ATP:

$$X + ATP \rightarrow Y + ADP + P_i$$

A. In this case, which molecule or molecules would be analogous to (i) rocks at the top of the cliff, (ii) broken debris at the bottom of the cliff, (iii) the bucket at its highest point, and (iv) the bucket on the ground?

B. What would be analogous to (i) the rocks hitting the ground in the absence of the paddle wheel in Figure 3–29A and (ii) the hydraulic machine in Figure 3–29C?

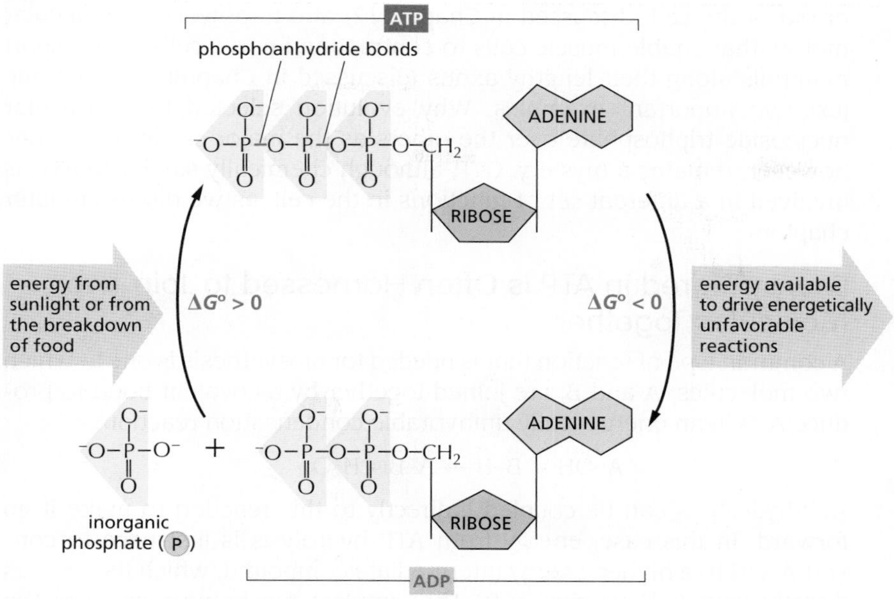

Figure 3–30 The interconversion of ATP and ADP occurs in a cycle. The two outermost phosphate groups in ATP are held to the rest of the molecule by "high-energy" phosphoanhydride bonds and are readily transferred to other organic molecules. Water can be added to ATP to form ADP and inorganic phosphate (P_i). Inside a cell, this hydrolysis of the terminal phosphate of ATP yields between 46 and 54 kJ/mole of usable energy. (Although the $\Delta G°$ of this reaction is –30.5 kJ/mole, its ΔG inside cells is much more negative, because the ratio of ATP to the products ADP and P_i is kept so high.)

The formation of ATP from ADP and P_i reverses the hydrolysis reaction; because this condensation reaction is energetically unfavorable, it must be coupled to a highly energetically favorable reaction to occur.

The large negative $\Delta G°$ of the ATP hydrolysis reaction arises from a number of factors. Release of the terminal phosphate group removes an unfavorable repulsion between adjacent negative charges; in addition, the inorganic phosphate ion (P_i) released is stabilized by favorable hydrogen-bond formation with water.

The energetically favorable reaction of ATP hydrolysis is coupled to many otherwise unfavorable reactions through which other molecules are synthesized. We will encounter several of these reactions in this chapter, where we will see exactly how this coupling is carried out. ATP hydrolysis is often accompanied by a transfer of the terminal phosphate in ATP to another molecule, as illustrated in **Figure 3–31**. Any reaction that involves the transfer of a phosphate group to a molecule is termed a *phosphorylation* reaction. Phosphorylation reactions are examples of condensation reactions (see Figure 2–19), and they occur in many important cell processes: they activate substrates for a subsequent reaction, mediate movement, and serve as key constituents of intracellular signaling pathways (discussed in Chapter 16).

ATP is the most abundant activated carrier in cells. It is used to supply energy for many of the pumps that actively transport substances into

The phosphoanhydride bond that links two phosphate groups in ATP in a high-energy linkage has a $\Delta G°$ of –30.5 kJ/mole. Hydrolysis of this bond in a cell liberates from 46 to 54 kJ/mole of usable energy. How can this be? Why do you think a range of energies is given, rather than a precise number as for $\Delta G°$?

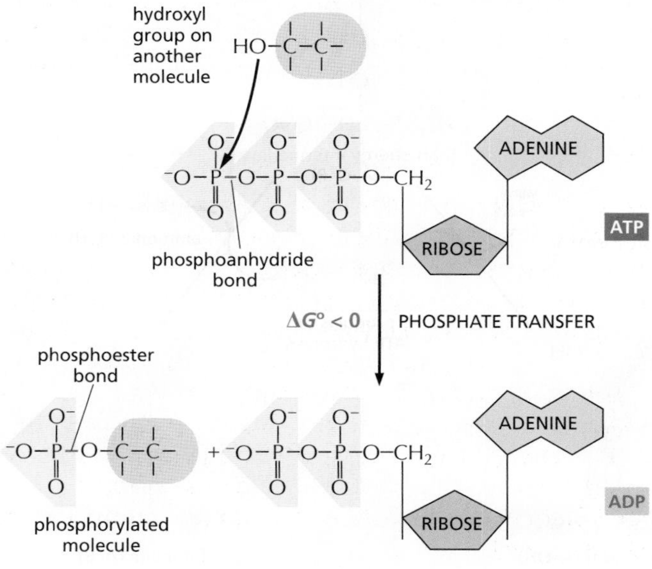

Figure 3–31 The terminal phosphate of ATP can be readily transferred to other molecules. Because an energy-rich phosphoanhydride bond in ATP is converted to a less energy-rich phosphoester bond in the phosphate-accepting molecule, this reaction is energetically favorable, having a large negative $\Delta G°$ (see Panel 3–1, pp. 94–95). Phosphorylation reactions of this type are involved in the synthesis of phospholipids and in the initial steps of the breakdown of sugars, as well as in many other metabolic and intracellular signaling pathways.

or out of the cell (discussed in Chapter 12) and to power the molecular motors that enable muscle cells to contract and nerve cells to transport materials along their lengthy axons (discussed in Chapter 17), to name just two important examples. Why evolution selected this particular nucleoside triphosphate over the others as the major carrier of energy, however, remains a mystery. GTP, although chemically similar to ATP, is involved in a different set of functions in the cell, as we discuss in later chapters.

Energy Stored in ATP Is Often Harnessed to Join Two Molecules Together

A common type of reaction that is needed for biosynthesis is one in which two molecules, A and B, are joined together by a covalent bond to produce A–B in an energetically unfavorable condensation reaction:

$$A\text{–}OH + B\text{–}H \rightarrow A\text{–}B + H_2O$$

ATP hydrolysis can be coupled indirectly to this reaction to make it go forward. In this case, energy from ATP hydrolysis is first used to convert A–OH to a higher-energy intermediate compound, which then reacts directly with B–H to give A–B. The simplest mechanism involves the transfer of a phosphate from ATP to A–OH to make A–O–PO₃, in which case the reaction pathway contains only two steps (**Figure 3–32A**). The condensation reaction, which by itself is energetically unfavorable, has been forced to occur by being coupled to ATP hydrolysis in an enzyme-catalyzed reaction pathway.

A biosynthetic reaction of exactly this type is employed to synthesize the amino acid glutamine, as illustrated in **Figure 3–32B**. We will see later in the chapter that very similar (but more complex) mechanisms are also used to produce nearly all of the large molecules of the cell.

NADH and NADPH Are Both Activated Carriers of Electrons

Other important activated carriers participate in oxidation–reduction reactions and are also commonly part of coupled reactions in cells. These

Figure 3–32 An energetically unfavorable biosynthetic reaction can be driven by ATP hydrolysis. (A) Schematic illustration of the condensation reaction described in the text. In this set of reactions, a phosphate group is first donated by ATP to form a high-energy intermediate, A–O–PO₃, which then reacts with the other substrate, B–H, to form the product A–B. (B) Reaction showing the biosynthesis of the amino acid glutamine from glutamic acid. Glutamic acid, which corresponds to the A–OH shown in (A), is first converted to a high-energy phosphorylated intermediate, which corresponds to A–O–PO₃. This intermediate then reacts with ammonia (which corresponds to B–H) to form glutamine. In this example, both steps occur on the surface of the same enzyme, glutamine synthetase (not shown). ATP hydrolysis can drive this energetically unfavorable reaction because it produces a favorable free-energy change ($\Delta G°$ of –30.5 kJ/mole) that is larger in magnitude than the energy required for the synthesis of glutamine from glutamic acid plus NH₃ ($\Delta G°$ of +14.2 kJ/mole). For clarity, the glutamic acid side chain is shown in its uncharged form.

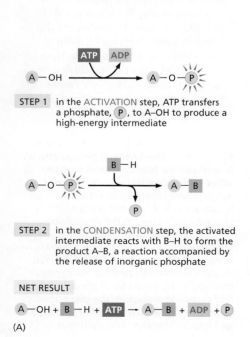

STEP 1 in the ACTIVATION step, ATP transfers a phosphate, (P), to A–OH to produce a high-energy intermediate

STEP 2 in the CONDENSATION step, the activated intermediate reacts with B–H to form the product A–B, a reaction accompanied by the release of inorganic phosphate

NET RESULT

A–OH + B–H + ATP → A–B + ADP + P

(A)

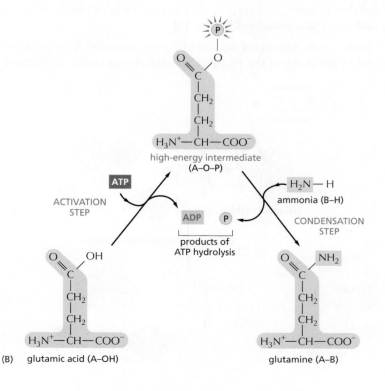

(B)   glutamic acid (A–OH)   glutamine (A–B)

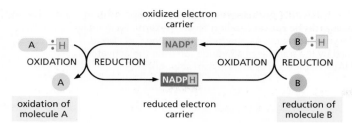

oxidized electron
carrier

A ∷H   NADP⁺   B ∷H

OXIDATION   REDUCTION   OXIDATION   REDUCTION

A   NADPH   B

oxidation of
molecule A   reduced electron
carrier   reduction of
molecule B

Figure 3–33 NADPH is an activated carrier of electrons that participates in oxidation–reduction reactions. NADPH is produced in reactions of the general type shown on the left, in which two electrons are removed from a substrate (A–H). The oxidized form of the carrier molecule, NADP⁺, receives these two electrons as one hydrogen atom plus an electron (a hydride ion). Because NADPH holds its hydride ion in a high-energy linkage, this ion can easily be transferred to other molecules, such as B, as shown on the right. In this reaction, NADPH is re-oxidized to yield NADP⁺, thus completing the cycle.

activated carriers are specialized to carry both high-energy electrons and hydrogen atoms. The most important of these *electron carriers* are **NADH** (nicotinamide adenine dinucleotide) and the closely related molecule **NADPH** (nicotinamide adenine dinucleotide phosphate). Both NADH and NADPH carry energy in the form of two high-energy electrons plus a proton (H⁺), which together form a hydride ion (H⁻). When these activated carriers pass their hydride ion to a donor molecule, they become oxidized to form **NAD⁺** and **NADP⁺**, respectively.

Like ATP, NADPH is an activated carrier that participates in many important biosynthetic reactions that would otherwise be energetically unfavorable. NADPH is produced according to the general scheme shown in **Figure 3–33**. During a special set of energy-yielding catabolic reactions, a hydride ion is removed from the substrate molecule and added to the nicotinamide ring of NADP⁺ to form NADPH. This is a typical oxidation–reduction reaction: the substrate is oxidized and NADP⁺ is reduced.

The hydride ion carried by NADPH is given up readily in a subsequent oxidation–reduction reaction, because the nicotinamide ring can achieve a more stable arrangement of electrons without it (**Figure 3–34**). In this subsequent reaction, which regenerates NADP⁺, the NADPH becomes oxidized and the substrate becomes reduced—thus completing the NADPH cycle (see Figure 3–33). NADPH is efficient at donating its hydride ion to other molecules for the same reason that ATP readily transfers a phosphate: in both cases, the transfer is accompanied by a large negative free-energy change. One example of the use of NADPH in biosynthesis is shown in **Figure 3–35**.

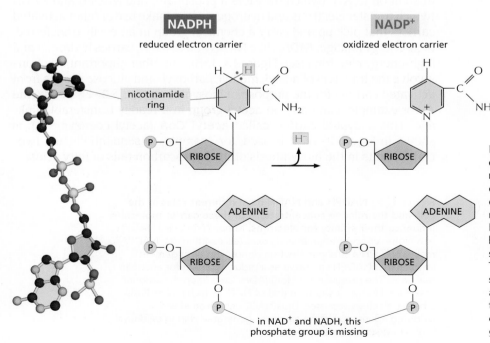

NADPH

reduced electron carrier

nicotinamide
ring

H   ·H   O
    C
      NH₂
N

P—O— RIBOSE

H⁻

ADENINE

P—O— RIBOSE

O

P

NADP⁺

oxidized electron carrier

H   O
   C
    NH₂
⁺N

P—O— RIBOSE

ADENINE

P—O— RIBOSE

O

P

in NAD⁺ and NADH, this
phosphate group is missing

Figure 3–34 NADPH accepts and donates electrons via its nicotinamide ring. NADPH donates its high-energy electrons together with a proton (the equivalent of a hydride ion, H⁻). This reaction, which oxidizes NADPH to NADP⁺, is energetically favorable because the nicotinamide ring is more stable when these electrons are absent. The ball-and-stick model on the left shows the structure of NADP⁺. NAD⁺ and NADH are identical in structure to NADP⁺ and NADPH, respectively, except that they lack the phosphate group, as indicated.

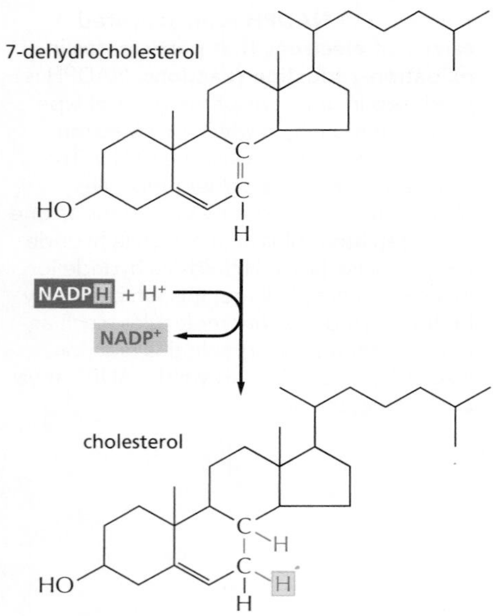

7-dehydrocholesterol

HO

NADP**H** + H$^+$

NADP$^+$

cholesterol

HO

Figure 3–35 **NADPH participates in the final stage of one of the biosynthetic routes leading to cholesterol.** As in many other biosynthetic reactions, the reduction of the C=C bond is achieved by the transfer of a hydride ion from the activated carrier NADPH, plus a proton (H$^+$) from solution.

NADPH and NADH Have Different Roles in Cells

NADPH and NADH differ in a single phosphate group, which is located far from the region involved in electron transfer in NADPH (see Figure 3–34). Although this phosphate group has no effect on the electron-transfer properties of NADPH compared with NADH, it is nonetheless crucial for their distinctive roles, as it gives NADPH a slightly different shape from NADH. This subtle difference in conformation makes it possible for the two carriers to bind as substrates to different sets of enzymes and thereby deliver electrons (in the form of hydride ions) to different target molecules.

Why should there be this division of labor? The answer lies in the need to regulate two sets of electron-transfer reactions independently. NADPH operates chiefly with enzymes that catalyze anabolic reactions, supplying the high-energy electrons needed to synthesize energy-rich biological molecules. NADH, by contrast, has a special role as an intermediate in the catabolic system of reactions that generate ATP through the oxidation of food molecules, as we discuss in Chapter 13. The genesis of NADH from NAD$^+$ and that of NADPH from NADP$^+$ occurs by different pathways that are independently regulated, so that the cell can adjust the supply of electrons for these two contrasting purposes. Inside the cell, the ratio of NAD$^+$ to NADH is kept high, whereas the ratio of NADP$^+$ to NADPH is kept low. This arrangement provides plenty of NAD$^+$ to act as an oxidizing agent and plenty of NADPH to act as a reducing agent—as required for their special roles in catabolism and anabolism, respectively (**Figure 3–36**).

Cells Make Use of Many Other Activated Carriers

In addition to ATP (which transfers a phosphate) and NADPH and NADH (which transfer electrons and hydrogen), cells make use of other activated carriers that pick up and carry a chemical group in an easily transferred, high-energy linkage. *FADH$_2$*, like NADH and NADPH, carries hydrogen and high-energy electrons (see Figure 13–13B). But other important reactions involve the transfers of acetyl, methyl, carboxyl, and glucose groups from activated carriers for the purpose of biosynthesis (**Table 3–2**). Coenzyme A, for example, can carry an acetyl group in a readily transferable linkage. This activated carrier, called **acetyl CoA** (acetyl coenzyme A), is shown in **Figure 3–37**. It is used, for example, to sequentially add two-carbon units in the biosynthesis of the hydrocarbon tails of fatty acids.

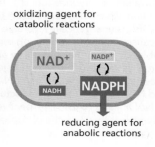

oxidizing agent for
catabolic reactions

NAD$^+$ NADP$^+$

( )   ( )

NADH   **NADPH**

reducing agent for
anabolic reactions

Figure 3–36 **NADPH and NADH have different roles in the cell, and the relative concentrations of these carrier molecules influence their affinity for electrons.** Keeping reduced NADPH at a higher concentration than its oxidized counterpart, NADP$^+$, makes NADPH a stronger electron donor. This arrangement ensures that NADPH can serve as a reducing agent for anabolic reactions. The reverse is true for NADH. Cells keep the amount of reduced NADH lower than that of NAD$^+$, which makes NAD$^+$ a better electron acceptor. Thus NAD$^+$ acts as an effective oxidizing agent, accepting electrons generated during oxidative breakdown of food molecules.

TABLE 3–2 SOME ACTIVATED CARRIERS WIDELY USED IN METABOLISM	
Activated Carrier	Group Carried in High-Energy Linkage
ATP	phosphate
NADH, NADPH, FADH$_2$	electrons and hydrogens
Acetyl CoA	acetyl group
Carboxylated biotin	carboxyl group
S-adenosylmethionine	methyl group
Uridine diphosphate glucose	glucose

In acetyl CoA and the other activated carriers in Table 3–2, the transferable group makes up only a small part of the molecule. The rest consists of a large organic portion that serves as a convenient "handle," facilitating the recognition of the carrier molecule by specific enzymes. As with acetyl CoA, this handle portion very often contains a nucleotide. This curious fact may be a relic from an early stage of cell evolution. It is thought that the main catalysts for early life-forms on Earth were RNA molecules (or their close relatives) and that proteins were a later evolutionary addition. It is therefore tempting to speculate that many of the activated carriers that we find today originated in an earlier RNA world, where their nucleotide portions would have been useful for binding these carriers to RNA-based catalysts, or *ribozymes* (discussed in Chapter 7).

Activated carriers are usually generated in reactions coupled to ATP hydrolysis, as shown for biotin in **Figure 3–38**. Therefore, the energy that enables their groups to be used for biosynthesis ultimately comes from the catabolic reactions that generate ATP. The same principle applies to the synthesis of large macromolecules—nucleic acids, proteins, and polysaccharides—as we discuss next.

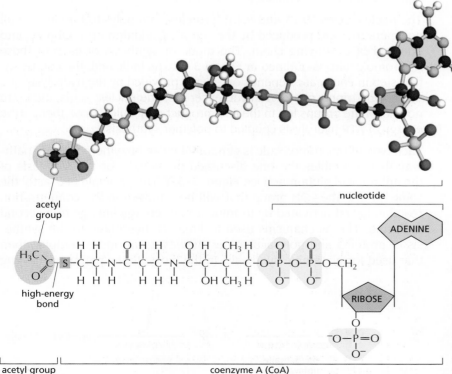

Figure 3–37 Acetyl coenzyme A (CoA) is another important activated carrier. A ball-and-stick model is shown above the structure of acetyl CoA. The sulfur atom (*orange*) forms a thioester bond to acetate. Because the thioester bond is a high-energy linkage, it releases a large amount of free energy when it is hydrolyzed. Thus the acetyl group carried by CoA can be readily transferred to other molecules.

Figure 3–38 Biotin transfers a carboxyl group to a substrate. Biotin is a vitamin that is used by a number of enzymes to transfer a carboxyl group to a substrate. Shown here is the reaction in which biotin, held by the enzyme *pyruvate carboxylase*, *accepts* a carboxyl group from bicarbonate and transfers it to pyruvate, producing oxaloacetate, a molecule required in the citric acid cycle (discussed in Chapter 13). Other enzymes use biotin to transfer carboxyl groups to other molecules. Note that the synthesis of carboxylated biotin requires energy derived from ATP hydrolysis—a general feature that applies to many activated carriers.

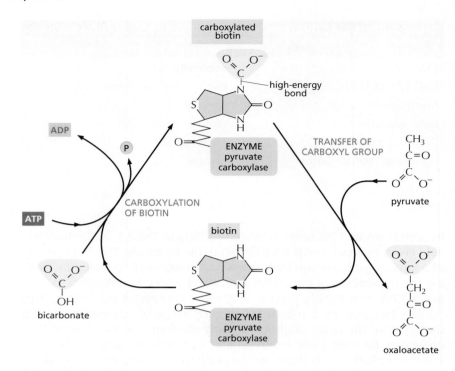

The Synthesis of Biological Polymers Requires an Energy Input

The macromolecules of the cell constitute the vast majority of its dry mass—that is, the mass not due to water. These molecules are made from *subunits* (or monomers) that are linked together by bonds formed during an enzyme-catalyzed *condensation* reaction. The reverse reaction—the breakdown of polymers—occurs through enzyme-catalyzed *hydrolysis* reactions. These hydrolysis reactions are energetically favorable, whereas the corresponding biosynthetic reactions require an energy input and are more complex (**Figure 3–39**).

The nucleic acids (DNA and RNA), proteins, and polysaccharides are all polymers that are produced by the repeated addition of a subunit onto one end of a growing chain. The mode of synthesis of each of these macromolecules is outlined in **Figure 3–40**. As indicated, the condensation step in each case depends on energy provided by the hydrolysis of a nucleoside triphosphate. And yet, except for the nucleic acids, there are no phosphate groups left in the final product molecules. How, then, is the energy of ATP hydrolysis coupled to polymer synthesis?

Each type of macromolecule is generated by an enzyme-catalyzed pathway that resembles the one discussed previously for the synthesis of the amino acid glutamine (see Figure 3–32). The principle is exactly the same, in that the –OH group that will be removed in the condensation reaction is first activated by forming a high-energy linkage to a second molecule. The mechanisms used to link ATP hydrolysis to the synthesis of proteins and polysaccharides, however, are more complex than that used for glutamine synthesis. In the biosynthetic pathways leading

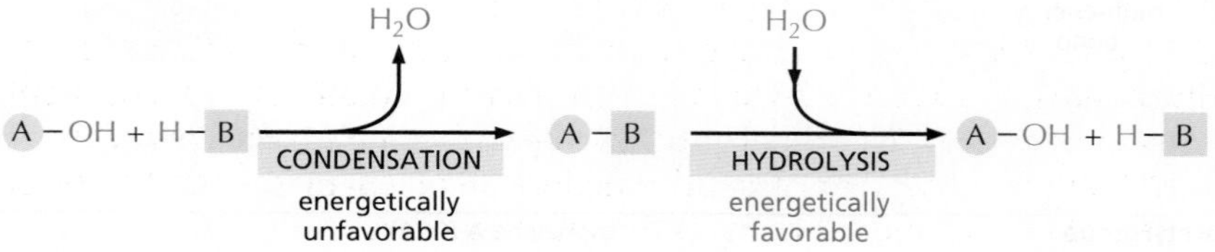

Figure 3–39 In cells, macromolecules are synthesized by condensation reactions and broken down by hydrolysis reactions. Condensation reactions are all energetically unfavorable, whereas hydrolysis reactions are all energetically favorable.

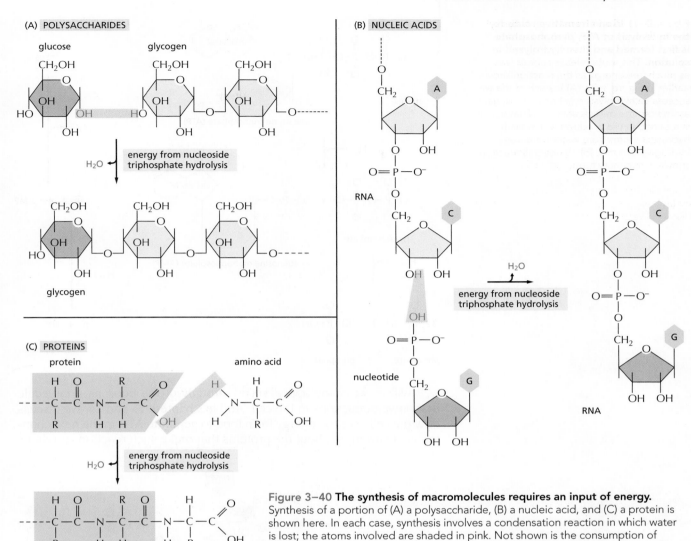

Figure 3–40 The synthesis of macromolecules requires an input of energy. Synthesis of a portion of (A) a polysaccharide, (B) a nucleic acid, and (C) a protein is shown here. In each case, synthesis involves a condensation reaction in which water is lost; the atoms involved are shaded in pink. Not shown is the consumption of high-energy nucleoside triphosphates that is required to activate each subunit prior to its addition. In contrast, the reverse reaction—the breakdown of all three types of polymers—occurs through the simple addition of water, or hydrolysis (not shown).

to these macromolecules, several high-energy intermediates are consumed in series to generate the final high-energy bond that will be broken during the condensation step. One important example of such a biosynthetic reaction, that of protein synthesis, is discussed in detail in Chapter 7.

There are limits to what each activated carrier can do in driving biosynthesis. For example, the ΔG for the hydrolysis of ATP to ADP and inorganic phosphate (P_i) depends on the concentrations of all of the reactants, and under the usual conditions in a cell, it is between –46 and –54 kJ/mole. In principle, this hydrolysis reaction can be used to drive an unfavorable reaction with a ΔG of, perhaps, +40 kJ/mole, provided that a suitable reaction path is available. For some biosynthetic reactions, however, even –54 kJ/mole may be insufficient. In these cases, the path of ATP hydrolysis can be altered so that it initially produces AMP and pyrophosphate (PP_i), which is itself then hydrolyzed in solution in a subsequent step (**Figure 3–41**). The whole process makes available a total ΔG of about –109 kJ/mole. The biosynthetic reaction involved in the synthesis of nucleic acids (polynucleotides) is driven in this way (**Figure 3–42**).

QUESTION 3–9

Which of the following reactions will occur only if coupled to a second, energetically favorable reaction?
A. glucose + O_2 → CO_2 + H_2O
B. CO_2 + H_2O → glucose + O_2
C. nucleoside triphosphates → DNA
D. nucleotide bases → nucleoside triphosphates
E. ADP + P_i → ATP

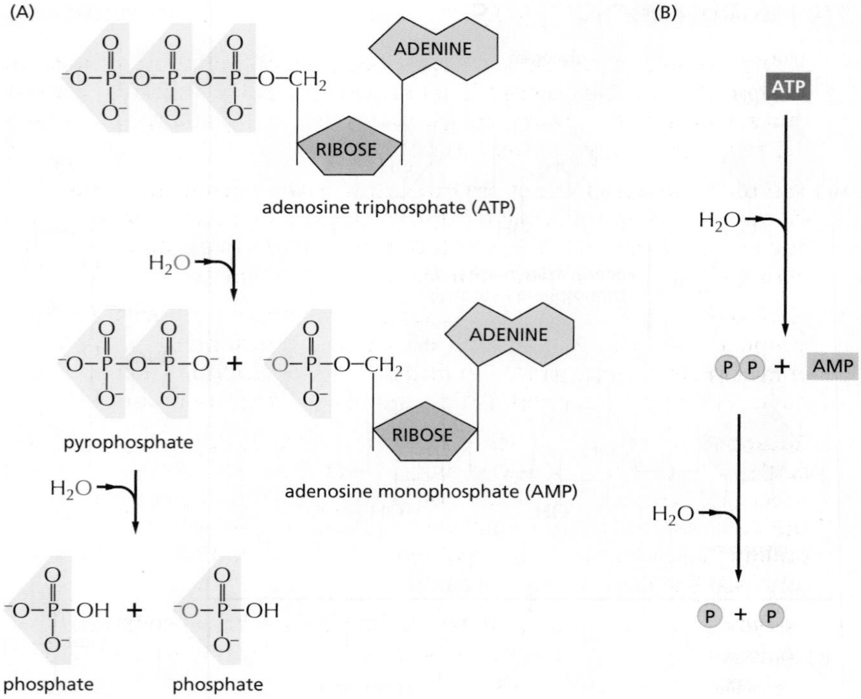

Figure 3–41 In an alternative route for the hydrolysis of ATP, pyrophosphate is first formed and then hydrolyzed in solution. This route releases about twice as much free energy as the reaction shown earlier in Figure 3–30. (A) In each of the two successive hydrolysis reactions, an oxygen atom from the participating water molecule is retained in the products, whereas the hydrogen atoms from water form free hydrogen ions, H⁺. (B) The overall reaction shown in summary form.

ATP will make many appearances throughout the book as a molecule that powers reactions in the cell. And in Chapters 13 and 14, we discuss how the cell uses the energy from food to generate ATP. In the next chapter, we learn more about the proteins that make such reactions possible.

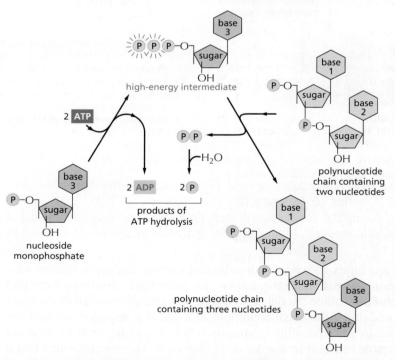

Figure 3–42 Synthesis of a polynucleotide, RNA or DNA, is a multistep process driven by ATP hydrolysis. In the first step, a nucleoside monophosphate is activated by the sequential transfer of the terminal phosphate groups from two ATP molecules. The high-energy intermediate formed—a nucleoside triphosphate—exists free in solution until it reacts with the growing end of an RNA or a DNA chain, with release of pyrophosphate. Hydrolysis of the pyrophosphate to inorganic phosphate is highly favorable and helps to drive the overall reaction in the direction of polynucleotide synthesis.

ESSENTIAL CONCEPTS

- Living organisms are able to exist because of a continual input of energy. Part of this energy is used to carry out essential reactions that support cell metabolism, growth, movement, and reproduction; the remainder is lost in the form of heat.

- The ultimate source of energy for most living organisms is the sun. Plants, algae, and photosynthetic bacteria use solar energy to produce organic molecules from carbon dioxide. Animals obtain food by eating plants or by eating animals that feed on plants.

- Each of the many hundreds of chemical reactions that occur in a cell is specifically catalyzed by an enzyme. Large numbers of different enzymes work in sequence to form chains of reactions, called metabolic pathways, each performing a different function in the cell.

- Catabolic reactions release energy by breaking down organic molecules, including foods, through oxidative pathways. Anabolic reactions generate the many complex organic molecules needed by the cell, and they require an energy input. In animal cells, both the building blocks and the energy required for the anabolic reactions are obtained through catabolic reactions.

- Enzymes catalyze reactions by binding to particular substrate molecules in a way that lowers the activation energy required for making and breaking specific covalent bonds.

- The rate at which an enzyme catalyzes a reaction depends on how rapidly it finds its substrates and how quickly the product forms and then diffuses away. These rates vary widely from one enzyme to another.

- The only chemical reactions possible are those that increase the total amount of disorder in the universe. The free-energy change for a reaction, ΔG, measures this disorder, and it must be less than zero for a reaction to proceed spontaneously.

- The ΔG for a chemical reaction depends on the concentrations of the reacting molecules, and it may be calculated from these concentrations if the equilibrium constant (K) of the reaction (or the standard free-energy change, $\Delta G°$, for the reactants) is known.

- Equilibrium constants govern all of the associations (and dissociations) that occur between macromolecules and small molecules in the cell. The larger the binding energy between two molecules, the larger the equilibrium constant and the more likely that these molecules will be found bound to each other.

- By creating a reaction pathway that couples an energetically favorable reaction to an energetically unfavorable one, enzymes can make otherwise impossible chemical transformations occur. Large numbers of such coupled reactions make life possible.

- A small set of activated carriers, particularly ATP, NADH, and NADPH, plays a central part in these coupled reactions in cells. ATP carries high-energy phosphate groups, whereas NADH and NADPH carry high-energy electrons.

- Food molecules provide the carbon skeletons for the formation of macromolecules. The covalent bonds of these larger molecules are produced by condensation reactions that are coupled to energetically favorable bond changes in activated carriers such as ATP and NADPH.

KEY TERMS

acetyl CoA	equilibrium
activated carrier	equilibrium constant, K
activation energy	free energy, G
ADP, ATP	free-energy change, ΔG
anabolism	metabolism
biosynthesis	NAD$^+$, NADH
catabolism	NADP$^+$, NADPH
catalyst	oxidation
cell respiration	photosynthesis
coupled reaction	reduction
diffusion	standard free-energy change, $\Delta G°$
entropy	substrate
enzyme	

QUESTIONS

QUESTION 3–10

Which of the following statements are correct? Explain your answers.

A. Some enzyme-catalyzed reactions cease completely if their enzyme is absent.

B. High-energy electrons (such as those found in the activated carriers NADH and NADPH) move faster around the atomic nucleus.

C. Hydrolysis of ATP to AMP can provide about twice as much energy as hydrolysis of ATP to ADP.

D. A partially oxidized carbon atom has a somewhat smaller diameter than a more reduced one.

E. Some activated carrier molecules can transfer both energy and a chemical group to a second molecule.

F. The rule that oxidations release energy, whereas reductions require energy input, applies to all chemical reactions, not just those that occur in living cells.

G. Cold-blooded animals have an energetic disadvantage because they release less heat to the environment than warm-blooded animals do. This slows their ability to make ordered macromolecules.

H. Linking the reaction X → Y to a second, energetically favorable reaction Y → Z will shift the equilibrium constant of the first reaction.

QUESTION 3–11

Consider a transition of X → Y. Assume that the only difference between X and Y is the presence of three hydrogen bonds in Y that are absent in X. What is the ratio of X to Y when the reaction is in equilibrium? Approximate your answer by using Table 3–1 (p. 96), with 4.2 kJ/mole as the energy of each hydrogen bond. If Y instead has six hydrogen bonds that distinguish it from X, how would that change the ratio?

QUESTION 3–12

Protein A binds to protein B to form a complex, AB. At equilibrium in a cell the concentrations of A, B, and AB are all at 1 μM.

A. Referring to Figure 3–19, calculate the equilibrium constant for the reaction A + B ↔ AB.

B. What would the equilibrium constant be if A, B, and AB were each present in equilibrium at the much lower concentrations of 1 nM each?

C. How many extra hydrogen bonds would be needed to hold A and B together at this lower concentration so that a similar proportion of the molecules are found in the AB complex? (Remember that each hydrogen bond contributes about 4.2 kJ/mole.)

QUESTION 3–13

Discuss the following statement: "Whether the ΔG for a reaction is larger, smaller, or the same as $\Delta G°$ depends on the concentration of the compounds that participate in the reaction."

QUESTION 3–14

A. How many ATP molecules could maximally be generated from one molecule of glucose, if the complete oxidation of 1 mole of glucose to CO_2 and H_2O yields 2867 kJ of free energy and the useful chemical energy available in the high-energy phosphate bond of 1 mole of ATP is 50 kJ?

B. As we will see in Chapter 14 (Table 14–1), respiration produces 30 moles of ATP from 1 mole of glucose. Compare this number with your answer in part (A). What is the overall efficiency of ATP production from glucose?

C. If the cells of your body oxidize 1 mole of glucose, by how much would the temperature of your body (assume that your body consists of 75 kg of water) increase if the heat were not dissipated into the environment? [Recall that a kilocalorie (kcal) is defined as that amount of energy that heats 1 kg of water by 1°C. And 1 kJ equals 0.24 kcal.]

D. What would the consequences be if the cells of your body could convert the energy in food substances with only 20% efficiency? Would your body—as it is presently constructed—work just fine, overheat, or freeze?

E. A resting human hydrolyzes about 40 kg of ATP every 24 hours. The oxidation of how much glucose would produce this amount of energy? (Hint: Look up the structure of ATP in Figure 2–26 to calculate its molecular weight; the atomic weights of H, C, N, O, and P are 1, 12, 14, 16, and 31, respectively.)

QUESTION 3–15

A prominent scientist claims to have isolated mutant cells that can convert 1 molecule of glucose into 57 molecules of ATP. Should this discovery be celebrated, or do you suppose that something might be wrong with it? Explain your answer.

QUESTION 3–16

In a simple reaction A ↔ A*, a molecule is interconvertible between two forms that differ in standard free energy $G°$ by 18 kJ/mole, with A* having the higher $G°$.

A. Use Table 3–1 (p. 96) to find how many more molecules will be in state A* compared with state A at equilibrium.

B. If an enzyme lowered the activation energy of the reaction by 11.7 kJ/mole, how would the ratio of A to A* change?

QUESTION 3–17

In a mushroom, a reaction in a single-step biosynthetic pathway that converts a metabolite into a particularly vicious poison (metabolite ↔ poison) is energetically highly unfavorable. The reaction is normally driven by ATP hydrolysis. Assume that a mutation in the enzyme that catalyzes the reaction prevents it from utilizing ATP, but still allows it to catalyze the reaction.

A. Do you suppose it might be safe for you to eat a mushroom that bears this mutation? Base your answer on an estimation of how much less poison the mutant mushroom would produce, assuming the reaction is in equilibrium and most of the energy stored in ATP is used to drive the unfavorable reaction in nonmutant mushrooms.

B. Would your answer be different for another mutant mushroom whose enzyme couples the reaction to ATP hydrolysis but works 100 times more slowly?

QUESTION 3–18

Consider the effects of two enzymes, A and B. Enzyme A catalyzes the reaction

$$ATP + GDP \leftrightarrow ADP + GTP$$

and enzyme B catalyzes the reaction

$$NADH + NADP^+ \leftrightarrow NAD^+ + NADPH$$

Discuss whether the enzymes would be beneficial or detrimental to cells.

QUESTION 3–19

Discuss the following statement: "Enzymes and heat are alike in that both can speed up reactions that—although thermodynamically feasible—do not occur at an appreciable rate because they require a high activation energy. Diseases that seem to benefit from the careful application of heat—in the form of hot chicken soup, for example—are therefore likely to be due to the insufficient function of an enzyme."

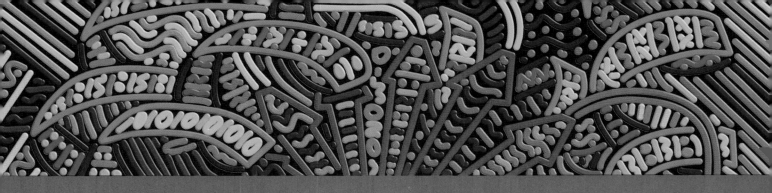

CHAPTER **FOUR**

4

Protein Structure and Function

When we look at a cell in a microscope or analyze its electrical or biochemical activity, we are, in essence, observing the handiwork of proteins. **Proteins** are the main building blocks from which cells are assembled, and they constitute most of the cell's dry mass. In addition to providing the cell with shape and structure, proteins also execute nearly all its myriad functions. *Enzymes* promote intracellular chemical reactions by providing intricate molecular surfaces contoured with particular bumps and crevices that can cradle or exclude specific molecules. Transporters and channels embedded in the plasma membrane control the passage of nutrients and other small molecules into and out of the cell. Other proteins carry messages from one cell to another, or act as signal integrators that relay information from the plasma membrane to the nucleus of individual cells. Some proteins act as motors that propel organelles through the cytosol, and others function as components of tiny molecular machines with precisely calibrated moving parts. Specialized proteins also act as antibodies, toxins, hormones, antifreeze molecules, elastic fibers, or luminescence generators. To understand how muscles contract, how nerves conduct electricity, how embryos develop, or how our bodies function, we must first understand how proteins operate.

The multiplicity of functions carried out by these remarkable macromolecules, a few of which are represented in **Panel 4–1**, p. 118, arises from the huge number of different shapes proteins adopt. We therefore begin our description of proteins by discussing their three-dimensional structures and the properties that these structures confer. We next look at how proteins work: how enzymes catalyze chemical reactions, how some proteins act as molecular switches, and how others generate orderly movement. We then examine how cells control the activity and location

THE SHAPE AND STRUCTURE
OF PROTEINS

HOW PROTEINS WORK

HOW PROTEINS ARE
CONTROLLED

HOW PROTEINS ARE STUDIED

ENZYMES

function: Catalyze covalent bond breakage or formation

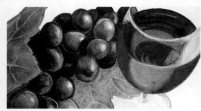

examples: Living cells contain thousands of different enzymes, each of which catalyzes (speeds up) one particular reaction. Examples include: *alcohol dehydrogenase*—makes the alcohol in wine; *pepsin*—degrades dietary proteins in the stomach; *ribulose bisphosphate carboxylase*—helps convert carbon dioxide into sugars in plants; *DNA polymerase*—copies DNA; *protein kinase*—adds a phosphate group to a protein molecule.

STRUCTURAL PROTEINS

function: Provide mechanical support to cells and tissues

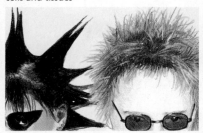

examples: Outside cells, *collagen* and *elastin* are common constituents of extracellular matrix and form fibers in tendons and ligaments. Inside cells, *tubulin* forms long, stiff microtubules, and *actin* forms filaments that underlie and support the plasma membrane; *keratin* forms fibers that reinforce epithelial cells and is the major protein in hair and horn.

TRANSPORT PROTEINS

function: Carry small molecules or ions

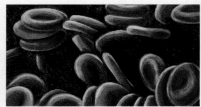

examples: In the bloodstream, *serum albumin* carries lipids, *hemoglobin* carries oxygen, and *transferrin* carries iron. Many proteins embedded in cell membranes transport ions or small molecules across the membrane. For example, the bacterial protein *bacteriorhodopsin* is a light-activated proton pump that transports H+ ions out of the cell; *glucose transporters* shuttle glucose into and out of cells; and a *Ca2+ pump* clears Ca^{2+} from a muscle cell's cytosol after the ions have triggered a contraction.

MOTOR PROTEINS

function: Generate movement in cells and tissues

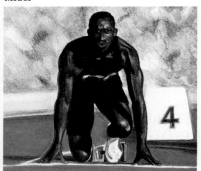

examples: *Myosin* in skeletal muscle cells provides the motive force for humans to move; *kinesin* interacts with microtubules to move organelles around the cell; *dynein* enables eukaryotic cilia and flagella to beat.

STORAGE PROTEINS

function: Store amino acids or ions

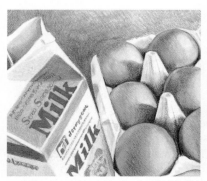

examples: Iron is stored in the liver by binding to the small protein *ferritin*; *ovalbumin* in egg white is used as a source of amino acids for the developing bird embryo; *casein* in milk is a source of amino acids for baby mammals.

SIGNAL PROTEINS

function: Carry extracellular signals from cell to cell

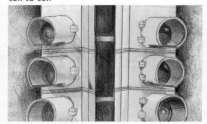

examples: Many of the hormones and growth factors that coordinate physiological functions in animals are proteins. *Insulin*, for example, is a small protein that controls glucose levels in the blood; *netrin* attracts growing nerve cell axons to specific locations in the developing spinal cord; *nerve growth factor* (NGF) stimulates some types of nerve cells to grow axons; *epidermal growth factor* (EGF) stimulates the growth and division of epithelial cells.

RECEPTOR PROTEINS

function: Detect signals and transmit them to the cell's response machinery

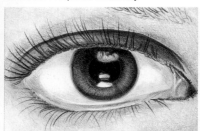

examples: *Rhodopsin* in the retina detects light; the *acetylcholine receptor* in the membrane of a muscle cell is activated by acetylcholine released from a nerve ending; the *insulin receptor* allows a cell to respond to the hormone insulin by taking up glucose; the *adrenergic receptor* on heart muscle increases the rate of the heartbeat when it binds to epinephrine secreted by the adrenal gland.

TRANSCRIPTION REGULATORS

function: Bind to DNA to switch genes on or off

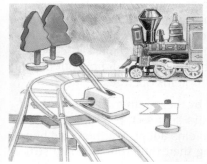

examples: The *Lac repressor* in bacteria silences the genes for the enzymes that degrade the sugar lactose; many different *DNA-binding proteins* act as genetic switches to control development in multicellular organisms, including humans.

SPECIAL-PURPOSE PROTEINS

function: Highly variable

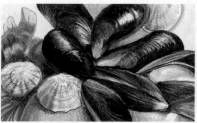

examples: Organisms make many proteins with highly specialized properties. These molecules illustrate the amazing range of functions that proteins can perform. The *antifreeze proteins* of Arctic and Antarctic fishes protect their blood against freezing; *green fluorescent protein* from jellyfish emits a green light; *monellin*, a protein found in an African plant, has an intensely sweet taste; mussels and other marine organisms secrete *glue proteins* that attach them firmly to rocks, even when immersed in seawater.

of the proteins they contain. Finally, we present a brief description of the techniques that biologists use to work with proteins, including methods for purifying them—from tissues or cultured cells—and for determining their structures.

THE SHAPE AND STRUCTURE OF PROTEINS

From a chemical point of view, proteins are by far the most structurally complex and functionally sophisticated molecules known. This is perhaps not surprising, considering that the structure and activity of each protein has developed and been fine-tuned over billions of years of evolution. We start by considering how the position of each amino acid in the long string of amino acids that forms a protein determines its three-dimensional conformation, a shape that is stabilized by noncovalent interactions between different parts of the molecule. Understanding the structure of a protein at the atomic level allows us to see how the precise shape of the protein determines its function.

The Shape of a Protein Is Specified by Its Amino Acid Sequence

Proteins, as you may recall from Chapter 2, are assembled mainly from a set of 20 different amino acids, each with different chemical properties. A protein molecule is made from a long chain of these amino acids, held together by covalent **peptide bonds** (**Figure 4–1**). Proteins are therefore referred to as **polypeptides**, or **polypeptide chains**. In each type of protein, the amino acids are present in a unique order, called the **amino acid sequence**, which is exactly the same from one molecule of that protein to the next. One molecule of human insulin, for example, should have the same amino acid sequence as every other molecule of human insulin. Many thousands of different proteins have been identified, each with its own distinct amino acid sequence.

Each polypeptide chain consists of a backbone that is adorned with a variety of chemical side chains. The **polypeptide backbone** is formed from a repeating sequence of the core atoms (–N–C–C–) found in every

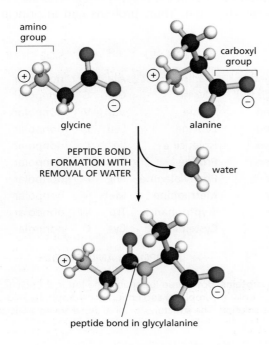

amino group

carboxyl group

glycine   alanine

PEPTIDE BOND
FORMATION WITH
REMOVAL OF WATER

water

peptide bond in glycylalanine

Figure 4–1 Amino acids are linked together by peptide bonds. A covalent peptide bond forms when the carbon atom of the carboxyl group of one amino acid (such as glycine) shares electrons with the nitrogen atom from the amino group of a second amino acid (such as alanine). Because a molecule of water is eliminated, peptide bond formation is classified as a condensation reaction (see Figure 2–31). In this diagram, carbon atoms are *black*, nitrogen *blue*, oxygen *red*, and hydrogen *white*.

Figure 4–2 A protein is made of amino acids linked together into a polypeptide chain. The amino acids are linked by peptide bonds (see Figure 4–1) to form a polypeptide backbone of repeating structure (*gray boxes*), from which the side chain of each amino acid projects. The sequence of these chemically distinct side chains—which can be nonpolar (*green*), polar uncharged (*yellow*), positively charged (*red*), or negatively charged (*blue*)—gives each protein its distinct, individual properties. A small polypeptide of just four amino acids is shown here. Proteins are typically made up of chains of several hundred amino acids, whose sequence is always presented starting with the N-terminus and read from left to right.

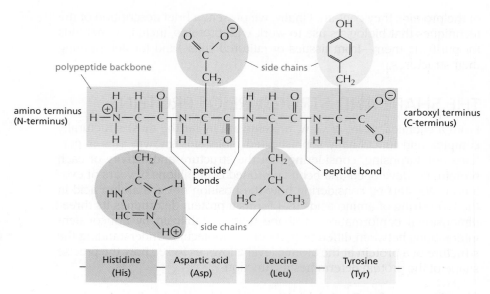

amino acid (**Figure 4–2**). Because the two ends of each amino acid are chemically different—one sports an amino group (NH_3^+, also written NH_2) and the other a carboxyl group (COO^-, also written $COOH$)—each polypeptide chain has a directionality: the end carrying the amino group is called the amino terminus, or **N-terminus**, and the end carrying the free carboxyl group is the carboxyl terminus, or **C-terminus**.

Projecting from the polypeptide backbone are the amino acid **side chains**—the part of the amino acid that is not involved in forming peptide bonds (see Figure 4–2). The side chains give each amino acid its unique properties: some are nonpolar and hydrophobic ("water-fearing"), some are negatively or positively charged, some can be chemically reactive, and so on. The atomic formula for each of the 20 amino acids in proteins is presented in Panel 2–6 (pp. 76–77), and a brief list of the 20 common amino acids, with their abbreviations, is provided in **Figure 4–3**.

Long polypeptide chains are very flexible, as many of the covalent bonds that link the carbon atoms in the polypeptide backbone allow free rotation of the atoms they join. Thus, proteins can in principle fold in an

AMINO ACID			SIDE CHAIN	AMINO ACID			SIDE CHAIN
Aspartic acid	Asp	D	negatively charged	Alanine	Ala	A	nonpolar
Glutamic acid	Glu	E	negatively charged	Glycine	Gly	G	nonpolar
Arginine	Arg	R	positively charged	Valine	Val	V	nonpolar
Lysine	Lys	K	positively charged	Leucine	Leu	L	nonpolar
Histidine	His	H	positively charged	Isoleucine	Ile	I	nonpolar
Asparagine	Asn	N	uncharged polar	Proline	Pro	P	nonpolar
Glutamine	Gln	Q	uncharged polar	Phenylalanine	Phe	F	nonpolar
Serine	Ser	S	uncharged polar	Methionine	Met	M	nonpolar
Threonine	Thr	T	uncharged polar	Tryptophan	Trp	W	nonpolar
Tyrosine	Tyr	Y	uncharged polar	Cysteine	Cys	C	nonpolar
── POLAR AMINO ACIDS ──				── NONPOLAR AMINO ACIDS ──			

Figure 4–3 Twenty different amino acids are commonly found in proteins. Both three-letter and one-letter abbreviations are given, as well as the character of the side chain. There are equal numbers of polar (hydrophilic) and nonpolar (hydrophobic) side chains, and half of the polar side chains are charged at neutral pH in an aqueous solution. The structures of all of these amino acids are shown in Panel 2–6, pp. 76–77.

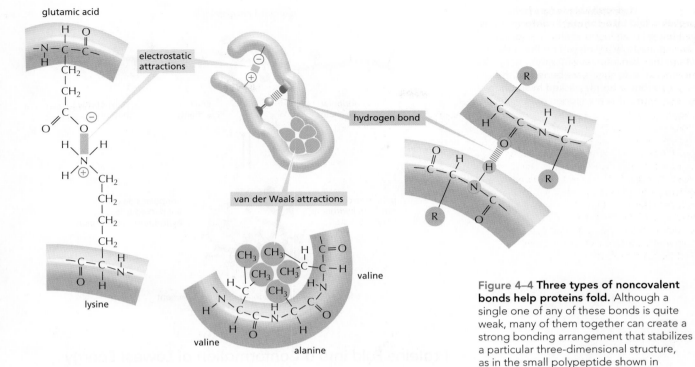

Figure 4–4 **Three types of noncovalent bonds help proteins fold.** Although a single one of any of these bonds is quite weak, many of them together can create a strong bonding arrangement that stabilizes a particular three-dimensional structure, as in the small polypeptide shown in the center. R is often used as a general designation for an amino acid side chain. Protein folding is also aided by hydrophobic forces, as shown in Figure 4–5.

enormous number of ways. The shape of each of these folded chains, however, is constrained by many sets of weak noncovalent bonds that form within proteins. These bonds involve atoms in the polypeptide backbone, as well as atoms within the amino acid side chains. The noncovalent bonds that help proteins fold up and maintain their shape include hydrogen bonds, electrostatic attractions, and van der Waals attractions, which are described in Chapter 2 (see Panel 2–3, pp. 70–71). Because a noncovalent bond is much weaker than a covalent bond, it takes many noncovalent bonds to hold two regions of a polypeptide chain tightly together. The stability of each folded shape is largely determined by the combined strength of large numbers of noncovalent bonds (**Figure 4–4**).

A fourth weak interaction, the *hydrophobic force*, also has a central role in determining the shape of a protein. In an aqueous environment, hydrophobic molecules, including the nonpolar side chains of particular amino acids, tend to be forced together to minimize their disruptive effect on the hydrogen-bonded network of the surrounding water molecules (see Panel 2–3, pp. 70–71). Therefore, an important factor governing the folding of any protein is the distribution of its polar and nonpolar amino acids. The nonpolar (hydrophobic) side chains—which belong to amino acids such as phenylalanine, leucine, valine, and tryptophan (see Figure 4–3)—tend to cluster in the interior of the folded protein (just as hydrophobic oil droplets coalesce to form one large drop). Tucked away inside the folded protein, hydrophobic side chains can avoid contact with the aqueous environment that surrounds them inside a cell. In contrast, polar side chains—such as those belonging to arginine, glutamine, and histidine—tend to arrange themselves near the outside of the folded protein, where they can form hydrogen bonds with water and with other polar molecules (**Figure 4–5**). When polar amino acids are buried within the protein, they are usually hydrogen-bonded to other polar amino acids or to the polypeptide backbone (**Figure 4–6**).

Figure 4–5 Hydrophobic forces help proteins fold into compact conformations. In a folded protein, polar amino acid side chains tend to be displayed on the surface, where they can interact with water; nonpolar amino acid side chains are buried on the inside to form a tightly packed hydrophobic core of atoms that are hidden from water.

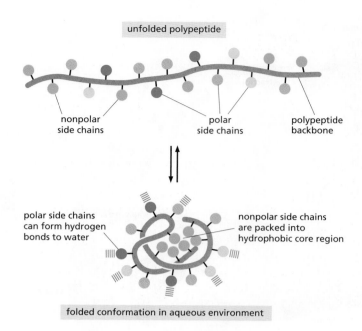

unfolded polypeptide

nonpolar side chains   polar side chains   polypeptide backbone

polar side chains can form hydrogen bonds to water   nonpolar side chains are packed into hydrophobic core region

folded conformation in aqueous environment

Proteins Fold into a Conformation of Lowest Energy

Each type of protein has a particular three-dimensional structure, which is determined by the order of the amino acids in its polypeptide chain. The final folded structure, or **conformation**, adopted by any polypeptide chain is determined by energetic considerations: a protein generally folds into the shape in which its free energy (G) is minimized. The folding process is thus energetically favorable, as it releases heat and increases the disorder of the universe (see Panel 3–1, pp. 94–95).

Figure 4–6 Hydrogen bonds within a protein molecule help stabilize its folded shape. Large numbers of hydrogen bonds form between adjacent regions of a folded polypeptide chain. The structure shown is a portion of the enzyme lysozyme, between amino acids 42 and 63. Hydrogen bonds between two atoms in the polypeptide backbone are shown in *red*; those between the backbone and a side chain are shown in *yellow*; and those between atoms of two side chains are shown in *blue*. Note that the same amino acid side chain can make multiple hydrogen bonds (*red* arrow). In this diagram, nitrogen atoms are *blue*, oxygen atoms are *red*, and carbon atoms are *gray*; hydrogen atoms are not shown. (After C.K. Mathews, K.E. van Holde, and K.G. Ahern, Biochemistry, 3rd ed. San Francisco: Benjamin Cummings, 2000.)

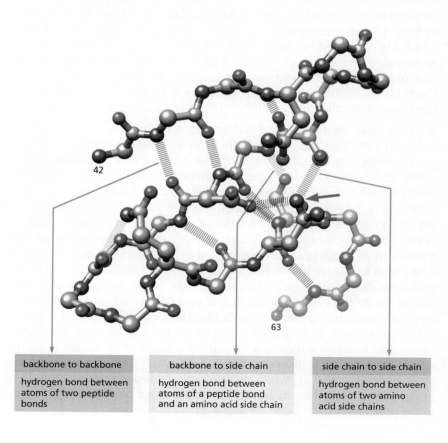

42

63

backbone to backbone
hydrogen bond between atoms of two peptide bonds

backbone to side chain
hydrogen bond between atoms of a peptide bond and an amino acid side chain

side chain to side chain
hydrogen bond between atoms of two amino acid side chains

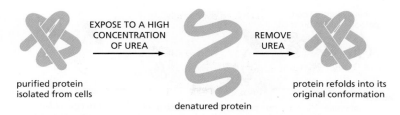

purified protein
isolated from cells

EXPOSE TO A HIGH
CONCENTRATION
OF UREA

denatured protein

REMOVE
UREA

protein refolds into its
original conformation

Figure 4–7 Denatured proteins can often recover their natural shapes. This type of experiment demonstrates that the conformation of a protein is determined solely by its amino acid sequence. Renaturation requires the correct conditions and works best for small proteins.

Protein folding has been studied in the laboratory using highly purified proteins. A protein can be unfolded, or *denatured*, by treatment with solvents that disrupt the noncovalent interactions holding the folded chain together. This treatment converts the protein into a flexible polypeptide chain that has lost its natural shape. Under the right conditions, when the denaturing solvent is removed, the protein often refolds spontaneously into its original conformation—a process called *renaturation* (**Figure 4–7**). The fact that a denatured protein can, on its own, refold into the correct conformation indicates that all the information necessary to specify the three-dimensional shape of a protein is contained in its amino acid sequence.

Although a protein chain can fold into its correct conformation without outside help, protein folding in a living cell is generally assisted by a large set of special proteins called *chaperone proteins*. Some of these chaperones bind to partly folded chains and help them to fold along the most energetically favorable pathway (**Figure 4–8**). Others form "isolation chambers" in which single polypeptide chains can fold without the risk of forming aggregates in the crowded conditions of the cytoplasm (**Figure 4–9**). In either case, the final three-dimensional shape of the protein is still specified by its amino acid sequence; chaperones merely make the folding process more efficient and reliable.

Each protein normally folds into a single, stable conformation. This conformation, however, often changes slightly when the protein interacts with other molecules in the cell. Such changes in shape are crucial to the function of the protein, as we discuss later.

QUESTION 4–1

Urea, used in the experiment shown in Figure 4–7, is a molecule that disrupts the hydrogen-bonded network of water molecules. Why might high concentrations of urea unfold proteins? The structure of urea is shown here.

$$\begin{array}{c} O \\ \| \\ C \\ / \quad \backslash \\ H_2N \quad NH_2 \end{array}$$

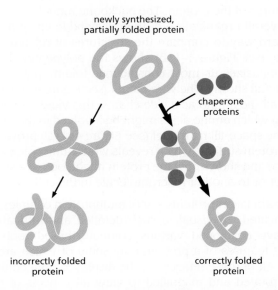

newly synthesized,
partially folded protein

chaperone
proteins

incorrectly folded
protein

correctly folded
protein

Figure 4–8 Chaperone proteins can guide the folding of a newly synthesized polypeptide chain. The chaperones bind to newly synthesized or partially folded chains and help them to fold along the most energetically favorable pathway. The function of these chaperones requires ATP binding and hydrolysis.

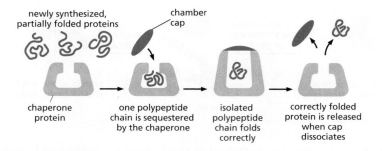

newly synthesized,
partially folded proteins

chamber
cap

chaperone
protein

one polypeptide
chain is sequestered
by the chaperone

isolated
polypeptide
chain folds
correctly

correctly folded
protein is released
when cap
dissociates

Figure 4–9 Some chaperone proteins act as isolation chambers that help a polypeptide fold. In this case, the barrel of the chaperone provides an enclosed chamber in which a newly synthesized polypeptide chain can fold without the risk of aggregating with other polypeptides in the crowded conditions of the cytoplasm. This system also requires an input of energy from ATP hydrolysis, mainly for the association and subsequent dissociation of the cap that closes off the chamber.

Proteins Come in a Wide Variety of Complicated Shapes

Proteins are the most structurally diverse macromolecules in the cell. Although they range in size from about 30 amino acids to more than 10,000, the vast majority are between 50 and 2000 amino acids long. Proteins can be globular or fibrous, and they can form filaments, sheets, rings, or spheres (**Figure 4–10**). We will encounter many of these structures throughout the book.

To date, the structures of about 100,000 different proteins have been determined (using techniques we discuss later in the chapter). Most proteins have a three-dimensional conformation so intricate and irregular that their structure would require the rest of the chapter to describe in detail. But we can get some sense of the intricacies of polypeptide structure by looking at the conformation of a relatively small protein, such as the bacterial transport protein *HPr*.

This small protein, only 88 amino acids long, facilitates the transport of sugar into bacterial cells. In **Figure 4–11**, we present HPr's three-dimensional structure in four different ways, each of which emphasizes different features of the protein. The backbone model (see Figure 4–11A) shows the overall organization of the polypeptide chain and provides a straightforward way to compare the structures of related proteins. The ribbon model (see Figure 4–11B) shows the polypeptide backbone in a way that emphasizes its most conspicuous folding patterns, which we describe in detail shortly. The wire model (see Figure 4–11C) includes the positions of all the amino acid side chains; this view is especially useful for predicting which amino acids might be involved in the protein's activity. Finally, the space-filling model (see Figure 4–11D) provides a contour map of the protein surface, which reveals which amino acids are exposed on the surface and shows how the protein might look to a small molecule such as water or to another macromolecule in the cell.

The structures of larger proteins—or of multiprotein complexes—are even more complicated. To visualize such detailed and intricate structures, scientists have developed various computer-based tools to emphasize different features of a protein, only some of which are depicted in Figure 4–11. All of these images can be displayed on a computer screen and readily rotated and magnified to view all aspects of the structure (Movie 4.1).

When the three-dimensional structures of many different protein molecules are compared, it becomes clear that, although the overall

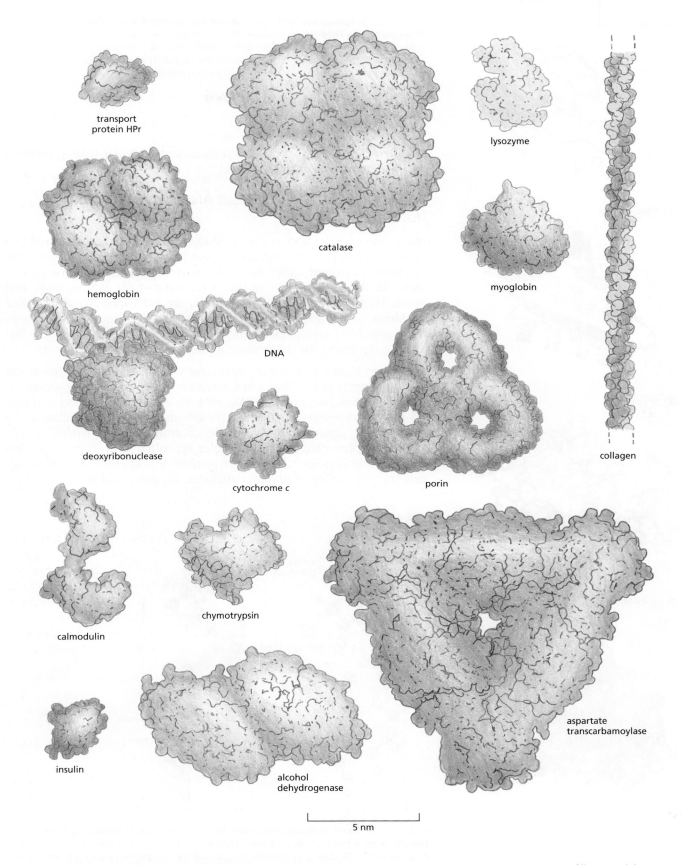

transport
protein HPr

lysozyme

catalase

hemoglobin

myoglobin

DNA

deoxyribonuclease

collagen

cytochrome c

porin

calmodulin

chymotrypsin

aspartate
transcarbamoylase

insulin

alcohol
dehydrogenase

5 nm

Figure 4–10 Proteins come in a wide variety of shapes and sizes. Each folded polypeptide is shown as a space-filling model, represented at the same scale. In the top-left corner is HPr, the small transport protein featured in detail in Figure 4–11. The protein deoxyribonuclease is shown bound to a portion of a DNA molecule (*gray*) for comparison.

(A) backbone model

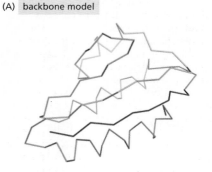

Figure 4–11 Protein conformation can be represented in a variety of ways. Shown here is the structure of the small bacterial transport protein HPr. The images are colored to make it easier to trace the path of the polypeptide chain. In these models, the region of polypeptide chain carrying the protein's N-terminus is *purple* and that near its C-terminus is *red*.

conformation of each protein is unique, some regular folding patterns can be detected, as we discuss next.

The α Helix and the β Sheet Are Common Folding Patterns

More than 60 years ago, scientists studying hair and silk discovered two regular folding patterns that are present in many different proteins. The first to be discovered, called the **α helix**, was found in the protein *α-keratin*, which is abundant in skin and its derivatives—such as hair, nails, and horns. Within a year of that discovery, a second folded structure, called a **β sheet**, was found in the protein *fibroin*, the major constituent of silk. (Biologists often use Greek letters to name their discoveries, with the first example receiving the designation α, the second β, and so on.)

These two folding patterns are particularly common because they result from hydrogen bonds that form between the N–H and C=O groups in the polypeptide backbone (see Figure 4–6). Because the amino acid side chains are not involved in forming these hydrogen bonds, α helices and β sheets can be generated by many different amino acid sequences. In each case, the protein chain adopts a regular, repeating form. These structural features, and the shorthand cartoon symbols that are often used to represent them in models of protein structures, are presented in **Figures 4–12** and **4–13**.

(B) ribbon model

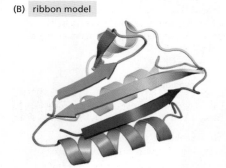

(C) wire model

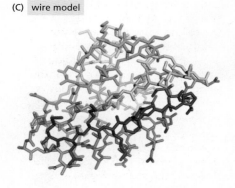

(D) space-filling model

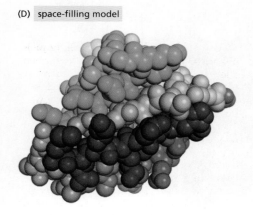

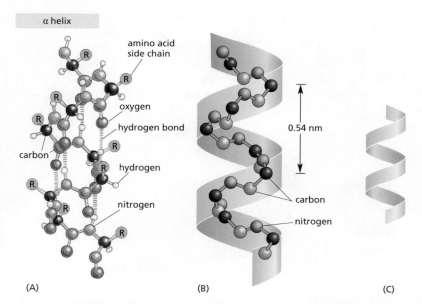

α helix

Figure 4–12 Some polypeptide chains fold into an orderly repeating form known as an α helix. (A) In an α helix, the N–H of every peptide bond is hydrogen-bonded to the C=O of a neighboring peptide bond located four amino acids away in the same chain. All of the atoms in the polypeptide backbone are shown; the amino acid side chains are denoted by R. (B) The same polypeptide, showing only the carbon (*black and gray*) and nitrogen (*blue*) atoms. (C) Cartoon symbol used to represent an α helix in ribbon models of proteins (see Figure 4–11B).

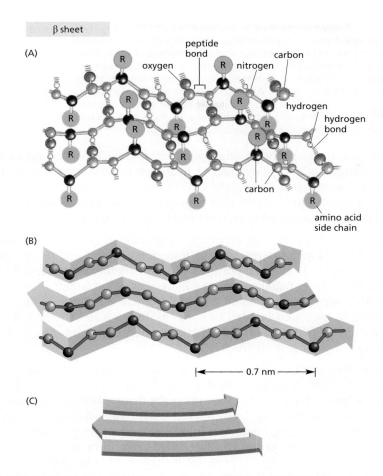

β sheet

(A)

peptide bond

oxygen | R nitrogen | carbon

R | hydrogen

hydrogen bond

carbon

amino acid side chain

(B)

|← 0.7 nm →|

(C)

Figure 4–13 Some polypeptide chains fold into an orderly pattern called a β sheet. (A) In a β sheet, several segments (strands) of an individual polypeptide chain are held together by hydrogen-bonding between peptide bonds in adjacent strands. The amino acid side chains in each strand project alternately above and below the plane of the sheet. In the example shown, the adjacent chains run in opposite directions, forming an *antiparallel* β sheet. All of the atoms in the polypeptide backbone are shown; the amino acid side chains are denoted by R. (B) The same polypeptide, showing only the carbon (*black* and *gray*) and nitrogen (*blue*) atoms. (C) Cartoon symbol used to represent β sheets in ribbon models of proteins (see Figure 4–11B).

QUESTION 4–2

Remembering that the amino acid side chains projecting from each polypeptide backbone in a β sheet point alternately above and below the plane of the sheet (see Figure 4–13A), consider the following protein sequence: Leu-Lys-Val-Asp-Ile-Ser-Leu-Arg-Leu-Lys-Ile-Arg-Phe-Glu. Do you find anything remarkable about the arrangement of the amino acids in this sequence when incorporated into a β sheet? Can you make any predictions as to how the β sheet might be arranged in a protein? (Hint: consult the properties of the amino acids listed in Figure 4–3.)

Helices Form Readily in Biological Structures

The abundance of helices in proteins is, in a way, not surprising. A **helix** is generated simply by placing many similar subunits next to one another, each in the same strictly repeated relationship to the one before. Because it is very rare for subunits to join up in a straight line, this arrangement will generally result in a structure that resembles a spiral staircase (**Figure 4–14**). Depending on the way it twists, a helix is said to be either right-handed or left-handed (see Figure 4–14E). Handedness is not affected by turning the helix upside down, but it is reversed if the helix is reflected in a mirror.

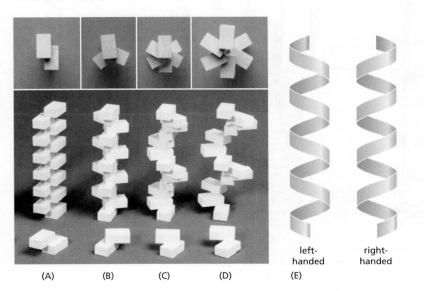

(A) (B) (C) (D) (E)

left-handed | right-handed

Figure 4–14 A helix is a common, regular, biological structure. A helix will form when a series of similar subunits bind to each other in a regular way. At the bottom, the interaction between two subunits is shown; behind them are the helices that result. These helices have (A) two, (B) three, or (C and D) six subunits per helical turn. At the top, the arrangement of subunits has been photographed from directly above the helix. Note that the helix in (D) has a wider path than that in (C), but the same number of subunits per turn. (E) A helix can be either right-handed or left-handed. As a reference, it is useful to remember that standard metal screws, which advance when turned clockwise, are right-handed. So to judge the handedness of a helix, imagine screwing it into a wall. Note that a helix preserves the same handedness when it is turned upside down. In proteins, α helices are almost always right-handed.

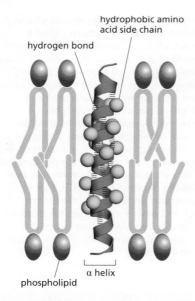

Figure 4–15 **Many membrane-bound proteins cross the lipid bilayer as an α helix.** The hydrophobic side chains of the amino acids that form the α helix make contact with the hydrophobic hydrocarbon tails of the phospholipid molecules, while the hydrophilic parts of the polypeptide backbone form hydrogen bonds with one another along the interior of the helix. About 20 amino acids are required to span a membrane in this way. Note that, despite the appearance of a space along the interior of the helix in this schematic diagram, the helix is not a channel: no ions or small molecules can pass through it.

An α helix is generated when a single polypeptide chain turns around itself to form a structurally rigid cylinder. A hydrogen bond is made between every fourth amino acid, linking the C=O of one peptide bond to the N–H of another (see Figure 4–12A). This pattern gives rise to a regular right-handed helix with a complete turn every 3.6 amino acids (Movie 4.2).

Short regions of α helix are especially abundant in proteins that are embedded in cell membranes, such as transport proteins and receptors. We see in Chapter 11 that the portions of a transmembrane protein that cross the lipid bilayer usually form an α helix, composed largely of amino acids with nonpolar side chains. The polypeptide backbone, which is hydrophilic, is hydrogen-bonded to itself inside the α helix, where it is shielded from the hydrophobic lipid environment of the membrane by the protruding nonpolar side chains (Figure 4–15).

Sometimes two (or three) α helices will wrap around one another to form a particularly stable structure called a **coiled-coil**. This structure forms when the α helices have most of their nonpolar (hydrophobic) side chains along one side, so they can twist around each other with their hydrophobic side chains facing inward—minimizing contact with the aqueous cytosol (Figure 4–16). Long, rodlike coiled-coils form the structural framework for many elongated proteins, including the α-keratin found in hair and the outer layer of the skin, as well as myosin, the motor protein responsible for muscle contraction (discussed in Chapter 17).

Figure 4–16 **Intertwined α helices can form a stiff coiled-coil.** (A) A single α helix is shown, with successive amino acid side chains labeled in a sevenfold repeating sequence "abcdefg." Amino acids "a" and "d" in such a sequence lie close together on the cylinder surface, forming a stripe (shaded in *green*) that winds slowly around the α helix. Proteins that form coiled-coils typically have nonpolar amino acids at positions "a" and "d." Consequently, as shown in (B), two α helices can wrap around each other, with the nonpolar side chains of one α helix interacting with the nonpolar side chains of the other, while the more hydrophilic amino acid side chains (shaded in *red*) are left exposed to the aqueous environment. (C) A portion of the atomic structure of a coiled-coil made by two α helices, as determined by x-ray crystallography. In this structure, the backbones of the helices are shown in *red*, the interacting, nonpolar side chains are *green*, and the remaining side chains are *light gray*. Coiled-coils can also form from three α helices (Movie 4.3).

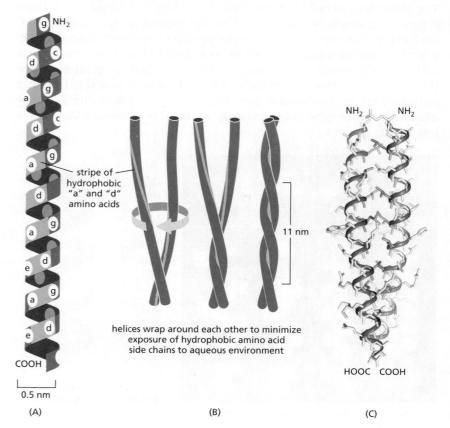

stripe of hydrophobic "a" and "d" amino acids

helices wrap around each other to minimize exposure of hydrophobic amino acid side chains to aqueous environment

11 nm

(A)   (B)   (C)

β Sheets Form Rigid Structures at the Core of Many Proteins

A β sheet is made when hydrogen bonds form between segments of a polypeptide chain that lie side by side (see Figure 4–13A). When the neighboring segments run in the same orientation (say, from the N-terminus to the C-terminus), the structure forms a *parallel β sheet*; when they run in opposite directions, the structure forms an *antiparallel β sheet* (Figure 4–17). Both types of β sheet produce a very rigid, pleated structure, and they form the core of many proteins. Even the small bacterial transport protein HPr (see Figure 4–11) contains several β sheets.

β sheets have remarkable properties. They give silk fibers their extraordinary tensile strength. They also form the basis of *amyloid structures*, in which β sheets are stacked together in long rows with their amino acid side chains interdigitated like the teeth of a zipper (Figure 4–18). Such structures play an important role in cells, as we discuss later in this chapter. However, they can also precipitate disease, as we see next.

Misfolded Proteins Can Form Amyloid Structures That Cause Disease

When proteins fold incorrectly, they sometimes form amyloid structures that can damage cells and even whole tissues. These amyloid struc-tures are thought to contribute to a number of neurodegenerative disorders, such as Alzheimer's disease and Huntington's disease. Some infectious neurodegenerative diseases—including scrapie in sheep, bovine spongiform encephalopathy (BSE, or "mad cow" disease) in cattle, and Creutzfeldt–Jakob disease (CJD) in humans—are caused by misfolded proteins called *prions*. The misfolded prion form of a protein can convert the properly folded version of the protein in an infected brain into the abnormal conformation. This allows the misfolded prions to form aggregates (Figure 4–19), which can spread rapidly from cell to cell, eventually causing the death of the affected animal or human. Prions are considered "infectious" because they can also spread from an affected individual to a normal individual via contaminated food, blood, or surgical instruments, for example.

Proteins Have Several Levels of Organization

A protein's structure does not begin and end with α helices and β sheets. Its complete conformation includes several interdependent levels of organization, which build one upon the next. Because a protein's structure begins with its amino acid sequence, this is considered its **primary structure**. The next level of organization includes the α helices and β sheets that form within certain segments of the polypeptide chain; these folds are elements of the protein's **secondary structure**. The full, three-dimensional conformation formed by an entire polypeptide chain—including the α helices, β sheets, and all other loops and folds that form between the N- and C-termini—is sometimes referred to as the **tertiary structure**. Finally, if the protein molecule exists as a complex of more than one polypeptide chain, then these interacting polypeptides form its **quaternary structure**.

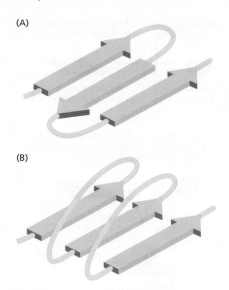

Figure 4–17 β sheets come in two varieties. (A) Antiparallel β sheet (see also Figure 4–13A). (B) Parallel β sheet. Both of these structures are common in proteins. By convention, the arrows point toward the C-terminus of the polypeptide chain (Movie 4.4).

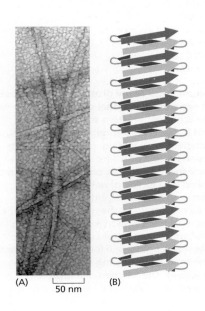

Figure 4–18 β sheets can stack to form an amyloid structure. (A) Electron micrograph showing an amyloid structure from a yeast. This structure resembles the type of insoluble aggregates observed in the neurons of individuals with different neurodegenerative diseases (see Figure 4–19). (B) Schematic representation shows the stacking of β sheets that stabilizes an individual amyloid strand. (A, from M.R. Sawaya et al., *Nature* 447:453–457, 2007. With permission from Macmillan Publishers Ltd.)

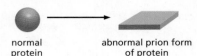

(A) normal protein can, on occasion, adopt an abnormal, misfolded prion form

normal protein   abnormal prion form of protein

(B) the prion form of the protein can bind to the normal form, inducing conversion to the abnormal conformation

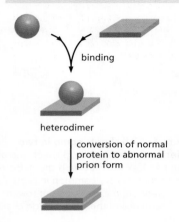

binding

heterodimer

conversion of normal protein to abnormal prion form

(C) abnormal prion proteins propagate and aggregate to form amyloid fibrils

amyloid fibril

Figure 4–19 Prion diseases are caused by proteins whose misfolding is infectious. (A) A protein undergoes a rare conformational change to produce an abnormally folded prion form. (B) The abnormal form causes the conversion of normal proteins in the host's brain into the misfolded prion form. (C) The prions aggregate into amyloid fibrils, which can disrupt brain-cell function, causing a neurodegenerative disorder (see also Figure 4–18). Some of the abnormal amyloid fibrils that form in major neurodegenerative disorders such as Alzheimer's disease may be able to propagate from cell to cell in this way.

Studies of the conformation, function, and evolution of proteins have also revealed the importance of a level of organization distinct from the four just described. This organizational unit is the **protein domain**, which is defined as any segment of a polypeptide chain that can fold independently into a compact, stable structure. A protein domain usually contains between 40 and 350 amino acids—folded into α helices and β sheets and other elements of structure—and it is the modular unit from which many larger proteins are constructed (**Figure 4–20**).

Different domains of a protein are often associated with different functions. For example, the bacterial *catabolite activator protein* (*CAP*), illustrated in Figure 4–20, has two domains: a small domain that binds to DNA and a large domain that binds cyclic AMP, a small intracellular signaling molecule. When the large domain binds cyclic AMP, it causes a conformational change in the protein that enables the small domain to bind to a specific DNA sequence and thereby promote the expression of an adjacent gene. To provide a sense of the many different domain structures observed in proteins, ribbon models of three different domains are shown in **Figure 4–21**.

Proteins Also Contain Unstructured Regions

Small protein molecules, such as the oxygen-carrying muscle protein myoglobin, contain only a single domain (see Figure 4–10). Larger proteins can contain as many as several dozen domains, which are often

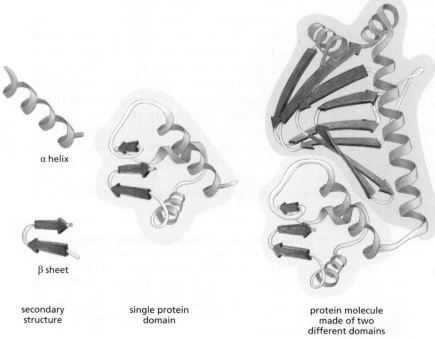

Figure 4–20 Many proteins are composed of separate functional domains. Elements of secondary structure such as α helices and β sheets pack together into stable, independently folding, globular elements called protein domains. A typical protein molecule is built from one or more domains, linked by a region of polypeptide chain that is often relatively unstructured. The ribbon diagram on the right represents the bacterial transcription regulatory protein CAP, which consists of one large cyclic AMP-binding domain (outlined in *blue*) and one small DNA-binding domain (outlined in *yellow*). The function of this protein is described in Chapter 8 (see Figure 8–9).

α helix

β sheet

secondary structure

single protein domain

protein molecule made of two different domains

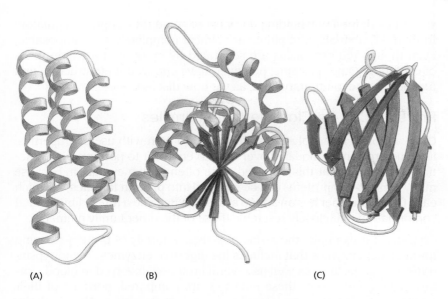

Figure 4–21 **Ribbon models show three different protein domains.** (A) Cytochrome b_{562} is a single-domain protein involved in electron transfer in *E. coli*. It is composed almost entirely of α helices. (B) The NAD-binding domain of the enzyme lactate dehydrogenase is composed of a mixture of α helices and β sheets. (C) An immunoglobulin domain of an antibody molecule is composed of a sandwich of two antiparallel β sheets. In these examples, the α helices are shown in *green*, while strands organized as β sheets are *red*. The protruding loop regions (*yellow*) are often unstructured and can provide binding sites for other molecules.

(A)   (B)   (C)

connected by relatively short, unstructured lengths of polypeptide chain. The ubiquity of such **intrinsically disordered sequences**, which continually bend and flex due to thermal buffeting, became appreciated only after bioinformatics methods were developed that could recognize them from their amino acid sequences. Present estimates suggest that a third of all eukaryotic proteins also possess longer, unstructured regions—greater than 30 amino acids in length—in their polypeptide chains. These unstructured sequences can have a variety of important functions in cells, as we discuss later in the chapter.

Few of the Many Possible Polypeptide Chains Will Be Useful

In theory, a vast number of different polypeptide chains could be made from 20 different amino acids. Because each amino acid is chemically distinct and could, in principle, occur at any position, a polypeptide chain four amino acids long has $20 \times 20 \times 20 \times 20 = 160,000$ different possible sequences. For a typical protein with a length of 300 amino acids, that means that more than 20^{300} (that's 10^{390}) different polypeptide chains could theoretically be produced. And that's just one protein.

Of the unimaginably large collection of potential polypeptide sequences, only a minuscule fraction is actually made by cells. That's because most biological functions depend on proteins with stable, well-defined three-dimensional conformations. This requirement greatly restricts the list of polypeptide sequences present in living cells. Another constraint is that functional proteins must be "well-behaved" and not engage in unwanted associations with other proteins in the cell—forming insoluble protein aggregates, for example. Many potential protein sequences would therefore have been eliminated by natural selection through the long trial-and-error process that underlies evolution (discussed in Chapter 9).

Thanks to natural selection, the amino acid sequences of many present-day polypeptides have evolved to adopt a stable conformation—one that bestows upon the protein the exact chemical properties that will enable it to perform a particular function. Such proteins are so precisely built that a change in even a few atoms in one amino acid can sometimes disrupt the structure of a protein and thereby eliminate its function. In fact, the conformations of many proteins—and their constituent domains—are so stable and effective that they have been conserved throughout the evolution of a diverse array of organisms. For example, the three-dimensional structures of the DNA-binding domains of some transcription regulators from yeast, animals, and plants are almost completely superimposable, even though the organisms are separated by more than a billion years of evolution. Other proteins, however, have changed their structure and function over evolutionary time, as we now discuss.

Proteins Can Be Classified into Families

Once a protein has evolved a stable conformation with useful properties, its structure can be modified over time to enable it to perform new functions. We know that this occurred quite often during evolution, because many present-day proteins can be grouped into **protein families**, in which each family member has an amino acid sequence and a three-dimensional conformation that closely resemble those of the other family members.

Consider, for example, the *serine proteases*, a family of protein-cleaving (proteolytic) enzymes that includes the digestive enzymes chymotrypsin, trypsin, and elastase, as well as several proteases involved in blood clotting. When any two of these enzymes are compared, portions of their amino acid sequences are found to be nearly the same. The similarity of their three-dimensional conformations is even more striking: most of the detailed twists and turns in their polypeptide chains, which are several hundred amino acids long, are virtually identical (**Figure 4–22**). The various serine proteases nevertheless have distinct enzymatic activities, each cleaving different proteins or the peptide bonds between different types of amino acids.

Large Protein Molecules Often Contain More than One Polypeptide Chain

The same type of weak noncovalent bonds that enable a polypeptide chain to fold into a specific conformation also allow proteins to bind to each other to produce larger structures in the cell. Any region on a protein's surface that interacts with another molecule through sets of noncovalent bonds is termed a *binding site*. A protein can contain binding sites for a variety of molecules, large and small. If a binding site recognizes the surface of a second protein, the tight binding of two folded polypeptide chains at this site will create a larger protein, whose quaternary structure has a precisely defined geometry. Each polypeptide chain in such a protein is called a **subunit**, and each of these subunits may contain more than one domain.

Figure 4–22 Serine proteases constitute a family of proteolytic enzymes. Backbone models of two serine proteases, elastase and chymotrypsin, are illustrated. Although only those amino acid sequences in the polypeptide chain shaded in *green* are the same in the two proteins, the two conformations are very similar nearly everywhere. Nonetheless, the two proteases act on different substrates.

The active site of each enzyme—where its substrates are bound and cleaved—is circled in *red*. The amino acid serine directly participates in the cleavage reaction, which is why the enzymes are called serine proteases. The *black* dots on the right side of the chymotrypsin molecule mark the two ends created where the enzyme has cleaved its own backbone.

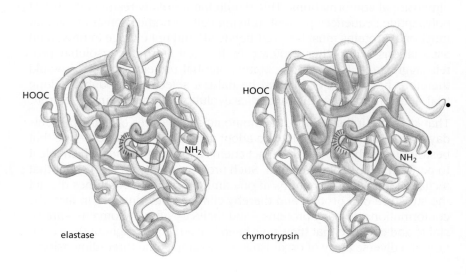

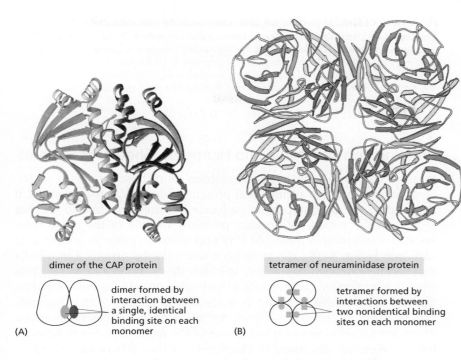

dimer of the CAP protein

dimer formed by interaction between a single, identical binding site on each monomer

(A)

tetramer of neuraminidase protein

tetramer formed by interactions between two nonidentical binding sites on each monomer

(B)

Figure 4–23 Many protein molecules contain multiple copies of the same protein subunit. (A) A symmetrical dimer. The protein CAP is a complex of two identical polypeptide chains (see also Figure 4–20). (B) A symmetrical homotetramer. The enzyme neuraminidase exists as a ring of four identical polypeptide chains. For both (A) and (B), a small schematic below the structure emphasizes how the repeated use of the same binding interaction forms the structure. In (A), the use of the same binding site on each monomer (represented by *brown* and *green* ovals) causes the formation of a symmetrical dimer. In (B), a pair of nonidentical binding sites (represented by *orange* circles and *blue* squares) causes the formation of a symmetrical tetramer.

In the simplest case, two identical, folded polypeptide chains form a symmetrical complex of two protein subunits (called a dimer) that is held together by interactions between two identical binding sites. CAP, the bacterial protein we discussed earlier, is such a dimer (**Figure 4–23A**); it is composed of two identical copies of the protein subunit, each of which contains two domains, as shown previously in Figure 4–20. Many other symmetrical protein complexes, formed from multiple copies of the same polypeptide chain, are commonly found in cells. The enzyme *neuraminidase*, for example, consists of a ring of four identical protein subunits (**Figure 4–23B**).

Other proteins contain two or more different polypeptide chains. *Hemoglobin*, the protein that carries oxygen in red blood cells, is a particularly well-studied example. The protein contains two identical α-globin subunits and two identical β-globin subunits, symmetrically arranged (**Figure 4–24**). Many proteins contain multiple subunits, and they can be very large (Movie 4.5).

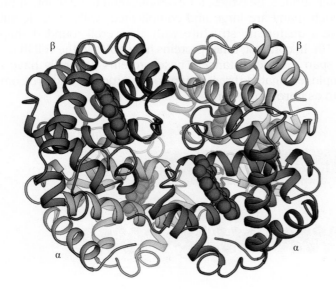

Figure 4–24 Some proteins are formed as a symmetrical assembly of two different subunits. Hemoglobin, an oxygen-carrying protein abundant in red blood cells, contains two copies of α-globin (*green*) and two copies of β-globin (*blue*). Each of these four polypeptide chains cradles a molecule of heme (*red*), where oxygen (O_2) is bound. Thus, each hemoglobin protein can carry four molecules of oxygen.

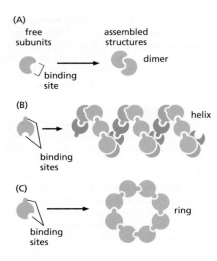

(A) free subunits → assembled structures
dimer
binding site

(B) binding sites → helix

(C) binding sites → ring

Figure 4–25 Identical protein subunits can assemble into complex structures. (A) A protein with just one binding site can form a dimer with another identical protein. (B) Identical proteins with two different binding sites will often form a long, helical filament. (C) If the two binding sites are positioned appropriately in relation to each other, the protein subunits will form a closed ring instead of a helix (see also Figure 4–23B).

Proteins Can Assemble into Filaments, Sheets, or Spheres

Proteins can form even larger assemblies than those discussed so far. Most simply, a chain of identical protein molecules can be formed if the binding site on one protein molecule is complementary to another region on the surface of another protein molecule of the same type. Because each protein molecule is bound to its neighbor in an identical way (see Figure 4–14), the molecules will often be arranged in a helix that can be extended indefinitely in either direction (Figure 4–25). This type of arrangement can produce an extended protein filament. An actin filament, for example, is a long, helical structure formed from many molecules of the protein actin (Figure 4–26). Actin is extremely abundant in eukaryotic cells, where it forms one of the major filament systems of the cytoskeleton (discussed in Chapter 17). Other sets of identical proteins associate to form tubes, as in the microtubules of the cytoskeleton (Figure 4–27), or cagelike spherical shells, as in the protein coats of virus particles (Figure 4–28).

Many large structures, such as viruses and ribosomes, are built from a mixture of one or more types of protein plus RNA or DNA molecules. These structures can be isolated in pure form and dissociated into their constituent macromolecules. It is often possible to mix the isolated components back together and watch them reassemble spontaneously into the original structure. This demonstrates that all the information needed for assembly of the complicated structure is contained in the macromolecules themselves. Experiments of this type show that much of the structure of a cell is self-organizing: if the required proteins are produced in the right amounts, the appropriate structures will form automatically.

Some Types of Proteins Have Elongated Fibrous Shapes

Most of the proteins we have discussed so far are **globular proteins**, in which the polypeptide chain folds up into a compact shape like a ball with an irregular surface. Enzymes, for example, tend to be globular proteins: even though many are large and complicated, with multiple subunits, most have a quaternary structure with an overall rounded shape (see Figure 4–10). In contrast, other proteins have roles in the cell that require them to span a large distance. These proteins generally have a relatively simple, elongated three-dimensional structure and are commonly referred to as **fibrous proteins**.

Figure 4–26 An actin filament is composed of identical protein subunits. (A) Transmission electron micrograph of an actin filament. (B) The helical array of actin molecules in an actin filament often contains thousands of molecules and extends for micrometers in the cell; 1 micrometer = 1000 nanometers. (A, courtesy of Roger Craig.)

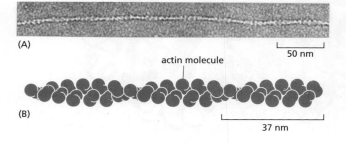

(A)

50 nm

actin molecule

(B)

37 nm

Figure 4–27 A single type of protein subunit can pack together to form a filament, a hollow tube, or a spherical shell. Actin subunits, for example, form actin filaments (see Figure 4–26), whereas tubulin subunits form hollow microtubules, and some virus proteins form a spherical shell (capsid) that encloses the viral genome (see Figure 4–28).

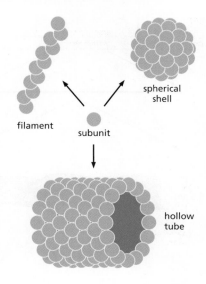

spherical shell

filament

subunit

hollow tube

One large class of intracellular fibrous proteins resembles α-keratin, which we met earlier when we introduced the α helix. Keratin filaments are extremely stable: long-lived structures such as hair, horns, and nails are composed mainly of this protein. An α-keratin molecule is a dimer of two identical subunits, with the long α helices of each subunit forming a coiled-coil (see Figure 4–16). These coiled-coil regions are capped at either end by globular domains containing binding sites that allow them to assemble into ropelike *intermediate filaments*—a component of the cytoskeleton that gives cells mechanical strength (discussed in Chapter 17).

Fibrous proteins are especially abundant outside the cell, where they form the gel-like *extracellular matrix* that helps bind cells together to form tissues. These proteins are secreted by the cells into their surroundings, where they often assemble into sheets or long fibrils. Collagen is the most abundant of these fibrous extracellular proteins in animal tissues. A collagen molecule consists of three long polypeptide chains, each containing the nonpolar amino acid glycine at every third position. This regular structure allows the chains to wind around one another to generate a long, regular, triple helix with glycine at its core (**Figure 4–29A**). Many such collagen molecules bind to one another, side-by-side and end-to-end, to create long, overlapping arrays called *collagen fibrils*, which are extremely strong and help hold tissues together, as described in Chapter 20.

In complete contrast to collagen is another fibrous protein in the extracellular matrix, *elastin*. Elastin molecules are formed from relatively loose and unstructured polypeptide chains that are covalently cross-linked into a rubberlike elastic meshwork. The resulting *elastic fibers* enable skin and other tissues, such as arteries and lungs, to stretch and recoil without tearing. As illustrated in **Figure 4–29B**, the elasticity is due to the ability of the individual protein molecules to uncoil reversibly whenever they are stretched.

Extracellular Proteins Are Often Stabilized by Covalent Cross-Linkages

Many protein molecules are attached to the surface of a cell's plasma membrane or secreted as part of the extracellular matrix, which exposes them to the potentially harsh conditions outside the cell. To help maintain their structures, the polypeptide chains in such proteins are often stabilized by covalent cross-linkages. These linkages can either tie together two amino acids in the same polypeptide chain or join together many polypeptide chains in a large protein complex—as for the collagen fibrils and elastic fibers just described. A variety of different types of cross-links exist.

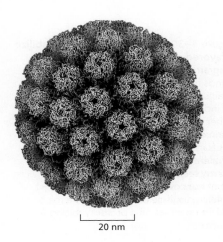

20 nm

Figure 4–28 Many viral capsids are essentially spherical protein assemblies. They are formed from many copies of a small set of protein subunits. The nucleic acid of the virus (DNA or RNA) is packaged inside. The structure of the simian virus SV40, shown here, was determined by x-ray crystallography and is known in atomic detail. (Courtesy of Robert Grant, Stephan Crainic, and James M. Hogle.)

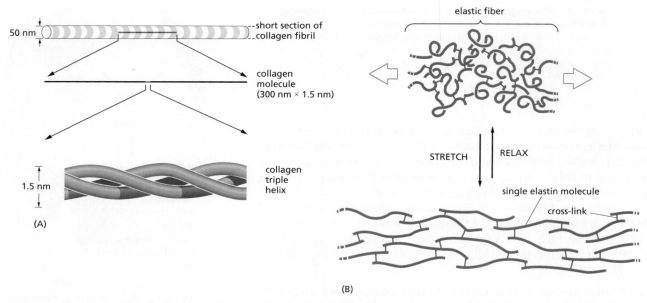

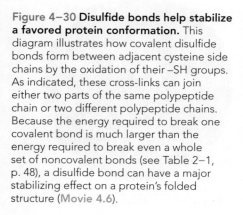

Figure 4–29 Fibrous proteins collagen and elastin form very different structures. (A) A collagen molecule is a triple helix formed by three extended protein chains that wrap around one another. Many rodlike collagen molecules are cross-linked together in the extracellular space to form collagen fibrils (*top*), which have the tensile strength of steel. The striping on the collagen fibril is caused by the regular repeating arrangement of the collagen molecules within the fibril. (B) Elastin molecules are cross-linked together by covalent bonds (*red*) to form rubberlike, elastic fibers. Each elastin polypeptide chain uncoils into a more extended conformation when the fiber is stretched, and recoils spontaneously as soon as the stretching force is relaxed.

The most common covalent cross-links in proteins are sulfur–sulfur bonds. These **disulfide bonds** (also called *S–S bonds*) are formed, before a protein is secreted, by an enzyme in the endoplasmic reticulum that links together two –SH groups from cysteine side chains that are adjacent in the folded protein (**Figure 4–30**). Disulfide bonds do not change a protein's conformation, but instead act as a sort of "atomic staple" to reinforce the protein's most favored conformation. Lysozyme—an enzyme in tears, saliva, and other secretions that can disrupt bacterial cell walls—retains its antibacterial activity for a long time because it is stabilized by such disulfide cross-links.

Disulfide bonds generally do not form in the cell cytosol, where a high concentration of reducing agents converts such bonds back to cysteine –SH groups. Apparently, proteins do not require this type of structural reinforcement in the relatively mild conditions inside the cell.

Figure 4–30 Disulfide bonds help stabilize a favored protein conformation. This diagram illustrates how covalent disulfide bonds form between adjacent cysteine side chains by the oxidation of their –SH groups. As indicated, these cross-links can join either two parts of the same polypeptide chain or two different polypeptide chains. Because the energy required to break one covalent bond is much larger than the energy required to break even a whole set of noncovalent bonds (see Table 2–1, p. 48), a disulfide bond can have a major stabilizing effect on a protein's folded structure (Movie 4.6).

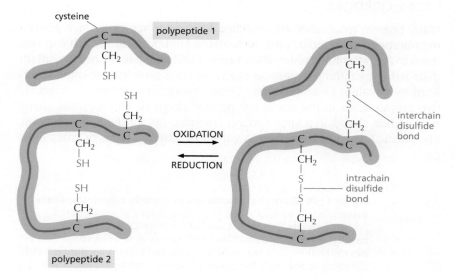

HOW PROTEINS WORK

For proteins, form and function are inextricably linked. Dictated by the surface topography of a protein's side chains, this union of structure, chemistry, and activity gives proteins the extraordinary ability to orchestrate the large number of dynamic processes that occur in cells. But the fundamental question remains: How do proteins actually work? In this section, we will see that the activity of proteins depends on their ability to bind specifically to other molecules, allowing them to act as catalysts, structural supports, tiny motors, and so on. The examples we review here by no means exhaust the vast functional repertoire of proteins. However, the specialized functions of the proteins you will encounter elsewhere in this book are based on the same principles.

All Proteins Bind to Other Molecules

The biological properties of a protein molecule depend on its physical interaction with other molecules. Antibodies attach to viruses or bacteria as part of the body's defenses; the enzyme hexokinase binds glucose and ATP to catalyze a reaction between them; actin molecules bind to one another to assemble into long filaments; and so on. Indeed, all proteins stick, or bind, to other molecules in a specific manner. In some cases, this binding is very tight; in others, it is weak and short-lived.

The binding of a protein to other biological molecules always shows great *specificity*: each protein molecule can bind to just one or a few molecules out of the many thousands of different molecules it encounters. Any substance that is bound by a protein—whether it is an ion, a small organic molecule, or a macromolecule—is referred to as a **ligand** for that protein (from the Latin *ligare*, "to bind").

The ability of a protein to bind selectively and with high affinity to a ligand is due to the formation of a set of weak, noncovalent interactions—hydrogen bonds, electrostatic attractions, and van der Waals attractions—plus favorable hydrophobic forces (see Panel 2–3, pp. 70–71). Each individual noncovalent interaction is weak, so that effective binding requires many such bonds to be formed simultaneously. This is possible only if the surface contours of the ligand molecule fit very closely to the protein, matching it like a hand in a glove (**Figure 4–31**).

When molecules have poorly matching surfaces, few noncovalent interactions occur, and the two molecules dissociate as rapidly as they come together. This is what prevents incorrect and unwanted associations from forming between mismatched molecules. At the other extreme, when many noncovalent interactions are formed, the association will persist (see Movie 2.4). Strong binding between molecules occurs in cells whenever a biological function requires that the molecules remain tightly associated for a long time—for example, when a group of macromolecules come together to form a functional subcellular structure such as a ribosome.

The region of a protein that associates with a ligand, known as its **binding site**, usually consists of a cavity in the protein surface formed by a particular arrangement of amino acid side chains. These side chains can belong to amino acids that are widely separated on the linear polypeptide chain, but are brought together when the protein folds (**Figure 4–32**). Other regions on the surface often provide binding sites for different ligands that regulate the protein's activity, as we discuss later. Still other parts of the protein may be required to attract or attach the protein to a particular location in the cell—for example, the hydrophobic α helix of a membrane-spanning protein allows it to be inserted into the lipid bilayer of a cell membrane (see Figure 4–15 and discussed in Chapter 11).

QUESTION 4–4

Hair is composed largely of fibers of the protein keratin. Individual keratin fibers are covalently cross-linked to one another by many disulfide (S–S) bonds. If curly hair is treated with mild reducing agents that break a few of the cross-links, pulled straight, and then oxidized again, it remains straight. Draw a diagram that illustrates the three different stages of this chemical and mechanical process at the level of the keratin filaments, focusing on the disulfide bonds. What do you think would happen if hair were treated with strong reducing agents that break all the disulfide bonds?

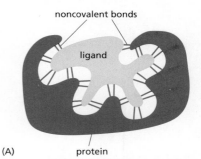

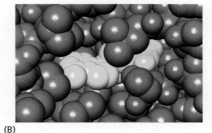

Figure 4–31 The binding of a protein to another molecule is highly selective. Many weak interactions are needed to enable a protein to bind tightly to a second molecule (a ligand). The ligand must therefore fit precisely into the protein's binding site, so that a large number of noncovalent interactions can be formed between the protein and the ligand. (A) Schematic drawing showing the binding of a hypothetical protein and ligand; (B) space-filling model of the ligand–protein interaction shown in Figure 4–32.

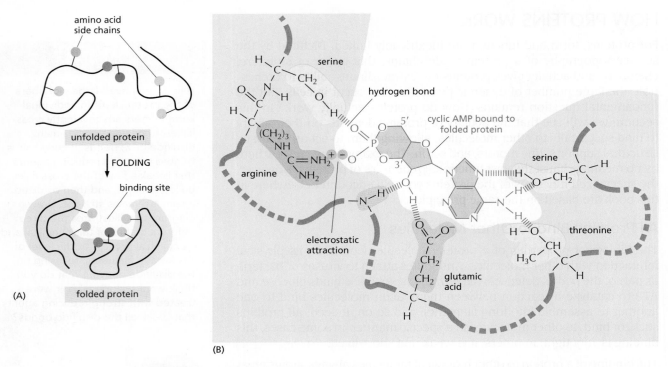

Figure 4–32 Binding sites allow proteins to interact with specific ligands. (A) The folding of the polypeptide chain typically creates a crevice or cavity on the folded protein's surface, where specific amino acid side chains are brought together in such a way that they can form a set of noncovalent bonds only with certain ligands. (B) Close-up view of an actual binding site showing the hydrogen bonds and an electrostatic interaction formed between a protein and its ligand (in this example, the bound ligand is cyclic AMP, shown in *dark yellow*).

Although the atoms buried in the interior of a protein have no direct contact with the ligand, they provide an essential framework that gives the surface its contours and chemical properties. Even tiny changes to the amino acids in the interior of a protein can change the protein's three-dimensional shape and destroy its function.

Humans Produce Billions of Different Antibodies, Each with a Different Binding Site

All proteins must bind to specific ligands to carry out their various functions. For antibodies, the universe of possible ligands is limitless and includes molecules found on bacteria, viruses, and other agents of infection. How does the body manage to produce antibodies capable of recognizing and binding tightly to such a diverse collection of ligands?

Antibodies are immunoglobulin proteins produced by the immune system in response to foreign molecules, especially those on the surface of an invading microorganism. Each antibody binds to a particular target molecule extremely tightly, either inactivating the target directly or marking it for destruction. An antibody recognizes its target molecule, called an **antigen**, with remarkable specificity. And because there are potentially billions of different antigens we might encounter, humans must be able to produce billions of different antibodies—one of which will be specific for almost any antigen imaginable.

Antibodies are Y-shaped molecules with two identical antigen-binding sites, each of which is complementary to a small portion of the surface of the antigen molecule. A detailed examination of antibody structure reveals that the antigen-binding sites are formed from several loops of polypeptide chain that protrude from the ends of a pair of closely

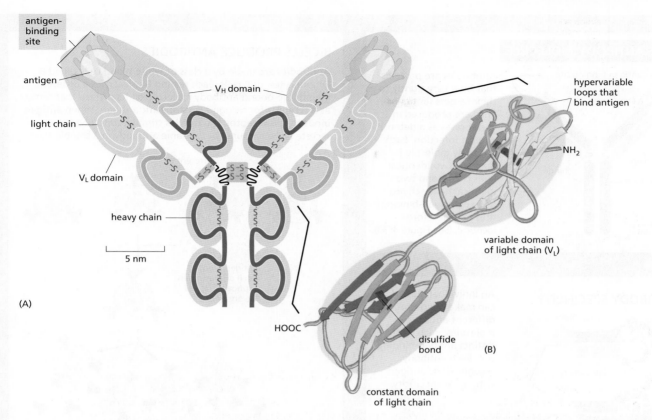

Figure 4–33 An antibody is Y-shaped and has two identical antigen-binding sites, one on each arm of the Y. (A) Schematic drawing of a typical antibody molecule. The protein is composed of four polypeptide chains (two identical heavy chains and two identical, smaller light chains), stabilized and held together by disulfide bonds (*red*). Each chain is made up of several similar domains, here shaded with *blue*, for the variable domains, or *gray*, for the constant domains. The antigen-binding site is formed where a heavy-chain variable domain (V_H) and a light-chain variable domain (V_L) come close together. These are the domains that differ most in their amino acid sequence in different antibodies—hence their name. (B) Ribbon drawing of a single light chain showing that the most variable parts of the polypeptide chain (*orange*) extend as loops at one end of the variable domain (V_L) to form half of one antigen-binding site of the antibody molecule shown in (A). Note that both the constant and variable domains are composed of a sandwich of two antiparallel β sheets connected by a disulfide bond (*red*).

juxtaposed protein domains (**Figure 4–33**). The amino acid sequence in these loops can vary greatly without altering the basic structure of the antibody. An enormous diversity of antigen-binding sites can therefore be generated by changing only the length and amino acid sequence of these "hypervariable loops," which is how the wide variety of different antibodies is formed (Movie 4.7).

With their unique combination of specificity and diversity, antibodies are not only indispensable for fighting off infections, they are also invaluable in the laboratory, where they can be used to identify, purify, and study other molecules (**Panel 4–2**, pp. 140–141).

Enzymes Are Powerful and Highly Specific Catalysts

For many proteins, binding to another molecule is their main function. An actin molecule, for example, need only associate with other actin molecules to form a filament. There are proteins, however, for which ligand binding is simply a necessary first step in their function. This is the case for the large and very important class of proteins called **enzymes**. These remarkable molecules are responsible for nearly all of the chemical transformations that occur in cells. Enzymes bind to one or more ligands, called **substrates**, and convert them into chemically modified products,

THE ANTIBODY MOLECULE

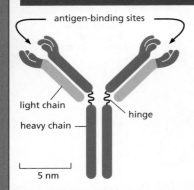

antigen-binding sites

light chain

hinge

heavy chain

5 nm

Antibodies are proteins that bind very tightly to their targets (antigens). They are produced in vertebrates as a defense against infection. Each antibody molecule is made of two identical light chains and two identical heavy chains. Its two antigen-binding sites are therefore identical. (See Figure 4–33).

ANTIBODY SPECIFICITY

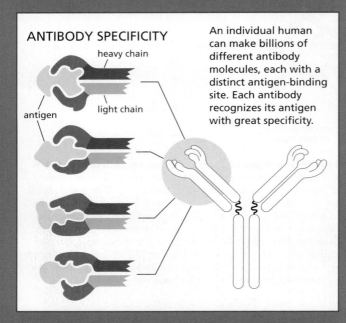

heavy chain

light chain

antigen

An individual human can make billions of different antibody molecules, each with a distinct antigen-binding site. Each antibody recognizes its antigen with great specificity.

ANTIBODIES DEFEND US AGAINST INFECTION

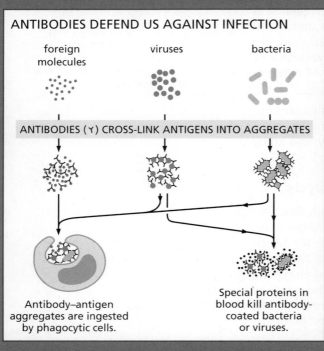

foreign molecules

viruses

bacteria

ANTIBODIES (Y) CROSS-LINK ANTIGENS INTO AGGREGATES

Antibody–antigen aggregates are ingested by phagocytic cells.

Special proteins in blood kill antibody-coated bacteria or viruses.

B CELLS PRODUCE ANTIBODIES

Antibodies are made by a class of white blood cells called B lymphocytes, or B cells. Each resting B cell carries a different membrane-bound antibody molecule on its surface that serves as a receptor for recognizing a specific antigen. When antigen binds to this receptor, the B cell is stimulated to divide and to secrete large amounts of the same antibody in a soluble form.

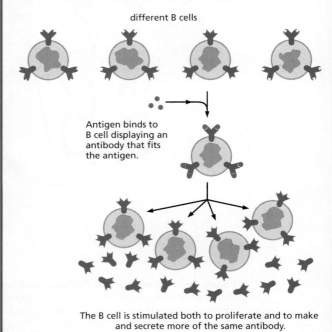

different B cells

Antigen binds to B cell displaying an antibody that fits the antigen.

The B cell is stimulated both to proliferate and to make and secrete more of the same antibody.

RAISING ANTIBODIES IN ANIMALS

Antibodies can be made in the laboratory by injecting an animal (usually a mouse, rabbit, sheep, or goat) with antigen A.

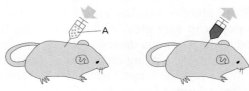

A

inject antigen A

take blood later

Repeated injections of the same antigen at intervals of several weeks stimulate specific B cells to secrete large amounts of anti-A antibodies into the bloodstream.

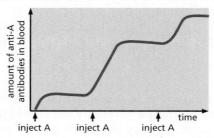

amount of anti-A antibodies in blood

time

inject A   inject A   inject A

Because many different B cells are stimulated by antigen A, the blood will contain a variety of anti-A antibodies, each of which binds A in a slightly different way.

USING ANTIBODIES TO PURIFY MOLECULES

IMMUNOPRECIPITATION

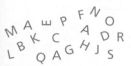

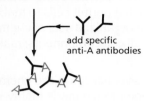

mixture of molecules

add specific
anti-A antibodies

collect aggregate of A molecules and
anti-A antibodies by centrifugation

IMMUNOAFFINITY COLUMN CHROMATOGRAPHY

bead coated with
anti-A antibodies

column packed
with these beads

mixture of molecules

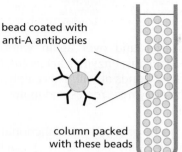

elute antigen A
from beads

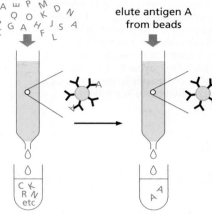

discard flow-through   collect pure antigen A

MONOCLONAL ANTIBODIES

Large quantities of a single type of antibody
molecule can be obtained by fusing a B cell
(taken from an animal injected with antigen A)
with a tumor cell. The resulting hybrid cell
divides indefinitely and secretes anti-A
antibodies of a single (monoclonal) type.

B cell from animal
injected with antigen
A makes anti-A
antibody but does
not divide forever.

Tumor cells in
culture divide
indefinitely but
do not make
antibody.

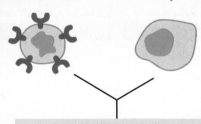

FUSE ANTIBODY-SECRETING
B CELL WITH TUMOR CELL

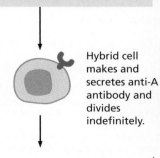

Hybrid cell
makes and
secretes anti-A
antibody and
divides
indefinitely.

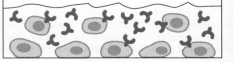

USING ANTIBODIES AS MOLECULAR TAGS

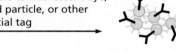

couple to fluorescent dye,
gold particle, or other
special tag

specific antibodies
against antigen A

labeled antibodies

MICROSCOPIC DETECTION

50 μm

200 nm

cell wall

Fluorescent antibody binds to
antigen A in tissue and is detected
in a fluorescence microscope. The
antigen here is pectin in the cell
walls of a slice of plant tissue.

Gold-labeled antibody binds to
antigen A in tissue and is detected
in an electron microscope. The
antigen is pectin in the cell wall
of a single plant cell.

BIOCHEMICAL DETECTION

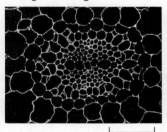

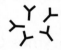

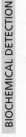

Antigen A is
separated from
other molecules
by electrophoresis.

Incubation with the
labeled antibodies
that bind to antigen A
allows the position of the
antigen to be determined.

Labeled second antibody
(*blue*) binds to first
antibody (*black*).

antigen

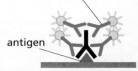

Note: In all cases, the sensitivity can
be greatly increased by using multiple
layers of antibodies. This "sandwich"
method enables smaller numbers of
antigen molecules to be detected.

Figure 4–34 Enzymes convert substrates to products while remaining unchanged themselves. Each enzyme has a site to which substrate molecules bind, forming an enzyme–substrate complex. There, a covalent bond making and/or breaking reaction occurs, generating an enzyme–product complex. The product is then released, allowing the enzyme to bind additional substrate molecules and repeat the reaction. An enzyme thus serves as a catalyst, and it usually forms or breaks a single covalent bond in a substrate molecule.

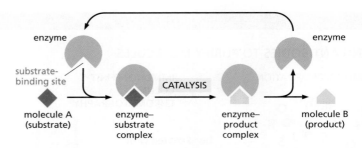

doing this over and over again without themselves being changed (**Figure 4–34**). Thus, enzymes act as *catalysts* that permit cells to make or break covalent bonds at will. This catalysis of organized sets of chemical reactions by enzymes creates and maintains all cell components, making life possible.

Enzymes can be grouped into functional classes based on the chemical reactions they catalyze (**Table 4–1**). Each type of enzyme is highly specific, catalyzing only a single type of reaction. Thus, *hexokinase* adds a phosphate group to D-glucose but not to its optical isomer L-glucose; the blood-clotting enzyme *thrombin* cuts one type of blood-clotting protein between a particular arginine and its adjacent glycine and nowhere else. As discussed in detail in Chapter 3, enzymes often work in sets, with the product of one enzyme becoming the substrate for the next. The result is an elaborate network of *metabolic pathways* that provides the cell with energy and generates the many large and small molecules that the cell needs.

Enzymes Greatly Accelerate the Speed of Chemical Reactions

The affinities of enzymes for their substrates, and the rates at which they convert bound substrate to product, vary widely from one enzyme to another. Both values can be determined experimentally by mixing purified enzymes and substrates together in a test tube. At a low concentration

TABLE 4–1 SOME COMMON FUNCTIONAL CLASSES OF ENZYMES	
Enzyme Class	**Biochemical Function**
Hydrolase	General term for enzymes that catalyze a hydrolytic cleavage reaction
Nuclease	Breaks down nucleic acids by hydrolyzing bonds between nucleotides
Protease	Breaks down proteins by hydrolyzing peptide bonds between amino acids
Ligase	Joins two molecules together; DNA ligase joins two DNA strands together end-to-end
Isomerase	Catalyzes the rearrangement of bonds within a single molecule
Polymerase	Catalyzes polymerization reactions such as the synthesis of DNA and RNA
Kinase	Catalyzes the addition of phosphate groups to molecules. Protein kinases are an important group of kinases that attach phosphate groups to proteins
Phosphatase	Catalyzes the hydrolytic removal of a phosphate group from a molecule
Oxido-reductase	General name for enzymes that catalyze reactions in which one molecule is oxidized while the other is reduced. Enzymes of this type are often called oxidases, reductases, or dehydrogenases
ATPase	Hydrolyzes ATP. Many proteins have an energy-harnessing ATPase activity as part of their function, including motor proteins such as myosin (discussed in Chapter 17) and membrane transport proteins such as the Na^+ pump (discussed in Chapter 12)

Enzyme names typically end in "-ase," with the exception of some enzymes, such as pepsin, trypsin, thrombin, lysozyme, and so on, which were discovered and named before the convention became generally accepted, at the end of the nineteenth century. The name of an enzyme usually indicates the nature of the reaction catalyzed. For example, citrate synthase catalyzes the synthesis of citrate by a reaction between acetyl CoA and oxaloacetate.

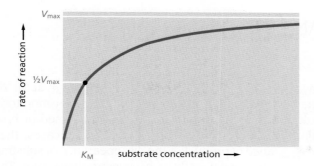

Figure 4–35 **An enzyme's performance depends on how rapidly it can process its substrate.** The rate of an enzyme reaction (*V*) increases as the substrate concentration increases, until a maximum value (V_{max}) is reached. At this point, all substrate-binding sites on the enzyme molecules are fully occupied, and the rate of the reaction is limited by the rate of the catalytic process on the enzyme surface. For most enzymes, the concentration of substrate at which the reaction rate is half-maximal (K_M) is a direct measure of how tightly the substrate is bound, with a large value of K_M (a large amount of substrate needed) corresponding to weak binding.

of substrate, the amount of enzyme–substrate complex—and the rate at which product is formed—will depend solely on the concentration of the substrate. If the concentration of substrate added is large enough, however, all of the enzyme molecules will be filled with substrate. When this happens, the rate of product formation depends on how rapidly the substrate molecule can undergo the reaction that will convert it to product. At this point, the enzymes are working as fast as they can, a value termed V_{max}. For many enzymes operating at V_{max}, the number of substrate molecules converted to product is in the vicinity of 1000 per second, although **turnover numbers** ranging from 1 to 100,000 molecules per second have been measured for different enzymes. Enzymes can speed up the rate of a chemical reaction by a factor of a million or more.

The same type of experiment can be used to gauge how tightly an enzyme interacts with its substrate, a value that is related to how much substrate it takes to fully saturate a sample of enzyme. Because it is difficult to determine at what point an enzyme sample is "fully occupied," biochemists instead determine the concentration of substrate at which an enzyme works at half its maximum speed. This value, called the **Michaelis constant**, K_M, was named after one of the biochemists who worked out the relationship (**Figure 4–35**). In general, a small K_M indicates that a substrate binds very tightly to the enzyme—due to a large number of noncovalent interactions (see Figure 4–31A); a large K_M, on the other hand, indicates weak binding. We describe the methods used to analyze enzyme performance in **How We Know**, pp. 144–145.

Lysozyme Illustrates How an Enzyme Works

We have discussed how enzymes recognize their substrates. But how do they catalyze the chemical conversion of these substrates into products? To find out, we take a closer look at **lysozyme**—an enzyme that acts as a natural antibiotic in egg white, saliva, tears, and other secretions. Lysozyme severs the polysaccharide chains that form the cell walls of bacteria. Because the bacterial cell is under pressure due to intracellular osmotic forces, cutting even a small number of polysaccharide chains causes the cell wall to rupture and the bacterium to burst, or lyse—hence the enzyme's name. Because lysozyme is a relatively small and stable protein, and can be isolated easily in large quantities, it has been studied intensively. It was the first enzyme to have its structure worked out at the atomic level by x-ray crystallography, and its mechanism of action is understood in great detail.

The reaction catalyzed by lysozyme is a hydrolysis: the enzyme adds a molecule of water to a single bond between two adjacent sugar groups in the polysaccharide chain, thereby causing the bond to break (see Figure 2–19). This reaction is energetically favorable because the free energy of the severed polysaccharide chains is lower than the free energy of the intact chain. However, the pure polysaccharide can sit for years in water

HOW WE KNOW

MEASURING ENZYME PERFORMANCE

At first glance, it seems that a cell's metabolic pathways have been pretty well mapped out, with each reaction proceeding predictably to the next. So why would anyone need to know exactly how tightly a particular enzyme clutches its substrate or whether it can process 100 or 1000 substrate molecules every second?

In reality, metabolic maps merely suggest which pathways a cell might follow as it converts nutrients into small molecules, chemical energy, and the larger building blocks of life. Like a road map, they do not predict the density of traffic under a particular set of conditions; that is, which pathways the cell will use when it is starving, when it is well fed, when oxygen is scarce, when it is stressed, or when it decides to divide. The study of an enzyme's *kinetics*—how fast it operates, how it handles its substrate, how its activity is controlled—allows us to predict how an individual catalyst will perform, and how it will interact with other enzymes in a network. Such knowledge leads to a deeper understanding of cell biology, and it opens the door to learning how to harness enzymes to perform desired reactions, including the large-scale production of specific chemicals.

Speed

The first step to understanding how an enzyme performs involves determining the maximal velocity, V_{max}, for the reaction it catalyzes. This is accomplished by measuring, in a test tube, how rapidly the reaction proceeds in the presence of a fixed amount of enzyme and different concentrations of substrate (**Figure 4–36A**): the rate should increase as the amount of substrate rises until the reaction reaches its V_{max} (**Figure 4–36B**). The velocity of the reaction can be measured by monitoring either how quickly the substrate is consumed or how rapidly the product accumulates. In many cases, the appearance of product or the disappearance of substrate can be observed directly with a spectrophotometer. This instrument detects the presence of molecules that absorb light at a particular wavelength; NADH, for example, absorbs light at 340 nm, while its oxidized counterpart, NAD^+, does not. So, a reaction that generates NADH (by reducing NAD^+) can be monitored by following the formation of NADH at 340 nm in a spectrophotometer.

Looking at the plot in Figure 4–36B, however, it is difficult to determine the exact value of V_{max}, as it is not clear where the reaction rate will reach its plateau. To get around this problem, the data are converted to their reciprocals and graphed in a "double-reciprocal plot," where the inverse of the velocity ($1/v$) appears on the y axis and the inverse of the substrate concentration ($1/[S]$) on the x axis (**Figure 4–36C**). This graph yields a straight line whose y intercept (the point where the line crosses the y axis) represents $1/V_{max}$ and whose x intercept corresponds to $-1/K_M$. These values are then converted to values for V_{max} and K_M.

Control

Substrates are not the only molecules that can influence how well or how quickly an enzyme works. In many cases, products, substrate lookalikes, inhibitors, and other small molecules can also increase or decrease

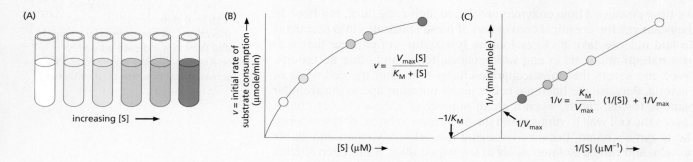

Figure 4–36 Measured reaction rates are plotted to determine the V_{max} and K_M of an enzyme-catalyzed reaction. (A) Test tubes containing a series of increasing substrate concentrations are prepared, a fixed amount of enzyme is added, and initial reaction rates (velocities) are determined. (B) The initial velocities (v) plotted against the substrate concentrations [S] give a curve described by the general equation $y = ax/(b + x)$. Substituting our kinetic terms, the equation becomes $v = V_{max}[S]/(K_M + [S])$, where V_{max} is the asymptote of the curve (the value of y at an infinite value of x), and K_M is equal to the substrate concentration where v is one-half V_{max}. This is called the *Michaelis–Menten equation*, named for the biochemists who provided evidence for this enzymatic relationship. (C) In a double-reciprocal plot, $1/v$ is plotted against $1/[S]$. The equation describing this straight line is $1/v = (K_M/V_{max})(1/[S]) + 1/V_{max}$. When $1/[S] = 0$, the y intercept ($1/v$) is $1/V_{max}$. When $1/v = 0$, the x intercept ($1/[S]$) is $-1/K_M$. Plotting the data this way allows V_{max} and K_M to be calculated more precisely. By convention, lowercase letters are used for variables (hence v for velocity) and uppercase letters are used for constants (hence V_{max}).

enzyme activity. Such regulation allows cells to control when and how rapidly various reactions occur, a process we discuss in detail in this chapter.

The effect of an inhibitor on an enzyme's activity is monitored in the same way that we measured the enzyme's kinetics. A curve is first generated showing the velocity of the uninhibited reaction between enzyme and substrate. Additional curves are then produced for reactions in which the inhibitor molecule has been included in the mix.

Comparing these curves, with and without inhibitor, can also reveal how a particular inhibitor impedes enzyme activity. For example, some inhibitors bind to the same site on an enzyme as its substrate. These *competitive inhibitors* block enzyme activity by competing directly with the substrate for the enzyme's attention. They resemble the substrate enough to tie up the enzyme, but they differ enough in structure to avoid getting converted to product. This blockage can be overcome by adding enough substrate so that enzymes are more likely to encounter a substrate molecule than an inhibitor molecule. From the kinetic data, we can see that competitive inhibitors do not change the V_{max} of a reaction; in other words, add enough substrate and the enzyme will encounter mostly substrate molecules and will reach its maximum velocity (**Figure 4–37**).

Competitive inhibitors can be used to treat patients who have been poisoned by ethylene glycol, an ingredient in commercially available antifreeze. Although ethylene glycol is itself not fatally toxic, a by-product of its metabolism—oxalic acid—can be lethal. To prevent oxalic acid from forming, the patient is given a large (though not quite intoxicating) dose of ethanol. Ethanol competes with the ethylene glycol for binding to alcohol dehydrogenase, the first enzyme in the pathway to oxalic acid formation. As a result, the ethylene glycol remains mostly unmetabolized and is safely eliminated from the body.

Other types of inhibitors may interact with sites on the enzyme distant from where the substrate binds. Many biosynthetic enzymes are regulated by feedback inhibition, whereby an enzyme early in a pathway will be shut down by a product generated later in the pathway (see, for example, Figure 4–43). Because this type of inhibitor binds to a separate, regulatory site on the enzyme, the substrate can still bind, but it might do so more slowly than it would in the absence of inhibitor. Such *noncompetitive inhibition* is not overcome by the addition of more substrate.

Design

With the kinetic data in hand, we can use computer modeling programs to predict how an enzyme will perform, and even how a cell will respond, when exposed to different conditions—such as the addition of a particular sugar or amino acid to the culture medium, or the addition of a poison or a pollutant. Seeing how a cell manages its resources—which pathways it favors for dealing with particular biochemical challenges—can also suggest strategies for designing better catalysts for reactions of medical or commercial importance (e.g., for producing drugs or detoxifying industrial waste). Using such tactics, bacteria have even been genetically engineered to produce large amounts of indigo—the dye, originally extracted from plants, that makes your blue jeans blue. We discuss the methods that enable such genetic manipulation in detail in Chapter 10.

Harnessing the power of cell biology for commercial purposes—even to produce something as simple as the amino acid tryptophan—is currently a multibillion-dollar industry. And, as more genome data come in, presenting us with more enzymes to exploit, vats of custom-made bacteria are increasingly churning out drugs and chemicals that represent the biological equivalent of pure gold.

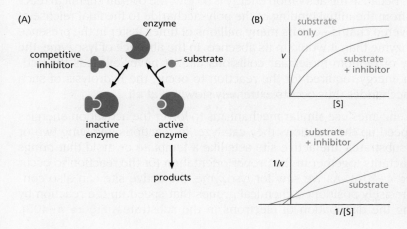

Figure 4–37 A competitive inhibitor directly blocks substrate binding to an enzyme. (A) The active site of the enzyme can bind either the competitive inhibitor or the substrate, but not both together. (B) The upper plot shows that inhibition by a competitive inhibitor can be overcome by increasing the substrate concentration. The double-reciprocal plot below shows that the V_{max} of the reaction is not changed in the presence of the competitive inhibitor: the *y* intercept is identical for both the curves.

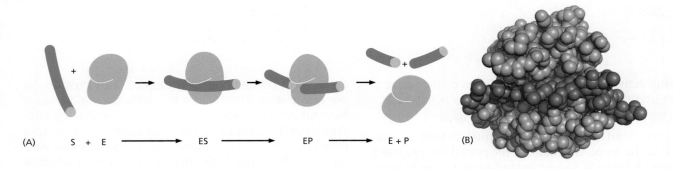

Figure 4–38 Lysozyme cleaves a polysaccharide chain. (A) Schematic view of the enzyme lysozyme (E), which catalyzes the cutting of a polysaccharide substrate molecule (S). The enzyme first binds to the polysaccharide to form an enzyme–substrate complex (ES), then it catalyzes the cleavage of a specific covalent bond in the backbone of the polysaccharide. The resulting enzyme–product complex (EP) rapidly dissociates, releasing the products (P) and leaving the enzyme free to act on another substrate molecule. (B) A space-filling model of lysozyme bound to a short length of polysaccharide chain prior to cleavage.

without being hydrolyzed to any detectable degree. This is because there is an energy barrier to such reactions, called the *activation energy* (discussed in Chapter 3, pp. 89–90). For a colliding water molecule to break a bond linking two sugars, the polysaccharide molecule has to be distorted into a particular shape—the **transition state**—in which the atoms around the bond have an altered geometry and electron distribution. To distort the polysaccharide in this way requires a large input of energy—which is where the enzyme comes in.

Like all enzymes, lysozyme has a binding site on its surface, termed an **active site**, which is where catalysis takes place. Because its substrate is a polymer, lysozyme's active site is a long groove that cradles six of the linked sugars in the polysaccharide chain at the same time. Once this enzyme–substrate complex forms, the enzyme cuts the polysaccharide by catalyzing the addition of a water molecule to one of its sugar–sugar bonds, and the severed chains are then quickly released, freeing the enzyme for further cycles of cleavage (**Figure 4–38**).

Like any protein binding to its ligand, lysosome recognizes its substrate through the formation of multiple noncovalent bonds (see Figure 4–32). However, lysozyme holds its polysaccharide substrate in such a way that one of the two sugars involved in the bond to be broken is distorted from its normal, most stable conformation. Conditions are thereby created in the microenvironment of the lysozyme active site that greatly reduce the activation energy necessary for the hydrolysis to take place (**Figure 4–39**). Because the activation energy is so low, the overall chemical reaction—from the initial binding of the polysaccharide to the final release of the severed chains—occurs many millions of times faster in the presence of lysozyme than it would in its absence. In the absence of lysozyme, the energy of random molecular collisions almost never exceeds the activation energy required for the reaction to occur; the hydrolysis of such polysaccharides thus occurs extremely slowly, if at all.

Other enzymes use similar mechanisms to lower the activation energies and speed up the reactions they catalyze. In reactions involving two or more substrates, the active site acts like a template or mold that brings the reactants together in the proper orientation for the reaction to occur (**Figure 4–40A**). As we saw for lysozyme, the active site can also contain precisely positioned chemical groups that speed up the reaction by altering the distribution of electrons in the substrates (**Figure 4–40B**).

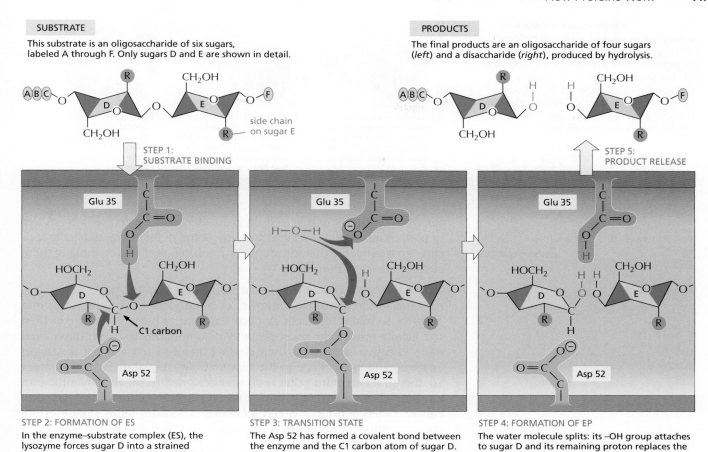

SUBSTRATE

This substrate is an oligosaccharide of six sugars, labeled A through F. Only sugars D and E are shown in detail.

PRODUCTS

The final products are an oligosaccharide of four sugars (*left*) and a disaccharide (*right*), produced by hydrolysis.

STEP 1: SUBSTRATE BINDING

STEP 5: PRODUCT RELEASE

STEP 2: FORMATION OF ES

In the enzyme–substrate complex (ES), the lysozyme forces sugar D into a strained conformation. The Glu 35 in the active site is positioned to serve as an acid that attacks the adjacent sugar–sugar bond by donating a proton (H⁺) to sugar E; Asp 52 is poised to attack the C1 carbon atom of sugar D.

STEP 3: TRANSITION STATE

The Asp 52 has formed a covalent bond between the enzyme and the C1 carbon atom of sugar D. The Glu 35 then polarizes a water molecule (*red*), so that its oxygen can readily attack the C1 carbon atom of sugar D and displace Asp 52.

STEP 4: FORMATION OF EP

The water molecule splits: its –OH group attaches to sugar D and its remaining proton replaces the proton donated by Glu 35 in step 2. This completes the hydrolysis and returns the enzyme to its initial state, forming the final enzyme–product complex (EP).

Figure 4–39 Enzymes bind to, and chemically alter, substrate molecules. In the active site of lysozyme, a covalent bond in a polysaccharide molecule is bent and then broken. The top row shows the free substrate and the free products. The three lower panels depict sequential events at the enzyme active site, during which a sugar–sugar covalent bond is broken. Note the change in the conformation of sugar D in the enzyme–substrate complex compared with the free substrate. This conformation favors the formation of the transition state shown in the middle panel, greatly lowering the activation energy required for the reaction. The reaction, and the structure of lysozyme bound to its product, are shown in Movie 4.8 and Movie 4.9. (Based on D.J. Vocadlo et al., *Nature* 412:835–838, 2001.)

Binding to the enzyme also changes the shape of the substrate, bending bonds so as to drive the bound molecule toward a particular transition state (**Figure 4–40C**). Finally, like lysozyme, many enzymes participate intimately in the reaction by briefly forming a covalent bond between the substrate and an amino acid side chain in the active site. Subsequent steps in the reaction restore the side chain to its original state, so that the enzyme remains unchanged after the reaction and can go on to catalyze many more reactions.

Many Drugs Inhibit Enzymes

Many of the drugs we take to treat or prevent illness work by blocking the activity of a particular enzyme. Cholesterol-lowering *statins* inhibit HMG-CoA reductase, an enzyme involved in the synthesis of cholesterol by the liver. *Methotrexate* kills some types of cancer cells by shutting down dihydrofolate reductase, an enzyme that produces a compound required

Figure 4–40 **Enzymes can encourage a reaction in several ways.** (A) Holding reacting substrates together in a precise alignment. (B) Rearranging the distribution of charge in a reaction intermediate. (C) Altering bond angles in the substrate to increase the rate of a particular reaction. A single enzyme may use any of these mechanisms in combination.

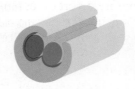
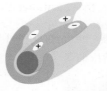
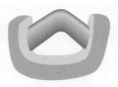

(A) enzyme binds to two substrate molecules and orients them precisely to encourage a reaction to occur between them

(B) binding of substrate to enzyme rearranges electrons in the substrate, creating partial negative and positive charges that favor a reaction

(C) enzyme strains the bound substrate molecule, forcing it toward a transition state that favors a reaction

for DNA synthesis during cell division. Because cancer cells have lost important intracellular control systems, some of them are unusually sensitive to treatments that interrupt chromosome replication, making them susceptible to methotrexate.

Pharmaceutical companies often develop drugs by first using automated methods to screen massive libraries of compounds to find chemicals that are able to inhibit the activity of an enzyme of interest. They can then chemically modify the most promising compounds to make them even more effective, enhancing their binding affinity, specificity for the target enzyme, and persistence in the human body. As we discuss in Chapter 20, the anticancer drug Gleevec® was designed to specifically inhibit an enzyme whose aberrant behavior is required for the growth of a type of cancer called chronic myeloid leukemia. The drug binds tightly in the substrate-binding pocket of that enzyme, blocking its activity.

Tightly Bound Small Molecules Add Extra Functions to Proteins

Although the precise order of their amino acids gives proteins their shape and functional versatility, sometimes amino acids by themselves are not enough for a protein to do its job. Just as we use tools to enhance and extend the capabilities of our hands, so proteins often employ small, nonprotein molecules to perform functions that would be difficult or impossible using amino acids alone. Thus, the photoreceptor protein *rhodopsin*, which is the light-sensitive protein made by the rod cells in the retina of our eyes, detects light by means of a small molecule, *retinal*, which is attached to the protein by a covalent bond to a lysine side chain (**Figure 4–41A**). Retinal changes its shape when it absorbs a photon of light, and this change is amplified by rhodopsin to trigger a cascade of reactions that eventually leads to an electrical signal being carried to the brain.

Figure 4–41 **Retinal and heme are required for the function of certain proteins.** (A) The structure of retinal, the light-sensitive molecule covalently attached to the rhodopsin protein in our eyes. (B) The structure of a heme group, shown with the carbon-containing heme ring colored *red* and the iron atom at its center in *orange*. A heme group is tightly, but noncovalently, bound to each of the four polypeptide chains in hemoglobin, the oxygen-carrying protein whose structure was shown in Figure 4–24.

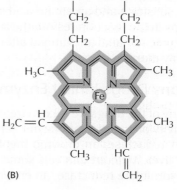

(A)

(B)

Another example of a protein that contains a nonprotein portion essential for its function is *hemoglobin* (see Figure 4–24). A molecule of hemoglobin carries four noncovalently bound *heme* groups, ring-shaped molecules each with a single central iron atom (**Figure 4–41B**). Heme gives hemoglobin—and blood—its red color. By binding reversibly to dissolved oxygen gas through its iron atom, heme enables hemoglobin to pick up oxygen in the lungs and release it in tissues that need it.

Enzymes, too, make use of nonprotein molecules: they frequently have a small molecule or metal atom associated with their active site that assists with their catalytic function. *Carboxypeptidase*, an enzyme that cuts polypeptide chains, carries a tightly bound zinc ion in its active site. During the cleavage of a peptide bond by carboxypeptidase, the zinc ion forms a transient bond with one of the substrate atoms, thereby assisting the hydrolysis reaction. In other enzymes, a small organic molecule—often referred to as a **coenzyme**—serves a similar purpose. *Biotin*, for example, is found in enzymes that transfer a carboxyl group ($-COO^-$) from one molecule to another (see Figure 3–38). Biotin participates in these reactions by forming a covalent bond to the $-COO^-$ group to be transferred, thereby producing an activated carrier (see Table 3–2, p. 109). This small molecule is better suited for this function than any of the amino acids used to make proteins.

Because biotin cannot be synthesized by humans, it must be provided in the diet; thus biotin is classified as a *vitamin*. Other vitamins are similarly needed to make small molecules that are essential components of our proteins; vitamin A, for example, is needed in the diet to make retinal, the light-sensitive part of rhodopsin.

HOW PROTEINS ARE CONTROLLED

Thus far, we have examined how binding to other molecules allows proteins to perform their specific functions. But inside the cell, most proteins and enzymes do not work continuously, or at full speed. Instead, their activities are regulated in a coordinated fashion so the cell can maintain itself in an optimal state, producing only those molecules it requires to thrive under current conditions. By coordinating not only when—and how vigorously—proteins perform, but also where in the cell they act, the cell ensures that it does not deplete its energy reserves by accumulating molecules it does not need or waste its stockpiles of critical substrates. We now consider how cells control the activity of their enzymes and other proteins.

The regulation of protein activity occurs at many levels. At the most fundamental level, the cell controls the amount of each protein it contains. It can do so by controlling the expression of the gene that encodes that protein (discussed in Chapter 8). It can also regulate the rate at which the protein is degraded (discussed in Chapter 7). The cell also controls protein activities by confining the participating proteins to particular subcellular compartments. Some of these compartments are enclosed by membranes (as discussed in Chapters 11, 12, 14, and 15); others are created by the proteins that are drawn there, as we discuss shortly. Finally, the activity of an individual protein can be rapidly adjusted at the level of the protein itself.

All of these mechanisms rely on the ability of proteins to interact with other molecules—including other proteins. These interactions can cause proteins to adopt different conformations, and thereby alter their function, as we see next.

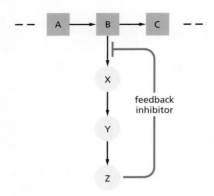

Figure 4–42 Feedback inhibition regulates the flow through biosynthetic pathways. B is the first metabolite in a pathway that gives the end product Z. Z inhibits the first enzyme that is specific to its own synthesis and thereby limits its own concentration in the cell. This form of negative regulation is called feedback inhibition.

QUESTION 4–6

Consider the drawing in Figure 4–42. What will happen if, instead of the indicated feedback,
A. feedback inhibition from Z affects the step B → C only?
B. feedback inhibition from Z affects the step Y → Z only?
C. Z is a positive regulator of the step B → X?
D. Z is a positive regulator of the step B → C?
For each case, discuss how useful these regulatory schemes would be for a cell.

Figure 4–43 Feedback inhibition at multiple points regulates connected metabolic pathways. The biosynthetic pathways for four different amino acids in bacteria are shown, starting from the amino acid aspartate. The *red* lines indicate points at which products feed back to inhibit enzymes and the blank boxes represent intermediates in each pathway. In this example, each amino acid controls the first enzyme specific to its own synthesis, thereby limiting its own concentration and avoiding a wasteful buildup of intermediates. Some of the products also separately inhibit the initial set of reactions common to all the syntheses. Three different enzymes catalyze the initial reaction from aspartate to aspartyl phosphate, and each of these enzymes is inhibited by a different product.

The Catalytic Activities of Enzymes Are Often Regulated by Other Molecules

A living cell contains thousands of different enzymes, many of which are operating at the same time in the same small volume of the cytosol. By their catalytic action, enzymes generate a complex web of metabolic pathways, each composed of chains of chemical reactions in which the product of one enzyme becomes the substrate of the next. In this maze of pathways, there are many branch points where different enzymes compete for the same substrate. The system is so complex that elaborate controls are required to regulate when and how rapidly each reaction occurs.

A common type of control occurs when a molecule other than a substrate specifically binds to an enzyme at a special *regulatory site*, altering the rate at which the enzyme converts its substrate to product. In **feedback inhibition**, for example, an enzyme acting early in a reaction pathway is inhibited by a molecule produced later in that pathway. Thus, whenever large quantities of the final product begin to accumulate, the product binds to an earlier enzyme and slows down its catalytic action, limiting further entry of substrates into that reaction pathway (**Figure 4–42**). Where pathways branch or intersect, there are usually multiple points of control by different final products, each of which regulates its own synthesis (**Figure 4–43**). Feedback inhibition can work almost instantaneously and is rapidly reversed when product levels fall.

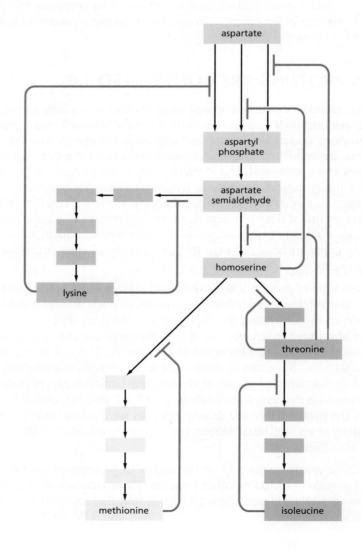

Feedback inhibition is a form of *negative regulation*: it prevents an enzyme from acting. Enzymes can also be subject to *positive regulation*, in which the enzyme's activity is stimulated by a regulatory molecule rather than being suppressed. Positive regulation occurs when a product in one branch of the metabolic maze stimulates the activity of an enzyme in another pathway. But how do these regulatory molecules change an enzyme's activity?

Allosteric Enzymes Have Two or More Binding Sites That Influence One Another

Feedback inhibition was initially puzzling to those who discovered it, in part because the regulatory molecule often has a shape that is totally different from the shape of the enzyme's preferred substrate. Indeed, when this form of regulation was discovered in the 1960s, it was termed *allostery* (from the Greek *allo*, "other," and *stere*, "solid" or "shape"). Given the numerous, specific, noncovalent interactions that allow enzymes to interact with their substrates within the active site, it seemed likely that these regulatory molecules were binding somewhere else on the surface of the protein. As more was learned about feedback inhibition, researchers realized that many enzymes must contain at least two different binding sites: an active site that recognizes the substrates and one or more sites that recognize regulatory molecules. These sites must somehow "communicate" to allow the catalytic events at the active site to be influenced by the binding of the regulatory molecule at a separate location.

The interaction between sites that are located in different regions on a protein molecule is now known to depend on a *conformational change* in the protein. The binding of a ligand to one of the sites causes a shift in the protein's structure from one folded shape to a slightly different folded shape, and this alters the shape of a second binding site that can be far away. Many enzymes have two conformations that differ in activity, each of which can be stabilized by the binding of a different ligand. During feedback inhibition, for example, the binding of an inhibitor at a regulatory site on a protein causes the protein to spend more time in a conformation in which its active site—located elsewhere in the protein—becomes less accommodating to the substrate molecule (**Figure 4–44**).

As schematically illustrated in **Figure 4–45A**, many—if not most—protein molecules are **allosteric**: they can adopt two or more slightly different conformations, and their activity can be regulated by a shift from one to another. This is true not only for enzymes, but also for many other proteins as well. The chemistry involved here is extremely simple in concept. Because each protein conformation will have somewhat different contours on its surface, the protein's binding sites for ligands will be

Figure 4–44 Feedback inhibition triggers a conformational change in an enzyme. Aspartate transcarbamoylase from *E. coli*, a large multisubunit enzyme used in early studies of allosteric regulation, catalyzes an important reaction that begins the synthesis of the pyrimidine ring of C, U, and T nucleotides (see Panel 2–7, pp. 78–79). One of the final products of this pathway, cytidine triphosphate (CTP), binds to the enzyme to turn it off whenever CTP is plentiful. This diagram shows the conformational change that occurs when the enzyme is turned off by CTP binding to its four regulatory sites, which are distinct from the active site where the substrate binds. Figure 4–10 shows the structure of aspartate transcarbamoylase as seen from the top. This figure depicts the enzyme as seen from the side.

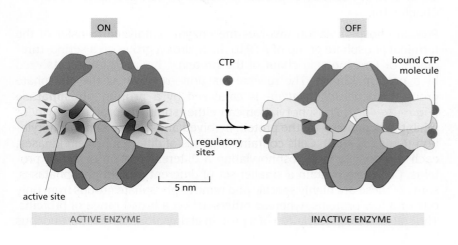

Figure 4–45 The binding of a regulatory ligand can change the equilibrium between two protein conformations. (A) Schematic diagram of a hypothetical, allosterically regulated enzyme for which a rise in the concentration of ADP molecules (*red* wedges) increases the rate at which the enzyme catalyzes the oxidation of sugar molecules (*blue* hexagons). (B) Due to thermal motions, the enzyme will spontaneously interconvert between the open (inactive) and closed (active) conformations shown in (A). But when ADP is absent, only a small fraction of the enzyme molecules will be present in the active conformation at any given time. As illustrated, most remain in the inactive conformation. (C) Because ADP can bind to the protein only in its closed, active conformation, an increase in ADP concentration locks nearly all of the enzyme molecules in the active form—an example of positive regulation. In cells, rising concentrations of ADP signal a depletion of ATP reserves; increased oxidation of sugars—in the presence of ADP—thus provides more energy for the synthesis of ATP from ADP.

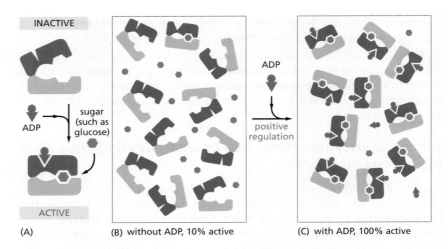

(A)   (B) without ADP, 10% active   (C) with ADP, 100% active

altered when the protein changes shape. Each ligand will stabilize the conformation that it binds to most strongly. Therefore, at high enough concentrations, a ligand will tend to "switch" the population of proteins to the conformation that it favors (**Figure 4–45B and C**).

Phosphorylation Can Control Protein Activity by Causing a Conformational Change

Another method that eukaryotic cells use to regulate protein activity involves attaching a phosphate group covalently to one or more of the protein's amino acid side chains. Because each phosphate group carries two negative charges, the enzyme-catalyzed addition of a phosphate group can cause a conformational change by, for example, attracting a cluster of positively charged amino acid side chains from somewhere else in the same protein. This structural shift can, in turn, affect the binding of ligands elsewhere on the protein surface, thereby altering the protein's activity. Removal of the phosphate group by a second enzyme will return the protein to its original conformation and restore its initial activity.

Reversible **protein phosphorylation** controls the activity of many types of proteins in eukaryotic cells. This form of regulation is used so extensively that more than one-third of the 10,000 or so proteins in a typical mammalian cell are phosphorylated at any one time. The addition and removal of phosphate groups from specific proteins often occur in response to signals that specify some change in a cell's state. For example, the complicated series of events that takes place as a eukaryotic cell divides is timed largely in this way (discussed in Chapter 18). And many of the intracellular signaling pathways activated by extracellular signals depend on a network of protein phosphorylation events (discussed in Chapter 16).

Protein phosphorylation involves the enzyme-catalyzed transfer of the terminal phosphate group of ATP to the hydroxyl group on a serine, threonine, or tyrosine side chain of the protein. This reaction is catalyzed by a **protein kinase**. The reverse reaction—removal of the phosphate group, or *dephosphorylation*—is catalyzed by a **protein phosphatase** (**Figure 4–46A**). Phosphorylation can either stimulate protein activity or inhibit it, depending on the protein involved and the site of phosphorylation (**Figure 4–46B**). Cells contain hundreds of different protein kinases, each responsible for phosphorylating a different protein or set of proteins. Cells also contain a smaller set of different protein phosphatases; some of these are highly specific and remove phosphate groups from only one or a few proteins, whereas others act on a broad range of proteins. The state of phosphorylation of a protein at any moment in time, and thus

Figure 4–46 **Protein phosphorylation is a very common mechanism for regulating protein activity.** Many thousands of proteins in a typical eukaryotic cell are modified by the covalent addition of one or more phosphate groups. (A) The general reaction, shown here, entails transfer of a phosphate group from ATP to an amino acid side chain of the target protein by a protein kinase. Removal of the phosphate group is catalyzed by a second enzyme, a protein phosphatase. In this example, the phosphate is added to a serine side chain; in other cases, the phosphate is instead linked to the –OH group of a threonine or tyrosine side chain. (B) Phosphorylation can either increase or decrease the protein's activity, depending on the site of phosphorylation and the structure of the protein.

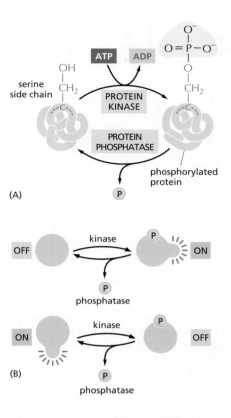

its activity, will depend on the relative activities of the protein kinases and phosphatases that act on it.

Phosphorylation can take place in a continuous cycle, in which a phosphate group is rapidly added to—and rapidly removed from—a particular side chain. Such phosphorylation cycles allow proteins to switch quickly from one state to another. The more swiftly the cycle is "turning," the faster the concentration of a phosphorylated protein can change in response to a sudden stimulus. Although keeping the cycle turning costs energy—because ATP is hydrolyzed with each phosphorylation—many enzymes in the cell undergo this speedy, cyclic form of regulation.

Covalent Modifications Also Control the Location and Interaction of Proteins

Phosphorylation can do more than control a protein's activity; it can create docking sites where other proteins can bind, thus promoting the assembly of proteins into larger complexes. For example, when extracellular signals stimulate a class of cell-surface, transmembrane proteins called *receptor tyrosine kinases*, they cause the receptor proteins to phosphorylate themselves on certain tyrosines. The phosphorylated tyrosines then serve as docking sites for the binding and activation of a set of intracellular signaling proteins, which transmits the message to the cell interior and changes the behavior of the cell (see Figure 16–29).

Phosphorylation is not the only form of covalent modification that can affect a protein's function. Many proteins are modified by the addition of an acetyl group to a lysine side chain, including the histones discussed in Chapter 5. And the addition of the fatty acid palmitate to a cysteine side chain drives a protein to associate with cell membranes. Attachment of ubiquitin, a 76-amino-acid polypeptide, can target a protein for degradation, as we discuss in Chapter 7. More than 100 types of covalent modifications can occur in the cell, each playing its own role in regulating protein function. Each of these modifying groups is enzymatically added or removed depending on the needs of the cell.

A large number of proteins are modified on more than one amino acid side chain. The p53 protein, which plays a central part in controlling how a cell responds to DNA damage and other stresses, can be covalently modified at 20 sites (**Figure 4–47**). Because an enormous number of combinations of these 20 modifications is possible, the protein's behavior can in principle be altered in a huge number of ways.

Figure 4–47 **The modification of a protein at multiple sites can control the protein's behavior.** This diagram shows some of the covalent modifications that control the activity and degradation of p53, a protein of nearly 400 amino acids. p53 is an important transcription regulator that regulates a cell's response to damage (discussed in Chapter 18). Not all of these modifications will be present at the same time. Colors along the body of the protein represent distinct protein domains, including one that binds to DNA (*green*) and one that activates gene transcription (*pink*). All of the modifications shown are located within relatively unstructured regions of the polypeptide chain.

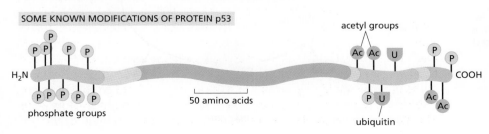

SOME KNOWN MODIFICATIONS OF PROTEIN p53

The set of covalent modifications that a protein contains at any moment constitutes an important form of regulation. The attachment or removal of these modifying groups can change a protein's activity or stability, its binding partners, or its location inside the cell. Covalent modifications thus enable the cell to make optimal use of the proteins it produces, and they allow the cell to respond rapidly to changes in its environment.

Regulatory GTP-Binding Proteins Are Switched On and Off by the Gain and Loss of a Phosphate Group

Eukaryotic cells have a second way to regulate protein activity by phosphate addition and removal. In this case, however, the phosphate is not enzymatically transferred from ATP to the protein. Instead, the phosphate is part of a guanine nucleotide—guanosine triphosphate (GTP)—that binds tightly various types of **GTP-binding proteins**. These proteins act as molecular switches: they are in their active conformation when GTP is bound, but they can hydrolyze this GTP to GDP—which releases a phosphate and flips the protein to an inactive conformation (Movie 4.10). As with protein phosphorylation, this process is reversible: the active conformation is regained by dissociation of the GDP, followed by the binding of a fresh molecule of GTP (Figure 4–48).

Hundreds of GTP-binding proteins function as molecular switches in cells. The dissociation of GDP and its replacement by GTP, which turns the switch on, is often stimulated in response to cell signals. The GTP-binding proteins activated in this way in turn bind to other proteins to regulate their activities. The crucial role GTP-binding proteins play in intracellular signaling pathways is discussed in detail in Chapter 16.

ATP Hydrolysis Allows Motor Proteins to Produce Directed Movements in Cells

We have seen how conformational changes in proteins play a central part in enzyme regulation and cell signaling. But conformational changes also play another important role in the operation of the eukaryotic cell: they enable certain specialized proteins to drive directed movements of cells and their components. These **motor proteins** generate the forces responsible for muscle contraction and most other eukaryotic cell movements. They also power the intracellular movements of organelles and macromolecules. For example, they help move chromosomes to opposite ends of the cell during mitosis (discussed in Chapter 18), and they move organelles along cytoskeletal tracks (discussed in Chapter 17).

Figure 4–48 Many different GTP-binding proteins function as molecular switches. A GTP-binding protein requires the presence of a tightly bound GTP molecule to be active. The active protein can shut itself off by hydrolyzing its bound GTP to GDP and inorganic phosphate (P_i), which converts the protein to an inactive conformation. To reactivate the protein, the tightly bound GDP must dissociate. As explained in Chapter 16, this dissociation is a slow step that can be greatly accelerated by important regulatory proteins called guanine nucleotide exchange factors (GEFs). As indicated, once the GDP dissociates, a molecule of GTP quickly replaces it, returning the protein to its active conformation.

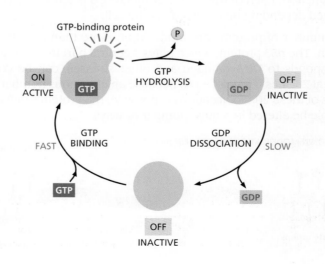

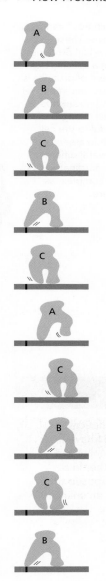

Figure 4–49 **Changes in conformation can allow a protein to "walk" along a cytoskeletal filament.** This protein cycles between three different conformations (A, B, and C) as it moves along the filament. But, without an input of energy to drive its movement in a single direction, the protein can only wander randomly back and forth, ultimately getting nowhere.

But how can the changes in shape experienced by proteins be used to generate such orderly movements? A protein that is required to walk along a cytoskeletal fiber, for example, can move by undergoing a series of conformational changes. However, with nothing to drive these changes in one direction or the other, the shape changes will be reversible and the protein will wander randomly back and forth (**Figure 4–49**).

To force the protein to proceed in a single direction, the conformational changes must be unidirectional. To achieve such directionality, one of the steps must be made irreversible. For most proteins that are able to move in a single direction for long distances, this irreversibility is achieved by coupling one of the conformational changes to the hydrolysis of an ATP molecule that is tightly bound to the protein—which is why motor proteins are also ATPases. A great deal of free energy is released when ATP is hydrolyzed, making it very unlikely that the protein will undergo a reverse shape change—as required for moving backward. (Such a reversal would require that the ATP hydrolysis be reversed, by adding a phosphate molecule to ADP to form ATP.) As a consequence, the protein moves steadily forward (**Figure 4–50**).

Many different motor proteins generate directional movement by using the hydrolysis of a tightly bound ATP molecule to drive an orderly series of conformational changes. These movements can be rapid: the muscle motor protein *myosin* walks along actin filaments at about 6 μm/sec during muscle contraction (discussed in Chapter 17).

Proteins Often Form Large Complexes That Function as Machines

As proteins progress from being small, with a single domain, to being larger with multiple domains, the functions they can perform become more elaborate. The most complex tasks are carried out by large protein assemblies formed from many protein molecules. Now that it is possible to reconstruct biological processes in cell-free systems in a test tube, it is clear that each central process in a cell—including DNA replication, gene transcription, protein synthesis, vesicle budding, and transmembrane signaling—is catalyzed by a highly coordinated, linked set of many proteins. For most such **protein machines**, the hydrolysis of bound nucleoside triphosphates (ATP or GTP) drives an ordered series of conformational changes in some of the individual protein subunits, enabling

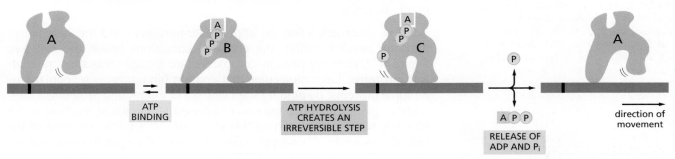

Figure 4–50 **A schematic model of how a motor protein uses ATP hydrolysis to move in one direction along a cytoskeletal filament.** An orderly transition among three conformations is driven by the hydrolysis of a bound ATP molecule and the release of the products, ADP and inorganic phosphate (P_i). Because these transitions are coupled to the hydrolysis of ATP, the entire cycle is essentially irreversible. Through repeated cycles, the protein moves continuously to the right along the filament.

Figure 4–51 "Protein machines" can carry out complex functions. These machines are made of individual proteins that collaborate to perform a specific task (Movie 4.11). The movement of proteins is often coordinated and made unidirectional by the hydrolysis of a bound nucleotide such as ATP. Conformational changes of this type are especially useful to the cell if they occur in a large protein assembly in which the activities of several different protein molecules can be coordinated by the movements within the complex, as schematically illustrated here.

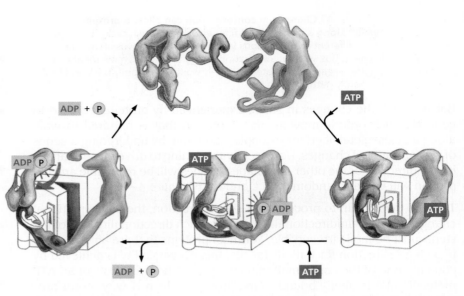

QUESTION 4–8

Explain why the hypothetical enzymes in Figure 4–51 have a great advantage in opening the safe if they work together in a protein complex, as opposed to working individually in an unlinked, sequential manner.

the ensemble of proteins to move coordinately (Figure 4–51). In these machine-like complexes, the appropriate enzymes can be positioned to carry out successive reactions in a series—as during the synthesis of proteins on a ribosome, for example (discussed in Chapter 7). And during cell division, a large protein machine moves rapidly along DNA to replicate the DNA double helix (discussed in Chapter 6 and shown in Movie 6.3 and Movie 6.4).

A large number of different protein machines have evolved to perform many critical biological tasks. Cells make wide use of protein machines for the same reason that humans have invented mechanical and electronic machines: for almost any job, manipulations that are spatially and temporally coordinated through linked processes are much more efficient than is the sequential use of individual tools.

Many Interacting Proteins Are Brought Together by Scaffolds

We have seen that proteins rely on interactions with other molecules to carry out their biological functions. Enzymes bind substrates and regulatory ligands—many of which are generated by other enzymes in the same reaction pathway. Receptor proteins in the plasma membrane, when activated by extracellular ligands, can recruit a set of intracellular signaling proteins that interact with and activate one another, propagating the signal to the cell interior. In addition, the proteins involved in DNA replication, gene transcription, DNA repair, and protein synthesis form protein machines that carry out these complex and crucial tasks with great efficiency.

But how do proteins find the appropriate partners—and the sites where they are needed—within the crowded conditions inside the cell (see Figure 3–22)? Many protein complexes are brought together by **scaffold proteins**, large molecules that contain binding sites recognized by multiple proteins. By binding a specific set of interacting proteins, a scaffold can greatly enhance the rate of a particular chemical reaction or cell process, while also confining this chemistry to a particular area of the cell—for example, drawing signaling proteins to the plasma membrane.

Although some scaffolds are rigid, the most abundant scaffolds in cells are very elastic. Because they contain long unstructured regions that allow them to bend and sway, these scaffolds serve as flexible tethers that greatly enhance the collisions between the proteins that are bound

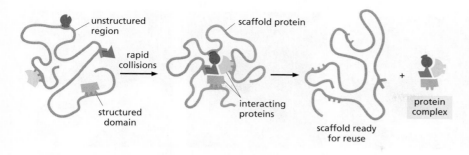

Figure 4–52 Scaffold proteins can concentrate interacting proteins in the cell. In this hypothetical example, each of a set of interacting proteins is bound to a specific structured domain within a long, otherwise unstructured scaffold protein. The unstructured regions of the scaffold act as flexible tethers, and they enhance the rate of formation of the functional complex by promoting the rapid, random collision of the proteins bound to the scaffold.

to them (**Figure 4–52**). Some other scaffolds are not proteins but long molecules of RNA. We encounter these RNA scaffolds when we discuss RNA synthesis and processing in Chapter 7.

Scaffolds allow proteins to be assembled and activated only when and where they are needed. Nerve cells, for example, deploy large, flexible scaffold proteins—some more than 1000 amino acids in length—to organize the specialized proteins involved in transmitting and receiving the signals that carry information from one nerve cell to the next. These proteins cluster beneath the plasma membranes of communicating nerve cells (see Figure 4–54), allowing them both to transmit and to respond to the appropriate messages when stimulated to do so.

Weak Interactions Between Macromolecules Can Produce Large Biochemical Subcompartments in Cells

The aggregates formed by sets of proteins, RNAs, and protein machines can grow quite large, producing distinct biochemical compartments within the cell. The largest of these is the *nucleolus*—the nuclear compartment in which ribosomal RNAs are transcribed and ribosomal subunits are assembled. This cell structure, which is formed when the chromosomes that carry the ribosomal genes come together during interphase (see Figure 5–17), is large enough to be seen in a light microscope. Smaller, transient structures assemble as needed in the nucleus to generate "factories" that carry out DNA replication, DNA repair, or mRNA production (see Figure 7–24). In addition, specific mRNAs are sequestered in cytoplasmic granules that help to control their use in protein synthesis.

The general term used to describe such assemblies, many of which contain both protein and RNA, is an **intracellular condensate**. Some of these condensates, including the nucleolus, can take the form of spherical, liquid droplets that can be seen to break up and fuse (**Figure 4–53**). Although these condensates resemble the sort of phase-separated compartments that form when oil and water mix, their interior makeup is complex and structured. Some are based on amyloid structures, reversible assemblies of stacked β sheets that come together to produce a

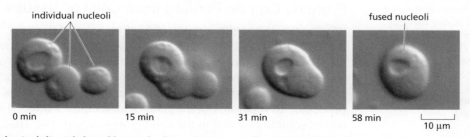

Figure 4–53 Spherical, liquid-drop-like nucleoli can be seen to fuse in the light microscope. In these experiments, the nucleoli are present inside a nucleus that has been dissected from *Xenopus* oocytes and placed under oil on a microscope slide. Here, three nucleoli are seen fusing to form one larger nucleolus (Movie 4.12). A very similar process occurs following each round of division, when small nucleoli initially form on multiple chromosomes, but then coalesce to form a single, large nucleolus. (From C.P. Brangwynne, T.J. Mitchison, and A.A. Hyman, *Proc. Natl. Acad. Sci. USA* 108:4334–4339, 2011.)

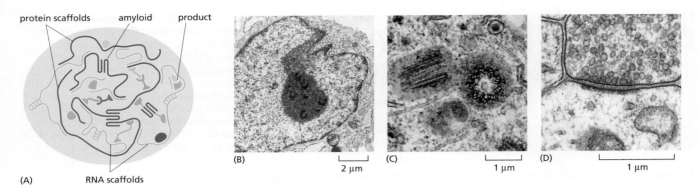

(A)

Figure 4–54 Intracellular condensates can form biochemical subcompartments in cells. These large aggregates form as a result of multiple weak binding interactions between scaffolds and other macromolecules. When these macromolecule–macromolecule interactions become sufficiently strong, a "phase separation" occurs. This creates two distinct aqueous compartments, in one of which the interacting molecules are densely aggregated. Such intracellular condensates concentrate a select set of macromolecules, thereby producing regions with a special biochemistry without the use of an encapsulating membrane.

(A) Schematic illustration of a phase-separated intracellular condensate. These condensates can create a factory that catalyzes the formation of a specific type of product, or they can serve to store important entities, such as specific mRNA molecules, for later use. As shown, reversible amyloid structures often help to create these aggregates. These β-sheet structures form between regions of unstructured amino acid sequence within the larger protein scaffolds.

(B–D) Three examples that illustrate how intracellular condensates (*colorized* regions) are thought to be used by cells. (B) Inside the interphase nucleus, the nucleolus is a large factory that produces ribosomes. In addition, many scattered RNA production factories concentrate the protein machines that transcribe the genome. (C) In the cytoplasm, a matrix forms the centrosome that nucleates the assembly of microtubules. (D) In a patch underlying the plasma membrane at the synapse where communicating nerve cells touch, multiple interacting scaffolds produce large protein assemblies; these create a local biochemistry that makes possible memory formation and storage in the nerve cell network. (B, courtesy of E.G. Jordan and J. McGovern; C, from M. McGill, D.P. Highfield, T.M. Monahan, and B.R. Brinkley, *J. Ultrastruct. Res.* 57:43–53, 1976. With permission from Elsevier; D, courtesy of Cedric Raine.)

"hydrogel" that pulls other molecules into the condensate (**Figure 4–54**). Amyloid-forming proteins thus have functional roles in cells. But for a handful of these amyloid-forming proteins, mutation or perturbation can lead to neurological disease, which is how some of them were initially discovered.

HOW PROTEINS ARE STUDIED

Understanding how a particular protein functions calls for detailed structural and biochemical analyses—both of which require large amounts of pure protein. But isolating a single type of protein from the thousands of other proteins present in a cell is a formidable task. For many years, proteins had to be purified directly from the source—the tissues in which they are most plentiful. That approach was inconvenient, entailing, for example, early-morning trips to the slaughterhouse. More importantly, the complexity of intact tissues and organs is a major disadvantage when trying to purify particular molecules, because a long series of chromatography steps is generally required. These procedures not only take weeks to perform, but they also yield only a few milligrams of pure protein.

Nowadays, proteins are more often isolated from cells that are grown in a laboratory (see, for example, Figure 1–39). Often these cells have been "tricked" into making large quantities of a given protein using the genetic engineering techniques discussed in Chapter 10. Such engineered cells frequently allow large amounts of pure protein to be obtained in only a few days.

In this section, we outline how proteins are extracted and purified from cultured cells and other sources. We describe how these proteins are analyzed to determine their amino acid sequence and their three-dimensional structure. Finally, we discuss how technical advances are allowing proteins to be analyzed, cataloged, manipulated, and even designed from scratch.

Proteins Can Be Purified from Cells or Tissues

Whether starting with a piece of liver or a vat of bacteria, yeast, or animal cells that have been engineered to produce a protein of interest, the first step in any purification procedure involves breaking open the cells to release their contents. The resulting slurry is called a *cell homogenate* or *extract*. This physical disruption is followed by an initial fractionation procedure to separate out the class of molecules of interest—for example, all the soluble proteins in the cell (**Panel 4–3**, pp. 164–165).

With this collection of proteins in hand, the job is then to isolate the desired protein. The standard approach involves purifying the protein through a series of **chromatography** steps, which use different materials to separate the individual components of a complex mixture into portions, or *fractions*, based on the properties of the protein—such as size, shape, or electrical charge. After each separation step, the resulting fractions are examined to determine which ones contain the protein of interest. These fractions are then pooled and subjected to additional chromatography steps until the desired protein is obtained in pure form.

The most efficient forms of protein chromatography separate polypeptides on the basis of their ability to bind to a particular molecule—a process called *affinity chromatography* (**Panel 4–4**, p. 166). If large amounts of antibodies that recognize the protein are available, for example, they can be attached to the matrix of a chromatography column and used to help extract the protein from a mixture (see Panel 4–2, pp. 140–141).

Affinity chromatography can also be used to isolate proteins that interact physically with a protein being studied. In this case, the purified protein of interest is attached tightly to the column matrix; the proteins that bind to it will remain in the column and can then be removed by changing the composition of the washing solution (**Figure 4–55**).

Proteins can also be separated by **electrophoresis**. In this technique, a mixture of proteins is loaded onto a polymer gel and subjected to an electric field; the polypeptides will then migrate through the gel at different speeds depending on their size and net charge (**Panel 4–5**, p. 167). If too many proteins are present in the sample, or if the proteins are very similar in their migration rate, they can be resolved further using two-dimensional gel electrophoresis (see Panel 4–5). These electrophoretic approaches yield a number of bands or spots that can be visualized by staining; each band or spot contains a different protein. Chromatography and electrophoresis—both developed more than 70 years ago but greatly improved since—continue to be instrumental in building an understanding of what proteins look like and how they behave. These and other historical breakthroughs are described in **Table 4–2**.

Once a protein has been obtained in pure form, it can be used in biochemical assays to study the details of its activity. It can also be subjected to techniques that reveal its amino acid sequence and, ultimately, its precise three-dimensional structure.

Determining a Protein's Structure Begins with Determining Its Amino Acid Sequence

The task of determining a protein's primary structure—its amino acid sequence—can be accomplished in several ways. For many years, sequencing a protein was done by directly analyzing the amino acids in the purified protein. First, the protein was broken down into smaller pieces using a selective protease; the enzyme trypsin, for example, cleaves polypeptide chains on the carboxyl side of a lysine or an arginine. Then the identities of the amino acids in each fragment were determined chemically. The first protein sequenced in this way was the hormone *insulin* in 1955.

A much faster way to determine the amino acid sequence of proteins that have been isolated from organisms for which the full genome sequence is known is a method called **mass spectrometry**. This technique determines the exact mass of every peptide fragment in a purified protein, which then allows the protein to be identified from a database that contains a list of every protein thought to be encoded by the genome of the relevant organism. Such lists are computed by taking the organism's genome sequence and applying the genetic code (discussed in Chapter 7).

To perform mass spectrometry, the peptides derived from digestion with trypsin are blasted with a laser. This treatment heats the peptides, causing them to become electrically charged (ionized) and ejected in the

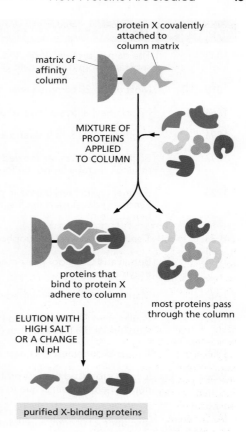

Figure 4–55 Affinity chromatography can be used to isolate the binding partners of a protein of interest. The purified protein of interest (protein X) is covalently attached to the matrix of a chromatography column. An extract containing a mixture of proteins is then loaded onto the column. Those proteins that associate with protein X inside the cell will usually bind to it on the column. Proteins not bound to the column pass right through, and the proteins that are bound tightly to protein X can then be released by changing the pH or ionic composition of the washing solution.

TABLE 4–2 HISTORICAL LANDMARKS IN OUR UNDERSTANDING OF PROTEINS

1838	The name "protein" (from the Greek *proteios*, "primary") was suggested by Berzelius for the complex nitrogen-rich substance found in the cells of all animals and plants
1819–1904	Most of the 20 common amino acids found in proteins were discovered
1864	Hoppe-Seyler crystallized, and named, the protein hemoglobin
1894	Fischer proposed a lock-and-key analogy for enzyme–substrate interactions
1897	Buchner and Buchner showed that cell-free extracts of yeast can break down sucrose to form carbon dioxide and ethanol, thereby laying the foundations of enzymology
1926	Sumner crystallized urease in pure form, demonstrating that proteins could possess the catalytic activity of enzymes; Svedberg developed the first analytical ultracentrifuge and used it to estimate the correct molecular weight of hemoglobin
1933	Tiselius introduced electrophoresis for separating proteins in solution
1934	Bernal and Crowfoot presented the first detailed x-ray diffraction patterns of a protein, obtained from crystals of the enzyme pepsin
1942	Martin and Synge developed chromatography, a technique now widely used to separate proteins
1951	Pauling and Corey proposed the structure of a helical conformation of a chain of amino acids—the α helix—and the structure of the β sheet, both of which were later found in many proteins
1955	Sanger determined the order of amino acids in insulin, the first protein whose amino acid sequence was determined
1956	Ingram produced the first protein fingerprints, showing that the difference between sickle-cell hemoglobin and normal hemoglobin is due to a change in a single amino acid (Movie 4.13)
1960	Kendrew described the first detailed three-dimensional structure of a protein (sperm whale myoglobin) to a resolution of 0.2 nm, and Perutz proposed a lower-resolution structure for hemoglobin
1963	Monod, Jacob, and Changeux recognized that many enzymes are regulated through allosteric changes in their conformation
1966	Phillips described the three-dimensional structure of lysozyme by x-ray crystallography, the first enzyme to be analyzed in atomic detail
1973	Nomura reconstituted a functional bacterial ribosome from purified components
1975	Henderson and Unwin determined the first three-dimensional structure of a transmembrane protein (bacteriorhodopsin), using a computer-based reconstruction from electron micrographs
1976	Neher and Sakmann developed patch-clamp recording to measure the activity of single ion-channel proteins
1984	Wüthrich used nuclear magnetic resonance (NMR) spectroscopy to solve the three-dimensional structure of a soluble sperm protein
1988	Tanaka and Fenn separately developed methods for using mass spectrometry to analyze proteins and other biological macromolecules
1996–2013	Mann, Aebersold, Yates, and others refine methods for using mass spectrometry to identify proteins in complex mixtures, exploiting the availability of complete genome sequences
1975–2013	Frank, Dubochet, Henderson and others develop computer-based methods for single-particle cryoelectron microscopy (cryo-EM), enabling determination of the structures of large protein complexes at atomic resolution

form of a gas. Accelerated by a powerful electric field, the peptide ions then fly toward a detector; the time it takes them to arrive is related to their mass and their charge. (The larger the peptide is, the more slowly it moves; the more highly charged it is, the faster it moves.) The set of very exact masses of the protein fragments produced by trypsin cleavage then serves as a "fingerprint" that can be used to identify the protein—and its corresponding gene—from publicly accessible databases (Figure 4–56).

This approach can even be applied to complex mixtures of proteins; for example, starting with an extract containing all the proteins made by yeast cells grown under a particular set of conditions. To obtain the increased resolution required to distinguish individual proteins, such

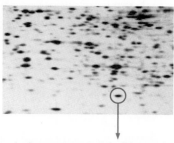

single protein spot excised from gel

Figure 4–56 Mass spectrometry can be used to identify proteins by determining the precise masses of peptides derived from them. As indicated, this in turn allows proteins of interest to be produced in the large amounts needed for determining their three-dimensional structure. In this example, a protein of interest is excised from a polyacrylamide gel after two-dimensional electrophoresis (see Panel 4–5, p. 167) and then digested with trypsin. The peptide fragments are loaded into the mass spectrometer, and their exact masses are measured. Genome sequence databases are then searched to find the protein encoded by the organism in question whose profile matches this peptide fingerprint. Mixtures of proteins can also be analyzed in this way. (Image courtesy of Patrick O'Farrell.)

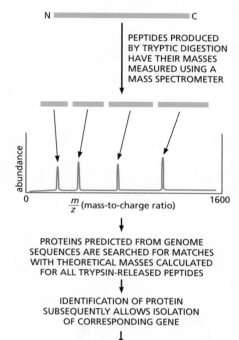

mixtures are frequently analyzed using *tandem mass spectrometry*. In this case, after the peptides pass through the first mass spectrometer, they are broken into even smaller fragments and analyzed by a second mass spectrometer.

Although all the information required for a polypeptide chain to fold is contained in its amino acid sequence, only in special cases can we reliably predict a protein's detailed three-dimensional conformation—the spatial arrangement of its atoms—from its sequence alone. Today, the predominant way to discover the precise folding pattern of any protein is by experiment, using **x-ray crystallography**, **nuclear magnetic resonance (NMR) spectroscopy**, or most recently **cryoelectron microscopy (cryo-EM)**, as described in Panel 4–6 (pp. 168–169).

Genetic Engineering Techniques Permit the Large-Scale Production, Design, and Analysis of Almost Any Protein

Advances in genetic engineering techniques now permit the production of large quantities of almost any desired protein. In addition to making life much easier for biochemists interested in purifying specific proteins, this ability to churn out huge quantities of a protein has given rise to an entire biotechnology industry (Figure 4–57). Bacteria, yeast, and cultured mammalian cells are now used to mass-produce a variety of therapeutic proteins, such as insulin, human growth hormone, and even the fertility-enhancing drugs used to boost egg production in women undergoing *in vitro* fertilization treatment. Preparing these proteins previously required the collection and processing of vast amounts of tissue and other biological products—including, in the case of the fertility drugs, the urine of postmenopausal nuns.

The same sorts of genetic engineering techniques can also be employed to produce new proteins and enzymes that contain novel structures or perform unusual tasks: metabolizing toxic wastes or synthesizing lifesaving drugs, for example. Most synthetic catalysts are nowhere near as effective as naturally occurring enzymes in terms of their ability to speed

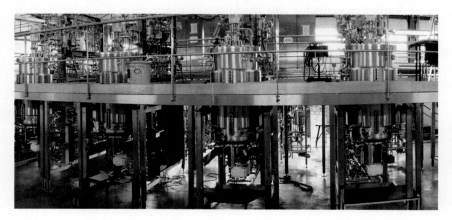

Figure 4–57 Biotechnology companies produce mass quantities of useful proteins. Shown in this photograph are the large, turnkey microbial fermenters used to produce a whooping cough vaccine. (Courtesy of Pierre Guerin Technologies.)

the rate of selected chemical reactions. But, as we continue to learn more about how proteins and enzymes exploit their unique conformations to carry out their biological functions, our ability to make novel proteins with useful functions can only improve.

The Relatedness of Proteins Aids the Prediction of Protein Structure and Function

Biochemists have made enormous progress over the past 150 years in understanding the structure and function of proteins (see Table 4–2, p. 160). These advances are the fruits of decades of painstaking research on isolated proteins, performed by individual scientists working tirelessly on single proteins or protein families, one by one, sometimes for their entire careers. In the future, however, more and more of these investigations of protein conformation and activity will likely take place on a larger scale.

Improvements in our ability to rapidly sequence whole genomes, and the development of methods such as mass spectrometry, have fueled our ability to determine the amino acid sequences of enormous numbers of proteins. Millions of unique protein sequences from thousands of different species have thereby been deposited into publicly available databases, and the collection is expected to double in size every two years. Comparing the amino acid sequences of all of these proteins reveals that the majority belong to protein families that share specific "sequence patterns"—stretches of amino acids that fold into distinct structural domains. In some of these families, the proteins contain only a single structural domain. In others, the proteins include multiple domains arranged in novel combinations (**Figure 4–58**).

Although the number of multidomain families is growing rapidly, the discovery of novel single domains appears to be leveling off. This plateau suggests that the vast majority of proteins may fold up into a limited number of structural domains—perhaps as few as 10,000 to 20,000. For many single-domain families, the structure of at least one family member is known. And knowing the structure of one family member allows us to say something about the structure of its relatives. By this account, we have some structural information for almost three-quarters of the proteins archived in databases (Movie 4.14).

A future goal is to acquire the ability to look at a protein's amino acid sequence and be able to deduce its structure and gain insight into its function. We are coming closer to being able to predict protein structure based on sequence information alone, but we still have a considerable way to go. To date, computational methods that take an amino acid sequence and search for the protein conformations with the lowest energy have been successful for proteins less than 100 amino acids long, or for longer proteins for which additional information is available (such as homology with proteins whose structure is known).

Looking at an amino acid sequence and predicting how a protein will function—alone or as part of a complex in the cell—is more challenging still. But the closer we get to accomplishing these goals, the closer we will be to understanding the fundamental basis of life.

ESSENTIAL CONCEPTS

- Living cells contain an enormously diverse set of protein molecules, each made as a linear chain of amino acids linked together by covalent peptide bonds.

- Each type of protein has a unique amino acid sequence, which

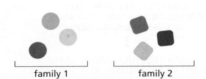

family 1   family 2

(A) single-domain protein families

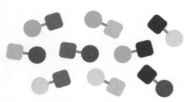

(B) a two-domain protein family

Figure 4–58 Most proteins belong to structurally related families. (A) More than two-thirds of all well-studied proteins contain a single structural domain. The members of these single-domain families can have different amino acid sequences but fold into a protein with a similar shape. (B) During evolution, structural domains have been combined in different ways to produce families of multidomain proteins. Almost all novelty in protein structure comes from the way these single domains are arranged. Unlike the number of novel single domains, the number of multidomain families being added to the public databases is still rapidly increasing.

determines both its three-dimensional shape and its biological activity.

- The folded structure of a protein is stabilized by multiple noncovalent interactions between different parts of the polypeptide chain.

- Hydrogen bonds between neighboring regions of the polypeptide backbone often give rise to regular folding patterns, known as α helices and β sheets.

- The structure of many proteins can be subdivided into smaller globular regions of compact three-dimensional structure, known as protein domains.

- The biological function of a protein depends on the detailed chemical properties of its surface and how it binds to other molecules called ligands.

- When a protein catalyzes the formation or breakage of a specific covalent bond in a ligand, the protein is called an enzyme and the ligand is called a substrate.

- At the active site of an enzyme, the amino acid side chains of the folded protein are precisely positioned so that they favor the formation of the high-energy transition states that the substrates must pass through to be converted to product.

- The three-dimensional structure of many proteins has evolved so that the binding of a small ligand outside of the active site can induce a significant change in protein shape.

- Most enzymes are allosteric proteins that can exist in two conformations that differ in catalytic activity, and the enzyme can be turned on or off by ligands that bind to a distinct regulatory site to stabilize either the active or the inactive conformation.

- The activities of most enzymes within the cell are strictly regulated. One of the most common forms of regulation is feedback inhibition, in which an enzyme early in a metabolic pathway is inhibited by the binding of one of the pathway's end products.

- Many thousands of proteins in a typical eukaryotic cell are regulated by cycles of phosphorylation and dephosphorylation.

- GTP-binding proteins also regulate protein function in eukaryotes; they act as molecular switches that are active when GTP is bound and inactive when GDP is bound, turning themselves off by hydrolyzing their bound GTP to GDP.

- Motor proteins produce directed movement in eukaryotic cells through conformational changes linked to the hydrolysis of a tightly bound molecule of ATP to ADP.

- Highly efficient protein machines are formed by assemblies of allosteric proteins in which the various conformational changes are coordinated to perform complex functions.

- Covalent modifications added to a protein's amino acid side chains can control the location and function of the protein and can serve as docking sites for other proteins.

- Biochemical subcompartments often form as phase-separated intracellular condensates, speeding important reactions and confining them to specific regions of the cell.

- Starting from crude cell or tissue homogenates, individual proteins can be obtained in pure form by using a series of chromatography steps.

- The function of a purified protein can be discovered by biochemical analyses, and its exact three-dimensional structure can be determined by x-ray crystallography, NMR spectroscopy, or cryoelectron microscopy.

BREAKING OPEN CELLS AND TISSUES

The first step in the purification of most proteins is to disrupt tissues and cells in a controlled fashion.

Using gentle mechanical procedures, called homogenization, the plasma membranes of cells can be ruptured so that the cell contents are released. Four commonly used procedures are shown here.

The resulting thick soup (called a homogenate or an extract) contains large and small molecules from the cytosol, such as enzymes, ribosomes, and metabolites, as well as all of the membrane-enclosed organelles.

cell
suspension
or
tissue

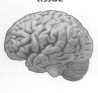

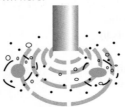

1 Break apart cells with high-frequency sound (ultrasound).

2 Use a mild detergent to make holes in the plasma membrane.

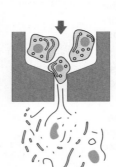

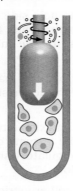

3 Force cells through a small hole using high pressure.

4 Shear cells between a close-fitting rotating plunger and the thick walls of a glass vessel.

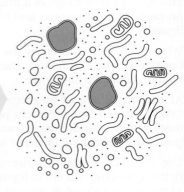

When carefully conducted, homogenization leaves most of the membrane-enclosed organelles largely intact.

THE CENTRIFUGE

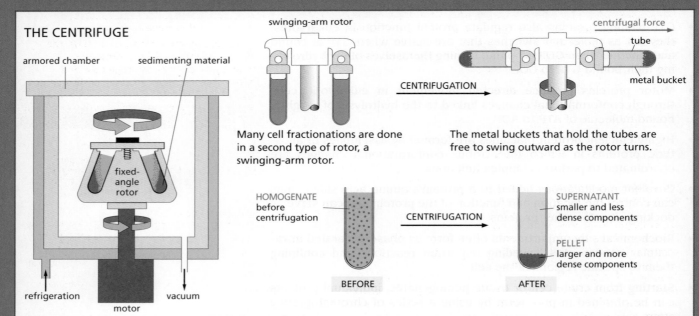

armored chamber

sedimenting material

fixed-angle rotor

refrigeration

motor

vacuum

swinging-arm rotor

CENTRIFUGATION

centrifugal force

tube

metal bucket

Many cell fractionations are done in a second type of rotor, a swinging-arm rotor.

The metal buckets that hold the tubes are free to swing outward as the rotor turns.

HOMOGENATE before centrifugation

CENTRIFUGATION

SUPERNATANT smaller and less dense components

PELLET larger and more dense components

BEFORE

AFTER

Centrifugation is the most widely used procedure to separate a homogenate into different parts, or fractions. The homogenate is placed in test tubes and rotated at high speed in a centrifuge or ultracentrifuge. Present-day ultracentrifuges rotate at speeds up to 100,000 revolutions per minute and produce enormous forces, as high as 600,000 times gravity.

Such speeds require centrifuge chambers to be refrigerated and have the air evacuated so that friction does not heat up the homogenate. The centrifuge is surrounded by thick armor plating, because an unbalanced rotor can shatter with an explosive release of energy. A fixed-angle rotor can hold larger volumes than a swinging-arm rotor, but the pellet forms less evenly, as shown.

DIFFERENTIAL CENTRIFUGATION

Repeated centrifugation at progressively higher speeds will fractionate cell homogenates into their components.

Centrifugation separates cell components on the basis of size and density. The larger and denser components experience the greatest centrifugal force and move most rapidly. They sediment to form a pellet at the bottom of the tube, while smaller, less dense components remain in suspension above, a portion called the supernatant.

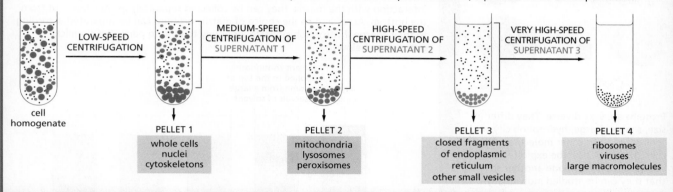

cell homogenate

LOW-SPEED CENTRIFUGATION

MEDIUM-SPEED CENTRIFUGATION OF SUPERNATANT 1

HIGH-SPEED CENTRIFUGATION OF SUPERNATANT 2

VERY HIGH-SPEED CENTRIFUGATION OF SUPERNATANT 3

PELLET 1
whole cells
nuclei
cytoskeletons

PELLET 2
mitochondria
lysosomes
peroxisomes

PELLET 3
closed fragments
of endoplasmic
reticulum
other small vesicles

PELLET 4
ribosomes
viruses
large macromolecules

VELOCITY SEDIMENTATION

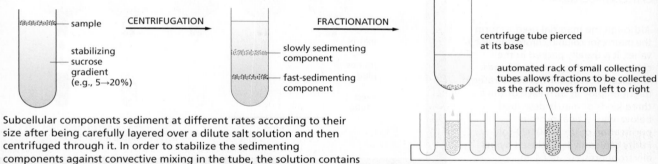

sample

CENTRIFUGATION

stabilizing sucrose gradient (e.g., 5→20%)

slowly sedimenting component

fast-sedimenting component

FRACTIONATION

centrifuge tube pierced at its base

automated rack of small collecting tubes allows fractions to be collected as the rack moves from left to right

rack movement ⟶

Subcellular components sediment at different rates according to their size after being carefully layered over a dilute salt solution and then centrifuged through it. In order to stabilize the sedimenting components against convective mixing in the tube, the solution contains a continuous shallow gradient of sucrose that increases in concentration toward the bottom of the tube. The gradient is typically 5→20% sucrose. When sedimented through such a dilute sucrose gradient, using a swinging-arm rotor, different cell components separate into distinct bands that can be collected individually.

After an appropriate centrifugation time, the bands may be collected, most simply by puncturing the plastic centrifuge tube and collecting drops from the bottom, as shown here.

EQUILIBRIUM SEDIMENTATION

The ultracentrifuge can also be used to separate cell components on the basis of their buoyant density, independently of their size or shape. The sample is usually either layered on top of, or dispersed within, a steep density gradient that contains a very high concentration of sucrose or cesium chloride. Each subcellular component will move up or down when centrifuged until it reaches a position where its density matches its surroundings and then will move no further. A series of distinct bands will eventually be produced, with those nearest the bottom of the tube containing the components of highest buoyant density. The method is also called density gradient centrifugation.

The sample is distributed throughout the sucrose density gradient.

At equilibrium, components have migrated to a region in the gradient that matches their own density.

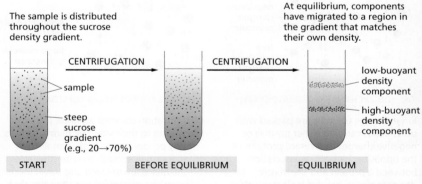

CENTRIFUGATION

sample

steep sucrose gradient (e.g., 20→70%)

START

CENTRIFUGATION

BEFORE EQUILIBRIUM

low-buoyant density component

high-buoyant density component

EQUILIBRIUM

A sucrose gradient is shown here, but denser gradients can be formed with cesium chloride that are particularly useful for separating nucleic acids (DNA and RNA).

The final bands can be collected from the base of the tube, as shown above for velocity sedimentation.

PROTEIN SEPARATION

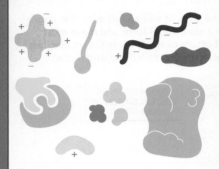

Proteins are very diverse. They differ in size, shape, charge, hydrophobicity, and their affinity for other molecules. All of these properties can be exploited to separate them from one another so that they can be studied individually.

THREE KINDS OF CHROMATOGRAPHY

Although the material used to form the matrix for column chromatography varies, it is usually packed in the column in the form of small beads. A typical protein purification strategy might employ in turn each of the three kinds of matrix described below, with a final protein purification of up to 10,000-fold. Purity can easily be assessed by gel electrophoresis (Panel 4–5).

COLUMN CHROMATOGRAPHY

Proteins are often fractionated by column chromatography. A mixture of proteins in solution is applied to the top of a cylindrical column filled with a permeable solid matrix immersed in solvent. A large amount of solvent is then pumped through the column. Because different proteins are retarded to different extents by their interaction with the matrix, they can be collected separately as they flow out from the bottom. According to the choice of matrix, proteins can be separated according to their charge, hydrophobicity, size, or ability to bind to particular chemical groups (see below).

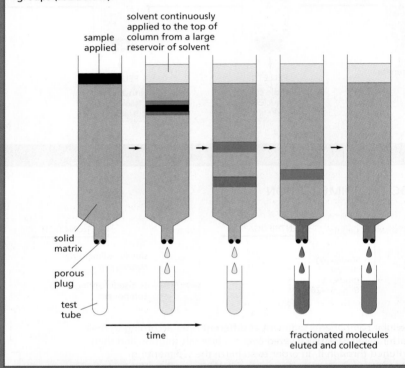

(A) ION-EXCHANGE CHROMATOGRAPHY

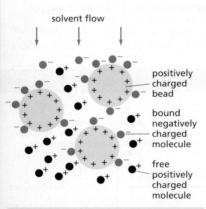

Ion-exchange columns are packed with small beads carrying either positive or negative charges that retard proteins of the opposite charge. The association between a protein and the matrix depends on the pH and ionic strength of the solution passing down the column. These can be varied in a controlled way to achieve an effective separation.

(B) GEL-FILTRATION CHROMATOGRAPHY

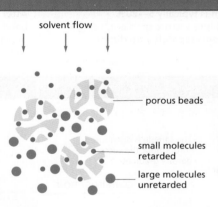

Gel-filtration columns separate proteins according to their size. The matrix consists of tiny porous beads. Protein molecules that are small enough to enter the holes in the beads are delayed and travel more slowly through the column. Proteins that cannot enter the beads are washed out of the column first. Such columns also allow an estimate of protein size.

(C) AFFINITY CHROMATOGRAPHY

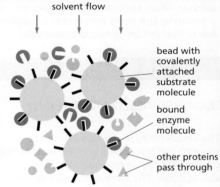

Affinity columns contain a matrix covalently coupled to a molecule that interacts specifically with the protein of interest (e.g., an antibody or an enzyme substrate). Proteins that bind specifically to such a column can subsequently be released by a pH change or by concentrated salt solutions, and they emerge highly purified (see Figure 4–55).

GEL ELECTROPHORESIS

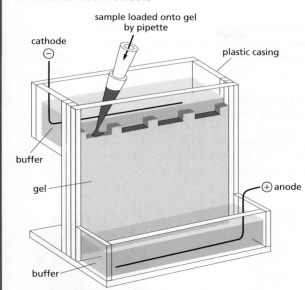

When an electric field is applied to a solution containing protein molecules, the proteins will migrate in a direction and at a speed that reflects their size and net charge. This forms the basis of the technique called electrophoresis.

The detergent sodium dodecyl sulfate (SDS) is used to solubilize proteins for SDS polyacrylamide-gel electrophoresis.

SDS

ISOELECTRIC FOCUSING

For any protein there is a characteristic pH, called the isoelectric point, at which the protein has no net charge and therefore will not move in an electric field. In isoelectric focusing, proteins are electrophoresed in a narrow tube of polyacrylamide gel in which a pH gradient is established by a mixture of special buffers. Each protein moves to a point in the pH gradient that corresponds to its isoelectric point and stays there.

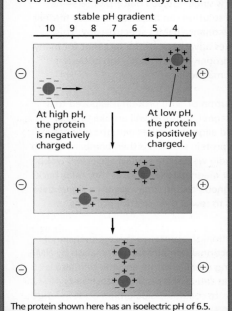

At high pH, the protein is negatively charged.

At low pH, the protein is positively charged.

The protein shown here has an isoelectric pH of 6.5.

SDS polyacrylamide-gel electrophoresis (SDS-PAGE)

Individual polypeptide chains form a complex with negatively charged molecules of sodium dodecyl sulfate (SDS) and therefore migrate as negatively charged SDS–protein complexes through a slab of porous polyacrylamide gel. The apparatus used for this electrophoresis technique is shown above (*left*). A reducing agent (mercaptoethanol) is usually added to break any S–S linkages within or between proteins. Under these conditions, unfolded polypeptide chains migrate at a rate that reflects their molecular weight, with the smallest proteins migrating most quickly.

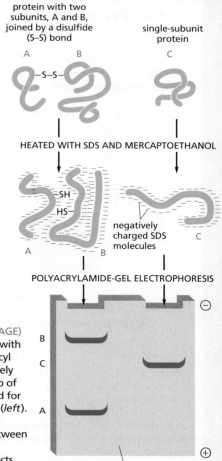

protein with two subunits, A and B, joined by a disulfide (S–S) bond

single-subunit protein

HEATED WITH SDS AND MERCAPTOETHANOL

negatively charged SDS molecules

POLYACRYLAMIDE-GEL ELECTROPHORESIS

slab of polyacrylamide gel

TWO-DIMENSIONAL POLYACRYLAMIDE-GEL ELECTROPHORESIS

Complex mixtures of proteins cannot be resolved well on one-dimensional gels, but two-dimensional gel electrophoresis, combining two different separation methods, can be used to resolve more than 1000 proteins in a two-dimensional protein map. In the first step, native proteins are separated in a narrow gel on the basis of their intrinsic charge using isoelectric focusing (see *left*). In the second step, this gel is placed on top of a gel slab, and the proteins are subjected to SDS-PAGE (see *above*) in a direction perpendicular to that used in the first step. Each protein migrates to form a discrete spot.

All the proteins in an *E. coli* bacterial cell are separated in this two-dimensional gel, in which each spot corresponds to a different polypeptide chain. They are separated according to their isoelectric point from left to right and to their molecular weight from top to bottom. (Courtesy of Patrick O'Farrell.)

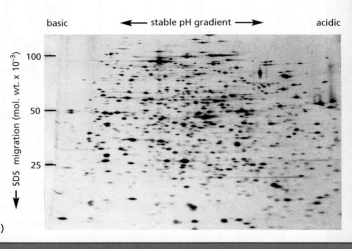

X-RAY CRYSTALLOGRAPHY

To determine a protein's **three-dimensional structure**—and assess how this conformation changes as the protein functions—one must be able to "see" the relative positions of the protein's individual atoms. Since the 1930s, x-ray crystallography has been the gold standard for the determination of protein structure. This method uses x rays—which have a wavelength approximately equal to the diameter of a hydrogen atom—to probe the structure of proteins at an atomic level.

To begin, the purified protein is first coaxed into forming crystals: large, highly ordered arrays in which every protein molecule has the same conformation and is perfectly aligned with its neighbors. The process can take years of trial and error to find the right conditions to produce high-quality protein crystals. When a narrow beam of x-rays is directed at this crystal, the atoms in the protein molecules scatter the incoming x-rays. These scattered waves either reinforce or cancel one another, producing a complex diffraction pattern that is collected by electronic detectors. The position and intensity of each spot in the x-ray diffraction pattern contain information about the position of the atoms in the protein crystal.

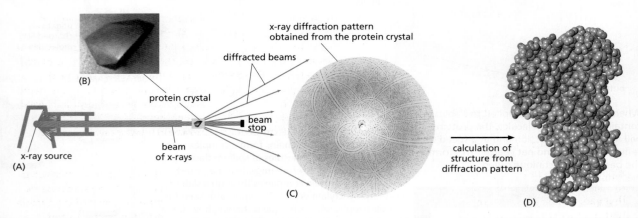

Computers then transform these patterns into maps of the relative spatial positions of the atoms. By combining this information with the amino acid sequence of the protein, an atomic model of the protein's structure can be generated. The protein shown here is ribulose bisphosphate carboxylase (Rubisco), an enzyme that plays a central role in CO_2 fixation during photosynthesis (discussed in Chapter 14). The protein illustrated is approximately 450 amino acids in length. Nitrogen atoms are shown in *blue*, oxygen in *red*, phosphorus in *yellow*; and carbon in *gray*. (B, courtesy of C. Branden; C, courtesy of J. Hajdu and I. Andersson.)

NMR SPECTROSCOPY

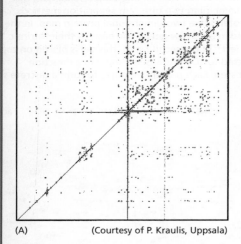

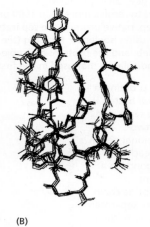

(A)   (Courtesy of P. Kraulis, Uppsala)   (B)

If a protein is small—50,000 daltons or less—its structure in solution can be determined by **nuclear magnetic resonance (NMR) spectroscopy.** This method takes advantage of the fact that for many atoms—hydrogen in particular—the nucleus is intrinsically magnetic.

When a solution of pure protein is exposed to a powerful magnet, its nuclei will act like tiny bar magnets and align themselves with the magnetic field. If the protein solution is then bombarded with a blast of radio waves, the excited nuclei will wobble around their magnetic axes, and, as they relax back into the aligned position, they give off a signal that can be used to reveal their relative positions.

Again, combined with an amino acid sequence, an NMR spectrum can allow the computation of a protein's three-dimensional structure. Proteins larger than 50,000 daltons can be broken up into their constituent functional domains before analysis by NMR spectroscopy. In (A), a two-dimensional NMR spectrum derived from the C-terminal binding domain of the enzyme cellulase is shown. The spots represent interactions between neighboring H atoms. The structures that satisfy the distance constraints presented by the NMR spectrum are shown superimposed in (B). This domain, which binds to cellulose, is 36 amino acids in length.

CRYOELECTRON MICROSCOPY

X-ray crystallography remains the first port of call when determining proteins' structures. However, large macromolecular machines are often hard to crystallize, as are many integral membrane proteins, and for dynamic proteins and assemblies it is hard to access different conformations through crystallography alone. To get around these problems, investigators are increasingly turning to **cryoelectron microscopy** (cryo-EM) to solve macromolecular structures.

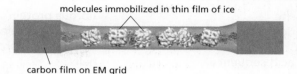

molecules immobilized in thin film of ice

carbon film on EM grid

In this technique, a droplet of the pure protein in water is placed on a small EM grid that is plunged into a vat of liquid ethane at −180°C. This freezes the proteins in a thin film of ice and the rapid freezing ensures that the surrounding water molecules have no time to form ice crystals, which would damage the protein's shape.

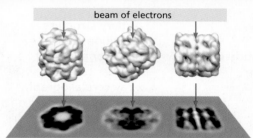

beam of electrons

electron detector captures projected image of molecules

The sample is examined, still frozen, by transmission electron microscopy (see Panel 1–1, p. 13). To avoid damage, it is important that only a few electrons pass through each part of the specimen, sensitive detectors are therefore deployed to capture every electron that passes through the specimen. Much EM specimen preparation and data collection is now fully automated and many thousands of micrographs are typically captured, each of which will contain hundreds or thousands of individual molecules all arranged in random orientations within the ice.

Algorithms then sort the particles into sets that each contains particles that are all oriented in the same direction. The thousands of images in each set are all then superimposed and averaged to improve the signal to noise ratio.

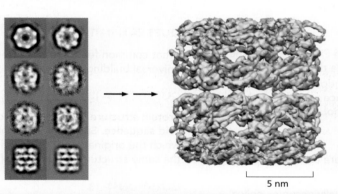

This crisper two-dimensional image set, which represents different views of the particle, are then combined and converted via a series of complex iterative steps into a high resolution three-dimensional structure.

Model of GroEL
(Courtesy of Gabriel Lander.)

5 nm

CRYO-EM STRUCTURE OF THE RIBOSOME

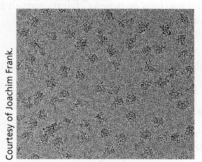

Courtesy of Joachim Frank.

60S ribosomal subunits randomly oriented in a thin film of ice

100 nm

60S large ribosomal subunit at 0.25 nm resolution

path of a rRNA loop fitted into the electron density map

Mg^{2+}

G   C
RNA bases

5 nm

1 nm

Although by no means routine, big improvements in image processing algorithms, modeling tools and sheer computing power all mean that structures of macromolecular complexes are now becoming attainable with resolutions in the 0.2 to 0.3 nm range.

This resolving power now approaches that of x-ray crystallography, and the two techniques thrive together, each bootstrapping the other to obtain ever more useful and dynamic structural information. A good example is the structure of the ribosome shown here at a resolution of 0.25 nm.

KEY TERMS

active site	fibrous protein	protein
allosteric	globular protein	protein domain
α helix	GTP-binding protein	protein family
amino acid sequence	helix	protein kinase
antibody	intracellular condensate	protein machine
antigen	intrinsically disordered sequence	protein phosphatase
β sheet	ligand	protein phosphorylation
binding site	lysozyme	quaternary structure
C-terminus	mass spectrometry	scaffold protein
chromatography	Michaelis constant (K_M)	secondary structure
coenzyme	motor protein	side chain
coiled-coil	N-terminus	substrate
conformation	nuclear magnetic resonance	subunit
cryoelectron microscopy (cryo-EM)	(NMR) spectroscopy	tertiary structure
disulfide bond	peptide bond	transition state
electrophoresis	polypeptide, polypeptide chain	turnover number
enzyme	polypeptide backbone	V_{max}
feedback inhibition	primary structure	x-ray crystallography

QUESTIONS

QUESTION 4–9

Look at the models of the protein in Figure 4–11. Is the *red* α helix right- or left-handed? Are the three strands that form the large β sheet parallel or antiparallel? Starting at the N-terminus (the *purple* end), trace your finger along the peptide backbone. Are there any knots? Why, or why not?

QUESTION 4–10

Which of the following statements are correct? Explain your answers.

A. The active site of an enzyme usually occupies only a small fraction of the enzyme surface.

B. Catalysis by some enzymes involves the formation of a covalent bond between an amino acid side chain and a substrate molecule.

C. A β sheet can contain up to five strands, but no more.

D. The specificity of an antibody molecule is contained exclusively in loops on the surface of the folded light-chain domain.

E. The possible linear arrangements of amino acids are so vast that new proteins almost never evolve by alteration of old ones.

F. Allosteric enzymes have two or more binding sites.

G. Noncovalent bonds are too weak to influence the three-dimensional structure of macromolecules.

H. Affinity chromatography separates molecules according to their intrinsic charge.

I. Upon centrifugation of a cell homogenate, smaller organelles experience less friction and thereby sediment faster than larger ones.

QUESTION 4–11

What common feature of α helices and β sheets makes them universal building blocks for proteins?

QUESTION 4–12

Protein structure is determined solely by a protein's amino acid sequence. Should a genetically engineered protein in which the original order of all amino acids is reversed have the same structure as the original protein?

QUESTION 4–13

Consider the following protein sequence as an α helix: Leu-Lys-Arg-Ile-Val-Asp-Ile-Leu-Ser-Arg-Leu-Phe-Lys-Val. How many turns does this helix make? Do you find anything remarkable about the arrangement of the amino acids in this sequence when folded into an α helix? (Hint: consult the properties of the amino acids in Figure 4–3.)

QUESTION 4–14

Simple enzyme reactions often conform to the equation:

$$E + S \leftrightarrow ES \rightarrow EP \leftrightarrow E + P$$

where E, S, and P are enzyme, substrate, and product, respectively.

A. What does ES represent in this equation?

B. Why is the first step shown with bidirectional arrows and the second step as a unidirectional arrow?

C. Why does E appear at both ends of the equation?

D. One often finds that high concentrations of P inhibit the enzyme. Suggest why this might occur.

E. If compound X resembles S and binds to the active site

of the enzyme but cannot undergo the reaction catalyzed by it, what effects would you expect the addition of X to the reaction to have? Compare the effects of X and of the accumulation of P.

QUESTION 4–15

Which of the following amino acids would you expect to find more often near the center of a folded globular protein? Which ones would you expect to find more often exposed to the outside? Explain your answers. Ser, Ser-P (a Ser residue that is phosphorylated), Leu, Lys, Gln, His, Phe, Val, Ile, Met, Cys–S–S–Cys (two cysteines that are disulfide-bonded), and Glu. Where would you expect to find the most N-terminal amino acid and the most C-terminal amino acid?

QUESTION 4–16

Assume you want to make and study fragments of a protein. Would you expect that any fragment of the polypeptide chain would fold the same way as it would in the intact protein? Consider the protein shown in Figure 4–20. Which fragments do you suppose are most likely to fold correctly?

QUESTION 4–17

Neurofilament proteins assemble into long, intermediate filaments (discussed in Chapter 17), found in abundance running along the length of nerve cell axons. The C-terminal region of these proteins is an unstructured polypeptide, hundreds of amino acids long and heavily modified by the addition of phosphate groups. The term "polymer brush" has been applied to this part of the neurofilament. Can you suggest why?

QUESTION 4–18

An enzyme isolated from a mutant bacterium grown at 20°C works in a test tube at 20°C but not at 37°C (37°C is the temperature of the gut, where this bacterium normally lives). Furthermore, once the enzyme has been exposed to the higher temperature, it no longer works at the lower one. The same enzyme isolated from the normal bacterium works at both temperatures. Can you suggest what happens (at the molecular level) to the mutant enzyme as the temperature increases?

QUESTION 4–19

A motor protein moves along protein filaments in the cell. Why are the elements shown in the illustration not sufficient to mediate directed movement (Figure Q4–19)? With reference to Figure 4–50, modify the illustration shown here to include other elements that are required to create a unidirectional motor, and justify each modification you make to the illustration.

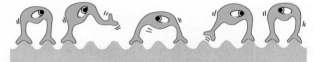

Figure Q4–19

QUESTION 4–20

Gel-filtration chromatography separates molecules according to their size (see Panel 4–4, p. 166). Smaller molecules diffuse faster in solution than larger ones, yet smaller molecules migrate more slowly through a gel-filtration column than larger ones. Explain this paradox. What should happen at very rapid flow rates?

QUESTION 4–21

As shown in Figure 4–16, both α helices and the coiled-coil structures that can form from them are helical structures, but do they have the same handedness in the figure? Explain why?

QUESTION 4–22

How is it possible that a change in a single amino acid in a protein of 1000 amino acids can destroy protein function, even when that amino acid is far away from any ligand-binding site?

QUESTION 4–23

The curve shown in Figure 4–35 is described by the Michaelis–Menten equation:

$$\text{rate } (v) = V_{max} [S]/(K_M + [S])$$

Can you convince yourself that the features qualitatively described in the text are accurately represented by this equation? In particular, how can the equation be simplified when the substrate concentration [S] is in one of the following ranges: (A) [S] is much smaller than the K_M, (B) [S] equals the K_M, and (C) [S] is much larger than the K_M?

QUESTION 4–24

The rate of a simple enzyme reaction is given by the standard Michaelis–Menten equation:

$$\text{rate} = V_{max} [S]/(K_M + [S])$$

If the V_{max} of an enzyme is 100 μmole/sec and the K_M is 1 mM, at what substrate concentration is the rate 50 μmole/sec? Plot a graph of rate versus substrate (S) concentration for [S] = 0 to 10 mM. Convert this to a plot of 1/rate versus 1/[S]. Why is the latter plot a straight line?

QUESTION 4–25

Select the correct options in the following and explain your choices. If [S] is very much smaller than K_M, the active site of the enzyme is mostly occupied/unoccupied. If [S] is very much greater than K_M, the reaction rate is limited by the enzyme/substrate concentration.

QUESTION 4–26

A. The reaction rates of the reaction S → P, catalyzed by enzyme E, were determined under conditions in which only very little product was formed. The data in the table below were measured, plot the data as a graph. Use this graph to estimate the K_M and the V_{max} for this enzyme.

B. To determine the K_M and V_{max} values more precisely, a trick is generally used in which the Michaelis–Menten equation is transformed so that it is possible to plot the data as a straight line. A simple rearrangement yields

$$1/\text{rate} = (K_M/V_{max}) (1/[S]) + 1/V_{max}$$

which is an equation of the form $y = ax + b$. Calculate 1/rate and 1/[S] for the data given in part (A) and then plot

Substrate Concentration (μM)	Reaction Rate (μmole/min)
0.08	0.15
0.12	0.21
0.54	0.7
1.23	1.1
1.82	1.3
2.72	1.5
4.94	1.7
10.00	1.8

1/rate versus 1/[S] as a new graph. Determine K_M and V_{max} from the intercept of the line with the axis, where 1/[S] = 0, combined with the slope of the line. Do your results agree with the estimates made from the first graph of the raw data?

C. It is stated in part (A) that only very little product was formed under the reaction conditions. Why is this important?

D. Assume the enzyme is regulated such that upon phosphorylation its K_M increases by a factor of 3 without changing its V_{max}. Is this an activation or inhibition? Plot the data you would expect for the phosphorylated enzyme in both the graph for (A) and the graph for (B).

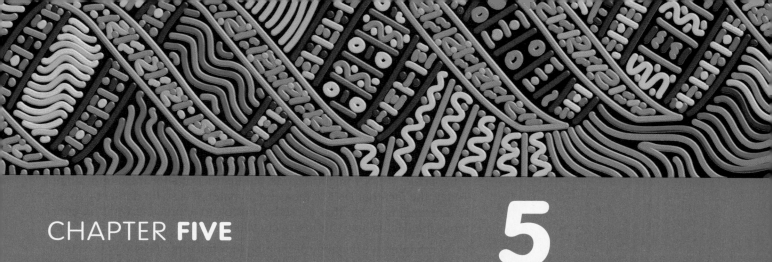

DNA and Chromosomes

Life depends on the ability of cells to store, retrieve, and translate the genetic instructions required to make and maintain a living organism. These instructions are stored within every living cell in its *genes*—the information-bearing elements that determine the characteristics of a species as a whole and of the individuals within it.

At the beginning of the twentieth century, when genetics emerged as a science, scientists became intrigued by the chemical nature of genes. The information in genes is copied and transmitted from a cell to its daughter cells millions of times during the life of a multicellular organism, and passed from generation to generation through the reproductive cells—eggs and sperm. Genes survive this process of replication and transmission essentially unchanged. What kind of molecule could be capable of such accurate and almost unlimited replication, and also be able to direct the development of an organism and the daily life of a cell? What kind of instructions does the genetic information contain? How are these instructions physically organized so that the enormous amount of information required for the development and maintenance of even the simplest organism can be contained within the tiny space of a cell?

The answers to some of these questions began to emerge in the 1940s, when it was discovered from studies in simple fungi that genetic information consists primarily of instructions for making proteins. As described in the previous chapter, proteins perform most of the cell's functions: they serve as building blocks for cell structures; they form the enzymes that catalyze the cell's chemical reactions; they regulate the activity of genes; and they enable cells to move and to communicate with one another. With hindsight, it is hard to imagine what other type of instructions the genetic information could have contained.

THE STRUCTURE OF DNA

THE STRUCTURE OF
EUKARYOTIC CHROMOSOMES

THE REGULATION OF
CHROMOSOME STRUCTURE

The other crucial advance made in the 1940s was the recognition that deoxyribonucleic acid (DNA) is the carrier of the cell's genetic information. But the mechanism whereby the information could be copied for transmission from one generation of cells to the next, and how proteins might be specified by instructions in DNA, remained completely mysterious until 1953, when the structure of DNA was determined by James Watson and Francis Crick. The structure immediately revealed how DNA might be copied, or replicated, and it provided the first clues about how a molecule of DNA might encode the instructions for making proteins. Today, the fact that DNA is the genetic material is so fundamental to our understanding of life that it can be difficult to appreciate what an enormous intellectual gap this discovery filled.

In this chapter, we begin by describing the structure of DNA. We see how, despite its chemical simplicity, the structure and chemical properties of DNA make it ideally suited for carrying genetic information. We then consider how genes and other important segments of DNA are arranged in the single, long DNA molecule that forms each chromosome in the cell. Finally, we discuss how eukaryotic cells fold these long DNA molecules into compact chromosomes inside the nucleus. This packing has to be done in an orderly fashion so that the chromosomes can be apportioned correctly between the two daughter cells at each cell division. At the same time, chromosomal packaging must allow DNA to be accessed by the large number of proteins that replicate and repair it, and that determine the activity of the cell's many genes.

This is the first of five chapters that deal with basic genetic mechanisms—the ways in which the cell maintains and makes use of the genetic information carried in its DNA. In Chapter 6, we discuss the mechanisms by which the cell accurately replicates and repairs its DNA. In Chapter 7, we consider gene expression—how genes are used to produce RNA and protein molecules. In Chapter 8, we describe how a cell controls gene expression to ensure that each of the many thousands of proteins encoded in its DNA is manufactured at the proper time and place. In Chapter 9, we discuss how present-day genes evolved, and, in Chapter 10, we consider some of the ways that DNA can be experimentally manipulated to study fundamental cell processes.

An enormous amount has been learned about these subjects in the past 60 years. Much less obvious, but equally important, is the fact that our knowledge is very incomplete; thus a great deal still remains to be discovered about how DNA provides the instructions to build living things.

THE STRUCTURE OF DNA

Long before biologists understood the structure of DNA, they had recognized that inherited traits and the genes that determine them were associated with chromosomes. Chromosomes (named from the Greek *chroma*, "color," because of their staining properties) were discovered in the nineteenth century as threadlike structures in the nucleus of eukaryotic cells that become visible as the cells begin to divide (**Figure 5–1**). As biochemical analyses became possible, researchers learned that chromosomes contain both DNA and protein. But which of these components encoded the organism's genetic information was not immediately clear.

We now know that the DNA carries the genetic information of the cell and that the protein components of chromosomes function largely to package and control the enormously long DNA molecules. But biologists in the 1940s had difficulty accepting DNA as the genetic material because of the apparent simplicity of its chemistry (see **How We Know**, pp. 193–195).

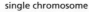
single chromosome

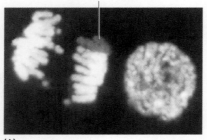
(A)

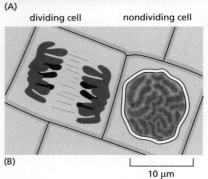
dividing cell   nondividing cell
(B)
10 μm

Figure 5–1 Chromosomes become visible as eukaryotic cells prepare to divide. (A) Two adjacent plant cells photographed using a fluorescence microscope. The DNA, which is labeled with a fluorescent dye (DAPI), is packaged into multiple chromosomes; these become visible as distinct structures only when they condense in preparation for cell division, as can be seen in the cell on the *left*. For clarity, a single chromosome has been shaded (*brown*) in the dividing cell. The cell on the *right*, which is not dividing, contains the identical chromosomes, but they cannot be distinguished as individual entities because the DNA is in a much more extended conformation at this phase in the cell's division cycle. (B) Schematic diagram of the outlines of the two cells and their chromosomes. (A, courtesy of Peter Shaw.)

DNA, after all, is simply a long polymer composed of only four types of nucleotide subunits, which are chemically very similar to one another.

Then, early in the 1950s, Maurice Wilkins and Rosalind Franklin examined DNA using x-ray diffraction analysis, a technique for determining the three-dimensional atomic structure of a molecule (see Panel 4–6, pp. 168–169). Their results provided one of the crucial pieces of evidence that led, in 1953, to Watson and Crick's model of the double-helical structure of DNA. This structure—in which two strands of DNA are wound around each other to form a helix—immediately suggested how DNA could encode the instructions necessary for life, and how these instructions could be copied and passed along when cells divide. In this section, we examine the structure of DNA and explain in general terms how it is able to store hereditary information.

A DNA Molecule Consists of Two Complementary Chains of Nucleotides

A molecule of **deoxyribonucleic acid** (**DNA**) consists of two long polynucleotide chains. Each *chain*, or *strand*, is composed of four types of nucleotide subunits, and the two strands are held together by hydrogen bonds between the base portions of the nucleotides (**Figure 5–2**).

As we saw in Chapter 2 (Panel 2–7, pp. 78–79), nucleotides are composed of a nitrogen-containing base and a five-carbon sugar, to which a phosphate group is attached. For the nucleotides in DNA, the sugar is deoxyribose (hence the name deoxyribonucleic acid) and the base can be either *adenine* (A), *cytosine* (C), *guanine* (G), or *thymine* (T). The

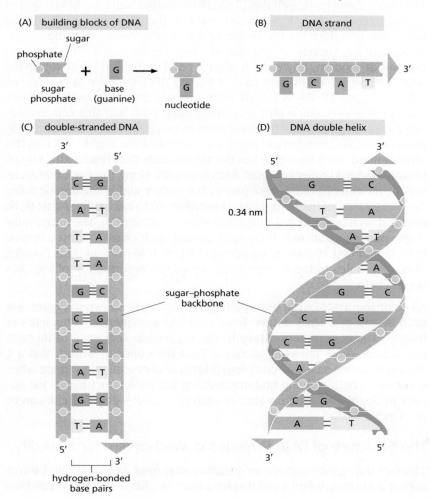

Figure 5–2 DNA is made of four nucleotide building blocks. (A) Each nucleotide is composed of a sugar phosphate covalently linked to a base—guanine (G) in this figure. (B) The nucleotides are covalently linked together into polynucleotide chains, with a sugar–phosphate backbone from which the bases—adenine, cytosine, guanine, and thymine (A, C, G, and T)—extend. (C) A DNA molecule is composed of two polynucleotide chains (DNA strands) held together by hydrogen bonds between the paired bases. The *arrows* on the DNA strands indicate the polarities of the two strands, which run *antiparallel* to each other (with opposite chemical polarities) in the DNA molecule. (D) Although the DNA is shown straightened out in (C), in reality, it is wound into a double helix, as shown here.

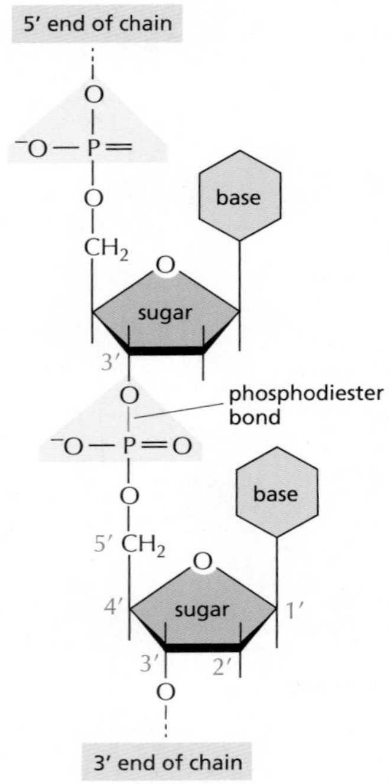

5′ end of chain

phosphodiester bond

3′ end of chain

Figure 5–3 The nucleotide subunits within a DNA strand are held together by phosphodiester bonds. These bonds connect one sugar to the next. The chemical differences in the ester linkages—between the 5′ carbon of one sugar and the 3′ carbon of the other—give rise to the polarity of the resulting DNA strand. For simplicity, only two nucleotides are shown here.

nucleotides are covalently linked together in a chain through the sugars and phosphates, which form a backbone of alternating sugar–phosphate–sugar–phosphate (see Figure 5–2B). Because only the base differs in each of the four types of subunits, each polynucleotide chain resembles a necklace: a sugar–phosphate backbone strung with four types of tiny beads (the four bases A, C, G, and T). These same symbols (A, C, G, and T) are also commonly used to denote the four different nucleotides—that is, the bases with their attached sugar phosphates.

The nucleotide subunits within a DNA strand are held together by phosphodiester bonds that link the 5′ end of one sugar with the 3′ end of the next (**Figure 5–3**). Because the ester linkages to the sugar molecules on either side of the bond are different, each DNA strand has a chemical polarity. If we imagine that each nucleotide has a phosphate "knob" and a hydroxyl "hole" (see Figure 5–2A), each strand, formed by interlocking knobs with holes, will have all of its subunits lined up in the same orientation. Moreover, the two ends of the strand can be easily distinguished, as one will have a hole (the 3′ hydroxyl) and the other a knob (the 5′ phosphate). This polarity in a DNA strand is indicated by referring to one end as the *3′ end* and the other as the *5′ end* (see Figure 5–3).

The two polynucleotide chains in the DNA **double helix** are held together by hydrogen-bonding between the bases on the different strands. All the bases are therefore on the inside of the double helix, with the sugar–phosphate backbones on the outside (see Figure 5–2D). The bases do not pair at random, however; A always pairs with T, and G always pairs with C (**Figure 5–4**). In each case, a bulkier two-ring base (a purine, see Panel 2–7, pp. 78–79) is paired with a single-ring base (a pyrimidine). Each purine–pyrimidine pair is called a **base pair**, and this *complementary base-pairing* enables the base pairs to be packed in the energetically most favorable arrangement along the interior of the double helix. In this arrangement, each base pair has the same width, thus holding the sugar–phosphate backbones an equal distance apart along the DNA molecule. For the members of each base pair to fit together within the double helix, the two strands of the helix must run *antiparallel* to each other—that is, be oriented with opposite polarities (see Figure 5–2C and D). The antiparallel sugar–phosphate strands then twist around each other to form a double helix containing 10 base pairs per helical turn (**Figure 5–5**). This twisting also contributes to the energetically favorable conformation of the DNA double helix.

As a consequence of the base-pairing arrangement shown in Figure 5–4, each strand of a DNA double helix contains a sequence of nucleotides that is exactly **complementary** to the nucleotide sequence of its partner strand—an A always matches a T on the opposite strand, and a C always matches a G. This complementarity is of crucial importance when it comes to both copying and maintaining the DNA structure, as we discuss in Chapter 6. An animated version of the DNA double helix can be seen in Movie 5.1.

The Structure of DNA Provides a Mechanism for Heredity

The fact that genes encode information that must be copied and transmitted accurately when a cell divides raised two fundamental issues: how

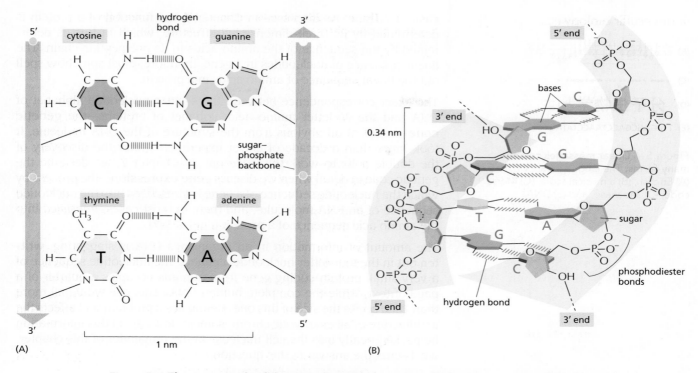

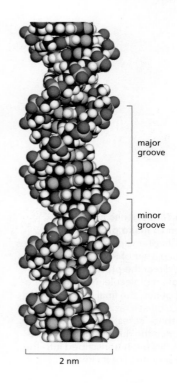

Figure 5–4 The two strands of the DNA double helix are held together by hydrogen bonds between complementary base pairs. (A) Schematic illustration showing how the shapes and chemical structures of the bases allow hydrogen bonds to form efficiently only between A and T and between G and C. The atoms that form the hydrogen bonds between these nucleotides (see Panel 2–3, pp. 70–71) can be brought close together without perturbing the double helix. As shown, two hydrogen bonds form between A and T, whereas three form between G and C. The bases can pair in this way only if the two polynucleotide chains that contain them are antiparallel—that is, oriented in opposite directions. (B) A short section of the double helix viewed from its side. Four base pairs are illustrated; note that they lie perpendicular to the axis of the helix, unlike the schematic shown in (A). As shown in Figure 5–3, the nucleotides are linked together covalently by phosphodiester bonds that connect the 3'-hydroxyl (–OH) group of one sugar and the 5' phosphate (–PO₃) attached to the next (see Panel 2–7, pp. 78–79, to review how the carbon atoms in the sugar ring are numbered). This linkage gives each polynucleotide strand a chemical polarity; that is, its two ends are chemically different. The 3' end carries an unlinked –OH group attached to the 3' position on the sugar ring; the 5' end carries a free phosphate group attached to the 5' position on the sugar ring.

can the information for specifying an organism be carried in chemical form, and how can the information be accurately copied? The structure of DNA provides the answer to both questions.

Information is encoded in the order, or sequence, of the nucleotides along each DNA strand. Each base—A, C, T, or G—can be considered a letter in a four-letter alphabet that is used to spell out biological messages (**Figure 5–6**). Organisms differ from one another because their respective DNA molecules have different *nucleotide sequences* and, consequently, carry different biological messages. But how is the nucleotide alphabet used to make up messages, and what do they spell out?

Before the structure of DNA was determined, investigators had established that genes contain the instructions for producing proteins. Thus, it was clear that DNA messages must somehow be able to encode proteins. Consideration of the chemical character of proteins makes the problem

Figure 5–5 A space-filling model shows the conformation of the DNA double helix. The two DNA strands wind around each other to form a right-handed helix (see Figure 4–14) with 10 bases per turn. Shown here are 1.5 turns of the DNA double helix. The coiling of the two strands around each other creates two grooves in the double helix. The wider groove is called the major groove and the smaller one the minor groove. The colors of the atoms are: N, *blue*; O, *red*; P, *yellow*; H, *white*; and C, *black*. (See Movie 5.1.)

(A) 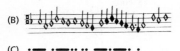molecular biology is...

(B) [musical score]

(C) ● ━ ● ●━●● ●● ━ ● ━ ● ●

(D) 分子生物学とは

(E) TTCGAGCGACCTAACCTATAG

Figure 5–6 Linear messages come in many forms. The languages shown are (A) English, (B) a musical score, (C) Morse code, (D) Japanese, and (E) DNA.

easier to define. As discussed in Chapter 4, the function of a protein is determined by its three-dimensional structure, which in turn is determined by the sequence of the amino acids in its polypeptide chain. The linear sequence of nucleotides in a gene, therefore, must somehow spell out the linear sequence of amino acids in a protein.

The exact correspondence between the 4-letter nucleotide alphabet of DNA and the 20-letter amino acid alphabet of proteins—the **genetic code**—is not at all obvious from the structure of the DNA molecule. It took more than a decade of clever experiments after the discovery of the double helix to work this code out. In Chapter 7, we describe the genetic code in detail when we discuss **gene expression**—the process by which the nucleotide sequence of a gene is *transcribed* into the nucleotide sequence of an RNA molecule—and then, in most cases, *translated* into the amino acid sequence of a protein (**Figure 5–7**).

The amount of information in an organism's DNA is staggering: written out in the four-letter nucleotide alphabet, the nucleotide sequence of a very small protein-coding gene from humans occupies a quarter of a page of text, while the complete human DNA sequence would fill more than 1000 books the size of this one. Herein lies a problem that affects the architecture of all eukaryotic chromosomes: How can all this information be packed neatly into the cell nucleus? In the remainder of this chapter, we discuss the answer to this question.

THE STRUCTURE OF EUKARYOTIC CHROMOSOMES

Large amounts of DNA are required to encode all the information needed to make a single-celled bacterium, and far more DNA is needed to encode the information to make a multicellular organism like you. Each human cell contains about 2 meters (m) of DNA; yet the cell nucleus is only 5–8 μm in diameter. Tucking all this material into such a small space is the equivalent of trying to fold 40 km (24 miles) of extremely fine thread into a tennis ball.

In eukaryotic cells, very long, double-stranded DNA molecules are packaged into **chromosomes**. These chromosomes not only fit handily inside the nucleus, but, after they are duplicated, they can be accurately apportioned between the two daughter cells at each cell division. The complex task of packaging DNA is accomplished by specialized proteins that bind to and fold the DNA, generating a series of coils and loops that provide increasingly higher levels of organization and prevent the DNA from becoming a tangled, unmanageable mess. Amazingly, this DNA is folded in a way that allows it to remain accessible to all of the enzymes and other proteins that replicate and repair it, and that cause the expression of its genes.

Figure 5–7 Most genes contain information to make proteins. As we discuss in Chapter 7, protein-coding genes each produce a set of RNA molecules, which then direct the production of a specific protein molecule. Note that for a minority of genes, the final product is the RNA molecule itself, as shown here for gene C. In these cases, gene expression is complete once the nucleotide sequence of the DNA has been transcribed into the nucleotide sequence of its RNA.

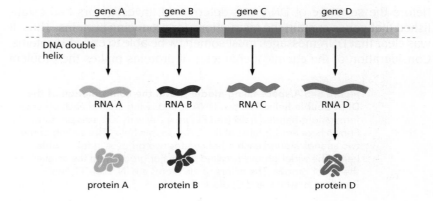

Bacteria typically carry their genes on a single, circular DNA molecule. This molecule is also associated with proteins that condense the DNA, but these bacterial proteins differ from the ones that package eukaryotic DNA. Although this prokaryotic DNA is called a bacterial "chromosome," it does not have the same structure as eukaryotic chromosomes, and less is known about how it is packaged. Our discussion of chromosome structure in this chapter will therefore focus entirely on eukaryotic chromosomes.

Eukaryotic DNA Is Packaged into Multiple Chromosomes

In eukaryotes, such as ourselves, nuclear DNA is distributed among a set of different chromosomes. The DNA in a human nucleus, for example, is parceled out into 23 or 24 different types of chromosome, depending on an individual's sex (males, with their *Y chromosome*, have an extra type of chromosome that females do not). Each of these chromosomes consists of a single, enormously long, linear DNA molecule associated with proteins that fold and pack the fine thread of DNA into a more compact structure. This complex of DNA and protein is called *chromatin*. In addition to the proteins involved in packaging the DNA, chromosomes also associate with many other proteins involved in DNA replication, DNA repair, and gene expression.

With the exception of the gametes (sperm and eggs) and highly specialized cells that lack DNA entirely (such as mature red blood cells), human cells each contain two copies of every chromosome, one inherited from the mother and one from the father. The maternal and paternal versions of each chromosome are called *homologous chromosomes* (*homologs*). The only nonhomologous chromosome pairs in humans are the sex chromosomes in males, where a Y chromosome is inherited from the father and an *X chromosome* from the mother. (Females inherit one X chromosome from each parent and have no Y chromosome.) Each full set of human chromosomes contains a total of approximately 3.2×10^9 nucleotide pairs of DNA—which together comprise the *human genome*.

In addition to being different sizes, the different human chromosomes can be distinguished from one another by a variety of techniques. Each chromosome can be "painted" a different color using sets of chromosome-specific DNA molecules coupled to different fluorescent dyes (**Figure 5–8A**). An earlier and more traditional way of distinguishing one chromosome from another involves staining the chromosomes with dyes that bind to certain types of DNA sequences. These dyes mainly distinguish between DNA that is rich in A-T nucleotide pairs and DNA that is G-C rich, and they produce a predictable pattern of bands along each type of chromosome. The resulting patterns allow each chromosome to be identified and numbered.

Figure 5–8 Each human chromosome can be "painted" a different color to allow its unambiguous identification. The chromosomes shown here were isolated from a cell undergoing nuclear division (mitosis) and are therefore in a highly compact (condensed) state. Chromosome painting is carried out by exposing the chromosomes to a collection of single-stranded DNA molecules that have been coupled to a combination of fluorescent dyes. For example, single-stranded DNA molecules that match sequences in chromosome 1 are labeled with one specific dye combination, those that match sequences in chromosome 2 with another, and so on. Because the labeled DNA can form base pairs (hybridize) only with its specific chromosome (discussed in Chapter 10), each chromosome is differently colored. For such experiments, the chromosomes are treated so that the individual strands of its double-helical DNA partly separate to enable base-pairing with the labeled, single-stranded DNA.
(A) Micrograph showing the array of chromosomes as they originally spilled from the lysed cell. (B) The same chromosomes artificially lined up in their numerical order. This arrangement of the full chromosome set is called a karyotype. (Adapted from N. McNeil and T. Ried, *Expert Rev. Mol. Med.* 2:1–14, 2000. With permission from Cambridge University Press.)

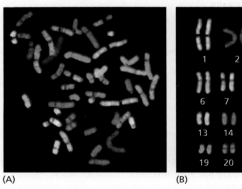
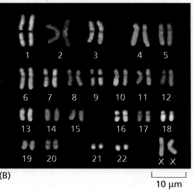

(A)   (B)

10 μm

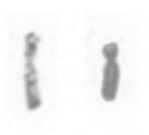

(A)   chromosome 6   chromosome 4

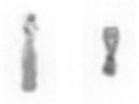

(B)   reciprocal chromosomal translocation

Figure 5–9 Abnormal chromosomes are associated with some inherited genetic disorders. (A) Two normal human chromosomes, chromosome 6 and chromosome 4, have been subjected to chromosome painting as described in Figure 5–8. (B) In an individual with a reciprocal chromosomal translocation, a segment of one chromosome has been swapped with a segment from the other. Such chromosomal translocations are a frequent event in cancer cells. (Courtesy of Zhenya Tang and the NIGMS Human Genetic Cell Repository at the Coriell Institute for Medical Research.)

An ordered display of the full set of 46 human chromosomes is called the human **karyotype** (Figure 5–8B). If parts of a chromosome are lost, or switched between chromosomes, these changes can be detected. Cytogeneticists analyze karyotypes to detect chromosomal abnormalities that are associated with some inherited disorders (Figure 5–9) and with certain types of cancer (as we see in Chapter 20).

Chromosomes Organize and Carry Genetic Information

The most important function of chromosomes is to carry genes—the functional units of heredity. A **gene** is often defined as a segment of DNA that contains the instructions for making a particular protein or RNA molecule. Most of the RNA molecules encoded by genes are subsequently used to produce a protein. In some cases, however, the RNA molecule is the final product (see Figure 5–7). Like proteins, these RNA molecules have diverse functions in the cell, including structural, catalytic, and gene regulatory roles, as we discuss in later chapters.

Together, the total genetic information carried by a complete set of the chromosomes present in a cell or organism constitutes its **genome**. Complete genome sequences have been determined for thousands of organisms, from *E. coli* to humans. As might be expected, some correlation exists between the complexity of an organism and the number of genes in its genome. For example, the total number of genes is about 500 for the simplest bacterium and about 24,000 for humans. Bacteria and some single-celled eukaryotes, including the budding yeast *S. cerevisiae*, have especially compact genomes: the DNA molecules that make up their chromosomes are little more than strings of closely packed genes (Figure 5–10). However, chromosomes from many eukaryotes—including humans—contain, in addition to genes and the specific nucleotide sequences required for normal gene expression, a large excess of interspersed DNA (Figure 5–11). This extra DNA is sometimes erroneously called "junk DNA," because its usefulness to the cell has not yet been demonstrated. Although this spare DNA does not code for protein, much of it may serve some other biological function. Comparisons of the genome sequences from many different species reveal that small portions of this extra DNA are highly conserved among related species, suggesting their importance for these organisms.

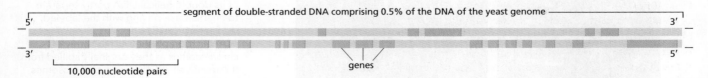

Figure 5–10 In yeast, genes are closely packed along chromosomes. This figure shows a small region of the DNA double helix in one chromosome from the budding yeast *S. cerevisiae*. The *S. cerevisiae* genome contains about 12.5 million nucleotide pairs and 6600 genes—spread across 16 chromosomes. Note that, for each gene, only one of the two DNA strands actually encodes the information to make an RNA molecule. This coding region can fall on either strand, as indicated by the *light red* bars. However, each "gene" is considered to include both the "coding strand" and its complement. The high density of genes is characteristic of *S. cerevisiae*.

Figure 5–11 In many eukaryotes, genes include an excess of interspersed, noncoding DNA. Presented here is the nucleotide sequence of the human β-globin gene. This gene carries the information that specifies the amino acid sequence of one of the two types of subunits found in hemoglobin, a protein that carries oxygen in the blood. Only the sequence of the coding strand is shown here; the noncoding strand of the double helix carries the complementary sequence. Starting from its 5′ end, such a sequence is read from left to right, like any piece of English text. The segments of the DNA sequence that encode the amino acid sequence of β-globin are highlighted in *yellow*. We will see in Chapter 7 how this information is transcribed and translated to produce a full-length β-globin protein.

In general, the more complex an organism, the larger is its genome. But this relationship does not always hold true. The human genome, for example, is 200 times larger than that of the yeast *S. cerevisiae*, but 30 times smaller than that of some plants and at least 60 times smaller than some species of amoeba (see Figure 1–41). Furthermore, how the DNA is apportioned over chromosomes also differs from one species to another. Humans have a total of 46 chromosomes (including both maternal and paternal sets), but a species of small deer has only 7, while some carp species have more than 100. Even closely related species with similar genome sizes can have very different chromosome numbers and sizes (Figure 5–12). Thus, although gene number is roughly correlated with species complexity, there is no simple relationship between gene number, chromosome number, and total genome size. The genomes and chromosomes of modern species have each been shaped by a unique history of seemingly random genetic events, acted on by specific selection pressures, as we discuss in Chapter 9.

Specialized DNA Sequences Are Required for DNA Replication and Chromosome Segregation

To form a functional chromosome, a DNA molecule must do more than simply carry genes: it must be able to be replicated, and the replicated copies must be separated and partitioned equally and reliably into the two daughter cells at each cell division. These processes occur through an ordered series of events, known collectively as the **cell cycle**. This cycle of cell growth and division is summarized—very briefly—in **Figure 5–13** and will be discussed in detail in Chapter 18. Only two broad stages of the cell cycle need concern us in this chapter: *interphase*, when chromosomes are duplicated, and *mitosis*, the much more brief stage when the duplicated chromosomes are distributed, or segregated, to the two daughter nuclei.

During interphase, chromosomes are extended as long, thin, tangled threads of DNA in the nucleus and cannot be easily distinguished in the light microscope (see Figure 5–1). We refer to chromosomes in this extended state as *interphase chromosomes*. It is during interphase that DNA replication takes place. As we discuss in Chapter 6, two specialized DNA sequences, found in all eukaryotes, ensure that this process occurs efficiently. One type of nucleotide sequence, called a **replication origin**, is where DNA replication begins; eukaryotic chromosomes contain many replication origins to allow the long DNA molecules to be replicated rapidly (**Figure 5–14**). Another DNA sequence forms the **telomeres** that mark the ends of each chromosome. Telomeres contain repeated nucleotide sequences that are required for the ends of chromosomes to be fully replicated. They also serve as a protective cap that keeps the chromosome tips from being mistaken by the cell as broken DNA in need of repair.

```
CCCTGTGGAGCCACACCCTAGGGTTGGCCA
ATCTACTCCCAGGAGCAGGGAGGGCAGGAG
CCAGGGCTGGGCATAAAAGTCAGGGCAGAG
CCATCTATTGCTTACATTTGCTTCTGACAC
AACTGTGTTCACTAGCAACTCAAACAGACA
CCATGGTGCACCTGACTCCTGAGGAGAAGT
CTGCCGTTACTGCCCTGTGGGGCAAGGTGA
ACGTGGATGAAGTTGGTGGTGAGGCCCTGG
GCAGGTTGGTATCAAGGTTACAAGACAGGT
TTAAGGAGACCAATAGAAACTGGGCATGTG
GAGACAGAGAAGACTCTTGGGTTTCTGATA
GGCACTGACTCTCTCTGCCTATTGGTCTAT
TTTCCCACCCTTAGGCTGCTGGTGGTCTAC
CCTTGGACCCAGAGGTTCTTTGAGTCCTTT
GGGGATCTGTCCACTCCTGATGCTGTTATG
GGCAACCCTAAGGTGAAGGCTCATGGCAAG
AAAGTGCTCGGTGCCTTTAGTGATGGCCTG
GCTCACCTGGACAACCTCAAGGGCACCTTT
GCCACACTGAGTGAGCTGCACTGTGACAAG
CTGCACGTGGATCCTGAGAACTTCAGGGTG
AGTCTATGGGACCCTTGATGTTTTCTTTCC
CCTTCTTTTCTATGGTTAAGTTCATGTCAT
AGGAAGGGGAGAAGTAACAGGGTACAGTTT
AGAATGGGAAACAGACGAATGATTGCATCA
GTGTGGAAGTCTCAGGATCGTTTTAGTTTC
TTTTATTTGCTGTTCATAACAATTGTTTTC
TTTTGTTTAATTCTTGCTTTCTTTTTTTTT
CTTCTCCGCAATTTTTACTATTATACTTAA
TGCCTTAACATTGTGTATAACAAAAGGAAA
TATCTCTGAGATACATTAAGTAACTTAAAA
AAAAACTTTACACAGTCTGCCTAGTACATT
ACTATTTGGAATATATGTGTGCTTATTTGC
ATATTCATAATCTCCCTACTTTATTTTCTT
TTATTTTTAATTGATACATAATCATTATAC
ATATTTATGGGTTAAAGTGTAATGTTTTAA
TATGTGTACACATATTGACCAAATCAGGGT
AATTTTGCATTTGTAATTTTAAAAAATGCT
TTCTTCTTTTAATATACTTTTTTGTTTATC
TTATTTCTAATACTTTCCCTAATCTCTTTC
TTTCAGGGCAATAATGATACAATGTATCAT
GCCTCTTTGCACCATTCTAAAGAATAACAG
TGATAATTTCTGGGTTAAGGCAATAGCAAT
ATTTCTGCATATAAATATTTCTGCATATAA
ATTGTAACTGATGTAAGAGGTTTCATATTG
CTAATAGCAGCTACAATCCAGCTACCATTC
TGCTTTTATTTTATGGTTGGGATAAGGCTG
GATTATTCTGAGTCCAAGCTAGGCCCTTTT
GCTAATCATGTTCATACCTCTTATCTTCCT
CCCACAGCTCCTGGGCAACGTGCTGGTCTG
TGTGCTGGCCCATCACTTTGGCAAAGAATT
CACCCCACCAGTGCAGGCTGCCTATCAGAA
AGTGGTGGCTGGTGTGGCTAATGCCCTGGC
CCACAAGTATCACTAAGCTCGCTTTCTTGC
TGTCCAATTTCTATTAAAGGTTCCTTTGTT
CCCTAAGTCCAACTACTAAACTGGGGGATA
TTATGAAGGGCCTTGAGCATCTGGATTCTG
CCTAATAAAAAACATTTATTTTCATTGCAA
TGATGTATTTAAATTATTTCTGAATATTTT
ACTAAAAAGGGAATGTGGGAGGTCAGTGCA
TTTAAAACATAAAGAAATGATGAGCTGTTC
AAACCTTGGGAAAATACACTATATCTTAAA
CTCCATGAAAGAAGGTGAGGCTGCAACCAG
CTAATGCACATTGGCAACAGCCCCTGATGC
CTATGCCTTATTCATCCCTCAGAAAAGGAT
TCTTGTAGAGGCTTGATTTGCAGGTTAAAG
TTTTGCTATGCTGTATTTTACATTACTTAT
TGTTTTAGCTGTCCTCATGAATGTCTTTTC
```

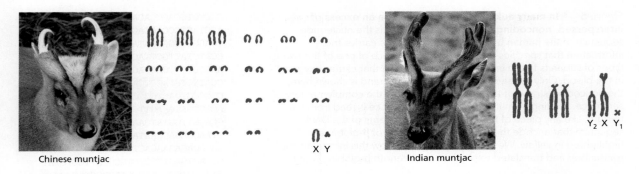

Chinese muntjac   Indian muntjac

Figure 5–12 Two closely related species can have similar genome sizes but very different chromosome numbers. In the evolution of the Indian muntjac deer, chromosomes that were initially separate, and that remain separate in the Chinese species, fused without having a major effect on the number of genes—or the animal. (Image left, courtesy of Deborah Carreno, Natural Wonders Photography; image right, courtesy of Beatrice Bourgery.)

Eukaryotic chromosomes also contain a third type of specialized DNA sequence, called the **centromere**, that allows duplicated chromosomes to be separated during M phase (see Figure 5–14). During this stage of the cell cycle, the DNA coils up, adopting a more and more compact structure, ultimately forming highly compacted, or condensed, *mitotic chromosomes* (**Figure 5–15**). This is the state in which the duplicated chromosomes can be most easily visualized (see Figure 5–1). Once the chromosomes have condensed, the centromere allows the mitotic spindle to attach to each duplicated chromosome in a way that directs one copy of each chromosome to be segregated to each of the two daughter cells (see Figure 5–13). We describe the central role that centromeres play in cell division in Chapter 18.

Interphase Chromosomes Are Not Randomly Distributed Within the Nucleus

Interphase chromosomes are much longer and finer than mitotic chromosomes. They are nevertheless organized within the nucleus in several ways. First, although interphase chromosomes are constantly undergoing dynamic rearrangements, each tends to occupy a particular region, or territory, of the interphase nucleus (**Figure 5–16**). This loose organization prevents interphase chromosomes from becoming extensively

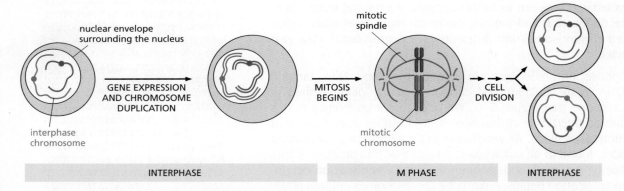

Figure 5–13 The duplication and segregation of chromosomes occurs through an ordered cell cycle in proliferating cells. During interphase, the cell expresses many of its genes, and—during part of this phase—it duplicates its chromosomes. Once chromosome duplication is complete, the cell can enter *M phase*, during which nuclear division, or mitosis, occurs. In mitosis, the duplicated chromosomes condense, gene expression largely ceases, the nuclear envelope breaks down, and the mitotic spindle forms from microtubules and other proteins. The condensed chromosomes are then captured by the mitotic spindle, one complete set is pulled to each end of the cell, and a nuclear envelope forms around each chromosome set. In the final step of M phase, the cell divides to produce two daughter cells. Only two different chromosomes are shown here for simplicity.

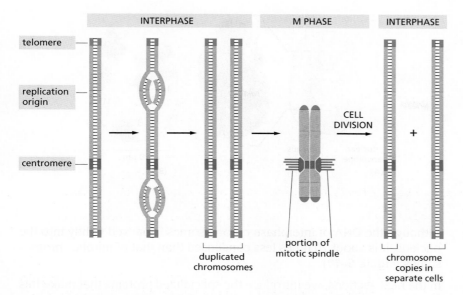

| INTERPHASE | M PHASE | INTERPHASE |

telomere

replication origin

centromere

CELL DIVISION

portion of mitotic spindle

duplicated chromosomes

chromosome copies in separate cells

Figure 5–14 Three DNA sequence elements are needed to produce a eukaryotic chromosome that can be duplicated and then segregated at mitosis. Each chromosome has multiple origins of replication, one centromere, and two telomeres. The sequence of events that a typical chromosome follows during the cell cycle is shown schematically. The DNA replicates in interphase, beginning at the origins of replication and proceeding bidirectionally from each origin along the chromosome. In M phase, the centromere attaches the compact, duplicated chromosomes to the mitotic spindle so that one copy will be distributed to each daughter cell when the cell divides. Prior to cell division, the centromere also helps to hold the duplicated chromosomes together until they are ready to be pulled apart. Telomeres contain DNA sequences that allow for the complete replication of chromosome ends.

entangled, like spaghetti in a bowl. In addition, some chromosomal regions are physically attached to particular sites on the *nuclear envelope*—the pair of concentric membranes that surround the nucleus—or to the underlying *nuclear lamina*, the protein meshwork that supports the envelope (discussed in Chapter 17). These attachments also help interphase chromosomes remain within their distinct territories.

The most obvious example of chromosomal organization in the interphase nucleus is the **nucleolus**—a structure large enough to be seen in the light microscope (**Figure 5–17A**). During interphase, the parts of different chromosomes that carry genes encoding ribosomal RNAs come together to form the nucleolus. In human cells, several hundred copies of these genes are distributed in 10 clusters, located near the tips of five different chromosome pairs (**Figure 5–17B**). In the nucleolus, ribosomal RNAs are synthesized and combine with proteins to form ribosomes, the cell's protein-synthesizing machines. As we discuss in Chapter 7, ribosomal RNAs play both structural and catalytic roles in the ribosome.

The DNA in Chromosomes Is Always Highly Condensed

As we have seen, all eukaryotic cells, whether in interphase or mitosis, package their DNA tightly into chromosomes. Human chromosome 22, for example, contains about 48 million nucleotide pairs; stretched out end-to-end, its DNA would extend about 1.5 cm. Yet, during mitosis, chromosome 22 measures only about 2 μm in length—that is, nearly 10,000 times more compact than the DNA would be if it were extended to its full length. This remarkable feat of compression is performed by proteins that coil and fold the DNA into higher and higher levels of organization.

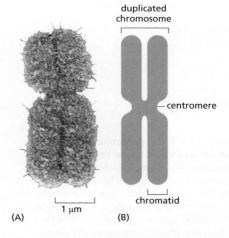

duplicated chromosome

centromere

1 μm

chromatid

(A)   (B)

Figure 5–15 A typical duplicated mitotic chromosome is highly compact. Because DNA is replicated during interphase, each mitotic chromosome contains two identical duplicated DNA molecules (see Figure 5–14). Each of these very long DNA molecules, with its associated proteins, is called a *chromatid*; as soon as the two sister chromatids separate, they are considered individual chromosomes. (A) A scanning electron micrograph of a mitotic chromosome. The two chromatids are tightly joined together. The constricted region reveals the position of the centromere. (B) A cartoon representation of a mitotic chromosome. (A, courtesy of Terry D. Allen.)

Figure 5–16 **Interphase chromosomes occupy their own distinct territories within the nucleus.** DNA probes coupled with different fluorescent markers are used to paint individual interphase chromosomes in a human cell. (A) Viewed in a fluorescence microscope, the nucleus is seen to be filled with a patchwork of discrete colors. (B) To highlight their distinct locations, three sets of chromosomes are singled out: chromosomes 3, 5, and 11. Note that pairs of homologous chromosomes, such as the two copies of chromosome 3, are not generally located in the same position. (Adapted from M.R. Hübner and D.L. Spector, *Annu. Rev. Biophys.* 39:471–489, 2010.)

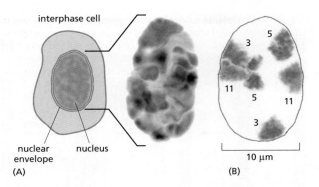

Although the DNA of interphase chromosomes is packed tightly into the nucleus, it is about 20 times less condensed than that of mitotic chromosomes (**Figure 5–18**).

In the next sections, we introduce the specialized proteins that make this compression possible. Bear in mind, though, that chromosome structure is dynamic. Not only do chromosomes condense and decondense during the cell cycle, but chromosome packaging must be flexible enough to allow rapid, on-demand access to different regions of the interphase chromosome, unpacking enough to allow protein complexes access to specific, localized nucleotide sequences for DNA replication, DNA repair, or gene expression.

Nucleosomes Are the Basic Units of Eukaryotic Chromosome Structure

The proteins that bind to DNA to form eukaryotic chromosomes are traditionally divided into two general classes: the **histones** and the *nonhistone chromosomal proteins*. Histones are present in enormous quantities (more than 60 million molecules of several different types in each human cell), and their total mass in chromosomes is about equal to that of the DNA itself. Nonhistone chromosomal proteins are also present in large numbers; they include hundreds of different chromatin-associated proteins. In contrast, only a handful of different histone proteins are present in eukaryotic cells. The complex of both classes of protein with nuclear DNA is called **chromatin**.

Histones are responsible for the first and most fundamental level of chromatin packing: the formation of the **nucleosome**. Nucleosomes convert the DNA molecules in an interphase nucleus into a *chromatin fiber* that

Figure 5–17 **The nucleolus is the most prominent structure in the interphase nucleus.** (A) Electron micrograph of a thin section through the nucleus of a human fibroblast. The nucleus is surrounded by the nuclear envelope. Inside the nucleus, the chromatin appears as a diffuse speckled mass; regions that are especially dense are called heterochromatin (dark staining). Heterochromatin contains few genes and is located mainly around the periphery of the nucleus, immediately under the nuclear envelope. The large, dark region within the nucleus is the nucleolus, which contains the genes for ribosomal RNAs. (B) Schematic illustration showing how ribosomal RNA genes, which are clustered near the tips of five different human chromosomes (13, 14, 15, 21, and 22), come together to form the nucleolus, which is a biochemical subcompartment produced by the aggregation of a set of macromolecules—DNA, RNAs, and proteins (see Figure 4–54). (A, courtesy of E.G. Jordan and J. McGovern.)

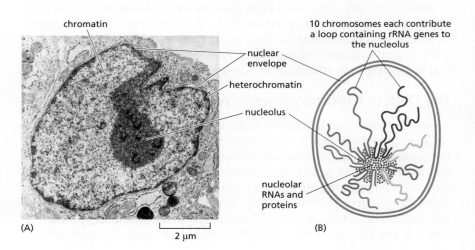

Figure 5–18 DNA in interphase chromosomes is less compact than in mitotic chromosomes. (A) An electron micrograph showing an enormous tangle of chromatin (DNA with its associated proteins) spilling out of a lysed interphase nucleus. (B) For comparison, a compact, human mitotic chromosome is shown at the same scale. (A, courtesy of Victoria Foe; B, courtesy of Terry D. Allen.)

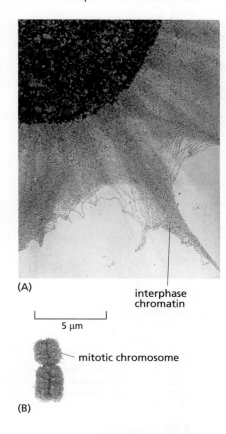

(A)

interphase chromatin

5 µm

mitotic chromosome

(B)

is approximately one-third the length of the initial DNA. These chromatin fibers, when examined with an electron microscope, contain clusters of closely packed nucleosomes (**Figure 5–19A**). If this chromatin is then subjected to treatments that cause it to unfold partially, it can then be seen in the electron microscope as a series of "beads on a string" (**Figure 5–19B**). The string is DNA, and each bead is a *nucleosome core particle*, which consists of DNA wound around a core of histone proteins.

To determine the structure of the nucleosome core particle, investigators treated chromatin in its unfolded, "beads-on-a-string" form with enzymes called nucleases, which cut the DNA by breaking the phosphodiester bonds between nucleotides. When this nuclease digestion is carried out for a short time, only the exposed DNA between the core particles—the *linker DNA*—will be cleaved, allowing the core particles to be isolated. An individual nucleosome core particle consists of a complex of eight histone proteins—two molecules each of histones H2A, H2B, H3, and H4—along with a segment of double-stranded DNA, 147 nucleotide pairs long, that winds around this *histone octamer* (**Figure 5–20**). The high-resolution structure of the nucleosome core particle was solved in 1997, revealing in atomic detail the disc-shaped histone octamer around which the DNA is tightly wrapped, making 1.7 turns in a left-handed coil (**Figure 5–21**). The linker DNA between each nucleosome core particle can vary in length from a few nucleotide pairs up to about 80. Technically speaking, a "nucleosome" consists of a nucleosome core particle plus one of its adjacent DNA linkers, as shown in Figure 5–20; however, the term is often used to refer to the nucleosome core particle itself.

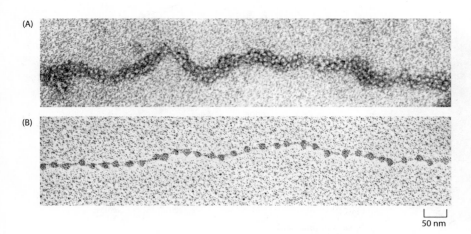

(A)

(B)

50 nm

Figure 5–19 Nucleosomes can be seen in the electron microscope. (A) Chromatin isolated directly from an interphase nucleus can appear in the electron microscope as a chromatin fiber, composed of packed nucleosomes. (B) Another electron micrograph shows a length of a chromatin fiber that has been experimentally unpacked, or decondensed, after isolation to show the "beads-on-a-string" appearance of the nucleosomes. (A, courtesy of Barbara Hamkalo; B, courtesy of Victoria Foe.)

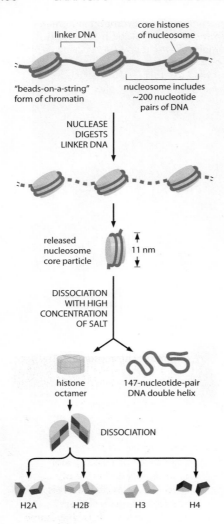

"beads-on-a-string" form of chromatin

linker DNA

core histones of nucleosome

nucleosome includes ~200 nucleotide pairs of DNA

NUCLEASE DIGESTS LINKER DNA

released nucleosome core particle

11 nm

DISSOCIATION WITH HIGH CONCENTRATION OF SALT

histone octamer

147-nucleotide-pair DNA double helix

DISSOCIATION

H2A   H2B   H3   H4

Figure 5–20 Nucleosomes contain DNA wrapped around a protein core of eight histone molecules. In a test tube, the nucleosome core particle can be released from chromatin by digestion of the linker DNA with a nuclease, which cleaves the exposed linker DNA but not the DNA wound tightly around the nucleosome core. When the DNA around each isolated nucleosome core particle is released, its length is found to be 147 nucleotide pairs; this DNA wraps around the histone octamer that forms the nucleosome core nearly twice.

All four of the histones that make up the octamer are relatively small proteins with a high proportion of positively charged amino acids (lysine and arginine). The positive charges help the histones bind tightly to the negatively charged sugar–phosphate backbone of DNA. These numerous electrostatic interactions explain in part why DNA of virtually any sequence can bind to a histone octamer. Each of the histones in the octamer also has a long, unstructured N-terminal amino acid "tail" that extends out from the nucleosome core particle (see the H3 tail in Figure 5–21). These histone tails are subject to several types of reversible, covalent chemical modifications that control many aspects of chromatin structure.

The histones that form the nucleosome core are among the most highly conserved of all known eukaryotic proteins: there are only two differences between the amino acid sequences of histone H4 from peas and cows, for example. This extreme evolutionary conservation reflects the vital role of histones in controlling eukaryotic chromosome structure.

Chromosome Packing Occurs on Multiple Levels

Although long strings of nucleosomes form on most chromosomal DNA, chromatin in the living cell rarely adopts the extended beads-on-a-string form seen in Figure 5–19B. Instead, the nucleosomes are further packed on top of one another to generate a more compact structure, such as the chromatin fiber shown in Figure 5–19A and Movie 5.2. This additional packing of nucleosomes into a chromatin fiber depends on a fifth

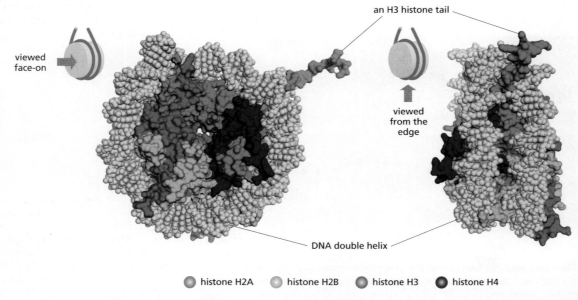

viewed face-on

an H3 histone tail

viewed from the edge

DNA double helix

● histone H2A   ● histone H2B   ● histone H3   ● histone H4

Figure 5–21 The structure of the nucleosome core particle, as determined by x-ray diffraction analysis, reveals how DNA is tightly wrapped around a disc-shaped histone octamer. Two views of a nucleosome core particle are shown here. The two strands of the DNA double helix are shown in *gray*. A portion of an H3 histone tail (*green*) can be seen extending from the nucleosome core particle, but the tails of the other histones have been truncated. (From K. Luger et al., *Nature* 389:251–260, 1997.)

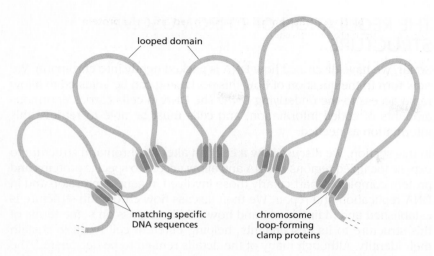

looped domain

matching specific
DNA sequences

chromosome
loop-forming
clamp proteins

Figure 5–22 The chromatin in human chromosomes is folded into looped domains. These loops are established by special nonhistone chromosomal proteins that bind to specific DNA sequences, creating a clamp at the base of each loop.

histone called histone H1, which is thought to pull adjacent nucleosomes together into a regular repeating array. This "linker" histone changes the path the DNA takes as it exits the nucleosome core, allowing it to form a more condensed chromatin fiber.

We saw earlier that, during mitosis, chromatin becomes so highly condensed that individual chromosomes can be seen in the light microscope. How is a chromatin fiber folded to produce mitotic chromosomes? Although the answer is not yet known in detail, it is known that specialized nonhistone chromosomal proteins fold the chromatin into a series of loops (**Figure 5–22**). These loops are further condensed to produce the interphase chromosome. Finally, this compact string of loops is thought to undergo at least one more level of packing to form the mitotic chromosome (**Figure 5–23**).

QUESTION 5–2

Assuming that the histone octamer (shown in Figure 5–20) forms a cylinder 9 nm in diameter and 5 nm in height and that the human genome forms 32 million nucleosomes, what volume of the nucleus (6 μm in diameter) is occupied by histone octamers? (Volume of a cylinder is $\pi r^2 h$; volume of a sphere is $4/3\ \pi r^3$.) What fraction of the total volume of the nucleus do the histone octamers occupy? How does this compare with the volume of the nucleus occupied by human DNA?

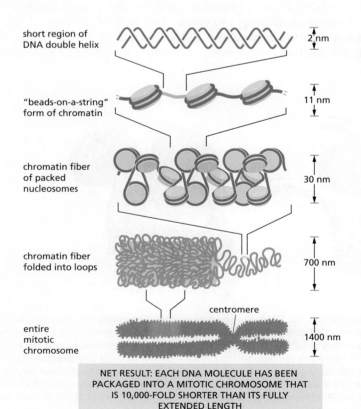

short region of
DNA double helix — 2 nm

"beads-on-a-string"
form of chromatin — 11 nm

chromatin fiber
of packed
nucleosomes — 30 nm

chromatin fiber
folded into loops — 700 nm

centromere

entire
mitotic
chromosome — 1400 nm

NET RESULT: EACH DNA MOLECULE HAS BEEN PACKAGED INTO A MITOTIC CHROMOSOME THAT IS 10,000-FOLD SHORTER THAN ITS FULLY EXTENDED LENGTH

Figure 5–23 DNA packing occurs on several levels in chromosomes. This schematic drawing shows some of the levels thought to give rise to the highly condensed mitotic chromosome. Both histone H1 and a set of specialized nonhistone chromosomal proteins are known to help drive these condensations, including the chromosome loop-forming clamp proteins and the abundant non-histone protein condensin (see Figure 18–18). However, the actual structures are still uncertain.

THE REGULATION OF CHROMOSOME STRUCTURE

So far, we have discussed how DNA is packed tightly into chromatin. We now turn to the question of how this packaging can be adjusted to allow rapid access to the underlying DNA. The DNA in cells carries enormous amounts of coded information, and cells must be able to retrieve this information as needed.

In this section, we discuss how a cell can alter its chromatin structure to expose localized regions of DNA and allow access to specific proteins and protein complexes, particularly those involved in gene expression and in DNA replication and repair. We then discuss how chromatin structure is established and maintained—and how a cell can pass on some forms of this structure to its descendants, helping different cell types to sustain their identity. Although many of the details remain to be deciphered, the regulation and inheritance of chromatin structure play crucial roles in the development of eukaryotic organisms.

Changes in Nucleosome Structure Allow Access to DNA

Eukaryotic cells have several ways to adjust rapidly the local structure of their chromatin. One way takes advantage of a set of ATP-dependent **chromatin-remodeling complexes**. These protein machines use the energy of ATP hydrolysis to change the position of the DNA wrapped around nucleosomes (**Figure 5–24**). By interacting with both the histone octamer and the DNA wrapped around it, chromatin-remodeling complexes can locally alter the arrangement of the nucleosomes, rendering the DNA more accessible (or less accessible) to other proteins in the cell. During mitosis, many of these complexes are inactivated, which may help mitotic chromosomes maintain their tightly packed structure.

Another way of altering chromatin structure relies on the reversible chemical modification of histones, catalyzed by a large number of different **histone-modifying enzymes**. The tails of all four of the core histones are particularly subject to these covalent modifications, which include the addition (and removal) of acetyl, phosphate, or methyl groups

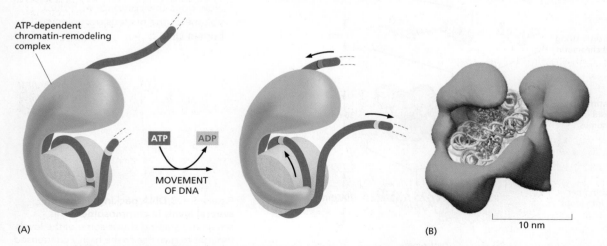

Figure 5–24 Chromatin-remodeling complexes locally reposition the DNA wrapped around nucleosomes. (A) The complexes use energy derived from ATP hydrolysis to loosen the nucleosomal DNA and push it along the histone octamer. In this way, the enzyme can expose or hide a sequence of DNA, controlling its availability to other DNA-binding proteins. The *blue* stripes have been added to show how the DNA shifts its position. Many cycles of ATP hydrolysis are required to produce such a shift. (B) The structure of a chromatin-remodeling complex, showing how the enzyme cradles a nucleosome core particle, including a histone octamer (*orange*) and the DNA wrapped around it (*light green*). This large complex, purified from yeast, contains 15 subunits, including one that hydrolyzes ATP and four that recognize specific covalently modified histones. (B, adapted from A.E. Leschziner et al., *Proc. Natl. Acad. Sci. USA* 104:4913–4918, 2007.)

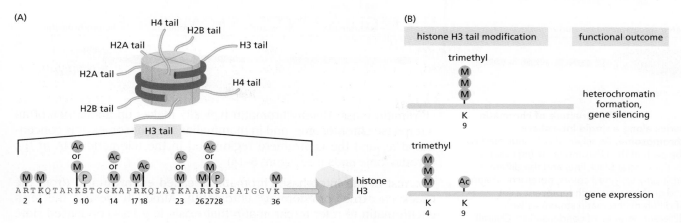

Figure 5–25 **The pattern of modification of histone tails can determine how a stretch of chromatin is handled by the cell.** (A) Schematic drawing showing the positions of the histone tails that extend from each nucleosome core particle. Each histone can be modified by the covalent attachment of a number of different chemical groups, mainly to the tails. The tail of histone H3, for example, can receive acetyl groups (Ac), methyl groups (M), or phosphate groups (P). The numbers denote the positions of the modified amino acids in the histone tail, with each amino acid designated by its one-letter code. Note that some amino acids, such as the lysine (K) at positions 9, 14, 23, and 27, can be modified by acetylation or methylation (but not by both at once). Lysines, in addition, can be modified with either one, two, or three methyl groups; trimethylation, for example, is shown in (B). Note that histone H3 contains 135 amino acids, most of which are in its globular portion (represented by the wedge); most modifications occur on the N-terminal tail, for which 36 amino acids are shown. (B) Different combinations of histone tail modifications can confer a specific meaning on the stretch of chromatin on which they occur, as indicated. Only a few of these functional outcomes are known.

(Figure 5–25A). These and other modifications can have important consequences for the packing of the chromatin fiber. Acetylation of lysines, for instance, can reduce the affinity of the tails for adjacent nucleosomes, thereby loosening chromatin structure and allowing access to particular nuclear proteins.

Most importantly, however, these modifications generally serve as docking sites on the histone tails for a variety of regulatory proteins. Different patterns of modifications attract specific sets of non-histone chromosomal proteins to a particular stretch of chromatin. Some of these proteins promote chromatin condensation, whereas others promote chromatin expansion and thus facilitate access to the DNA. Specific combinations of tail modifications, and the proteins that bind to them, have different functional outcomes for the cell: one pattern, for example, might mark a particular stretch of chromatin as newly replicated; another might indicate that the genes in that stretch of chromatin are being actively expressed; still others are associated with genes that are silenced (Figure 5–25B).

Both ATP-dependent chromatin-remodeling complexes and histone-modifying enzymes are tightly regulated. These enzymes are often brought to particular chromatin regions by interactions with proteins that bind to a specific nucleotide sequence in the DNA—or in an RNA transcribed from this DNA (a topic we return to in Chapter 8). Histone-modifying enzymes work in concert with the chromatin-remodeling complexes to condense and relax stretches of chromatin, allowing local chromatin structure to change rapidly according to the needs of the cell.

Interphase Chromosomes Contain both Highly Condensed and More Extended Forms of Chromatin

The localized alteration of chromatin packing by remodeling complexes and histone modification has important effects on the large-scale structure of interphase chromosomes. Interphase chromatin is not uniformly packed. Instead, regions of the chromosome containing genes that are being actively expressed are generally more extended, whereas those that contain silent genes are more condensed. Thus, the detailed structure of an interphase chromosome can differ from one cell type to the next, helping to determine which genes are switched on and which are shut down. Most cell types express only about half of the genes they contain, and many of these are active only at very low levels.

The most highly condensed form of interphase chromatin is called **heterochromatin** (from the Greek *heteros*, "different," chromatin). This highly compact form of chromatin was first observed in the light microscope in the 1930s as discrete, strongly staining regions within the total

QUESTION 5–3

Histone proteins are among the most highly conserved proteins in eukaryotes. Histone H4 proteins from a pea and a cow, for example, differ in only 2 of 102 amino acids. Comparison of the gene sequences shows many more differences, but only two change the amino acid sequence. These observations indicate that mutations that change amino acids must have been selected against during evolution. Why do you suppose that amino-acid-altering mutations in histone genes are deleterious?

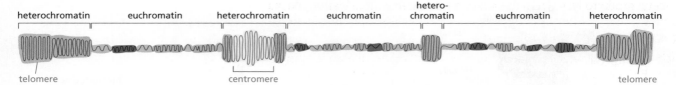

Figure 5–26 **The structure of chromatin varies along a single interphase chromosome.** As schematically indicated by the path of the DNA molecule (represented by the central *black* line) and the different arbitrarily assigned colors, heterochromatin and euchromatin each represent a set of different chromatin structures with different degrees of condensation. Overall, heterochromatin is more condensed than euchromatin.

chromatin mass. Heterochromatin typically makes up about 10% of an interphase chromosome, and in mammalian chromosomes, it is concentrated around the centromere region and in the telomeric DNA at the chromosome ends (see Figure 5–14).

The rest of the interphase chromatin is called **euchromatin** (from the Greek *eu*, "true" or "normal," chromatin). Although we use the term euchromatin to refer to chromatin that exists in a less condensed state than heterochromatin, it is now clear that both euchromatin and heterochromatin are composed of mixtures of different chromatin structures (Figure 5–26).

Each type of chromatin structure is established and maintained by different sets of histone tail modifications, which attract distinct sets of nonhistone chromosomal proteins. The modifications that direct the formation of the most common type of heterochromatin, for example, include the methylation of lysine 9 in the tail of histone H3 (see Figure 5–25B). Once heterochromatin has been established, it can spread to neighboring regions of DNA, because its histone tail modifications attract a set of heterochromatin-specific proteins, including histone-modifying enzymes, which then add the same histone tail modifications on adjacent nucleosomes. These modifications in turn recruit more of the heterochromatin-specific proteins, causing a wave of condensed chromatin to propagate along the chromosome. This extended region of heterochromatin will continue to spread until it encounters a barrier DNA sequence that stops the propagation (Figure 5–27). As an example, some barrier sequences contain binding sites for histone-modifying enzymes that add

Figure 5–27 **Heterochromatin-specific histone modifications allow heterochromatin to form and to spread.** These modifications attract heterochromatin-specific proteins that reproduce the same histone modifications on neighboring nucleosomes. In this manner, heterochromatin can spread until it encounters a barrier DNA sequence that blocks further propagation into regions of euchromatin.

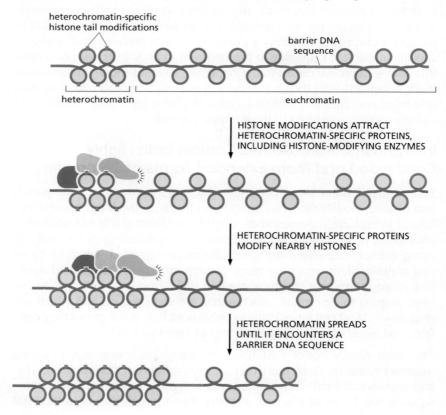

an acetyl group to lysine 9 of the histone H3 tail; this modification blocks the methylation of that lysine, preventing any further spread of heterochromatin (see Figure 5–25B).

Much of the DNA that is folded into heterochromatin does not contain genes. Because heterochromatin is so compact, genes that accidentally become packaged into heterochromatin usually fail to be expressed. Such inappropriate packaging of genes in heterochromatin can cause disease: in humans, the gene that encodes β-globin—a protein that forms part of the oxygen-carrying hemoglobin molecule—is situated near a region of heterochromatin. In an individual with an inherited deletion of its barrier DNA, that heterochromatin spreads and deactivates the β-globin gene, causing severe anemia.

Perhaps the most striking example of the use of heterochromatin to keep genes shut down, or *silenced*, is found in the interphase X chromosomes of female mammals. In mammals, female cells contain two X chromosomes, whereas male cells contain one X and one Y. A double dose of X-chromosome products could be lethal, and female mammals have evolved a mechanism for permanently inactivating one of the two X chromosomes in each cell. At random, one or other of the two X chromosomes in each nucleus becomes highly condensed into heterochromatin early in embryonic development. Thereafter, the condensed and inactive state of that X chromosome is inherited in all of the many descendants of those cells (**Figure 5–28**). This process of X-inactivation is responsible for the patchwork coloration of calico cats (**Figure 5–29**).

X-inactivation is an extreme example of a process that takes place in all eukaryotic cells—one that operates on a much finer scale to help control gene expression. When a cell divides, it can pass along its histone modifications, chromatin structure, and gene expression patterns to the two daughter cells. Such "cell memory" transmits information about which

Figure 5–28 One of the two X chromosomes is inactivated in the cells of mammalian females by heterochromatin formation.
(A) Each female cell contains two X chromosomes, one from the mother (X_m) and one from the father (X_p). At an early stage in embryonic development, one of these two chromosomes becomes condensed into heterochromatin in each cell, apparently at random. At each cell division, the same X chromosome becomes condensed (and inactivated) in all the descendants of that original cell. Thus, all mammalian females end up as mixtures (mosaics) of cells bearing either inactivated maternal or inactivated paternal X chromosomes. In most of their tissues and organs, about half the cells will be of one type, and the rest will be of the other. (B) In the nucleus of a female cell, the inactivated X chromosome can be seen as a small, discrete mass of chromatin called a Barr body, named after the physician who first observed it. In these micrographs of the nuclei of human fibroblasts, the inactivated X chromosome in the female nucleus (*bottom* micrograph) has been visualized by use of an antibody that recognizes proteins associated with the Barr body. The male nucleus (*top*) contains only a single X chromosome, which is not inactivated and thus not recognized by this antibody. Below the micrographs, a cartoon shows the locations of both the active and the inactive X chromosomes in the female nucleus. (B, adapted from B. Hong et al. *Proc. Natl Acad. Sci. USA* 98:8703–8708, 2001.)

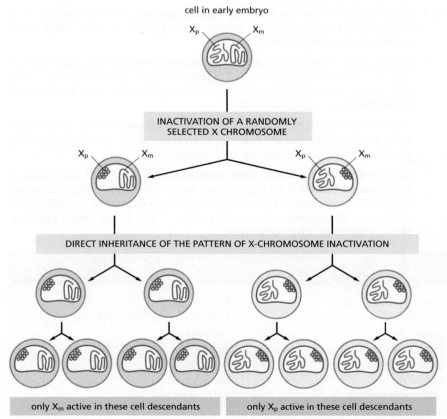

cell in early embryo

X_p X_m

INACTIVATION OF A RANDOMLY SELECTED X CHROMOSOME

X_p X_m X_p X_m

DIRECT INHERITANCE OF THE PATTERN OF X-CHROMOSOME INACTIVATION

only X_m active in these cell descendants   only X_p active in these cell descendants

(A)

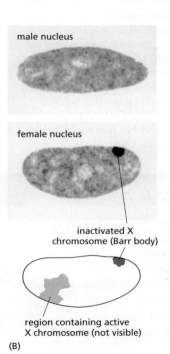

male nucleus

female nucleus

inactivated X chromosome (Barr body)

region containing active X chromosome (not visible)

(B)

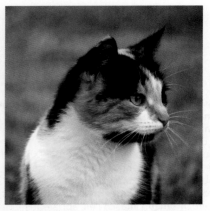

Figure 5–29 The coat color of a calico cat is dictated in large part by patterns of X-inactivation. In cats, one of the genes specifying coat color is located on the X chromosome. In female calicos, one X chromosome carries the form of the gene that specifies black fur, the other carries the form of the gene that specifies orange fur. Skin cells in which the X chromosome carrying the gene for black fur is inactivated will produce orange fur; those in which the X chromosome carrying the gene for orange fur is inactivated will produce black fur. The size of each patch will depend on the number of skin cells that have descended from an embryonic cell in which one or the other of the X chromosomes was randomly inactivated during development (see Figure 5–28). (bluecaterpillar/Depositphotos.)

QUESTION 5–4

Mutations in a particular gene on the X chromosome result in color blindness in men. By contrast, most women carrying the mutation have proper color vision but see colored objects with reduced resolution, as though functional cone cells (the photoreceptor cells responsible for color vision) are spaced farther apart than normal in the retina. Can you give a plausible explanation for this observation? If a woman is color-blind, what could you say about her father? About her mother? Explain your answers.

genes are active and which are not—a process critical for the establishment and maintenance of different cell types during the development of a complex multicellular organism. We discuss some of the mechanisms involved in cell memory in Chapter 8, when we consider how cells control gene expression.

ESSENTIAL CONCEPTS

- Life depends on the stable storage, maintenance, and inheritance of genetic information.

- Genetic information is carried by very long DNA molecules and is encoded in the linear sequence of four nucleotides: A, T, G, and C.

- Each molecule of DNA is a double helix composed of a pair of antiparallel, complementary DNA strands, which are held together by hydrogen bonds between G-C and A-T base pairs.

- The genetic material of a eukaryotic cell—its genome—is contained in a set of chromosomes, each formed from a single, enormously long DNA molecule that contains many genes.

- When a gene is expressed, part of its nucleotide sequence is transcribed into RNA molecules, most of which are translated to produce a protein.

- The DNA that forms each eukaryotic chromosome contains, in addition to genes, many replication origins, one centromere, and two telomeres. These special DNA sequences ensure that, before cell division, each chromosome can be duplicated efficiently, and that the resulting daughter chromosomes can be parceled out equally to the two daughter cells.

- In eukaryotic chromosomes, the DNA is tightly folded by binding to a set of histone and nonhistone chromosomal proteins. This complex of DNA and protein is called chromatin.

- Histones pack the DNA into a repeating array of DNA–protein particles called nucleosomes, which further fold up into even more compact chromatin structures.

- A cell can regulate its chromatin structure—temporarily decondensing or condensing particular regions of its chromosomes—using chromatin-remodeling complexes and enzymes that covalently modify histone tails in various ways.

- The loosening of chromatin to a more decondensed state allows proteins involved in gene expression, DNA replication, and DNA repair to gain access to the necessary DNA sequences.

- Some forms of chromatin have a pattern of histone tail modification that causes the DNA to become so highly condensed that its genes cannot be expressed to produce RNA; a high degree of condensation occurs on all chromosomes during mitosis and in the heterochromatin of interphase chromosomes.

KEY TERMS

base pair	double helix	histone
cell cycle	euchromatin	histone-modifying enzyme
centromere	gene	karyotype
chromatin	gene expression	nucleolus
chromatin-remodeling complex	genetic code	nucleosome
chromosome	genome	replication origin
complementary	heterochromatin	telomere
deoxyribonucleic acid (DNA)		

HOW WE KNOW

GENES ARE MADE OF DNA

By the 1920s, scientists generally agreed that genes reside on chromosomes. And studies in the late nineteenth century had demonstrated that chromosomes are composed of both DNA and proteins. But because DNA is so chemically simple, biologists naturally assumed that genes had to be made of proteins, which are much more chemically diverse than DNA molecules. Even when the experimental evidence suggested otherwise, this assumption proved hard to shake.

Messages from the dead

The case for DNA began to emerge in the late 1920s, when a British medical officer named Fred Griffith made an astonishing discovery. He was studying *Streptococcus pneumoniae* (pneumococcus), a bacterium that causes pneumonia. As antibiotics had not yet been discovered, infection with this organism was usually fatal. When grown in the laboratory, pneumococci come in two

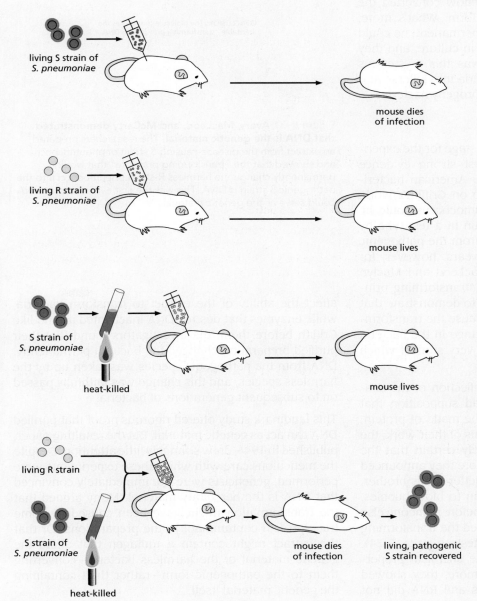

living S strain of
S. pneumoniae

mouse dies
of infection

living R strain of
S. pneumoniae

mouse lives

S strain of
S. pneumoniae

heat-killed

mouse lives

living R strain

S strain of
S. pneumoniae

heat-killed

mouse dies
of infection

living, pathogenic
S strain recovered

Figure 5–30 Griffith showed that heat-killed infectious bacteria can transform harmless live bacteria into pathogens. The bacterium *Streptococcus pneumoniae* comes in two forms that differ in their microscopic appearance and in their ability to cause disease. Cells of the pathogenic strain, which are lethal when injected into mice, are encased in a slimy, glistening polysaccharide capsule. When grown on a plate of nutrients in the laboratory, this disease-causing bacterium forms colonies that look dome-shaped and smooth; hence it is designated the S form. The harmless strain of the pneumococcus, on the other hand, lacks this protective coat; it forms colonies that appear flat and rough—hence, it is referred to as the R form. As illustrated in this diagram, Griffith found that a substance present in the pathogenic S strain could permanently change, or transform, the nonlethal R strain into the deadly S strain.

forms: a pathogenic form that causes a lethal infection when injected into animals, and a harmless form that is easily conquered by the animal's immune system and does not produce an infection.

In the course of his investigations, Griffith injected various preparations of these bacteria into mice. He showed that pathogenic pneumococci that had been killed by heating were no longer able to cause infection. The surprise came when Griffith injected both heat-killed pathogenic bacteria and live harmless bacteria into the same mouse. This combination proved unexpectedly lethal: not only did the animals die of pneumonia, but Griffith found that their blood was teeming with live bacteria of the pathogenic form (**Figure 5–30**). The heat-killed pneumococci had somehow converted the harmless bacteria into the lethal form. What's more, Griffith found that the change was permanent: he could grow these "transformed" bacteria in culture, and they remained pathogenic. But what was this mysterious material that turned harmless bacteria into killers? And how was this change passed on to progeny bacteria?

Transformation

Griffith's remarkable finding set the stage for the experiments that would provide the first strong evidence that genes are made of DNA. The American bacteriologist Oswald Avery, following up on Griffith's work, discovered that the harmless pneumococcus could be transformed into a pathogenic strain in a test tube by exposing it to an extract prepared from the pathogenic strain. It would take another 15 years, however, for Avery and his colleagues Colin MacLeod and Maclyn McCarty to successfully purify the "transforming principle" from this soluble extract and to demonstrate that the active ingredient was DNA. Because the transforming principle caused a heritable change in the bacteria that received it, DNA must be the very stuff of which genes are made.

The 15-year delay was in part a reflection of the academic climate—and the widespread supposition that the genetic material was likely to be made of protein. Because of the potential ramifications of their work, the researchers wanted to be absolutely certain that the transforming principle was DNA before they announced their findings. As Avery noted in a letter to his brother, also a bacteriologist, "It's lots of fun to blow bubbles, but it's wiser to prick them yourself before someone else tries to." So the researchers subjected the transforming material to a battery of chemical tests (**Figure 5–31**). They found that it exhibited all the chemical properties characteristic of DNA; furthermore, they showed that enzymes that destroy proteins and RNA did not

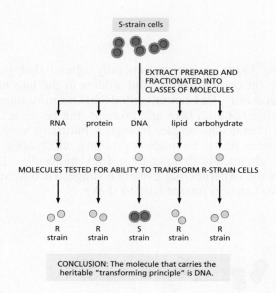

Figure 5–31 Avery, MacLeod, and McCarty demonstrated that DNA is the genetic material. The researchers prepared an extract from the disease-causing S strain of pneumococci and showed that the "transforming principle" that would permanently change the harmless R-strain pneumococci into the pathogenic S strain is DNA. This was the first evidence that DNA could serve as the genetic material.

affect the ability of the extract to transform bacteria, while enzymes that destroy DNA inactivated it. And like Griffith before them, the investigators found that their purified preparation changed the bacteria permanently: DNA from the pathogenic species was taken up by the harmless species, and this change was faithfully passed on to subsequent generations of bacteria.

This landmark study offered rigorous proof that purified DNA can act as genetic material. But the resulting paper, published in 1944, drew strangely little attention. Despite the meticulous care with which these experiments were performed, geneticists were not immediately convinced that DNA is the hereditary material. Many argued that the transformation might have been caused by some trace protein contaminant in the preparations. Or that the extract might contain a mutagen that alters the genetic material of the harmless bacteria—converting them to the pathogenic form—rather than containing the genetic material itself.

Virus cocktails

The debate was not settled definitively until 1952, when Alfred Hershey and Martha Chase fired up their laboratory blender and demonstrated, once and for all, that genes are made of DNA. The researchers were studying T2—a virus that infects and eventually destroys the bacterium *E. coli*. These bacteria-killing viruses behave like tiny molecular syringes: they inject their genetic material into the bacterial host cell, while the empty virus heads remain attached outside (Figure 5–32A). Once inside the bacterial cell, the viral genes direct the formation of new virus particles. In less than an hour, the infected cells explode, spewing thousands of new viruses into the medium. These then infect neighboring bacteria, and the process begins again.

The beauty of T2 is that these viruses contain only two kinds of molecules: DNA and protein. So the genetic material had to be one or the other. But which? The experiment was fairly straightforward. Because the viral genes enter the bacterial cell, while the rest of the virus particle remains outside, the researchers decided to radioactively label the protein in one batch of virus and the DNA in another. Then, all they had to do was follow the radioactivity to see whether viral DNA or viral protein wound up inside the bacteria. To do this, Hershey and Chase incubated their radiolabeled viruses with *E. coli*; after allowing a few minutes for infection to take place, they poured the mix into a Waring blender and hit "puree." The blender's spinning blades sheared the empty virus heads from the surfaces of the bacterial cells. The researchers then centrifuged the sample to separate the heavier, infected bacteria, which formed a pellet at the bottom of the centrifuge tube, from empty viral coats, which remained in suspension (Figure 5–32B).

As you have probably guessed, Hershey and Chase found that the radioactive DNA entered the bacterial cells, while the radioactive proteins remained outside with the empty virus heads. They found that the radioactive DNA was also incorporated into the next generation of virus particles.

This experiment demonstrated conclusively that viral DNA enters bacterial host cells, whereas viral protein does not. Thus, the genetic material in this virus had to be made of DNA. Together with the studies done by Avery, MacLeod, and McCarty, this evidence clinched the case for DNA as the agent of heredity.

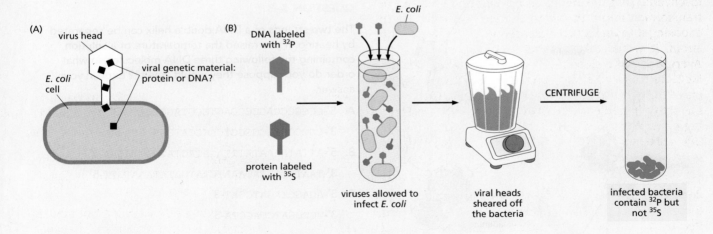

Figure 5–32 **Hershey and Chase showed definitively that genes are made of DNA.** (A) The researchers worked with T2 viruses, which are made entirely of protein and DNA. Each virus acts as a molecular syringe, injecting its genetic material into a bacterium; the empty viral capsule remains attached to the outside of the cell. (B) To determine whether the genetic material of the virus is made of protein or DNA, the researchers labeled the DNA in one batch of viruses with radioactive phosphorous (^{32}P) and the proteins in a second batch of viruses with radioactive sulfur (^{35}S). Because DNA lacks sulfur and the proteins lack phosphorus, these radioactive isotopes allowed the researchers to distinguish these two types of molecules. The radioactively labeled viruses were allowed to infect *E. coli*, and the mixture was then disrupted by brief pulsing in a Waring blender and centrifuged to separate the infected bacteria from the empty viral heads. When the researchers measured the radioactivity, they found that much of the ^{32}P-labeled DNA had entered the bacterial cells, while the vast majority of the ^{35}S-labeled proteins remained in solution with the spent viral particles. Furthermore, the radioactively labeled DNA also made its way into subsequent generations of virus particles, confirming that DNA is the heritable, genetic material.

QUESTIONS

QUESTION 5–5

A. The nucleotide sequence of one DNA strand of a DNA double helix is 5'-GGATTTTTGTCCACAATCA-3'.

What is the sequence of the complementary strand?

B. In the DNA of certain bacterial cells, 13% of the nucleotides contain adenine. What are the percentages of the other nucleotides?

C. How many possible nucleotide sequences are there for a stretch of single-stranded DNA that is N nucleotides long?

D. Suppose you had a method of cutting DNA at specific sequences of nucleotides. How many nucleotides long (on average) would such a sequence have to be in order to make just one cut in a bacterial genome of 3×10^6 nucleotide pairs? How would the answer differ for the genome of an animal cell that contains 3×10^9 nucleotide pairs?

QUESTION 5–6

An A-T base pair is stabilized by only two hydrogen bonds. Hydrogen-bonding schemes of very similar strengths can also be drawn between other base combinations that normally do not occur in DNA molecules, such as the A-C and the A-G pairs shown in Figure Q5–6. What would happen if these pairs formed during DNA replication and the inappropriate bases were incorporated? Discuss why this does not often happen. (Hint: see Figure 5–4.)

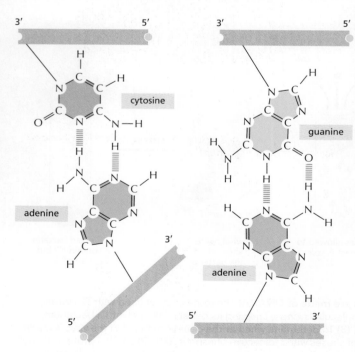

Figure Q5–6

QUESTION 5–7

A. A macromolecule isolated from an extraterrestrial source superficially resembles DNA, but closer analysis reveals that the bases have quite different structures (Figure Q5–7). Bases V, W, X, and Y have replaced bases A, T, G, and C. Look at these structures closely. Could these DNA-like molecules have been derived from a living organism that uses principles of genetic inheritance similar to those used by organisms on Earth?

B. Simply judged by their potential for hydrogen-bonding, could any of these extraterrestrial bases replace terrestrial A, T, G, or C in terrestrial DNA? Explain your answer.

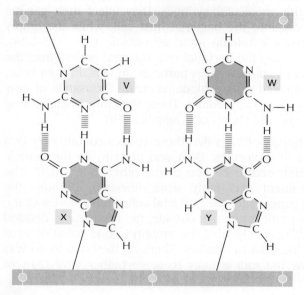

Figure Q5–7

QUESTION 5–8

The two strands of a DNA double helix can be separated by heating. If you raised the temperature of a solution containing the following three DNA molecules, in what order do you suppose they would "melt"? Explain your answer.

A. 5'-GCGGGCCAGCCCGAGTGGGTAGCCCAGG-3'

    3'-CGCCCGGTCGGGCTCACCCATCGGGTCC-5'

B. 5'-ATTATAAAATATTTAGATACTATATTTACAA-3'

    3'-TAATATTTTATAAATCTATGATATAAATGTT-5'

C. 5'-AGAGCTAGATCGAT-3'

    3'-TCTCGATCTAGCTA-5'

QUESTION 5–9

The total length of DNA in one copy of the human genome is about 1 m, and the diameter of the double helix is about 2 nm. Nucleotides in a DNA double helix are stacked (see Figure 5–4B) at an interval of 0.34 nm. If the DNA were enlarged so that its diameter equaled that of an electrical extension cord (5 mm), how long would the extension cord be from one end to the other (assuming that it is completely stretched out)? How close would the bases be to each other? How long would a gene of 1000 nucleotide pairs be?

QUESTION 5–10

A compact disc (CD) stores about 4.8×10^9 bits of information in a 96 cm² area. This information is stored as a binary code—that is, every bit is either a 0 or a 1.

A. How many bits would it take to specify each nucleotide pair in a DNA sequence?

B. How many CDs would it take to store the information contained in the human genome?

QUESTION 5–11

Which of the following statements are correct? Explain your answers.

A. Each eukaryotic chromosome must contain the following DNA sequence elements: multiple origins of replication, two telomeres, and one centromere.

B. Nucleosome core particles are 30 nm in diameter.

QUESTION 5–12

Define the following terms and their relationships to one another:

A. Interphase chromosome

B. Mitotic chromosome

C. Chromatin

D. Heterochromatin

E. Histones

F. Nucleosome

QUESTION 5–13

Carefully consider the result shown in Figure Q5–13. Each of the two colonies shown on the *left* is a clump of approximately 100,000 yeast cells that has grown up from a single cell, which is now somewhere in the middle of the colony. The two yeast colonies are genetically different, as shown by the chromosomal maps on the right. The yeast *Ade2* gene encodes one of the enzymes required for adenine biosynthesis, and the absence of the *Ade2* gene product leads to the accumulation of a red pigment. At its normal chromosome location, *Ade2* is expressed in all cells. When it is positioned near the telomere, which is highly condensed, *Ade2* is no longer expressed. How do you think the white sectors arise? What can you conclude about the propagation of the transcriptional state of the *Ade2* gene from mother to daughter cells?

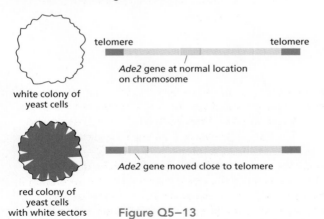

telomere   telomere

Ade2 gene at normal location on chromosome

white colony of yeast cells

Ade2 gene moved close to telomere

red colony of yeast cells with white sectors

Figure Q5–13

QUESTION 5–14

The two electron micrographs in Figure Q5–14 show nuclei of two different cell types. Can you tell from these pictures which of the two cells is transcribing more of its genes? Explain how you arrived at your answer. (Micrographs courtesy of Don W. Fawcett.)

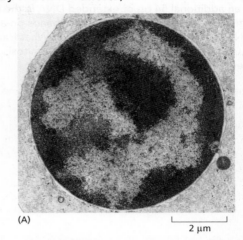

(A)
⊢──────⊣
2 μm

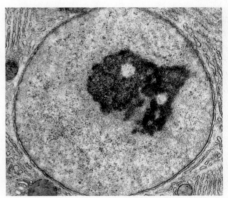

(B)

Figure Q5–14

QUESTION 5–15

DNA forms a right-handed helix. Pick out the right-handed helix from those shown in Figure Q5–15.

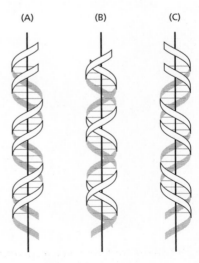

(A)   (B)   (C)

Figure Q5–15

QUESTION 5–16

A single nucleosome core particle is 11 nm in diameter and contains 147 base pairs (bp) of DNA (the DNA double helix measures 0.34 nm/bp). What packing ratio (ratio of DNA length to nucleosome diameter) has been achieved by wrapping DNA around the histone octamer? Assuming that there are an additional 54 bp of extended DNA in the linker between nucleosomes, how condensed is "beads-on-a-string" DNA relative to fully extended DNA? What fraction of the 10,000-fold condensation that occurs at mitosis does this first level of packing represent?

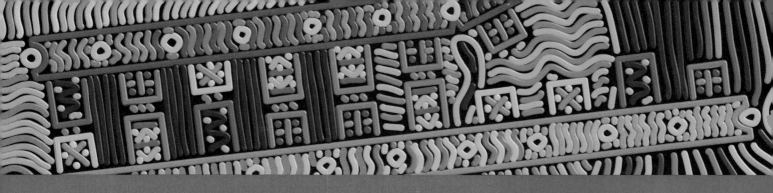

CHAPTER SIX

6

DNA Replication and Repair

For a cell to survive and proliferate in a chaotic environment, it must be able to accurately copy the vast quantity of genetic information carried in its DNA. This fundamental process, called **DNA replication**, must occur before a cell can divide to produce two genetically identical daughter cells. In addition to carrying out this painstaking task with stunning accuracy and efficiency, a cell must also continuously monitor and repair its genetic material, as DNA is subjected to unavoidable damage by chemicals and radiation in the environment and by reactive molecules that are generated inside the cell.

Yet despite the molecular safeguards that have evolved to protect a cell's DNA from copying errors and accidental damage, permanent changes— or **mutations**—sometimes do occur. Although most mutations do not affect the organism in any noticeable way, some have profound consequences. Occasionally, these changes can benefit the organism: for example, mutations can make bacteria resistant to antibiotics that are used to kill them. What is more, changes in DNA sequence can produce small variations that underlie the differences between individuals of the same species (Figure 6–1); such changes, when they accumulate over hundreds of millions of years, provide the variety in genetic material that makes one species distinct from another, as we discuss in Chapter 9.

Unfortunately, as mutations occur randomly, they are more likely to be detrimental than beneficial: they are responsible for thousands of human diseases, including cancer. The survival of a cell or organism, therefore, depends on keeping the changes in its DNA to a minimum. Without the systems that are continually inspecting and repairing damage to DNA, it is questionable whether life could exist at all. In this chapter, we describe the protein machines that replicate and repair the cell's DNA. These

DNA REPLICATION

DNA REPAIR

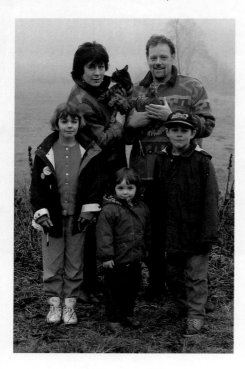

Figure 6–1 Differences in DNA can produce the variations that underlie the differences between individuals of the same species—even within the same family. Over evolutionary time, these genetic changes give rise to the differences that distinguish one species from another.

machines catalyze some of the most rapid and elegant processes that take place within cells, and uncovering the strategies they employ to achieve these marvelous feats represents a triumph of scientific investigation.

DNA REPLICATION

At each cell division, a cell must copy its genome with extraordinary accuracy. In this section, we explore how the cell achieves this feat, while replicating its DNA at rates as high as 1000 nucleotides per second.

Base-Pairing Enables DNA Replication

In the preceding chapter, we saw that each strand of a DNA double helix contains a sequence of nucleotides that is exactly complementary to the nucleotide sequence of its partner strand. Each strand can therefore serve as a **template**, or mold, for the synthesis of a new complementary strand. In other words, if we designate the two DNA strands as S and S′, strand S can serve as a template for making a new strand S′, while strand S′ can serve as a template for making a new strand S (Figure 6–2). Thus, the genetic information in DNA can be accurately copied by the beautifully simple process in which strand S separates from strand S′, and each separated strand then serves as a template for the production of a new complementary partner strand that is identical to its former partner.

The ability of each strand of a DNA molecule to act as a template for producing a complementary strand enables a cell to copy, or *replicate*, its genes before passing them on to its descendants. Although simple in principle, the process is awe-inspiring, as it can involve the copying of billions of nucleotide pairs with incredible speed and accuracy: a human cell undergoing division will copy the equivalent of 1000 books like this one in about 8 hours and, on average, get no more than a few letters wrong. This impressive feat is performed by a cluster of proteins that together form a *replication machine*.

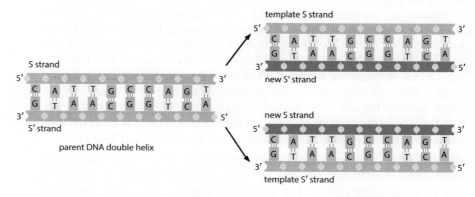

Figure 6–2 DNA acts as a template for its own replication. Because the nucleotide A will successfully pair only with T, and G with C, each strand of a DNA double helix—labeled here as the S strand and its complementary S′ strand—can serve as a template to specify the sequence of nucleotides in its complementary strand. In this way, both strands of a DNA double helix can be copied with precision.

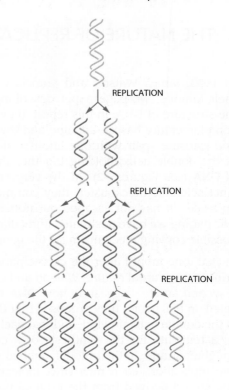

Figure 6–3 **In each round of DNA replication, each of the two strands of DNA is used as a template for the formation of a new, complementary strand.** DNA replication is "semiconservative" because each daughter DNA double helix is composed of one conserved (old) strand and one newly synthesized strand.

DNA replication produces two complete double helices from the original DNA molecule, with each new DNA helix being identical in nucleotide sequence (except for rare copying errors) to the original DNA double helix (see Figure 6–2). Because each parental strand serves as the template for one new strand, each of the daughter DNA double helices ends up with one of the original (old) strands plus one strand that is completely new; this style of replication is said to be *semiconservative* (**Figure 6–3**). We describe the inventive experiments that revealed this feature of DNA replication in **How We Know**, pp. 202–204.

DNA Synthesis Begins at Replication Origins

The DNA double helix is normally very stable: the two DNA strands are locked together firmly by the large numbers of hydrogen bonds between the bases on both strands (see Figure 5–2). As a result, only temperatures approaching those of boiling water provide enough thermal energy to separate the two strands. To be used as a template, however, the double helix must first be opened up and the two strands separated to expose the nucleotide bases. How does this separation occur at the temperatures found in living cells?

The process of DNA synthesis is begun by *initiator proteins* that bind to specific DNA sequences called **replication origins**. Here, the initiator proteins pry the two DNA strands apart, breaking the hydrogen bonds between the bases (**Figure 6–4**). Although the hydrogen bonds collectively make the DNA helix very stable, individually each hydrogen bond is weak (as discussed in Chapter 2). Separating a short length of DNA a few base pairs at a time therefore does not require a large energy input, and the initiator proteins can readily unzip short regions of the double helix at normal temperatures.

In simple cells such as bacteria or yeast, replication origins span approximately 100 nucleotide pairs. They are composed of DNA sequences that attract the initiator proteins and are especially easy to open. We saw in Chapter 5 that an A-T base pair is held together by fewer hydrogen bonds than is a G-C base pair. Therefore, DNA rich in A-T base pairs is easier to pull apart, and A-T-rich stretches of DNA are typically found at replication origins.

A bacterial genome, which is typically contained in a circular DNA molecule of several million nucleotide pairs, has a single replication origin. The human genome, which is very much larger, has approximately 10,000 such origins—an average of 220 origins per chromosome. Beginning DNA replication at many places at once greatly shortens the time a cell needs to copy its entire genome.

Once an initiator protein binds to DNA at a replication origin and locally opens up the double helix, it attracts a group of proteins that carry out DNA replication. These proteins form a replication machine, in which each protein carries out a specific function.

Two Replication Forks Form at Each Replication Origin

DNA molecules in the process of being replicated contain Y-shaped junctions called **replication forks**. Two replication forks are formed at each

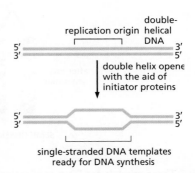

single-stranded DNA templates
ready for DNA synthesis

Figure 6–4 **A DNA double helix is opened at replication origins.** DNA sequences at replication origins are recognized by initiator proteins (not shown), which locally pull apart the two strands of the double helix. The exposed single strands can then serve as templates for copying the DNA.

HOW WE KNOW

THE NATURE OF REPLICATION

In 1953, James Watson and Francis Crick published their famous two-page paper describing a model for the structure of DNA. In this report, they proposed that complementary bases—adenine and thymine, guanine and cytosine—pair with one another along the center of the double helix, holding together the two strands of DNA (see Figure 5–2). At the very end of this succinct scientific blockbuster, they comment, almost as an aside, "It has not escaped our notice that the specific pairing we have postulated immediately suggests a possible copying mechanism for the genetic material."

Indeed, one month after the classic paper appeared in print in the journal *Nature*, Watson and Crick published a second article, suggesting how DNA might be replicated. In this paper, they proposed that the two strands of the double helix unwind, and that each strand serves as a template for the synthesis of a complementary daughter strand. In their model, dubbed semiconservative replication, each new DNA molecule consists of one strand derived from the original parent molecule and one newly synthesized strand (Figure 6–5A).

We now know that Watson and Crick's model for DNA replication was correct—but it was not universally accepted at first. Respected physicist-turned-geneticist Max Delbrück, for one, got hung up on what he termed "the untwiddling problem"; that is: How could the two strands of a double helix, twisted around each other so many times all along their great length, possibly be unwound without making a big tangled mess? Watson and Crick's conception of the DNA helix opening up like a zipper seemed, to Delbrück, physically unlikely and simply "too inelegant to be efficient."

Instead, Delbrück proposed that DNA replication proceeds through a series of breaks and reunions, in which the DNA backbone is broken and the strands are copied in short segments—perhaps only 10 nucleotides at a time—before being rejoined. In this model, which was later dubbed dispersive, the resulting copies would be patchwork collections of old and new DNA, each strand containing a mixture of both (Figure 6–5B). No unwinding was necessary.

Yet a third camp promoted the idea that DNA replication might be *conservative*: that the parent helix would somehow remain entirely intact after copying, and the daughter molecule would contain two entirely new DNA strands (Figure 6–5C). To determine which of these models was correct, an experiment was needed—one that would reveal the composition of the newly synthesized DNA strands. That's where Matt Meselson and Frank Stahl came in.

Heavy DNA

As a graduate student working with Linus Pauling, Meselson was toying with a method for telling the difference between old and new proteins. After chatting with Delbrück about Watson and Crick's replication

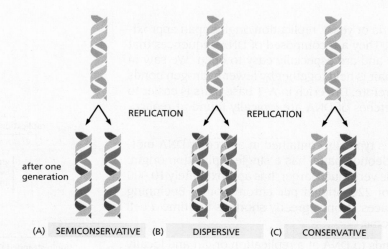

Figure 6–5 Three models for DNA replication make different predictions. (A) In the semiconservative model, each parent strand serves as a template for the synthesis of a new daughter strand. The first round of replication would produce two hybrid molecules, each containing one strand from the original parent and one newly synthesized strand. A subsequent round of replication would yield two hybrid molecules and two molecules that contain none of the original parent DNA (see Figure 6–3). (B) In the dispersive model, each generation of replicated DNA molecules will be a mosaic of DNA from the parent strands and the newly synthesized DNA. (C) In the conservative model, the parent molecule remains intact after being copied. In this case, the first round of replication would yield the original parent double helix and an entirely new double helix. For each model, parent DNA molecules are shown in *orange*; newly replicated DNA is *red*. Note that only a very small segment of DNA is shown for each model.

model, it occurred to Meselson that the approach he'd envisaged for exploring protein synthesis might also work for studying DNA. In the summer of 1954, Meselson met Stahl, who was then a graduate student in Rochester, NY, and they agreed to collaborate. It took a few years to get everything working, but the two eventually performed what has come to be known as "the most beautiful experiment in biology."

Their approach, in retrospect, was stunningly straightforward. They started by growing two batches of *Escherichia coli* bacteria, one in a medium containing a heavy isotope of nitrogen, ^{15}N, the other in a medium containing the normal, lighter ^{14}N. The nitrogen in the nutrient medium gets incorporated into the nucleotide bases and, from there, makes its way into the DNA of the organism. After growing bacterial cultures for many generations in either the ^{15}N- or ^{14}N-containing medium, the researchers had two flasks of bacteria, one with heavy DNA (containing *E. coli* that had incorporated the heavy isotope), the other with DNA that was light. Meselson and Stahl then broke open the bacterial cells and loaded the DNA into tubes containing a high concentration of the salt cesium chloride. When these tubes are centrifuged at high speed, the cesium chloride forms a density gradient, and the DNA molecules float or sink within the solution until they reach the point at which their density equals that of the salt solution that surrounds them (see Panel 4–3, pp. 164–165). Using this method, called equilibrium density centrifugation,

Meselson and Stahl found that they could distinguish between heavy (^{15}N-containing) DNA and light (^{14}N-containing) DNA by observing the positions of the DNA within the cesium chloride gradient. Because the heavy DNA was denser than the light DNA, it collected at a position nearer to the bottom of the centrifuge tube (**Figure 6–6**).

And the winner is...

Once they had established this method for differentiating between light and heavy DNA, Meselson and Stahl set out to test the various hypotheses proposed for DNA replication. To do this, they took a flask of bacteria that had been grown in heavy nitrogen and transferred the bacteria into a medium containing the light isotope. At the start of the experiment, all the DNA would be heavy. But, as the bacteria divided, the newly synthesized DNA would be light. They could then monitor the accumulation of light DNA and see which model, if any, best fit their data. After one generation of growth, the researchers found that the parental, heavy DNA molecules—those made of two strands containing ^{15}N—had disappeared and were replaced by a new species of DNA that banded at a density halfway between those of ^{15}N-DNA and ^{14}N-DNA (**Figure 6–7**). These newly synthesized daughter helices, Meselson and Stahl reasoned, must be hybrids—containing both heavy and light isotopes.

Right away, this observation ruled out the conservative model of DNA replication, which predicted that the

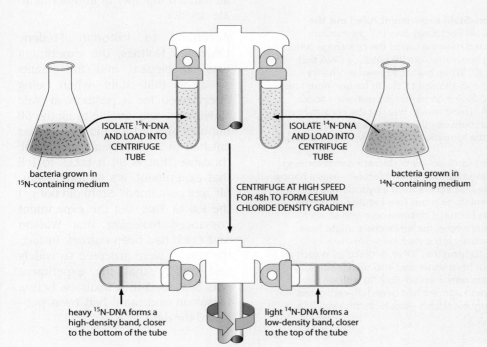

ISOLATE ^{15}N-DNA AND LOAD INTO CENTRIFUGE TUBE

ISOLATE ^{14}N-DNA AND LOAD INTO CENTRIFUGE TUBE

bacteria grown in ^{15}N-containing medium

bacteria grown in ^{14}N-containing medium

CENTRIFUGE AT HIGH SPEED FOR 48h TO FORM CESIUM CHLORIDE DENSITY GRADIENT

heavy ^{15}N-DNA forms a high-density band, closer to the bottom of the tube

light ^{14}N-DNA forms a low-density band, closer to the top of the tube

Figure 6–6 Centrifugation in a cesium chloride gradient allows the separation of heavy and light DNA. Bacteria are grown for several generations in a medium containing either ^{15}N (the heavy isotope) or ^{14}N (the light isotope) to label their DNA. The cells are then broken open, and the DNA is loaded into an ultracentrifuge tube containing a cesium chloride salt solution (*yellow*). These tubes are centrifuged at high speed for two days to allow the cesium chloride to form a gradient with low density at the top of the tube and high density at the bottom. As the gradient forms, the DNA will migrate to the region where its density matches that of the salt surrounding it. The heavy and light DNA molecules thus collect in different positions in the tube.

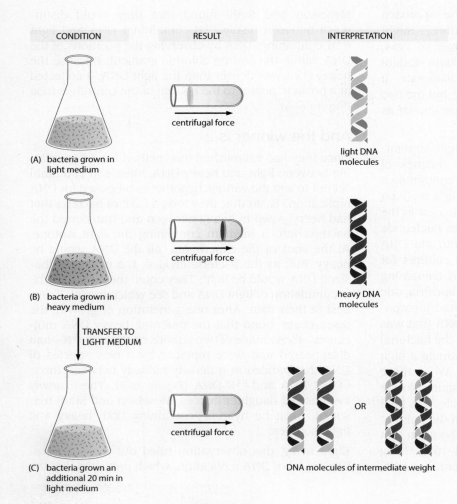

CONDITION	RESULT	INTERPRETATION
(A) bacteria grown in light medium	centrifugal force	light DNA molecules
(B) bacteria grown in heavy medium	centrifugal force	heavy DNA molecules
TRANSFER TO LIGHT MEDIUM		
(C) bacteria grown an additional 20 min in light medium	centrifugal force	OR — DNA molecules of intermediate weight

Figure 6–7 The first part of the Meselson–Stahl experiment ruled out the conservative model of DNA replication. (A) Bacteria grown in light medium (containing ^{14}N) yield DNA that forms a band near the top of the centrifuge tube, whereas bacteria grown in ^{15}N-containing heavy medium (B) produce DNA that reaches a position further down the tube. (C) When bacteria grown in a heavy medium are transferred to a light medium and allowed to divide for one hour (the time needed for one generation), they produce a band that is positioned about midway between the heavy and light DNA. These results rule out the conservative model of replication but do not distinguish between the semiconservative and dispersive models, both of which predict the formation of daughter DNA molecules with intermediate densities.

The fact that the results came out looking so clean—with discrete bands forming at the expected positions for newly replicated hybrid DNA molecules—was a happy accident of the experimental protocol. The researchers used a hypodermic syringe to load their DNA samples into the ultracentrifuge tubes (see Figure 6–6). In the process, they unwittingly sheared the large bacterial chromosome into smaller fragments. Had the chromosomes remained whole, the researchers might have isolated DNA molecules that were only partially replicated, because many cells would have been caught in the middle of copying their DNA. Molecules in such an intermediate stage of replication would not have separated into such beautifully discrete bands. But because the researchers were instead working with smaller pieces of DNA, the likelihood that any given fragment had been fully replicated—and contained a complete parent and daughter strand—was high, thus yielding clean, easy-to-interpret results.

parental DNA would remain entirely heavy, while the daughter DNA would be entirely light (see Figure 6–5C). The data supported the semiconservative model, which predicted the formation of hybrid molecules containing one strand of heavy DNA and one strand of light (see Figure 6–5A). The results, however, were also consistent with the dispersive model, in which hybrid DNA strands would contain a mixture of heavy and light DNA (see Figure 6–5B).

To distinguish between the remaining two models, Meselson and Stahl turned up the heat. When DNA is subjected to high temperature, the hydrogen bonds holding the two strands together break and the helix comes apart, leaving a collection of single-stranded DNAs. When the researchers heated the hybrid molecules before centrifuging, they discovered that one strand of the DNA was heavy, whereas the other was light. This observation ruled out the dispersive model; if this model were correct, the resulting strands, each containing a mottled assembly of heavy and light DNA, would have all banded together at an intermediate density.

According to historian Frederic Lawrence Holmes, the experiment was so elegant and the results so clean that Stahl—when being interviewed for a position at Yale University—was unable to fill the 50 minutes allotted for his talk. "I was finished in 25 minutes," said Stahl, "because that is all it takes to tell that experiment. It's so totally simple and contained." Stahl did not get the job at Yale, but the experiment convinced biologists that Watson and Crick had been correct. In fact, the results were accepted so widely and rapidly that the experiment was described in a textbook before Meselson and Stahl had even published the data.

replication origin (**Figure 6–8**). At each fork, a replication machine moves along the DNA, opening up the two strands of the double helix and using each strand as a template to make a new daughter strand. The two forks move away from the origin in opposite directions, unzipping the DNA double helix and copying the DNA as they go (**Figure 6–9**). DNA replication—in both bacterial and eukaryotic chromosomes—is therefore termed *bidirectional*. The forks move very rapidly: at about 1000 nucleotide pairs per second in bacteria and 100 nucleotide pairs per second in humans. The slower rate of fork movement in humans (indeed, in all eukaryotes) may be due to the difficulties in replicating DNA through the more complex chromatin structure of eukaryotic chromosomes (discussed in Chapter 5).

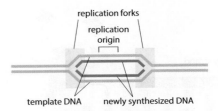

Figure 6–8 DNA synthesis occurs at Y-shaped junctions called replication forks. Two replication forks form at each replication origin and subsequently move away from each other as replication proceeds.

DNA Polymerase Synthesizes DNA Using a Parental Strand as a Template

The movement of a replication fork is driven by the action of the replication machine, at the heart of which is an enzyme called **DNA polymerase**. This enzyme catalyzes the addition of nucleotides to the 3′ end of a growing DNA strand, using one of the original, parental DNA strands as a template. Base-pairing between an incoming nucleotide and the template strand determines which of the four nucleotides (A, G, T, or C) will be selected. The final product is a new strand of DNA that is complementary in nucleotide sequence to the template (**Figure 6–10**).

The polymerization reaction involves the formation of a phosphodiester bond between the 3′ end of the growing DNA chain and the 5′-phosphate group of the incoming nucleotide, which enters the reaction as a *deoxyribonucleoside triphosphate*. The energy for polymerization is provided

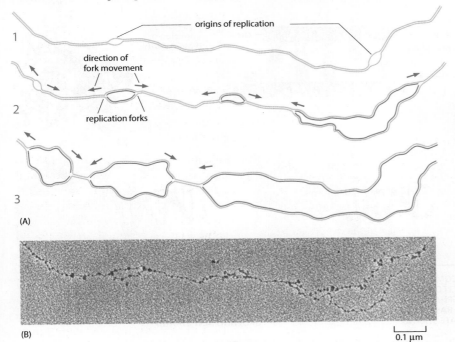

Figure 6–9 The two replication forks formed at a replication origin move away in opposite directions. (A) These drawings represent the same portion of a DNA molecule as it might appear at different times during replication. The *orange* lines represent the two parental DNA strands; the *red* lines represent the newly synthesized DNA strands. (B) An electron micrograph showing DNA replicating in an early fly embryo. The particles visible along the DNA are nucleosomes, structures made of DNA and the histone protein complexes around which the DNA is wrapped (discussed in Chapter 5). The chromosome in this micrograph is the same one that was redrawn in sketch (2) of (A). (B, courtesy of Victoria Foe.)

QUESTION 6–1

Look carefully at the micrograph and corresponding sketch (2) in Figure 6–9.
A. Using the scale bar, estimate the lengths of the DNA double helices between the replication forks. Numbering the replication forks sequentially from the left, how long will it take until forks 4 and 5, and forks 7 and 8, respectively, collide with each other? (Recall that the distance between the bases in DNA is 0.34 nm, and eukaryotic replication forks move at about 100 nucleotides per second.) For this question, disregard the nucleosomes seen in the micrograph and assume that the DNA is fully extended.
B. The fly genome is about 1.8×10^8 nucleotide pairs in size. What fraction of the genome is shown in the micrograph?

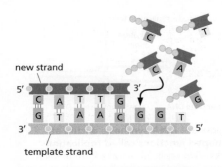

Figure 6–10 A new DNA strand is synthesized in the 5′-to-3′ direction. At each step, the appropriate incoming nucleoside triphosphate is selected by forming base pairs with the next nucleotide in the template strand: A with T, T with A, C with G, and G with C. Each is added to the 3′ end of the growing new strand, as indicated.

by the incoming deoxyribonucleoside triphosphate itself: hydrolysis of one of its high-energy phosphate bonds fuels the reaction that links the nucleotide monomer to the chain, releasing pyrophosphate (Figure 6–11). Pyrophosphate is further hydrolyzed to inorganic phosphate (P_i), which makes the polymerization reaction effectively irreversible (see Figure 3–42).

DNA polymerase does not dissociate from the DNA each time it adds a new nucleotide to the growing strand; rather, it stays associated with the DNA and moves along the template strand stepwise for many cycles of the polymerization reaction (Movie 6.1). We will see later that a special protein keeps the polymerase attached to DNA as it repeatedly adds new nucleotides to the growing strand.

The Replication Fork Is Asymmetrical

The 5′-to-3′ direction of the DNA polymerization reaction poses a problem at the replication fork. As illustrated in Figure 5–2, the sugar–phosphate backbone of each strand of a DNA double helix has a unique chemical direction, or polarity, determined by the way each sugar residue is linked to the next, and the two strands in the double helix are antiparallel; that is, they run in opposite directions. As a consequence, at each replication fork, one new DNA strand is being made on a template that runs in one direction (3′ to 5′), whereas the other new strand is being made on a template that runs in the opposite direction (5′ to 3′). The replication fork is therefore asymmetrical (Figure 6–12). Figure 6–9A, however, makes it look like both of the new DNA strands are growing in the same direction;

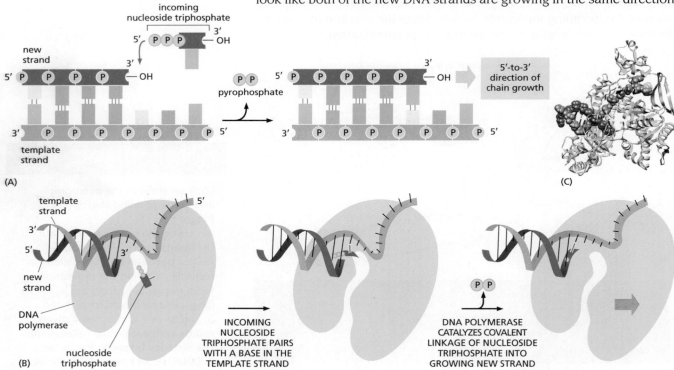

Figure 6–11 DNA polymerase adds a deoxyribonucleotide to the 3′ end of a growing DNA strand. (A) Nucleotides enter the reaction as deoxyribonucleoside triphosphates. An incoming nucleoside triphosphate forms a base pair with its partner in the template strand. It is then covalently attached to the free 3′ hydroxyl on the growing DNA strand. The new DNA strand is therefore synthesized in the 5′-to-3′ direction. The energy for the polymerization reaction comes from the hydrolysis of a high-energy phosphate bond in the incoming nucleoside triphosphate and the release of pyrophosphate, which is subsequently hydrolyzed to yield two molecules of inorganic phosphate (not shown). (B) The reaction is catalyzed by the enzyme DNA polymerase (*light green*). The polymerase guides the incoming nucleoside triphosphate to the template strand and positions it such that its 5′ triphosphate will be able to react with the 3′-hydroxyl group on the newly synthesized strand. The *gray* arrow indicates the direction of polymerase movement. (C) Structure of DNA polymerase, as determined by x-ray crystallography, also showing the replicating DNA. The template strand is the longer, *orange* strand, and the newly synthesized DNA strand is colored *red* (Movie 6.1).

that is, the direction in which the replication fork is moving. For that to be true, one strand would have to be synthesized in the 5'-to-3' direction and the other in the 3'-to-5' direction.

Does the cell have two types of DNA polymerase, one for each direction? The answer is no: all DNA polymerases add new subunits only to the 3' end of a DNA strand (see Figure 6–11A). As a result, a new DNA chain can be synthesized only in a 5'-to-3' direction. This can easily account for the synthesis of one of the two strands of DNA at the replication fork, but what happens on the other? This conundrum is solved by the use of a "backstitching" maneuver. The DNA strand that appears to grow in the incorrect 3'-to-5' direction is actually made *discontinuously*, in successive, separate, small pieces—with the DNA polymerase moving backward with respect to the direction of replication-fork movement so that each new DNA fragment can be polymerized in the 5'-to-3' direction.

The resulting small DNA pieces—called **Okazaki fragments** after the pair of biochemists who discovered them—are later joined together to form a continuous new strand. The DNA strand that is made discontinuously in this way is called the **lagging strand**, because the cumbersome backstitching mechanism imparts a slight delay to its synthesis; the other strand, which is synthesized continuously, is called the **leading strand** (**Figure 6–13**).

Although they differ in subtle details, the replication forks of all cells, prokaryotic and eukaryotic, have leading and lagging strands. This common feature arises from the fact that all DNA polymerases work only in the 5'-to-3' direction—a restriction that allows DNA polymerase to "check its work," as we discuss next.

DNA Polymerase Is Self-correcting

DNA polymerase is so accurate that it makes only about one error in every 10^7 nucleotide pairs it copies. This error rate is much lower than can be explained simply by the accuracy of complementary base-pairing. Although A-T and C-G are by far the most stable base pairs, other, less stable base pairs—for example, G-T and C-A—can also be formed. Such incorrect base pairs are formed much less frequently than correct ones, but, if allowed to remain, they would result in an accumulation of

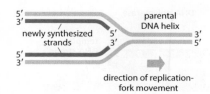

Figure 6–12 At a replication fork, the two newly synthesized DNA strands are of opposite polarities. This is because the two template strands are oriented in opposite directions.

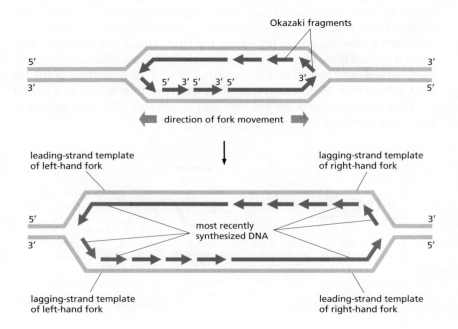

Figure 6–13 At each replication fork, the lagging DNA strand is synthesized in pieces. Because both of the new strands at a replication fork are synthesized in the 5'-to-3' direction, the lagging strand of DNA must be made initially as a series of short DNA strands, which are later joined together. The upper diagram shows two replication forks moving in opposite directions; the lower diagram shows the same forks a short time later. To replicate the lagging strand, DNA polymerase uses a backstitching mechanism: it synthesizes short pieces of DNA (called Okazaki fragments) in the 5'-to-3' direction and then moves back along the template strand (toward the fork) before synthesizing the next fragment.

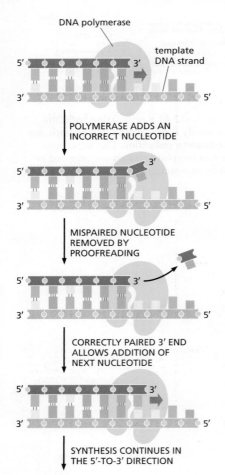

Figure 6–14 During DNA synthesis, DNA polymerase proofreads its own work. If an incorrect nucleotide is accidentally added to a growing strand, the DNA polymerase cleaves it from the strand and replaces it with the correct nucleotide before continuing.

Figure 6–15 DNA polymerase contains separate sites for DNA synthesis and proofreading. The diagrams are based on the structure of an *E. coli* DNA polymerase molecule, as determined by x-ray crystallography. The DNA polymerase, which cradles the DNA molecule being replicated, is shown in the polymerizing mode (*left*) and in the proofreading, or editing, mode (*right*). The catalytic sites for the polymerization activity (P) and editing activity (E) are indicated. When the polymerase adds an incorrect nucleotide, the newly synthesized DNA strand (*red*) transiently unpairs from the template strand (*orange*), and its 3′ end moves into the editing site (E) to allow the incorrect nucleotide to be removed.

mutations. This disaster is avoided because DNA polymerase has two special qualities that greatly increase the accuracy of DNA replication. First, the enzyme carefully monitors the base-pairing between each incoming nucleoside triphosphate and the template strand. Only when the match is correct does DNA polymerase undergo a small structural rearrangement that allows it to catalyze the nucleotide-addition reaction. Second, when DNA polymerase does make a rare mistake and adds the wrong nucleotide, it can correct the error through an activity called **proofreading**.

Proofreading takes place at the same time as DNA synthesis. Before the enzyme adds the next nucleotide to a growing DNA strand, it checks whether the previously added nucleotide is correctly base-paired to the template strand. If so, the polymerase adds the next nucleotide; if not, the polymerase clips off the mispaired nucleotide and tries again (**Figure 6–14**). Polymerization and proofreading are tightly coordinated, and the two reactions are carried out by different catalytic domains in the same polymerase molecule (**Figure 6–15**).

This proofreading mechanism is possible only for DNA polymerases that synthesize DNA exclusively in the 5′-to-3′ direction. If a DNA polymerase were able to synthesize in the 3′-to-5′ direction (circumventing the need for backstitching on the lagging strand), it would be unable to proofread. That's because if this "backward" polymerase were to remove an incorrectly paired nucleotide from the 5′ end, it would create a chemical dead end—a strand that could no longer be elongated (**Figure 6–16**). Thus, for a DNA polymerase to function as a self-correcting enzyme that removes its own polymerization errors as it moves along the DNA, it must proceed only in the 5′-to-3′ direction. The cumbersome backstitching mechanism on the lagging strand can be seen as a necessary consequence of maintaining this crucial proofreading activity.

Short Lengths of RNA Act as Primers for DNA Synthesis

We have seen that the accuracy of DNA replication depends on the requirement of the DNA polymerase for a correctly base-paired 3′ end before it can add more nucleotides to a growing DNA strand. How then can the polymerase begin a completely new DNA strand? To get the process started, a different enzyme is needed—one that can begin a new polynucleotide strand simply by joining two nucleotides together without the need for a base-paired end. This enzyme does not, however, synthesize DNA. It makes a short length of a closely related type of nucleic acid—**RNA** (**ribonucleic acid**)—using the DNA strand as a template. This short length of RNA, about 10 nucleotides long, is base-paired to the template strand and provides a base-paired 3′ end as a starting point for DNA polymerase (**Figure 6–17**). An RNA fragment thus serves as a *primer* for DNA synthesis, and the enzyme that synthesizes the RNA primer is known as **primase**.

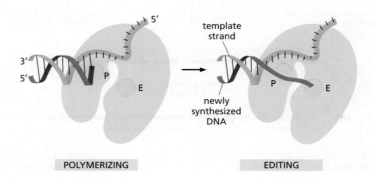

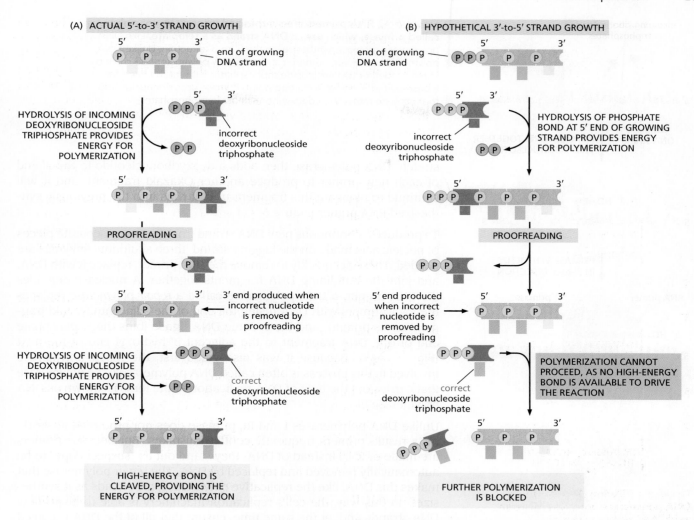

(A) ACTUAL 5'-to-3' STRAND GROWTH

end of growing DNA strand

HYDROLYSIS OF INCOMING DEOXYRIBONUCLEOSIDE TRIPHOSPHATE PROVIDES ENERGY FOR POLYMERIZATION

incorrect deoxyribonucleoside triphosphate

PROOFREADING

3' end produced when incorrect nucleotide is removed by proofreading

HYDROLYSIS OF INCOMING DEOXYRIBONUCLEOSIDE TRIPHOSPHATE PROVIDES ENERGY FOR POLYMERIZATION

correct deoxyribonucleoside triphosphate

HIGH-ENERGY BOND IS CLEAVED, PROVIDING THE ENERGY FOR POLYMERIZATION

(B) HYPOTHETICAL 3'-to-5' STRAND GROWTH

end of growing DNA strand

HYDROLYSIS OF PHOSPHATE BOND AT 5' END OF GROWING STRAND PROVIDES ENERGY FOR POLYMERIZATION

incorrect deoxyribonucleoside triphosphate

PROOFREADING

5' end produced when incorrect nucleotide is removed by proofreading

POLYMERIZATION CANNOT PROCEED, AS NO HIGH-ENERGY BOND IS AVAILABLE TO DRIVE THE REACTION

correct deoxyribonucleoside triphosphate

FURTHER POLYMERIZATION IS BLOCKED

Figure 6–16 For proofreading to take place, DNA polymerization must proceed in the 5'-to-3' direction. (A) Polymerization in the normal 5'-to-3' direction allows the DNA strand to continue to be elongated after an incorrectly added nucleotide (*gray*) has been removed by proofreading (see Figure 6–14). (B) If DNA synthesis instead proceeded in the backward 3'-to-5' direction, the energy for polymerization would come from the hydrolysis of the phosphate groups at the 5' end of the growing chain (*orange*), rather than the 5' end of the incoming nucleoside triphosphate. Removal of an incorrect nucleotide would block the addition of the correct nucleotide (*red*), as there are no high-energy phosphodiester bonds remaining at the 5' end of the growing strand.

Primase is an example of an *RNA polymerase*, an enzyme that synthesizes RNA using DNA as a template. A strand of RNA is very similar chemically to a single strand of DNA except that it is made of ribonucleotide subunits, in which the sugar is ribose, not deoxyribose; RNA also differs from DNA in that it contains the base uracil (U) instead of thymine (T) (see Panel 2–7, pp. 78–79). However, because U can form a base pair with A, the RNA primer is synthesized on the DNA strand by complementary base-pairing in exactly the same way as is DNA.

For the leading strand, an RNA primer is needed only to start replication at a replication origin; at that point, the DNA polymerase simply takes over, extending this primer with DNA synthesized in the 5'-to-3' direction. But on the lagging strand, where DNA synthesis is discontinuous, new primers are continuously needed to keep polymerization going (see Figure 6–13). The movement of the replication fork continually exposes unpaired bases on the lagging-strand template, and new RNA primers must be laid down at intervals along the newly exposed, single-stranded

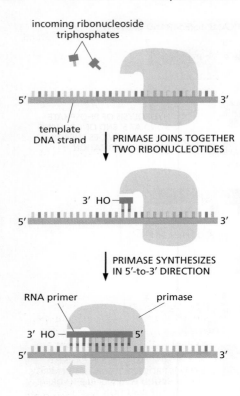

incoming ribonucleoside triphosphates

template DNA strand

PRIMASE JOINS TOGETHER TWO RIBONUCLEOTIDES

3′ HO

PRIMASE SYNTHESIZES IN 5′-to-3′ DIRECTION

RNA primer   primase

3′ HO   5′

Figure 6–17 RNA primers are synthesized by an RNA polymerase called primase, which uses a DNA strand as a template. Like DNA polymerase, primase synthesizes in the 5′-to-3′ direction. Unlike DNA polymerase, however, primase can start a new polynucleotide chain by joining together two nucleoside triphosphates without the need for a base-paired 3′ end as a starting point. Primase uses ribonucleoside triphosphate rather than deoxyribonucleoside triphosphate.

stretch. DNA polymerase then adds a deoxyribonucleotide to the 3′ end of each new primer to produce another Okazaki fragment, and it will continue to elongate this fragment until it runs into the previously synthesized RNA primer (**Figure 6–18**).

To produce a continuous new DNA strand from the many separate pieces of nucleic acid made on the lagging strand, three additional enzymes are needed. These act quickly to remove the RNA primer, replace it with DNA, and join the remaining DNA fragments together. A nuclease degrades the RNA primer, a DNA polymerase called a *repair polymerase* replaces the RNA primers with DNA (using the end of the adjacent Okazaki fragment as its primer), and the enzyme **DNA ligase** joins the 5′-phosphate end of one DNA fragment to the adjacent 3′-hydroxyl end of the next (**Figure 6–19**). Because it was discovered first, the repair polymerase involved in this process is often called DNA polymerase I; the polymerase that carries out the bulk of DNA replication at the forks is known as DNA polymerase III.

Unlike DNA polymerases I and III, primase does not proofread its work. As a result, primers frequently contain mistakes. But because primers are made of RNA instead of DNA, they stand out as "suspect copy" to be automatically removed and replaced by DNA. The repair polymerase that makes this DNA, like the replicative polymerase, proofreads as it synthesizes. In this way, the cell's replication machinery is able to begin new DNA strands and, at the same time, ensure that all of the DNA is copied faithfully.

Proteins at a Replication Fork Cooperate to Form a Replication Machine

DNA replication requires the cooperation of a large number of proteins that act in concert to synthesize new DNA. These proteins form part of a remarkably complex replication machine. The first problem faced by the replication machine is accessing the nucleotides that lie ahead of the replication fork and are thus buried within the double helix. For DNA replication to occur, the double helix must be continuously pried apart so that the incoming nucleoside triphosphates can form base pairs with

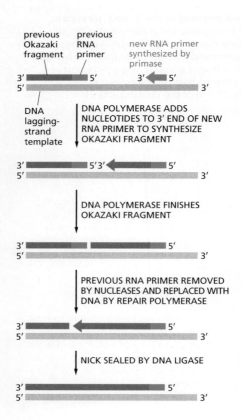

previous Okazaki fragment | previous RNA primer | new RNA primer synthesized by primase

DNA lagging-strand template

DNA POLYMERASE ADDS NUCLEOTIDES TO 3′ END OF NEW RNA PRIMER TO SYNTHESIZE OKAZAKI FRAGMENT

DNA POLYMERASE FINISHES OKAZAKI FRAGMENT

PREVIOUS RNA PRIMER REMOVED BY NUCLEASES AND REPLACED WITH DNA BY REPAIR POLYMERASE

NICK SEALED BY DNA LIGASE

Figure 6–18 Multiple enzymes are required to synthesize the lagging DNA strand. In eukaryotes, RNA primers are made at intervals of about 200 nucleotides on the lagging strand, and each RNA primer is approximately 10 nucleotides long. These primers are extended by a replicative DNA polymerase to produce Okazaki fragments. The primers are subsequently removed by nucleases that recognize the RNA strand in an RNA–DNA hybrid helix and degrade it; this leaves gaps that are filled in by a repair DNA polymerase that can proofread as it fills in the gaps. The completed DNA fragments are finally joined together by an enzyme called DNA ligase, which catalyzes the formation of a phosphodiester bond between the 3′-hydroxyl end of one fragment and the 5′-phosphate end of the next, thus linking up the sugar–phosphate backbones. This nick-sealing reaction requires an input of energy in the form of ATP (see Figure 6–19).

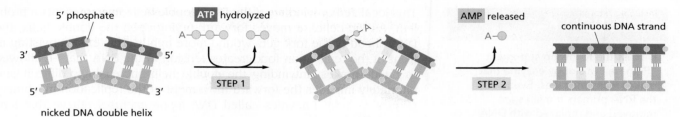

Figure 6–19 DNA ligase joins together Okazaki fragments on the lagging strand during DNA synthesis. The ligase enzyme uses a molecule of ATP to activate the 5' phosphate of one fragment (step 1) before forming a new bond with the 3' hydroxyl of the other fragment (step 2).

each template strand. Two types of replication proteins—*DNA helicases* and *single-strand DNA-binding proteins*—cooperate to carry out this task. A helicase sits at the very front of the replication machine, where it uses the energy of ATP hydrolysis to propel itself forward, prying apart the double helix as it speeds along the DNA (**Figure 6–20** and Movie 6.2). Single-strand DNA-binding proteins then latch onto the single-stranded DNA exposed by the helicase, preventing the strands from re-forming base pairs and keeping them in an elongated form so that they can serve as efficient templates.

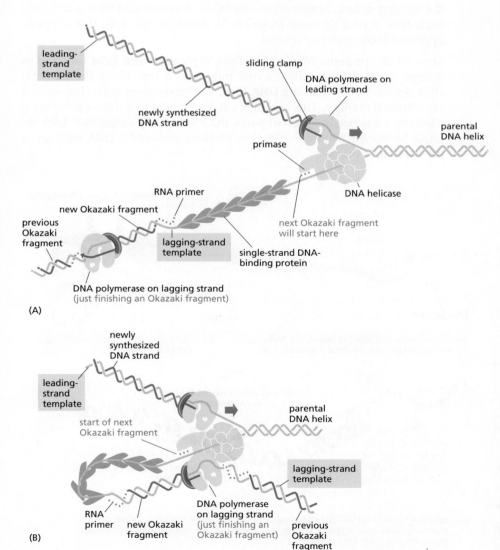

Figure 6–20 DNA synthesis is carried out by a group of proteins that act together as a replication machine. (A) DNA polymerases are held on the leading- and lagging-strand templates by circular protein clamps that allow the polymerases to slide. On the lagging-strand template, the clamp detaches each time the polymerase completes an Okazaki fragment. A clamp loader (not shown) is required to attach a sliding clamp each time a new Okazaki fragment is synthesized. At the head of the fork, a DNA helicase unwinds the strands of the parental DNA double helix. Single-strand DNA-binding proteins keep the DNA strands apart to provide access for the primase and polymerase. For simplicity, this diagram shows the proteins working independently; in the cell, they are held together in a large replication machine, as shown in (B).

(B) This diagram shows a current view of how the replication proteins are arranged when a replication fork is moving. To generate this structure, the lagging strand shown in (A) has been folded to bring its DNA polymerase in contact with the leading-strand DNA polymerase. This folding process also brings the 3' end of each completed Okazaki fragment close to the start site for the next Okazaki fragment. Because the lagging-strand DNA polymerase is bound to the rest of the replication proteins, the same polymerase can be reused to synthesize successive Okazaki fragments; in this diagram, the lagging-strand DNA polymerase is about to let go of its completed Okazaki fragment and move to the next RNA primer being synthesized by the nearby primase. To watch the replication complex in action, see Movie 6.3 and Movie 6.4.

QUESTION 6–2

Discuss the following statement: "Primase is a sloppy enzyme that makes many mistakes. Eventually, the RNA primers it makes are removed and replaced with DNA synthesized by a polymerase with higher fidelity. This is wasteful. It would be more energy-efficient if a DNA polymerase were used to make an accurate primer in the first place."

This localized unwinding of the DNA double helix itself presents a problem. As the helicase moves forward, prying open the double helix, the DNA ahead of the fork gets wound more tightly. This excess twisting in front of the replication fork creates tension in the DNA that—if allowed to build—makes unwinding the double helix increasingly difficult and ultimately impedes the forward movement of the replication machinery (**Figure 6–21A**). Enzymes called *DNA topoisomerases* relieve this tension. A DNA topoisomerase produces a transient, single-strand nick in the DNA backbone, which temporarily releases the built-up tension; the enzyme then reseals the nick before falling off the DNA (**Figure 6–21B**).

Back at the replication fork, an additional protein, called a *sliding clamp*, keeps DNA polymerase firmly attached to the template while it is synthesizing new strands of DNA. Left on their own, most DNA polymerase molecules will synthesize only a short string of nucleotides before falling off the DNA template strand. The sliding clamp forms a ring around the newly formed DNA double helix and, by tightly gripping the polymerase, allows the enzyme to move along the template strand without falling off as it synthesizes new DNA (see Figure 6–20A and Movie 6.5).

Assembly of the clamp around DNA requires the activity of another replication protein, the *clamp loader*, which hydrolyzes ATP each time it locks a sliding clamp around a newly formed DNA double helix. This loading needs to occur only once per replication cycle on the leading strand; on the lagging strand, however, the clamp is removed and then reattached each time a new Okazaki fragment is made. In bacteria, this happens approximately once per second.

Most of the proteins involved in DNA replication are held together in a large multienzyme complex that moves as a unit along the parental DNA double helix, enabling DNA to be synthesized on both strands in a coordinated manner. This complex can be likened to a miniature sewing machine composed of protein parts and powered by nucleoside triphosphate hydrolysis (Figure 6–20B). The proteins involved in DNA replication are listed in **Table 6–1**.

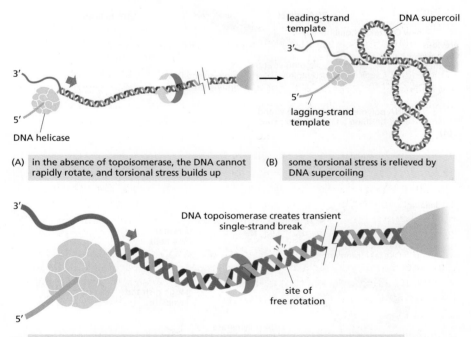

Figure 6–21 DNA topoisomerases relieve the tension that builds up in front of a replication fork. (A) As a DNA helicase moves forward, unwinding the DNA double helix, it generates a section of overwound DNA ahead of it. Tension builds up because the rest of the chromosome (shown in *brown*) is too large to rotate fast enough to relieve the buildup of torsional stress. The broken bars represent approximately 20 turns of DNA. (B) Some of this torsional stress is relieved by additional coiling of the DNA double helix to form supercoils. (C) DNA topoisomerases relieve this stress by generating temporary nicks in the DNA, which allow rapid rotation around the single strands opposite the nicks.

(A) in the absence of topoisomerase, the DNA cannot rapidly rotate, and torsional stress builds up

(B) some torsional stress is relieved by DNA supercoiling

(C) torsional stress ahead of the helicase relieved by free rotation of DNA around the phosphodiester bond opposite the single-strand break; the same DNA topoisomerase that produced the break reseals it

TABLE 6–1 PROTEINS INVOLVED IN DNA REPLICATION

Protein	Activity
DNA polymerase	catalyzes the addition of nucleotides to the 3′ end of a growing strand of DNA using a parental DNA strand as a template
DNA helicase	uses the energy of ATP hydrolysis to unwind the DNA double helix ahead of the replication fork
Single-strand DNA-binding protein	binds to single-stranded DNA exposed by DNA helicase, preventing base pairs from re-forming before the lagging strand can be replicated
DNA topoisomerase	produces transient nicks in the DNA backbone to relieve the tension built up by the unwinding of DNA ahead of the DNA helicase
Sliding clamp	keeps DNA polymerase attached to the template, allowing the enzyme to move along without falling off as it synthesizes new DNA
Clamp loader	uses the energy of ATP hydrolysis to lock the sliding clamp onto DNA
Primase	synthesizes RNA primers along the lagging-strand template
DNA ligase	uses the energy of ATP hydrolysis to join Okazaki fragments made on the lagging-strand template

Telomerase Replicates the Ends of Eukaryotic Chromosomes

Having discussed how DNA replication begins at origins and continues as the replication forks proceed, we now turn to the special problem of replicating the very ends of chromosomes. As we discussed previously, because DNA replication proceeds only in the 5′-to-3′ direction, the lagging strand of the replication fork must be synthesized in the form of discontinuous DNA fragments, each of which is initiated from an RNA primer laid down by a primase (see Figure 6–18). A serious problem arises, however, as the replication fork approaches the end of a chromosome: although the leading strand can be replicated all the way to the chromosome tip, the lagging strand cannot. When the final RNA primer on the lagging strand is removed, there is no enzyme that can replace it with DNA (**Figure 6–22**). Without a strategy to deal with this problem, the lagging strand would become shorter with each round of DNA replication and, after repeated cell divisions, the chromosomes themselves would shrink—eventually losing valuable genetic information.

Bacteria avoid this "end-replication" problem by having circular DNA molecules as chromosomes. Eukaryotes get around it by adding long, repetitive nucleotide sequences to the ends of every chromosome. These sequences, which are incorporated into structures called **telomeres**, attract an enzyme called **telomerase** to the chromosome ends. Telomerase carries its own RNA template, which it uses to add multiple copies of the same repetitive DNA sequence to the lagging-strand template. In many dividing cells, telomeres are continuously replenished, and the resulting extended templates can then be copied by conventional DNA replication, ensuring that no peripheral chromosomal sequences are lost (**Figure 6–23**).

In addition to allowing replication of chromosome ends, telomeres form structures that mark the true ends of a chromosome. These structures allow the cell to distinguish unambiguously between the natural ends of

QUESTION 6–3

A gene encoding one of the proteins involved in DNA replication has been inactivated by a mutation in a cell. In the absence of this protein, the cell attempts to replicate its DNA. What would happen during the DNA replication process if each of the following proteins were missing?
A. DNA polymerase
B. DNA ligase
C. Sliding clamp
D. Nuclease that removes RNA primers
E. DNA helicase
F. Primase

Figure 6–22 Without a special mechanism to replicate the ends of linear chromosomes, DNA would be lost during each round of cell division. DNA synthesis begins at origins of replication and continues until the replication machinery reaches the ends of the chromosome. The leading strand is synthesized in its entirety. But the ends of the lagging strand can't be completed, because once the final RNA primer has been removed, there is no mechanism for replacing it with DNA. Complete replication of the lagging strand requires a special mechanism to keep the chromosome ends from shrinking with each cell division.

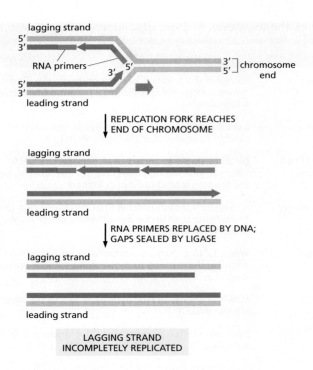

chromosomes and the double-strand DNA breaks that sometimes occur accidentally in the middle of chromosomes. These breaks are dangerous and must be immediately repaired, as we will see shortly.

Telomere Length Varies by Cell Type and with Age

In addition to attracting telomerase, the repetitive DNA sequences found within telomeres attract other telomere-binding proteins that not only physically protect chromosome ends, but help maintain telomere length.

Cells that divide at a rapid rate throughout the life of the organism—those that line the gut or generate blood cells in the bone marrow, for example—keep their telomerase fully active. Many other cell types, however, gradually turn down their telomerase activity. After many rounds

Figure 6–23 Telomeres and telomerase prevent linear eukaryotic chromosomes from shortening with each cell division. To complete the replication of the lagging strand at the ends of a chromosome, the template strand (*orange*) is first extended beyond the DNA that is to be copied. To achieve this, the enzyme telomerase adds to the telomere repeat sequences at the 3′ end of the template strand, which then allows the newly synthesized lagging strand (*red*) to be lengthened by DNA polymerase, as shown. The telomerase enzyme itself carries a short piece of RNA (*blue*) with a sequence that is complementary to the DNA repeat sequence; this RNA acts as the template for telomere DNA synthesis. After the lagging-strand replication is complete, a short stretch of single-stranded DNA remains at the ends of the chromosome; however, the newly synthesized lagging strand, at this point, contains all the information present in the original DNA. To see telomerase in action, view Movie 6.6.

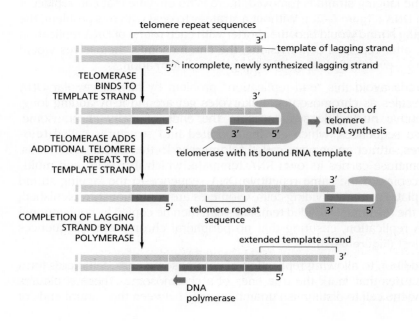

of cell division, the telomeres in these descendent cells will shrink, until they essentially disappear. At this point, these cells will cease dividing. In theory, such a mechanism could provide a safeguard against the uncontrolled proliferation of cells—including abnormal cells that have accumulated mutations that could promote the development of cancer.

DNA REPAIR

The diversity of living organisms and their success in colonizing almost every part of the Earth's surface depend on genetic changes accumulated gradually over billions of years. A small subset of these changes will be beneficial, allowing the affected organisms to adapt to changing conditions and to thrive in new habitats. However, most of these changes will be of little consequence or even deleterious.

In the short term, and from the perspective of an individual organism, such genetic alterations—called mutations—are kept to a minimum: to survive and reproduce, individuals must be genetically stable. This stability is achieved not only through the extremely accurate mechanism for replicating DNA that we have just discussed, but also through the work of a variety of protein machines that continually scan the genome for DNA damage and fix it when it occurs. Although some changes arise from rare mistakes in the replication process, the majority of DNA damage is an unintended consequence of the vast number of chemical reactions that occur inside cells.

Most DNA damage is only temporary, because it is immediately corrected by processes collectively called **DNA repair**. The importance of these DNA repair processes is evident from the consequences of their malfunction. Humans with the genetic disease *xeroderma pigmentosum*, for example, cannot mend the damage done by ultraviolet (UV) radiation because they have inherited a defective gene for one of the proteins involved in this repair process. Such individuals develop severe skin lesions, including skin cancer, because of the DNA damage that accumulates in cells exposed to sunlight and the consequent mutations that arise in these cells.

In this section, we describe a few of the specialized mechanisms cells use to repair DNA damage. We then consider examples of what happens when these mechanisms fail—and we discuss how the evolutionary history of DNA replication and repair is reflected in our genome.

DNA Damage Occurs Continually in Cells

Just like any other molecule in the cell, DNA is continually undergoing thermal collisions with other molecules, often resulting in major chemical changes in the DNA. For example, in the time it takes to read this sentence, a total of about a trillion (10^{12}) purine bases (A and G) will be lost from DNA in the cells of your body by a spontaneous reaction called *depurination* (**Figure 6–24A**). Depurination does not break the DNA phosphodiester backbone but instead removes a purine base from a nucleotide, giving rise to lesions that resemble missing teeth (see Figure 6–26B). Another common reaction is the spontaneous loss of an amino group (*deamination*) from a cytosine in DNA to produce the base uracil (**Figure 6–24B**).

The ultraviolet radiation in sunlight is also damaging to DNA; it promotes covalent linkage between two adjacent pyrimidine bases, forming, for example, the *thymine dimer* shown in **Figure 6–25**. It is the failure to repair thymine dimers that spells trouble for individuals with the disease xeroderma pigmentosum.

QUESTION 6–4

Discuss the following statement: "The DNA repair enzymes that fix deamination and depurination damage must preferentially recognize such damage on newly synthesized DNA strands."

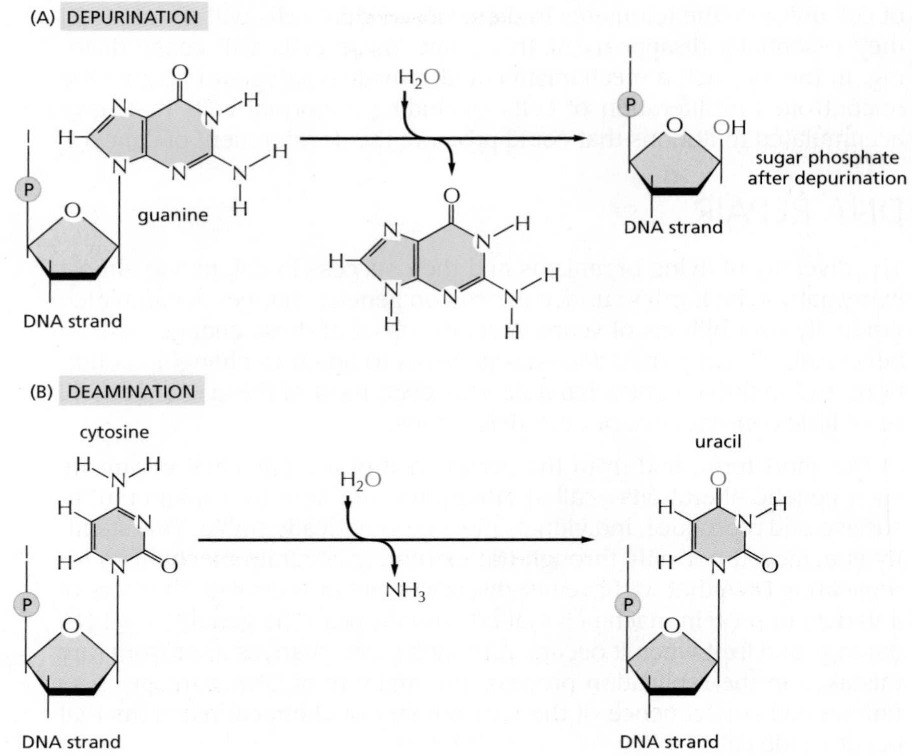

Figure 6–24 Depurination and deamination are the most frequent chemical reactions known to create serious DNA damage in cells. (A) Depurination can remove guanine (or adenine) from DNA. (B) The major type of deamination reaction converts cytosine to uracil, which, as we have seen, is not normally found in DNA. However, deamination can occur on other bases as well. Both depurination and deamination take place on double-helical DNA, and neither break the phosphodiester backbone.

(A) DEPURINATION

(B) DEAMINATION

These are only a few of many chemical changes that can occur in our DNA. Others are caused by reactive chemicals produced as a normal part of cell metabolism. If left unrepaired, DNA damage leads either to the substitution of one nucleotide pair for another as a result of incorrect base-pairing during replication (**Figure 6–26A**) or to deletion of one or more nucleotide pairs in the daughter DNA strand after DNA replication (**Figure 6–26B**). Some types of DNA damage (thymine dimers, for example) can stall the DNA replication machinery at the site of the damage.

In addition to this chemical damage, DNA can also be altered by replication itself. The replication machinery that copies the DNA can—albeit rarely—incorporate an incorrect nucleotide that it fails to correct via proofreading (see Figure 6–14).

For each of these forms of DNA damage, cells possess a mechanism for repair, as we discuss next.

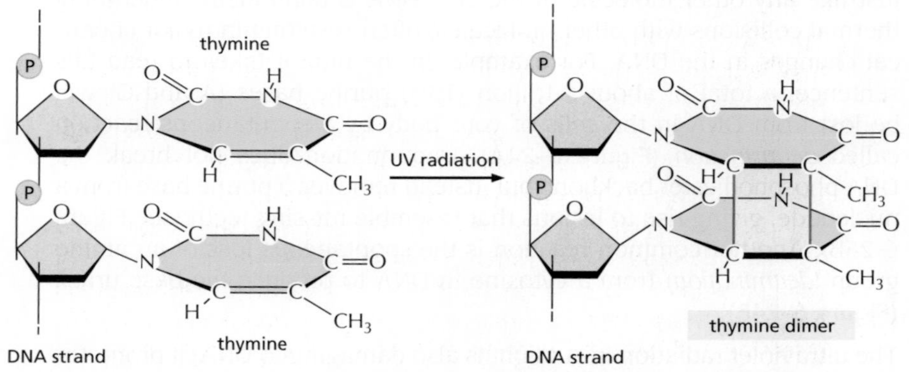

Figure 6–25 The ultraviolet radiation in sunlight can cause the formation of thymine dimers. Two adjacent thymine bases have become covalently attached to each other to form a thymine dimer. Skin cells that are exposed to sunlight are especially susceptible to this type of DNA damage.

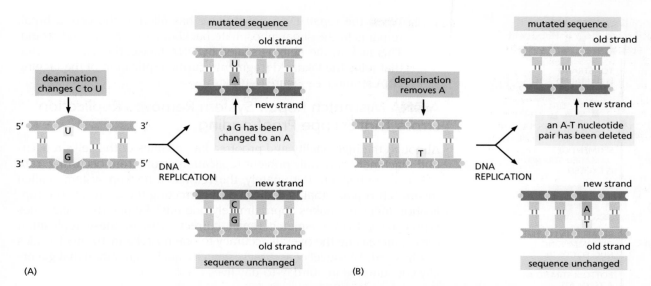

Figure 6–26 Chemical modifications of nucleotides, if left unrepaired, produce mutations. (A) Deamination of cytosine, if uncorrected, results in the substitution of one base for another when the DNA is replicated. As shown in Figure 6–24B, deamination of cytosine produces uracil. Uracil differs from cytosine in its base-pairing properties and preferentially base-pairs with adenine. The DNA replication machinery therefore inserts an adenine when it encounters a uracil on the template strand. (B) Depurination, if uncorrected, can lead to the loss of a nucleotide pair. When the replication machinery encounters a missing purine on the template strand, it can skip to the next complete nucleotide, as shown, thus producing a daughter DNA molecule that is missing one nucleotide pair. In other cases, the replication machinery places an incorrect nucleotide across from the missing base, again resulting in a mutation (not shown).

Cells Possess a Variety of Mechanisms for Repairing DNA

The thousands of random chemical changes that occur every day in the DNA of a human cell—through thermal collisions or exposure to reactive metabolic by-products, DNA-damaging chemicals, or radiation—are repaired by a variety of mechanisms, each catalyzed by a different set of enzymes. Nearly all these repair mechanisms depend on the double-helical structure of DNA, which provides two copies of the genetic information—one in each strand of the double helix. Thus, if the sequence in one strand is accidentally damaged, information is not lost irretrievably, because a backup version of the altered strand remains in the complementary sequence of nucleotides in the other, undamaged strand. Most DNA damage creates structures that are never encountered in an undamaged DNA strand; thus the good strand is easily distinguished from the bad.

The basic pathway for repairing damage to DNA, illustrated schematically in Figure 6–27, involves three basic steps:

1. The damaged DNA is recognized and removed by one of a variety of mechanisms. These involve nucleases, which cleave the covalent bonds that join the damaged nucleotides to the rest of the DNA strand, leaving a small gap on one strand of the DNA double helix.

2. A *repair DNA polymerase* binds to the 3'-hydroxyl end of the cut DNA strand. The enzyme then fills in the gap by making a complementary copy of the information present in the undamaged strand. Although they differ from the DNA polymerase that replicates DNA, repair DNA polymerases synthesize DNA strands in the same way. For example, they elongate chains in the 5'-to-3' direction and have the same type of proofreading activity to ensure that the template strand is copied accurately. In many cells, the repair polymerase is the same enzyme that fills in the gaps left after the RNA primers are removed during the normal DNA replication process (see Figure 6–18).

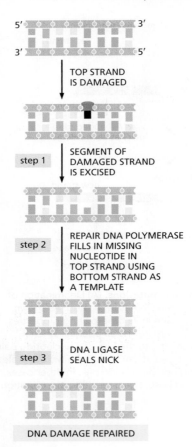

Figure 6–27 The basic mechanism of DNA repair involves three steps. In step 1 (excision), the damage is cut out by one of a series of nucleases, each specialized for a certain type of DNA damage. In step 2 (resynthesis), the original DNA sequence is restored by a repair DNA polymerase, which fills in the gap created by the excision events. In step 3 (ligation), DNA ligase seals the nick left in the sugar–phosphate backbone of the repaired strand. Nick sealing, which requires energy from ATP hydrolysis, remakes the broken phosphodiester bond between the adjacent nucleotides (see Figure 6–19).

3. When the repair DNA polymerase has filled in the gap, a break remains in the sugar–phosphate backbone of the repaired strand. This nick in the helix is sealed by DNA ligase, the same enzyme that joins the Okazaki fragments during replication of the lagging DNA strand (see Figure 6–19).

A DNA Mismatch Repair System Removes Replication Errors That Escape Proofreading

Although the high fidelity and proofreading abilities of the cell's replication machinery generally prevent replication errors from occurring, rare mistakes do happen. Fortunately, the cell has a backup system—called **mismatch repair**—that is dedicated to correcting these errors. The replication machine makes approximately one mistake per 10^7 nucleotides synthesized; DNA mismatch repair corrects 99% of these replication errors, increasing the overall accuracy to one mistake in 10^9 nucleotides synthesized. This level of accuracy is much, much higher than that generally encountered in our day-to-day lives (Table 6–2).

Whenever the replication machinery makes a copying mistake, it leaves behind a mispaired nucleotide (commonly called a *mismatch*). If left uncorrected, the mismatch will result in a permanent mutation in the next round of DNA replication (Figure 6–28). In most cases, however, a complex of mismatch repair proteins will detect the DNA mismatch, remove a portion of the DNA strand containing the error, and then resynthesize the missing DNA. This repair mechanism restores the correct sequence (Figure 6–29).

To be effective, the mismatch repair system must be able to recognize which of the DNA strands contains the error. Removing a segment from the strand that contains the correct sequence would only compound the mistake. The way the mismatch system solves this problem is by recognizing and removing only the newly made DNA. In bacteria, newly synthesized DNA lacks a type of chemical modification (a methyl group added to certain adenines) that is present on the preexisting parent DNA. Newly synthesized DNA is unmethylated for a short time, during which the new and template strands can be easily distinguished. Other cells use different strategies for distinguishing their parent DNA from a newly replicated strand.

In humans, mismatch repair plays an important role in preventing cancer. An inherited predisposition to certain cancers (especially some types of colon cancer) is caused by mutations in genes that encode mismatch repair proteins. Human cells have two copies of these genes (one from each parent), and individuals who inherit one damaged mismatch

TABLE 6–2 ERROR RATES	
A professional typist typing at 120 words per minute	1 mistake per 250 characters
Airline luggage system	1 bag lost, damaged, or delayed per 400 passengers
Driving a car in the United States	1 death per 10^4 people per year
DNA replication (without proofreading)	1 mistake per 10^5 nucleotides copied
DNA replication (with proofreading; without mismatch repair)	1 mistake per 10^7 nucleotides copied
DNA replication (with mismatch repair)	1 mistake per 10^9 nucleotides copied

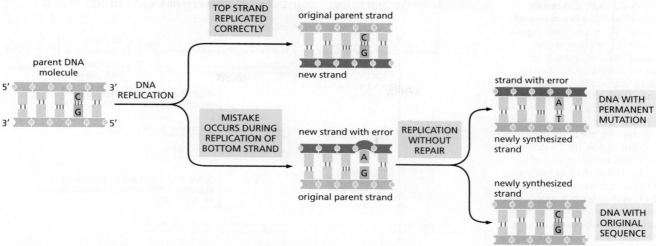

repair gene are unaffected until the undamaged copy of the same gene is randomly mutated in a somatic cell. This mutant cell—and all of its progeny—are then deficient in mismatch repair; they therefore accumulate mutations more rapidly than do normal cells. Because cancers arise from cells that have accumulated multiple mutations, a cell deficient in mismatch repair has a greatly enhanced chance of becoming cancerous. Thus, inheriting a single damaged mismatch repair gene strongly predisposes an individual to cancer.

Figure 6–28 Errors made during DNA replication must be corrected to avoid mutations. If uncorrected, a mismatch will lead to a permanent mutation in one of the two DNA molecules produced during the next round of DNA replication.

Double-Strand DNA Breaks Require a Different Strategy for Repair

The repair mechanisms we have discussed thus far rely on the genetic redundancy built into every DNA double helix. If nucleotides on one strand are damaged, they can be repaired using the information present in the complementary strand. This feature makes the DNA double helix especially well-suited for stably carrying genetic information from one generation to the next.

But what happens when both strands of the double helix are damaged at the same time? Mishaps at the replication fork, radiation, and various chemical assaults can all fracture DNA, creating a *double-strand break*. Such lesions are particularly dangerous, because they can lead to the fragmentation of chromosomes and the subsequent loss of genes.

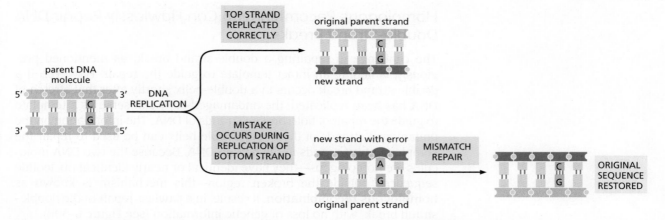

Figure 6–29 Mismatch repair eliminates replication errors and restores the original DNA sequence. When mistakes occur during DNA replication, the repair machinery must replace the incorrect nucleotide on the newly synthesized strand, using the original parent strand as its template. This mechanism eliminates the error, and allows the original sequence to be copied during subsequent rounds of replication.

Figure 6–30 Cells can repair double-strand breaks in one of two ways. (A) In nonhomologous end joining, the break is first "cleaned" by a nuclease that chews back the broken ends to produce flush ends. The flush ends are then stitched together by a DNA ligase. Some nucleotides are usually lost in the repair process, as indicated by the *black* lines in the repaired DNA. (B) If a double-strand break occurs in one of two duplicated DNA double helices after DNA replication has occurred, but before the chromosome copies have been separated, the undamaged double helix can be readily used as a template to repair the damaged double helix through homologous recombination. Although more complicated than nonhomologous end joining, this process accurately restores the original DNA sequence at the site of the break. The detailed mechanism is presented in Figure 6–31.

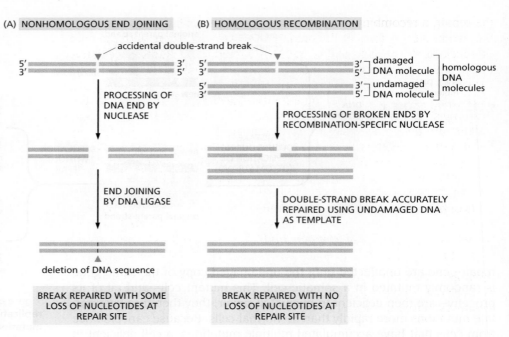

This type of damage is especially difficult to repair. Every chromosome contains unique information; if a chromosome experiences a double-strand break, and the broken pieces become separated, the cell has no spare copy it can use to reconstruct the information that is now missing.

To handle this potentially disastrous type of DNA damage, cells have evolved two basic strategies. The first involves hurriedly sticking the broken ends back together, before the DNA fragments drift apart and get lost. This repair mechanism, called **nonhomologous end joining**, occurs in many cell types and is carried out by a specialized group of enzymes that "clean" the broken ends and rejoin them by DNA ligation. This "quick and dirty" mechanism rapidly seals the break, but it comes with a price: in "cleaning" the break to make it ready for ligation, nucleotides are often lost at the site of repair (**Figure 6–30A** and Movie 6.7). If this imperfect repair disrupts the activity of a gene, the cell could suffer serious consequences. Thus, nonhomologous end joining can be a risky strategy for fixing broken chromosomes. Fortunately, cells have an alternative, error-free strategy for repairing double-strand breaks, called *homologous recombination* (**Figure 6–30B**), as we discuss next.

Homologous Recombination Can Flawlessly Repair DNA Double-Strand Breaks

The challenge in repairing a double-strand break, as mentioned previously, is finding an intact template to guide the repair. However, if a double-strand break occurs in a double helix shortly after that stretch of DNA has been replicated, the undamaged copy can serve as a template to guide the repair of both broken strands of DNA. The information on the undamaged strands of the intact double helix can be used to repair the complementary strands in the broken DNA. Because the two DNA molecules are homologous—they have identical or nearly identical nucleotide sequences outside the broken region—this mechanism is known as **homologous recombination**. It results in a flawless repair of the double-strand break, with no loss of genetic information (see Figure 6–30B).

Homologous recombination most often occurs shortly after a cell's DNA has been replicated before cell division, when the duplicated helices are still physically close to each other (**Figure 6–31A**). To initiate the repair, a recombination-specific nuclease chews back the 5′ ends of the two broken strands at the break (Figure 6–31B). Then, with the help of specialized enzymes (called recA in bacteria and Rad52 in eukaryotes), one of the broken 3′ ends "invades" the unbroken homologous DNA duplex and searches for a complementary sequence through base-pairing (Figure 6–31C). Once an extensive, accurate match is made, the invading strand is elongated by a repair DNA polymerase, using the complementary undamaged strand as a template (Figure 6–31D). After the repair polymerase has passed the point where the break occurred, the newly elongated strand rejoins its original partner, forming base pairs that hold the two strands of the broken double helix together (Figure 6–31E). Repair is then completed by additional DNA synthesis at the 3′ ends of both strands of the broken double helix (Figure 6–31F), followed by DNA ligation (Figure 6–31G). The net result is two intact DNA helices, for which the genetic information from one was used as a template to repair the other.

Homologous recombination can also be used to repair many other types of DNA damage, making it perhaps the most handy DNA repair mechanism available to the cell: all that is needed is an intact homologous

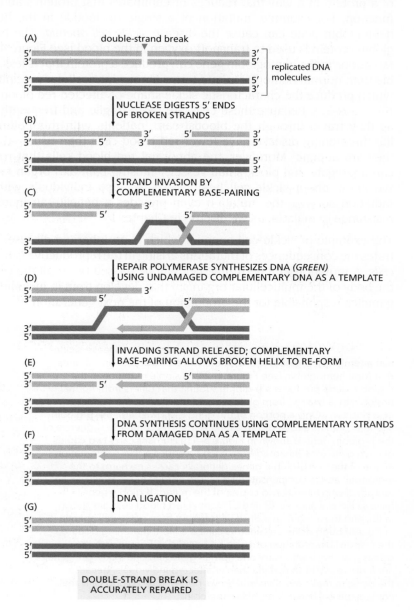

Figure 6–31 **Homologous recombination flawlessly repairs DNA double-strand breaks.** This is the preferred method for repairing double-strand breaks that arise shortly after the DNA has been replicated but before the cell has divided. See text for details. (Adapted from M. McVey et al., *Proc. Natl. Acad. Sci. U.S.A.* 101: 15694–15699, 2004.)

chromosome to use as a partner—a situation that occurs transiently each time a chromosome is duplicated. The "all-purpose" nature of homologous recombinational repair probably explains why this mechanism, and the proteins that carry it out, have been conserved in virtually all cells on Earth.

Homologous recombination is versatile, and it also has a crucial role in the exchange of genetic information that occurs during the formation of the gametes—sperm and eggs. This exchange, during the specialized form of cell division called *meiosis*, enhances the generation of genetic diversity within a species during sexual reproduction. We will discuss it when we talk about sex in Chapter 19.

Failure to Repair DNA Damage Can Have Severe Consequences for a Cell or Organism

On occasion, the cell's DNA replication and repair processes fail and allow a mutation to arise. This permanent change in the DNA sequence can have profound consequences. If the change occurs in a particular position in the DNA sequence, it could alter the amino acid sequence of a protein in a way that reduces or eliminates that protein's ability to function. For example, mutation of a single nucleotide in the human hemoglobin gene can cause the disease *sickle-cell anemia*. The hemoglobin protein is used to transport oxygen in the blood (see Figure 4–24). Mutations in the hemoglobin gene can produce a protein that is less soluble than normal hemoglobin and forms fibrous intracellular precipitates, which produce the characteristic sickle shape of affected red blood cells (**Figure 6–32**). Because these cells are more fragile and frequently tear as they travel through the bloodstream, patients with this potentially life-threatening disease have fewer red blood cells than usual—that is, they are anemic. Moreover, the abnormal red blood cells that remain can aggregate and block small vessels, causing pain and organ failure. We know about sickle-cell hemoglobin because individuals with the mutation survive; the mutation even provides a benefit—an increased resistance to malaria, as we discuss in Chapter 19.

The example of sickle-cell anemia, which is an inherited disease, illustrates the consequences of mutations arising in the reproductive *germ-line cells*. A mutation in a germ-line cell will be passed on to all the cells in the body of the multicellular organism that develop from it, including the gametes responsible for the production of the next generation.

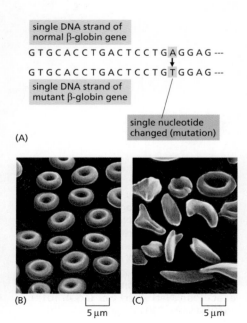

single DNA strand of normal β-globin gene

GTGCACCTGACTCCTGAGGAG ---

GTGCACCTGACTCCTGTGGAG ---

single DNA strand of mutant β-globin gene

single nucleotide changed (mutation)

(A)

(B)   (C)

5 μm   5 μm

Figure 6–32 **A single nucleotide change causes the disease sickle-cell anemia.** (A) β-globin is one of the two types of protein subunits that form hemoglobin (see Figure 4–24). A single mutation in the β-globin gene produces a β-globin subunit that differs from normal β-globin by a change from glutamic acid to valine at the sixth amino acid position. (Only a portion of the gene is shown here; the β-globin subunit contains a total of 146 amino acids. The complete sequence of the β-globin gene is shown in Figure 5–11.) Humans carry two copies of each gene (one inherited from each parent); a sickle-cell mutation in one of the two β-globin genes generally causes no harm to the individual, as it is compensated for by the normal gene. However, an individual who inherits two copies of the mutant β-globin gene will have sickle-cell anemia. (B and C) Normal red blood cells are shown in (B), and those from an individual suffering from sickle-cell anemia in (C). Although sickle-cell anemia can be a life-threatening disease, the responsible mutation can also be beneficial. People with the disease, or those who carry one normal gene and one sickle-cell gene, are more resistant to malaria than unaffected individuals, because the parasite that causes malaria grows poorly in red blood cells that contain the sickle-cell form of hemoglobin.

The many other cells in a multicellular organism (its *somatic cells*) must also be protected against mutation—in this case, against mutations that arise during the life of the individual. Nucleotide changes that occur in somatic cells can give rise to variant cells, some of which grow and divide in an uncontrolled fashion at the expense of the other cells in the organism. In the extreme case, an unchecked cell proliferation known as **cancer** results. Cancers are responsible for about 30% of the deaths that occur in Europe and North America, and they are caused primarily by a gradual accumulation of random mutations in a somatic cell and its descendants (**Figure 6–33**). Increasing the mutation frequency even two- or threefold could cause a disastrous increase in the incidence of cancer by accelerating the rate at which such somatic cell variants arise.

Thus, the high fidelity with which DNA sequences are replicated and maintained is important both for germ-line cells, which transmit the genes to the next generation, and for somatic cells, which normally function as carefully regulated members of the complex community of cells in a multicellular organism. We should therefore not be surprised to find that all cells possess a very sophisticated set of mechanisms to reduce the number of mutations that occur in their DNA, devoting hundreds of genes to these repair processes.

A Record of the Fidelity of DNA Replication and Repair Is Preserved in Genome Sequences

Although the majority of mutations do neither harm nor good to an organism, those that have severely harmful consequences are usually eliminated through natural selection; individuals carrying the altered DNA may die or experience decreased fertility, in which case these changes will be gradually lost from the population. By contrast, favorable changes will tend to persist and spread.

But even where no selection operates—at the many sites in the DNA where a change of nucleotide has no effect on the fitness of the organism—the genetic message has been faithfully preserved over tens of millions of years. Thus humans and chimpanzees, after about 5 million years of divergent evolution, still have DNA sequences that are at least 98% identical. Even humans and whales, after 10 or 20 times this amount of time, have chromosomes that are unmistakably similar in their DNA sequence (**Figure 6–34**). Thus our genome—and those of our relatives—contains a message from the distant past. Thanks to the faithfulness of DNA replication and repair, 100 million years of evolution have scarcely changed its essential content.

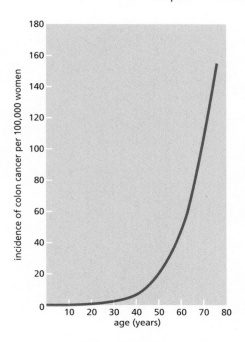

Figure 6–33 Cancer incidence increases dramatically with age. The number of newly diagnosed cases of colon cancer in women in England and Wales in a single year is plotted as a function of age at diagnosis. Colon cancer, like most human cancers, is caused by the accumulation of multiple mutations. Because cells are continually experiencing accidental changes to their DNA—which accumulate and are passed on to progeny cells when the mutated cells divide—the chance that a cell will become cancerous increases greatly with age. (Data from C. Muir et al., Cancer Incidence in Five Continents, Vol. V. Lyon: International Agency for Research on Cancer, 1987.)

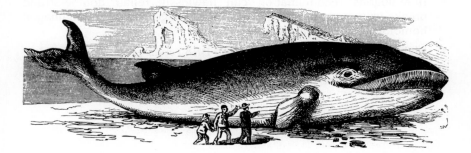

whale	GTGTGGTCTCGTGATCAAAGGCGAAAGGTGGCTCTAGAGAATCCC
human	GTGTGGTCTCGCGATCAGAGGCGCAAGATGGCTCTAGAGAATCCC

Figure 6–34 The sex-determination genes from humans and whales are noticeably similar. Despite the many millions of years that have passed since humans and whales diverged from a common ancestor, the nucleotide sequences of many of their genes remain closely related. The DNA sequences of a part of the gene that determines maleness in both humans and whales are lined up, one above the other; the positions where the two sequences are identical are shaded in *gray*.

ESSENTIAL CONCEPTS

- Before a cell divides, it must accurately replicate the vast quantity of genetic information carried in its DNA.

- Because the two strands of a DNA double helix are complementary, each strand can act as a template for the synthesis of the other. Thus DNA replication produces two identical, double-helical DNA molecules, enabling genetic information to be copied and passed on from a cell to its daughter cells and from a parent to its offspring.

- During replication, the two strands of a DNA double helix are pulled apart at a replication origin to form two Y-shaped replication forks. DNA polymerases at each fork produce a new, complementary DNA strand on each parental strand.

- DNA polymerase replicates a DNA template with remarkable fidelity, making only about one error in every 10^7 nucleotides copied. This accuracy is made possible, in part, by a proofreading process in which the enzyme corrects its own mistakes as it moves along the DNA.

- Because DNA polymerase synthesizes new DNA in the 5′-to-3′ direction, only the leading strand at the replication fork can be synthesized in a continuous fashion. On the lagging strand, DNA is synthesized in a discontinuous backstitching process, producing short fragments of DNA that are later joined together by DNA ligase.

- DNA polymerase is incapable of starting a new DNA strand from scratch. Instead, DNA synthesis is primed by an RNA polymerase called primase, which makes short lengths of RNA primers that are then elongated by DNA polymerase. These primers are subsequently removed and replaced with DNA.

- DNA replication requires the cooperation of many proteins that form a multienzyme replication machine that pries open the double helix and copies the information contained in both DNA strands.

- In eukaryotes, a special enzyme called telomerase replicates the DNA at the ends of the chromosomes, particularly in rapidly dividing cells.

- The rare copying mistakes that escape proofreading are dealt with by mismatch repair proteins, which increase the accuracy of DNA replication to one mistake per 10^9 nucleotides copied.

- Damage to one of the two DNA strands, caused by unavoidable chemical reactions, is repaired by a variety of DNA repair enzymes that recognize damaged DNA and excise a short stretch of the damaged strand. The missing DNA is then resynthesized by a repair DNA polymerase, using the undamaged strand as a template.

- If both DNA strands are broken, the double-strand break can be rapidly repaired by nonhomologous end joining. Nucleotides are often lost in the process, altering the DNA sequence at the repair site.

- Homologous recombination can flawlessly repair double-strand breaks (and many other types of DNA damage) using an undamaged homologous double helix as a template.

- Highly accurate DNA replication and DNA repair processes play a key role in protecting us from the uncontrolled growth of somatic cells known as cancer.

KEY TERMS

cancer	nonhomologous end joining
DNA ligase	Okazaki fragment
DNA polymerase	primase
DNA repair	proofreading
DNA replication	replication fork
homologous recombination	replication origin
lagging strand	RNA (ribonucleic acid)
leading strand	telomerase
mismatch repair	telomere
mutation	template

QUESTIONS

QUESTION 6–5

DNA mismatch repair enzymes preferentially repair bases on the newly synthesized DNA strand, using the old DNA strand as a template. If mismatches were simply repaired without regard for which strand served as template, would this reduce replication errors as effectively? Explain your answer.

QUESTION 6–6

Suppose a mutation affects an enzyme that is required to repair the damage to DNA caused by the loss of purine bases. The loss of a purine occurs about 5000 times in the DNA of each of your cells per day. As the average difference in DNA sequence between humans and chimpanzees is about 1%, how long will it take you to turn into an ape? Or would this transformation be unlikely to occur?

QUESTION 6–7

Which of the following statements are correct? Explain your answers.

A. A bacterial replication fork is asymmetrical because it contains two DNA polymerase molecules that are structurally distinct.

B. Okazaki fragments are removed by a nuclease that degrades RNA.

C. The error rate of DNA replication is reduced both by proofreading by DNA polymerase and by DNA mismatch repair.

D. In the absence of DNA repair, genes become less stable.

E. None of the aberrant bases formed by deamination occur naturally in DNA.

F. Cancer can result from the accumulation of mutations in somatic cells.

QUESTION 6–8

The speed of DNA replication at a replication fork is about 100 nucleotides per second in human cells. What is the minimum number of origins of replication that a human cell must have if it is to replicate its DNA once every 24 hours?

Recall that a human cell contains two copies of the human genome—one inherited from the mother, the other from the father—each consisting of 3×10^9 nucleotide pairs.

QUESTION 6–9

Look carefully at Figure 6–11 and at the structures of the compounds shown in Figure Q6–9.

A. What would you expect if ddCTP were added to a DNA replication reaction in large excess over the concentration of the available dCTP, the normal deoxycytidine triphosphate?

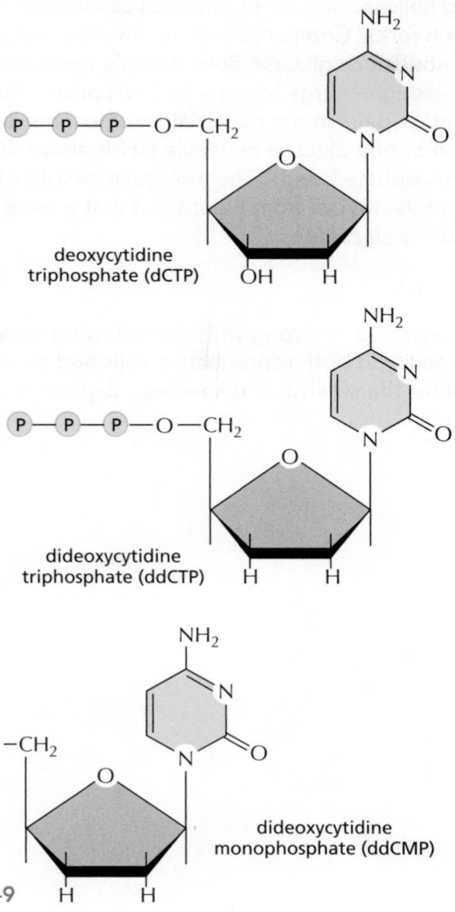

Figure Q6–9

B. What would happen if it were added at 10% of the concentration of the available dCTP?

C. What effects would you expect if ddCMP were added under the same conditions?

QUESTION 6–10

Figure Q6–10 shows a snapshot of a replication fork in which the RNA primer has just been added to the lagging strand. Using this diagram as a guide, sketch the path of the DNA as the next Okazaki fragment is synthesized. Indicate the sliding clamp and the single-strand DNA-binding protein as appropriate.

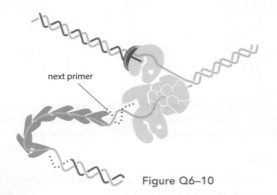

next primer

Figure Q6–10

QUESTION 6–11

Approximately how many high-energy bonds does DNA polymerase use to replicate a bacterial chromosome (ignoring helicase and other enzymes associated with the replication fork)? Compared with its own dry weight of 10^{-12} g, how much glucose does a single bacterium need to provide enough energy to copy its DNA once? The number of nucleotide pairs in the bacterial chromosome is 3×10^6. Oxidation of one glucose molecule yields about 30 high-energy phosphate bonds. The molecular weight of glucose is 180 g/mole. (Recall from Figure 2–3 that a mole consists of 6×10^{23} molecules.)

QUESTION 6–12

What, if anything, is wrong with the following statement: "DNA stability in both reproductive cells and somatic cells is essential for the survival of a species." Explain your answer.

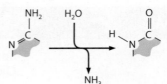

Figure Q6–13

QUESTION 6–13

A common type of chemical damage to DNA is produced by a spontaneous reaction termed *deamination*, in which a nucleotide base loses an amino group (NH_2). The amino group is replaced with a keto group (C=O) by the general reaction shown in Figure Q6–13. Write the structures of the bases A, G, C, T, and U and predict the products that will be produced by deamination. By looking at the products of this reaction—and remembering that, in the cell, these will need to be recognized and repaired—can you propose an explanation for why DNA does not contain uracil?

QUESTION 6–14

A. Explain why telomeres and telomerase are needed for replication of eukaryotic chromosomes but not for replication of circular bacterial chromosomes. Draw a diagram to illustrate your explanation.

B. Would you still need telomeres and telomerase to complete eukaryotic chromosome replication if primase always laid down the RNA primer at the very 3′ end of the template for the lagging strand?

QUESTION 6–15

Describe the consequences that would arise if a eukaryotic chromosome:

A. contained only one origin of replication:

    (i) at the exact center of the chromosome.

    (ii) at one end of the chromosome.

B. lacked telomeres.

C. lacked a centromere.

Assume that the chromosome is 150 million nucleotide pairs in length, a typical size for an animal chromosome, and that DNA replication in animal cells proceeds at about 100 nucleotides per second.

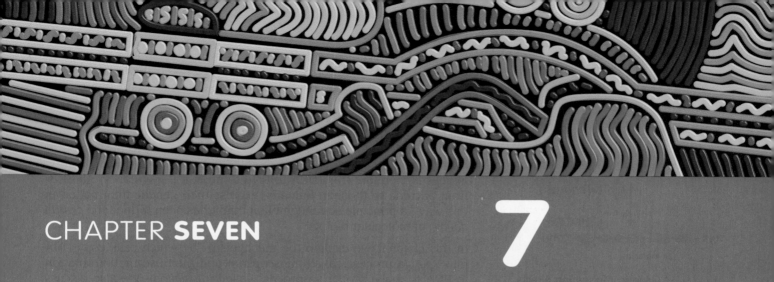

From DNA to Protein: How Cells Read the Genome

Once the double-helical structure of DNA (deoxyribonucleic acid) had been determined in the early 1950s, it became clear that the hereditary information in cells is encoded in the linear order—or *sequence*—of the four different nucleotide subunits that make up the DNA. We saw in Chapter 6 how this information can be passed on unchanged from a cell to its descendants through the process of DNA replication. But how does the cell decode and use the information? How do genetic instructions written in an alphabet of just four "letters" direct the formation of a bacterium, a fruit fly, or a human? We still have a lot to learn about how the information stored in an organism's genes produces even the simplest unicellular bacterium, let alone how it directs the development of complex multicellular organisms like ourselves. But the DNA code itself has been deciphered, and we have come a long way in understanding how cells read it.

Even before the code was broken, it was known that the information contained in genes somehow directed the synthesis of proteins. Proteins are the principal constituents of cells and determine not only cell structure but also cell function. In previous chapters, we encountered some of the thousands of different kinds of proteins that cells can make. We saw in Chapter 4 that the properties and function of a protein molecule are determined by the sequence of the 20 different amino acid subunits in its polypeptide chain: each type of protein has its own unique amino acid sequence, which dictates how the chain will fold to form a molecule with a distinctive shape and chemistry. The genetic instructions carried by DNA must therefore specify the amino acid sequences of proteins. We will see in this chapter exactly how this happens.

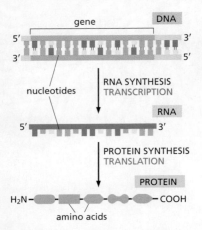

Figure 7–1 Genetic information directs the synthesis of proteins. The flow of genetic information from DNA to RNA (transcription) and from RNA to protein (translation) occurs in all living cells. DNA can also be copied—or replicated—to produce new DNA molecules, as we saw in Chapter 6. The segments of DNA that are transcribed into RNA are called genes (*orange*).

DNA does not synthesize proteins on its own: it acts more like a manager, delegating the various tasks to a team of workers. When a particular protein is needed by the cell, the nucleotide sequence of the appropriate segment of a DNA molecule is first copied into another type of nucleic acid—RNA (*ribonucleic acid*). That segment of DNA is called a **gene**, and the resulting RNA copies are then used to direct the synthesis of the protein. Many thousands of these conversions from DNA to protein occur every second in each cell in our body. The flow of genetic information in cells is therefore from DNA to RNA to protein (**Figure 7–1**). All cells, from bacteria to those in humans, express their genetic information in this way—a principle so fundamental that it has been termed the *central dogma* of molecular biology.

In this chapter, we explain the mechanisms by which cells copy DNA into RNA (a process called *transcription*) and then use the information in RNA to make protein (a process called *translation*). We also discuss a few of the key variations on this basic scheme. Principal among these is *RNA splicing*, a process in eukaryotic cells in which segments of an *RNA transcript* are removed—and the remaining segments stitched back together—before the RNA is translated into protein. We will also learn that, for some genes, it is the RNA, not a protein, that is the final product. In the final section, we consider how the present scheme of information storage, transcription, and translation might have arisen from much simpler systems in the earliest stages of cell evolution.

FROM DNA TO RNA

The first step in *gene expression*, the process by which cells read out the instructions in their *genes*, is transcription. Many identical RNA copies can be made from the same gene. For most genes, RNA serves solely as an intermediary on the pathway to making a protein. For these genes, each RNA molecule can direct the synthesis, or translation, of many identical protein molecules. This successive amplification enables cells to rapidly synthesize large amounts of protein whenever necessary. At the same time, each gene can be transcribed, and its RNA translated, at different rates, providing the cell with a way to make vast quantities of some proteins and tiny quantities of others (**Figure 7–2**). Moreover, as we discuss in Chapter 8, a cell can change (or regulate) the expression of each of its genes according to the needs of the moment. In this section, we focus on the production of RNA. We describe how the transcriptional machinery recognizes genes and copies the instructions they contain into molecules

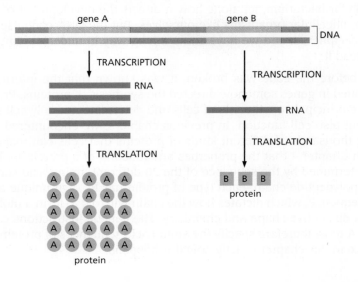

Figure 7–2 A cell can express different genes at different rates. In this and later figures, the portions of the DNA that are not transcribed are shown in *gray*.

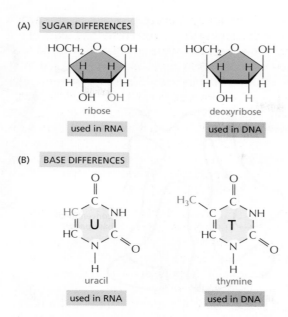

(A) **SUGAR DIFFERENCES**

ribose
used in RNA

deoxyribose
used in DNA

(B) **BASE DIFFERENCES**

uracil
used in RNA

thymine
used in DNA

Figure 7–3 The chemical structure of RNA differs slightly from that of DNA. (A) RNA contains the sugar ribose, which differs from deoxyribose, the sugar used in DNA, by the presence of an additional –OH group. (B) RNA contains the base uracil, which differs from thymine, the equivalent base in DNA, by the absence of a –CH$_3$ group. (C) A short length of RNA. The chemical linkage between nucleotides in RNA—a phosphodiester bond—is the same as that in DNA.

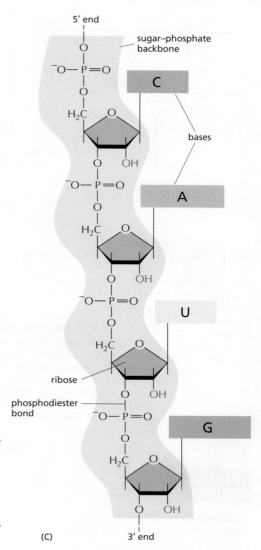

5′ end

sugar–phosphate backbone

C

bases

A

U

ribose

phosphodiester bond

G

(C)   3′ end

of RNA. We then discuss how these RNAs are processed, the variety of roles they play in the cell, and, ultimately, how they are removed from circulation.

Portions of DNA Sequence Are Transcribed into RNA

The first step a cell takes in expressing one of its many thousands of genes is to copy the nucleotide sequence of that gene into RNA. The process is called **transcription** because the information, though copied into another chemical form, is still written in essentially the same language—the language of nucleotides. Like DNA, **RNA** is a linear polymer made of four different nucleotide subunits, linked together by phosphodiester bonds. It differs from DNA chemically in two respects: (1) the nucleotides in RNA are *ribonucleotides*—that is, they contain the sugar ribose (hence the name *ribo*nucleic acid) rather than the deoxyribose found in DNA; and (2) although, like DNA, RNA contains the bases adenine (A), guanine (G), and cytosine (C), it contains uracil (U) instead of the thymine (T) found in DNA (**Figure 7–3**). Because U, like T, can base-pair by hydrogen-bonding with A (**Figure 7–4**), the complementary base-pairing properties described for DNA in Chapter 5 apply also to RNA.

Although their chemical differences are small, DNA and RNA differ quite dramatically in overall structure. Whereas DNA always occurs in cells as a double-stranded helix, RNA is largely single-stranded. This difference has important functional consequences. Because an RNA chain is single-stranded, it can fold up into a variety of shapes, just as a polypeptide chain folds up to form the final shape of a protein (**Figure 7–5**);

Figure 7–4 Uracil forms a base pair with adenine. The hydrogen bonds that hold the base pair together are shown in *red*. Uracil has the same base-pairing properties as thymine. Thus U-A base pairs in RNA closely resemble T-A base pairs in DNA (see Figure 5–4A).

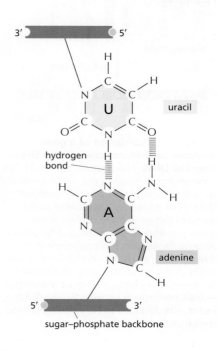

3′   5′

uracil

hydrogen bond

adenine

5′   3′

sugar–phosphate backbone

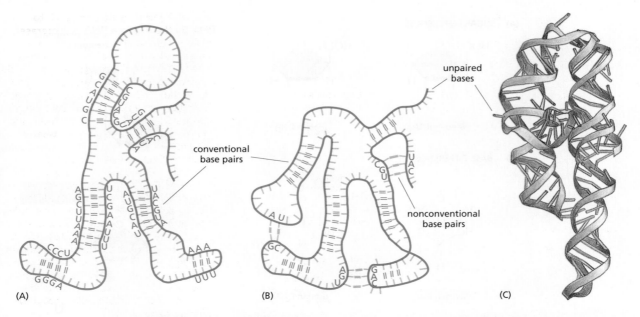

(A)   (B)   (C)

Figure 7–5 RNA molecules can fold into specific structures that are held together by hydrogen bonds between different base pairs. RNA is largely single-stranded, but it often contains short stretches of nucleotides that can base-pair with complementary sequences found elsewhere on the same molecule. These interactions—along with some "nonconventional" base-pair interactions (e.g., A-G)—allow an RNA molecule to fold into a three-dimensional structure that is determined by its sequence of nucleotides. (A) A diagram of a hypothetical, folded RNA structure showing only conventional (G-C and A-U) base-pair interactions (*red*). (B) Formation of nonconventional base-pair interactions (*green*) folds the structure of the hypothetical RNA shown in (A) even further. (C) Structure of an actual RNA molecule that is involved in RNA splicing. The considerable amount of double-helical structure displayed by this RNA is produced by conventional base pairing. For an additional view of RNA structure, see Movie 7.1.

double-stranded DNA cannot fold in this fashion. As we discuss later in the chapter, the ability to fold into a complex three-dimensional shape allows RNA to carry out various functions in cells, in addition to conveying information between DNA and protein. Whereas DNA functions solely as an information store, some RNAs have structural, regulatory, or catalytic roles.

Transcription Produces RNA That Is Complementary to One Strand of DNA

All the RNA in a cell is made by transcription, a process that has certain similarities to DNA replication (discussed in Chapter 6). Transcription begins with the opening of a small portion of the DNA double helix to expose the bases on each DNA strand. One of the two strands of the DNA double helix then serves as a template for the synthesis of RNA. Ribonucleotides are added, one by one, to the growing RNA chain; as in DNA replication, the nucleotide sequence of the RNA chain is determined by complementary base-pairing with the DNA template strand. When a good match is made, the incoming ribonucleoside triphosphate is covalently linked to the growing RNA chain by the enzyme *RNA polymerase*. The RNA chain produced by transcription—the **RNA transcript**—therefore has a nucleotide sequence exactly complementary to the strand of DNA used as the template (**Figure 7–6**).

Transcription differs from DNA replication, however, in several crucial respects. Unlike a newly formed DNA strand, the RNA strand does not remain hydrogen-bonded to the DNA template strand. Instead, just behind the region where the ribonucleotides are being added, the RNA chain is displaced and the DNA helix re-forms. For this reason—and because only one strand of the DNA molecule is transcribed—RNA molecules are

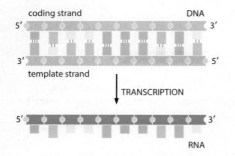

Figure 7–6 Transcription of a gene produces an RNA complementary to one strand of DNA. The *bottom* strand of DNA in this example is called the template strand because it is used to guide the synthesis of the RNA molecule. The nontemplate strand of the gene (here, shown at the *top*) is sometimes called the *coding strand* because its sequence is equivalent to the RNA product, as shown. Which DNA strand serves as the template varies, depending on the gene, as we discuss later. By convention, an RNA molecule is usually depicted with its 5′ end—the first part to be synthesized—to the left.

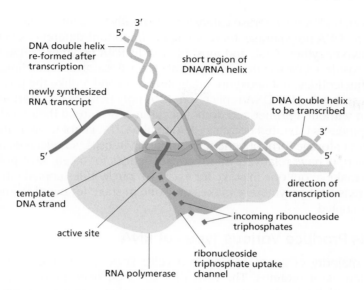

Figure 7–7 DNA is transcribed into RNA by the enzyme RNA polymerase. (A) RNA polymerase (*pale blue*) moves stepwise along the DNA, unwinding the DNA helix in front of it. As it progresses, the polymerase adds ribonucleotides one-by-one to the RNA chain, using an exposed DNA strand as a template. The resulting RNA transcript is thus single-stranded and complementary to the template strand (see Figure 7–6). As the polymerase moves along the DNA template, it displaces the newly formed RNA, allowing the two strands of DNA behind the polymerase to rewind. A short region of hybrid DNA/RNA helix (approximately nine nucleotides in length) therefore forms only transiently, causing a "window" of DNA/RNA helix to move along the DNA with the polymerase. Note that although the primase discussed in Chapter 6 and RNA polymerase both synthesize RNA using a DNA template, they are different enzymes, encoded by different genes.

single-stranded. Furthermore, a given RNA molecule is copied from only a limited region of DNA, making it much shorter than the DNA molecule from which it is made. A DNA molecule in a human chromosome can be up to 250 million nucleotide pairs long, whereas most mature RNAs are no more than a few thousand nucleotides long, and many are much shorter than that.

Like the DNA polymerase that carries out DNA replication (discussed in Chapter 6), **RNA polymerases** catalyze the formation of the phosphodiester bonds that link the nucleotides together and form the sugar–phosphate backbone of the RNA chain (see Figure 7–3). The RNA polymerase moves stepwise along the DNA, unwinding the DNA helix just ahead to expose a new region of the template strand for complementary base-pairing. In this way, the growing RNA chain is elongated by one nucleotide at a time in the 5'-to-3' direction (**Figure 7–7**). The incoming ribonucleoside triphosphates (ATP, CTP, UTP, and GTP) provide the energy needed to drive the reaction forward, analogous to the process of DNA synthesis (see Figure 6–11).

The almost immediate release of the RNA strand from the DNA as it is synthesized means that many RNA copies can be made from the same gene in a relatively short time; the synthesis of the next RNA is usually started before the first RNA has been completed (**Figure 7–8**). A medium-sized gene—say, 1500 nucleotide pairs—requires approximately 50 seconds for a molecule of RNA polymerase to transcribe it (Movie 7.2). At any given time, there could be dozens of polymerases speeding along this single stretch of DNA, hard on one another's heels, allowing more than 1000 transcripts to be synthesized in an hour. For most genes, however, the amount of transcription is much less than this.

QUESTION 7–2

In the electron micrograph in Figure 7–8, are the RNA polymerase molecules moving from right to left or from left to right? Why are the RNA transcripts so much shorter than the DNA segments (genes) that encode them?

Figure 7–8 Many molecules of RNA polymerase can simultaneously transcribe the same gene. Shown in this electron micrograph are two adjacent ribosomal genes on a single DNA molecule. Molecules of RNA polymerase are barely visible as a series of tiny dots along the spine of the DNA molecule; each polymerase has an RNA transcript (a short, fine thread) radiating from it. The RNA molecules being transcribed from the two ribosomal genes— ribosomal RNAs (rRNAs)—are not translated into protein, but are instead used directly as components of ribosomes, macromolecular machines made of RNA and protein. The large particles that can be seen at the free, 5' end of each rRNA transcript are ribosomal proteins that have assembled on the ends of the growing transcripts. These proteins will be discussed later in the chapter. (Courtesy of Ulrich Scheer.)

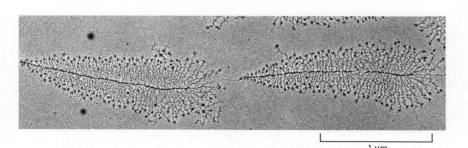

1 μm

Although RNA polymerase catalyzes essentially the same chemical reaction as DNA polymerase, there are some important differences between the two enzymes. First, and most obviously, RNA polymerase uses ribonucleoside triphosphates as substrates, so it catalyzes the linkage of ribonucleotides, not deoxyribonucleotides. Second, unlike the DNA polymerase involved in DNA replication, RNA polymerases can start an RNA chain without a primer and do not accurately proofread their work. This sloppiness is tolerated because RNA, unlike DNA, is not used as the permanent storage form of genetic information in cells, so mistakes in RNA transcripts have relatively minor consequences for a cell. RNA polymerases make about one mistake for every 10^4 nucleotides copied into RNA, whereas DNA polymerase makes only one mistake for every 10^7 nucleotides copied.

Cells Produce Various Types of RNA

The majority of genes carried in a cell's DNA specify the amino acid sequences of proteins. The RNA molecules encoded by these genes—which ultimately direct the synthesis of proteins—are called **messenger RNAs (mRNAs)**. In eukaryotes, each mRNA typically carries information transcribed from just one gene, which codes for a single protein; in bacteria, a set of adjacent genes is often transcribed as a single mRNA, which therefore carries the information for several different proteins.

The final product of other genes, however, is the RNA itself. As we see later, these *noncoding RNAs*, like proteins, have various roles, serving as regulatory, structural, and catalytic components of cells. They play key parts, for example, in translating the genetic message into protein: *ribosomal RNAs* (*rRNAs*) form the structural and catalytic core of the ribosomes, which translate mRNAs into protein, and *transfer RNAs* (*tRNAs*) act as adaptors that select specific amino acids and hold them in place on a ribosome for their incorporation into protein. Other small RNAs, called *microRNAs* (*miRNAs*), serve as key regulators of eukaryotic gene expression, as we discuss in Chapter 8. The most common types of RNA are summarized in Table 7–1.

In the broadest sense, the term **gene expression** refers to the process by which the information encoded in a DNA sequence is converted into a product, whether RNA or protein, that has some effect on a cell or organism. In cases where the final product of the gene is a protein, gene expression includes both transcription and translation. When an RNA molecule is the gene's final product, however, gene expression does not require translation.

TABLE 7–1 TYPES OF RNA PRODUCED IN CELLS	
Type of RNA	Function
messenger RNAs (mRNAs)	code for proteins
ribosomal RNAs (rRNAs)	form the core of the ribosome's structure and catalyze protein synthesis
microRNAs (miRNAs)	regulate gene expression
transfer RNAs (tRNAs)	serve as adaptors between mRNA and amino acids during protein synthesis
Other noncoding RNAs	used in RNA splicing, gene regulation, telomere maintenance, and many other processes

Signals in the DNA Tell RNA Polymerase Where to Start and Stop Transcription

The initiation of transcription is an especially critical process because it is the main point at which the cell selects which RNAs are to be produced. To begin transcription, RNA polymerase must be able to recognize the start of a gene and bind firmly to the DNA at this site. The way in which RNA polymerases recognize the *transcription start site* of a gene differs somewhat between bacteria and eukaryotes. Because the situation in bacteria is simpler, we describe it first.

When an RNA polymerase collides randomly with a DNA molecule, the enzyme sticks weakly to the double helix and then slides rapidly along its length. RNA polymerase latches on tightly only after it has encountered a gene region called a **promoter**, which contains a specific sequence of nucleotides that lies immediately upstream of the starting point for RNA synthesis. As it binds tightly to this sequence, the RNA polymerase opens up the double helix immediately in front of the promoter to expose the nucleotides on each strand of a short stretch of DNA. One of the two exposed DNA strands then acts as a template for complementary base-pairing with incoming ribonucleoside triphosphates, two of which are joined together by the polymerase to begin synthesis of the RNA strand. Elongation then continues until the enzyme encounters a second signal in the DNA, the *terminator* (or stop site), where the polymerase halts and releases both the DNA template and the newly made RNA transcript (**Figure 7–9**). The terminator sequence itself is also transcribed, and it is the interaction of this 3′ segment of RNA with the polymerase that causes the enzyme to let go of the template DNA.

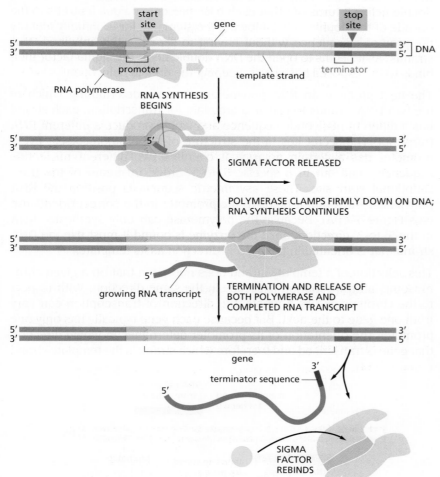

Figure 7–9 Signals in the nucleotide sequence of a gene tell bacterial RNA polymerase where to start and stop transcription. Bacterial RNA polymerase (*light blue*) contains a subunit called sigma factor (*yellow*) that recognizes the promoter of a gene (*green*). Once transcription has begun, sigma factor is released, and the polymerase moves forward and continues synthesizing the RNA. Elongation continues until the polymerase encounters a sequence in the gene called the terminator (*red*). After transcribing this sequence into RNA (*dark blue*), the enzyme halts and releases both the DNA template and the newly made RNA transcript. The polymerase then reassociates with a free sigma factor and searches for another promoter to begin the process again.

Figure 7–10 Bacterial promoters and terminators have specific nucleotide sequences that are recognized by RNA polymerase. (A) The *green*-shaded regions represent the nucleotide sequences that specify a promoter. The numbers above the DNA indicate the positions of nucleotides counting from the first nucleotide transcribed, which is designated +1. The polarity of the promoter orients the polymerase and determines which DNA strand is transcribed. All bacterial promoters contain DNA sequences at −10 and −35 that closely resemble those shown here. (B) The *red*-shaded regions represent sequences in the gene that signal the RNA polymerase to terminate transcription. Note that the regions transcribed into RNA contain the terminator but not the promoter nucleotide sequences.

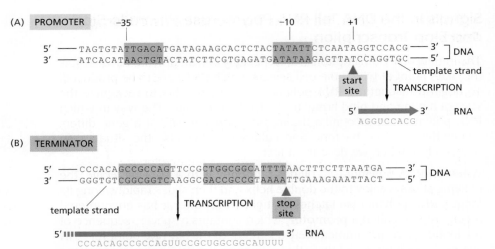

Because the polymerase must bind tightly to DNA before transcription can begin, a segment of DNA will be transcribed only if it is preceded by a promoter. This ensures that only those portions of a DNA molecule that contain a gene will be transcribed into RNA. The nucleotide sequences of a typical promoter—and a typical terminator—are presented in **Figure 7–10**.

In bacteria, it is a subunit of RNA polymerase, the *sigma* (σ) factor (see Figure 7–9), that is primarily responsible for recognizing the promoter sequence on the DNA. But how can this factor "see" the promoter, given that the base pairs in question are situated in the interior of the DNA double helix? It turns out that each base presents unique features to the outside of the double helix, allowing the sigma factor to initially identify the promoter sequence without having to separate the entwined DNA strands. As it begins to open the DNA double helix, the sigma factor then binds to the exposed base pairs, keeping the double helix open.

The next problem an RNA polymerase faces is determining which of the two DNA strands to use as a template for transcription: each strand has a different nucleotide sequence and would produce a different RNA transcript. The secret lies in the structure of the promoter itself. Every promoter has a certain polarity: it contains two different nucleotide sequences, laid out in a specific 5′-to-3′ order, upstream of the transcriptional start site. These asymmetric sequences position the RNA polymerase such that it binds to the promoter in the correct orientation (see Figure 7–10A). Because the polymerase can only synthesize RNA in the 5′-to-3′ direction, once the enzyme is bound it must use the DNA strand that is oriented in the 3′-to-5′ direction as its template.

This selection of a template strand does not mean that on a given chromosome, all transcription proceeds in the same direction. With respect to the chromosome as a whole, the direction of transcription can vary from one gene to the next. But because each gene typically has only one promoter, the orientation of its promoter determines in which direction that gene is transcribed and therefore which strand is the template strand (**Figure 7–11**).

Figure 7–11 On an individual chromosome, some genes are transcribed using one DNA strand as a template, and others are transcribed from the other DNA strand. RNA polymerase always moves in the 3′-to-5′ direction with respect to the template DNA strand. Which strand will serve as the template is determined by the polarity of the promoter sequences (*green* arrowheads) at the beginning of each gene. In this drawing, gene a, which is transcribed from left to right, uses the bottom DNA strand as its template (see Figure 7–10); gene b, which is transcribed from right to left, uses the top strand as its template.

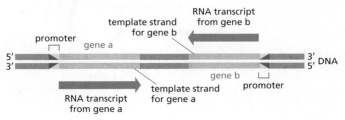

Initiation of Eukaryotic Gene Transcription Is a Complex Process

Many of the principles we just outlined for bacterial transcription also apply to eukaryotes. However, the initiation of transcription in eukaryotes differs in several important ways from the process in bacteria:

1. While bacteria use a single type of RNA polymerase for transcription, eukaryotic cells employ three: *RNA polymerase I*, *RNA polymerase II*, and *RNA polymerase III*. These polymerases are responsible for transcribing different types of genes. RNA polymerases I and III transcribe the genes encoding transfer RNA, ribosomal RNA, and various other RNAs that play structural and catalytic roles in the cell (Table 7–2). RNA polymerase II transcribes the rest, including all those that encode proteins—which constitutes the majority of genes in eukaryotes (Movie 7.3). Our subsequent discussion will therefore focus on RNA polymerase II.

2. Whereas the bacterial RNA polymerase (along with its sigma subunit) is able to initiate transcription on its own, eukaryotic RNA polymerases require the assistance of a large set of accessory proteins. Principal among these are the *general transcription factors*, which must assemble at each promoter, along with the polymerase, before transcription can begin.

3. The mechanisms that control the initiation of transcription in eukaryotes are much more elaborate than those that operate in prokaryotes—a point we discuss in detail in Chapter 8. In bacteria, genes tend to lie very close to one another, with only very short lengths of nontranscribed DNA between them. But in plants and animals, including humans, individual genes are spread out along the DNA, with stretches of up to 100,000 nucleotide pairs between one gene and the next. This architecture allows a single gene to be controlled by a large variety of *regulatory DNA sequences* scattered along the DNA, and it enables eukaryotes to engage in more complex forms of transcriptional regulation than do bacteria.

4. Eukaryotic transcription initiation must deal with the packing of DNA into *nucleosomes* and higher-order forms of chromatin structure, as we describe in Chapter 8.

To begin our discussion of eukaryotic transcription, we take a look at the general transcription factors and see how they help RNA polymerase II initiate the process.

Eukaryotic RNA Polymerase Requires General Transcription Factors

The initial finding that, unlike bacterial RNA polymerase, purified eukaryotic RNA polymerase II cannot initiate transcription on its own in a test tube led to the discovery and purification of the **general transcription**

QUESTION 7–3

Could the RNA polymerase used for transcription also be used to make the RNA primers required for DNA replication (discussed in Chapter 6)?

TABLE 7–2 THE THREE RNA POLYMERASES IN EUKARYOTIC CELLS

Type of Polymerase	Genes Transcribed
RNA polymerase I	most rRNA genes
RNA polymerase II	all protein-coding genes, miRNA genes, plus genes for other noncoding RNAs (e.g., those of the spliceosome)
RNA polymerase III	tRNA genes, 5S rRNA gene, genes for many other small RNAs

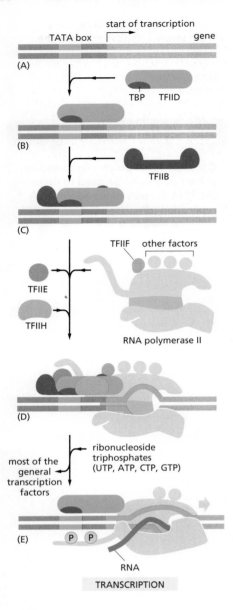

(A) TATA box — start of transcription — gene

(B) TBP TFIID

(C) TFIIB

TFIIF other factors

TFIIE

TFIIH

RNA polymerase II

(D)

most of the general transcription factors — ribonucleoside triphosphates (UTP, ATP, CTP, GTP)

(E) P P

RNA

TRANSCRIPTION

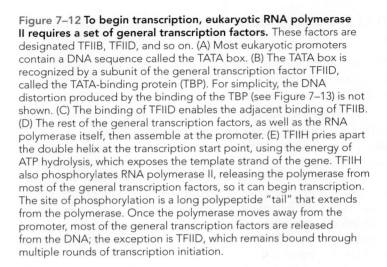

Figure 7–12 To begin transcription, eukaryotic RNA polymerase II requires a set of general transcription factors. These factors are designated TFIIB, TFIID, and so on. (A) Most eukaryotic promoters contain a DNA sequence called the TATA box. (B) The TATA box is recognized by a subunit of the general transcription factor TFIID, called the TATA-binding protein (TBP). For simplicity, the DNA distortion produced by the binding of the TBP (see Figure 7–13) is not shown. (C) The binding of TFIID enables the adjacent binding of TFIIB. (D) The rest of the general transcription factors, as well as the RNA polymerase itself, then assemble at the promoter. (E) TFIIH pries apart the double helix at the transcription start point, using the energy of ATP hydrolysis, which exposes the template strand of the gene. TFIIH also phosphorylates RNA polymerase II, releasing the polymerase from most of the general transcription factors, so it can begin transcription. The site of phosphorylation is a long polypeptide "tail" that extends from the polymerase. Once the polymerase moves away from the promoter, most of the general transcription factors are released from the DNA; the exception is TFIID, which remains bound through multiple rounds of transcription initiation.

factors. These accessory proteins assemble on the promoter, where they position the RNA polymerase and pull apart the DNA double helix to expose the template strand, allowing the polymerase to begin transcription. Thus, the general transcription factors have a similar role in eukaryotic transcription as sigma factor has in bacterial transcription.

Figure 7–12 shows the assembly of the general transcription factors at a promoter used by RNA polymerase II. The process begins with the binding of the general transcription factor TFIID to a short segment of DNA double helix composed primarily of T and A nucleotides; because of its composition, this part of the promoter is known as the *TATA box*. Upon binding to DNA, TFIID causes a dramatic local distortion in the DNA double helix (**Figure 7–13**); this structure helps to serve as a landmark for the subsequent assembly of other proteins at the promoter. The TATA box is a key component of many promoters used by RNA polymerase II, and it is typically located about 30 nucleotides upstream from the transcription start site. Once TFIID has bound to the TATA box, the other factors assemble, along with RNA polymerase II, to form a complete *transcription initiation complex*. Although Figure 7–12 shows the general transcription factors loading onto the promoter in a certain sequence, the actual order of assembly probably differs somewhat from one promoter to the next. Like bacterial promoters, eukaryotic promoters are composed of several distinct DNA sequences; these direct the general transcription factors where to assemble, and they orient the RNA polymerase so that it will begin transcription in the correct direction and on the correct DNA template strand (**Figure 7–14**).

Once RNA polymerase II has been positioned on the promoter, it must be released from the complex of general transcription factors to begin its task of making an RNA molecule. A key step in liberating the RNA polymerase is the addition of phosphate groups to its "tail" (see Figure

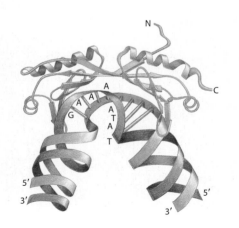

Figure 7–13 TATA-binding protein (TBP) binds to the TATA box (indicated by letters) and bends the DNA double helix. TBP, a subunit of TFIID (see Figure 7–12), distorts the DNA when it binds. TBP is a single polypeptide chain that is folded into two very similar domains (*blue* and *green*). The protein sits atop the DNA double helix like a saddle on a bucking horse (Movie 7.4).

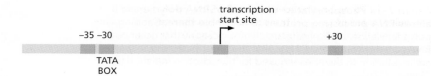

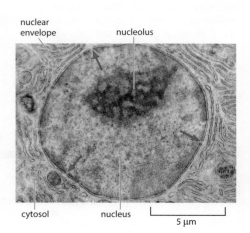

Figure 7–14 **Eukaryotic promoters contain sequences that promote the binding of the general transcription factors.** The location of each sequence and the general transcription factor that recognizes it are indicated. N stands for any nucleotide, and a *slash* (/) indicates that either nucleotide can be found at the indicated position. For most start sites transcribed by RNA polymerase II, only two or three of the four sequences are needed. Although most of these DNA sequences are located upstream of the transcription start site, one, at +30, is located within the transcribed region of the gene.

location	DNA sequence	general transcription factor
–35	G/C G/C G/A C G C C	TFIIB
–30	T A T A A/T A A/T	TBP subunit of TFIID
transcription start site	C/T C/T A N T/A C/T C/T	TFIID
+30	A/G G A/T C G T G	TFIID

7–12E). This action is initiated by the general transcription factor TFIIH, which contains a protein kinase as one of its subunits. Once transcription has begun, most of the general transcription factors dissociate from the DNA and then are available to initiate another round of transcription with a new RNA polymerase molecule. When RNA polymerase II finishes transcribing a gene, it too is released from the DNA; the phosphates on its tail are stripped off by protein phosphatases, and the polymerase is then ready to find a new promoter. Only the dephosphorylated form of RNA polymerase II can re-initiate RNA synthesis.

Eukaryotic mRNAs Are Processed in the Nucleus

The principle of templating, by which DNA is transcribed into RNA, is the same in all organisms; however, the way in which the resulting RNA transcripts are handled before they are translated into protein differs between bacteria and eukaryotes. Because bacteria lack a nucleus, their DNA is directly exposed to the cytosol, which contains the *ribosomes* on which protein synthesis takes place. As an mRNA molecule in a bacterium starts to be synthesized, ribosomes immediately attach to the free 5′ end of the RNA transcript and begin translating it into protein.

In eukaryotic cells, by contrast, DNA is enclosed within the *nucleus*, which is where transcription takes place. Translation, however, occurs on ribosomes that are located in the cytosol. So, before a eukaryotic mRNA can be translated into protein, it must be transported out of the nucleus through small pores in the nuclear envelope (**Figure 7–15**). And before it can be exported to the cytosol, a eukaryotic RNA must go through several **RNA processing** steps, which include *capping*, *splicing*, and *polyadenylation*, as we discuss shortly. These steps take place as the RNA is being synthesized. The enzymes responsible for RNA processing ride on the phosphorylated tail of eukaryotic RNA polymerase II as it synthesizes an RNA molecule (see Figure 7–12), and they process the transcript as it emerges from the polymerase (**Figure 7–16**).

Figure 7–15 **Before they can be translated, mRNA molecules made in the nucleus must be exported to the cytosol via pores in the nuclear envelope (*red arrows*).** Shown here is a section of a liver cell nucleus. The nucleolus is where ribosomal RNAs are synthesized and combined with proteins to form ribosomes, which are then exported to the cytosol. (From D.W. Fawcett, *A Textbook of Histology*, 12th ed. 1994. With permission from Taylor & Francis Books UK.)

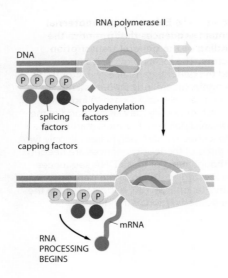

RNA polymerase II

DNA

splicing factors

polyadenylation factors

capping factors

mRNA

RNA PROCESSING BEGINS

Figure 7–16 Phosphorylation of the tail of RNA polymerase II allows RNA-processing proteins to assemble there. Capping, polyadenylation, and splicing are all modifications that occur as the RNA is being synthesized. Note that the phosphates shown here are in addition to the ones required for transcription initiation (see Figure 7–12).

Two of these processing steps, capping and polyadenylation, occur on all RNA transcripts destined to become mRNA molecules.

1. **RNA capping** modifies the 5′ end of the RNA transcript, the part of the RNA that is synthesized first. The RNA cap includes an atypical nucleotide: a guanine (G) nucleotide bearing a methyl group is attached to the 5′ end of the RNA in an unusual way (**Figure 7–17**). In bacteria, by contrast, the 5′ end of an mRNA molecule is simply the first nucleotide of the transcript. In eukaryotic cells, capping takes place after RNA polymerase II has produced about 25 nucleotides of RNA, long before it has completed transcribing the whole gene.

2. **Polyadenylation** provides a newly transcribed mRNA with a special structure at its 3′ end. In contrast with bacteria, where the 3′ end of an mRNA is simply the end of the chain synthesized by the RNA polymerase, the 3′ end of a eukaryotic mRNA is first trimmed by an enzyme that cuts the RNA chain at a particular sequence of nucleotides. The transcript is then finished off by a second enzyme that adds a series of repeated adenine (A) nucleotides to the trimmed end. This *poly-A tail* is generally a few hundred nucleotides long (see Figure 7–17A).

These two modifications—capping and polyadenylation—increase the stability of a eukaryotic mRNA molecule, facilitate its export from the nucleus to the cytosol, and generally mark the RNA molecule as an mRNA. They are also used by the protein-synthesis machinery to make sure that both ends of the mRNA are present and that the message is therefore complete before protein synthesis begins.

Figure 7–17 Eukaryotic mRNA molecules are modified by capping and polyadenylation. (A) A eukaryotic mRNA has a cap at the 5′ end and a poly-A tail at the 3′ end. In addition to the nucleotide sequences that code for protein, most mRNAs also contain extra, noncoding sequences, as shown. The noncoding portion at the 5′ end is called the 5′ untranslated region, or 5′ UTR, and that at the 3′ end is called the 3′ UTR. (B) The structure of the 5′ cap. Many eukaryotic mRNA caps carry an additional modification: the 2′-hydroxyl group on the second ribose sugar in the mRNA is methylated (not shown).

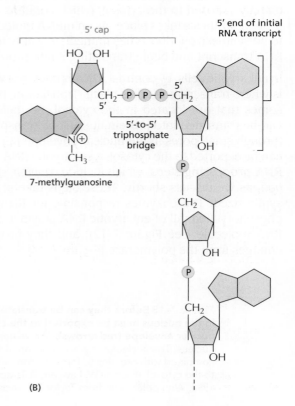

5′ cap

HO   OH

CH_2–P–P–P–CH_2

5′-to-5′ triphosphate bridge

7-methylguanosine

5′ end of initial RNA transcript

OH

P

CH_2

OH

P

CH_2

OH

RNA capping and polyadenylation

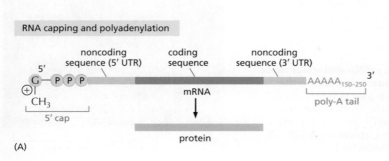

noncoding sequence (5′ UTR)   coding sequence   noncoding sequence (3′ UTR)

5′

G—P P P

CH₃

5′ cap

mRNA

$AAAAA_{150-250}$ 3′

poly-A tail

protein

(A)

(B)

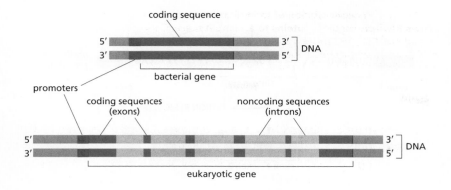

coding sequence

bacterial gene

promoters

coding sequences
(exons)

noncoding sequences
(introns)

eukaryotic gene

Figure 7–18 Eukaryotic and bacterial genes are organized differently. A bacterial gene consists of a single stretch of uninterrupted nucleotide sequence that encodes the amino acid sequence of a protein. In contrast, the protein-coding sequences of most eukaryotic genes (*exons*) are interrupted by noncoding sequences (*introns*). Promoter sequences are indicated in *green*.

In Eukaryotes, Protein-Coding Genes Are Interrupted by Noncoding Sequences Called Introns

Most eukaryotic mRNAs have to undergo an additional processing step before they become functional. This step involves a far more radical modification of the RNA transcript than capping or polyadenylation, and it is the consequence of a surprising feature of most eukaryotic genes. In bacteria, most proteins are encoded by an uninterrupted stretch of DNA sequence that is transcribed into an mRNA that, without any further processing, can be translated into protein. Most protein-coding eukaryotic genes, in contrast, have their coding sequences interrupted by long, noncoding, *intervening sequences* called **introns**. The scattered pieces of coding sequence—called *expressed sequences* or **exons**—are usually shorter than the introns, and they often represent only a small fraction of the total length of the gene (**Figure 7–18**). Introns range in length from a single nucleotide to more than 10,000 nucleotides. Some protein-coding eukaryotic genes lack introns altogether, some have only a few, but most have many (**Figure 7–19**). Note that the terms "exon" and "intron" apply to both the DNA and the corresponding RNA sequences.

Introns Are Removed from Pre-mRNAs by RNA Splicing

To produce an mRNA in a eukaryotic cell, the entire length of the gene, introns as well as exons, is transcribed into RNA. After capping, and as RNA polymerase II continues to transcribe the gene, **RNA splicing** begins. In this process, the introns are removed from the newly synthesized RNA and the exons are stitched together. Each transcript ultimately receives a poly-A tail; in many cases, this happens after splicing, whereas in other cases, it occurs before the final splicing reactions have been completed. Once a transcript has been spliced and its 5′ and 3′ ends have been modified, the RNA is now a functional mRNA molecule that can leave the nucleus and be translated into protein. Before these steps are completed, the RNA transcript is known as a *precursor-mRNA* or *pre-mRNA* for short.

How does the cell determine which parts of the RNA transcript to remove during splicing? Unlike the coding sequence of an exon, most of the nucleotide sequence of an intron is unimportant. Although there is little overall resemblance between the nucleotide sequences of different

Figure 7–19 Most protein-coding human genes are broken into multiple exons and introns. (A) The β-globin gene, which encodes one of the subunits of the oxygen-carrying protein hemoglobin, contains 3 exons. (B) The gene that encodes Factor VIII, a protein that functions in the blood-clotting pathway, contains 26 exons. Mutations in this large gene are responsible for the most prevalent form of the blood disorder hemophilia.

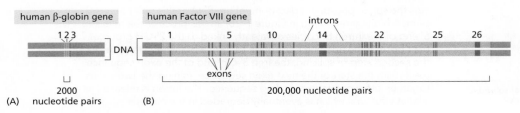

human β-globin gene

human Factor VIII gene

introns

exons

(A) 2000 nucleotide pairs

(B) 200,000 nucleotide pairs

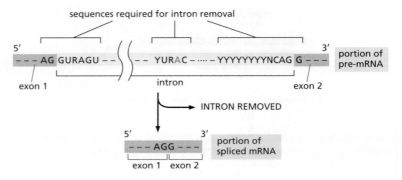

Figure 7–20 **Special nucleotide sequences in a pre-mRNA transcript signal the beginning and the end of an intron.** Only the nucleotide sequences shown are required to remove an intron; the other positions in an intron can be occupied by any nucleotide. The special sequences are recognized primarily by small nuclear ribonucleoproteins (snRNPs), which direct the cleavage of the RNA at the intron–exon borders and catalyze the covalent linkage of the exon sequences. Here, in addition to the standard symbols for nucleotides (A, C, G, U), R stands for either A or G; Y stands for either C or U; and N stands for any nucleotide. The A shown in *red* forms the branch point of the lariat produced in the splicing reaction shown in Figure 7–21. The distances along the RNA between the three splicing sequences are highly variable; however, the distance between the branch point and the 5′ splice junction is typically much longer than that between the 3′ splice junction and the branch point (see Figure 7–21). The splicing sequences shown are from humans; similar sequences direct RNA splicing in other eukaryotes.

introns, each intron contains a few short nucleotide sequences that act as cues for its removal from the pre-mRNA. These special sequences are found at or near each end of the intron and are the same or very similar in all introns (**Figure 7–20**). Guided by these sequences, an elaborate splicing machine cuts out the intron in the form of a "lariat" structure (**Figure 7–21**), formed by the reaction of an adenine nucleotide, highlighted in *red* in both Figures 7–20 and 7–21, with the beginning of the intron.

Although we will not describe the splicing process in detail, it is worthwhile to note that, unlike the other steps of mRNA production, RNA splicing is carried out largely by RNA molecules rather than proteins. These RNA molecules, called **small nuclear RNAs** (**snRNAs**), are packaged with additional proteins to form *small nuclear ribonucleoproteins* (*snRNPs*, pronounced "snurps"). The snRNPs recognize splice-site sequences through complementary base-pairing between their RNA components and the sequences in the pre-mRNA, and they carry out the chemistry of splicing (**Figure 7–22**). RNA molecules that catalyze reactions in this way are known as *ribozymes*, and we discuss them in more detail later in the chapter. Together, these snRNPs form the core of the **spliceosome**, the large assembly of RNA and protein molecules that carries out RNA splicing in the nucleus. To watch the spliceosome in action, see Movie 7.5.

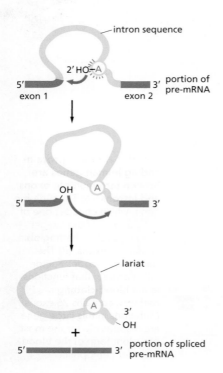

Figure 7–21 **An intron in a pre-mRNA molecule forms a branched structure during RNA splicing.** In the first step, the branch-point adenine (*red* A) in the intron sequence attacks the 5′ splice site and cuts the sugar–phosphate backbone of the RNA at this point (this is the same A highlighted in *red* in Figure 7–20). In this process, the released 5′ end of the intron becomes covalently linked to the 2′-OH group of the ribose of the adenine nucleotide to form a branched structure. In the second step of splicing, the free 3′-OH end of the exon sequence reacts with the start of the next exon sequence, joining the two exons together into a continuous coding sequence. The intron is released as a lariat structure, which is eventually degraded in the nucleus.

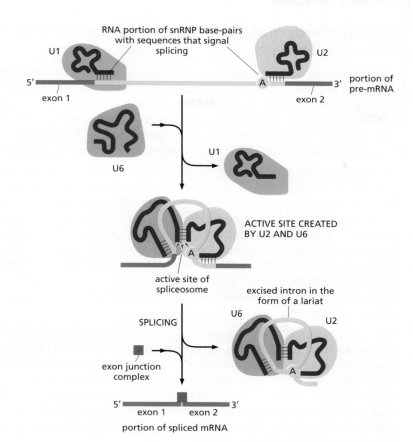

Figure 7–22 **Splicing is carried out by a collection of RNA–protein complexes called snRNPs.** Although there are five snRNPs and about 200 additional proteins required for splicing, only the three most important snRNPs—called U1, U2, and U6—are shown here. In the first steps of splicing, U1 recognizes the 5′ splice site and U2 recognizes the lariat branch-point site through complementary base-pairing. U6 then "re-checks" the 5′ splice site by displacing U1 and base-pairing with this intron sequence itself. This "re-reading" step improves the accuracy of splicing by double-checking the 5′ splice site before carrying out the splicing reaction. In the next steps, conformational changes in U2 and U6—triggered by the hydrolysis of ATP by spliceosomal proteins (not shown)—drive the formation of the spliceosome active site. Once the splicing reactions have occurred (see Figure 7–21), the spliceosome deposits a group of RNA-binding proteins, known as the exon junction complex (*red*), on the mRNA to mark the splice site as successfully completed.

The intron–exon type of gene arrangement in eukaryotes might seem wasteful, but it does provide some important benefits. First, the transcripts of many eukaryotic genes can be spliced in different ways, each of which can produce a distinct protein. Such **alternative splicing** thereby allows many different proteins to be produced from the same gene (**Figure 7–23**). About 95% of human genes are thought to undergo alternative splicing. Thus RNA splicing enables eukaryotes to increase the already enormous coding potential of their genomes. In Chapter 9, we will encounter another advantage of splicing—the production of novel proteins—when we discuss how proteins evolve.

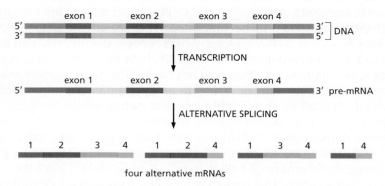

Figure 7–23 **Some pre-mRNAs undergo alternative RNA splicing to produce different mRNAs and proteins from the same gene.** Whereas all exons are transcribed, they can be skipped over by the spliceosome to produce alternatively spliced mRNAs, as shown. Such skipping occurs when the splicing signals at the 5′ end of one intron are paired up with the branch-point and 3′ end of a different intron. An important feature of alternative splicing is that exons can be skipped or included; however, their order—which is specified in the DNA sequence—cannot be rearranged.

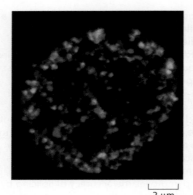

2 µm

Figure 7–24 RNAs are produced by factories within the nucleus. RNAs are synthesized and processed (*red*) and DNA is replicated (*green*) in intracellular condensates that form discrete compartments within a mammalian nucleus. In this micrograph, these loose aggregates of protein and nucleic acid were visualized by detecting newly synthesized DNA and RNA. In some instances, both replication and transcription are taking place at the same site (*yellow*). (From D.G. Wansink et al., *J. Cell Sci.* 107:1449–1456, 1994. With permission from The Company of Biologists.)

RNA Synthesis and Processing Takes Place in "Factories" Within the Nucleus

RNA synthesis and processing in eukaryotes requires the coordinated action of a large number of proteins, from the RNA polymerases and accessory proteins that carry out transcription to the enzymes responsible for capping, polyadenylation, and splicing. With so many components required to produce and process every one of the RNA molecules that are being transcribed, how do all these factors manage to find one another?

We have already seen that the enzymes responsible for RNA processing ride on the phosphorylated tail of eukaryotic RNA polymerase II as it synthesizes an RNA molecule, so that the RNA transcript can be processed as it is being synthesized (see Figure 7–16). In addition to this association, RNA polymerases and RNA-processing proteins also form loose molecular aggregates—generally termed *intracellular condensates*—that act as "factories" for the production of RNA. These factories, which bring together the numerous RNA polymerases, RNA-processing components, and the genes being expressed, are large enough to be seen microscopically (**Figure 7–24**).

The aggregation of components needed to perform a specific task is not unique to RNA transcription. Proteins involved in DNA replication and repair also converge to form functional factories dedicated to their specific tasks. And genes encoding ribosomal RNAs cluster together in the nucleolus (see Figure 5–17), where their RNA products are combined with proteins to form ribosomes. These ribosomes, along with the mature mRNAs they will decode, must then be exported to the cytosol, where translation will take place.

Mature Eukaryotic mRNAs Are Exported from the Nucleus

Of all the pre-mRNA that is synthesized by a cell, only a small fraction—the sequences contained within mature mRNAs—will be useful. The remaining RNA fragments—excised introns, broken RNAs, and aberrantly spliced transcripts—are not only useless, but they could be dangerous to the cell if allowed to leave the nucleus. How, then, does the cell distinguish between the relatively rare mature mRNA molecules it needs to export to the cytosol and the overwhelming amount of debris generated by RNA processing?

The answer is that the transport of mRNA from the nucleus to the cytosol is highly selective: only correctly processed mRNAs are exported and therefore available to be translated. This selective transport is mediated by *nuclear pore complexes*, which connect the nucleoplasm with the cytosol and act as gates that control which macromolecules can enter or leave the nucleus (discussed in Chapter 15). To be "export ready," an mRNA molecule must be bound to an appropriate set of proteins, each of which recognizes different parts of a mature mRNA molecule. These proteins include poly-A-binding proteins, a cap-binding complex, and proteins that bind to mRNAs that have been appropriately spliced (**Figure 7–25**). The entire set of bound proteins, rather than any single protein, ultimately determines whether an mRNA molecule will leave the nucleus. The "waste RNAs" that remain behind in the nucleus are degraded there, and their nucleotide building blocks are reused for transcription.

mRNA Molecules Are Eventually Degraded in the Cytosol

Because a single mRNA molecule can be translated into protein many times (see Figure 7–2), the length of time that a mature mRNA molecule persists in the cell greatly influences the amount of protein it produces.

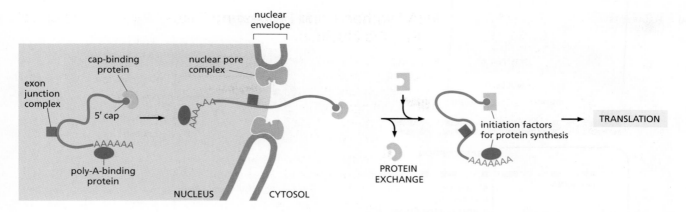

Figure 7–25 A specialized set of RNA-binding proteins signals that a completed mRNA is ready for export to the cytosol. As indicated on the *left*, the 5′ cap and poly-A tail of a mature mRNA molecule are "marked" by proteins that recognize these modifications. Successful splices are marked by exon junction complexes (see Figure 7–22). Once an mRNA is deemed "export ready," a nuclear transport receptor (discussed in Chapter 15) associates with the mRNA and guides it through the nuclear pore. In the cytosol, the mRNA can shed some of these proteins and bind new ones, which, along with poly-A-binding protein, act as initiation factors for protein synthesis, as we discuss in the next section of the chapter.

Each mRNA molecule is eventually degraded into nucleotides by ribonucleases (RNAses) present in the cytosol, but the lifespans of mRNA molecules differ considerably—depending on the nucleotide sequence of the mRNA and the type of cell. In bacteria, most mRNAs are degraded rapidly, having a typical lifespan of about 3 minutes. The mRNAs in eukaryotic cells usually persist longer: some, such as those encoding β-globin, have lifespans of more than 10 hours, whereas others stick around for less than 30 minutes.

These different lifespans are in part controlled by nucleotide sequences in the mRNA itself, most often in the portion of RNA called the 3′ *untranslated region*, which lies between the 3′ end of the coding sequence and the poly-A tail (see Figure 7–17). The lifespans of different mRNAs help the cell control how much protein will be produced. In general, proteins made in large amounts, such as β-globin, are translated from mRNAs that have long lifespans, whereas proteins made in smaller amounts, or whose levels must change rapidly in response to signals, are typically synthesized from short-lived mRNAs.

The synthesis, processing, and degradation of RNA in eukaryotes and prokaryotes is summarized and compared in **Figure 7–26**.

FROM RNA TO PROTEIN

By the end of the 1950s, biologists had demonstrated that the information encoded in DNA is copied first into RNA and then into protein. The debate then shifted to the "coding problem": How is the information in a linear sequence of nucleotides in an RNA molecule translated into the linear sequence of a chemically quite different set of subunits—the amino acids in a protein? This fascinating question intrigued scientists from many different disciplines, including physics, mathematics, and chemistry. Here was a cryptogram set up by nature that, after more than 3 billion years of evolution, could finally be solved by one of the products of evolution— the human brain! Indeed, scientists have not only cracked the code but have revealed, in atomic detail, the precise workings of the machinery by which cells read this code.

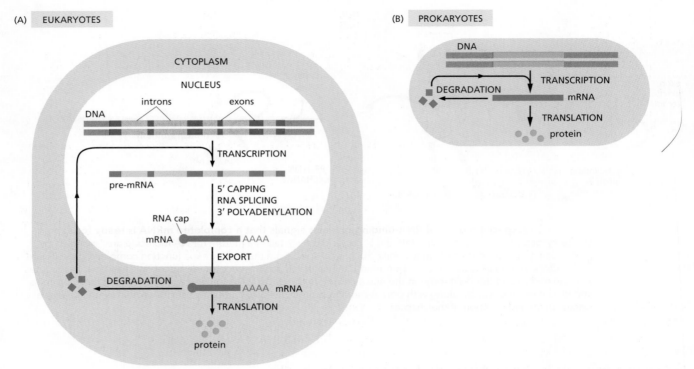

Figure 7–26 **Producing mRNA molecules is more complex in eukaryotes than it is in prokaryotes.** (A) In eukaryotic cells, the pre-mRNA molecule produced by transcription contains both intron and exon sequences. Its two ends are modified by capping and polyadenylation, and the introns are removed by RNA splicing. The completed mRNA is then transported from the nucleus to the cytosol, where it is translated into protein. Although these steps are depicted as occurring one after the other, in reality they occur simultaneously. For example, the RNA cap is usually added and splicing usually begins before transcription has been completed. Because of this overlap, transcripts of the entire gene (including all introns and exons) do not typically exist in the cell. Ultimately, mRNAs are degraded by RNAses in the cytosol and their nucleotide building blocks are reused for transcription. (B) In prokaryotes, the production of mRNA molecules is simpler. The 5′ end of an mRNA molecule is produced by the initiation of transcription by RNA polymerase, and the 3′ end is produced by the termination of transcription. Because prokaryotic cells lack a nucleus, transcription and translation—as well as degradation—take place in a common compartment. Translation of a prokaryotic mRNA can therefore begin before its synthesis has been completed. In both eukaryotes and prokaryotes, the amount of a protein in a cell depends on the rates of each of these steps, as well as on the rates of degradation of the mRNA and protein molecules.

An mRNA Sequence Is Decoded in Sets of Three Nucleotides

Transcription as a means of information transfer is simple to understand: DNA and RNA are chemically and structurally similar, and DNA can act as a direct template for the synthesis of RNA through complementary base-pairing. As the term transcription signifies, it is as if a message written out by hand were being converted, say, into a typewritten text. The language itself and the form of the message do not change, and the symbols used are closely related.

In contrast, the conversion of the information from RNA into protein represents a **translation** of the information into another language that uses different symbols. Because there are only 4 different nucleotides in mRNA but 20 different types of amino acids in a protein, this translation cannot be accounted for by a direct one-to-one correspondence between a nucleotide in RNA and an amino acid in protein. The set of rules by which the nucleotide sequence of a gene, through an intermediary mRNA molecule, is translated into the amino acid sequence of a protein is known as the **genetic code**.

In 1961, it was discovered that the sequence of nucleotides in an mRNA molecule is read consecutively in groups of three. And because RNA is made of 4 different nucleotides, there are $4 \times 4 \times 4 = 64$ possible combinations of three nucleotides: AAA, AUA, AUG, and so on. However, only 20 different amino acids are commonly found in proteins. Either some nucleotide triplets are never used, or the code is redundant, with some amino acids being specified by more than one triplet. The second possibility turned out to be correct, as shown by the completely deciphered genetic code shown in **Figure 7–27**. Each group of three consecutive nucleotides in RNA is called a **codon**, and each codon specifies one amino acid. The strategy by which this code was cracked is described in **How We Know**, pp. 246–247.

The same basic genetic code is used in all present-day organisms. Although a few slight differences have been found, these occur chiefly in

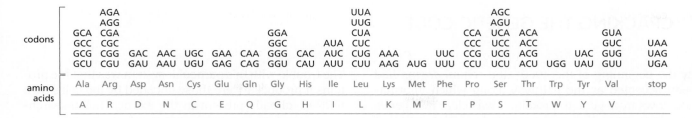

codons																				
		AGA									UUA					AGC				
		AGG									UUG					AGU				
	GCA	CGA					GGA				CUA				CCA	UCA	ACA			
	GCC	CGC					GGC		AUA	CUC				CCC	UCC	ACC		GUA		
	GCG	CGG	GAC	AAC	UGC	GAA	CAA	GGG	CAC	AUC	CUG	AAA		UUC	CCG	UCG	ACG		GUC	UAA
	GCU	CGU	GAU	AAU	UGU	GAG	CAG	GGU	CAU	AUU	CUU	AAG	AUG	UUU	CCU	UCU	ACU	UGG	UAC	GUU	UAG
																			UAU		UGA

amino acids																				
	Ala	Arg	Asp	Asn	Cys	Glu	Gln	Gly	His	Ile	Leu	Lys	Met	Phe	Pro	Ser	Thr	Trp	Tyr	Val	stop
	A	R	D	N	C	E	Q	G	H	I	L	K	M	F	P	S	T	W	Y	V	

Figure 7–27 The nucleotide sequence of an mRNA is translated into the amino acid sequence of a protein via the genetic code. All of the three-nucleotide codons in mRNAs that specify a given amino acid are listed above that amino acid, which is given in both its three-letter and one-letter abbreviations (see Panel 2–6, pp. 76–77, for the full name of each amino acid and its structure). Like RNA molecules, codons are usually written with the 5′-terminal nucleotide to the left. Note that most amino acids are represented by more than one codon, and there are some regularities in the set of codons that specify each amino acid. For example, codons for the same amino acid tend to contain the same nucleotides at the first and second positions and vary at the third position. There are three codons that do not specify any amino acid but act as termination sites (*stop codons*), signaling the end of the protein-coding sequence in an mRNA. One codon—AUG—acts both as an initiation codon, signaling the start of a protein-coding message, and as the codon that specifies the amino acid methionine.

the mRNA of mitochondria and of some fungi and protozoa. Mitochondria have their own DNA replication, transcription, and protein-synthesis machinery, which operates independently of the corresponding machinery in the rest of the cell (discussed in Chapter 14), and they have been able to accommodate minor changes to the otherwise universal genetic code. Even in fungi and protozoa, the similarities in the code far outweigh the differences.

In principle, an mRNA sequence can be translated in any one of three different **reading frames**, depending on where the decoding process begins (Figure 7–28). However, only one of the three possible reading frames in an mRNA specifies the correct protein. We discuss later how a special signal at the beginning of each mRNA molecule sets the correct reading frame.

tRNA Molecules Match Amino Acids to Codons in mRNA

The codons in an mRNA molecule do not directly recognize the amino acids they specify: the set of three nucleotides does not, for example, bind directly to the amino acid. Rather, the translation of mRNA into protein depends on adaptor molecules that bind to a codon with one part of the adaptor and to an amino acid with another. These adaptors consist of a set of small RNA molecules known as **transfer RNAs (tRNAs)**, each about 80 nucleotides in length.

We saw earlier that an RNA molecule generally folds into a three-dimensional structure by forming internal base pairs between different regions of the molecule. If the base-paired regions are sufficiently extensive, they will fold back on themselves to form a double-helical structure, like that of double-stranded DNA. Such is the case for the tRNA molecule. Four short segments of the folded tRNA are double-helical, producing a distinctive

Figure 7–28 In principle, an mRNA molecule can be translated in three possible reading frames. In the process of translating a nucleotide sequence (*blue*) into an amino acid sequence (*red*), the sequence of nucleotides in an mRNA molecule is read from the 5′ to the 3′ end in sequential sets of three nucleotides. In principle, therefore, the same mRNA sequence can specify three completely different amino acid sequences, depending on the nucleotide at which translation begins—that is, on the reading frame used. In reality, however, only one of these reading frames encodes the actual message, as we discuss later.

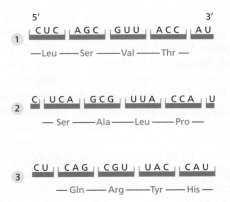

CRACKING THE GENETIC CODE

By the beginning of the 1960s, the *central dogma* had been accepted as the pathway along which information flows from gene to protein. It was clear that genes encode proteins, that genes are made of DNA, and that mRNA serves as an intermediary, carrying the information from DNA to the ribosome, where the RNA is translated into protein.

Even the general format of the genetic code had been worked out: each of the 20 amino acids found in proteins is represented by a triplet codon in an mRNA molecule. But an even greater challenge remained: biologists, chemists, and even physicists set their sights on breaking the genetic code—attempting to figure out which amino acid each of the 64 possible nucleotide triplets designates. The most straightforward path to the solution would have been to compare the sequence of a segment of DNA or of mRNA with its corresponding polypeptide product. Techniques for sequencing nucleic acids, however, would not be developed for another decade.

So researchers decided that, to crack the genetic code, they would have to synthesize their own simple RNA molecules. If they could feed these RNA molecules to ribosomes—the machines that make proteins—and then analyze the resulting polypeptide product, they would be on their way to deciphering which triplets encode which amino acids.

Losing the cells

Before researchers could test their synthetic mRNAs, they needed to perfect a cell-free system for protein synthesis. This would allow them to translate their messages into polypeptides in a test tube. (Generally speaking, when working in the laboratory, the simpler the system, the easier it is to interpret the results.) To isolate the molecular machinery they needed for such a cell-free translation system, researchers broke open *E. coli* cells and loaded their contents into a centrifuge tube. Spinning these samples at high speed caused the membranes and other large chunks of cellular debris to be dragged to the bottom of the tube; the lighter cellular components required for protein synthesis—including mRNA, the tRNA adaptors, ribosomes, enzymes, and other small molecules—were left floating near the top of the tube (see Panel 4-3, pp. 164–165). Researchers found that simply adding radioactive amino acids to this cell "soup" would trigger the production of radiolabeled polypeptides. By centrifuging this material again, at a higher speed, the researchers could force the ribosomes, and any newly synthesized peptides attached to them, to the bottom of the tube; the labeled polypeptides could then be detected by measuring the radioactivity in the sediment remaining in the tube after the fluid layer above it had been discarded.

The trouble with this particular system was that the proteins it produced were those encoded by the cell's own mRNAs, already present in the extract. But researchers wanted to use their own synthetic messages to direct protein synthesis. This problem was solved when Marshall Nirenberg discovered that he could destroy the cells' mRNA in the extract by adding a small amount of ribonuclease—an enzyme that degrades RNA—to the mix. Now all he needed to do was prepare large quantities of synthetic mRNA, add it to the cell-free system, and see what peptides came out.

Faking the message

Producing a synthetic polynucleotide with a defined sequence was not as simple as it sounds. Again, it would be years before chemists and bioengineers developed machines that could synthesize any given string of nucleic acids quickly and cheaply. Nirenberg decided to use polynucleotide phosphorylase, an enzyme that would join ribonucleotides together in the absence of a template. The sequence of the resulting RNA would then depend entirely on which nucleotides were presented to the enzyme. A mixture of nucleotides would be sewn into a random sequence; but a single type of nucleotide would yield a homogeneous polymer containing only that one nucleotide. Thus Nirenberg, working with his collaborator Heinrich Matthaei, first produced synthetic mRNAs made entirely of uracil—poly U.

Together, the researchers fed this poly U to their cell-free translation system. They then added a single type of radioactively labeled amino acid to the mix. After testing each amino acid—one at a time, in 20 different experiments—they determined that poly U directs the synthesis of a polypeptide containing only phenylalanine (**Figure 7–29**). With this electrifying result, the first word in the genetic code had been deciphered.

Nirenberg and Matthaei then repeated the experiment with poly A and poly C and determined that AAA codes for lysine and CCC for proline. The meaning of poly G could not be ascertained by this method because, as we now know, this polynucleotide forms an aberrant structure that gums up the system.

Feeding ribosomes with synthetic RNA seemed a fruitful technique. But with the single-nucleotide possibilities exhausted, researchers had nailed down only three codons; they had 61 still to go. The other codons, however, were harder to decipher, and a new synthetic approach was needed. In the 1950s, the organic chemist Gobind Khorana had been developing methods for preparing mixed polynucleotides of defined sequence—but his techniques worked only for DNA. When he learned of Nirenberg's work with synthetic RNAs, Khorana directed his energies and skills to producing

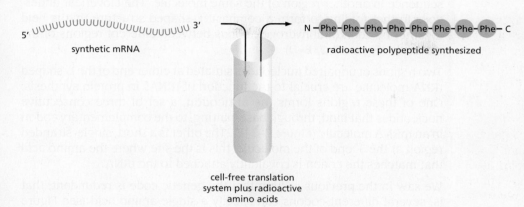

5′ UUUUUUUUUUUUUUUUUUUUUUUUUUUU 3′

synthetic mRNA

N – Phe-Phe-Phe-Phe-Phe-Phe-Phe-Phe – C

radioactive polypeptide synthesized

cell-free translation
system plus radioactive
amino acids

Figure 7–29 UUU codes for phenylalanine. Synthetic mRNAs are fed into a cell-free translation system containing bacterial ribosomes, tRNAs, enzymes, and other small molecules. Radioactive amino acids were added to this mix, one per experiment; when the "correct" amino acid was added, a radioactive polypeptide would be produced. In this case, poly U is shown to encode a polypeptide containing only phenylalanine.

polyribonucleotides. He found that if he started out by making DNAs of a defined sequence, he could then use RNA polymerase to produce RNAs from those. In this way, Khorana prepared a collection of different RNAs of defined repeating sequence: he generated sequences of repeating dinucleotides (such as poly UC), trinucleotides (such as poly UUC), or tetranucleotides (such as poly UAUC).

These mixed polynucleotides, however, yielded results that were much more difficult to decode than the mononucleotide messages that Nirenberg had used. Take poly UG, for example. When this repeating dinucleotide was added to the translation system, researchers discovered that it codes for a polypeptide of alternating cysteines and valines. The RNA, of course, contains two different, alternating codons: UGU and GUG. So the researchers could say that UGU and GUG code for cysteine and valine, although they could not tell which went with which. Thus these mixed messages provided useful information, but they did not definitively reveal which codons specified which amino acids (**Figure 7–30**).

Trapping the triplets

These final ambiguities in the code were resolved when Nirenberg and a young medical graduate named Phil Leder discovered that RNA fragments that were only three nucleotides in length—the size of a single codon—could bind to a ribosome and attract the appropriate amino-acid-containing tRNA molecule. These complexes—containing one ribosome, one mRNA codon, and one radiolabeled aminoacyl-tRNA—could then be captured on a piece of filter paper and the attached amino acid identified.

Their trial run with UUU—the first word—worked splendidly. Leder and Nirenberg primed the usual cell-free translation system with snippets of UUU. These trinucleotides bound to the ribosomes, and Phe-tRNAs bound to the UUU. The new system was up and running,

and the researchers had confirmed that UUU codes for phenylalanine.

All that remained was for researchers to produce all 64 possible codons—a task that was quickly accomplished in both Nirenberg's and Khorana's laboratories. Because these small trinucleotides were much simpler to synthesize chemically, and the triplet-trapping tests were easier to perform and analyze than the previous decoding experiments, the researchers were able to work out the complete genetic code within the next year.

MESSAGE	PEPTIDES PRODUCED	CODON ASSIGNMENTS	
poly UG	...Cys–Val–Cys–Val...	UGU GUG	Cys, Val*
poly AG	...Arg–Glu–Arg–Glu...	AGA GAG	Arg, Glu
poly UUC	...Phe–Phe–Phe... + ...Ser–Ser–Ser... + ...Leu–Leu–Leu...	UUC UCU CUU	Phe, Ser, Leu
poly UAUC	...Tyr–Leu–Ser–Ile...	UAU CUA UCU AUC	Tyr, Leu, Ser, Ile

* One codon specifies Cys, the other Val, but which is which? The same ambiguity exists for the other codon assignments shown here.

Figure 7–30 Using synthetic RNAs of mixed, repeating ribonucleotide sequences, scientists further narrowed the coding possibilities. Because these mixed messages produced mixed polypeptides, they did not permit the unambiguous assignment of a single codon to a specific amino acid. For example, the results of the poly-UG experiment cannot distinguish whether UGU or GUG encodes cysteine. As indicated, the same type of ambiguity confounded the interpretation of all the experiments using di-, tri-, and tetranucleotides.

structure that looks like a cloverleaf when drawn schematically (Figure 7–31A). As shown in the figure, for example, a 5′-GCUC-3′ sequence in one part of a polynucleotide chain can base-pair with a 5′-GAGC-3′ sequence in another region of the same molecule. The cloverleaf undergoes further folding to form a compact, L-shaped structure that is held together by additional hydrogen bonds between different regions of the molecule (Figure 7–31B–D).

Two regions of unpaired nucleotides situated at either end of the L-shaped tRNA molecule are crucial to the function of tRNAs in protein synthesis. One of these regions forms the **anticodon**, a set of three consecutive nucleotides that bind, through base-pairing, to the complementary codon in an mRNA molecule (Figure 7–31E). The other is a short, single-stranded region at the 3′ end of the molecule; this is the site where the amino acid that matches the codon is covalently attached to the tRNA.

We saw in the previous section that the genetic code is redundant; that is, several different codons can specify a single amino acid (see Figure 7–27). This redundancy implies either that there is more than one tRNA for many of the amino acids or that some tRNA molecules can base-pair with more than one codon. In fact, both situations occur. Some amino acids have more than one tRNA, and some tRNAs require accurate base-pairing only at the first two positions of the codon and can tolerate a mismatch (or *wobble*) at the third position. This wobble base-pairing explains why so many of the alternative codons for an amino acid differ only in their third nucleotide (see Figure 7–27). Wobble base-pairings make it possible to fit the 20 amino acids to their 61 codons with as few as 31 kinds of tRNA molecules. The exact number of different kinds of tRNAs, however, differs from one species to the next. For example, humans have approximately 500 different tRNA genes, but this collection includes only 48 different anticodons.

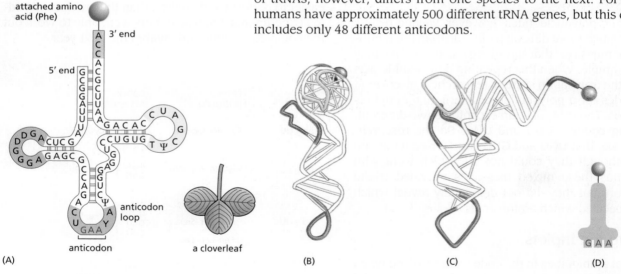

(E)

Figure 7–31 tRNA molecules are molecular adaptors, linking amino acids to codons. In this series of diagrams, the same tRNA molecule—in this case, a tRNA specific for the amino acid phenylalanine (Phe)—is depicted in various ways. (A) The conventional "cloverleaf" structure shows the complementary base-pairing (*red* lines) that creates the double-helical regions of the molecule. The anticodon loop (*blue*) contains the sequence of three nucleotides (*red* letters) that base-pairs with the Phe codon in mRNA. The amino acid matching the anticodon is attached at the 3′ end of the tRNA. tRNAs contain some unusual bases, which are produced by chemical modification after the tRNA has been synthesized. The bases denoted ψ (for pseudouridine) and D (for dihydrouridine) are derived from uracil. (B and C) Views of the actual L-shaped molecule, based on x-ray diffraction analysis. These two images are rotated 90° with respect to each other. (D) The schematic representation of tRNA that will be used in subsequent figures emphasizes the anticodon. (E) The linear nucleotide sequence of the tRNA molecule, color-coded to match (A), (B), and (C).

Specific Enzymes Couple tRNAs to the Correct Amino Acid

For a tRNA molecule to carry out its role as an adaptor, it must be linked—or charged—with the correct amino acid. How does each tRNA molecule recognize the one amino acid in 20 that is its proper partner? Recognition and attachment of the correct amino acid depend on enzymes called **aminoacyl-tRNA synthetases**, which covalently couple each amino acid to the appropriate set of tRNA molecules. In most organisms, there is a different synthetase enzyme for each amino acid. That means that there are 20 synthetases in all: one attaches glycine to all tRNAs that recognize codons for glycine, another attaches phenylalanine to all tRNAs that recognize codons for phenylalanine, and so on. Each synthetase enzyme recognizes its designated amino acid, as well as nucleotides in the anticodon loop and in the amino-acid-accepting arm that are specific to the correct tRNA (**Figure 7–32** and Movie 7.6). The synthetases are thus equal in importance to the tRNAs in the decoding process, because it is the combined action of the synthetases and tRNAs that allows each codon in the mRNA molecule to be correctly matched to its amino acid (**Figure 7–33**).

The synthetase-catalyzed reaction that attaches the amino acid to the 3′ end of the tRNA is one of many reactions in cells that is coupled to the energy-releasing hydrolysis of ATP (see Figure 3–32). The reaction produces a high-energy bond between the charged tRNA and the amino acid. The energy of this bond is later used to link the amino acid covalently to the growing polypeptide chain.

The mRNA Message Is Decoded on Ribosomes

The recognition of a codon by the anticodon on a tRNA molecule depends on the same type of complementary base-pairing used in DNA replication and transcription. However, accurate and rapid translation of mRNA into protein requires a molecular machine that can latch onto an mRNA, capture and position the correct tRNA molecules, and then covalently link the amino acids that they carry to form a polypeptide chain. In both

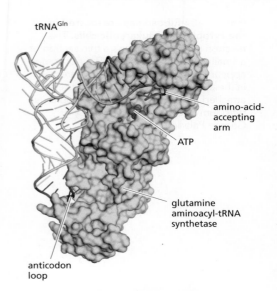

Figure 7–32 Each aminoacyl-tRNA synthetase makes multiple contacts with its tRNA molecule. For this tRNA, which is specific for the amino acid glutamine, nucleotides in both the anticodon loop (*dark blue*) and the amino-acid-accepting arm (*green*) are recognized by the synthetase (*yellow-green*). The ATP molecule that will be hydrolyzed to provide the energy needed to attach the amino acid to the tRNA is shown in *red*.

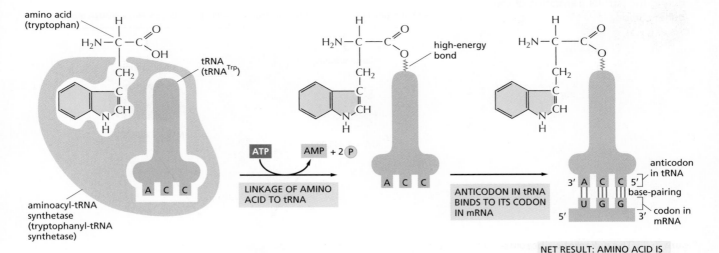

Figure 7–33 The genetic code is translated by aminoacyl-tRNA synthetases and tRNAs. Each synthetase couples a particular amino acid to its corresponding tRNAs, a process called charging. The anticodon on the charged tRNA molecule then forms base pairs with the appropriate codon on the mRNA. An error in either the charging step or the binding of the charged tRNA to its codon will cause the wrong amino acid to be incorporated into a polypeptide chain. In the sequence of events shown, the amino acid tryptophan (Trp) is specified by the codon UGG on the mRNA.

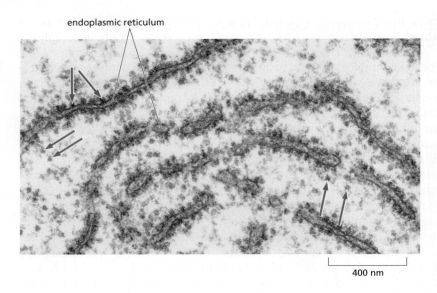

Figure 7–34 Ribosomes are located in the cytoplasm of eukaryotic cells. This electron micrograph shows a thin section of a small region of cytoplasm. The ribosomes appear as small *gray* blobs. Some are free in the cytoplasm (*red* arrows); others are attached to membranes of the endoplasmic reticulum (*green* arrows). (Courtesy of George Palade.)

endoplasmic reticulum

400 nm

QUESTION 7–4

In a clever experiment performed in 1962, a cysteine already attached to its tRNA was chemically converted to an alanine. These "hybrid" tRNA molecules were then added to a cell-free translation system from which the normal cysteine-tRNAs had been removed. When the resulting protein was analyzed, it was found that alanine had been inserted at every point in the polypeptide chain where cysteine was supposed to be. Discuss what this experiment tells you about the role of aminoacyl-tRNA synthetases and ribosomes during the normal translation of the genetic code.

prokaryotes and eukaryotes, the machine that gets the job done is the **ribosome**—a large complex made from dozens of small proteins (the *ribosomal proteins*) and several RNA molecules called **ribosomal RNAs (rRNAs)**. A typical eukaryotic cell contains millions of ribosomes in its cytosol (**Figure 7–34**).

Eukaryotic and prokaryotic ribosomes are very similar in structure and function. Both are composed of one large subunit and one small subunit, which fit together to form a complete ribosome with a mass of several million daltons (**Figure 7–35**); for comparison, an average-sized protein

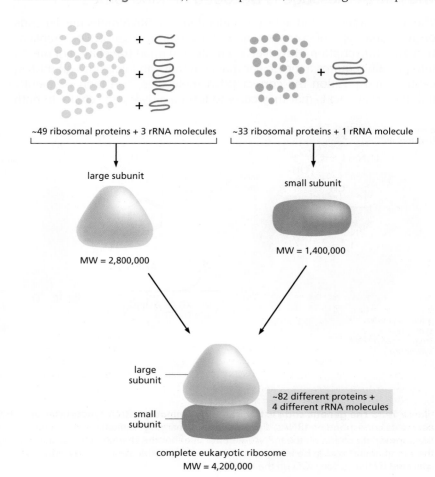

~49 ribosomal proteins + 3 rRNA molecules

~33 ribosomal proteins + 1 rRNA molecule

large subunit

small subunit

MW = 2,800,000

MW = 1,400,000

large subunit

small subunit

~82 different proteins + 4 different rRNA molecules

complete eukaryotic ribosome
MW = 4,200,000

Figure 7–35 The eukaryotic ribosome is a large complex of four rRNAs and more than 80 small proteins. Prokaryotic ribosomes are very similar: both are formed from a large and small subunit, which only come together after the small subunit has bound an mRNA. The RNAs account for most of the mass of the ribosome and give it its overall shape and structure.

has a mass of 30,000 daltons. The small ribosomal subunit matches the tRNAs to the codons of the mRNA, while the large subunit catalyzes the formation of the peptide bonds that covalently link the amino acids together into a polypeptide chain. These two subunits come together on an mRNA molecule near its 5′ end to start the synthesis of a protein. The mRNA is then pulled through the ribosome like a long piece of tape. As the mRNA inches forward in a 5′-to-3′ direction, the ribosome translates its nucleotide sequence into an amino acid sequence, one codon at a time, using the tRNAs as adaptors. Each amino acid is thereby added in the correct sequence to the end of the growing polypeptide chain (Movie 7.7). When synthesis of the protein is finished, the two subunits of the ribosome separate. Ribosomes operate with remarkable efficiency: a eukaryotic ribosome adds about 2 amino acids to a polypeptide chain each second; a bacterial ribosome operates even faster, adding about 20 amino acids per second.

How does the ribosome choreograph all the movements required for translation? In addition to a binding site for an mRNA molecule, each ribosome contains three binding sites for tRNA molecules, called the A site, the P site, and the E site (Figure 7–36). To add an amino acid to a growing peptide chain, a charged tRNA enters the A site by base-pairing with the complementary codon on the mRNA molecule. Its amino acid is then linked to the growing peptide chain, which is held in place by the tRNA in the neighboring P site. Next, the large ribosomal subunit shifts forward, moving the spent tRNA to the E site before ejecting it (Figure 7–37). This cycle of reactions is repeated each time an amino acid is added to the polypeptide chain, with the new protein growing from its amino to its carboxyl end until a stop codon in the mRNA is encountered and the protein is released.

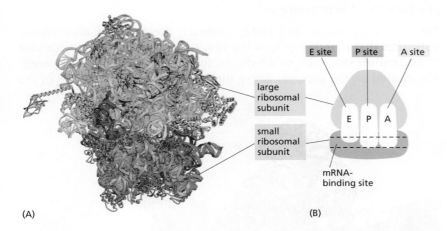

(A)   (B)

Figure 7–36 **Each ribosome has a binding site for an mRNA molecule and three binding sites for tRNAs.** The tRNA sites are designated the A, P, and E sites (short for aminoacyl-tRNA, peptidyl-tRNA, and exit, respectively). (A) Three-dimensional structure of a bacterial ribosome, as determined by x-ray crystallography, with the small subunit in *dark green* and the large subunit in *light green*. Both the rRNAs and the ribosomal proteins are shown in *green*. tRNAs are shown bound in the E site (*red*), the P site (*orange*), and the A site (*yellow*). Although all three of the tRNA sites shown here are filled, during protein synthesis only two of these sites are occupied by a tRNA at any one time (see Figure 7–37). (B) Highly schematized representation of a ribosome, in the same orientation as (A), which is used in subsequent figures. Note that both the large and small subunits are involved in forming the A, P, and E sites, while only the small subunit contains the binding site for an mRNA. (A, adapted from M.M. Yusupov et al., *Science* 292:883–896, 2001. Courtesy of Albion A. Bausom and Harry Noller.)

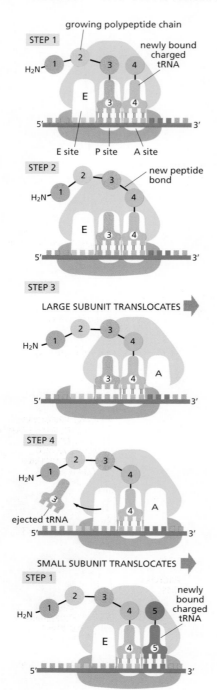

Figure 7–37 Translation takes place in a four-step cycle, which is repeated over and over during the synthesis of a protein. In *step 1*, a charged tRNA carrying the next amino acid to be added to the polypeptide chain binds to the vacant A site on the ribosome by forming base pairs with the mRNA codon that is exposed there. Only a matching tRNA molecule can base-pair with this codon, which determines the specific amino acid added. The A and P sites are sufficiently close together that their two tRNA molecules are forced to form base pairs with codons that are contiguous, with no stray bases in-between. This positioning of the tRNAs ensures that the correct reading frame will be preserved throughout the synthesis of the protein. In *step 2*, the carboxyl end of the polypeptide chain (amino acid 3 in step 1) is uncoupled from the tRNA at the P site and joined by a peptide bond to the free amino group of the amino acid linked to the tRNA at the A site. This reaction is carried out by a catalytic site in the large subunit. In *step 3*, a shift of the large subunit relative to the small subunit moves the two bound tRNAs into the E and P sites of the large subunit. In *step 4*, the small subunit moves exactly three nucleotides along the mRNA molecule, bringing it back to its original position relative to the large subunit. This movement ejects the spent tRNA and resets the ribosome with an empty A site so that the next charged tRNA molecule can bind (Movie 7.8).

As indicated, the mRNA is translated in the 5′-to-3′ direction, and the N-terminal end of a protein is made first, with each cycle adding one amino acid to the C-terminus of the polypeptide chain. To watch the translation cycle in atomic detail, see Movie 7.9.

The Ribosome Is a Ribozyme

The ribosome is one of the largest and most complex structures in the cell, composed of two-thirds RNA and one-third protein by weight. The determination of the entire three-dimensional structure of its large and small subunits in 2000 was a major triumph of modern biology. The structure confirmed earlier evidence that the rRNAs—not the proteins—are responsible for the ribosome's overall structure and its ability to choreograph and catalyze protein synthesis.

The rRNAs are folded into highly compact, precise three-dimensional structures that form the core of the ribosome (Figure 7–38). In contrast to the central positioning of the rRNAs, the ribosomal proteins are generally located on the surface, where they fill the gaps and crevices of the

Figure 7–38 Ribosomal RNAs give the ribosome its overall shape. Shown here are the detailed structures of the two rRNAs that form the core of the large subunit of a bacterial ribosome—the 23S rRNA (*blue*) and the 5S rRNA (*purple*). One of the protein subunits of the ribosome (L1) is included as a reference point, as this protein forms a characteristic protrusion on the ribosome surface. Ribosomal RNAs are commonly designated by their "S values," which refer to their rate of sedimentation in an ultracentrifuge. The larger the S value, the larger the size of the molecule. (Adapted from N. Ban et al., *Science* 289: 905–920, 2000.)

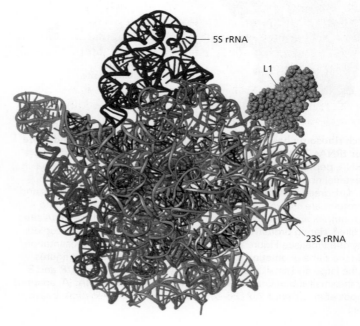

folded RNA. The main role of the ribosomal proteins seems to be to help fold and stabilize the RNA core, while permitting the changes in rRNA conformation that are necessary for this RNA to catalyze efficient protein synthesis.

Not only are the three tRNA-binding sites (the A, P, and E sites) on the ribosome formed primarily by the rRNAs, but the catalytic site for peptide bond formation is formed by the 23S rRNA of the large subunit; the nearest ribosomal protein is located too far away to make contact with the incoming amino acid or with the growing polypeptide chain. The catalytic site in this RNA—a peptidyl transferase—is similar in many respects to that found in some protein enzymes: it is a highly structured pocket that precisely orients the two reactants—the elongating polypeptide and the amino acid carried by the incoming tRNA—thereby greatly increasing the likelihood of a productive reaction.

RNA molecules that possess catalytic activity are called **ribozymes**. In the final section of this chapter, we will consider other ribozymes and discuss what the existence of RNA-based catalysis might mean for the early evolution of life on Earth. Here, we need only note that there is good reason to suspect that RNA rather than protein molecules served as the first catalysts for living cells. If so, the ribosome, with its catalytic RNA core, could be viewed as a relic of an earlier time in life's history, when cells were run almost entirely by RNAs.

Specific Codons in an mRNA Signal the Ribosome Where to Start and to Stop Protein Synthesis

In a test tube, ribosomes can be forced to translate any RNA molecule (see How We Know, pp. 246–247). In a cell, however, a specific start signal is required to initiate translation. The site at which protein synthesis begins on an mRNA is crucial, because it sets the reading frame for the entire message. An error of one nucleotide either way at this stage will cause every subsequent codon in the mRNA to be misread, resulting in a nonfunctional protein with a garbled sequence of amino acids (see Figure 7–28). Furthermore, the rate of initiation has a major impact on the overall rate at which the protein is synthesized from the mRNA.

The translation of an mRNA begins with the codon AUG, for which a special charged tRNA is required. This **initiator tRNA** always carries the amino acid methionine (or a modified form of methionine, formylmethionine, in bacteria). Thus newly made proteins all have methionine as the first amino acid at their N-terminal end, the end of a protein that is synthesized first. This methionine is usually removed later by a specific protease.

In eukaryotes, an initiator tRNA, charged with methionine, is first loaded into the P site of the small ribosomal subunit, along with additional proteins called **translation initiation factors** (Figure 7–39). The initiator tRNA is distinct from the tRNA that normally carries methionine. Of all the tRNAs in the cell, only a charged initiator tRNA molecule is capable of binding tightly to the P site in the absence of the large ribosomal subunit.

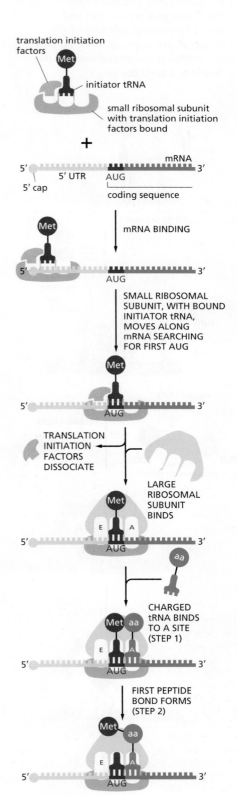

Figure 7–39 Initiation of protein synthesis in eukaryotes requires translation initiation factors and a special initiator tRNA. Although not shown here, efficient translation initiation also requires additional proteins that are bound at the 5′ cap and poly-A tail of the mRNA (see Figure 7–25). In this way, the translation apparatus can ascertain that both ends of the mRNA are intact before initiating translation. Following initiation, the protein is elongated by the reactions outlined in Figure 7–37.

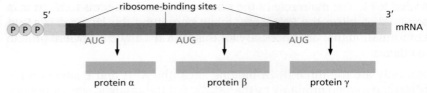

Figure 7–40 A single prokaryotic mRNA molecule can encode several different proteins. In prokaryotes, genes directing the different steps in a process are often organized into clusters (operons) that are transcribed together into a single mRNA. A prokaryotic mRNA does not have the same sort of 5′ cap as a eukaryotic mRNA, but instead has a triphosphate at its 5′ end. Prokaryotic ribosomes initiate translation at ribosome-binding sites (*dark blue*), which can be located in the interior of an mRNA molecule. This feature enables prokaryotes to simultaneously synthesize different proteins from a single mRNA molecule, with each protein made by a different ribosome.

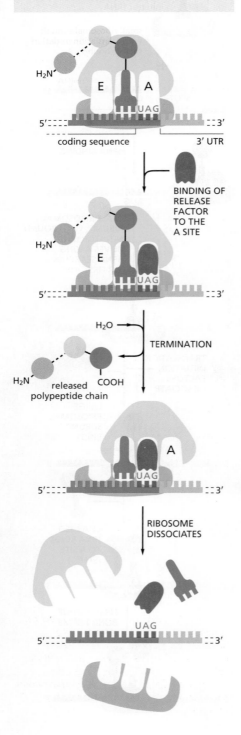

Next, the small ribosomal subunit loaded with the initiator tRNA binds to the 5′ end of an mRNA molecule, which is marked by the 5′ cap that is present on all eukaryotic mRNAs (see Figure 7–17). The small ribosomal subunit then scans the mRNA, in the 5′-to-3′ direction, until it encounters the first AUG. When this AUG is recognized by the initiator tRNA, several of the initiation factors dissociate from the small ribosomal subunit to make way for the large ribosomal subunit to bind and complete ribosomal assembly. Because the initiator tRNA is bound to the P site, protein synthesis is ready to begin with the addition of the next charged tRNA to the A site (see Figure 7–37).

The mechanism for selecting a start codon is different in bacteria. Bacterial mRNAs have no 5′ caps to tell the ribosome where to begin searching for the start of translation. Instead, each mRNA molecule contains a specific ribosome-binding sequence, approximately six nucleotides long, located a few nucleotides upstream of the AUG at which translation is to begin. Unlike a eukaryotic ribosome, a prokaryotic ribosome can readily bind directly to a start codon that lies in the interior of an mRNA, as long as a ribosome-binding site precedes it by several nucleotides. Such ribosome-binding sequences are necessary in bacteria, as prokaryotic mRNAs are often *polycistronic*—that is, they encode several different proteins on the same mRNA molecule; these transcripts contain a separate ribosome-binding site for each protein-coding sequence (**Figure 7–40**). In contrast, a eukaryotic mRNA usually carries the information for a single protein, and so it can rely on the 5′ cap—and the proteins that recognize it—to position the ribosome for its AUG search.

The end of translation in both prokaryotes and eukaryotes is signaled by the presence of one of several codons, called *stop codons*, in the mRNA (see Figure 7–27). The stop codons—UAA, UAG, and UGA—are not recognized by a tRNA and do not specify an amino acid, but instead signal to the ribosome to stop translation. Proteins known as *release factors* bind to any stop codon that reaches the A site on the ribosome; this binding alters the activity of the peptidyl transferase in the ribosome, causing it to catalyze the addition of a water molecule instead of an amino acid to the peptidyl-tRNA (**Figure 7–41**). This reaction frees the carboxyl end of the polypeptide chain from its attachment to a tRNA molecule; because this is the only attachment that holds the growing polypeptide to the

Figure 7–41 Translation halts at a stop codon. In the final phase of protein synthesis, the binding of release factor to an A site bearing a stop codon terminates translation of an mRNA molecule. The completed polypeptide is released, and the ribosome dissociates into its two separate subunits.

ribosome, the completed protein chain is immediately released. At this point, the ribosome also releases the mRNA and dissociates into its two separate subunits, which can then assemble on another mRNA molecule to begin a new round of protein synthesis.

Proteins Are Produced on Polyribosomes

The synthesis of most protein molecules takes between 20 seconds and several minutes. But even during this short period, multiple ribosomes usually bind to each mRNA molecule being translated. If an mRNA is being translated efficiently, a new ribosome will hop onto its 5′ end almost as soon as the preceding ribosome has translated enough of the nucleotide sequence to move out of the way. The mRNA molecules being translated are therefore usually found in the form of *polyribosomes*, also known as *polysomes*. These large cytosolic assemblies are made up of many ribosomes spaced as close as 80 nucleotides apart along a single mRNA molecule (Figure 7–42). With multiple ribosomes working simultaneously on a single mRNA, many more protein molecules can be made in a given time than would be possible if each polypeptide had to be completed before the next could be started.

Polysomes operate in both bacteria and eukaryotes, but bacteria can speed up the rate of protein synthesis even further. Because bacterial mRNA does not need to be processed and is also physically accessible to ribosomes while it is being synthesized, ribosomes will typically attach to the free end of a bacterial mRNA molecule and start translating it even before the transcription of that RNA is complete; these ribosomes follow closely behind the RNA polymerase as it moves along DNA.

Inhibitors of Prokaryotic Protein Synthesis Are Used as Antibiotics

The ability to translate mRNAs accurately into proteins is a fundamental feature of all life on Earth. Although the ribosome and other molecules that carry out this complex task are very similar among organisms, we have seen that there are some subtle differences in the way that bacteria and eukaryotes synthesize RNA and proteins. Although they represent a quirk of evolution, these differences form the basis of one of the most important advances in modern medicine.

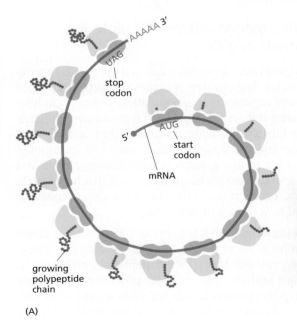

(A)

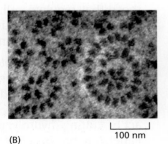

(B)

100 nm

Figure 7–42 Proteins are synthesized on polyribosomes. (A) Schematic drawing showing how a series of ribosomes can simultaneously translate the same mRNA molecule (Movie 7.10). (B) Electron micrograph of a polyribosome in the cytosol of a eukaryotic cell. (B, courtesy of John Heuser.)

TABLE 7–3 ANTIBIOTICS THAT INHIBIT BACTERIAL PROTEIN OR RNA SYNTHESIS	
Antibiotic	Specific Effect
Tetracycline	blocks binding of aminoacyl-tRNA to A site of ribosome (step 1 in Figure 7–37)
Streptomycin	prevents the transition from initiation complex to chain elongation (see Figure 7–39); also causes miscoding
Chloramphenicol	blocks the peptidyl transferase reaction on ribosomes (step 2 in Figure 7–37)
Cycloheximide	blocks the translocation step in translation (step 3 in Figure 7–37)
Rifamycin	blocks initiation of transcription by binding to and inhibiting RNA polymerase

Many of our most effective antibiotics are compounds that act by inhibiting bacterial, but not eukaryotic, gene expression. Some of these drugs exploit the small structural and functional differences between bacterial and eukaryotic ribosomes, so that they interfere preferentially with bacterial protein synthesis. These compounds can thus be taken in doses high enough to kill bacteria without being toxic to humans. Because different antibiotics bind to different regions of the bacterial ribosome, these drugs often inhibit different steps in protein synthesis. A few of the antibiotics that inhibit bacterial gene expression are listed in Table 7–3.

Many common antibiotics were first isolated from fungi. Fungi and bacteria often occupy the same ecological niches, and to gain a competitive edge, fungi have evolved, over time, potent toxins that kill bacteria but are harmless to themselves. Because fungi and humans are both eukaryotes, and are thus much more closely related to each other than either is to bacteria (see Figure 1–29), we have been able to borrow these weapons to combat our own bacterial foes. At the same time, bacteria have unfortunately evolved a resistance to many of these drugs, as we discuss in Chapter 9. Thus it remains a continual challenge for us to remain one step ahead of our microbial foes.

Controlled Protein Breakdown Helps Regulate the Amount of Each Protein in a Cell

After a protein is released from the ribosome, a cell can control its activity and longevity in various ways. The number of copies of a protein in a cell depends, like the number of organisms in a population, not only on how quickly new individuals arise but also on how long they survive. Proteins vary enormously in their lifespan. Structural proteins that become part of a relatively stable tissue such as bone or muscle may last for months or even years, whereas other proteins, such as metabolic enzymes and those that regulate cell growth and division (discussed in Chapter 18), last only for days, hours, or even seconds. But what determines the lifespan of a protein—and how does a protein "die"?

Cells produce many proteins whose job it is to break other proteins down into their constituent amino acids (a process termed *proteolysis*). These enzymes, which degrade proteins, first to short peptides and finally to individual amino acids, are known collectively as **proteases**. Proteases act by cutting (hydrolyzing) the peptide bonds between amino acids (see Panel 2–6, pp. 76–77). One function of proteolytic pathways is to rapidly degrade those proteins whose lifetime must be kept short. Another is to recognize and remove proteins that are damaged or misfolded. Eliminating improperly folded proteins is critical for an organism, as misfolded proteins tend to aggregate, and protein aggregates can damage cells and even trigger cell death. Eventually, all proteins—even long-lived ones—accumulate damage and are degraded by proteolysis. The amino acids produced by this proteolysis can then be re-used by the cell to make new proteins.

In eukaryotic cells, proteins are broken down by large protein machines called **proteasomes**, present in both the cytosol and the nucleus. A proteasome contains a central cylinder formed from proteases whose active sites face into an inner chamber. Each end of the cylinder is plugged by a large protein complex formed from at least 10 types of protein subunits (Figure 7–43). These stoppers bind the proteins destined for degradation and then—using ATP hydrolysis to fuel this activity—unfold the doomed proteins and thread them into the inner chamber of the cylinder. Once the proteins are inside, proteases chop them into short peptides, which are then jettisoned from either end of the proteasome. Housing proteases inside these molecular destruction chambers makes sense, as it prevents the enzymes from running rampant in the cell.

How do proteasomes select which proteins in the cell should be degraded? In eukaryotes, proteasomes act primarily on proteins that have been marked for destruction by the covalent attachment of a small protein called *ubiquitin*. Specialized enzymes tag those proteins that are destined for rapid degradation with a short chain of ubiquitin molecules; these ubiquitylated proteins are then recognized, unfolded, and fed into proteasomes by proteins within the stopper (Figure 7–44).

Proteins that are meant to be short-lived often contain a short amino acid sequence that identifies the protein as one to be ubiquitylated and degraded in proteasomes. Damaged or misfolded proteins, as well as proteins containing oxidized or otherwise abnormal amino acids, are also recognized and degraded by this ubiquitin-dependent proteolytic system. The enzymes that add a polyubiquitin chain to such proteins recognize signals that become exposed on these proteins as a result of the misfolding or chemical damage—for example, amino acid sequences or conformational motifs that are typically buried and inaccessible in a "healthy" protein.

There Are Many Steps Between DNA and Protein

We have seen that many steps are required to produce a functional protein from the information contained in a gene. In a eukaryotic cell, mRNAs must be synthesized, processed, and exported to the cytosol

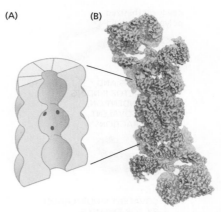

Figure 7–43 Proteins are degraded by the proteasome. The structures depicted here were determined by x-ray crystallography. (A) This drawing shows a cut-away view of the central cylinder of the proteasome, with the active sites of the proteases indicated by *red* dots. (B) The structure of the entire proteasome, in which access to the central cylinder (*yellow*) is regulated by a stopper (*blue*) at each end. (B, from P.C.A. da Fonseca et al., *Mol. Cell* 46:54–66, 2012. With permission from Elsevier.)

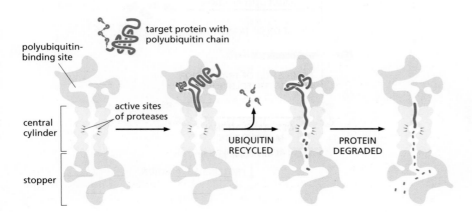

Figure 7–44 Proteins marked by a polyubiquitin chain are degraded by the proteasome. Proteins in the stopper of a proteasome (*blue*) recognize proteins marked by a specific type of polyubiquitin chain (*red*). The stopper unfolds the target protein and threads it into the proteasome's central cylinder (*yellow*), which is lined with proteases that chop the protein to pieces.

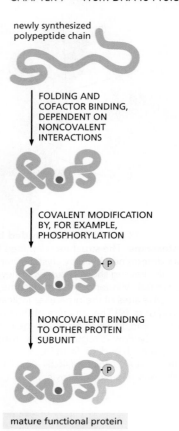

newly synthesized
polypeptide chain

FOLDING AND
COFACTOR BINDING,
DEPENDENT ON
NONCOVALENT
INTERACTIONS

COVALENT MODIFICATION
BY, FOR EXAMPLE,
PHOSPHORYLATION

NONCOVALENT BINDING
TO OTHER PROTEIN
SUBUNIT

mature functional protein

Figure 7–45 Many proteins require post-translational modifications to become fully functional. To be useful to the cell, a completed polypeptide must fold correctly into its three-dimensional conformation and then bind any required cofactors (*red*) and protein partners—all via noncovalent bonding. Many proteins also require one or more covalent modifications to become active—or to be recruited to specific membranes or organelles (not shown). Although phosphorylation and glycosylation are the most common, more than 100 types of covalent modifications of proteins are known.

Figure 7–46 Protein production in a eukaryotic cell requires many steps. The final concentration of each protein depends on the rate of each step depicted. Even after an mRNA and its corresponding protein have been produced, their concentrations can be regulated by degradation.

where they are translated to produce a protein. But the process does not end there. Proteins must then fold into the correct, three-dimensional shape (as we discuss in Chapter 4). Some proteins do so spontaneously, as they emerge from the ribosome. Most, however, require the assistance of *chaperone proteins*, which steer them along productive folding pathways and prevent them from aggregating inside the cell (see Figures 4–8 and 4–9).

In addition to folding properly, many proteins—once they leave the ribosome—require further adjustments before they are useful to the cell. As we discussed in Chapter 4, some proteins are covalently modified—for example, by phosphorylation or glycosylation. Others bind to small-molecule cofactors or associate with additional protein subunits. Such *post-translational modifications* are often needed for a newly synthesized protein to become fully functional (**Figure 7–45**). The final concentration of a protein, therefore, depends on the rate at which each of these steps—from DNA to mature, functional protein—is carried out (**Figure 7–46**).

In principle, any one of these steps can be controlled by cells as they adjust the concentrations of their proteins to suit their needs. However,

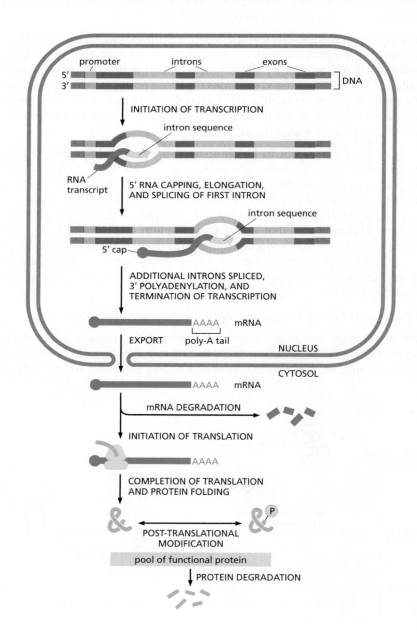

promoter   introns   exons

5′
3′   DNA

INITIATION OF TRANSCRIPTION

intron sequence

RNA
transcript   5′ RNA CAPPING, ELONGATION,
AND SPLICING OF FIRST INTRON

intron sequence

5′ cap

ADDITIONAL INTRONS SPLICED,
3′ POLYADENYLATION, AND
TERMINATION OF TRANSCRIPTION

AAAA   mRNA

EXPORT   poly-A tail

NUCLEUS

CYTOSOL

AAAA   mRNA

mRNA DEGRADATION

INITIATION OF TRANSLATION

AAAA

COMPLETION OF TRANSLATION
AND PROTEIN FOLDING

POST-TRANSLATIONAL
MODIFICATION

pool of functional protein

PROTEIN DEGRADATION

as we will discuss thoroughly in the next chapter, the initiation of transcription is the most common point for a cell to regulate the expression of its genes.

RNA AND THE ORIGINS OF LIFE

The central dogma—that DNA makes RNA, which makes protein—presented evolutionary biologists with a knotty puzzle: if nucleic acids are required to direct the synthesis of proteins, and proteins are required to synthesize nucleic acids, how could this system of interdependent components have arisen? The prevailing view is that an **RNA world** existed on Earth before cells containing DNA and proteins appeared. According to this hypothesis, RNA—which today serves largely as an intermediate between genes and proteins—both stored genetic information and catalyzed chemical reactions in primitive cells. Only later in evolutionary time did DNA take over as the genetic material and proteins become the major catalysts and structural components of cells (**Figure 7–47**). As we have seen, RNA still catalyzes several fundamental reactions in modern cells, including protein synthesis and RNA splicing. These ribozymes are like molecular fossils, holdovers from an earlier RNA world.

Life Requires Autocatalysis

The origin of life requires molecules that possess, if only to a small extent, one crucial property: the ability to catalyze reactions that lead—directly or indirectly—to the production of more molecules like themselves. Catalysts with this self-reproducing property, once they had arisen by chance, would divert raw materials from the production of other substances to make more of themselves. In this way, one can envisage the gradual development of an increasingly complex chemical system of organic monomers and polymers that function together to generate more molecules of the same types, fueled by a supply of simple raw materials in the primitive environment on Earth. Such an *autocatalytic* system would have many of the properties we think of as characteristic of living matter: the system would contain a far-from-random selection of interacting molecules; it would tend to reproduce itself; it would compete with other systems dependent on the same raw materials; and, if deprived of its raw materials or maintained at a temperature that upset the balance of reaction rates, it would decay toward chemical equilibrium and "die."

But what molecules could have had such autocatalytic properties? In present-day living cells, the most versatile catalysts are proteins, which are able to adopt diverse three-dimensional forms that bristle with chemically reactive sites on their surface. However, there is no known way in which a protein can reproduce itself directly. RNA molecules, by contrast, possess properties that—at least, in principle—could be exploited to catalyze their own synthesis.

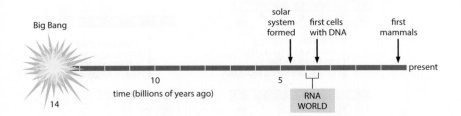

Figure 7–47 An RNA world may have existed before modern cells arose.

RNA Can Store Information and Catalyze Chemical Reactions

We have seen that complementary base-pairing enables one nucleic acid to act as a template for the formation of another. Thus a single strand of RNA or DNA contains the information needed to specify the sequence of a complementary polynucleotide, which, in turn, can specify the sequence of the original molecule, allowing the original nucleic acid to be replicated (Figure 7–48). Such complementary templating mechanisms lie at the heart of both DNA replication and transcription in modern-day cells.

But the efficient synthesis of polynucleotides by such complementary templating mechanisms also requires catalysts to promote the polymerization reaction: without catalysts, polymer formation is slow, error-prone, and inefficient. Today, nucleotide polymerization is catalyzed by protein enzymes—such as DNA and RNA polymerases. But how could this reaction be catalyzed before proteins with the appropriate catalytic ability existed? The beginnings of an answer were obtained in 1982, when it was discovered that RNA molecules themselves can act as catalysts.

In present-day cells, RNA is synthesized as a single-stranded molecule, and we have seen that complementary base-pairing can occur between nucleotides in the same chain. This base-pairing, along with nonconventional hydrogen bonds, can cause each RNA molecule to fold up in a unique way that is determined by its nucleotide sequence (see Figure 7–5). Such associations produce complex three-dimensional shapes.

Protein enzymes are able to catalyze biochemical reactions because they have surfaces with unique contours and chemical properties, as we discuss in Chapter 4. In the same way, RNA molecules, with their unique folded shapes, can serve as catalysts (Figure 7–49). Catalytic RNAs do not have the same structural and functional diversity as do protein enzymes; they are, after all, built from only four different subunits. Nonetheless, ribozymes can catalyze many types of chemical reactions. Although relatively few catalytic RNAs operate in present-day cells, they play major roles in some of the most fundamental steps in the expression of genetic information—specifically those steps where RNA molecules themselves are spliced or translated into protein. Additional ribozymes, with other catalytic capabilities, have been generated in the laboratory and selected for their activity in a test tube (Table 7–4).

RNA, therefore, has all the properties required of an information-containing molecule that could also catalyze its own synthesis (Figure 7–50). Although self-replicating systems of RNA molecules have not been found in nature, scientists appear to be well on the way to constructing them in the laboratory. This achievement would not prove that self-replicating RNA molecules were essential to the origin of life on Earth, but it would demonstrate that such a scenario is possible.

Figure 7–48 An RNA molecule can in principle guide the formation of an exact copy of itself. In the first step, the original RNA molecule acts as a template to produce an RNA molecule of complementary sequence. In the second step, this complementary RNA molecule itself acts as a template to produce an RNA molecule of the original sequence. Since each template molecule can produce many copies of the complementary strand, these reactions can result in the amplification of the original sequence.

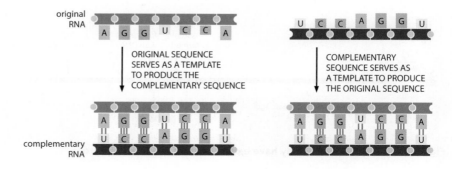

TABLE 7–4 BIOCHEMICAL REACTIONS THAT CAN BE CATALYZED BY RIBOZYMES

Activity	Ribozymes
Peptide bond formation in protein synthesis	ribosomal RNA
RNA splicing	small nuclear RNAs (snRNAs), self-splicing RNAs
DNA ligation	*in vitro* selected RNA
RNA polymerization	*in vitro* selected RNA
RNA phosphorylation	*in vitro* selected RNA
RNA aminoacylation	*in vitro* selected RNA
RNA alkylation	*in vitro* selected RNA
C–C bond rotation (isomerization)	*in vitro* selected RNA

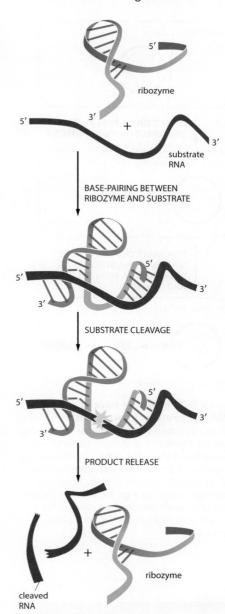

Figure 7–49 A ribozyme is an RNA molecule that possesses catalytic activity. The RNA molecule shown catalyzes the cleavage of a second RNA at a specific site. Such ribozymes are found embedded in large RNA genomes—called viroids— that infect plants, where the cleavage reaction is one step in the replication of the viroid. (Adapted from T.R. Cech and O.C. Uhlenbeck, *Nature* 372:39–40, 1994. With permission from Macmillan Publishers Ltd.)

RNA Is Thought to Predate DNA in Evolution

If the evolutionary role for RNA proposed above is correct, the first cells on Earth would have stored their genetic information in RNA rather than DNA. And based on the chemical differences between these polynucleotides, it appears that RNA could indeed have arisen before DNA. Ribose (see Figure 7–3A), like glucose and other simple carbohydrates, is readily formed from formaldehyde (HCHO), which is one of the principal products of experiments simulating conditions on the primitive Earth. The sugar deoxyribose is harder to make, and in present-day cells it is produced from ribose in a reaction catalyzed by a protein enzyme, suggesting that ribose predates deoxyribose in cells. Presumably, DNA appeared on the scene after RNA, and then proved better suited than RNA as a permanent repository of genetic information. In particular, the deoxyribose in its sugar–phosphate backbone makes chains of DNA chemically much more stable than chains of RNA, so that DNA can grow to greater lengths without breakage.

The other differences between RNA and DNA—the double-helical structure of DNA and the use of thymine rather than uracil—further enhance DNA stability by making the molecule easier to repair. We saw in Chapter 6 that a damaged nucleotide on one strand of the double helix can be repaired by using the other strand as a template. Furthermore, deamination, one of the most common detrimental chemical changes occurring

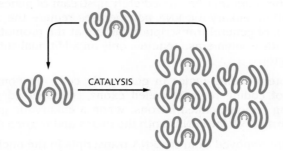

CATALYSIS

Figure 7–50 Could an RNA molecule catalyze its own synthesis? The process would require that the RNA catalyze the self-templated amplification steps shown in Figure 7–48. The *red* rays represent the active site of this hypothetical ribozyme.

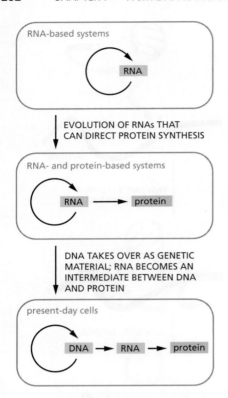

Figure 7–51 RNA may have preceded DNA and proteins in evolution. According to this hypothesis, RNA molecules provided genetic, structural, and catalytic functions in the earliest cells. DNA is now the repository of genetic information, and proteins carry out almost all catalysis in cells. RNA now functions mainly as a go-between in protein synthesis, while remaining a catalyst for a few crucial reactions (including protein synthesis).

QUESTION 7–6

Discuss the following: "During the evolution of life on Earth, RNA lost its glorious position as the first self-replicating catalyst. Its role now is as a mere messenger in the information flow from DNA to protein."

in polynucleotides, is easier to detect and repair in DNA than in RNA (see Figure 6–24). This is because the product of the deamination of cytosine is, by chance, uracil, which already exists in RNA, so that such damage would be impossible for repair enzymes to detect in an RNA molecule. However, in DNA, which has thymine rather than uracil, any uracil produced by the accidental deamination of cytosine is easily detected and repaired.

Taken together, the evidence we have discussed supports the idea that RNA—with its ability to provide genetic, structural, and catalytic functions—preceded DNA in evolution. As cells more closely resembling present-day cells appeared, it is believed that RNAs were relieved of many of the duties they had originally performed: DNA took over the primary storage of genetic information, and proteins became the major catalysts, while RNA remained primarily as the intermediary connecting the two (**Figure 7–51**). With the rise of DNA, cells were able to become more complex, for they could then carry and transmit more genetic information than could be stably maintained by RNA alone. Because of the greater chemical complexity of proteins and the variety of chemical reactions they can catalyze, the shift from RNA to proteins (albeit incomplete) also provided a much richer source of structural components and enzymes, enabling cells to evolve the great diversity of appearance and function that we see today.

ESSENTIAL CONCEPTS

- The flow of genetic information in all living cells is DNA → RNA → protein. The conversion of the genetic instructions in DNA into RNAs and proteins is termed gene expression.

- To express the genetic information carried in DNA, the nucleotide sequence of a gene is first transcribed into RNA. Transcription is catalyzed by the enzyme RNA polymerase, which uses nucleotide sequences in the DNA molecule to determine which strand to use as a template, and where to start and stop transcribing.

- RNA differs in several respects from DNA. It contains the sugar ribose instead of deoxyribose and the base uracil (U) instead of thymine (T). RNAs in cells are synthesized as single-stranded molecules, which often fold up into complex three-dimensional shapes.

- Cells make several functional types of RNAs, including messenger RNAs (mRNAs), which carry the instructions for making proteins; ribosomal RNAs (rRNAs), which are the crucial components of ribosomes; and transfer RNAs (tRNAs), which act as adaptor molecules in protein synthesis.

- To begin transcription, RNA polymerase binds to specific DNA sites called promoters that lie immediately upstream of genes. To initiate transcription, eukaryotic RNA polymerases require the assembly of a complex of general transcription factors at the promoter, whereas bacterial RNA polymerase requires only an additional subunit, called sigma factor.

- Most protein-coding genes in eukaryotic cells are composed of a number of coding regions, called exons, interspersed with larger, noncoding regions, called introns. When a eukaryotic gene is transcribed from DNA into RNA, both the exons and introns are copied.

- Introns are removed from the RNA transcripts in the nucleus by RNA splicing, a reaction catalyzed by small ribonucleoprotein complexes known as snRNPs. Splicing removes the introns from the RNA and joins together the exons—often in a variety of combinations, allowing multiple proteins to be produced from the same gene.

- Eukaryotic pre-mRNAs go through several additional RNA processing steps before they leave the nucleus as mRNAs, including 5' RNA capping and 3' polyadenylation. These reactions, along with splicing, take place as the pre-mRNA is being transcribed.

- Translation of the nucleotide sequence of an mRNA into a protein takes place in the cytoplasm on large ribonucleoprotein assemblies called ribosomes. As the mRNA moves through the ribosome, its message is translated into protein.

- The nucleotide sequence in mRNA is read in consecutive sets of three nucleotides called codons; each codon corresponds to one amino acid.

- The correspondence between amino acids and codons is specified by the genetic code. The possible combinations of the 4 different nucleotides in RNA give 64 different codons in the genetic code. Most amino acids are specified by more than one codon.

- tRNAs act as adaptor molecules in protein synthesis. Enzymes called aminoacyl-tRNA synthetases covalently link amino acids to their appropriate tRNAs. Each tRNA contains a sequence of three nucleotides, the anticodon, which recognizes a codon in an mRNA through complementary base-pairing.

- Protein synthesis begins when a ribosome assembles at an initiation codon (AUG) in an mRNA molecule, a process that depends on proteins called translation initiation factors. The completed protein chain is released from the ribosome when a stop codon (UAA, UAG, or UGA) in the mRNA is reached.

- The stepwise linking of amino acids into a polypeptide chain is catalyzed by an rRNA molecule in the large ribosomal subunit, which thus acts as a ribozyme.

- The concentration of a protein in a cell depends on the rates at which the mRNA and protein are synthesized and degraded. Protein degradation in the cytosol and nucleus occurs inside large protein complexes called proteasomes.

- From our knowledge of present-day organisms and the molecules they contain, it seems likely that life on Earth began with the evolution of RNA molecules that could catalyze their own replication.

- It has been proposed that RNA served as both the genome and the catalysts in the first cells, before DNA replaced RNA as a more stable molecule for storing genetic information, and proteins replaced RNAs as the major catalytic and structural components. RNA catalysts in modern cells are thought to provide a glimpse into an ancient, RNA-based world.

KEY TERMS

alternative splicing	messenger RNA (mRNA)	RNA polymerase
aminoacyl-tRNA synthetase	polyadenylation	RNA processing
anticodon	promoter	RNA splicing
codon	protease	RNA transcript
exon	proteasome	RNA world
gene	reading frame	small nuclear RNA (snRNA)
gene expression	ribosomal RNA (rRNA)	spliceosome
general transcription factors	ribosome	transcription
genetic code	ribozyme	transfer RNA (tRNA)
initiator tRNA	RNA	translation
intron	RNA capping	translation initiation factor

QUESTIONS

QUESTION 7–7

Which of the following statements are correct? Explain your answers.

A. An individual ribosome can make only one type of protein.

B. All mRNAs fold into particular three-dimensional structures that are required for their translation.

C. The large and small subunits of an individual ribosome always stay together and never exchange partners.

D. Ribosomes are cytoplasmic organelles that are encapsulated by a single membrane.

E. Because the two strands of DNA are complementary, the mRNA of a given gene can be synthesized using either strand as a template.

F. An mRNA may contain the sequence
ATTGACCCCGGTCAA.

G. The amount of a protein present in a cell depends on its rate of synthesis, its catalytic activity, and its rate of degradation.

QUESTION 7–8

The Lacheinmal protein is a hypothetical protein that causes people to smile more often. It is inactive in many chronically unhappy people. The mRNA isolated from a number of different unhappy individuals in the same family was found to lack an internal stretch of 173 nucleotides that is present in the Lacheinmal mRNA isolated from happy members of the same family. The DNA sequences of the *Lacheinmal* genes from the happy and unhappy family members were determined and compared. They differed by a single nucleotide substitution, which lay in an intron. What can you say about the molecular basis of unhappiness in this family?

(Hints: [1] Can you hypothesize a molecular mechanism by which a single nucleotide substitution in a gene could cause the observed deletion in the mRNA? Note that the deletion is *internal* to the mRNA. [2] Assuming the 173-base-pair deletion removes coding sequences from the Lacheinmal mRNA, how would the Lacheinmal protein differ between the happy and unhappy people?)

QUESTION 7–9

Use the genetic code shown in Figure 7–27 to identify which of the following nucleotide sequences would code for the polypeptide sequence arginine-glycine-aspartate:

1. 5′-AGA–GGA–GAU-3′

2. 5′-ACA–CCC–ACU-3′

3. 5′-GGG–AAA–UUU-3′

4. 5′-CGG–GGU–GAC-3′

QUESTION 7–10

"The bonds that form between the anticodon of a tRNA molecule and the three nucleotides of a codon in mRNA are _____." Complete this sentence with each of the following options and explain whether each of the resulting statements is correct or incorrect.

A. covalent bonds formed by GTP hydrolysis

B. hydrogen bonds that form when the tRNA is at the A site

C. broken by the translocation of the ribosome along the mRNA

QUESTION 7–11

List the ordinary, dictionary definitions of the terms *replication*, *transcription*, and *translation*. By their side, list the special meaning each term has when applied to the living cell.

QUESTION 7–12

In an alien world, the genetic code is written in pairs of nucleotides. How many amino acids could such a code specify? In a different world, a triplet code is used, but the order of nucleotides is not important; it only matters which nucleotides are present. How many amino acids could this code specify? Would you expect to encounter any problems translating these codes?

QUESTION 7–13

One remarkable feature of the genetic code is that amino acids with similar chemical properties often have similar codons. Thus codons with U or C as the second nucleotide tend to specify hydrophobic amino acids. Can you suggest a possible explanation for this phenomenon in terms of the early evolution of the protein-synthesis machinery?

QUESTION 7–14

A mutation in DNA generates a UGA stop codon in the middle of the mRNA coding for a particular protein. A second mutation in the cell's DNA leads to a single nucleotide change in a tRNA that allows the correct translation of this protein; that is, the second mutation "suppresses" the defect caused by the first. The altered tRNA translates the UGA as tryptophan. What nucleotide change has probably occurred in the mutant tRNA molecule? What consequences would the presence of such a mutant tRNA have for the translation of the normal genes in this cell?

QUESTION 7–15

The charging of a tRNA with an amino acid can be represented by the following equation:

amino acid + tRNA + ATP → aminoacyl-tRNA + AMP + PP$_i$

where PP$_i$ is pyrophosphate (see Figure 3–41). In the aminoacyl-tRNA, the amino acid and tRNA are linked with a high-energy covalent bond; a large portion of the energy derived from the hydrolysis of ATP is thus stored in this bond and is available to drive peptide bond formation during the later stages of protein synthesis. The free-energy change of the charging reaction shown in the equation is close to zero and therefore would not be expected to favor attachment of the amino acid to tRNA. Can you suggest a further step that could drive the reaction to completion?

QUESTION 7–16

A. The average molecular weight of a protein in the cell is about 30,000 daltons. A few proteins, however, are much larger. The largest known polypeptide chain made by any cell is a protein called titin (made by mammalian muscle cells), and it has a molecular weight of 3,000,000 daltons. Estimate how long it will take a muscle cell to translate an mRNA coding for titin (assume the average molecular weight of an amino acid to be 120, and a translation rate of two amino acids per second for eukaryotic cells).

B. Protein synthesis is very accurate: for every 10,000 amino acids joined together, only one mistake is made. What is the fraction of average-sized protein molecules and of titin molecules that are synthesized without any errors? [Hint: the probability P of obtaining an error-free protein is given by $P = (1 - E)^n$, where E is the error frequency and n the number of amino acids.]

C. The combined molecular weight of the eukaryotic ribosomal proteins is about 2.5×10^6 daltons. Would it be advantageous to synthesize them as a single protein?

D. Transcription occurs at a rate of about 30 nucleotides per second. Is it possible to calculate the time required to synthesize a titin mRNA from the information given here?

QUESTION 7–17

Which of the following types of mutations would be predicted to harm an organism? Explain your answers.

A. Insertion of a single nucleotide near the end of the coding sequence.

B. Removal of a single nucleotide near the beginning of the coding sequence.

C. Deletion of three consecutive nucleotides in the middle of the coding sequence.

D. Deletion of four consecutive nucleotides in the middle of the coding sequence.

E. Substitution of one nucleotide for another in the middle of the coding sequence.

QUESTION 7–18

Figure 7–8 shows many molecules of RNA polymerase simultaneously transcribing two adjacent genes on a single DNA molecule. Looking at this figure, label the 5′ and 3′ ends of the DNA template strand and the sets of RNA molecules being transcribed.

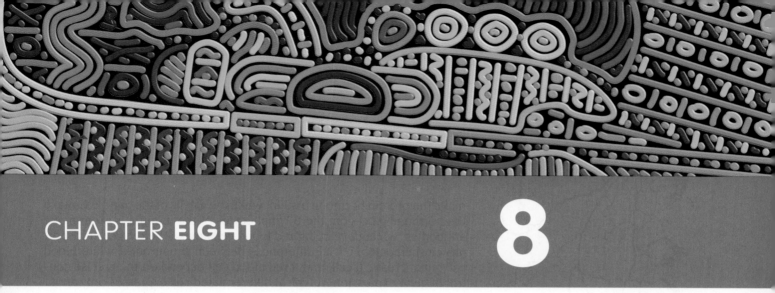

Control of Gene Expression

An organism's DNA encodes all of the RNA and protein molecules that are needed to make its cells. Yet a complete description of the DNA sequence of an organism—be it the few million nucleotides of a bacterium or the few billion nucleotides in each human cell—does not enable us to reconstruct that organism any more than a list of all the English words in a dictionary enables us to reconstruct a Shakespeare play. We need to know how the elements in the DNA sequence or the words on a list work together to produce the masterpiece.

For cells, the answer comes down to *gene expression*. Even the simplest single-celled bacterium can use its genes selectively—for example, switching genes on and off to make the enzymes needed to digest whatever food sources are available. In multicellular plants and animals, gene expression is even more elaborate. Over the course of embryonic development, a fertilized egg cell gives rise to many cell types that differ dramatically in both structure and function. The differences between an information-processing nerve cell and toxin-neutralizing liver cell, for example, are so extreme that it is difficult to imagine that the two cells contain the same DNA (**Figure 8–1**). For this reason, and because cells in an adult organism rarely lose their distinctive characteristics, biologists originally suspected that certain genes might be selectively eliminated from cells as they become specialized. We now know, however, that nearly all the cells of a multicellular organism contain the same genome. Cell *differentiation* is instead achieved by changes in gene expression.

In mammals, hundreds of different cell types carry out a range of specialized functions that depend upon genes that are switched on in that cell type but not in most others: for example, the β cells of the pancreas

AN OVERVIEW OF GENE EXPRESSION

HOW TRANSCRIPTION IS REGULATED

GENERATING SPECIALIZED CELL TYPES

POST-TRANSCRIPTIONAL CONTROLS

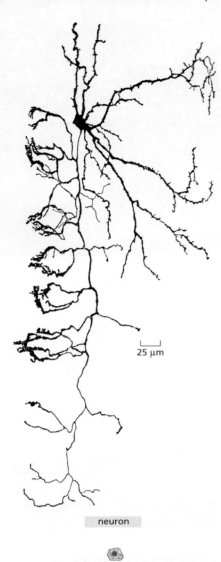

neuron

liver cell

Figure 8–1 A neuron and a liver cell share the same genome.
The long branches of this neuron from the retina enable it to receive electrical signals from numerous other neurons and pass these signals along to many neighboring neurons. The liver cell, which is drawn to the same scale, is involved in many metabolic processes, including digestion and the detoxification of alcohol and other drugs. Both of these mammalian cells contain the same genome, but they express different RNAs and proteins. (Neuron adapted from S. Ramón y Cajal, Histologie du Système Nerveux de l'Homme et de Vertébrés, 1909–1911. Paris: Maloine; reprinted, Madrid: C.S.I.C., 1972.)

make the protein hormone insulin, while the α cells of the pancreas make the hormone glucagon; the B lymphocytes of the immune system make antibodies, while developing red blood cells make the oxygen-transport protein hemoglobin. The differences between a neuron, a white blood cell, a pancreatic β cell, and a red blood cell depend on the precise control of gene expression. A typical differentiated cell expresses only about half the genes in its total repertoire. This selection, which differs from one cell type to the next, is the basis for the specialized properties of each cell type.

In this chapter, we discuss the main ways in which gene expression is regulated, with a focus on those genes that encode proteins as their final product. Although some of these control mechanisms apply to both eukaryotes and prokaryotes, eukaryotic cells—with their larger number of genes and more complex chromosomes—have some additional ways of controlling gene expression that are not found in bacteria.

AN OVERVIEW OF GENE EXPRESSION

Gene expression is a complex process by which cells selectively direct the synthesis of the many thousands of proteins and RNAs encoded in their genome. But how do cells coordinate and control such an intricate process—and how does an individual cell specify which of its genes to express? This decision is an especially important problem for animals because, as they develop, their cells become highly specialized, ultimately producing an array of muscle, nerve, and blood cells, along with the hundreds of other cell types seen in the adult. Such cell **differentiation** arises because cells make and accumulate different sets of RNA and protein molecules: that is, they express different genes.

The Different Cell Types of a Multicellular Organism Contain the Same DNA

The evidence that cells have the ability to change which genes they express without altering the nucleotide sequence of their DNA comes from experiments in which the genome from a differentiated cell is made to direct the development of a complete organism. If the chromosomes of the differentiated cell were altered irreversibly during development—for example, by jettisoning some of their genes—they would not be able to accomplish this feat.

Consider, for example, an experiment in which the nucleus is taken from a skin cell in an adult frog and injected into a frog egg from which the nucleus has been removed. In at least some cases, that doctored egg will develop into a normal tadpole (**Figure 8–2**). Thus, the nucleus from the transplanted skin cell cannot have lost any critical DNA sequences. Nuclear transplantation experiments carried out with differentiated cells taken from adult mammals—including sheep, cows, pigs, goats, and mice—have shown similar results. And in plants, individual cells removed from a carrot, for example, can regenerate an entire adult carrot plant.

25 µm

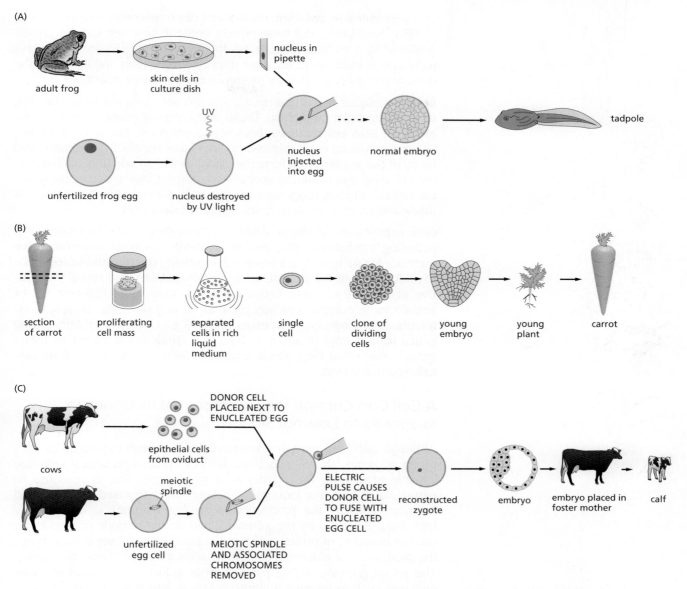

Figure 8–2 Differentiated cells contain all the genetic instructions needed to direct the formation of a complete organism. (A) The nucleus of a skin cell from an adult frog transplanted into an "enucleated" egg—one whose nucleus has been destroyed—can give rise to an entire tadpole. The broken arrow indicates that to give the transplanted genome time to adjust to an embryonic environment, a further transfer step is required in which one of the nuclei is taken from the early embryo that begins to develop and is put back into a second enucleated egg. (B) In many types of plants, differentiated cells retain the ability to "de-differentiate," so that a single cell can proliferate to form a clone of progeny cells that later give rise to an entire plant. (C) A nucleus removed from a differentiated cell of an adult cow can be introduced into an enucleated egg from a different cow to give rise to a calf. Different calves produced from the same differentiated cell donor are all clones of the donor and are therefore genetically identical. The cloned sheep Dolly was produced by this type of nuclear transplantation. (A, modified from J.B. Gurdon, *Sci. Am.* 219:24–35, 1968.)

These experiments all demonstrate that the DNA in specialized cell types of multicellular organisms still contains the entire set of instructions needed to form a whole organism. The various cell types of an organism therefore differ not because they contain different genes, but because they express them differently.

Different Cell Types Produce Different Sets of Proteins

The extent of the differences in gene expression between different cell types may be roughly gauged by comparing the protein composition of cells in liver, heart, brain, and so on. In the past, such analysis was performed by two-dimensional gel electrophoresis (see Panel 4–5, p. 167). Nowadays, the total protein content of a cell can be rapidly analyzed by a method called mass spectrometry (see Figure 4–56). This technique is much more sensitive than electrophoresis and it enables the detection of proteins that are produced even in minor quantities.

Both techniques reveal that many proteins are common to all the cells of a multicellular organism. These *housekeeping* proteins include, for example, RNA polymerases, DNA repair enzymes, ribosomal proteins, enzymes involved in glycolysis and other basic metabolic processes, and many of the proteins that form the cytoskeleton. In addition, each different cell type also produces specialized proteins that are responsible for the cell's distinctive properties. In mammals, for example, hemoglobin is made almost exclusively in developing red blood cells.

Gene expression can also be studied by cataloging a cell's RNA molecules, including the mRNAs that encode protein. The most comprehensive methods for such analyses involve determining the nucleotide sequence of all RNAs made by the cell, an approach that can also reveal the relative abundance of each. Estimates of the number of different mRNA sequences in human cells suggest that, at any one time, a typical differentiated human cell expresses perhaps 5000–15,000 protein-coding genes from a total of about 19,000. And studies of a variety of tissue types confirm that the collection of expressed mRNAs differs from one cell type to the next.

A Cell Can Change the Expression of Its Genes in Response to External Signals

Although each cell type in a multicellular organism expresses its own group of genes, these collections are not static. Specialized cells are capable of altering their patterns of gene expression in response to extracellular cues. For example, if a liver cell is exposed to the steroid hormone cortisol, the production of several proteins is dramatically increased. Released by the adrenal gland during periods of starvation, intense exercise, or prolonged stress, cortisol signals liver cells to boost the production of glucose from amino acids and other small molecules. The set of proteins whose production is induced by cortisol includes enzymes such as tyrosine aminotransferase, which helps convert tyrosine to glucose. When the hormone is no longer present, the production of these proteins returns to its resting level.

Other cell types respond to cortisol differently. In fat cells, for example, the production of tyrosine aminotransferase is reduced; some other cell types do not respond to cortisol at all. The fact that different cell types often respond in different ways to the same extracellular signal contributes to the specialization that gives each cell type its distinctive character.

Gene Expression Can Be Regulated at Various Steps from DNA to RNA to Protein

If differences among the various cell types of an organism depend on the particular genes that each cell expresses, at what level is this control of gene expression exercised? As we discussed in the previous chapter, there are many steps in the pathway leading from DNA to protein, and each of them can in principle be regulated. Thus a cell can control the proteins it contains by (1) controlling when and how often a given gene is transcribed, (2) controlling how an RNA transcript is spliced or otherwise processed, (3) selecting which mRNAs are exported from the nucleus to the cytosol, (4) regulating how quickly certain mRNA molecules are

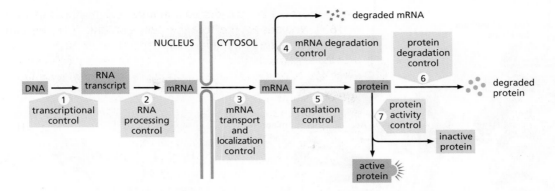

degraded, (5) selecting which mRNAs are translated into protein by ribosomes, or (6) regulating how rapidly specific proteins are destroyed after they have been made; in addition, the activity of individual proteins, once they have been synthesized, can be further regulated in a variety of ways.

In eukaryotic cells, gene expression can be regulated at each of these steps (Figure 8–3). For most genes, however, the control of transcription (shown in step 1) is paramount. This makes sense because only transcriptional control can ensure that no unnecessary intermediates are synthesized. Thus it is the regulation of transcription—and the DNA and protein components that determine which genes a cell transcribes into RNA—that we address first.

Figure 8–3 Gene expression in eukaryotic cells can be controlled at various steps. Examples of regulation at each of these steps are known, although for most genes the main site of control is step 1: transcription of a DNA sequence into RNA.

HOW TRANSCRIPTION IS REGULATED

Until 50 years ago, the idea that genes could be switched on and off was revolutionary. This concept was a major advance, and it came originally from studies of how *E. coli* bacteria adapt to changes in the composition of their growth medium. Many of the same principles apply to eukaryotic cells. However, the enormous complexity of gene regulation in organisms that possess a nucleus, combined with the packaging of their DNA into chromatin, creates special challenges and some novel opportunities for control—as we will see. We begin with a discussion of the *transcription regulators* (often loosely referred to as transcription factors), proteins that bind to specific DNA sequences and control gene transcription.

Transcription Regulators Bind to Regulatory DNA Sequences

Nearly all genes, whether bacterial or eukaryotic, contain sequences that direct and control their transcription. In Chapter 7, we saw that the **promoter** region of a gene binds the enzyme *RNA polymerase* and correctly orients the enzyme to begin its task of making an RNA copy of the gene. The promoters of both bacterial and eukaryotic genes include a *transcription initiation site*, where RNA synthesis begins, plus nearby sequences that contain recognition sites for proteins that associate with RNA polymerase: sigma factor in bacteria (see Figure 7–9) or the general transcription factors in eukaryotes (see Figure 7–12).

In addition to the promoter, the vast majority of genes include **regulatory DNA sequences** that are used to switch the gene on or off. Some regulatory DNA sequences are as short as 10 nucleotide pairs and act as simple switches that respond to a single signal; such simple regulatory switches predominate in bacteria. Other regulatory DNA sequences, especially those in eukaryotes, are very long (sometimes spanning more than 100,000 nucleotide pairs) and act as molecular microprocessors,

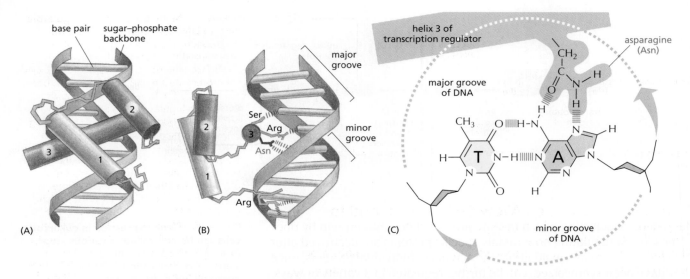

Figure 8–4 A transcription regulator interacts with the DNA double helix. (A) The regulator shown recognizes DNA via three α helices, drawn as numbered cylinders, which allow the protein to fit into the major groove and form tight associations with the base pairs in a short stretch of DNA. This particular structural motif, called a *homeodomain*, is found in many eukaryotic DNA-binding proteins (Movie 8.1). (B) Most of the contacts with the DNA bases are made by helix 3 (*red*), which is shown here end-on. (C) An asparagine side chain from helix 3 forms two hydrogen bonds with the adenine in an A-T base pair. The view is end-on, looking down the center of the DNA double helix, and the protein contacts the base pair from the major-groove side. Note that the interactions between the protein and DNA take place along the edges of the nucleotide base and do not disrupt the hydrogen bonds that hold the base pairs together. For simplicity, only one amino acid–base contact is shown; in reality, transcription regulators form hydrogen bonds (as shown here), ionic bonds, and hydrophobic interactions with multiple bases. Most of these contacts occur in the major groove, but some proteins also interact with bases in the minor groove, as shown in (B). Typically, the protein–DNA interface would consist of 10–20 such contacts, each involving a different amino acid and each contributing to the overall strength of the protein–DNA interaction.

integrating information from a variety of signals into a command that determines how often transcription of the gene is initiated.

Regulatory DNA sequences do not work by themselves. To have any effect, these sequences must be recognized by proteins called **transcription regulators**. It is the binding of a transcription regulator to a regulatory DNA sequence that acts as the switch to control transcription. The simplest bacterium produces several hundred different transcription regulators, each of which recognizes a different DNA sequence and thereby regulates a distinct set of genes. Humans make many more—2000 or so—indicating the importance and complexity of this form of gene regulation in the development and function of a complex organism.

Proteins that recognize a specific nucleotide sequence do so because the surface of the protein fits tightly against the surface features of the DNA double helix in that region. Because these surface features will vary depending on the nucleotide sequence, different DNA-binding proteins will recognize different nucleotide sequences. In most cases, the protein inserts into the major groove of the DNA double helix and makes a series of intimate, noncovalent molecular contacts with the nucleotide pairs within the groove (**Figure 8–4**, Movie 8.2). Although each individual contact is weak, the 10 to 20 contacts that typically form at the protein–DNA interface combine to ensure that the interaction is both highly specific and very strong; indeed, protein–DNA interactions are among the tightest and most specific molecular interactions known in biology.

Many transcription regulators bind to the DNA helix as dimers. Such dimerization roughly doubles the area of contact with the DNA, thereby greatly increasing the potential strength and specificity of the protein–DNA interaction (**Figure 8–5**, Movie 8.3).

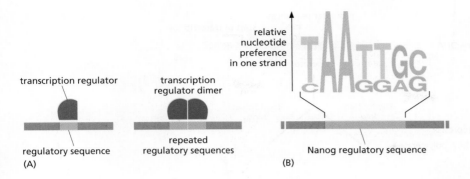

relative
nucleotide
preference
in one strand

transcription regulator

regulatory sequence
(A)

transcription
regulator dimer

repeated
regulatory sequences

Nanog regulatory sequence

(B)

Figure 8–5 Many transcription regulators bind to DNA as dimers. (A) As shown, such dimerization doubles the number of protein–DNA contacts. Here, and throughout the book, regulatory sequences are represented by colored bars; each bar represents a double-helical segment of DNA, as in Figure 8–4. (B) Shown here is a regulatory sequence recognized by Nanog, a homeodomain family member that is a key regulator in embryonic stem cells. This diagram, called a "logo," represents the preferred nucleotide at each position of the sequence; the height of each letter is proportional to the frequency with which this base is found at that position in the regulatory sequence. In the first position, for example, T is found more often than C, while A is the only nucleotide found in the second and third position of the sequence. Although regulatory sequences in the cell are double-stranded, a logo typically shows the sequence of only one DNA strand; the other strand is simply the complementary sequence. Logos are useful because they reveal at a glance the range of DNA sequences to which a given transcription regulator will bind.

Transcription Switches Allow Cells to Respond to Changes in Their Environment

The simplest and best-understood examples of gene regulation occur in bacteria. The genome of the bacterium *E. coli* consists of a single, circular DNA molecule of about 4.6×10^6 nucleotide pairs. This DNA encodes approximately 4300 proteins, although only a fraction of these are made at any one time. Bacteria regulate the expression of many of their genes according to the food sources that are available in the environment. In *E. coli*, for example, five genes code for enzymes that manufacture tryptophan when this amino acid is scarce. These genes are arranged in a cluster on the chromosome and are transcribed from a single promoter as one long mRNA molecule; such coordinately transcribed clusters are called *operons* (**Figure 8–6**). Although operons are common in bacteria (see Figure 7–40), they are rare in eukaryotes, where genes are transcribed and regulated individually.

When tryptophan concentrations are low, the operon is transcribed; the resulting mRNA is translated to produce a full set of biosynthetic enzymes, which work in tandem to synthesize the amino acid. When tryptophan is abundant, however—for example, when the bacterium is in the gut of a mammal that has just eaten a protein-rich meal—the amino acid is imported into the cell and shuts down production of the enzymes, which are no longer needed.

We understand in considerable detail how this repression of the tryptophan operon comes about. Within the operon's promoter is a short DNA sequence, called the operator (see Figure 8–6), that is recognized by a transcription regulator. When this regulator binds to the *operator*, it blocks access of RNA polymerase to the promoter, thus preventing transcription of the operon and, ultimately, the production of the tryptophan-synthesizing enzymes. The transcription regulator is known as the *tryptophan repressor*, and it is controlled in an ingenious way: the repressor can bind to DNA only if it is also bound to tryptophan (**Figure 8–7**).

The tryptophan repressor is an allosteric protein (see Figure 4–44): the binding of tryptophan causes a subtle change in its three-dimensional

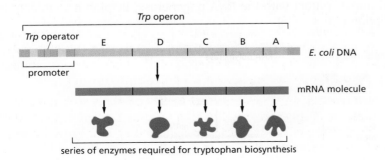

Trp operon

Trp operator

E   D   C   B   A

promoter

E. coli DNA

mRNA molecule

series of enzymes required for tryptophan biosynthesis

Figure 8–6 A cluster of bacterial genes can be transcribed from a single promoter. Each of these five genes encodes a different enzyme; all of the enzymes are needed to synthesize the amino acid tryptophan from simpler molecular building blocks. The genes are transcribed as a single mRNA molecule, a feature that allows their expression to be coordinated. Such clusters of genes, called operons, are common in bacteria. In this case, the entire operon is controlled by a single regulatory DNA sequence, called the *Trp operator* (*green*), situated within the promoter. The *yellow* blocks in the promoter represent DNA sequences that bind RNA polymerase.

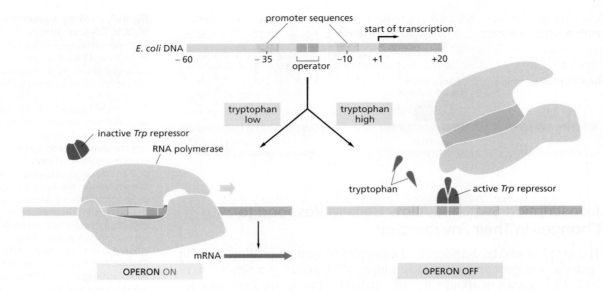

Figure 8–7 Genes can be switched off by repressor proteins. If the concentration of tryptophan inside a bacterium is low (*left*), RNA polymerase (*blue*) binds to the promoter and transcribes the five genes of the tryptophan operon. However, if the concentration of tryptophan is high (*right*), the repressor protein (*dark green*) becomes active and binds to the operator (*light green*), where it blocks the binding of RNA polymerase to the promoter. Whenever the concentration of intracellular tryptophan drops, the repressor falls off the DNA, allowing the polymerase to again transcribe the operon. The promoter contains two key blocks of DNA sequence information, the –35 and –10 regions, highlighted in *yellow*, which are recognized by RNA polymerase (see Figure 7–10). The complete operon is shown in Figure 8–6.

structure so that the protein can bind to the operator sequence. When the concentration of free tryptophan in the bacterium drops, the repressor no longer binds to DNA, and the tryptophan operon is transcribed. The repressor is thus a simple device that switches production of a set of biosynthetic enzymes on and off according to the availability of tryptophan—a form of feedback inhibition (see Figure 4–42).

The tryptophan repressor protein itself is always present in the cell. The gene that encodes it is continuously transcribed at a low level, so that a small amount of the repressor protein is always being made. Thus the bacterium can respond very rapidly to increases and decreases in tryptophan concentration.

Repressors Turn Genes Off and Activators Turn Them On

The tryptophan repressor, as its name suggests, is a **transcriptional repressor** protein: in its active form, it switches genes off, or *represses* them. Some bacterial transcription regulators do the opposite: they switch genes on, or *activate* them. These **transcriptional activator** proteins work on promoters that—in contrast to the promoter for the tryptophan operon—are only marginally able to bind and position RNA polymerase on their own. These inefficient promoters can be made fully functional by activator proteins that bind to a nearby regulatory sequence and make contact with the RNA polymerase, helping it to initiate transcription (**Figure 8–8**).

Figure 8–8 Genes can be switched on by activator proteins. An activator protein binds to a regulatory sequence on the DNA and then interacts with the RNA polymerase to help it initiate transcription. Without the activator, the promoter fails to initiate transcription efficiently. In bacteria, the binding of the activator to DNA is often controlled by the interaction of a metabolite or other small molecule (*red* circle) with the activator protein.

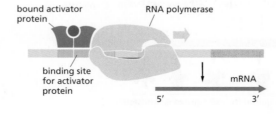

Like the tryptophan repressor, activator proteins often have to interact with a second molecule to be able to bind DNA. For example, the bacterial activator protein *CAP* has to bind cyclic AMP (cAMP) before it can bind to DNA (see Figure 4–20). Genes activated by CAP are switched on in response to an increase in intracellular cAMP concentration, which occurs when glucose, the bacterium's preferred carbon source, is no longer available; as a result, CAP drives the production of enzymes that allow the bacterium to digest other sugars.

The Lac Operon Is Controlled by an Activator and a Repressor

In many instances, the activity of a single promoter is controlled by two different transcription regulators. The *Lac operon* in *E. coli*, for example, is controlled by both the *Lac repressor* and the CAP activator that we just discussed. The *Lac* operon encodes proteins required to import and digest the disaccharide lactose. In the absence of glucose, the bacterium makes cAMP, which activates CAP to switch on genes that allow the cell to utilize alternative sources of carbon—including lactose. It would be wasteful, however, for CAP to induce expression of the *Lac* operon if lactose itself were not present. Thus the *Lac* repressor shuts off the operon in the absence of lactose. This arrangement enables the control region of the *Lac* operon to integrate two different signals, so that the operon is highly expressed only when two conditions are met: glucose must be absent and lactose must be present (**Figure 8–9**). This circuit thus behaves much like a switch that carries out a logic operation in a computer. When lactose is present AND glucose is absent, the cell executes the appropriate program—in this case, transcription of the genes that permit the uptake and utilization of lactose. None of the other combinations of conditions produce this result.

The elegant logic of the *Lac* operon first attracted the attention of biologists more than 50 years ago. The molecular basis of the switch in *E. coli* was uncovered by a combination of genetics and biochemistry, providing the first insight into how transcription is controlled. In a eukaryotic

QUESTION 8–1

Bacterial cells can take up the amino acid tryptophan (Trp) from their surroundings or, if there is an insufficient external supply, they can synthesize tryptophan from other small molecules. The *Trp* repressor is a transcription regulator that shuts off the transcription of genes that code for the enzymes required for the synthesis of tryptophan (see Figure 8–7).
A. What would happen to the regulation of the tryptophan operon in cells that express a mutant form of the tryptophan repressor that (1) cannot bind to DNA, (2) cannot bind tryptophan, or (3) binds to DNA even in the absence of tryptophan?
B. What would happen in scenarios (1), (2), and (3) if the cells, in addition, produced normal tryptophan repressor protein from a second, normal gene?

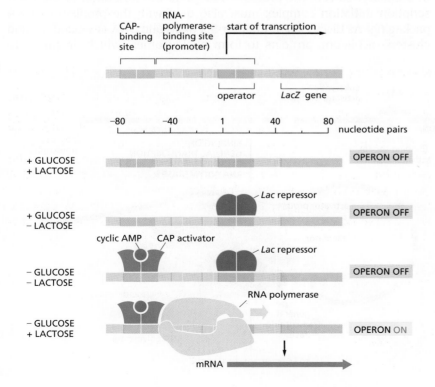

Figure 8–9 The *Lac* operon is controlled by two transcription regulators, the *Lac* repressor and CAP. When lactose is absent, the *Lac* repressor binds to the *Lac* operator and shuts off expression of the operon. Addition of lactose increases the intracellular concentration of a related compound, allolactose; allolactose binds to the *Lac* repressor, causing it to undergo a conformational change that releases its grip on the operator DNA (not shown). When glucose is absent, cyclic AMP (*red* circle) is produced by the cell, and CAP binds to DNA. For the operon to be transcribed, glucose must be absent (allowing the CAP activator to bind) and lactose must be present (releasing the *Lac* repressor). *LacZ*, the first gene of the operon, encodes the enzyme β-galactosidase, which breaks down lactose to galactose and glucose (Movie 8.4).

cell, similar transcription regulatory devices are combined to generate increasingly complex circuits, including those that enable a fertilized egg to form the tissues and organs of a multicellular organism.

Eukaryotic Transcription Regulators Control Gene Expression from a Distance

Eukaryotes, too, use transcription regulators—both activators and repressors—to regulate the expression of their genes. The DNA sites to which eukaryotic gene activators bind are termed *enhancers*, because their presence dramatically enhances the rate of transcription. However, biologists discovered that eukaryotic activator proteins could enhance transcription even when they are bound thousands of nucleotide pairs upstream—or downstream—of the gene's promoter. These observations raised several questions. How do enhancer sequences and the proteins bound to them function over such long distances? How do they communicate with a gene's promoter?

Many models for this "action at a distance" have been proposed, but the simplest of these seems to apply in most cases. The DNA between the enhancer and the promoter loops out, bringing the activator protein into close proximity with the promoter (**Figure 8–10**). The DNA thus acts as a tether, allowing a protein that is bound to an enhancer—even one that is thousands of nucleotide pairs away—to interact with the proteins in the vicinity of the promoter (see Figure 7–12). Often, additional proteins serve as adaptors to close the loop; the most important of these is a large complex of proteins known as *Mediator*. Together, all of these proteins ultimately attract and position the general transcription factors and RNA polymerase at the promoter, forming a *transcription initiation complex* (see Figure 8–10). Eukaryotic repressor proteins do the opposite: they decrease transcription by preventing the assembly of this complex.

Eukaryotic Transcription Regulators Help Initiate Transcription by Recruiting Chromatin-Modifying Proteins

In a eukaryotic cell, the proteins that guide the formation of the transcription initiation complex must also deal with the problem of DNA packaging. As discussed in Chapter 5, eukaryotic DNA is wound around clusters of histone proteins to form nucleosomes, which, in turn, are

QUESTION 8–2

Explain how DNA-binding proteins can make sequence-specific contacts to a double-stranded DNA molecule without breaking the hydrogen bonds that hold the bases together. Indicate how, through such contacts, a protein can distinguish a T-A from a C-G pair. Indicate the parts of the nucleotide base pairs that could form noncovalent interactions—hydrogen bonds, electrostatic attractions, or hydrophobic interactions (see Panel 2–3, pp. 70–71)—with a DNA-binding protein. The structures of all the base pairs in DNA are given in Figure 5–4.

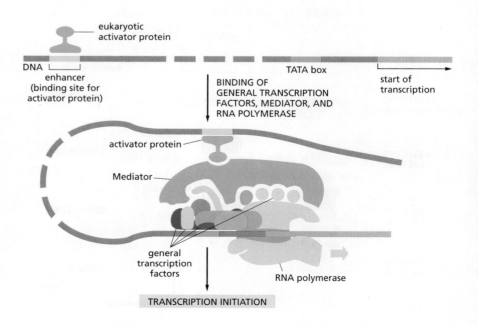

Figure 8–10 In eukaryotes, gene activation can occur at a distance. An activator protein bound to a distant enhancer attracts RNA polymerase and the general transcription factors to the promoter. Looping of the intervening DNA permits contact between the activator and the transcription initiation complex bound to the promoter. In the case shown here, a large protein complex called Mediator serves as a go-between. The broken stretch of DNA signifies that the segment of DNA between the enhancer and the start of transcription varies in length, sometimes reaching tens of thousands of nucleotide pairs. The TATA box is a DNA recognition sequence for the first general transcription factor that binds to the promoter (see Figure 7–12). Some eukaryotic activator proteins bind to DNA as dimers, but others bind DNA as monomers, as shown.

folded into higher-order structures. How do transcription regulators, general transcription factors, and RNA polymerase gain access to the underlying DNA? Although some of these proteins can bind efficiently to DNA that is wrapped up in nucleosomes, others are thwarted by these compact structures. More critically, nucleosomes that are positioned over a promoter can inhibit the initiation of transcription by physically blocking the assembly of the general transcription factors and RNA polymerase on the promoter. Such packaging may have evolved in part to prevent leaky gene expression by blocking the initiation of transcription in the absence of the proper activator proteins.

In eukaryotic cells, activator and repressor proteins can exploit the mechanisms used to package DNA to help turn genes on and off. As we saw in Chapter 5, chromatin structure can be altered by *chromatin-remodeling complexes* and by enzymes that covalently modify the histone proteins that form the core of the nucleosome (see Figures 5–24 and 5–25). Many gene activators take advantage of these mechanisms by attracting such chromatin-modifying proteins to promoters. For example, the recruitment of *histone acetyltransferases* promotes the attachment of acetyl groups to selected lysines in the tail of histone proteins; these acetyl groups themselves attract proteins that promote transcription, including some of the general transcription factors (**Figure 8–11**). And the recruitment of chromatin-remodeling complexes makes nearby DNA more accessible. These actions enhance the efficiency of transcription initiation.

In a similar way, gene repressor proteins can modify chromatin in ways that reduce the efficiency of transcription initiation. For example, many repressors attract *histone deacetylases*—enzymes that remove the acetyl groups from histone tails, thereby reversing the positive effects that acetylation has on transcription initiation. Although some eukaryotic repressor proteins work on a gene-by-gene basis, others can orchestrate the formation of large swathes of transcriptionally inactive chromatin. As discussed in Chapter 5, these transcription-resistant regions of DNA include the heterochromatin found in interphase chromosomes and the inactive X chromosome in the cells of female mammals.

QUESTION 8–3

Some transcription regulators bind to DNA and cause the double helix to bend at a sharp angle. Such "bending proteins" can stimulate the initiation of transcription without contacting either the RNA polymerase, any of the general transcription factors, or any other transcription regulators. Can you devise a plausible explanation for how these proteins might work to modulate transcription? Draw a diagram that illustrates your explanation.

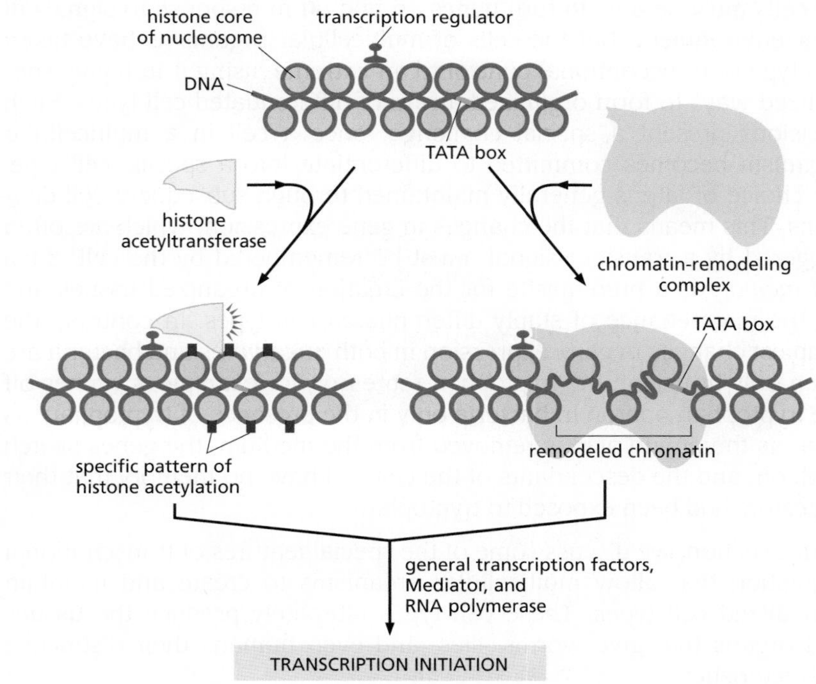

Figure 8–11 Eukaryotic transcriptional activators can recruit chromatin-modifying proteins to help initiate gene transcription. On the left, the recruitment of histone-modifying enzymes such as histone acetyltransferases adds acetyl groups to specific histones, which can then serve as binding sites for proteins that stimulate transcription initiation (not shown). On the right, chromatin-remodeling complexes render the DNA packaged in nucleosomes more accessible to other proteins in the cell, including those required for transcription initiation; notice, for example, the increased exposure of the TATA box.

Figure 8–12 Animal and plant chromosomes are arranged in DNA loops. In this schematic diagram, specialized proteins (*green*) hold chromosomal DNA in loops, thereby favoring the association of each gene with its proper enhancer. The loops, sometimes called *topological associated domains* (TADs), range in size between thousands and millions of nucleotide pairs and are typically much larger than the loops that form between regulatory sequences and promoters (see Figure 8–10).

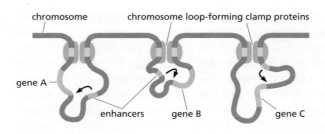

The Arrangement of Chromosomes into Looped Domains Keeps Enhancers in Check

We have seen that all genes have regulatory regions, which dictate at which times, under what conditions, and in what tissues the gene will be expressed. We have also seen that eukaryotic transcription regulators can act across very long stretches of DNA, with the intervening DNA looped out. What, then, prevents a transcripton regulator—bound to the control region of one gene—from looping in the wrong direction and inappropriately influencing the transcription of a neighboring gene?

To avoid such unwanted cross-talk, the chromosomal DNA of plants and animals is arranged in a series of loops that hold individual genes and their regulatory regions in rough proximity. This localization restricts the action of enhancers, preventing them from wandering across to adjacent genes. The chromosomal loops are formed by specialized proteins that bind to sequences that are then drawn together to form the base of the loop (Figure 8–12).

The importance of these loops is highlighted by the effects of mutations that prevent the loops from properly forming. Such mutations, which lead to genes being expressed at the wrong time and place, are found in numerous cancers and inherited diseases.

GENERATING SPECIALIZED CELL TYPES

All cells must be able to turn genes on and off in response to signals in their environment. But the cells of multicellular organisms have taken this type of transcriptional control to an extreme, using it in highly specialized ways to form organized arrays of differentiated cell types. Such decisions present a special challenge: once a cell in a multicellular organism becomes committed to differentiate into a specific cell type, the choice of fate is generally maintained through subsequent cell divisions. This means that the changes in gene expression, which are often triggered by a transient signal, must be remembered by the cell. Such *cell memory* is a prerequisite for the creation of organized tissues and for the maintenance of stably differentiated cell types. In contrast, the simplest changes in gene expression in both eukaryotes and bacteria are often only transient; the tryptophan repressor, for example, switches off the tryptophan operon in bacteria only in the presence of tryptophan; as soon as the amino acid is removed from the medium, the genes switch back on, and the descendants of the cell will have no memory that their ancestors had been exposed to tryptophan.

In this section, we discuss some of the special features of transcriptional regulation that allow multicellular organisms to create and maintain specialized cell types. These cell types ultimately produce the tissues and organs that give worms, flies, and even humans their distinctive characteristics.

Eukaryotic Genes Are Controlled by Combinations of Transcription Regulators

The genes we have examined thus far have all been controlled by a small number of transcription regulators. While this is true for many simple bacterial systems, most eukaryotic transcription regulators work as part of a large "committee" of regulatory proteins, all of which cooperate to express the gene in the right cell type, in response to the right conditions, at the right time, and in the required amount.

The term **combinatorial control** refers to the process by which groups of transcription regulators work together to determine the expression of a single gene. The bacterial *Lac* operon we discussed earlier provides a simple example of the use of multiple regulators to control transcription (see Figure 8–9). In eukaryotes, such regulatory inputs have been amplified, so that a typical gene is controlled by dozens of transcription regulators that bind to regulatory sequences that may be spread over tens of thousands of nucleotide pairs. Together, these regulators direct the assembly of the Mediator, chromatin-remodeling complexes, histone-modifying enzymes, general transcripton factors, and, ultimately, RNA polymerase (**Figure 8–13**). In many cases, multiple repressors and activators are bound to the DNA that controls transcription of a given gene; how the cell integrates the effects of all of these proteins to determine the final level of gene expression is only now beginning to be understood. An example of such a complex regulatory system—one that participates in the development of a fruit fly from a fertilized egg—is described in **How We Know**, pp. 280–281.

The Expression of Different Genes Can Be Coordinated by a Single Protein

In addition to being able to switch individual genes on and off, all cells—whether prokaryote or eukaryote—need to coordinate the expression of different genes. When a eukaryotic cell receives a signal to proliferate, for example, a number of hitherto unexpressed genes are turned on together to set in motion the events that lead eventually to cell division (discussed in Chapter 18). As discussed earlier, bacteria often coordinate the expression of a set of genes by having them clustered together in an operon under the control of a single promoter (see Figure 8–6). Such clustering is

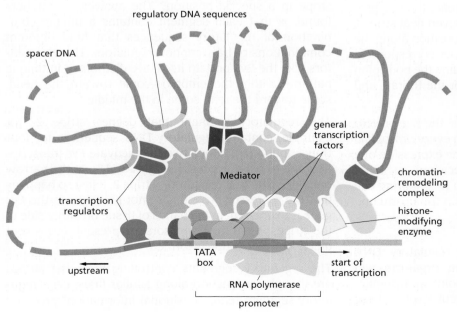

Figure 8–13 **Transcription regulators work together as a "committee" to control the expression of a eukaryotic gene.** Whereas the general transcription factors that assemble at the promoter are the same for all genes transcribed by RNA polymerase (see Figure 7–12), the transcription regulators and the locations of their DNA binding sites relative to the promoters are different for different genes. These regulators, along with chromatin-modifying proteins, are assembled at the promoter by the Mediator. The effects of multiple transcription regulators combine to determine the final rate of transcription initiation. The "spacer" DNA sequences that separate the regulatory DNA sequences are not recognized by any transcription regulators.

HOW WE KNOW

GENE REGULATION—THE STORY OF *EVE*

The ability to regulate gene expression is crucial to the proper development of a multicellular organism from a fertilized egg to an adult. Beginning at the earliest moments in development, a succession of transcriptional programs guides the differential expression of genes that allows an animal to form a proper body plan—helping to distinguish its back from its belly, and its head from its tail. These programs ultimately direct the correct placement of a wing or a leg, a mouth or an anus, a neuron or a liver cell.

A central challenge in developmental biology, then, is to understand how an organism generates these patterns of gene expression, which are laid down within hours of fertilization. Among the most important genes involved in these early stages of development are those that encode transcription regulators. By interacting with different regulatory DNA sequences, these proteins instruct every cell in the embryo to switch on the genes that are appropriate for that cell at each time point during development. How can a protein binding to a piece of DNA help direct the development of a complex multicellular organism? To see how we can address that large question, we review the story of *Eve*.

Seeing *Eve*

Even-skipped—*Eve*, for short—is a gene whose expression plays an important part in the development of the *Drosophila* embryo. If this gene is inactivated by mutation, many parts of the embryo fail to form and the fly larva dies early in development. But *Eve* is not expressed uniformly throughout the embryo. Instead, the Eve protein is produced in a striking series of seven neat stripes, each of which occupies a very precise position along the length of the embryo. These seven stripes correspond to seven of the fourteen segments that define the body plan of the fly—three for the head, three for the thorax, and eight for the abdomen.

This pattern of expression never varies: the Eve protein can be found in the very same places in every *Drosophila* embryo (see Figure 8–14B). How can the expression of a gene be regulated with such spatial precision—such that one cell will produce a protein while a neighboring cell does not? To find out, researchers took a trip upstream.

Dissecting the DNA

As we have seen in this chapter, regulatory DNA sequences control which cells in an organism will express a particular gene, and at what point during development that gene will be turned on. In eukaryotes, these regulatory sequences are frequently located upstream of the gene itself. One way to locate a regulatory DNA sequence—and study how it operates—is to remove a piece of DNA from the region upstream of a gene of interest and insert that DNA upstream of a **reporter gene**—one that encodes a protein with an activity that is easy to monitor experimentally. If the piece of DNA contains a regulatory sequence, it will drive the expression of the reporter gene. When this patchwork piece of DNA is subsequently introduced into a cell or organism, the reporter gene will be expressed in the same cells and tissues that normally express the gene from which the regulatory sequence was derived (see Figure 10–24).

By excising various segments of the DNA sequences upstream of *Eve*, and coupling them to a reporter gene, researchers found that the expression of the gene is controlled by a series of seven regulatory modules—each of which specifies a single stripe of *Eve* expression. In this way, researchers identified, for example, a single segment of regulatory DNA that specifies stripe 2. They could excise this regulatory segment, link it to a reporter gene, and introduce the resulting DNA segment into the fly. When they examined embryos that carried this engineered DNA, they found that the reporter gene is expressed in the precise position of stripe 2 (**Figure 8–14**). Similar experiments revealed the existence of six other regulatory modules, one for each of the other Eve stripes.

The next question was: How does each of these seven regulatory segments direct the formation of a single stripe in a specific position? The answer, researchers found, is that each segment contains a unique combination of regulatory sequences that bind different combinations of transcription regulators. These regulators, like the Eve protein itself, are distributed in unique patterns within the embryo—some toward the head, some toward the rear, some in the middle.

The regulatory segment that defines stripe 2, for example, contains regulatory DNA sequences for four transcription regulators: two that activate *Eve* transcription and two that repress it (**Figure 8–15**). In the narrow band of tissue that constitutes stripe 2, it just so happens that the repressor proteins are not present—so the *Eve* gene is expressed; in the bands of tissue on either side of the stripe, where the repressors are present, *Eve* is kept quiet. And so a stripe is formed.

The regulatory segments controlling the other stripes are thought to function along similar lines; each regulatory segment reads "positional information" provided

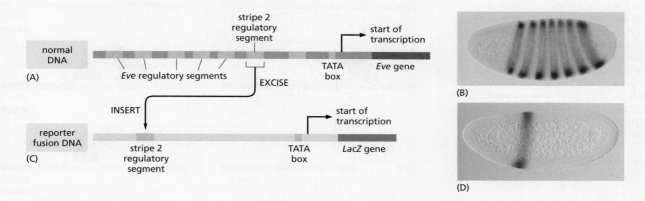

(A)

normal
DNA

Eve regulatory segments

stripe 2
regulatory
segment

EXCISE

start of
transcription

TATA
box

Eve gene

(B)

INSERT

(C)

reporter
fusion DNA

stripe 2
regulatory
segment

start of
transcription

TATA
box

LacZ gene

(D)

Figure 8–14 An experimental approach using a reporter gene reveals the modular construction of the *Eve* gene regulatory region. (A) Expression of the *Eve* gene is controlled by a series of regulatory segments (*orange*) that direct the production of Eve protein in stripes along the embryo. (B) Embryos stained with antibodies to the Eve protein show the seven characteristic stripes of *Eve* expression. (C) In the laboratory, the regulatory segment that directs the formation of stripe 2 can be excised from the DNA shown in part (A) and inserted upstream of the *E. coli LacZ* gene, which encodes the enzyme β-galactosidase (see Figure 8–9). (D) When the engineered DNA containing the stripe 2 regulatory segment is introduced into the genome of a fly, the resulting embryo expresses β-galactosidase mRNA precisely in the position of the second *Eve* stripe. This mRNA is visualized by *in situ* hybridization (see p. 352) using a labeled RNA probe that base pairs only with the *lacZ* mRNA. (B and D, courtesy of Stephen Small and Michael Levine.)

by some unique combination of transcription regulators and expresses *Eve* on the basis of this information. The entire regulatory region is strung out over 20,000 nucleotide pairs of DNA and, altogether, binds more than 20 transcription regulators. This large regulatory region is built from a series of smaller regulatory segments, each of which consists of a unique arrangement of regulatory DNA sequences recognized by specific transcription regulators. In this way, the *Eve* gene can respond to an enormous combination of inputs.

The Eve protein is itself a transcription regulator, and it—in combination with many other regulatory proteins—controls key events in the development of the fly. This complex organization of a discrete number of regulatory elements begins to explain how the development of an entire organism can be orchestrated by repeated applications of a few basic principles.

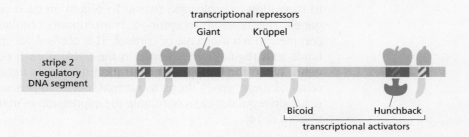

transcriptional repressors

Giant   Krüppel

stripe 2
regulatory
DNA segment

Bicoid

Hunchback

transcriptional activators

Figure 8–15 The regulatory segment that specifies *Eve* stripe 2 contains binding sites for four different transcription regulators. All four regulators are responsible for the proper expression of *Eve* in stripe 2. Flies that are deficient in the two activators, called Bicoid and Hunchback, fail to form stripe 2 efficiently; in flies deficient in either of the two repressors, called Giant and Krüppel, stripe 2 expands and covers an abnormally broad region of the embryo. As indicated in the diagram, in some cases the binding sites for the transcription regulators overlap, and the proteins compete for binding to the DNA. For example, the binding of Bicoid and Krüppel to the site at the far right is thought to be mutually exclusive. The regulatory segment is 480 base pairs in length.

Figure 8–16 A single transcription regulator can coordinate the expression of many different genes. The action of the cortisol receptor is illustrated. On the left is a series of genes, each of which has a different activator protein bound to its respective regulatory DNA sequences. However, these bound proteins are not sufficient on their own to activate transcription efficiently. On the right is shown the effect of adding an additional transcription regulator—the cortisol–receptor complex—that binds to the same regulatory DNA sequence in each gene. The activated cortisol receptor completes the combination of transcription regulators required for efficient initiation of transcription, and all three genes are now switched on as a set.

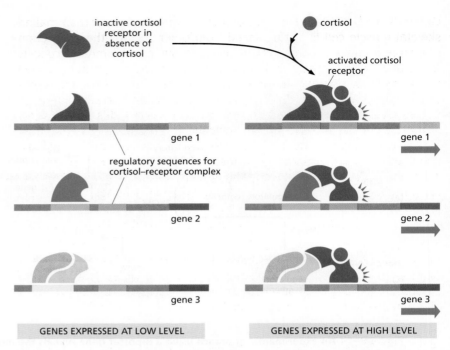

inactive cortisol receptor in absence of cortisol

cortisol

activated cortisol receptor

gene 1

regulatory sequences for cortisol–receptor complex

gene 2

gene 3

GENES EXPRESSED AT LOW LEVEL

gene 1

gene 2

gene 3

GENES EXPRESSED AT HIGH LEVEL

rarely seen in eukaryotic cells, where each gene is transcribed and regulated individually. So how do eukaryotic cells coordinate the expression of multiple genes? In particular, given that a eukaryotic cell uses a committee of transcription regulators to control each of its genes, how can it rapidly and decisively switch whole groups of genes on or off?

The answer is that even though control of gene expression is combinatorial, the effect of a single transcription regulator can still be decisive in switching any particular gene on or off, simply by completing the combination needed to activate or repress that gene. This is like dialing in the final number of a combination lock: the lock will spring open if the other numbers have been previously entered. And just as the same number can complete the combination for different locks, the same protein can complete the combination for several different genes. As long as different genes contain regulatory DNA sequences that are recognized by the same transcription regulator, they can be switched on or off together as a coordinated unit.

An example of such coordinated regulation in humans is seen in response to cortisol (see Table 16–1, p. 536). As discussed earlier in this chapter, when this hormone is present, liver cells increase the expression of many genes, including those that allow the liver to produce glucose in response to starvation or prolonged stress. To switch on such cortisol-responsive genes, the cortisol receptor—a transcription regulator—first forms a complex with a molecule of cortisol. This cortisol–receptor complex then binds to a regulatory sequence in the DNA of each cortisol-responsive gene. When the cortisol concentration decreases again, the expression of all of these genes drops to normal levels. In this way, a single transcription regulator can coordinate the expression of many different genes (**Figure 8–16**).

Combinatorial Control Can Also Generate Different Cell Types

The ability to switch many different genes on or off using a limited number of transcription regulators is not only useful in the day-to-day regulation of cell function. It is also one of the means by which eukaryotic cells diversify into particular types of cells during embryonic development.

One striking example is the development of muscle cells. A mammalian skeletal muscle cell is distinguished from other cells by the production of a large number of characteristic proteins, such as the muscle-specific forms of actin and myosin that make up the contractile apparatus, as well as the receptor proteins and ion channel proteins in the plasma membrane that allow the muscle cell to contract in response to stimulation by nerves (discussed in Chapter 17). The genes encoding this unique array of muscle-specific proteins are all switched on coordinately as the muscle cell differentiates. Studies of developing muscle cells in culture have identified a small number of key transcription regulators, expressed only in potential muscle cells, that coordinate muscle-specific gene expression and are thus crucial for muscle-cell differentiation. This set of regulators activates the transcription of the genes that code for muscle-specific proteins by binding to specific DNA sequences present in their regulatory regions.

In the same way, other sets of transcription regulators can activate the expression of genes that are specific for other cell types. How different combinations of transcription regulators can tailor the development of different cell types is illustrated schematically in **Figure 8–17**.

Still other transcription regulators can maintain cells in an undifferentiated state, like the precursor cell shown in Figure 8–17. Some undifferentiated cells are so developmentally flexible they are capable of giving rise to all the specialized cell types in the body. The *embryonic stem (ES) cells* we discuss in Chapter 20 retain this remarkable quality, a property called *pluripotency*.

The differentiation of a particular cell type involves changes in the expression of thousands of genes: genes that encode products needed by the cell are expressed at high levels, while those that are not needed are expressed at low levels or shut down completely. A given transcription regulator, therefore, often controls the expression of hundreds or even

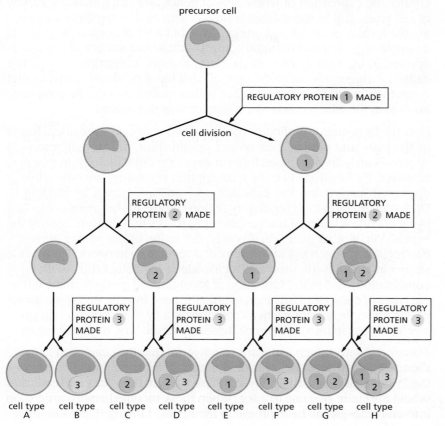

Figure 8–17 Combinations of a few transcription regulators can generate many cell types during development. In this simple scheme, a "decision" to make a new transcription regulator (shown as a numbered circle) is made after each cell division. Repetition of this simple rule can generate eight cell types (A through H) using only three transcription regulators. Each of these hypothetical cell types would then express different sets of genes, as dictated by the combination of transcription regulators that each cell type produces.

Figure 8–18 A set of three transcription regulators forms the regulatory network that specifies an embryonic stem cell. (A) The three transcription regulators—Klf4, Oct4, and Sox2—are shown in large *colored* circles. The genes whose regulatory sequences contain binding sites for each of these regulators are indicated by small *green* dots. The lines that link each regulator to a gene represent the binding of that regulator to the regulatory region of the gene. Note that although each regulator controls the expression of a unique set of genes, many of these target genes are bound by more than one transcription regulator—and a substantial set interacts with all three. (B) These three regulators also control their own expression. As shown here, each regulator binds to the regulatory region of its own gene, as indicated by the feedback loops (*red*). In addition, the regulators also bind to each other's regulatory regions (*blue*). Positive feedback loops, a common form of regulation, are discussed later in the chapter.

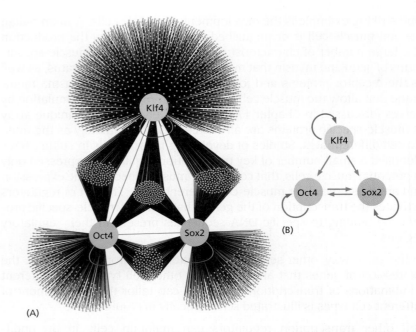

(A)

(B)

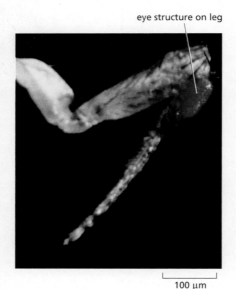

eye structure on leg

100 μm

Figure 8–19 A master transcription regulator can direct the formation of an entire organ. Artificially induced expression of the *Drosophila Ey* gene in the precursor cells of the leg triggers the misplaced development of an eye on a fly's leg. The experimentally induced organ appears to be structurally normal, containing the various types of cells found in a typical fly eye. It does not, however, communicate with the fly's brain. (Walter Gehring, courtesy of Biozentrum, University of Basel.)

thousands of genes (**Figure 8–18**). Because each gene, in turn, is typically controlled by many different transcription regulators, a relatively small number of regulators acting in different combinations can form the enormously complex regulatory networks that generate specialized cell types. It is estimated that approximately 1000 transcription regulators are sufficient to control the 24,000 genes that give rise to an individual human.

The Formation of an Entire Organ Can Be Triggered by a Single Transcription Regulator

We have seen that transcription regulators, working in combination, can control the expression of whole sets of genes and can produce a variety of cell types. But in some cases a single transcription regulator can initiate the formation of not just one cell type but a whole organ. A stunning example of such transcriptional control comes from studies of eye development in the fruit fly *Drosophila*. Here, a single transcription regulator called Ey triggers the differentiation of all of the specialized cell types that come together to form the eye. Flies with a mutation in the *Ey* gene have no eyes at all, which is how the regulator was discovered.

How the Ey protein coordinates the specification of each type of cell found in the eye—and directs their proper organization in three-dimensional space—is an actively studied topic in developmental biology. In essence, however, Ey functions like the transcription regulators we have already discussed, controlling the expression of multiple genes by binding to DNA sequences in their regulatory regions. Some of the genes controlled by Ey encode additional transcription regulators that, in turn, control the expression of other genes. In this way, the action of this *master transcription regulator*, which sits at the apex of a regulatory network like the one shown in Figure 8–18, produces a cascade of regulators that, working in combination, lead to the formation of an organized group of many different types of cells. One can begin to imagine how, by repeated applications of this principle, an organism as complex as a fly—or a human—progressively self-assembles, cell by cell, tissue by tissue, and organ by organ.

Master regulators such as Ey are so powerful that they can even activate their regulatory networks outside the normal location. In the laboratory, the *Ey* gene has been artificially expressed in fruit fly embryos in cells that would normally give rise to a leg. When these modified embryos develop into adult flies, some have an eye in the middle of a leg (**Figure 8–19**).

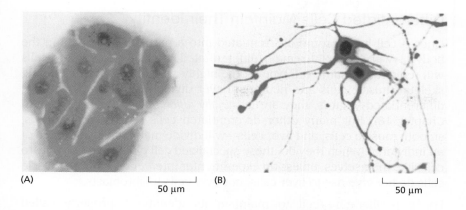

(A) ⊢ 50 µm ⊣ (B) ⊢ 50 µm ⊣

Figure 8–20 A small number of transcription regulators can convert one differentiated cell type directly into another. In this experiment, liver cells grown in culture (A) were converted into neuronal cells (B) via the artificial introduction of three nerve-specific transcription regulators. The cells are labeled with a fluorescent dye. Such interconversion would never take place during normal development. The result shown here depends on an experimenter expressing several nerve-specific regulators in liver cells, where these regulators would, during normal development, be tightly shut off. (From S. Marro et al., *Cell Stem Cell* 9:374–382, 2011. With permission from Elsevier.)

Transcription Regulators Can Be Used to Experimentally Direct the Formation of Specific Cell Types in Culture

We have seen that the *Ey* gene, when introduced into a fly embryo, can produce an eye in an unnatural location; this somewhat unusual outcome is made possible by the cooperation of numerous transcription regulators in a variety of cell types—a situation that is common in a developing embryo. Perhaps even more surprising is that some transcription regulators can convert one specialized cell type to another in a culture dish. For example, when the gene encoding the transcription regulator MyoD is artificially introduced into fibroblasts cultured from skin, the fibroblasts form musclelike cells. It appears that the fibroblasts, which are derived from the same broad class of embryonic cells as muscle cells, have already accumulated many of the other necessary transcription regulators required for the combinatorial control of the muscle-specific genes, and that addition of MyoD completes the unique combination required to direct the cells to become muscle.

This same type of *reprogramming* can produce even more impressive transformations. For example, a set of nerve-specific transcription regulators, when artificially expressed in cultured liver cells, can convert them into functional neurons (**Figure 8–20**). And the combination of transcription regulators shown in Figure 8–18 can be used in the laboratory to coax differentiated cells to *de-differentiate* into **induced pluripotent stem (iPS) cells**; these reprogrammed cells behave much like naturally occurring ES cells, and they can be directed to generate a variety of specialized differentiated cells (**Figure 8–21**). This approach, initially performed using cultured fibroblasts, has been adapted to produce iPS cells from a variety of specialized cell types, including those taken from humans. Differentiated cells produced from human iPS cells are currently being used in the study or treatment of disease, as we discuss in Chapter 20. Taken together, these dramatic demonstrations suggest that it may someday be possible to produce in the laboratory any cell type for which the correct combination of transcription regulators can be identified.

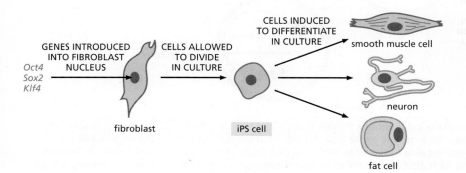

Figure 8–21 A combination of transcription regulators can induce a differentiated cell to de-differentiate into a pluripotent iPS cell. The artificial expression of a set of three genes, each of which encodes a transcription regulator, can reprogram a fibroblast into a pluripotent cell with ES cell-like properties. Like ES cells, such iPS cells can proliferate indefinitely in culture and can be stimulated by appropriate extracellular signal molecules to differentiate into almost any cell type in the body.

Differentiated Cells Maintain Their Identity

Once a cell has become differentiated into a particular cell type in the body, it will generally remain differentiated, and all its progeny cells will remain that same cell type. Some highly specialized cells, including skeletal muscle cells and neurons, never divide again once they have differentiated—that is, they are *terminally differentiated* (as discussed in Chapter 18). But many other differentiated cells—such as fibroblasts, smooth muscle cells, and liver cells—will divide many times in the life of an individual. When they do, these specialized cell types give rise only to cells like themselves: unless an experimenter intervenes, smooth muscle cells do not give rise to liver cells, nor liver cells to fibroblasts.

For a proliferating cell to maintain its identity—a property called **cell memory**—the patterns of gene expression responsible for that identity must be "remembered" and passed on to its daughter cells through all subsequent cell divisions. Thus, in the model illustrated in Figure 8–17, the production of each transcription regulator, once begun, has to be continued in the daughter cells of each cell division. How is such perpetuation accomplished?

Cells have several ways of ensuring that their daughters remember what kind of cells they should be. One of the simplest and most important is through a **positive feedback loop**, where a master transcription regulator activates transcription of its own gene, in addition to that of other cell-type-specific genes. Each time a cell divides, the regulator is distributed to both daughter cells, where it continues to stimulate the positive feedback loop (**Figure 8–22**). The continued stimulation ensures that the regulator will continue to be produced in subsequent cell generations. The Ey protein and the transcription regulators involved in the generation of ES cells and iPS cells take part in such positive feedback loops (see Figure 8–18B). Positive feedback is crucial for establishing the "self-sustaining" circuits of gene expression that allow a cell to commit to a particular fate—and then to transmit that decision to its progeny.

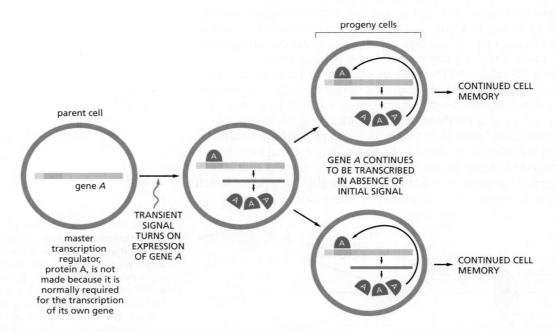

Figure 8–22 A positive feedback loop can generate cell memory. Protein A is a master transcription regulator that activates the transcription of its own gene—as well as other cell-type-specific genes (not shown). All of the descendants of the original cell will therefore "remember" that the progenitor cell had experienced a transient signal that initiated the production of protein A. As shown in Figure 8–18, each of the regulators needed to form iPS cells influences its own expression using this type of positive feedback loop.

Although positive feedback loops are probably the most prevalent way of ensuring that daughter cells remember what kind of cells they are meant to be, there are other ways of reinforcing cell identity. One involves the methylation of DNA. In vertebrate cells, **DNA methylation** occurs on certain cytosine bases (**Figure 8–23**). This covalent modification generally turns off the affected genes by attracting proteins that bind to methylated cytosines and block gene transcription. DNA methylation patterns are passed on to progeny cells by the action of an enzyme that copies the methylation pattern on the parent DNA strand to the daughter DNA strand as it is synthesized (**Figure 8–24**).

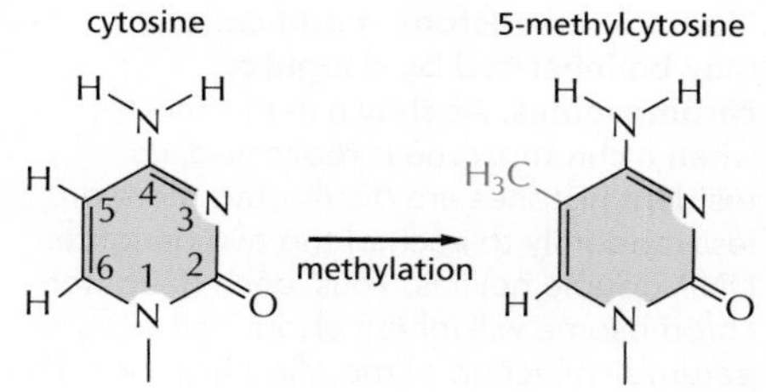

Another mechanism for inheriting gene expression patterns involves the modification of histones. When a cell replicates its DNA, each daughter double helix receives half of its parent's histone proteins, which contain the covalent modifications that were present on the parent chromosome. Enzymes responsible for these modifications may bind to the parental histones and confer the same modifications to the new histones nearby. It has been proposed that this cycle of modification helps reestablish the pattern of chromatin structure found in the parent chromosome (**Figure 8–25**).

Because all of these cell-memory mechanisms transmit patterns of gene expression from parent to daughter cell without altering the actual nucleotide sequence of the DNA, they are considered to be forms of **epigenetic inheritance**. These mechanisms, which work together, play an important part in maintaining patterns of gene expression, allowing transient signals from the environment to be remembered by our cells—a fact that has important implications for understanding how cells operate and how they malfunction in disease.

POST-TRANSCRIPTIONAL CONTROLS

We have seen that transcription regulators control gene expression by promoting or hindering the transcription of specific genes. The vast majority of genes in all organisms are regulated in this way. But many additional points of control can come into play later in the pathway from DNA to protein, giving cells a further opportunity to regulate the amount or activity of the gene products that they make (see Figure 8–3). These

cytosine   5-methylcytosine

Figure 8–23 Formation of 5-methylcytosine occurs by methylation of a cytosine base in the DNA double helix. In vertebrates, this modification is confined to selected cytosine (C) nucleotides that fall next to a guanine (G) in the sequence 5'-CG-3'.

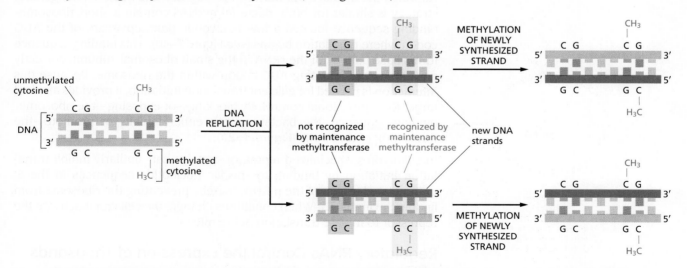

Figure 8–24 DNA methylation patterns can be faithfully inherited when a cell divides. An enzyme called a maintenance methyltransferase guarantees that once a pattern of DNA methylation has been established, it is inherited by newly made DNA. Immediately after DNA replication, each daughter double helix will contain one methylated DNA strand—inherited from the parent double helix—and one unmethylated, newly synthesized strand. The maintenance methyltransferase interacts with these hybrid double helices and methylates only those CG sequences that are base-paired with a CG sequence that is already methylated.

Figure 8–25 Histone modifications may be inherited by daughter chromosomes. As shown in this model, when a chromosome is replicated, its resident histones are distributed more or less randomly to each of the two daughter DNA double helices. Thus, each daughter chromosome will inherit about half of its parent's collection of modified histones. The remaining stretches of DNA receive newly synthesized, not-yet-modified histones. If the enzymes responsible for each type of modification bind to the specific modification they create, they can catalyze the "filling in" of this modification on the new histones. This cycle of modification and recognition can restore the parental histone modification pattern and, ultimately, allow the inheritance of the parental chromatin structure.

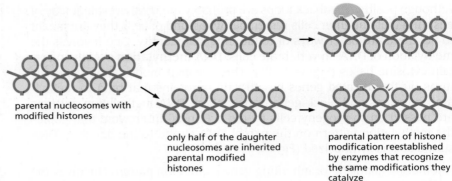

parental nucleosomes with modified histones

only half of the daughter nucleosomes are inherited parental modified histones

parental pattern of histone modification reestablished by enzymes that recognize the same modifications they catalyze

post-transcriptional controls, which operate after transcription has begun, play a crucial part in further fine-tuning the expression of almost all genes.

We have already encountered a few examples of such post-transcriptional control. For example, alternative RNA splicing allows different forms of a protein, encoded by the same gene, to be made in different tissues (Figure 7–23). And we saw that various post-translational modifications of a protein can regulate its concentration and activity (see Figure 4–47). In the remainder of this chapter, we consider several other examples—some only recently discovered—of the many ways in which cells can manipulate the expression of a gene after transcription has commenced.

mRNAs Contain Sequences That Control Their Translation

We saw in Chapter 7 that an mRNA's lifespan is dictated by specific nucleotide sequences within the untranslated regions that lie both upstream and downstream of the protein-coding sequence. These sequences often contain binding sites for proteins that are involved in RNA degradation. But they also carry information specifying whether—and how often—the mRNA is to be translated into protein.

Although the details differ between eukaryotes and bacteria, the general strategy is similar for both. Bacterial mRNAs contain a short ribosome-binding sequence located a few nucleotide pairs upstream of the AUG codon where translation begins (see Figure 7–40). This binding sequence forms base pairs with the rRNA in the small ribosomal subunit, correctly positioning the initiating AUG codon within the ribosome. Because this interaction is needed for efficient translation initiation, it provides an ideal target for translational control. By blocking—or exposing—the ribosome-binding sequence, the bacterium can either inhibit—or promote—the translation of an mRNA (Figure 8–26).

In eukaryotes, specialized repressor proteins can similarly inhibit translation initiation by binding to specific nucleotide sequences in the 5′ untranslated region of the mRNA, thereby preventing the ribosome from finding the first AUG. When conditions change, the cell can inactivate the repressor to initiate translation of the mRNA.

Regulatory RNAs Control the Expression of Thousands of Genes

As we saw in Chapter 7, RNAs perform many critical biological tasks. In addition to the mRNAs, which code for proteins, *noncoding RNAs* have a variety of functions. Some, such as transfer RNAs (tRNAs) and ribosomal

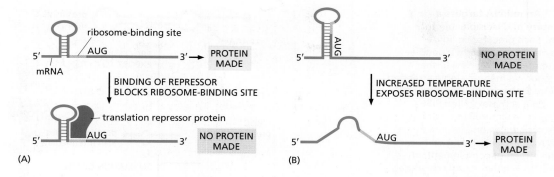

Figure 8–26 A bacterial gene's expression can be controlled by regulating translation of its mRNA.
(A) Sequence-specific RNA-binding proteins can repress the translation of specific mRNAs by keeping the ribosome from binding to the ribosome-binding sequence (*orange*) in the mRNA. Some bacteria exploit this mechanism to inhibit the translation of ribosomal proteins. If a ribosomal protein is accidentally produced in excess over other ribosomal components, the free protein will inhibit translation of its own mRNA, thereby blocking its own synthesis. As new ribosomes are assembled, the levels of the free protein decrease, allowing the mRNA to again be translated and the ribosomal protein to be produced. (B) An mRNA from the pathogen *Listeria monocytogenes* contains a "thermosensor" RNA sequence that controls the translation of a set of mRNAs that code for proteins the bacterium needs to successfully infect its host. At the warmer temperatures inside a host, base pairs within the thermosensor come apart, exposing the ribosome-binding sequence, so the necessary protein is made.

RNAs (rRNAs) play key structural and catalytic roles in the cell, particularly in protein synthesis (see pp. 252–253). And the RNA component of telomerase is crucial for the complete duplication of eukaryotic chromosomes (see Figure 6–23). But we now know that many organisms, particularly animals and plants, produce thousands of additional noncoding RNAs.

Many of these noncoding RNAs have crucial roles in regulating gene expression and are therefore referred to as **regulatory RNAs**. These regulatory RNAs include *microRNAs*, *small interfering RNAs*, and *long noncoding RNAs*, and we discuss each in the remaining sections of the chapter.

MicroRNAs Direct the Destruction of Target mRNAs

MicroRNAs, or **miRNAs**, are tiny RNA molecules that control gene expression by base-pairing with specific mRNAs and reducing both their stability and their translation into protein. Like other RNAs, miRNAs also undergo processing to produce the mature, functional miRNA molecule. The mature miRNA, about 22 nucleotides in length, is packaged with specialized proteins to form an *RNA-induced silencing complex (RISC)*, which patrols the cytosol in search of mRNAs that are complementary in sequence to its bound miRNA (Figure 8–27). Once a target mRNA base-pairs with an miRNA, it is either destroyed immediately—by a nuclease that is part of the RISC—or its translation is blocked. In the latter case, the bound mRNA molecule is delivered to a region of the cytosol where other nucleases eventually degrade it. Destruction of the mRNA releases the miRNA-bearing RISC, allowing it to seek out additional mRNA targets. Thus, a single miRNA—as part of a RISC—can eliminate one mRNA molecule after another, thereby efficiently blocking production of the encoded protein.

There are thought to be around 1000 different miRNAs encoded by the human genome; these RNAs may regulate as many as one-third of our protein-coding genes. Although we are only beginning to understand the full impact of these miRNAs, it is clear that they play a critical part in regulating gene expression and thereby influence many cell functions.

Figure 8–27 An miRNA targets a complementary mRNA molecule for destruction. Each precursor miRNA transcript is processed to form a double-stranded intermediate, which is further processed to form a mature, single-stranded miRNA. This miRNA assembles with a set of proteins into a complex called RISC, which then searches for mRNAs that have a nucleotide sequence complementary to its bound miRNA. Depending on how extensive the region of complementarity is, the target mRNA is either rapidly degraded by a nuclease within the RISC (shown on the *left*) or transferred to an area of the cytoplasm where other nucleases destroy it (shown on the *right*).

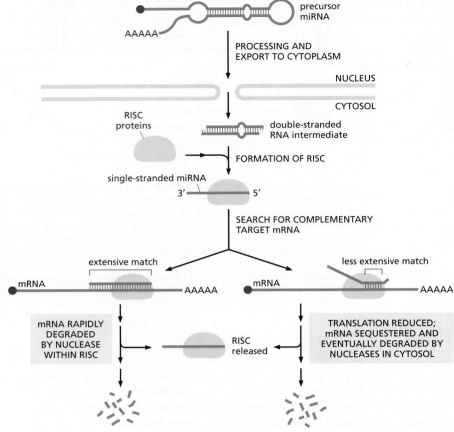

Small Interfering RNAs Protect Cells From Infections

Some of the same components that process and package miRNAs also play another crucial part in the life of a cell: they serve as a powerful cell defense mechanism. In this case, the system is used to eliminate "foreign" RNA molecules—in particular, long, double-stranded RNA molecules. Such RNAs are rarely produced by normal genes, but they often serve as intermediates in the life cycles of viruses and in the movement of some transposable genetic elements (discussed in Chapter 9). This form of RNA targeting, called **RNA interference** (**RNAi**), keeps these potentially destructive elements in check.

In the first step of RNAi, double-stranded, foreign RNAs are cut into short fragments (approximately 22 nucleotide pairs in length) in the cytosol by a protein called Dicer—the same protein used to generate the double-stranded RNA intermediate in miRNA production (see Figure 8–27). The resulting double-stranded RNA fragments, called **small interfering RNAs** (**siRNAs**), are then taken up by the same RISC proteins that carry miRNAs. The RISC discards one strand of the siRNA duplex and uses the remaining single-stranded RNA to seek and destroy complementary RNA molecules (**Figure 8–28**). In this way, the infected cell effectively turns the foreign RNA against itself.

Figure 8–28 siRNAs are produced from double-stranded, foreign RNAs during the process of RNA interference. Double-stranded RNAs from a virus or transposable genetic element are first cleaved by a nuclease called Dicer. The resulting double-stranded fragments (known as siRNAs) are incorporated into RISCs, which discard one strand of the duplex and use the other strand to locate and destroy foreign RNAs that contain a complementary sequence.

At the same time, RNAi can also selectively shut off the synthesis of foreign RNAs by the host's RNA polymerase. In this case, the siRNAs produced by Dicer are packaged into a protein complex called RITS (for RNA-induced transcriptional silencing). Using its single-stranded siRNA as a guide, the RITS complex attaches itself to complementary RNA sequences as they emerge from an actively transcribing RNA polymerase (**Figure 8–29**). Positioned along a gene in this way, the RITS complex then attracts proteins that covalently modify nearby histones in a way that promotes the localized formation of heterochromatin (see Figure 5–27). This heterochromatin then blocks further transcription initiation at that site. Such RNAi-directed heterochromatin formation helps limit the spread of transposable genetic elements throughout the host genome.

RNAi operates in a wide variety of organisms, including single-celled fungi, plants, and worms, indicating that it is an evolutionarily ancient defense mechanism, particularly against viral infection. In some organisms, including many plants, the RNAi defense response can spread from tissue to tissue, allowing an entire organism to become resistant to a virus after only a few of its cells have been infected. In this sense, RNAi resembles certain aspects of the adaptive immune responses of vertebrates; in both cases, an invading pathogen elicits the production of molecules—either siRNAs or antibodies—that are custom-made to inactivate the specific invader and thereby protect the host.

Thousands of Long Noncoding RNAs May Also Regulate Mammalian Gene Activity

At the other end of the size spectrum are the **long noncoding RNAs**, a class of RNA molecules that are defined as being more than 200 nucleotides in length. There are thought to be upward of 5000 of these lengthy RNAs encoded in the human and mouse genomes. Yet, with few exceptions, their roles in the biology of the organism, if any, are not entirely clear.

One of the best understood of the long noncoding RNAs is *Xist*. This enormous RNA molecule, some 17,000 nucleotides long, is a key player in X-inactivation—the process by which one of the two X chromosomes in the cells of female mammals is permanently silenced (see Figure 5–28). Early in development, Xist is produced by only one of the X chromosomes in each female nucleus. The transcript then "sticks around," coating the chromosome and attracting the enzymes and chromatin-remodeling complexes that promote the formation of highly condensed heterochromatin. Other long noncoding RNAs may promote the silencing of specific genes in a similar manner.

Some long noncoding RNAs fold into specific, three-dimensional structures via complementary base pairing, as discussed in Chapter 7 (see for example Figure 7–5). These structures can serve as scaffolds, which bring together proteins that function together in a particular cell process (**Figure 8–30**). For example, one of the roles of the RNA molecule in telomerase—the enzyme that duplicates the ends of eukaryotic chromosomes (see

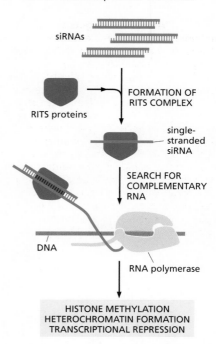

Figure 8–29 RNAi can also trigger transcriptional silencing. In this case, a single-stranded siRNA is incorporated into a RITS complex, which uses the single-stranded siRNA to search for complementary RNA sequences as they emerge from a transcribing RNA polymerase. The binding of the RITS complex attracts proteins that promote the modification of histones and the formation of tightly packed heterochromatin. This change in chromatin structure, directed by complementary base-pairing, causes transcriptional repression. Such silencing is used in plants, animals, and fungi to hold transposable elements in check.

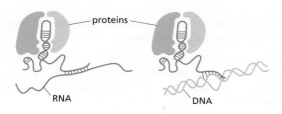

Figure 8–30 Long noncoding RNAs can serve as scaffolds, bringing together proteins that function in the same cell process. As described in Chapter 7, RNAs can fold into three-dimensional structures that can be recognized by specific proteins. By engaging in complementary base-pairing with other RNA molecules, these long noncoding RNAs can, in principle, localize proteins to specific sequences in RNA or DNA molecules, as shown.

Figure 6–23)—is to hold its different protein subunits together. By bringing together protein subunits, long noncoding RNAs can play important roles in many cell activities.

Regardless of how the various long noncoding RNAs operate—or what exactly each of them does—the discovery of this large class of RNAs reinforces the idea that a eukaryotic genome contains information that provides not only an inventory of the molecules and structures every cell must make, but also a set of instructions for how and when to assemble these parts to guide the growth and development of a complete organism.

ESSENTIAL CONCEPTS

- A typical eukaryotic cell expresses only a fraction of its genes, and the distinct types of cells in multicellular organisms arise because different sets of genes are expressed as cells differentiate.

- In principle, gene expression can be controlled at any of the steps between a gene and its ultimate functional product. For the majority of genes, however, the initiation of transcription is the most important point of control.

- The transcription of individual genes is switched on and off in cells by transcription regulators, proteins that bind to short stretches of DNA called regulatory DNA sequences.

- In bacteria, transcription regulators usually bind to regulatory DNA sequences close to where RNA polymerase binds. This binding can either activate or repress transcription of the gene. In eukaryotes, regulatory DNA sequences are often separated from the promoter by many thousands of nucleotide pairs.

- Eukaryotic transcription regulators act in two main ways: (1) they can directly affect the assembly process that requires RNA polymerase and the general transcription factors at the promoter, and (2) they can locally modify the chromatin structure of promoter regions.

- In eukaryotes, the expression of a gene is generally controlled by a combination of different transcription regulators.

- In multicellular plants and animals, the production of different transcription regulators in different cell types ensures the expression of only those genes appropriate to the particular type of cell.

- A master transcription regulator, if expressed in the appropriate precursor cell, can trigger the formation of a specialized cell type or even an entire organ.

- One differentiated cell type can be converted to another by artificially expressing an appropriate set of transcription regulators. A differentiated cell can also be reprogrammed into a stem cell by artificially expressing a different, specific set of such regulators.

- Cells in multicellular organisms have mechanisms that enable their progeny to "remember" what type of cell they should be. A prominent mechanism for propagating cell memory relies on transcription regulators that perpetuate transcription of their own gene—a form of positive feedback.

- The pattern of DNA methylation can be transmitted from one cell generation to the next, producing a form of epigenetic inheritance that helps a cell remember the state of gene expression in its parent cell. There is also evidence for a form of epigenetic inheritance based on transmitted chromatin structures.

- Cells can regulate gene expression by controlling events that occur after transcription has begun. Many of these post-transcriptional mechanisms rely on RNA molecules that can influence their own stability or translation.

- MicroRNAs (miRNAs) control gene expression by base-pairing with specific mRNAs and inhibiting their stability and translation.

- Cells have a defense mechanism for destroying "foreign" double-stranded RNAs, many of which are produced by viruses. It makes use of small interfering RNAs (siRNAs) that are produced from the foreign RNAs in a process called RNA interference (RNAi).

- The recent discovery of thousands of long noncoding RNAs in mammals has revealed new roles for RNAs in assembling protein complexes and regulating gene expression.

KEY TERMS

cell memory	post-transcriptional control
combinatorial control	promoter
differentiation	regulatory DNA sequence
DNA methylation	regulatory RNA
epigenetic inheritance	reporter gene
gene expression	RNA interference (RNAi)
induced pluripotent stem (iPS) cells	small interfering RNA (siRNA)
	transcription regulator
long noncoding RNA	transcriptional activator
microRNA (miRNA)	transcriptional repressor
positive feedback loop	

QUESTIONS

QUESTION 8–4

A virus that grows in bacteria (bacterial viruses are called bacteriophages) can replicate in one of two ways. In the prophage state, the viral DNA is inserted into the bacterial chromosome and is copied along with the bacterial genome each time the cell divides. In the lytic state, the viral DNA is released from the bacterial chromosome and replicates many times in the cell. This viral DNA then produces viral coat proteins that together with the replicated viral DNA form many new virus particles that burst out of the bacterial cell. These two forms of growth are controlled by two transcription regulators, the repressor (product of the *cI* gene) and Cro, both of which are encoded by the virus. In the prophage state, *cI* is expressed; in the lytic state, *Cro* is expressed. In addition to regulating the expression of other genes, cI represses the *Cro* gene, and Cro represses the *cI* gene (Figure Q8–4). When bacteria containing a phage in the prophage state are briefly irradiated with UV light, cI protein is degraded.

A. What will happen next?

B. Will the change in (A) be reversed when the UV light is switched off?

C. What advantage might this response to UV light provide to the virus?

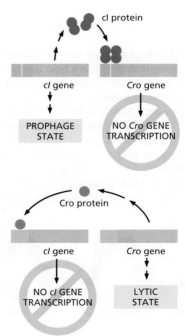

Figure Q8–4

QUESTION 8–5

Which of the following statements are correct? Explain your answers.

A. In bacteria, but not in eukaryotes, many mRNAs contain the coding region for more than one gene.

B. Most DNA-binding proteins bind to the major groove of the DNA double helix.

C. Of the major control points in gene expression (transcription, RNA processing, RNA transport, translation, and control of a protein's activity), transcription initiation is one of the most common.

QUESTION 8–6

Your task in the laboratory of Professor Quasimodo is to determine how far an enhancer (a binding site for an activator protein) can be moved from the promoter of the *straightspine* gene and still activate transcription. You systematically vary the number of nucleotide pairs between these two sites and then determine the amount of transcription by measuring the production of Straightspine mRNA. At first glance, your data look confusing (**Figure Q8–6**). What would you have expected for the results of this experiment? Can you save your reputation and explain these results to Professor Quasimodo?

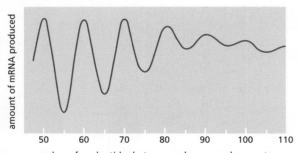

Figure Q8–6

QUESTION 8–7

The λ repressor binds as a dimer to critical sites on the λ genome to repress the virus's lytic genes. This is necessary to maintain the prophage (integrated) state. Each molecule of the repressor consists of an N-terminal DNA-binding domain and a C-terminal dimerization domain (**Figure Q8–7**). Upon viral induction (for example, by irradiation with UV light), the genes for lytic growth are expressed, λ progeny are produced, and the bacterial cell is lysed (see Question 8–4). Induction is initiated by cleavage of the λ repressor at a site between the DNA-binding domain and the dimerization domain, which causes the

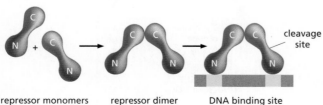

repressor monomers   repressor dimer   DNA binding site

Figure Q8–7

repressor to dissociate from the DNA. In the absence of bound repressor, RNA polymerase binds and initiates lytic growth. Given that the number (concentration) of DNA-binding domains is unchanged by cleavage of the repressor, why do you suppose its cleavage results in its dissociation from the DNA?

QUESTION 8–8

The *Arg* genes that encode the enzymes for arginine biosynthesis are located at several positions around the genome of *E. coli*, and they are regulated coordinately by a transcription regulator encoded by the *ArgR* gene. The activity of the ArgR protein is modulated by arginine. Upon binding arginine, ArgR alters its conformation, dramatically changing its affinity for the DNA sequences in the promoters of the genes for the arginine biosynthetic enzymes. Given that ArgR is a repressor protein, would you expect that ArgR would bind more tightly or less tightly to the DNA sequences when arginine is abundant? If ArgR functioned instead as an activator protein, would you expect the binding of arginine to increase or to decrease its affinity for its regulatory DNA sequences? Explain your answers.

QUESTION 8–9

When enhancers were initially found to influence transcription from many thousands of nucleotide pairs away from the promoters they control, two principal models were invoked to explain this action at a distance. In the "DNA looping" model, direct interactions between proteins bound at enhancers and promoters were proposed to stimulate transcription initiation. In the "scanning" or "entry-site" model, RNA polymerase (or another component of the transcription machinery) was proposed to bind at the enhancer and then scan along the DNA until it reached the promoter. These two models were tested using an enhancer on one piece of DNA and a β-globin gene and promoter on a separate piece of DNA (**Figure Q8–9**). The β-globin gene was not expressed when these two separate pieces of DNA were introduced together. However, when the two segments of DNA were joined via a linker (made of a protein that binds to a small molecule called biotin), the β-globin gene was expressed.

Does this experiment distinguish between the DNA looping model and the scanning model? Explain your answer.

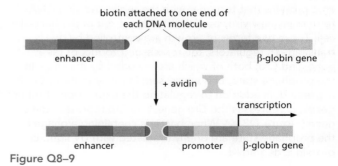

Figure Q8–9

QUESTION 8–10

Differentiated cells of an organism contain the same genes. (Among the few exceptions to this rule are the cells of the mammalian immune system, in which the formation of specialized cells is based on limited rearrangements of the genome.) Describe an experiment that substantiates the first sentence of this question, and explain why it does.

Figure 8–17 shows a simple scheme by which three transcription regulators are used during development to create eight different cell types. How many cell types could you create, using the same rules, with four different transcription regulators? As described in the text, MyoD is a transcription regulator that by itself is sufficient to induce muscle-specific gene expression in fibroblasts. How does this observation fit the scheme in Figure 8–17?

Imagine the two situations shown in Figure Q8–12. In cell I, a transient signal induces the synthesis of protein A, which is a transcriptional activator that turns on many genes including its own. In cell II, a transient signal induces the synthesis of protein R, which is a transcriptional repressor that turns off many genes including its own. In which, if either, of these situations will the descendants of the original cell "remember" that the progenitor cell had experienced the transient signal? Explain your reasoning.

(A) CELL I

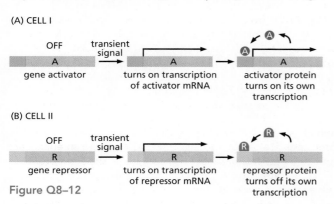

(B) CELL II

Figure Q8–12

Discuss the following argument: "If the expression of every gene depends on a set of transcription regulators, then the expression of these regulators must also depend on the expression of other regulators, and their expression must depend on the expression of still other regulators, and so on. Cells would therefore need an infinite number of genes, most of which would code for transcription regulators." How does the cell get by without having to achieve the impossible?

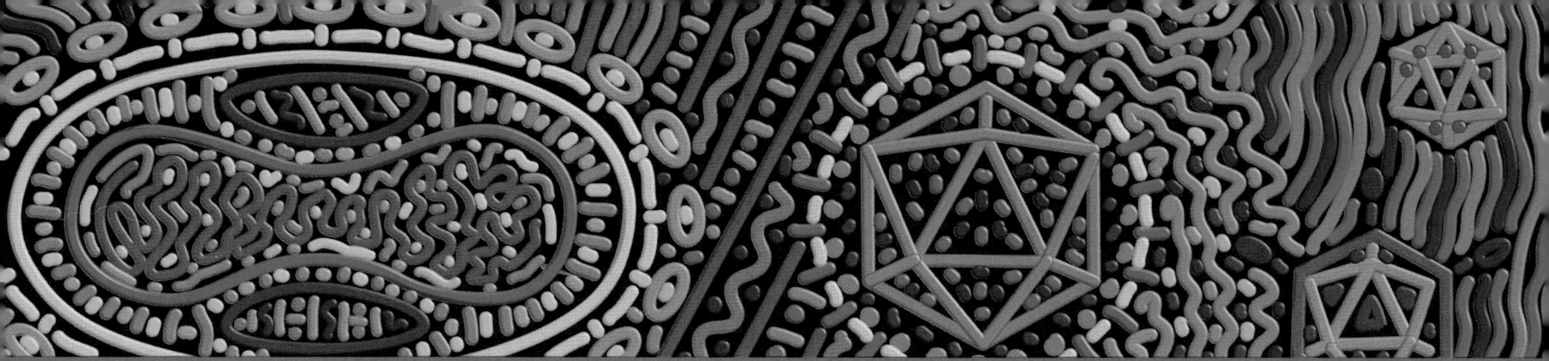

How Genes and Genomes Evolve

For a given individual, the nucleotide sequence of the genome in every one of its cells is virtually the same. But compare the DNA of two individuals—even parent and child—and that is no longer the case: the genomes of individuals within a species contain slightly different information. And between members of different species, the deviations are even more extensive.

Such differences in DNA sequence are responsible for the diversity of life on Earth, from the subtle variations in hair color, eye color, and skin color that characterize members of our own species (Figure 9–1) to the dramatic differences in phenotype that distinguish a fish from a fungus or a robin from a rose. But if all life emerged from a common ancestor—a single-celled organism that existed some 3.5 billion years ago—where did these genetic improvisations come from? How did they arise, why were they preserved, and how do they contribute to the breathtaking biological diversity that surrounds us?

Improvements in the methods used to sequence and analyze whole genomes—from pufferfish to people—are now allowing us to address some of these questions. In Chapter 10, we describe these revolutionary technologies, which continue to transform the modern era of genomics. In this chapter, we present some of the fruits of these technological innovations. We discuss how genes and genomes have been sculpted over billions of years to give rise to the spectacular menagerie of life-forms that crowd every corner of the planet. We examine the molecular mechanisms that generate genetic diversity, and we consider how the information in present-day genomes can be deciphered to yield a historical record of the evolutionary processes that have shaped these DNA

GENERATING GENETIC VARIATION

RECONSTRUCTING LIFE'S FAMILY TREE

MOBILE GENETIC ELEMENTS AND VIRUSES

EXAMINING THE HUMAN GENOME

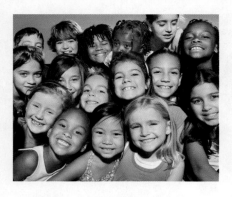

Figure 9–1 Small differences in DNA sequence account for differences in appearance between one individual and the next. A group of schoolchildren displays a sampling of the characteristics that define the unity and diversity of our own species. (joSon/Getty Images.)

sequences. We also take a brief look at mobile genetic elements and consider how these elements, along with modern-day viruses, can carry genetic information from place to place and from organism to organism. Finally, we end the chapter by taking a closer look at the human genome to see what the DNA sequences from individuals all around the world tell us about who we are and where we come from.

GENERATING GENETIC VARIATION

There is no natural mechanism for making long stretches of entirely novel nucleotide sequences. Thus evolution is more a tinkerer than an inventor: it uses as its raw materials the DNA sequences that each organism inherits from its ancestors. In this sense, no gene or genome is ever entirely new. Instead, the astonishing diversity in form and function in the living world is all the result of variations on preexisting themes. As genetic variations pile up over millions of generations, they can produce radical change.

Several basic types of genetic change are especially crucial in evolution (**Figure 9–2**):

- *Mutation within a gene:* An existing gene can be modified by a mutation that changes a single nucleotide or deletes or duplicates one or more nucleotides. These mutations can alter the splicing of a gene's RNA transcript or change the stability, activity, location, or interactions of its encoded protein or RNA product.

- *Mutation within regulatory DNA sequences:* When and where a gene is expressed can be affected by a mutation in the stretches of DNA sequence that regulate the gene's activity (described in Chapter 8). For example, humans and fish have a surprisingly large number of genes in common, but changes in the regulation of those shared genes underlie many of the most dramatic differences between those species.

- *Gene duplication and divergence:* An existing gene, or even a whole genome, can be duplicated. As the cell containing this duplication, and its progeny, continue to divide, the original DNA sequence and the duplicate sequence can acquire different mutations and thereby assume new functions and patterns of expression.

- *Exon shuffling:* Two or more existing genes can be broken and rejoined to make a hybrid gene containing DNA segments that originally belonged to separate genes. In eukaryotes, such breaking and rejoining often occurs within the long intron sequences, which do not encode protein. Because these intron sequences are removed by RNA splicing, the breaking and joining do not have to be precise to produce a functional gene.

- *Transposition of mobile genetic elements:* Specialized DNA sequences that can move from one chromosomal location to another can alter the activity or regulation of a gene; they can also promote gene duplication, exon shuffling, and other genome rearrangements.

- *Horizontal gene transfer:* A piece of DNA can be passed from the genome of one cell to that of another—even to that of another species. This process, which is rare among eukaryotes but common among bacteria, differs from the usual "vertical" transfer of genetic information from parent to progeny.

Each of these forms of genetic variation has played an important part in the evolution of modern organisms. And they still play that part today, as organisms continue to evolve. In this section, we discuss these basic mechanisms of genetic change, and we consider their consequences for

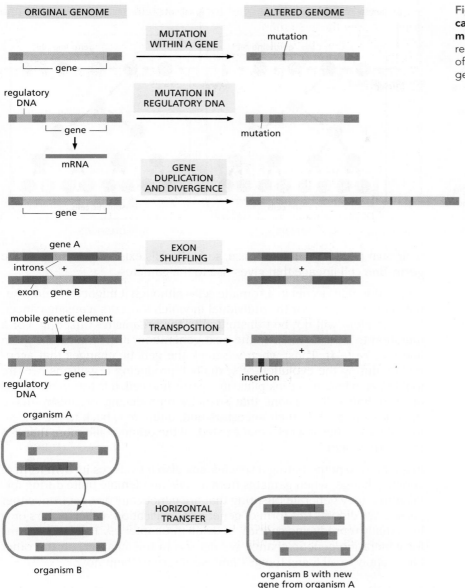

Figure 9–2 Genes and genomes can be altered by several different mechanisms. Small mutations, duplications, rearrangements, and even the infusion of fresh genetic material all contribute to genome evolution.

genome evolution. But first, we pause to consider the contribution of sex—the mechanism that many organisms use to pass genetic information on to future generations.

In Sexually Reproducing Organisms, Only Changes to the Germ Line Are Passed On to Progeny

For bacteria and unicellular organisms that reproduce asexually, the inheritance of genetic information is fairly straightforward. Each individual duplicates its genome and donates one copy to each daughter cell when the individual divides in two. The family tree of such unicellular organisms is simply a branching diagram of cell divisions that directly links each individual to its progeny and to its ancestors.

For a multicellular organism that reproduces sexually, however, the family connections are considerably more complex. Although individual cells within that organism divide, only the specialized reproductive cells—the **gametes**—carry a copy of its genome to the next generation of organisms (discussed in Chapter 19). All the other cells of the body—the **somatic cells**—are doomed to die without leaving evolutionary descendants of

Figure 9–3 Germ-line cells and somatic cells have fundamentally different functions. In sexually reproducing organisms, genetic information is propagated into the next generation exclusively by germ-line cells (*red*). This cell lineage includes the specialized reproductive cells—the gametes (eggs and sperm, half circles)—which contain only half the number of chromosomes than do the other cells in the body (full circles). When two gametes come together during fertilization, they form a fertilized egg or zygote (*purple*), which once again contains a full set of chromosomes (discussed in Chapter 19). The zygote gives rise to both germ-line cells and to somatic cells (*blue*). Somatic cells form the body of the organism but do not contribute their DNA to the next generation.

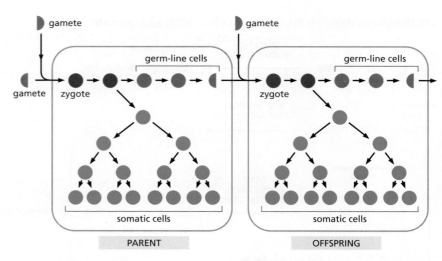

their own (**Figure 9–3**). In a sense, somatic cells exist only to support the **germ-line** cell lineage that gives rise to the gametes.

A mutation that occurs in a somatic cell—although it might have unfortunate consequences for the individual in which it occurs (causing cancer, for example)—will not be transmitted to the organism's offspring. For a mutation to be passed on to the next generation, it must alter the germ line (**Figure 9–4**). Thus, when we track the genetic changes that accumulate during the evolution of sexually reproducing organisms, we are looking at events that took place in a germ-line cell. It is through a series of germ-line cell divisions that sexually reproducing organisms trace their descent back to their ancestors and, ultimately, back to the ancestors of us all—the first cells that existed, at the origin of life more than 3.5 billion years ago.

In addition to perpetuating a species, sex also introduces its own form of genetic change: when gametes from a male and female unite during fertilization, they generate offspring that are genetically distinct from either parent. We discuss this form of genetic diversification, which occurs only in sexually reproducing species, in detail in Chapter 19. The mechanisms for generating genetic change we discuss in this chapter, on the other hand, apply to all living things—and we return to them now.

Point Mutations Are Caused by Failures of the Normal Mechanisms for Copying and Repairing DNA

Despite the elaborate mechanisms that exist to faithfully copy and repair DNA sequences, every nucleotide pair in an organism's genome runs a

Figure 9–4 Mutations in germ-line cells and somatic cells have different consequences. A mutation that occurs in a germ-line cell (A) can be passed on to the next generation (*green*). By contrast, a mutation that arises in a somatic cell (B) affects only the progeny of that cell (*orange*) and will not be passed on to the organism's offspring. As we discuss in Chapter 20, somatic mutations are responsible for most human cancers (see pp. 720–721).

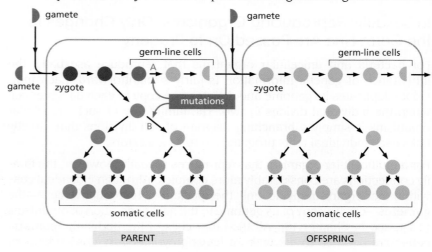

small risk of changing each time a cell divides. Changes that affect a single nucleotide pair are called **point mutations**. These typically arise from rare errors in DNA replication or repair (discussed in Chapter 6).

The point mutation rate has been determined directly in experiments with bacteria such as *E. coli*. Under laboratory conditions, *E. coli* divides about once every 20–25 minutes; in less than a day, a single *E. coli* can produce more descendants than there are humans on Earth—enough to provide a good chance for almost any conceivable point mutation to occur. A culture containing 10^9 *E. coli* cells thus harbors millions of mutant cells whose genomes differ subtly from a single ancestor cell. A few of these mutations may confer a selective advantage on individual cells: resistance to a poison, for example, or the ability to survive when deprived of a standard nutrient. By exposing the culture to a selective condition— adding an antibiotic or removing an essential nutrient, for example—one can find these needles in the haystack; that is, the cells that have undergone a specific mutation enabling them to survive in conditions where the original cells cannot (**Figure 9–5**). Such experiments have revealed that the overall point mutation frequency in *E. coli* is about 3 changes for each 10^{10} nucleotide pairs replicated. With a genome size of 4.6 million nucleotide pairs, this mutation rate means that approximately 99.99% of the time, the two daughter cells produced in a round of cell division will inherit exactly the same genome sequence of the parent *E. coli* cell; mutant cells are therefore produced only rarely.

The overall mutation rate in humans, as determined by comparing the DNA sequences of children and their parents (and estimating how many times the parental germ cells divided before producing gametes), is about one-third that of *E. coli*—which suggests that the mechanisms that

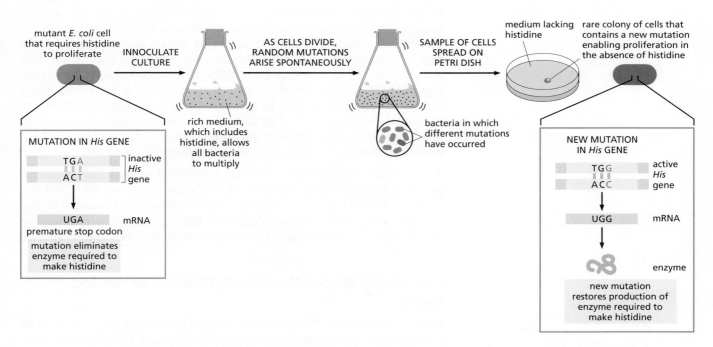

Figure 9–5 Mutation rates can be measured in the laboratory. In this experiment, an *E. coli* strain that carries a deleterious point mutation in the *His* gene—which is needed to manufacture the amino acid histidine—is used. The mutation has converted a G-C nucleotide pair to an A-T, resulting in a premature stop signal in the mRNA produced from the mutant gene (*left* box). As long as histidine is supplied in the growth medium, this strain can grow and divide normally. If a large number of mutant cells (say 10^{10}) is spread on an agar plate that lacks histidine, the great majority will die. The rare survivors will contain a new mutation in which the A-T is changed back to a G-C. This "reversion" corrects the original defect and allows the bacterium to make the enzyme it needs to survive in the absence of histidine. Such mutations happen by chance and only rarely, but the ability to work with very large numbers of *E. coli* cells makes it possible to detect this change and to accurately measure its frequency.

evolved to maintain genome integrity operate with an efficiency that does not greatly differ between even distantly related species.

Point mutations can destroy a gene's activity or—very rarely—improve it (as shown in Figure 9–5). More often, however, they do neither of these things. At many sites in the genome, a point mutation has absolutely no effect on the organism's appearance, viability, or ability to reproduce. Such *neutral mutations* often fall in regions of the gene where the DNA sequence is unimportant, including most of an intron's sequence. In cases where they occur within an exon, neutral mutations can change the third position of a codon such that the amino acid it specifies is unchanged—or is so similar that the protein's function is unaffected.

Mutations Can Also Change the Regulation of a Gene

Point mutations that lie outside the coding sequences of genes can sometimes affect regulatory DNA sequences—elements that control the timing, location, and level of gene expression. Such mutations in regulatory DNA sequences can have a profound effect on the protein's production and thereby on the organism. For example, a small number of people are resistant to malaria because of a point mutation that affects the expression of a cell-surface receptor to which the malaria parasite *Plasmodium vivax* binds. The mutation prevents the receptor from being produced in red blood cells, rendering the individuals who carry this mutation immune to malarial infection.

Point mutations in regulatory DNA sequences also have a role in our ability to digest lactose, the main sugar in milk. Our earliest ancestors were lactose intolerant, because the enzyme that breaks down lactose—called lactase—was made only during infancy. Adults, who were no longer exposed to breast milk, did not need the enzyme. When humans began to get milk from domesticated cattle some 10,000 years ago, variant genes—the product of random mutation—enabled those who carried the variation to continue to express lactase as adults, and thus take advantage of nutrition provided by cow's milk. We now know that people who retain the ability to digest milk as adults contain a point mutation in the regulatory DNA sequence of the lactase gene, allowing it to be efficiently transcribed throughout life. In a sense, these milk-drinking adults are "mutants" with respect to their ancestors. It is remarkable how quickly this adaptation spread through the human population, especially in societies that depended heavily on milk for nutrition (Figure 9–6).

These evolutionary changes in the regulatory DNA sequence of the lactase gene occurred relatively recently (10,000 years ago), well after humans became a distinct species. However, much more ancient changes in regulatory DNA sequences have occurred in other genes, and some of these are thought to underlie many of the profound differences among species (Figure 9–7).

DNA Duplications Give Rise to Families of Related Genes

Point mutations can influence the activity of an existing gene, but how do new genes with new functions come into being? Gene duplication is perhaps the most important mechanism for generating new genes from old ones. Once a gene has been duplicated, each of the two copies is free to accumulate mutations—as long as whatever activities the original gene may have had are not lost. Over time, as mutations continue to accumulate in the descendants of the original cell in which gene duplication occurred, some of these genetic changes allow one of the gene copies to perform a different function.

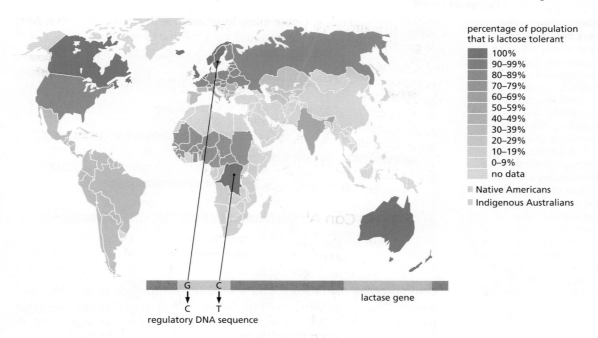

Figure 9–6 The widespread ability of adult humans to digest milk followed the domestication of cattle. Approximately 10,000 years ago, humans in northern Europe and central Africa began to raise cattle. The subsequent availability of cow's milk—particularly during periods of starvation—gave a selective advantage to those humans able to digest lactose as adults. Two independent point mutations that allow the expression of lactase in adults arose in human populations—one in northern Europe and another in central Africa. These mutations have since spread through different regions of the world.

By repeated rounds of this process of **gene duplication and divergence** over many millions of years, one gene can give rise to a whole family of genes, each with a specialized function, within a single genome. Analysis of genome sequences reveals many examples of such **gene families**: in *Bacillus subtilis*, for example, nearly half of the genes have one or more obvious relatives elsewhere in the genome. And in vertebrates, the globin family of genes, which encode oxygen-carrying proteins, clearly arose from a single primordial gene, as we see shortly. But how does gene duplication occur in the first place?

Many gene duplications are believed to be generated by *homologous recombination*. As discussed in Chapter 6, homologous recombination provides an important mechanism for mending a broken double helix; it allows an intact chromosome to be used as a template to repair a damaged sequence on its homolog. But as we discuss in Chapter 19, homologous recombination can also catalyze *crossovers* in which two

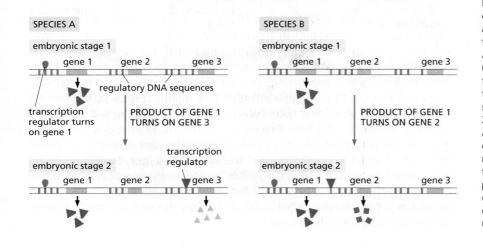

Figure 9–7 Changes in regulatory DNA sequences can have dramatic consequences for the development of an organism. In this hypothetical example, the genomes of two closely related species A and B contain the same three genes (1, 2, and 3) and encode the same two transcription regulators (*red oval, brown triangle*). However, the regulatory DNA sequences controlling expression of genes 2 and 3 are different in the two species. Although both express gene 1 during embryonic stage 1, the differences in their regulatory DNA sequences cause them to express different genes in stage 2. In principle, a collection of such regulatory changes can have profound effects on an organism's developmental program—and, ultimately, on the appearance of the adult.

Figure 9–8 Gene duplication can be caused by crossovers between short, repeated DNA sequences in adjacent homologous chromosomes. The two chromosomes shown here undergo homologous recombination at short repeated sequences (*red*), that bracket a gene (*orange*). For simplicity, only one gene is shown on each homolog. The repeated sequences can be remnants of mobile genetic elements, which are present in many copies in the human genome, as we discuss shortly. When crossing-over occurs unequally, as shown, one chromosome will get two copies of the gene, while the other will get none. The type of homologous recombination that produces gene duplications is called *unequal crossing-over* because the resulting products are unequal in size. If this process occurs in the germ line, some progeny will inherit the long chromosome, while others will inherit the short one.

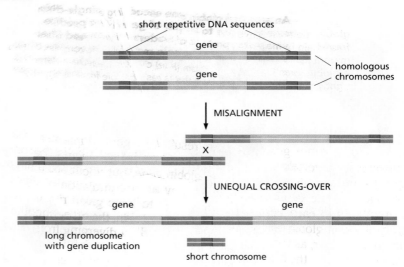

chromosomes are broken and joined up to produce hybrid chromosomes. Crossovers take place only between regions of chromosomes that have nearly identical DNA sequences; for this reason, they usually occur between homologous chromosomes and generate hybrid chromosomes in which the order of genes is exactly the same as on the original chromosomes. This process occurs extensively during meiosis, as we see in Chapter 19.

On rare occasions, however, a crossover can occur between a pair of short DNA sequences—identical or very similar—that fall on either side of a gene. If these short sequences are not aligned properly during recombination, a lopsided exchange of genetic information can occur. Such unequal crossovers can generate one chromosome that has an extra copy of the gene and another with no copy (**Figure 9–8**); this shorter chromosome will eventually be lost.

Once a gene has been duplicated in this way, extra copies of the gene can be added by the same mechanism. As a result, entire sets of closely related genes, arranged in series, are commonly found in genomes.

Duplication and Divergence Produced the Globin Gene Family

The evolutionary history of the globin gene family provides a striking example of how gene duplication and divergence has generated new proteins. The unmistakable similarities in amino acid sequence and structure among present-day globin proteins indicate that all the globin genes must derive from a single ancestral gene.

The simplest globin protein has a single polypeptide chain of about 150 amino acids, and is found in many marine worms, insects, and primitive fish. Like our hemoglobin, this protein transports oxygen molecules throughout the animal's body. The oxygen-carrying protein in the blood of adult mammals and most other vertebrates, however, is more complex; it is composed of four globin chains of two distinct types—α globin and β globin (**Figure 9–9**). The four oxygen-binding sites in the $\alpha_2\beta_2$ molecule interact, allowing an allosteric change in the molecule as it binds and releases oxygen. This structural shift enables the four-chain hemoglobin molecule to efficiently take up and release four oxygen molecules in an all-or-none fashion, a feat not possible for the single-chain version. Such efficiency is particularly important for large multicellular animals, which cannot rely on the simple diffusion of oxygen through the body to oxygenate their tissues adequately.

Figure 9–9 An ancestral globin gene encoding a single-chain globin molecule gave rise to the pair of genes that produce four-chain hemoglobin proteins of modern humans and other mammals. The mammalian hemoglobin molecule is a complex of two α-globin (*green*) and two β-globin (*blue*) chains. Each chain contains a tightly bound heme group (*red*) that is responsible for binding oxygen.

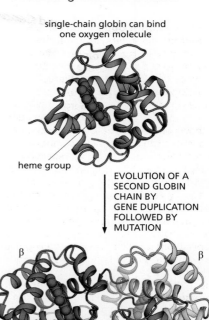

single-chain globin can bind one oxygen molecule

heme group

EVOLUTION OF A SECOND GLOBIN CHAIN BY GENE DUPLICATION FOLLOWED BY MUTATION

four-chain hemoglobin can bind four oxygen molecules in a cooperative way

The α- and β-globin genes are the result of a gene duplication that occurred early in vertebrate evolution. Genome analyses suggest that one of our distant ancestors had a single globin gene. But about 500 million years ago, a gene duplication followed by an accumulation of different mutations in each gene copy is thought to have given rise to two slightly different globin genes, one encoding α globin, the other encoding β globin. Still later, as the different mammals began diverging from their common ancestor, the β-globin gene underwent its own duplication and divergence to give rise to a second β-like globin gene that is expressed specifically in the fetus (**Figure 9–10**). The resulting fetal hemoglobin molecule has a higher affinity for oxygen compared with adult hemoglobin, a property that helps transfer oxygen from mother to fetus.

Subsequent rounds of duplication and divergence in both the α- and β-globin genes gave rise to additional members of these families. Each of these duplicated genes has been modified by point mutations that affect the properties of the final hemoglobin molecule, and by changes in regulatory DNA sequences that determine when—and how strongly—each gene is expressed. As a result, each globin differs slightly in its ability to bind and release oxygen and in the stage of development during which it is expressed.

In addition to these specialized globin genes, there are several duplicated DNA sequences in the α- and β-globin gene clusters that are not functional genes. They are similar in DNA sequence to the functional globin genes, but they have been disabled by the accumulation of many inactivating mutations. The existence of such *pseudogenes* makes it clear that not every DNA duplication leads to a new functional gene. In fact, most gene duplication events are unsuccessful in that one copy is gradually inactivated by mutation. Although we have focused here on the evolution of the globin genes, similar rounds of gene duplication and divergence have clearly taken place in many other gene families present in the human genome.

Figure 9–10 Repeated rounds of duplication and mutation generated the globin gene family in humans. About 500 million years ago, an ancestral globin gene duplicated and gave rise to both the β-globin gene family (including the five genes shown) and the α-globin gene family. In most vertebrates, a molecule of hemoglobin (see Figure 9–9) is formed from two chains of α globin and two chains of β globin—which can be any one of the five subtypes of the β family listed here.

The evolutionary scheme shown was worked out by comparing globin genes from many different organisms. The nucleotide sequences of the γG and γA genes—which produce the β-globin-like chains that form fetal hemoglobin—are much more similar to each other than either of them is to the adult β gene. The δ-globin gene encodes a minor form of adult β-globin. In humans, the β-globin genes are located in a cluster on Chromosome 11.

A subsequent chromosome breakage event, which occurred about 300 million years ago, is believed to have separated the α- and β-globin genes; the α-globin genes now reside on human Chromosome 16 (not shown).

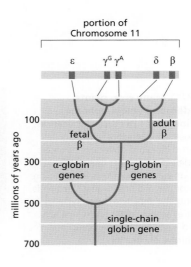

portion of Chromosome 11

ε   γG γA   δ β

millions of years ago

100

fetal β

adult β

300   α-globin genes   β-globin genes

500

single-chain globin gene

700

Whole-Genome Duplications Have Shaped the Evolutionary History of Many Species

Almost every gene in the genomes of vertebrates exists in multiple versions, suggesting that, rather than single genes being duplicated in a piecemeal fashion, the whole vertebrate genome was long ago duplicated in one fell swoop. Early in vertebrate evolution, it appears that the entire genome actually underwent duplication twice in succession, giving rise to four copies of every gene. In some groups of vertebrates, such as the salmon and carp families (including the zebrafish; see Figure 1–38), there may have been yet another duplication, creating an eightfold multiplicity of genes.

The precise history of whole-genome duplications in vertebrate evolution is difficult to chart because many other changes, including the loss of genes, have occurred since these ancient evolutionary events. In some organisms, however, full genome duplications are especially obvious, as they have occurred relatively recently, evolutionarily speaking. The frog genus *Xenopus*, for example, includes closely related species that differ dramatically in DNA content: some are diploid—containing two complete sets of chromosomes—whereas others are tetraploid or octoploid. Such large-scale duplications can happen if cell division fails to occur following a round of genome replication in the germ line of a particular individual. Once an accidental doubling of the genome occurs in a germ-line cell, it will be faithfully passed on to germ-line progeny cells in that individual and, ultimately, to any offspring these cells might produce.

Whole-genome duplications are also common in plants, including many of those that we eat. These genome duplications generally make the plant easier to cultivate and its fruit more palatable. In some cases, genome duplication renders the plant sterile so that it cannot produce seeds; such is the case with seedless grapes. Apples, leeks, and potatoes are all tetraploid, whereas strawberries and sugarcane are octoploid (**Figure 9–11**).

Novel Genes Can Be Created by Exon Shuffling

As we discussed in Chapter 4, many proteins are composed of smaller functional *domains*. In eukaryotes, each of these protein domains is usually encoded by a separate exon, which is surrounded by long stretches of noncoding introns (see Figures 7–18 and 7–19). This organization of eukaryotic genes can facilitate the evolution of new proteins by allowing exons from one gene to be added to another—a process called **exon shuffling**.

Such duplication and movement of exons is promoted by the same type of recombination that gives rise to gene duplications (see Figure 9–8). In this case, recombination occurs within the introns that surround the exons.

Figure 9–11 Many crop plants have undergone whole-genome duplication. Many of these duplications, which arose spontaneously, were propagated by plant breeders because they rendered the plants easier to cultivate or made their fruits larger, more flavorful, or devoid of indigestible seeds. N indicates the ploidy of each type of plant: for example, wheat and kiwi are hexaploid—possessing six complete sets of chromosomes (6N).

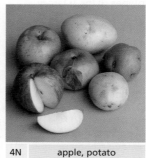
4N   apple, potato

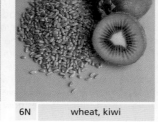
6N   wheat, kiwi

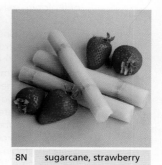
8N   sugarcane, strawberry

If the introns in question are from two different genes, this recombination can generate a hybrid gene that includes complete exons from both. The results of such exon shuffling are seen in many present-day proteins, which contain a patchwork of many different protein domains (**Figure 9–12**).

It has been proposed that nearly all the proteins encoded by the human genome (approximately 19,000) arose from the duplication and shuffling of a few thousand distinct exons, each encoding a protein domain of approximately 30–50 amino acids. This remarkable idea suggests that the great diversity of protein structures is generated from a fairly small universal "parts list," pieced together in different combinations.

The Evolution of Genomes Has Been Profoundly Influenced by Mobile Genetic Elements

Mobile genetic elements—DNA sequences that can move from one chromosomal location to another—are an important source of genomic change and have profoundly affected the structure of modern genomes. These parasitic DNA sequences can colonize a genome and then spread within it. In the process, they often disrupt the function or alter the regulation of existing genes; sometimes they even create novel genes through fusions between mobile sequences and segments of existing genes.

The insertion of a mobile genetic element into the coding sequence of a gene or into its regulatory DNA sequence can cause the "spontaneous" mutations that are observed in many of today's organisms. Mobile genetic elements can severely disrupt a gene's activity if they land directly within its coding sequence. Such an insertion mutation destroys the gene's capacity to encode a useful protein—as is the case for a number of mutations that cause hemophilia in humans, for example.

The activity of mobile genetic elements can also change the way existing genes are regulated. An insertion of an element into a regulatory DNA sequence, for instance, will often have a striking effect on where or when genes are expressed (**Figure 9–13**). Many mobile genetic elements carry DNA sequences that are recognized by specific transcription regulators; if these elements insert themselves near a gene, that gene can be brought under the control of these transcription regulators, thereby changing the gene's expression pattern. Thus, mobile genetic elements can be a major source of developmental changes: they have been particularly important in the evolution of domesticated plants. For example, the development of modern corn from a wild, grassy plant called teosinte required only a small number of genetic alterations. One of these changes was the insertion of a mobile genetic element upstream of a gene active in seed development, which transformed the small, hard seeds of teosinte into the plentiful soft kernels of modern corn (**Figure 9–14**).

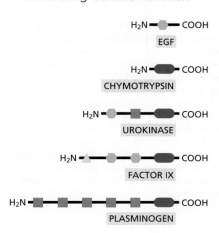

Figure 9–12 Exon shuffling during evolution can generate proteins with new combinations of protein domains. Each type of colored symbol represents a different protein domain. These different domains were joined together by exon shuffling during evolution to create the modern-day human proteins shown here. EGF, epidermal growth factor.

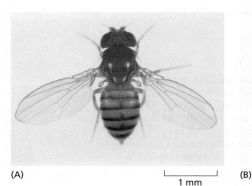
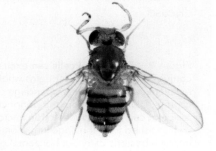

(A) |— 1 mm —| (B)

Figure 9–13 Mutation due to a mobile genetic element can induce dramatic alterations in the body plan of an organism. (A) A normal fruit fly (*Drosophila melanogaster*). (B) A mutant fly in which the antennae have been replaced by legs because of a mutation in a regulatory DNA sequence that causes genes for leg formation to be activated in the positions normally reserved for antennae. Although this particular change is not advantageous to the fly, it illustrates how the movement of a transposable element can produce a major change in the appearance of an organism. (A, Edward B. Lewis. Courtesy of the Archives, California Institute of Technology; B, courtesy of Matthew Scott.)

Figure 9–14 The insertion of a mobile genetic element helped produce modern corn. Today's corn plants were originally bred from a wild plant called teosinte (A). This wild ancestor produced numerous ears that contained small, hard seeds. (B) Modern corn, by contrast, produces fewer cobs—but they contain numerous plump, sweet kernels. The insertion of a mobile genetic element near a gene involved in seed development helped drive the change. Here, the two plants are drawn to the same scale; for simplicity, the leaves are not shown.

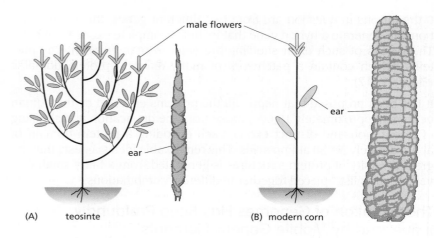

(A) teosinte   (B) modern corn

Finally, mobile genetic elements provide opportunities for genome rearrangements by serving as targets of homologous recombination (see Figure 9–8). For example, the duplications that gave rise to the β-globin gene cluster are thought to have occurred by crossovers between the abundant mobile genetic elements sprinkled throughout the human genome. Later in the chapter, we describe these elements in more detail and discuss the mechanisms that have allowed them to establish a stronghold within our genome.

Genes Can Be Exchanged Between Organisms by Horizontal Gene Transfer

So far we have considered genetic changes that take place within the genome of an individual organism. However, genes and other portions of genomes can also be exchanged between individuals of different species. This mechanism of **horizontal gene transfer** is rare among eukaryotes but common among bacteria, which can exchange DNA by the process of conjugation (**Figure 9–15** and Movie 9.1).

E. coli, for example, has acquired about one-fifth of its genome from other bacterial species within the past 100 million years. And such genetic exchanges are currently responsible for the rise of new and potentially dangerous strains of drug-resistant bacteria. Genes that confer resistance to antibiotics are readily transferred from species to species, providing the recipient bacterium with an enormous selective advantage in evading the antimicrobial compounds that constitute modern medicine's frontline attack against bacterial infection. As a result, many antibiotics are no longer effective against the common bacterial infections for which they were originally used; as an example, most strains of *Neisseria gonorrhoeae*, the bacterium that causes gonorrhea, are now resistant to penicillin, which is therefore no longer the primary drug used to treat this disease.

QUESTION 9–2

Why do you suppose that horizontal gene transfer is more prevalent in single-celled organisms than in multicellular organisms?

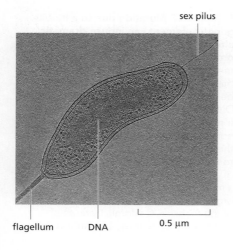

sex pilus

flagellum   DNA   0.5 μm

Figure 9–15 Bacterial cells can exchange DNA through conjugation. Conjugation begins when a donor cell captures a recipient cell using a fine appendage called a sex pilus. Following capture, DNA moves from the donor cell, through the pilus, into the recipient cell. In this cryoelectron micrograph, the sex pilus is clearly distinguished from the flagellum. Conjugation is one of several ways in which bacteria carry out horizontal gene transfer. (From C.M. Oikonomou and G.J. Jensen, *Nat. Rev. Microbiol.* 14:205–220, 2016. With permission from Macmillan Publishers Ltd.)

RECONSTRUCTING LIFE'S FAMILY TREE

The nucleotide sequences of present-day genomes provide a record of those genetic changes that have survived the test of time. By comparing the genomes of a variety of living organisms, we can thus begin to decipher our evolutionary history and see how our ancestors veered off in adventurous new directions that led us to where we are today.

The most astonishing revelation of such genome comparisons has been that **homologous genes**—those that are similar in nucleotide sequence because of their common ancestry—can be recognized across vast evolutionary distances. Unmistakable homologs of many human genes are easy to detect in organisms such as worms, fruit flies, yeasts, and even bacteria. Although the lineage that led to the evolution of vertebrates is thought to have diverged from the one that led to nematode worms and insects more than 600 million years ago, when we compare the genomes of the nematode *Caenorhabditis elegans* and the fruit fly *Drosophila melanogaster* with that of *Homo sapiens*, we find that about 50% of the genes in each of these species have clear homologs in one or both of the other two species. In other words, clearly recognizable versions of at least half of all human genes must have already been present in the common ancestor of worms, flies, and humans.

By tracing such relationships among genes, we can begin to define the evolutionary relationships among different species, placing each bacterium, animal, plant, or fungus in a single vast family tree of life. In this section, we discuss how these relationships are determined and what they tell us about our genetic heritage.

Genetic Changes That Provide a Selective Advantage Are Likely to Be Preserved

Evolution is commonly thought of as progressive, but at the molecular level the process is random. Consider the fate of a point mutation that occurs in a germ-line cell. On rare occasions, the mutation might cause a change for the better. But most often it will either have no consequence or cause serious damage. Mutations of the first type will tend to be perpetuated, because the organism that inherits them will have an increased likelihood of reproducing itself. Mutations that are deleterious will usually be lost. And mutations that are *selectively neutral* may or may not persist, depending on factors such as the size of the population, or whether the individual carrying the neutral mutation also harbors a favorable mutation located nearby. Through endless repetition of such cycles of mutation and natural selection—a molecular form of trial and error—organisms gradually evolve. Their genomes change and they develop new ways to exploit the environment—to outcompete others and to reproduce successfully.

Clearly, some parts of the genome can accumulate mutations more easily than others in the course of evolution. A segment of DNA that does not code for protein or RNA and has no significant regulatory role is free to change at a rate limited only by the frequency of random mutation. In contrast, deleterious alterations in a gene that codes for an essential protein or RNA molecule cannot be accommodated so easily: when mutations occur, the faulty organism will almost always be eliminated or fail to reproduce. Genes of this latter sort are therefore *highly conserved*; that is, the products they encode, whether RNA or protein, are very similar from organism to organism. Throughout the 3.5 billion years or more of evolutionary history, the most highly conserved genes remain perfectly recognizable in all living species. They encode crucial proteins such as DNA and RNA polymerases, and they are the ones we turn to

QUESTION 9–3

Highly conserved genes such as those for ribosomal RNA are present as clearly recognizable relatives in all organisms on Earth; thus, they have evolved very slowly over time. Were such genes "born" perfect?

Figure 9–16 **Phylogenetic trees display the relationships among modern life-forms.** In this family tree of higher primates, humans fall closer to chimpanzees than to gorillas or orangutans, as there are fewer differences between human and chimp DNA sequences than there are between those of humans and gorillas, or of humans and orangutans. As indicated, the genome sequences of each of these four species are estimated to differ from the sequence of the last common ancestor of higher primates by about 1.5%. Because changes occur independently in each lineage after two species diverge from a common ancestor, the genetic differences between any two species will be twice as much as the amount of change between each of the species and the common ancestor. For example, although humans and orangutans each differ from their common ancestor by about 1.5% in terms of nucleotide sequence, they typically differ from one another by slightly more than 3%; human and chimp genomes differ by about 1.2%. This phylogenetic tree is based solely on nucleotide sequences of species alive today, as indicated on the *left* side of the graph; the estimated dates of divergence, shown on the *right* side of the graph, are derived from analysis of the fossil record. (Modified from F.C. Chen and W.H. Li, *Am. J. Hum. Genet.* 68:444–456, 2001.)

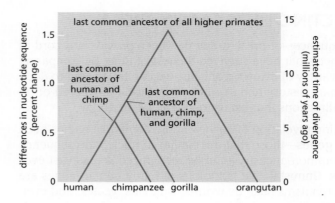

when we wish to trace family relationships among the most distantly related organisms in the tree of life.

Closely Related Organisms Have Genomes That Are Similar in Organization as Well as Sequence

For species that are closely related, it is often most informative to focus on selectively neutral mutations. Because they accumulate steadily at a rate that is unconstrained by selection pressures, these mutations provide a metric for gauging how much modern species have diverged from their common ancestor. Such sequence comparisons allow the construction of a **phylogenetic tree**, a diagram that depicts the evolutionary relationships among a group of organisms. As an example, Figure 9–16 presents a phylogenetic tree that lays out the relationships among higher primates.

As indicated in this figure, chimpanzees are our closest living relative among the higher primates. Not only do chimpanzees seem to have essentially the same set of genes as we do, but their genes are arranged in nearly the same way on their chromosomes. The only substantial exception is human Chromosome 2, which arose from a fusion of two chromosomes that remain separate in the chimpanzee, gorilla, and orangutan. Humans and chimpanzees are so closely related that it is possible to use DNA sequence comparisons to reconstruct the amino acid sequences of proteins that must have been present in the now-extinct, common ancestor of the two species (Figure 9–17).

Even the rearrangement of genomes by crossing over, which we described earlier, has produced only minor differences between the human and chimp genomes. For example, both the chimp and human genomes contain a million copies of a type of mobile genetic element called an *Alu* sequence. More than 99% of these elements are in corresponding positions in both genomes, indicating that most of the *Alu* sequences in our genome were in place before humans and chimpanzees diverged.

Functionally Important Genome Regions Show Up as Islands of Conserved DNA Sequence

As we delve back further into our evolutionary history and compare our genomes with those of more distant relatives, the picture begins to change. The lineages of humans and mice, for example, diverged about 75 million years ago. These genomes are about the same size, contain practically the same genes, and are both riddled with mobile genetic elements. However, the mobile genetic elements found in mouse and human DNA, although similar in nucleotide sequence, are distributed

```
                        gorilla CAA
                                Q
human DNA  GTGCCCATCCAAAAAGTCCAAGATGACACCAAAACCCTCATCAAGACAATTGTCACCAGG
chimp DNA  GTGCCCATCCAAAAAGTCCAAGATGACACCAAAACCCTCATCAAGACAATTGTCACCAGG
  protein   V  P  I  Q  K  V  Q  D  D  T  K  T  L  I  K  T  I  V  T  R


                                                       K
human DNA  ATCAATGACATTTCACACACGCAGTCAGTCTCCTCCAAACAGAAAGTCACCGGTTTGGAC
chimp DNA  ATCAATGACATTTCACACACGCAGTCAGTCTCCTCCAAACAGAAGGTCACCGGTTTGGAC
  protein   I  N  D  I  S  H  T  Q  S  V  S  S  K  Q  K  V  T  G  L  D
                                                 gorilla AAG


             gorilla CCC
                     P
human DNA  TTCATTCCTGGGCTCCACCCCATCCTGACCTTATCCAAGATGGACCAGACACTGGCAGTC
chimp DNA  TTCATTCCTGGGCTCCACCCTATCCTGACCTTATCCAAGATGGACCAGACACTGGCAGTC
  protein   F  I  P  G  L  H  P  I  L  T  L  S  K  M  D  Q  T  L  A  V


                               *
                               V
human DNA  TACCAACAGATCCTCACCAGTATGCCTTCCAGAAACGTGATCCAAATATCCAACGACCTG
chimp DNA  TACCAACAGATCCTCACCAGTATGCCTTCCAGAAACATGATCCAAATATCCAACGACCTG
  protein   Y  Q  Q  I  L  T  S  M  P  S  R  N  M  I  Q  I  S  N  D  L
                                            gorilla ATG


                   D
human DNA  GAGAACCTCCGGGATCTTCTTCAGGTGCTGGCCTTCTCTAAGAGCTGCCACTTGCCCTGG
chimp DNA  GAGAACCTCCGGGACCTTCTTCAGGTGCTGGCCTTCTCTAAGAGCTGCCACTTGCCCTGG
  protein   E  N  L  R  D  L  L  H  V  L  A  F  S  K  S  C  H  L  P  W
             gorilla GAC
```

Figure 9–17 Ancestral gene sequences can be reconstructed by comparing closely related present-day species. Shown here, in five contiguous segments of DNA, are the nucleotide sequences that encode the mature leptin protein from humans and chimpanzees. Leptin is a hormone that regulates food intake and energy utilization. As indicated by the codons boxed in *green*, only five nucleotides differ between the chimp and human sequences. Only one of these changes (marked with an asterisk) results in a change in the amino acid sequence.

The nucleotide sequence of the last common ancestor was probably the same as the human and chimp sequences where they agree; in the few places where they disagree, the gorilla sequence (*red*) can be used as a "tiebreaker," as the gorilla sequence is evolutionarily more distant than those of chimp and human (see Figure 9–16). Thus, the amino acid indicated by the asterisk was a methionine in the common ancestor of humans and chimpanzees and is changed to a valine in the human lineage. For convenience, only the first 300 nucleotides of the coding sequences for the mature leptin protein are shown; the last 141 nucleotides of that sequence are identical between humans and chimpanzees.

differently, as they have had more time to proliferate and move around the two genomes after these species diverged (**Figure 9–18**).

In addition to the movement of mobile genetic elements, the large-scale organization of the human and mouse genomes has been scrambled by many episodes of chromosome breakage and recombination over the past 75 million years: it is estimated that about 180 such "break-and-join" events have dramatically altered chromosome organization. For example, in humans most centromeres lie near the middle of the chromosome, whereas those of mouse are located at the chromosome ends.

Regardless of this significant degree of genetic shuffling, one can nevertheless still recognize many blocks of **conserved synteny**, regions in which corresponding genes are strung together in the same order in both species. These genes were neighbors in the ancestral species and, despite all the chromosomal upheavals, they remain neighbors in the two present-day species. More than 90% of the mouse and human genomes can be partitioned into such corresponding regions of conserved synteny. Within these regions, we can align the DNA of mouse with that of humans so that we can compare the nucleotide sequences in detail. Such genome-wide sequence comparisons reveal that, in the roughly

Figure 9–18 Differences in the positions of mobile genetic elements in the human and mouse genomes reflect the long evolutionary time separating the two species. This stretch of human Chromosome 11 (seen also in Figure 9–10) contains five functional β-globin-like genes (*orange*); the comparable region from the mouse genome contains only four. The positions of two types of mobile genetic element—*Alu* sequences (*green*) and *L1* sequences (*red*)—are shown in each genome. Although the mobile genetic elements in human (*circles*) and mouse (*triangles*) are not identical, they are closely related. The absence of these elements within the globin genes can be attributed to *purifying selection*, which would have eliminated any insertion that compromised gene function. (The mobile genetic element that falls inside the human β-globin gene (*far right*) is located within an intron, not in a coding sequence.) (Courtesy of Ross Hardison and Webb Miller.)

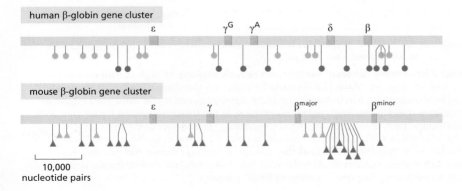

human β-globin gene cluster

ε   γ^G   γ^A   δ   β

mouse β-globin gene cluster

ε   γ   β^major   β^minor

10,000
nucleotide pairs

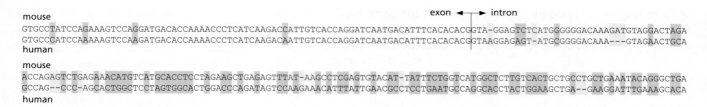

```
mouse                                                                           exon ◀─▶ intron
GTGCCTATCCAGAAAGTCCAGGATGACACCAAAACCCTCATCAAGACCATTGTCACCAGGATCAATGACATTTCACACACGGTA-GGAGTCTCATGGGGGGACAAAGATGTAGGACTAGA
GTGCCCATCCAAAAAGTCCAAGATGACACCAAAACCCTCATCAAGACAATTGTCACCAGGATCAATGACATTTCACACACGGTAAGGAGAGT-ATGCGGGGACAAA---GTAGAACTGCA
human

mouse
ACCAGAGTCTGAGAAACATGTCATGCACCTCCTAGAAGCTGAGAGTTTAT-AAGCCTCGAGTGTACAT-TATTTCTGGTCATGGCTCTTGTCACTGCTGCCTGCTGAAATACAGGGCTGA
GCCAG--CCC-AGCACTGGCTCCTAGTGGCACTGGACCCAGATAGTCCAAGAAACATTTATTGAACGCCTCCTGAATGCCAGGCACCTACTGGAAGCTGA--GAAGGATTTGAAAGCACA
human
```

Figure 9–19 Accumulated mutations have resulted in considerable divergence in the nucleotide sequences of the human and the mouse genomes. Shown here in two contiguous segments of DNA are portions of the human and mouse leptin gene sequences. Positions where the sequences differ by a single nucleotide substitution are boxed in *green*, and positions where they differ by the addition or deletion of nucleotides are boxed in *yellow*. Note that the coding sequence of the exon is much more conserved than the adjacent intron sequence.

75 million years since humans and mice diverged from their common ancestor, about 50% of the nucleotides have changed. However, these differences are not dispersed evenly across the genome. By observing where the human and mouse sequences have remained nearly the same, one can thus see very clearly the regions where genetic changes are not tolerated (**Figure 9–19**). These sequences have been conserved by **purifying selection**—that is, by the elimination of individuals carrying mutations that interfere with important functions.

The power of *comparative genomics* can be further increased by stacking our genome up against the genomes of additional animals, including the rat, chicken, and dog. Such comparisons take advantage of the results of the "natural experiment" that has lasted for hundreds of millions of years, and they highlight some of the most important regions of these genomes. These comparisons reveal that roughly 4.5% of the human genome consists of DNA sequences that are highly conserved in many other mammals (**Figure 9–20**). Surprisingly, only about one-third

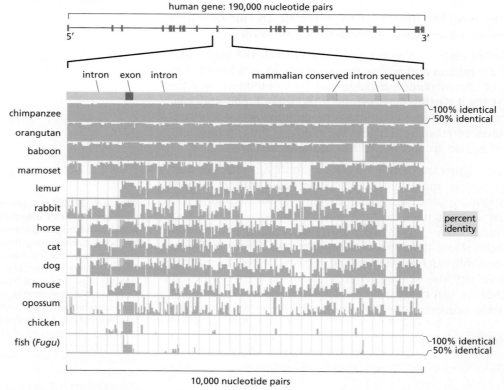

Figure 9–20 Comparison of nucleotide sequences from many different vertebrates reveals regions of high conservation. The nucleotide sequence examined in this diagram is a small segment of the human gene for a plasma membrane transporter protein. The upper part of the diagram shows the location of the exons (*red*) in both the complete gene (*top*) and in the expanded region of the gene. Three blocks of intron sequence that are conserved in mammals are shown in *blue*. In the lower part of the figure, the DNA sequence of the expanded segment of 10,000 nucleotide pairs is aligned with the corresponding sequences of different vertebrates; the percent identity with the human sequences for successive stretches of 100 nucleotide pairs is plotted in *green*, with only identities above 50% shown. Note that the sequence of the exon is highly conserved in all the species, including chicken and fish, but the three intron sequences that are conserved in mammals are not conserved in chickens or fish. The functions of most conserved intron sequences in the human genome (including these three) are not known. (Courtesy of Eric D. Green.)

of these sequences code for proteins. Some of the conserved noncoding sequences correspond to regulatory DNA, whereas others are transcribed to produce RNA molecules that are not translated into protein but serve a variety of functions (see Chapter 8). The functions of many of these conserved noncoding sequences, however, remain unknown. The unexpected discovery of these mysterious conserved DNA sequences suggests that we understand much less about the cell biology of mammals than we had previously imagined. With the plummeting cost and accelerating speed of whole-genome sequencing, we can expect many more surprises that will lead to an increased understanding in the years ahead.

Genome Comparisons Show That Vertebrate Genomes Gain and Lose DNA Rapidly

Going back even further in evolution, we can compare our genome with those of more distantly related vertebrates. The lineages of fish and mammals diverged about 400 million years ago. This stretch of time is long enough for random sequence changes and differing selection pressures to have obliterated almost every trace of similarity in nucleotide sequence—except where purifying selection has operated to prevent change. Regions of the genome conserved between humans and fishes thus stand out even more strikingly than those conserved between different mammals. In fishes, one can still recognize most of the same genes as in humans and even many of the same regulatory DNA sequences. On the other hand, the extent of duplication of any given gene is often different, resulting in different numbers of members of gene families in the two species.

Even more striking is the finding that although all vertebrate genomes contain roughly the same number of genes, their overall size varies considerably. Whereas human, dog, and mouse are all in the same size range (around 3×10^9 nucleotide pairs), the chicken genome is only one-third this size. An extreme example of genome compression is the pufferfish *Fugu rubripes* (Figure 9–21). The fish's tiny genome is about one-eighth the size of mammalian genomes, largely because of the small size of its intergenic regions, which are missing nearly all of the repetitive DNA that makes up a large portion of most mammalian genomes. The *Fugu* introns are also short in comparison to human introns. Nonetheless, the positions of most *Fugu* introns are perfectly conserved when compared with their positions in the genomes of mammals. Clearly, the intron structure of most vertebrate genes was already in place in the common ancestor of fish and mammals.

What factors could be responsible for the size differences among modern vertebrate genomes? Detailed comparisons of many genomes have led to the unexpected finding that small blocks of sequence are being lost from and added to genomes at a surprisingly rapid rate. It seems likely, for example, that the *Fugu* genome is so tiny because it lost DNA sequences faster than it gained them. Over long periods, this imbalance apparently cleared out those DNA sequences whose loss could be tolerated. This "cleansing" process has been enormously helpful to biologists: by "trimming the fat" from the *Fugu* genome, evolution has provided a conveniently slimmed-down version of a vertebrate genome in which the only DNA sequences that remain are those that are very likely to have important functions.

Sequence Conservation Allows Us to Trace Even the Most Distant Evolutionary Relationships

As we go back further still to the genomes of our even more distant relatives—beyond apes, mice, fish, flies, worms, plants, and yeasts, all

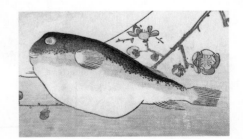

Figure 9–21 The pufferfish, *Fugu rubripes*, has a remarkably compact genome. At 400 million nucleotide pairs, the *Fugu* genome is only one-quarter the size of the zebrafish genome, even though the two species have nearly the same genes. (From a woodcut by Hiroshige, courtesy of Arts and Designs of Japan.)

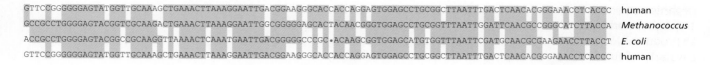

Figure 9–22 **Some genetic information has been conserved since the beginnings of life.** A part of the gene for the small ribosomal subunit rRNA (see Figure 7–35) is shown. Corresponding segments of nucleotide sequence from this gene in three distantly related species (*Methanococcus jannaschii* and *Escherichia coli*, both prokaryotes, and *Homo sapiens*, a eukaryote) are aligned in parallel. Sites where the nucleotides are identical between any two species are indicated by *green* shading; the human sequence is repeated at the bottom of the alignment so that all three two-way comparisons can be seen. The *red dot* halfway along the *E. coli* sequence denotes a site where a nucleotide has been either deleted from the bacterial lineage in the course of evolution or inserted in the other two lineages. Note that the three sequences have all diverged from one another to a roughly similar extent, while still retaining unmistakable similarities.

the way to bacteria—we find fewer and fewer resemblances to our own genome. Yet even across this enormous evolutionary divide, purifying selection has maintained a few hundred fundamentally important genes. By comparing the sequences of these genes in different organisms and seeing how far they have diverged, we can attempt to construct a phylogenetic tree that goes all the way back to the ultimate ancestors—the cells at the very origins of life, from which we all derive.

To construct such a tree, biologists have focused on one particular gene that is conserved in all living species: the gene that codes for the ribosomal RNA (rRNA) of the small ribosomal subunit (shown schematically in Figure 7–35). Because the process of translation is fundamental to all living cells, this component of the ribosome has been highly conserved since early in the history of life on Earth (**Figure 9–22**).

By applying the same principles used to construct the primate family tree (see Figure 9–16), the small-subunit rRNA nucleotide sequences have been used to create a single, all-encompassing tree of life. Although many aspects of this phylogenetic tree were anticipated by classical taxonomy (which is based on the outward appearance of organisms), there were also many surprises. Perhaps the most important was the realization that some of the organisms that were traditionally classed as "bacteria" are as widely divergent in their evolutionary origins as is any prokaryote from any eukaryote. As discussed in Chapter 1, it is now apparent that the prokaryotes comprise two distinct groups—the *bacteria* and the *archaea*—that diverged early in the history of life on Earth. The living world therefore has three major divisions or *domains*: bacteria, archaea, and eukaryotes (**Figure 9–23**).

Although we humans have been classifying the visible world since antiquity, we now realize that most of life's genetic diversity lies in the world of microscopic organisms. These microbes have tended to go unnoticed, unless they cause disease or rot the timbers of our houses. Yet they make up most of the total mass of living matter on our planet. Many of these

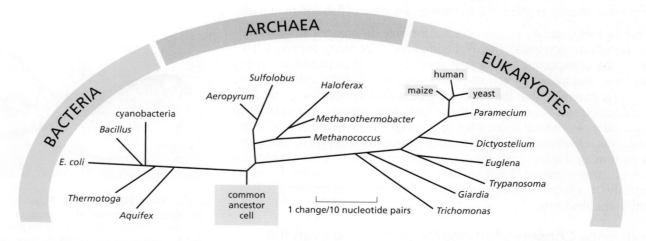

Figure 9–23 **The tree of life has three major divisions.** Each branch on the tree is labeled with the name of a representative member of that group, and the length of each branch corresponds to the degree of difference in the DNA sequences that encode their small-subunit rRNAs (see Figure 9–22). Note that all the organisms we can see with the unaided eye—animals, plants, and some fungi (highlighted in *yellow*)—represent only a small subset of the diversity of life.

organisms cannot be grown under laboratory conditions. Thus it is only through the analysis of DNA sequences, obtained from around the globe, that we are beginning to obtain a more detailed understanding of all life on Earth—knowledge that is less distorted by our biased perspective as large animals living on dry land.

MOBILE GENETIC ELEMENTS AND VIRUSES

The tree of life depicted in Figure 9–23 includes representatives from life's most distant branches, from the cyanobacteria that release oxygen into Earth's atmosphere to the animals, like us, that use that oxygen to boost their metabolism. What the diagram does not encompass, however, are the parasitic genetic elements that operate on the outskirts of life. Although these elements are built from the same nucleic acids contained in all life-forms and can multiply and move from place to place, they do not cross the threshold of actually being alive. Yet because of their prevalence and their penchant for propagating themselves, these diminutive genetic parasites have major implications for the evolution of species and for human health.

We briefly discussed these **mobile genetic elements**, earlier in the chapter, and here we consider them in greater detail. Known informally as jumping genes, mobile genetic elements are found in virtually all cells. Their DNA sequences make up almost half of the human genome. Although they can insert themselves into virtually any region of the genome, most mobile genetic elements lack the ability to leave the cell in which they reside. This is not the case for their relatives, the *viruses*. Not much more than strings of genes wrapped in a protective coat, viruses can escape from one cell and infect another.

In this section, we discuss mobile genetic elements and viruses. We review their structure and outline how they operate—and we consider the effects they have on gene expression, genome evolution, and the transmission of disease.

Mobile Genetic Elements Encode the Components They Need for Movement

Mobile genetic elements, also called **transposons,** are typically classified according to the mechanism by which they move or *transpose*. In bacteria, the most common mobile genetic elements are the *DNA-only transposons*. The name is derived from the fact that the element moves from one place to another as a piece of DNA, as opposed to being converted into an RNA intermediate—which is the case for another type of mobile element we discuss shortly. Bacteria contain many different DNA-only transposons. Some move to the target site using a simple cut-and-paste mechanism, whereby the element is simply excised from the genome and inserted into a different site. Other DNA-only transposons replicate before transposing; in this case, the new copy of the transposon inserts into a second chromosomal site, while the original copy remains intact at its previous location (**Figure 9–24**).

Each mobile genetic element typically encodes a specialized enzyme, called a *transposase*, that mediates its movement. These enzymes recognize and act on unique DNA sequences that are present on the mobile genetic elements that code for the transposase. Many mobile genetic elements also harbor additional genes: some mobile genetic elements, for example, carry antibiotic-resistance genes, which have contributed greatly to the widespread dissemination of antibiotic resistance in bacterial populations (**Figure 9–25**).

Figure 9–24 **The most common mobile genetic elements in bacteria, DNA-only transposons, move by two types of mechanism.** (A) In cut-and-paste transposition, the element is cut out of the donor DNA and inserted into the target DNA, leaving behind a broken donor DNA molecule, which is subsequently repaired. (B) In replicative transposition, the mobile genetic element is copied by DNA replication. The donor molecule remains unchanged, and the target molecule receives a copy of the mobile genetic element. In general, a particular type of transposon moves by only one of these mechanisms. However, the two mechanisms have many enzymatic similarities, and a few transposons can move by either mechanism. The donor and target DNAs can be part of the same DNA molecule or reside on different DNA molecules.

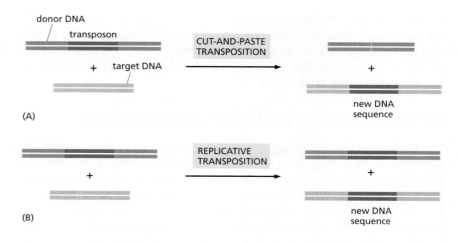

(A)

(B)

In addition to relocating themselves, mobile genetic elements occasionally rearrange the DNA sequences of the genome in which they are embedded. For example, if two mobile genetic elements that are recognized by the same transposase integrate into neighboring regions of the same chromosome, the DNA between them can be accidentally excised and inserted into a different gene or chromosome (**Figure 9–26**). In eukaryotic genomes, such accidental transposition provides a pathway for generating novel genes, both by altering gene expression and by duplicating existing genes.

The Human Genome Contains Two Major Families of Transposable Sequences

The sequencing of human genomes has revealed many surprises, as we describe in detail in the next section. But one of the most stunning was the finding that a large part of our DNA is not entirely our own. Nearly half of the human genome is made up of mobile genetic elements, which number in the millions. Some of these elements have moved from place to place within the human genome using the cut-and-paste mechanism discussed earlier (see Figure 9–24A). However, most have moved not as DNA, but via an RNA intermediate. These **retrotransposons** appear to be unique to eukaryotes.

One abundant human retrotransposon, the **L1 element** (sometimes referred to as *LINE-1, a long interspersed nuclear element*), is transcribed into RNA by a host cell's RNA polymerase. A double-stranded DNA copy of this RNA is then made using an enzyme called **reverse transcriptase**, an unusual DNA polymerase that can use RNA as a template. The reverse transcriptase is encoded by the *L1* element itself. The DNA copy of the element is then free to reintegrate into another site in the genome (**Figure 9–27**).

L1 elements constitute about 15% of the human genome. Although most copies have been immobilized by the accumulation of deleterious

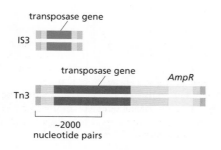

Figure 9–25 **Transposons contain the components they need for transposition.** Shown here are two types of bacterial DNA-only transposons. Each carries a gene that encodes a transposase (*blue* and *red*)—the enzyme that catalyzes the element's movement—as well as DNA sequences (*red*) that are recognized by each transposase.

Some transposons carry additional genes (*yellow*) that encode enzymes that inactivate antibiotics such as ampicillin (*AmpR*). The spread of these transposons is a serious problem in medicine, as it has allowed many disease-causing bacteria to become resistant to antibiotics developed during the twentieth century.

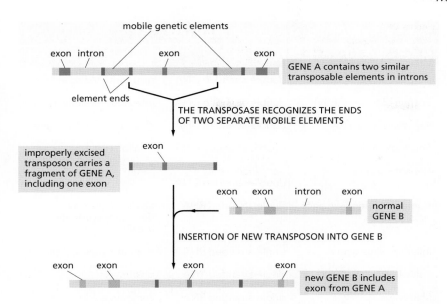

mobile genetic elements

exon intron exon exon

GENE A contains two similar transposable elements in introns

element ends

THE TRANSPOSASE RECOGNIZES THE ENDS OF TWO SEPARATE MOBILE ELEMENTS

improperly excised transposon carries a fragment of GENE A, including one exon

exon

exon exon intron exon

normal GENE B

INSERTION OF NEW TRANSPOSON INTO GENE B

exon exon exon exon

new GENE B includes exon from GENE A

Figure 9–26 Mobile genetic elements can move exons from one gene to another. When two mobile genetic elements of the same type (*red*) happen to insert near each other in a chromosome, the transposition mechanism occasionally recognizes the ends of two different elements (instead of the two ends of the same element). As a result, the chromosomal DNA that lies between the mobile genetic elements gets excised and moved to a new site. Such inadvertent transposition of chromosomal DNA can either generate novel genes, as shown, or alter gene regulation (not shown).

mutations, a few still retain the ability to transpose. Their movement can sometimes precipitate disease: for example, movement in the germline of an *L1* element into the gene that encodes Factor VIII—a protein essential for proper blood clotting—caused hemophilia in a child with no family history of the disease.

Another type of retrotransposon, the ***Alu* sequence**, is present in about 1 million copies, making up about 10% of our genome. *Alu* elements do not encode their own reverse transcriptase and thus depend on enzymes already present in the cell to help them move.

Comparisons of the sequence and locations of the *L1* and *Alu* elements in different mammals suggest that these sequences have proliferated in primates relatively recently in evolutionary history (see Figure 9–18). Given that the placement of mobile genetic elements can have profound effects on gene expression, it is humbling to contemplate how many of our uniquely human qualities we might owe to these prolific genetic parasites.

Viruses Can Move Between Cells and Organisms

Viruses are also mobile, but unlike the transposons we have discussed so far, they can actually escape from cells and move to other cells and organisms. Viruses were first categorized as disease-causing agents that, by virtue of their tiny size, passed through ultrafine filters that can hold back even the smallest bacterial cell. We now know that viruses are essentially small genomes enclosed by a protective protein coat, and that they must enter a cell and coopt its molecular machinery to express their genes, make their proteins, and reproduce. Although the first viruses that were discovered attack mammalian cells, it is now recognized that many types of viruses exist, and virtually all organisms—including plants, animals, and bacteria—can serve as viral hosts.

Viral reproduction is often lethal to the host cells; in many cases, the infected cell breaks open (lyses), releasing progeny viruses, which can then infect neighboring cells. Many of the symptoms of viral infections reflect this lytic effect of the virus. The cold sores formed by herpes simplex virus and the blisters caused by the chickenpox virus, for example, reflect the localized killing of human skin cells.

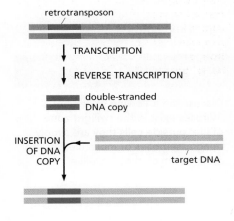

retrotransposon

TRANSCRIPTION

REVERSE TRANSCRIPTION

double-stranded DNA copy

INSERTION OF DNA COPY

target DNA

Figure 9–27 Retrotransposons move via an RNA intermediate. These transposable elements are first transcribed into an RNA intermediate (not shown). Next, a double-stranded DNA copy of this RNA is synthesized by the enzyme reverse transcriptase. This DNA copy is then inserted into the target location, which can be on either the same or a different DNA molecule. The donor retrotransposon remains at its original location, so each time it transposes, it duplicates itself. These mobile genetic elements are called retrotransposons because at one stage in their transposition their genetic information flows backward, from RNA to DNA.

TABLE 9–1 VIRUSES THAT CAUSE HUMAN DISEASE

Virus	Genome Type	Disease
Herpes simplex virus	double-stranded DNA	recurrent cold sores
Epstein–Barr virus (EBV)	double-stranded DNA	infectious mononucleosis
Varicella-zoster virus	double-stranded DNA	chickenpox and shingles
Smallpox virus	double-stranded DNA	smallpox
Hepatitis B virus	part single-, part double-stranded DNA	serum hepatitis
Human immunodeficiency virus (HIV)	single-stranded RNA	acquired immune deficiency syndrome (AIDS)
Influenza virus type A	single-stranded RNA	respiratory disease (flu)
Poliovirus	single-stranded RNA	poliomyelitis
Rhinovirus	single-stranded RNA	common cold
Hepatitis A virus	single-stranded RNA	infectious hepatitis
Hepatitis C virus	single-stranded RNA	non-A, non-B type hepatitis
Yellow fever virus	single-stranded RNA	yellow fever
Rabies virus	single-stranded RNA	rabies encephalitis
Mumps virus	single-stranded RNA	mumps
Measles virus	single-stranded RNA	measles

QUESTION 9–5

Discuss the following statement: "Viruses exist in the twilight zone of life: outside cells they are simply dead assemblies of molecules; inside cells, however, they are alive."

Most viruses that cause human disease have genomes made of either double-stranded DNA or single-stranded RNA (Table 9–1). However, viral genomes composed of single-stranded DNA and of double-stranded RNA are also known. The simplest viruses found in nature have a small genome, composed of as few as three genes, enclosed by a protein coat built from many copies of a single polypeptide chain. More complex viruses have larger genomes of up to several hundred genes, surrounded by an elaborate shell composed of many different proteins (Figure 9–28). The amount of genetic material that can be packaged inside a viral protein shell is limited. Because these shells are too small to encase the genes needed to encode the many enzymes and other proteins that are required to replicate even the simplest virus, viruses must hijack their host's biochemical machinery to reproduce themselves (Figure 9–29). A viral genome will typically encode both viral coat proteins and proteins that help the virus to commandeer the host enzymes needed to replicate its genetic material.

Retroviruses Reverse the Normal Flow of Genetic Information

Although there are many similarities between bacterial and eukaryotic viruses, one important class of viruses—the **retroviruses**—is found only in eukaryotic cells. In many respects, retroviruses resemble the retrotransposons we just discussed. A key feature of the replication cycle of both is a step in which DNA is synthesized using RNA as a template— hence the prefix *retro,* which refers to the reversal of the usual flow of information from DNA to RNA. Retroviruses are thought to have derived from a retrotransposon that long ago acquired additional genes encoding

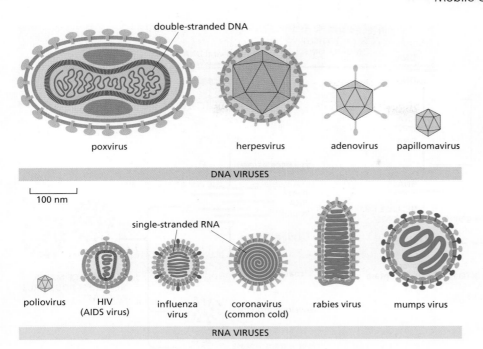

double-stranded DNA

poxvirus   herpesvirus   adenovirus   papillomavirus

DNA VIRUSES

100 nm

single-stranded RNA

poliovirus   HIV
(AIDS virus)   influenza
virus   coronavirus
(common cold)   rabies virus   mumps virus

RNA VIRUSES

Figure 9–28 Viruses come in different shapes and sizes. Some of the viruses are shown in cross section (such as poxvirus and HIV). For others, the outer structure is emphasized. Some viruses (such as papilloma and polio) contain an outer surface that is composed solely of viral-encoded proteins. Others (such as poxvirus and HIV) bear a lipid-bilayer envelope (*gray*) in which viral-encoded proteins are embedded.

the coat proteins and other proteins required to make a virus particle. The RNA stage of its replicative cycle could then be packaged into a viral particle that could leave the cell.

Like retrotransposons, retroviruses use the enzyme reverse transcriptase to convert RNA into DNA. The enzyme is encoded by the retroviral genome, and a few molecules of the enzyme are packaged along with the RNA genome in each virus particle. When the single-stranded RNA genome of the retrovirus enters a cell, the reverse transcriptase brought in with it makes a complementary DNA strand to form a DNA/RNA hybrid double helix. The RNA strand is removed, and the reverse transcriptase (which can use either DNA or RNA as a template) now synthesizes a complementary DNA strand to produce a DNA double helix. This DNA is then inserted, or integrated, into a randomly selected site in the host genome by a virally encoded *integrase* enzyme. In this integrated state, the virus is *latent*: each time the host cell divides, it passes on a copy of the integrated viral genome, which is known as a *provirus*, to its progeny cells.

The next step in the replication of a retrovirus—which can take place long after its integration into the host genome—is the copying of the integrated viral DNA into RNA by a host-cell RNA polymerase, which produces large numbers of single-stranded RNAs identical to the original infecting genome. These viral RNAs are then translated by the host-cell ribosomes to produce the viral shell proteins, the envelope proteins, and reverse transcriptase—all of which are assembled with the RNA genome into new virus particles. The steps involved in the integration and replication of a retrovirus are shown in **Figure 9–30**.

Figure 9–29 Viruses commandeer the host cell's molecular machinery to reproduce. The hypothetical virus illustrated here consists of a small, double-stranded DNA molecule that encodes just a single type of viral coat protein. To reproduce, the viral genome must first enter a host cell, where it is replicated to produce multiple copies, which are transcribed and translated to produce the viral coat protein. The viral genomes can then assemble spontaneously with the coat protein to form new virus particles, which escape from the cell by lysing it.

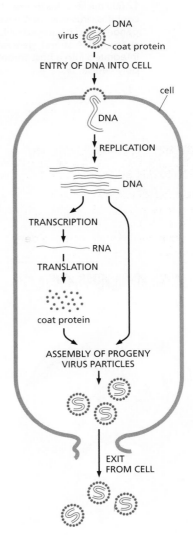

virus   DNA
coat protein

ENTRY OF DNA INTO CELL

cell

DNA

REPLICATION

DNA

TRANSCRIPTION

RNA

TRANSLATION

coat protein

ASSEMBLY OF PROGENY VIRUS PARTICLES

EXIT FROM CELL

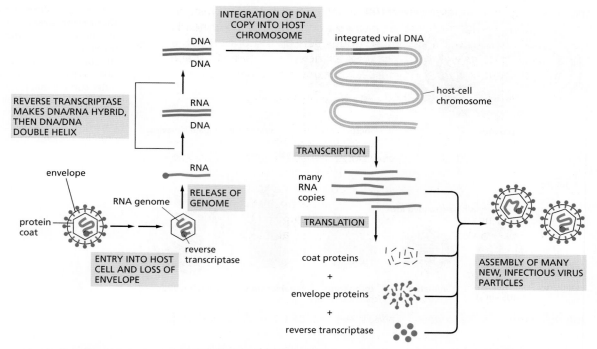

Figure 9–30 Infection by a retrovirus includes reverse transcription and integration of the viral genome into the host cell's DNA. The retrovirus genome consists of an RNA molecule (*blue*) that is typically between 7000 and 12,000 nucleotides in size. It is packaged inside a protein coat, which is surrounded by a lipid-bilayer envelope that contains virus-encoded envelope proteins (*green*). The enzyme reverse transcriptase (*red circle*), encoded by the viral genome and packaged with its RNA, first makes a single-stranded DNA copy of the viral RNA molecule and then a second DNA strand, generating a double-stranded DNA copy of the RNA genome. This DNA double helix is then integrated into a host chromosome, a step required for the synthesis of new viral RNA molecules by a host-cell RNA polymerase.

The human immunodeficiency virus (HIV), which is the cause of AIDS, is a retrovirus. As with other retroviruses, the HIV genome can persist in a latent state as a provirus embedded in the chromosomes of an infected cell. This ability to hide in host cells complicates attempts to treat the infection with antiviral drugs. But because the HIV reverse transcriptase is not used by cells for any purpose of their own, it is one of the prime targets of drugs currently used to treat AIDS.

EXAMINING THE HUMAN GENOME

The human genome contains an enormous amount of information about who we are and where we came from (**Figure 9–31**). Its 3.2×10^9 nucleotide pairs, spread out over 23 sets of chromosomes—22 autosomes and a pair of sex chromosomes (X and Y)—provide the instructions needed to build a human being. Yet, 25 years ago, biologists actively debated the value of determining the *human genome sequence*—the complete list of nucleotides contained in our chromosomes.

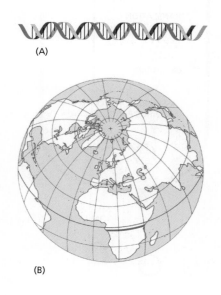

Figure 9–31 The 3 billion nucleotide pairs of the human genome contain a vast amount of information, including clues about our origins. If each nucleotide pair is drawn to span 1 mm, as shown in (A), the human genome would extend 3200 km (approximately 2000 miles)—far enough to stretch across central Africa, where humans first arose (*red* line in B). At this scale, there would be, on average, a protein-coding gene every 150 m. An average gene would extend for about 30 m, but the coding sequences (exons) in this gene would add up to only just over a meter; the rest would be introns.

The task was not simple. An international consortium of investigators labored tirelessly for the better part of a decade—and spent nearly $3 billion—to give us our first glimpse of this genetic blueprint. But the effort turned out to be well worth the cost, as the data continue to shape our thinking about how our genome functions and how it has evolved.

The first human genome sequence was just the beginning. The spectacular improvements in sequencing technologies (which we discuss in Chapter 10), coupled with powerful new tools for handling massive amounts of data, are taking genomics to a whole new level. The cost of DNA sequencing has dropped enormously since the Human Genome Project was launched in 1990, such that a whole human genome can now be sequenced in a few days for about $1000. Investigators around the world are collaborating to collect and compare the nucleotide sequences of thousands of human genomes. This resulting deluge of data offers tantalizing clues as to what makes us human, and what makes each of us unique.

Although it will take many years to analyze the rapidly accumulating genome data, the recent findings have already influenced the content of every chapter in this book. In this section, we describe some of the most striking features of the human genome—many of which were entirely unexpected. We review what genome comparisons can tell us about how we evolved, and we discuss some of the mysteries that still remain.

The Nucleotide Sequences of Human Genomes Show How Our Genes Are Arranged

When the DNA sequence of human Chromosome 22, one of the smallest human chromosomes, was completed in 1999, it became possible for the first time to see exactly how genes are arranged along an entire vertebrate chromosome (Figure 9–32). The subsequent publication of the

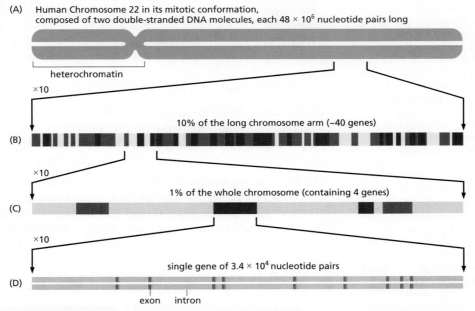

Figure 9–32 The sequence of Chromosome 22 shows how human chromosomes are organized. (A) Chromosome 22, one of the smallest human chromosomes, contains 48×10^6 nucleotide pairs and makes up approximately 1.5% of the human genome. Most of the short arm of Chromosome 22 consists of short repeated sequences of DNA that are packaged in a particularly compact form of chromatin (heterochromatin), as discussed in Chapter 5. (B) A tenfold expansion of a portion of Chromosome 22 shows about 40 genes. Those in *dark brown* are known genes, and those in *red* are predicted genes. (C) An expanded portion of (B) shows the entire length of several genes. (D) The intron–exon arrangement of a typical gene is shown after a further tenfold expansion. Each exon (*red*) codes for a portion of the protein, while the DNA sequence of the introns (*yellow*) is relatively unimportant. (Adapted from The International Human Genome Sequencing Consortium, *Nature* 409:860–921, 2001.)

TABLE 9–2 SOME VITAL STATISTICS FOR THE HUMAN GENOME	
DNA Length	3.2 × 10⁹ Nucleotide Pairs*
Number of protein-coding genes	approximately 19,000
Number of non-protein-coding genes**	approximately 5000
Largest gene	2.4×10^6 nucleotide pairs
Mean gene size	27,000 nucleotide pairs
Smallest number of exons per gene	1
Largest number of exons per gene	178
Mean number of exons per gene	10.4
Largest exon size	17,106 nucleotide pairs
Mean exon size	145 nucleotide pairs
Number of pseudogenes***	approximately 11,000
Percentage of DNA sequence in exons (protein-coding sequences)	1.5%
Percentage of DNA conserved with other mammals that does not encode protein****	3.0%
Percentage of DNA in high-copy repetitive elements	approximately 50%

*The sequence of 2.85 billion nucleotide pairs is known precisely (error rate of only about one in 100,000 nucleotides). The remaining DNA consists primarily of short, highly repeated sequences that are tandemly repeated, with repeat numbers differing from one individual to the next.

**These include genes that encode structural, catalytic, and regulatory RNAs.

***A pseudogene is a DNA sequence that closely resembles that of a functional gene but contains numerous mutations that prevent its proper expression. Most pseudogenes arise from the duplication of a functional gene, followed by the accumulation of damaging mutations in one copy.

****This includes DNA encoding 5′ and 3′ UTRs (untranslated regions of mRNAs), regulatory DNA sequences, and conserved regions of unknown function.

Figure 9–33 The bulk of the human genome is made of repetitive nucleotide sequences and other noncoding DNA. About half of our genome consists of repeated sequences. These include the LINEs (long interspersed nuclear elements, such as *L1*), SINEs (short interspersed nuclear elements, such as *Alu*), other retrotransposons, and DNA-only transposons—mobile genetic elements that have multiplied in our genome by replicating themselves and inserting the new copies in different positions. Most of these mobile genetic elements are fossils—remnants that are no longer capable of transposition. Simple repeats are short nucleotide sequences (less than 14 nucleotide pairs) that are repeated again and again for long stretches. Segment duplications are large blocks of the genome (1000–200,000 nucleotide pairs) that are present at two or more locations in the genome. These, too, represent repeated DNA sequences. The most highly repeated blocks of DNA in heterochromatin have not yet been completely sequenced; these comprise about 10% of human DNA sequences and are not represented in this diagram.

The unique sequences that are not part of any introns or exons (*dark green*) include regulatory DNA sequences, sequences that code for functional RNA, and sequences whose functions are not known. (Data courtesy of E.H. Margulies.)

whole human genome sequence—a first draft in 2001 and a finished draft in 2004—provided a more panoramic view of the complete genetic landscape, including how many genes we have, what those genes look like, and how they are distributed across the genome (Table 9–2).

The first striking feature of the human genome is how little of it—less than 2%—codes for proteins (Figure 9–33). In addition, almost half of our DNA is made up of mobile genetic elements that have colonized our genome over evolutionary time. Because these elements have accumulated

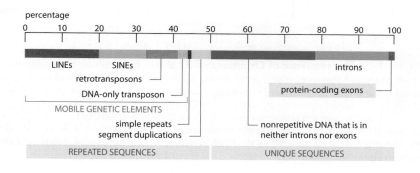

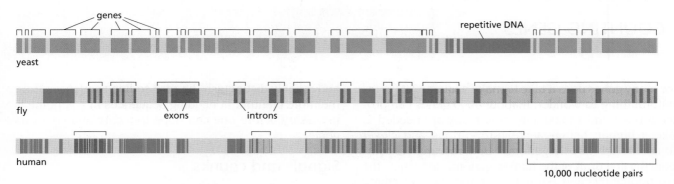

mutations, most can no longer move; rather, they are relics from an earlier evolutionary era when mobile genetic elements ran rampant through our genome.

It was a surprise to discover how few protein-coding genes our genome actually contains. Earlier estimates had been in the neighborhood of 100,000 (as discussed in How We Know, pp. 324–325). Although the exact count is still being refined, current estimates place the number of human protein-coding genes at about 19,000, with perhaps another 5000 genes encoding functional RNAs that are not translated into proteins. This estimate brings us much closer to the gene numbers for simpler multicellular animals—for example, 14,000 protein-coding genes for *Drosophila*, 22,000 for *C. elegans*, and 28,000 for the small weed *Arabidopsis* (see Table 1–2).

The number of protein-coding genes we have may be unexpectedly small, but their relative size is unusually large. Only about 1300 nucleotide pairs are needed to encode an average-sized human protein of about 430 amino acids. Yet the average length of a human gene is 27,000 nucleotide pairs. Most of this DNA is in noncoding introns. In addition to the voluminous introns (see Figure 9–32D), each gene is associated with regulatory DNA sequences that ensure that the gene is expressed at the proper level, time, and place. In humans, these regulatory DNA sequences are typically interspersed along tens of thousands of nucleotide pairs, much of which seems to be "spacer" DNA. Indeed, compared to many other eukaryotic genomes, the human genome is much less densely packed (Figure 9–34).

Although exons and their associated regulatory DNA sequences comprise less than 2% of the human genome, comparative studies indicate that about 4.5% of the human genome is highly conserved when compared with other mammalian genomes (see Figure 9–20). An additional 5% of the genome shows reduced variation in the human population, as determined by comparing the DNA sequence of thousands of individuals. This reduced variation reflects the relative importance of these sequences compared with the majority of the genome. Taken together, such analyses suggest that only about 10% of the human genome contains sequences that truly matter—but we do not yet know the function of much of this DNA.

Differences in Gene Regulation May Help Explain How Animals with Similar Genomes Can Be So Different

We now have the complete genome sequences for many different mammals, including humans, chimpanzees, gorillas, orangutans, dogs, cats, and mice. All of these species contain essentially the same protein-coding genes, which raises a fundamental question: What makes these creatures so different from one another? And what makes humans different from other animals?

Figure 9–34 Genes are sparsely distributed in the human genome. Compared to some other eukaryotic genomes, the human genome is less gene-dense. Shown here are DNA segments about 50,000 nucleotide pairs in length from bakers yeast, *Drosophila*, and human. The human segment contains only 4 genes, compared to 26 in the yeast and 11 in the fly. Exons are shown in *orange*, introns in *yellow*, repetitive elements in *blue*, and intergenic DNA in *gray*. The genes of yeast and flies are generally more compact, with fewer introns, than the genes of humans.

HOW WE KNOW

COUNTING GENES

How many genes does it take to make a human? It seems a natural thing to wonder. If about 6000 genes can produce a yeast and 14,000 a fly, how many are needed to make a human being—a creature curious and clever enough to study its own genome? Until researchers completed the first draft of the human genome sequence, the most frequently cited estimate was 100,000. But where did that figure come from? And how was the revised estimate of only 19,000 protein-coding genes derived?

Walter Gilbert, a physicist-turned-biologist who won a Nobel Prize for developing techniques for sequencing DNA, was one of the first to throw out a ballpark estimate of the number of human genes. In the mid-1980s, Gilbert suggested that humans could have 100,000 genes, an estimate based on the average size of the few human genes known at the time (about 3×10^4 nucleotide pairs) and the size of our genome (about 3×10^9 nucleotide pairs). This back-of-the-envelope calculation yielded a number with such a pleasing roundness that it wound up being quoted widely in articles and textbooks.

The calculation provides an estimate of the number of genes a human could have in principle, but it does not address the question of how many genes we actually have. As it turns out, that question is not so easy to answer, even with the complete human genome sequence in hand. The problem is, how does one identify a gene? Consider protein-coding genes, which comprise only 1.5% of the human genome. Looking at a given piece of raw DNA sequence—an apparently random string of As, Ts, Gs, and Cs—how can one tell which parts represent protein-coding segments? Being able to accurately and reliably distinguish the rare coding sequences from the more plentiful noncoding sequences in a genome is necessary before one can hope to locate and count its genes.

Signals and chunks

As always, the situation is simplest in bacteria and simple eukaryotes such as yeasts. In these genomes, genes that encode proteins are identified by searching through the entire DNA sequence looking for **open reading frames** (**ORFs**). These are long sequences—say, 100 codons or more—that lack stop codons. A random sequence of nucleotides will by chance encode a stop codon about once every 20 codons (as there are three stop codons in the set of 64 possible codons—see Figure 7–27). So finding an ORF—a continuous nucleotide sequence that encodes more than 100 amino acids—is the first step in identifying a good candidate for a protein-coding gene. Today, computer programs are used to search for such ORFs, which begin with an initiation codon, usually ATG, and end with a termination codon, TAA, TAG, or TGA (**Figure 9–35**).

In animals and plants, the process of identifying ORFs is complicated by the presence of large intron sequences, which interrupt the protein-coding portions of genes. As we have seen, these introns are generally much larger than the exons, which might represent only a few percent of the gene. In human DNA, exons sometimes contain as few as 50 codons (150 nucleotide pairs), while introns may exceed 10,000 nucleotide pairs in length. Fifty codons is too short to generate a statistically significant

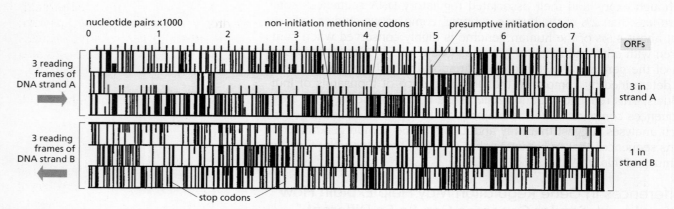

Figure 9–35 Computer programs are used to identify protein-coding genes. In this example, a DNA sequence of 7500 nucleotide pairs from the pathogenic yeast *Candida albicans* was fed into a computer, which then calculated the proteins that could, in theory, be produced from each of its six possible reading frames—three on each of the two strands (see Figure 7–28). The output shows the location of start and stop codons for each reading frame. The reading frames are laid out in horizontal columns. Stop, or termination, codons (TGA, TAA, and TAG) are represented by tall, vertical black lines, and methionine codons (ATG) are represented by shorter black lines. Four open reading frames, or ORFs (shaded *yellow*), can be clearly identified by the statistically significant absence of stop codons. For each ORF, the presumptive initiation codon (ATG) is indicated in *red*. The additional ATG codons (*black*) in the ORFs code for methionine in the protein.

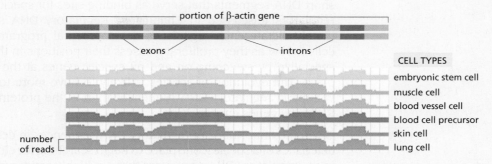

Figure 9–36 RNA sequencing can be used to characterize protein-coding genes.
Presented here is a set of data corresponding to RNAs produced from a segment of the gene for β-actin, which is depicted schematically at the top. Millions of RNA "sequence reads," each approximately 200 nucleotides long, were collected from a variety of cell types (*right*) and matched to DNA sequences within the β-actin gene. The height of each trace is proportional to how often each sequence appears in a read. Exon sequences are present at high levels, reflecting their presence in mature β-actin mRNAs. Intron sequences are present at low levels, most likely reflecting their presence in pre-mRNA molecules that have not yet been spliced or spliced introns that have not yet been degraded.

"ORF signal," as it is not all that unusual for 50 random codons to lack a stop signal. Moreover, introns are so long that they are likely to contain by chance quite a bit of "ORF noise," numerous stretches of sequence lacking stop signals. Finding the true ORFs in this sea of information in which the noise often outweighs the signal can be difficult. To make the task more manageable, computers are used to search for other distinctive features that mark the presence of a protein-coding gene. These include the splicing sequences that signal an intron–exon boundary (see Figure 7–20), regulatory DNA sequences, or conservation with coding sequences from other organisms.

In 1992, researchers used a computer program to predict protein-coding regions in a preliminary human sequence. They found two genes in a 58,000-nucleotide-pair segment of Chromosome 4, and five genes in a 106,000-nucleotide-pair segment of Chromosome 19. That works out to an average of 1 gene every 23,000 nucleotide pairs. Extrapolating from that density to the whole genome would give humans nearly 130,000 genes. It turned out, however, that the chromosomes the researchers analyzed had been chosen for sequencing precisely because they appeared to be gene-rich. When the estimate was adjusted to take into account the gene-poor regions of the human genome—guessing that half of the human genome had maybe one-tenth of that gene-rich density—the estimated number dropped to 71,000.

Matching RNAs

Of course, these estimates are based on what we think genes look like; to get around this bias, we must employ more direct, experiment-based methods for locating genes. Because genes are transcribed into RNA, the preferred strategy for finding genes involves isolating all of the RNAs produced by a particular cell type and determining their nucleotide sequence—a technique called RNA-Seq. These sequences are then mapped back to the genome to locate their genes. For protein-coding genes, exon segments are more highly represented among the sequenced transcripts, as intron sequences tend to be spliced out and destroyed. Because different cell types express different genes, and splice their RNA transcripts differently, a variety of cell types are used in the analysis (**Figure 9–36**).

Thanks to RNA-Seq, the number of predicted protein-coding genes has dropped even further, because the technique detects only those genes that are actively transcribed. At the same time, the approach also allowed the detection of genes that do not code for proteins, but instead encode functional or regulatory RNAs. Many noncoding RNAs were first identified through RNA-Seq.

Human gene countdown

Based on a combination of all of these computational and experimental techniques, current estimates of the total number of human genes are now converging around 24,000, of which approximately 19,000 are protein-coding. It could be many years, however, before we have the final answer to how many genes it takes to make a human. In the end, having an exact count will not be nearly as important as understanding the functions of each gene and how they interact to build the living organism.

The instructions needed to produce a multicellular animal from a fertilized egg are provided, in large part, by the regulatory DNA sequences associated with each gene. These noncoding DNA sequences contain, scattered within them, dozens of separate regulatory elements, including short DNA segments that serve as binding sites for specific transcription regulators (discussed in Chapter 8). Regulatory DNA sequences ultimately dictate each organism's developmental program—the rules its cells follow as they proliferate, assess their positions in the embryo, and specialize by switching on and off specific genes at the right time and place. The evolution of species is likely to have more to do with innovations in regulatory DNA sequences than in the proteins or functional RNAs the genes encode.

Given the importance of regulatory DNA sequences in defining the characteristics of a species, one place to begin searching for clues to identity is in the regulatory DNA sequences that are highly conserved across mammalian species, but are altered or absent in our own genome. One study identified more than 500 such sequences, providing some intriguing clues as to what makes us human. One of these regulatory DNA sequences, missing in humans, seems to suppress the proliferation of neurons in the brain. Although further investigation is required, it is possible that the loss of this sequence—or changes in other neural-specific regulatory DNA sequences—played an instrumental role in the evolution of the human brain.

Another regulatory DNA sequence lost in the human lineage directs the formation of penile spines—structures present in a wide variety of mammals including chimpanzees, bonobos, gorillas, orangutans, gibbons, rhesus monkeys, and bushbabies. Whether the loss of these structures provides some advantage to humans is not known; it could be that the change is neutral—neither advantageous nor harmful. Regardless, it is a characteristic that makes us unique.

Thanks to such genetic comparisons, we are beginning to unravel the secrets of how our genome evolved to produce the qualities that define us as a species. But these analyses can only provide information about our distant evolutionary past. To learn about the more recent events in the history of modern *Homo sapiens*, we are turning to the genomes of our closest extinct relations, as we see next.

The Genome of Extinct Neanderthals Reveals Much about What Makes Us Human

In 2010, investigators completed their analysis of the first Neanderthal genome. One of our closest evolutionary relatives, Neanderthals lived side-by-side with the ancestors of modern humans in Europe and Western Asia. By comparing the Neanderthal genome sequence—obtained from DNA that was extracted from a fossilized bone fragment found in a cave in Croatia—with those of people from different parts of the world, researchers identified a handful of genomic regions that have undergone a sudden spurt of changes in modern humans. These regions include genes involved in metabolism, brain development, the voice box, and the shape of the skeleton, particularly the rib cage and brow—all features thought to differ between modern humans and our extinct cousins.

Remarkably, these studies also revealed that many modern humans—particularly those that hail from Europe and Asia—share about 2% of their genomes with Neanderthals. This genetic overlap indicates that our ancestors mated with Neanderthals—before outcompeting or actively exterminating them—on the way out of Africa (**Figure 9–37**). This ancient relationship left a permanent mark in the human genome.

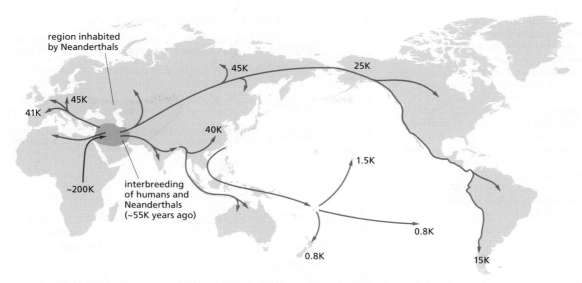

region inhabited
by Neanderthals

45K

45K

41K

25K

40K

1.5K

~200K

interbreeding
of humans and
Neanderthals
(~55K years ago)

0.8K

0.8K

15K

Figure 9–37 Ancestral humans encountered Neanderthals on their way out of Africa. Modern humans descended from a relatively small population—perhaps as few as 10,000 individuals—that existed in Africa approximately 200,000 (200 K) years ago. Among that small group of ancestors, some migrated northward, and their descendants spread across the globe. As ancestral humans left Africa, around 130,000 years ago (*purple* arrows), they encountered Neanderthals who inhabited the region indicated in *light blue*. As a result of interbreeding (in the region shown in *dark blue*), the humans that subsequently spread throughout Europe and Asia (*red* arrows) carried with them traces of Neanderthal DNA. Ultimately, ancestral humans continued their global spread to the New World, reaching North America approximately 25,000 years ago and the southern regions of South America 15,000 years later. This scenario is based on many types of data, including fossil records, anthropological studies, and the genome sequences of Neanderthals and of humans from around the world. (Adapted from M.A. Jobling et al., *Human Evolutionary Genetics*, 2nd ed. New York: Garland Science, 2014.)

Genome Variation Contributes to Our Individuality—But How?

With the possible exception of some identical twins, no two people have exactly the same genome sequence. When the same region of the genome from two different humans is compared, the nucleotide sequences typically differ by about 0.1%. This degree of variation represents about 1 difference in every 1000 nucleotide pairs—or some 3 million genetic differences between the genome of one person and the next. Detailed analyses of human genetic variation suggest that the bulk of this variation was already present early in our evolution, perhaps 200,000 years ago, when the human population was still small. Yet much of this variation has been reshuffled as more and more generations of humans have arisen. Thus, although a great deal of the genetic diversity in present-day humans was inherited from our early human ancestors, each individual inherits a unique combination of this ancient genetic variation.

Sprinkled on top of this "tossed salad" of ancient variation are mutations that are much more recent. At birth, each human's genome contains approximately 70 new mutations that were not present in the genomes of either parent. Combined with the jumbled collection of ancient variation we acquired from our ancestors, these recent mutations further distinguish one individual from another. Most of the variation in the human genome takes the form of single base-pair changes. Although some of these base-pair changes are unique to individual humans, many more are preserved from our distant ancestors and are therefore widespread in the human population. Those single-base changes that are present in at least 1% of the population are called **single-nucleotide polymorphisms** (**SNPs**, pronounced "snips"). These polymorphisms are simply points in the genome that differ in nucleotide sequence between one portion of the population and another—positions where, for example, more than 1%

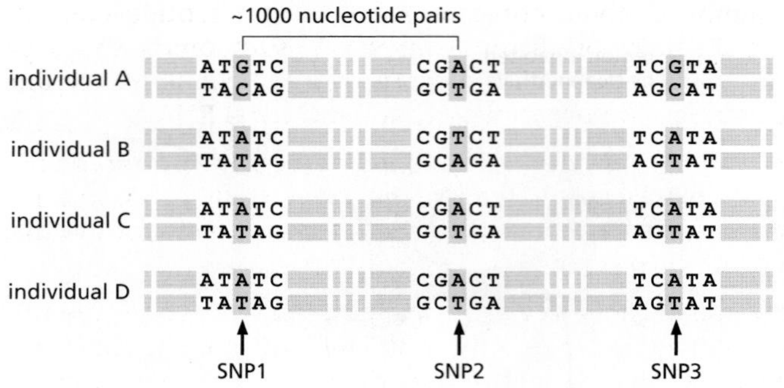

Figure 9–38 **Single-nucleotide polymorphisms (SNPs) are points in the genome that differ by a single nucleotide pair between one portion of the population and another.** Here, the differences are highlighted in *green* and *blue*. By convention, to count as a polymorphism, a genetic difference must be present in at least 1% of the total population of the species. Most, but not all, SNPs in the human genome occur in regions where they do not affect the function of a gene. As indicated by the bracket, when comparing any two humans one finds, on average, about one SNP per every 1000 nucleotide pairs.

of the population has a G-C nucleotide pair, while the rest have an A-T (Figure 9–38). Two human genomes chosen at random from the world's population will differ by approximately 2.5×10^6 SNPs that are scattered throughout the genome.

Most of these SNPs are genetically silent, as they fall within noncritical regions of the genome. Such variations have no effect on how we look or how our cells function. This means that only a small subset of the variation we observe in our DNA is responsible for the heritable differences from one human to the next. We discussed one such difference—that responsible for the ability of some adults to digest milk—earlier in the chapter. However, it remains a major challenge to identify the thousands of other genetic variations that are functionally important—a problem we return to in Chapter 19.

Genome sequences hold the secrets to why humans look, think, and act the way we do—and why one human differs from another. Our genome contains the instructions that guide the countless decisions made by all of our cells as they interact with one another to build our tissues and organs. But we are only just beginning to learn the grammar and rules by which this genetic information orchestrates our biology and our behavior. Deciphering this code—which has been shaped by evolution and refined by individual variation—is one of the great challenges facing the next generation of cell biologists.

ESSENTIAL CONCEPTS

- By comparing the DNA and protein sequences of contemporary organisms, we are beginning to reconstruct how genomes have evolved in the billions of years that have elapsed since the appearance of the first cells.

- Genetic variation—the raw material for evolutionary change—arises through a variety of mechanisms that alter the nucleotide sequence of genomes. These changes in sequence range from simple point mutations to larger-scale deletions, duplications, and rearrangements.

- Genetic changes that give an organism a selective advantage are likely to be perpetuated. Changes that compromise an organism's fitness or ability to reproduce are eliminated through natural selection.

- Gene duplication is one of the most important sources of genetic diversity. Once duplicated, the two genes can accumulate different mutations and thereby diversify to perform different roles.

- Repeated rounds of gene duplication and divergence during evolution have produced many large gene families.

- The evolution of new proteins is thought to have been greatly facilitated by the swapping of exons between genes to create hybrid proteins with new functions.

- The human genome contains 3.2×10^9 nucleotide pairs distributed among 23 pairs of chromosomes—22 autosomes and a pair of sex chromosomes. Less than a tenth of this DNA is transcribed to produce protein-coding or otherwise functional RNAs.

- Individual humans differ from one another by an average of 1 nucleotide pair in every 1000; this and other genetic variation underlies most of our individuality and provides the basis for identifying individuals by DNA analysis.

- Nearly half of the human genome consists of mobile genetic elements that can move from one site to another within a genome. Two classes of these elements have multiplied to especially high copy numbers.

- Viruses are genes packaged in protective coats that can move from cell to cell and organism to organism, but they require host cells to reproduce.

- Some viruses have RNA instead of DNA as their genetic material. To reproduce, retroviruses copy their RNA genomes into DNA, and integrate into the host-cell genome.

- Comparing genome sequences of different species provides a powerful way to identify conserved, functionally important DNA sequences.

- Related species, such as human and mouse, have many genes in common; evolutionary changes in the regulatory DNA sequences that affect how these genes are expressed are especially important in determining the differences between species.

- A comparison of genome sequences from people around the world has helped reveal how humans have evolved and spread across the globe.

KEY TERMS

Alu sequence	horizontal gene transfer	retrotransposon
conserved synteny	*L1* element	retrovirus
exon shuffling	mobile genetic element	reverse transcriptase
gamete	open reading frame (ORF)	single-nucleotide polymorphism (SNP)
gene duplication and divergence	phylogenetic tree	somatic cell
gene family	point mutation	transposon
germ line	purifying selection	virus
homologous gene		

QUESTIONS

QUESTION 9–7

Discuss the following statement: "Mobile genetic elements are parasites. They are always harmful to the host organism."

QUESTION 9–8

Human Chromosome 22 (48×10^6 nucleotide pairs in length) has about 700 protein-coding genes, which average 19,000 nucleotide pairs in length and contain an average of 5.4 exons, each of which averages 266 nucleotide pairs. What fraction of the average protein-coding gene is converted into mRNA? What fraction of the chromosome do these genes occupy?

QUESTION 9–9

(True or False?) The DNA sequence of most of the human genome is unimportant. Explain your answer.

QUESTION 9–10

Mobile genetic elements make up nearly half of the human genome and are inserted more or less randomly throughout it. However, in some spots these elements are rare, as illustrated for a cluster of genes called HoxD, which lies on Chromosome 2 (Figure Q9–10). This cluster is about 100 kb in length and contains nine genes whose differential expression along the length of the developing

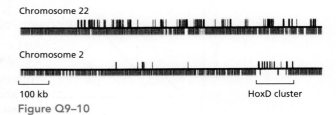

Chromosome 22

Chromosome 2

100 kb

HoxD cluster

Figure Q9–10

embryo helps establish the basic body plan for humans (and other animals). In Figure Q9–10, lines that project *upward* indicate exons of known genes. Lines that project *downward* indicate mobile genetic elements; they are so numerous they merge into nearly a solid block outside the HoxD cluster. For comparison, an equivalent region of Chromosome 22 is shown. Why do you suppose that mobile genetic elements are so rare in the HoxD cluster?

QUESTION 9–11

An early graphical method for comparing nucleotide sequences—the so-called diagon plot—still yields one of the best visual comparisons of sequence relatedness. An example is illustrated in Figure Q9–11, in which the human β-globin gene is compared with the human cDNA for β globin (which contains only the coding portion of the gene; Figure Q9–11A) and with the mouse β-globin gene (Figure Q9–11B). Diagon plots are generated by comparing blocks of sequence, in this case blocks of 11 nucleotides at a time. If 9 or more of the nucleotides match, a dot is placed on the diagram at the coordinates corresponding to the blocks being compared. A comparison of all possible blocks generates diagrams such as the ones shown in Figure Q9–11, in which sequence similarities show up as diagonal lines.

A. From the comparison of the human β-globin gene with the human β-globin cDNA (Figure Q9–11A), can you deduce the positions of exons and introns in the β-globin gene?

B. Are the exons of the human β-globin gene (indicated by shading in Figure Q9–11B) similar to those of the mouse β-globin gene? Identify and explain any key differences.

C. Is there any sequence similarity between the human and mouse β-globin genes that lies outside the exons? If so, identify its location and offer an explanation for its preservation during evolution.

D. Did the mouse or human gene undergo a change of intron length during their evolutionary divergence? How can you tell?

QUESTION 9–12

Your advisor suggests that you write a computer program that will identify the exons of protein-coding genes directly from the sequence of the human genome. In preparation for that task, you decide to write down a list of the features that might distinguish protein-coding sequences from intronic DNA and from other sequences in the genome. What features would you list? (You may wish to review basic aspects of gene expression in Chapter 7.)

QUESTION 9–13

You are interested in finding out the function of a particular gene in the mouse genome. You have determined the nucleotide sequence of the gene, defined the portion that codes for its protein product, and searched the relevant database for similar sequences; however, neither the gene nor the encoded protein resembles anything previously described. What types of additional information about the gene and the encoded protein would you like to know in order to narrow down its function, and why? Focus on the information you would want, rather than on the techniques you might use to get that information.

QUESTION 9–14

Why do you expect to encounter a stop codon about every 20 codons or so in a random sequence of DNA?

QUESTION 9–15

Which of the processes listed below contribute significantly to the evolution of new protein-coding genes?

A. Duplication of genes to create extra copies that can acquire new functions.

B. Formation of new genes *de novo* from noncoding DNA in the genome.

C. Horizontal transfer of DNA between cells of different species.

D. Mutation of existing genes to create new functions.

E. Shuffling of protein domains by gene rearrangement.

QUESTION 9–16

Some protein sequences evolve more rapidly than others. But how can this be demonstrated? One approach is to compare several genes from the same two species, as shown for rat and human in the table. Two measures of rates of nucleotide substitution are indicated in the table. Nonsynonymous changes refer to single-nucleotide changes in the DNA sequence that alter the encoded amino acid (for example, ATC → TTC, which gives isoleucine → phenylalanine). Synonymous changes refer

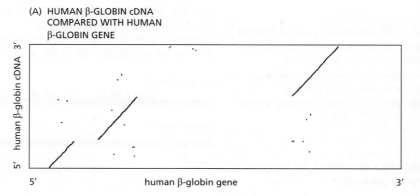

(A) HUMAN β-GLOBIN cDNA COMPARED WITH HUMAN β-GLOBIN GENE

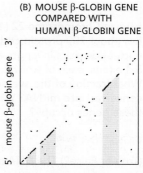

(B) MOUSE β-GLOBIN GENE COMPARED WITH HUMAN β-GLOBIN GENE

Figure Q9–11

Gene	Amino Acids	Rates of Change	
		Nonsynonymous	Synonymous
Histone H3	135	0.0	4.5
Hemoglobin α	141	0.6	4.4
Interferon γ	136	3.1	5.5

Rates were determined by comparing rat and human sequences and are expressed as nucleotide changes per site per 10^9 years. The average rate of nonsynonymous changes for several dozen rat and human genes is about 0.8.

to those that do not alter the encoded amino acid (ATC → ATT, which gives isoleucine → isoleucine, for example). (As is apparent in the genetic code, Figure 7–27, there are many cases where several codons correspond to the same amino acid.)

A. Why are there such large differences between the synonymous and nonsynonymous rates of nucleotide substitution?

B. Considering that the rates of synonymous changes are about the same for all three genes, how is it possible for the histone H3 gene to resist so effectively those nucleotide changes that alter its amino acid sequence?

C. In principle, a protein might be highly conserved because its gene exists in a "privileged" site in the genome that is subject to very low mutation rates. What feature of the data in the table argues against this possibility for the histone H3 protein?

QUESTION 9–17

Hemoglobin-like proteins were discovered in legumes, where they function in root nodules to lower the oxygen concentration, allowing the resident bacteria to fix nitrogen. These plant "hemoglobins" impart a characteristic pink color to the root nodules. The discovery of hemoglobin in plants was initially surprising because scientists regarded hemoglobin as a distinctive feature of animal blood. It was hypothesized that the plant hemoglobin gene was acquired by horizontal transfer from an animal. Many more hemoglobin-like genes have now been discovered and sequenced from a variety of organisms, and a phylogenetic tree of hemoglobins is shown in Figure Q9–17.

A. Does the evidence in the tree support or refute the hypothesis that the plant hemoglobins arose by horizontal gene transfer from animals?

B. Supposing that the plant hemoglobin genes were originally derived by horizontal transfer (from a parasitic nematode, for example), what would you expect the phylogenetic tree to look like?

QUESTION 9–18

The accuracy of DNA replication in the human germ-cell line is such that on average only about 0.6 out of the 6 billion nucleotides is altered at each cell division. Because most of our DNA is not subject to any precise constraint on its sequence, most of these changes are selectively neutral. Any two modern humans chosen at random will

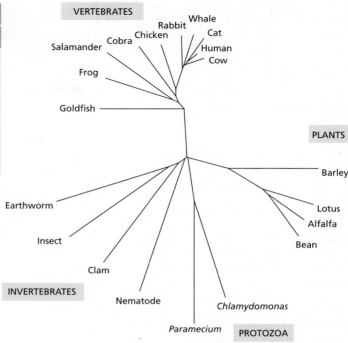

Figure Q9–17

differ by about 1 nucleotide pair per 1000. Suppose we are all descended from a single pair of ancestors (an "Adam and Eve") who were genetically identical and homozygous (each chromosome was identical to its homolog). Assuming that all germ-line mutations that arise are preserved in descendants, how many cell generations must have elapsed since the days of our original ancestor parents for 1 difference per 1000 nucleotides to have accumulated in modern humans? Assuming that each human generation corresponds on average to 200 cell-division cycles in the germ-cell lineage and allowing 30 years per human generation, how many years ago would this ancestral couple have lived?

QUESTION 9–19

Reverse transcriptases do not proofread as they synthesize DNA using an RNA template. What do you think the consequences of this are for the treatment of AIDS?

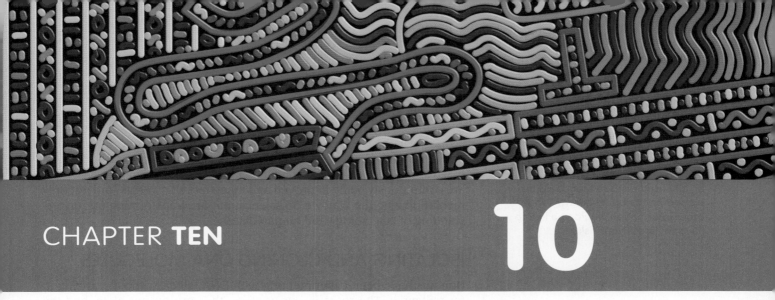

Analyzing the Structure and Function of Genes

Since the turn of the century, biologists have amassed an unprecedented wealth of information about the genes that direct the development and behavior of living things. Thanks to advances in our ability to rapidly determine the nucleotide sequence of entire genomes, we now have access to the complete molecular blueprints for thousands of different organisms, from the platypus to the plague bacterium, and for thousands of different people from all over the world.

This information explosion was ignited by technological advances that allowed the isolation and manipulation of a selected piece of DNA from among the many millions of nucleotide pairs in a typical chromosome. Investigators then developed powerful techniques for replicating, sequencing, and modifying this DNA—and even introducing it into other organisms that can then be studied in the laboratory.

These technical breakthroughs have had a dramatic impact on all aspects of cell biology. They have advanced our understanding of the organization and evolutionary history of complex eukaryotic genomes (as discussed in Chapter 9) and have led to the discovery of whole new classes of genes, RNAs, and proteins. They continue to generate new ways of determining the functions of genes and proteins in living organisms, and they provide an important set of tools for unraveling the mechanisms—still poorly understood—by which a complex organism can develop from a single fertilized egg.

At the same time, our ability to manipulate DNA has had a profound influence on our understanding and treatment of disease: using these techniques, we can now detect the mutations in human genes that are responsible for inherited disorders or that predispose us to a variety of

ISOLATING AND CLONING DNA MOLECULES

DNA CLONING BY PCR

SEQUENCING DNA

EXPLORING GENE FUNCTION

QUESTION 10–1

DNA sequencing of your own two β-globin genes (one from each of your two Chromosome 11s) reveals a mutation in one of the genes. Given this information alone, should you worry about being a carrier of an inherited disease that could be passed on to your children? What other information would you like to have to assess your risk?

common diseases, including cancer. We can also produce an increasing number of pharmaceuticals, such as insulin for diabetics and blood-clotting proteins for hemophiliacs.

In this chapter, we present a brief overview of how we can manipulate DNA, identify genes, and produce many copies of any given nucleotide sequence in the laboratory. We discuss several ways to explore gene function, including recent approaches to DNA sequencing and to modifying or inactivating genes in cells, animals, and plants. These methods—which are continuously being improved and made more powerful—are not only revolutionizing the way we do science, but are transforming our understanding of cell biology and human disease.

ISOLATING AND CLONING DNA MOLECULES

Humans have been experimenting with DNA, albeit without realizing it, for millennia. The roses in our gardens, the corn on our plate, and the dogs in our yards are all the product of selective breeding that has taken place over many, many generations (Figure 10–1). But it wasn't until the 1970s that we could begin to engineer organisms with desired properties by directly tinkering with their genes.

Isolating and manipulating individual genes is not a trivial matter. Unlike a protein, a gene does not exist as a discrete entity in cells; it is a small part of a much larger DNA molecule. Even bacterial genomes, which are much less expansive and complex than the chromosomes of eukaryotes, are still enormously long. The *E. coli* genome, for example, contains 4.6 million nucleotide pairs.

How, then, can we go about separating a single gene from a eukaryotic genome—which is considerably larger than that of a bacterium—so that it can be handled in the laboratory? The solution to this problem emerged, in large part, with the discovery of a class of bacterial enzymes that cut double-stranded DNA at particular sequences. These enzymes can be used to produce a reproducible set of specific DNA fragments from any genome—including fragments that harbor genes. The desired fragment is then amplified, producing many identical copies, by a process called **DNA cloning**. It is this amplification that makes it possible to separate a gene of interest from the rest of the genome.

In this section, we describe how specific DNA fragments can be generated, isolated, and produced in large quantities in bacteria—the classical approach to DNA cloning. In the next section of the chapter, we present

Figure 10–1 Selective breeding is, in essence, a form of genetic manipulation.
(A) The oldest known depiction of a rose in Western art, from the palace of Knossos in Crete, around 2000 BC. Modern roses are the result of centuries of breeding between such wild roses. (B) Dogs have been bred to exhibit a wide variety of characteristics, including different head shapes, coat colors, and of course size. All dogs, regardless of breed, belong to a single species that was domesticated from the gray wolf some 10,000 to 15,000 years ago. (B, from A.L. Shearin & E.A. Ostrander, *PLoS Biol.* 8:e1000310, 2010.)

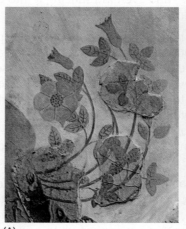

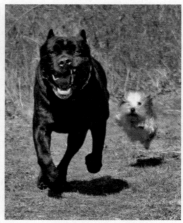

(A)   (B)

an alternative approach to cloning DNA: this method, which is carried out in a test tube, uses a special form of DNA polymerase to make copies of the desired nucleotide sequence.

Restriction Enzymes Cut DNA Molecules at Specific Sites

Like many of the tools of DNA technology, the enzymes used to prepare DNA fragments for cloning were discovered by researchers trying to understand an intriguing biological phenomenon. It had been observed that certain bacteria always degraded "foreign" DNA that was introduced into them experimentally. A search for the underlying mechanism revealed a novel class of enzymes that cleave DNA at specific nucleotide sequences. Because these enzymes function to restrict the transfer of DNA between strains of bacteria, they were called **restriction enzymes**, or *restriction nucleases*. The pursuit of this seemingly arcane biological puzzle set off the development of technologies that have forever changed the way cell and molecular biologists study living things.

Different bacterial species produce different restriction enzymes, each cutting at a different, specific nucleotide sequence (**Figure 10–2**). The bacteria's own DNA is protected from cleavage by chemical modification of these specific sequences. Because these target sequences are short— generally four to eight nucleotide pairs—many sites of cleavage will occur, purely by chance, in any long DNA molecule. The reason restriction enzymes are so useful in the laboratory is that each enzyme will cut a particular DNA molecule at the same sites. Thus for a given sample of DNA, a particular restriction enzyme will reliably generate the same set of DNA fragments.

The size of the resulting fragments depends on the target sequences of the restriction enzymes. As shown in Figure 10–2, the enzyme HaeIII cuts at a sequence of four nucleotide pairs; a sequence this long would be expected to occur purely by chance approximately once every 256 nucleotide pairs (1 in 4^4). In comparison, a restriction enzyme with a target sequence that is eight nucleotides long would be expected to cleave DNA on average once every 65,536 nucleotide pairs (1 in 4^8). This difference in sequence selectivity makes it possible to cleave a long DNA molecule into the fragment sizes that are most suitable for a given application.

Gel Electrophoresis Separates DNA Fragments of Different Sizes

After a large DNA molecule is cleaved into smaller pieces with a restriction enzyme, the DNA fragments can be separated from one another on the basis of their length by gel electrophoresis—the same method used to separate mixtures of proteins (see Panel 4–5, p. 167). A mixture of DNA

Figure 10–2 Restriction enzymes cleave both strands of the DNA double helix at specific nucleotide sequences. Target sequences (*orange*) are often palindromic— that is, the nucleotide sequence is symmetrical around a central point. Some enzymes, such as HaeIII, cut straight across the double helix and leave two blunt-ended DNA molecules; with others, such as EcoRI and HindIII, the cuts on each strand are staggered. These staggered cuts generate "sticky ends"—short, single-stranded overhangs that help the cut DNA molecules join back together through complementary base-pairing. This rejoining of DNA molecules becomes important for DNA cloning, as we discuss shortly. Restriction enzymes are usually obtained from bacteria, and their names reflect their origins: for example, the enzyme EcoRI comes from *E. coli*.

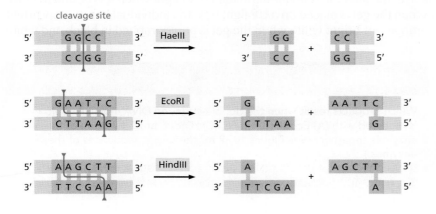

Figure 10–3 DNA molecules can be separated by size using gel electrophoresis. (A) Schematic illustration compares the results of cutting the same DNA molecule (in this case, the genome of a virus that infects parasitic wasps) with two different restriction enzymes, EcoRI (*middle*) and HindIII (*right*). The fragments are then separated by gel electrophoresis. Because larger fragments migrate more slowly than smaller ones, the lowermost bands on the gel contain the smallest DNA fragments. The sizes of the fragments can be estimated by comparing them to a set of DNA fragments of known sizes (*left*). (B) Photograph of an actual gel shows the positions of DNA bands that have been labeled with a fluorescent dye. (B, from U. Albrecht et al., *J. Gen. Virol.* 75: 3353–3363, 1994. With permission from the Microbiology Society.)

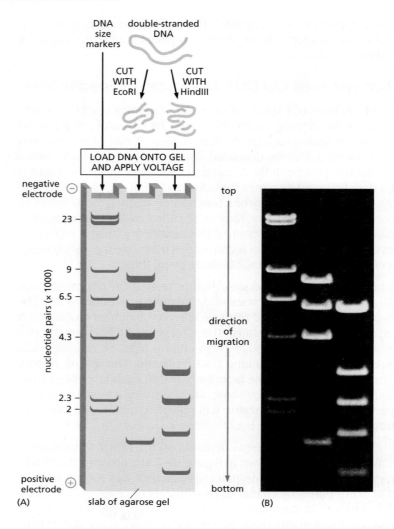

fragments is loaded at one end of a slab of agarose or polyacrylamide gel, which contains a microscopic network of pores. When a voltage is applied across the gel, the negatively charged DNA fragments migrate toward the positive electrode; larger fragments migrate more slowly because their progress is impeded to a greater extent by the gel matrix. Over several hours, the DNA fragments become spread out across the gel according to size, forming a ladder of discrete bands, each composed of a collection of DNA molecules of identical length (**Figure 10–3**).

The separated DNA bands on an agarose or polyacrylamide gel are not, by themselves, visible. To see these bands, the DNA must be labeled or stained in some way. One sensitive method involves exposing the gel to a dye that fluoresces under ultraviolet (UV) light when it is bound to DNA. When the gel is placed on a UV light box, the individual bands glow bright orange—or bright white when the gel is photographed in black and white

QUESTION 10–2

Which products result when the double-stranded DNA molecule *below* is digested with (A) EcoRI, (B) HaeIII, (C) HindIII, or (D) all three of these enzymes together? (See Figure 10–2 for the target sequences of these enzymes.)

5′-AAGAATTGCGGAATTCGGGCCTTAAGCGCCGCGTCGAGGCCTTAAA-3′
3′-TTCTTAACGCCTTAAGCCCGGAATTCGCGGCGCAGCTCCGGAATTT-5′

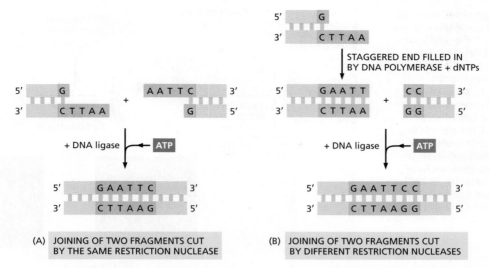

Figure 10–4 DNA ligase can join together any two DNA fragments *in vitro* to produce recombinant DNA molecules. The fragments joined by DNA ligase can be from different cells, tissues, or even different organisms. ATP provides the energy necessary to reseal the sugar–phosphate backbone of the DNA. (A) DNA ligase can readily join two DNA fragments produced by the same restriction enzyme, in this case EcoRI. Note that the staggered ends produced by this enzyme enable the ends of the two fragments to base-pair correctly with each other, greatly facilitating their rejoining. (B) DNA ligase can also be used to join DNA fragments produced by different restriction enzymes—for example, EcoRI and HaeIII. In this case, before the fragments undergo ligation, DNA polymerase plus a mixture of deoxyribonucleoside triphosphates (dNTPs) are used to fill in the staggered cut produced by EcoRI prior to ligation.

(see Figure 10–3B). To isolate a desired DNA fragment, the small section of the gel that contains the band is excised with a scalpel, and the DNA is then extracted.

DNA Cloning Begins with the Production of Recombinant DNA

Once a genome has been broken into smaller, more manageable pieces, the resulting fragments must then be prepared for cloning. This process involves inserting the DNA fragments into a carrier, or *vector*—another piece of DNA that can be copied inside cells. Because this union involves "recombining" DNA from different sources, the resulting molecules are called **recombinant DNA**. The production of recombinant DNA molecules in this way is a key step in the classical approach to DNA cloning.

Like the cutting of DNA by restriction enzymes, the joining together of DNA fragments to produce recombinant DNA molecules is made possible by an enzyme produced by cells. In this case, the enzyme is **DNA ligase**. In cells, DNA ligase reseals the nicks that arise in the DNA backbone during DNA replication and DNA repair (see Figure 6–19). In the laboratory, DNA ligase can be used to link together any two pieces of DNA in a test tube, producing recombinant DNA molecules that are not found in nature (**Figure 10–4**).

Recombinant DNA Can Be Copied Inside Bacterial Cells

The vectors used to carry the DNA that is to be cloned are small, circular DNA molecules called **plasmids** (**Figure 10–5**). Each plasmid contains its own replication origin, which enables it to replicate in a bacterial cell independently of the bacterial chromosome. This feature allows the DNA of interest to be produced in large amounts, even within a single bacterial cell. The plasmid also has cleavage sites for common restriction enzymes, so that it can be conveniently opened and a foreign DNA fragment inserted.

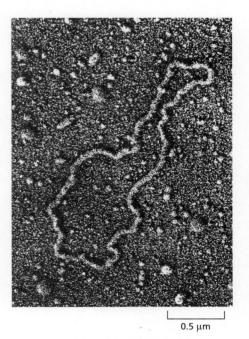

0.5 μm

Figure 10–5 Bacterial plasmids are commonly used as cloning vectors. This circular, double-stranded DNA molecule was the first plasmid for DNA cloning; it contains about nine thousand nucleotide pairs. The staining procedure used to make the DNA visible in this electron micrograph causes the DNA to appear much thicker than it actually is. (Courtesy of Stanley N. Cohen, Stanford University.)

Figure 10–6 A DNA fragment is inserted into a bacterial plasmid using the enzyme DNA ligase. The plasmid is first cut open at a single site with a restriction enzyme (in this case, one that produces staggered ends). It is then mixed with the DNA fragment to be cloned, which has been cut with the same restriction enzyme. The staggered ends base-pair, and when DNA ligase and ATP are added, the nicks in the DNA backbone are sealed to produce a complete recombinant DNA molecule. In the accompanying micrographs, we have colored the DNA fragment *red* to make it easier to see. (Micrographs courtesy of Huntington Potter and David Dressler.)

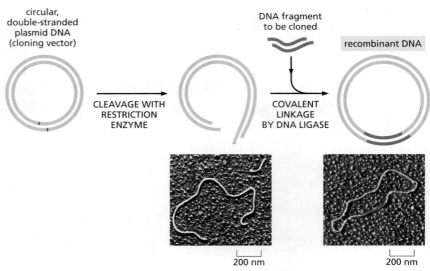

The vectors used for cloning are streamlined versions of plasmids that occur naturally in many bacteria. Bacterial plasmids were first recognized by physicians and scientists because they often carry genes that render their microbial host resistant to one or more antibiotics. Indeed, historically potent antibiotics—penicillin, for example—are no longer effective against many of today's bacterial infections because plasmids that confer resistance to the antibiotic have spread among bacterial species by horizontal gene transfer (see Figure 9–15).

To insert a piece of DNA into a plasmid vector, the purified plasmid DNA is opened up by a restriction enzyme that cleaves it at a single site, and the DNA fragment to be cloned is then spliced into that site using DNA ligase (**Figure 10–6**). This recombinant DNA molecule is now ready to be introduced into a bacterium, where it will be copied and amplified.

To accomplish this feat, investigators take advantage of the fact that some bacteria naturally take up DNA molecules present in their surroundings. The mechanism that controls this uptake is called **transformation**, because early observations suggested it could "transform" one bacterial strain into another. Indeed, the first proof that genes are made of DNA came from an experiment in which DNA purified from a pathogenic strain of pneumococcus was used to transform a harmless bacterium into a deadly one (see How We Know, pp. 192–194).

In a natural bacterial population, a source of DNA for transformation is provided by bacteria that have died and released their contents, including DNA, into the environment. In a test tube, however, bacteria such as *E. coli* can be coaxed to take up recombinant DNA that has been created in the laboratory. These bacteria are then suspended in a nutrient-rich broth and allowed to proliferate.

Each time the bacterial population doubles—every 30 minutes or so—the number of copies of the recombinant DNA molecule also doubles. Thus, in 24 hours, the engineered cells will produce hundreds of millions of copies of the plasmid, along with the DNA fragment it contains. The bacteria can then be split open (lysed) and the plasmid DNA purified from the rest of the cell contents, including the large bacterial chromosome (**Figure 10–7**).

The DNA fragment can be readily recovered by cutting it out of the plasmid DNA with the same restriction enzyme that was used to insert it, and then separating it from the plasmid DNA by gel electrophoresis (see Figure 10–3). Together, these steps allow the amplification and purification of any segment of DNA from the genome of any organism.

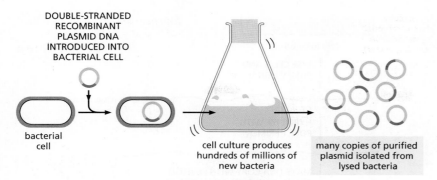

DOUBLE-STRANDED RECOMBINANT PLASMID DNA INTRODUCED INTO BACTERIAL CELL

bacterial cell

cell culture produces hundreds of millions of new bacteria

many copies of purified plasmid isolated from lysed bacteria

Figure 10–7 A DNA fragment can be replicated inside a bacterial cell. To clone a particular fragment of DNA, it is first inserted into a plasmid vector, as shown in Figure 10–6. The resulting recombinant plasmid DNA is then introduced into a bacterium, where it is replicated many millions of times as the bacterium multiplies. For simplicity, the genome of the bacterial cell is not shown.

An Entire Genome Can Be Represented in a DNA Library

When a whole genome is cut by a restriction enzyme, a large number of different DNA fragments is generated. This collection of DNA fragments can be ligated into plasmid vectors, under conditions that favor the insertion of a single DNA fragment into each plasmid molecule. These recombinant plasmids are then introduced into *E. coli* at a concentration that ensures that no more than one plasmid molecule is taken up by each bacterium. The resulting collection of cloned DNA fragments, present in the bacterial culture, is known as a **DNA library**. Because the DNA fragments were derived by digesting chromosomal DNA directly from an organism, the resulting collection—called a **genomic library**—should represent the entire genome of that organism (**Figure 10–8**). Such genomic libraries often provide the starting material for determining the complete nucleotide sequence of an organism's genome.

For other applications, however, it can be advantageous to work with a different type of library—one that includes only the coding sequences of genes; that is, a library that lacks intronic and other noncoding sequences that make up most eukaryotic DNA. For some genes, the complete genomic clone—including introns and exons—is too large and unwieldy to handle conveniently in the laboratory (see, for example, Figure 7–19B). What's more, the bacterial cells typically used to amplify cloned DNA are unable to remove introns from mammalian RNA transcripts. So if the goal is to use a cloned mammalian gene to produce a large amount of the protein it encodes, for example, it is essential to use only the coding sequence of the gene.

In this case, investigators generate a **cDNA library**. A cDNA library is similar to a genomic library in that it also contains numerous clones containing many different DNA sequences. But it differs in one important respect. The DNA that goes into a cDNA library is not genomic DNA; it is DNA copied from the mRNAs present in a particular type of cell. To prepare a cDNA library, all of the mRNAs are extracted, and double-stranded DNA copies of these mRNAs are produced by the enzymes *reverse transcriptase* and DNA polymerase (**Figure 10–9**). The resulting **complementary DNA**—or **cDNA**—molecules are then introduced into bacteria and amplified, as described for genomic DNA fragments (see Figure 10–8).

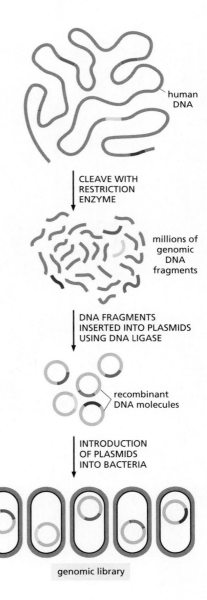

human DNA

CLEAVE WITH RESTRICTION ENZYME

millions of genomic DNA fragments

DNA FRAGMENTS INSERTED INTO PLASMIDS USING DNA LIGASE

recombinant DNA molecules

INTRODUCTION OF PLASMIDS INTO BACTERIA

genomic library

Figure 10–8 Human genomic libraries containing DNA fragments representing the whole human genome can be constructed using restriction enzymes and DNA ligase. Such a genomic library consists of a set of bacteria, each carrying a different small fragment of human DNA. For simplicity, only the *colored* DNA fragments are shown in the library; in reality, all of the different *gray* fragments will also be represented.

Figure 10–9 Complementary DNA (cDNA) is prepared from mRNA. Total mRNA is extracted from a selected type of cell, and double-stranded complementary DNA (cDNA) is produced using reverse transcriptase (see Figure 9–30) and DNA polymerase. For simplicity, the copying of just one of these mRNAs into cDNA is illustrated here. Following synthesis of the first cDNA strand by reverse transcriptase, treatment with RNAse leaves a few RNA fragments on the cDNA. The RNA fragment that is base-paired to the 3′ end of the first DNA strand acts as the primer for DNA polymerase to synthesize the second, complementary DNA strand. Any remaining RNA is degraded during subsequent cloning steps. As a result, the nucleotide sequences at the extreme 5′ ends of the original mRNA molecules are often absent from cDNA libraries.

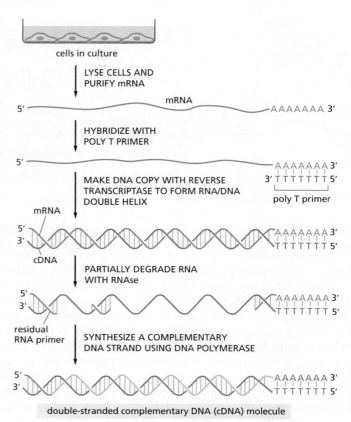

double-stranded complementary DNA (cDNA) molecule

There are several important differences between genomic DNA clones and cDNA clones. Genomic clones represent a random sample of all of the DNA sequences found in an organism's genome and, with very rare exceptions, will contain the same sequences regardless of the cell type from which the DNA came. Also, genomic clones from eukaryotes contain large amounts of noncoding DNA, repetitive DNA sequences, introns, regulatory DNA, and spacer DNA; sequences that code for proteins will make up only a few percent of the library (see Figure 9–33). By contrast, cDNA clones contain predominantly protein-coding sequences, and only those sequences that have been transcribed into mRNA in the cells from which the cDNA was made.

As different types of cells produce distinct sets of mRNA molecules, each yields a different cDNA library. Furthermore, patterns of gene expression change during development, so cells at different stages in their development will also yield different cDNA libraries. Thus, cDNAs can be used to assess which genes are expressed in specific cells, at particular times in development, or under a particular set of conditions.

Hybridization Provides a Sensitive Way to Detect Specific Nucleotide Sequences

Thus far, we have been talking about large collections of DNA fragments. For many studies, however, investigators wish to identify or examine an individual gene or RNA. Fortunately, an intrinsic property of nucleic acids—their ability to form complementary base pairs—provides a convenient and powerful technique for detecting a specific nucleotide sequence.

To see how, let's look at a molecule of double-stranded DNA. Under normal conditions, the two strands of a DNA double helix are held together by hydrogen bonds between the complementary base pairs (see Figure 5–4).

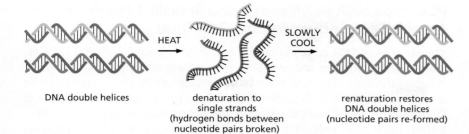

DNA double helices   denaturation to single strands (hydrogen bonds between nucleotide pairs broken)   renaturation restores DNA double helices (nucleotide pairs re-formed)

Figure 10–10 A molecule of DNA can undergo denaturation and renaturation (hybridization). For two single-stranded molecules to hybridize, they must have complementary nucleotide sequences that allow base-pairing. In this example, the *red* and *orange* strands are complementary to each other, and the *blue* and *green* strands are complementary to each other. Although denaturation by heating is shown, DNA can also be denatured by alkali treatment. The 1961 discovery that single strands of DNA could readily re-form a double helix in this way was a big surprise to scientists. Hybridization can also occur between complementary strands of DNA and RNA or between two RNAs.

But these relatively weak, noncovalent bonds can be fairly easily broken—for example, by heating the DNA to around 90°C. Such treatment will cause *DNA denaturation*, releasing the two strands from each other. When the conditions are reversed—by slowly lowering the temperature—the complementary strands will readily come back together to re-form a double helix. This *DNA renaturation*, or **hybridization**, is driven by the re-formation of the hydrogen bonds between complementary base pairs **(Figure 10–10)**.

Hybridization can be employed for detecting any nucleotide sequence of interest, whether DNA or RNA. One simply designs a short, single-stranded *DNA probe* that is complementary to that sequence. Because the nucleotide sequences of so many genomes are known—and are stored in publicly accessible databases—designing such a probe is straightforward. The desired probe can then be synthesized in the laboratory—usually by a commercial organization or a centralized academic facility.

Hybridization with DNA probes has many uses in cell and molecular biology. As we will see later in this chapter, for example, DNA probes that carry a fluorescent or radioactive label can be used to detect complementary RNA molecules in tissue preparations. But one of the most powerful applications of hybridization is in the cloning of DNA by the polymerase chain reaction, as we discuss next.

DNA CLONING BY PCR

Genomic and cDNA libraries were once the only route to gene cloning, and they are still used for cloning very large genes and for sequencing whole genomes. However, a powerful and versatile method for amplifying DNA, known as the **polymerase chain reaction** (**PCR**), provides a more rapid and straightforward approach, particularly in organisms whose complete genome sequence is known. Today, most genes are cloned via PCR.

Invented in the 1980s, PCR revolutionized the way that DNA and RNA are analyzed. The technique can amplify any nucleotide sequence quickly and selectively. Unlike the traditional approach of cloning using vectors—which relies on bacteria to make copies of the desired DNA sequences—PCR is performed entirely in a test tube. Eliminating the need for bacteria makes PCR convenient and fast—billions of copies of a nucleotide sequence can be generated in a matter of hours. At the same time, PCR is remarkably sensitive: the method can be used to amplify and detect the trace amounts of DNA in a drop of blood left at a crime scene or in a few copies of a viral genome in a patient's blood sample. Because of its sensitivity, speed, and ease of use, PCR has many applications in addition to DNA cloning, including forensics and diagnostics.

In this section, we provide a brief overview of how PCR works and how it is used for a range of purposes that require the amplification of specific DNA sequences.

QUESTION 10–3

Discuss the following statement: "From the nucleotide sequence of a cDNA clone, the complete amino acid sequence of a protein can be deduced by applying the genetic code. Thus, protein biochemistry has become superfluous because there is nothing more that can be learned by studying the protein."

PCR Uses DNA Polymerase and Specific DNA Primers to Amplify DNA Sequences in a Test Tube

The success of PCR depends on the exquisite selectivity of DNA hybridization, along with the ability of DNA polymerase to copy a DNA template reliably, through repeated rounds of replication *in vitro*. The enzyme works by adding nucleotides to the 3′ end of a growing strand of DNA (see Figure 6–11). To initiate the reaction, the polymerase requires a primer—a short nucleotide sequence that provides a 3′ end from which synthesis can begin. The beauty of PCR is that the primers that are added to the reaction mixture not only serve as starting points, but they also direct the polymerase to the specific DNA sequence to be amplified. These primers are designed by the experimenter based on the DNA sequence of interest and then synthesized chemically. Thus, PCR can only be used to clone a DNA segment for which the sequence is known in advance. However, with the large and growing number of genome sequences available in public databases, this requirement is rarely a drawback.

The power of PCR comes from repetition: the cycle of amplification is carried out dozens of times over the course of a few hours. At the start of each cycle, the two strands of the double-stranded DNA template are separated and a unique primer is hybridized, or annealed, to each. DNA polymerase is then allowed to replicate each strand independently (**Figure 10–11**). In subsequent cycles, all the newly synthesized DNA molecules produced by the polymerase serve as templates for the next round of replication (**Figure 10–12**). Through this iterative process of amplification, many copies of the original sequence can be made—billions after about 20 to 30 cycles.

PCR is the method of choice for cloning relatively short DNA fragments (say, under 10,000 nucleotide pairs). Because the original template for PCR can be either DNA or RNA, the method can be used to obtain either a full genomic clone (complete with introns and exons) or a cDNA copy of an mRNA (**Figure 10–13**). A major benefit of PCR is that genes can be cloned directly from any piece of DNA or RNA without the time and effort needed to first construct a DNA library.

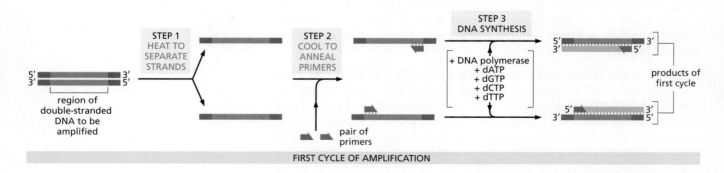

Figure 10–11 A pair of PCR primers directs the amplification of a desired segment of DNA in a test tube. Each cycle of PCR includes three steps: (1) The double-stranded DNA is heated briefly to separate the two strands. (2) The DNA is exposed to a large excess of a pair of specific primers—designed to bracket the region of DNA to be amplified—and the sample is cooled to allow the primers to hybridize to complementary sequences in the two DNA strands. (3) This mixture is incubated with DNA polymerase and the four deoxyribonucleoside triphosphates so that DNA can be synthesized, starting from the two primers. The process can then be repeated by reheating the sample to separate the double-stranded products of the previous cycle (see Figure 10–12).
    The technique depends on the use of a special DNA polymerase isolated from a thermophilic bacterium; this polymerase is stable at much higher temperatures than eukaryotic DNA polymerases, so it is not denatured by the heat treatment shown in step 1. The enzyme therefore does not have to be added again after each cycle.

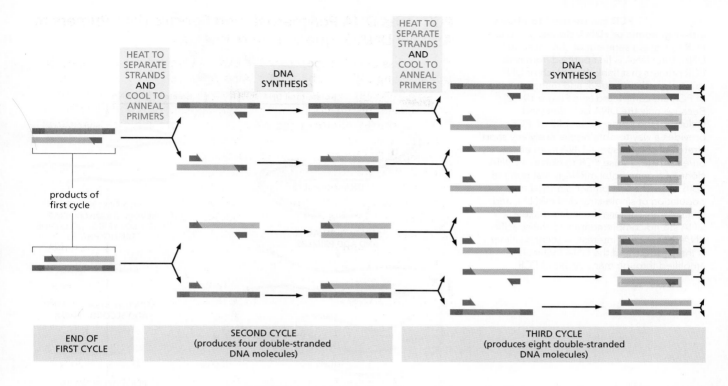

HEAT TO SEPARATE STRANDS AND COOL TO ANNEAL PRIMERS

DNA SYNTHESIS

HEAT TO SEPARATE STRANDS AND COOL TO ANNEAL PRIMERS

DNA SYNTHESIS

products of first cycle

| END OF FIRST CYCLE | SECOND CYCLE (produces four double-stranded DNA molecules) | THIRD CYCLE (produces eight double-stranded DNA molecules) |

Figure 10–12 PCR uses repeated rounds of strand separation, hybridization, and synthesis to amplify DNA. As the procedure outlined in Figure 10–11 is repeated, all the newly synthesized fragments serve as templates in their turn. Because the polymerase and the primers remain in the sample after the first cycle, PCR involves simply heating and then cooling the same sample, in the same test tube, again and again. Each cycle doubles the amount of DNA synthesized in the previous cycle, so that within a few cycles, the predominant DNA is identical to the sequence bracketed by and including the two primers in the original template. In the example illustrated here, three cycles of reaction produce 16 DNA chains, 8 of which (boxed in *yellow*) correspond exactly to one or the other strand of the original bracketed sequence. After four more cycles, 240 of the 256 DNA chains will correspond exactly to the original sequence, and after several more cycles, essentially all of the DNA strands will be this length. The whole procedure is shown in Movie 10.1.

PCR Can Be Used for Diagnostic and Forensic Applications

In addition to its use in cloning, PCR is frequently employed to amplify DNA for other, more practical purposes. Because of its extraordinary sensitivity, PCR can be used to detect an infection at its earliest stages. In this case, short sequences complementary to the suspected pathogen's genome are used as primers, and following many cycles of amplification, even a few copies of an invading bacterial or viral genome in a patient sample can be detected (Figure 10–14). PCR can also be used to track epidemics, detect bioterrorist attacks, and test food products for the presence of potentially harmful microbes. It is also used to verify the authenticity of a food source—for example, whether a sample of beef actually came from a cow.

Finally, PCR is widely used in forensic medicine. The method's extreme sensitivity allows forensic investigators to isolate DNA from even the smallest traces of human blood or other tissue to obtain a *DNA fingerprint* of the person who left the sample behind. With the possible exception of identical twins, the genome of each human differs in DNA sequence from that of every other person on Earth. Using primer pairs targeted at genome sequences that are known to be highly variable in the human

QUESTION 10–4

A. If the PCR shown in Figure 10–12 is carried through an additional two rounds of amplification, how many of the DNA fragments (gray, green, red, or outlined in yellow) will be produced? If many additional cycles are carried out, which fragments will predominate?

B. Assume you start with one double-stranded DNA molecule and amplify a 500-nucleotide-pair sequence contained within it. Approximately how many cycles of PCR amplification will you need to produce 100 ng of this DNA? 100 ng is an amount that can be easily detected after staining with a fluorescent dye. (Hint: for this calculation, you need to know that each nucleotide has an average molecular mass of 330 g/mole.)

Figure 10–13 PCR can be used to obtain either genomic or cDNA clones. (A) To use PCR to clone a segment of chromosomal DNA, total DNA is first purified from cells. PCR primers that flank the stretch of DNA to be cloned are added, and many cycles of PCR are completed (see Figure 10–12). Because only the DNA between (and including) the primers is amplified, PCR provides a way to obtain selectively any short stretch of chromosomal DNA in an effectively pure form. (B) To use PCR to obtain a cDNA clone of a gene, total mRNA is first purified from cells. The first primer is added to a population of single-stranded mRNAs, and reverse transcriptase is used to make a DNA strand complementary to the specific RNA sequence of interest. A second primer is then added, and the DNA molecule is amplified through many cycles of PCR.

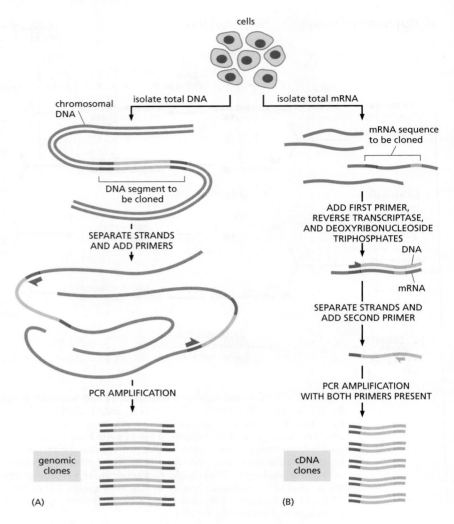

population, PCR makes it possible to generate a distinctive DNA finger-print for any individual (**Figure 10–15**). Such forensic analyses can be used not only to point the finger at those who have done wrong, but—equally important—to help exonerate those who have been wrongfully convicted.

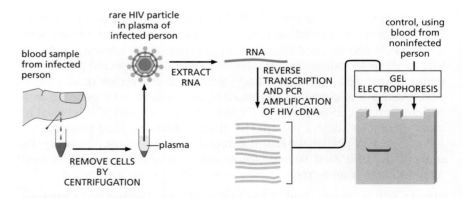

Figure 10–14 PCR can be used to detect the presence of a viral genome in a sample of blood. Because of its ability to amplify enormously the signal from every single molecule of nucleic acid, PCR is an extraordinarily sensitive method for detecting trace amounts of virus in a sample of blood or tissue without the need to purify the virus. For HIV, the virus that causes AIDS, the genome is a single-stranded molecule of RNA, as illustrated here. In addition to HIV, many other viruses that infect humans are now detected in this way.

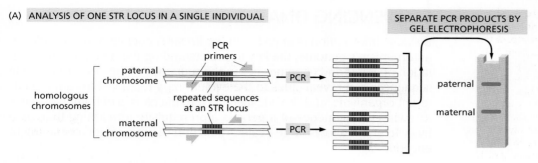

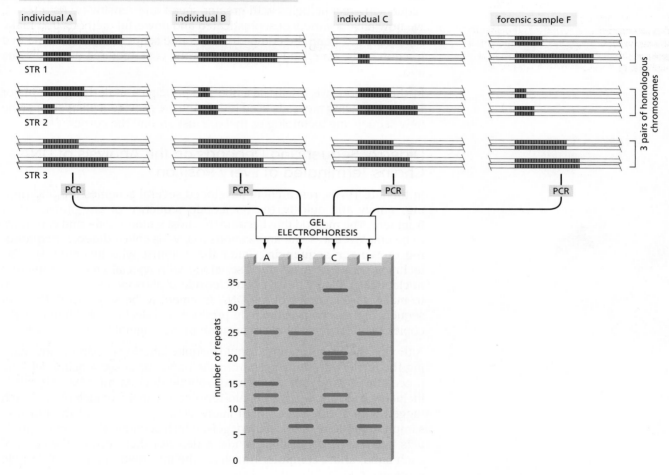

Figure 10–15 **PCR is used in forensic science to distinguish one individual from another.** The DNA sequences typically analyzed are short tandem repeats (STRs). These sequences, composed of stretches of CACA… or GTGT…, for example, are found in various positions (loci) in the human genome. The number of repeats in each STR locus is highly variable in the population, ranging from 4 to 40 in different individuals. Because of the variability in these sequences, individuals will usually inherit a different number of repeats at each STR locus from their mother and from their father; two unrelated individuals, therefore, rarely contain the same pair of repeat sequences at a given STR locus. (A) PCR using primers that recognize unique sequences on either side of one particular STR locus produces a pair of bands of amplified DNA from each individual, one band representing the maternal STR variant and the other representing the paternal STR variant. The length of the amplified DNA, and thus its position after gel electrophoresis, will depend on the exact number of repeats at the locus. (B) In the schematic example shown here, the same three STR loci are analyzed in samples from three suspects (individuals A, B, and C), producing six bands for each individual. Although different people can have several bands in common, the overall pattern is quite distinctive for each person. The band pattern can therefore serve as a *DNA fingerprint* to identify an individual nearly uniquely. The fourth lane in the gel (lane F) contains the products of the same PCR amplifications carried out on a hypothetical forensic DNA sample, which could have been obtained from a single hair or a tiny spot of blood left at a crime scene.

   The more loci that are examined, the more confidence we can have about the results. When examining the variability at 5–10 different STR loci, the odds that two random individuals would share the same fingerprint by chance are approximately one in 10 billion. In the case shown here, individuals A and C can be eliminated from inquiries, while B is a clear suspect. A similar approach is now used routinely in paternity testing.

SEQUENCING DNA

Because information is encoded in the linear sequence of nucleotides in an organism's genome, the key to understanding the function and regulation of genes and genomes lies in the sequence of the DNA. Nucleotide sequences can reveal clues to the evolutionary relationships among different organisms, and provide insights into the causes of human disease. Knowing the sequence of a gene is a prerequisite for cloning that gene by PCR, and it allows large-scale production of any protein a gene might encode.

Because sequence information is so valuable, a great deal of effort has been dedicated over the past few decades to the development of DNA sequencing technologies with greater speed and sensitivity. As a result, we now have a variety of sophisticated and powerful methods that make it possible to obtain the complete nucleotide sequence of a genome in a fraction of the time, and at a fraction of the cost, required even 10 years ago.

In this section, we briefly describe the principles underlying the major DNA sequencing methods used today, and we provide a glimpse of some new sequencing technologies that are just around the corner.

Dideoxy Sequencing Depends on the Analysis of DNA Chains Terminated at Every Position

In the late 1970s, researchers developed several schemes for determining, simply and quickly, the nucleotide sequence of any purified DNA fragment. The method that became the most widely used—and continues to be employed in some applications today—is called **dideoxy sequencing** or **Sanger sequencing** (after the scientist who invented it). This technique uses DNA polymerase, along with special chain-terminating nucleotides called dideoxyribonucleoside triphosphates (**Figure 10–16**), to make partial copies of the DNA fragment to be sequenced. Dideoxy sequencing reactions ultimately produce a collection of different DNA copies that terminate at every position in the original DNA sequence.

Although the original method could be quite laborious—particularly reading the nucleotide sequences from the bands on a sequencing gel—the procedure is now fully automated: robotic devices mix the reagents—including the four different chain-terminating dideoxynucleotides, each tagged with a different-colored fluorescent dye—and load the reaction samples onto long, thin capillary gels, which separate the reaction products into a series of distinct bands. A detector then records the color of each band, and a computer translates the information into a nucleotide sequence (**Figure 10–17**).

The automated dideoxy method made it possible to sequence the first genomes of humans and of many other organisms, including most of those discussed in this book. How such sequence information was analyzed to assemble a complete genome sequence—for example, the initial draft of the human genome—is described in **How We Know**, pp. 348–349.

Figure 10–16 The dideoxy method of sequencing DNA relies on chain-terminating dideoxynucleoside triphosphates (ddNTPs). These ddNTPs are derivatives of the normal deoxyribonucleoside triphosphates that lack the 3′ hydroxyl group. When incorporated into a growing DNA strand, they block further elongation of that strand.

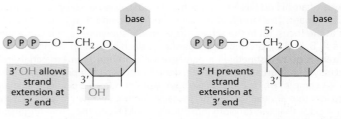

normal deoxyribonucleoside triphosphate (dNTP)

chain-terminating dideoxyribonucleoside triphosphate (ddNTP)

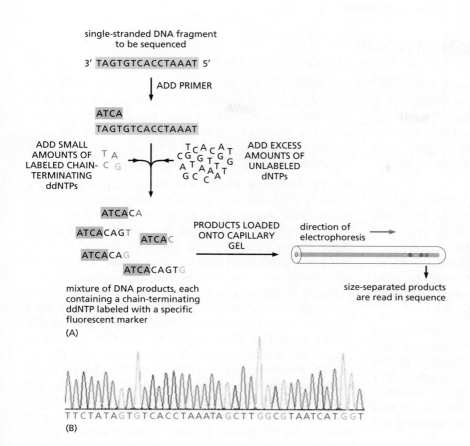

single-stranded DNA fragment
to be sequenced

3′ TAGTGTCACCTAAAT 5′

ADD PRIMER

ATCA
TAGTGTCACCTAAAT

ADD SMALL
AMOUNTS OF
LABELED CHAIN-
TERMINATING
ddNTPs

ADD EXCESS
AMOUNTS OF
UNLABELED
dNTPs

ATCACA
ATCACAGT
ATCAC
ATCACAG
ATCACAGTG

PRODUCTS LOADED
ONTO CAPILLARY
GEL

direction of
electrophoresis

size-separated products
are read in sequence

mixture of DNA products, each
containing a chain-terminating
ddNTP labeled with a specific
fluorescent marker

(A)

TTCTATAGTGTCACCTAAATAGCTTGGCGTAATCATGGT

(B)

Figure 10–17 Automated dideoxy sequencing relies on a set of four ddNTPs, each bearing a uniquely colored fluorescent tag. (A) To determine the complete sequence of a single-stranded fragment of DNA (*gray*), the DNA is first hybridized with a short DNA primer (*orange*). The DNA is then mixed with DNA polymerase (not shown), an excess amount of normal dNTPs, and a mixture containing small amounts of all four chain-terminating ddNTPs, each of which is labeled with a fluorescent tag of a different color. Because the chain-terminating ddNTPs will be incorporated only occasionally, each reaction produces a diverse set of DNA copies that terminate at different points in the sequence. The reaction products are loaded onto a long, thin capillary gel and separated by electrophoresis. A camera reads the color of each band on the gel and feeds the data to a computer that assembles the sequence (not shown). The sequence read from the gel will be complementary to the sequence of the original DNA molecule. (B) A tiny part of the data from such an automated sequencing run. Each colored peak represents a nucleotide in the DNA sequence.

Next-Generation Sequencing Techniques Make Genome Sequencing Faster and Cheaper

Newer methods for the determination of nucleotide sequence, developed over the past decade or so, have made genome sequencing much more rapid—and much cheaper. As the cost of sequencing DNA has plummeted, the number of genomes that have been sequenced has skyrocketed. These rapid methods allow multiple genomes to be sequenced in parallel in a matter of weeks. With these techniques—collectively referred to as *second-generation sequencing methods*—investigators have been able to examine thousands of human genomes, catalog the variation in nucleotide sequences from people around the world, and uncover the mutations that increase the risk of various diseases—from cancer to autism—as we discuss in Chapter 19.

Although each method differs in detail, many rely on the sequencing of libraries of DNA fragments that, taken together, represent the DNA of the entire genome. Instead of using bacterial cells to generate these libraries (as seen in Figure 10–8), however, the libraries are synthesized by PCR amplification of a collection of DNA fragments, each attached to a solid support such as a glass slide or bead. The resulting PCR-generated copies, instead of drifting away in solution, remain bound in proximity to their original "parent" DNA fragment. The process thus generates DNA clusters, each containing about 1000 identical copies of a single DNA fragment. All of these clusters are then sequenced at the same time. One of the most common methods for doing so is called *Illumina sequencing*. Like automated dideoxy sequencing, Illumina sequencing is based on the use of chain-terminating nucleotides with uniquely colored fluorescent tags. In the Illumina method, however, the fluorescent tags and the chemical group that blocks elongation are removable. Once DNA

SEQUENCING THE HUMAN GENOME

When DNA sequencing techniques became fully automated, determining the order of the nucleotides in a piece of DNA went from being an elaborate Ph.D. thesis project to a routine laboratory chore. Feed DNA into the sequencing machine, add the necessary reagents, and out comes the sought-after result: the order of As, Ts, Gs, and Cs. Nothing could be simpler.

So why was sequencing the human genome such a formidable task? Largely because of its size. The DNA sequencing methods employed at the time were limited by the physical size of the gel used to separate the labeled fragments (see, for example, Figure Q10–9). At most, only a few hundred nucleotides could be read from a single gel. How, then, do you handle a genome that contains billions of nucleotide pairs?

The solution is to break the genome into fragments and sequence these smaller pieces. The main challenge then comes in piecing the short fragments together in the correct order to yield a comprehensive sequence of a whole chromosome, and ultimately a whole genome. There are two main strategies for accomplishing this genomic breakage and reassembly: the shotgun method and the clone-by-clone approach.

Shotgun sequencing

The most straightforward approach to sequencing a genome is to break it into random fragments, separate and sequence each of the single-stranded fragments, and then use a powerful computer to order these pieces using sequence overlaps to guide the assembly (**Figure 10–18**). This approach is called the shotgun sequencing strategy. As an analogy, imagine shredding several copies of *Essential Cell Biology* (*ECB*), mixing up the pieces,

and then trying to put one whole copy of the book back together again by matching up the words or phrases or sentences that appear on each piece. (Several copies would be needed to generate enough overlap for reassembly.) It could be done, but it would be much easier if the book were, say, only two pages long.

For this reason, a straight-out shotgun approach is the strategy of choice only for sequencing small genomes. The method proved its worth in 1995, when it was used to sequence the genome of the infectious bacterium *Haemophilus influenzae*, the first organism to have its complete genome sequence determined. The trouble with shotgun sequencing is that the reassembly process can be derailed by repetitive nucleotide sequences. Although rare in bacteria, these sequences make up a large fraction of vertebrate genomes (see Figure 9–33). Highly repetitive DNA segments make it difficult to piece DNA sequences back together accurately (**Figure 10–19**). Returning to the *ECB* analogy, this chapter alone contains more than a few instances of the phrase "the human genome." Imagine that one slip of paper from the shredded *ECB*s contains the information: "So why was sequencing the human genome" (which appears at the start of this section); another contains the information: "the human genome sequence consortium combined shotgun sequencing with a clone-by-clone approach" (which appears below). You might be tempted to join these two segments together based on the overlapping phrase "the human genome." But you would wind up with the nonsensical statement: "So why was sequencing the human genome sequence consortium combined shotgun sequencing with a clone-by-clone approach." You would also lose the several paragraphs of important text that originally appeared between these two instances of "the human genome."

And that's just in this section. The phrase "the human genome" appears in many chapters of this book. Such repetition compounds the problem of placing each fragment in its correct context. To circumvent these assembly problems, researchers in the human genome sequence consortium combined shotgun sequencing with a clone-by-clone approach.

Clone-by-clone

In this approach, researchers started by preparing a genomic DNA library. They broke the human genome into overlapping fragments, 100–200 kilobase pairs in size. They then plugged these segments into bacterial artificial chromosomes (BACs) and inserted them into *E. coli*. (BACs are similar to the bacterial plasmids discussed earlier, except they can carry much larger pieces of DNA.) As the bacteria divided, they copied the BACs, thus producing a collection of overlapping cloned fragments (see Figure 10–8).

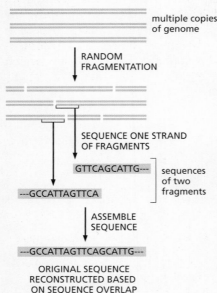

Figure 10–18 **Shotgun sequencing is the method of choice for small genomes.** The genome is first broken into much smaller, overlapping fragments. Each fragment is then sequenced, and the genome is assembled based on overlapping sequences.

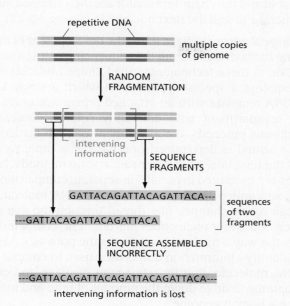

repetitive DNA

multiple copies
of genome

↓ RANDOM
FRAGMENTATION

intervening
information

SEQUENCE
FRAGMENTS

GATTACAGATTACAGATTACA---

---GATTACAGATTACAGATTACA

↓ SEQUENCE ASSEMBLED
INCORRECTLY

---GATTACAGATTACAGATTACAGATTACA---

intervening information is lost

sequences
of two
fragments

Figure 10–19 Repetitive DNA sequences in a genome make it difficult to accurately assemble its fragments. In this example, the DNA contains two segments of repetitive DNA, each made of many copies of the sequence GATTACA. When the resulting sequences are examined, two fragments from different parts of the DNA appear to overlap. Assembling these sequences incorrectly would result in a loss of the information (in brackets) that lies between the original repeats.

The researchers then determined where each of these DNA fragments fit into the existing map of the human genome. To do this, different restriction enzymes were used to cut each clone to generate a unique restriction-site "signature." The locations of the restriction sites in each fragment allowed researchers to map each BAC clone onto a restriction map of a whole human genome that had been generated previously using the same set of restriction enzymes (**Figure 10–20**).

Knowing the relative positions of the cloned fragments, the researchers then selected some 30,000 BACs, sheared each into smaller fragments, and determined the nucleotide sequence of each BAC separately using the shotgun method. They could then assemble the whole genome

sequence by stitching together the sequences of thousands of individual BACs that span the length of the genome.

The beauty of this approach was that it was relatively easy to accurately determine where the BAC fragments belong in the genome. This mapping step reduced the likelihood that regions containing repetitive sequences were assembled incorrectly, and it virtually eliminated the possibility that sequences from different chromosomes were mistakenly joined together. Returning to the textbook analogy, the BAC-based approach is akin to first separating your copies of *ECB* into individual pages and then shredding each page into its own separate pile. It should be much easier to put the book back together when one pile of fragments contains words from page 1, a second pile from page 2, and so on. And there's virtually no chance of mistakenly sticking a sentence from page 40 into the middle of a paragraph on page 412.

All together now

The clone-by-clone approach produced the first draft of the human genome sequence in 2000 and the completed sequence in 2004. As the set of instructions that specify all of the RNA and protein molecules needed to build a human being, this string of genetic bits holds the secrets to human development and physiology. But the sequence was also of great value to researchers interested in comparative genomics or in the physiology of other organisms: it eased the assembly of nucleotide sequences from other mammalian genomes—mice, rats, dogs, and other primates. It also made it much easier to determine the nucleotide sequences of the genomes of individual humans by providing a framework on which the new sequences could be simply superimposed.

The first human sequence was the only mammalian genome completed in this methodical way. But the Human Genome Project was an unqualified success in that it provided the techniques, confidence, and momentum that drove the development of the next generation of DNA sequencing methods, which are now rapidly transforming all areas of biology.

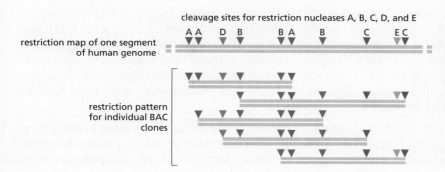

cleavage sites for restriction nucleases A, B, C, D, and E

A A   D B   B A   B   C   E C

restriction map of one segment
of human genome

restriction pattern
for individual BAC
clones

Figure 10–20 Individual BAC clones are positioned on the physical map of the human genome sequence on the basis of their restriction-site "signatures." Clones are digested with five different restriction enzymes, and the sites at which the different enzymes cut each clone are recorded. The distinctive pattern of restriction sites allows investigators to order the fragments and place them on a restriction map of a human genome that had been previously generated using the same nucleases.

polymerase has added the labeled, chain-terminating nucleotide, a photo of the slide is taken and the identity of the nucleotide added at each cluster is recorded; the label and the chain-terminator are then stripped away, allowing DNA polymerase to add the next nucleotide (**Figure 10–21**).

More recent technological advances have led to the development of *third-generation sequencing methods* that permit the sequencing of just a single molecule of DNA. One of these techniques, called Single Molecule Real Time sequencing, employs a special apparatus in which a single DNA polymerase and a DNA template with an attached primer are anchored together in a tiny compartment with differently colored fluorescent dNTPs. As DNA synthesis proceeds, the attachment of each nucleotide to the growing DNA strand is determined one base at a time, revealing the sequence of the template; as in other sequencing methods, large numbers of reactions are measured in parallel in separate compartments. In another method, still under development, a single DNA molecule is pulled slowly through a tiny channel, like thread through the eye of a needle. Because each of the four nucleotides has different, characteristic chemical properties, the way a nucleotide obstructs the pore as it passes through reveals its identity—information that is then used to compile the sequence of the DNA molecule. Further refinement of these and other technologies will continue to drive down the amount of time and money required to sequence a human genome.

Comparative Genome Analyses Can Identify Genes and Predict Their Function

Strings of nucleotides, at first glance, reveal nothing about how that genetic information directs the development of a living organism—or even what type of organism it might encode. One way to learn something about the function of a particular nucleotide sequence is to compare it with the multitude of sequences available in public databases. Using a computer program to search for sequence similarity, one can determine whether a nucleotide sequence contains a gene and what that gene is likely to do—based on the gene's known activity in other organisms.

Comparative analyses have revealed that the coding regions of genes from a wide variety of organisms show a large degree of sequence conservation (see Figure 9–20). The sequences of noncoding regions, however, tend to diverge rapidly over evolutionary time (see Figure 9–19). Thus, a search for sequence similarity can often indicate from which organism a particular piece of DNA was derived, and which species are most closely related. Such information is particularly useful when the origin of a DNA sample is unknown—because it was extracted, for example, from a sample of soil or seawater or the blood of a patient with an undiagnosed infection.

EXPLORING GENE FUNCTION

Knowing where a nucleotide sequence comes from—or even what activity it might have—is only the first step toward determining what role it has in the development or physiology of an organism. The knowledge that a particular DNA sequence encodes a transcription regulator, for example, does not reveal when and where that protein is produced, or which genes it might regulate. To learn that, investigators must head back to the laboratory.

This is where creativity comes in. There are as many ways to study how genes function as there are scientists with an interest in studying the question. The techniques an investigator chooses often depend on his or

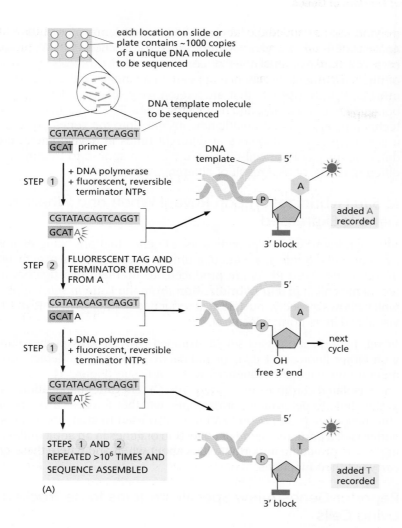

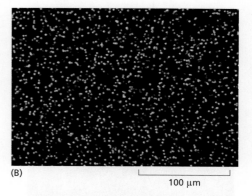

100 μm

Figure 10–21 Illumina sequencing is based on the basic principles of automated dideoxy sequencing.
(A) A genome or other large DNA sample of interest is broken into millions of short fragments. These fragments are attached to a glass surface and amplified by PCR to generate DNA clusters, each containing about a thousand copies of a single DNA fragment. The large number of clusters provides complete coverage of the genome. In the first step, the anchored DNA clusters are incubated with DNA polymerase and a special set of four nucleoside triphosphates (NTPs) with two reversible chemical modifications: a uniquely colored fluorescent marker and a 3' chemical group that terminates DNA synthesis. No normal dNTPs are present in the reaction. After a nucleotide is added by DNA polymerase, a high-resolution digital camera records the color of the fluorescence at each DNA cluster. In the second step, the DNA is chemically treated to remove the fluorescent markers and chemical blockers. A new batch of fluorescent, reversible terminator NTPs is then added to initiate another round of DNA synthesis. These steps are repeated until the sequence is complete. The snapshots of each round of synthesis are compiled by computer to yield the sequence of each DNA fragment. The sequence of the millions of overlapping DNA fragments can then be used to reconstruct the complete genome sequence. (B) An image of a glass slide showing individual DNA clusters after a round of DNA synthesis with colored NTPs. (B, courtesy of Illumina, Inc.)

her background and training: a geneticist might, for example, engineer mutant organisms in which the activity of the gene has been disrupted, whereas a biochemist might take the same gene and produce large amounts of its protein to determine its three-dimensional structure.

In this section, we present a few of the approaches that investigators currently use to study gene function. We explore a variety of techniques for investigating when and where a gene is expressed. We then describe how disrupting the activity of a gene in a cell, tissue, or whole plant or animal can provide insights into what that gene normally does. Finally, we explain how proteins can be produced in large amounts for biochemical and structural studies.

Analysis of mRNAs Provides a Snapshot of Gene Expression

As we discuss in Chapter 8, a cell expresses only a subset of the thousands of genes available in its genome. This subset of genes differs from one cell type to another, and under different conditions in the same cell type. One way to determine which genes are being expressed in a population of cells or in a tissue is to analyze which mRNAs are being produced.

To sequence all the RNAs produced by a cell, investigators make use of the next-generation sequencing technologies described earlier. In most cases, a collection of RNAs is converted into complementary DNA (cDNA) by reverse transcriptase, and these cDNAs are then sequenced. This

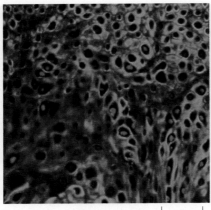

50 μm

Figure 10–22 In situ hybridization can be used to detect the presence of a virus in cells. In this micrograph, the nuclei of cultured epithelial cells infected with the human papillomavirus (HPV) are stained *pink* by a fluorescent probe that recognizes a viral DNA sequence. The cytoplasm of all cells is stained *green*. (Courtesy of Hogne Røed Nilsen.)

method, called **RNA-Seq** or deep RNA sequencing, provides a quantitative analysis of the *transcriptome*—the complete collection of RNAs produced by a cell under a certain set of conditions. It also reveals the number of times a particular sequence appears in a sample and can detect rare mRNAs, RNA transcripts that are alternatively spliced, mRNAs that harbor sequence variations, and noncoding RNAs. This remarkably powerful technology has led to dramatic new insights into the genes expressed in a variety of cells and tissues at different times in development, during different stages of the cell-division cycle, in response to treatment with different drugs, or as a result of different mutations.

In Situ Hybridization Can Reveal When and Where a Gene Is Expressed

Although RNA-Seq can provide a list of genes that are being expressed by a particular tissue at a particular time, it does not reveal exactly where in the tissue those RNAs are produced. To do that, investigators use a technique called *in situ* **hybridization** (from the Latin *in situ*, "in place"), which allows a specific nucleic acid sequence—either DNA or RNA—to be visualized in its normal location.

In situ hybridization uses single-stranded DNA or RNA probes, labeled with either fluorescent dyes or radioactive isotopes, to detect complementary nucleic acid sequences within a tissue (**Figure 10–22**) or even on an isolated chromosome (**Figure 10–23**). The latter application is used in the clinic to determine, for example, whether fetuses carry abnormal chromosomes. *In situ* hybridization is also used to study the expression patterns of a particular gene or collection of genes in an adult or developing tissue, providing important clues about when and where these genes carry out their functions.

Reporter Genes Allow Specific Proteins to Be Tracked in Living Cells

For a gene that encodes a protein, the location of the protein within the cell, tissue, or organism yields clues to the gene's function. Traditionally, the most effective way to visualize a protein within a cell or tissue involved using a labeled antibody. That approach requires the generation of an antibody that specifically recognizes the protein of interest—a process that can be time-consuming and offers no guarantee of success.

An alternative approach is to use the regulatory DNA sequences of the protein-coding gene to drive the expression of some type of **reporter gene**, which encodes a protein that can be easily monitored by its fluorescence or enzymatic activity. A recombinant gene of this type usually mimics the expression of the gene of interest, producing the reporter

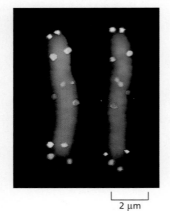

2 μm

Figure 10–23 In situ hybridization can be used to locate genes on isolated chromosomes. Here, six different DNA probes have been used to mark the locations of their respective nucleotide sequences on human Chromosome 5 isolated from a mitotic cell in metaphase (see Figure 5–15 and Panel 18–1, pp. 628–629). The DNA probes have been labeled with different chemical groups and are detected using fluorescent antibodies specific for those groups. Both the maternal and paternal copies of Chromosome 5 are shown, aligned side-by-side. Each probe produces two dots on each chromosome because chromosomes undergoing mitosis have already replicated their DNA; therefore, each chromosome contains two identical DNA helices. The technique employed here is nicknamed FISH, for fluorescence *in situ* hybridization. (Courtesy of David C. Ward.)

(A) CONSTRUCTING A REPORTER GENE

normal gene

coding sequence for protein X

1   2   3

regulatory DNA sequences that determine the expression of gene X

start site for RNA synthesis

	A	B	C	D	E	F

expression pattern of gene X

REPLACE CODING SEQUENCE OF GENE X WITH THAT OF REPORTER GENE Y

recombinant reporter gene

coding sequence for reporter protein Y

1   2   3

expression pattern of reporter gene Y

(B) USING A REPORTER GENE TO STUDY GENE X REGULATORY SEQUENCES

	A	B	C	D	E	F

3

2

1

1   2

expression pattern of reporter gene Y

CONCLUSIONS —regulatory sequence 3 turns on gene X in cell B
—regulatory sequence 2 turns on gene X in cells D, E, and F
—regulatory sequence 1 turns off gene X in cell D

Figure 10–24 **Reporter genes can be used to determine the pattern of a gene's expression.** (A) Suppose the goal is to find out which cell types (A–F) express protein X, but it is difficult to detect the protein directly—with antibodies, for example. Using recombinant DNA techniques, the coding sequence for protein X can be replaced with the coding sequence for reporter protein Y, which can be easily monitored visually; two commonly used reporter proteins are the enzyme β-galactosidase (see Figure 8–14C) and green fluorescent protein (GFP, see Figure 10–25). The expression of the reporter protein Y will now be controlled by the regulatory sequences (here labeled 1, 2, and 3) that control the expression of the normal protein X. (B) To determine which regulatory sequences normally control expression of gene X in particular cell types, reporters with various combinations of the regulatory regions associated with gene X can be constructed. These recombinant DNA molecules are then tested for expression after their introduction into the different cell types.

protein when, where, and in the same amounts as the normal protein would be made (**Figure 10–24A**). This approach can also be used to study the regulatory DNA sequences that control the gene's expression (**Figure 10–24B**).

One of the most popular reporter proteins is **green fluorescent protein** (**GFP**), the molecule that gives luminescent jellyfish their greenish glow. If the gene that encodes GFP is fused to the regulatory sequences of a gene of interest, the expression of the resulting reporter gene can be monitored by fluorescence microscopy (**Figure 10–25**). The use of multiple GFP variants that fluoresce at different wavelengths can provide insights into how different cells interact in a living tissue (**Figure 10–26**).

In some cases, the DNA encoding GFP is attached directly to the protein-coding region of the gene of interest, resulting in a GFP fusion protein

Figure 10–25 **Green fluorescent protein (GFP) can be used to identify specific cells in a living animal.** For this experiment, carried out in the fruit fly, recombinant DNA techniques were used to join the gene encoding GFP to the regulatory DNA sequences that direct the production of a particular *Drosophila* protein. Both the GFP and the normal fly protein are made only in a specialized set of neurons. This image of a live fly larva was captured by a fluorescence microscope and shows approximately 20 neurons, each with long extensions (axons and dendrites) that communicate with other (nonfluorescent) cells. These neurons, located just under the body surface, allow the organism to sense its immediate environment. (Courtesy of Samantha Galindo/Grueber Lab/Columbia University's Zuckerman Institute.)

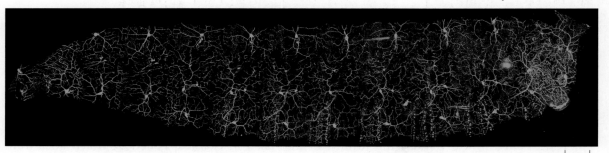

200 μm

Figure 10–26 GFPs that fluoresce at different wavelengths help reveal the connections that individual neurons make within the brain. This image shows differently colored neurons in one region of a mouse brain. The neurons express different combinations of differently colored GFPs, making it possible to distinguish and trace many individual neurons within a population. The stunning appearance of these labeled neurons earned the animals that bear them the colorful nickname "brainbow mice." (From J. Livet et al., *Nature* 450:56–62, 2007. With permission from Macmillan Publishers Ltd.)

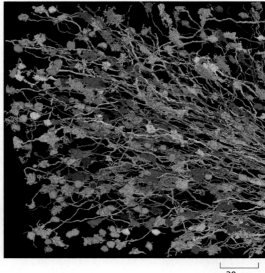

30 μm

that often behaves in the same way as the normal protein produced by the gene. GFP fusion has become a standard strategy for tracking not only the location but also the movement of specific proteins in living cells (see How We Know, pp. 520–521).

The Study of Mutants Can Help Reveal the Function of a Gene

Although it may seem counterintuitive, one of the best ways to determine a gene's function is to see what happens to an organism when the gene is inactivated by a mutation. Before the advent of gene cloning, geneticists would often study the mutant organisms that arise at random in a population. The mutants of most interest were often selected because of their unusual *phenotype*—fruit flies with white eyes or curly wings, for example. The gene responsible for the mutant phenotype could then be studied by breeding experiments, as Gregor Mendel did with peas in the nineteenth century (discussed in Chapter 19).

Although mutant organisms can arise spontaneously, they do so infrequently. The process can be accelerated by treating organisms with radiation or chemical mutagens, which randomly disrupt gene activity. Such random mutagenesis generates large numbers of mutant organisms, each of which can then be studied individually. This "classical genetic approach," which we discuss in detail in Chapter 19, is most applicable to organisms that reproduce rapidly and can be analyzed genetically in the laboratory—such as bacteria, yeasts, nematode worms, and fruit flies—although it has also been used to study zebrafish and mice, which require more time to reproduce and develop.

RNA Interference (RNAi) Inhibits the Activity of Specific Genes

DNA technology has made possible more targeted genetic approaches to studying gene function. Instead of beginning with a randomly generated mutant and then identifying the responsible gene, a gene of known sequence can be inactivated deliberately, and the effects on the cell or organism's phenotype can be observed. Because this strategy is essentially the reverse of that used in classical genetics—which goes from mutants to genes—it is often referred to as *reverse genetics*.

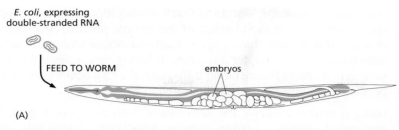

(A)

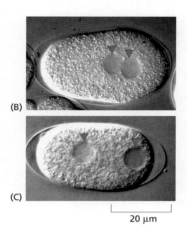

(B)

(C)

20 μm

One of the fastest and easiest ways to silence genes in cells and organisms is via **RNA interference** (**RNAi**). Discovered in 1998, RNAi exploits a natural mechanism used in a wide variety of plants and animals to protect themselves against infection with certain viruses and the proliferation of mobile genetic elements (discussed in Chapter 9). The technique involves introducing into a cell or organism double-stranded RNA molecules with a nucleotide sequence that matches the gene to be inactivated. The double-stranded RNA is cleaved and processed by special RNAi machinery to produce shorter, double-stranded fragments called small interfering RNAs (siRNAs). These siRNAs are separated to form single-stranded RNA fragments that hybridize with the target gene's mRNAs and direct their degradation (see Figure 8–28). In some organisms, the same fragments can direct the production of more siRNAs, allowing continued inactivation of the target mRNAs.

RNAi is frequently used to inactivate genes in cultured mammalian cell lines, *Drosophila*, and the nematode *C. elegans*. Introducing double-stranded RNAs into *C. elegans* is particularly easy: the worm can be fed with *E. coli* that have been genetically engineered to produce the double-stranded RNAs that trigger RNAi (**Figure 10–27**). These RNAs are converted into siRNAs, which are then distributed throughout the animal's body to inhibit expression of the target gene in various tissues. For the many organisms whose genomes have been completely sequenced, RNAi can, in principle, be used to explore the function of any gene, and large collections of DNA vectors that produce these double-stranded RNAs are available for several species.

Figure 10–27 Gene function can be tested by RNA interference. (A) Double-stranded RNA (dsRNA) can be introduced into *C. elegans* by feeding the worms *E. coli* that express the dsRNA. Gene function is reduced in all tissues, including the reproductive tissues where embryos are produced by self-fertilization. (B) In a wild-type worm embryo, the egg and sperm pronuclei (*red* arrowheads) come together in the posterior half of the embryo shortly after fertilization. (C) In an embryo in which a particular gene has been silenced by RNAi, the pronuclei fail to migrate. This experiment revealed an important but previously unknown function of this gene in embryonic development. (B and C, from P. Gönczy et al., *Nature* 408:331–336, 2000. With permission from Macmillan Publishers Ltd.)

A Known Gene Can Be Deleted or Replaced with an Altered Version

Despite its usefulness, RNAi has some limitations. Non-target genes are sometimes inhibited along with the gene of interest, and certain cell types are resistant to RNAi entirely. Even for cell types in which the mechanism functions effectively, gene inactivation by RNAi is often temporary, earning the description "gene knockdown."

Fortunately, there are other, more specific and effective means of eliminating gene activity in cells and organisms. The coding sequence of a cloned gene can be mutated *in vitro* to change the functional properties of its protein product. Alternatively, the coding region can be left intact and the regulatory region of the gene changed, so that the amount of protein made will be altered or the gene will be expressed in a different type of cell or at a different time during development. By re-introducing this altered gene back into the organism from which it originally came, one can produce a mutant organism that can be studied to determine the gene's function. Often the altered gene is inserted into the genome of reproductive cells so that it can be stably inherited by subsequent generations. Organisms whose genomes have been altered in this way are known as **transgenic organisms**, or *genetically modified organisms* (*GMOs*); the introduced gene is called a *transgene*.

To study the function of a gene that has been altered *in vitro*, ideally one would like to generate an organism in which the normal gene has been replaced by the altered one. In this way, the function of the mutant protein can be analyzed in the absence of the normal protein. A common way of doing this in mice makes use of cultured mouse embryonic stem (ES) cells (discussed in Chapter 20). These cells are first subjected to targeted gene replacement before being transplanted into a developing embryo to produce a mutant mouse, as illustrated in **Figure 10–28**.

Using a similar strategy, the activities of both copies of a gene can be eliminated entirely, creating a "**gene knockout**." To do this, one can either introduce an inactive, mutant version of the gene into cultured ES cells or delete the gene altogether. The ability to use ES cells to produce such "knockout mice" revolutionized the study of gene function, and the

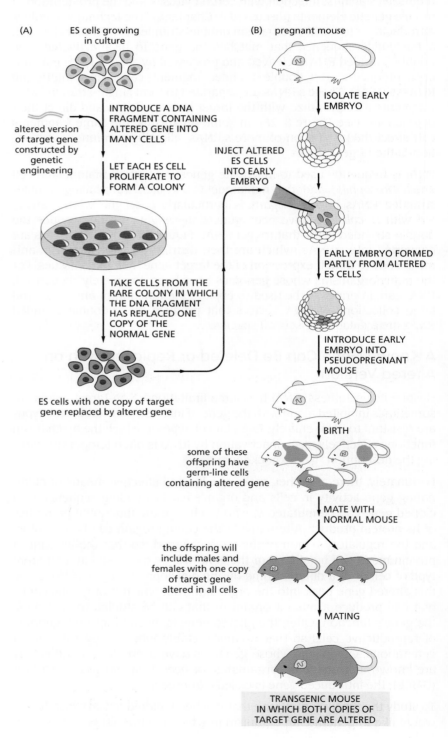

Figure 10–28 Targeted gene replacement in mice utilizes embryonic stem (ES) cells. (A) First, an altered version of the gene is introduced into cultured ES cells. In a few rare ES cells, the altered gene will replace the corresponding normal gene through homologous recombination (as described in Chapter 6, pp. 220–222 and Figure 6–31). Although the procedure is often laborious, these rare cells can be identified and cultured to produce many descendants, each of which carries an altered gene in place of one of its two normal corresponding genes. (B) Next, the altered ES cells are injected into a very early mouse embryo; the cells are incorporated into the growing embryo, which then develops into a mouse that contains some somatic cells (colored *orange*) that carry the altered gene. Some of these mice may also have germ-line cells that contain the altered gene; when bred with a normal mouse, some of the progeny of these mice will contain the altered gene in all of their cells. Such a mouse is called a "knock-in" mouse. If two such mice are bred, one can obtain progeny that contain two copies of the altered gene—one on each chromosome—in all of their cells.

(A) ES cells growing in culture

altered version of target gene constructed by genetic engineering

INTRODUCE A DNA FRAGMENT CONTAINING ALTERED GENE INTO MANY CELLS

LET EACH ES CELL PROLIFERATE TO FORM A COLONY

TAKE CELLS FROM THE RARE COLONY IN WHICH THE DNA FRAGMENT HAS REPLACED ONE COPY OF THE NORMAL GENE

ES cells with one copy of target gene replaced by altered gene

(B) pregnant mouse

ISOLATE EARLY EMBRYO

INJECT ALTERED ES CELLS INTO EARLY EMBRYO

EARLY EMBRYO FORMED PARTLY FROM ALTERED ES CELLS

INTRODUCE EARLY EMBRYO INTO PSEUDOPREGNANT MOUSE

BIRTH

some of these offspring have germ-line cells containing altered gene

MATE WITH NORMAL MOUSE

the offspring will include males and females with one copy of target gene altered in all cells

MATING

TRANSGENIC MOUSE IN WHICH BOTH COPIES OF TARGET GENE ARE ALTERED

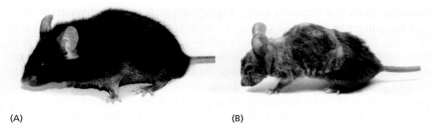

(A)   (B)

Figure 10–29 Transgenic mice with a mutant DNA helicase show premature aging. The helicase, encoded by the *Xpd* gene, is involved in both transcription and DNA repair. Compared with a wild-type mouse (A), a transgenic mouse that expresses a defective version of *Xpd* (B) exhibits many of the symptoms of premature aging, including osteoporosis, emaciation, early graying, infertility, and reduced lifespan. The mutation in *Xpd* used here impairs the activity of the helicase and mimics a human mutation that causes trichothiodystrophy, a disorder characterized by brittle hair, skeletal abnormalities, and a greatly reduced life expectancy. These results support the hypothesis that an accumulation of DNA damage contributes to the aging process in both humans and mice. (From J. de Boer et al., *Science* 296:1276–1279, 2002. With permission from AAAS.)

technique is now being used to systematically determine the function of every mouse gene (**Figure 10–29**).

A variation of this technique can be used to produce *conditional knockout mice*, in which a known gene can be disrupted more selectively—only in a particular cell type or at a certain time in development. The strategy involves the introduction of an enzyme, called a recombinase, that can be directed to selectively excise—and thus disable—a gene of interest (**Figure 10–30**). Such conditional knockouts are useful for studying genes with a critical function during development, because mice missing these crucial genes often die before birth.

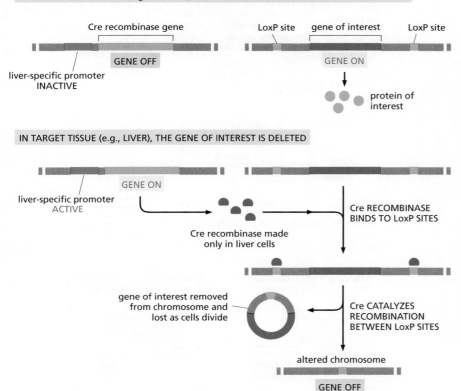

Figure 10–30 In conditional knockouts, a gene can be selectively disabled in a particular target tissue. The approach requires the insertion of two engineered segments of DNA into an animal's germ-line cells. The first contains the gene encoding a recombinase (in this case, Cre recombinase) that is under the control of a tissue-specific promoter. This promoter ensures that recombinase will be produced only in the target tissue. The second DNA molecule contains the gene of interest flanked by nucleotide sequences (in this case, LoxP recombination sites) that are recognized by the recombinase. The mouse is engineered so that this version of the gene of interest is the only copy the animal has.

In non-target tissues, no recombinase will be produced and the gene of interest will be expressed normally. In the target tissue, however, the tissue-specific promoter will be activated, allowing the recombinase to be produced. The enzyme will then bind to the LoxP sites and catalyze a recombination reaction that will excise the gene of interest—thus disabling it specifically in the target tissue.

Genes Can Be Edited with Great Precision Using the Bacterial CRISPR System

Bacteria employ several mechanisms to protect themselves from foreign DNA. One line of defense is provided by the restriction enzymes, as previously discussed. Recently, the discovery of another bacterial defense system led to the development of a powerful new method for editing genes in a variety of cells, tissues, and organisms. This system, called **CRISPR**, relies on a bacterial enzyme called Cas9, which produces a double-strand break in a molecule of DNA. Unlike restriction enzymes, Cas9 is not sequence-specific; to direct Cas9 to its target sequence, investigators provide the enzyme with a guide RNA molecule. This guide RNA, carried by Cas9, allows the enzyme to search the genome and bind to a segment of DNA with a complementary sequence (**Figure 10–31A**). The gene coding for Cas9 has been genetically engineered into a variety of organisms; thus, to use the CRISPR system to target a gene—or multiple genes—researchers need only introduce the appropriate guide RNAs (Movie 10.2).

As we saw in Chapter 6, double-strand breaks, like the one induced by Cas9, are often repaired by homologous recombination—a process that uses the information on an undamaged segment of DNA to repair the break. Thus, to replace a target gene using CRISPR, investigators simply provide an altered version of the gene to serve as a template for the homologous repair. In this way, a target gene can be selectively cut by the CRISPR system and replaced at high efficiency by an experimentally altered version of the gene (**Figure 10–31B**). The CRISPR system therefore provides another means of generating transgenic organisms.

Researchers are also adapting the CRISPR system for turning selected genes on or off. In this case, a catalytically inactive Cas9 protein can be

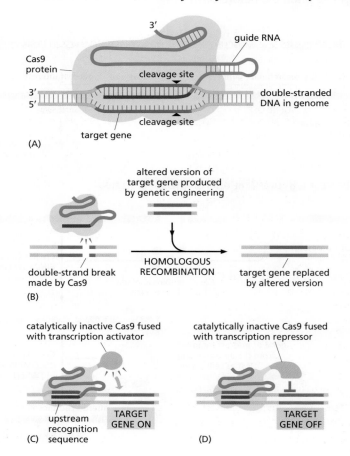

Figure 10–31 The CRISPR system can be used to study gene function in a variety of species. (A) The Cas9 protein, along with a guide RNA designed by the experimenter, are both artificially expressed in the cell or species of interest. One portion of the guide RNA (*light blue*) associates with Cas9, and another segment (*dark blue*) is designed to match a particular target sequence in the genome. (B) Once Cas9 has made a double-strand break in the target gene, that gene can be replaced with an experimentally altered gene by the enzymes that repair double-strand breaks through homologous recombination (see Figure 6–31). In this way, the CRISPR system promotes the precise and rapid replacement of a target gene. (C and D) By using a mutant form of Cas9 that can no longer cleave DNA, Cas9 can be used to activate a normally dormant gene (C) or turn off an actively expressed gene (D). (Adapted from P. Mali et al., *Nat. Methods* 10:957–963, 2013.)

fused to a transcription activator or repressor; this hybrid transcription regulator can then be directed to a target gene by the appropriate guide RNA (**Figure 10–31C and D**).

The transfer of the CRISPR system from bacteria to virtually all other experimental organisms—including mice, zebrafish, worms, flies, rice, and wheat—has revolutionized the study of gene function. Like the earlier discoveries of restriction enzymes and RNAi, this incredible breakthrough came from the work of scientists who were studying a fascinating biological phenomenon without—at first—realizing the enormous impact these discoveries would have on all aspects of biology, including human health. Such unintentional application highlights the fundamental importance of basic research.

Mutant Organisms Provide Useful Models of Human Disease

Technically speaking, transgenic approaches—including CRISPR—could be used to alter genes in the human germ line. Such manipulations would be unethical. However, transgenic technologies are currently being used to generate animal models of human diseases in which mutant genes play a major part.

With the explosion of DNA sequencing technologies, investigators can rapidly search the genomes of patients for mutations that cause or greatly increase the risk of their disease (discussed in Chapter 19). These mutations can then be introduced into animals, such as mice, that can be studied in the laboratory. The resulting transgenic animals, which often mimic some of the phenotypic abnormalities associated with the condition in patients, can be used to explore the cellular and molecular basis of the disease and to screen for drugs that could potentially be used therapeutically in humans.

An encouraging example is provided by *fragile X syndrome*, a neuropsychiatric disorder associated with intellectual impairment, neurological abnormalities, and often autism. The disease is caused by a mutation in the *fragile X mental retardation gene* (*FMR1*), which encodes a protein that inhibits the translation of mRNAs into proteins at synapses—the junctions where nerve cells communicate with one another (see Figure 12–39). Transgenic mice in which the *FMR1* gene has been disabled show many of the same neurological and behavioral abnormalities seen in patients with the disorder, and drugs that return synaptic protein synthesis to near-normal levels also reverse many of the problems seen in these mutant mice. Preliminary studies suggest that at least one of these drugs may benefit patients with the disease.

Transgenic Plants Are Important for both Cell Biology and Agriculture

Although we tend to think of DNA technology in terms of animal biology, these techniques have also had a profound impact on the study of plants. In fact, certain features of plants make them especially amenable to these methods.

When a piece of plant tissue is cultured in a sterile medium containing nutrients and appropriate growth regulators, some of the cells are stimulated to proliferate indefinitely in a disorganized manner, producing a mass of relatively undifferentiated cells called a *callus*. If the nutrients and growth regulators are carefully manipulated, one can induce the formation of a shoot within the callus, and in many species a whole new plant can be regenerated from such shoots. In a number of plants—including

Figure 10–32 Transgenic plants can be made using recombinant DNA techniques optimized for plants. A disc is cut out of a leaf and incubated in a culture of *Agrobacterium* that carries a recombinant plasmid with both a selectable marker and a desired genetically engineered gene. The wounded plant cells at the edge of the disc release substances that attract the bacteria, which inject their DNA into the plant cells. Only those plant cells that take up the appropriate DNA and express the selectable marker gene survive and proliferate and form a callus. The manipulation of growth factors supplied to the callus induces it to form shoots, which subsequently root and grow into adult plants carrying the engineered gene.

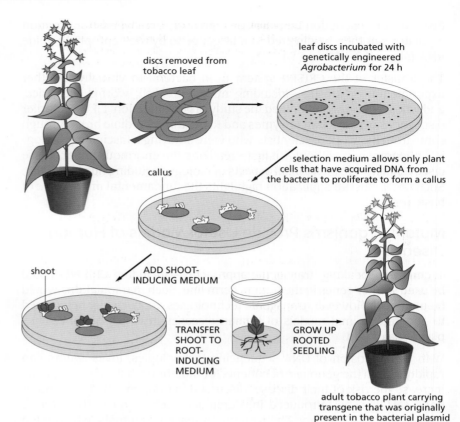

Figure 10–33 DNA technology allows the production of rice grains with high levels of β-carotene. To help reduce vitamin A deficiency in the developing world, a strain of rice, called "golden rice," was developed in which the edible part of the grain (called the endosperm) contains large amounts of β-carotene, which is converted in the human gut to vitamin A. (A) Rice plants, like most other plants, can synthesize β-carotene in their leaves from an abundant precursor (geranylgeranyl pyrophosphate) found in all plant tissues. However, the genes that code for two of the enzymes that act early in this biosynthetic pathway are turned off in the endosperm, preventing the production of β-carotene in rice grains. To produce golden rice, the genes for these two enzymes in the pathway were obtained from organisms that produce large amounts of β-carotene: one from maize and the other from a bacterium. Using DNA technology, these genes were connected to a promoter that drives gene expression in rice endosperm. Using the method outlined in Figure 10–32, this engineered DNA was then used to generate a transgenic rice plant that expresses these enzymes in endosperm, resulting in rice grains that contain high levels of β-carotene. Compared to the milled grains of wild-type rice (B), the grains of the transgenic rice are a deep yellow/orange due to the presence of β-carotene (C). (B and C, from J.A. Paine et al., *Nature Biotechnology*, Letters 23: 482–487, 2005. With permission from Macmillan Publishers Ltd.)

tobacco, petunia, carrot, potato, and *Arabidopsis*—a single cell from such a callus can be grown into a small clump of cells from which a whole plant can be regenerated (see Figure 8–2B). Just as mutant mice can be derived by the genetic manipulation of embryonic stem cells in culture, transgenic plants can be created from plant cells transfected with DNA in culture (**Figure 10–32**).

The ability to produce transgenic plants has greatly accelerated progress in many areas of plant cell biology. It has played an important part, for example, in isolating receptors for growth regulators and in analyzing the mechanisms of morphogenesis and of gene expression in plants. These techniques have also opened up many new possibilities in agriculture that could benefit both the farmer and the consumer. They have made it possible, for example, to modify the ratio of lipid, starch, and protein in seeds, to impart pest and virus resistance to plants, and to create modified plants that tolerate extreme habitats such as salt marshes or water-stressed soil. One variety of rice has been genetically engineered to produce β-carotene, the precursor of vitamin A (**Figure 10–33**). If it replaced conventional rice, this "golden rice"—so called because of its

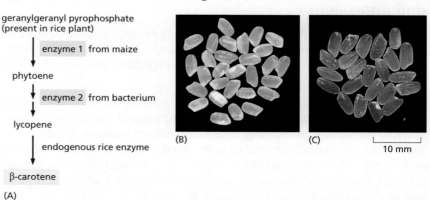

Figure 10–34 Large amounts of a protein can be produced from a protein-coding DNA sequence inserted into an expression vector and introduced into cells. Here, a plasmid vector has been engineered to contain a highly active promoter, which causes unusually large amounts of mRNA to be produced from the inserted protein-coding gene. Depending on the characteristics of the cloning vector, the plasmid is introduced into bacterial, yeast, insect, or mammalian cells, where the inserted gene is efficiently transcribed and translated into protein.

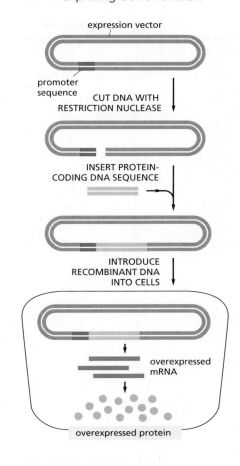

yellow/orange color—could help to alleviate severe vitamin A deficiency, which causes blindness in hundreds of thousands of children in the developing world each year.

Even Rare Proteins Can Be Made in Large Amounts Using Cloned DNA

One of the most important contributions of DNA cloning and genetic engineering to cell biology is that they make it possible to produce any protein, including the rare ones, in large amounts. Such high-level production is usually accomplished by using specially designed vectors known as *expression vectors*. These vectors include transcription and translation signals that direct an inserted gene to be expressed at high levels. Different expression vectors are designed for use in bacterial, yeast, insect, or mammalian cells, each containing the appropriate regulatory sequences for transcription and translation in these cells (**Figure 10–34**). The expression vector is replicated at each round of cell division, so that the transfected cells in the culture are able to synthesize large amounts of the protein of interest—sometimes comprising 1–10% of the total cell protein. It is usually a simple matter to purify this protein away from the other proteins made by the host cell.

This technology is now used to make large amounts of many medically useful proteins, including hormones (such as insulin), growth factors, therapeutic antibodies, and viral coat proteins for use in vaccines. Expression vectors also allow scientists to produce many proteins of biological interest in large enough amounts for detailed structural and functional studies that were once impossible—especially for proteins that are normally present in very small amounts, such as some receptors and transcription regulators. Recombinant DNA techniques thus allow scientists to move with ease from protein to gene, and vice versa, so that the functions of both can be explored from multiple directions (**Figure 10–35**).

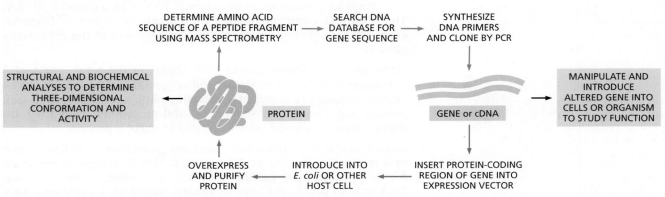

Figure 10–35 Recombinant DNA techniques make it possible to move experimentally from gene to protein or from protein to gene. A small quantity of a purified protein or peptide fragment is used to obtain a partial amino acid sequence, which is used to search a DNA database for the corresponding nucleotide sequence. This sequence is used to synthesize DNA primers, which can be used to clone the gene by PCR from a sequenced genome (see Figure 10–13). Once the gene has been isolated and sequenced, its protein-coding sequence can be inserted into an expression vector to produce large quantities of the protein (see Figure 10–34), which can then be studied biochemically or structurally. In addition to producing protein, the gene or DNA can also be manipulated and introduced into cells or organisms to study its function.

KEY TERMS

complementary DNA (cDNA)	hybridization
cDNA library	*in situ* hybridization
CRISPR	plasmid
dideoxy (Sanger) sequencing	polymerase chain reaction (PCR)
DNA cloning	recombinant DNA
DNA library	reporter gene
DNA ligase	restriction enzyme
gene knockout	RNA interference (RNAi)
genomic library	RNA-Seq
green fluorescent protein	transformation
(GFP)	transgenic organism

ESSENTIAL CONCEPTS

- DNA technology has revolutionized the study of cells, making it possible to pick out any gene at will from the thousands of genes in a cell and to determine its nucleotide sequence.

- A crucial element in this technology is the ability to cut a large DNA molecule into a specific and reproducible set of DNA fragments using restriction enzymes, each of which cuts the DNA double helix only at a particular nucleotide sequence.

- DNA fragments can be separated from one another on the basis of size by gel electrophoresis.

- DNA cloning techniques enable any DNA sequence to be selected from millions of other sequences and produced in unlimited amounts in pure form.

- DNA fragments can be joined together *in vitro* by using DNA ligase to form recombinant DNA molecules that are not found in nature.

- DNA fragments can be maintained and amplified by inserting them into a larger DNA molecule capable of replication, such as a plasmid. This recombinant DNA molecule is then introduced into a rapidly dividing host cell, usually a bacterium, so that the DNA is replicated at each cell division.

- A collection of cloned fragments of chromosomal DNA representing the complete genome of an organism is known as a genomic library. The library is often maintained as millions of clones of bacteria, each different clone carrying a different fragment of the organism's genome.

- cDNA libraries contain cloned DNA copies of the total mRNA of a particular type of cell or tissue. Unlike genomic DNA clones, cDNA clones contain predominantly protein-coding sequences; they lack introns, regulatory DNA sequences, and promoters. Thus they are useful when the cloned gene is needed to make a protein.

- Nucleic acid hybridization can detect any given DNA or RNA sequence in a mixture of nucleic acid fragments. This technique depends on highly specific base-pairing between a labeled, single-stranded DNA or RNA probe and another nucleic acid with a complementary sequence.

- The polymerase chain reaction (PCR) is a powerful form of DNA amplification that is carried out *in vitro* using a purified DNA polymerase. Cloning via PCR requires prior knowledge of the sequence to be amplified, because two synthetic oligonucleotide primers must be synthesized that bracket the portion of DNA to be replicated.

- DNA sequencing techniques have become increasingly fast and cheap, so that the entire genome sequences of thousands of different organisms are now known, including thousands of individual humans.

- Using DNA technology, a protein can be joined to a molecular tag, such as green fluorescent protein (GFP), which allows its movement to be tracked inside a cell and, in some cases, inside a living organism.

- *In situ* nucleic acid hybridization can be used to detect the precise location of genes on chromosomes and of RNAs in cells and tissues.

- RNA-Seq can be used to monitor the expression of all of the genes in a cell or tissue.

- Cloned genes can be altered *in vitro* and stably inserted into the genome of a cell or an organism to study their function. Such mutants are called transgenic organisms.

- The expression of particular genes can be inhibited in cells or organisms by the technique of RNA interference (RNAi), which prevents an mRNA from being translated into protein.

- Genes can be deleted or modified with high specificity by the CRISPR system, which uses guide mRNAs to promote DNA cleavage at a specific nucleotide sequence in the genome.

- Bacteria, yeasts, and mammalian cells can be engineered to synthesize large quantities of any protein whose gene has been cloned, making it possible to study proteins that are otherwise rare or difficult to isolate.

QUESTIONS

QUESTION 10–5

What are the consequences for a dideoxy DNA sequencing reaction if the ratio of dideoxyribonucleoside triphosphates to deoxyribonucleoside triphosphates is increased? What happens if this ratio is decreased?

QUESTION 10–6

Almost all the cells in an individual animal contain identical genomes. In an experiment, a tissue composed of several different cell types is fixed and subjected to *in situ* hybridization with a DNA probe to a particular gene. To your surprise, the hybridization signal is much stronger in some cells than in others. How might you explain this result?

QUESTION 10–7

After decades of work, Dr. Ricky M. isolated a small amount of attractase—an enzyme that produces a powerful human pheromone—from hair samples of Hollywood celebrities. To take advantage of attractase for his personal use, he obtained a complete genomic clone of the attractase gene, connected it to a strong bacterial promoter on an expression plasmid, and introduced the plasmid into *E. coli* cells. He was devastated to find that no attractase was produced in the cells. What is a likely explanation for his failure?

QUESTION 10–8

Which of the following statements are correct? Explain your answers.

A. Restriction enzymes cut DNA at specific sites that are always located between genes.

B. DNA migrates toward the positive electrode during electrophoresis.

C. Clones isolated from cDNA libraries contain promoter sequences.

D. PCR utilizes a heat-stable DNA polymerase because for each amplification step, double-stranded DNA must be heat-denatured.

E. Digestion of genomic DNA with AluI, a restriction enzyme that recognizes a four-nucleotide sequence, produces fragments that are all exactly 256 nucleotides in length.

F. To make a cDNA library, both a DNA polymerase and a reverse transcriptase must be used.

G. DNA fingerprinting by PCR relies on the fact that different individuals have different numbers of repeats in STR regions in their genome.

H. It is possible for a coding region of a gene to be present in a genomic library prepared from a particular tissue but to be absent from a cDNA library prepared from the same tissue.

QUESTION 10–9

A. What is the sequence of the DNA that was used in the sequencing reaction shown in Figure Q10–9? The four lanes show the products of sequencing reactions that contained ddG (lane 1), ddA (lane 2), ddT (lane 3), and ddC (lane 4). The numbers to the right of the autoradiograph represent the positions of marker DNA fragments of 50 and 116 nucleotides.

lanes
1 2 3 4 — 116

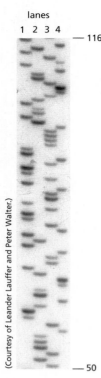

— 50

(Courtesy of Leander Lauffer and Peter Walter.)

Figure Q10–9

B. This DNA was derived from the middle of a cDNA clone of a mammalian protein. Using the genetic code table (see Figure 7–27), can you determine the amino acid sequence of this portion of the protein?

QUESTION 10–10

A. How many different DNA fragments would you expect to obtain if you cleaved human genomic DNA with HaeIII? (Recall that there are 3×10^9 nucleotide pairs per haploid genome.) How many fragments would you expect with EcoRI?

B. Human genomic libraries used for DNA sequencing are often made from fragments obtained by cleaving human DNA with HaeIII in such a way that the DNA is only partially digested; that is, not all the possible HaeIII sites have been cleaved. What is a possible reason for doing this?

QUESTION 10–11

A molecule of double-stranded DNA was cleaved with restriction enzymes, and the resulting products were separated by gel electrophoresis (Figure Q10–11). You do not know if the molecule is linear DNA or a DNA circle. DNA fragments of known sizes were electrophoresed on the same gel for use as size markers (*left* lane). The size of the DNA markers is given in kilobase pairs (kb), where 1 kb = 1000 nucleotide pairs. Using the size markers as a guide, estimate the length of each restriction fragment obtained. From this information, construct a map of the original DNA molecule indicating the relative positions of all the restriction enzyme cleavage sites.

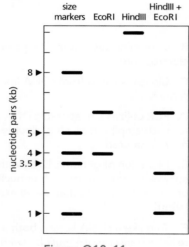

Figure Q10–11

QUESTION 10–12

There has been a colossal snafu in the maternity ward of your local hospital. Four sets of male twins, born within an hour of each other, were inadvertently shuffled in the excitement occasioned by that unlikely event. You have been called in to set things straight. As a first step, you would like to match each baby with his twin. (Many

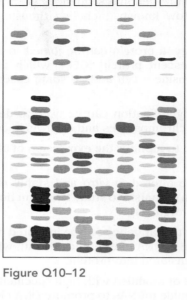

Figure Q10–12

newborns look alike so you don't want to rely on appearance alone.) To that end you analyze a small blood sample from each infant using a hybridization probe that detects short tandem repeats (STRs) located in widely scattered regions of the genome. The results are shown in Figure Q10–12.

A. Which infants are twins? Which are identical twins?

B. How could you match a pair of twins to the correct parents?

QUESTION 10–13

One of the first organisms that was genetically modified using recombinant DNA technology was a bacterium that normally lives on the surface of strawberry plants. This bacterium makes a protein, called ice-protein, that causes the efficient formation of ice crystals around it when the temperature drops to just below freezing. Thus, strawberries harboring this bacterium are particularly susceptible to frost damage because their cells are destroyed by the ice crystals. Consequently, strawberry farmers have a considerable interest in preventing ice crystallization.

A genetically engineered version of this bacterium was constructed in which the ice-protein gene was knocked out. The mutant bacteria were then introduced in large numbers into strawberry fields, where they displaced the normal bacteria by competition for their ecological niche. This approach has been successful: strawberries bearing the mutant bacteria show a much reduced susceptibility to frost damage.

At the time they were first carried out, the initial open-field trials triggered an intense debate because they represented the first release into the environment of an organism that had been genetically engineered using recombinant DNA technology. Indeed, all preliminary experiments were carried out with extreme caution and in strict containment.

Do you think that bacteria lacking the ice-protein could be isolated without the use of modern DNA technology? Is it likely that such mutations have already occurred in nature? Would the use of a mutant bacterial strain isolated from nature be of lesser concern? Should we be concerned about the risks posed by the application of recombinant DNA techniques in agriculture and medicine? Do the potential benefits outweigh the risks? Explain your answers.

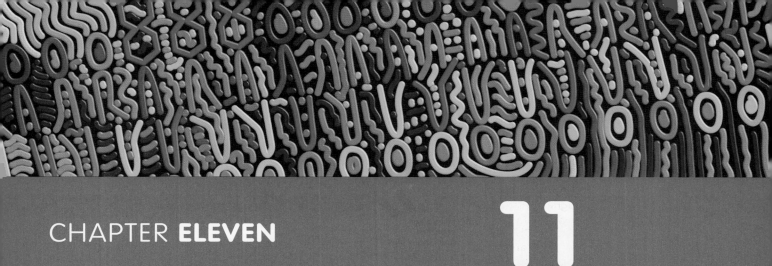

CHAPTER **ELEVEN**

11

Membrane Structure

A living cell is a self-reproducing system of molecules held inside a container. That container is the **plasma membrane**—a protein-studded, fatty film so thin that it cannot be seen directly in the light microscope. Every cell on Earth uses such a membrane to separate and protect its chemical components from the outside environment. Without membranes, there would be no cells, and thus no life.

The structure of the plasma membrane is simple: it consists of a two-ply sheet of lipid molecules about 5 nm—or 50 atoms—thick, into which proteins have been inserted. Its properties, however, are unlike those of any sheet of material we are familiar with in the everyday world. Although it serves as a barrier to prevent the contents of the cell from escaping and mixing with molecules in the surrounding environment (**Figure 11–1**), the plasma membrane does much more than that. If a cell is to survive and grow, nutrients must pass inward across the plasma membrane, and waste products must make their way out. To facilitate this

THE LIPID BILAYER

MEMBRANE PROTEINS

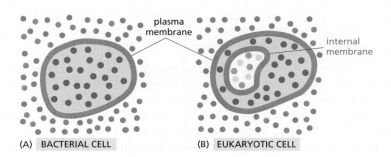

Figure 11–1 **Cell membranes act as selective barriers.** The plasma membrane separates a cell from its surroundings, enabling the molecular composition of a cell to differ from that of its environment. (A) In some bacteria, the plasma membrane is the only membrane. (B) In addition to a plasma membrane, eukaryotic cells also have internal membranes that enclose individual organelles. All cell membranes prevent molecules on one side from freely mixing with those on the other, as indicated schematically by the colored dots.

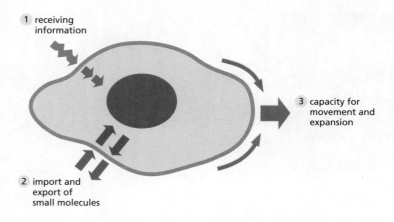

Figure 11–2 The plasma membrane is involved in cell communication, import and export of molecules, and cell growth and motility. (1) Receptor proteins in the plasma membrane enable the cell to receive signals from the environment; (2) channels and transporters in the membrane enable the import and export of small molecules; (3) the flexibility of the membrane and its capacity for expansion allow the cell to grow, change shape, and move.

exchange, the membrane is penetrated by highly selective channels and transporters—proteins that allow specific, small molecules and ions to be imported and exported. Other proteins in the membrane act as sensors, or receptors, that enable the cell to receive information about changes in its environment and respond to them in appropriate ways. The mechanical properties of the plasma membrane are equally impressive. When a cell grows, so does its membrane: this remarkable structure enlarges in area by adding new membrane without ever losing its continuity, and it can deform without tearing, allowing the cell to move or change shape (**Figure 11–2**). The membrane is also self-healing: if it is pierced, it neither collapses like a balloon nor remains torn; instead, the membrane quickly reseals.

As shown in Figure 11–1, many bacteria have only a single membrane—the plasma membrane—whereas eukaryotic cells also contain *internal membranes* that enclose intracellular compartments. The internal membranes form various organelles, including the endoplasmic reticulum, Golgi apparatus, endosomes, and mitochondria (**Figure 11–3**). Although these internal membranes are constructed on the same principles as the plasma membrane, they differ subtly in composition, especially in their resident proteins.

Regardless of their location, all cell membranes are composed of lipids and proteins and share a common general structure (**Figure 11–4**). The lipids are arranged in two closely apposed sheets, forming a *lipid bilayer* (see Figure 11–4B). This lipid bilayer serves as a permeability barrier to most water-soluble molecules, while the proteins embedded within it carry out the other functions of the membrane and give different membranes their individual characteristics.

In this chapter, we consider the structure of biological membranes and the organization of their two main constituents: lipids and proteins. Although we focus mainly on the plasma membrane, most of the concepts we discuss also apply to internal membranes. The functions of cell membranes, including their role in cell communication, the transport of small molecules, and energy generation, are considered in later chapters.

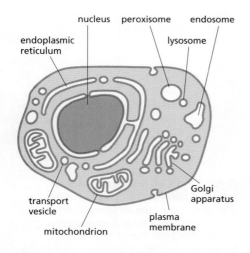

Figure 11–3 Internal membranes form many different compartments in a eukaryotic cell. Some of the main membrane-enclosed organelles in a typical animal cell are shown here. Note that the nucleus and mitochondria are each enclosed by two membranes.

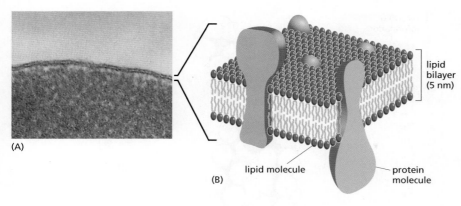

(A)

(B)

lipid molecule

protein molecule

lipid bilayer (5 nm)

Figure 11–4 **A cell membrane consists of a lipid bilayer in which proteins are embedded.** (A) An electron micrograph of a plasma membrane of a human red blood cell seen in cross section. In this image, the proteins that extend from either side of the bilayer form the two closely spaced dark lines indicated by the brackets; the thin, white layer between them is the lipid bilayer. (B) Schematic drawing showing a three-dimensional view of a cell membrane. (A, by permission of E.L. Bearer.)

THE LIPID BILAYER

Because cells are filled with—and surrounded by—water, the structure of cell membranes is determined by the way membrane lipids behave in a watery (aqueous) environment. Lipid molecules are not very soluble in water, although they do dissolve readily in organic solvents such as benzene. It was this property that scientists exploited in 1925, when they set out to investigate how lipids are arranged in cell membranes.

Using benzene, investigators extracted all the lipids from the plasma membranes of purified red blood cells. These lipids were then spread out in a film on the surface of a trough filled with water, like an oil slick on a puddle. Using a movable barrier, the researchers then pushed the floating lipids together until they formed a continuous sheet only one molecule thick. When the investigators measured the surface area of this monolayer, they found that it occupied twice the area of the original, intact cells. Based on this observation, they deduced that, in an intact cell membrane, lipid molecules must double up to form a bilayer—a finding that had a profound influence on cell biology.

In this section, we take a closer look at this **lipid bilayer**, which constitutes the fundamental structure of all cell membranes. We consider how lipid bilayers form, how they are maintained, and how their properties establish the general properties of all cell membranes.

Membrane Lipids Form Bilayers in Water

The lipids found in cell membranes combine two very different properties in a single molecule: each lipid has a hydrophilic ("water-loving") head and a hydrophobic ("water-fearing") tail. The most abundant lipids in cell membranes are the **phospholipids**, which have a phosphate-containing, hydrophilic head linked to a pair of hydrophobic, hydrocarbon tails (**Figure 11–5**). For example, **phosphatidylcholine**, one of the most abundant phospholipids in the membranes of animals and plants, has the small molecule choline attached to a phosphate group as its hydrophilic head (**Figure 11–6**).

Phospholipids are not the only membrane lipids that are **amphipathic**, a term used to describe molecules with both hydrophilic and hydrophobic parts. Cholesterol, which is found in animal cell membranes, and *glycolipids*, which have sugars as part of their hydrophilic head, are also amphipathic (**Figure 11–7**).

Having both hydrophilic and hydrophobic parts plays a crucial part in driving lipid molecules to assemble into bilayers in an aqueous environment.

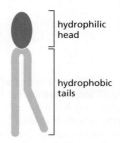

hydrophilic head

hydrophobic tails

Figure 11–5 **Cell membranes are packed with phospholipids.** A typical membrane phospholipid molecule has a hydrophilic head and two hydrophobic tails.

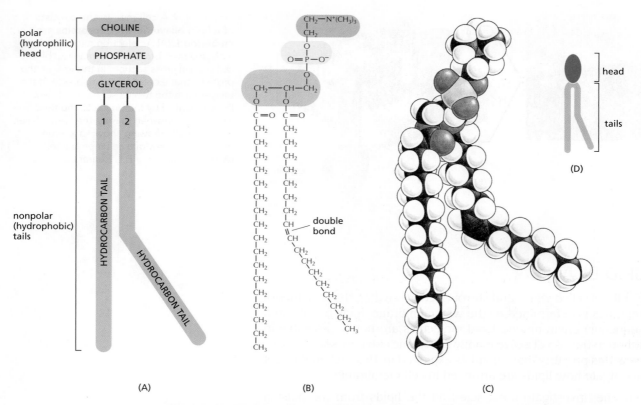

(A) (B) (C) (D)

Figure 11–6 Phosphatidylcholine is the most common phospholipid in cell membranes. It is represented schematically in (A), as a chemical formula in (B), as a space-filling model in (C), and as a symbol in (D). This particular phospholipid is built from five parts: the hydrophilic head, which consists of *choline* linked to a *phosphate* group; two *hydrocarbon chains*, which form the hydrophobic tails; and a molecule of glycerol, which links the head to the tails. Each of the hydrophobic tails is a *fatty acid*—a hydrocarbon chain with a carboxyl (–COOH) group at one end; glycerol attaches via this carboxyl group, as shown in (B). A kink in one of the hydrocarbon chains occurs where there is a double bond between two carbon atoms. (The "phosphatidyl" part of the name of a phospholipid refers to the phosphate–glycerol–fatty acid portion of the molecule.)

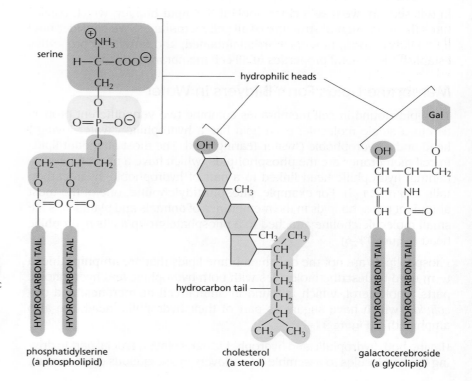

Figure 11–7 Different types of membrane lipids are all amphipathic. Each of the three types shown here has a hydrophilic head and one or two hydrophobic tails. The hydrophilic head is serine phosphate (shaded *blue* and *yellow*) in phosphatidylserine, an –OH group (*blue*) in cholesterol, and the sugar galactose plus an –OH group (both *blue*) in galactocerebroside. See also Panel 2–4, pp. 72–73.

phosphatidylserine (a phospholipid)

cholesterol (a sterol)

galactocerebroside (a glycolipid)

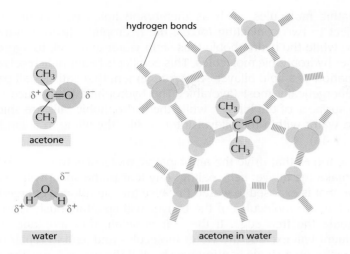

hydrogen bonds

acetone

water

acetone in water

Figure 11–8 A hydrophilic molecule attracts water molecules. Both acetone and water are polar molecules: thus acetone readily dissolves in water. Polar atoms are shown in *red* and *blue*, with δ^- indicating a partial negative charge, and δ^+ indicating a partial positive charge. Hydrogen bonds (*red*) and an electrostatic attraction (*yellow*) form between acetone and the surrounding water molecules. Nonpolar groups are shown in *gray*.

As discussed in Chapter 2 (see Panel 2–2, pp. 68–69), hydrophilic molecules dissolve readily in water because they contain either charged groups or uncharged polar groups that can form electrostatic attractions or hydrogen bonds with water molecules (**Figure 11–8**). Hydrophobic molecules, by contrast, are insoluble in water because all—or almost all—of their atoms are uncharged and nonpolar; they therefore cannot form favorable interactions with water molecules. Instead, they force adjacent water molecules to reorganize into a cagelike structure around them (**Figure 11–9**). Because this cagelike structure is more highly ordered than the rest of the water, its formation requires free energy. This energy cost is minimized when the hydrophobic molecules cluster together, limiting their contacts with the surrounding water molecules. Thus, purely hydrophobic molecules, like the fats found in the oils of plant seeds and the adipocytes (fat cells) of animals (**Figure 11–10**), coalesce into large **fat droplets** when dispersed in water.

2-methylpropane

water

2-methylpropane in water

QUESTION 11–1

Water molecules are said "to reorganize into a cagelike structure" around hydrophobic compounds (e.g., see Figure 11–9). This seems paradoxical because water molecules do not interact with the hydrophobic compound. So how could they "know" about its presence and change their behavior to interact differently with one another? Discuss this argument and, in doing so, develop a clear concept of what is meant by a "cagelike" structure. How does it compare to ice? Why would this cagelike structure be energetically unfavorable?

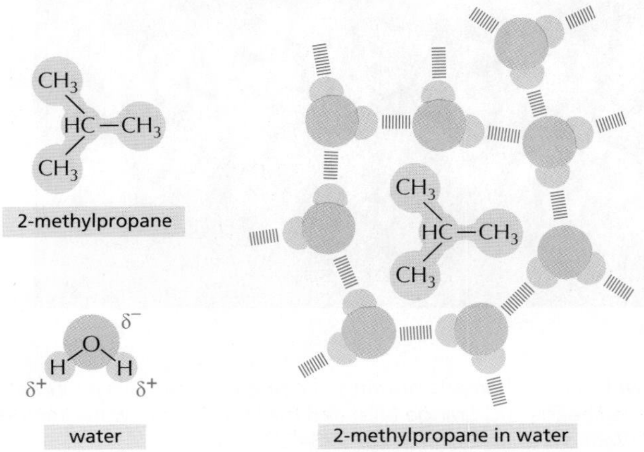

Figure 11–9 A hydrophobic molecule tends to avoid water. Because the 2-methylpropane molecule is entirely hydrophobic, it cannot form favorable interactions with water. This causes the adjacent water molecules to reorganize into a cagelike structure around it, to maximize their hydrogen bonds with each other.

triacylglycerol

hydrocarbon tail

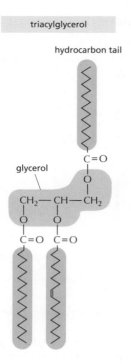

glycerol

Figure 11–10 Fat molecules are entirely hydrophobic. Unlike phospholipids, triacylglycerols, which are the main constituents of animal fats and plant oils, are entirely hydrophobic. Here, the third hydrophobic tail of the triacylglycerol molecule is drawn facing upward for comparison with the structure of a phospholipid (see Figure 11–6), although normally it is depicted facing down (see Panel 2–5, pp. 74–75).

Amphipathic molecules, such as membrane lipids (see Figure 11–7), are subject to two conflicting forces: the hydrophilic head is attracted to water, while the hydrophobic tails shun water and seek to aggregate with other hydrophobic molecules. This conflict is beautifully resolved by the formation of a lipid bilayer—an arrangement that satisfies all parties and is energetically most favorable. The hydrophilic heads face water on both surfaces of the bilayer, while the hydrophobic tails are shielded from the water within the bilayer interior, like the filling in a sandwich (Figure 11–11).

The same forces that drive the amphipathic molecules to form a bilayer help to make the bilayer self-sealing. Any tear in the sheet will create a free edge that is exposed to water. Because this situation is energetically unfavorable, the molecules of the bilayer will spontaneously rearrange to eliminate the free edge. If the tear is small, this spontaneous re-arrangement will exclude the water molecules and lead to repair of the bilayer, restoring a single continuous sheet. If the tear is large, the sheet may begin to fold in on itself and break up into separate closed vesicles. In either case, the overriding principle is that free edges are quickly eliminated.

The prohibition on free edges has a profound consequence: the only way an amphipathic sheet can avoid having free edges is to bend and seal, forming a boundary around a closed space (Figure 11–12). Therefore, amphipathic molecules such as phospholipids necessarily assemble into self-sealing containers that define closed compartments—from vesicles and organelles to entire cells. This remarkable behavior, fundamental to the creation of a living cell, is essentially a by-product of the nature of membrane lipids: hydrophilic at one end and hydrophobic at the other.

The Lipid Bilayer Is a Flexible Two-dimensional Fluid

The aqueous environment inside and outside a cell prevents membrane lipids from escaping from the bilayer, but nothing stops these molecules from moving about and changing places with one another within the plane of the membrane. The lipid bilayer therefore behaves as a two-dimensional fluid, a fact that is crucial for membrane function and integrity (Movie 11.1; "laser tweezers" are explained in Movie 11.2).

At the same time, the lipid bilayer is also flexible—that is, it is able to bend. Like fluidity, flexibility is important for membrane function, and it

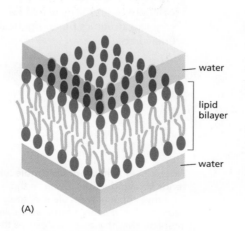

(A)

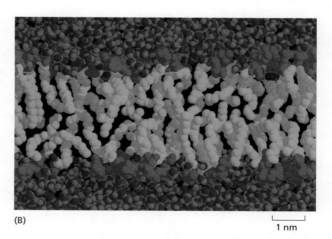

(B)

1 nm

Figure 11–11 Amphipathic phospholipids form a bilayer in water. (A) Schematic drawing of a phospholipid bilayer in water. (B) Computer simulation showing the phospholipid molecules (*red* heads and *orange* tails) and the surrounding water molecules (*blue*) in a cross section of a lipid bilayer. (B, adapted from R.M. Venable et al., *Science* 262:223–228, 1993.)

sets a lower limit of about 25 nm to the vesicle diameter that cell membranes can form.

The fluidity of lipid bilayers can be studied using synthetic lipid bilayers, which are easily produced by the spontaneous aggregation of amphipathic lipid molecules in water. Pure phospholipids, for example, will form closed, spherical vesicles, called *liposomes*, when added to water; these vesicles vary in size from about 25 nm to 1 mm in diameter (Figure 11–13).

Using such simple synthetic bilayers, investigators can measure the movements of the lipid molecules in a lipid bilayer. These measurements reveal that some types of movement are rare, while others are frequent and rapid. Thus, in synthetic lipid bilayers, phospholipid molecules very rarely tumble from one half of the bilayer, or monolayer, to the other. Without proteins to facilitate the process, it is estimated that this event, called "flip-flop," occurs less than once a month for any individual lipid molecule under conditions similar to those in a cell. On the other hand, as the result of random thermal motions, lipid molecules continuously exchange places with their neighbors within the same monolayer. This exchange leads to rapid lateral diffusion of lipid molecules within the plane of each monolayer, so that, for example, a lipid in an artificial bilayer may diffuse a length equal to that of an entire bacterial cell (~2 μm) in about one second.

Similar studies show that individual lipid molecules not only flex their hydrocarbon tails, but they also rotate rapidly about their long axis—some reaching speeds of 500 revolutions per second. Studies of whole cells—and of isolated cell membranes—indicate that lipid molecules in cell membranes undergo the same movements as they do in synthetic bilayers. The movements of membrane phospholipid molecules are summarized in Figure 11–14.

The Fluidity of a Lipid Bilayer Depends on Its Composition

The fluidity of a cell membrane—the ease with which its lipid molecules move within the plane of the bilayer—is important for membrane function and has to be maintained within certain limits. Just how fluid a lipid bilayer is at a given temperature depends on its phospholipid composition and, in particular, on the nature of the hydrocarbon tails: the closer and more regular the packing of the tails, the more viscous and less fluid the bilayer will be.

Two major properties of hydrocarbon tails affect how tightly they pack in the bilayer: their length and the number of double bonds they contain. A shorter chain length reduces the tendency of the hydrocarbon tails to interact with one another and therefore increases the fluidity of the bilayer. The hydrocarbon tails of membrane phospholipids vary in length between 14 and 24 carbon atoms, with 18 or 20 atoms being the most common. For most phospholipids, one of these hydrocarbon tails contains only single bonds between its adjacent carbon atoms, whereas the other tail includes one or more double bonds (see Figure 11–6). The chain that harbors a double bond does not contain the maximum number of hydrogen atoms that could, in principle, be attached to its carbon backbone; it is thus said to be **unsaturated** with respect to hydrogen. The

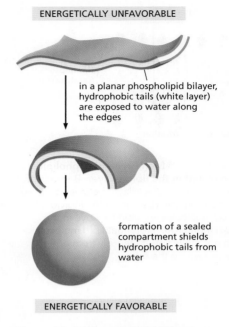

in a planar phospholipid bilayer, hydrophobic tails (white layer) are exposed to water along the edges

formation of a sealed compartment shields hydrophobic tails from water

ENERGETICALLY FAVORABLE

Figure 11–12 **Phospholipid bilayers spontaneously close in on themselves to form sealed compartments.** The closed structure is stable because it avoids the exposure of the hydrophobic hydrocarbon tails to water, which would be energetically unfavorable.

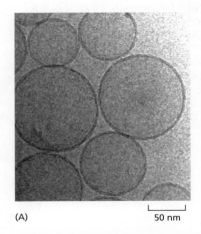

(A)   50 nm

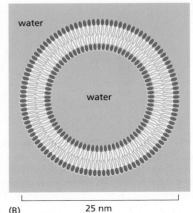

water

water

(B)   25 nm

Figure 11–13 **Pure phospholipids can form closed, spherical liposomes.** (A) An electron micrograph of phospholipid vesicles, or liposomes. (B) A drawing of a small, spherical liposome seen in cross section. (A, courtesy of Jean Lepault.)

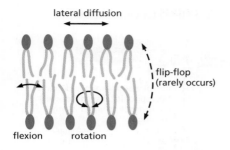

Figure 11–14 Membrane phospholipids move within the lipid bilayer. Because of these motions, the bilayer behaves as a two-dimensional fluid, in which the individual lipid molecules are able to move in their own monolayer. Note that lipid molecules do not move spontaneously from one monolayer to the other.

QUESTION 11–2

Five students in your class always sit together in the front row. This could be because (A) they really like each other or (B) nobody else in your class wants to sit next to them. Which explanation holds for the assembly of a lipid bilayer? Explain. Suppose, instead, that the other explanation held for lipid molecules. How would the properties of the lipid bilayer be different?

hydrocarbon tail with no double bonds has a full complement of hydrogen atoms and is said to be **saturated**. Each double bond in an unsaturated tail creates a small kink in the tail (see Figure 11–6), which makes it more difficult for the tails to pack against one another. For this reason, lipid bilayers that contain a large proportion of unsaturated hydrocarbon tails are more fluid than those with lower proportions.

In bacterial and yeast cells, which have to adapt to varying temperatures, both the lengths and the degree of saturation of the hydrocarbon tails in the bilayer are adjusted constantly to maintain a membrane with a relatively consistent fluidity: at higher temperatures, for example, the cell makes membrane lipids with tails that are longer and that contain fewer double bonds. A similar trick is used in the manufacture of margarine from vegetable oils. The fats produced by plants are generally unsaturated and therefore liquid at room temperature, unlike animal fats such as butter or lard, which are generally saturated and therefore solid at room temperature. To produce margarine, vegetable oils are "hydrogenated": this addition of hydrogen removes their double bonds, making the oils more solid and butterlike at room temperature.

In animal cells, membrane fluidity is modulated by the inclusion of the sterol **cholesterol**. This molecule is present in especially large amounts in the plasma membrane, where it constitutes approximately 20% of the lipids in the membrane by weight. With its short and rigid steroid ring structure, cholesterol can fill the spaces between neighboring phospholipid molecules left by the kinks in their unsaturated hydrocarbon tails (**Figure 11–15**). In this way, cholesterol tends to stiffen the bilayer, making it less flexible, as well as less permeable. The chemical properties of membrane lipids—and how they affect membrane fluidity—are reviewed in Movie 11.3 and Movie 11.4.

For all cells, membrane fluidity is important for a number of reasons. It enables many membrane proteins to diffuse rapidly in the plane of the bilayer and to interact with one another, as is crucial, for example, in cell signaling (discussed in Chapter 16). It permits membrane lipids and proteins to diffuse from sites where they are inserted into the bilayer after their synthesis to other regions of the cell. It ensures that membrane molecules are distributed evenly between daughter cells when a cell divides. And, under appropriate conditions, it allows membranes to fuse with one another and mix their molecules (discussed in Chapter 15). If biological

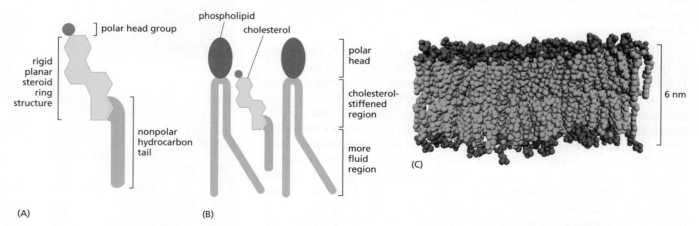

Figure 11–15 Cholesterol tends to stiffen cell membranes. (A) The shape of a cholesterol molecule. The chemical formula of cholesterol is shown in Figure 11–7. (B) How cholesterol fits into the gaps between phospholipid molecules in a lipid bilayer. (C) Space-filling model of the bilayer, with cholesterol molecules in *green*. Although the nonpolar hydrocarbon tail of cholesterol is shown in *green*—to visually distinguish it from the hydrocarbon tails of the membrane phospholipids—in reality, the hydrophobic tail of cholesterol is chemically equivalent to the hydrophobic tails of the phospholipids. (C, from H.L. Scott, *Curr. Opin. Struct. Biol.* 12:495–502, 2002.)

Figure 11–16 Newly synthesized phospholipids are added to the cytosolic side of the ER membrane and then redistributed by transporters that transfer them from one half of the lipid bilayer to the other. Biosynthetic enzymes bound to the cytosolic monolayer of the ER membrane (not shown) produce new phospholipids from free fatty acids and insert them into the cytosolic monolayer. Transporters called scramblases then randomly transfer phospholipid molecules from one monolayer to the other, allowing the membrane to grow as a bilayer in which the two leaflets even out continuously in size and lipid composition.

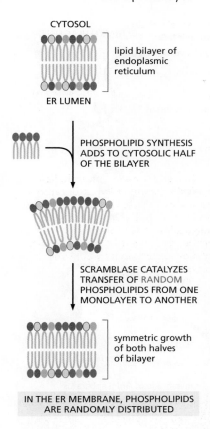

membranes were not fluid, it is hard to imagine how cells could live, grow, and reproduce.

Membrane Assembly Begins in the ER

In eukaryotic cells, new phospholipids are manufactured by enzymes bound to the cytosolic surface of the *endoplasmic reticulum* (*ER*). Using free fatty acids as substrates (see Panel 2–5, pp. 74–75), these enzymes deposit the newly made phospholipids exclusively in the cytosolic half of the bilayer.

Despite the unbalanced addition of newly made phospholipids, cell membranes manage to grow evenly. So how do new phospholipids make it to the opposite monolayer? As we saw in Figure 11–14, flip-flops that move lipids from one monolayer to the other rarely occur spontaneously. Instead, phospholipid transfers are catalyzed by a *scramblase*, a type of transporter protein that removes randomly selected phospholipids from one half of the lipid bilayer and inserts them in the other. (Transporters and their functions are discussed in detail in Chapter 12.) As a result of this scrambling, newly made phospholipids are redistributed equally between each monolayer of the ER membrane (**Figure 11–16**).

Some of this newly assembled membrane will remain in the ER; the rest will be used to supply fresh membrane to other compartments in the cell, including the Golgi apparatus and plasma membrane (see Figure 11–3). We discuss this dynamic process—in which membranes bud from one organelle and fuse with another—in detail in Chapter 15.

Certain Phospholipids Are Confined to One Side of the Membrane

Most cell membranes are asymmetric: the two halves of the bilayer often include strikingly different sets of phospholipids. But if membranes emerge from the ER with an evenly assorted set of phospholipids, where does this asymmetry arise? It begins in the Golgi apparatus.

The Golgi membrane contains another family of phospholipid-handling transporters, called *flippases*. Unlike scramblases, which move random phospholipids from one half of the bilayer to the other, flippases remove specific phospholipids from the side of the bilayer facing the exterior space and flip them into the monolayer that faces the cytosol (**Figure 11–17**).

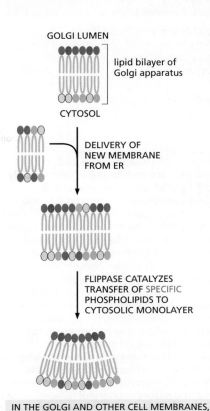

Figure 11–17 Flippases help to establish and maintain the asymmetric distribution of phospholipids characteristic of animal cell membranes. When membranes leave the ER and are incorporated in the Golgi, they encounter a different set of transporters called flippases, which selectively remove phosphatidylserine (*light green*) and phosphatidylethanolamine (*yellow*) from the noncytosolic monolayer and flip them to the cytosolic side. This transfer leaves phosphatidylcholine (*red*) and sphingomyelin (*brown*) concentrated in the noncytosolic monolayer. The resulting curvature of the membrane may help drive subsequent vesicle budding.

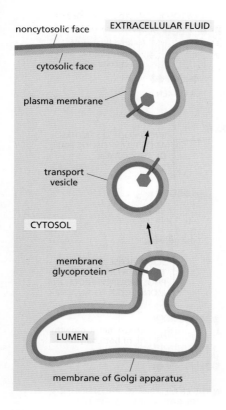

noncytosolic face

EXTRACELLULAR FLUID

cytosolic face

plasma membrane

transport vesicle

CYTOSOL

membrane glycoprotein

LUMEN

membrane of Golgi apparatus

QUESTION 11–3

It seems paradoxical that a lipid bilayer can be fluid yet asymmetrical. Explain.

Figure 11–19 Phospholipids and glycolipids are distributed asymmetrically in the lipid bilayer of an animal cell plasma membrane. Phosphatidylcholine (*red*) and sphingomyelin (*brown*) are concentrated in the noncytosolic monolayer, whereas phosphatidylserine (*light green*) and phosphatidylethanolamine (*yellow*) are found mainly on the cytosolic side. In addition to these phospholipids, phosphatidylinositols (*dark green* head group), a minor constituent of the plasma membrane, are shown in the cytosolic monolayer, where they participate in cell signaling. Glycolipids are drawn with hexagonal *blue* head groups to represent sugars; these are found exclusively in the noncytosolic monolayer of the membrane. Within the bilayer, cholesterol (*green*) is distributed almost equally in both monolayers.

Figure 11–18 Membranes retain their orientation during transfer between cell compartments. Membranes are transported by a process of vesicle budding and fusing. Here, a vesicle is shown budding from the Golgi apparatus and fusing with the plasma membrane. Note that the orientations of both the membrane lipids and proteins are preserved during the process: the original cytosolic surface of the lipid bilayer (*pink*) remains facing the cytosol, and the noncytosolic surface (*red*) continues to face away from the cytosol, toward the lumen of the Golgi and the transport vesicle—or toward the extracellular fluid. Similarly, the glycoprotein shown here (*blue* and *green*) remains in the same orientation, with its attached sugar facing the noncytosolic side.

The action of these flippases—and of similar transporters in the plasma membrane—initiates and maintains the asymmetric arrangement of phospholipids that is characteristic of the membranes of animal cells. This asymmetry is preserved as membranes bud from one organelle and fuse with another—or with the plasma membrane. This means that all cell membranes have distinct "inside" and "outside" faces: the cytosolic monolayer always faces the cytosol, while the noncytosolic monolayer is exposed to either the cell exterior—in the case of the plasma membrane—or the interior space (*lumen*) of an organelle. This conservation of orientation applies not only to the phospholipids that make up the membrane, but also to any proteins that might be inserted in the membrane (**Figure 11–18**). This positioning is very important, as a protein's orientation within the lipid bilayer is crucial for its function (see Figure 11–20).

Among lipids, those that show the most dramatically lopsided distribution in cell membranes are the glycolipids, which are located mainly in the plasma membrane, and only in the noncytosolic half of the bilayer (**Figure 11–19**). The sugar groups of these membrane lipids face the cell exterior, where they form part of a continuous coat of carbohydrate that surrounds and protects animal cells. Glycolipid molecules acquire their sugar groups in the Golgi apparatus, where the enzymes that engineer this chemical modification are confined. These enzymes are oriented such that sugars are added only to lipid molecules in the noncytosolic half of the bilayer. Once a glycolipid molecule has been created in this way, it remains trapped in this monolayer, as there are no flippases that transfer glycolipids to the cytosolic side. Thus, when a glycolipid molecule is finally delivered to the plasma membrane, it displays its sugars to the exterior of the cell.

Other lipid molecules show different types of asymmetric distributions, which relate to their specific functions. For example, the inositol phospholipids—a minor component of the plasma membrane—have a special role in relaying signals from the cell surface into the cell interior (discussed in Chapter 16); thus they are concentrated in the cytosolic half of the lipid bilayer.

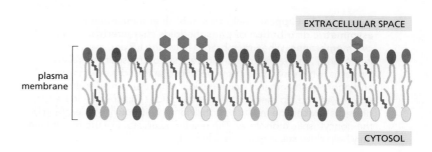

EXTRACELLULAR SPACE

plasma membrane

CYTOSOL

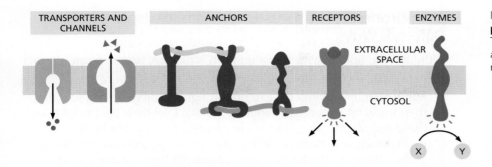

MEMBRANE PROTEINS

Although the lipid bilayer provides the basic structure of all cell membranes and serves as a permeability barrier to the hydrophilic molecules on either side of it, most membrane functions are carried out by **membrane proteins**. In animals, proteins constitute about 50% of the mass of most plasma membranes, the remainder being lipid plus the relatively small amounts of carbohydrate found on some of the lipids (glycolipids) and many of the proteins (glycoproteins). Because lipid molecules are much smaller than proteins, however, a cell membrane typically contains about 50 times the number of lipid molecules compared to protein molecules (see Figure 11–4B).

Membrane proteins serve many functions. Some transport particular nutrients, metabolites, and ions across the lipid bilayer. Others anchor the membrane to macromolecules on either side. Still others function as receptors that detect chemical signals in the cell's environment and relay them into the cell interior, or work as enzymes to catalyze specific reactions at the membrane (**Figure 11–20** and **Table 11–1**). Each type of cell membrane contains a different set of proteins, reflecting the specialized functions of the particular membrane. In this section, we discuss the structure of membrane proteins and how they associate with the lipid bilayer.

TABLE 11–1 SOME EXAMPLES OF PLASMA MEMBRANE PROTEINS AND THEIR FUNCTIONS		
Functional Class	**Protein Example**	**Specific Function**
Transporters	Na$^+$ pump	actively pumps Na$^+$ out of cells and K$^+$ in (discussed in Chapter 12)
Ion channels	K$^+$ leak channel	allows K$^+$ ions to leave cells, thereby influencing cell excitability (discussed in Chapter 12)
Anchors	integrins	link intracellular actin filaments to extracellular matrix proteins (discussed in Chapter 20)
Receptors	platelet-derived growth factor (PDGF) receptor	binds extracellular PDGF and, as a consequence, generates intracellular signals that direct the cell to grow and divide (discussed in Chapters 16 and 18)
Enzymes	adenylyl cyclase	catalyzes the production of the small intracellular signaling molecule cyclic AMP in response to extracellular signals (discussed in Chapter 16)

Membrane Proteins Associate with the Lipid Bilayer in Different Ways

Although the lipid bilayer has a uniform structure, proteins can interact with a cell membrane in a number of different ways.

- Many membrane proteins extend through the bilayer, with part of their mass on either side (**Figure 11–21A**). Like their lipid neighbors, these *transmembrane proteins* are amphipathic, having both hydrophobic and hydrophilic regions. Their hydrophobic regions lie in the interior of the bilayer, nestled against the hydrophobic tails of the lipid molecules. Their hydrophilic regions are exposed to the aqueous environment on either side of the membrane.

- Other membrane proteins are located almost entirely in the cytosol and are associated with the cytosolic half of the lipid bilayer by an amphipathic α helix exposed on the surface of the protein (**Figure 11–21B**).

- Some proteins lie entirely outside the bilayer, on one side or the other, attached to the membrane by one or more covalently attached lipid groups (**Figure 11–21C**).

- Yet other proteins are bound indirectly to one face of the membrane or the other, held in place only by their interactions with other membrane proteins (**Figure 11–21D**).

Proteins that are directly attached to the lipid bilayer—whether they are transmembrane, associated with the lipid monolayer, or lipid-linked—can be removed only by disrupting the bilayer with detergents, as discussed shortly. Such proteins are known as *integral membrane proteins*. The remaining membrane proteins are classified as *peripheral membrane proteins*; they can be released from the membrane by more gentle extraction procedures that interfere with protein–protein interactions but leave the lipid bilayer intact.

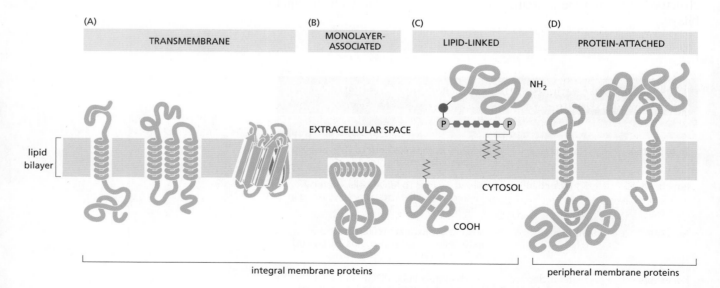

Figure 11–21 Membrane proteins can associate with the lipid bilayer in different ways. (A) Transmembrane proteins can extend across the bilayer as a single α helix, as multiple α helices, or as a rolled-up β sheet (called a β barrel). (B) Some membrane proteins are anchored to the cytosolic half of the lipid bilayer by an amphipathic α helix. (C) Others are linked to either side of the bilayer solely by a covalently attached lipid molecule (*red* zigzag lines). (D) Many proteins are attached to the membrane only by relatively weak, noncovalent interactions with other membrane proteins. (A–C) are examples of integral membrane proteins; the proteins shown in (D) are considered peripheral membrane proteins.

A Polypeptide Chain Usually Crosses the Lipid Bilayer as an α Helix

All membrane proteins have a unique orientation in the lipid bilayer, which is essential for their function. For a transmembrane receptor protein, for example, the part of the protein that receives a signal from the environment must be on the outside of the cell, whereas the part that passes along the signal must be in the cytosol (see Figure 11–20). This orientation is a consequence of the way in which membrane proteins are synthesized (discussed in Chapter 15). The portions of a transmembrane protein located on either side of the lipid bilayer are connected by specialized membrane-spanning segments of the polypeptide chain (see Figure 11–21A). These segments, which run through the hydrophobic environment of the interior of the lipid bilayer, are composed largely of amino acids with hydrophobic side chains. Because these side chains cannot form favorable interactions with water molecules, they prefer to interact with the hydrophobic tails of the lipid molecules, where no water is present.

In contrast to the hydrophobic side chains, however, the peptide bonds that join the successive amino acids in a protein are normally polar, making the polypeptide backbone itself hydrophilic (**Figure 11–22**). Because water is absent from the interior of the bilayer, atoms that are part of the polypeptide backbone are thus driven to form hydrogen bonds with one another. Hydrogen-bonding is maximized if the polypeptide chain forms a regular α helix, and so the great majority of the membrane-spanning segments of polypeptide chains traverse the bilayer as α helices (see Figure 4–12). In these membrane-spanning α helices, the hydrophobic side chains are exposed on the outside of the helix, where they contact the hydrophobic lipid tails, while the atoms of the hydrophilic polypeptide backbone form hydrogen bonds with one another within the helix (**Figure 11–23**).

For many transmembrane proteins, the polypeptide chain crosses the membrane only once (see Figure 11–21A, *left*). Many of these *single-pass* transmembrane proteins are receptors for extracellular signals. Other transmembrane proteins function as channels, forming aqueous pores across the lipid bilayer to allow small, water-soluble molecules to cross the membrane. Such channels cannot be formed by proteins with a single transmembrane α helix. Instead, they usually consist of a series of α helices that cross the bilayer a number of times (see Figure 11–21A, *center*). For many of these *multipass* transmembrane proteins, one or more of the membrane-spanning regions are amphipathic—formed from α helices that contain both hydrophobic and hydrophilic amino acid side chains. These amino acids tend to be arranged so that the hydrophobic side chains fall on one side of the helix, while the hydrophilic side chains are concentrated on the other side. In the hydrophobic environment of the lipid bilayer, α helices of this type pack side by side in a ring, with the hydrophobic side chains exposed to the hydrophobic lipid tails and the hydrophilic side chains forming the lining of a hydrophilic pore

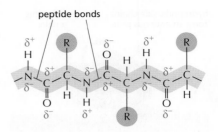

Figure 11–22 The backbone of a polypeptide chain is hydrophilic. The atoms on either side of a peptide bond (*red line*) are polar and carry partial positive or negative charges (δ^+ or δ^-). These charges allow these atoms to hydrogen-bond with one another when the polypeptide folds into an α helix that spans the lipid bilayer (see Figure 11–23).

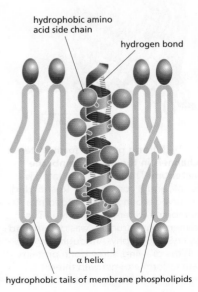

Figure 11–23 A transmembrane polypeptide chain usually crosses the lipid bilayer as an α helix. In this segment of a transmembrane protein, the hydrophobic side chains (*light green*) of the amino acids forming the α helix contact the hydrophobic hydrocarbon tails of the phospholipid molecules, while the hydrophilic parts of the polypeptide backbone form hydrogen bonds with one another (dashed *red* lines) along the interior of the helix. An α helix containing about 20 amino acids is required to completely traverse a cell membrane.

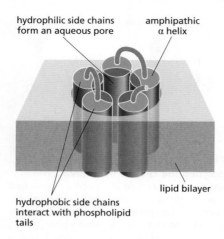

hydrophilic side chains
form an aqueous pore

amphipathic
α helix

hydrophobic side chains
interact with phospholipid
tails

lipid bilayer

Figure 11–24 A transmembrane hydrophilic pore can be formed by multiple amphipathic α helices. In this example, five amphipathic transmembrane α helices form a water-filled channel across the lipid bilayer. The hydrophobic amino acid side chains on one side of each helix (*green*) come in contact with the hydrophobic lipid tails of the lipid bilayer, while the hydrophilic side chains on the opposite side of the helices (*red*) form a water-filled pore.

through the membrane (**Figure 11–24**). How such channels function in the selective transport of small, water-soluble molecules, especially inorganic ions, is discussed in Chapter 12.

Although the α helix is by far the most common form in which a polypeptide chain crosses a lipid bilayer, the polypeptide chain of some transmembrane proteins crosses the lipid bilayer as a β sheet that is rolled into a cylinder, forming a keglike structure called a β barrel (see Figure 11–21A, *right*). As expected, the amino acid side chains that face the inside of the barrel, and therefore line the aqueous channel, are mostly hydrophilic, while those on the outside of the barrel, which contact the hydrophobic core of the lipid bilayer, are exclusively hydrophobic. A striking example of a β-barrel structure is found in the *porin* proteins, which form large, water-filled pores in mitochondrial and bacterial outer membranes (**Figure 11–25**). Mitochondria and some bacteria are surrounded by a double membrane, and porins allow the passage of small nutrients, metabolites, and inorganic ions across their outer membranes, while preventing unwanted larger molecules from crossing.

Membrane Proteins Can Be Solubilized in Detergents

To understand a protein fully, one needs to know its structure in detail. For membrane proteins, this presents special problems. Most biochemical procedures are designed for studying molecules in aqueous solution. Membrane proteins, however, are built to operate in an environment that is partly aqueous and partly fatty, and taking them out of this environment to study in isolation—while preserving their essential structure—is no easy task.

Before an individual protein can be examined in detail, it must be separated from all the other cell proteins. For most membrane proteins, the first step in this purification process involves solubilizing the membrane with agents that destroy the lipid bilayer by disrupting hydrophobic associations. The most widely used disruptive agents are **detergents** (Movie 11.5). These small, amphipathic, lipidlike molecules differ from membrane phospholipids in that they have only a single hydrophobic tail (**Figure 11–26**). Because they have one tail, detergent molecules are shaped like cones; in water, these conical molecules tend to aggregate into small clusters called *micelles*, rather than forming a bilayer as do the phospholipids, which—with their two tails—are more cylindrical in shape.

When mixed in great excess with membranes, the hydrophobic ends of detergent molecules interact with the membrane-spanning hydrophobic regions of the transmembrane proteins, as well as with the hydrophobic tails of the phospholipid molecules, thereby disrupting the lipid bilayer and separating the proteins from most of the phospholipids. Because the other end of the detergent molecule is hydrophilic, these interactions draw the membrane proteins into the aqueous solution as protein–detergent complexes; at the same time, the detergent

QUESTION 11–4

Explain why the polypeptide chain of most transmembrane proteins crosses the lipid bilayer as an α helix or a β barrel.

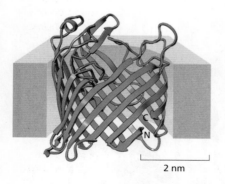

2 nm

Figure 11–25 Porin proteins form water-filled channels in the outer membrane of a bacterium. The protein illustrated is from *E. coli*, and it consists of a 16-stranded β sheet curved around on itself to form a transmembrane water-filled channel. The three-dimensional structure was determined by x-ray crystallography. Although not shown in the drawing, three porin proteins associate to form a trimer with three separate channels.

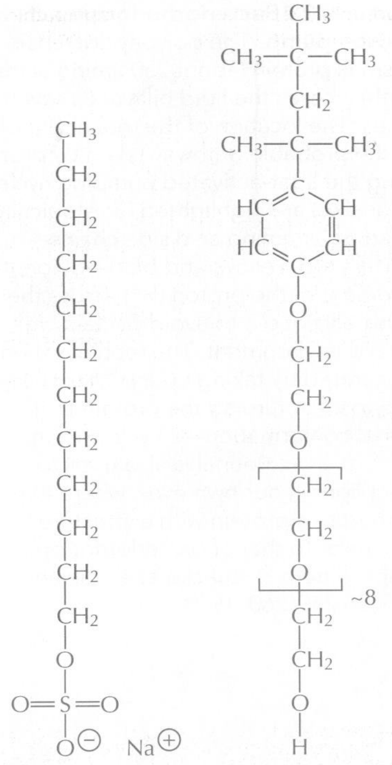

Figure 11–26 **SDS and Triton X-100 are two commonly used detergents.** Sodium dodecyl sulfate (SDS) is a strong ionic detergent—that is, it has an ionized (charged) group at its hydrophilic end (*blue*). Triton X-100 is a mild nonionic detergent—that is, it has a nonionized but polar structure at its hydrophilic end (*blue*). The hydrophobic portion of each detergent is shown in *red*. The bracketed portion of Triton X-100 is repeated about eight times. Strong ionic detergents like SDS not only displace lipid molecules from proteins but also unfold the proteins (see Panel 4–5, p. 167).

also solubilizes the phospholipids (**Figure 11–27**). The protein–detergent complexes can then be separated from one another and from the lipid–detergent complexes for further analysis.

We Know the Complete Structure of Relatively Few Membrane Proteins

For many years, much of what we knew about the structure of membrane proteins was learned by indirect means. The standard method for determining a protein's three-dimensional structure directly has been x-ray crystallography, but this approach requires ordered crystalline arrays of the molecule. Because membrane proteins have to be purified in detergent micelles that are often heterogeneous in size, they are harder to crystallize than the soluble proteins that inhabit the cell cytosol or extracellular fluids. Nevertheless, with recent advances in x-ray crystallography, along with powerful new approaches such as cryoelectron microscopy, the structures of an increasing number of membrane proteins have now been determined to high resolution (see Panel 4–6, pp. 168–169).

One example is bacteriorhodopsin, the structure of which first revealed exactly how α helices cross the lipid bilayer. **Bacteriorhodopsin** is a small protein found in large amounts in the plasma membrane of *Halobacterium halobium*, an archaean that lives in salt marshes. Bacteriorhodopsin acts as a membrane transport protein that pumps H⁺ (protons) out of the cell. Each bacteriorhodopsin molecule contains a single chromophore, a light-absorbing, nonprotein molecule called *retinal*, that gives the protein—and

sodium dodecyl sulfate (SDS)   Triton X-100

QUESTION 11–5

For the two detergents shown in Figure 11–26, explain why the blue portions of the molecules are hydrophilic and the red portions hydrophobic. Draw a short stretch of a polypeptide chain made up of three amino acids with hydrophobic side chains (see Panel 2–6, pp. 76–77) and apply a similar color scheme. Indicate which portions of your polypeptide would form hydrogen bonds with water.

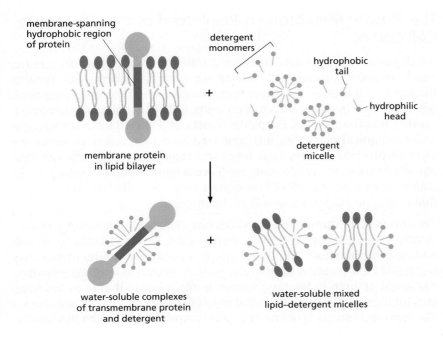

membrane-spanning hydrophobic region of protein

detergent monomers

hydrophobic tail

hydrophilic head

membrane protein in lipid bilayer

detergent micelle

water-soluble complexes of transmembrane protein and detergent

water-soluble mixed lipid–detergent micelles

Figure 11–27 **Membrane proteins can be solubilized by a mild detergent such as Triton X-100.** The detergent molecules (*gold*) are shown as both monomers and micelles, the form in which these molecules tend to aggregate in water. The detergent disrupts the lipid bilayer and interacts with the membrane-spanning hydrophobic portion of the protein (*dark green*). These actions bring the proteins into solution as protein–detergent complexes. As illustrated, the phospholipids in the membrane are also solubilized by the detergents, forming lipid–detergent micelles.

Figure 11–28 Bacteriorhodopsin acts as a proton pump. The polypeptide chain of this small protein (about 250 amino acids in length) crosses the lipid bilayer as seven α helices. The location of the retinal (*purple*) and the probable pathway taken by protons during the light-activated pumping cycle (*red arrows*) are highlighted. Strategically placed polar amino acid side chains—shown in *red*, *yellow*, and *blue*—guide the movement of the proton (H⁺) across the bilayer, allowing it to avoid contact with the lipid environment. The retinal is then regenerated by taking up a H⁺ from the cytosol, returning the protein to its original conformation—a cycle shown in Movie 11.6. Retinal is also used to detect light in our own eyes, where it is attached to a protein with a structure very similar to that of bacteriorhodopsin. (Adapted from H. Luecke et al., *Science* 286:5438 255–260, 1999.)

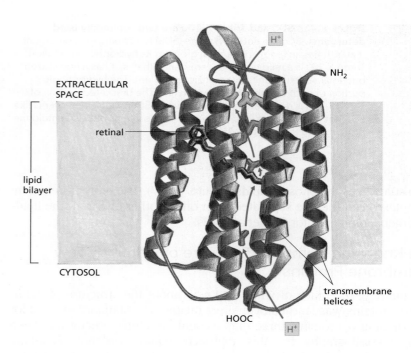

the entire organism—a deep purple color. When retinal, which is covalently attached to one of bacteriorhodopsin's transmembrane α helices, absorbs a photon of light, it changes shape. This shape change causes the surrounding helices to undergo a series of small conformational changes, which pump one proton from the retinal to the outside of the organism (Figure 11–28).

In the presence of sunlight, thousands of bacteriorhodopsin molecules pump H⁺ out of the cell, generating a concentration gradient of H⁺ across the plasma membrane. The cell uses this proton gradient to store energy and convert it into ATP, as we discuss in detail in Chapter 14. Bacteriorhodopsin is a *pump*, a class of transmembrane protein that actively moves small organic molecules and inorganic ions into and out of cells. We will discuss the action of other important transmembrane pumps in Chapter 12.

The Plasma Membrane Is Reinforced by the Underlying Cell Cortex

A cell membrane by itself is extremely thin and fragile. It would require nearly 10,000 cell membranes laid on top of one another to achieve the thickness of this paper. Most cell membranes are therefore strengthened and supported by a framework of proteins, attached to the membrane via transmembrane proteins. For plants, yeasts, and bacteria, the cell's shape and mechanical properties are conferred by a rigid *cell wall*—a fibrous layer of proteins, sugars, and other macromolecules that encases the plasma membrane. By contrast, the plasma membrane of animal cells is stabilized by a meshwork of filamentous proteins, called the **cell cortex**, that is attached to the underside of the membrane.

The cortex of the human red blood cell has a relatively simple and regular structure and has been especially well studied. Red blood cells are small and have a distinctive flattened shape (Figure 11–29A). The main component of their cortex is the dimeric protein *spectrin*, a long, thin, flexible rod about 100 nm in length. Spectrin forms a lattice that provides support for the plasma membrane and maintains the cell's biconcave shape. The spectrin network is connected to the membrane through intracellular

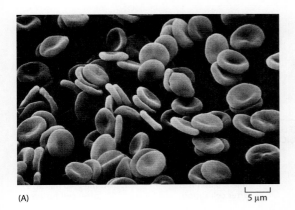

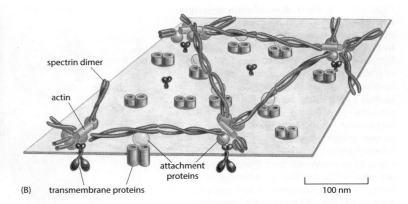

(A)   5 µm

(B)   transmembrane proteins   100 nm

spectrin dimer

actin

attachment proteins

Figure 11–29 A cortex made largely of spectrin gives human red blood cells their characteristic shape. (A) Scanning electron micrograph showing human red blood cells, which have a flattened, biconcave shape. These cells lack a nucleus and other intracellular organelles. (B) In the cortex of a red blood cell, spectrin dimers (*red*) are linked end-to-end to form longer tetramers. The spectrin tetramers, together with a smaller number of actin molecules, are linked together into a mesh. This network is attached to the plasma membrane by the binding of at least two types of attachment proteins (shown here in *yellow* and *blue*) to two kinds of transmembrane proteins (shown here in *green* and *brown*). (A, courtesy of Bernadette Chailley.)

attachment proteins that link spectrin to specific transmembrane proteins (**Figure 11–29B** and Movie 11.7). The importance of this meshwork is seen in mice and humans that, due to genetic alterations, produce a form of spectrin with an abnormal structure. These individuals are anemic: they have fewer red blood cells than normal. The red cells they do have are spherical instead of flattened and are abnormally fragile.

Proteins similar to spectrin, and to its associated attachment proteins, are present in the cortex of most animal cells. But the cortex in these cells is especially rich in actin and the motor protein *myosin*, and it is much more complex than that of red blood cells. Whereas red blood cells need their cortex mainly to provide mechanical strength as they are pumped through blood vessels, other cells also use their cortex to selectively take up materials from their environment, to change their shape, and to move, as we discuss in Chapter 17. In addition, cells also use their cortex to restrain the diffusion of proteins within the plasma membrane, as we see next.

A Cell Can Restrict the Movement of Its Membrane Proteins

Because a membrane is a two-dimensional fluid, many of its proteins, like its lipids, can move freely within the plane of the bilayer. This lateral diffusion was initially demonstrated by experimentally fusing a mouse cell with a human cell to form a double-sized hybrid cell and then monitoring the distribution of certain mouse and human plasma membrane proteins. At first, the mouse and human proteins are confined to their own halves of the newly formed hybrid cell, but within half an hour or so the two sets of proteins become evenly mixed over the entire cell surface (**Figure 11–30**). We describe some other techniques for studying the movement of membrane proteins in How We Know, pp. 384–385.

The picture of a cell membrane as a sea of lipid in which all proteins float freely is too simple, however. Cells have ways of confining particular proteins to localized areas within the bilayer, thereby creating functionally specialized regions, or **membrane domains**, on the surface of the cell or organelle.

Figure 11–30 Formation of mouse–human hybrid cells shows that some plasma membrane proteins can move laterally in the lipid bilayer. When the mouse and human cells are first fused, their proteins are confined to their own halves of the newly formed hybrid-cell plasma membrane. Within a short time, however, the membrane proteins—and lipids—completely intermix. To monitor the movement of a selected sampling of the proteins, the cells are labeled with antibodies that bind to either human or mouse proteins; the antibodies are coupled to two different fluorescent tags—for example, rhodamine (*red*) and fluorescein (shown here in *blue*)—so they can be distinguished in a fluorescence microscope (see Panel 4–2, pp. 140–141). (Based on observations of L.D. Frye and M. Edidin, *J. Cell Sci.* 7:319–335, 1970.)

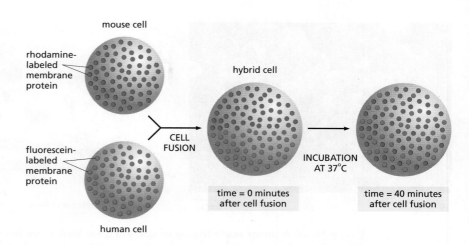

As illustrated in **Figure 11–31**, plasma membrane proteins can be tethered to structures outside the cell—for example, to molecules in the extracellular matrix or on an adjacent cell (discussed in Chapter 20)—or to relatively immobile structures inside the cell, especially to the cell cortex (see Figure 11–29B). Additionally, cells can create barriers that restrict particular membrane components to one membrane domain. In epithelial cells that line the gut, for example, it is important that transport proteins involved in the uptake of nutrients from the gut be confined to the *apical* surface of the cells (which faces the gut contents) and that other transport proteins—including those involved in the export of solutes out of the epithelial cell into the tissues and bloodstream—be confined to the *basal* and *lateral* surfaces (see Figure 12–17). This asymmetric distribution of membrane proteins is maintained by a barrier formed along the line where the cell is sealed to adjacent epithelial cells by a so-called *tight junction* (**Figure 11–32**). At this site, specialized junctional proteins form a continuous belt around the cell where the cell contacts its neighbors, creating a seal between adjacent plasma membranes (see Figure 20–22). Membrane proteins are unable to diffuse past the junction.

The Cell Surface Is Coated with Carbohydrate

We saw earlier that some of the lipids in the outer layer of the plasma membrane have sugars covalently attached to them. The same is true for most of the proteins in the plasma membrane. The great majority of these proteins have short chains of sugars, called *oligosaccharides*, linked to them; they are called *glycoproteins*. Other membrane proteins, the *proteoglycans*, contain one or more long polysaccharide chains. All of

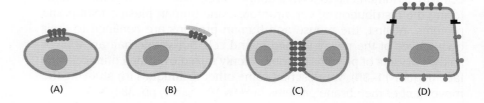

Figure 11–31 The lateral mobility of plasma membrane proteins can be restricted in several ways. Proteins can be tethered (A) to the cell cortex inside the cell, (B) to extracellular matrix molecules outside the cell, or (C) to proteins on the surface of another cell. (D) Diffusion barriers (shown as *black* bars) can restrict proteins to a particular membrane domain.

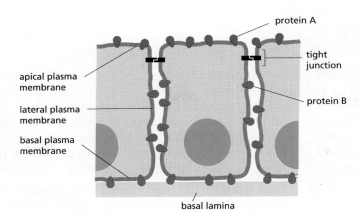

apical plasma membrane

lateral plasma membrane

basal plasma membrane

protein A

tight junction

protein B

basal lamina

Figure 11–32 Membrane proteins are restricted to particular domains of the plasma membrane of epithelial cells in the gut. Protein A (*green*) and protein B (*red*) can diffuse laterally in their own membrane domains but are prevented from entering the other domain by a specialized cell junction called a tight junction. The basal lamina (*yellow*) is a mat of extracellular matrix that supports all epithelial sheets (discussed in Chapter 20).

the carbohydrate on the glycoproteins, proteoglycans, and glycolipids is located on the outside of the plasma membrane, where it forms a sugar coating called the *carbohydrate layer* or **glycocalyx** (Figure 11–33).

This layer of carbohydrate helps protect the cell surface from mechanical damage. And because the oligosaccharides and polysaccharides attract water molecules, they also give the cell a slimy surface, which helps motile cells such as white blood cells squeeze through narrow spaces and prevents blood cells from sticking to one another or to the walls of blood vessels.

Cell-surface carbohydrates do more than just protect and lubricate the cell, however. They have an important role in cell–cell recognition and adhesion. Transmembrane proteins called *lectins* are specialized to bind to particular oligosaccharide side chains. The oligosaccharide side chains of glycoproteins and glycolipids, although short (typically fewer than 15 sugar units), are enormously diverse. Unlike proteins, in which the amino acids are all joined together in a linear chain by identical peptide bonds, sugars can be joined together in many different arrangements, often forming elaborate branched structures (see Panel 2–4, pp. 72–73). Using a variety of covalent linkages, even three different sugars can form hundreds of different trisaccharides.

The carbohydrate layer on the surface of cells in a multicellular organism serves as a kind of distinctive clothing, like a police officer's uniform. It is characteristic of each cell type and is recognized by other cell types that

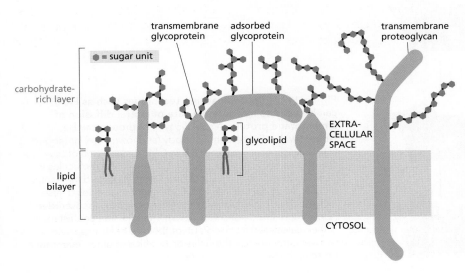

transmembrane glycoprotein

adsorbed glycoprotein

transmembrane proteoglycan

= sugar unit

carbohydrate-rich layer

glycolipid

EXTRA-CELLULAR SPACE

lipid bilayer

CYTOSOL

Figure 11–33 Eukaryotic cells are coated with sugars. This carbohydrate-rich layer is made of the oligosaccharide side chains attached to membrane glycolipids and glycoproteins, and of the polysaccharide chains on membrane proteoglycans. As shown, glycoproteins that have been secreted by the cell and then adsorbed back onto its surface can also contribute. Note that all the carbohydrate is on the external (noncytosolic) surface of the plasma membrane.

HOW WE KNOW

MEASURING MEMBRANE FLOW

An essential feature of the lipid bilayer is its fluidity, which is crucial for cell membrane integrity and function. This property allows many membrane-embedded proteins to move laterally in the plane of the bilayer, so that they can engage in the various protein–protein interactions on which cells depend. The fluid nature of cell membranes is so central to their proper function that it may seem surprising that this property was not recognized until the early 1970s.

Given its importance for membrane structure and function, how do we measure and study the fluidity of cell membranes? The most common methods are visual: simply label some of the molecules native to the membrane and then watch where they go. Such an approach first demonstrated the lateral movement of membrane proteins that had been tagged with labeled antibodies (see Figure 11–30). This experiment seemed to suggest that membrane proteins diffuse freely, without restriction, in an open sea of lipids. We now know that this image is not entirely accurate. To probe membrane fluidity more thoroughly, researchers had to invent more precise methods for tracking the movement of proteins within a membrane such as the plasma membrane of a living cell.

The FRAP attack

One such technique, called *fluorescence recovery after photobleaching* (*FRAP*), involves uniformly labeling the components of the cell membrane—its lipids or, more often, its proteins—with some sort of fluorescent marker. Labeling membrane proteins can be accomplished by incubating cells with a fluorescent antibody or by covalently attaching a fluorescent protein such as green fluorescent protein (GFP) to a membrane protein using the DNA techniques discussed in Chapter 10.

Once a protein has been labeled, a small patch of membrane is irradiated with an intense pulse of light from a sharply focused laser beam. This treatment irreversibly "bleaches" the fluorescence from the labeled proteins in that small patch of membrane, typically an area about 1 μm square. The fluorescence of this irradiated membrane is monitored in a fluorescence microscope, and the amount of time it takes for the neighboring, unbleached fluorescent proteins to migrate into the bleached region of the membrane is measured (**Figure 11–34**). The rate of this "fluorescence recovery" is a direct measure of the rate at which the protein molecules can diffuse within the membrane (Movie 11.8). Such experiments have revealed that, generally speaking, cell membranes are about as viscous as olive oil.

One-by-one

One drawback to the FRAP approach is that the technique monitors the movement of fairly large populations of proteins—hundreds or thousands—across a relatively large area of the membrane. With this technique

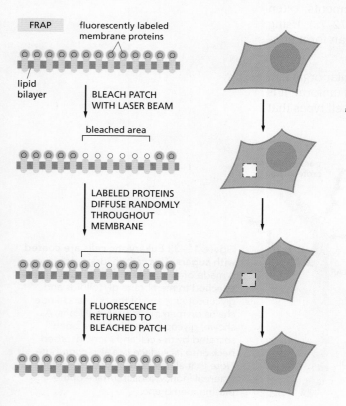

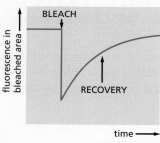

Figure 11–34 Photobleaching techniques such as FRAP can be used to measure the rate of lateral diffusion of a membrane protein. A specific type of protein can be labeled with a fluorescent antibody (as shown here) or tagged with a fluorescent protein, such as GFP. A small area of the membrane containing these fluorescent protein molecules is then bleached using a laser beam. As the bleached molecules diffuse away, and unbleached, fluorescent molecules diffuse into the area, the intensity of the fluorescence is recovered (shown here in side and top views). The diffusion coefficient is then calculated from a graph of the rate of fluorescence recovery: the greater the diffusion coefficient of the membrane protein, the faster the recovery.

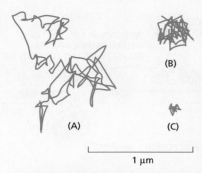

Figure 11–35 Proteins show different patterns of diffusion.
Single-particle tracking studies reveal some of the pathways that single proteins follow on the surface of a living cell. Shown here are some trajectories representative of different kinds of proteins in the plasma membrane. (A) Tracks made by a protein that is free to diffuse randomly in the lipid bilayer. (B) Tracks made by a protein that is corralled within a small membrane domain by other proteins. (C) Tracks made by a protein that is tethered to the cytoskeleton and hence is essentially immobile. The movement of the proteins is monitored over a period of seconds.

it is impossible to track the motion of individual molecules, which can make analysis of the results difficult. If the labeled proteins fail to migrate into the bleached zone over the course of a FRAP study, for example, is it because they are immobile, essentially anchored in one place in the membrane? Or, alternatively, are they restricted to movement within a very small region—fenced in by cytoskeletal proteins—and thus only appear motionless?

To get around this problem, researchers have developed methods for labeling and observing the movement of individual molecules or small clusters of molecules. One such technique, dubbed *single-particle tracking (SPT) microscopy*, relies on tagging protein molecules with antibody-coated gold nanoparticles. The gold particles look like tiny black dots when seen with a light microscope, and their movement, and thus the movement of individually tagged protein molecules, can be followed using video microscopy.

From the studies carried out to date, it appears that membrane proteins can display a variety of patterns of movement, from random diffusion to complete immobility (**Figure 11–35**). Some proteins rapidly switch between these different kinds of motion.

Freed from cells

In many cases, researchers wish to study the behavior of a particular type of membrane protein in a synthetic lipid bilayer, in the absence of other proteins that might restrain its movement or alter its activity. For such studies, membrane proteins can be isolated from cells and the protein of interest purified and reconstituted in artificial phospholipid vesicles (**Figure 11–36**). The lipids

allow the purified protein to maintain its proper structure and function, so that its activity and behavior can be analyzed in detail.

It is apparent from such studies that membrane proteins diffuse more freely and rapidly in artificial lipid bilayers than in cell membranes. The fact that most proteins show reduced mobility in a cell membrane makes sense, as these membranes are crowded with many types of proteins and contain a greater variety of lipids than an artificial lipid bilayer. Furthermore, many membrane proteins in a cell are tethered to proteins in the extracellular matrix, or anchored to the cell cortex just under the plasma membrane, or both (as illustrated in Figure 11–31).

Taken together, such studies have revolutionized our understanding of membrane proteins and of the architecture and organization of cell membranes.

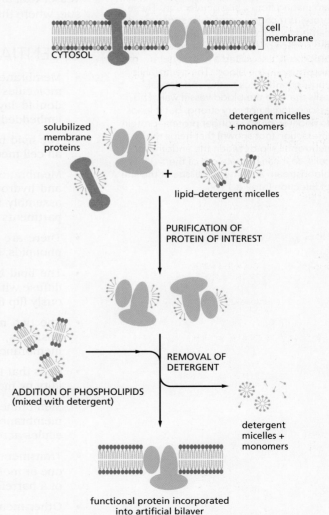

Figure 11–36 Mild detergents can be used to solubilize and reconstitute functional membrane proteins. Proteins incorporated into artificial lipid bilayers generally diffuse more freely and rapidly than they do in cell membranes.

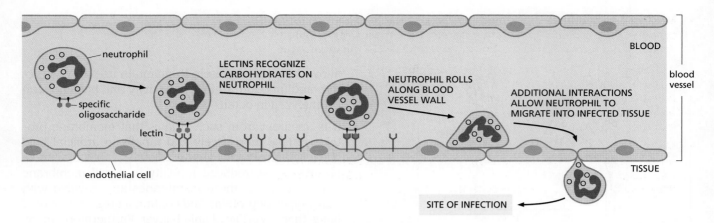

Figure 11–37 The recognition of cell-surface carbohydrates on neutrophils allows these immune cells to begin to migrate out of the blood and into infected tissues. Specialized transmembrane proteins (called lectins) are made by the endothelial cells lining the blood vessel in response to chemical signals emanating from a site of infection. These proteins recognize particular sugar groups carried by glycolipids and glycoproteins on the surface of neutrophils (a type of white blood cell, also called a leukocyte) circulating in the blood. The neutrophils consequently stick to the endothelial cells that line the blood vessel wall. This association is not very strong, but it leads to another, much stronger protein–protein interaction (not shown) that helps the neutrophil slip between the endothelial cells, so it can migrate out of the bloodstream and into the tissue at the site of infection (Movie 11.9).

interact with it. Specific oligosaccharides in the carbohydrate layer are involved, for example, in the recognition of an egg by sperm (discussed in Chapter 19). Similarly, in the early stages of a bacterial infection, carbohydrates on the surface of white blood cells called *neutrophils* are recognized by a lectin on the cells lining the blood vessels at the site of infection; this recognition causes the neutrophils to adhere to the blood vessel wall and then migrate from the bloodstream into the infected tissue, where they help destroy the invading bacteria (Figure 11–37).

ESSENTIAL CONCEPTS

- Membranes enable cells to create barriers that confine particular molecules to specific compartments. They consist of a continuous double layer—a bilayer—of lipid molecules in which proteins are embedded.

- The lipid bilayer provides the basic structure and barrier function of all cell membranes.

- Membrane lipid molecules are amphipathic, having both hydrophobic and hydrophilic regions. This property promotes their spontaneous assembly into bilayers when placed in water, forming closed compartments that reseal if torn.

- There are three major classes of membrane lipid molecules: phospholipids, sterols, and glycolipids.

- The lipid bilayer is fluid, and individual lipid molecules are able to diffuse within their own monolayer; they do not, however, spontaneously flip from one monolayer to the other.

- The two monolayers of a cell membrane have different lipid compositions, reflecting the different functions of the two faces of the membrane.

- Cells that live at different temperatures maintain their membrane fluidity by modifying the lipid composition of their membranes.

- Membrane proteins are responsible for most of the functions of cell membranes, including the transport of small, water-soluble molecules across the lipid bilayer.

- Transmembrane proteins extend across the lipid bilayer, usually as one or more α helices but sometimes as a β sheet rolled into the form of a barrel.

- Other membrane proteins do not extend across the lipid bilayer but are attached to one or the other side of the membrane, either by noncovalent association with other membrane proteins, by covalent attachment of lipids, or by association of an exposed amphipathic α helix with a single lipid monolayer.

- Most cell membranes are supported by an attached framework of proteins. An especially important example is the meshwork of fibrous proteins that forms the cell cortex underneath the plasma membrane.

- Although many membrane proteins can diffuse rapidly in the plane of the membrane, cells have ways of confining proteins to specific membrane domains. They can also immobilize particular membrane proteins by attaching them to intracellular or extracellular macromolecules.

- Many of the proteins and some of the lipids exposed on the surface of cells have attached sugar chains, which form a carbohydrate layer that helps protect and lubricate the cell surface, while also being involved in specific cell–cell recognition.

KEY TERMS

amphipathic	membrane domain
bacteriorhodopsin	membrane protein
cell cortex	phosphatidylcholine
cholesterol	phospholipid
detergent	plasma membrane
fat droplet	saturated
glycocalyx	unsaturated
lipid bilayer	

QUESTIONS

QUESTION 11–7

Describe the different methods that cells use to restrict proteins to specific regions of the plasma membrane. Can a membrane with many of its proteins restricted still be fluid?

QUESTION 11–8

Which of the following statements are correct? Explain your answers.

A. Lipids in a lipid bilayer spin rapidly around their long axis.

B. Lipids in a lipid bilayer rapidly exchange positions with one another in their own monolayer.

C. Lipids in a lipid bilayer do not flip-flop readily from one lipid monolayer to the other.

D. Hydrogen bonds that form between lipid head groups and water molecules are continually broken and re-formed.

E. Glycolipids move between different membrane-enclosed compartments during their synthesis but remain restricted to one side of the lipid bilayer.

F. Margarine contains more saturated lipids than the vegetable oil from which it is made.

G. Some membrane proteins are enzymes.

H. The sugar layer that surrounds all cells makes cells more slippery.

QUESTION 11–9

What is meant by the term "two-dimensional fluid"?

QUESTION 11–10

The structure of a lipid bilayer is determined by the particular properties of its lipid molecules. What would happen if:

A. phospholipids had only one hydrocarbon tail instead of two?

B. the hydrocarbon tails were shorter than normal, say, about 10 carbon atoms long?

C. all of the hydrocarbon tails were saturated?

D. all of the hydrocarbon tails were unsaturated?

E. the bilayer contained a mixture of two kinds of phospholipid molecules, one with two saturated hydrocarbon tails and the other with two unsaturated hydrocarbon tails?

F. each phospholipid molecule were covalently linked through the end carbon atom of one of its hydrocarbon tails to a phospholipid tail in the opposite monolayer?

QUESTION 11–11

What are the differences between a phospholipid molecule and a detergent molecule? How would the structure of a phospholipid molecule need to change to make it a detergent?

QUESTION 11–12

A. Membrane lipid molecules exchange places with their lipid neighbors every 10^{-7} second. A lipid molecule diffuses from one end of a 2-μm-long bacterial cell to the other in about 0.2 seconds. Are these two numbers in agreement (assume that the diameter of a lipid head group is about 0.5 nm)? If not, can you think of a reason for the difference?

B. To get an appreciation for the great speed of molecular diffusion, assume that a lipid head group is about the size of a ping-pong ball (4 cm in diameter) and that the floor of your living room (6 m × 6 m) is covered wall-to-wall with these balls. If two neighboring balls exchanged positions once every 10^{-7} second, what would their speed be in kilometers per hour? How long would it take for a ball to move from one side of the room to the opposite side?

QUESTION 11–13

Why does a red blood cell plasma membrane need transmembrane proteins?

QUESTION 11–14

Consider a transmembrane protein that forms a hydrophilic pore across the plasma membrane of a eukaryotic cell. When this protein is activated by binding a specific ligand on its extracellular side it allows Na^+ to enter the cell. The protein is made of five similar transmembrane subunits, each containing a membrane-spanning α helix with hydrophilic amino acid side chains on one surface of the helix and hydrophobic amino acid side chains on the opposite surface. Considering the function of the protein as a channel for Na^+ ions to enter the cell, propose a possible arrangement of the five membrane-spanning α helices in the membrane.

QUESTION 11–15

In the membrane of a human red blood cell, the ratio of the mass of protein (average molecular weight 50,000) to phospholipid (molecular weight 800) to cholesterol (molecular weight 386) is about 2:1:1. How many lipid molecules are there for every protein molecule?

QUESTION 11–16

Draw a schematic diagram that shows a close-up view of two plasma membranes as they come together during cell fusion, as shown in Figure 11–30. Show membrane proteins in both cells that were labeled from the outside by the binding of differently colored fluorescent antibody molecules. Indicate in your drawing the fates of these color tags as the cells fuse. Will the fluorescent labels remain on the outside of the hybrid cell after cell fusion and still be there after the mixing of membrane proteins that occurs during the incubation at 37°C? How would the experimental outcome be different if the incubation were done at 0°C?

QUESTION 11–17

Compare the hydrophobic forces that hold a membrane protein in the lipid bilayer with those that help proteins fold into a unique three-dimensional structure (described in Chapter 4, pp. 121–122 and pp. 127–128).

QUESTION 11–18

Predict which one of the following organisms will have the highest percentage of unsaturated phospholipids in its membranes. Explain your answer.

A. Antarctic fish

B. Desert snake

C. Human being

D. Polar bear

E. Thermophilic bacterium that lives in hot springs at 100°C.

QUESTION 11–19

Which of the three 20-amino-acid sequences listed below in the single-letter amino acid code is the most likely candidate to form a transmembrane region (α helix) of a transmembrane protein? Explain your answer.

A. I T L I Y F G N M S S V T Q T I L L I S

B. L L L I F F G V M A L V I V V I L L I A

C. L L K K F F R D M A A V H E T I L E E S

QUESTION 11–20

Figure Q11–20 shows the structure of triacylglycerol. Would you expect this molecule to be incorporated into the lipid bilayer? If so, which part of the molecule would face the interior of the bilayer and which would face the water on either side of the bilayer? If not, what sort of structure would these molecules form in the aqueous environment inside a cell?

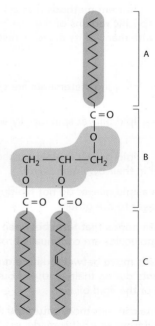

Figure Q11–20   triacylglycerol

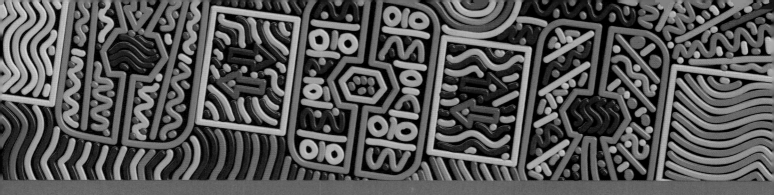

CHAPTER **TWELVE**

12

Transport Across Cell Membranes

To survive and grow, cells must be able to exchange molecules with their environment. They must import nutrients such as sugars and amino acids and eliminate metabolic waste products. They must also regulate the concentrations of a variety of inorganic ions in their cytosol and organelles. A few molecules, such as CO_2 and O_2, can simply diffuse across the lipid bilayer of the plasma membrane. But the vast majority cannot. Instead, their movement depends on specialized **membrane transport proteins** that span the lipid bilayer, providing private passageways across the membrane for select substances (**Figure 12–1**).

In this chapter, we consider how cell membranes control the traffic of inorganic ions and small, water-soluble molecules into and out of the cell and its membrane-enclosed organelles. Cells can also selectively transfer large macromolecules such as proteins across their membranes, but this transport requires more elaborate machinery and is discussed in Chapter 15.

We begin by outlining some of the general principles that guide the passage of ions and small molecules through cell membranes. We then examine, in turn, the two main classes of membrane proteins that mediate this transfer: transporters and channels. *Transporters* shift small organic molecules or inorganic ions from one side of the membrane to the other by changing shape. *Channels*, in contrast, form tiny hydrophilic pores across the membrane through which substances can pass by diffusion. Most channels only permit passage of ions and are therefore called *ion channels*. Because these ions are electrically charged, their movements can create a powerful electric force—or voltage—across the membrane. In the final part of the chapter, we discuss how these voltage differences enable nerve cells to communicate—and, ultimately, to shape how we behave.

PRINCIPLES OF
TRANSMEMBRANE TRANSPORT

TRANSPORTERS AND THEIR
FUNCTIONS

ION CHANNELS AND THE
MEMBRANE POTENTIAL

ION CHANNELS AND NERVE
CELL SIGNALING

Figure 12–1 Cell membranes contain specialized membrane transport proteins that facilitate the passage of selected small, water-soluble molecules. (A) Protein-free, artificial lipid bilayers such as liposomes (see Figure 11–13) are impermeable to most water-soluble molecules. (B) Cell membranes, by contrast, contain membrane transport proteins (*light green*), each of which transfers a particular substance across the membrane. This selective transport can facilitate the passive diffusion of specific molecules or ions across the membrane (*blue* circles), as well as the active pumping of specific substances either out of (*purple* triangles) or into (*green* bars) the cell. For other molecules, the membrane is impermeable (*red* squares). The combined action of different membrane transport proteins allows a specific set of solutes to build up inside a membrane-enclosed compartment, such as the cytosol or an organelle.

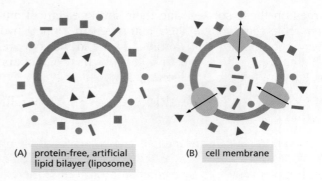

(A)   protein-free, artificial lipid bilayer (liposome)

(B)   cell membrane

PRINCIPLES OF TRANSMEMBRANE TRANSPORT

As we saw in Chapter 11, the hydrophobic interior of the lipid bilayer creates a barrier to the passage of most hydrophilic molecules, including all ions. These molecules are as reluctant to enter a fatty environment as hydrophobic molecules are reluctant to interact with water. But cells and organelles must allow the passage of many hydrophilic, water-soluble molecules, such as inorganic ions, sugars, amino acids, nucleotides, and other cell metabolites. These molecules cross lipid bilayers far too slowly by *simple diffusion*, so their passage across cell membranes must be accelerated by specialized membrane transport proteins—a process called *facilitated transport*. In this section, we review the basic principles of such facilitated transmembrane transport and introduce the various types of membrane transport proteins that mediate this movement. We also discuss why the transport of inorganic ions, in particular, is of such fundamental importance for all cells.

Lipid Bilayers Are Impermeable to Ions and Most Uncharged Polar Molecules

Given enough time, virtually any molecule will diffuse across a lipid bilayer. The rate at which it diffuses, however, varies enormously depending on the size of the molecule and its solubility properties. In general, the smaller the molecule and the more hydrophobic, or nonpolar, it is, the more rapidly it will diffuse across the lipid bilayer.

Of course, many of the molecules that are of interest to cells are polar and water-soluble. These *solutes*—substances that, in this case, are dissolved in water—are unable to cross the lipid bilayer without the aid of membrane transport proteins. The relative ease with which a variety of solutes can cross a lipid bilayer that lacks membrane transport proteins is shown in **Figure 12–2**.

1. *Small, nonpolar molecules,* such as molecular oxygen (O_2, molecular mass 32 daltons) and carbon dioxide (CO_2, 44 daltons), dissolve readily in lipid bilayers and therefore diffuse rapidly across them; indeed, cells depend on this permeability to gases for the *cell respiration* processes discussed in Chapter 14.

2. *Uncharged polar molecules* (those with an uneven distribution of electric charge) also diffuse readily across a bilayer, but only if they are small enough. Water (H_2O, 18 daltons) and ethanol (46 daltons), for example, cross at a measurable rate, whereas glycerol (92 daltons) crosses less rapidly. Larger uncharged polar molecules, such as glucose (180 daltons), cross hardly at all.

3. In contrast, lipid bilayers are highly impermeable to all charged substances, including all inorganic ions, no matter how small. The

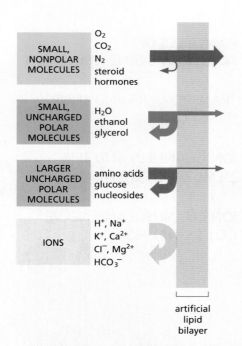

SMALL, NONPOLAR MOLECULES	O_2 CO_2 N_2 steroid hormones
SMALL, UNCHARGED POLAR MOLECULES	H_2O ethanol glycerol
LARGER UNCHARGED POLAR MOLECULES	amino acids glucose nucleosides
IONS	H^+, Na^+ K^+, Ca^{2+} Cl^-, Mg^{2+} HCO_3^-

artificial lipid bilayer

Figure 12–2 The rate at which a solute crosses a protein-free, artificial lipid bilayer by simple diffusion depends on its size and solubility. Many of the organic molecules that a cell uses as nutrients (*red*) are too large and polar to pass efficiently through an artificial lipid bilayer that does not contain the appropriate membrane transport proteins.

charges on these solutes, and their strong electrical attraction to water molecules, inhibit their entry into the inner, hydrocarbon phase of the bilayer. Thus protein-free lipid bilayers are a billion (10^9) times more permeable to water, which is polar but uncharged, than they are to even small ions such as Na^+ or K^+.

The Ion Concentrations Inside a Cell Are Very Different from Those Outside

Because lipid bilayers are impermeable to inorganic ions, living cells are able to maintain internal ion concentrations that are very different from the concentrations of ions in the medium that surrounds them. These differences in ion concentration are crucial for a cell's survival and function. Among the most important inorganic ions for cells are Na^+, K^+, Ca^{2+}, Cl^-, and H^+ (protons). The movement of these ions across cell membranes plays an essential part in many biological processes, but is perhaps most striking in the production of ATP by all cells (discussed in Chapter 14) and in the communication of nerve cells (discussed later in this chapter).

Na^+ is the most plentiful positively charged ion (cation) outside the cell, whereas K^+ is the most abundant inside (Table 12–1). For a cell to avoid being torn apart by electrical forces, the quantity of positive charge inside the cell must be balanced by an almost exactly equal quantity of negative charge, and the same is true for the charge in the surrounding fluid. The high concentration of Na^+ outside the cell is electrically balanced chiefly by extracellular Cl^-, whereas the high concentration of K^+ inside is balanced by a variety of negatively charged inorganic and organic ions (anions), including nucleic acids, proteins, and many cell metabolites (see Table 12–1).

Differences in the Concentration of Inorganic Ions Across a Cell Membrane Create a Membrane Potential

Although the electrical charges inside and outside the cell are generally kept in balance, tiny excesses of positive or negative charge, concentrated in the neighborhood of the plasma membrane, do occur. Such electrical imbalances generate a voltage difference across the membrane called the **membrane potential**.

When a cell is "unstimulated," the movement of anions and cations across the membrane will be precisely balanced. In such steady-state

TABLE 12–1 A COMPARISON OF ION CONCENTRATIONS INSIDE AND OUTSIDE A TYPICAL MAMMALIAN CELL

Ion	Intracellular Concentration (mM)	Extracellular Concentration (mM)
Cations		
Na^+	5–15	145
K^+	140	5
Mg^{2+}	0.5*	1–2
Ca^{2+}	10^{-4}*	1–2
H^+	7×10^{-5} ($10^{-7.2}$ M or pH 7.2)	4×10^{-5} ($10^{-7.4}$ M or pH 7.4)
Anions**		
Cl^-	5–15	110

*The concentrations of Mg^{2+} and Ca^{2+} given are for the free ions. There is a total of about 20 mM Mg^{2+} and 1–2 mM Ca^{2+} in cells, but most of these ions are bound to proteins and other organic molecules and, for Ca^{2+}, stored within various organelles.
**In addition to Cl^-, a cell contains many other anions not listed in this table. In fact, most cell constituents are negatively charged (HCO_3^-, PO_4^{3-}, proteins, nucleic acids, metabolites carrying phosphate and carboxyl groups, and so on).

conditions, the voltage difference across the cell membrane—called the *resting membrane potential*—holds steady. But it is not zero. In animal cells, for example, the resting membrane potential can be anywhere between –20 and –200 millivolts (mV), depending on the organism and cell type. The value is expressed as a negative number because the interior of the cell is more negatively charged than the exterior.

The membrane potential allows cells to power the transport of certain metabolites, and it provides cells that are excitable with a means to communicate with their neighbors. As we discuss shortly, it is the activity of different membrane transport proteins, embedded in the bilayer, that enables cells to establish and maintain their characteristic membrane potential.

Cells Contain Two Classes of Membrane Transport Proteins: Transporters and Channels

Membrane transport proteins occur in many forms and are present in all cell membranes. Each provides a private portal across the membrane for a particular small, water-soluble substance—an ion, sugar, or amino acid, for example. Most of these membrane transport proteins allow passage of only select members of a particular type: some permit transit of Na^+ but not K^+, others K^+ but not Na^+, and so on. Each type of cell membrane has its own characteristic set of transport proteins, which determines exactly which solutes can pass into and out of that cell or organelle.

As discussed in Chapter 11, most membrane transport proteins have polypeptide chains that traverse the lipid bilayer multiple times—that is, they are multipass transmembrane proteins (see Figure 11–24). When these transmembrane segments cluster together, they establish a continuous protein-lined pathway that allows selected small, hydrophilic molecules to cross the membrane without coming into direct contact with the hydrophobic interior of the lipid bilayer.

Cells contain two main classes of membrane transport proteins: transporters and channels. These proteins differ in the way they discriminate between solutes, transporting some but not others (**Figure 12–3**). *Channels* discriminate mainly on the basis of size and electric charge: when the channel is open, only ions of an appropriate size and charge can pass through. A *transporter*, on the other hand, transfers only those molecules or ions that fit into specific binding sites on the protein. Transporters bind their solutes with great specificity, in the same way an enzyme binds its substrate, and it is this requirement for specific binding that gives transporters their selectivity.

Solutes Cross Membranes by Either Passive or Active Transport

Transporters and channels allow small, hydrophilic molecules and ions to cross the cell membrane, but what controls whether these substances move into the cell (or organelle)—or out of it? In many cases, the direction

Figure 12–3 Inorganic ions and small, polar organic molecules can cross a cell membrane through either a transporter or a channel. (A) A channel forms a pore across the bilayer through which specific inorganic ions or, in some cases, polar organic molecules can diffuse. Ion channels can exist in either an open or a closed conformation, and they transport only in the open conformation, as shown here. Channel opening and closing is usually controlled by an external stimulus or by conditions within the cell. (B) A transporter undergoes a series of conformational changes to transfer small solutes across the lipid bilayer. Transporters are very selective for the solutes that they bind, and they transfer them at a much slower rate than do channels.

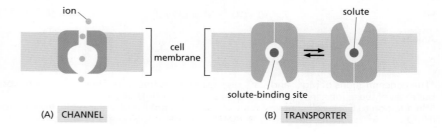

of transport depends only on the relative concentrations of the solute on either side of the membrane. Substances will spontaneously flow "downhill" from a region of high concentration to a region of low concentration, provided a pathway exists. Such movements are called passive, because they need no additional driving force. If, for example, a solute is present at a higher concentration outside the cell than inside, and an appropriate channel or transporter is present in the plasma membrane, the solute will move into the cell by **passive transport**, without expenditure of energy by the membrane transport protein. This is because even though the solute can move in either direction across the membrane, more solute will move in than out until the two concentrations equilibrate. All channels—and many transporters—act as conduits for such passive transport.

To move a solute against its concentration gradient, however, a membrane transport protein must do work: it has to drive the flow of the substance "uphill" from a region of low concentration to a region of higher concentration. To do so, it couples the transport to some other process that provides an input of energy (as discussed in Chapter 3). The movement of a solute against its concentration gradient in this way is termed **active transport**, and it is carried out by special types of transporters called *pumps*, which harness an energy source to power the transport process (**Figure 12–4**). As discussed later, this energy can come from ATP hydrolysis, a transmembrane ion gradient, or sunlight.

Both the Concentration Gradient and Membrane Potential Influence the Passive Transport of Charged Solutes

For an uncharged molecule, the direction of passive transport is determined solely by its concentration gradient, as we have outlined above. But for electrically charged substances, whether inorganic ions or small organic molecules, an additional force comes into play. As mentioned earlier, most cell membranes have a voltage across them—a difference in charge referred to as a membrane potential. This membrane potential exerts a force on any substance that carries an electric charge. The cytosolic side of the plasma membrane is usually at a negative potential relative to the extracellular side, so the membrane potential tends to pull positively charged ions and molecules into the cell and drive negatively charged solutes out.

At the same time, a charged solute—like an uncharged one—will also tend to move down its concentration gradient. The net force driving a charged solute across a cell membrane is therefore a composite of two forces, one due to the concentration gradient and the other due to the membrane potential. This net driving force, called the solute's **electrochemical gradient**, determines the direction in which each solute will flow across the membrane by passive transport.

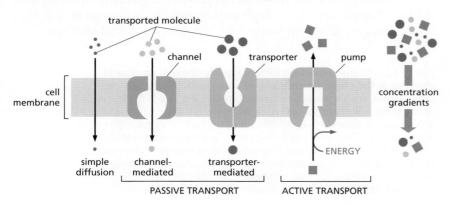

Figure 12–4 Solutes cross cell membranes by either passive or active transport. Some small, nonpolar molecules such as CO_2 (see Figure 12–2) can move passively down their concentration gradient across the lipid bilayer by simple diffusion, without the help of a membrane transport protein. Most solutes, however, require the assistance of a channel or transporter. Passive transport, which allows solutes to move down their concentration gradients, occurs spontaneously; active transport against a concentration gradient requires an input of energy. Only transporters can carry out active transport, and the transporters that perform this function are called pumps.

Figure 12–5 An electrochemical gradient has two components. The net driving force tending to move a charged solute across a cell membrane—its electrochemical gradient—is the sum of a force from the concentration gradient of the solute and a force from the membrane potential. The membrane potential is represented here by the + and – signs on opposite sides of the membrane. The width of the *green* arrow represents the magnitude of the electrochemical gradient. (A) The concentration gradient and membrane potential work together to increase the driving force for movement of the solute. Such is the case for Na^+. (B) The membrane potential acts against the concentration gradient, decreasing the electrochemical driving force. Such is the case for K^+.

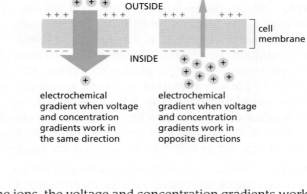

For some ions, the voltage and concentration gradients work in the same direction, creating a relatively steep electrochemical gradient (**Figure 12–5A**). This is the case for Na^+, which is positively charged and at a higher concentration outside cells than inside (see Table 12–1). Na^+ therefore tends to enter cells when given an opportunity. If, however, the voltage and concentration gradients have opposing effects, the resulting electrochemical gradient can be small (**Figure 12–5B**). This is the case for K^+, which is present at a much higher concentration inside cells, where the resting membrane potential is negative. Because its electrochemical gradient across the plasma membrane of resting cells is small, there is little net movement of K^+ across the membrane even when K^+ channels are open.

Water Moves Across Cell Membranes Down Its Concentration Gradient—a Process Called Osmosis

Cells are mostly water (generally about 70% by weight), and so the movement of water across cell membranes is crucially important for living things. Because water molecules are small and uncharged, they can diffuse directly across the lipid bilayer (see Figure 12–2). However, this movement is relatively slow. To facilitate the flow of water, some cells contain specialized channels called aquaporins in their plasma membrane (**Figure 12–6** and Movie 12.1). For many cells, such as those in the kidney or in various secretory glands, aquaporins are essential for their function.

But for water-filled cells in an aqueous environment, does water tend to enter the cell or leave it? As we saw in Table 12–1, cells contain a high concentration of solutes, including many charged molecules and ions. Thus the total concentration of solute particles inside the cell—also called its *osmolarity*—generally exceeds the solute concentration outside the cell. The resulting osmotic gradient tends to "pull" water into the cell. This movement of water down its concentration gradient—from an area of low solute concentration (high water concentration) to an area of high solute concentration (low water concentration)—is called **osmosis**.

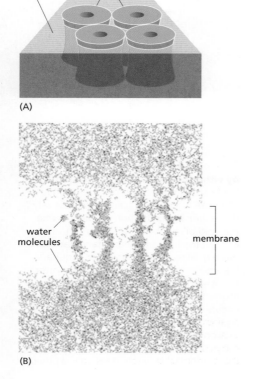

Figure 12–6 Water molecules diffuse rapidly through aquaporin channels in the plasma membrane of some cells. (A) Shaped like an hourglass, each aquaporin channel forms a pore across the bilayer, allowing the selective passage of water molecules. Shown here is an aquaporin tetramer, the biologically active form of the protein. (B) In this snapshot, taken from a real-time, molecular dynamics simulation, four columns of water molecules (*blue*) can be seen passing through the pores of an aquaporin tetramer (not shown). The space where the membrane would be located is indicated. (B, adapted from B. de Groot and H. Grubmüller, *Science* 294:2353–2357, 2001.)

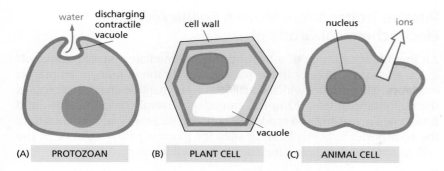

(A)   PROTOZOAN   (B)   PLANT CELL   (C)   ANIMAL CELL

Figure 12–7 Cells use different tactics to avoid osmotic swelling. (A) A freshwater amoeba avoids swelling by periodically ejecting the water that moves into the cell and accumulates in contractile vacuoles. The contractile vacuole first accumulates solutes, which cause water to follow by osmosis; it then pumps most of the solutes back into the cytosol before emptying its contents at the cell surface. (B) The plant cell's tough cell wall prevents swelling. (C) The animal cell reduces its intracellular solute concentration by pumping out ions.

Osmosis, if it occurs without constraint, can make a cell swell. Different cells cope with this osmotic challenge in different ways. Some freshwater protozoans, such as amoebae, eliminate excess water using contractile vacuoles that periodically discharge their contents to the exterior (**Figure 12–7A**). Plant cells are prevented from swelling by their tough cell walls and so can tolerate a large osmotic difference across their plasma membrane (**Figure 12–7B**); indeed, plant cells make use of osmotic swelling pressure, or turgor pressure, to keep their cell walls tense, so that the stems of the plant are rigid and its leaves are extended. If turgor pressure is lost, plants wilt. Animal cells maintain osmotic equilibrium by using transmembrane pumps to expel solutes, such as the Na^+ ions that tend to leak into the cell (**Figure 12–7C**).

TRANSPORTERS AND THEIR FUNCTIONS

Transporters are responsible for the movement of most small, water-soluble, organic molecules and a handful of inorganic ions across cell membranes. Each transporter is highly selective, often transferring just one type of solute. To guide and propel the complex traffic of substances into and out of the cell, and between the cytosol and the different membrane-enclosed organelles, each cell membrane contains a characteristic set of different transporters appropriate to that particular membrane. For example, the plasma membrane contains transporters that import nutrients such as sugars, amino acids, and nucleotides; the lysosome membrane contains an H^+ transporter that imports H^+ to acidify the lysosome interior and other transporters that move digestion products out of the lysosome into the cytosol; the inner membrane of mitochondria contains transporters for importing the pyruvate that mitochondria use as fuel for generating ATP, as well as transporters for exporting ATP once it is synthesized (**Figure 12–8**).

In this section, we describe the general principles that govern the function of transporters, and we present a more detailed view of the molecular mechanisms that drive the movement of a few key solutes.

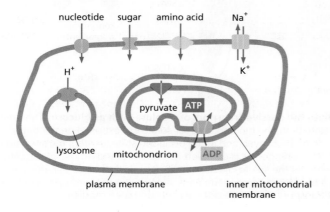

Figure 12–8 Each cell membrane has its own characteristic set of transporters. These transporters allow each membrane to carry out its unique functions. Only a few of these transporters are shown here.

Passive Transporters Move a Solute Along Its Electrochemical Gradient

An important example of a transporter that mediates passive transport is the *glucose transporter* in the plasma membrane of many mammalian cell types. The protein, which consists of a polypeptide chain that crosses the membrane at least 12 times, can adopt several conformations—and it switches reversibly and randomly between them. In one conformation, the transporter exposes binding sites for glucose to the exterior of the cell; in another, it exposes the sites to the cell interior.

Because glucose is uncharged, the electrical component of its electrochemical gradient is zero. Thus the direction in which it is transported is determined by its concentration gradient alone. When glucose is plentiful outside cells, as it is after a meal, the sugar binds to the transporter's externally displayed binding sites; if the protein then switches conformation—spontaneously and at random—it will carry the bound sugar inward and release it into the cytosol, where the glucose concentration is low (**Figure 12–9**). Conversely, when blood glucose levels are low—as they are when you are hungry—the hormone glucagon stimulates liver cells to produce large amounts of glucose by the breakdown of glycogen. As a result, the glucose concentration is higher inside liver cells than outside. This glucose can bind to the internally displayed binding sites on the transporter. When the protein then switches conformation in the opposite direction—again spontaneously and randomly—the glucose will be transported out of the cells and made available for import by other, energy-requiring cells. The net flow of glucose can thus go either way, according to the direction of the glucose concentration gradient across the plasma membrane: inward if more glucose is binding to the transporter's externally displayed sites, and outward if the opposite is true.

Although passive transporters themselves play no part in controlling the direction of solute transport, they are highly selective in terms of which solutes they will move. For example, the binding sites in the glucose transporter bind only D-glucose and not its mirror image L-glucose, which the cell cannot use as an energy source.

Pumps Actively Transport a Solute Against Its Electrochemical Gradient

Cells cannot rely solely on passive transport to maintain the proper balance of solutes. The active transport of solutes against their electrochemical gradient is essential to achieving the appropriate intracellular

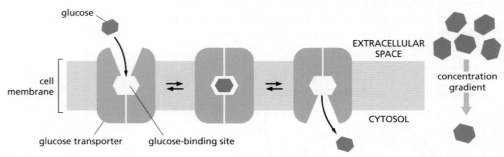

Figure 12–9 Conformational changes in a transporter mediate the passive transport of a solute such as glucose. The transporter is shown in three conformational states: in the outward-open state (*left*), the binding sites for solute are exposed on the outside; in the inward-open state (*right*), the sites are exposed on the inside of the bilayer; and in the occluded state (*center*), the sites are not accessible from either side. The transition between the states occurs randomly, is completely reversible, and—most importantly for the function of the transporter shown—does not depend on whether the solute-binding site is occupied. Therefore, if the solute concentration is higher on the outside of the bilayer, solute will bind more often to the transporter in the outward-open conformation than in the inward-open conformation, and there will be a net transport of glucose down its concentration gradient.

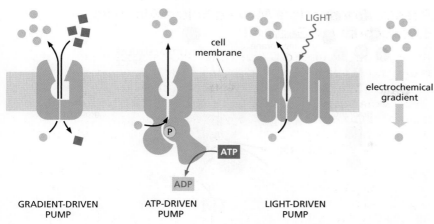

GRADIENT-DRIVEN PUMP   ATP-DRIVEN PUMP   LIGHT-DRIVEN PUMP

Figure 12–10 **Pumps carry out active transport in three main ways.** The actively transported solute is shown in *gold*, and the energy source is shown in *red*.

ionic composition and for importing solutes that are at a lower concentration outside the cell than inside. For these purposes, cells depend on transmembrane **pumps**, which can carry out active transport in three main ways (**Figure 12–10**): (i) *gradient-driven pumps* link the uphill transport of one solute across a membrane to the downhill transport of another; (ii) *ATP-driven pumps* use the energy released by the hydrolysis of ATP to drive uphill transport; and (iii) *light-driven pumps*, which are found mainly in bacterial cells, use energy derived from sunlight to drive uphill transport, as discussed in Chapter 11 for bacteriorhodopsin (see Figure 11–28).

These different forms of active transport are often linked. Thus, in the plasma membrane of an animal cell, an ATP-driven *Na+ pump* transports Na^+ out of the cell against its electrochemical gradient; this Na^+ can then flow back into the cell, down its electrochemical gradient, through various Na^+ gradient-driven pumps. The influx of Na^+ through these gradient-driven pumps provides the energy for the active transport of many other substances into the cell against their electrochemical gradients. If the ATP-driven Na^+ pump ceased operating, the Na^+ gradient would soon run down, and transport through Na^+ gradient-driven pumps would come to a halt. For this reason, the ATP-driven Na^+ pump has a central role in the active transport of small molecules across the plasma membrane of animal cells. Plant cells, fungi, and many bacteria use ATP-driven H^+ pumps in an analogous way: in pumping H^+ out of the cell, these proteins create an electrochemical gradient of H^+ across the plasma membrane that is subsequently harnessed for solute transport, as we discuss later.

The Na+ Pump in Animal Cells Uses Energy Supplied by ATP to Expel Na+ and Bring in K+

The ATP-driven **Na+ pump** plays such a central part in the energy economy of animal cells that it typically accounts for 30% or more of their total ATP consumption. This pump uses the energy derived from ATP hydrolysis to transport Na^+ out of the cell as it carries K^+ in. The pump is therefore sometimes called the *Na+-K+ ATPase* or the *Na+-K+ pump*.

During the pumping process, the energy from ATP hydrolysis fuels a stepwise series of protein conformational changes that drives the exchange of Na^+ and K^+ ions. As part of the process, the phosphate group removed from ATP gets transferred to the pump itself (**Figure 12–11**).

The transport of Na^+ ions out, and K^+ ions in, takes place in a cycle in which each step depends on the one before (**Figure 12–12**). If any of the individual steps is prevented from occurring, the entire cycle halts. The toxin *ouabain*, for example, inhibits the Na^+ pump by preventing the binding of extracellular K^+, arresting the cycle.

Figure 12–11 The Na⁺ pump uses the energy of ATP hydrolysis to pump Na⁺ out of animal cells and K⁺ in. In this way, the pump helps keep the cytosolic concentrations of Na⁺ low and K⁺ high.

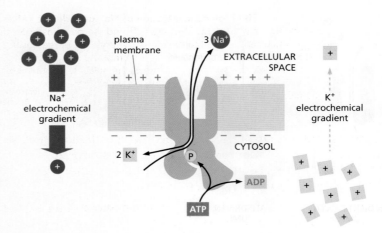

The Na⁺ pump is very efficient: the whole pumping cycle takes only 10 milliseconds. Furthermore, the tight coupling between steps in the cycle ensures that the pump operates only when the appropriate ions—both Na⁺ and K⁺—are available to be transported, thereby avoiding a wasteful hydrolysis of ATP.

The Na⁺ Pump Generates a Steep Concentration Gradient of Na⁺ Across the Plasma Membrane

The Na⁺ pump functions like a bilge pump in a leaky ship, ceaselessly expelling the Na⁺ that is constantly slipping into the cell through other

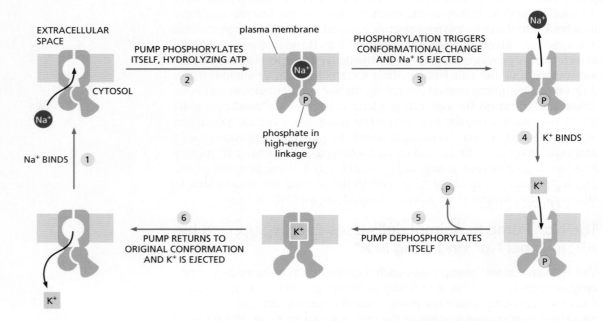

Figure 12–12 The Na⁺ pump undergoes a series of conformational changes as it exchanges Na⁺ ions for K⁺. The binding of cytosolic Na⁺ (1) and the subsequent phosphorylation by ATP of the cytosolic face of the pump (2) induce the protein to undergo conformational changes that transfer the Na⁺ across the membrane and release it outside the cell (3). The high-energy linkage of the phosphate to the protein provides the energy to drive the conformational changes. The binding of K⁺ from the extracellular space (4) and the subsequent dephosphorylation (5) allow the protein to return to its original conformation, which transfers the K⁺ across the membrane and releases it into the cytosol (6). The cycle is shown in Movie 12.2. The changes in conformation are analogous to those shown for the glucose transporter in Figure 12–9, except that here the Na⁺-dependent phosphorylation and K⁺-dependent dephosphorylation of the protein cause the conformational changes to occur in an orderly fashion, enabling the protein to do useful work. For simplicity, only one binding site is shown for each ion. The real pump in mammalian cells contains three binding sites for Na⁺ and two for K⁺. The net result of one cycle of the pump is therefore the transport of three Na⁺ out and two K⁺ in. Ouabain inhibits the pump by preventing K⁺ binding (4).

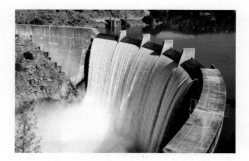

Figure 12–13 The high concentration of Na$^+$ outside the cell is like water behind a high dam. The water behind the dam has potential energy, which can be used to drive energy-requiring processes. In the same way, an ion gradient across a membrane can be used to drive active processes in a cell, including the active transport of other molecules across the plasma membrane. Shown here is the Table Rock Dam in Branson, Missouri, USA. (Gary Saxe/Shutterstock.)

transporters and ion channels in the plasma membrane. In this way, the pump keeps the Na$^+$ concentration in the cytosol about 10–30 times lower than that in the extracellular fluid and the K$^+$ concentration about 10–30 times higher (see Table 12–1, p. 391).

This steep concentration gradient of Na$^+$ across the plasma membrane acts together with the membrane potential to create a large Na$^+$ electrochemical gradient (see Figure 12–5A). This high concentration of Na$^+$ outside the cell, on the uphill side of its electrochemical gradient, is like a large volume of water behind a high dam: it represents a very large store of energy (Figure 12–13). Even if one artificially halts the operation of the Na$^+$ pump with ouabain, this stored energy is sufficient to sustain for many minutes the various gradient-driven pumps in the plasma membrane that are fueled by the downhill flow of Na$^+$, which we discuss shortly.

Ca^{2+} Pumps Keep the Cytosolic Ca^{2+} Concentration Low

Ca^{2+}, like Na$^+$, is also kept at a low concentration in the cytosol compared with its concentration in the extracellular fluid. But Ca^{2+} is much less plentiful than Na$^+$, both inside and outside cells (see Table 12–1). The movement of this ion across cell membranes is nonetheless crucial, because Ca^{2+} can bind tightly to a variety of proteins in the cell, altering their activities. An influx of Ca^{2+} into the cytosol through Ca^{2+} channels, for example, is used by different cells as an intracellular signal to trigger various complex processes, such as muscle contraction (discussed in Chapter 17), fertilization (discussed in Chapters 16 and 19), and nerve cell communication, which is discussed later.

The lower the background concentration of free Ca^{2+} in the cytosol, the more sensitive the cell is to an increase in cytosolic Ca^{2+}. Thus eukaryotic cells in general maintain a very low concentration of free Ca^{2+} in their cytosol (about 10^{-4} mM) compared to the much higher concentration of Ca^{2+} outside of the cell (typically 1–2 mM). This huge concentration difference is achieved mainly by means of ATP-driven **Ca^{2+} pumps** in both the plasma membrane and the endoplasmic reticulum membrane, which actively remove Ca^{2+} from the cytosol.

Ca^{2+} pumps are ATPases that work in much the same way as the Na$^+$ pump depicted in Figure 12–12. The main difference is that Ca^{2+} pumps return to their original conformation without a requirement for binding and transporting a second ion (Figure 12–14). The Na$^+$ and Ca^{2+} pumps have similar amino acid sequences and structures, indicating that they share a common evolutionary origin.

Gradient-driven Pumps Exploit Solute Gradients to Mediate Active Transport

A gradient of any solute across a membrane, like the electrochemical Na$^+$ gradient generated by the Na$^+$ pump, can be used to drive the active transport of a second molecule. The downhill movement of the first solute down its gradient provides the energy to power the uphill transport of the second solute. The active transporters that work in this way are

Figure 12–14 The Ca²⁺ pump in the sarcoplasmic reticulum was the first ATP-driven ion pump to have its three-dimensional structure determined by x-ray crystallography. When a muscle cell is stimulated, Ca²⁺ floods into the cytosol from the sarcoplasmic reticulum—a specialized form of endoplasmic reticulum. The influx of Ca²⁺ stimulates the cell to contract; to recover from the contraction, Ca²⁺ must be pumped back into the sarcoplasmic reticulum by this Ca²⁺ pump.

The Ca²⁺ pump uses ATP to phosphorylate itself, inducing a series of conformational changes (similar to the ones of the Na⁺ pump shown in Figure 12–12); when the pump is open to the lumen of the sarcoplasmic reticulum, the Ca²⁺-binding sites are eliminated, ejecting the two Ca²⁺ ions into the organelle (Movie 12.3).

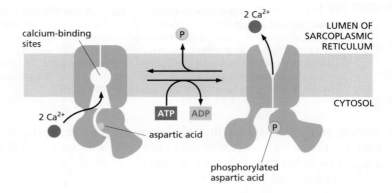

called **gradient-driven pumps** (see Figure 12–10). They can couple the movement of one inorganic ion to that of another, the movement of an inorganic ion to that of a small organic molecule, or the movement of one small organic molecule to that of another. If the pump moves both solutes in the same direction across the membrane, it is called a *symport*. If it moves them in opposite directions, it is called an *antiport*. A transporter that ferries only one type of solute across the membrane down its concentration gradient (and is therefore not a pump) is called a *uniport* (Figure 12–15). The glucose transporter described earlier (see Figure 12–9) is an example of a uniport.

The Electrochemical Na⁺ Gradient Drives the Transport of Glucose Across the Plasma Membrane of Animal Cells

Symports that make use of the inward flow of Na⁺ down its steep electrochemical gradient have an especially important role in driving the import of solutes into animal cells. The epithelial cells that line the gut, for example, transport glucose from the gut lumen across the gut epithelium and, ultimately, into the blood. If these cells had only a passive glucose uniport (the transporter shown in Figure 12–9), they would release glucose into the gut lumen after fasting just as freely as they take it up from the gut after a feast. However, these epithelial cells also possess a *glucose–Na⁺ symport*, which they can use to take up glucose from the gut lumen, even when the concentration of glucose is higher in the epithelial cell's cytosol than it is inside the gut. As the electrochemical gradient for Na⁺ is so steep, when Na⁺ moves into the cell down its gradient, glucose is, in a sense, "dragged" into the cell along with it. Because the binding of Na⁺ and glucose is cooperative—the binding of one enhances the binding of the other—if one of the two solutes is missing, the other fails to bind; therefore both molecules must be present for this gradient-driven

Figure 12–15 Gradient-driven pumps can act as symports or antiports. They transfer solutes either in the same direction, in which case they are called symports, or in opposite directions, which are antiports (Movie 12.4). Uniports, by contrast, only facilitate the movement of a solute down its concentration gradient. Because such movement does not require an additional energy source, uniports are not pumps.

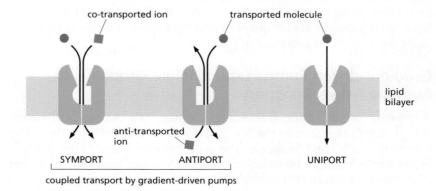

coupled transport by gradient-driven pumps

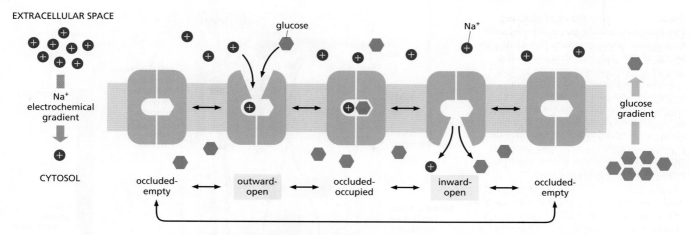

EXTRACELLULAR SPACE

glucose

Na⁺

Na⁺
electrochemical
gradient

glucose
gradient

CYTOSOL

occluded-
empty

outward-
open

occluded-
occupied

inward-
open

occluded-
empty

Figure 12–16 A glucose–Na⁺ symport uses the electrochemical Na⁺ gradient to drive the active import of glucose. The pump oscillates randomly between alternate states. In one state ("outward-open") the pump is open to the extracellular space; in another state ("inward-open") it is open to the cytosol. Although Na⁺ and glucose can each bind to the pump in either of these "open" states, the pump can transition between them only through an "occluded" state in which both glucose and Na⁺ are bound ("occluded-occupied") or neither is bound ("occluded-empty"). Because the Na⁺ concentration is high in the extracellular space, the Na⁺-binding site is readily occupied in the outward-open state, and the transporter must wait for a rare glucose molecule to bind. At that point, the pump flips to the occluded-occupied state, trapping both solutes.

Because conformational transitions are reversible, one of two things can happen to the pump in the occluded-occupied state. The transporter could flip back to the outward-open state; in this case, the solutes would dissociate, and nothing would be gained. Alternatively, it could flip into the inward-open state, exposing the solute-binding sites to the cytosol where the Na⁺ concentration is very low. Thus sodium readily dissociates (and will be subsequently pumped back out of the cell by the Na⁺ pump, shown in Figure 12–11, to maintain the steep Na⁺ gradient). The transporter is now trapped with a partially occupied binding site until the glucose molecule also dissociates. At this point, with no solute bound, it can transition into the occluded-empty state and from there back to the outward-open state to repeat the transport cycle.

transport to occur and Na⁺ will not leak into the cell without doing useful work (**Figure 12–16**).

If the gut epithelial cells had *only* this symport, however, they would take up glucose and never release it for use by the other cells of the body. These epithelial cells, therefore, have two types of glucose transporters located at opposite ends of the cell. In the apical domain of the plasma membrane, which faces the gut lumen, they have the glucose–Na⁺ symports. These use the energy of the Na⁺ gradient to actively import glucose, creating a high concentration of the sugar in the cytosol. In the basal and lateral domains of the plasma membrane, the cells have passive glucose uniports, which release the glucose down its concentration gradient for use by other tissues (**Figure 12–17**). As shown in Figure 12–17, the two types of glucose transporters are kept segregated in their proper domains of the plasma membrane by a diffusion barrier formed by a tight junction around the apex of the cell. This prevents mixing of membrane components between the two domains, as discussed in Chapter 11 (see Figure 11–32).

Cells in the lining of the gut and in many other organs, including the kidney, contain a variety of symports in their plasma membrane that are similarly driven by the electrochemical gradient of Na⁺; each of these gradient-driven pumps specifically imports a small group of related sugars or amino acids into the cell. At the same time, Na⁺-driven pumps that operate as **antiports** are also important for cells. For example, the *Na⁺–H⁺ exchanger* in the plasma membrane of many animal cells uses the downhill influx of Na⁺ to pump H⁺ out of the cell; it is one of the main devices that animal cells use to control the pH in their cytosol—preventing the cell interior from becoming too acidic.

Figure 12–17 Two types of glucose transporters enable gut epithelial cells to transfer glucose across the epithelial lining of the gut. Na^+ that enters the cell via the Na^+-driven glucose symport is subsequently pumped out by Na^+ pumps in the basal and lateral plasma membranes, keeping the concentration of Na^+ in the cytosol low—and the Na^+ electrochemical gradient steep. The diet provides ample Na^+ in the gut lumen to drive the Na^+ gradient-driven glucose symport. The process is shown in Movie 12.5.

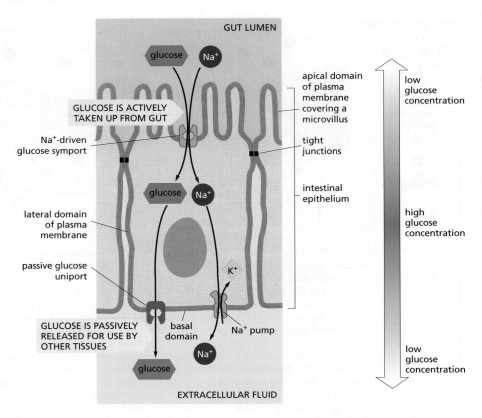

Electrochemical H^+ Gradients Drive the Transport of Solutes in Plants, Fungi, and Bacteria

Plant cells, bacteria, and fungi (including yeasts) do not have Na^+ pumps in their plasma membrane. Instead of an electrochemical Na^+ gradient, they rely mainly on an electrochemical gradient of H^+ to import solutes into the cell. The gradient is created by **H^+ pumps** in the plasma membrane that pump H^+ out of the cell, thus setting up an electrochemical proton gradient across this membrane and creating an acid pH in the medium surrounding the cell. The import of many sugars and amino acids into bacterial cells is then mediated by H^+ symports, which use the electrochemical H^+ gradient in much the same way that animal cells use the electrochemical Na^+ gradient to import these nutrients.

In some photosynthetic bacteria, the H^+ gradient is created by the activity of light-driven H^+ pumps such as bacteriorhodopsin (see Figure 11–28). In other bacteria, fungi, and plants, the H^+ gradient is generated by H^+ pumps in the plasma membrane that use the energy of ATP hydrolysis to pump H^+ out of the cell; these H^+ pumps resemble the Na^+ pumps and Ca^{2+} pumps of animal cells discussed earlier.

A different type of ATP-dependent H^+ pump is found in the membranes of some intracellular organelles, such as the lysosomes of animal cells and the central vacuole of plant and fungal cells. These pumps—which resemble the turbine-like enzyme that synthesizes ATP in mitochondria and chloroplasts (discussed in Chapter 14)—actively transport H^+ out of the cytosol into the organelle, thereby helping to keep the pH of the cytosol neutral and the pH of the interior of the organelle acidic. An acid environment is crucial to the function of many organelles, as we discuss in Chapter 15.

Some of the transmembrane pumps considered in this chapter are shown in **Figure 12–18** and are listed in **Table 12–2**.

QUESTION 12–2

A rise in the intracellular Ca^{2+} concentration causes muscle cells to contract. In addition to an ATP-driven Ca^{2+} pump, muscle cells that contract quickly and regularly, such as those of the heart, have an additional type of Ca^{2+} pump—an antiport that exchanges Ca^{2+} for extracellular Na^+ across the plasma membrane. The majority of the Ca^{2+} ions that have entered the cell during contraction are rapidly pumped back out of the cell by this antiport, thus allowing the cell to relax. Ouabain and digitalis are used for treating patients with heart disease because they make heart muscle cells contract more strongly. Both drugs function by partially inhibiting the Na^+ pump in the plasma membrane of these cells. Can you propose an explanation for the effects of the drugs in the patients? What will happen if too much of either drug is taken?

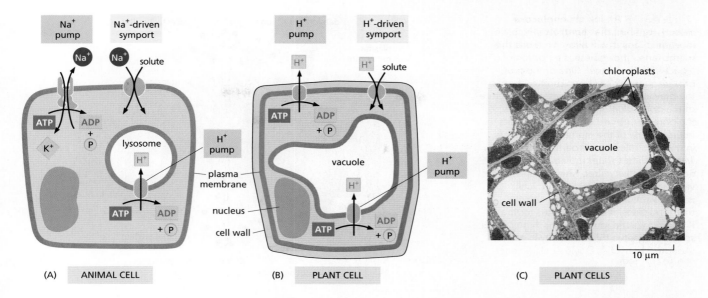

(A)   ANIMAL CELL   (B)   PLANT CELL   (C)   PLANT CELLS

ION CHANNELS AND THE MEMBRANE POTENTIAL

In principle, the simplest way to allow a small, water-soluble substance to cross from one side of a membrane to the other is to create a hydrophilic channel through which the solute can pass. Channel proteins, or **channels**, perform this function in cell membranes, forming transmembrane pores that allow the passive movement of small, water-soluble molecules and ions into or out of the cell or organelle.

A few channels form relatively large, aqueous pores; examples are the proteins that form *gap junctions* between two adjacent cells (see Figure 20–28) and the *porins* that form pores in the outer membrane of mitochondria and some bacteria (see Figure 11–25). But such large, permissive channels would lead to disastrous leaks if they directly connected the cytosol of a cell to the extracellular space. Thus most of the channels in the plasma membrane form narrow, highly selective pores.

Figure 12–18 Animal and plant cells use a variety of transmembrane pumps to drive the active transport of solutes. (A) In animal cells, an electrochemical Na^+ gradient across the plasma membrane, generated by the Na^+ pump, is used by symports to import various solutes. (B) In plant cells, an electrochemical gradient of H^+, set up by an H^+ pump, is often used for this purpose; a similar strategy is used by bacteria and fungi (not shown). The lysosomes in animal cells and the vacuoles in plant and fungal cells contain a similar H^+ pump in their membranes that pumps in H^+, helping to keep the internal environment of these organelles acidic. (C) An electron micrograph shows the vacuole in plant cells in a young tobacco leaf. (C, courtesy of J. Burgess.)

TABLE 12–2 SOME EXAMPLES OF TRANSMEMBRANE PUMPS

Pump	Location	Energy Source	Function
Na^+-driven glucose pump (glucose–Na^+ symport)	apical plasma membrane of kidney and intestinal cells	Na^+ gradient	active import of glucose
Na^+–H^+ exchanger	plasma membrane of animal cells	Na^+ gradient	active export of H^+ ions, pH regulation
Na^+ pump (Na^+-K^+ ATPase)	plasma membrane of most animal cells	ATP hydrolysis	active export of Na^+ and import of K^+
Ca^{2+} pump (Ca^{2+} ATPase)	plasma membrane of eukaryotic cells	ATP hydrolysis	active export of Ca^{2+}
Ca^{2+} pump (Ca^{2+} ATPase)	sarcoplasmic reticulum membrane of muscle cells and endoplasmic reticulum membrane of most animal cells	ATP hydrolysis	active import of Ca^{2+} into sarcoplasmic reticulum or endoplasmic reticulum
H^+ pump (H^+ ATPase)	plasma membrane of plant cells, fungi, and some bacteria	ATP hydrolysis	active export of H^+
H^+ pump (H^+ ATPase)	membranes of lysosomes in animal cells and of vacuoles in plant and fungal cells	ATP hydrolysis	active export of H^+ from cytosol into lysosome or vacuole
Bacteriorhodopsin	plasma membrane of some bacteria	light	active export of H^+

Figure 12–19 An ion channel has a selectivity filter that controls which inorganic ions it will allow to cross the membrane. Shown here is a portion of a bacterial K⁺ channel. One of the four protein subunits has been omitted from the drawing to expose the interior structure of the pore (*blue*). From the cytosolic side, the pore opens into a vestibule that sits in the middle of the membrane. K⁺ ions in the vestibule are still partially cloaked with associated water molecules. The narrow selectivity filter, which connects the vestibule with the outside of the cell, is lined with polar groups (not shown) that form transient binding sites for the K⁺ ions once the ions have shed their water shell. To observe this selectivity in action. (Adapted from D.A. Doyle et al., *Science* 280:69–77, 1998.)

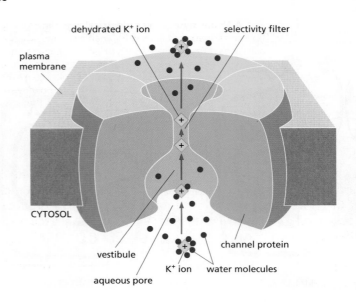

The aquaporins discussed earlier, for example, facilitate the flow of water across the plasma membrane of some prokaryotic and eukaryotic cells. These pores are structured in such a way that they allow the passive diffusion of uncharged water molecules, while prohibiting the movement of ions, including even the smallest ion, H^+.

The bulk of a cell's channels facilitate the passage of select inorganic ions. It is these ion channels that we discuss in this section.

Ion Channels Are Ion-selective and Gated

Two important properties distinguish **ion channels** from simple holes in the membrane. First, they show *ion selectivity*, permitting some inorganic ions to pass but not others. Ion selectivity depends on the diameter and shape of the ion channel and on the distribution of the charged amino acids that line it. Each ion in aqueous solution is surrounded by a small shell of water molecules, most of which have to be shed for the ions to pass, in single file, through the selectivity filter in the narrowest part of the ion channel (**Figure 12–19**). An ion channel is narrow enough in places to force ions into contact with the channel wall, so that only those ions of appropriate size and charge are able to pass (**Movie 12.6**).

The second important distinction between ion channels and simple holes in the membrane is that ion channels are not continuously open. Ion transport would be of no value to the cell if the many thousands of ion channels in a cell membrane were open all the time and there were no means of controlling the flow of ions through them. Instead, ion channels open only briefly and then close again (**Figure 12–20**). As we discuss later, most ion channels are *gated*: a specific stimulus triggers them to switch between a closed and an open state by inducing a change in their conformation.

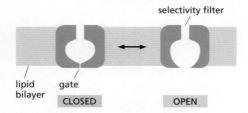

Figure 12–20 A typical ion channel fluctuates between closed and open conformations. The channel shown here in cross section forms a hydrophilic pore across the lipid bilayer only in the "open" conformation. As illustrated in Figure 12–19, the pore narrows to atomic dimensions in the selectivity filter, where the ion selectivity of the channel is largely determined.

Unlike a transporter, an ion channel does not need to undergo conformational changes for each ion it passes, and so it has a large advantage over a transporter with respect to its maximum rate of transport. More than a million ions can pass through an open channel each second, which is 1000 times greater than the fastest rate of transfer known for any transporter. On the other hand, channels cannot couple the ion flow to an energy source to carry out active transport; they simply make the membrane transiently permeable to selected inorganic ions, mainly Na^+, K^+, Ca^{2+}, or Cl^-.

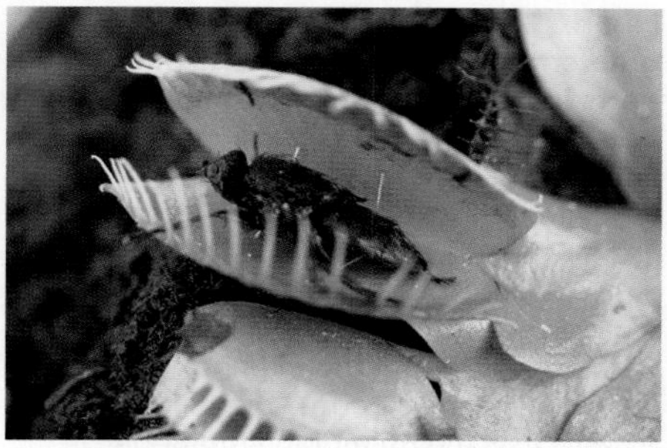

Figure 12–21 **A Venus flytrap uses electrical signaling to capture**

Figure 12–21 **A Venus flytrap uses electrical signaling to capture its prey.** The leaves snap shut in less than half a second when an insect moves across them. The response is triggered by touching any two of the three trigger hairs in succession in the center of each leaf. This mechanical stimulation opens ion channels in the plasma membrane and thereby sets off an electrical signal, which, by an unknown mechanism, leads to a rapid change in turgor pressure that closes the leaf. (Gabor Izso/Getty Images.)

Thanks to active transport by pumps, the concentrations of many ions are far from equilibrium across a cell membrane. When an ion channel opens, therefore, ions usually flow through it, moving rapidly down their electrochemical gradients. This rapid shift of ions changes the membrane potential, as we discuss next.

Membrane Potential Is Governed by the Permeability of a Membrane to Specific Ions

Changes in membrane potential are the basis of electrical signaling in many types of cells, whether they are the nerve or muscle cells in animals, or the touch-sensitive cells of a carnivorous plant (**Figure 12–21**). Such electrical changes are mediated by alterations in the permeability of membranes to ions. As we saw earlier, in an animal cell that is in an unstimulated, or "resting," state, the negative charges on the many types of organic molecules found inside the cell are largely balanced by K^+, the predominant intracellular ion (see Table 12–1). K^+ is continuously imported into the cell by the Na^+ pump, which generates a K^+ gradient across the plasma membrane as it pumps Na^+ out and K^+ in (see Figure 12–11).

The plasma membrane, however, also contains a set of K^+ channels, known as **K^+ leak channels**, that allow K^+ to move freely across the membrane. In a resting cell, these are the main ion channels open in the plasma membrane, rendering the membrane much more permeable to K^+ than to other ions. When K^+ flows out of the cell—down the concentration gradient generated by the ceaseless operation of the Na^+ pump—the loss of positive charge inside the cell creates a voltage difference, or membrane potential (**Figure 12–22**). Because this charge imbalance will oppose any further movement of K^+ out of the cell, an equilibrium condition is established in which the membrane potential keeping K^+ inside the cell is just strong enough to counteract the tendency of K^+ to move down its concentration gradient and out of the cell. In this state of equilibrium,

Figure 12–22 **The distribution of ions on either side of a cell membrane gives rise to its membrane potential.** The membrane potential results from a thin (<1 nm) layer of ions close to the membrane, held in place by their electrical attraction to oppositely charged ions on the other side of the membrane. (A) When there is an exact balance of charges on either side of the membrane, there is no membrane potential. (B) When ions of one type cross the membrane, they establish a charge difference across the two sides of the membrane that creates a membrane potential. The number of ions that must move across the membrane to set up a membrane potential is a tiny fraction of all those present on either side. In the case of the plasma membrane in animal cells, for example, 6000 K^+ ions crossing 1 μm^2 of membrane are enough to shift the membrane potential by about 100 mV; the number of K^+ ions in 1 μm^3 of cytosol is 70,000 times larger than this.

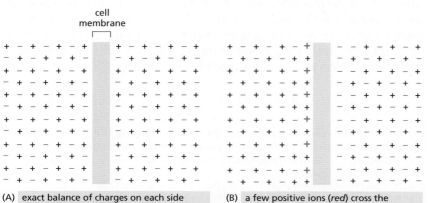

cell membrane

(A) exact balance of charges on each side of the membrane: membrane potential = 0

(B) a few positive ions (*red*) cross the membrane from right to left, setting up a nonzero membrane potential

Figure 12–23 The K$^+$ concentration gradient and K$^+$ leak channels play major parts in generating the resting membrane potential across the plasma membrane in animal cells. (A) A hypothetical situation in which the K$^+$ leak channels are closed and the membrane potential is zero. (B) As soon as the channels open, K$^+$ will tend to leave the cell, moving down its concentration gradient. Assuming the membrane contains no open channels permeable to other ions, K$^+$ will cross the membrane but negative ions will be unable to follow. The resulting charge imbalance gives rise to a membrane potential that tends to drive K$^+$ back into the cell. At equilibrium, the effect of the K$^+$ concentration gradient is exactly balanced by the effect of the membrane potential, and there is no net movement of K$^+$ across the membrane.

The Na$^+$ pump (not shown here) also contributes to the resting potential—both by helping to establish the K$^+$ gradient and by pumping 3 Na$^+$ ions out of the cell for every 2 K$^+$ ions it pumps in (see Figure 12–11). Moving one more positively charged ion out of the cell with each pumping cycle helps to keep the inside of the cell more negative than the outside.

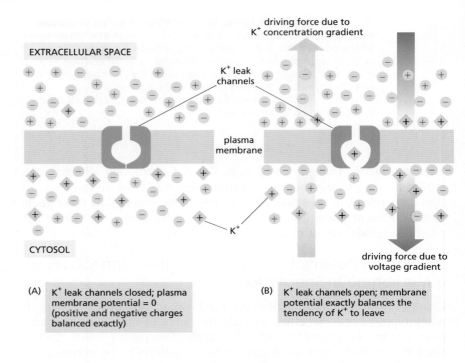

EXTRACELLULAR SPACE

driving force due to K$^+$ concentration gradient

K$^+$ leak channels

plasma membrane

driving force due to voltage gradient

K$^+$

CYTOSOL

(A)   K$^+$ leak channels closed; plasma membrane potential = 0 (positive and negative charges balanced exactly)

(B)   K$^+$ leak channels open; membrane potential exactly balances the tendency of K$^+$ to leave

the electrochemical gradient for K$^+$ is zero, even though there is still a much higher concentration of K$^+$ inside the cell than out (**Figure 12–23**).

The membrane potential in such steady-state conditions—in which the flow of positive and negative ions across the plasma membrane is precisely balanced, so that no further difference in charge accumulates across the membrane—is called the **resting membrane potential**. A simple formula called the **Nernst equation** expresses this equilibrium quantitatively and makes it possible to calculate the theoretical resting membrane potential if the ion concentrations on either side of the membrane are known (**Figure 12–24**). In animal cells, the resting membrane potential—which varies between –20 and –200 mV—is chiefly a reflection of the electrochemical K$^+$ gradient across the plasma membrane, because, at rest, the plasma membrane is chiefly permeable to K$^+$, and K$^+$ is the main positive ion inside the cell.

When a cell is stimulated, other ion channels in the plasma membrane open, changing the membrane's permeability to those ions. Whether the ions enter or leave the cell depends on the direction of their electrochemical gradients. Thus the membrane potential at any time depends on both the state of the membrane's ion channels and the ion concentrations on either side of the plasma membrane. Bulk changes in ion concentrations cannot occur quickly enough to drive the rapid changes in membrane potential that are associated with electrical signaling. Instead, it is the rapid opening and closing of ion channels, which occurs within milliseconds, that matters most for this type of cell signaling.

The force tending to drive an ion across a membrane is made up of two components: one due to the electrical membrane potential and one due to the concentration gradient of the ion. At equilibrium, the two forces are balanced and satisfy a simple mathematical relationship given by the

Nernst equation

$$V = 62 \log_{10}(C_o / C_i)$$

where V is the membrane potential in millivolts, and C_o and C_i are the outside and inside concentrations of the ion, respectively. This form of the equation assumes that the ion carries a single positive charge and that the temperature is 37°C.

Figure 12–24 The Nernst equation can be used to calculate the contribution of each ion to the resting potential of the membrane. The relevant ion concentrations are those on either side of the membrane. From this equation, we see that each tenfold change in the ion concentration ratio (C_o/C_i) across the membrane alters the membrane potential by 62 millivolts. The resting potential can then be calculated by combining the individual ion gradient contributions and adjusting for the relative permeability for each ion.

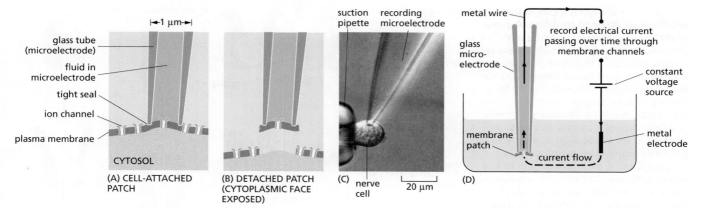

(A) CELL-ATTACHED PATCH

(B) DETACHED PATCH (CYTOPLASMIC FACE EXPOSED)

(C) nerve cell 20 μm

(D)

Figure 12–25 **Patch-clamp recording is used to monitor ion channel activity.** First, a microelectrode is filled with an aqueous conducting solution, and its tip is pressed against the surface of the cell. (A) With gentle suction, a tight seal is formed where the cell membrane contacts the mouth of the microelectrode. Because of the extremely tight seal, current can enter or leave the microelectrode only by passing through the ion channel or channels in the patch of membrane covering its tip. (B) To expose the cytosolic face of the membrane, the patch of membrane held in the microelectrode can be torn from the cell. This technique makes it easy to alter the composition of the solution on either side of the membrane to test the effect of various solutes on channel activity. (C) A micrograph showing an isolated nerve cell held in a suction pipette (the tip of which is shown on the left), while a microelectrode is being used for patch-clamp recording. (D) The circuitry for patch-clamp recording. At the open end of the microelectrode, a metal wire is inserted. Current that enters the microelectrode through ion channels in the small patch of membrane covering its tip passes via the wire, through measuring instruments, back into the bath of medium surrounding the cell or the detached patch. (C, from T.D. Lamb, H.R. Matthews, and V. Torre, *J. Physiol.* 372:315–349, 1986. With permission from Blackwell Publishing.)

Ion Channels Randomly Snap Between Open and Closed States

Measuring changes in electrical current is the main method used to study ion movements and ion channels in living cells. Amazingly, electrical recording techniques can detect and measure the current flowing through a single channel molecule. The procedure developed for doing this is known as **patch-clamp recording**, and it provides a direct and surprising picture of how individual ion channels behave.

In patch-clamp recording, a fine glass tube is used as a *microelectrode* to isolate and make electrical contact with a small area of the membrane at the surface of the cell (**Figure 12–25**). When a sufficiently small area of membrane is trapped in the patch, sometimes only a single ion channel will be present. Modern electrical instruments are sensitive enough to monitor the ion flow through this single channel, detected as a minute electric current (of the order of 10^{-12} ampere or 1 picoampere).

Monitoring individual ion channels in this way revealed something surprising about the way they behave: even when conditions are held constant, the currents abruptly appear and disappear, as though an on/ off switch were being jiggled randomly (**Figure 12–26**). This behavior

Figure 12–26 **The behavior of a single ion channel can be observed using the patch-clamp technique.** The voltage (the membrane potential) across the isolated patch of membrane is held constant during the recording. (A) In this example, the neurotransmitter acetylcholine is present, and the membrane patch from a muscle cell contains a single channel protein that is responsive to acetylcholine (discussed later, see Figure 12–42). This ion channel opens to allow passage of positive ions when acetylcholine binds to the exterior face of the channel. But even when acetylcholine is bound to the channel, as is the case during the three channel openings shown here, the channel does not remain open all the time. Instead, it flickers between open and closed states. Note that how long the channel remains open is variable. (B) When acetylcholine is not present, the channel opens very rarely. (Courtesy of David Colquhoun.)

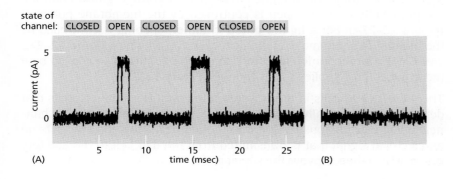

state of channel: CLOSED OPEN CLOSED OPEN CLOSED OPEN

current (pA)

5

0

5   10   15   20   25
time (msec)

(A)   (B)

Figure 12–27 Different types of gated ion channels respond to different types of stimuli. Depending on the type of channel, the probability of gate opening is controlled by (A) a change in the voltage difference across the membrane, (B) the binding of a chemical ligand to the extracellular face of a channel, (C) ligand binding to the intracellular face of a channel, or (D) mechanical stress. In the case of the voltage-gated channels, positively charged amino acids (*white* plus signs) in the channel's voltage sensor domains become attracted to negative charges on the extracellular surface of the depolarized plasma membrane, pulling the channel into its open conformation.

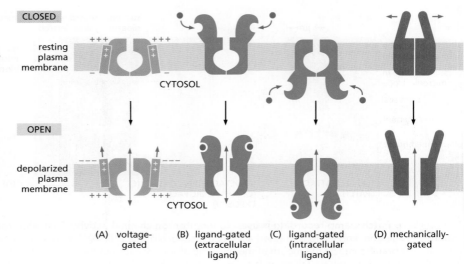

(A) voltage-gated   (B) ligand-gated (extracellular ligand)   (C) ligand-gated (intracellular ligand)   (D) mechanically-gated

indicates that the channel has moving parts and is snapping back and forth between open and closed conformations as the channel is knocked from one conformation to the other by the random thermal movements of the molecules in its environment. Patch-clamp recording was the first technique that could detect such conformational changes, and the picture it paints—of a jerky piece of machinery subjected to constant external buffeting—is now known to apply also to other proteins with moving parts.

The activity of each ion channel is very much "all-or-none": when an ion channel is open, it is fully open; when it is closed, it is fully closed. That raises a fundamental question: If ion channels randomly snap between open and closed conformations even when conditions on each side of the membrane are held constant, how can their state be regulated by conditions inside or outside the cell? The answer is that when the appropriate conditions change, the random behavior continues but with a greatly changed bias: if the altered conditions tend to open the channel, for example, the channel will now spend a much greater proportion of its time in the open conformation, although it will not remain open continuously (see Figure 12–26).

Different Types of Stimuli Influence the Opening and Closing of Ion Channels

There are more than a hundred types of ion channels, and even simple organisms can possess many different types. The human genome contains 80 genes that encode different but related K^+ channels alone. Ion channels differ from one another primarily with respect to their *ion selectivity*—the type of ions they allow to pass—and their *gating*—the conditions that influence their opening and closing. For a **voltage-gated channel**, the probability of being open is controlled by the membrane potential (Figure 12–27A). For a **ligand-gated channel**, opening is controlled by the binding of some molecule (a ligand) to the channel (Figure 12–27B and C). For a **mechanically-gated channel**, opening is controlled by a mechanical force applied to the channel (Figure 12–27D).

The *auditory hair* cells in the ear are an important example of cells that depend on mechanically-gated channels. Sound vibrations pull the channels open, causing ions to flow into the hair cells; this ion flow sets up an electrical signal that is transmitted from the hair cell to the auditory nerve, which then conveys the signal to the brain (Figure 12–28).

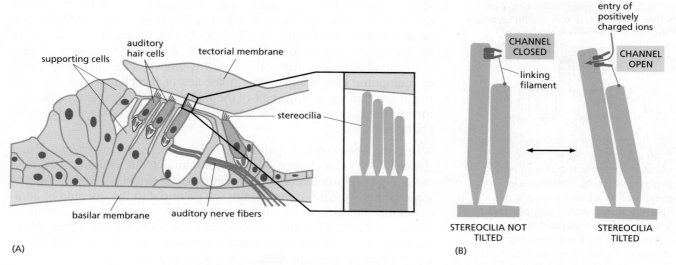

(A)

(B)

Figure 12–28 Mechanically-gated ion channels allow us to hear. (A) A section through the organ of Corti, which runs the length of the cochlea, the auditory portion of the inner ear. Each auditory hair cell has a tuft of spiky extensions called stereocilia projecting from its upper surface. The hair cells are embedded in an epithelial sheet of supporting cells, which is sandwiched between the *basilar membrane* below and the *tectorial membrane* above. (These are not lipid bilayer membranes but sheets of extracellular matrix.) (B) Sound vibrations cause the basilar membrane to vibrate up and down, causing the stereocilia to tilt. Each stereocilium in the staggered array of stereocilia on a hair cell is attached to the next, shorter stereocilium by a fine filament. The tilting stretches the filaments, which pull open mechanically-gated ion channels in the stereocilium plasma membrane, allowing positively charged ions to enter from the surrounding fluid (Movie 12.7). The influx of ions activates the hair cells, which stimulate underlying nerve endings of the auditory nerve fibers that relay the auditory signal to the brain.

The hair-cell mechanism is astonishingly sensitive: the faintest sounds we can hear have been estimated to stretch the filaments by an average of about 0.04 nm, which is less than the diameter of a hydrogen ion (Movie 12.8).

Voltage-gated Ion Channels Respond to the Membrane Potential

Voltage-gated ion channels play a major role in propagating electrical signals along all nerve cell extensions, such as those that relay signals from our brain to our toe muscles. But voltage-gated ion channels are present in many other cell types, too, including muscle cells, egg cells, protozoans, and even plant cells, where they enable electrical signals to travel from one part of the plant to another, as in the leaf-closing response of a *Mimosa pudica* plant (Figure 12–29).

Voltage-gated ion channels have domains called *voltage sensors* that are extremely sensitive to changes in the membrane potential: changes

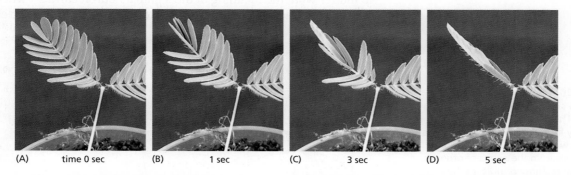

(A) time 0 sec (B) 1 sec (C) 3 sec (D) 5 sec

Figure 12–29 Both mechanically-gated and voltage-gated ion channels underlie the leaf-closing response in the touch-sensitive plant *Mimosa pudica*. (A) Resting leaf. (B–D) Successive leaflet closures in response to touch. A few seconds after the leaf on the left is touched, its leaflets snap shut. The response involves the opening of mechanically-gated ion channels in touch-sensitive sensory cells, which then pass a signal to cells containing voltage-gated ion channels, generating an electric impulse. When the impulse reaches specialized hinge cells at the base of each leaflet, a rapid loss of water by these cells occurs, causing the leaflets to fold into a closed conformation suddenly and progressively down the leaf stalk (Movie 12.9).

QUESTION 12–3

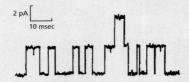

The figure above shows a recording from a patch-clamp experiment in which the electrical current passing across a patch of membrane is measured as a function of time. The membrane patch was plucked from the plasma membrane of a muscle cell by the technique shown in Figure 12–25 and contains molecules of the acetylcholine receptor, which is a ligand-gated cation channel that is opened by the binding of acetylcholine to the extracellular face of the channel. To obtain a recording, acetylcholine was added to the solution inside the microelectrode. (A) Describe what you can learn about the channels from this recording. (B) How would the recording differ if acetylcholine were (i) omitted or (ii) added to the solution outside the microelectrode only?

above a certain threshold value exert sufficient electrical force on these domains to encourage the channel to switch from its closed to its open conformation (see Figure 12–27A). As discussed earlier, a change in the membrane potential does not affect how wide the channel is open, but instead alters the probability that it will open. Thus, in a large patch of membrane containing many molecules of the channel protein, one might find that on average 10% of them are open at any instant when the membrane is at one potential, whereas 90% are open after this potential changes.

When one type of voltage-gated ion channel opens, the membrane potential of the cell can change. This in turn can activate or inactivate other voltage-gated ion channels. Such circuits, which couple the opening of ion channels to changes in membrane potential to the opening of additional ion channels, are fundamental to all electrical signaling in cells. In the next section, we consider the special case of nerve cells: they—more than any other cell type—have made a profession of electrical signaling, and they employ ion channels in very sophisticated ways.

ION CHANNELS AND NERVE CELL SIGNALING

The fundamental task of a nerve cell, or **neuron**, is to receive, integrate, and transmit signals. Neurons carry signals from sense organs, such as eyes and ears, to the *central nervous system*—the brain and spinal cord. In the central nervous system, neurons signal from one to another through networks of enormous complexity, allowing the brain and spinal cord to analyze, interpret, and respond to the signals coming in from the sense organs.

Every neuron consists of a *cell body*, which contains the nucleus and has a number of long, thin extensions radiating outward from it. Usually, a neuron has one long extension called an **axon**, which conducts electrical signals away from the cell body toward distant target cells; it also usually has several shorter, branching extensions called **dendrites**, which radiate from the cell body like antennae and provide an enlarged surface area to receive signals from the axons of other neurons (**Figure 12–30**). The axon commonly divides at its far end into many branches, each of which ends in a **nerve terminal**, so that the neuron's message can be passed simultaneously to many target cells—muscle or gland cells or other neurons. Likewise, the branching of the dendrites can be extensive, in some cases sufficient to receive as many as 100,000 inputs on a single neuron (see Figure 12–43A).

No matter what the meaning of the signal a neuron carries—whether it is visual information from the eye, a motor command to a muscle, or one

Figure 12–30 A typical neuron has a cell body, a single axon, and multiple dendrites. The axon conducts electrical signals away from the cell body toward its target cells, while the multiple dendrites receive signals from the axons of other neurons. The *red* arrows indicate the direction in which signals travel. During brain development, neurons probe their environment for guidance clues to extend axons and dendrites in appropriate directions to make useful connections (**Movies 12.10 and 12.11**).

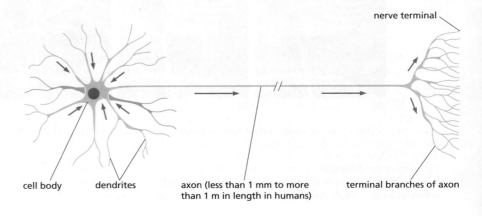

Figure 12–31 **The squid *Loligo* has a nervous system that is adept at responding rapidly to threats in the animal's environment.** Among the nerve cells that make up this escape system is one that possesses a "giant axon," with a very large diameter. Long before patch clamping allowed recordings from single ion channels in small cells (see Figure 12–25), the squid giant axon was routinely used to record and study action potentials. (NOAA.)

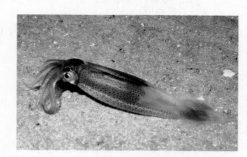

step in a complex network of neural processing in the brain—the form of the signal is always the same: it consists of changes in the electrical potential across the neuron's plasma membrane.

Action Potentials Allow Rapid Long-Distance Communication Along Axons

A neuron is stimulated by a signal—typically from another neuron—delivered to a localized site on its surface. This signal initiates a change in the membrane potential at that site. To transmit the signal onward, this local change in membrane potential has to spread from this initial site, which is usually on a dendrite or the cell body, to the axon terminals. There, the signal is relayed to the next cells in the pathway—forming a *neural circuit*. The distances covered by such circuits can be substantial: a signal that leaves a motor neuron in your spinal cord may have to travel a meter or more before it reaches a muscle in your foot.

The local change in membrane potential generated by a signal will spread passively along an axon or a dendrite to adjacent regions of the plasma membrane. Over long distances, such *passive spread* is inadequate, as the signal rapidly becomes weaker with increasing distance from the source. Neurons solve this long-distance communication problem by employing an active signaling mechanism. In this case, a local electrical stimulus of sufficient strength triggers a burst of electrical activity in the plasma membrane that propagates rapidly along the membrane of the axon, continuously renewing itself all along the way. This traveling wave of electrical excitation, known as an **action potential**, or a *nerve impulse*, can carry a message, without weakening, all the way from one end of a neuron to the other, at speeds of up to 100 meters per second.

The early research that established this mechanism of electrical signaling along axons was done on the giant axon of the squid (**Figure 12–31**). This axon has such a large diameter that it is possible to record its electrical activity from an electrode inserted directly into it (**How We Know**, pp. 412–413). From such studies, it was deduced how action potentials are the direct consequence of the properties of voltage-gated ion channels in the axonal plasma membrane, as we now explain.

Action Potentials Are Mediated by Voltage-gated Cation Channels

When a neuron is stimulated, the membrane potential of the plasma membrane shifts to a less negative value (that is, toward zero). If this **depolarization** is sufficiently large, it will cause **voltage-gated Na⁺ channels** in the membrane to open transiently at the site. As these channels flicker open, they allow a small amount of Na^+ to enter the cell down its steep electrochemical gradient. The influx of positive charge depolarizes the membrane further (that is, it makes the membrane potential even less negative), thereby opening additional voltage-gated Na⁺ channels and causing still further depolarization. This process continues in an explosive, self-amplifying fashion until, within about a millisecond, the membrane potential in the local region of the neuron's plasma

---

QUESTION 12–4

Using the Nernst equation and the ion concentrations given in Table 12–1 (p. 391), calculate the equilibrium membrane potential of K^+ and Na^+—that is, the membrane potential where there would be no net movement of the ion across the plasma membrane (assume that the concentration of intracellular Na^+ is 10 mM). What membrane potential would you predict in a resting animal cell? Explain your answer. What would happen if a large number of Na⁺ channels suddenly opened, making the membrane much more permeable to Na^+ than to K^+? (Note that because few ions need to move across the membrane to change drastically the charge distribution across that membrane, you can safely assume that the ion concentrations on either side of the membrane do not change significantly.) What would you predict would happen next if the Na⁺ channels closed again?

HOW WE KNOW

SQUID REVEAL SECRETS OF MEMBRANE EXCITABILITY

Each spring, *Loligo pealei* migrate to the shallow waters off Cape Cod on the eastern coast of the United States. There they spawn, launching the next generation of squid. But more than just meeting and breeding, these animals provide neuroscientists summering at the Marine Biological Laboratory in Woods Hole, Massachusetts, with a golden opportunity to study the mechanism of electrical signaling along nerve axons.

Like most animals, squid survive by catching prey and escaping predators. Fast reflexes and an ability to accelerate rapidly and make sudden changes in swimming direction help them avoid danger while chasing down a decent meal. Squid derive their speed and agility from a specialized biological jet propulsion system: they draw water into their mantle cavity and then contract their muscular body wall to expel the collected water rapidly through a tubular siphon, thus propelling themselves through the water.

Controlling such quick and coordinated muscle contraction requires a nervous system that can convey signals with great speed down the length of the animal's body. Indeed, *Loligo pealei* possesses some of the largest nerve cell axons found in nature. Squid giant axons can reach 10 cm in length and are over 100 times the diameter of a mammalian axon—about the width of a pencil lead. Generally speaking, the larger the diameter of an axon, the more rapidly signals can travel along its length.

In the 1930s, scientists first started to take advantage of the squid giant axon for studying the electrophysiology of the nerve cell. Because of its relatively large size, an investigator can isolate an individual axon and insert an electrode into it to measure the axon's membrane potential and monitor its electrical activity. This experimental system allowed researchers to address a variety of questions, including which ions are important for establishing the resting membrane potential and for initiating and propagating an action potential, and how changes in the membrane potential control ion permeability.

Set-up for action

Because the squid axon is so long and wide, an electrode made from a glass capillary tube containing a conducting solution can be thrust down the axis of the isolated axon so that its tip lies deep in the cytoplasm. This set-up allowed investigators to measure the voltage difference between the inside and the outside of the axon—that is, the membrane potential—as an action potential sweeps past the tip of the electrode (**Figure 12–32**). The action potential itself would be triggered by applying a brief electrical stimulus to one end of the axon. It didn't matter which end was stimulated, as the action potential could travel in either direction; it also didn't matter how big the stimulus was, as long as it exceeded a certain threshold (see Figure 12–35), indicating that an action potential is an "all or nothing" response.

Once researchers could reliably generate and measure an action potential, they could use the preparation to answer other questions about membrane excitability. For example, which ions are critical for an action potential? The three most plentiful ions, both inside and outside an axon, are Na$^+$, K$^+$, and Cl$^-$. Do they have

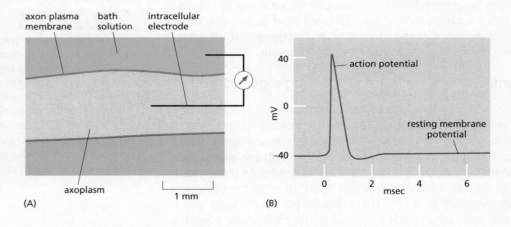

Figure 12–32 Scientists can study nerve cell excitability using an isolated axon from squid. (A) An electrode can be inserted into the cytoplasm (axoplasm) of a squid giant axon to (B) measure the resting membrane potential and monitor action potentials induced when the axon is electrically stimulated.

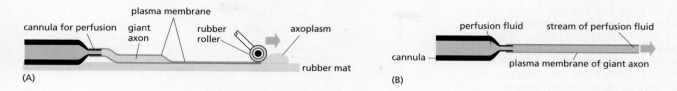

Figure 12–33 The cytoplasm in a squid axon can be removed and replaced with an artificial solution of pure ions. (A) The axon cytoplasm (axoplasm) is extruded using a rubber roller. (B) A perfusion fluid containing the desired concentration of ions is pumped gently through the emptied-out axon.

equal importance when it comes to the action potential? Because the squid axon is so large and strong, investigators could extrude the cytoplasm from the axon like toothpaste from a tube (**Figure 12–33A**). The emptied-out axon could then be reinflated by filling it with a pure solution of Na^+, K^+, or Cl^- (**Figure 12–33B**). Thus, the ions inside the axon and in the bath solution could be varied independently (see Figure 12–32A). Using this set-up, the researchers discovered that the axon would generate a normal action potential if, and only if, the concentrations of Na^+ and K^+ approximated the natural concentrations found inside and outside the cell. Thus, they concluded that the cell components crucial to the action potential are the plasma membrane, Na^+ and K^+ ions, and the energy provided by the concentration gradients of these ions across the membrane; all other components, including other sources of metabolic energy, were presumably removed when the axon was emptied and refilled.

Channel traffic

Once Na^+ and K^+ had been singled out as critical for an action potential, the questions then became: What does each of these ions contribute to the action potential? How permeable is the membrane to each, and how does the membrane permeability change as an action potential sweeps by? Again, the squid giant axon provided some answers. The concentrations of Na^+ and K^+ inside and outside the axon could be altered, and the effects of these changes on the membrane potential could be measured directly. From such studies, it was determined that, at rest, the membrane potential of an axon is close to the equilibrium potential for K^+: when the external concentration of K^+ was varied, the resting potential of the axon changed roughly in accordance with the Nernst equation (see Figure 12–24). The results suggested that at rest, the membrane is chiefly permeable to K^+; we now know that K^+ leak channels provide the main pathway that these ions can take through the resting plasma membrane.

The situation for Na^+ is very different. When the external concentration of Na^+ was varied, there was no effect on the resting potential of the axon. However, the height of the peak of the action potential varied with the concentration of Na^+ outside the axon (**Figure 12–34**). During the action potential, therefore, the membrane appeared to be chiefly permeable to Na^+, presumably as the result of the opening of Na^+ channels. In the aftermath of the action potential, the Na^+ permeability decreased and the membrane potential reverted to a negative value, which depended on the external concentration of K^+. As the membrane lost its permeability to Na^+, it became even more permeable to K^+ than before, presumably because additional K^+ channels opened, accelerating the resetting of the membrane potential to the resting state, and readying the membrane for the next action potential.

These studies on the squid giant axon made an enormous contribution to our understanding of nerve cell excitability, and the researchers who made these discoveries in the 1940s and 1950s—Alan Hodgkin and Andrew Huxley—received a Nobel Prize in 1963. However, it was years before the various ion channel proteins that they had hypothesized to exist would be biochemically identified. We now know the three-dimensional structures of many of these channel proteins, allowing us to marvel at the fundamental beauty of these molecular machines.

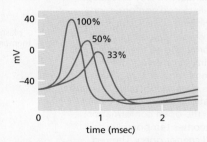

Figure 12–34 The shape of the action potential depends on the concentration of Na^+ outside the squid axon. Shown here are action potentials recorded when the external medium contains 100%, 50%, or 33% of the normal extracellular concentration of Na^+.

Figure 12–35 An action potential is triggered by a depolarization of a neuron's plasma membrane. The resting membrane potential in this neuron is –60 mV, and a stimulus that depolarizes the plasma membrane to about –40 mV (the threshold potential) is applied. This depolarizing stimulus is sufficient to open voltage-gated Na⁺ channels in the membrane and thereby trigger an action potential. As the membrane rapidly depolarizes further, the membrane potential (*red* curve) swings past zero, reaching +40 mV before it returns to its resting negative value as the action potential terminates. The *green* curve shows how the membrane potential would simply have relaxed back to the resting value after the initial depolarizing stimulus if there had been no amplification by voltage-gated ion channels in the plasma membrane.

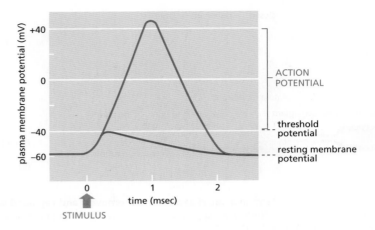

Figure 12–36 A voltage-gated Na⁺ channel can flip from one conformation to another, depending on the membrane potential. When the membrane is at rest and highly polarized, positively charged amino acids in the voltage sensors of the channel (*red* bars) are oriented by the membrane potential in a way that keeps the channel in its closed conformation. When the membrane is depolarized, the voltage sensors shift, changing the channel's conformation so the channel has a high probability of opening. But in the depolarized membrane, the inactivated conformation is even more stable than the open conformation, and so, after a brief period spent in the open conformation, the channel becomes temporarily inactivated and cannot open. The *red* arrows indicate the sequence that follows a sudden depolarization, and the *black* arrow indicates the return to the original conformation after the membrane has repolarized.

membrane has shifted from its resting value of about –60 mV to about +40 mV (**Figure 12–35**).

The voltage of +40 mV is close to the membrane potential at which the electrochemical driving force for movement of Na⁺ across the membrane is zero—that is, the effects of the membrane potential and the concentration gradient for Na⁺ are equal and opposite; therefore Na⁺ has no further tendency to enter or leave the cell.

If these voltage-gated channels continued to respond to the depolarized membrane potential, the cell would get stuck with most of its Na⁺ channels open. The cell is saved from this fate because voltage-gated Na⁺ channels have an automatic inactivating mechanism—a kind of "timer" that causes them to rapidly adopt (within a millisecond or so) a special inactivated conformation in which the channel is closed, even though the membrane is still depolarized. The Na⁺ channels remain in this *inactivated state* until the membrane potential has returned to its resting, negative value. A schematic illustration of these three distinct states of the voltage-gated Na⁺ channel—*closed*, *open*, and *inactivated*—is shown in **Figure 12–36**. How they contribute to the rise and fall of an action potential is shown in **Figure 12–37**.

During an action potential, voltage-gated Na⁺ channels do not act alone. The depolarized axonal membrane is helped to return to its resting potential by the opening of *voltage-gated K⁺ channels*. These also open in response to depolarization, but not as promptly as the Na⁺ channels, and they stay open as long as the membrane remains depolarized. As the local depolarization reaches its peak, K⁺ ions (carrying positive charge) therefore start to flow out of the cell, down their electrochemical gradient,

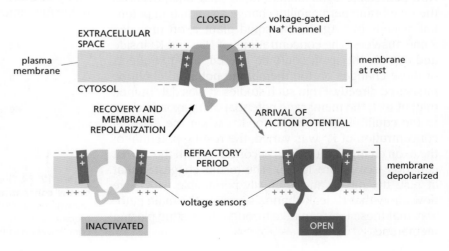

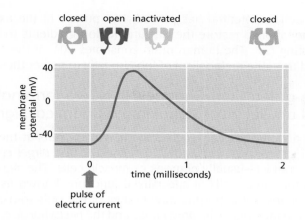

Figure 12–37 Voltage-gated Na⁺ channels change their conformation during an action potential. In this example, the action potential is triggered by a brief pulse of electric current (arrow), which partially depolarizes the membrane, as shown in the plot of membrane potential versus time. The course of the action potential reflects the opening and subsequent inactivation of voltage-gated Na⁺ channels, as shown (*top*). Even if restimulated, the plasma membrane cannot produce a second action potential until the Na⁺ channels have returned from the inactivated to the closed conformation (see Figure 12–36). Until then, the membrane is resistant, or refractory, to stimulation.

through these newly opened K⁺ channels—temporarily unhindered by the negative membrane potential that normally restrains them in the resting cell. The rapid outflow of K⁺ through the voltage-gated K⁺ channels brings the membrane back to its resting state much more quickly than could be achieved by K⁺ outflow through the K⁺ leak channels alone.

Once it begins, the self-amplifying depolarization of a small patch of plasma membrane quickly spreads outward: the Na⁺ flowing in through open Na⁺ channels begins to depolarize the neighboring region of the membrane, which then goes through the same self-amplifying cycle. In this way, an action potential spreads outward as a traveling wave from the initial site of depolarization, eventually reaching the axon terminals (**Figure 12–38**).

QUESTION 12–5

Explain as precisely as you can, but in no more than 100 words, the ionic basis of an action potential and how it is passed along an axon.

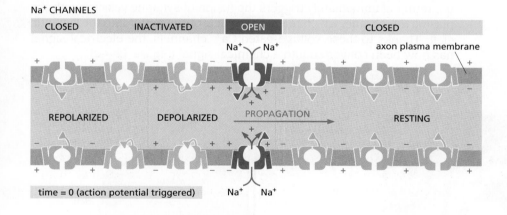

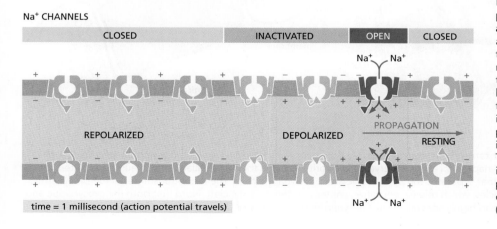

Figure 12–38 An action potential propagates along the length of an axon. The changes in the Na⁺ channels and the consequent flow of Na⁺ across the membrane (*red* arrows) alters the membrane potential and gives rise to the traveling action potential, as shown here and in **Movie 12.12**. The region of the axon with a depolarized membrane is shaded in *blue*. Note that an action potential can only travel forward; that is, away from the site of depolarization. This is because Na⁺ channel inactivation in the aftermath of an action potential prevents the advancing front of depolarization from spreading backward (see also Figure 12–37).

Once an action potential has passed, Na$^+$ pumps in the axon plasma membrane labor to restore the Na$^+$ and K$^+$ ion gradients to their levels in the resting cell. The human brain consumes 20% of the total energy generated from the metabolism of food, mostly to power these pumps.

Voltage-gated Ca^{2+} Channels in Nerve Terminals Convert an Electrical Signal into a Chemical Signal

When an action potential reaches the *nerve terminals* at the end of an axon, the signal must somehow be relayed to the *target cells* that the terminals contact—usually neurons or muscle cells. The signal is transmitted to the target cells at specialized junctions known as **synapses**. At most synapses, the plasma membranes of the cells transmitting and receiving the message—the *presynaptic* and the *postsynaptic* cells, respectively—are separated from each other by a narrow *synaptic cleft* (typically 20 nm across), which the electrical signal cannot cross. To transmit the message across this gap, the electrical signal is converted into a chemical signal, in the form of a small, secreted signal molecule called a **neurotransmitter**. Neurotransmitters are stored in the nerve terminals within membrane-enclosed **synaptic vesicles** (**Figure 12–39**).

When an action potential reaches the nerve terminal, some of the synaptic vesicles fuse with the plasma membrane, releasing their neurotransmitter into the synaptic cleft. This link between the arrival of an action potential and the secretion of neurotransmitter involves the activation of yet another type of voltage-gated cation channel: *voltage-gated Ca^{2+} channels* located in the plasma membrane of the presynaptic nerve terminal. Because the Ca^{2+} concentration outside the nerve terminal is more than 1000 times greater than the free Ca^{2+} concentration in its cytosol (see Table 12–1), Ca^{2+} rushes into the nerve terminal through the open channels. The resulting increase in Ca^{2+} concentration in the cytosol of the terminal immediately triggers the fusion of synaptic vesicles with the plasma membrane, which releases the neurotransmitter into the synaptic cleft. Thanks to these voltage-gated Ca^{2+} channels, the electrical signal has now been converted into a chemical signal (**Figure 12–40**).

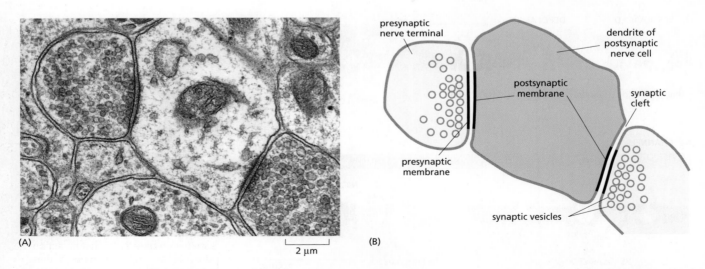

(A)   2 µm   (B)

Figure 12–39 Neurons connect to their target cells at synapses. (A) An electron micrograph and (B) a drawing of a cross section of two nerve terminals (*yellow*) forming synapses on a single nerve cell dendrite (*blue*) in the mammalian brain. Neurotransmitters carry the signal across the synaptic cleft that separates the presynaptic and postsynaptic cells. The neurotransmitter in the presynaptic terminal is contained within synaptic vesicles, which release neurotransmitter into the synaptic cleft. Note that both the presynaptic and postsynaptic membranes are thickened and highly specialized at the synapse. (A, courtesy of Cedric Raine.)

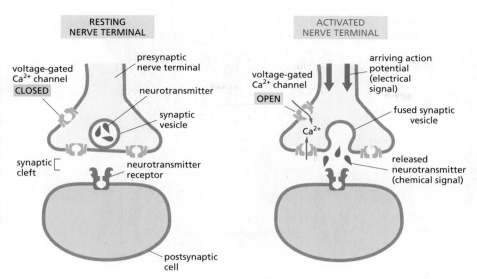

Figure 12–40 An electrical signal is converted into a secreted chemical signal at a nerve terminal. When an action potential reaches a nerve terminal, it opens voltage-gated Ca²⁺ channels in the plasma membrane, allowing Ca²⁺ to flow into the terminal. The increased Ca²⁺ in the nerve terminal stimulates the synaptic vesicles to fuse with the plasma membrane, releasing their neurotransmitter into the synaptic cleft—a process called exocytosis (discussed in Chapter 15).

Transmitter-gated Ion Channels in the Postsynaptic Membrane Convert the Chemical Signal Back into an Electrical Signal

The released neurotransmitter rapidly diffuses across the synaptic cleft and binds to *neurotransmitter receptors* concentrated in the plasma membrane of the postsynaptic target cell. Once released, neurotransmitters are rapidly removed from the synaptic cleft—either by enzymes that destroy them or by pumps that return them to the nerve terminal or that transport them into neighboring non-neuronal cells. This rapid removal of the neurotransmitter limits the duration and spread of the signal and ensures that when the presynaptic cell falls quiet, the postsynaptic cell will do the same.

Neurotransmitter receptors can be of various types; some mediate relatively slow effects in the target cell, whereas others trigger more rapid responses. Rapid responses—on a time scale of milliseconds—depend on receptors that are **transmitter-gated ion channels** (also called ion-channel-coupled receptors). These constitute a subclass of ligand-gated ion channels (see Figure 12–27B), and their function is to convert the chemical signal carried by a neurotransmitter back into an electrical signal. The channels open transiently in response to the binding of the neurotransmitter, thus changing the ion permeability of the postsynaptic membrane. This in turn causes a change in the membrane potential (**Figure 12–41**).

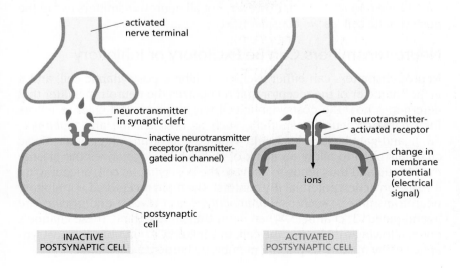

Figure 12–41 A chemical signal is converted into an electrical signal by postsynaptic transmitter-gated ion channels at a synapse. The released neurotransmitter binds to and opens the transmitter-gated ion channels in the plasma membrane of the postsynaptic cell. The resulting ion flows alter the membrane potential of the postsynaptic cell, thereby converting the chemical signal back into an electrical one (Movie 12.13).

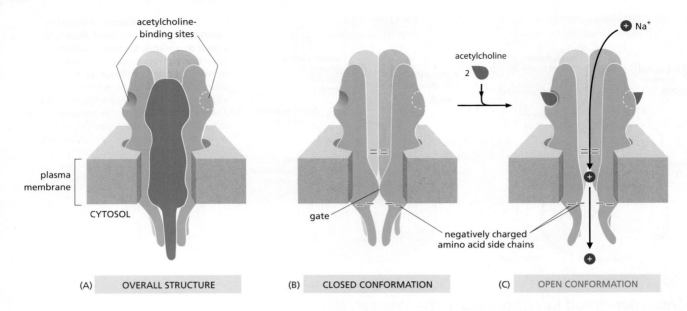

plasma membrane

CYTOSOL

(A) OVERALL STRUCTURE

(B) CLOSED CONFORMATION

(C) OPEN CONFORMATION

acetylcholine-binding sites

acetylcholine

gate

negatively charged amino acid side chains

Figure 12–42 The acetylcholine receptor in the plasma membrane of vertebrate skeletal muscle cells opens when it binds the neurotransmitter acetylcholine. (A) This transmitter-gated ion channel is composed of five transmembrane protein subunits, two of which (*green*) are identical. The subunits combine to form a transmitter-gated aqueous pore across the lipid bilayer. There are two acetylcholine-binding sites, one formed by parts of a *green* and *blue* subunit, the other by parts of a *green* and *orange* subunit, as shown. (B) The closed conformation. The *blue* subunit has been removed here and in (C) to show the interior of the pore. Negatively charged amino acid side chains at either end of the pore (indicated here by *red* minus signs) ensure that only positively charged ions, mainly Na^+ and K^+, can pass. But when acetylcholine is not bound and the channel is in its closed conformation, the pore is occluded (blocked) by hydrophobic amino acid side chains in the region called the gate. (C) The open conformation. When acetylcholine, released by a motor neuron, binds to both binding sites, the channel undergoes a conformational change; the hydrophobic side chains move apart and the gate opens, allowing Na^+ to flow across the membrane down its electrochemical gradient, depolarizing the membrane. Even with acetylcholine bound, the channel flickers randomly between the open and closed states (see Figure 12–26); without acetylcholine bound, the channel rarely opens.

QUESTION 12–6

In the disease myasthenia gravis, the human body makes—by mistake—antibodies to its own acetylcholine receptor molecules. These antibodies bind to and inactivate acetylcholine receptors on the plasma membrane of muscle cells. The disease leads to a devastating progressive weakening of the muscles of people affected. Early on, they may have difficulty opening their eyelids, for example, and, in an animal model of the disease, rabbits have difficulty holding their ears up. As the disease progresses, most muscles weaken, and people with myasthenia gravis have difficulty speaking and swallowing. Eventually, impaired breathing can cause death. Explain which step of muscle function is affected.

If the change is large enough, the postsynaptic membrane will depolarize and trigger an action potential in the postsynaptic cell.

A well-studied example of a neurotransmitter in action is found at the *neuromuscular junction*—the specialized synapse formed between a motor neuron and a skeletal muscle cell. In vertebrates, the neurotransmitter *acetylcholine* stimulates muscle contraction by binding to the *acetylcholine receptor*, a transmitter-gated ion channel in the muscle cell's membrane (**Figure 12–42**). However, not all neurotransmitters excite the postsynaptic cell, as we consider next.

Neurotransmitters Can Be Excitatory or Inhibitory

Neurotransmitters can either excite or inhibit a postsynaptic cell, and it is the character of the receptor that recognizes the neurotransmitter that determines how the postsynaptic cell will respond. The chief receptors for excitatory neurotransmitters, such as *acetylcholine* and *glutamate*, are ligand-gated cation channels. When a neurotransmitter binds, these channels open to allow an influx of Na^+, which depolarizes the plasma membrane and thus tends to activate the postsynaptic cell, encouraging it to fire an action potential. By contrast, the main receptors for inhibitory neurotransmitters, such as γ-*aminobutyric acid* (*GABA*) and *glycine*, are ligand-gated Cl^- channels. When neurotransmitters bind, these channels open, allowing Cl^- to enter the cell; this influx of Cl^- inhibits the postsynaptic cell by making its plasma membrane harder to depolarize.

TABLE 12–3 SOME EXAMPLES OF ION CHANNELS

Ion Channel	Typical Location	Function
K⁺ leak channel	plasma membrane of most animal cells	maintenance of resting membrane potential
Voltage-gated Na⁺ channel	plasma membrane of nerve cell axon	generation of action potentials
Voltage-gated K⁺ channel	plasma membrane of nerve cell axon	return of membrane to resting potential after initiation of an action potential
Voltage-gated Ca²⁺ channel	plasma membrane of nerve terminal	stimulation of neurotransmitter release
Acetylcholine receptor (acetylcholine-gated cation channel)	plasma membrane of muscle cell (at neuromuscular junction)	excitatory synaptic signaling
Glutamate receptor (glutamate-gated cation channel)	plasma membrane of many neurons (at synapses)	excitatory synaptic signaling
GABA receptor (GABA-gated Cl⁻ channel)	plasma membrane of many neurons (at synapses)	inhibitory synaptic signaling
Glycine receptor (glycine-gated Cl⁻ channel)	plasma membrane of many neurons (at synapses)	inhibitory synaptic signaling
Mechanically-gated cation channel	auditory hair cell in inner ear	detection of sound vibrations

Toxins that bind to any of these excitatory or inhibitory neurotransmitter receptors can have dramatic effects on an animal—or a human. *Curare*, for example, causes muscle paralysis by blocking excitatory acetylcholine receptors at the neuromuscular junction. This drug was used by South American Indians to make poison arrows and is still used by surgeons to relax muscles during an operation. By contrast, *strychnine*—a common ingredient in rat poisons—causes muscle spasms, convulsions, and death by blocking inhibitory glycine receptors on neurons in the brain and spinal cord.

The locations and functions of the ion channels discussed in this chapter are summarized in Table 12–3.

Most Psychoactive Drugs Affect Synaptic Signaling by Binding to Neurotransmitter Receptors

Many drugs used in the treatment of insomnia, anxiety, depression, and schizophrenia act by binding to transmitter-gated ion channels in the brain. Sedatives and tranquilizers such as barbiturates, Valium, Ambien, and Restoril, for example, bind to GABA-gated Cl⁻ channels. Their binding makes the channels easier to open by GABA, rendering the neuron more sensitive to GABA's inhibitory action. By contrast, the antidepressant Prozac blocks the Na⁺-driven symport responsible for the reuptake of the excitatory neurotransmitter *serotonin*, increasing the amount of serotonin available in the synapses that use it. This drug has changed the lives of many people who suffer from depression—although why boosting serotonin can elevate mood is still unknown.

QUESTION 12–7

When an inhibitory neurotransmitter such as GABA opens Cl⁻ channels in the plasma membrane of a postsynaptic neuron, why does this make it harder for an excitatory neurotransmitter to excite the neuron?

The number of distinct types of neurotransmitter receptors is very large, although they fall into a small number of families. There are, for example, many subtypes of acetylcholine, glutamate, GABA, glycine, and serotonin receptors; they are usually located on different neurons and often differ only subtly in their electrophysiological properties. With such a large variety of receptors, it may be possible to design a new generation of psychoactive drugs that will act more selectively on specific sets of neurons to mitigate the mental illnesses that devastate so many people's lives. One percent of the human population, for example, have schizophrenia, another 1% have bipolar disorder, about 1% have an autistic disorder, and many more suffer from anxiety or depressive disorders. The fact that these disorders are so prevalent suggests that the complexity of synaptic signaling may make the brain especially vulnerable to genetic alterations. But complexity also provides some distinct advantages, as we discuss next.

The Complexity of Synaptic Signaling Enables Us to Think, Act, Learn, and Remember

For a process so critical for animal survival, the mechanism that governs synaptic signaling seems unnecessarily cumbersome, as well as error-prone. For a signal to pass from one neuron to the next, the nerve terminal of the presynaptic cell must convert an electrical signal into a secreted chemical. This chemical signal must then diffuse across the synaptic cleft so that a postsynaptic cell can convert it back into an electric one. Why would evolution have favored such an apparently inefficient and vulnerable method for passing a signal between two cells? It would seem more efficient and robust to have a direct electrical connection between them—or to do away with the synapse altogether and use a single continuous cell.

The value of synapses that rely on secreted chemical signals becomes clear when we consider how they function in the context of the nervous system—an elaborate network of neurons, interconnected by many branching circuits, performing complex computations, storing memories, and generating plans for action. To carry out these functions, neurons have to do more than merely generate and relay signals: they must also combine them, interpret them, and record them. Chemical synapses make these activities possible. A motor neuron in the spinal cord, for example, receives inputs from hundreds or thousands of other neurons that make synapses on it (Figure 12–43). Some of these signals tend to

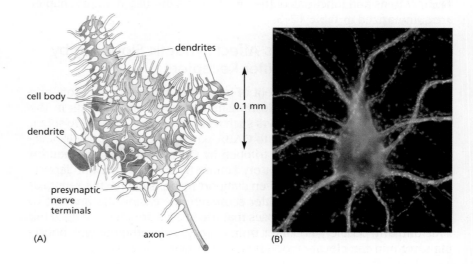

Figure 12–43 Thousands of synapses form on the cell body and dendrites of a motor neuron in the spinal cord. (A) Many thousands of nerve terminals synapse on this neuron, delivering signals from other parts of the animal to control the firing of action potentials along the neuron's axon. (B) A rat nerve cell in culture. Its cell body and dendrites (*green*) are stained with a fluorescent antibody that recognizes a cytoskeletal protein. Thousands of axon terminals (*red*) from other nerve cells (not visible) make synapses on the cell's surface; they are stained with a fluorescent antibody that recognizes a protein in synaptic vesicles, which are located in the nerve terminals (see Figure 12–39). (B, courtesy of Olaf Mundigl and Pietro de Camilli.)

dendrites

cell body

dendrite

presynaptic nerve terminals

axon

0.1 mm

(A)

(B)

stimulate the neuron, while others inhibit it. The motor neuron has to combine all of the information it receives and react, either by stimulating a muscle to contract or by remaining quiet.

This task of computing an appropriate output from a babble of inputs is achieved by a complicated interplay between different types of ion channels in the neuron's plasma membrane. Each of the hundreds of types of neurons in the brain has its own characteristic set of receptors and ion channels that enables the cell to respond in a particular way to a certain set of inputs and thus to perform its specialized task.

Ion channels are thus critical components of the machinery that enables us to act, think, feel, speak, learn, and remember. Given that these channels operate within neuronal circuits that are dauntingly complex, will we ever be able to deeply understand the molecular mechanisms that direct the complex behaviors of organisms such as ourselves? Although cracking this problem in humans is still far in the future, we now have increasingly powerful ways to study the neural circuits—and molecules—that underlie behavior in experimental animals. One of the most promising techniques makes use of a different type of ion channel, a light-gated ion channel borrowed from unicellular algae, as we now discuss.

Light-gated Ion Channels Can Be Used to Transiently Activate or Inactivate Neurons in Living Animals

Photosynthetic green algae use light-gated channels to sense and navigate toward sunlight. In response to blue light, one of these channels—called *channelrhodopsin*—allows Na^+ to flow into the cell. This depolarizes the plasma membrane and, ultimately, modulates the beating of the flagella that the organism uses to swim. Although these channels are peculiar to unicellular green algae, they function perfectly well when they are artificially transferred into other cell types, thereby rendering the recipient cells responsive to light.

Because nerve cells are also activated by a depolarizing influx of Na^+, as we have discussed (see Figure 12–38), channelrhodopsin can be used to manipulate the activity of neurons and neural circuits—including those in living animals. In one particularly stunning experiment, the channelrhodopsin gene was introduced into a select subpopulation of neurons in the mouse hypothalamus—a brain region involved in many functions, including aggression. The activity of these neurons could then be controlled by light that was provided by a thin, optic fiber implanted in the animal's brain. When the channels were illuminated, the mouse would launch an attack on any object in its path—including other mice or, in one comical instance, an inflated rubber glove. When the light was switched off, the neurons once again fell silent, and the mouse's behavior would immediately return to normal (**Figure 12–44** and Movie 12.14).

Because the approach relies on a light-gated channel that is introduced into cells by genetic engineering techniques (discussed in Chapter 10), the method has been dubbed **optogenetics**. This tool is revolutionizing neurobiology, allowing investigators to dissect the neural circuits that govern even the most complex behaviors in a variety of experimental animals, from fruit flies to monkeys. But its implications extend beyond the laboratory. As genetic studies continue to identify genes associated with various human neurological and psychiatric disorders, the ability to exploit light-gated ion channels to study where and how these genes function in model organisms promises to greatly advance our understanding of the molecular and cellular basis of our own behavior.

Figure 12–44 Light-gated ion channels can control the activity of specific neurons in a living animal. (A) In this experiment, the gene encoding channelrhodopsin was introduced into a subset of neurons in the mouse hypothalamus. (B) When the neurons are exposed to blue light using a tiny fiber-optic cable implanted into the animal's brain, channelrhodopsin opens, depolarizing and stimulating the channel-containing neurons. (C) When the light is switched on, the mouse immediately becomes aggressive; when the light is switched off, its behavior immediately returns to normal. (C, from D. Lin et al., *Nature* 470:221–226, 2011.)

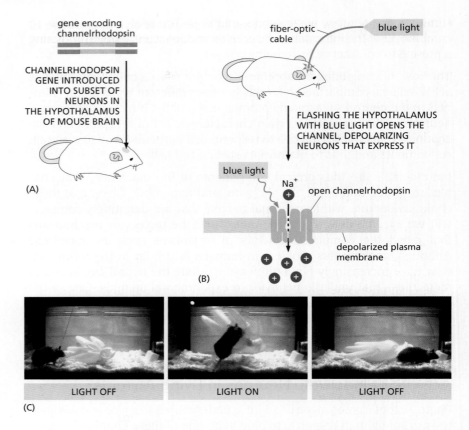

ESSENTIAL CONCEPTS

- The lipid bilayer of cell membranes is highly permeable to small, non-polar molecules such as oxygen and carbon dioxide and, to a lesser extent, to very small, polar molecules such as water. It is highly impermeable to most large, water-soluble molecules and to all ions.

- Transfer of nutrients, metabolites, and inorganic ions across cell membranes depends on membrane transport proteins.

- Cell membranes contain a variety of transport proteins that function either as transporters or channels, each responsible for the transfer of a particular type of solute.

- Channel proteins form pores across the lipid bilayer through which solutes can passively diffuse.

- Both transporters and channels can mediate passive transport, in which an uncharged solute moves spontaneously down its concentration gradient.

- For the passive transport of a charged solute, its electrochemical gradient determines its direction of movement, rather than its concentration gradient alone.

- Transporters can act as pumps to mediate active transport, in which solutes are moved uphill against their concentration or electrochemical gradients; this process requires energy that is provided by ATP hydrolysis, a downhill flow of Na^+ or H^+ ions, or sunlight.

- Transporters transfer specific solutes across a membrane by undergoing conformational changes that expose the solute-binding site first on one side of the membrane and then on the other.

- The Na^+ pump in the plasma membrane of animal cells is an ATPase; it actively transports Na^+ out of the cell and K^+ in, maintaining a steep Na^+ gradient across the plasma membrane that is used to drive other active transport processes and to convey electrical signals.

- Ion channels allow inorganic ions of appropriate size and charge to cross the membrane. Most are gated and open transiently in response to a specific stimulus.

- Even when activated by a specific stimulus, ion channels do not remain continuously open: they flicker randomly between open and closed conformations. An activating stimulus increases the proportion of time that the channel spends in the open state.

- The membrane potential is determined by the unequal distribution of charged ions on the two sides of a cell membrane; it is altered when these ions flow through open ion channels in the membrane.

- In most animal cells, the negative value of the resting membrane potential across the plasma membrane depends mainly on the K^+ gradient and the operation of K^+-selective leak channels; at this resting potential, the driving force for the movement of K^+ across the membrane is almost zero.

- Neurons produce electrical impulses in the form of action potentials, which can travel long distances along an axon without weakening. Action potentials are propagated by voltage-gated Na^+ and K^+ channels that open sequentially in response to depolarization of the plasma membrane.

- Voltage-gated Ca^{2+} channels in a nerve terminal couple the arrival of an action potential to neurotransmitter release at a synapse. Transmitter-gated ion channels convert this chemical signal back into an electrical one in the postsynaptic target cell.

- Excitatory neurotransmitters open transmitter-gated cation channels that allow the influx of Na^+, which depolarizes the postsynaptic cell's plasma membrane and encourages the cell to fire an action potential. Inhibitory neurotransmitters open transmitter-gated Cl^- channels in the postsynaptic cell's plasma membrane, making it harder for the membrane to depolarize and fire an action potential.

- Complex sets of nerve cells in the human brain exploit all of the above mechanisms to make human behaviors possible.

KEY TERMS

action potential	Nernst equation
active transport	nerve terminal
antiport	neuron
axon	neurotransmitter
Ca^{2+} pump (or Ca^{2+} ATPase)	optogenetics
channel	osmosis
dendrite	passive transport
depolarization	patch-clamp recording
electrochemical gradient	pump
gradient-driven pump	resting membrane potential
H^+ pump (or H^+ ATPase)	symport
ion channel	synapse
K^+ leak channel	synaptic vesicle
ligand-gated channel	transmitter-gated ion channel
mechanically-gated channel	transporter
membrane potential	voltage-gated channel
membrane transport protein	voltage-gated Na^+ channel
Na^+ pump (or Na^+-K^+ ATPase)	

QUESTIONS

QUESTION 12–8

The diagram in Figure 12–9 shows a transporter that mediates the passive transfer of a solute down its concentration gradient across the membrane. How would you need to change the diagram to convert the transporter into a pump that moves the solute up its concentration gradient by hydrolyzing ATP? Explain the need for each of the steps in your new illustration.

QUESTION 12–9

Which of the following statements are correct? Explain your answers.

A. The plasma membrane is highly impermeable to all charged molecules.

B. Channels have specific binding pockets for the solute molecules they allow to pass.

C. Transporters allow solutes to cross a membrane at much faster rates than do channels.

D. Certain H^+ pumps are fueled by light energy.

E. The plasma membrane of many animal cells contains open K^+ channels, yet the K^+ concentration in the cytosol is much higher than outside the cell.

F. A symport would function as an antiport if its orientation in the membrane were reversed (i.e., if the portion of the molecule normally exposed to the cytosol faced the outside of the cell instead).

G. The membrane potential of an axon temporarily becomes more negative when an action potential excites it.

QUESTION 12–10

List the following compounds in order of decreasing lipid-bilayer permeability: RNA, Ca^{2+}, glucose, ethanol, N_2, water.

QUESTION 12–11

Name at least one similarity and at least one difference between the following (it may help to review the definitions of the terms using the Glossary):

A. Symport and antiport

B. Active transport and passive transport

C. Membrane potential and electrochemical gradient

D. Pump and transporter

E. Axon and telephone wire

F. Solute and ion

QUESTION 12–12

Discuss the following statement: "The differences between a channel and a transporter are like the differences between a bridge and a ferry."

QUESTION 12–13

The neurotransmitter acetylcholine is made in the cytosol and then transported into synaptic vesicles, where its concentration is more than 100-fold higher than in the cytosol. When synaptic vesicles are isolated from neurons, they can take up additional acetylcholine added to the solution in which they are suspended, but only when ATP is present. Na^+ ions are not required for the uptake, but, curiously, raising the pH of the solution in which the synaptic vesicles are suspended increases the rate of uptake. Furthermore, transport is inhibited when drugs are added that make the membrane permeable to H^+ ions. Suggest a mechanism that is consistent with all of these observations.

QUESTION 12–14

The resting membrane potential of a typical animal cell is about –70 mV, and the thickness of a lipid bilayer is about 4.5 nm. What is the strength of the electric field across the membrane in V/cm? What do you suppose would happen if you applied this field strength to two metal electrodes separated by a 1-cm air gap?

QUESTION 12–15

Phospholipid bilayers form sealed, spherical vesicles in water (discussed in Chapter 11). Assume you have constructed lipid vesicles that contain Na^+ pumps as the sole membrane protein, and assume for the sake of simplicity that each pump transports one Na^+ one way and one K^+ the other way in each pumping cycle. All the Na^+ pumps have the portion of the molecule that normally faces the cytosol oriented toward the outside of the vesicles. With the help of Figures 12–11 and 12–12, determine what would happen in each of the following cases.

A. Your vesicles were suspended in a solution containing both Na^+ and K^+ ions and had a solution with the same ionic composition inside them.

B. You add ATP to the suspension described in (A).

C. You add ATP, but the solution—outside as well as inside the vesicles—contains only Na^+ ions and no K^+ ions.

D. The concentrations of Na^+ and K^+ were as in (A), but half of the pump molecules embedded in the membrane of each vesicle were oriented the other way around, so that the normally cytosolic portions of these molecules faced the inside of the vesicles. You then add ATP to the suspension.

E. You add ATP to the suspension described in (A), but in addition to Na^+ pumps, the membrane of your vesicles also contains K^+ leak channels.

QUESTION 12–16

Name the three ways in which an ion channel can be gated.

QUESTION 12–17

One thousand Ca^{2+} channels open in the plasma membrane of a cell that is 1000 μm^3 in size and has a cytosolic Ca^{2+} concentration of 100 nM. For how long would the channels need to stay open in order for the cytosolic Ca^{2+} concentration to rise to 5 μM? There is virtually unlimited Ca^{2+} available in the outside medium (the extracellular Ca^{2+} concentration in which most animal cells live is a few millimolar), and each channel passes 10^6 Ca^{2+} ions per second.

QUESTION 12–18

Amino acids are taken up by animal cells using a symport in the plasma membrane. What is the most likely ion whose electrochemical gradient drives the import? Is ATP consumed in the process? If so, how?

QUESTION 12–19

We will see in Chapter 15 that endosomes, which are membrane-enclosed intracellular organelles, need an acidic lumen in order to function. Acidification is achieved by an H^+ pump in the endosomal membrane, which also contains Cl^- channels. If the channels do not function properly (e.g., because of a mutation in the genes encoding the channel proteins), acidification is also impaired.

A. Can you explain how Cl^- channels might help acidification?

B. According to your explanation, would the Cl^- channels be absolutely required to lower the pH inside the endosome?

QUESTION 12–20

Some bacterial cells can grow on either ethanol (CH_3CH_2OH) or acetate (CH_3COO^-) as their only carbon source. Dr. Schwips measured the rate at which the two compounds traverse the bacterial plasma membrane but, due to excessive inhalation of one of the compounds (which one?), failed to label his data accurately.

A. Plot the data from the table below.

Concentration of Carbon Source (mM)	Rate of Transport (μmol/min)	
	Compound A	Compound B
0.1	2.0	18
0.3	6.0	46
1.0	20	100
3.0	60	150
10.0	200	182

B. Determine from your graph whether the data describing compound A correspond to the uptake of ethanol or acetate.

Explain your answers.

QUESTION 12–21

Acetylcholine-gated cation channels do not discriminate between Na^+, K^+, and Ca^{2+} ions, allowing all to pass through them freely. So why is it that when acetylcholine binds to this protein in the plasma membrane of muscle cells, the channel opens and there is a large net influx of primarily Na^+ ions?

QUESTION 12–22

The ion channels that are regulated by binding of neurotransmitters, such as acetylcholine, glutamate, GABA, or glycine, have a similar overall structure. Yet each class of these channels consists of a very diverse set of subtypes with different transmitter affinities, different channel conductances, and different rates of opening and closing. Do you suppose that such extreme diversity is a good or a bad thing from the standpoint of the pharmaceutical industry?

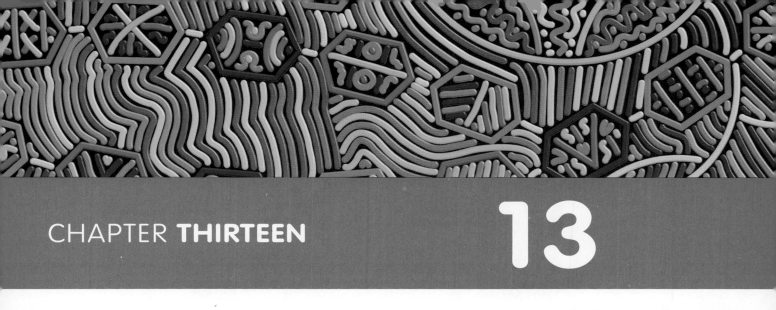

How Cells Obtain Energy from Food

To be able to grow, divide, and carry out day-to-day activities, cells require a constant supply of energy. This energy comes from the chemical-bond energy in food molecules, which thereby serve as fuel for cells.

Perhaps the most important fuel molecules are the sugars (too much of which can, unfortunately, lead to obesity and type 2 diabetes). Plants make their own sugars from CO_2 by photosynthesis. Animals obtain sugars—and other organic molecules that can be chemically transformed into sugars—by eating plants and other organisms. Nevertheless, the process whereby all these sugars are broken down to generate energy is very similar in both animals and plants. In both cases, the organism's cells harvest useful energy from the chemical-bond energy locked in sugars as the sugar molecule is broken down and oxidized to carbon dioxide (CO_2) and water (H_2O)—a process called **cell respiration**. The energy released during these reactions is captured in the form of "high-energy" chemical bonds—covalent bonds that release large amounts of energy when hydrolyzed—in *activated carriers* such as ATP and NADH. These carriers in turn serve as portable sources of the chemical groups and electrons needed for biosynthesis (discussed in Chapter 3).

In this chapter, we trace the major steps in the breakdown of sugars and show how ATP, NADH, and other activated carriers are produced along the way. We concentrate on the breakdown of glucose because it generates most of the energy produced in the majority of animal cells. A very similar pathway operates in plants, fungi, and many bacteria. Other molecules, such as fatty acids and proteins, can also serve as energy sources if they are funneled through appropriate enzymatic pathways. We will see how cells use many of the molecules generated from the breakdown of sugars and fats as starting points to make other organic molecules.

THE BREAKDOWN AND
UTILIZATION OF SUGARS
AND FATS

REGULATION OF METABOLISM

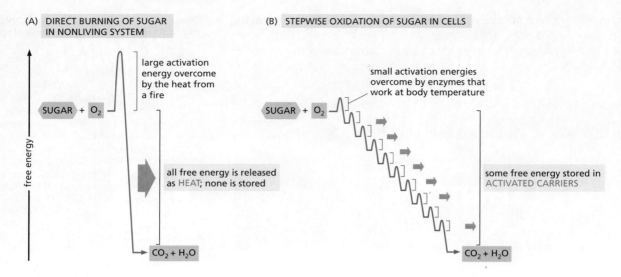

(A) DIRECT BURNING OF SUGAR IN NONLIVING SYSTEM

large activation energy overcome by the heat from a fire

SUGAR + O_2

free energy

all free energy is released as HEAT; none is stored

$CO_2 + H_2O$

(B) STEPWISE OXIDATION OF SUGAR IN CELLS

small activation energies overcome by enzymes that work at body temperature

SUGAR + O_2

some free energy stored in ACTIVATED CARRIERS

$CO_2 + H_2O$

Figure 13–1 The controlled, stepwise oxidation of sugar in cells captures useful energy, unlike the simple burning of the same fuel molecule. (A) The direct burning of sugar in nonliving conditions releases a large amount of energy all at once. This quantity is too large to be captured by any carrier molecule, and all of the energy is released as heat. (B) In a cell, enzymes catalyze the breakdown of sugars via a series of small steps, in which a portion of the free energy released is captured by the formation of activated carriers—most often ATP and NADH. Each step is catalyzed by an enzyme that lowers the activation-energy barrier that must be surmounted by the random collision of molecules at the temperature of cells (body temperature), so as to allow the reaction to occur (see Figures 3–12 and 3–13). Note that the total free energy released by the complete oxidative breakdown of glucose to CO_2 and H_2O—2880 kJ/mole—is exactly the same in (A) and (B).

Finally, we examine how cells regulate their metabolism and how they store food molecules for their future metabolic needs. We will save our discussion of the elaborate mechanism cells use to produce the bulk of their ATP for Chapter 14.

THE BREAKDOWN AND UTILIZATION OF SUGARS AND FATS

If a fuel molecule such as glucose were oxidized to CO_2 and H_2O in a single step—by, for example, the direct application of fire—it would release an amount of energy many times larger than any carrier molecule could capture (**Figure 13–1A**). Instead, cells use enzymes to carry out the oxidation of sugars in a tightly controlled series of reactions. Thanks to the action of enzymes—which operate at temperatures typical of living things—cells degrade each glucose molecule step by step, paying out energy in small packets to activated carriers by means of coupled reactions (**Figure 13–1B**). In this way, much of the energy released by the oxidative breakdown of glucose is saved in the high-energy bonds of ATP and other activated carriers, which can then be made available to do useful work for the cell.

Animal cells make ATP in two ways. First, certain energetically favorable, enzyme-catalyzed reactions involved in the breakdown of food-derived molecules are coupled directly to the energetically unfavorable reaction **ADP** + P_i → **ATP**. Thus the oxidation of food molecules can provide energy for the immediate production of ATP. Most ATP synthesis, however, requires an intermediary. In this second pathway to ATP production, the energy from other activated carriers is used to drive ATP synthesis. This process, called *oxidative phosphorylation*, takes place on the inner mitochondrial membrane of eukaryotic cells (**Figure 13–2**)—or on the plasma membrane of aerobic prokaryotes—and it is described in detail in Chapter 14. In this chapter, we focus on the first sequence of reactions by which food molecules are oxidized—both in the cytosol and in the mitochondrial matrix (see Figure 13–2). These reactions produce both ATP and the additional activated carriers that can subsequently help drive the production of much larger amounts of ATP by oxidative phosphorylation.

Food Molecules Are Broken Down in Three Stages

The proteins, fats, and polysaccharides that make up most of the food we eat must be broken down into smaller molecules before our cells can

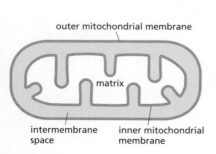

outer mitochondrial membrane

matrix

intermembrane space

inner mitochondrial membrane

Figure 13–2 A mitochondrion has two membranes and a large internal space called the matrix. Most of the energy from food molecules is harvested in mitochondria—both in the matrix and in the inner mitochondrial membrane.

use them—either as a source of energy or as building blocks for making other organic molecules. This breakdown process—in which enzymes degrade complex organic molecules into simpler ones—is called **catabolism**. The process takes place in three stages, as illustrated in Figure 13–3.

In *stage 1* of catabolism, enzymes convert the large polymeric molecules in food into simpler monomeric subunits: proteins into amino acids, polysaccharides into sugars, and fats into fatty acids and glycerol. This

Figure 13–3 In animals, the breakdown of food molecules occurs in three stages. (A) Stage 1 mostly occurs outside cells, with the breakdown of large food molecules in the mouth and the gut—although intracellular lysosomes can also digest such large molecules. Stage 2 starts intracellularly with *glycolysis* in the cytosol, and ends with the conversion of pyruvate to acetyl groups on acetyl CoA in the mitochondrial matrix. Stage 3 begins with the *citric acid cycle* in the mitochondrial matrix and concludes with *oxidative phosphorylation* on the mitochondrial inner membrane. The NADH generated in stage 2 adds to the NADH produced by the citric acid cycle to drive the production of large amounts of ATP by oxidative phosphorylation.

(B) The net products of the complete oxidation of food include ATP, NADH, CO_2, and H_2O. The ATP and NADH provide the energy and electrons needed for biosynthesis; the CO_2 and H_2O are waste products.

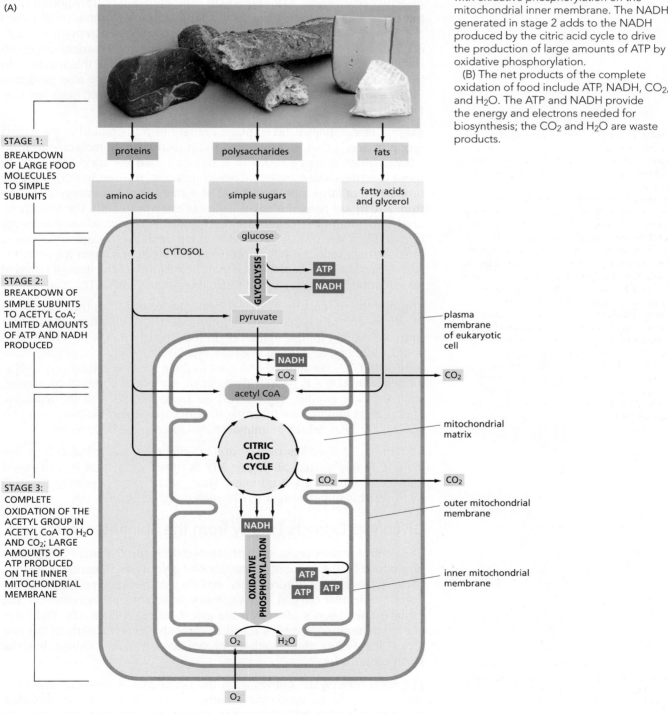

stage—also called *digestion*—occurs either outside cells (mainly in the intestine) or in specialized organelles within cells (called lysosomes, as discussed in Chapter 15). After digestion, the small organic molecules derived from food enter the cytosol of a cell, where their gradual oxidative breakdown begins.

In *stage 2* of catabolism, a chain of reactions called *glycolysis* splits each molecule of *glucose* into two smaller molecules of *pyruvate*. Sugars other than glucose can also be used, after first being converted into one of the intermediates in this sugar-splitting pathway. Glycolysis takes place in the cytosol and, in addition to producing pyruvate, it generates two types of activated carriers: ATP and NADH. The pyruvate is transported from the cytosol into the mitochondrion's large, internal compartment called the *matrix*. There, a giant enzyme complex converts each pyruvate molecule into CO_2 plus *acetyl CoA*, another of the activated carriers discussed in Chapter 3 (see Figure 3–37). NADH is also produced in this reaction. In the same compartment, large amounts of acetyl CoA are also produced by the stepwise oxidative breakdown of fatty acids derived from fats (see Figure 13–3).

Stage 3 of catabolism takes place entirely in mitochondria. The acetyl group in acetyl CoA is transferred to an oxaloacetate molecule to form citrate, which enters a series of reactions called the *citric acid cycle*. In these reactions, the transferred acetyl group is oxidized to CO_2, with the production of large amounts of NADH. Finally, the high-energy electrons from NADH are passed along a series of enzymes within the mitochondrial inner membrane called an *electron-transport chain*, where the energy released by their transfer is used to drive oxidative phosphorylation—a process that produces ATP and consumes molecular oxygen (O_2 gas). It is in these final steps of catabolism that the majority of the energy released by oxidation is harnessed to produce most of the cell's ATP.

Through the production of ATP, the energy derived from the breakdown of sugars and fats is redistributed into packets of chemical energy in a form convenient for use in the cell. In total, nearly 50% of the energy that could, in theory, be derived from the breakdown of glucose or fatty acids to H_2O and CO_2 is captured and used to drive the energetically unfavorable reaction ADP + P_i → ATP. By contrast, a modern combustion engine, such as a car engine, can convert no more than 20% of the available energy in its fuel into useful work. In both cases, the remaining energy is released as heat, which in animals helps to keep the body warm.

Roughly 10^9 molecules of ATP are in solution in a typical cell at any instant. In many cells, all of this ATP is turned over (that is, consumed and replaced) every 1–2 minutes. Thus, an average person at rest will hydrolyze his or her weight in ATP molecules every 24 hours.

Glycolysis Extracts Energy from the Splitting of Sugar

The central process in stage 2 of catabolism is the oxidative breakdown of **glucose** by the sequential reactions of **glycolysis.** The reactions take place in the cytosol of most cells, and they do not require the participation of molecular oxygen. Indeed, many anaerobic microorganisms that thrive in the absence of oxygen use glycolysis to produce ATP. Thus, this energy-generating series of reactions probably evolved early in the history of life, before photosynthetic organisms introduced oxygen into the Earth's atmosphere.

The term "glycolysis" comes from the Greek *glykys*, "sweet," and *lysis*, "splitting." It is an appropriate name, as glycolysis splits a molecule of glucose, which has six carbon atoms, to form two molecules of **pyruvate**, each of which contains three carbon atoms. The series of

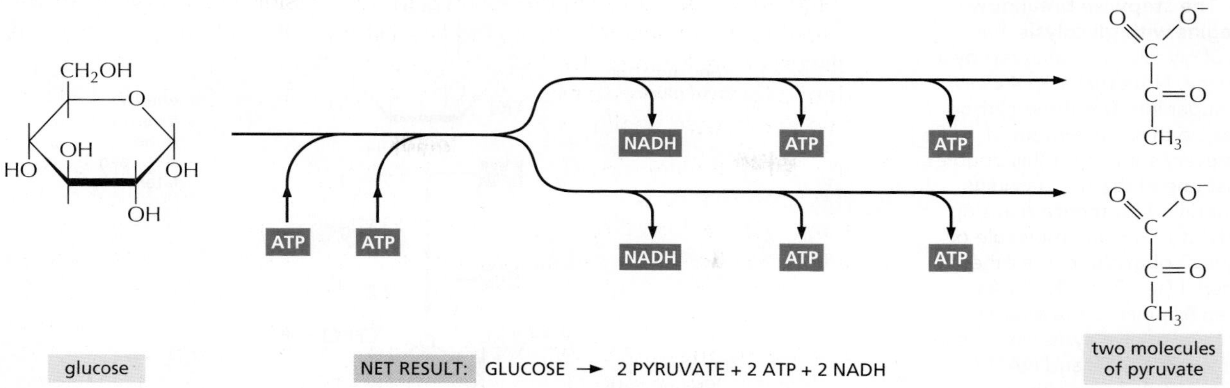

glucose

NET RESULT: GLUCOSE → 2 PYRUVATE + 2 ATP + 2 NADH

two molecules of pyruvate

chemical re-arrangements that ultimately generate pyruvate release energy because the electrons in a molecule of pyruvate are, overall, at a lower energy state than those in a molecule of glucose. Nevertheless, for each molecule of glucose that enters glycolysis, two molecules of ATP are initially consumed to provide the energy needed to prepare the sugar to be split. This investment of energy is more than recouped in the later steps of glycolysis, when four molecules of ATP are produced. During this "payoff phase," energy is also captured in the form of NADH. Thus, at the end of glycolysis, there is a net gain of two molecules of ATP and two molecules of NADH for each molecule of glucose that is oxidized (**Figure 13–4**).

Figure 13–4 Glycolysis splits a molecule of glucose to form two molecules of pyruvate. The process requires an input of energy, in the form of ATP, at the start. This energy investment is later recouped by the production of two NADHs and four ATPs.

Glycolysis Produces both ATP and NADH

Piecing together the complete glycolytic pathway in the 1930s was a major triumph of biochemistry, as the pathway consists of a sequence of 10 separate reactions, each producing a different sugar intermediate and each catalyzed by a different enzyme. These reactions are presented in outline in **Figure 13–5** and in detail in **Panel 13–1** (pp. 436–437). The different enzymes participating in the reactions of glycolysis, like most enzymes, all have names ending in -ase—like *isomerase* and *dehydrogenase*—which specify the type of reaction they catalyze (**Table 13–1**).

Much of the energy released by the breakdown of glucose is used to drive the synthesis of ATP molecules from ADP and P_i. This form of ATP

TABLE 13–1 SOME TYPES OF ENZYMES INVOLVED IN GLYCOLYSIS		
Enzyme Type	General Function	Role in Glycolysis
Kinase	catalyzes the addition of a phosphate group to molecules	a kinase transfers a phosphate group from ATP to a substrate in steps 1 and 3; other kinases transfer a phosphate to ADP to form ATP in steps 7 and 10
Isomerase	catalyzes the rearrangement of bonds within a single molecule	isomerases in steps 2 and 5 prepare molecules for the chemical alterations to come
Dehydrogenase	catalyzes the oxidation of a molecule by removing a hydrogen atom plus an electron (a hydride ion, H⁻)	the enzyme glyceraldehyde 3-phosphate dehydrogenase generates NADH in step 6
Mutase	catalyzes the shifting of a chemical group from one position to another within a molecule	the movement of a phosphate by phosphoglycerate mutase in step 8 helps prepare the substrate to transfer this group to ADP to make ATP in step 10

Figure 13–5 The stepwise breakdown of sugars begins with glycolysis. Each of the 10 steps of glycolysis is catalyzed by a different enzyme. Note that step 4 cleaves a six-carbon sugar into two three-carbon intermediates, so that the number of molecules at every stage after this doubles. Note also that one of the two products of step 4 is modified (isomerized) in step 5 to convert it into a second molecule of glyceraldehyde 3-phosphate, the other product of step 4 (see Panel 13–1). As indicated, step 6 launches the energy-generation phase of glycolysis, which results in the net synthesis of ATP and NADH (see also Figure 13–4). Glycolysis is also sometimes referred to as the Embden–Meyerhof pathway, named for the chemists who first described it. All the steps of glycolysis are reviewed in Movie 13.1.

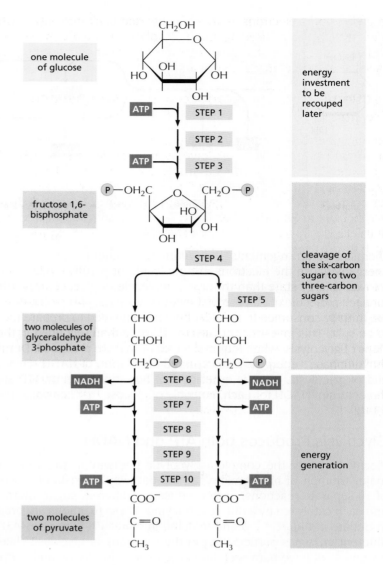

synthesis, which takes place in steps 7 and 10 in glycolysis, is known as *substrate-level phosphorylation* because it occurs by the transfer of a phosphate group directly from a substrate molecule—one of the sugar intermediates—to ADP. By contrast, most phosphorylations in cells occur by the transfer of a phosphate group from ATP to a substrate molecule.

The remainder of the useful energy harnessed by the cell during glycolysis is stored in the electrons in the **NADH** molecule produced in step 6 by an oxidation reaction. As discussed in Chapter 3, oxidation does not always involve oxygen; it occurs in any reaction in which electrons are lost from one atom and transferred to another. So, although no molecular oxygen is involved in glycolysis, oxidation does occur: in step 6, a hydrogen atom plus an electron (a hydride ion, H^-) is removed from the sugar intermediate, glyceraldehyde 3-phosphate, and transferred to **NAD$^+$**, producing NADH (see Panel 13–1, p. 437).

Over the course of glycolysis, two molecules of NADH are formed per molecule of glucose consumed. In eukaryotic organisms, these NADH molecules are transported into mitochondria, where they donate their electrons to an electron-transport chain that produces ATP by oxidative phosphorylation in the inner mitochondrial membrane, as described in detail in Chapter 14. These electrons pass along the electron-transport chain to O_2, eventually forming water.

In giving up its electrons, NADH is converted back into NAD⁺, which is then available to be used again for glycolysis. In the absence of oxygen, NAD⁺ can be regenerated by an alternate type of energy-yielding reaction called a fermentation, as we discuss next.

Fermentations Can Produce ATP in the Absence of Oxygen

For most animal and plant cells, glycolysis is only a prelude to the third and final stage of the breakdown of food molecules, in which large amounts of ATP are generated in mitochondria by oxidative phosphorylation, a process that requires the consumption of oxygen. However, for many anaerobic microorganisms, which can grow and divide in the absence of oxygen, glycolysis is the principal source of ATP. Certain animal cells also rely on ATP produced by glycolysis when oxygen levels fall, such as skeletal muscle cells during vigorous exercise.

In these anaerobic conditions, the pyruvate and NADH made by glycolysis remain in the cytosol (see Figure 13–3). There, pyruvate is converted into products that are excreted from the cell: lactate in muscle cells, for example, or ethanol and CO_2 in the yeast cells used in brewing and breadmaking. In the process, the NADH gives up its electrons and is converted back to the NAD⁺ required to maintain the reactions of glycolysis. Such energy-yielding pathways that break down sugar in the absence of oxygen are called **fermentations** (Figure 13–6). Scientific studies of the commercially important fermentations carried out by yeasts laid the foundations for early biochemistry.

QUESTION 13–1

At first glance, the final steps in fermentation appear to be unnecessary: the generation of lactate or ethanol does not produce any additional energy for the cell. Explain why cells growing in the absence of oxygen could not simply discard pyruvate as a waste product. Which products derived from glucose would accumulate in cells unable to generate either lactate or ethanol by fermentation?

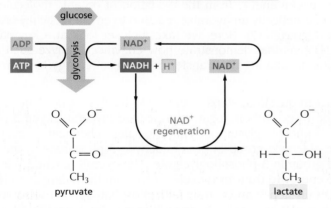

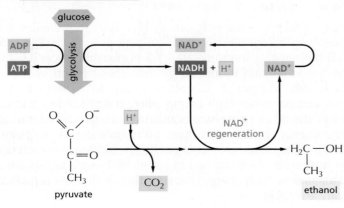

Figure 13–6 Pyruvate is broken down in the absence of oxygen by fermentation. (A) When inadequate oxygen is present, for example in a muscle cell undergoing repeated contraction, glycolysis produces pyruvate, which is converted to lactate in the cytosol. This reaction restores the NAD⁺ consumed in step 6 of glycolysis. The whole pathway yields much less energy overall than if the pyruvate were oxidized in mitochondria. (B) In some microorganisms that can grow anaerobically, pyruvate is converted into carbon dioxide and ethanol. Again, this pathway regenerates NAD⁺ from NADH, as required to enable glycolysis to continue. In both (A) and (B), for each molecule of glucose that enters glycolysis, two molecules of pyruvate are generated (only a single pyruvate is shown here); these two pyruvates subsequently yield two molecules of lactate—or two molecules of CO_2 and ethanol—plus two molecules of NAD⁺.

Figure 13–7 A pair of coupled reactions drives the energetically unfavorable formation of NADH and ATP in steps 6 and 7 of glycolysis. In this diagram, energetically favorable reactions are represented by *blue* arrows (see Figure 3–17) and energetically costly reactions by *red* arrows. In step 6, the energy released by the energetically favorable oxidation of a C–H bond in glyceraldehyde 3-phosphate (*blue* arrow) is large enough to drive two energetically costly reactions: the formation of both NADH and a high-energy phosphate bond in 1,3-bisphosphoglycerate (*red* arrows). The subsequent energetically favorable hydrolysis of that high-energy phosphate bond in step 7 then drives the formation of ATP. The formation of 1,3-bisphosphoglycerate (in step 6) and of ATP (in step 7) both represent a substrate-level phosphorylation.

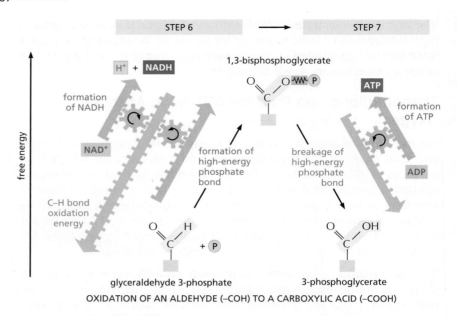

TOTAL ENERGY CHANGE ($\Delta G°$) for step 6 followed by step 7 is a favorable –12.5 kJ/mole

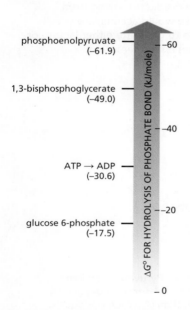

Figure 13–8 Differences in the energies of different phosphate bonds allow the formation of ATP by substrate-level phosphorylation. Examples of molecules formed during glycolysis that contain different types of phosphate bonds are shown, along with the free-energy change for hydrolysis of those bonds in kJ/mole. The transfer of a phosphate group from one molecule to another is energetically favorable if the standard free-energy change ($\Delta G°$) for hydrolysis of the phosphate bond is more negative for the donor molecule than for the acceptor. (The hydrolysis reactions can be thought of as the transfer of the phosphate group to water.) Thus, a phosphate group is readily transferred from 1,3-bisphosphoglycerate to ADP to form ATP. Transfer reactions involving the phosphate groups in these molecules are detailed in Panel 13–1 (pp. 436–437).

Many bacteria and archaea can also generate ATP in the absence of oxygen by *anaerobic respiration*, a process that uses a molecule other than oxygen as a final electron acceptor. Anaerobic respiration differs from fermentation in that it involves an electron-transport chain embedded in a membrane—in this case, the plasma membrane of the prokaryote.

Glycolytic Enzymes Couple Oxidation to Energy Storage in Activated Carriers

Cells harvest useful energy from the oxidation of organic molecules by coupling an energetically unfavorable reaction to an energetically favorable one (see Figure 3–17). Here, we take a closer look at a key pair of glycolytic reactions that demonstrate how enzymes catalyze such coupled reactions, facilitating the transfer of chemical energy to form ATP and NADH.

The reactions in question, steps 6 and 7 of glycolysis (see Panel 13–1), transform the three-carbon sugar intermediate glyceraldehyde 3-phosphate into 3-phosphoglycerate. This two-step chemical conversion oxidizes the aldehyde group in glyceraldehyde 3-phosphate to the carboxylic acid group in 3-phosphoglycerate. The overall reaction releases enough free energy to transfer two electrons from the aldehyde to NAD⁺ to form NADH (in step 6) and to transfer a phosphate group to a molecule of ADP to form ATP (in step 7). It also releases enough heat to the environment to make the overall reaction energetically favorable: the $\Delta G°$ for step 6 followed by step 7 is –12.5 kJ/mole (**Figure 13–7**).

The reaction in step 6 is the only one in glycolysis that creates a high-energy phosphate linkage directly from inorganic phosphate. This reaction generates a high-energy intermediate—1,3-bisphosphoglycerate—whose phosphate bonds contain more energy than those found in ATP. Such molecules readily transfer a phosphate group to ADP to form ATP. **Figure 13–8** compares the high-energy phosphoanhydride bond in ATP with a few of the other phosphate bonds that are generated during glycolysis. The energy contained in these phosphate bonds is determined by measuring the standard free-energy change ($\Delta G°$) when each bond is broken by hydrolysis. As explained in Panel 13–1, such bonds are often described as having "high energy" because their hydrolysis is particularly energetically favorable.

The important substrate-level phosphorylation reaction at the center of glycolysis, in which a high-energy linkage in 1,3-bisphosphoglycerate is generated in step 6—and then consumed in step 7 to produce ATP—is presented in detail in **Figure 13–9**.

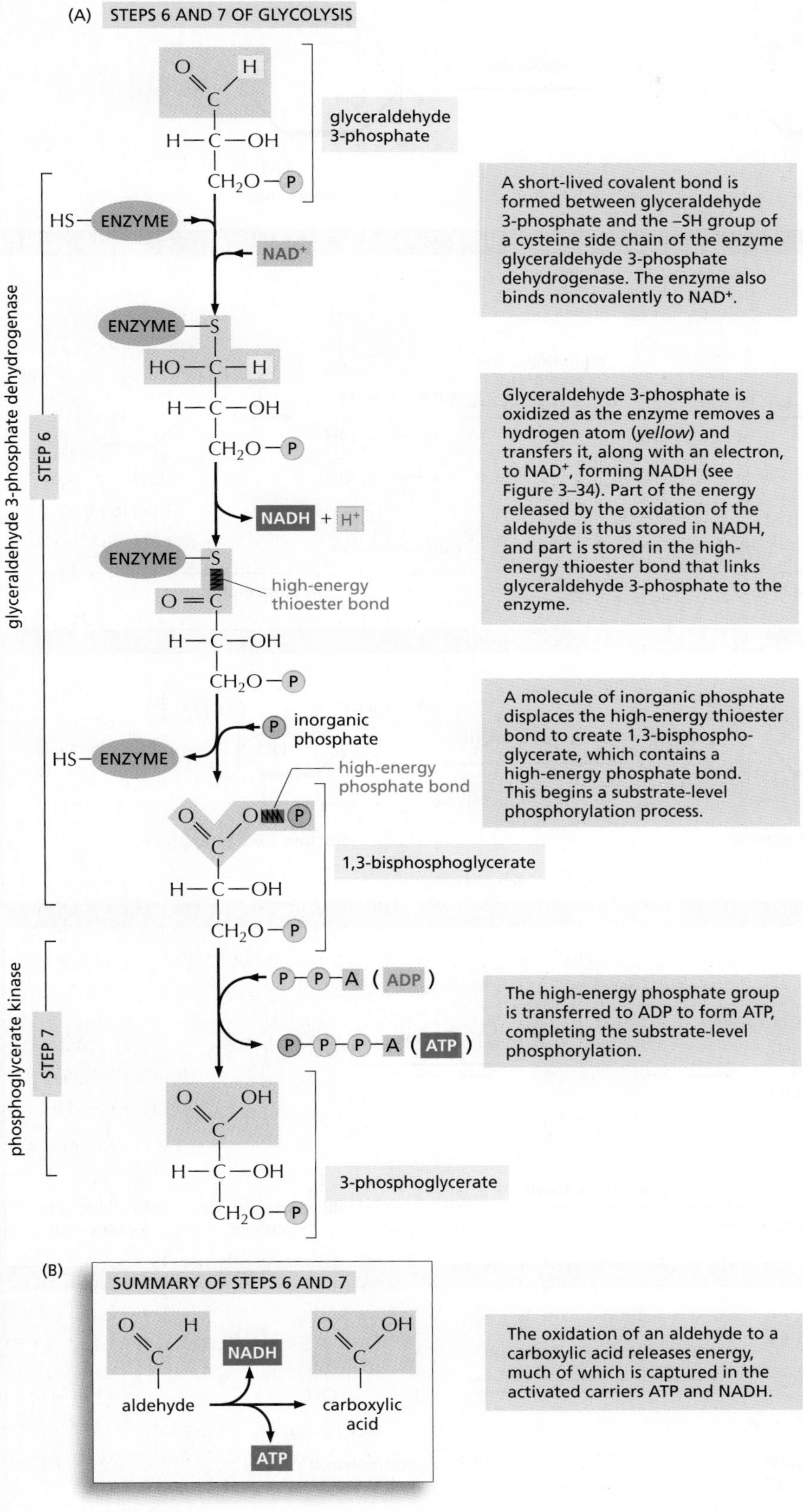

(A)   STEPS 6 AND 7 OF GLYCOLYSIS

A short-lived covalent bond is formed between glyceraldehyde 3-phosphate and the –SH group of a cysteine side chain of the enzyme glyceraldehyde 3-phosphate dehydrogenase. The enzyme also binds noncovalently to NAD^+.

Glyceraldehyde 3-phosphate is oxidized as the enzyme removes a hydrogen atom (*yellow*) and transfers it, along with an electron, to NAD^+, forming NADH (see Figure 3–34). Part of the energy released by the oxidation of the aldehyde is thus stored in NADH, and part is stored in the high-energy thioester bond that links glyceraldehyde 3-phosphate to the enzyme.

A molecule of inorganic phosphate displaces the high-energy thioester bond to create 1,3-bisphospho-glycerate, which contains a high-energy phosphate bond. This begins a substrate-level phosphorylation process.

The high-energy phosphate group is transferred to ADP to form ATP, completing the substrate-level phosphorylation.

(B)   SUMMARY OF STEPS 6 AND 7

The oxidation of an aldehyde to a carboxylic acid releases energy, much of which is captured in the activated carriers ATP and NADH.

QUESTION 13–2

Arsenate ($AsO_4{}^{3-}$) is chemically very similar to phosphate ($PO_4{}^{3-}$) and can be used as an alternative substrate by many phosphate-requiring enzymes. In contrast to phosphate, however, an anhydride bond between arsenate and carbon is very quickly hydrolyzed nonenzymatically in water. Knowing this, suggest why arsenate is a compound of choice for murderers but not for cells. Formulate your explanation in the context of Figure 13–7.

Figure 13–9 The oxidation of glyceraldehyde 3-phosphate is coupled to the formation of ATP and NADH in steps 6 and 7 of glycolysis. (A) In step 6, the enzyme glyceraldehyde 3-phosphate dehydrogenase couples the energetically favorable oxidation of an aldehyde to the energetically unfavorable formation of a high-energy phosphate bond. At the same time, it enables energy to be stored in NADH. In step 7, the newly formed high-energy phosphate bond in 1,3-bisphosphoglycerate is transferred to ADP, forming a molecule of ATP and leaving a free carboxylic acid group on the oxidized sugar. The part of the molecule that undergoes a change is shaded in *blue*; the rest of the molecule remains unchanged throughout all these reactions. (B) Summary of the overall chemical change produced by the reactions of steps 6 and 7.

For each step, the part of the molecule that undergoes a change is shadowed in *blue*, and the name of the enzyme that catalyzes the reaction is in a *yellow* box. Reactions represented by double arrows ($\rightleftarrows$) are readily reversible, whereas those represented by single arrows ($\longrightarrow$) are effectively irreversible. To watch a video of the reactions of glycolysis, see Movie 13.1.

STEP 1

Glucose is phosphorylated by ATP to form a sugar phosphate. The negative charge of the phosphate prevents passage of the sugar phosphate through the plasma membrane, trapping glucose inside the cell.

glucose + ATP → hexokinase → glucose 6-phosphate + ADP + H⁺

STEP 2

A readily reversible rearrangement of the chemical structure (isomerization) moves the carbonyl oxygen from carbon 1 to carbon 2, forming a ketose from an aldose sugar. (See Panel 2–4, pp. 72–73.)

glucose 6-phosphate (ring form) ⇌ (open-chain form) → phosphoglucose isomerase → (open-chain form) ⇌ fructose 6-phosphate (ring form)

STEP 3

The new hydroxyl group on carbon 1 is phosphorylated by ATP, in preparation for the formation of two three-carbon sugar phosphates. The entry of sugars into glycolysis is controlled at this step, through regulation of the enzyme *phosphofructokinase*.

fructose 6-phosphate + ATP → phosphofructokinase → fructose 1,6-bisphosphate + ADP + H⁺

STEP 4

The six-carbon sugar is cleaved to produce two three-carbon molecules. Only the glyceraldehyde 3-phosphate can proceed immediately through glycolysis.

fructose 1,6-bisphosphate (ring form) ⇌ (open-chain form) → aldolase → dihydroxyacetone phosphate + glyceraldehyde 3-phosphate

STEP 5

The other product of step 4, dihydroxyacetone phosphate, is isomerized to form a second molecule of glyceraldehyde 3-phosphate.

dihydroxyacetone phosphate → triose phosphate isomerase → glyceraldehyde 3-phosphate

STEP 6

The two molecules of glyceraldehyde 3-phosphate produced in steps 4 and 5 are oxidized. The energy-generation phase of glycolysis begins, as NADH and a new high-energy anhydride linkage to phosphate are formed (see Figure 13–5).

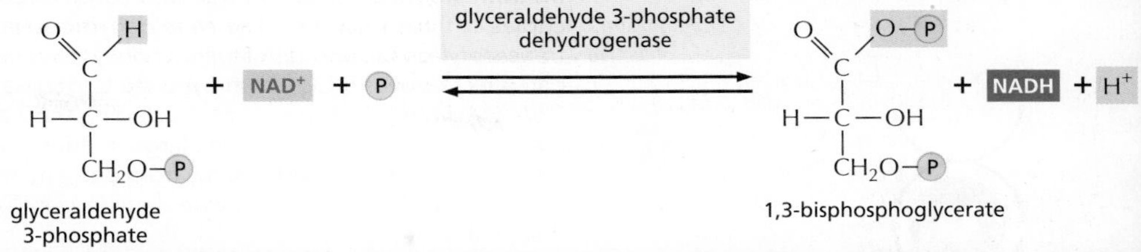

glyceraldehyde 3-phosphate dehydrogenase

glyceraldehyde 3-phosphate

1,3-bisphosphoglycerate

+ NAD⁺ + P ⇌ + NADH + H⁺

STEP 7

The transfer to ADP of the high-energy phosphate group that was generated in step 6 forms ATP.

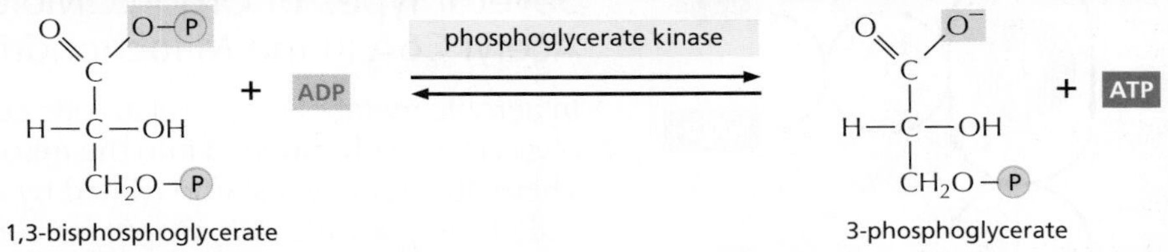

phosphoglycerate kinase

1,3-bisphosphoglycerate + ADP ⇌ 3-phosphoglycerate + ATP

STEP 8

The remaining phosphate ester linkage in 3-phosphoglycerate, which has a relatively low free energy of hydrolysis, is moved from carbon 3 to carbon 2 to form 2-phosphoglycerate.

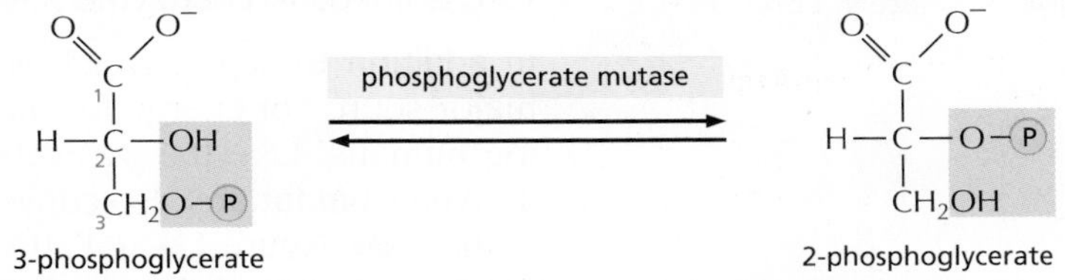

phosphoglycerate mutase

3-phosphoglycerate ⇌ 2-phosphoglycerate

STEP 9

The removal of water from 2-phosphoglycerate creates a high-energy enol phosphate linkage.

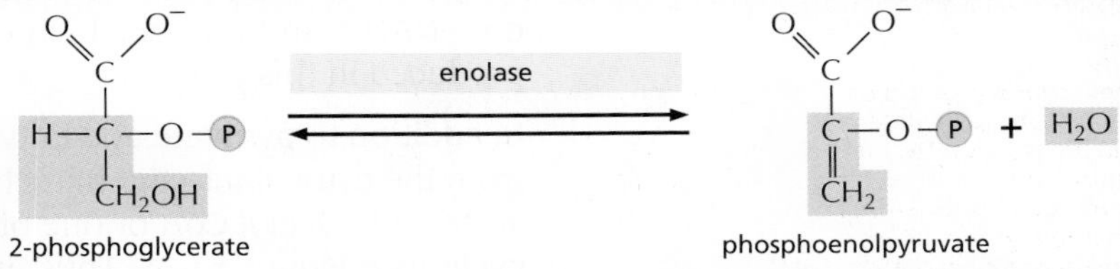

enolase

2-phosphoglycerate ⇌ phosphoenolpyruvate + H_2O

STEP 10

The transfer to ADP of the high-energy phosphate group that was generated in step 9 forms ATP, completing glycolysis.

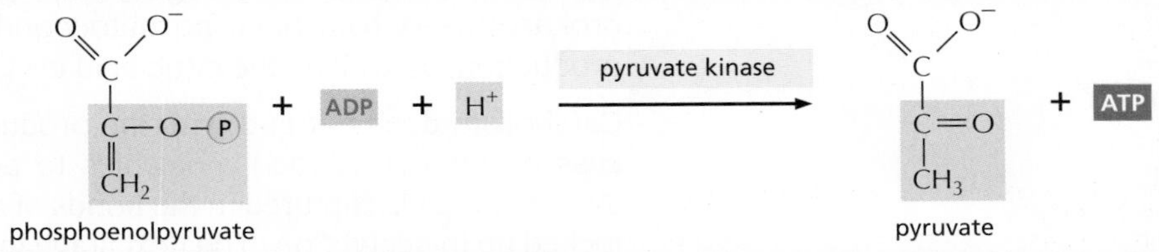

pyruvate kinase

phosphoenolpyruvate + ADP + H⁺ → pyruvate + ATP

NET RESULT OF GLYCOLYSIS

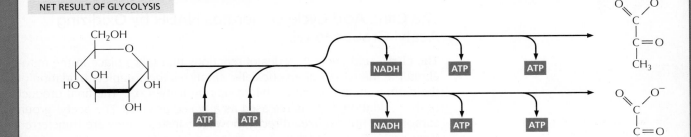

one molecule of glucose

In addition to the pyruvate, the net products of glycolysis are two molecules of ATP and two molecules of NADH.

two molecules of pyruvate

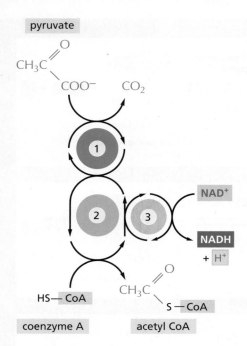

pyruvate

coenzyme A

acetyl CoA

Figure 13–10 Pyruvate is converted into acetyl CoA and CO$_2$ by the pyruvate dehydrogenase complex in the mitochondrial matrix. The pyruvate dehydrogenase complex contains multiple copies of three enzymes—*pyruvate dehydrogenase* (1), *dihydrolipoyl transacetylase* (2), and *dihydrolipoyl dehydrogenase* (3). This enzyme complex removes a CO$_2$ from pyruvate to generate NADH and acetyl CoA. Pyruvate and its products—including the waste product, CO$_2$— are shown in *red* lettering. In the large multienzyme complex, reaction intermediates are passed directly from one enzyme to another. To get a sense of scale, a single pyruvate dehydrogenase complex is larger than a ribosome.

Several Types of Organic Molecules Are Converted to Acetyl CoA in the Mitochondrial Matrix

In aerobic metabolism in eukaryotic cells, the pyruvate produced by glycolysis is actively pumped into the mitochondrial matrix (see Figure 13–3). There, it is rapidly decarboxylated by a giant complex of three enzymes, called the *pyruvate dehydrogenase complex*. The products of this set of reactions are CO$_2$ (a waste product), NADH, and **acetyl CoA** (**Figure 13–10**). The latter is produced when the acetyl group derived from pyruvate is linked to coenzyme A (CoA).

In addition to sugar, which is broken down during glycolysis, **fat** is a major source of energy for most nonphotosynthetic organisms, including humans. Like the pyruvate derived from glycolysis, the fatty acids derived from fat are also converted into acetyl CoA in the mitochondrial matrix (see Figure 13–3). Fatty acids are first activated by covalent linkage to CoA and are then broken down completely by a cycle of reactions that trims two carbons at a time from their carboxyl end, generating one molecule of acetyl CoA for each turn of the cycle; two activated carriers—NADH and another high-energy electron carrier, *FADH$_2$*—are also produced in this process (**Figure 13–11**).

In addition to pyruvate and fatty acids, some amino acids are transported from the cytosol into the mitochondrial matrix, where they are also converted into acetyl CoA or one of the other intermediates of the citric acid cycle (see Figure 13–3). Thus, in the eukaryotic cell, the mitochondrion represents the center toward which all energy-yielding catabolic processes lead, whether they begin with sugars, fats, or proteins. In aerobic prokaryotes—which have no mitochondria—glycolysis and acetyl CoA production, as well as the citric acid cycle, take place in the cytosol.

Catabolism does not end with the production of acetyl CoA. In the process of converting food molecules to acetyl CoA, only a part of their stored energy is captured in the bonds of activated carriers: most remains locked up in acetyl CoA. The next stage in cell respiration is the citric acid cycle, in which the acetyl group in acetyl CoA is oxidized to CO$_2$ in the mitochondrial matrix, as we now discuss.

The Citric Acid Cycle Generates NADH by Oxidizing Acetyl Groups to CO$_2$

The **citric acid cycle**, a series of reactions that takes place in the mitochondrial matrix of eukaryotic cells, catalyzes the complete oxidation of the carbon atoms of the acetyl groups in acetyl CoA. The final product of this oxidation, CO$_2$, is released as a waste product. The acetyl-group carbons are not oxidized directly, however. Instead, they are transferred from acetyl CoA to a larger four-carbon molecule, *oxaloacetate*, to form the six-carbon tricarboxylic acid, *citric acid*, for which the subsequent cycle of reactions is named. The citric acid molecule (also called citrate) is then progressively oxidized, and the energy of this oxidation is harnessed

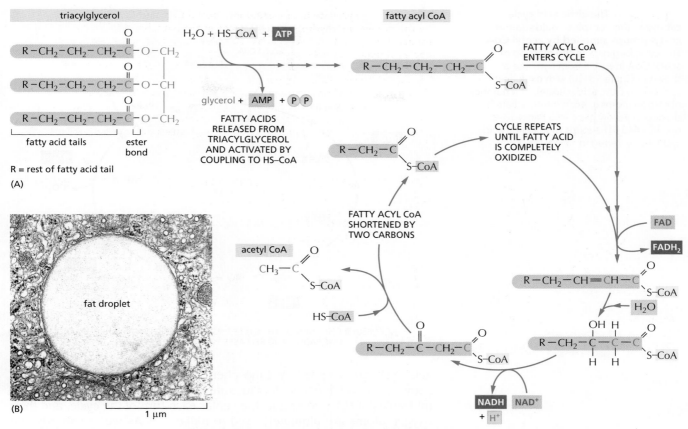

Figure 13–11 Fatty acids derived from fats are also converted to acetyl CoA in the mitochondrial matrix.
(A) Fats are stored in the form of triacylglycerol, the glycerol portion of which is shown in *blue*. Three fatty acid chains (shaded in *red*) are linked to this glycerol through ester bonds. Enzymes called lipases can hydrolyze these ester bonds when fatty acids are needed for energy (not shown). The released fatty acids are then coupled to coenzyme A in a reaction requiring ATP. These activated fatty acids (fatty acyl CoA) are subsequently oxidized in a cycle containing four enzymes, which are not shown. Each turn of the cycle shortens the fatty acyl CoA molecule by two carbons (*red*) and generates one molecule each of $FADH_2$, NADH, and acetyl CoA. (B) Fats are insoluble in water and spontaneously form large lipid droplets in specialized fat cells called adipocytes. This electron micrograph shows a lipid droplet in the cytoplasm of an adipocyte. (B, courtesy of Daniel S. Friend.)

to produce activated carriers, including NADH, in much the same manner as we described for glycolysis. This series of eight reactions forms a cycle, because the oxaloacetate that began the process is regenerated at the end (**Figure 13–12**). The citric acid cycle—which is also called the *tricarboxylic acid cycle* or the *Krebs cycle*—is presented in detail in **Panel 13–2** (pp. 442–443), and the experiments that first revealed its cyclic nature are described in **How We Know**, pp. 444–445.

Although the citric acid cycle accounts for about two-thirds of the total oxidation of carbon compounds in most cells, none of its steps use molecular oxygen. The cycle, however, requires O_2 to proceed because the NADH generated passes its high-energy electrons to an electron-transport chain in the inner mitochondrial membrane, and this chain uses O_2 as its final electron acceptor. Oxygen thus allows NADH to hand off its high-energy electrons, regenerating the NAD^+ needed to keep the citric acid cycle going. Although living organisms have inhabited Earth for more than 3.5 billion years, the planet is thought to have developed an atmosphere containing O_2 gas only some 1 to 2 billion years ago (see Figure 14–46). Many of the energy-generating reactions of the citric acid cycle, which is now used by all aerobic organisms, are therefore likely to be of relatively recent origin.

A common misconception about the citric acid cycle is that the oxygen atoms required to make CO_2 from the acetyl groups entering the citric

QUESTION 13–3

Many catabolic and anabolic reactions are based on reactions that are similar but work in opposite directions, such as the hydrolysis and condensation reactions described in Figure 3–39. This is true for fatty acid breakdown and fatty acid synthesis. From what you know about the mechanism of fatty acid breakdown outlined in Figure 13–11, would you expect the fatty acids found in cells to most commonly have an even or an odd number of carbon atoms?

Figure 13–12 The citric acid cycle catalyzes the complete oxidation of acetyl groups supplied by acetyl CoA. The cycle begins with the reaction of acetyl CoA (derived from pyruvate as shown in Figure 13–10) with oxaloacetate to produce citric acid (citrate). The number of carbon atoms in each intermediate is shaded in *yellow*. (See also Panel 13–2, pp. 442–443.) The steps of the citric acid cycle are reviewed in Movie 13.2.

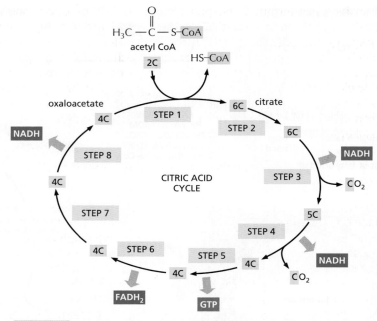

NET RESULT: ONE TURN OF THE CYCLE PRODUCES THREE NADH, ONE GTP, AND ONE FADH$_2$, AND RELEASES TWO MOLECULES OF CO$_2$

acid cycle are supplied by atmospheric O$_2$. In fact, these oxygen atoms come from water (H$_2$O). As illustrated at the top of Panel 13–2, three molecules of H$_2$O are split as they enter each turn of the cycle, and their oxygen atoms are ultimately used to make CO$_2$. As we see shortly, the O$_2$ that we breathe is actually reduced to H$_2$O by the electron-transport chain; it does not form the CO$_2$ that we exhale.

Thus far, we have discussed only one of the three types of activated carriers that are produced by the citric acid cycle—NADH. In addition to three molecules of NADH, each turn of the cycle also produces one molecule of **FADH$_2$ (reduced flavin adenine dinucleotide)** from FAD and one molecule of the ribonucleoside triphosphate **GTP (guanosine triphosphate)** from **GDP** (see Figure 13–12). The structures of these two activated carriers are illustrated in **Figure 13–13**. GTP is a close relative of ATP, and

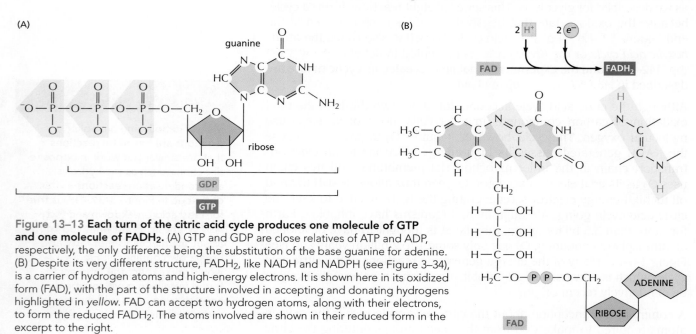

Figure 13–13 Each turn of the citric acid cycle produces one molecule of GTP and one molecule of FADH$_2$. (A) GTP and GDP are close relatives of ATP and ADP, respectively, the only difference being the substitution of the base guanine for adenine. (B) Despite its very different structure, FADH$_2$, like NADH and NADPH (see Figure 3–34), is a carrier of hydrogen atoms and high-energy electrons. It is shown here in its oxidized form (FAD), with the part of the structure involved in accepting and donating hydrogens highlighted in *yellow*. FAD can accept two hydrogen atoms, along with their electrons, to form the reduced FADH$_2$. The atoms involved are shown in their reduced form in the excerpt to the right.

the transfer of its terminal phosphate group to ADP produces one ATP molecule in each cycle. Like NADH, FADH$_2$ is a carrier of high-energy electrons. And like NADH, FADH$_2$ transfers its high-energy electrons to the electron-transport chain in the inner mitochondrial membrane. As we discuss shortly, the movement of energy stored in these readily transferrable electrons is subsequently used to produce ATP through oxidative phosphorylation on the inner mitochondrial membrane, the only step in the oxidative catabolism of foodstuffs that directly requires O$_2$ from the atmosphere.

Many Biosynthetic Pathways Begin with Glycolysis or the Citric Acid Cycle

Catabolic reactions, such as those of glycolysis and the citric acid cycle, produce both energy for the cell and the building blocks from which many other organic molecules are made. Thus far, we have emphasized energy production rather than the provision of starting materials for biosynthesis. But many of the intermediates formed in glycolysis and the citric acid cycle are siphoned off by such **anabolic pathways**, in which the intermediates are converted by a series of enzyme-catalyzed reactions into amino acids, nucleotides, lipids, and other small organic molecules that the cell needs. The oxaloacetate and α-ketoglutarate produced during the citric acid cycle, for example (see Panel 13–2), are transferred from the mitochondrial matrix back to the cytosol, where they serve as precursors for the production of many essential molecules, such as the amino acids aspartate and glutamate, respectively. An idea of the extent of these anabolic pathways can be gathered from **Figure 13–14**, which illustrates some of the branches leading from the central catabolic reactions to biosyntheses. How cells control the flow of intermediates through anabolic and catabolic pathways is discussed in the final section of the chapter.

QUESTION 13–4

Looking at the chemistry detailed in the overview of the citric acid cycle at the top of the first page of Panel 13–2 (p. 442), why do you suppose it is useful to link the two-carbon acetyl group to another, larger carbon skeleton, oxaloacetate, before completely oxidizing both of the acetyl-group carbons to CO$_2$? (See also Figure 13–12.)

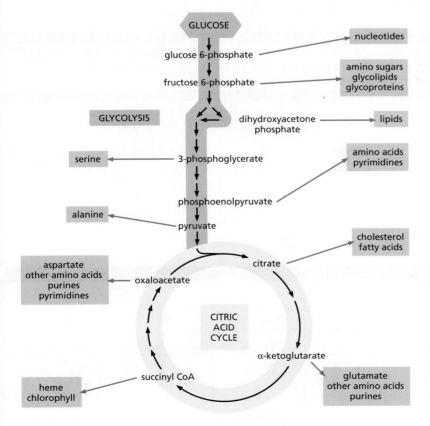

Figure 13–14 Glycolysis and the citric acid cycle provide the precursors needed for cells to synthesize many important organic molecules. The amino acids, nucleotides, lipids, sugars, and other molecules—shown here as products—in turn serve as the precursors for many of the cell's macromolecules. Each *black* arrow in this diagram denotes a single enzyme-catalyzed reaction; the *red* arrows generally represent pathways with many steps that are required to produce the indicated products.

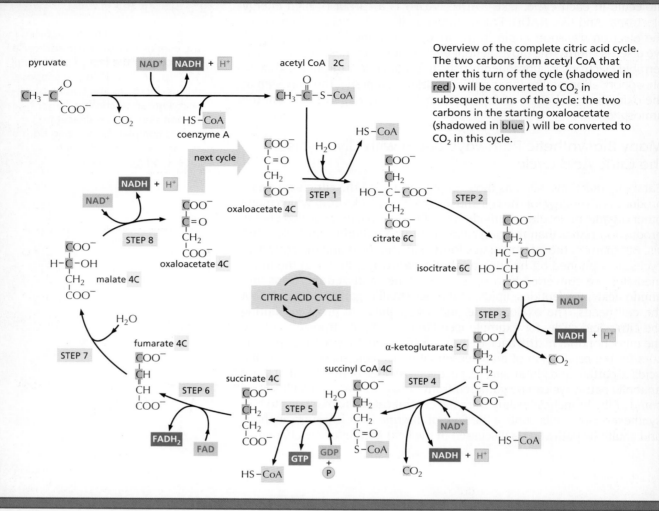

Overview of the complete citric acid cycle. The two carbons from acetyl CoA that enter this turn of the cycle (shadowed in red) will be converted to CO_2 in subsequent turns of the cycle: the two carbons in the starting oxaloacetate (shadowed in blue) will be converted to CO_2 in this cycle.

Details of these eight steps are shown below. In this part of the panel, for each step, the part of the molecule that undergoes a change is shadowed in blue, and the name of the enzyme that catalyzes the reaction is in a yellow box.
To watch a video of the reactions of the citric acid cycle, see Movie 13.2.

STEP 1

After the enzyme removes a proton from the CH_3 group on acetyl CoA, the negatively charged CH_2^- forms a bond to a carbonyl carbon of oxaloacetate. The subsequent loss of the coenzyme A (HS–CoA) by hydrolysis drives the reaction strongly forward.

acetyl CoA   oxaloacetate   citrate synthase   S-cityl-CoA intermediate   citrate

STEP 2

An isomerization reaction, in which water is first removed and then added back, moves the hydroxyl group from one carbon atom to its neighbor.

citrate   aconitase   cis-aconitate intermediate   isocitrate

STEP 3

In the first of four oxidation steps in the cycle, the carbon carrying the hydroxyl group is converted to a carbonyl group. The immediate product is unstable, losing CO_2 while still bound to the enzyme.

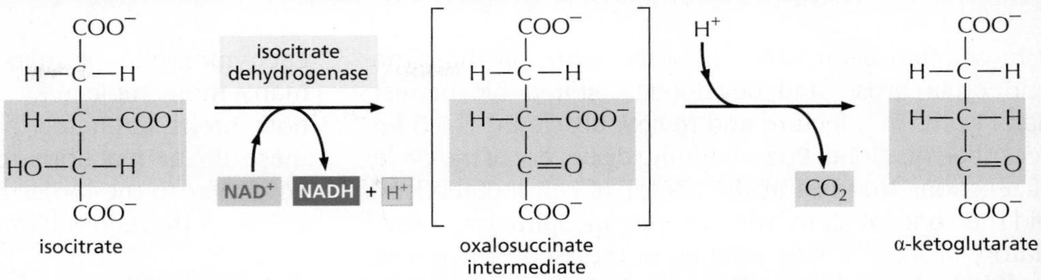

isocitrate — isocitrate dehydrogenase (NAD^+ → $NADH$ + H^+) — oxalosuccinate intermediate — (H^+, CO_2) — α-ketoglutarate

STEP 4

The α-*ketoglutarate dehydrogenase complex* closely resembles the large enzyme complex that converts pyruvate to acetyl CoA, the pyruvate dehydrogenase complex in Figure 13–10. It likewise catalyzes an oxidation that produces NADH, CO_2, and a high-energy thioester bond to coenzyme A (CoA).

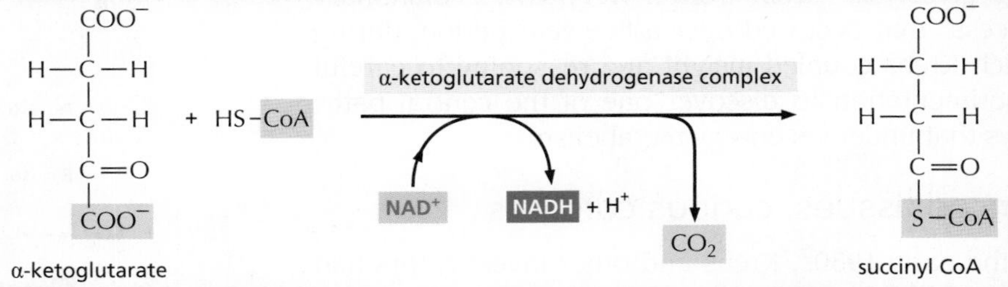

α-ketoglutarate + HS–CoA — α-ketoglutarate dehydrogenase complex (NAD^+ → $NADH$ + H^+, CO_2) — succinyl CoA

STEP 5

An inorganic phosphate displaces the CoA, forming a high-energy phosphate linkage to succinate. This phosphate is then passed to GDP to form GTP. (In bacteria and plants, ATP is formed instead.)

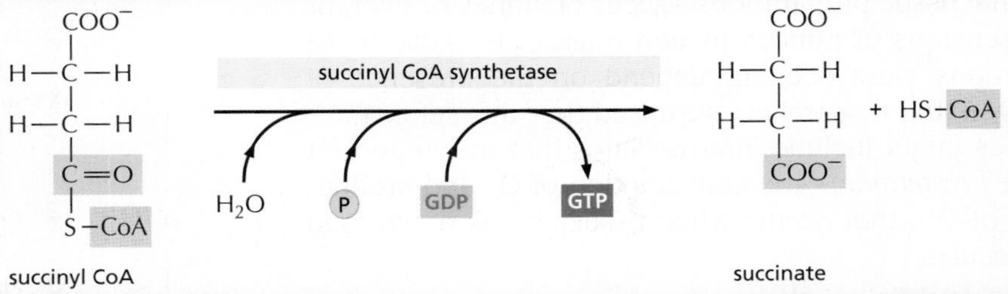

succinyl CoA — succinyl CoA synthetase (H_2O, P, GDP → GTP) — succinate + HS–CoA

STEP 6

In the third oxidation step of the cycle, FAD accepts two hydrogen atoms from succinate.

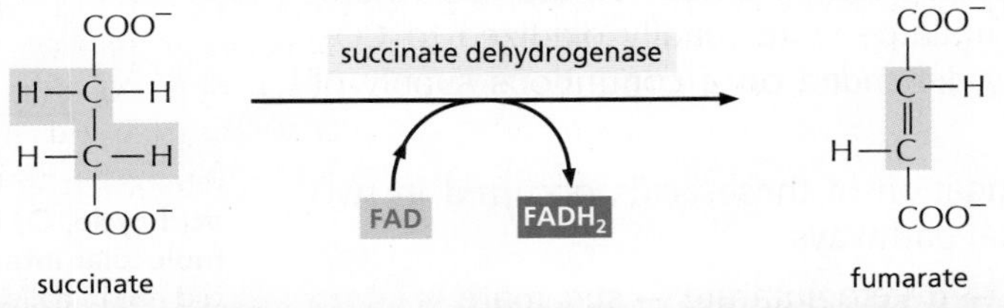

succinate — succinate dehydrogenase (FAD → $FADH_2$) — fumarate

STEP 7

The addition of water to fumarate places a hydroxyl group next to a carbonyl carbon.

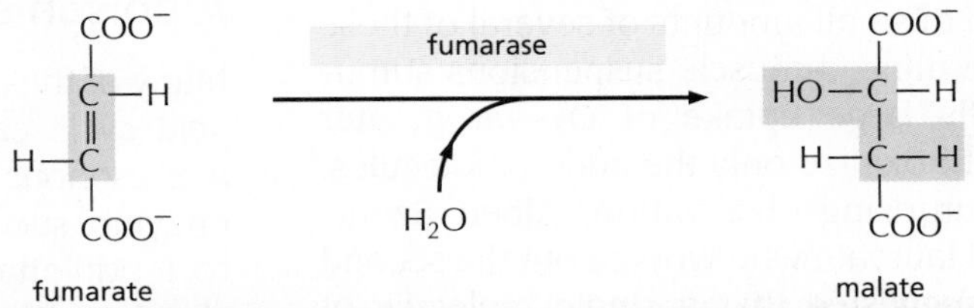

fumarate — fumarase (H_2O) — malate

STEP 8

In the last of four oxidation steps in the cycle, the carbon carrying the hydroxyl group is converted to a carbonyl group, regenerating the oxaloacetate needed for step 1.

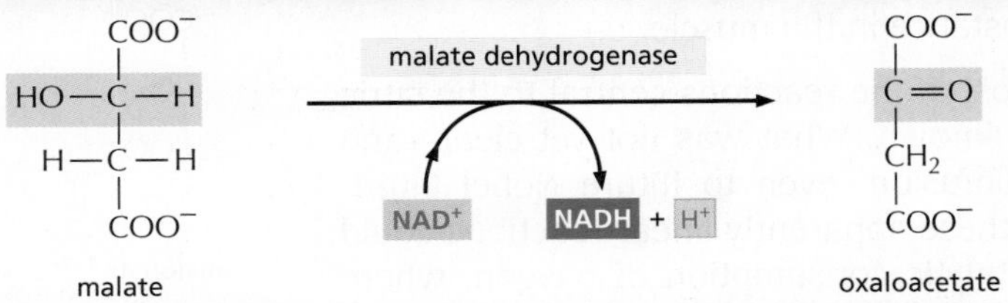

malate — malate dehydrogenase (NAD^+ → $NADH$ + H^+) — oxaloacetate

HOW WE KNOW

UNRAVELING THE CITRIC ACID CYCLE

"I have often been asked how the work on the citric acid cycle arose and developed," stated biochemist Hans Krebs in a lecture and review article in which he described his Nobel Prize-winning discovery of the cycle of reactions that lies at the center of cell metabolism. Did the concept stem from a sudden inspiration, a revelatory vision? "It was nothing of the kind," answered Krebs. Instead, his realization that these reactions occur in a cycle—rather than a set of linear pathways, as in glycolysis—arose from a "very slow evolutionary process" that occurred over a five-year period, during which Krebs coupled insight and reasoning to careful experimentation to discover one of the central pathways that underlies energy metabolism.

Minced tissues, curious catalysis

By the early 1930s, Krebs and other investigators had discovered that a select set of small organic molecules is oxidized extraordinarily rapidly in various types of animal tissue preparations—slices of kidney or liver, or suspensions of minced pigeon muscle. Because these reactions were seen to depend on the presence of oxygen, the researchers surmised that this set of molecules might include intermediates that are important in *cell respiration*—the consumption of O_2 and production of CO_2 that occurs when tissues break down food molecules.

Using the minced-tissue preparations, Krebs and others made the following observations. First, in the presence of oxygen, certain organic acids—citrate, succinate, fumarate, and malate—were readily oxidized to CO_2. These reactions depended on a continuous supply of oxygen.

Second, the oxidation of these acids occurred in two linear, sequential pathways:

$$\text{citrate} \rightarrow \alpha\text{-ketoglutarate} \rightarrow \text{succinate}$$

and

$$\text{succinate} \rightarrow \text{fumarate} \rightarrow \text{malate} \rightarrow \text{oxaloacetate}$$

Third, the addition of small amounts of several of these compounds to the minced-muscle suspensions stimulated an unusually large uptake of O_2—far greater than that needed to oxidize only the added molecules. To explain this surprising observation, Albert Szent-Györgyi (the Nobel laureate who worked out the second pathway above) suggested that a single molecule of each compound must somehow act catalytically to stimulate the oxidation of many molecules of some endogenous substance in the muscle.

At this point, most of the reactions central to the citric acid cycle were known. What was not yet clear—and caused great confusion, even to future Nobel laureates—was how these apparently linear reactions could drive such a catalytic consumption of oxygen, where

each molecule of metabolite fuels the oxidation of many more molecules. To simplify the discussion of how Krebs ultimately solved this puzzle—by linking these linear reactions together into a circle—we will now refer to the molecules involved by a sequence of letters, A through H (Figure 13–15).

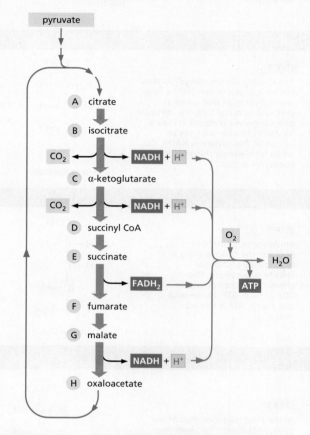

Figure 13–15 In this simplified representation of the citric acid cycle, O_2 is consumed and CO_2 is liberated as the molecular intermediates become oxidized. Krebs and others did not initially realize that these oxidation reactions occur in a cycle, as shown here.

A poison suggests a cycle

Many of the clues that Krebs used to work out the citric acid cycle came from experiments using malonate—a poisonous compound that specifically inhibits the enzyme succinate dehydrogenase, which converts E to F. Malonate closely resembles succinate (E) in its structure (Figure 13–16), and it serves as a competitive

$$
\begin{array}{cc}
\text{COO}^- & \text{COO}^- \\
| & | \\
\text{CH}_2 & \text{CH}_2 \\
| & | \\
\text{COO}^- & \text{CH}_2 \\
& | \\
& \text{COO}^- \\
\text{malonate} & \text{succinate}
\end{array}
$$

Figure 13–16 The structure of malonate closely resembles that of succinate.

inhibitor of the enzyme. Because the addition of malonate poisons cell respiration in tissues, Krebs concluded that succinate dehydrogenase (and the entire pathway linked to it) must play a critical role in the cell respiration process.

Krebs then determined that when A, B, or C was added to malonate-poisoned tissue suspensions, E accumulated (Figure 13–17A). This observation reinforced the importance of succinate dehydrogenase for successful cell respiration. However, he found that E also accumulated when F, G, or H was added to malonate-poisoned muscle (Figure 13–17B). The latter result suggested that an additional set of reactions must exist that can convert F, G, and H molecules into E, since E was previously shown to be a precursor for F, G, and H, rather than a product of their reaction pathway.

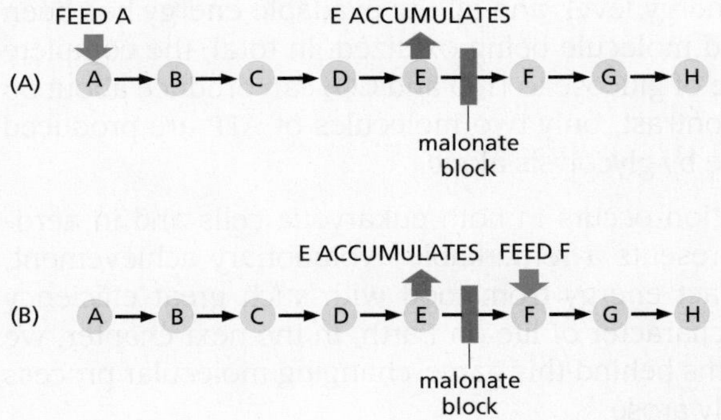

FEED A   E ACCUMULATES

(A)   A → B → C → D → E ▐ F → G → H

malonate block

E ACCUMULATES   FEED F

(B)   A → B → C → D → E ▐ F → G → H

malonate block

Figure 13–17 Poisoning muscle preparations with malonate provided clues to the cyclic nature of these oxidative reactions. (A) Adding A (or B or C—not shown) to malonate-poisoned muscle causes an accumulation of E. (B) Addition of F (or G or H—not shown) to a malonate-poisoned preparation also causes an accumulation of E, suggesting that enzymatic reactions can convert these molecules into E. The discovery that citrate (A) can be formed from oxaloacetate (H) and pyruvate allowed Krebs to join these two reaction pathways into a complete circle.

At about this time, Krebs also determined that when muscle suspensions were incubated with pyruvate and oxaloacetate, citrate formed: pyruvate + H → A.

This observation led Krebs to postulate that when oxygen is present, pyruvate and H condense to form A, converting the previously delineated string of linear reactions into a cyclic sequence (see Figure 13–15).

Explaining the mysterious stimulatory effects

The cycle of reactions that Krebs proposed clearly explained how the addition of small amounts of any of the intermediates A through H could cause the large increase in the uptake of O_2 that had been observed. Pyruvate is abundant in these minced tissues, being readily produced by glycolysis (see Figure 13–4), using glucose derived from the breakdown of stored glycogen (as discussed later in this chapter). The oxidation of pyruvate requires a functioning citric acid cycle, in which each turn of the cycle results in the oxidation of one molecule of pyruvate. If the intermediates A through H are in small enough supply, the rate at which the entire cycle turns will be restricted. Adding a supply of any one of these intermediates will then have a dramatic effect on the rate at which the entire cycle operates. Thus, it is easy to see how a large number of pyruvate molecules can be oxidized, and a great deal of oxygen consumed, for every molecule of a citric acid cycle intermediate that is added (Figure 13–18).

Krebs went on to demonstrate that all of the individual enzymatic reactions in his postulated cycle took place in tissue preparations. Furthermore, the reactions occurred at rates high enough to account for the rate of pyruvate and oxygen consumption in these tissues. Krebs therefore concluded that this series of reactions is the major, if not the sole, pathway for the oxidation of pyruvate—at least in muscle. By fitting together pieces of information like a jigsaw puzzle, he arrived at a coherent picture of the intricate metabolic processes that underlie the oxidation—and took home a share of the 1953 Nobel Prize in Physiology or Medicine.

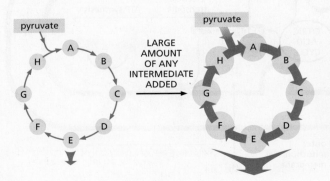

Figure 13–18 Replenishing the supply of any single intermediate has a dramatic effect on the rate at which the entire citric acid cycle operates. When the concentrations of intermediates are limiting, the cycle turns slowly and little pyruvate is used. O_2 uptake is low because only small amounts of NADH and $FADH_2$ are produced to feed oxidative phosphorylation (see Figure 13–19). But when a large amount of any one intermediate is added, the cycle turns rapidly; more of all the intermediates is made, and O_2 uptake is high.

Electron Transport Drives the Synthesis of the Majority of the ATP in Most Cells

We now return briefly to the final stage in the oxidation of food molecules: **oxidative phosphorylation**. It is in this stage that the chemical energy captured by the activated carriers produced during glycolysis and the citric acid cycle is used to generate ATP. During oxidative phosphorylation, NADH and $FADH_2$ transfer their high-energy electrons to the **electron-transport chain**—a series of electron carriers embedded in the inner mitochondrial membrane in eukaryotic cells (and in the plasma membrane of aerobic prokaryotes). As the electrons pass through the series of electron acceptor and donor molecules that form the chain, they fall to successively lower energy states. At specific sites in the chain, the energy released is used to drive protons (H^+) across the inner membrane, from the mitochondrial matrix to the intermembrane space (see Figure 13–2). This movement generates a proton gradient across the inner membrane, which serves as a source of energy (like a battery) that can be tapped to drive a variety of energy-requiring reactions (discussed in Chapter 12). The most prominent of these reactions is the phosphorylation of ADP to generate ATP on the matrix side of the inner membrane (**Figure 13–19**).

At the end of the transport chain, the electrons are added to molecules of O_2 that have diffused into the mitochondrion, and the resulting reduced oxygen molecules immediately combine with protons from the surrounding solution to produce water (see Figure 13–19). The electrons have now reached their lowest energy level, and all the available energy has been extracted from the food molecule being oxidized. In total, the complete oxidation of a molecule of glucose to H_2O and CO_2 can produce about 30 molecules of ATP. In contrast, only two molecules of ATP are produced per molecule of glucose by glycolysis alone.

Oxidative phosphorylation occurs in both eukaryotic cells and in aerobic prokaryotes. It represents a remarkable evolutionary achievement, and the ability to extract energy from food with such great efficiency has shaped the entire character of life on Earth. In the next chapter, we describe the mechanisms behind this game-changing molecular process and discuss how it likely arose.

QUESTION 13–5

What, if anything, is wrong with the following statement? "The oxygen consumed during the complete oxidation of glucose in animal cells is returned as part of CO_2 to the atmosphere." How could you support your answer experimentally?

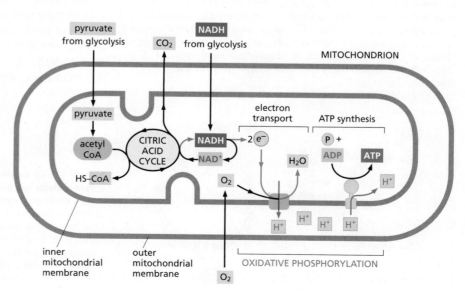

Figure 13–19 Oxidative phosphorylation completes the catabolism of food molecules and generates the bulk of the ATP made by the cell. Electron-bearing activated carriers produced by the citric acid cycle and glycolysis donate their high-energy electrons to an electron-transport chain in the inner mitochondrial membrane (or in the plasma membrane of aerobic prokaryotes). This electron transfer pumps protons (H^+) across the inner membrane (*red* arrows). The resulting proton gradient is then used to drive the synthesis of ATP through the process of oxidative phosphorylation, as we discuss in detail in the next chapter.

REGULATION OF METABOLISM

A cell is an intricate chemical machine, and our discussion of metabolism—with a focus on glycolysis and the citric acid cycle—has reviewed only a tiny fraction of the many enzymatic reactions that can take place in a cell at any time (Figure 13–20). For all these pathways to work together smoothly, as is required to allow the cell to survive and to respond to its environment, the choice of which pathway each metabolite will follow must be carefully regulated at every branch point.

Many sets of reactions need to be coordinated and controlled. For example, to maintain order within their cells, all organisms need to replenish their ATP pools continuously through the oxidation of sugars or fats. Yet animals have only periodic access to food, and plants need to survive without sunlight overnight, when they are unable to produce sugar through photosynthesis. Animals and plants have evolved several ways to cope with this transient deprivation. One way is to synthesize food reserves in times of plenty that can later be consumed when other energy sources are scarce. Thus, depending on conditions, a cell must decide whether to route key metabolites into anabolic or catabolic pathways—in other words, whether to use them to build other molecules or burn them to provide immediate energy. In this section, we discuss how a cell regulates its intricate web of interconnected metabolic pathways to best serve both its immediate and long-term needs.

Catabolic and Anabolic Reactions Are Organized and Regulated

All the reactions shown in Figure 13–20 occur in a cell that is less than 0.1 mm in diameter, and each step requires a different enzyme. To add to the complexity, the same substrate is often a part of many different pathways. Pyruvate, for example, is a substrate for half a dozen or more different enzymes, each of which modifies it chemically in a different way. We have already seen that the pyruvate dehydrogenase complex uses pyruvate to produce acetyl CoA (see Figure 13–10), and that, during fermentation, lactate dehydrogenase can convert pyruvate to lactate (see Figure 13–6A). A third enzyme converts pyruvate to the amino acid alanine (see Figure 13–14), a fourth to oxaloacetate, and so on. All these pathways compete for pyruvate molecules, and similar competitions for thousands of other small molecules go on in cells all the time.

To balance the activities of these interrelated reactions—and to allow organisms to adapt swiftly to changes in food availability or energy expenditure—an elaborate network of *control mechanisms* regulates and coordinates the activity of the enzymes that catalyze the myriad metabolic reactions that go on in a cell. As we discuss in Chapter 4, the activity of enzymes can be controlled by covalent modification—such as the addition or removal of a phosphate group (see Figure 4–46)—and by the binding of small regulatory molecules, often a metabolite (see pp. 150–152). Such regulation can either enhance the activity of the enzyme or inhibit it. As we see next, both types of regulation—positive and negative—control the activity of key enzymes involved in the breakdown and synthesis of glucose.

Feedback Regulation Allows Cells to Switch from Glucose Breakdown to Glucose Synthesis

Animals need an ample supply of glucose. Active muscles need glucose to power their contraction, and brain cells depend almost exclusively on glucose for energy. During periods of fasting or intense physical exercise,

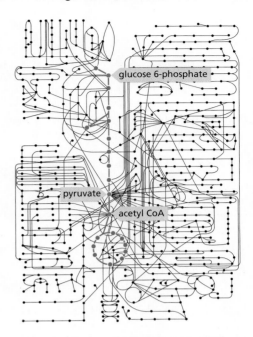

Figure 13–20 Glycolysis and the citric acid cycle constitute a small fraction of the reactions that occur in a cell. In this diagram, the filled circles represent molecules in some of the best-characterized metabolic pathways, and the lines that connect them represent the enzymatic reactions that convert one metabolite to another. The reactions of glycolysis and the citric acid cycle are shown in *red*. Many other reactions either lead into these two central catabolic pathways—delivering small organic molecules to be oxidized for energy—or lead outward to the anabolic pathways that supply carbon compounds for biosynthesis.

QUESTION 13–6

A cyclic reaction pathway requires that the starting material be regenerated and available at the end of each cycle. If compounds of the citric acid cycle are siphoned off as building blocks to make other organic molecules via a variety of metabolic reactions (see Figure 13–14), why does the citric acid cycle not quickly grind to a halt?

the body's glucose reserves get used up faster than they can be replenished from food. One way to increase available glucose is to synthesize it from pyruvate by a process called **gluconeogenesis**.

Gluconeogenesis is, in many ways, a reversal of glycolysis: it builds glucose from pyruvate, whereas glycolysis breaks down glucose and produces pyruvate. Indeed, gluconeogenesis makes use of many of the same enzymes as glycolysis; it simply runs them in reverse. For example, the isomerase that converts glucose 6-phosphate to fructose 6-phosphate in step 2 of glycolysis will readily catalyze the reverse reaction (see Panel 13–1, pp. 436–437). There are, however, three steps in glycolysis that so strongly favor glucose breakdown that they are effectively irreversible: steps 1, 3, and 10. To get around these one-way steps, gluconeogenesis uses a special set of enzymes that catalyze a set of bypass reactions. In step 3 of glycolysis, for example, the enzyme phosphofructokinase uses ATP to phosphorylate fructose 6-phosphate, producing the intermediate fructose 1,6-bisphosphate. In gluconeogenesis, an enzyme called fructose 1,6-bisphosphatase simply removes a phosphate from this intermediate to generate fructose 6-phosphate (Figure 13–21).

How does a cell determine whether to synthesize glucose or to degrade it? Part of the decision centers on the three irreversible glycolytic reactions. The activity of the enzyme phosphofructokinase, for example, is allosterically regulated by the binding of a variety of metabolites, which provide both positive and negative **feedback regulation**. Such feedback loops, in which a product in a chain of enzymatic reactions reduces or stimulates its own production by altering the activity of an enzyme earlier in the pathway, regulate many biological processes (see Figure 4–42). Phosphofructokinase is activated by by-products of ATP hydrolysis—including ADP, AMP, and inorganic phosphate—and it is inhibited by ATP. Thus, when ATP is depleted and its metabolic by-products accumulate, phosphofructokinase is turned on and glycolysis proceeds, generating ATP; when ATP is abundant, the enzyme is turned off and glycolysis shuts down. The enzyme that catalyzes the reverse reaction during gluconeogenesis, fructose 1,6-bisphosphatase (see Figure 13–21), is regulated by the same molecules but in the opposite direction. This enzyme is thus activated when phosphofructokinase is turned off, allowing gluconeogenesis to proceed. Many such coordinated feedback mechanisms enable a cell to respond rapidly to changing conditions and to adjust its metabolism accordingly.

Some of the biosynthetic bypass reactions required for gluconeogenesis are energetically costly. Reversal of step 10 alone consumes one molecule of ATP and one of GTP. Altogether, producing a single molecule of glucose by gluconeogenesis consumes four molecules of ATP and two molecules of GTP. Thus a cell must tightly regulate the balance between glycolysis and gluconeogenesis. If both processes were to proceed simultaneously, they would shuttle metabolites back and forth in a futile cycle that would consume large amounts of energy and generate heat for no purpose.

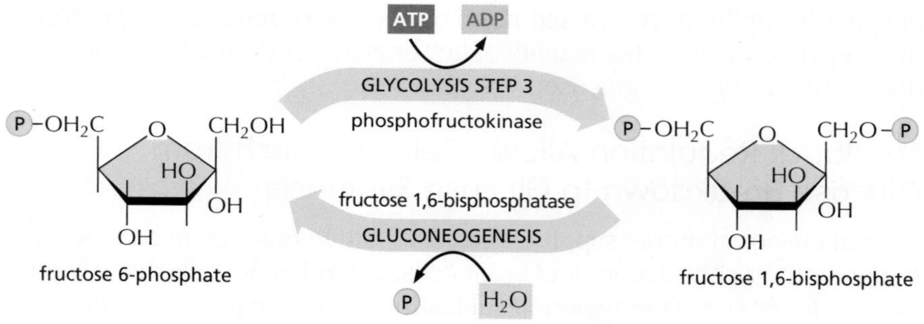

Figure 13–21 Gluconeogenesis uses specific enzymes to bypass those steps in glycolysis that are essentially irreversible. The enzyme phosphofructokinase catalyzes the phosphorylation of fructose 6-phosphate to form fructose 1,6-bisphosphate in step 3 of glycolysis. This reaction is so energetically favorable that the enzyme will not work in reverse (see step 3 in Panel 13–1). To produce fructose 6-phosphate during gluconeogenesis, the enzyme fructose 1,6-bisphosphatase removes the phosphate from fructose 1,6-bisphosphate in a simple hydrolysis reaction. Coordinated feedback regulation of these two enzymes helps a cell control the flow of metabolites toward glucose synthesis or glucose breakdown.

Cells Store Food Molecules in Special Reservoirs to Prepare for Periods of Need

As we have seen, gluconeogenesis is a costly process, requiring substantial amounts of energy from the hydrolysis of ATP and GTP. During periods when food is scarce, this expensive way of producing glucose is suppressed if alternatives are available. Fasting cells, for example, can mobilize glucose that has been stored in the form of **glycogen**, a branched polymer of glucose (**Figure 13–22A** and see Panel 2–4, pp. 72–73). This large polysaccharide is stored as small granules in the cytoplasm of many animal cells, but mainly in liver and muscle cells (**Figure 13–22B**). The synthesis and degradation of glycogen occur by separate metabolic pathways, which can be rapidly and coordinately regulated to suit an organism's needs. When more ATP is needed than can be generated from food-derived molecules available in the bloodstream, cells break down glycogen in a reaction that is catalyzed by the enzyme *glycogen phosphorylase*. This enzyme produces *glucose 1-phosphate*, which is then converted to the glucose 6-phosphate that feeds into the glycolytic pathway (**Figure 13–22C**).

Like glycolysis and gluconeogenesis, the glycogen degradative and synthetic pathways are coordinated by feedback regulation. In this case, enzymes in each pathway are allosterically regulated by glucose 6-phosphate, but in opposite directions: in the synthetic pathway, *glycogen synthetase* is activated by glucose 6-phosphate, whereas *glycogen phosphorylase,* which breaks down glycogen (see Figure 13–22C), is inhibited by glucose 6-phosphate, as well as by ATP. This regulation helps to prevent glycogen breakdown when ATP is plentiful and to favor glycogen

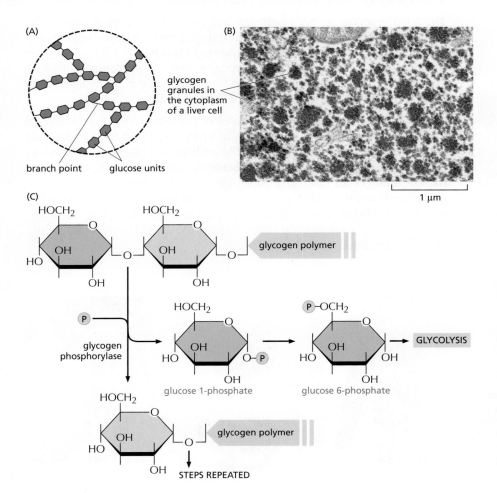

Figure 13–22 Animal cells store glucose in the form of glycogen to provide energy in times of need. (A) The structure of glycogen; starch in plants is a very similar branched polymer of glucose, but has many fewer branch points. (B) An electron micrograph showing glycogen granules in the cytoplasm of a liver cell; each granule contains both glycogen and the enzymes required for glycogen synthesis and breakdown. (C) The enzyme glycogen phosphorylase breaks down glycogen when cells need more glucose. (B, courtesy of Robert Fletterick and Daniel S. Friend, by permission of E.L. Bearer.)

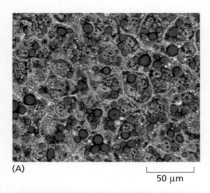

(A)   50 μm

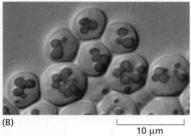

(B)   10 μm

Figure 13–23 Fats are stored in the form of lipid droplets in cells. (A) Fat droplets (stained *red*) in the cytoplasm of developing adipocytes. (B) Lipid droplets (*red*) in yeast cells, which also use them as a reservoir of energy and building blocks for membrane lipid biosynthesis. (A, courtesy of Peter Tontonoz and Ronald M. Evans; B, courtesy of Sepp D. Kohlwein.)

QUESTION 13–7

After looking at the structures of sugars and fatty acids (discussed in Chapter 2), give an intuitive explanation as to why oxidation of a sugar yields only about half as much energy as the oxidation of an equivalent dry weight of a fatty acid.

synthesis when the glucose 6-phosphate concentration is high. The balance between glycogen synthesis and breakdown is further regulated by intracellular signaling pathways that are controlled by the hormones insulin, epinephrine, and glucagon (see Table 16–1, p. 536 and Figure 16–21).

Quantitatively, fat is a far more important storage material than glycogen, in part because the oxidation of a gram of fat releases about twice as much energy as the oxidation of a gram of glycogen. Moreover, glycogen binds a great deal of water, producing a sixfold difference in the actual mass of glycogen required to store the same amount of energy as fat. An average adult human stores enough glycogen for only about a day of normal activity, but we store enough fat to last nearly a month. If our main fuel reserves had to be carried as glycogen instead of fat, our body weight would need to be increased by an average of about 60 pounds (nearly 30 kilograms).

Fats are generally stored as droplets of water-insoluble triacylglycerols inside cells (**Figure 13–23** and see Figure 13–11). Most animal species possess specialized fat-storing cells called *adipocytes*. In response to hormonal signals, fatty acids can be released from these depots into the bloodstream for other cells to use as required. Such a need arises after a period of not eating. Even a normal overnight fast results in the mobilization of fat: in the morning, most of the acetyl CoA that enters the citric acid cycle is derived from fatty acids rather than from glucose. After a meal, however, most of the acetyl CoA entering the citric acid cycle comes from glucose derived from food, and any excess glucose is used to make glycogen or fat. (Although animal cells can readily convert sugars to fats, they cannot convert fatty acids to sugars.)

The food reserves in both animals and plants form a vital part of the human diet. Plants convert some of the sugars they make through photosynthesis during daylight into fats and into **starch**, a branched polymer of glucose very similar to animal glycogen. The fats in plants are triacylglycerols, as they are in animals, and they differ only in the types of fatty acids that predominate (see Figures 2–21 and 2–22).

The embryo inside a plant seed must live on stored food reserves for a long time, until the seed germinates to produce a plant with leaves that can harvest the energy in sunlight. The embryo uses these food stores as sources of energy and of small molecules to build cell walls and to synthesize many other biological molecules as it develops. For this reason, plant seeds often contain especially large amounts of fats and starch—which make them a major food source for animals, including ourselves (**Figure 13–24**). Germinating seeds convert the stored fat and starch into glucose as needed.

Figure 13–24 Some plant seeds serve as important foods for humans. Corn, nuts, and peas all contain rich stores of starch and fats, which provide the plant embryo in the seed with energy and building blocks for biosynthesis. (Courtesy of the John Innes Foundation.)

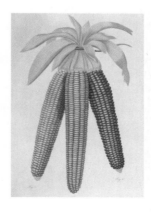
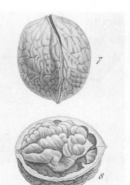
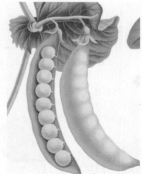

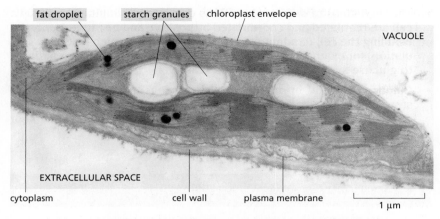

fat droplet   starch granules   chloroplast envelope

VACUOLE

EXTRACELLULAR SPACE

cytoplasm   cell wall   plasma membrane

1 µm

Figure 13–25 Plant cells store both starch and fats in their chloroplasts.
An electron micrograph of a single chloroplast in a plant cell shows the starch granules and fat droplets that have been synthesized in the organelle. (Courtesy of K. Plaskitt.)

In plant cells, fats and starch are both stored in chloroplasts—specialized organelles that carry out photosynthesis (**Figure 13–25**). These energy-rich molecules serve as food reservoirs that are mobilized by the cell to produce ATP in mitochondria during periods of darkness. In the next chapter, we take a closer look at chloroplasts and mitochondria, and review the elaborate mechanisms by which they harvest energy from sunlight and from food.

ESSENTIAL CONCEPTS

- Food molecules are broken down in successive steps, in which energy is captured in the form of activated carriers such as ATP and NADH.

- In plants and animals, these catabolic reactions occur in different cell compartments: glycolysis in the cytosol, the citric acid cycle in the mitochondrial matrix, and oxidative phosphorylation on the inner mitochondrial membrane.

- During glycolysis, the six-carbon sugar glucose is split to form two molecules of the three-carbon sugar pyruvate, producing small amounts of ATP and NADH.

- In the presence of oxygen, eukaryotic cells convert pyruvate into acetyl CoA plus CO_2 in the mitochondrial matrix. The citric acid cycle then converts the acetyl group in acetyl CoA to CO_2 and H_2O, capturing much of the energy released as high-energy electrons in the activated carriers NADH and $FADH_2$.

- Fatty acids produced from the digestion of fats are also imported into mitochondria and converted to acetyl CoA molecules, which are then further oxidized through the citric acid cycle.

- In the mitochondrial matrix, NADH and $FADH_2$ pass their high-energy electrons to an electron-transport chain in the inner mitochondrial membrane, where a series of electron transfers is used to drive the formation of ATP. Most of the energy captured during the breakdown of food molecules is harvested during this process of oxidative phosphorylation (described in detail in Chapter 14).

- Many intermediates of glycolysis and the citric acid cycle are starting points for the anabolic pathways that lead to the synthesis of proteins, nucleic acids, and the many other organic molecules of the cell.

- The thousands of different reactions carried out simultaneously by a cell are regulated and coordinated by positive and negative feedback, enabling the cell to adapt to changing conditions; such feedback regulation, for example, allows a cell to switch from glucose breakdown to glucose synthesis when food is scarce.

- Glucose is stored in animal cells as glycogen, whereas plant cells store glucose as starch; both animal and plant cells store fatty acids as fats (triacylglycerols). The food reserves stored by plants are major sources of food for animals, including humans.

KEY TERMS

acetyl CoA	fermentation
ADP, ATP	GDP, GTP
anabolic pathway	gluconeogenesis
catabolism	glucose
cell respiration	glycogen
citric acid cycle	glycolysis
electron-transport chain	NAD⁺, NADH
FAD, FADH₂	oxidative phosphorylation
fat	pyruvate
feedback regulation	starch

QUESTIONS

QUESTION 13–8

The complete oxidation of sugar molecules by the cell takes place according to the general reaction $C_6H_{12}O_6$ (glucose) $+ 6O_2 \rightarrow 6CO_2 + 6H_2O$ + energy. Which of the following statements are correct? Explain your answers.

A. All of the energy produced is in the form of heat.

B. None of the produced energy is in the form of heat.

C. The energy is produced by a process that involves the oxidation of carbon atoms.

D. The reaction supplies the cell with essential water.

E. In cells, the reaction takes place in more than one step.

F. Many steps in the oxidation of sugar molecules involve reaction with oxygen gas.

G. Some organisms carry out the reverse reaction.

H. Some cells that grow in the absence of O_2 produce CO_2.

QUESTION 13–9

An exceedingly sensitive instrument (yet to be devised) shows that one of the carbon atoms in Charles Darwin's last breath is resident in your bloodstream, where it forms part of a hemoglobin molecule. Suggest how this carbon atom might have traveled from Darwin to you, and list some of the molecules it could have entered en route.

QUESTION 13–10

Yeast cells can proliferate both in the presence of O_2 (aerobically) and in its absence (anaerobically). Under which of the two conditions could you expect the cells to proliferate better? Explain your answer.

QUESTION 13–11

During movement, muscle cells require large amounts of ATP to fuel their contractile apparatus. These cells contain high levels of creatine phosphate (Figure Q13–11), which has a standard free-energy change ($\Delta G°$) for hydrolysis of its phosphate bond of –43 kJ/mole. Why is this a useful compound to store energy? Justify your answer with the information shown in Figure 13–8.

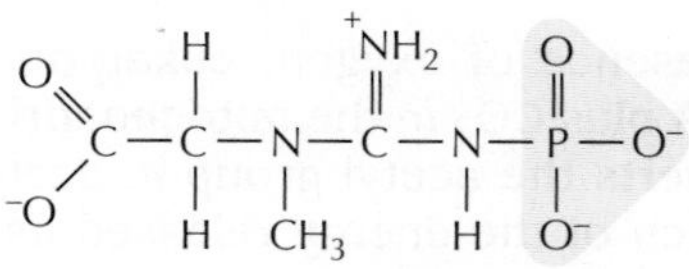

creatine phosphate

Figure Q13–11

QUESTION 13–12

Identical pathways that make up the complicated sequence of reactions of glycolysis, shown in Panel 13–1 (pp. 436–437), are found in most living cells, from bacteria to humans. One could envision, however, countless alternative chemical reaction mechanisms that would allow the oxidation of sugar molecules and that could, in principle, have evolved to take the place of glycolysis. Discuss this fact in the context of evolution.

QUESTION 13–13

An animal cell, roughly cubical in shape with a side length of 10 μm, uses 10^9 ATP molecules every minute. Assume that the cell replaces this ATP by the oxidation of glucose according to the overall reaction $6O_2 + C_6H_{12}O_6 \rightarrow 6CO_2 + 6H_2O$ and that complete oxidation of each glucose molecule produces 30 ATP molecules. How much oxygen does the cell consume every minute? How long will it take before the cell has used up an amount of oxygen gas equal to its own volume? (Recall that one mole of a gas has a volume of 22.4 liters.)

QUESTION 13–14

Under the conditions existing in the cell, the free energies of the first few reactions in glycolysis (in Panel 13–1, pp. 436–437) are:

step 1 $\Delta G = -33.5$ kJ/mole

step 2 $\Delta G = -2.5$ kJ/mole

step 3 $\Delta G = -22.2$ kJ/mole

step 4 $\Delta G = -1.3$ kJ/mole

Are these reactions energetically favorable? Using these values, draw to scale an energy diagram (A) for the overall reaction and (B) for the pathway composed of the four individual reactions.

QUESTION 13–15

The chemistry of most metabolic reactions was deciphered by synthesizing metabolites containing atoms that are different isotopes from those occurring naturally. The products of reactions starting with isotopically labeled metabolites can be analyzed to determine precisely which atoms in the products are derived from which atoms in the starting material. The methods of detection exploit, for example, the fact that different isotopes have different masses that can be distinguished using biophysical techniques such as mass spectrometry. Moreover, some isotopes are radioactive and can therefore be readily recognized with electronic counters or photographic film that becomes exposed by radiation.

A. Assume that pyruvate containing radioactive ^{14}C in its carboxyl group is added to a cell extract that can support oxidative phosphorylation. Which of the molecules produced should contain the vast majority of the ^{14}C that was added?

B. Assume that oxaloacetate containing radioactive ^{14}C in its keto group (refer to Panel 13–2, pp. 442–443) is added to the extract. Where should the ^{14}C atom be located after precisely one turn of the citric acid cycle?

QUESTION 13–16

In cells that can proliferate both aerobically and anaerobically, fermentation is inhibited in the presence of O_2. Suggest a reason for this observation.

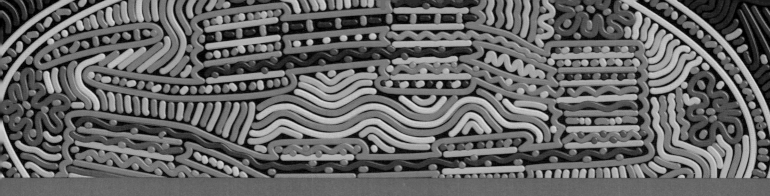

CHAPTER **FOURTEEN**

14

Energy Generation in Mitochondria and Chloroplasts

The fundamental need to generate energy efficiently has had a profound influence on the history of life on Earth. Much of the structure, function, and evolution of cells and organisms can be traced to their quest for energy. Oxygen did not appear in the atmosphere until more than a billion years after the first cells appeared on Earth. It is therefore thought that the earliest cells may have produced ATP by breaking down organic molecules that had been generated by geochemical processes. Such fermentation reactions, discussed in Chapter 13, can occur in the cytosol of present-day cells, when they use the energy derived from the partial oxidation of energy-rich food molecules to form ATP.

But very early in the history of life, a much more efficient mechanism for generating energy and synthesizing ATP appeared—one based on the transport of electrons along membranes. This mechanism is so central to the survival of life on Earth that we devote this entire chapter to it. Membrane-based electron transport first appeared in bacteria more than 3 billion years ago, and the progeny of these pioneering cells currently crowd every crevice of our planet's land and oceans in a wild menagerie of living forms. Perhaps most remarkably, remnants of these energy-generating electron-transport systems can be found in the bacterial descendants that labor within living eukaryotic cells: chloroplasts and mitochondria.

In this chapter, we consider the molecular mechanisms that enable electron-transport systems to generate the energy that cells need to survive. We begin with a brief overview of the general principles central to the generation of energy in all living things: the use of a membrane to harness the energy of moving electrons. We describe how such processes

MITOCHONDRIA AND
OXIDATIVE PHOSPHORYLATION

MOLECULAR MECHANISMS OF
ELECTRON TRANSPORT AND
PROTON PUMPING

CHLOROPLASTS AND
PHOTOSYNTHESIS

THE EVOLUTION OF ENERGY-
GENERATING SYSTEMS

Figure 14–1 Membrane-based mechanisms use the energy provided by food or sunlight to generate ATP. In oxidative phosphorylation, which occurs in mitochondria, an electron-transport system uses energy derived from the oxidation of food to generate a proton (H⁺) gradient across a membrane. In photosynthesis, which occurs in chloroplasts, an electron-transport system uses energy derived from the sun to generate a proton gradient across a membrane. In both cases, this proton gradient is then used to drive ATP synthesis.

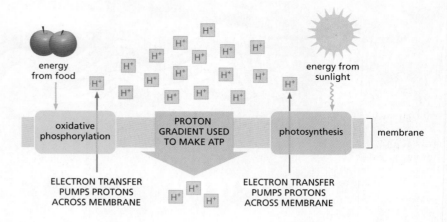

operate in both mitochondria and chloroplasts, and we review the chemical principles that allow the transfer of electrons to release large amounts of energy. Finally, we trace the evolutionary pathways that most likely gave rise to these marvelous mechanisms.

Cells Obtain Most of Their Energy by a Membrane-based Mechanism

The main chemical energy currency in cells is ATP (see Figure 3–31). Although small amounts of ATP are generated during glycolysis in the cell cytosol (discussed in Chapter 13), most of the ATP needed by cells is produced by *oxidative phosphorylation*. The generation of ATP by oxidative phosphorylation differs from the way ATP is produced during glycolysis, in that it requires a membrane-bound compartment. In eukaryotic cells, oxidative phosphorylation takes place in mitochondria, and it depends on an electron-transport process that drives the transport of protons (H^+) across the inner mitochondrial membrane. A related membrane-based process produces ATP during photosynthesis in plants, algae, and photosynthetic bacteria (**Figure 14–1**).

This membrane-based process for making ATP consists of two linked stages: one sets up an electrochemical proton gradient, and the other uses that gradient to generate ATP. Both stages are carried out by special protein complexes embedded in a membrane.

1. In stage 1, high-energy electrons—derived from the oxidation of food molecules (discussed in Chapter 13) or from sunlight or other chemical sources (discussed later)—are transferred along a series of electron carriers, called an **electron-transport chain**, embedded in a membrane. These electron transfers release energy that is used to pump protons, derived from the water that is ubiquitous in cells, across the membrane and thus generate an electrochemical proton gradient (**Figure 14–2A**). An ion gradient across a membrane is a form of stored energy that can be harnessed to do useful work when the ions are allowed to flow back across the membrane, down their electrochemical gradient (discussed in Chapter 12).

2. In stage 2, protons flow back down their electrochemical gradient through a membrane-embedded protein complex called *ATP synthase*, which catalyzes the energy-requiring synthesis of ATP from ADP and inorganic phosphate (P_i). This ubiquitous enzyme functions like a turbine that couples the movement of protons across the membrane to the production of ATP (**Figure 14–2B**).

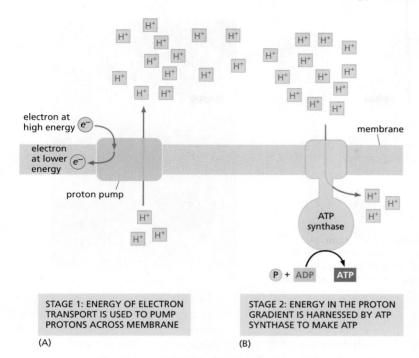

STAGE 1: ENERGY OF ELECTRON TRANSPORT IS USED TO PUMP PROTONS ACROSS MEMBRANE

(A)

STAGE 2: ENERGY IN THE PROTON GRADIENT IS HARNESSED BY ATP SYNTHASE TO MAKE ATP

(B)

Figure 14–2 Membrane-based systems use the energy stored in an electrochemical proton gradient to synthesize ATP. The process occurs in two stages. (A) In the first stage, a proton pump harnesses the energy of electron transfer (described later in the chapter) to pump protons (H^+) across a membrane, creating a proton gradient. The *blue* arrow shows the direction of electron movement. These high-energy electrons can come from organic or inorganic molecules, or they can be produced by the action of light on special molecules such as chlorophyll. The protons are derived from water, which is ubiquitous in the aqueous environment of the cell. (B) The proton gradient produced in (A) serves as a versatile energy store that can be used to drive a variety of energy-requiring reactions in mitochondria, chloroplasts, and prokaryotes—most importantly, the synthesis of ATP by ATP synthase.

QUESTION 14–1

Dinitrophenol (DNP) is a small molecule that renders membranes permeable to protons. In the 1940s, small amounts of this highly toxic compound were given to patients to induce weight loss. DNP was effective in melting away the pounds, especially promoting the loss of fat reserves. Can you explain how it might cause such loss? As an unpleasant side reaction, however, patients had an elevated temperature and sweated profusely during the treatment. Provide an explanation for these symptoms.

When it was first proposed in 1961, this mechanism for generating energy was called the *chemiosmotic hypothesis*, because it linked the chemical bond-forming reactions that synthesize ATP ("chemi-") with the membrane transport processes that pump protons ("osmotic," from the Greek *osmos*, "to push"). Thanks to this chemiosmotic mechanism, now known as **chemiosmotic coupling**, cells can harness the energy of electron transfers in much the same way that the energy stored in a battery can be harnessed to do useful work (**Figure 14–3**).

Chemiosmotic Coupling Is an Ancient Process, Preserved in Present-Day Cells

The membrane-based, chemiosmotic mechanism for making ATP arose very early in life's history, more than 3 billion years ago. The exact same type of ATP-generating processes occur in the plasma membrane of modern bacteria and archaea. The mechanism was so successful that its essential features have been retained in the long evolutionary journey from early prokaryotes to present-day cells.

The remarkable resemblance of the mechanism in prokaryotes and eukaryotes can be attributed in part to the fact that the organelles that produce ATP in eukaryotic cells—the chloroplasts and mitochondria—evolved from bacteria that were engulfed by ancestral cells more than a billion years ago (see Figures 1–19 and 1–21). As evidence of their bacterial ancestry, both chloroplasts and mitochondria reproduce in a manner

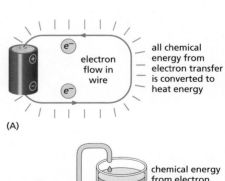

all chemical energy from electron transfer is converted to heat energy

(A)

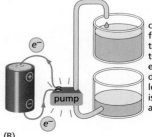

chemical energy from electron transfer is converted to the potential energy stored in a difference in water levels; less energy is therefore lost as heat energy

(B)

Figure 14–3 Batteries can use the energy of electron transfer to perform work. (A) If a battery's terminals are directly connected to each other, the energy released by electron transfer is all converted into heat. (B) If the battery is connected to a pump, much of the energy released by electron transfer can be harnessed to do work instead (in this case, to pump water). Cells can similarly harness the energy of electron transfer to do work—for example, pumping H^+ across a membrane (see Figure 14–2A).

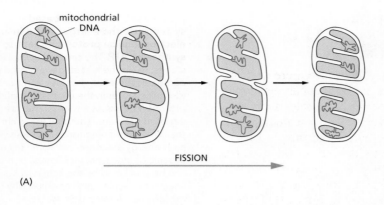

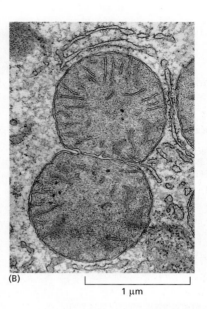

Figure 14–4 A mitochondrion can divide like a bacterium. (A) It undergoes a fission process that is conceptually similar to bacterial division. (B) An electron micrograph of a dividing mitochondrion in a liver cell. (B, courtesy of Daniel S. Friend, by permission of E.L. Bearer.)

similar to that of most prokaryotes (**Figure 14–4**). The organelles also harbor bacterial-like biosynthetic machinery for making RNA and proteins, and they possess DNA-based genomes (**Figure 14–5**). Not surprisingly, many chloroplast genes are strikingly similar to those of cyanobacteria—the photosynthetic bacteria from which these organelles were derived.

Although mitochondria and chloroplasts retain their own genomes, the bacteria from which they arose gave up many of the genes required for independent living as they developed their symbiotic relationships with eukaryotic animal and plant cells. Many of these jettisoned genes were not lost, however; they were relocated to the cell nucleus, where they continue to direct the production of proteins that mitochondria and chloroplasts import to carry out their specialized functions—including the generation of ATP.

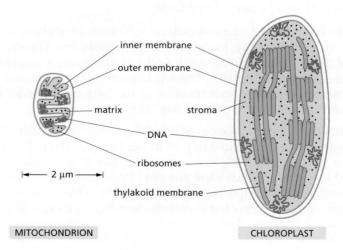

Figure 14–5 Mitochondria and chloroplasts share many of the features of their bacterial ancestors. Both organelles contain their own DNA-based genome and the machinery to replicate this DNA and to make RNA and protein. The inner compartments of these organelles—the mitochondrial matrix and the chloroplast stroma—contain the DNA (*red*) and a special set of ribosomes. Membranes in both organelles—the mitochondrial inner membrane and the chloroplast thylakoid membrane—contain the protein complexes involved in ATP production.

MITOCHONDRIA AND OXIDATIVE PHOSPHORYLATION

Mitochondria are present in nearly all eukaryotic cells, where they produce the bulk of the cell's ATP. Without mitochondria, eukaryotes would have to rely on the relatively inefficient process of glycolysis for all of their ATP production. When glucose is converted to pyruvate by glycolysis in the cytosol, the net result is that only two molecules of ATP are produced per glucose molecule, which is less than 10% of the total free energy potentially available from oxidizing the sugar. By contrast, about 30 molecules of ATP are produced when mitochondria are recruited to complete the oxidation of glucose that begins in glycolysis. Had ancestral cells not established the relationship with the bacteria that gave rise to modern mitochondria, it seems unlikely that complex multicellular organisms could have evolved.

The importance of mitochondria is further highlighted by the dire consequences of mitochondrial dysfunction. Defects in the proteins required for electron transport, for example, are responsible for an inherited disorder called *myoclonic epilepsy and ragged red fiber disease* (MERRF). Because muscle and nerve cells need large amounts of ATP to function normally, individuals with this condition typically experience muscle weakness, heart problems, epilepsy, and often dementia.

MERFF, like many of the disorders that affect mitochondrial function, stems from mutations that disable genes present in mitochondrial DNA (see Figure 14–5). Because mitochondria are passed down from mother to child (sperm mitochondria are lost after fertilization), such mutations are transmitted by the egg. To prevent the transmission of these life-threatening defects, reproductive biologists have developed methods for removing the nucleus from an egg that carries faulty mitochondria and transferring it to a donor egg that has healthy mitochondria. Although a baby boy produced using this form of *mitochondrial replacement therapy* was born in 2016, the approach remains controversial, in part because the effects of having genetic material from three "parents"—mother, father, and mitochondrial donor—are unknown.

In this section, we review the structure and function of mitochondria. We outline how this organelle makes use of an electron-transport chain, embedded in its inner membrane, to generate the proton gradient needed to drive the synthesis of ATP. And we consider the overall efficiency with which this membrane-based system converts the energy stored in food molecules into the energy contained in the phosphate bonds of ATP.

Mitochondria Are Dynamic in Structure, Location, and Number

Isolated mitochondria are generally similar in appearance to their bacterial ancestors. Inside a cell, however, mitochondria are remarkably adaptable and can adjust their location, shape, and number to suit that particular cell's needs. In some cell types, mitochondria remain fixed in one location, where they supply ATP directly to a site of unusually high energy consumption. In a heart muscle cell, for example, mitochondria are located close to the contractile apparatus, whereas in a sperm they are wrapped tightly around the motile flagellum (**Figure 14–6**). In other cells, mitochondria fuse to form elongated, tubular networks, which are diffusely distributed through the cytoplasm (**Figure 14–7**). These networks are dynamic, continually breaking apart by fission (see Figure 14–4) and fusing again (Movie 14.1 and Movie 14.2).

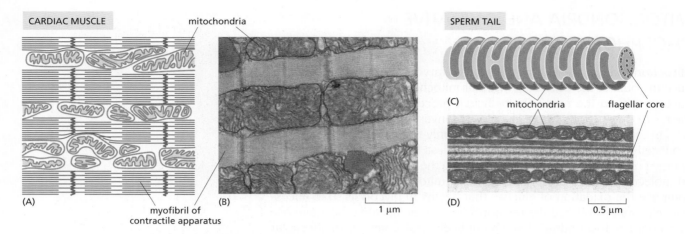

Figure 14–6 Mitochondria are located near sites of high ATP utilization. (A) In a cardiac muscle cell, mitochondria are located close to the contractile apparatus, where ATP hydrolysis provides the energy for contraction. The structure of the contractile apparatus is discussed in Chapter 17. (B) An electron micrograph of cardiac muscle shows a preponderance of mitochondria. (C) In a sperm, mitochondria are located in the tail, wrapped around a portion of the motile flagellum that requires ATP for its movement. The internal structure of the flagellar core is discussed in Chapter 17. (D) Micrograph showing a flagellum that has been thinly sliced to reveal the internal core structure as well as the surrounding mitochondria. (B, Keith Porter papers, Center for Biological Sciences Archives, University of Maryland, Baltimore Country; D, from W. Bloom and D.W. Fawcett, *A Textbook of Histology*, 10th ed. Philadelphia: W.B. Saunders Company, 1975. Reprinted with permission from the Estate of D.W. Fawcett.)

Mitochondria are present in large numbers—1000 to 2000 in a liver cell, for example. But their numbers vary depending on the cell type and can change with the energy needs of the cell. In skeletal muscle cells that have been repeatedly stimulated to contract, mitochondria can divide until their numbers increase five- to tenfold. Marathon runners, for example, may have twice the volume of mitochondria in their leg muscles than do individuals who are more sedentary.

Regardless of their varied appearance, location, and number, however, all mitochondria have the same basic internal structure—a design that supports the efficient production of ATP, as we see next.

A Mitochondrion Contains an Outer Membrane, an Inner Membrane, and Two Internal Compartments

An individual mitochondrion is bounded by two highly specialized membranes—one inside the other. These membranes, called the inner and outer mitochondrial membranes, create two mitochondrial

Figure 14–7 Mitochondria often form elongated, tubular networks, which can extend throughout the cytoplasm. (A) Mitochondria (*red*) are fluorescently labeled in this cultured mouse fibroblast. (B) In a yeast cell, the mitochondria (*red*) form a continuous network, tucked against the plasma membrane. (A, courtesy of Carl Zeiss Microscopy, LLC; B, from J. Nunnari et al., *Mol. Biol. Cell* 8:1233–1242, 1997. With permission from The American Society for Cell Biology.)

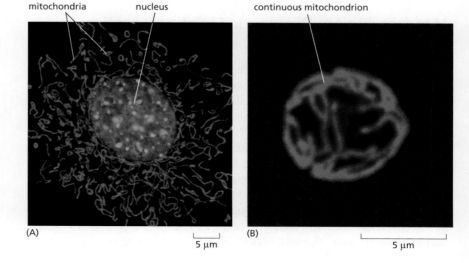

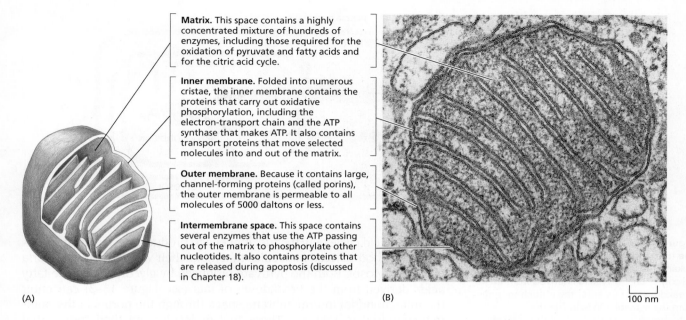

Matrix. This space contains a highly concentrated mixture of hundreds of enzymes, including those required for the oxidation of pyruvate and fatty acids and for the citric acid cycle.

Inner membrane. Folded into numerous cristae, the inner membrane contains the proteins that carry out oxidative phosphorylation, including the electron-transport chain and the ATP synthase that makes ATP. It also contains transport proteins that move selected molecules into and out of the matrix.

Outer membrane. Because it contains large, channel-forming proteins (called porins), the outer membrane is permeable to all molecules of 5000 daltons or less.

Intermembrane space. This space contains several enzymes that use the ATP passing out of the matrix to phosphorylate other nucleotides. It also contains proteins that are released during apoptosis (discussed in Chapter 18).

(A)

(B)

100 nm

compartments: a large internal space called the **matrix** and a much narrower *intermembrane space* (**Figure 14–8**). When purified mitochondria are gently fractionated into separate components and their contents analyzed (see Panel 4–3, pp. 164–165), each of the membranes, and the spaces they enclose, are found to contain a unique collection of proteins.

The *outer membrane* contains many molecules of a transport protein called *porin*, which forms wide, aqueous channels through the lipid bilayer (described in Chapter 11). As a result, the outer membrane is like a sieve that is permeable to all molecules of 5000 daltons or less, including small proteins. This makes the intermembrane space chemically equivalent to the cytosol with respect to the small molecules and inorganic ions it contains. In contrast, the *inner membrane*, like other membranes in the cell, is impermeable to the passage of ions and most small molecules, except where a path is provided by the specific membrane transport proteins that it contains. The mitochondrial matrix thus contains only those molecules that are selectively transported into the matrix across the inner membrane, and its contents are highly specialized.

The inner mitochondrial membrane is the site of oxidative phosphorylation, and it is here that the proteins of the electron-transport chain and the ATP synthase required for ATP production are concentrated. This membrane is highly convoluted, forming a series of infoldings—known as *cristae*—that project into the matrix space (see Figure 14–8 and Movie 14.3). These folds greatly increase the surface area of the membrane. In a liver cell, the inner membranes of all the mitochondria make up about one-third of the total membranes of the cell.

The Citric Acid Cycle Generates High-Energy Electrons Required for ATP Production

The generation of ATP is powered by the flow of electrons that are derived from the burning of carbohydrates, fats, and other foodstuffs during glycolysis and the citric acid cycle. These "high-energy" electrons are provided by activated carriers generated during these two sets of catabolic reactions, with the majority being churned out by the citric acid cycle that operates in the mitochondrial matrix (discussed in Chapter 13).

Figure 14–8 A mitochondrion is organized into four separate compartments. (A) A schematic drawing and (B) an electron micrograph of a mitochondrion. Each compartment contains a unique set of proteins, enabling it to perform its distinct functions. In liver mitochondria, an estimated 67% of the total mitochondrial protein is located in the matrix, 21% in the inner membrane, 6% in the outer membrane, and 6% in the intermembrane space. (B, courtesy of Daniel S. Friend, by permission of E.L. Bearer.)

QUESTION 14–2

Electron micrographs show that mitochondria in heart muscle have a much higher density of cristae than mitochondria in skin cells. Suggest an explanation for this observation.

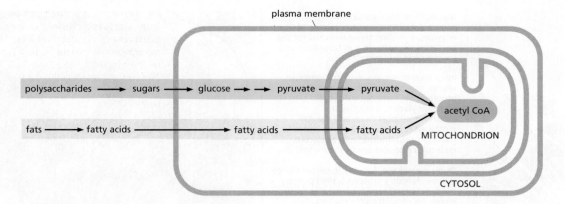

plasma membrane

polysaccharides → sugars → glucose → pyruvate → pyruvate ↘
                                                              acetyl CoA
fats → fatty acids → fatty acids → fatty acids ↗

MITOCHONDRION

CYTOSOL

Figure 14–9 Acetyl CoA is produced in the mitochondria. In animal cells and other eukaryotes, pyruvate produced during glycolysis and fatty acids derived from the breakdown of fats enter the mitochondrion from the cytosol. Once inside the mitochondrial matrix, both of these food-derived molecules are converted to acetyl CoA and then oxidized to CO_2.

The citric acid cycle gets the fuel it needs to produce these activated carriers from food-derived molecules that make their way into mitochondria from the cytosol. Both the pyruvate produced by glycolysis and the fatty acids derived from the breakdown of fats (see Figure 13–3) can enter the mitochondrial intermembrane space through the porins in the outer mitochondrial membrane. These fuel molecules are then transported across the inner mitochondrial membrane into the matrix, where they are converted into the crucial metabolic intermediate, acetyl CoA (**Figure 14–9**). The acetyl groups in acetyl CoA are then oxidized to CO_2 via the citric acid cycle (see Figure 13–12). Some of the energy derived from this oxidation is saved in the form of high-energy electrons, held by the activated carriers NADH and $FADH_2$. These two activated carriers can then donate their electrons to the electron-transport chain in the inner mitochondrial membrane (**Figure 14–10**).

The Movement of Electrons Is Coupled to the Pumping of Protons

The chemiosmotic generation of energy begins when the activated carriers NADH and $FADH_2$ donate their electrons to the electron-transport chain in the inner mitochondrial membrane, becoming oxidized to NAD^+ and FAD, respectively, in the process (see Figure 14–10). The electrons are quickly passed along the chain to molecular oxygen (O_2) to form water (H_2O). The stepwise movement of these electrons through the components of the electron-transport chain releases energy that can then be used to pump protons across the inner mitochondrial membrane (**Figure 14–11**). The resulting proton gradient, in turn, is used to drive the synthesis of ATP. The full sequence of reactions is shown in **Figure 14–12**. The inner mitochondrial membrane thus serves as a device that converts the energy contained in the high-energy electrons of NADH (and $FADH_2$) into the phosphate bond of ATP molecules (**Figure 14–13**). This chemiosmotic

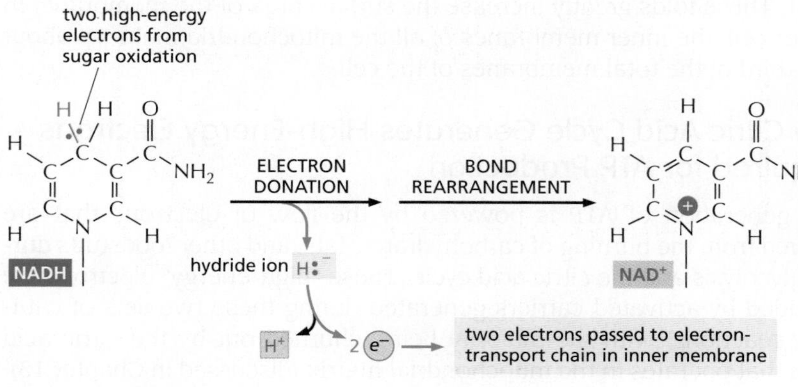

Figure 14–10 NADH donates its "high-energy" electrons to an electron-transport chain. A hydride ion (a hydrogen atom with two electrons, *red*) is removed from NADH and is converted into a proton and two electrons (*blue*). Only the part of NADH that carries these high-energy electrons is shown; for the complete structure and the conversion of NAD^+ back to NADH, see the structure of the closely related NADPH in Figure 3–34. Electrons are also carried in a similar way by $FADH_2$, whose structure is shown in Figure 13–13B.

two high-energy electrons from sugar oxidation

NADH   → ELECTRON DONATION → BOND REARRANGEMENT → NAD^+

hydride ion H:⁻

H^+ 2 e^- → two electrons passed to electron-transport chain in inner membrane

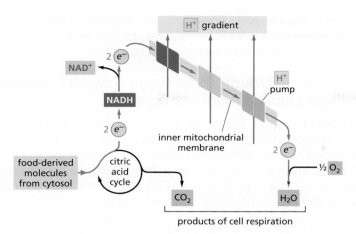

products of cell respiration

Figure 14–11 As electrons are transferred from activated carriers to oxygen, protons are pumped across the inner mitochondrial membrane. This is stage 1 of chemiosmotic coupling (see Figure 14–2). The path of electron flow is indicated by *blue* arrows. Only the pathway for NADH is shown here.

mechanism for ATP synthesis is called **oxidative phosphorylation** because it involves both the consumption of O_2 and the addition of a phosphate group to ADP to form ATP.

The source of the high-energy electrons that power the proton pumping differs widely between different organisms and different processes. During cell respiration—the energy-generating process that takes place in both mitochondria and aerobic bacteria—these electrons are ultimately derived from sugars or fats. In photosynthesis, the high-energy electrons come from the organic green pigment *chlorophyll*, which captures energy from sunlight. And many single-celled organisms (archaea and bacteria) use inorganic substances such as hydrogen, iron, and sulfur as the source of the high-energy electrons that they need to make ATP (see, for example, Figure 1–13).

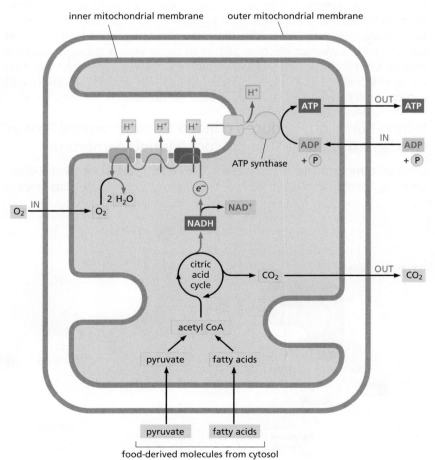

food-derived molecules from cytosol

Figure 14–12 Activated carriers generated during the citric acid cycle power the production of ATP. Pyruvate and fatty acids enter the mitochondrial matrix (*bottom*), where they are converted to acetyl CoA. The acetyl CoA is then metabolized by the citric acid cycle, which produces NADH (and $FADH_2$, not shown). During oxidative phosphorylation, high-energy electrons donated by NADH (and $FADH_2$) are then passed along the electron-transport chain in the inner membrane and ultimately handed off to oxygen (O_2); this electron transport generates a proton gradient across the inner membrane, which is used to drive the production of ATP by ATP synthase. The exact ratios of "reactants" and "products" are not indicated in this diagram: for example, we will see shortly that it requires four electrons from NADH molecules to convert O_2 to two H_2O molecules.

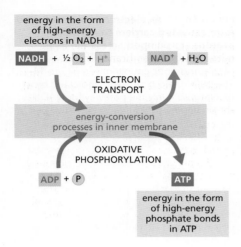

Figure 14–13 To produce ATP, mitochondria catalyze a major conversion of energy. In oxidative phosphorylation, the energy released by the oxidation of NADH to NAD$^+$ is harnessed—through energy-conversion processes in the inner mitochondrial membrane—to drive the energy-requiring phosphorylation of ADP to form ATP. The net equation for this process, in which four electrons pass from NADH to oxygen, is $2NADH + O_2 + 2H^+ \rightarrow 2NAD^+ + 2H_2O$. A smaller amount of ATP is similarly generated from energy released by the oxidation of FADH$_2$ to FAD (not shown).

Regardless of the electron source, the vast majority of living organisms use a chemiosmotic mechanism to generate ATP. In the following sections, we describe in detail how this process occurs.

Electrons Pass Through Three Large Enzyme Complexes in the Inner Mitochondrial Membrane

The electron-transport chain—or *respiratory chain*—that carries out oxidative phosphorylation is present in many copies in the inner mitochondrial membrane. Each chain contains over 40 proteins, grouped into three large **respiratory enzyme complexes**. These complexes each contain multiple individual proteins, including transmembrane proteins that anchor the complex firmly in the inner mitochondrial membrane.

The three respiratory enzyme complexes, in the order in which they receive electrons, are (1) *NADH dehydrogenase complex*, (2) *cytochrome* c *reductase complex*, and (3) *cytochrome* c *oxidase complex* (**Figure 14–14**). Each complex contains metal ions and other chemical groups that act as stepping stones to enable the passage of electrons through the complex. The movement of electrons through these respiratory complexes is accompanied by the pumping of protons from the mitochondrial matrix to the intermembrane space. Thus each complex can be thought of as a proton pump.

The first respiratory complex in the chain, NADH dehydrogenase, accepts electrons from NADH. These electrons are extracted from NADH in the form of a hydride ion (H$^-$), which is then converted into a proton and two high-energy electrons (see Figure 14–10). That reaction, $H^- \rightarrow H^+ + 2e^-$, is catalyzed by the NADH dehydrogenase complex itself. After passing through this complex, the electrons move along the chain to each of the other enzyme complexes in turn, using mobile electron carriers to ferry them between the complexes (see Figure 14–14). This transfer of electrons is energetically favorable: the electrons are passed from electron carriers with a weaker electron affinity to those with a stronger electron affinity, until they combine with a molecule of O$_2$ to form water. The final electron transfer is the only oxygen-requiring step in cell respiration, and it consumes nearly all of the oxygen that we breathe.

Proton Pumping Produces a Steep Electrochemical Proton Gradient Across the Inner Mitochondrial Membrane

Without a mechanism for harnessing the energy released by the energetically favorable transfer of electrons from NADH to O$_2$, this energy

Figure 14–14 High-energy electrons are transferred through three respiratory enzyme complexes in the inner mitochondrial membrane. The relative size and shape of each complex are indicated, but the numerous individual protein components that form each complex are not. During the transfer of electrons from NADH to oxygen (*blue* lines), protons derived from water are pumped across the membrane from the matrix into the intermembrane space by each of the complexes (**Movie 14.4**). Ubiquinone (Q) and cytochrome *c* (c) serve as mobile carriers that ferry electrons from one complex to the next.

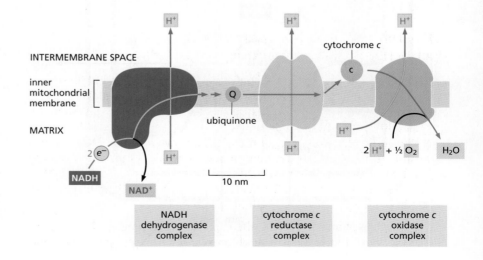

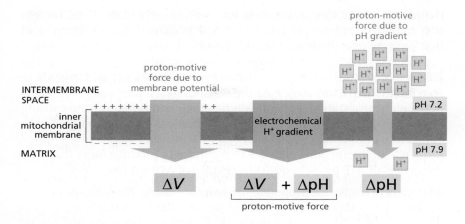

Figure 14–15 The electrochemical H⁺ **gradient across the inner mitochondrial membrane includes a large force due to the membrane potential (ΔV) and a smaller force due to the H⁺ concentration gradient—that is, the pH gradient (ΔpH).** The intermembrane space is slightly more acidic than the matrix, because the higher the concentration of protons, the more acidic the solution (see Panel 2–2, pp. 68–69). Both the membrane potential and the pH gradient combine to generate the proton-motive force, which pulls H⁺ back into the mitochondrial matrix. The exact, mathematical relationship between these forces is expressed by the Nernst equation (see Figure 12–24).

would simply be liberated as heat. Cells are able to recover much of this energy because each of the respiratory enzyme complexes in the electron-transport chain uses it to pump protons across the inner mitochondrial membrane, from the matrix into the intermembrane space (see Figure 14–14). Later, we will outline the molecular mechanisms involved. For now, we focus on the consequences of this nifty maneuver. First, the pumping of protons generates an H⁺ gradient—or pH gradient—across the inner membrane. As a result, the pH in the matrix (around 7.9) is about 0.7 unit higher than it is in the intermembrane space (which is 7.2, the same pH as the cytosol). Second, proton pumping generates a voltage gradient—or membrane potential—across the inner membrane; as H⁺ flows outward, the matrix side of the membrane becomes negative and the side facing the intermembrane space becomes positive.

As discussed in Chapter 12, the force that drives the passive flow of an ion across a membrane is proportional to the ion's *electrochemical gradient*. The strength of that electrochemical gradient depends both on the voltage across the membrane, as measured by the membrane potential, and on the ion's concentration gradient (see Figure 12–5). Because protons are positively charged, they will more readily cross a membrane if there is an excess of negative charge on the other side. In the case of the inner mitochondrial membrane, the pH gradient and membrane potential work together to create a steep electrochemical proton gradient that makes it energetically very favorable for H⁺ to flow back into the mitochondrial matrix. The membrane potential contributes significantly to this *proton-motive force*, which pulls H⁺ back across the membrane; the greater the membrane potential, the more energy is stored in the proton gradient (**Figure 14–15**).

ATP Synthase Uses the Energy Stored in the Electrochemical Proton Gradient to Produce ATP

If protons in the intermembrane space were simply allowed to flow back into the mitochondrial matrix, the energy stored in the electrochemical proton gradient would be lost as heat. Such a seemingly wasteful process allows hibernating bears to stay warm, as we discuss further in How We Know (pp. 476–477). In most cells, however, the electrochemical proton gradient across the inner mitochondrial membrane is used to drive the synthesis of ATP from ADP and P_i (see Figure 2–27). The device that makes this possible is **ATP synthase**, a large, multisubunit protein embedded in the inner mitochondrial membrane.

ATP synthase is of ancient origin; the same enzyme generates ATP in the mitochondria of animal cells, the chloroplasts of plants and algae, and

QUESTION 14–3

When the drug dinitrophenol (DNP) is added to mitochondria, the inner membrane becomes permeable to protons (H⁺). In contrast, when the drug nigericin is added to mitochondria, the inner membrane becomes permeable to K⁺. (A) How does the electrochemical proton gradient change in response to DNP? (B) How does it change in response to nigericin?

the plasma membrane of bacteria and archaea. The part of the protein that catalyzes the phosphorylation of ADP is shaped like a lollipop head that projects into the mitochondrial matrix; it is penetrated by a central stalk that is attached to a transmembrane H^+ carrier (**Figure 14–16**). The passage of protons through the carrier causes the carrier and its stalk to spin rapidly, like a tiny motor. As the stalk rotates, it rubs against proteins in the enzyme's stationary head, altering their conformation and causing them to produce ATP. In this way, a mechanical deformation gets converted into the chemical-bond energy of ATP (Movie 14.5). This fine-tuned sequence of interactions allows ATP synthase to produce more than 100 molecules of ATP per second—3 molecules of ATP per revolution.

ATP synthase can also operate in reverse—using the energy of ATP hydrolysis to pump protons "uphill," against their electrochemical gradient (**Figure 14–17**). In this mode, ATP synthase functions like the H^+ pumps described in Chapter 12. Whether ATP synthase primarily makes ATP—or consumes it to pump protons—depends on the magnitude of the electrochemical proton gradient across the membrane in which the enzyme is embedded. In many bacteria that can grow either aerobically or anaerobically, the direction in which the ATP synthase works is routinely reversed when the bacterium runs out of O_2. Under these conditions, the ATP synthase uses some of the ATP generated inside the cell by glycolysis to pump protons out of the cell, creating the proton gradient that the bacterial cell needs to import its essential nutrients by coupled transport. A proton gradient is similarly used to drive the transport of small molecules in and out of the mitochondrial matrix, as we discuss next.

The Electrochemical Proton Gradient Also Drives Transport Across the Inner Mitochondrial Membrane

The synthesis of ATP is not the only process driven by the electrochemical proton gradient in mitochondria. Many small, charged molecules, such as pyruvate, ADP, and inorganic phosphate (P_i), are imported into the

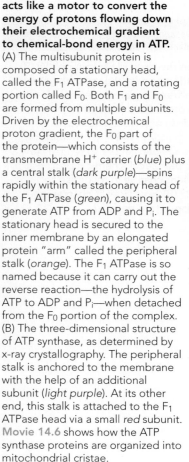

Figure 14–16 ATP synthase acts like a motor to convert the energy of protons flowing down their electrochemical gradient to chemical-bond energy in ATP. (A) The multisubunit protein is composed of a stationary head, called the F_1 ATPase, and a rotating portion called F_0. Both F_1 and F_0 are formed from multiple subunits. Driven by the electrochemical proton gradient, the F_0 part of the protein—which consists of the transmembrane H^+ carrier (*blue*) plus a central stalk (*dark purple*)—spins rapidly within the stationary head of the F_1 ATPase (*green*), causing it to generate ATP from ADP and P_i. The stationary head is secured to the inner membrane by an elongated protein "arm" called the peripheral stalk (*orange*). The F_1 ATPase is so named because it can carry out the reverse reaction—the hydrolysis of ATP to ADP and P_i—when detached from the F_0 portion of the complex. (B) The three-dimensional structure of ATP synthase, as determined by x-ray crystallography. The peripheral stalk is anchored to the membrane with the help of an additional subunit (*light purple*). At its other end, this stalk is attached to the F_1 ATPase head via a small *red* subunit. Movie 14.6 shows how the ATP synthase proteins are organized into mitochondrial cristae.

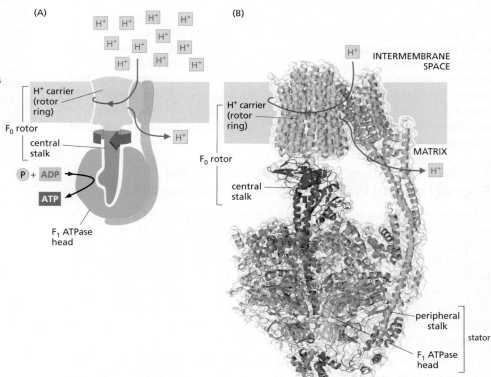

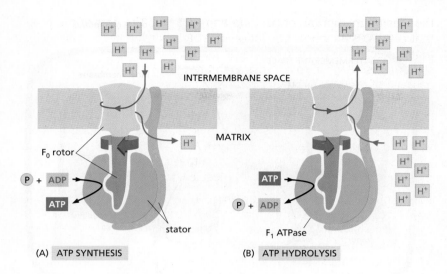

INTERMEMBRANE SPACE

MATRIX

F_0 rotor

P + ADP

ATP

stator

(A) ATP SYNTHESIS

ATP

P + ADP

F_1 ATPase

(B) ATP HYDROLYSIS

Figure 14–17 ATP synthase is a reversible coupling device. The protein can either (A) synthesize ATP by harnessing the electrochemical H^+ gradient or (B) pump protons against this gradient by hydrolyzing ATP. The direction of operation (and of rotation) at any given instant depends on the net free-energy change (ΔG, discussed in Chapter 3) for the coupled processes of H^+ translocation across the membrane and the synthesis of ATP from ADP and P_i. For example, if the electrochemical proton gradient falls below a certain level, the ΔG for H^+ transport into the matrix will no longer be large enough to drive ATP production; instead, ATP will be hydrolyzed by the ATP synthase to rebuild the proton gradient. A tribute to the activity of this all-important protein complex is shown in Movie 14.7.

mitochondrial matrix from the cytosol, while others, such as ATP, must be transported in the opposite direction. Carrier proteins that bind some of these molecules couple their transport to the energetically favorable flow of H^+ into the matrix (see the "coupled transporters" in Figure 12–15). Pyruvate and P_i, for example, are each co-transported inward, along with protons, as the protons move down their electrochemical gradient into the matrix.

Other transporters take advantage of the membrane potential generated by the electrochemical proton gradient, which makes the matrix side of the inner mitochondrial membrane more negatively charged than the side that faces the intermembrane space (see Figure 14–15). A special antiport carrier protein exploits this voltage gradient to export ATP from the mitochondrial matrix and to bring ADP in. This exchange allows the ATP synthesized in the mitochondrion to be exported rapidly, which is important for energizing the rest of the cell (**Figure 14–18**).

The electrochemical proton gradient is also required for the translocation of proteins across the inner mitochondrial membrane and into the matrix. As mentioned earlier, although mitochondria retain their own genome—and synthesize some of their own proteins—most of the proteins required for mitochondrial function are made in the cytosol and must be actively imported into the organelle. We discuss this transport process—which requires energy supplied by the electrochemical proton gradient as well as ATP hydrolysis—in Chapter 15.

In eukaryotic cells, therefore, the electrochemical proton gradient is used to drive both the generation of ATP and the transport of selected metabolites and proteins across the inner mitochondrial membrane. In bacteria, the proton gradient across the plasma membrane is similarly used to drive ATP synthesis and metabolite transport. But it also serves as an important source of directly usable energy: in motile bacteria, for instance, the flow of protons into the cell drives the rapid rotation of the bacterial flagellum, which propels the bacterium along (Movie 14.8).

The Rapid Conversion of ADP to ATP in Mitochondria Maintains a High ATP/ADP Ratio in Cells

As a result of the nucleotide exchange shown in Figure 14–18, ADP molecules—produced by hydrolysis of ATP in the cytosol—are rapidly drawn back into mitochondria for recharging, while the bulk of the ATP molecules

QUESTION 14–4

The remarkable properties that allow ATP synthase to run in either direction allow the interconversion of energy stored in the H^+ gradient and energy stored in ATP to proceed in either direction. (A) If ATP synthase making ATP can be likened to a water-driven turbine producing electricity, what would be an appropriate analogy when it works in the opposite direction? (B) Under what conditions would one expect the ATP synthase to stall, running neither forward nor backward? (C) What determines the direction in which the ATP synthase operates?

Figure 14–18 The electrochemical proton gradient across the inner mitochondrial membrane is used to drive some coupled transport processes. The charge on each of the transported molecules is indicated for comparison with the membrane potential, which is negative inside, as shown. Pyruvate and inorganic phosphate (P_i) are moved into the matrix along with protons, as the protons move down their electrochemical gradient. Both are negatively charged, so their movement is opposed by the negative membrane potential; however, the H^+ concentration gradient—the pH gradient—is harnessed in a way that nevertheless drives their inward transport. ADP is pumped into the matrix and ATP is pumped out by an antiport process that uses the voltage gradient across the membrane to drive the exchange. The outer mitochondrial membrane is freely permeable to all of these compounds due to the presence of porins in the membrane (not shown). The active transport of molecules across membranes by carrier proteins and the generation of a membrane potential are discussed in Chapter 12.

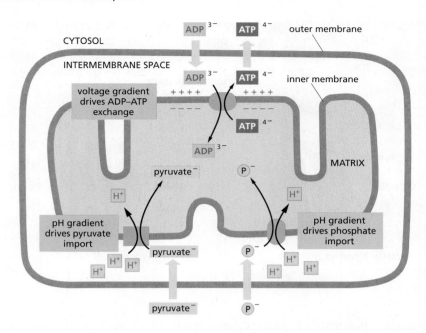

produced in mitochondria are exported into the cytosol, where they are most needed. (A small amount of ATP is used within the mitochondrion itself to power DNA replication, protein synthesis and translocation, and other energy-consuming reactions that occur there.) With all of this back-and-forth, a typical ATP molecule in a human cell will shuttle out of a mitochondrion, then back in as ADP, more than once every minute.

As discussed in Chapter 3, most biosynthetic enzymes drive energetically unfavorable reactions by coupling them to the energetically favorable hydrolysis of ATP (see Figure 3–32). The pool of ATP in a cell is thus used to drive a huge variety of cell processes in much the same way that a battery is used to drive an electric engine. To serve as a readily available energy source, the concentration of ATP in the cytosol must be kept about 10 times higher than that of ADP. When the activity of mitochondria is halted, ATP levels fall dramatically and the cell's battery runs down. Eventually, energetically unfavorable reactions can no longer take place and the cell dies. The poison cyanide, which blocks electron transport in the inner mitochondrial membrane, causes cell death in exactly this way.

Cell Respiration Is Amazingly Efficient

The oxidation of sugars to produce ATP may seem unnecessarily complex. Surely the process could be accomplished more directly—perhaps by eliminating the citric acid cycle or some of the steps in the respiratory chain. Such simplification would certainly make the chemistry easier to learn—but it would not be as helpful for the cell. As discussed in Chapter 13, the oxidative pathways that allow cells to extract energy from food in a usable form involve many intermediates, each differing only slightly from its predecessor. In this way, the huge amount of energy locked up in food molecules can be parceled out into small packets that can be captured in activated carriers such as NADH and $FADH_2$ (see Figure 13–1).

Much of the energy carried by NADH and $FADH_2$ is ultimately converted into the bond energy of ATP. How much ATP each of these activated carriers can produce depends on several factors, including where its electrons enter the respiratory chain. The NADH molecules produced in the mitochondrial matrix during the citric acid cycle pass their high-energy electrons to the NADH dehydrogenase complex—the first complex in the chain. As the electrons pass from one enzyme complex to the next, they promote the pumping of protons across the inner mitochondrial membrane. In this way, each NADH molecule provides enough net energy to generate about 2.5 molecules of ATP (see Question 14–5 and its answer).

$FADH_2$ molecules, on the other hand, bypass the NADH dehydrogenase complex and pass their electrons to the membrane-embedded mobile carrier ubiquinone (see Figure 14–14). Because these electrons enter further down the respiratory chain than those donated by NADH, they promote the pumping of fewer protons: each molecule of $FADH_2$ thus produces only 1.5 molecules of ATP. Table 14–1 provides a full accounting of the ATP produced by the complete oxidation of glucose.

Although the biological oxidation of glucose to CO_2 and H_2O consists of many interdependent steps, the overall process—known as **cell respiration**—is remarkably efficient. Almost 50% of the total energy that could be released by burning sugars or fats is captured and stored in the phosphate bonds of ATP during cell respiration. That might not seem impressive, but it is considerably better than most nonbiological energy-conversion devices. Electric motors and gasoline engines operate at about 10–20% efficiency. If cells operated at this efficiency, an organism would have to eat voraciously just to maintain itself. Moreover, because the wasted energy is liberated as heat, large organisms (including humans) would need far better mechanisms for cooling themselves. It is hard to imagine how animals could have evolved without the elaborate yet economical mechanisms that allow cells to extract a maximum amount of energy from food.

MOLECULAR MECHANISMS OF ELECTRON TRANSPORT AND PROTON PUMPING

For many years, biochemists struggled to understand why electron-transport chains had to be embedded in membranes to function in ATP production. The puzzle was essentially solved in the 1960s, when it was discovered that transmembrane proton gradients drive the process. The concept of chemiosmotic coupling was so novel, however, that it was not widely accepted until more than a decade later, when experiments with artificial energy-generating systems put the power of proton gradients to the test, as described in How We Know (pp. 476–477).

Although investigators are still unraveling some of the details of chemiosmotic coupling at the atomic level, the fundamentals are now clear. In this section, we examine the basic principles that underlie the movement of electrons, and we explain in molecular detail how electron transport can drive the generation of a proton gradient. Because very similar mechanisms are used by mitochondria, chloroplasts, and prokaryotes, these principles apply to nearly all living things.

Protons Are Readily Moved by the Transfer of Electrons

Although protons resemble other positive ions such as Na^+ and K^+ in the way they move across membranes, in some respects they are unique. Hydrogen atoms are by far the most abundant atom in living organisms: they are plentiful not only in all carbon-containing biological molecules but also in the water molecules that surround them. The protons in water are highly mobile: by rapidly dissociating from one water molecule and then associating with its neighbor, they can quickly flit through a hydrogen-bonded network of water molecules (see Figure 2–15B). Thus water, which is everywhere in cells, serves as a ready reservoir for the donation

TABLE 14–1 PRODUCT YIELDS FROM GLUCOSE OXIDATION

Process	Direct Product	Final ATP Yield per Glucose
Glycolysis	2 NADH (cytosolic)	3*
	2 ATP	2
Pyruvate oxidation to acetyl CoA (two per glucose)	2 NADH (mitochondrial matrix)	5
Complete oxidation of the acetyl group of acetyl CoA (two per glucose)	6 NADH (mitochondrial matrix)	15
	2 $FADH_2$	3
	2 GTP	2
	TOTAL	30

*NADH produced in the cytosol yields fewer ATP molecules than NADH produced in the mitochondrial matrix because the mitochondrial inner membrane is impermeable to NADH. Transporting NADH into the mitochondrial matrix—where it can pass electrons to NADH dehydrogenase—thus requires energy.

QUESTION 14–5

Calculate the number of usable ATP molecules produced per pair of electrons transferred from NADH to oxygen if (i) five protons are pumped across the inner mitochondrial membrane for each electron passed through the three respiratory enzyme complexes, (ii) three protons must pass through the ATP synthase for each ATP molecule that it produces from ADP and inorganic phosphate inside the mitochondrion, and (iii) one proton is used to produce the voltage gradient needed to transport each ATP molecule out of the mitochondrion to the cytosol where it is used.

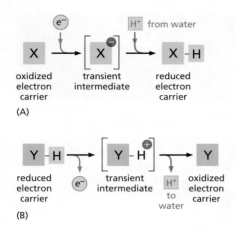

(A)

(B)

Figure 14–19 Electron transfers can cause the movement of entire hydrogen atoms, because protons are readily accepted from or donated to water. In these examples, (A) an oxidized electron carrier molecule, X, picks up an electron plus a proton when it is reduced, and (B) a reduced electron carrier molecule, Y, loses an electron plus a proton when it is oxidized.

and acceptance of protons. These nomadic protons often accompany the electrons that are transferred during oxidation and reduction. An isolated electron (e^-) bears a negative charge. But when a molecule is reduced by acquiring an electron, in many cases, this charge is immediately neutralized by the addition of a proton from water. Thus the net effect of the reduction is to transfer an entire hydrogen atom, $H^+ + e^-$ (**Figure 14–19A**).

Similarly, when a molecule is oxidized, it often loses an electron belonging to one of its hydrogen atoms: in most instances, when this electron is transferred to an electron carrier, the proton that is left behind is passed on to water (**Figure 14–19B**). Therefore, in a membrane in which electrons are being passed along an electron-transport chain, it is a relatively simple matter, in principle, to move protons from one side of the membrane to the other. All that is required is that the electron carrier be oriented in the membrane in such a way that it accepts an electron—along with a proton from water—on one side of the membrane, and then releases a proton on the other side of the membrane when it passes an electron on to the next electron carrier molecule in the chain (**Figure 14–20**).

The Redox Potential Is a Measure of Electron Affinities

The proteins of the respiratory chain guide the electrons so that they move sequentially from one enzyme complex to the next. Each of these electron transfers is an oxidation–reduction reaction: as described in Chapter 3, the molecule or atom donating the electron becomes oxidized, while the receiving molecule or atom becomes reduced (see pp. 87–88). These reactions are necessarily coupled: electrons removed from one molecule are always passed to another, so that whenever one molecule is oxidized, another is reduced.

Like any other chemical reaction, the tendency of such oxidation–reduction reactions, or **redox reactions**, to proceed spontaneously depends on the free-energy change (ΔG) for the electron transfer, which in turn depends on the relative electron affinities of the participating molecules. Electrons will pass spontaneously from molecules that have a relatively low affinity for some of their electrons, and thus lose them easily, to molecules that have a higher affinity for electrons. For example, NADH has a low electron affinity, so that its electrons are readily passed to the NADH dehydrogenase complex (see Figure 14–14). The batteries that power our electronic gadgets are based on similar electron transfers between chemical substances with different electron affinities.

Because electron transfers provide most of the energy in living things, it is worth taking time to understand them. We saw in Chapter 2 that molecules that donate protons are known as acids; those that accept protons are called bases (see Panel 2–2, pp. 68–69). These molecules exist in conjugate acid–base pairs, in which the acid is readily converted into the base by the loss of a proton. For example, acetic acid (CH_3COOH) is converted into its conjugate base (CH_3COO^-) in the reaction

$$CH_3COOH \rightleftharpoons CH_3COO^- + H^+$$

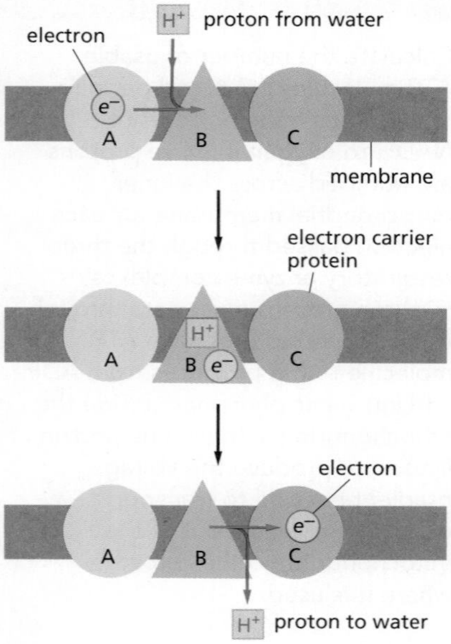

Figure 14–20 The orientation of a membrane-embedded electron carrier allows electron transfer to drive proton pumping. As an electron passes along an electron-transport chain, it can bind and release a proton at each step. In this schematic diagram, the electron carrier, protein B, picks up a proton (H^+) from one side of the membrane when it accepts an electron (e^-) from protein A; protein B releases the proton to the other side of the membrane when it donates its electron to the electron carrier, protein C. In this example, the transfer of a single electron thereby pumps the equivalent of one proton across a membrane.

In a similar way, pairs of compounds such as NADH and NAD^+ are called **redox pairs**, because NADH is converted to NAD^+ by the loss of electrons in the reaction

$$NADH \rightleftharpoons NAD^+ + H^+ + 2e^-$$

NADH is a strong electron donor. Its electrons can be said to be held at "high energy" because the ΔG for passing them to many other molecules is highly favorable. Conversely, because it is difficult to produce the high-energy electrons in NADH, its partner, NAD^+, is a weak electron acceptor.

The tendency for a redox pair such as NADH/NAD^+ to donate or accept electrons can be determined experimentally by measuring its **redox potential** (Panel 14–1, p. 472). The lower the redox potential, the lower the molecules' affinity for electrons—and the more likely they are to act as electron donors. Redox potentials are expressed in units of volts, as for a standard battery.

Electrons will move spontaneously from a redox pair with a low redox potential (or low affinity for electrons), such as NADH/NAD^+, to a redox pair with a high redox potential (or high affinity for electrons), such as O_2/H_2O. Thus, NADH is an excellent molecule to donate electrons to the respiratory chain, while O_2 is well suited to act as an electron "sink" at the end of the pathway. As explained in Panel 14–1, the difference in redox potential, $\Delta E_0'$, is a direct measure of the standard free-energy change ($\Delta G°$) for the transfer of an electron from one molecule to another.

Electron Transfers Release Large Amounts of Energy

The amount of energy that can be released by an electron transfer can be determined by comparing the redox potentials of the molecules involved. Again, let's look at the transfer of electrons from NADH and to O_2. As shown in Panel 14–1, a 1:1 mixture of NADH and NAD^+ has a redox potential of –320 mV, indicating that NADH has a weak affinity for electrons—and a strong tendency to donate them; a 1:1 mixture of H_2O and $\frac{1}{2}O_2$ has a redox potential of +820 mV, indicating that O_2 has a strong affinity for electrons—and a strong tendency to accept them. The difference in redox potential between these two pairs is 1.14 volts (1140 mV), which means that the transfer of each electron from NADH to O_2 under these standard conditions is enormously favorable: the $\Delta G°$ for that electron transfer is –109.6 kJ/mole per electron—or –219.2 kJ/mole for the two electrons that are donated from each NADH molecule (see Panel 14–1). If we compare this free-energy change with that needed for the formation of the terminal phosphoanhydride bond of ATP in cells (about 54 kJ/mole), we see that enough energy is released by the oxidization of one NADH molecule to synthesize several molecules of ATP.

Living systems could have evolved enzymes that would allow NADH to donate electrons directly to O_2 to make water. But because of the huge drop in free energy, this reaction would proceed with almost explosive force and nearly all of the energy would be released as heat. Instead, as we have seen, the transfer of electrons from NADH to O_2 is made in many small steps along the electron-transport chain, enabling nearly half of the released energy to be stored in the proton gradient across the inner mitochondrial membrane rather than getting lost to the environment as heat.

Metals Tightly Bound to Proteins Form Versatile Electron Carriers

Each of the three respiratory enzyme complexes includes metal atoms that are tightly bound to the proteins. Once an electron has been donated

HOW REDOX POTENTIALS ARE MEASURED

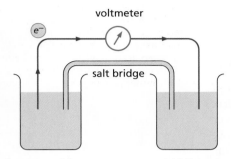

voltmeter

e⁻

salt bridge

$A_{reduced}$ and $A_{oxidized}$ in equimolar amounts

1 M H⁺ and 1 atmosphere H_2 gas

One beaker (*left*) contains substance A with an equimolar mixture of the reduced ($A_{reduced}$) and oxidized ($A_{oxidized}$) members of its redox pair. The other beaker contains the hydrogen reference standard ($2H^+ + 2e^- \rightleftharpoons H_2$), whose redox potential is arbitrarily assigned as zero by international agreement. (A salt bridge formed from a concentrated KCl solution allows K⁺ and Cl⁻ to move between the beakers as required to neutralize the charges when electrons flow between the beakers.) The metal wire (*dark blue*) provides a resistance-free path for electrons, and a voltmeter then measures the redox potential of substance A. If electrons flow from $A_{reduced}$ to H⁺, as indicated here, the redox pair formed by substance A is said to have a negative redox potential. If they instead flow from H_2 to $A_{oxidized}$, the redox pair is said to have a positive redox potential.

THE STANDARD REDOX POTENTIAL, E_0'

The standard redox potential for a redox pair, defined as E_0, is measured for a standard state where all of the reactants are at a concentration of 1 M, including H⁺. Since biological reactions occur at pH 7, biologists instead define the standard state as $A_{reduced} = A_{oxidized}$ and $H^+ = 10^{-7}$ M. This standard redox potential is designated by the symbol E_0', in place of E_0.

examples of redox reactions		standard redox potential E_0'
NADH $\rightleftharpoons$ NAD⁺ + H⁺ + 2e⁻		–320 mV
reduced ubiquinone $\rightleftharpoons$ oxidized ubiquinone + 2H⁺ + 2e⁻		+30 mV
reduced cytochrome c $\rightleftharpoons$ oxidized cytochrome c + e⁻		+230 mV
$H_2O \rightleftharpoons \frac{1}{2}O_2 + 2H^+ + 2e^-$		+820 mV

CALCULATION OF $\Delta G°$ FROM REDOX POTENTIALS

To determine the energy change for an electron transfer, the $\Delta G°$ of the reaction (kJ/mole) is calculated as follows:

$\Delta G° = -n(0.096)\,\Delta E_0'$, where n is the number of electrons transferred across a redox potential change of $\Delta E_0'$ millivolts (mV), and

$\Delta E_0' = E_0'(\text{acceptor}) - E_0'(\text{donor})$

EXAMPLE:

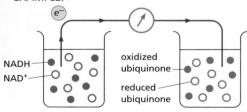

e⁻

NADH
NAD⁺

oxidized ubiquinone
reduced ubiquinone

1:1 mixture of NADH and NAD⁺

1:1 mixture of oxidized and reduced ubiquinone

For the transfer of one electron from NADH to ubiquinone:

$$\Delta E_0' = +30 - (-320) = +350 \text{ mV}$$

$\Delta G° = -n(0.096)\Delta E_0' = -1(0.096)(350) = -34$ kJ/mole

A similar calculation reveals that the transfer of one electron from ubiquinone to oxygen has an even more favorable $\Delta G°$ of –76 kJ/mole. The $\Delta G°$ value for the transfer of one electron from NADH to oxygen is the sum of these two values, –110 kJ/mole.

EFFECT OF CONCENTRATION CHANGES

As explained in Chapter 3 (see p. 93), the actual free-energy change for a reaction, ΔG, depends on the concentrations of the reactants and generally will be different from the standard free-energy change, $\Delta G°$. The standard redox potentials are for a 1:1 mixture of the redox pair. For example, the standard redox potential of –320 mV is for a 1:1 mixture of NADH and NAD⁺. But when there is an excess of NADH over NAD⁺, electron transfer from NADH to an electron acceptor becomes more favorable. This is reflected by a more negative redox potential and a more negative ΔG for electron transfer.

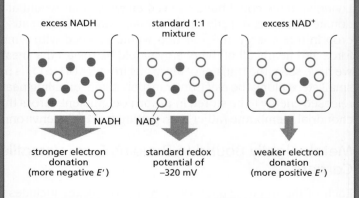

excess NADH

standard 1:1 mixture

excess NAD⁺

NADH   NAD⁺

stronger electron donation (more negative E')

standard redox potential of –320 mV

weaker electron donation (more positive E')

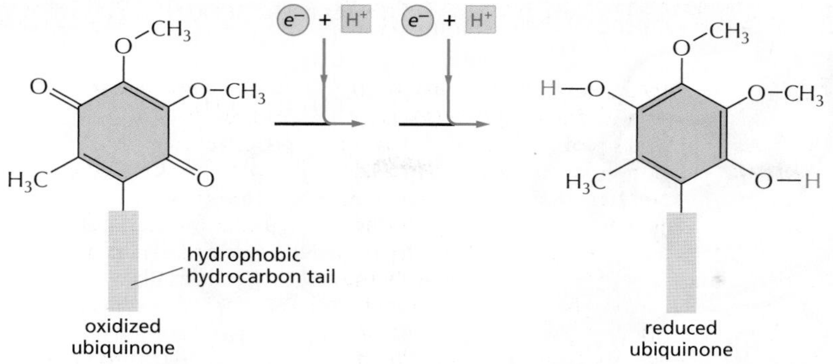

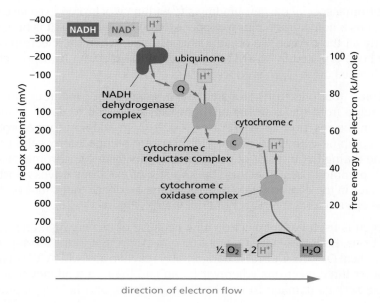

oxidized
ubiquinone

reduced
ubiquinone

hydrophobic
hydrocarbon tail

Figure 14–21 Quinones carry electrons within the lipid bilayer. The quinone in the mitochondrial electron-transport chain is called ubiquinone. It picks up one H^+ from the aqueous environment for every electron it accepts, and it can carry two electrons as part of its hydrogen atoms (*red*). When this reduced ubiquinone donates its electrons to the next carrier in the chain, the protons are released. Its long, hydrophobic hydrocarbon tail confines ubiquinone to the inner mitochondrial membrane.

to a respiratory complex, it can move within the complex by skipping from one embedded metal ion to another ion with an even greater affinity for electrons.

When electrons pass from one respiratory complex to the next, in contrast, they are ferried by electron carriers that can diffuse freely within or along the lipid bilayer. These mobile molecules pick up electrons from one complex and deliver them to the next in line. In the mitochondrial respiratory chain, for example, a small, hydrophobic molecule called ubiquinone picks up electrons from the NADH dehydrogenase complex and delivers them to the cytochrome *c* reductase complex (see Figure 14–14). A related **quinone** functions similarly during electron transport in photosynthesis. A ubiquinone molecule can accept or donate either one or two electrons, and it picks up one H^+ from water with each electron that it carries (**Figure 14–21**). Its redox potential of +30 mV places ubiquinone between the NADH dehydrogenase complex and the cytochrome *c* reductase complex in terms of its tendency to gain or lose electrons— which explains why ubiquinone receives electrons from the former and donates them to the latter (**Figure 14–22**). Ubiquinone also serves as the entry point for electrons donated by the $FADH_2$ that is generated both during the citric acid cycle and from fatty acid oxidation (see Figures 13–11 and 13–12).

The redox potentials of different metal complexes influence where they are used along the electron-transport chain. **Iron–sulfur centers** have relatively low affinities for electrons and thus are prominent in the electron carriers that operate in the early part of the chain. An iron–sulfur center

QUESTION 14–6

At many steps in the electron-transport chain, Fe ions are used as part of heme or FeS clusters to bind the electrons in transit. Why do these functional groups that carry out the chemistry of electron transfer need to be bound to proteins? Provide several reasons why this is necessary.

Figure 14–22 Redox potential increases along the mitochondrial electron-transport chain. The biggest increases in redox potential occur across each of the three respiratory enzyme complexes, which allows each of them to pump protons.

Figure 14–23 The iron in a heme group can serve as an electron acceptor. (A) Ribbon structure showing the position of the heme group (*red*) associated with cytochrome *c* (*green*). (B) The porphyrin ring of the heme group (*light red*) is attached covalently to side chains in the protein. The heme groups of different cytochromes have different electron affinities because they differ slightly in structure and are held in different local environments within each protein.

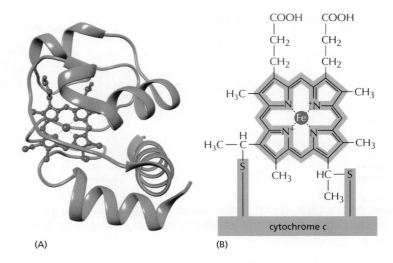

(A)   (B)

in the NADH dehydrogenase complex, for example, passes electrons to ubiquinone. Later in the pathway, iron atoms that are held in the heme groups bound to cytochrome proteins are commonly used as electron carriers (**Figure 14–23**). These heme groups give **cytochromes,** such as the cytochrome *c* reductase and cytochrome *c* oxidase complexes, their color ("cytochrome" from the Greek *chroma*, "color"). Like other electron carriers, the cytochrome proteins increase in redox potential the further down the mitochondrial electron-transport chain they are located. For example, cytochrome *c*, a small protein that accepts electrons from the cytochrome *c* reductase complex and transfers them to the cytochrome *c* oxidase complex, has a redox potential of +230 mV—a value about midway between those of the cytochromes with which it interacts (see Figure 14–22).

Cytochrome *c* Oxidase Catalyzes the Reduction of Molecular Oxygen

Cytochrome *c* oxidase, the final electron carrier in the respiratory chain, has the highest redox potential of all. This protein complex removes electrons from cytochrome *c*, thereby oxidizing it—hence the name "cytochrome *c* oxidase." The exceptionally high electron affinity stems in part from a special oxygen-binding site within cytochrome *c* oxidase that contains a heme group plus a copper atom (**Figure 14–24**). It is here that nearly all the oxygen we breathe is consumed, when the electrons that had been donated by NADH at the start of the electron-transport chain are handed off to O_2 to produce H_2O.

In total, four electrons donated by cytochrome *c* and four protons extracted from the aqueous environment are added to each O_2 molecule in the reaction $4e^- + 4H^+ + O_2 \rightarrow 2H_2O$. In addition to the protons that combine with O_2, four other protons are pumped across the membrane during the transfer of the four electrons from cytochrome *c* to O_2. This pumping occurs because the transfer of electrons drives allosteric changes in the conformation of cytochrome *c* oxidase that cause protons to be ejected from the mitochondrial matrix (**Figure 14–25**).

Oxygen is useful as an electron sink because of its very high affinity for electrons. However, once O_2 picks up one electron, it forms the superoxide radical O_2^-; this radical is dangerously reactive and will avidly take up another three electrons wherever it can find them, a tendency that can cause serious damage to nearby DNA, proteins, and lipid membranes.

QUESTION 14–7

Two different diffusible electron carriers, ubiquinone and cytochrome *c*, shuttle electrons between the three protein complexes of the electron-transport chain. Could the same diffusible carrier, in principle, be used for both steps? Explain your answer.

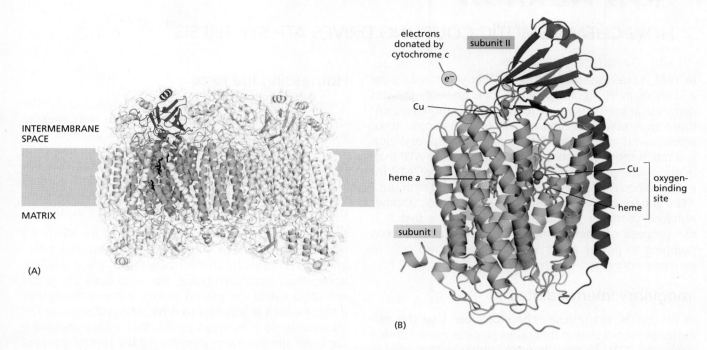

Figure 14–24 Cytochrome c oxidase is a finely tuned protein machine. The protein is a dimer formed from a monomer with 13 different protein subunits. (A) The entire protein is shown positioned in the inner mitochondrial membrane. The three colored subunits that form the functional core of the complex are encoded by the mitochondrial genome; the remaining subunits are encoded by the nuclear genome. (B) As electrons pass through this protein on the way to its bound O_2 molecule, they cause the protein to pump protons across the membrane. As indicated, a heme and a copper atom (Cu) form the site where a tightly bound O_2 molecule will receive four electrons to produce H_2O. Only two of the 13 subunits are shown.

The active site of cytochrome c oxidase therefore holds on tightly to an oxygen molecule until it receives all four of the electrons needed to convert it to two molecules of H_2O. This retention is critical, because it prevents superoxide radicals from attacking macromolecules throughout the cell—a type of damage that has been postulated to contribute to human aging.

The evolution of cytochrome c oxidase allowed cells to use O_2 as an electron acceptor, and this protein complex is essential for all aerobic life. Poisons such as cyanide are extremely toxic because they bind tightly to cytochrome c oxidase complexes, thereby halting electron transport and the production of ATP.

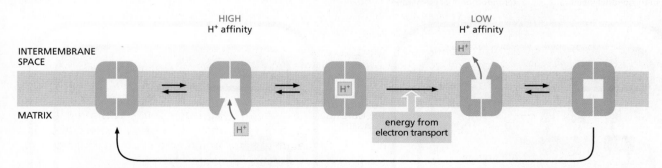

Figure 14–25 Proton pumping is coupled to electron transport. This type of mechanism is thought to be used by the NADH dehydrogenase complex and by cytochrome c oxidase, as well as by many other proton pumps. The protein is driven through a cycle of three conformations. In one of these conformations, the protein has a high affinity for H^+, causing it to pick up an H^+ on the matrix side of the membrane. In another conformation, the protein has a low affinity for H^+, causing it to release an H^+ on the other side of the membrane. As indicated, the cycle goes only in one direction—releasing the proton into the intermembrane space—because one of the steps is driven by allosteric change in conformation driven by the energetically favorable transport of electrons.

HOW WE KNOW

HOW CHEMIOSMOTIC COUPLING DRIVES ATP SYNTHESIS

In 1861, Louis Pasteur discovered that yeast cells grow and divide more vigorously when air is present—the first demonstration that aerobic metabolism is more efficient than anaerobic metabolism. His observations make sense now that we know that oxidative phosphorylation is a much more efficient means of generating ATP than is glycolysis, producing about 30 molecules of ATP for each molecule of glucose oxidized, compared with the 2 ATPs generated by glycolysis alone. But it took another hundred years for researchers to determine that it is the process of chemiosmotic coupling—using proton pumping to power ATP synthesis—that allows cells to generate energy with such efficiency.

Imaginary intermediates

In the 1950s, many researchers believed that the oxidative phosphorylation that takes place in mitochondria generated ATP via a mechanism similar to that used in glycolysis. During glycolysis, ATP is produced when a molecule of ADP receives a phosphate group directly from a "high-energy" intermediate. Such substrate-level phosphorylation occurs in steps 7 and 10 of glycolysis, where the high-energy phosphate groups from 1,3-bisphosphoglycerate and phosphoenolpyruvate, respectively, are transferred to ADP to form ATP (see Panel 13–1, pp. 436–437). It was assumed that the electron-transport chain in mitochondria would similarly generate some phosphorylated intermediate that could then donate its phosphate group directly to ADP. This assumption inspired a long and frustrating search for this mysterious high-energy intermediate. Investigators occasionally claimed to have discovered the missing intermediate, but the compounds turned out to be either unrelated to electron transport or, as one researcher put it in a review of the history of bioenergetics, "products of high-energy imagination."

Harnessing the force

It wasn't until 1961 that Peter Mitchell suggested that the "high-energy intermediate" his colleagues were seeking was, in fact, the electrochemical proton gradient generated by the electron-transport system. His proposal, dubbed the chemiosmotic hypothesis, stated that the energy of an electrochemical proton gradient formed during the transfer of electrons through the electron-transport chain could be tapped to drive ATP synthesis.

Several lines of evidence offered support for Mitchell's proposed mechanism. First, it was known that mitochondria do generate an electrochemical proton gradient across their inner membrane. But what does this gradient—also called the proton-motive force—actually do? If the gradient is required to drive ATP synthesis, as the chemiosmotic hypothesis posits, then either disrupting the inner membrane or eliminating the proton gradient across it should inhibit ATP production. In fact, researchers found both these predictions to be true. Physical disruption of the inner mitochondrial membrane halts ATP synthesis in that organelle. Similarly, dissipation of the proton gradient by a chemical "uncoupling" agent such as 2,4-dinitrophenol (DNP) also inhibits mitochondrial ATP production. Such gradient-busting chemicals carry H^+ across the inner mitochondrial membrane, forming a shuttle system for the movement of H^+ that bypasses the ATP synthase that generates ATP (**Figure 14–26**). In this way, compounds such as DNP uncouple electron transport from ATP synthesis. As a result of this short-circuiting, the proton-motive force is dissipated completely, and the organelle can no longer make ATP.

Such uncoupling occurs naturally in some specialized fat cells. In these cells, called *brown fat cells*, most of the energy from the oxidation of fat is dissipated as heat rather than being converted into ATP. The inner

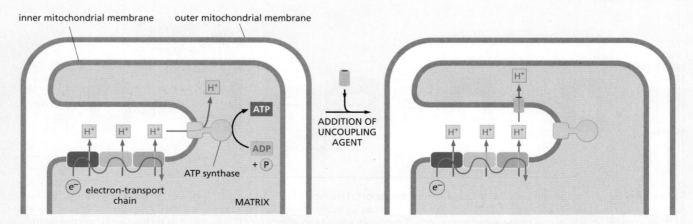

Figure 14–26 Uncoupling agents are H^+ carriers that can insert into the inner mitochondrial membrane. They render the membrane permeable to protons, allowing H^+ to flow into the mitochondrial matrix without passing through ATP synthase. This short-circuit effectively uncouples electron transport from ATP synthesis.

membranes of the mitochondria in these cells contain a carrier protein that allows protons to move down their electrochemical gradient, circumventing ATP synthase. As a result, the cells oxidize their fat stores at a rapid rate and produce much more heat than ATP. Tissues containing brown fat serve as biological heating pads, helping to revive hibernating animals and to protect sensitive areas of newborn human babies (such as the backs of their necks) from the cold.

Artificial ATP generation

If disrupting the electrochemical proton gradient across the mitochondrial inner membrane terminates ATP synthesis, then, conversely, generating an artificial proton gradient should stimulate ATP synthesis. Again, this is exactly what happens. When a proton gradient is imposed artificially by lowering the pH on the outside of the mitochondrial inner membrane, out pours ATP.

How does the electrochemical proton gradient drive ATP production? This is where the ATP synthase comes in. In 1974, Efraim Racker and Walther Stoeckenius demonstrated that they could assemble an artificial ATP-generating system by combining an ATP synthase isolated from the mitochondria of cow heart muscle with a proton pump purified from the purple membrane of the archaean *Halobacterium halobium*. As discussed in

Chapter 11, the plasma membrane of this prokaryote is packed with bacteriorhodopsin, a protein that pumps H⁺ out of the cell in response to sunlight (see Figure 11–28).

When bacteriorhodopsin alone was reconstituted into artificial lipid vesicles (liposomes), Racker and Stoeckenius showed that, in the presence of light, the protein pumps H⁺ into the vesicles, generating a proton gradient. (The orientation of the protein is reversed in these membranes, so that protons are transported into the vesicles; in the organism, protons are pumped out.) When the bovine ATP synthase was then incorporated into these vesicles, much to the amazement of many biochemists, the system catalyzed the synthesis of ATP from ADP and inorganic phosphate in response to light. This ATP formation showed an absolute dependence on an intact proton gradient, as either eliminating bacteriorhodopsin from the system or adding uncoupling agents such as DNP abolished ATP synthesis (**Figure 14–27**).

This remarkable experiment demonstrated without a doubt that a proton gradient can cause ATP synthase to make ATP. Thus, although biochemists had initially hoped to discover a high-energy intermediate involved in oxidative phosphorylation, the experimental evidence eventually convinced them that their search was in vain and that the chemiosmotic hypothesis was correct. Mitchell was awarded a Nobel Prize in 1978.

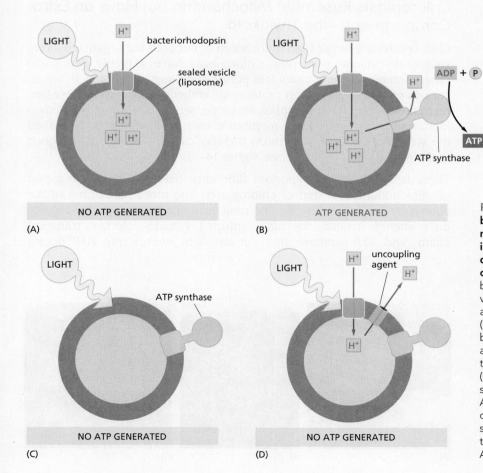

Figure 14–27 Experiments in which bacteriorhodopsin and bovine mitochondrial ATP synthase were introduced into liposomes provided direct evidence that proton gradients can power ATP production. (A) When bacteriorhodopsin is added to artificial lipid vesicles (liposomes), the protein generates a proton gradient in response to light. (B) In artificial vesicles containing both bacteriorhodopsin and an ATP synthase, a light-generated proton gradient drives the formation of ATP from ADP and P_i. (C) Artificial vesicles containing only ATP synthase do not on their own produce ATP in response to light. (D) In vesicles containing both bacteriorhodopsin and ATP synthase, uncoupling agents that abolish the proton gradient eliminate light-induced ATP synthesis.

CHLOROPLASTS AND PHOTOSYNTHESIS

Virtually all the organic material in present-day cells is produced by **photosynthesis**—the series of light-driven reactions that creates organic molecules from atmospheric carbon dioxide (CO_2). Plants, algae, and photosynthetic bacteria such as cyanobacteria use electrons from water and the energy of sunlight to perform this chemical feat. In the process, water molecules are split, releasing vast quantities of O_2 gas into the atmosphere. This oxygen in turn supports oxidative phosphorylation—not only in animals but also in plants and aerobic bacteria. As we discuss in detail at the end of the chapter, it was the activity of photosynthetic bacteria that eventually filled the atmosphere with oxygen, enabling the subsequent evolution of the myriad life-forms that today use aerobic metabolism to make their ATP (**Figure 14–28**).

For most plants, photosynthesis occurs mainly in the leaves. There, specialized intracellular organelles called **chloroplasts** capture light energy and use it to produce ATP and NADPH. These activated carriers are used to convert CO_2 into organic molecules that serve as the precursors for sugars—a process called *carbon fixation*.

Given the chloroplast's central role in photosynthesis, we begin this section by describing the structure of this highly specialized organelle. We then provide an overview of photosynthesis, followed by a detailed accounting of the mechanism by which chloroplasts harvest energy from sunlight to produce huge amounts of ATP and NADPH. Finally, we explain how plants use these two activated carriers to synthesize the sugars and other food molecules that sustain them, as well as the huge number of organisms that subsequently consume plants as part of their diet.

Chloroplasts Resemble Mitochondria but Have an Extra Compartment—the Thylakoid

Chloroplasts are larger than mitochondria, but both are organized along structurally similar principles. Chloroplasts have a highly permeable outer membrane and a much less permeable inner membrane, in which various membrane transport proteins are embedded. Together, these two membranes form the chloroplast envelope, separated by a narrow, inter-membrane space. The inner membrane surrounds a large space called the **stroma**, which contains many metabolic enzymes and is analogous to the mitochondrial matrix (see Figure 14–5).

There is, however, an important difference between the organization of mitochondria and that of chloroplasts. The inner membrane of the chloroplast does not contain the molecular machinery needed to produce energy. Instead, the light-capturing systems, electron-transport chain, and ATP synthase that convert light energy into ATP during

Figure 14–28 Microorganisms that carry out oxygen-producing photosynthesis changed Earth's atmosphere. (A) Living stromatolites from a lagoon in Western Australia. These structures are formed in specialized environments by large colonies of oxygen-producing photosynthetic cyanobacteria, which form mats that trap sand or minerals in thin layers. (B) Cross section of a modern stromatolite, showing its stratification. (C) A similar, layered structure can be seen in a fossilized stromatolite. These ancient accretions, some more than 3.5 billion years old, contain the remnants of the photosynthetic bacteria whose O_2-liberating activities ultimately transformed the Earth's atmosphere. (A, courtesy of Cambridge Carbonates Ltd.; B, courtesy of Roger Perkins, Virtual Fossil Museum, https://creativecommons.org/licenses/by-nc/4.0/; C, courtesy of S.M. Awramik, University of California/Biological Photo Service.)

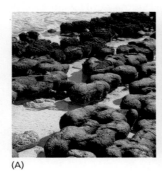
(A)

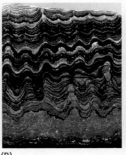
(B)

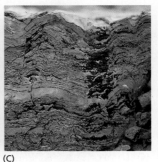
(C)

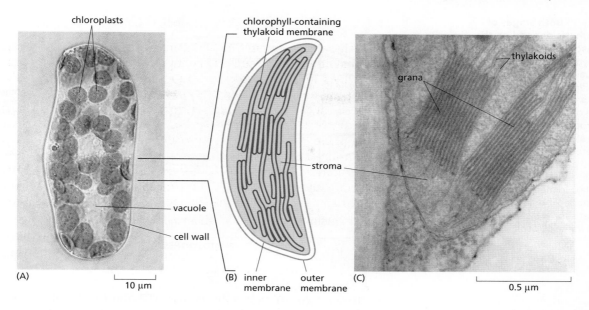

Figure 14–29 Chloroplasts, like mitochondria, are composed of a set of specialized membranes and compartments. (A) Light micrograph showing chloroplasts (*green*) in the cell of a flowering plant. (B) Drawing of a single chloroplast showing the organelle's three sets of membranes, including the thylakoid membrane (*dark green*), which contains the light-capturing and ATP-generating systems. (C) A high-magnification view of an electron micrograph shows the thylakoids arranged in stacks called *grana*; a single thylakoid stack is called a *granum* (Movie 14.9). (A, courtesy of Preeti Dahiya; C, courtesy of K. Plaskitt.)

photosynthesis are all contained in the *thylakoid membrane*. This third membrane is folded to form a set of flattened, disclike sacs, called the **thylakoids**, which are arranged in stacks called grana (**Figure 14–29**). The interior of each thylakoid is thought to be connected with that of other thylakoids, creating the *thylakoid space*—a compartment that is separate from the chloroplast stroma.

Photosynthesis Generates—and Then Consumes—ATP and NADPH

The chemistry carried out by photosynthesis can be summarized in one simple equation:

$$\text{light energy} + CO_2 + H_2O \rightarrow \text{sugars} + O_2 + \text{heat energy}$$

On its surface, the equation accurately represents the process by which light energy drives the production of sugars from CO_2. But this superficial accounting leaves out two of the most important players in photosynthesis: the activated carriers ATP and NADPH. In the first stage of photosynthesis, the energy from sunlight is used to produce ATP and NADPH; in the second stage, these activated carriers are consumed to fuel the synthesis of sugars.

1. *Stage 1* of photosynthesis resembles the oxidative phosphorylation that takes place on the mitochondrial inner membrane. In this stage, an electron-transport chain in the thylakoid membrane harnesses the energy of electron transport to pump protons into the thylakoid space; the resulting proton gradient then drives the synthesis of ATP by ATP synthase. What makes photosynthesis very different is that the high-energy electrons donated to the *photosynthetic electron-transport chain* come from a molecule of **chlorophyll** that has absorbed energy from sunlight. Thus the energy-producing reactions of stage 1 are sometimes called the **light reactions** (**Figure 14–30**). Another major difference between photosynthesis and oxidative phosphorylation is where the high-energy electrons ultimately wind up: those that make their way down the photosynthetic electron-transport chain in chloroplasts are donated not to O_2 but to $NADP^+$, to produce NADPH.

QUESTION 14–8

Chloroplasts have a third internal compartment, the thylakoid space, bounded by the thylakoid membrane. This membrane contains the photosystems, reaction centers, electron-transport chain, and ATP synthase. In contrast, mitochondria use their inner membrane for electron transport and ATP synthesis. In both organelles, protons are pumped out of the largest internal compartment (the matrix in mitochondria and the stroma in chloroplasts). The thylakoid space is completely sealed off from the rest of the cell. Why does this arrangement allow a larger H^+ gradient in chloroplasts than can be achieved for mitochondria?

Figure 14–30 Both stages of photosynthesis depend on the chloroplast. In stage 1, a series of photosynthetic electron-transfer reactions produce ATP and NADPH; in the process, electrons are extracted from water and oxygen is released as a by-product, as we discuss shortly. In stage 2, carbon dioxide is assimilated (fixed) to produce sugars and a variety of other organic molecules. Stage 1 occurs in the thylakoid membrane, whereas stage 2 begins in the chloroplast stroma (as shown) and continues in the cytosol.

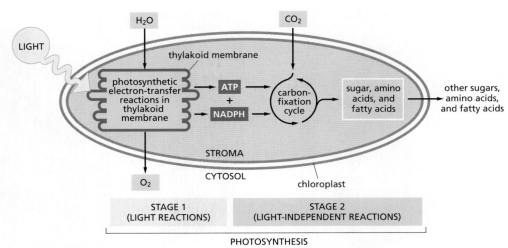

2. In *stage 2* of photosynthesis, the ATP and the NADPH produced by the photosynthetic electron-transfer reactions of stage 1 are used to drive the manufacture of sugars from CO_2 (see Figure 14–30). These *carbon-fixation reactions,* which do not directly require sunlight, begin in the chloroplast stroma. There they generate a three-carbon sugar called *glyceraldehyde 3-phosphate.* This simple sugar is exported to the cytosol, where it is used to produce a large number of organic molecules in the leaves of the plant, including the disaccharide sucrose, which is exported from the leaves to nourish the rest of the plant.

Although the formation of ATP and NADPH during stage 1, and the conversion of CO_2 to carbohydrate during stage 2, are mediated by two separate sets of reactions, they are linked by elaborate feedback mechanisms that allow a plant to manufacture sugars only when it is appropriate to do so. Several of the enzymes required for carbon fixation, for example, are inactivated in the dark and reactivated by light-stimulated electron transport.

Chlorophyll Molecules Absorb the Energy of Sunlight

Visible light is a form of electromagnetic radiation composed of many wavelengths, ranging from violet (wavelength 400 nm) to deep red (700 nm). Most chlorophylls absorb light best in the blue and red wavelengths, and they absorb green light poorly (**Figure 14–31**). Plants look green to us because the green light that is not absorbed is reflected back to our eyes.

Chlorophyll's ability to harness energy derived from sunlight stems from its unique structure. The electrons in a chlorophyll molecule are distributed in a decentralized cloud around the molecule's light-absorbing porphyrin ring (**Figure 14–32**). When light of an appropriate wavelength hits a molecule of chlorophyll, it excites electrons within this diffuse network. This high-energy state is unstable, and an excited chlorophyll molecule will rapidly release this excess energy and return to its more stable, unexcited state.

A molecule of chlorophyll, on its own in solution, would simply release its absorbed energy in the form of light or heat—accomplishing nothing useful. However, the chlorophyll molecules in a chloroplast are able to convert light energy into a form of energy useful to the cell because they are associated with a special set of photosynthetic proteins in the thylakoid membrane, as we see next.

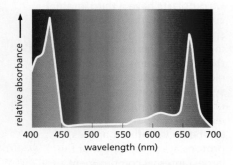

Figure 14–31 Chlorophylls absorb light of blue and red wavelengths. As shown in this absorption spectrum, one form of chlorophyll preferentially absorbs light around wavelengths of 430 nm (blue) and 660 nm (red). Green light, in contrast, is absorbed poorly by this pigment. Other chlorophylls can absorb light of slightly different wavelengths.

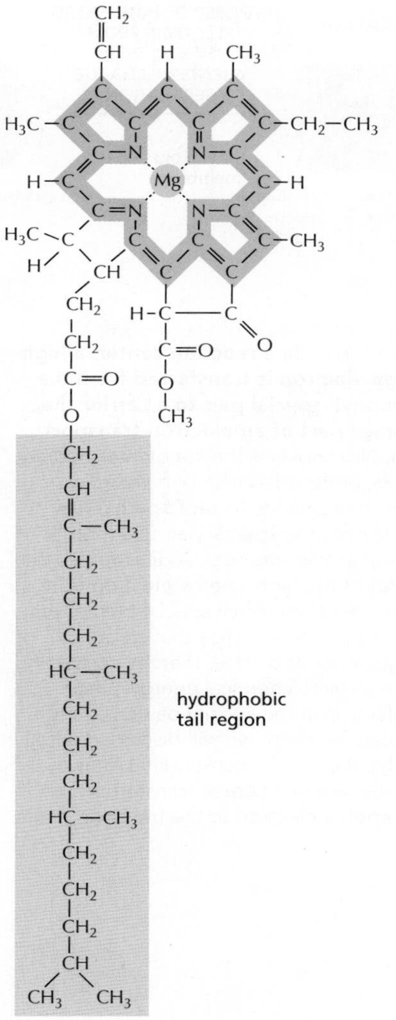

Figure 14–32 Chlorophyll's structure allows it to absorb energy from light. Each chlorophyll molecule contains a porphyrin ring with a magnesium atom (*pink*) at its center. This porphyrin ring is structurally similar to the one that binds iron in heme (see Figure 14–25). Light is absorbed by electrons within the bond network shown in *blue*, while the long, hydrophobic tail (*gray*) helps hold the chlorophyll in the thylakoid membrane.

Excited Chlorophyll Molecules Funnel Energy into a Reaction Center

In the thylakoid membrane of plants—and the plasma membrane of photosynthetic bacteria—chlorophyll molecules are held in large multiprotein complexes called **photosystems**. Each photosystem consists of a set of *antenna complexes*, which capture light energy, and a *reaction center*, which converts that light energy into chemical energy.

In an **antenna complex**, hundreds of chlorophyll molecules are arranged so that the light energy captured by one chlorophyll molecule can be transferred to a neighboring chlorophyll molecule in the network. In this way, energy jumps randomly from one chlorophyll molecule to the next—either within the same antenna or in an adjacent antenna. At some point, this wandering energy will encounter a chlorophyll dimer called the *special pair*, which holds its electrons at a slightly lower energy than do the other chlorophyll molecules. When energy is accepted by this special pair, it becomes effectively trapped there.

The chlorophyll special pair is not located in an antenna complex. Instead, it is part of the **reaction center**—a transmembrane complex of proteins and pigments that is thought to have first evolved more than 3 billion years ago in primitive photosynthetic bacteria (Movie 14.10). Within the reaction center, the special pair is positioned directly next to a set of electron carriers that are poised to accept a high-energy electron from the excited chlorophyll special pair (**Figure 14–33**). This electron transfer converts the light energy that entered the special pair into the chemical energy of a transferable electron—a transformation that lies at the heart of photosynthesis.

As soon as a high-energy electron is passed from chlorophyll to an electron carrier, the chlorophyll special pair becomes positively charged, and the electron carrier that accepts the electron becomes negatively charged. The rapid movement of this electron along a set of intermediary electron carriers within the reaction center then creates a *charge separation* that sets in motion the flow of high-energy electrons from the reaction center to the electron-transport chain (**Figure 14–34**).

hydrophobic tail region

Figure 14–33 A photosystem consists of a reaction center surrounded by chlorophyll-containing antenna complexes. Once light energy has been captured by a chlorophyll molecule in an antenna complex, it will pass randomly from one chlorophyll molecule to another (*red* lines), until it gets trapped by a chlorophyll dimer called the *special pair*, located in the reaction center. The chlorophyll special pair holds its electrons at a somewhat lower energy than the antenna chlorophylls, so the energy transferred to it from the antenna gets trapped there. Note that in the antenna complex, it is energy that moves from one chlorophyll molecule to another, not electrons.

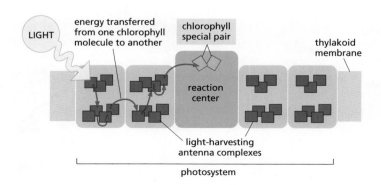

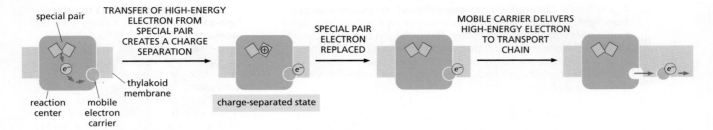

Figure 14–34 In a reaction center, a high-energy electron is transferred from the chlorophyll special pair to a carrier that becomes part of an electron-transport chain. Not shown is the set of intermediary carriers, embedded within the reaction center, that provides a rapid path (*blue arrows*) from the special pair to a mobile electron carrier (*orange*). As illustrated, the transfer of the high-energy electron from the excited chlorophyll special pair leaves behind a positive charge that creates a charge-separated state, thereby converting light energy to chemical energy. Once the electron in the special pair has been replaced (an event we will discuss in detail shortly), the mobile carrier diffuses away from the reaction center, transferring the high-energy electron to the transport chain.

A Pair of Photosystems Cooperate to Generate both ATP and NADPH

Photosynthesis is ultimately a biosynthetic process. Building organic molecules from CO_2 requires a huge input of energy, in the form of ATP, and a very large amount of reducing power, in the form of the activated carrier NADPH (see Figure 3–34). To generate both ATP and NADPH, plant cells—and free-living photosynthetic organisms such as cyanobacteria—make use of two different photosystems, which operate in series. Although they are similar in structure, these two photosystems do different things with the high-energy electrons that leave their reaction-center chlorophylls.

When the first photosystem (which, paradoxically, is called photosystem II for historical reasons) absorbs light energy, its reaction center passes electrons to a mobile electron carrier called *plastoquinone*, which is part of the photosynthetic electron-transport chain. This carrier transfers the high-energy electrons to a proton pump, which—like the proton pumps in the mitochondrial inner membrane—uses the movement of electrons to generate an electrochemical proton gradient. The electrochemical proton gradient then drives the production of ATP by an ATP synthase located in the thylakoid membrane (**Figure 14–35**).

At the same time, a second, nearby photosystem—called photosystem I—has been also busy capturing the energy from sunlight. The reaction center of this photosystem passes its high-energy electrons to a different mobile electron carrier, called *ferredoxin*, which brings them to an enzyme that uses the electrons to reduce NADP+ to NADPH (**Figure 14–36**). It is the combined action of these two photosystems that produces both the ATP (photosystem II) and the NADPH (photosystem I) required for carbon fixation in stage 2 of photosynthesis (see Figure 14–30).

Figure 14–35 Photosystem II feeds electrons to a photosynthetic proton pump, leading to the generation of ATP by ATP synthase. When light energy is captured by photosystem II, a high-energy electron is transferred to a mobile electron carrier called plastoquinone (Q), which closely resembles the ubiquinone of mitochondria. This carrier transfers its electrons to a proton pump called the cytochrome b_6-f complex, which resembles the cytochrome c reductase complex of mitochondria and is the sole site of active proton pumping in the chloroplast electron-transport chain. As in mitochondria, an ATP synthase embedded in the membrane then uses the energy of the electrochemical proton gradient to produce ATP.

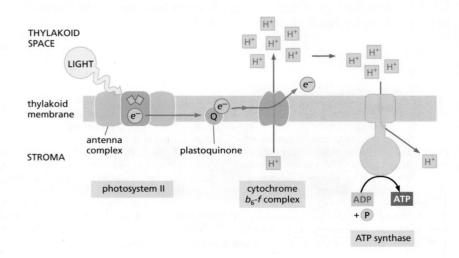

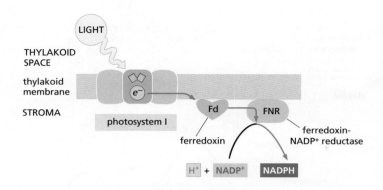

Figure 14–36 Photosystem I transfers high-energy electrons to an enzyme that produces NADPH. When light energy is captured by photosystem I, a high-energy electron is passed to a mobile electron carrier called ferredoxin (Fd), a small protein that contains an iron–sulfur center. Ferredoxin carries its electrons to ferredoxin-NADP$^+$ reductase (FNR), the final protein in the electron-transport chain that catalyzes the production of NADPH.

Oxygen Is Generated by a Water-Splitting Complex Associated with Photosystem II

The scheme that we have thus far described for photosynthesis has ignored a major chemical conundrum. When a mobile electron carrier removes an electron from a reaction center (whether in photosystem I or photosystem II), it leaves behind a positively charged chlorophyll special pair (see Figure 14–34). To reset the system and allow photosynthesis to proceed, this missing electron must be replaced.

For photosystem II, the missing electron is replaced by a special manganese-containing protein complex that removes the electrons from water. The cluster of manganese atoms in this *water-splitting enzyme* holds onto two water molecules from which electrons are extracted one at a time. Once four electrons have been removed from these two water molecules—and used to replace the electrons lost by four excited chlorophyll special pairs—O_2 is released (**Figure 14–37**). It is by this means that all of the O_2 in our atmosphere—all of the O_2 we breathe—is produced. Life on Earth would be a very different affair without the water-splitting enzyme of photosystem II.

> ### QUESTION 14–9
>
> Both NADPH and the related carrier molecule NADH are strong electron donors. Why might plant cells have evolved to rely on NADPH, rather than NADH, to provide the reducing power for biosynthesis?

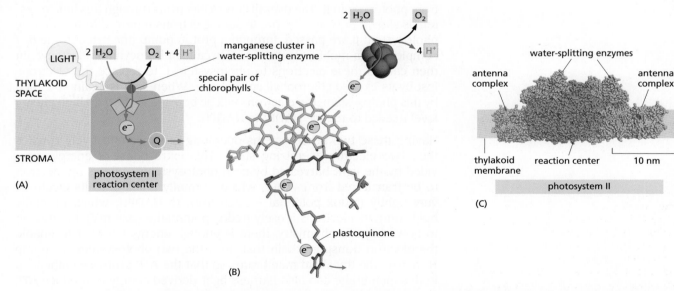

Figure 14–37 The reaction center of photosystem II includes a water-splitting enzyme that catalyzes the extraction of electrons from water. (A) Schematic diagram showing the flow of electrons through the reaction center of photosystem II. When light energy excites the chlorophyll special pair, an electron is passed to the mobile electron carrier plastoquinone (Q). An electron is then returned to the special pair by a water-splitting enzyme that extracts electrons from water. The manganese (Mn) cluster that participates in the electron extraction is shown as a *red spot*. Once four electrons have been withdrawn from two water molecules, O_2 is released into the atmosphere. (B) The structure and position of some of the electron carriers involved. (C) Structure of a membrane-embedded photosystem II (PSII) complex, including a reaction center and several light-harvesting antenna complexes. This structure, obtained from spinach, was determined by cryoelectron microscopy (see Panel 4–6, pp. 168–169). Note that this complex exists as a dimer in the membrane, and thus contains two copies of the water-splitting enzyme.

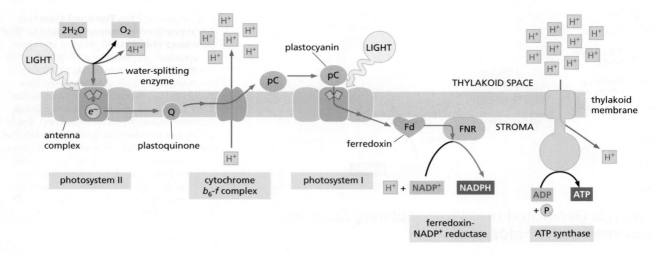

Figure 14–38 The serial movement of electrons through two photosystems powers the production of both ATP and NADPH. Electrons are supplied to photosystem II by a water-splitting enzyme that extracts four electrons from two molecules of water, producing O_2 as a by-product. Their energy is raised by the absorption of light to power the pumping of protons by the cytochrome b_6-f complex. Electrons that pass through this complex are then donated to a copper-containing protein, the mobile electron carrier plastocyanin (pC), which ferries them to the reaction center of photosystem I. After a second energy boost from light, these electrons are used to generate NADPH. An overview of these reactions is shown in Movie 14.11.

The "waiting for four electrons" maneuver executed by the water-splitting enzyme ensures that no partly oxidized water molecules are released as dangerous, highly reactive chemicals. As we discussed earlier, that same trick is used by the cytochrome c oxidase that catalyzes the reverse reaction—the transfer of electrons to O_2 to produce water—during oxidative phosphorylation (see Figure 14–24).

The Special Pair in Photosystem I Receives its Electrons from Photosystem II

We have seen that photosystem II replaces electrons lost by its chlorophyll special pair with electrons extracted from water. But where does photosystem I get the electrons it needs to reset its special pair? These electrons come from photosystem II: the two photosystems work in series, such that the chlorophyll special pair in photosystem I serves as the final electron acceptor for the electron-transport chain that carries electrons from photosystem II. The overall flow of electrons through this linked system is shown in **Figure 14–38**. In sum, electrons removed from water by photosystem II are passed, through a proton pump (the cytochrome b_6-f complex), to a mobile electron carrier called plastocyanin. Plastocyanin then carries these electrons to photosystem I, to replace the electrons lost by its excited chlorophyll special pair. When light is again absorbed by this photosystem, the electrons will be boosted to the very high energy level needed to reduce NADP$^+$ to NADPH.

Having these two photosystems operating in series effectively couples their two electron-energizing steps. This extra boost of energy—provided by the light harvested by both photosystems—allows an electron to be transferred from water, which normally holds onto its electrons very tightly (redox potential = +820 mV), to NADPH, which normally holds onto its electrons loosely (redox potential = –320 mV). In addition to powering this chemistry, there is enough energy left over to enable the electron-transport chain that links the two photosystems to pump H$^+$ across the thylakoid membrane, so that the ATP synthase embedded in this membrane can also harness light-derived energy to produce ATP (**Figure 14–39**).

Carbon Fixation Uses ATP and NADPH to Convert CO_2 into Sugars

The light reactions of photosynthesis generate ATP and NADPH in the chloroplast stroma, as we have just seen. But the inner membrane of the chloroplast is impermeable to both of these compounds, which means

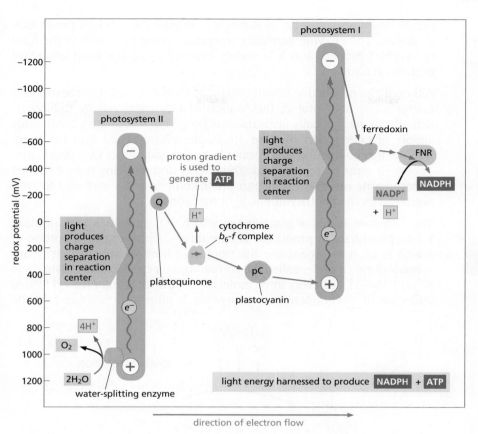

Figure 14–39 The combined actions of photosystems I and II boost electrons to the energy level needed to produce both ATP and NADPH. The redox potential for each molecule is indicated by its position on the vertical axis. Electron transfers are shown with non-wavy *blue* arrows. Photosystem II passes electrons from its excited chlorophyll special pair to an electron-transport chain in the thylakoid membrane that leads to photosystem I (see Figure 14–38). The net electron flow through these two photosystems linked in series is from water to $NADP^+$, to form NADPH.

that they cannot be exported directly to the cytosol. To provide energy and reducing power for the rest of the cell, the ATP and NADPH are instead used within the chloroplast stroma to produce a simple three-carbon sugar that can be exported to the cytosol by specific carrier proteins in the chloroplast inner membrane. This production of sugar from CO_2 and water, which occurs during stage 2 of photosynthesis, is called **carbon fixation**.

In the central reaction of photosynthetic carbon fixation, CO_2 from the atmosphere is attached to a five-carbon sugar derivative, ribulose 1,5-bisphosphate, to yield two molecules of the three-carbon compound *3-phosphoglycerate*. This carbon-fixing reaction, which was discovered in 1948, is catalyzed in the chloroplast stroma by a large enzyme called ribulose bisphosphate carboxylase or *Rubisco* (**Figure 14–40**). Rubisco works much more slowly than most other enzymes: it processes about three molecules of substrate per second—compared with 1000 molecules per second for a typical enzyme. To compensate for this sluggish behavior,

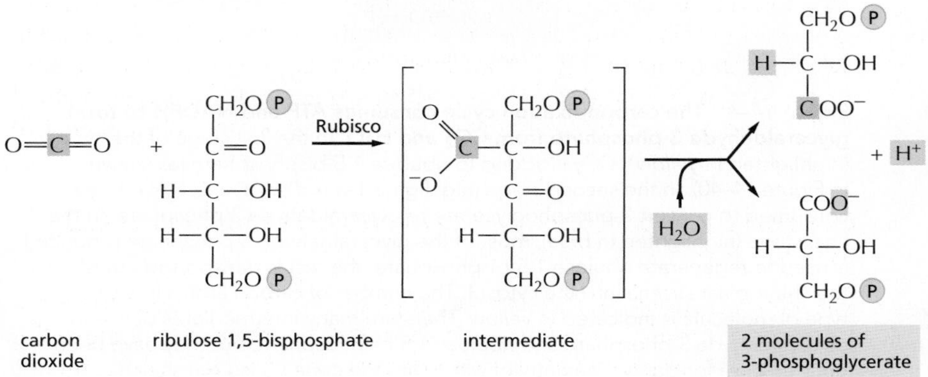

Figure 14–40 Carbon fixation is catalyzed by the enzyme ribulose bisphosphate carboxylase, also called Rubisco. In this reaction, which takes place in the chloroplast stroma, a covalent bond is formed between carbon dioxide and an energy-rich molecule of ribulose 1,5-bisphosphate. This union generates a chemical intermediate that then reacts with water (highlighted in *blue*) to generate two molecules of 3-phosphoglycerate.

plants maintain a surplus of Rubisco to ensure the efficient production of sugars. The enzyme generally represents more than 50% of the total chloroplast protein, and it is widely claimed to be the most abundant protein on Earth.

Although the production of carbohydrates from CO_2 and H_2O is extremely energetically unfavorable, the fixation of CO_2 catalyzed by Rubisco is actually an energetically favorable reaction. That's because a continuous supply of energy-rich ribulose 1,5-bisphosphate is fed into the reaction. As this compound is consumed—by the addition of CO_2 (see Figure 14–40)—it must be replenished. The energy and reducing power needed to regenerate ribulose 1,5-bisphosphate come from the ATP and NADPH produced by the photosynthetic light reactions.

The elaborate series of reactions in which CO_2 combines with ribulose 1,5-bisphosphate to produce a simple three-carbon sugar—a portion of which is used to regenerate the ribulose 1,5-bisphosphate that's consumed—forms a cycle, called the *carbon-fixation cycle*, or the *Calvin cycle* (**Figure 14–41**). For every three molecules of CO_2 that enter the cycle, one molecule of glyceraldehyde 3-phosphate is ultimately produced, at the

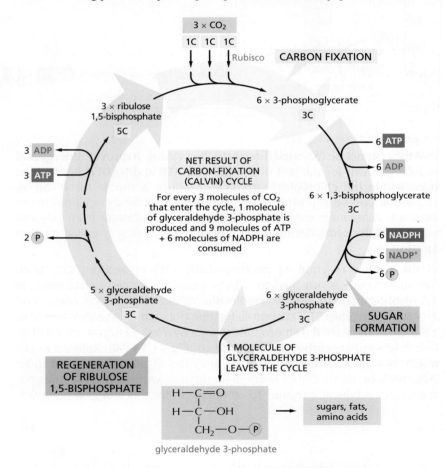

Figure 14–41 **The carbon-fixation cycle consumes ATP and NADPH to form glyceraldehyde 3-phosphate from CO_2 and H_2O.** In the first stage of the cycle (highlighted in *yellow*), CO_2 is added to ribulose 1,5-bisphosphate (as shown in Figure 14–40). In the second stage (highlighted in *red*), ATP and NADPH are consumed to convert 3-phosphoglycerate to glyceraldehyde 3-phosphate. In the final stage (highlighted in *blue*), most of the glyceraldehyde 3-phosphate produced is used to regenerate ribulose 1,5-bisphosphate; the rest is transported out of the chloroplast stroma into the cytosol. The number of carbon atoms in each type of molecule is indicated in *yellow*. There are many intermediates between glyceraldehyde 3-phosphate and ribulose 1,5-bisphosphate, but they have been omitted here for clarity. The entry of water into the cycle is also not shown.

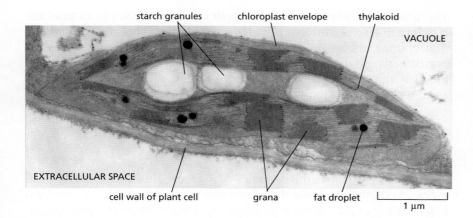

Figure 14–42 Chloroplasts often contain large stores of carbohydrates and fatty acids. An electron micrograph of a thin section of a single chloroplast shows the chloroplast envelope and the starch granules and fat droplets that have accumulated in the stroma as a result of the biosynthetic processes that occur there. (Courtesy of K. Plaskitt.)

expense of nine molecules of ATP and six molecules of NADPH, which are consumed in the process. *Glyceraldehyde 3-phosphate*, the three-carbon sugar that is the final product of the cycle, provides the starting material for the synthesis of the many other sugars and other organic molecules that the plant needs.

Sugars Generated by Carbon Fixation Can Be Stored as Starch or Consumed to Produce ATP

The glyceraldehyde 3-phosphate generated by carbon fixation in the chloroplast stroma can be used in a number of ways, depending on the needs of the plant. During periods of excess photosynthetic activity, much of the sugar is retained in the chloroplast stroma and converted to *starch*. Like glycogen in animal cells, starch is a large polymer of glucose that serves as a carbohydrate reserve, and it is stored as large granules in the chloroplast stroma. Starch forms an important part of the diet of all animals that eat plants. Other glyceraldehyde 3-phosphate molecules are converted to fat in the stroma. This material, which accumulates as fat droplets, likewise serves as an energy reserve (Figure 14–42).

At night, this stored starch and fat can be broken down to sugars and fatty acids, which are exported to the cytosol to help support the metabolic needs of the plant. Some of the exported sugar enters the glycolytic pathway (see Figure 13–5), where it is converted to pyruvate. Most of that pyruvate, along with the fatty acids, enters the plant cell mitochondria and is fed into the citric acid cycle, ultimately leading to the production of ATP by oxidative phosphorylation (Figure 14–43). Plants use this ATP to power a huge variety of metabolic reactions, just as animal cells and other nonphotosynthetic organisms do.

Figure 14–43 In plants, the chloroplasts and mitochondria collaborate to supply cells with metabolites and ATP. The chloroplast's inner membrane is impermeable to the ATP and NADPH that are produced in the stroma during the light reactions of photosynthesis. These molecules are funneled into the carbon-fixation cycle, where they are used to make sugars. The resulting sugars and their metabolites are either stored within the chloroplast—in the form of starch or fat—or exported to the rest of the plant cell. There, they can enter the energy-generating pathway that ends in ATP synthesis in the mitochondria. Unlike those chloroplasts, mitochondrial membranes are permeable to ATP, as indicated. Note that some of the O_2 released to the atmosphere by photosynthesis in chloroplasts is used for oxidative phosphorylation in mitochondria; similarly, some of the CO_2 released by the citric acid cycle in mitochondria is used for carbon fixation in chloroplasts.

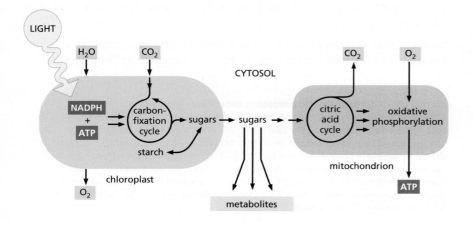

The glyceraldehyde 3-phosphate exported from chloroplasts into the cytosol can also be converted into many other metabolites, including the disaccharide *sucrose*. Sucrose is the major form in which sugar is transported between the cells of a plant: just as glucose is transported in the blood of animals, so sucrose is exported from the leaves via the vascular system to provide carbohydrate to the rest of the plant.

THE EVOLUTION OF ENERGY-GENERATING SYSTEMS

The ability to sequence the genomes of microorganisms that are difficult, if not impossible, to grow in culture has made it possible to identify a huge variety of previously mysterious life-forms. Some of these unicellular organisms thrive in the most inhospitable habitats on the planet, including sulfurous hot springs and hydrothermal vents that lie deep on the ocean floor. In these remarkable microbes, we are finding clues to life's history. Like fingerprints left at the scene of a crime, the proteins and small molecules these organisms produce provide evidence that allows us to trace the history of ancient biological events, including those that gave rise to the ATP-generating systems present in the mitochondria and chloroplasts of modern eukaryotic cells. We therefore end this chapter with a brief review of what has been learned about the origins of present-day energy-harvesting systems, which have played such a critical part in fueling the evolution of life on Earth.

Oxidative Phosphorylation Evolved in Stages

As we mentioned earlier, the first living cells on Earth may have consumed geochemically produced organic molecules and generated ATP by fermentation. Because oxygen was not yet present in the atmosphere, such anaerobic fermentation reactions would have dumped organic acids—such as lactic or formic acids, for example—into the environment (see Figure 13–6A).

A buildup of such acids would have lowered the pH of the environment, favoring the survival of cells that evolved transmembrane proteins that could pump H^+ out of the cytosol, preventing the cell interior from becoming too acidic. Some of these pumps may have used the energy available from ATP hydrolysis to eject H^+ from the cell (stage 1 in **Figure 14–44**). Such a proton pump could have been the ancestor of present-day ATP synthases. Other pumps, like those in modern respiratory chain complexes, eventually evolved to use the movement of electrons between molecules of different redox potentials as a source of energy for pumping H^+ across the plasma membrane (stage 2 in Figure 14–44). Indeed, some present-day bacteria that grow on formic acid use the small amount of redox energy derived from the transfer of electrons from formic acid to fumarate to pump H^+.

When these H^+-pumping electron-transport systems became efficient enough, cells could harvest more redox energy than they needed to

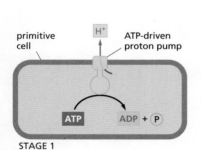

STAGE 1

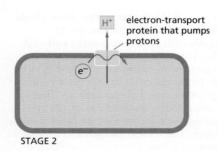

STAGE 2

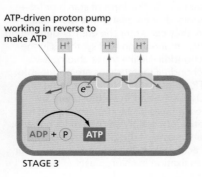

STAGE 3

Figure 14–44 Chemiosmotic processes most likely evolved in stages. The first stage might have involved the evolution of an ATPase that pumped protons out of the cell using the energy of ATP hydrolysis. Stage 2 could have involved the evolution of a different proton pump, driven by an electron-transport chain. Stage 3 could then link these two systems together to generate an ATP synthase that uses the protons pumped by the electron-transport chain to synthesize ATP. An early cell with this final system would have had a large selective advantage over cells with neither of the systems or only one.

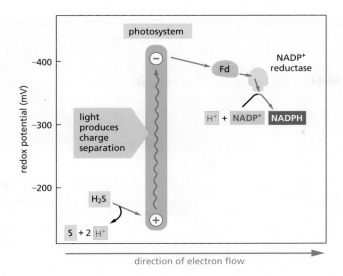

direction of electron flow

Figure 14–45 Photosynthesis in green sulfur bacteria uses hydrogen sulfide (H$_2$S) as an electron donor rather than water. Electrons are easier to extract from H$_2$S than from H$_2$O, because H$_2$S has a much higher redox potential (compare with Figure 14–39). Therefore, only one photosystem is needed to produce NADPH, and elemental sulfur is formed as a by-product instead of O$_2$. The photosystem in green sulfur bacteria resembles photosystem I in plants and cyanobacteria. These photosystems all use a series of iron–sulfur centers as the electron carriers that eventually donate their high-energy electrons to ferredoxin (Fd). A bacterium of this type is *Chlorobium tepidum*, which can thrive at high temperatures and low light intensities in hot springs.

maintain their internal pH. These cells could then generate large electrochemical proton gradients, which they could couple to the production of ATP (stage 3 in Figure 14–44). Because such cells would require much less of the dwindling supply of fermentable nutrients, they would have proliferated at the expense of their neighbors.

Photosynthetic Bacteria Made Even Fewer Demands on Their Environment

The major evolutionary breakthrough in energy metabolism, however, was almost certainly the formation of photochemical reaction centers that could use the energy of sunlight to produce molecules such as NADPH. It is thought that this development occurred early in the process of evolution—more than 3 billion years ago, in the ancestors of green sulfur bacteria. Present-day green sulfur bacteria use light energy to transfer hydrogen atoms (as an electron plus a proton) from H$_2$S to NADPH, thereby creating the strong reducing power required for carbon fixation (**Figure 14–45**).

The next step is thought to have involved the evolution of organisms capable of using water instead of H$_2$S as the electron source for photosynthesis. This entailed the evolution of a water-splitting enzyme and the addition of a second photosystem, acting in conjunction with the first, to bridge the enormous gap in redox potential between H$_2$O and NADPH (see Figure 14–39).

The biological consequences of this evolutionary step were far-reaching. For the first time, there were organisms that made only minimal chemical demands on their environment. These cells—including the first cyanobacteria (see Figure 14–28)—could spread and evolve in ways denied to the earlier photosynthetic bacteria, which needed H$_2$S, organic acids, or other sources of electrons. Consequently, large amounts of fermentable organic materials—produced by these cells and their ancestors—began to accumulate. Moreover, O$_2$ began to enter the atmosphere in large amounts (**Figure 14–46**).

The availability of O$_2$ made possible the development of bacteria that relied on aerobic metabolism to make their ATP. As explained previously, these organisms could harness the large amount of energy released when carbohydrates and other reduced organic molecules are broken down all the way to CO$_2$ and H$_2$O.

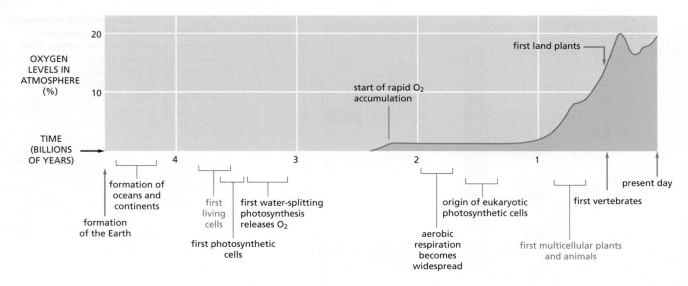

Figure 14–46 Oxygen entered Earth's atmosphere billions of years ago. With the evolution of photosynthesis in prokaryotes more than 3 billion years ago, organisms would have no longer depended on preformed organic chemicals: they could make their own organic molecules from CO_2. Note that there was a delay of about a billion years between the appearance of photosynthetic bacteria that split water and released O_2 and the accumulation of high levels of O_2 in the atmosphere. This delay is thought to have been due to the initial reaction of the O_2 with abundant ferrous iron (Fe^{2+}) dissolved in the early oceans. Only when the iron was used up could large amounts of O_2 begin to accumulate in the atmosphere. In response to rising amounts of O_2 in the atmosphere, nonphotosynthetic, aerobic organisms appeared, and the concentration of O_2 in the atmosphere eventually leveled out.

As organic materials accumulated as a by-product of photosynthesis, some photosynthetic bacteria—including the ancestors of the bacterium *Escherichia coli*—lost their ability to survive on light energy alone and came to rely entirely on cell respiration. Mitochondria arose when a pre-eukaryotic cell engulfed such an aerobic bacterium (see Figure 1–19). Plants arose somewhat later, when a descendant of this early aerobic eukaryote captured a photosynthetic bacterium, which became the precursor of chloroplasts (see Figure 1–21). Once eukaryotes had acquired the bacterial symbionts that became mitochondria and chloroplasts, they could then embark on the spectacular pathway of evolution that eventually led to complex multicellular organisms, including ourselves.

The Lifestyle of *Methanococcus* Suggests That Chemiosmotic Coupling Is an Ancient Process

The conditions today that most resemble those under which cells are thought to have lived 3.5–3.8 billion years ago may be those near deep-ocean hydrothermal vents. These vents represent places where the Earth's molten mantle is breaking through the overlying crust, expanding the width of the ocean floor. Indeed, the modern organisms that appear to be most closely related to the hypothetical cells from which all life evolved live at 75°C to 95°C, temperatures approaching that of boiling water. This ability to thrive at such extreme temperatures suggests that life's common ancestor—the cell that gave rise to bacteria, archaea, and eukaryotes—lived under very hot, anaerobic conditions.

One of the archaea that live in this environment today is *Methanococcus jannaschii*. Originally isolated from a hydrothermal vent more than a mile beneath the ocean surface, the organism grows in the complete absence of light and gaseous oxygen, using as nutrients the inorganic gases—hydrogen (H_2), CO_2, and nitrogen (N_2)—that bubble up from the vent (**Figure 14–47**). Its mode of existence gives us a hint of how early cells might have used electron transport to derive energy and to extract carbon molecules from inorganic materials that were freely available on the hot early Earth.

Methanococcus relies on N_2 gas as its source of nitrogen for making organic molecules such as amino acids. The organism reduces N_2 to ammonia (NH_3) by the addition of hydrogen, a process called **nitrogen fixation**. Nitrogen fixation requires a large amount of energy, as does the carbon-fixation process that converts CO_2 and H_2O into sugars. Much

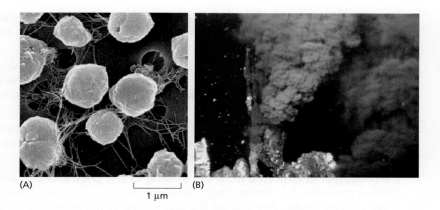

(A)   (B)

|⊢——— ⊣|
1 µm

Figure 14–47 *Methanococcus* represents life-forms that might have existed early in Earth's history. (A) Scanning electron micrograph showing individual *Methanococcus* cells. These deep-sea archaea use the hydrogen gas (H_2) that bubbles from deep-sea vents (B) as the source of reducing power to generate energy via chemiosmotic coupling. (A, from C.B. Park & D.S. Clark, *Appl. Environ. Microbiol.* 68:1458–1463, 2002. With permission from the American Society for Microbiology; B, National Oceanic and Atmospheric Administration's Pacific Marine Environmental Laboratory Vents Program.)

of the energy that *Methanococcus* requires for both processes is derived from the transfer of electrons from H_2 to CO_2, with the release of large amounts of methane (CH_4) as a waste product (thus producing natural gas and giving the organism its name). Part of this electron transfer occurs in the plasma membrane and results in the pumping of protons (H^+) across it. The resulting electrochemical proton gradient drives an ATP synthase in the same membrane to make ATP.

The fact that such chemiosmotic coupling exists in an organism like *Methanococcus* suggests that the storage of energy in a proton gradient derived from electron transport is an extremely ancient process. Thus, chemiosmotic coupling may have fueled the evolution of nearly all life-forms on Earth.

ESSENTIAL CONCEPTS

- Mitochondria, chloroplasts, and many prokaryotes generate energy by a membrane-based mechanism known as chemiosmotic coupling, which involves using an electrochemical proton gradient to drive the synthesis of ATP.

- In animal cells, mitochondria produce most of the ATP, using energy derived from the oxidation of sugars and fatty acids.

- Mitochondria have an inner and an outer membrane. The inner membrane encloses the mitochondrial matrix; there, the citric acid cycle produces large amounts of NADH and $FADH_2$ from the oxidation of acetyl CoA derived from sugars and fats.

- In the inner mitochondrial membrane, high-energy electrons donated by NADH and $FADH_2$ move along an electron-transport chain and eventually combine with molecular oxygen (O_2) to form water.

- Much of the energy released by electron transfers along the electron-transport chain is harnessed to pump protons (H^+) out of the matrix, creating an electrochemical proton gradient. The proton pumping is carried out by three large respiratory enzyme complexes embedded in the inner membrane.

- The electrochemical proton gradient across the inner mitochondrial membrane is harnessed to make ATP when protons move back into the matrix through an ATP synthase located in the inner membrane.

- The electrochemical proton gradient also drives the active transport of selected metabolites into and out of the mitochondrial matrix.

- During photosynthesis in chloroplasts and photosynthetic bacteria, the energy of sunlight is captured by chlorophyll molecules embedded in large protein complexes known as photosystems; in plants, these photosystems are located in the thylakoid membranes of chloroplasts in leaf cells.

- Electron-transport chains associated with photosystems transfer electrons from water to $NADP^+$ to form NADPH, which produces O_2 as a by-product.

- The photosynthetic electron-transport chains in chloroplasts also generate a proton gradient across the thylakoid membrane, which is used by an ATP synthase embedded in that membrane to generate ATP.

- The ATP and the NADPH made by photosynthesis are used within the chloroplast stroma to drive the carbon-fixation cycle, which produces carbohydrate from CO_2 and water.

- Carbohydrate is exported from the stroma to the plant cell cytosol; there it provides the starting material used for the synthesis of many other organic molecules and for the production of the materials used by plant cell mitochondria to produce ATP.

- Both mitochondria and chloroplasts are thought to have evolved from bacteria that were endocytosed by other cells. Each retains its own genome and divides by processes that resemble bacterial cell division.

- Chemiosmotic coupling mechanisms are of ancient origin. Modern microorganisms that live in environments similar to those thought to have been present on the early Earth also use chemiosmotic coupling to produce ATP.

KEY TERMS

antenna complex	mitochondrion
ATP synthase	nitrogen fixation
carbon fixation	oxidative phosphorylation
cell respiration	photosynthesis
chemiosmotic coupling	photosystem
chlorophyll	quinone
chloroplast	reaction center
cytochrome	redox pair
cytochrome *c* oxidase	redox potential
electron-transport chain	redox reaction
iron–sulfur center	respiratory enzyme complex
light reactions	stroma
matrix	thylakoid

QUESTIONS

QUESTION 14–11

Which of the following statements are correct? Explain your answers.

A. After an electron has been removed by light, the positively charged chlorophyll in the reaction center of the first photosystem (photosystem II) has a greater affinity for electrons than O_2 has.

B. Photosynthesis is the light-driven transfer of an electron from chlorophyll to a second molecule that normally has a much lower affinity for electrons.

C. Because it requires the removal of four electrons to release one O_2 molecule from two H_2O molecules, the

water-splitting enzyme in photosystem II has to keep the reaction intermediates tightly bound so as to prevent partly reduced, and therefore hazardous, superoxide radicals from escaping.

QUESTION 14–12

Which of the following statements are correct? Explain your answers.

A. Many, but not all, electron-transfer reactions involve metal ions.

B. The electron-transport chain generates an electrical potential across the membrane because it moves electrons from the intermembrane space into the matrix.

C. The electrochemical proton gradient consists of two components: a pH difference and an electrical potential.

D. Ubiquinone and cytochrome *c* are both diffusible electron carriers.

E. Plants have chloroplasts and therefore can live without mitochondria.

F. Both chlorophyll and heme contain an extensive system of double bonds that allows them to absorb visible light.

G. The role of chlorophyll in photosynthesis is equivalent to that of heme in mitochondrial electron transport.

H. Most of the dry weight of a tree comes from the minerals that are taken up by the roots.

QUESTION 14–13

A single proton moving down its electrochemical gradient into the mitochondrial matrix space liberates 19.2 kJ/mole of free energy (ΔG). How many protons have to flow across the inner mitochondrial membrane to synthesize one molecule of ATP if the ΔG for ATP synthesis under intracellular conditions is between 46 and 54 kJ/ mole? (ΔG is discussed in Chapter 3, pp. 88–98.) Why is a range given for this latter value and not a precise number? Under which conditions would the lower value apply?

QUESTION 14–14

In the following statement, choose the correct one of the alternatives in italics and justify your answers. "If no O_2 is available, all components of the mitochondrial electron-transport chain will accumulate in their *reduced/oxidized* form. If O_2 is suddenly added again, the electron carriers in cytochrome *c* oxidase will become *reduced/oxidized before/after* those in NADH dehydrogenase."

QUESTION 14–15

Assume that the conversion of oxidized ubiquinone to reduced ubiquinone by NADH dehydrogenase occurs on the matrix side of the inner mitochondrial membrane and that its oxidation by cytochrome *c* reductase occurs on the intermembrane-space side of the membrane (see Figures 14–14 and 14–21). What are the consequences of this arrangement for the generation of the H^+ gradient across the membrane?

QUESTION 14–16

If a voltage is applied to two platinum wires (electrodes) immersed in water, then water molecules become split into H_2 and O_2 gas. At the negative electrode, electrons are donated and H_2 gas is released; at the positive electrode, electrons are accepted and O_2 gas is produced. When photosynthetic bacteria and plant cells split water, they produce O_2 but no H_2. Why?

QUESTION 14–17

In an insightful experiment performed in the 1960s, chloroplasts were first soaked in an acidic solution at pH 4, so that the stroma and thylakoid space became acidified (Figure Q14–17). They were then transferred to a basic solution (pH 8). This quickly increased the pH of the stroma to 8, while the thylakoid space temporarily remained at

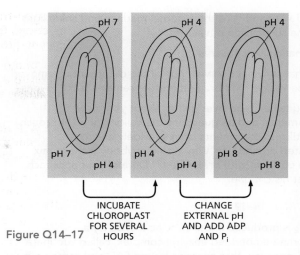

Figure Q14–17

INCUBATE CHLOROPLAST FOR SEVERAL HOURS

CHANGE EXTERNAL pH AND ADD ADP AND P_i

pH 4. A burst of ATP synthesis was observed, and the pH difference between the thylakoid and the stroma then disappeared.

A. Explain why these conditions lead to ATP synthesis.

B. Is light needed for the experiment to work?

C. What would happen if the solutions were switched, so that the first incubation is in the pH 8 solution and the second one in the pH 4 solution?

D. Does the experiment support or question the chemiosmotic model?

Explain your answers.

QUESTION 14–18

As your first experiment in the laboratory, your adviser asks you to reconstitute purified bacteriorhodopsin, a light-driven H^+ pump from the plasma membrane of photosynthetic bacteria, and purified ATP synthase from ox-heart mitochondria together into the same membrane vesicles—as shown in Figure Q14–18. You are then asked

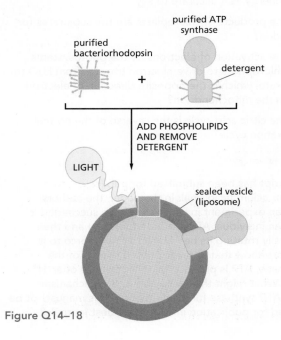

purified bacteriorhodopsin

purified ATP synthase

detergent

ADD PHOSPHOLIPIDS AND REMOVE DETERGENT

LIGHT

sealed vesicle (liposome)

Figure Q14–18

to add ADP and P_i to the external medium and shine light into the suspension of vesicles.

A. What do you observe?

B. What do you observe if not all the detergent is removed and the vesicle membrane therefore remains leaky to ions?

C. You tell a friend over dinner about your new experiments, and he questions the validity of an approach that utilizes components from so widely divergent, unrelated organisms: "Why would anybody want to mix vanilla pudding with brake fluid?" Defend your approach against his critique.

QUESTION 14–19

$FADH_2$ is produced in the citric acid cycle by a membrane-embedded enzyme complex, called succinate dehydrogenase, that contains bound FAD and carries out the reactions

$$\text{succinate} + \text{FAD} \rightarrow \text{fumarate} + FADH_2$$

and

$$FADH_2 \rightarrow \text{FAD} + 2H^+ + 2e^-$$

The redox potential of $FADH_2$, however, is only –220 mV. Referring to Panel 14–1 (p. 472) and Figure 14–22, suggest a plausible mechanism by which its electrons could be fed into the electron-transport chain. Draw a diagram to illustrate your proposed mechanism.

QUESTION 14–20

Some bacteria have become specialized to live in an environment of high pH (pH ~10). Do you suppose that these bacteria use a proton gradient across their plasma membrane to produce their ATP? (Hint: all cells must maintain their cytoplasm at a pH close to neutrality.)

QUESTION 14–21

Figure Q14–21 summarizes the circuitry used by mitochondria and chloroplasts to interconvert different forms of energy. Is it accurate to say

A. that the products of chloroplasts are the substrates for mitochondria?

B. that the activation of electrons by the photosystems enables chloroplasts to drive electron transfer from H_2O to carbohydrate, which is the opposite direction of electron transfer in the mitochondrion?

C. that the citric acid cycle is the reverse of the normal carbon-fixation cycle?

QUESTION 14–22

A manuscript has been submitted for publication to a prestigious scientific journal. In the paper, the authors describe an experiment in which they have succeeded in trapping an individual ATP synthase molecule and then mechanically rotating its head by applying a force to it. The authors show that upon rotating the head of the ATP synthase, ATP is produced, in the absence of an H^+ gradient. What might this mean about the mechanism whereby ATP synthase functions? Should this manuscript be considered for publication in one of the best journals?

QUESTION 14–23

You mix the following components in a reconstituted membrane-bound system. Assuming that the electrons must follow the path specified in Figure 14–14, in which experiments would you expect a net transfer of electrons to cytochrome *c*? Discuss why electron transfer does not occur in the other experiments.

A. reduced ubiquinone and oxidized cytochrome *c*

B. oxidized ubiquinone and oxidized cytochrome *c*

C. reduced ubiquinone and reduced cytochrome *c*

D. oxidized ubiquinone and reduced cytochrome *c*

E. reduced ubiquinone, oxidized cytochrome *c*, and cytochrome *c* reductase complex

F. oxidized ubiquinone, oxidized cytochrome *c*, and cytochrome *c* reductase complex

G. reduced ubiquinone, reduced cytochrome *c*, and cytochrome *c* reductase complex

H. oxidized ubiquinone, reduced cytochrome *c*, and cytochrome *c* reductase complex

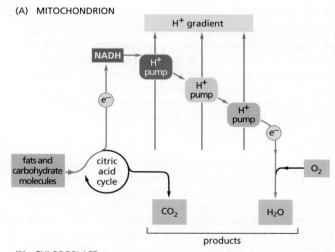

(A) MITOCHONDRION

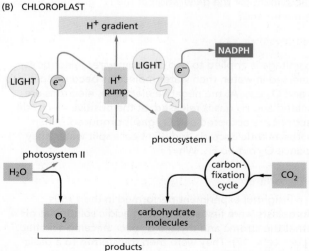

(B) CHLOROPLAST

Figure Q14–21

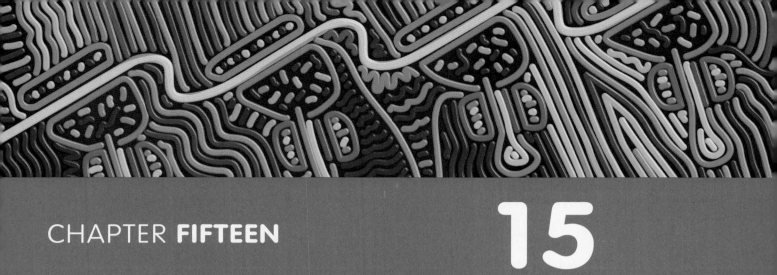

Intracellular Compartments and Protein Transport

At any one time, a typical eukaryotic cell carries out thousands of different chemical reactions, many of which are mutually incompatible. One series of reactions makes glucose, for example, while another breaks it down; some enzymes synthesize peptide bonds, whereas others hydrolyze them, and so on. Indeed, if the cells of an organ such as the liver are broken apart and their contents are mixed together in a test tube, the result is chemical chaos, and the cells' enzymes and other proteins are quickly degraded by their own proteolytic enzymes. For a cell to operate effectively, the different intracellular processes that occur simultaneously must somehow be segregated.

Cells have evolved several strategies for isolating and organizing their chemical reactions. One strategy used by both prokaryotic and eukaryotic cells is to aggregate the different enzymes required to catalyze a particular sequence of reactions into large, multicomponent complexes. Such complexes—which can form large biochemical subcompartments with distinct functions—are involved in many important cell processes, including the synthesis of DNA and RNA, and the assembly of ribosomes (as discussed in Chapter 4, pp. 155–158). A second strategy, which is most highly developed in eukaryotic cells, is to confine different metabolic processes—and the proteins required to perform them—within different membrane-enclosed compartments. As discussed in Chapters 11 and 12, cell membranes provide selectively permeable barriers through which the transport of most molecules can be controlled. In this chapter, we consider this strategy of membrane-dependent compartmentalization.

In the first section, we describe the principal membrane-enclosed compartments, or *membrane-enclosed organelles*, of eukaryotic cells and

MEMBRANE-ENCLOSED
ORGANELLES

PROTEIN SORTING

VESICULAR TRANSPORT

SECRETORY PATHWAYS

ENDOCYTIC PATHWAYS

Figure 15–1 In eukaryotic cells, internal membranes create enclosed compartments that segregate different metabolic processes. Examples of many of the major membrane-enclosed organelles can be identified in this electron micrograph of part of a liver cell, seen in cross section. The small, black granules between the compartments are aggregates of glycogen and the enzymes that control its synthesis and breakdown. (By permission of E.L. Bearer and Daniel S. Friend.)

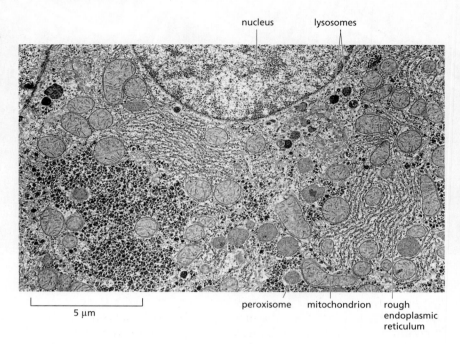

nucleus   lysosomes

peroxisome   mitochondrion   rough
endoplasmic
reticulum

5 μm

briefly consider their main functions. In the second section, we discuss how the protein composition of the different compartments is set up and maintained. Each compartment contains a unique set of proteins that have to be transferred selectively from the cytosol, where they are made, to the compartment where they will be used. This transfer process, called *protein sorting*, depends on signals built into the amino acid sequence of the proteins. In the third section, we describe how certain membrane-enclosed compartments in a eukaryotic cell communicate with one another by forming small, membrane-enclosed sacs, or *vesicles*. These vesicles pinch off from one compartment, move through the cytosol, and fuse with another compartment in a process called *vesicular transport*. In the last two sections, we discuss how this constant vesicular traffic also provides the main routes for releasing proteins from the cell by the process of *exocytosis* and for importing them by the process of *endocytosis*.

MEMBRANE-ENCLOSED ORGANELLES

Whereas a prokaryotic cell usually consists of a single compartment enclosed by the plasma membrane, eukaryotic cells are elaborately subdivided by internal membranes. When a cross section through a plant or an animal cell is examined in the electron microscope, numerous small, membrane-enclosed sacs, tubes, spheres, and irregularly shaped structures can be seen, often arranged without much apparent order (**Figure 15–1**). Most of these structures are **membrane-enclosed organelles**, or parts of such organelles, each of which contains a unique set of large and small molecules and carries out a specialized function. In this section, we review these functions and discuss how different membrane-enclosed organelles may have evolved.

Eukaryotic Cells Contain a Basic Set of Membrane-enclosed Organelles

The major membrane-enclosed organelles of an animal cell are illustrated in **Figure 15–2**, and their functions are summarized in **Table 15–1**. These organelles are surrounded by the *cytosol*, which is enclosed by the plasma membrane. The *nucleus* is generally the most prominent organelle in eukaryotic cells. It is surrounded by a double membrane,

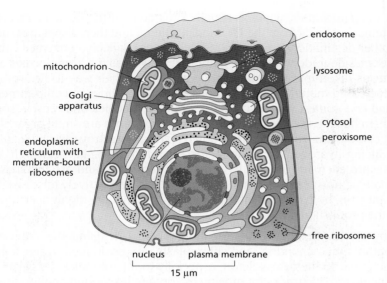

mitochondrion

Golgi
apparatus

endoplasmic
reticulum with
membrane-bound
ribosomes

endosome

lysosome

cytosol

peroxisome

free ribosomes

nucleus   plasma membrane

15 μm

Figure 15–2 **A cell from the lining of the intestine contains the basic set of membrane-enclosed organelles found in most animal cells.** The nucleus, endoplasmic reticulum (ER), Golgi apparatus, lysosomes, endosomes, mitochondria, and peroxisomes are distinct compartments separated from the cytosol by at least one selectively permeable membrane. Ribosomes are shown bound to the cytosolic surface of portions of the ER, called the rough ER; the ER that lacks ribosomes is called smooth ER. Additional ribosomes can be found free in the cytosol.

known as the *nuclear envelope*, and communicates with the cytosol via *nuclear pores* that perforate the envelope. The outer nuclear membrane is continuous with the membrane of the *endoplasmic reticulum (ER)*, a system of interconnected membranous sacs and tubes that often extends throughout most of the cell. The ER is the major site of synthesis of new membranes in the cell. Large areas of the ER have ribosomes attached to the cytosolic surface and are designated *rough endoplasmic reticulum (rough ER)*. The ribosomes are actively synthesizing proteins that are inserted into the ER membrane or delivered to the ER interior, a space called the *lumen*. The *smooth endoplasmic reticulum (smooth ER)* lacks ribosomes. It is scanty in most cells but is highly developed for performing particular functions in others: for example, it is the site of steroid hormone synthesis in some endocrine cells of the adrenal gland and the site where a variety of organic molecules, including alcohol, are detoxified in liver cells. In many eukaryotic cells, the smooth ER also sequesters Ca^{2+} from the cytosol; the release and reuptake of Ca^{2+} from the ER is involved in muscle contraction and other responses to extracellular signals (discussed in Chapters 16 and 17).

TABLE 15–1 THE MAIN FUNCTIONS OF MEMBRANE-ENCLOSED ORGANELLES OF A EUKARYOTIC CELL

Compartment	Main Function
Cytosol	contains many metabolic pathways (Chapters 3 and 13); protein synthesis (Chapter 7); the cytoskeleton (Chapter 17)
Nucleus	contains main genome (Chapter 5); DNA and RNA synthesis (Chapters 6 and 7)
Endoplasmic reticulum (ER)	synthesis of most lipids (Chapter 11); synthesis of proteins for distribution to many organelles and to the plasma membrane (this chapter)
Golgi apparatus	modification, sorting, and packaging of proteins and lipids for either secretion or delivery to another organelle (this chapter)
Lysosomes	intracellular degradation (this chapter)
Endosomes	sorting of endocytosed material (this chapter)
Mitochondria	ATP synthesis by oxidative phosphorylation (Chapter 14)
Chloroplasts (in plant cells)	ATP synthesis and carbon fixation by photosynthesis (Chapter 14)
Peroxisomes	oxidative breakdown of toxic molecules (this chapter)

The *Golgi apparatus*, which is usually situated near the nucleus, receives proteins and lipids from the ER, modifies them, and then dispatches them to other destinations in the cell. Small sacs of digestive enzymes called *lysosomes* degrade worn-out organelles, as well as macromolecules and particles taken into the cell by endocytosis. On their way to lysosomes, endocytosed materials must first pass through a series of compartments called *endosomes*, which sort the ingested molecules and recycle some of them back to the plasma membrane. *Peroxisomes* are small organelles that contain enzymes that break down lipids and destroy toxic molecules, producing hydrogen peroxide. *Mitochondria* and (in plant cells) *chloroplasts* are each surrounded by a double membrane and are the sites of oxidative phosphorylation and photosynthesis, respectively (discussed in Chapter 14); both contain internal membranes that are highly specialized for the production of ATP.

Many of the membrane-enclosed organelles, including the ER, Golgi apparatus, mitochondria, and chloroplasts, are positioned in the cell by attachment to the cytoskeleton, especially to microtubules. Cytoskeletal filaments provide tracks for moving the organelles around and for directing the traffic of vesicles between one organelle and another. These movements are driven by motor proteins that use the energy of ATP hydrolysis to propel the organelles and vesicles along the filaments, as discussed in Chapter 17.

On average, the membrane-enclosed organelles together occupy nearly half the volume of a eukaryotic cell (Table 15–2), and the total amount of membrane associated with them is enormous. In a typical mammalian cell, for example, the area of the endoplasmic reticulum membrane is 20–30 times greater than that of the plasma membrane. In terms of its area and mass, the plasma membrane is only a minor membrane in most eukaryotic cells.

Much can be learned about the composition and function of an organelle once it has been isolated from other cell structures. For the most part, organelles are far too small to be isolated by hand, but it is possible to separate one type of organelle from another by differential centrifugation (described in Panel 4–3, pp. 164–165). Once a purified sample of one type of organelle has been obtained, the organelle's proteins can be identified. In many cases, the organelle itself can be incubated in a test tube under conditions that allow its functions to be studied. Isolated mitochondria, for example, can produce ATP from the oxidation of pyruvate to CO_2 and water, provided they are adequately supplied with ADP, inorganic phosphate, and O_2.

TABLE 15–2 THE RELATIVE VOLUMES AND NUMBERS OF THE MAJOR MEMBRANE-ENCLOSED ORGANELLES IN A LIVER CELL (HEPATOCYTE)		
Intracellular Compartment	Percentage of Total Cell Volume	Approximate Number per Cell
Cytosol	54	1
Mitochondria	22	1700
Endoplasmic reticulum	12	1
Nucleus	6	1
Golgi apparatus	3	1
Peroxisomes	1	400
Lysosomes	1	300
Endosomes	1	200

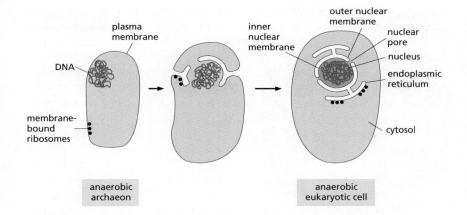

In modern bacteria and archaea, a single DNA molecule is typically attached to the plasma membrane. It is possible that, in a very ancient anaerobic archaeon, the plasma membrane, with its attached DNA, could have invaginated and, in subsequent generations, formed a two-layered envelope of membrane completely surrounding the DNA. This envelope is presumed to have eventually pinched off completely from the plasma membrane, ultimately producing a nuclear compartment penetrated by channels called nuclear pores, which enable communication with the cytosol. Other portions of the invaginated membrane may have formed the ER, which would explain why the space between the inner and outer nuclear membranes is continuous with the ER lumen.

Membrane-enclosed Organelles Evolved in Different Ways

In trying to understand the relationships between the different compartments of a modern eukaryotic cell, it is helpful to consider how they evolved. The precursors of the first eukaryotic cells are thought to have been simple microorganisms, resembling present-day archaea, which had a plasma membrane but no internal membranes. The plasma membrane in such cells would have provided all membrane-dependent functions, including ATP synthesis and lipid synthesis, as does the plasma membrane in most modern prokaryotes. Archaea and bacteria can get by with this arrangement because of their small size, which gives them a high surface-to-volume ratio: their plasma membrane area is thus sufficient to sustain all the vital functions for which membranes are required. Present-day eukaryotic cells, by contrast, have volumes that are 1000 to 10,000 times greater. Such a large cell has a small surface-to-volume ratio and presumably could not survive with a plasma membrane as its only membrane. Thus, the increase in size typical of eukaryotic cells probably could not have occurred without the development of internal membranes.

Membrane-enclosed organelles are thought to have arisen in evolution in stages. The nuclear membranes and the membranes of the ER, Golgi apparatus, endosomes, and lysosomes most likely originated by invagination of the plasma membrane, as illustrated for the nuclear and ER membranes in **Figure 15–3**. The ER, Golgi apparatus, peroxisomes, endosomes, and lysosomes are all part of what is collectively called the **endomembrane system**. As we discuss later, the interiors of these organelles communicate extensively with one another and with the outside of the cell by means of small vesicles that bud off from one of these organelles and fuse with another. Consistent with this proposed evolutionary origin, the interiors of these organelles are treated by the cell in many ways as "extracellular," as we will see. The hypothetical scheme shown in Figure 15–3 also explains why the nucleus is surrounded by two membranes.

Mitochondria and chloroplasts are thought to have originated in a different way. They differ from all other organelles in that they possess their own small genomes and can make some of their own proteins, as discussed in Chapter 14. The similarity of their genomes to those of bacteria and the close resemblance of some of their proteins to bacterial proteins strongly suggest that both these organelles evolved from bacteria that were engulfed by primitive eukaryotic cells with which they initially lived in symbiosis (**Figure 15–4**). As might be expected from their origins, mitochondria and chloroplasts remain isolated from the extensive vesicular

Figure 15–4 Mitochondria are thought to have originated when an aerobic bacterium was engulfed by a larger anaerobic eukaryotic cell. Chloroplasts are thought to have originated later in a similar way, when a eukaryotic cell with mitochondria engulfed a photosynthetic bacterium. This theory would explain why these organelles have two membranes, possess their own genomes, and do not participate in the vesicular traffic that connects the compartments of the endomembrane system.

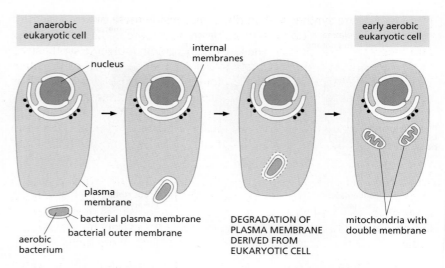

traffic that connects the interiors of most of the other membrane-enclosed organelles to one another and to the outside of the cell.

PROTEIN SORTING

Before a eukaryotic cell divides, it must duplicate its membrane-enclosed organelles. As cells grow, membrane-enclosed organelles enlarge by incorporation of new molecules; the organelles then divide and, during cell division, are distributed between the two daughter cells. Organelle growth requires a supply of new lipids to make more membrane and a supply of the appropriate proteins—both membrane proteins and the soluble proteins that will occupy the interior of the organelle. Even in cells that are not dividing, proteins are being produced continually. These newly synthesized proteins must be accurately delivered to their appropriate organelle—some for eventual secretion from the cell and some to replace organelle proteins that have been degraded. Directing newly made proteins to their correct organelle is therefore necessary for any cell to grow and divide, or just to function properly.

For some organelles, including mitochondria, chloroplasts, and the interior of the nucleus, proteins are delivered directly from the cytosol. For others, including the Golgi apparatus, lysosomes, endosomes, and the inner nuclear membrane, proteins and lipids are delivered indirectly via the ER, which is itself a major site of lipid and protein synthesis. Proteins enter the ER directly from the cytosol: some are retained there, but most are transported by vesicles to the Golgi apparatus and then onward to the plasma membrane or to other organelles. Peroxisomes make use of both pathways. Although these organelles acquire some of their membrane proteins from the ER, the bulk of their digestive enzymes enter directly from the cytosol.

In this section, we discuss the mechanisms by which proteins enter membrane-enclosed organelles from the cytosol. Proteins made in the cytosol are dispatched to different locations in the cell according to specific address labels contained in their amino acid sequence. Once at the correct address, the protein enters either the membrane or the interior lumen of its designated organelle.

Proteins Are Transported into Organelles by Three Mechanisms

The synthesis of virtually all proteins in the cell begins on ribosomes in the cytosol. The exceptions are the few mitochondrial and chloroplast proteins that are synthesized on ribosomes inside these organelles; most mitochondrial and chloroplast proteins, however, are made in the cytosol and subsequently imported. The fate of any protein molecule synthesized in the cytosol depends on its amino acid sequence, which can contain a *sorting signal* that directs the protein to the organelle in which it is required. Proteins that lack such signals remain as permanent residents of the cytosol; those that possess a sorting signal move from the cytosol to the appropriate organelle. Different sorting signals direct proteins into the nucleus, mitochondria, chloroplasts (in plants), peroxisomes, and the ER.

When a membrane-enclosed organelle imports a water-soluble protein to its interior—either from the cytosol or from another organelle—it faces a problem: the protein must be transported across its membrane (or membranes), which is normally impermeable to hydrophilic macromolecules. How this task is accomplished depends on the organelle.

1. Proteins moving from the cytosol into the nucleus are transported through the nuclear pores, which penetrate both the inner and outer nuclear membranes. The pores function as selective gates that actively transport specific macromolecules but also allow free diffusion of smaller molecules (mechanism 1 in **Figure 15–5**).

2. Proteins moving from the cytosol into the ER, mitochondria, or chloroplasts are transported across the organelle membrane by *protein translocators* located in the membrane. Unlike the transport through nuclear pores, the transported protein must usually unfold for the translocator to guide it across the hydrophic interior of the membrane (mechanism 2 in Figure 15–5). Bacteria have similar protein translocators in their plasma membrane, which they use to export proteins from the cytosol to the cell exterior.

3. Proteins moving onward from the ER—and from one compartment of the endomembrane system to another—are transported by a mechanism that is fundamentally different than the ones just

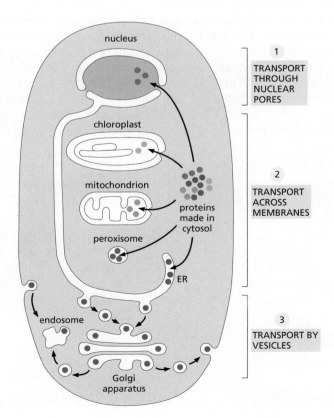

Figure 15–5 **Membrane-enclosed organelles import proteins by one of three mechanisms.** All of these processes require energy. The protein remains folded during transport in mechanisms 1 and 3 but usually has to be unfolded during mechanism 2.

TABLE 15–3 SOME TYPICAL SIGNAL SEQUENCES

Function of Signal	Example of Signal Sequence
Import into ER	^+H_3N-Met-Met-Ser-Phe-Val-Ser-Leu-Leu-Leu-Val-Gly-Ile-Leu-Phe-Trp-Ala-Thr-Glu-Ala-Glu-Gln-Leu-Thr-Lys-Cys-Glu-Val-Phe-Gln-
Retention in lumen of ER	-Lys-Asp-Glu-Leu-COO$^-$
Import into mitochondria	^+H_3N-Met-Leu-Ser-Leu-Arg-Gln-Ser-Ile-Arg-Phe-Phe-Lys-Pro-Ala-Thr-Arg-Thr-Leu-Cys-Ser-Ser-Arg-Tyr-Leu-Leu-
Import into nucleus	-Pro-Pro-Lys-Lys-Lys-Arg-Lys-Val-
Export from nucleus	-Met-Glu-Glu-Leu-Ser-Gln-Ala-Leu-Ala-Ser-Ser-Phe-
Import into peroxisomes	-Ser-Lys-Leu-

Positively charged amino acids are shown in *red* and negatively charged amino acids in *blue*. Important hydrophobic amino acids are shown in *green*. ^+H_3N indicates the N-terminus of a protein; COO$^-$ indicates the C-terminus.

described. These proteins are ferried by *transport vesicles*, which pinch off from the membrane of one compartment and then fuse with the membrane of a second compartment (mechanism 3 in Figure 15–5). In this process, transport vesicles deliver soluble cargo proteins, as well as the proteins and lipids that are part of the vesicle membrane.

Signal Sequences Direct Proteins to the Correct Compartment

The typical sorting signal on a protein is a continuous stretch of amino acid sequence, typically 15–60 amino acids long. This **signal sequence** is often (but not always) removed from the finished protein once it has been sorted. Some of the signal sequences used to specify different destinations in the cell are shown in **Table 15–3**.

Signal sequences are both necessary and sufficient to direct a protein to a particular destination. This has been shown by experiments in which the sequence is either deleted or transferred from one protein to another by genetic engineering techniques (discussed in Chapter 10). Deleting a signal sequence from an ER protein, for example, converts it into a cytosolic protein, while placing an ER signal sequence at the beginning of a cytosolic protein redirects the protein to the ER (**Figure 15–6**). The signal sequences specifying the same destination can vary greatly even though

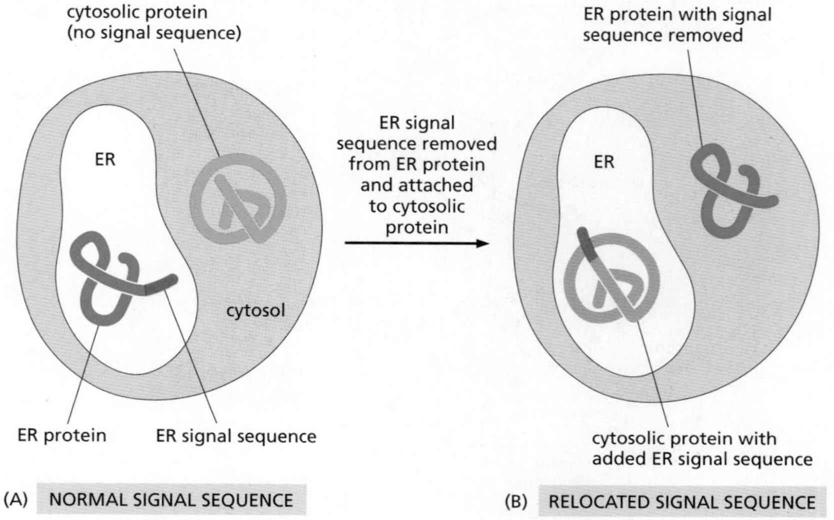

Figure 15–6 Signal sequences direct proteins to the correct destination. (A) Proteins destined for the ER possess an N-terminal signal sequence that directs them to that organelle, whereas those destined to remain in the cytosol lack any such signal sequence. (B) Recombinant DNA techniques can be used to change the destination of the two proteins: if the signal sequence is removed from an ER protein and attached to a cytosolic protein, both proteins are reassigned to the expected, inappropriate location.

(A) NORMAL SIGNAL SEQUENCE

(B) RELOCATED SIGNAL SEQUENCE

they have the same function: physical properties such as hydrophobicity or the placement of charged amino acids often appear to be more important for the function of these signals than the exact amino acid sequence.

Proteins Enter the Nucleus Through Nuclear Pores

The **nuclear envelope**, which encloses the nuclear DNA and defines the nuclear compartment, is formed from two concentric membranes. The *inner nuclear membrane* contains some proteins that act as binding sites for the chromosomes (discussed in Chapter 5) and others that provide anchorage for the *nuclear lamina*, a finely woven meshwork of protein filaments that lines the inner face of this membrane and provides structural support for the nuclear envelope (discussed in Chapter 17). The composition of the *outer nuclear membrane* closely resembles the membrane of the ER, with which it is continuous (**Figure 15–7**).

The nuclear envelope in all eukaryotic cells is perforated by **nuclear pores** that form the gates through which molecules enter or leave the nucleus. A nuclear pore is a large, elaborate structure composed of a complex of about 30 different proteins, each present in multiple copies (**Figure 15–8**). Many of the proteins that line the nuclear pore contain extensive, unstructured regions in which the polypeptide chains are largely disordered. These disordered segments form a soft, tangled meshwork—like a kelp forest—that fills the center of the channel, preventing the passage of large molecules but allowing small, water-soluble molecules to pass freely and nonselectively between the nucleus and the cytosol.

Selected larger molecules and macromolecular complexes also need to pass through nuclear pores. RNA molecules, which are synthesized in the nucleus, and ribosomal subunits, which are assembled there, must be exported to the cytosol (discussed in Chapter 7). Newly made proteins

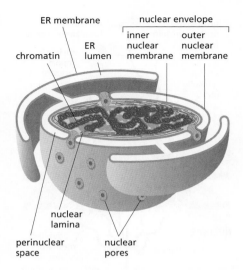

Figure 15–7 The outer nuclear membrane is continuous with the ER membrane. The double membrane of the nuclear envelope is penetrated by nuclear pores. The ribosomes that are normally bound to the cytosolic surface of the ER membrane and outer nuclear membrane are not shown.

Figure 15–8 The nuclear pore complex forms a gate through which selected macromolecules and larger complexes enter or exit the nucleus. (A) Drawing of a small region of the nuclear envelope showing two pores. Protein fibrils protrude from both sides of the pore complex; on the nuclear side, they converge to form a basketlike structure. The spacing between the fibrils is wide enough that the fibrils do not obstruct access to the pores. (B) Electron micrograph of a region of nuclear envelope showing a side view of two nuclear pores (brackets). (C) Electron micrograph showing a face-on view of nuclear pore protein complexes; the membranes have been extracted with detergent. (B, courtesy of Werner W. Franke; C, courtesy of Ron Milligan.)

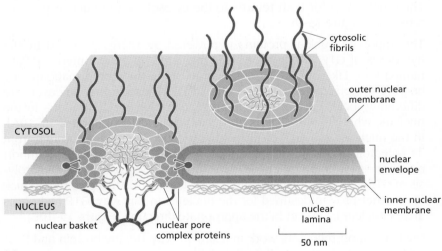

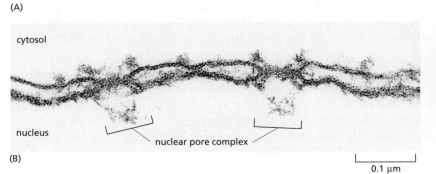

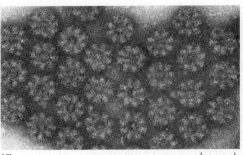

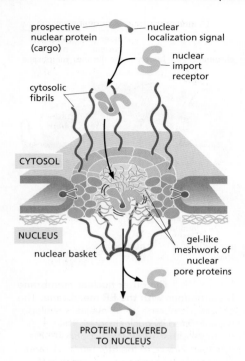

prospective nuclear protein (cargo)

nuclear localization signal

nuclear import receptor

cytosolic fibrils

CYTOSOL

NUCLEUS

nuclear basket

gel-like meshwork of nuclear pore proteins

PROTEIN DELIVERED TO NUCLEUS

Figure 15–9 Prospective nuclear proteins are imported from the cytosol through nuclear pores. The proteins contain a nuclear localization signal that is recognized by nuclear import receptors, which interact with the cytosolic fibrils that extend from the rim of the pore. After being captured, the receptors with their cargo jostle their way through the gel-like meshwork formed from the unstructured regions of the nuclear pore proteins until nuclear entry triggers cargo release. After cargo delivery, the receptors return to the cytosol via nuclear pores for reuse. Similar types of transport receptors, operating in the reverse direction, export mRNAs from the nucleus (see Figure 7–25). These sets of import and export receptors have a similar basic structure.

that are destined for the nucleus must also be imported from the cytosol (Movie 15.1). To gain entry to a pore, these large molecules and macromolecular complexes must display an appropriate sorting signal. The signal sequence that directs a protein from the cytosol into the nucleus, called a *nuclear localization signal*, typically consists of one or two short sequences containing several positively charged lysines or arginines (see Table 15–3).

The nuclear localization signal on proteins destined for the nucleus is recognized by cytosolic proteins called *nuclear import receptors*. These receptors help direct a newly synthesized protein to a nuclear pore by interacting with the tentacle-like fibrils that extend from the rim of the pore into the cytosol (Figure 15–9). Once there, the nuclear import receptor penetrates the pore by grabbing onto short, repeated amino acid sequences within the tangle of nuclear pore proteins that fill the center of the pore. When the nuclear pore is empty, these repeated sequences bind to one another, forming a loosely packed gel. Nuclear import receptors interrupt these interactions, and they open a local passageway through the meshwork. The import receptors then bump along from one repeat sequence to the next, until they enter the nucleus and deliver their cargo. The empty receptor then returns to the cytosol via the nuclear pore for reuse (see Figure 15–9).

The import of nuclear proteins is powered by energy provided by the hydrolysis of GTP. This hydrolysis is mediated by a monomeric GTPase named Ran. Like other GTPases, Ran exists in two conformations: one bearing a molecule of GTP, the other GDP. These forms, however, are differently localized: Ran-GTP is present in high concentrations in the nucleus, whereas Ran-GDP is produced in the cytosol (Figure 15–10A). In the nucleus, Ran-GTP displaces the prospective nuclear protein from its receptor, allowing the imported protein to be released. The import receptor—now bearing Ran–GTP—returns to the cytosol, where hydrolysis of GTP allows Ran-GDP to dissociate, leaving the receptor free to pick up another protein destined for the nucleus. In this way, GTP hydrolysis drives nuclear transport in the appropriate direction (Figure 15–10B).

Nuclear export receptors work in a similar way, driving protein and RNA traffic from the nucleus to the cytosol. They recognize nuclear export signals, which are different from those specifying import (see Table 15–3), and they also use Ran to couple the transport to an energy source.

Nuclear pore proteins operate this molecular gate at an amazing speed, rapidly pumping macromolecules in both directions through each pore. Proteins are transported into the nucleus in their fully folded conformation and ribosomal components as assembled particles. This feature distinguishes the nuclear transport mechanism from the mechanisms that transport proteins into most other organelles. Proteins have to unfold to cross the membranes of mitochondria and chloroplasts, as we discuss next.

QUESTION 15–2

Why do eukaryotic cells require a nucleus as a separate compartment when prokaryotic cells can manage perfectly well without?

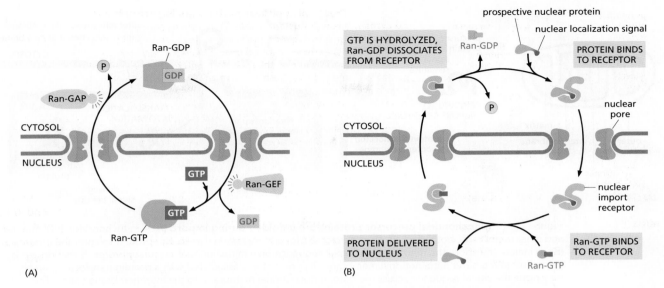

Figure 15–10 Energy supplied by GTP hydrolysis drives nuclear transport. (A) The small monomeric GTPase, Ran, exists in two conformations—one carrying GTP, the other GDP (see Figure 4–48 or 16–12). Ran is converted from one conformation to the other with the help of accessory proteins that are differently localized. The accessory protein that triggers GTP hydrolysis, called Ran-GAP (GTPase-activating protein), is found exclusively in the cytosol, where it converts Ran-GTP to Ran-GDP. The accessory protein that causes Ran-GDP to release its GDP and take up GTP, called Ran-GEF (guanine nucleotide exchange factor), is found exclusively in the nucleus. The localization of these accessory proteins guarantees that the concentration of Ran-GTP is higher in the nucleus, thus driving the nuclear import cycle in the desired direction. (B) A nuclear import receptor picks up a prospective nuclear protein in the cytosol and enters the nucleus. There it encounters Ran-GTP, which binds to the import receptor, causing it to release the nuclear protein. Having discharged its cargo in the nucleus, the receptor—still carrying Ran-GTP—is transported back through the pore to the cytosol, where Ran hydrolyzes its bound GTP. Ran-GDP falls off the import receptor, which is then free to bind another protein destined for the nucleus. Ran-GDP is carried into the nucleus by its own unique import receptor (not shown).

Proteins Unfold to Enter Mitochondria and Chloroplasts

Both mitochondria and chloroplasts are surrounded by inner and outer membranes, and both organelles specialize in the synthesis of ATP. Chloroplasts also contain a third membrane system, the thylakoid membrane (discussed in Chapter 14). Although both organelles contain their own genomes and make some of their own proteins, most mitochondrial and chloroplast proteins are encoded by genes in the nucleus and are imported from the cytosol. These proteins usually have a signal sequence at their N-terminus that allows them to enter their specific organelle. Proteins destined for either organelle are translocated simultaneously across both the inner and outer membranes at specialized sites where the two membranes are closely apposed. Each protein is unfolded as it is transported, and its signal sequence is removed after translocation is complete (**Figure 15–11**).

Chaperone proteins (discussed in Chapter 4) inside the organelles help to pull the protein across the two membranes and to fold it once it is inside. Subsequent transport to a particular site within the organelle, such as the inner or outer membrane or the thylakoid membrane in chloroplasts, usually requires further sorting signals in the protein, which are often only exposed after the first signal sequence has been removed. The insertion of transmembrane proteins into the inner membrane, for example, is guided by signal sequences in the protein that start and stop the transfer process across the membrane, as we describe later for the insertion of transmembrane proteins in the ER membrane.

The growth and maintenance of mitochondria and chloroplasts require not only the import of new proteins but also the incorporation of new

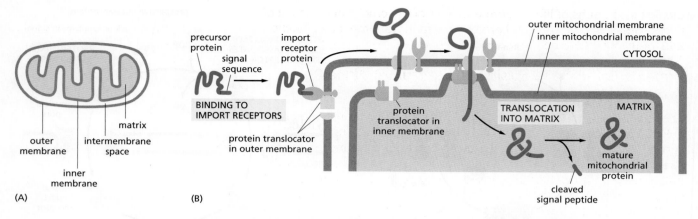

Figure 15–11 Mitochondrial precursor proteins are unfolded during import. (A) A mitochondrion has an outer and inner membrane, both of which must be crossed for a mitochondrial precursor protein to enter the organelle. (B) To initiate transport, the mitochondrial signal sequence on a mitochondrial precursor protein is recognized by a receptor in the outer mitochondrial membrane. This receptor is associated with a protein translocator, which transports the signal sequence across the outer mitochondrial membrane to the intermembrane space. The complex of receptor, precursor protein, and translocator then diffuses laterally in the outer membrane until the signal sequence is recognized by a second translocator in the inner membrane. Together, the two translocators transport the protein across both the outer and inner membranes, unfolding the protein in the process (Movie 15.2). The signal sequence is finally cleaved off by a signal peptidase in the mitochondrial matrix. Proteins are imported into chloroplasts by a similar mechanism. The chaperone proteins that help pull the protein across the membranes and help it to refold are not shown. Some of the energy needed for this protein translocation comes from the hydrolysis of ATP, which allows the chaperones to function.

lipids into the organelle membranes. Most of their membrane phospholipids are thought to be imported from the ER, which is the main site of lipid synthesis in the cell. Phospholipids are transported to these organelles by lipid-carrying proteins that extract a phospholipid molecule from one membrane and deliver it into another. Such transport frequently occurs at specific junctions where the membranes of different organelles are held in close proximity. By controlling which lipids are transported, the different cell membranes are able to maintain different lipid compositions.

Proteins Enter Peroxisomes from both the Cytosol and the Endoplasmic Reticulum

Peroxisomes are packed with enzymes that digest toxins and synthesize certain phospholipids, including those present in the myelin sheath surrounding nerve cell axons. These organelles acquire the bulk of their proteins via selective transport from the cytosol. A short sequence of only three amino acids serves as an import signal for many peroxisomal proteins (see Table 15–3, p. 502). This sequence is recognized by receptor proteins in the cytosol, at least one of which escorts its cargo protein all the way into the peroxisome before returning to the cytosol. Like the membranes of mitochondria and chloroplasts, the peroxisomal membrane contains a translocator that aids in protein transport. Unlike the mechanism that operates in mitochondria and chloroplasts, however, proteins do not need to unfold to enter the peroxisome—and the transport mechanism is still mysterious.

Although most peroxisomal proteins come from the cytosol, a few of the proteins embedded in the peroxisomal membrane arrive via vesicles that bud from the ER. The vesicles either fuse with preexisting peroxisomes or import additional peroxisomal proteins from the cytosol to grow into mature peroxisomes.

Mutations that block peroxisomal protein import can cause severe illness. Individuals with Zellweger syndrome, for example, are born with severe abnormalities in their brain, liver, and kidneys. Most do not survive past the first six months of life—a grim reminder of the crucial importance of peroxisomes, and peroxisomal protein transport, for proper cell function and for the health of the organism.

Proteins Enter the Endoplasmic Reticulum While Being Synthesized

The **endoplasmic reticulum** is the most extensive membrane system in a eukaryotic cell (Figure 15–12A). Unlike the organelles discussed so far, it serves as an entry point for proteins destined for other organelles, as well as for the ER itself. Proteins destined for the Golgi apparatus, endosomes, and lysosomes, as well as proteins destined for the cell surface, all first enter the ER from the cytosol. Once inside the ER lumen, or embedded in the ER membrane, individual proteins will not re-enter the cytosol during their onward journey. They will instead be ferried by transport vesicles from organelle to organelle within the endomembrane system, or to the plasma membrane (see Figure 15–5).

Two kinds of proteins are transferred from the cytosol to the ER: (1) water-soluble proteins are completely translocated across the ER membrane and are released into the ER lumen; (2) prospective transmembrane proteins are only partly translocated across the ER membrane and become embedded in it. The water-soluble proteins are destined either for secretion (by release at the cell surface) or for the lumen of an organelle of the endomembrane system. The transmembrane proteins are destined to reside in the membrane of one of these organelles or in the plasma membrane. All of these proteins are initially directed to the ER by an *ER signal sequence*, a segment of eight or more hydrophobic amino acids (see Table 15–3, p. 502), which is also involved in the process of translocation across the membrane.

Unlike the proteins that enter the nucleus, mitochondria, chloroplasts, or peroxisomes, most of the proteins that enter the ER begin to be threaded across the ER membrane before the polypeptide chain has been completely synthesized. This requires that the ribosome synthesizing the protein be attached to the ER membrane. These membrane-bound ribosomes coat the surface of the ER, creating regions termed **rough endoplasmic reticulum** because of its characteristic beaded appearance when viewed in an electron microscope (Figure 15–12B).

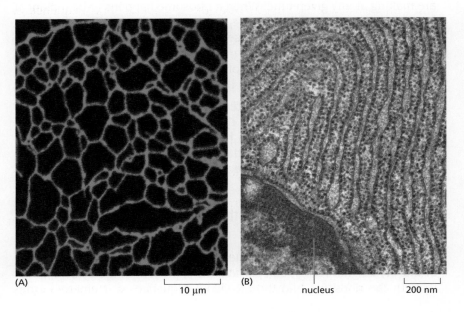

(A)   10 μm

(B)   nucleus   200 nm

Figure 15–12 The endoplasmic reticulum is the most extensive membrane network in eukaryotic cells. (A) Fluorescence micrograph of a living plant cell showing the ER as a complex network of tubes. The cell shown here has been genetically engineered so that it contains a fluorescent protein in the ER lumen. Only part of the ER network in the cell is shown. (B) An electron micrograph showing the rough ER in a cell from a dog's pancreas, which makes and secretes large amounts of digestive enzymes. The cytosol is filled with closely packed sheets of ER, studded with ribosomes. A portion of the nucleus and its nuclear envelope can be seen at the bottom left; note that the outer nuclear membrane, which is continuous with the ER, is also studded with ribosomes. For a dynamic view of the ER network, watch Movie 15.3. (A, from P. Boevink et al., *The Plant Journal* 15:441–447, 1998. With permission from John Wiley & Sons; B, courtesy of Lelio Orci.)

Figure 15–13 A common pool of ribosomes is used to synthesize all the proteins encoded by the nuclear genome. Ribosomes that are translating proteins with no ER signal sequence remain free in the cytosol. Ribosomes that are translating proteins containing an ER signal sequence (*red*) on the growing polypeptide chain will be directed to the ER membrane. Many ribosomes bind to each mRNA molecule, forming a polyribosome. At the end of each round of protein synthesis, the ribosomal subunits are released and rejoin the common pool in the cytosol. As we see shortly, how the ribosome and signal sequence bind to the ER and translocation channel is more complicated than illustrated here.

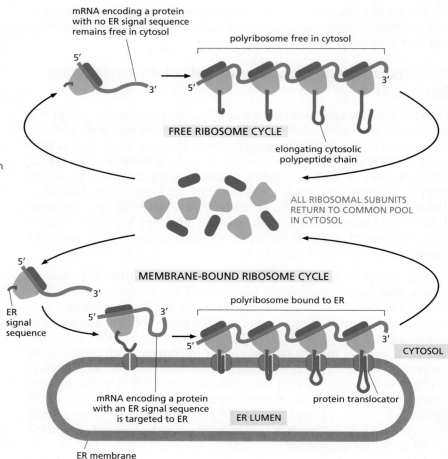

There are, therefore, two separate populations of ribosomes in the cytosol. *Membrane-bound ribosomes* are attached to the cytosolic side of the ER membrane (and outer nuclear membrane) and are making proteins that are being translocated into the ER. *Free ribosomes* are unattached to any membrane and are making all of the other proteins encoded by the nuclear DNA. Membrane-bound ribosomes and free ribosomes are structurally and functionally identical; they differ only in the proteins they are making at any given time. When a ribosome happens to be making a protein with an ER signal sequence, the signal sequence directs the ribosome to the ER membrane. Because proteins with an ER signal sequence are translocated as they are being made, no additional energy is required for their transport; the elongation of each polypeptide provides the thrust needed to push the growing chain through the ER membrane.

As an mRNA molecule is translated, many ribosomes bind to it, forming a *polyribosome* (discussed in Chapter 7). In the case of an mRNA molecule directing synthesis of a protein with an ER signal sequence, the polyribosome becomes riveted to the ER membrane by the growing polypeptide chains, which have become inserted into the ER membrane (**Figure 15–13**).

Soluble Proteins Made on the ER Are Released into the ER Lumen

Two protein components help guide ER signal sequences to the ER membrane: (1) a *signal-recognition particle* (*SRP*), present in the cytosol, binds to both the ribosome and the ER signal sequence as it emerges from

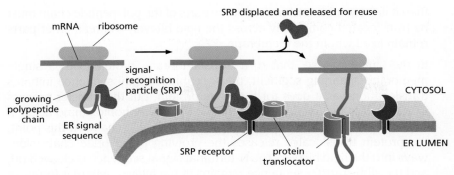

Figure 15–14 An ER signal sequence and an SRP direct a ribosome to the ER membrane. The SRP (*brown*) binds to both the exposed ER signal sequence and the ribosome, thereby slowing protein synthesis by the ribosome. The SRP–ribosome complex then binds to an SRP receptor (*dark blue*) in the ER membrane. The SRP is released, and the ribosome passes from the SRP receptor to a protein translocator (*light blue*) in the ER membrane. Protein synthesis resumes, and the translocator starts to transfer the growing polypeptide across the lipid bilayer.

the ribosome; and (2) an *SRP receptor*, embedded in the ER membrane, recognizes the SRP. Binding of an SRP to a ribosome that displays an ER signal sequence slows protein synthesis by that ribosome until the SRP engages with an SRP receptor on the ER. Once bound, the SRP is released, the receptor passes the ribosome to a *protein translocator* in the ER membrane, and protein synthesis recommences. The polypeptide is then threaded across the ER membrane through a *channel* in the translocator (**Figure 15–14**). The SRP and SRP receptor thus function as molecular matchmakers, bringing together ribosomes that are synthesizing proteins with an ER signal sequence and protein translocators within the ER membrane.

In addition to directing proteins to the ER, the signal sequence—which for soluble proteins is almost always at the N-terminus, the end synthesized first—functions to open the protein translocator. This sequence remains bound to the translocator, while the rest of the polypeptide chain is threaded through the membrane as a large loop. The signal sequence is removed by a transmembrane signal peptidase, which has an active site facing the lumenal side of the ER membrane. The cleaved signal sequence is then released from the protein translocator into the lipid bilayer and rapidly degraded.

Once the C-terminus of a soluble protein has passed through the translocator, the protein is released into the ER lumen (**Figure 15–15**).

Start and Stop Signals Determine the Arrangement of a Transmembrane Protein in the Lipid Bilayer

Not all proteins made by ER-bound ribosomes are released into the ER lumen. Some remain embedded in the ER membrane as transmembrane proteins. The translocation process for such proteins is more complicated

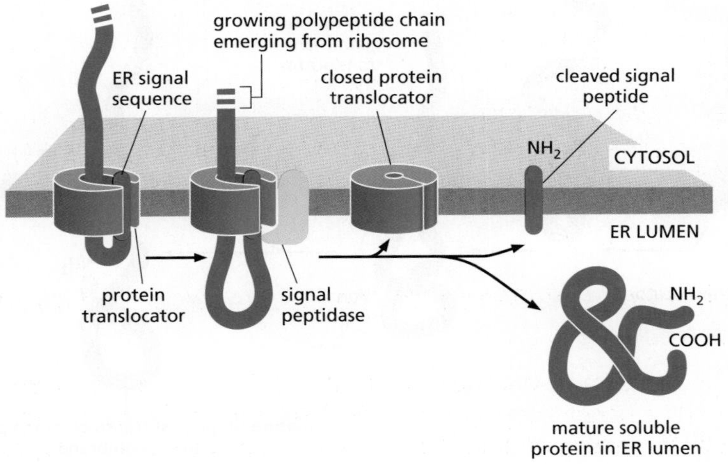

> ## QUESTION 15–3
>
> Explain how an mRNA molecule can remain attached to the ER membrane while individual ribosomes translating it are released and rejoin the cytosolic pool of ribosomes after each round of translation.

Figure 15–15 A soluble protein crosses the ER membrane and enters the lumen. The protein translocator binds the signal sequence and threads the rest of the polypeptide across the lipid bilayer as a loop. At some point during the translocation process, the signal peptide is cleaved from the growing protein by a signal peptidase (*yellow*). This cleaved signal sequence is ejected into the bilayer, where it is degraded. Once protein synthesis is complete, the translocated polypeptide is released as a soluble protein into the ER lumen, and the protein translocator closes. The membrane-bound ribosome is omitted from this and the following two figures for clarity.

than it is for soluble proteins, as some parts of the polypeptide chain must be translocated completely across the lipid bilayer, whereas other parts remain fixed within the membrane.

In the simplest case, that of a transmembrane protein with a single membrane-spanning segment, the N-terminal signal sequence initiates translocation—as it does for a soluble protein. But the transfer process is then halted by an additional sequence of hydrophobic amino acids, a *stop-transfer sequence*, further along the polypeptide chain. At this point, the protein translocator releases the growing polypeptide chain sideways into the lipid bilayer. The N-terminal signal sequence is cleaved off, and the stop-transfer sequence remains in the bilayer, where it forms an α-helical membrane-spanning segment that anchors the protein in the membrane. As a result, the protein ends up as a single-pass transmembrane protein inserted in the membrane with a defined orientation—the N-terminus on the lumenal side of the lipid bilayer and the C-terminus on the cytosolic side (Figure 15–16). Once inserted into the membrane, a transmembrane protein will never change its orientation; its cytosolic portion will always remain in the cytosol, even if the protein is subsequently transported to another organelle via vesicle budding and fusion (see Figure 11–18).

In some transmembrane proteins, an internal, rather than an N-terminal, signal sequence is used to start the protein transfer; this internal signal sequence, called a *start-transfer sequence*, is never removed from the polypeptide. This arrangement occurs in some transmembrane proteins in which the polypeptide chain passes back and forth across the lipid bilayer. In these cases, hydrophobic signal sequences are thought to work in pairs: an internal start-transfer sequence serves to initiate translocation, which continues until a stop-transfer sequence is reached; the two hydrophobic sequences are then released into the bilayer, where they remain as membrane-spanning α helices (Figure 15–17). In complex multipass proteins, in which many hydrophobic α helices span the bilayer, additional pairs of start- and stop-transfer sequences come into play: one sequence reinitiates translocation further down the polypeptide chain, and the other stops translocation and causes polypeptide release, and so on for subsequent starts and stops. In this way, multipass membrane proteins are stitched into the lipid bilayer as they are being synthesized, by a mechanism resembling the workings of a sewing machine.

QUESTION 15–4

A.   Predict the membrane orientation of a protein that is synthesized with an uncleaved, internal signal sequence (shown as the *red* start-transfer sequence in Figure 15–17) but does not contain a stop-transfer sequence.
B.   Similarly, predict the membrane orientation of a protein that is synthesized with an N-terminal cleaved signal sequence followed by a stop-transfer sequence, followed by a start-transfer sequence.
C.   What arrangement of signal sequences would enable the insertion of a multipass protein with an odd number of transmembrane segments?

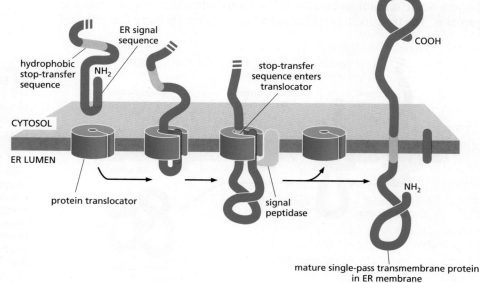

Figure 15–16 A single-pass transmembrane protein is retained in the lipid bilayer. An N-terminal ER signal sequence (*red*) initiates transfer as in Figure 15–15. In addition to this sequence, the protein also contains a second hydrophobic sequence, which acts as a stop-transfer sequence (*orange*). When this sequence enters the protein translocator, the growing polypeptide chain is discharged into the lipid bilayer. The N-terminal signal sequence is cleaved off, leaving the transmembrane protein anchored in the membrane (Movie 15.4). Protein synthesis on the cytosolic side then continues to completion.

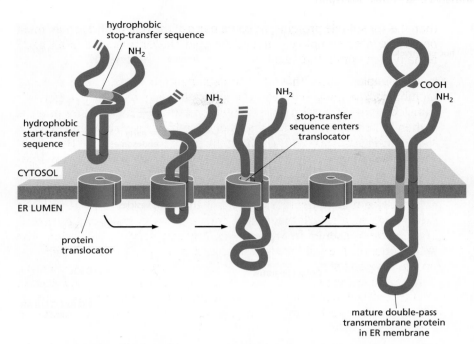

hydrophobic
stop-transfer sequence

NH₂

hydrophobic
start-transfer
sequence

CYTOSOL

ER LUMEN

protein
translocator

NH₂

NH₂

stop-transfer
sequence enters
translocator

COOH
NH₂

mature double-pass
transmembrane protein
in ER membrane

Figure 15–17 A double-pass transmembrane protein has an internal ER signal sequence. This internal sequence (*red*) not only acts as a start-transfer signal, it also helps to anchor the final protein in the membrane. Like the N-terminal ER signal sequence, the internal signal sequence is recognized by an SRP, which brings the ribosome to the ER membrane (not shown). When a stop-transfer sequence (*orange*) enters the protein translocator, the translocator discharges both sequences into the lipid bilayer. Neither the start-transfer nor the stop-transfer sequence is cleaved off, and the entire polypeptide chain remains anchored in the membrane as a double-pass transmembrane protein. Proteins that span the membrane more than twice contain additional pairs of start- and stop-transfer sequences, and the same process is repeated for each pair.

Having considered how proteins enter the ER lumen or become embedded in the ER membrane, we now discuss how they are carried onward by vesicular transport.

VESICULAR TRANSPORT

Entry into the ER lumen or membrane is usually only the first step on the pathway to another destination. That destination, initially at least, is generally the Golgi apparatus; there, proteins and lipids are modified and sorted for shipment to other sites. Transport from the ER to the Golgi apparatus—and from the Golgi apparatus to other compartments of the endomembrane system—is carried out by the continual budding and fusion of **transport vesicles**. This **vesicular transport** extends outward from the ER to the plasma membrane, where it allows proteins and other molecules to be secreted by exocytosis, and it reaches inward from the plasma membrane to lysosomes, allowing extracellular molecules to be imported by endocytosis (**Figure 15–18**). Together, these pathways thus provide routes of communication between the interior of the cell and its surroundings.

In this section, we discuss how vesicles shuttle proteins and membranes between intracellular compartments, allowing cells to eat, drink, and secrete. We also consider how these transport vesicles are directed to their proper destination, be it an organelle of the endomembrane system or the plasma membrane.

Transport Vesicles Carry Soluble Proteins and Membrane Between Compartments

Vesicular transport between membrane-enclosed compartments of the endomembrane system is highly organized. A major outward *secretory pathway* starts with the synthesis of proteins on the ER membrane and their entry into the ER, and it leads through the Golgi apparatus to the cell surface; at the Golgi apparatus, a side branch leads off through endosomes to lysosomes. A major inward *endocytic pathway,* which is responsible for the ingestion and degradation of extracellular molecules, moves materials from the plasma membrane, through endosomes, to lysosomes (**Figure 15–19**).

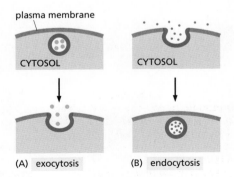

plasma membrane

CYTOSOL

CYTOSOL

(A) exocytosis

(B) endocytosis

Figure 15–18 Vesicular transport allows materials to exit or enter the cell. (A) During exocytosis, a vesicle fuses with the plasma membrane, releasing its content to the cell's surroundings. (B) During endocytosis, extracellular materials are captured by vesicles that bud inward from the plasma membrane and are carried into the cell.

Figure 15–19 Transport vesicles bud from one membrane and fuse with another, carrying membrane components and soluble proteins between compartments of the endomembrane system and the plasma membrane. The membrane of each compartment or vesicle maintains its orientation, so the cytosolic side always faces the cytosol and the noncytosolic side faces the lumen of the compartment or the outside of the cell (see Figure 11–18). The extracellular space and each of the membrane-enclosed compartments (shaded *gray*) communicate with one another by means of transport vesicles, as shown. In the inward endocytic pathway (*green* arrows), extracellular molecules are ingested (endocytosed) in vesicles derived from the plasma membrane and are delivered to early endosomes and, usually, on to lysosomes via late endosomes. In the outward secretory pathway (*red* arrows), protein molecules are transported from the ER, through the Golgi apparatus, to the plasma membrane or (via early and late endosomes) to lysosomes. Note that movement through the Golgi apparatus occurs by vesicles that shuttle between its individual cisternae and by a process of maturation, whereby the cisternae themselves move through the stack (central *red* arrows).

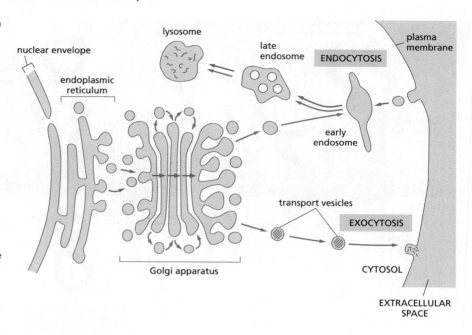

To function optimally, each transport vesicle that buds off from a compartment must take with it only the proteins appropriate to its destination and must fuse only with the appropriate target membrane. A vesicle carrying cargo from the Golgi apparatus to the plasma membrane, for example, must exclude proteins that are to stay in the Golgi apparatus, and it must fuse only with the plasma membrane and not with any other organelle. While participating in this constant flow of membrane components, each organelle must maintain its own distinct identity; that is, its own distinctive protein and lipid composition. All of these recognition events depend on proteins displayed on the surface of the transport vesicle. As we will see, different types of transport vesicles shuttle between the various organelles, each carrying a distinct set of molecules.

Vesicle Budding Is Driven by the Assembly of a Protein Coat

Vesicles that bud from membranes usually have a distinctive protein coat on their cytosolic surface and are therefore called **coated vesicles**. After budding from its parent organelle, the vesicle sheds its coat, allowing its membrane to interact directly with the membrane to which it will fuse. Cells produce several kinds of coated vesicles, each with a distinctive protein coat. The coat serves at least two functions: it helps shape the membrane into a bud and it captures molecules for onward transport.

The best-studied vesicles are those that have an outer coat made of the protein **clathrin**. These *clathrin-coated vesicles* bud from both the Golgi apparatus on the outward secretory pathway and from the plasma membrane on the inward endocytic pathway. At the plasma membrane, for example, each vesicle starts off as a *clathrin-coated pit*. Clathrin molecules assemble into a basketlike network on the cytosolic surface of the membrane, and it is this assembly process that starts shaping the membrane into a vesicle (Figure 15–20). A GTP-binding protein called *dynamin* assembles as a ring around the neck of each deeply invaginated clathrin-coated pit. Together with other proteins recruited to the neck of the vesicle, the dynamin causes the neck to constrict, thereby pinching off the vesicle from its parent membrane. Other kinds of transport vesicles, with different coat proteins, are also involved in vesicular transport. They form in a similar way and carry their own characteristic sets of molecules

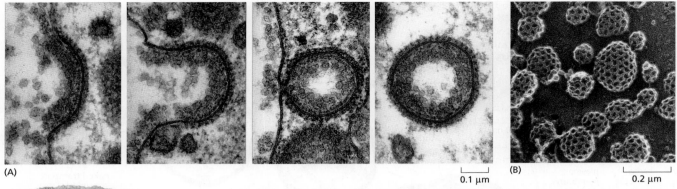

(A)

0.1 μm

(B)

0.2 μm

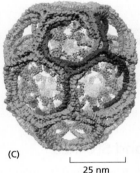

(C)

25 nm

Figure 15–20 **Clathrin molecules form basketlike cages that help shape membranes into vesicles.**
(A) Electron micrographs showing the sequence of events in the formation of a clathrin-coated vesicle from a clathrin-coated pit. The clathrin-coated pits and vesicles shown here are unusually large and are being formed at the plasma membrane of a hen oocyte. They are involved in taking up particles made of lipid and protein into the oocyte to form yolk. (B) Electron micrograph showing numerous clathrin-coated pits and vesicles budding from the inner surface of the plasma membrane of cultured skin cells. (C) In a test tube, clathrin molecules sometimes self-assemble into basketlike cages. The structure of one such clathrin cage was determined by cryoelectron microscopy. The positions of three of the constituent clathrin molecules, each of which has a characteristic three-armed shape, are highlighted in *red, green,* and *brown.* (A, from M.M. Perry and A.B. Gilbert, *J. Cell Sci.* 39:257–272, 1979. With permission from The Company of Biologists Ltd; B, from J. Heuser, *J. Cell Biol.* 84:560–583, 1980. With permission from Rockefeller University Press; C, from A. Fotin et al., *Nature* 432:573–579, 2004. With permission from Macmillan Publishers Ltd.)

between the endoplasmic reticulum, the Golgi apparatus, and the plasma membrane. But how does a transport vesicle select its particular cargo? The mechanism is best understood for clathrin-coated vesicles.

Clathrin itself plays no part in choosing specific molecules for transport. This is the function of a second class of coat proteins called *adaptins*, which both secure the clathrin coat to the vesicle membrane and help select cargo molecules for transport. Molecules for onward transport carry specific *transport signals* that are recognized by *cargo receptors* in the Golgi or plasma membrane. Adaptins help capture specific cargo molecules by trapping the cargo receptors that bind them. In this way, a selected set of cargo molecules, bound to their specific receptors, is incorporated into the lumen of each newly formed clathrin-coated vesicle (Figure 15–21). There are different types of adaptins: the adaptins that bind cargo receptors in the plasma membrane, for example, are not the same as those that bind cargo receptors in the Golgi apparatus, reflecting the differences in the cargo molecules to be transported from each of these sources.

Other classes of coated vesicles, called *COP-coated vesicles* (COP being shorthand for "coat protein"), are involved in transporting molecules between the ER and the Golgi apparatus and from one part of the Golgi apparatus to another (Table 15–4).

TABLE 15–4 SOME TYPES OF COATED VESICLES			
Type of Coated Vesicle	Coat Proteins	Origin	Destination
Clathrin-coated	clathrin + adaptin 1	Golgi apparatus	lysosome (via endosomes)
Clathrin-coated	clathrin + adaptin 2	plasma membrane	endosomes
COPII-coated	COPII proteins	ER	Golgi cisterna
COPI-coated	COPI proteins	Golgi cisterna	ER

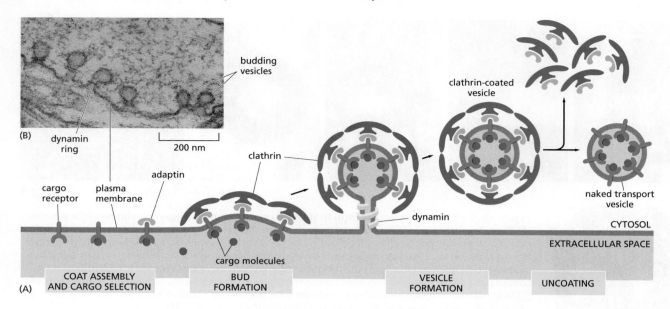

Figure 15–21 Clathrin-coated vesicles transport selected cargo molecules. Here, as in Figure 15–20, the vesicles are shown budding from the plasma membrane. (A) Cargo receptors, with their bound cargo molecules, are captured by adaptins, which also bind clathrin molecules to the cytosolic surface of the budding vesicle (Movie 15.5). Dynamin proteins assemble around the neck of budding vesicles; once assembled, the dynamin molecules hydrolyze their bound GTP and, with the help of other proteins recruited to the neck (not shown), pinch off the vesicle. After budding is complete, the coat proteins are removed, and the naked vesicle can fuse with its target membrane. Functionally similar coat proteins are found in other types of coated vesicles. (B) In flies that produce a mutant dynamin protein, clathrin-coated pits assemble and dynamin is recruited around the neck of budding vesicles but fail to pinch them off, as can be seen in this electron micrograph of the plasma membrane in a fly's nerve ending. Flies with this mutation become paralyzed, because clathrin-mediated endocytosis grinds to a halt, preventing the recycling of vesicles needed to release neurotransmitters (see Figure 12–40). (B, from J.H. Koenig and K. Ikeda, *J. Neurosci.* 9:3844–3860, 1989. With permission from the Society for Neuroscience.)

Vesicle Docking Depends on Tethers and SNAREs

After a transport vesicle buds from a membrane, it must find its way to the correct destination to deliver its contents. Often, the vesicle is actively transported by motor proteins that move along cytoskeletal fibers, as discussed in Chapter 17 (see Figure 17–20).

Once a transport vesicle has reached its target, it must recognize and dock with its specific organelle. Only then can the vesicle membrane fuse with the target membrane and unload the vesicle's cargo. The impressive specificity of vesicular transport suggests that each type of transport vesicle in the cell displays molecular markers on its surface that identify the vesicle according to its origin and cargo. These markers must be recognized by complementary receptors on the appropriate target membrane, including the plasma membrane.

The identification process depends on a diverse family of monomeric GTPases called **Rab proteins**. Specific Rab proteins on the surface of each type of vesicle are recognized by corresponding **tethering proteins** on the cytosolic surface of the target membrane. Each organelle and each type of transport vesicle carries a unique combination of Rab proteins, which serve as molecular markers for each membrane type. The coding system of matching Rab and tethering proteins helps to ensure that transport vesicles fuse only with the correct membrane.

Additional recognition is provided by a family of transmembrane proteins called **SNAREs**. Once the tethering protein has captured a vesicle by grabbing hold of its Rab protein, SNAREs on the vesicle (called v-SNAREs) interact with complementary SNAREs on the target membrane (called t-SNAREs), firmly docking the vesicle in place (Figure 15–22).

The same SNAREs involved in docking also play a central role in catalyzing the membrane fusion required for a transport vesicle to deliver its cargo. Fusion not only delivers the soluble contents of the vesicle into the interior of the target organelle or to the extracellular space, but it also adds the vesicle membrane to the membrane of the organelle (see Figure 15–22). After vesicle docking, the fusion of a vesicle with its target membrane sometimes requires a special stimulatory signal. Whereas docking requires only that the two membranes come close enough for the SNAREs protruding from the two lipid bilayers to

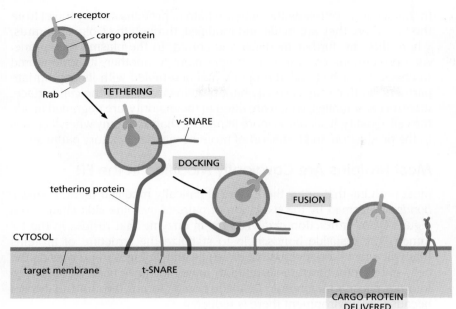

Figure 15–22 Rab proteins, tethering proteins, and SNAREs help direct transport vesicles to their target membranes. A filamentous tethering protein (*green*) on a membrane binds to a Rab protein (*yellow*) on the surface of a vesicle. This interaction allows the vesicle to dock on its particular target membrane. A v-SNARE (*red*) on the vesicle then binds to a complementary t-SNARE (*blue*) on the target membrane. Whereas Rab and tethering proteins provide the initial recognition between a vesicle and its target membrane, complementary SNARE proteins ensure that transport vesicles dock at their appropriate target membranes. These SNARE proteins also catalyze the final fusion of the two membranes (see Figure 15–23).

interact, fusion requires a much closer approach: the two bilayers must come within 1.5 nanometers (nm) of each other so that their lipids can intermix. For this close approach, water must be displaced from the hydrophilic surfaces of the membranes—a process that is energetically highly unfavorable and thus prevents membranes from fusing randomly. All membrane fusions in cells must therefore be catalyzed by specialized proteins that assemble to form a fusion complex that provides the means to cross this energy barrier. For vesicle fusion, the SNARE proteins themselves catalyze the process: when fusion is triggered, the v-SNAREs and t-SNAREs wrap around each other tightly, thereby acting like a winch that pulls the two lipid bilayers into close proximity (**Figure 15–23**).

SECRETORY PATHWAYS

Vesicular traffic is not confined to the interior of the cell. It extends to and from the plasma membrane. Newly made proteins, lipids, and carbohydrates are delivered from the ER, via the Golgi apparatus, to the cell surface by transport vesicles that fuse with the plasma membrane in the process of **exocytosis** (see Figure 15–19). Each molecule that travels along this secretory pathway passes through a fixed sequence of membrane-enclosed compartments and is often chemically modified en route.

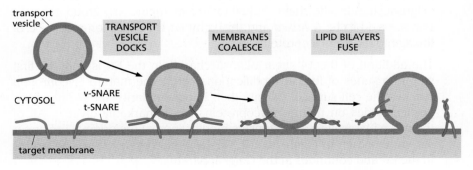

Figure 15–23 Following vesicle docking, SNARE proteins can catalyze the fusion of the vesicle and target membranes. Once appropriately triggered, the tight pairing of v-SNAREs and t-SNAREs draws the two lipid bilayers into close apposition. The force of the SNAREs winding together squeezes out any water molecules that remain trapped between the two membranes, allowing their lipids to flow together to form a continuous bilayer. In a cell, other proteins recruited to the fusion site help to complete the fusion process. After fusion, the SNAREs are pried apart so that they can be used again.

In this section, we follow the outward path of proteins as they travel from the ER, where they are made and modified, through the Golgi apparatus, where they are further modified and sorted, to the plasma membrane. As a protein passes from one compartment to another, it is monitored to check that it has folded properly and assembled with its appropriate partners, so that only correctly built proteins make it to the cell surface. Incorrect assemblies, which are often in the majority, are degraded inside the cell. Quality, it seems, is more important than economy when it comes to the production and transport of proteins via the secretory pathway.

Most Proteins Are Covalently Modified in the ER

Most proteins that enter the ER are chemically modified there. *Disulfide bonds* are formed by the oxidation of pairs of cysteine side chains (see Figure 4–30), a reaction catalyzed by an enzyme that resides in the ER lumen. The disulfide bonds help to stabilize the structure of proteins that will encounter degradative enzymes and changes in pH outside the cell—either after they are secreted or once they have been incorporated into the plasma membrane. Disulfide bonds do not form in the cytosol because the environment there is reducing.

Many of the proteins that enter the ER lumen or ER membrane are converted to glycoproteins in the ER by the covalent attachment of short, branched oligosaccharide side chains composed of multiple sugars. This process of *glycosylation* is carried out by glycosylating enzymes present in the ER but not in the cytosol. Very few proteins in the cytosol are glycosylated, and those that are have only a single sugar attached to them. The oligosaccharides on proteins can serve various functions. They can protect a protein from degradation, hold it in the ER until it is properly folded, or help guide it to the appropriate organelle by serving as a transport signal for packaging the protein into appropriate transport vesicles. When displayed on the cell surface, oligosaccharides form part of the cell's outer carbohydrate layer or *glycocalyx* (see Figure 11–33) and can function in the recognition of one cell by another.

In the ER, individual sugars are not added one-by-one to the protein to create an oligosaccharide side chain. Instead, a preformed, branched oligosaccharide containing a total of 14 sugars is attached *en bloc* to all proteins that carry the appropriate site for glycosylation. The oligosaccharide is originally attached to a specialized lipid, called *dolichol*, in the ER membrane; it is then transferred to the amino (NH$_2$) group of an asparagine side chain on the protein, immediately after a target asparagine emerges in the ER lumen during protein translocation (**Figure 15–24**). The addition takes place in a single enzymatic step that is catalyzed by a membrane-bound enzyme (an oligosaccharyl transferase) that has its active site exposed on the lumenal side of the ER membrane—which explains why cytosolic proteins are not glycosylated in this way. A simple sequence of three amino acids, of which the target asparagine is one, defines which sites in a protein receive the oligosaccharide. Oligosaccharide side chains linked to an asparagine NH$_2$ group in a protein are said to be *N-linked* and this is by far the most common type of linkage found on glycoproteins.

The addition of the 14-sugar oligosaccharide in the ER is only the first step in a series of further modifications before the mature glycoprotein reaches the cell surface. Despite their initial similarity, the *N*-linked oligosaccharides on mature glycoproteins are remarkably diverse. All of the diversity results from extensive modification of the original precursor structure shown in Figure 15–24. This *oligosaccharide processing* begins in the ER and continues in the Golgi apparatus.

QUESTION 15–6

Why might it be advantageous to add a preassembled block of 14 sugar residues to a protein in the ER, rather than building the sugar chains step-by-step on the surface of the protein by the sequential addition of sugars by individual enzymes?

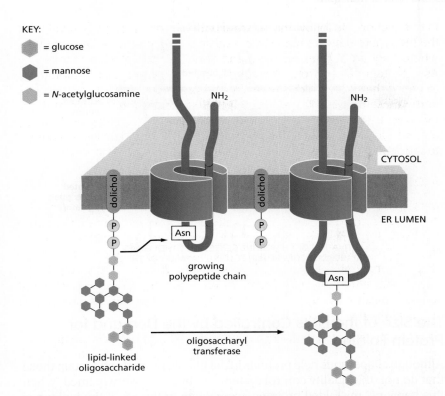

KEY:

= glucose

= mannose

= *N*-acetylglucosamine

NH₂

NH₂

CYTOSOL

ER LUMEN

dolichol

dolichol

P

P

P

P

Asn

growing
polypeptide chain

Asn

lipid-linked
oligosaccharide

oligosaccharyl
transferase

Figure 15–24 Many proteins are glycosylated on asparagines in the ER. When an appropriate asparagine in a growing polypeptide chain enters the ER lumen, it is glycosylated by addition of a branched oligosaccharide side chain. Each oligosaccharide chain is transferred as an intact unit to the asparagine from a lipid called dolichol, catalyzed by the enzyme oligosaccharyl transferase. Asparagines that are glycosylated are always present in the tripeptide sequences asparagine-X-serine or asparagine-X-threonine, where X can be almost any amino acid.

Exit from the ER Is Controlled to Ensure Protein Quality

Some proteins made in the ER are destined to function there. They are retained in the ER (and are returned to the ER should they manage to escape to the Golgi apparatus) by a C-terminal sequence of four amino acids called an *ER retention signal* (see Table 15–3, p. 502). This retention signal is recognized by a membrane-bound receptor protein in the ER and Golgi apparatus. Most proteins that enter the ER, however, are destined for other locations; they are packaged into transport vesicles that bud from the ER and fuse with the Golgi apparatus.

Exit from the ER is highly selective. Proteins that fail to fold correctly, and dimeric or multimeric proteins that do not assemble properly, are actively retained in the ER by binding to *chaperone proteins* that reside there. The chaperones hold these proteins in the ER until proper folding or assembly occurs. Chaperones prevent misfolded proteins from aggregating, which helps steer proteins along a path toward proper folding (see Figures 4–8 and 4–9); if proper folding and assembly still fail, the proteins are exported to the cytosol, where they are degraded by the proteasome (see Figure 7–43). Antibody molecules, for example, are composed of four polypeptide chains (see Figure 4–33) that assemble into the complete antibody molecule in the ER. Partially assembled antibodies are retained in the ER until all four polypeptide chains have assembled; any antibody molecule that fails to assemble properly is degraded. In this way, the ER controls the quality of the proteins that it exports to the Golgi apparatus.

Sometimes, however, this quality control mechanism can be detrimental to the organism. For example, the predominant mutation that causes the common genetic disease *cystic fibrosis*, which leads to severe lung damage, produces a plasma membrane transport protein that is slightly misfolded; even though the mutant protein could function normally as a chloride channel if it reached the plasma membrane, it is retained in the ER and then degraded, with dire consequences. This devastating disease comes about not because the mutation inactivates an important protein but because the active protein is discarded by the cells before it is given an opportunity to function.

Figure 15–25 Accumulation of misfolded proteins in the ER lumen triggers an unfolded protein response (UPR). The misfolded proteins are recognized by several types of transmembrane sensor proteins in the ER membrane, each of which activates a different component of the UPR. Some sensors stimulate the production of transcription regulators that activate genes encoding chaperones or other proteins involved in ER quality control. Another sensor can also inhibit protein synthesis, reducing the flow of proteins through the ER (Movie 15.6 and Movie 15.7).

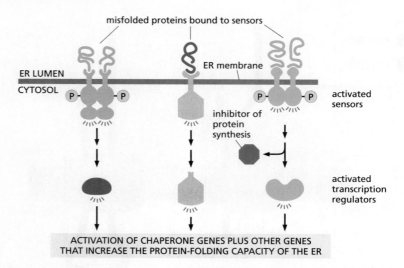

The Size of the ER Is Controlled by the Demand for Protein Folding

Although chaperones help proteins in the ER fold properly and retain those that do not, this quality control system can become overwhelmed. When this happens, misfolded proteins accumulate in the ER. If the buildup is large enough, it triggers a complex program called the **unfolded protein response (UPR)**. This program prompts the cell to produce more ER, including more chaperones and other proteins concerned with quality control (Figure 15–25).

The UPR allows a cell to adjust the size of its ER to properly handle the volume of proteins entering the secretory pathway. In some cases, however, even an expanded ER cannot keep up with the demand, and the UPR directs the cell to self-destruct by undergoing apoptosis. Such a situation may occur in adult-onset diabetes, where tissues gradually become resistant to the effects of insulin. To compensate for this resistance, the insulin-secreting cells in the pancreas produce more and more insulin. Eventually, their ER reaches a maximum capacity, at which point the UPR can trigger cell death. As more insulin-secreting cells are eliminated, the demand on the surviving cells increases, making it more likely that they will die as well, further exacerbating the disease.

Proteins Are Further Modified and Sorted in the Golgi Apparatus

The **Golgi apparatus** is usually located near the cell nucleus, and in animal cells it is often close to the centrosome, a small cytoskeletal structure near the cell center (see Figure 17–13). The Golgi apparatus consists of a collection of flattened, membrane-enclosed sacs called *cisternae*, which are piled like stacks of pita bread (Figure 15–26). Each stack contains 3–20 cisternae, and the number of Golgi stacks per cell varies greatly depending on the cell type: some cells contain one large stack, while others contain hundreds of very small ones.

Each Golgi stack has two distinct faces: an entry, or *cis*, face and an exit, or *trans,* face. The *cis* face is adjacent to the ER, while the *trans* face points toward the plasma membrane. The outermost cisterna at each face is connected to a network of interconnected membranous tubes and vesicles (see Figure 15–26A). Soluble proteins and pieces of membrane enter the *cis Golgi network* via transport vesicles derived from the ER.

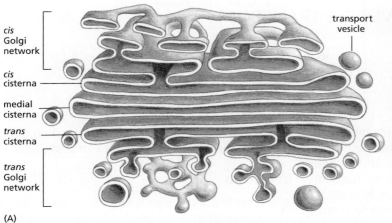

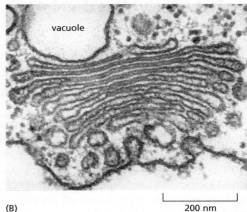

(A)   (B)   200 nm

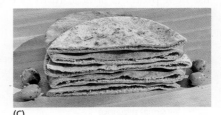

(C)

Figure 15–26 The Golgi apparatus consists of a stack of flattened, membrane-enclosed sacs. (A) A three-dimensional model of a Golgi stack reconstructed from a sequential series of electron micrographs of the Golgi apparatus in a secretory animal cell. To see how such models are assembled, watch Movie 15.8. (B) Electron micrograph of a Golgi stack from a plant cell, where the Golgi apparatus is especially distinct; the stack is oriented as in (A). (C) A pita-bread model of the Golgi apparatus. Vesicles are shown as olives. (B, courtesy of George Palade.)

The proteins travel through the cisternae in sequence in two ways: (1) by means of transport vesicles that bud from one cisterna and fuse with the next; and (2) by a maturation process in which the Golgi cisternae themselves migrate through the Golgi stack. Proteins finally exit from the *trans Golgi network* in transport vesicles destined for either the cell surface or another organelle of the endomembrane system (see Figure 15–19).

Both the *cis* and *trans* Golgi networks are thought to be important for protein sorting: proteins entering the *cis* Golgi network can either move onward through the Golgi stack or, if they contain an ER retention signal, be returned to the ER; proteins exiting from the *trans* Golgi network are sorted according to whether they are destined for lysosomes (via endosomes) or for the cell surface. We discuss some examples of sorting by the *trans* Golgi network later, and we present some of the methods for tracking proteins through the secretory pathways of the cell in How We Know, pp. 520–521.

Many of the oligosaccharide chains that are added to proteins in the ER (see Figure 15–24) undergo further modifications in the Golgi apparatus. On some proteins, for example, more complex oligosaccharide chains are created by a highly ordered process in which sugars are added and removed by a series of enzymes that act in a rigidly determined sequence as the protein passes through the Golgi stack. As would be expected, the enzymes that act early in the chain of processing events are located in cisternae close to the *cis* face, while enzymes that act late are located in cisternae near the *trans* face.

Secretory Proteins Are Released from the Cell by Exocytosis

In all eukaryotic cells, a steady stream of vesicles buds from the *trans* Golgi network and fuses with the plasma membrane in the process of exocytosis. This *constitutive exocytosis pathway* supplies the plasma

TRACKING PROTEIN AND VESICLE TRANSPORT

Over the years, biologists have taken advantage of a variety of techniques to untangle the pathways and mechanisms by which proteins are sorted and transported into and out of the cell and its resident organelles. Biochemical, genetic, molecular biological, and microscopic techniques all provide ways to monitor how proteins shuttle from one cell compartment to another. Some can even track the migration of proteins and transport vesicles in real time in living cells.

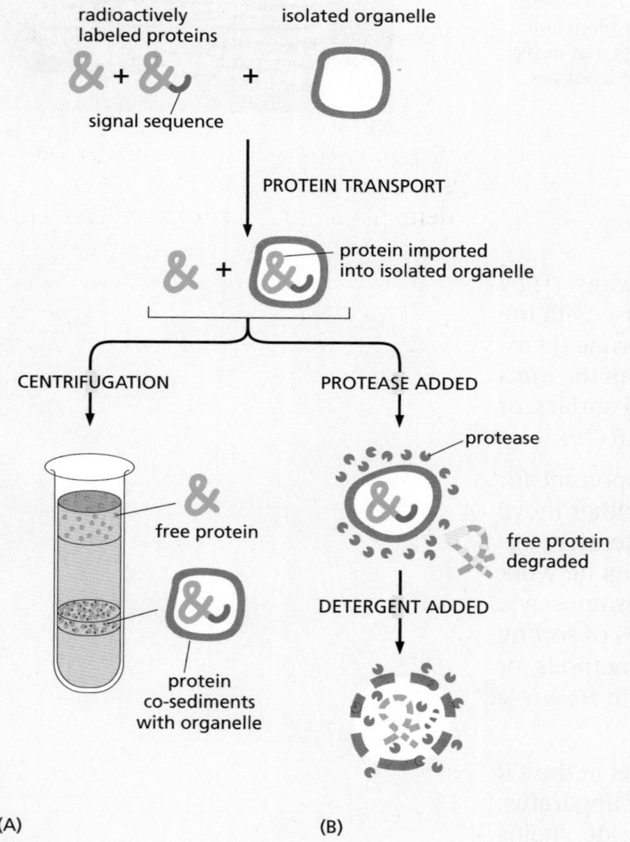

In a tube

A protein bearing a signal sequence can be introduced to a preparation of isolated organelles in a test tube. This mixture can then be tested to see whether the protein is taken up by the organelle. The protein is usually produced *in vitro* by cell-free translation of a purified mRNA encoding the polypeptide; in the process, radioactive amino acids can be used to label the protein so that it will be easy to isolate and to follow. The labeled protein is incubated with a selected organelle and its translocation is monitored by one of several methods (**Figure 15–27**).

Ask a yeast

Movement of proteins between different cell compartments via transport vesicles has been studied extensively using genetic techniques. Studies of mutant yeast cells that are defective for secretion at high temperatures have identified numerous genes involved in carrying proteins from the ER to the cell surface. Many of these mutant genes encode temperature-sensitive proteins (discussed in Chapter 19). These mutant proteins may function normally at 25°C, but, when the yeast cells are shifted to 35°C, the proteins are inactivated. As a result, when researchers raise the temperature, the various proteins destined for secretion instead accumulate inappropriately in the ER, Golgi apparatus, or transport vesicles—depending on the particular mutation (**Figure 15–28**).

At the movies

The most commonly used method for tracking a protein as it moves throughout the cell involves tagging the polypeptide with a fluorescent protein, such as green fluorescent protein (GFP). Using the genetic engineering techniques discussed in Chapter 10, this small protein can be fused to other cell proteins. Fortunately, for many proteins studied, the addition of GFP to one or other end does not perturb the protein's normal function or transport. The movement of a GFP-tagged protein can then be monitored in a living cell with a fluorescence microscope. In 2008, the Nobel Prize in Chemistry was awarded to Osamu Shimomura, Martin Chalfie, and Roger Tsien for the development and refinement of this technology.

Figure 15–27 **Several methods can be used to determine whether a labeled protein bearing a particular signal sequence is transported into a preparation of isolated organelles.** (A) The labeled protein with or without a signal sequence is incubated with the organelles, and the preparation is centrifuged. Only those labeled proteins that contained a signal sequence will be transported and therefore will co-fractionate with the organelle. (B) The labeled proteins are incubated with the organelle, and a protease is added to the preparation. A transported protein will be selectively protected from digestion by the organelle membrane; adding a detergent that disrupts the organelle membrane will eliminate that protection, and the transported protein will also be degraded.

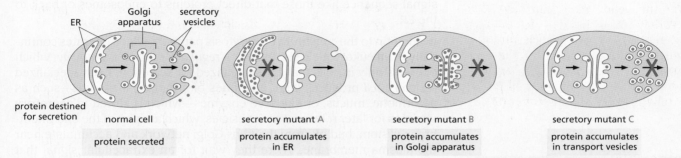

Figure 15–28 Temperature-sensitive mutants have been used to dissect the protein secretory pathway in yeast. Mutations in genes involved at different stages of the transport process, as indicated by the *red* X, result in the accumulation of proteins in the ER, the Golgi apparatus, or transport vesicles.

Such GFP fusion proteins are widely used to study the location and movement of proteins in cells (**Figure 15–29**). GFP fused to a protein that shuttles in and out of the nucleus, for example, can be used to study nuclear transport events. GFP fused to a plasma membrane protein can be used to measure the kinetics of its movement through the secretory pathway. Movies 15.1, 15.9, 15.10, and 15.13 demonstrate the power and beauty of this technique.

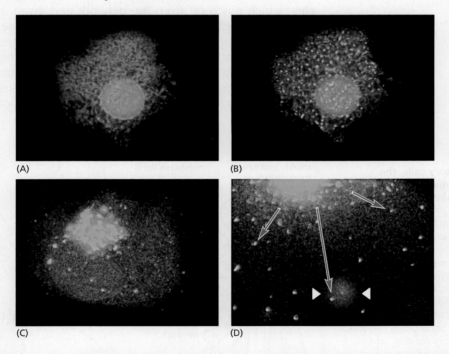

Figure 15–29 Tagging a protein with GFP allows the resulting fusion protein to be tracked throughout the cell. In this experiment, GFP is fused to a viral coat protein and expressed in cultured animal cells. In an infected cell, the viral protein moves through the secretory pathway from the ER to the cell surface, where the virus particles are assembled. *Red* arrows indicate the direction of protein movement. The viral coat protein used in this experiment contains a mutation that allows export from the ER only at a low temperature. (A) At high temperatures, the fusion protein labels the ER. (B) As the temperature is lowered, the GFP fusion protein rapidly accumulates at ER exit sites. (C) The fusion protein then moves to the Golgi apparatus. (D) Finally, the fusion protein is delivered to the plasma membrane, shown here in a more close-up view. The halo between the two *white* arrowheads marks the spot where a single vesicle has fused, allowing the fusion protein to incorporate into the plasma membrane. These images are stills taken from Movie 15.9. (A–D, courtesy of Jennifer Lippincott-Schwartz.)

membrane with newly made lipids and proteins (Movie 15.9), enabling the plasma membrane to expand prior to cell division and refreshing old lipids and proteins in nonproliferating cells. The constitutive pathway also carries soluble proteins to the cell surface to be released to the outside, a process called **secretion**. Some of these proteins remain attached to the cell surface; some are incorporated into the extracellular matrix; still others diffuse into the extracellular fluid to nourish or signal other cells. Entry into the constitutive pathway does not require a particular signal sequence like those that direct proteins to endosomes or back to the ER.

In addition to the constitutive exocytosis pathway, which operates continually in all eukaryotic cells, there is a *regulated exocytosis pathway*, which operates only in cells that are specialized for secretion. Each specialized *secretory cell* produces large quantities of a particular product—such as a hormone, mucus, or digestive enzymes—which is stored in **secretory vesicles** for later release. These vesicles, which are part of the endomembrane system, bud off from the *trans* Golgi network and accumulate near the plasma membrane. There they wait for an extracellular signal that will stimulate them to fuse with the plasma membrane and release their contents to the cell exterior by exocytosis (Figure 15–30). An increase in blood glucose, for example, signals insulin-producing endocrine cells in the pancreas to secrete the hormone (Figure 15–31).

Proteins destined for regulated secretion are sorted and packaged in the *trans* Golgi network. Proteins that travel by this pathway have special surface properties that cause them to aggregate with one another under the ionic conditions (acidic pH and high Ca^{2+}) that prevail in the *trans* Golgi network. The aggregated proteins are packaged into secretory vesicles, which pinch off from the network and await a signal instructing them to fuse with the plasma membrane. Proteins secreted by the constitutive pathway, on the other hand, do not aggregate and are therefore carried automatically to the plasma membrane by the transport vesicles of the constitutive pathway. Selective aggregation has another function: it allows secretory proteins to be packaged into secretory vesicles at concentrations much higher than the concentration of the unaggregated

QUESTION 15–7

What would you expect to happen in cells that secrete large amounts of protein through the regulated secretory pathway if the ionic conditions in the ER lumen could be changed to resemble those in the lumen of the *trans* Golgi network?

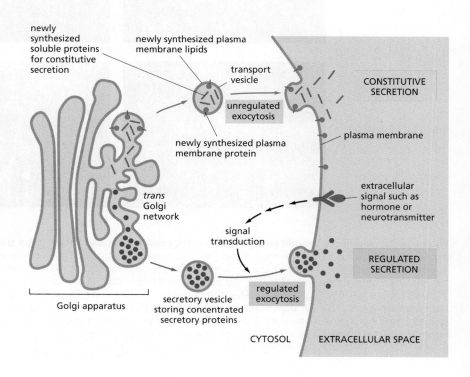

Figure 15–30 In secretory cells, the regulated and constitutive pathways of exocytosis diverge in the *trans* Golgi network. Many soluble proteins are continually secreted from the cell by the constitutive secretory pathway (*blue* arrows), which operates in all eukaryotic cells (Movie 15.10). This pathway also continually supplies the plasma membrane with newly synthesized lipids and proteins. Specialized secretory cells have, in addition, a regulated exocytosis pathway (*red* arrows) by which selected proteins in the *trans* Golgi network are diverted into secretory vesicles, where the proteins are concentrated and stored until an extracellular signal stimulates their secretion. It is unclear how these special aggregates of secretory proteins (*red*) are segregated into secretory vesicles. Secretory vesicles have unique proteins in their membranes; perhaps some of these proteins act as receptors for secretory protein aggregates in the *trans* Golgi network.

protein in the Golgi lumen. This increase in concentration can reach 200-fold, enabling secretory cells to release large amounts of the protein promptly when triggered to do so (see Figure 15–30).

When a secretory vesicle or transport vesicle fuses with the plasma membrane and discharges its contents by exocytosis, its membrane becomes part of the plasma membrane. Although this should greatly increase the surface area of the plasma membrane, it does so only transiently because membrane components are removed from other regions of the surface by endocytosis almost as fast as they are added by exocytosis. This removal returns both the lipids and the proteins of the vesicle membrane to the Golgi network, where they can be used again. Similar membrane retrieval pathways also operate in the Golgi apparatus to return lipids and selected proteins to the endoplasmic reticulum.

ENDOCYTIC PATHWAYS

Eukaryotic cells are continually taking up fluid, along with large and small molecules, by the process of **endocytosis**. Certain specialized cells are also able to internalize large particles and even other cells. The material to be ingested is progressively enclosed by a small portion of the plasma membrane, which first buds inward and then pinches off to form an intracellular *endocytic vesicle*. The ingested materials, including the membrane components, are delivered to *endosomes*, from which they can be recycled to the plasma membrane or sent to lysosomes for digestion. The metabolites generated by digestion are transferred directly out of the lysosome into the cytosol, where they can be used by the cell.

Two main types of endocytosis are distinguished on the basis of the size of the endocytic vesicles formed. *Pinocytosis* ("cellular drinking") involves the ingestion of fluid and molecules via small pinocytic vesicles (<150 nm in diameter). *Phagocytosis* ("cellular eating") involves the ingestion of large particles, such as microorganisms and cell debris, via large vesicles called *phagosomes* (generally >250 nm in diameter). Whereas all eukaryotic cells are continually ingesting fluid and molecules by pinocytosis, large particles are ingested mainly by specialized *phagocytic cells*.

In this final section, we trace the endocytic pathway from the plasma membrane to lysosomes. We start by considering the uptake of large particles by phagocytosis.

Specialized Phagocytic Cells Ingest Large Particles

The most dramatic form of endocytosis, **phagocytosis**, was first observed more than a hundred years ago. In protozoa, phagocytosis is a form of feeding: these unicellular eukaryotes ingest large particles such as bacteria by taking them up into phagosomes (Movie 15.11). The phagosomes then fuse with lysosomes, where the food particles are digested. Few cells in multicellular organisms are able to ingest large particles efficiently. In the animal gut, for example, large particles of food have to be broken down to individual molecules by extracellular enzymes before they can be taken up by the absorptive cells lining the gut.

Nevertheless, phagocytosis is important in most animals for purposes other than nutrition. **Phagocytic cells**—including *macrophages*, which are widely distributed in tissues, and other white blood cells, such as *neutrophils*—defend us against infection by ingesting invading microorganisms. To be taken up by macrophages or neutrophils, particles must first bind to the phagocytic cell surface and activate one of a variety of surface receptors. Some of these receptors recognize antibodies, the proteins that help protect us against infection by binding to the surface

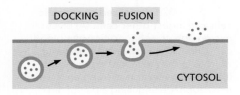

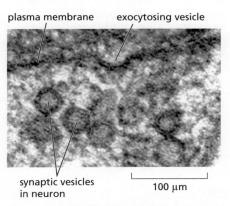

Figure 15–31 Secretory vesicles store and release concentrated proteins. The process, which takes place through vesicle docking and fusion (see Figure 15–23), requires a signal to initiate. The cryoelectron micrograph shows the release of concentrated neurotransmitter from a cultured mouse hippocampal neuron. The sample was rapidly frozen just 5 ms after the neuron was stimulated to fire. (From S. Watanabe, *Front. Synaptic. Neurosci.* 8:1–10, 2016.)

Figure 15–32 Specialized phagocytic cells can ingest other cells. (A) Electron micrograph of a phagocytic white blood cell (a neutrophil) ingesting a bacterium, which is in the process of dividing. (B) Scanning electron micrograph showing a macrophage engulfing a pair of red blood cells. The lines point to the edges of the pseudopods that the phagocytic cells are extending like collars to envelop their targets. (A, courtesy of Dorothy F. Bainton; B, courtesy of Jean Paul Revel.)

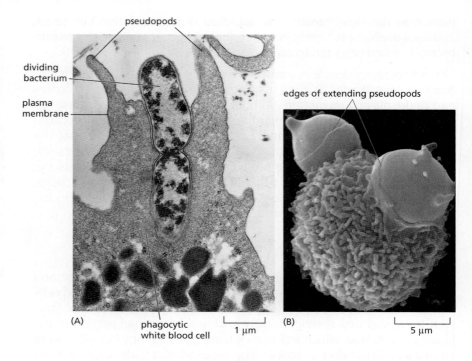

Figure 15–32 Specialized phagocytic cells can ingest other cells. (A) Electron micrograph of a phagocytic white blood cell (a neutrophil) ingesting a bacterium, which is in the process of dividing. (B) Scanning electron micrograph showing a macrophage engulfing a pair of red blood cells. The lines point to the edges of the pseudopods that the phagocytic cells are extending like collars to envelop their targets. (A, courtesy of Dorothy F. Bainton; B, courtesy of Jean Paul Revel.)

of microorganisms. Binding of antibody-coated bacteria to these receptors induces the phagocytic cell to extend sheetlike projections of the plasma membrane, called *pseudopods*, that engulf the bacterium (**Figure 15–32A**). These pseudopods fuse at their tips to form a phagosome, which then fuses with a lysosome, where the microbe is destroyed. Some pathogenic bacteria have evolved tricks for subverting the system: for example, *Mycobacterium tuberculosis*, the agent responsible for tuberculosis, can inhibit the membrane fusion that unites the phagosome with a lysosome. Instead of being destroyed, the engulfed organism survives and multiplies within the macrophage. Although the mechanism is not completely understood, identifying the proteins involved will provide therapeutic targets for drugs that could restore the macrophages' ability to eliminate the infection.

Phagocytic cells also play an important part in scavenging dead and damaged cells and cell debris. Macrophages, for example, ingest more than 10^{11} worn-out red blood cells in the human body each day (**Figure 15–32B**).

Fluid and Macromolecules Are Taken Up by Pinocytosis

Eukaryotic cells continually ingest bits of their plasma membrane, along with small amounts of extracellular fluid, in the process of **pinocytosis**. The rate at which plasma membrane is internalized in pinocytic vesicles varies from cell type to cell type, but it is usually surprisingly large. A macrophage, for example, swallows 25% of its own volume of fluid each hour. This means that it removes 3% of its plasma membrane each minute, or 100% in about half an hour. Pinocytosis occurs more slowly in fibroblasts, but even more rapidly in some phagocytic amoebae. Because a cell's total surface area and volume remain unchanged during this process, as much membrane is being added to the cell surface by exocytosis as is being removed by endocytosis (see Figure 15–19). It is not known how eukaryotic cells maintain this remarkable balance.

Pinocytosis is carried out mainly by the clathrin-coated pits and vesicles that we discussed earlier (see Figures 15–20 and 15–21). After they pinch off from the plasma membrane, clathrin-coated vesicles rapidly shed their coat and fuse with an endosome. Extracellular fluid is trapped in the coated pit as it invaginates to form a coated vesicle, and so substances dissolved in the extracellular fluid are internalized and delivered to endosomes. This fluid intake by clathrin-coated and other types of pinocytic vesicles is generally balanced by fluid loss during exocytosis.

Receptor-mediated Endocytosis Provides a Specific Route into Animal Cells

Pinocytosis, as just described, is indiscriminate. The endocytic vesicles simply trap any molecules that happen to be present in the extracellular fluid and carry them into the cell. However, pinocytosis can sometimes be more selective. In most animal cells, specific macromolecules can be taken up from the extracellular fluid via clathrin-coated vesicles. The macromolecules bind to complementary receptors on the cell surface and enter the cell as receptor–macromolecule complexes in clathrin-coated vesicles (see Figure 15–21). This process, called **receptor-mediated endocytosis**, provides a selective concentrating mechanism that increases the efficiency of internalization of particular macromolecules more than 1000-fold compared with ordinary pinocytosis, so that even minor components of the extracellular fluid can be taken up in large amounts without taking in a correspondingly large volume of extracellular fluid. Such is the case when animal cells import the cholesterol they need to make new membrane.

Cholesterol is a lipid that is extremely insoluble in water (see Figure 11–7). It is transported in the bloodstream bound to proteins in the form of particles called *low-density lipoproteins*, or *LDL*. Cholesterol-containing LDLs, which are secreted by the liver, bind to receptors located on the surface of cells. The resulting receptor–LDL complexes can then be ingested by receptor-mediated endocytosis and delivered to endosomes. The interior of endosomes is more acidic than the surrounding cytosol or the extracellular fluid, and in this acidic environment the LDL dissociates from its receptor: the empty receptors are returned, via transport vesicles, to the plasma membrane for reuse, while the LDL is delivered to lysosomes. In the lysosomes, the LDL is broken down by hydrolytic enzymes. Freed from the bulky LDLs, cholesterol escapes into the cytosol, where it can be used to synthesize new membrane (**Figure 15–33**).

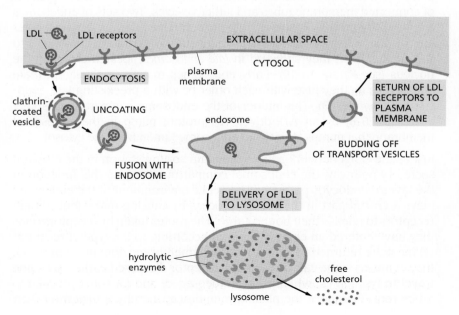

Figure 15–33 LDL enters cells via receptor-mediated endocytosis. LDL binds to LDL receptors on the cell surface and is internalized in clathrin-coated vesicles. The vesicles lose their coat and then fuse with endosomes. In the acidic environment of the endosome, LDL dissociates from its receptors. The LDL ends up in lysosomes, where it is degraded to release free cholesterol (*red* dots), while the LDL receptors are returned to the plasma membrane via transport vesicles to be used again (Movie 15.12). For simplicity, only one LDL receptor is shown entering the cell and returning to the plasma membrane. Whether it is occupied or not, an LDL receptor typically makes one round trip into the cell and back every 10 minutes, making a total of several hundred trips over its 20-hour life-span.

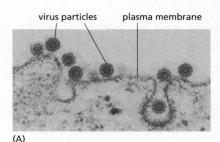

virus particles   plasma membrane

(A)

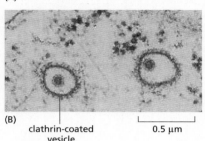

(B)

clathrin-coated vesicle

0.5 μm

Figure 15–34 **Viruses can enter cells via receptor-mediated endocytosis.** (A) Electron micrograph showing viruses bound to receptors on the surface of a T cell; one virus particle is being internalized in a clathrin-coated vesicle. (B) A pair of viruses have been taken up by receptor-mediated endocytosis. These vesicles will fuse with lysosomes, where the low pH will allow the release of the viral genome into the cytoplasm—a necessary step in viral replication. (A, from E. Fries and A. Helenius, *Eur. J. Biochem.* 97:213–220, 1979. With permission from John Wiley & Sons; B, from K. Simons, H. Garoff, A. Helenius, *Sci. Am.* 246:58–66, 1982. With permission from the authors.)

This pathway for cholesterol uptake is disrupted in individuals who inherit a defective version of the gene encoding the LDL receptor protein. In some cases, the receptors are missing; in others, they are present but nonfunctional. In either case, because the cells are deficient in taking up LDL, cholesterol accumulates in the blood and predisposes the individuals to develop atherosclerosis. Unless they take drugs (statins) to reduce their blood cholesterol, they will likely die at an early age of heart attacks, which result from cholesterol clogging the coronary arteries that supply the heart muscle.

Receptor-mediated endocytosis is also used to take up many other essential metabolites, such as vitamin B_{12} and iron, which cells cannot take up by the processes of transmembrane transport discussed in Chapter 12. Vitamin B_{12} and iron are both required, for example, to make hemoglobin, which is the major protein in red blood cells; these substances enter immature red blood cells as part of a complex with their respective receptor proteins. Many cell-surface receptors that bind extracellular signal molecules are also ingested by this pathway: some are recycled to the plasma membrane for reuse, whereas others are degraded in lysosomes. Unfortunately, receptor-mediated endocytosis can also be exploited by viruses (Figure 15–34). The influenza virus, which causes the flu, and HIV, which causes AIDS, gain entry into cells in this way.

Endocytosed Macromolecules Are Sorted in Endosomes

Because most extracellular material taken up by pinocytosis is rapidly delivered to **endosomes**, it is possible to visualize the endosomal compartment by incubating living cells in fluid containing a fluorescent marker that will show up when viewed in a fluorescence microscope. When examined in this way, the endosomal compartment reveals itself to be a complex set of connected membrane tubes and larger vesicles. Two sets of endosomes can be distinguished in such loading experiments: the marker molecules appear first in *early endosomes*, just beneath the plasma membrane; 5 to 15 minutes later, they show up in *late endosomes*, located closer to the nucleus (see Figure 15–19). Early endosomes mature gradually into late endosomes as they fuse with each other or with a preexisting late endosome (Movie 15.13). The interior of the endosome compartment is kept acidic (pH 5–6) by an ATP-driven H^+ (proton) pump in the endosomal membrane that pumps H^+ into the endosome lumen from the cytosol.

Just as the Golgi network acts as the main sorting station in the outward secretory pathway, the endosomal compartment serves this function in the inward endocytic pathway. The acidic environment of the endosome plays a crucial part in the sorting process by causing many (but not all) receptors to release their bound cargo. The routes taken by receptors once they have entered an endosome differ according to the type of receptor: (1) most are returned to the same plasma membrane domain from which they came, as is the case for the LDL receptor discussed earlier; (2) some travel to lysosomes, where they are degraded; and (3) some proceed to a different domain of the plasma membrane, thereby transferring their

QUESTION 15–8

Iron (Fe) is an essential trace metal that is needed by all cells. It is required, for example, for synthesis of the heme groups and iron–sulfur centers that are part of the active site of many proteins involved in electron-transfer reactions; it is also required in hemoglobin, the main protein in red blood cells. Iron is taken up by cells by receptor-mediated endocytosis. The iron-uptake system has two components: a soluble protein called transferrin, which circulates in the bloodstream; and a transferrin receptor—a transmembrane protein that, like the LDL receptor in Figure 15–33, is continually endocytosed and recycled to the plasma membrane. Fe ions bind to transferrin at neutral pH but not at acidic pH. Transferrin binds to the transferrin receptor at neutral pH only when it has an Fe ion bound, but it binds to the receptor at acidic pH even in the absence of bound iron. From these properties, describe how iron is taken up, and discuss the advantages of this elaborate scheme.

Figure 15–35 The fate of receptor proteins following their endocytosis depends on the type of receptor. Three pathways from the endosomal compartment in an epithelial cell are shown. Receptors that are not specifically retrieved from early endosomes follow the pathway from the endosomal compartment to lysosomes, where they are degraded. Retrieved receptors are returned either to the same plasma membrane domain from which they came (*recycling*) or to a different domain of the plasma membrane (*transcytosis*). Tight junctions separate the apical and basolateral plasma membranes, preventing their resident receptor proteins from diffusing from one domain to another (see Figure 11–32). If the ligand that is endocytosed with its receptor stays bound to the receptor in the acidic environment of the endosome, it will follow the same pathway as the receptor; otherwise it will be delivered to lysosomes for degradation.

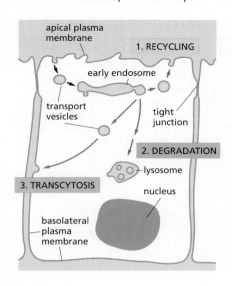

bound cargo molecules across the cell from one extracellular space to another, a process called *transcytosis* (**Figure 15–35**).

Cargo proteins that remain bound to their receptors share the fate of their receptors. Those that dissociate from their receptors in the endosome are doomed to destruction in lysosomes, along with most of the contents of the endosome lumen. Late endosomes contain some lysosomal enzymes, so digestion of cargo proteins and other macromolecules begins in the endosome and continues as the endosome gradually matures into a lysosome: once it has digested most of its ingested contents, the endosome takes on the dense, rounded appearance characteristic of a mature, "classical" lysosome.

Lysosomes Are the Principal Sites of Intracellular Digestion

Many extracellular particles and molecules ingested by cells end up in **lysosomes**, which are membranous sacs of hydrolytic enzymes that carry out the controlled intracellular digestion of both extracellular materials and worn-out organelles. They contain about 40 types of hydrolytic enzymes, including those that degrade proteins, nucleic acids, oligosaccharides, and lipids. All of these enzymes are optimally active in the acidic conditions (pH ~5) maintained within lysosomes. The membrane of the lysosome normally keeps these destructive enzymes out of the cytosol (whose pH is about 7.2), but the enzymes' acid dependence protects the contents of the cytosol against damage should some of them escape.

Like all other intracellular organelles, the lysosome not only contains a unique collection of enzymes but also has a unique surrounding membrane. The lysosomal membrane contains transporters that allow the final products of the digestion of macromolecules, such as amino acids, sugars, and nucleotides, to be transferred to the cytosol; from there, these materials can be either exported or utilized by the cell. The membrane also contains an ATP-driven H^+ pump, which, like the ATPase in the endosome membrane, pumps H^+ into the lysosome, thereby maintaining its contents at an acidic pH (**Figure 15–36**). Most of the lysosomal membrane proteins are unusually highly glycosylated; the sugars, which cover much of the protein surfaces facing the lysosome lumen, protect the proteins from digestion by the lysosomal proteases.

The specialized digestive enzymes and membrane proteins of the lysosome are synthesized in the ER and transported through the Golgi apparatus to the *trans* Golgi network. While in the ER and the *cis* Golgi network, the enzymes are tagged with a specific phosphorylated sugar group (mannose 6-phosphate), so that when they arrive in the *trans* Golgi network they can be recognized by an appropriate receptor, the mannose 6-phosphate receptor. This tagging permits the lysosomal enzymes to be

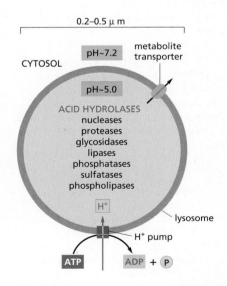

Figure 15–36 A lysosome contains a large variety of hydrolytic enzymes, which are only active under acidic conditions. The lumen of the lysosome is maintained at an acidic pH by an ATP-driven H^+ pump in the membrane that hydrolyzes ATP to pump H^+ into the lumen.

Figure 15–37 Materials destined for degradation in lysosomes follow different pathways to the lysosome. Each pathway leads to the intracellular digestion of materials derived from a different source. Early endosomes, phagosomes, and autophagosomes can fuse with either lysosomes or late endosomes, both of which contain acid-dependent hydrolytic enzymes. Where the membrane fragments that form the autophagosome originate is still actively investigated.

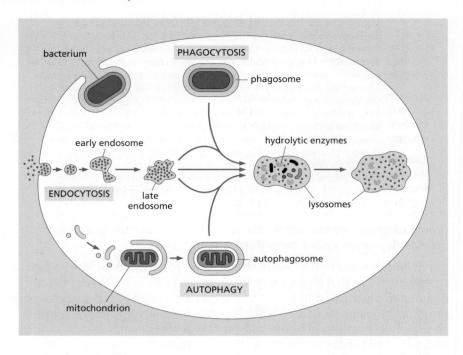

sorted and packaged into transport vesicles, which bud off and deliver their contents to lysosomes via endosomes (see Figure 15–19).

Depending on their source, materials follow different paths to lysosomes. We have seen that extracellular particles are taken up into phagosomes, which fuse with lysosomes, and that extracellular fluid and macromolecules are taken up into smaller endocytic vesicles, which deliver their contents to lysosomes via endosomes.

Cells have an additional pathway that supplies materials to lysosomes; this pathway, called **autophagy**, is used to degrade obsolete parts of the cell: as the term suggests, the cell literally eats itself. In electron micrographs of liver cells, for example, one often sees lysosomes digesting mitochondria, as well as other organelles. The process involves the enclosure of the organelle by a double membrane, creating an *autophagosome*, which then fuses with a lysosome (**Figure 15–37**). Autophagy of organelles and cytosolic proteins—some of which are marked for destruction by the attachment of ubiquitin tags (as discussed in Chapter 4)—increases when eukaryotic cells are starved or when they remodel themselves extensively during development. The amino acids generated by this cannibalistic form of digestion can then be recycled to allow continued protein synthesis.

ESSENTIAL CONCEPTS

- Eukaryotic cells contain many membrane-enclosed organelles, including a nucleus, an endoplasmic reticulum (ER), a Golgi apparatus, lysosomes, endosomes, mitochondria, chloroplasts (in plant cells), and peroxisomes. The ER, Golgi apparatus, peroxisomes, endosomes, and lysosomes are all part of the *endomembrane system*.

- Most organelle proteins are made in the cytosol and transported into the organelle where they function. Sorting signals in the amino acid sequence guide the proteins to the correct organelle; proteins that function in the cytosol have no such signals and remain where they are made.

- Nuclear proteins contain nuclear localization signals that help direct their active transport from the cytosol into the nucleus through nuclear pores, which penetrate the double membrane of the nuclear envelope. The proteins are transported in their fully folded conformation.

- Most mitochondrial and chloroplast proteins are made in the cytosol and are then transported into the organelles by protein translocators in their membranes. The proteins are unfolded during the transport process.

- The ER makes most of the cell's lipids and many of its proteins. The proteins are made by ribosomes that are directed to the ER by a signal-recognition particle (SRP) in the cytosol that recognizes an ER signal sequence on the growing polypeptide chain. The ribosome–SRP complex binds to a receptor on the ER membrane, which passes the ribosome to a protein translocator that threads the growing polypeptide across the ER membrane.

- Water-soluble proteins destined for secretion or for the lumen of an organelle of the endomembrane system pass completely into the ER lumen, while transmembrane proteins destined for either the membrane of these organelles or for the plasma membrane remain anchored in the lipid bilayer by one or more membrane-spanning α helices.

- In the ER lumen, proteins fold up, assemble with their protein partners, form disulfide bonds, and become decorated with oligosaccharide chains.

- Exit from the ER is an important quality-control step; proteins that either fail to fold properly or fail to assemble with their normal partners are retained in the ER by chaperone proteins, which prevent their aggregation and help them fold; proteins that still fail to fold or assemble are transported to the cytosol, where they are degraded.

- Excessive accumulation of misfolded proteins triggers an unfolded protein response that expands the ER, increases its capacity to fold new proteins properly, and reduces protein synthesis.

- Protein transport from the ER to the Golgi apparatus and from the Golgi apparatus to other destinations is mediated by transport vesicles that continually bud off from one membrane and fuse with another, a process called vesicular transport.

- Budding transport vesicles have distinctive coat proteins on their cytosolic surface; the assembly of the coat helps drive both the budding process and the incorporation of cargo receptors, with their bound cargo molecules, into the forming vesicle.

- Coated vesicles rapidly lose their protein coat, enabling them to dock and then fuse with a particular target membrane; docking and fusion are mediated by proteins on the surface of the vesicle and target membrane, including Rab, tethering, and SNARE proteins.

- The Golgi apparatus receives newly made proteins from the ER; it modifies their oligosaccharides, sorts the proteins, and dispatches them from the *trans* Golgi network to the plasma membrane, lysosomes (via endosomes), or secretory vesicles.

- In all eukaryotic cells, transport vesicles continually bud from the *trans* Golgi network and fuse with the plasma membrane; this process of constitutive exocytosis delivers proteins to the cell surface for secretion and incorporates lipids and proteins into the plasma membrane.

- Specialized secretory cells also have a regulated exocytosis pathway, in which molecules concentrated and stored in secretory vesicles are released from the cell by exocytosis when the cell is signaled to secrete.

- Cells ingest fluid, molecules, and sometimes even particles by endocytosis, in which regions of plasma membrane invaginate and pinch off to form endocytic vesicles.

- Much of the material that is endocytosed is delivered to endosomes, which mature into lysosomes, in which the material is degraded by hydrolytic enzymes; most of the components of the endocytic vesicle membrane, however, are recycled in transport vesicles back to the plasma membrane for reuse.

KEY TERMS

autophagy	phagocytic cell
clathrin	phagocytosis
coated vesicle	pinocytosis
endocytosis	Rab protein
endomembrane system	receptor-mediated endocytosis
endoplasmic reticulum (ER)	rough endoplasmic reticulum
endosome	secretion
exocytosis	secretory vesicle
Golgi apparatus	signal sequence
lysosome	SNARE
membrane-enclosed organelle	tethering protein
nuclear envelope	transport vesicle
nuclear pore	unfolded protein response (UPR)
peroxisome	vesicular transport

QUESTIONS

QUESTION 15–9

Which of the following statements are correct? Explain your answers.

A. Ribosomes are cytoplasmic structures that, during protein synthesis, become linked by an mRNA molecule to form polyribosomes.

B. The amino acid sequence Leu-His-Arg-Leu-Asp-Ala-Gln-Ser-Lys-Leu-Ser-Ser is a signal sequence that directs proteins to the ER.

C. All transport vesicles in the cell must have a v-SNARE protein in their membrane.

D. Transport vesicles deliver proteins and lipids to the cell surface.

E. If the delivery of prospective lysosomal proteins from the *trans* Golgi network to the late endosomes were blocked, lysosomal proteins would be secreted by the constitutive secretion pathways shown in Figure 15–30.

F. Lysosomes digest only substances that have been taken up by cells by endocytosis.

G. *N*-linked sugar chains are found on glycoproteins that face the cell surface, as well as on glycoproteins that face the lumen of the ER, *trans* Golgi network, and mitochondria.

H. Ribosomes bound to the outer nuclear membrane make proteins that are translocated co-translationally into the membrane.

QUESTION 15–10

Some proteins shuttle back and forth between the nucleus and the cytosol. They need a nuclear export signal to get out of the nucleus. How do you suppose they get into the nucleus?

QUESTION 15–11

Influenza viruses enter the cell by receptor-mediated endocytosis. The viruses are surrounded by a membrane that contains a fusion protein, which is activated by the acidic pH in the endosome. Upon activation, the protein causes the viral membrane to fuse with cell membranes. An old folk remedy against flu recommends that one should spend a night in a horse's stable. Odd as it may sound, there is a rational explanation for this advice. Air in stables contains ammonia (NH_3) generated by bacteria in the horse's urine. Sketch a diagram showing the pathway (in detail) by which flu virus enters cells, and speculate how NH_3 may protect cells from virus infection.
(Hint: NH_3 can neutralize acidic solutions by the reaction $NH_3 + H^+ \rightarrow NH_4^+$.)

QUESTION 15–12

Consider the v-SNAREs that direct transport vesicles from the *trans* Golgi network to the plasma membrane. They, like all other v-SNAREs, are membrane proteins that are integrated into the membrane of the ER during their biosynthesis and are then carried by transport vesicles to their destination. Thus, transport vesicles budding from the ER contain at least two kinds of v-SNAREs—those that target the vesicles to the *cis* Golgi cisternae, and those that are in transit to the *trans* Golgi network to be packaged in different transport vesicles destined for the plasma membrane. (A) Why might this be a problem? (B) Suggest possible ways in which the cell might solve it.

QUESTION 15–13

A particular type of *Drosophila* mutant becomes paralyzed when the temperature is raised. The mutation affects the structure of dynamin, causing it to be inactivated at the higher temperature. Indeed, the function of dynamin was discovered by analyzing the defect in these mutant fruit flies. The complete paralysis at the elevated temperature suggests that synaptic transmission between nerve and muscle cells (discussed in Chapter 12) is blocked. Suggest why signal transmission at a synapse might require dynamin.

QUESTION 15–14

Edit each of the following statements, if required, to make them true: "Because nuclear localization sequences are not cleaved off by proteases following protein import into the nucleus, they can be reused to import nuclear proteins after mitosis, when cytosolic and nuclear proteins have become intermixed. This is in contrast to ER signal sequences, which are cleaved off by a signal peptidase once they reach the lumen of the ER. ER signal sequences cannot therefore be reused to import ER proteins after mitosis, when cytosolic and ER proteins have become intermixed; these ER proteins must therefore be degraded and resynthesized."

QUESTION 15–15

Consider a protein that contains an ER signal sequence at its N-terminus and a nuclear localization sequence in its middle. What do you think the fate of this protein would be? Explain your answer.

QUESTION 15–16

Compare and contrast protein import into the ER and into the nucleus. List at least two major differences in the mechanisms, and speculate why the ER mechanism might not work for nuclear import and vice versa.

QUESTION 15–17

During mitosis, the nuclear envelope breaks down and intranuclear proteins completely intermix with cytosolic proteins. Is this consistent with the evolutionary scheme proposed in Figure 15–3? Explain your answer.

QUESTION 15–18

A protein that inhibits certain proteolytic enzymes (proteases) is normally secreted into the bloodstream by liver cells. This inhibitor protein, antitrypsin, is absent from the bloodstream of patients who carry a mutation that results in a single amino acid change in the protein. Antitrypsin deficiency causes a variety of severe problems, particularly in lung tissue, because of the uncontrolled activity of proteases. Surprisingly, when the mutant antitrypsin is synthesized in the laboratory, it is as active as the normal antitrypsin at inhibiting proteases.

Why, then, does the mutation cause the disease? Think of more than one possibility and suggest ways in which you could distinguish between them.

QUESTION 15–19

Dr. Outonalimb's claim to fame is her discovery of forgettin, a protein predominantly made by the pineal gland in human teenagers. The protein causes selective, short-term unresponsiveness and memory loss when the auditory system receives statements like "Please take out the garbage!" Her hypothesis is that forgettin has a hydrophobic ER signal sequence at its C-terminus that is recognized by an SRP and causes it to be translocated across the ER membrane by the mechanism shown in Figure 15–14. She predicts that the protein is secreted from pineal cells into the bloodstream, from where it exerts its devastating systemic effects. You are a member of the committee deciding whether she should receive a grant for further work on her hypothesis. Critique her proposal, and remember that grant reviews should be polite and constructive.

QUESTION 15–20

Taking the evolutionary scheme in Figure 15–3 one step further, suggest how the Golgi apparatus could have evolved. Sketch a simple diagram to illustrate your ideas. For the Golgi apparatus to be functional, what else would be needed?

QUESTION 15–21

If membrane proteins are integrated into the ER membrane by means of the ER protein translocator (which is itself composed of membrane proteins), how do the first protein translocation channels become incorporated into the ER membrane?

QUESTION 15–22

The sketch in Figure Q15–22 is a schematic drawing of the electron micrograph shown in the third panel of Figure 15–20A. Name the structures that are labeled in the sketch.

QUESTION 15–23

What would happen to proteins bound for the nucleus if there were insufficient energy to transport them?

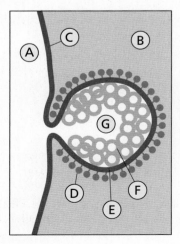

Figure Q15–22

CHAPTER **SIXTEEN**

16

Cell Signaling

Individual cells, like multicellular organisms, need to sense and respond to their environment. A free-living cell—even a humble bacterium—must be able to track down nutrients, tell the difference between light and dark, and avoid poisons and predators. And if such a cell is to have any kind of "social life," it must be able to communicate with other cells. When a yeast cell is ready to mate, for example, it secretes a small protein called a mating factor. Yeast cells of the opposite "sex" detect this chemical mating call and respond by halting their progress through the cell-division cycle and reaching out toward the cell that emitted the signal (Figure 16–1).

In a multicellular organism, things are much more complicated. Cells must interpret the multitude of signals they receive from other cells to help coordinate their behaviors. During animal development, for example, cells in the embryo exchange signals to determine which specialized role each cell will adopt, what position it will occupy in the animal, and whether it will survive, divide, or die. Later in life, a large variety of signals coordinates the animal's growth and its day-to-day physiology and behavior. In plants as well, cells are in constant communication with one another. These cell–cell interactions allow the plant to coordinate what happens in its roots, stems, and leaves.

In this chapter, we examine some of the most important mechanisms by which cells send signals and interpret the signals they receive. First, we present an overview of the general principles of cell signaling. We then consider two of the main systems animal cells use to receive and interpret signals. Finally, we describe a few signaling mechanisms that work in a different way—including one that operates in plants—before

GENERAL PRINCIPLES OF
CELL SIGNALING

G-PROTEIN-COUPLED
RECEPTORS

ENZYME-COUPLED RECEPTORS

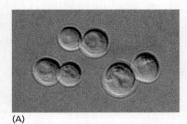

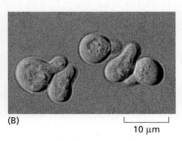

(A)

(B)

|— 10 µm —|

Figure 16–1 Yeast cells respond to mating factor. Budding yeast (*Saccharomyces cerevisiae*) cells are (A) normally spherical, but (B) when they are exposed to an appropriate mating factor produced by neighboring yeast cells, they extend a protrusion toward the source of the factor. (Courtesy of Michael Snyder.)

considering how these intricate signaling networks ultimately interact to control complex behaviors.

GENERAL PRINCIPLES OF CELL SIGNALING

Information can come in a variety of forms, and communication frequently involves converting the signals that carry that information from one form to another. When you receive a call from a friend on your mobile phone, for instance, the phone converts radio signals, which travel through the air, into sound waves, which you hear. This process of conversion is called **signal transduction** (Figure 16–2).

The signals that pass between cells are simpler than the sorts of messages that humans ordinarily exchange. In a typical communication between cells, the *signaling cell* produces a particular type of *extracellular signal molecule* that is detected by the *target cell*. As in human conversation, most animal cells both send and receive signals, and they can therefore act as both signaling cells and target cells.

Target cells possess proteins called *receptors* that recognize and respond specifically to the signal molecule. Signal transduction begins when the receptor on a target cell receives an incoming extracellular signal and then produces *intracellular signaling molecules* that alter cell behavior. Most of this chapter is concerned with signal reception and transduction—the events that cell biologists have in mind when they refer to **cell signaling**. First, however, we look briefly at a few of the different types of extracellular signals that cells send to one another—and what happens when target cells receive those signals.

Signals Can Act over a Long or Short Range

Cells in multicellular organisms use hundreds of kinds of **extracellular signal molecules** to communicate with one another. The signal molecules can be proteins, peptides, amino acids, nucleotides, steroids, fatty acid derivatives, or even dissolved gases—but they all rely on just a handful of basic styles of communication for getting the message across.

In multicellular organisms, the most "public" style of cell–cell communication involves broadcasting the signal throughout the whole body by secreting it into an animal's bloodstream or a plant's sap. Extracellular signal molecules used in this way are called **hormones**, and, in animals, the cells that produce hormones are called *endocrine* cells (Figure 16–3A). Part of the pancreas, for example, is an endocrine gland that produces several hormones—including insulin, which regulates glucose uptake in cells all over the body.

Somewhat less public is the process known as *paracrine signaling*. In this case, rather than entering the bloodstream, the signal molecules diffuse locally through the extracellular fluid, remaining in the neighborhood of

Figure 16–2 Signal transduction is the process whereby one type of signal is converted into another. (A) When a mobile telephone receives a radio signal, it converts it into a sound signal; when transmitting a signal, it does the reverse. (B) A target cell converts an extracellular signal into an intracellular signal.

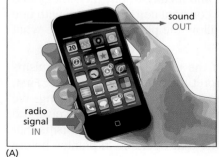

(A)

sound
OUT

radio
signal
IN

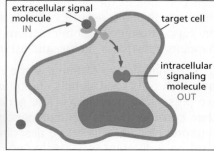

(B)

extracellular signal
molecule
IN

target cell

intracellular
signaling
molecule
OUT

the cell that secretes them. Thus, they act as **local mediators** on nearby cells (**Figure 16–3B**). Many of the signal molecules that regulate inflammation at the site of an infection or that control cell proliferation in a healing wound function in this way. In some cases, cells can respond to the local mediators that they themselves produce, a form of paracrine communication called *autocrine signaling*; cancer cells sometimes promote their own survival and proliferation in this way.

Neuronal signaling is a third form of cell communication. Like endocrine cells, nerve cells (neurons) can deliver messages over long distances. In the case of neuronal signaling, however, a message is not broadcast widely but is instead delivered quickly and specifically to individual target cells through private lines. As described in Chapter 12, the axon of a neuron terminates at specialized junctions (*synapses*) on target cells that can lie far from the neuronal cell body (**Figure 16–3C**). The axons that extend from the spinal cord to the big toe in an adult human, for example, can be more than a meter in length. When activated by signals from the environment or from other nerve cells, a neuron sends electrical impulses racing along its axon at speeds of up to 100 m/sec. On reaching the axon terminal, these electrical signals are converted into a chemical form: each electrical impulse stimulates the nerve terminal to release a pulse of an extracellular signal molecule called a **neurotransmitter**. The neurotransmitter then diffuses across the narrow (<100 nm) gap that separates the membrane of the axon terminal from that of the target cell, reaching its destination in less than 1 msec.

A fourth style of signal-mediated cell–cell communication—the most intimate and short-range of all—does not require the release of a secreted molecule. Instead, the cells make direct physical contact through signal molecules lodged in the plasma membrane of the signaling cell and receptor proteins embedded in the plasma membrane of the target cell (**Figure 16–3D**). During embryonic development, for example, such

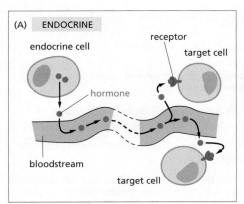

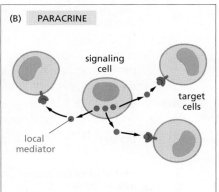

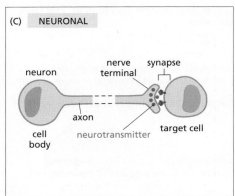

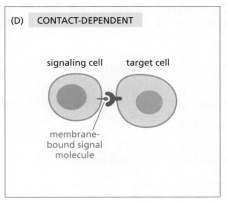

Figure 16–3 Animal cells use extracellular signal molecules to communicate with one another in various ways. (A) Hormones produced in endocrine glands are secreted into the bloodstream and are distributed widely throughout the body. (B) Paracrine signals are released by cells into the extracellular fluid in their neighborhood and act locally. (C) Neuronal signals are transmitted electrically along a nerve cell axon. When this electrical signal reaches the nerve terminal, it causes the release of neurotransmitters onto adjacent target cells. (D) In contact-dependent signaling, a cell-surface-bound signal molecule binds to a receptor protein on an adjacent cell. Many of the same types of signal molecules are used for endocrine, paracrine, and neuronal signaling. The crucial differences lie in the speed and selectivity with which the signals are delivered to their targets.

contact-dependent signaling allows adjacent cells that are initially similar to become specialized to form different cell types, as we discuss later in the chapter.

To get a better feel for these different signaling styles, imagine trying to publicize a potentially stimulating lecture—or a concert or sporting event. An endocrine signal would be akin to broadcasting the information over the radio. A more localized paracrine signal would be the equivalent of posting a flyer on selected notice boards near the arena—with an autocrine signal being a reminder you add to your own personal calendar.

Neuronal signals—long-distance but personal—would be similar to a phone call, text message, or e-mail, and contact-dependent signaling would be like a good old-fashioned, face-to-face conversation.

Table 16–1 lists some examples of hormones, local mediators, neurotransmitters, and contact-dependent signal molecules. The actions of several of these are discussed in greater detail throughout the chapter.

TABLE 16–1 SOME EXAMPLES OF SIGNAL MOLECULES

Signal Molecule	Site of Origin	Chemical Nature	Some Actions
Hormones			
Epinephrine (adrenaline)	adrenal gland	derivative of the amino acid tyrosine	increases blood pressure, heart rate, and metabolism
Cortisol	adrenal gland	steroid (derivative of cholesterol)	affects metabolism of proteins, carbohydrates, and lipids in most tissues
Estradiol	ovary	steroid (derivative of cholesterol)	induces and maintains secondary female sexual characteristics
Insulin	β cells of pancreas	protein	stimulates glucose uptake, protein synthesis, and lipid synthesis in various cell types
Testosterone	testis	steroid (derivative of cholesterol)	induces and maintains secondary male sexual characteristics
Thyroid hormone (thyroxine)	thyroid gland	derivative of the amino acid tyrosine	stimulates metabolism in many cell types
Local Mediators			
Epidermal growth factor (EGF)	various cells	protein	stimulates epidermal and many other cell types to proliferate
Platelet-derived growth factor (PDGF)	various cells, including blood platelets	protein	stimulates many cell types to proliferate
Nerve growth factor (NGF)	various innervated tissues	protein	promotes survival and axonal growth of certain classes of neurons
Histamine	mast cells	derivative of the amino acid histidine	causes blood vessels to dilate and become leaky, helping to cause inflammation
Nitric oxide (NO)	nerve cells; endothelial cells lining blood vessels	dissolved gas	causes smooth muscle cells to relax; regulates nerve-cell activity
Neurotransmitters			
Acetylcholine	nerve terminals	derivative of choline	excitatory neurotransmitter at many nerve–muscle synapses and in central nervous system
γ-Aminobutyric acid (GABA)	nerve terminals	derivative of the amino acid glutamic acid	inhibitory neurotransmitter in central nervous system
Contact-dependent Signal Molecules			
Delta	prospective neurons; various other developing cell types	transmembrane protein	inhibits neighboring cells from becoming specialized in same way as the signaling cell

A Limited Set of Extracellular Signals Can Produce a Huge Variety of Cell Behaviors

A typical cell in a multicellular organism is exposed to hundreds of different signal molecules in its environment. These may be free in the extracellular fluid, embedded in the extracellular matrix in which many cells reside, or bound to the surface of neighboring cells. Each cell must respond very selectively to this mixture of signals, disregarding some and reacting to others, according to the cell's specialized function.

Whether a cell responds to a signal molecule depends, first of all, on whether it possesses a **receptor** for that signal. Each receptor is usually activated by only one type of signal. Without the appropriate receptor, a cell will be deaf to the signal and will not respond to it.

Extracellular signal molecules can be divided into two major classes, depending on the type of receptor with which they interact. The first and largest class of signals consists of molecules that are too large or too hydrophilic to cross the plasma membrane of the target cell. These signal molecules rely on receptors on the surface of the target cell to relay their message across the plasma membrane (**Figure 16–4A**). The second class of signals consists of molecules that are small enough or hydrophobic enough to pass through the plasma membrane and into the cytosol of the target cell, where they bind to intracellular receptor proteins (**Figure 16–4B**). Here, we focus primarily on signaling through cell-surface receptors, but we will briefly describe signaling through intracellular receptors later in the chapter.

By producing only a limited set of receptors out of the thousands that are possible, a cell restricts the types of signals that can affect it. Of course, even this restricted set of extracellular signal molecules can change the behavior of a target cell in a large variety of ways, altering its shape, movement, metabolism, gene expression, or some combination of these. How a cell reacts to a signal depends on the set of intracellular signaling molecules each cell-surface receptor produces and how these molecules alter the activity of *effector proteins*, which have a direct effect on the behavior of the target cell. This intracellular relay system and the intracellular effector proteins on which it acts vary from one type of specialized cell to another, so that different types of cells respond to the same signal in different ways. For example, when a heart pacemaker cell is exposed to the neurotransmitter *acetylcholine*, its rate of firing decreases. When a salivary gland cell is exposed to the same signal, it secretes components of saliva, even though the receptors on both cell types are the same. In skeletal muscle, acetylcholine binds to a different receptor protein, causing the muscle cell to contract (**Figure 16–5**). Thus, the extracellular signal molecule alone is not the message: the information conveyed by the signal depends on how the target cell receives and interprets the signal.

A typical cell possesses many sorts of receptors—each present in tens to hundreds of thousands of copies. Such variety makes the cell simultaneously sensitive to many different extracellular signals and allows

QUESTION 16–1

To keep their action local, paracrine signal molecules must be prevented from straying too far from their points of origin. Suggest different ways by which this could be accomplished. Explain your answers.

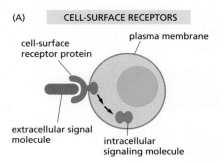

(A)   **CELL-SURFACE RECEPTORS**

plasma membrane

cell-surface receptor protein

extracellular signal molecule

intracellular signaling molecule

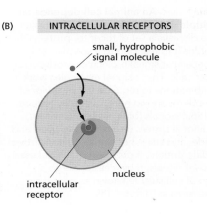

(B)   **INTRACELLULAR RECEPTORS**

small, hydrophobic signal molecule

nucleus

intracellular receptor

Figure 16–4 Extracellular signal molecules bind either to cell-surface receptors or to intracellular receptors. (A) Most extracellular signal molecules are large and hydrophilic and are therefore unable to cross the plasma membrane directly; instead, they bind to cell-surface receptors, which in turn generate one or more intracellular signaling molecules in the target cell. (B) Some small, hydrophobic, extracellular signal molecules pass through the target cell's plasma membrane and bind to intracellular receptors—in the cytosol or in the nucleus (as shown here)—that then regulate gene transcription or other functions.

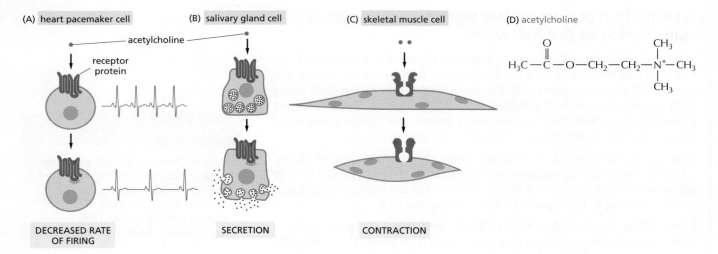

Figure 16–5 The same signal molecule can induce different responses in different target cells. Different cell types are configured to respond to the neurotransmitter acetylcholine in different ways. Acetylcholine binds to similar receptor proteins on (A) heart pacemaker cells and (B) salivary gland cells, but it evokes different responses in each cell type. (C) Skeletal muscle cells produce a different type of receptor protein for the same signal molecule. (D) For such a versatile molecule, acetylcholine has a fairly simple chemical structure.

a relatively small number of signal molecules, used in different combinations, to exert subtle and complex control over cell behavior. A combination of signals can evoke a response that is different from the sum of the effects that each signal would trigger on its own. As we discuss later, this "tailoring" of a cell's response occurs, in part, because the intracellular relay systems activated by the different signals interact. Thus the presence of one signal will often modify the effects of another. One combination of signals might enable a cell to survive; another might drive it to differentiate in some specialized way; and another might cause it to divide. In the absence of the proper signals, most animal cells are programmed to kill themselves (**Figure 16–6**).

A Cell's Response to a Signal Can Be Fast or Slow

The length of time a cell takes to respond to an extracellular signal can vary greatly, depending on what needs to happen once the message has

Figure 16–6 An animal cell depends on multiple extracellular signals. Every cell type displays a set of receptor proteins that enables it to respond to a specific set of extracellular signal molecules produced by other cells. These signal molecules work in combinations to regulate the behavior of the cell. As shown here, cells may require multiple signals (*blue* arrows) to survive, additional signals (*red* arrows) to grow and divide, and still other signals (*green* arrows) to differentiate. If deprived of the necessary survival signals, most cells undergo a form of cell suicide known as apoptosis (discussed in Chapter 18).

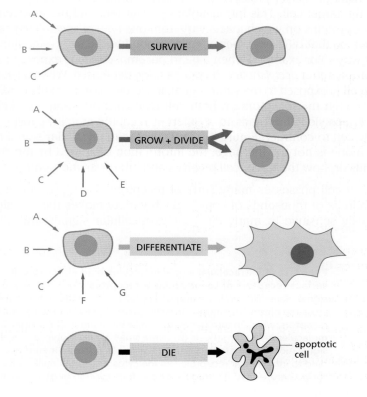

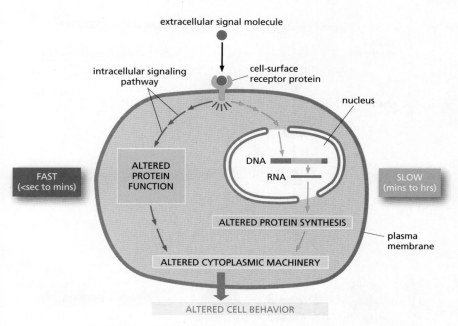

Figure 16–7 Extracellular signals can act slowly or rapidly. Certain types of cell responses—such as cell differentiation or increased cell growth and division (see Figure 16–6)—involve changes in gene expression and the synthesis of new proteins; they therefore occur relatively slowly. Other responses—such as changes in cell movement, secretion, or metabolism—need not involve changes in gene expression and therefore occur more quickly (see Figure 16–5).

been received. Some extracellular signals act swiftly: acetylcholine can stimulate a skeletal muscle cell to contract within milliseconds and a salivary gland cell to secrete within a minute or so. Such rapid responses are possible because, in each case, the signal affects the activity of proteins that are already present inside the target cell, awaiting their marching orders.

Other responses take more time. Cell growth and cell division, when triggered by the appropriate signal molecules, can take many hours to execute. This is because the response to these extracellular signals requires changes in gene expression and the production of new proteins (**Figure 16–7**). We will encounter additional examples of both fast and slow responses—and the signal molecules that stimulate them—later in the chapter.

Cell-Surface Receptors Relay Extracellular Signals via Intracellular Signaling Pathways

The majority of extracellular signal molecules are proteins, peptides, or small, hydrophilic molecules that bind to cell-surface receptors that span the plasma membrane (see Figure 16–4A). Transmembrane receptors detect a signal on the outside and relay the message, in a new form, across the membrane into the interior of the cell.

The receptor protein performs the primary step in signal transduction: it recognizes the extracellular signal and generates new intracellular signals in response (see Figure 16–2B). The resulting intracellular signaling process usually works like a molecular relay race, in which the message is passed "downstream" from one intracellular signaling molecule to another, each activating or generating the next signaling molecule in the pathway, until a metabolic enzyme is kicked into action, the cytoskeleton is tweaked into a new configuration, or a gene is switched on or off. This final outcome is called the response of the cell (**Figure 16–8**).

Figure 16–8 Many extracellular signals activate intracellular signaling pathways to change the behavior of the target cell. A cell-surface receptor protein activates one or more intracellular signaling pathways, each mediated by a series of intracellular signaling molecules, which can be proteins or small messenger molecules; only one pathway is shown. Signaling molecules eventually interact with specific *effector* proteins, altering them to change the behavior of the cell in various ways.

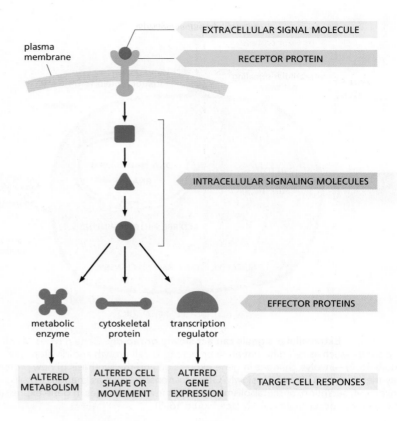

QUESTION 16–2

In principle, how might an intracellular signaling protein amplify a signal as it relays it onward?

The components of these **intracellular signaling pathways** perform one or more crucial functions (**Figure 16–9**):

1. They can *relay* the signal onward and thereby help spread it through the cell.
2. They can *amplify* the signal received, making it stronger, so that a few extracellular signal molecules are enough to evoke a large intracellular response.
3. They can detect signals from more than one intracellular signaling pathway and *integrate* them before relaying a signal onward.
4. They can *distribute* the signal to more than one effector protein, creating branches in the information flow diagram and evoking a complex response.
5. They can modulate the response to the signal by regulating the activity of components upstream in the signaling pathway, a process known as *feedback*.

Feedback regulation, although it is last on our list, is actually a very important feature of cell signaling. It can occur anywhere in the signaling pathway and can either boost or weaken the response to the signal. In positive feedback, a component that lies downstream in the pathway acts on an earlier component in the same pathway to enhance the response to the initial signal; in negative feedback, a downstream component acts to inhibit an earlier component in the pathway to diminish the response to the initial signal (**Figure 16–10**). Such feedback regulation is very common in biological systems and can lead to sophisticated responses: positive feedback can generate all-or-none, switchlike responses, for example, whereas negative feedback can generate responses that oscillate on and off as the activities or concentrations of the inhibitory components rise and fall.

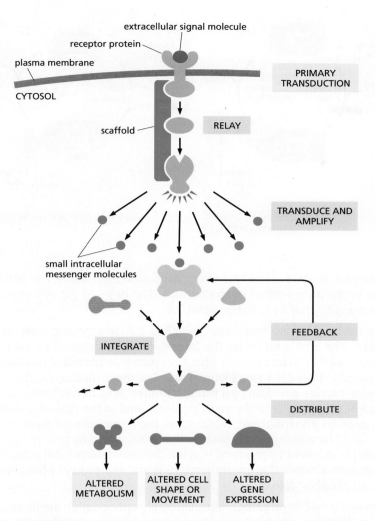

Figure 16–9 Intracellular signaling proteins can relay, amplify, integrate, distribute, and modulate via feedback an incoming signal. In this example, a receptor protein located on the cell surface transduces an extracellular signal into an intracellular signal, which initiates one or more intracellular signaling pathways that relay the signal into the cell interior. Each pathway includes intracellular signaling proteins that can function in one of the various ways shown; some, for example, integrate signals from other intracellular signaling pathways. Many of the steps in the process can be modulated via feedback by other molecules or events in the cell. Note that some proteins in the pathway may be held in close proximity by a scaffold protein, which allows them to be activated at a specific location in the cell and with greater speed, efficiency, and selectivity (discussed in Chapter 4; see Figure 4–52). We review the production and function of small intracellular messenger molecules, more commonly called second messenger molecules, later in the chapter.

Some Intracellular Signaling Proteins Act as Molecular Switches

Many intracellular signaling proteins behave as **molecular switches**: receipt of a signal causes them to toggle from an inactive to an active state. Once activated, these proteins can stimulate—or in some cases suppress—other proteins in the signaling pathway. They then persist in an active state until some other process switches them off again.

The importance of the switching-off process is often underappreciated: imagine the consequences if a signaling pathway that boosts your heart rate were to remain active indefinitely. If a signaling pathway is to recover after transmitting a signal and make itself ready to transmit another, every activated protein in the pathway must be reset to its original,

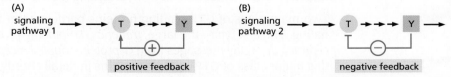

Figure 16–10 Feedback regulation within an intracellular signaling pathway can adjust the response to an extracellular signal. (A) In this simple example, a downstream protein in a signaling pathway, protein Y, acts to increase the activity of the protein that activated it—a form of positive feedback. Positive feedback loops can ignite an explosive response, such as the activation of the proteins that trigger cell division (discussed in Chapter 18). (B) In a simple example of negative feedback, protein Y inhibits the protein that activated it. Negative feedback loops can generate oscillations, similar to the way that populations of predators and prey can seesaw: an increase in prey (here, protein T) would promote the expansion of predators (protein Y); as the number of predators increases, the availability of prey will fall (via negative feedback), which will ultimately cause the predator population to decline. As the predators disappear, the prey populations will recover and multiply, providing food for more predators, and so on.

Figure 16–11 Many intracellular signaling proteins act as molecular switches. These proteins can be activated—or in some cases inhibited—by the addition or removal of a phosphate group. (A) In one class of switch protein, the phosphate is added covalently by a protein kinase, which transfers the terminal phosphate group from ATP to the signaling protein; the phosphate is then removed by a protein phosphatase. (B) In the other class of switch protein, a GTP-binding protein is activated when it exchanges its bound GDP for GTP (which, in a sense, adds a phosphate to the protein); the protein then switches itself off by hydrolyzing its bound GTP to GDP.

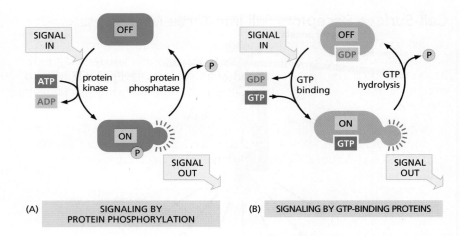

(A) **SIGNALING BY PROTEIN PHOSPHORYLATION**

(B) **SIGNALING BY GTP-BINDING PROTEINS**

unstimulated state. Thus, for every activation step along the pathway, there exists an inactivation mechanism. The two are equally important for a signaling pathway to be useful.

Proteins that act as molecular switches fall mostly into one of two classes. The first—and by far the largest—class consists of proteins that are activated or inactivated by phosphorylation, a chemical modification discussed in Chapter 4 (see Figure 4–46). For these molecules, the switch is thrown in one direction by a **protein kinase**, which covalently attaches a phosphate group onto the switch protein, and in the opposite direction by a **protein phosphatase**, which takes the phosphate off again (**Figure 16–11A**). The activity of any protein that is regulated by phosphorylation depends—moment by moment—on the balance between the activities of the protein kinases that phosphorylate it and the protein phosphatases that dephosphorylate it.

Many of the switch proteins controlled by phosphorylation are themselves protein kinases, and these are often organized into *phosphorylation cascades*: one protein kinase, activated by phosphorylation, phosphorylates the next protein kinase in the sequence, and so on, transmitting the signal onward and, in the process, amplifying, distributing, and regulating it. Two main types of protein kinases operate in intracellular signaling pathways: the most common are **serine/threonine kinases**, which—as the name implies—phosphorylate proteins on serines or threonines; others are **tyrosine kinases**, which phosphorylate proteins on tyrosines.

The other class of switch proteins involved in intracellular signaling pathways are **GTP-binding proteins**. These toggle between an active and an inactive state depending on whether they have GTP or GDP bound to them, respectively (**Figure 16–11B**). Once activated by GTP binding, many of these proteins have intrinsic GTP-hydrolyzing (*GTPase*) activity, and they shut themselves off by hydrolyzing their bound GTP to GDP.

Two main types of GTP-binding proteins participate in intracellular signaling. The first type—the large, *trimeric GTP-binding proteins* (also called *G proteins*)—relay messages from *G-protein-coupled receptors*. We discuss this major class of GTP-binding proteins in detail shortly.

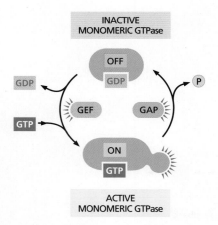

Figure 16–12 The activity of monomeric GTPases is controlled by two types of regulatory proteins. Guanine nucleotide exchange factors (GEFs) promote the exchange of GDP for GTP, thereby switching the protein on. GTPase-activating proteins (GAPs) stimulate the hydrolysis of GTP to GDP, thereby switching the protein off.

Other cell-surface receptors rely on a second type of GTP-binding protein—the small, *monomeric GTPases*—to help relay their signals. These switch proteins are generally aided by two sets of regulatory proteins that help them bind and hydrolyze GTP: *guanine nucleotide exchange factors* (*GEFs*) activate the switches by promoting the exchange of GDP for GTP, and *GTPase-activating proteins* (*GAPs*) turn them off by promoting GTP hydrolysis (**Figure 16–12**).

Cell-Surface Receptors Fall into Three Main Classes

All cell-surface receptor proteins bind to an extracellular signal molecule and transduce its message into one or more intracellular signaling molecules that alter the cell's behavior. Most of these receptors belong to one of three large classes, which differ in the transduction mechanism they use.

1. *Ion-channel-coupled receptors* change the permeability of the plasma membrane to selected ions, thereby altering the membrane potential and, if the conditions are right, producing an electrical current (**Figure 16–13A**).
2. *G-protein-coupled receptors* activate membrane-bound, trimeric GTP-binding proteins (G proteins), which then activate (or inhibit) an enzyme or an ion channel in the plasma membrane, initiating an intracellular signaling cascade (**Figure 16–13B**).
3. *Enzyme-coupled receptors* either act as enzymes or associate with enzymes inside the cell (**Figure 16–13C**); when stimulated, the enzymes can activate a wide variety of intracellular signaling pathways.

The number of different types of receptors in each of these three classes is even greater than the number of extracellular signals that act on them. This is because for many extracellular signal molecules there is more than one type of receptor, and these may belong to different receptor classes. The neurotransmitter acetylcholine, for example, acts on skeletal muscle cells via an ion-channel-coupled receptor, whereas in heart cells it acts through a G-protein-coupled receptor. These two types of receptors generate different intracellular signals and thus enable the two types

Figure 16–13 Cell-surface receptors fall into one of three main classes. (A) An ion-channel-coupled receptor opens in response to binding an extracellular signal molecule. These channels are also called transmitter-gated ion channels. (B) When a G-protein-coupled receptor binds its extracellular signal molecule, the activated receptor signals to a trimeric G protein on the cytosolic side of the plasma membrane, which then turns on (or off) an enzyme (or an ion channel; not shown) in the same membrane. (C) When an enzyme-coupled receptor binds its extracellular signal molecule, an enzyme activity is switched on at the other end of the receptor, inside the cell. Many enzyme-coupled receptors have their own enzyme activity (*left*), while others rely on an enzyme that becomes associated with the activated receptor (*right*).

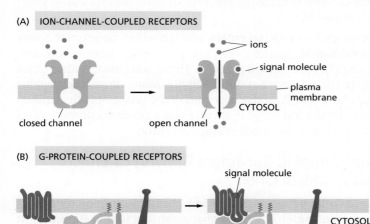

(A) ION-CHANNEL-COUPLED RECEPTORS

ions

signal molecule

plasma membrane

CYTOSOL

closed channel

open channel

(B) G-PROTEIN-COUPLED RECEPTORS

signal molecule

CYTOSOL

inactive receptor

inactive G protein

inactive enzyme

activated receptor binds to G protein

activated enzyme

activated G protein

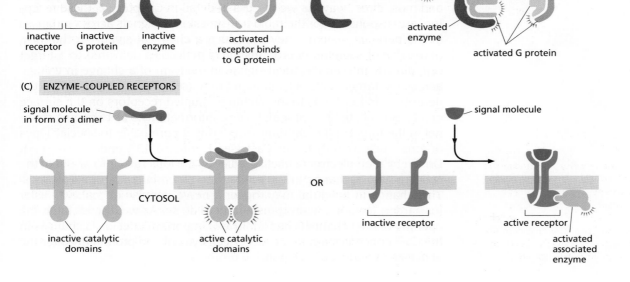

(C) ENZYME-COUPLED RECEPTORS

signal molecule in form of a dimer

CYTOSOL

inactive catalytic domains

active catalytic domains

OR

signal molecule

inactive receptor

active receptor

activated associated enzyme

TABLE 16–2 SOME FOREIGN SUBSTANCES THAT ACT ON CELL–SURFACE RECEPTORS

Substance	Normal Signal	Receptor Action	Effect
Barbiturates and benzodiazepines (Valium and Ambien)	γ-aminobutyric acid (GABA)	stimulate GABA-activated ion-channel-coupled receptors	relief of anxiety; sedation
Nicotine	acetylcholine	stimulates acetylcholine-activated ion-channel-coupled receptors	constriction of blood vessels; elevation of blood pressure
Morphine and heroin	endorphins and enkephalins	stimulate G-protein-coupled opiate receptors	analgesia (relief of pain); euphoria
Curare	acetylcholine	blocks acetylcholine-activated ion-channel-coupled receptors	blockage of neuromuscular transmission, resulting in paralysis
Strychnine	glycine	blocks glycine-activated ion-channel-coupled receptors	blockage of inhibitory synapses in spinal cord and brain, resulting in seizures and muscle spasm
Capsaicin	heat	stimulates temperature-sensitive ion-channel-coupled receptors	induces painful, burning sensation; prolonged exposure paradoxically leads to pain relief
Menthol	cold	stimulates temperature-sensitive ion-channel-coupled receptors	in moderate amounts, induces a cool sensation; in higher doses, can cause burning pain

of cells to react to acetylcholine in different ways, increasing contraction in skeletal muscle and decreasing the rate of contractions in the heart (see Figure 16–5A and C).

This plethora of cell-surface receptors also provides targets for many foreign substances that interfere with our physiology, from heroin and nicotine to tranquilizers and chili peppers. These substances either block or overstimulate the receptor's natural activity. Many drugs and poisons act in this way (Table 16–2), and a large part of the pharmaceutical industry is devoted to producing drugs that will exert a precisely defined effect by binding to a specific type of cell-surface receptor.

Ion-Channel-Coupled Receptors Convert Chemical Signals into Electrical Ones

Of all the types of cell-surface receptors, **ion-channel-coupled receptors** (also known as transmitter-gated ion channels) function in the simplest and most direct way. As we discuss in detail in Chapter 12, these receptors are responsible for the rapid transmission of signals across synapses in the nervous system. They transduce a chemical signal, in the form of a pulse of secreted neurotransmitter molecules delivered to a target cell, directly into an electrical signal, in the form of a change in voltage across the target cell's plasma membrane (see Figure 12–41). When the neurotransmitter binds to ion-channel-coupled receptors on the surface of a target cell, the receptor alters its conformation so as to open a channel in the target cell membrane, rendering it permeable to specific types of ions, such as Na^+, K^+, or Ca^{2+} (see Figure 16–13A and Movie 16.1). Driven by their electrochemical gradients, the ions rush into or out of the cell, creating a change in the membrane potential within milliseconds. This change in potential may trigger a nerve impulse or make it easier (or harder) for other neurotransmitters to do so. As we discuss later, the opening of Ca^{2+} channels has additional important effects, as changes in the Ca^{2+} concentration in the target-cell cytosol can profoundly alter the activities of many Ca^{2+}-responsive proteins.

Whereas ion-channel-coupled receptors are especially important in nerve cells and other electrically excitable cells such as muscle cells, G-protein-coupled receptors and enzyme-coupled receptors are important for practically every cell type in the body. Most of the remainder of this chapter deals with these two receptor families and with the signal transduction processes that they use.

G-PROTEIN-COUPLED RECEPTORS

G-protein-coupled receptors (**GPCRs**) form the largest family of cell-surface receptors. There are more than 700 GPCRs in humans, and mice have about 1000 involved in the sense of smell alone. These receptors mediate responses to an enormous diversity of extracellular signal molecules, including hormones, local mediators, and neurotransmitters. The signal molecules that bind GPCRs are as varied in structure as they are in function: they can be proteins, small peptides, or derivatives of amino acids or fatty acids, and for each one of them there is a different receptor or set of receptors. Because GPCRs are involved in such a large variety of cell processes, they are an attractive target for the development of drugs to treat many disorders. About one-third of all drugs used today work through GPCRs.

Despite the diversity of the signal molecules that bind to them, all GPCRs have a similar structure: each is made of a single polypeptide chain that threads back and forth across the lipid bilayer seven times (**Figure 16–14**). The GPCR superfamily includes rhodopsin (the light-activated photoreceptor protein in the vertebrate eye), the olfactory (smell) receptors in the vertebrate nose, and the receptors that participate in the mating rituals of single-celled yeasts (see Figure 16–1). Evolutionarily speaking, GPCRs are ancient: even prokaryotes possess structurally similar membrane proteins—such as the bacteriorhodopsin that functions as a light-driven H⁺ pump (see Figure 11–28). Although they resemble eukaryotic GPCRs, these prokaryotic proteins do not act through G proteins, but are coupled to other signal transduction systems.

We begin this section with a discussion of how G proteins are activated by GPCRs. We then consider how activated G proteins stimulate ion channels and how they regulate membrane-bound enzymes that control the concentrations of small intracellular messenger molecules, including cyclic AMP and Ca²⁺, which in turn control the activity of important intracellular signaling proteins. We end with a discussion of how light-activated GPCRs in photoreceptors in our eyes enable us to see.

Stimulation of GPCRs Activates G-Protein Subunits

When an extracellular signal molecule binds to a GPCR, the receptor protein undergoes a conformational change that enables it to activate a **G protein** located on the other side of the plasma membrane. To explain how this activation leads to the transmission of a signal, we must first consider how G proteins are constructed and how they operate.

There are several varieties of G proteins. Each is specific for a particular set of receptors and for a particular set of target enzymes or ion channels in the plasma membrane. All of these G proteins, however, have a similar general structure and operate in a similar way. They are composed of three protein subunits—α, β, and γ—two of which are tethered to the plasma membrane by short lipid tails. In the unstimulated state, the α subunit has GDP bound to it, and the G protein is idle (**Figure 16–15A**). When an extracellular signal molecule binds to its receptor, the altered receptor activates a G protein by causing the α subunit to decrease its

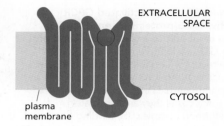

(A)

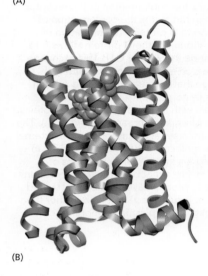

(B)

Figure 16–14 All GPCRs possess a similar structure. The polypeptide chain traverses the membrane as seven α helices. The cytoplasmic portions of the receptor bind to a G protein inside the cell. (A) For receptors that recognize small signal molecules, such as acetylcholine or epinephrine, the ligand (*red*) usually binds deep within the plane of the membrane to a pocket that is formed by amino acids from several transmembrane segments. Receptors that recognize signal molecules that are proteins usually have a large, extracellular domain that, together with some of the transmembrane segments, binds the protein ligand (not shown). (B) Shown here is the structure of a GPCR that binds to epinephrine (*red*). Stimulation of this receptor by epinephrine makes the heart beat faster.

Figure 16–15 An activated GPCR activates G proteins by encouraging the α subunit to expel its GDP and pick up GTP. (A) In the unstimulated state, the receptor and the G protein are both inactive. Although they are shown here as separate entities in the plasma membrane, in some cases they are associated in a preformed complex. (B) Binding of an extracellular signal molecule to the receptor changes the conformation of the receptor, which in turn alters the conformation of the bound G protein. The alteration of the α subunit of the G protein allows it to exchange its GDP for GTP. This exchange triggers an additional conformational change that activates both the α subunit and a βγ complex, which dissociate to interact with their preferred target proteins in the plasma membrane (**Movie 16.2**). The receptor stays active as long as the external signal molecule is bound to it, and it can therefore activate many molecules of G protein. Note that both the α and γ subunits of the G protein have covalently attached lipid molecules (*red*) that help anchor the subunits to the plasma membrane.

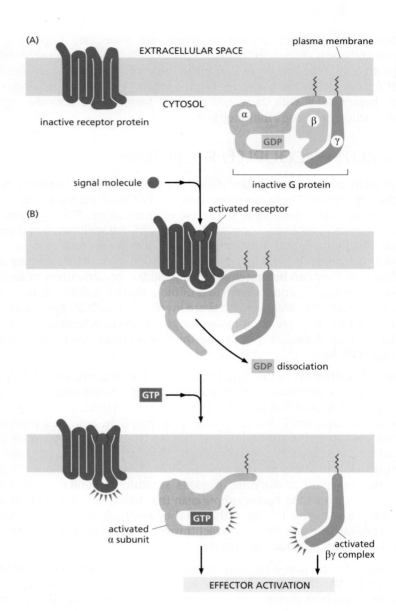

affinity for GDP, which is then exchanged for a molecule of GTP. In some cases, this activation breaks up the G-protein subunits, so that the activated α subunit, clutching its GTP, detaches from the βγ complex, which is also activated (**Figure 16–15B**). The two activated parts of the G protein—the α subunit and the βγ complex—can then each interact directly with target proteins in the plasma membrane, which in turn may relay the signal to other destinations in the cell. The longer these target proteins remain bound to an α subunit or a βγ complex, the more prolonged the relayed signal will be.

The amount of time that the α subunit and βγ complex remain "switched on"—and hence available to relay signals—also determines how long a response lasts. This timing is controlled by the behavior of the α subunit. The α subunit has an intrinsic GTPase activity, and it eventually hydrolyzes its bound GTP to GDP, returning the whole G protein to its original, inactive conformation (**Figure 16–16**). GTP hydrolysis and inactivation usually occur within seconds after the G protein has been activated. The inactive G protein is then ready to be reactivated by another activated receptor.

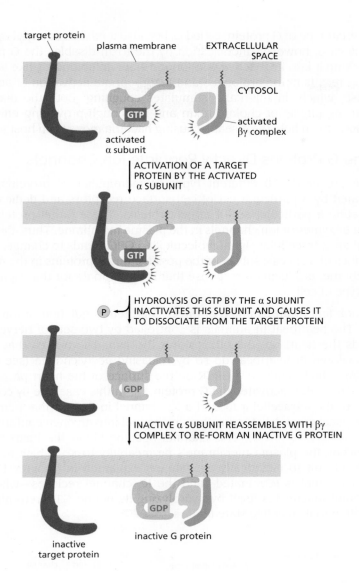

target protein

plasma membrane

EXTRACELLULAR SPACE

CYTOSOL

GTP

activated α subunit

activated βγ complex

ACTIVATION OF A TARGET PROTEIN BY THE ACTIVATED α SUBUNIT

GTP

HYDROLYSIS OF GTP BY THE α SUBUNIT INACTIVATES THIS SUBUNIT AND CAUSES IT TO DISSOCIATE FROM THE TARGET PROTEIN

P

GDP

INACTIVE α SUBUNIT REASSEMBLES WITH βγ COMPLEX TO RE-FORM AN INACTIVE G PROTEIN

GDP

inactive target protein

inactive G protein

Figure 16–16 The G protein α subunit switches itself off by hydrolyzing its bound GTP to GDP. When an activated α subunit interacts with its target protein, it activates that target protein for as long as the two remain in contact. (In some cases, the α subunit instead inactivates its target; not shown.) The α subunit then hydrolyzes its bound GTP to GDP—an event that takes place usually within seconds of G-protein activation. The hydrolysis of GTP inactivates the α subunit, which dissociates from its target protein and—if the α subunit had separated from the βγ complex (as shown)—reassociates with a βγ complex to re-form an inactive G protein. The G protein is now ready to couple to another activated receptor, as in Figure 16–15B. Both the activated α subunit and the activated βγ complex can interact with target proteins in the plasma membrane. See also Movie 16.2.

Some Bacterial Toxins Cause Disease by Altering the Activity of G Proteins

G proteins offer a striking example of the importance of being able to shut down a signal, as well as turn it on. Disrupting the activation—and deactivation—of G proteins can have dire consequences for a cell or organism. Consider cholera, for example. The disease is caused by a bacterium that multiplies in the human intestine, where it produces a protein called *cholera toxin*. This protein enters the cells that line the intestine and modifies the α subunit of a G protein called G_S—so named because it *stimulates* the enzyme adenylyl cyclase, which we discuss shortly. The modification prevents G_S from hydrolyzing its bound GTP, thus locking the G protein in an active state, in which it continuously stimulates adenylyl cyclase. In intestinal cells, this stimulation causes a prolonged and excessive outflow of Cl⁻ and water into the gut, resulting in catastrophic diarrhea and dehydration. The condition often leads to death unless urgent steps are taken to replace the lost water and ions.

A similar situation occurs in whooping cough (pertussis), a common respiratory infection against which infants are now routinely vaccinated. In this case, the disease-causing bacterium colonizes the lung, where it produces a protein called *pertussis toxin*. This protein alters the α subunit of

QUESTION 16–3

GPCRs activate G proteins by reducing the strength of GDP binding to the G protein. This results in rapid dissociation of bound GDP, which is then replaced by GTP, because GTP is present in the cytosol in much higher concentrations than GDP. What consequences would result from a mutation in the α subunit of a G protein that caused its affinity for GDP to be reduced without significantly changing its affinity for GTP? Compare the effects of this mutation with the effects of cholera toxin.

a different type of G protein, called G_i because it *inhibits* adenylyl cyclase. In this case, however, modification by the toxin disables the G protein by locking it into its inactive GDP-bound state. Inhibiting G_i, like activating G_s, results in the prolonged and inappropriate activation of adenylyl cyclase, which, in this case, stimulates coughing. Both the diarrhea-producing effects of cholera toxin and the cough-provoking effects of pertussis toxin help the disease-causing bacteria move from host to host.

Some G Proteins Directly Regulate Ion Channels

There are about 20 different types of mammalian G proteins, each activated by a particular set of cell-surface receptors and dedicated to activating a particular set of target proteins. These target proteins are either enzymes or ion channels in the plasma membrane. Thus, the binding of an extracellular signal molecule to a GPCR leads to changes in the activities of a specific subset of the possible target proteins in the plasma membrane, producing a response that is appropriate for that signal and that type of cell.

We look first at an example of direct G-protein regulation of ion channels. The heartbeat in animals is controlled by two sets of nerves: one speeds the heart up, the other slows it down. The nerves that signal a slowdown in heartbeat do so by releasing acetylcholine (see Figure 16–5A), which binds to a GPCR on the surface of the heart pacemaker cells. This GPCR activates the G protein, G_i. In this case, the βγ complex binds to the intracellular face of a K^+ channel in the plasma membrane of the pacemaker cell, forcing the ion channel into an open conformation (**Figure 16–17A and B**). This channel opening slows the heart rate by increasing the plasma membrane's permeability to K^+, which makes it more difficult to electrically activate, as explained in Chapter 12. The original signal is terminated—and the K^+ channel recloses—when the α subunit inactivates itself by hydrolyzing its bound GTP, returning the G protein to its inactive state (**Figure 16–17C**).

Figure 16–17 A G_i protein directly couples receptor activation to the opening of K^+ channels in the plasma membrane of heart pacemaker cells. (A) Binding of the neurotransmitter acetylcholine to its GPCR on the heart cells results in the activation of the G protein, G_i. (B) The activated βγ complex directly opens a K^+ channel in the plasma membrane, increasing its permeability to K^+ and thereby making the membrane harder to activate and slowing the heart rate. (C) Inactivation of the α subunit by hydrolysis of its bound GTP returns the G protein to its inactive state, allowing the K^+ channel to close.

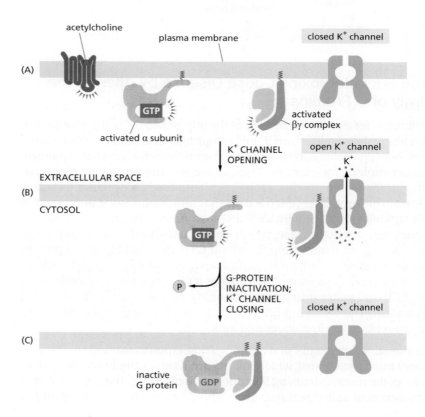

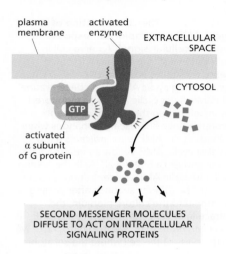

Figure 16–18 **Enzymes activated by G proteins increase the concentrations of small intracellular signaling molecules.** Because each activated enzyme generates many molecules of these second messengers, the signal is greatly amplified at this step in the pathway (see Figure 16–28). The signal is relayed onward by the second messenger molecules, which bind to specific signaling proteins in the cell and influence their activity.

Many G Proteins Activate Membrane-bound Enzymes That Produce Small Messenger Molecules

When G proteins interact with ion channels they cause an immediate change in the state and behavior of the cell. The interaction of activated G proteins with enzymes, in contrast, has consequences that are less rapid and more complex, as they lead to the production of additional intracellular signaling molecules. The two most frequent target enzymes for G proteins are *adenylyl cyclase*, which produces a small molecule called *cyclic AMP*, and *phospholipase C*, which generates small molecules called *inositol trisphosphate* and *diacylglycerol*. Inositol trisphosphate, in turn, promotes the accumulation of cytosolic Ca^{2+}—yet another intracellular signaling molecule.

Adenylyl cyclase and phospholipase C are activated by different types of G proteins, allowing cells to couple the production of the small molecules to different extracellular signals. Although the coupling may be either stimulatory or inhibitory—as we saw in our discussion of the actions of cholera toxin and pertussis toxin—we concentrate here on G proteins that stimulate enzyme activity.

The small molecules generated by these enzymes are often called *second messengers*—the "first messengers" being the extracellular signals that activated the enzymes in the first place. Once activated, the enzymes generate large quantities of second messengers, which rapidly diffuse away from their source, thereby amplifying and spreading the intracellular signal (**Figure 16–18**).

Different second messenger molecules produce different responses. We first examine the consequences of an increase in the cytosolic concentration of cyclic AMP. This will take us along one of the main types of signaling pathways that lead from the activation of GPCRs. We then discuss the actions of three other second messenger molecules—inositol trisphosphate, diacylglycerol, and Ca^{2+}—which will lead us along a different signaling route.

The Cyclic AMP Signaling Pathway Can Activate Enzymes and Turn On Genes

Many extracellular signals acting via GPCRs affect the activity of the enzyme **adenylyl cyclase** and thus alter the intracellular concentration of the second messenger molecule **cyclic AMP**. Most commonly, the activated G protein α subunit switches on the adenylyl cyclase, causing a dramatic and sudden increase in the synthesis of cyclic AMP from ATP (which is always present in the cell). To help terminate the signal, a second enzyme, called *cyclic AMP phosphodiesterase*, rapidly converts cyclic AMP to ordinary AMP (**Figure 16–19**). One way that caffeine acts as a stimulant is by inhibiting this phosphodiesterase in the nervous system, blocking cyclic AMP degradation and thereby keeping the concentration of this second messenger high.

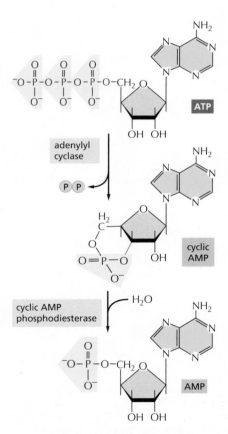

Figure 16–19 **Cyclic AMP is synthesized by adenylyl cyclase and degraded by cyclic AMP phosphodiesterase.** Cyclic AMP (abbreviated cAMP) is formed from ATP by a cyclization reaction that removes two phosphate groups from ATP and joins the "free" end of the remaining phosphate group to the sugar part of the AMP molecule (*red* bond). The degradation reaction breaks this new bond, forming AMP.

Figure 16–20 **The concentration of cyclic AMP rises rapidly in response to an extracellular signal.** A nerve cell in culture responds to the binding of the neurotransmitter serotonin to a GPCR by synthesizing cyclic AMP. The concentration of intracellular cyclic AMP was monitored by injecting into the cell a fluorescent protein whose fluorescence changes when it binds cyclic AMP. *Blue* indicates a low level of cyclic AMP, *yellow* an intermediate level, and *red* a high level. (A) In the resting cell, the cyclic AMP concentration is about 5×10^{-8} M. (B) Fifty seconds after adding serotonin to the culture medium, the intracellular concentration of cyclic AMP has risen more than twentyfold (to $>10^{-6}$ M) in the parts of the cell where the serotonin receptors are concentrated. (From B.J. Bacskai et al. *Science* 260:222–226, 1993.)

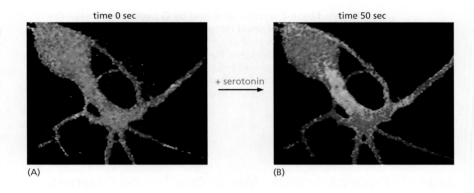

Cyclic AMP phosphodiesterase is continuously active inside the cell. Because it eliminates cyclic AMP so quickly, the cytosolic concentration of this second messenger can change rapidly in response to extracellular signals, rising or falling tenfold in a matter of seconds (**Figure 16–20**). Cyclic AMP is water-soluble, so it can, in some cases, carry the signal throughout the cell, traveling from the site on the membrane where it is synthesized to interact with proteins located in the cytosol, in the nucleus, or on other organelles.

Cyclic AMP exerts most of its effects by activating the enzyme **cyclic-AMP-dependent protein kinase** (**PKA**). This enzyme is normally held inactive in a complex with a regulatory protein. The binding of cyclic AMP to the regulatory protein forces a conformational change that releases the inhibition and unleashes the active kinase. Activated PKA then catalyzes the phosphorylation of particular serines or threonines on specific intracellular proteins, thus altering the activity of these target proteins. In different cell types, different sets of proteins are available to be phosphorylated, which largely explains why the effects of cyclic AMP vary with the type of target cell.

Many kinds of cell responses are mediated by cyclic AMP; a few are listed in **Table 16–3**. As the table shows, different target cells respond very differently to extracellular signals that change intracellular cyclic AMP concentrations. When we are frightened or excited, for example, the adrenal gland releases the hormone *epinephrine* (also called *adrenaline*), which circulates in the bloodstream and binds to a class of GPCRs called adrenergic receptors (see Figure 16–14B), which are present on many types of cells. The consequences of epinephrine binding vary from one cell type to another, but all the cell responses help prepare the body for

TABLE 16–3 SOME CELL RESPONSES MEDIATED BY CYCLIC AMP		
Extracellular Signal Molecule*	**Target Tissue**	**Major Response**
Epinephrine	heart	increase in heart rate and force of contraction
Epinephrine	skeletal muscle	glycogen breakdown
Epinephrine, glucagon	fat	fat breakdown
Adrenocorticotropic hormone (ACTH)	adrenal gland	cortisol secretion

*Although all of the signal molecules listed here are hormones, some responses to local mediators and to neurotransmitters are also mediated by cyclic AMP.

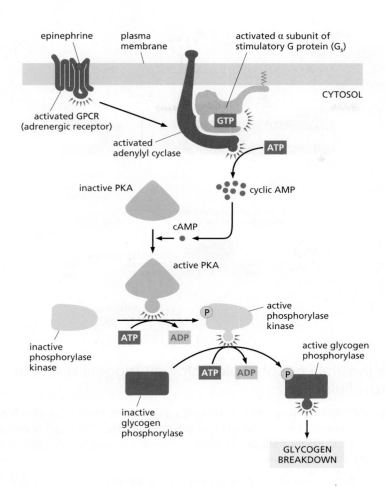

Figure 16–21 Epinephrine stimulates glycogen breakdown in skeletal muscle cells. The hormone activates a GPCR, which turns on a G protein (G_s) that activates adenylyl cyclase to boost the production of cyclic AMP. The increase in cyclic AMP activates PKA, which phosphorylates and activates an enzyme called phosphorylase kinase. This kinase activates glycogen phosphorylase, the enzyme that breaks down glycogen (see Figure 13–22). Because these reactions do not involve changes in gene transcription or new protein synthesis, they occur rapidly.

sudden action. In skeletal muscle, for instance, epinephrine increases intracellular cyclic AMP, causing the breakdown of glycogen—the polymerized storage form of glucose. It does so by activating PKA, which leads to both the activation of an enzyme that promotes glycogen breakdown (**Figure 16–21**) and the inhibition of an enzyme that drives glycogen synthesis. By stimulating glycogen breakdown and inhibiting its synthesis, the increase in cyclic AMP maximizes the amount of glucose available as fuel for anticipated muscular activity. Epinephrine also acts on fat cells, stimulating the breakdown of fat to fatty acids. These fatty acids can then be exported to fuel ATP production in other cells.

In some cases, the effects of increasing cyclic AMP are rapid; in skeletal muscle, for example, glycogen breakdown occurs within seconds of epinephrine binding to its receptor (see Figure 16–21). In other cases, cyclic AMP responses involve changes in gene expression that take minutes or hours to develop. In these slow responses, PKA typically phosphorylates transcription regulators, proteins that activate the transcription of selected genes (as discussed in Chapter 8). For example, an increase in cyclic AMP in certain neurons in the brain controls the production of proteins involved in some forms of learning. **Figure 16–22** illustrates a typical cyclic-AMP-mediated pathway from the plasma membrane to the nucleus.

We now turn to the other enzyme-mediated signaling pathway that leads from GPCRs—the pathway that begins with the activation of the membrane-bound enzyme *phospholipase C* and leads to an increase in the second messengers diacylglycerol, inositol trisphosphate, and Ca^{2+}.

QUESTION 16–4

Explain why cyclic AMP must be broken down rapidly in a cell to allow rapid signaling.

Figure 16–22 A rise in intracellular cyclic AMP can activate gene transcription. PKA, activated by a rise in intracellular cyclic AMP, can enter the nucleus and phosphorylate specific transcription regulators. Once phosphorylated, these proteins stimulate the transcription of a whole set of target genes (Movie 16.3). This type of signaling pathway controls many processes in cells, ranging from hormone synthesis in endocrine cells to the production of proteins involved in long-term memory in the brain. Activated PKA can also phosphorylate and thereby regulate other proteins and enzymes in the cytosol, as shown in Figure 16–21.

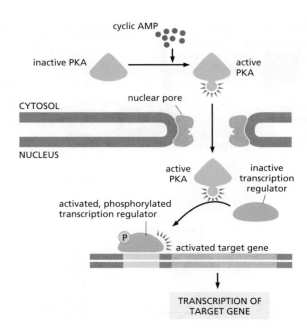

The Inositol Phospholipid Pathway Triggers a Rise in Intracellular Ca²⁺

Some GPCRs exert their effects through a G protein called G_q, which activates the membrane-bound enzyme **phospholipase C** instead of adenylyl cyclase. Examples of signal molecules that act through phospholipase C are given in Table 16–4.

Once activated, phospholipase C propagates the signal by cleaving a lipid molecule that is a component of the plasma membrane. The molecule is an **inositol phospholipid** (a phospholipid with the sugar inositol attached to its head) that is present in small quantities in the cytosolic leaflet of the membrane lipid bilayer (see Figure 11–19). Because of the involvement of this phospholipid, the signaling pathway that begins with the activation of phospholipase C is often referred to as the *inositol phospholipid pathway*. It operates in almost all eukaryotic cells and regulates a large number of different effector proteins.

The cleavage of a membrane inositol phospholipid by phospholipase C generates two second messenger molecules: **inositol 1,4,5-trisphosphate (IP_3)** and **diacylglycerol (DAG)**. Both molecules play a crucial part in relaying the signal (Figure 16–23).

IP_3 is a water-soluble sugar phosphate that is released into the cytosol; there it binds to and opens Ca²⁺ channels that are embedded in the endoplasmic reticulum (ER) membrane. Ca²⁺ stored inside the ER rushes out

TABLE 16–4 SOME CELL RESPONSES MEDIATED BY PHOSPHOLIPASE C ACTIVATION		
Signal Molecule	**Target Tissue**	**Major Response**
Vasopressin (a peptide hormone)	liver	glycogen breakdown
Acetylcholine	pancreas	secretion of amylase (a digestive enzyme)
Acetylcholine	skeletal muscle	contraction
Thrombin (a proteolytic enzyme)	blood platelets	aggregation

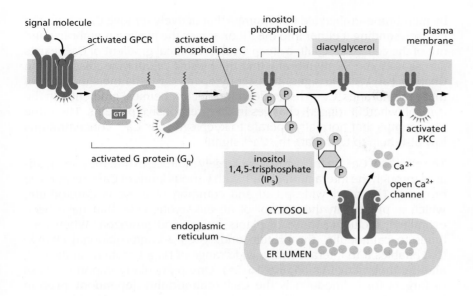

Figure 16–23 Phospholipase C activates two signaling pathways. Two messenger molecules are produced when a membrane inositol phospholipid is hydrolyzed by activated phospholipase C. Inositol 1,4,5-trisphosphate (IP$_3$) diffuses through the cytosol and triggers the release of Ca^{2+} from the ER by binding to and opening special Ca^{2+} channels in the ER membrane. The large electrochemical gradient for Ca^{2+} across this membrane causes Ca^{2+} to rush out of the ER and into the cytosol. Diacylglycerol remains in the plasma membrane and, together with Ca^{2+}, helps activate the enzyme protein kinase C (PKC), which is recruited from the cytosol to the cytosolic face of the plasma membrane (Movie 16.4). PKC then phosphorylates its own set of intracellular proteins, further propagating the signal. At the start of the pathway, both the α subunit and the βγ complex of the G protein G$_q$ are involved in activating phospholipase C.

into the cytosol through these open channels, causing a sharp rise in the cytosolic concentration of free Ca^{2+}, which is normally kept very low. This Ca^{2+} in turn signals to other proteins, as we discuss shortly.

Diacylglycerol is a lipid that remains embedded in the plasma membrane after it is produced by phospholipase C; there, it helps recruit and activate a protein kinase, which translocates from the cytosol to the plasma membrane. This enzyme is called **protein kinase C (PKC)** because it also needs to bind Ca^{2+} to become active (see Figure 16–23). Once activated, PKC phosphorylates a set of intracellular proteins that varies depending on the cell type.

A Ca^{2+} Signal Triggers Many Biological Processes

Ca^{2+} has such an important and widespread role as an intracellular messenger that we will digress to consider its functions more generally. A surge in the cytosolic concentration of free Ca^{2+} is triggered by many kinds of cell stimuli, not only those that act through GPCRs. When a sperm fertilizes an egg cell, for example, Ca^{2+} channels open, and the resulting rise in cytosolic Ca^{2+} triggers the egg to start development (Figure 16–24); for muscle cells, a signal from a nerve triggers a rise in cytosolic Ca^{2+} that initiates muscle contraction (discussed in Chapter 17; see Figure 17–45); and in many secretory cells, including nerve cells, Ca^{2+} triggers secretion (discussed in Chapter 12; see Figure 12–40). Ca^{2+} stimulates all these responses by binding to and influencing the activity of various Ca^{2+}-responsive proteins.

The concentration of free Ca^{2+} in the cytosol of an unstimulated cell is extremely low (10^{-7} M) compared with its concentration in the extracellular fluid (about 10^{-3} M) and in the ER. These differences are maintained

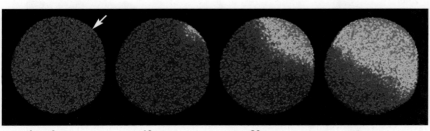

time 0 sec   10 sec   20 sec   40 sec

Figure 16–24 Fertilization of an egg by a sperm triggers an increase in cytosolic Ca^{2+} in the egg. This starfish egg was injected with a Ca^{2+}-sensitive fluorescent dye before it was fertilized. When a sperm enters the egg, a wave of cytosolic Ca^{2+} (*red*)—released from the ER—sweeps across the egg from the site of sperm entry (*arrow*). This Ca^{2+} wave provokes a change in the egg surface, preventing entry of other sperm, and it also initiates embryonic development. To catch this Ca^{2+} wave, go to Movie 16.5. (Adapted from S. Stricker, *Dev. Bio.* 166:34–58, 1994.)

by membrane-embedded Ca^{2+} pumps that actively remove Ca^{2+} from the cytosol, sending it either into the ER or across the plasma membrane and out of the cell. As a result, a steep electrochemical gradient of Ca^{2+} exists across both the ER membrane and the plasma membrane (discussed in Chapter 12). When a signal transiently opens Ca^{2+} channels in either of these membranes, Ca^{2+} rushes down its electrochemical gradient into the cytosol, where it triggers changes in Ca^{2+}-responsive proteins. The same Ca^{2+} pumps that normally operate to keep cytosolic Ca^{2+} concentrations low also help to terminate the Ca^{2+} signal.

The effects of Ca^{2+} in the cytosol are largely indirect, in that they are mediated through the interaction of Ca^{2+} with various kinds of Ca^{2+}-responsive proteins. The most widespread and common of these is **calmodulin**, which is present in the cytosol of all eukaryotic cells that have been examined, including those of plants, fungi, and protozoa. When Ca^{2+} binds to calmodulin, the protein undergoes a conformational change that enables it to interact with a wide range of target proteins in the cell, altering their activities (**Figure 16–25**). One particularly important class of targets for calmodulin is the **Ca^{2+}/calmodulin-dependent protein kinases** (**CaM-kinases**). When these kinases are activated by binding to calmodulin complexed with Ca^{2+}, they influence other processes in the cell by phosphorylating selected proteins. In the mammalian brain, for example, a neuron-specific CaM-kinase is abundant at synapses, where it is thought to play an important part in some forms of learning and memory. This CaM-kinase is activated by the pulses of Ca^{2+} signals that occur during neural activity, and mutant mice that lack the kinase show a marked inability to remember where things are.

A GPCR Signaling Pathway Generates a Dissolved Gas That Carries a Signal to Adjacent Cells

Second messengers like cyclic AMP and calcium are hydrophilic molecules that generally act within the cell where they are produced. But some molecules produced in response to GPCR activation are small enough or hydrophobic enough to pass across the membrane and carry a signal directly to nearby cells. An important example is the gas **nitric oxide** (**NO**), which acts as a signaling molecule in many tissues. NO diffuses readily from its site of synthesis and slips into neighboring cells. The distance the gas diffuses is limited by its reaction with oxygen and water in the extracellular environment, which converts NO into nitrates and nitrites within seconds.

Figure 16–25 Calcium binding changes the shape of the calmodulin protein. (A) Calmodulin has a dumbbell shape, with two globular ends connected by a long α helix. Each of the globular ends has two Ca^{2+}-binding sites. (B) Simplified representation of the structure, showing the conformational changes that occur when Ca^{2+}-bound calmodulin interacts with an isolated segment of a target protein (red). In this conformation, the α helix jackknifes to surround the target (Movie 16.6). (B, adapted from W.E. Meador, A.R. Means, and F.A. Quiocho, *Science* 257:1251–1255, 1992, and M. Ikura et al., *Science* 256:632–638, 1992.)

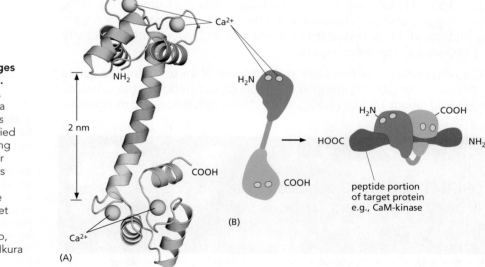

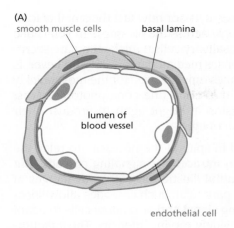

(A)

smooth muscle cells   basal lamina

lumen of
blood vessel

endothelial cell

Figure 16–26 Nitric oxide (NO) triggers smooth muscle relaxation in a blood-vessel wall. (A) Simplified drawing showing a cross section of a blood vessel with endothelial cells lining its lumen and smooth muscle cells surrounding the outside of the vessel. (B) The neurotransmitter acetylcholine causes the blood vessel to dilate by binding to a GPCR on the surface of the endothelial cells, thereby activating a G protein, G_q, to trigger Ca^{2+} release (as illustrated in Figure 16–23). Ca^{2+} activates nitric oxide synthase, stimulating the production of NO. NO then diffuses out of the endothelial cells and into adjacent smooth muscle cells, where it regulates the activity of specific proteins, causing the muscle cells to relax. One key target protein that can be activated by NO in smooth muscle cells is guanylyl cyclase, which catalyzes the production of cyclic GMP from GTP. Note that NO gas is highly toxic when inhaled and should not be confused with nitrous oxide (N_2O), also known as laughing gas.

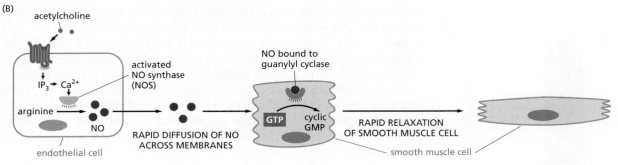

(B)

acetylcholine

$IP_3 \rightarrow Ca^{2+}$

arginine

NO

endothelial cell

activated
NO synthase
(NOS)

RAPID DIFFUSION OF NO
ACROSS MEMBRANES

NO bound to
guanylyl cyclase

GTP   cyclic
GMP

RAPID RELAXATION
OF SMOOTH MUSCLE CELL

smooth muscle cell

Endothelial cells—the flattened cells that line every blood vessel—release NO in response to acetylcholine secreted by nearby nerve endings. Acetylcholine binds to a GPCR on the endothelial cell surface, resulting in activation of G_q and the release of Ca^{2+} inside the cell (see Figure 16–23). Ca^{2+} then stimulates nitric oxide synthase, which produces NO from the amino acid arginine. This NO diffuses into smooth muscle cells in the adjacent vessel wall, causing the cells to relax; this relaxation allows the vessel to dilate, so that blood flows through it more freely (**Figure 16–26**). The effect of NO on blood vessels accounts for the action of nitroglycerin, which has been used for almost 100 years to treat patients with angina—pain caused by inadequate blood flow to the heart muscle. In the body, nitroglycerin is converted to NO, which rapidly relaxes blood vessels, thereby reducing the workload on the heart and decreasing the muscle's need for oxygen-rich blood. Many nerve cells also use NO to signal neighboring cells: NO released by nerve terminals in the penis, for instance, acts as a local mediator to trigger the blood-vessel dilation responsible for penile erection.

Inside many target cells, NO binds to and activates the enzyme *guanylyl cyclase*, stimulating the formation of *cyclic GMP* from the nucleotide GTP (see Figure 16–26B). Cyclic GMP, a second messenger similar in structure to cyclic AMP, is a key link in the NO signaling chain. The drug Viagra enhances penile erection by blocking the enzyme that degrades cyclic GMP, prolonging the NO signal.

GPCR-Triggered Intracellular Signaling Cascades Can Achieve Astonishing Speed, Sensitivity, and Adaptability

The steps in the *signaling cascades* associated with GPCRs take a long time to describe, but they often take only seconds to execute. Consider how quickly a thrill can make your heart race (when epinephrine stimulates the GPCRs in your cardiac pacemaker cells), or how fast the smell of food can make your mouth water (through the GPCRs for odors in your nose and the GPCRs for acetylcholine in salivary cells, which stimulate secretion). Among the fastest of all responses mediated by a GPCR, however, is the response of the eye to light: it takes only 20 msec for the most quickly responding photoreceptor cells of the retina (the cone photoreceptors, which are responsible for color vision in bright light) to produce their electrical response to a sudden flash of light.

This exceptional speed is achieved in spite of the necessity to relay the signal over the multiple steps of an intracellular signaling cascade. But photoreceptors also provide a beautiful illustration of the advantages of intracellular signaling cascades: in particular, such cascades allow spectacular amplification of the incoming signal and also allow cells to adapt so as to be able to detect signals of widely varying intensity. The quantitative details have been most thoroughly analyzed for the rod photoreceptor cells in the eye, which are responsible for noncolor vision in dim light (Figure 16–27). In this photoreceptor cell, light is sensed by rhodopsin, a G-protein-coupled light receptor. Rhodopsin, when stimulated by light, activates a G protein called transducin. The activated α subunit of transducin then activates an intracellular signaling cascade that causes cation channels to close in the plasma membrane of the photoreceptor cell. This produces a change in the voltage across the cell membrane, which alters neurotransmitter release and ultimately leads to a nerve impulse being sent to the brain.

The signal is repeatedly amplified as it is relayed along this intracellular signaling pathway (Figure 16–28). When lighting conditions are dim, as on a moonless night, the amplification is enormous: as few as a dozen photons absorbed across the entire retina will cause a perceptible signal to be delivered to the brain. In bright sunlight, when photons flood through each photoreceptor cell at a rate of billions per second, the signaling cascade undergoes a form of *adaptation*, stepping down the amplification more than 10,000-fold, so that the photoreceptor cells are not overwhelmed and can still register increases and decreases in the strong light. The adaptation depends on negative feedback: an intense response in the photoreceptor cell decreases the cytosolic Ca^{2+} concentration, inhibiting the enzymes responsible for signal amplification.

Adaptation frequently occurs in intracellular signaling pathways that respond to extracellular signal molecules, allowing cells to respond to fluctuations in the concentration of such molecules regardless of whether they are present in small or large amounts. By taking advantage of positive and negative feedback mechanisms (see Figure 16–10), adaptation thus allows a cell to respond equally well to the signaling equivalents of shouts and whispers.

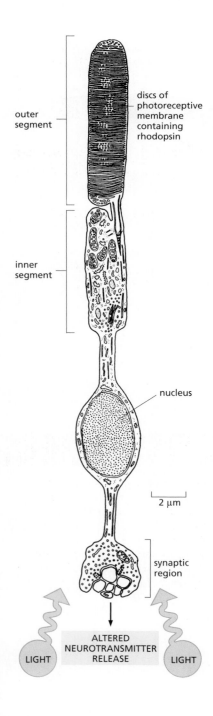

outer segment

discs of photoreceptive membrane containing rhodopsin

inner segment

nucleus

2 μm

synaptic region

LIGHT   ALTERED NEUROTRANSMITTER RELEASE   LIGHT

Figure 16–27 **A rod photoreceptor cell from the retina is exquisitely sensitive to light.** The light-absorbing rhodopsin proteins are embedded in many pancake-shaped vesicles (discs) of membrane inside the outer segment of the photoreceptor cell. When the rod cell is stimulated by light, a signal is relayed from the rhodopsin molecules in the discs, through the cytosol, to ion channels that allow positive ions to flow through the plasma membrane of the outer segment. These cation channels close in response to the cytosolic signal, producing a change in the membrane potential of the rod cell. By mechanisms similar to those that control neurotransmitter release in ordinary nerve cells, the change in membrane potential alters the rate of neurotransmitter release from the synaptic region of the cell. Released neurotransmitters then act on retinal nerve cells that pass the signal on to the brain. (From T.L. Lentz, *Cell Fine Structure*. Philadelphia: Saunders, 1971. With permission from Elsevier.)

Figure 16–28 The light-induced signaling cascade in rod photoreceptor cells greatly amplifies the light signal. When rod photoreceptors are adapted for dim light, the signal amplification is enormous. The intracellular signaling pathway from the G protein transducin uses components that differ from the ones in previous figures. The cascade functions as follows. In the absence of a light signal, the second messenger molecule cyclic GMP is continuously produced by guanylyl cyclase in the cytosol of the photoreceptor cell. The cyclic GMP then binds to cation channels in the photoreceptor cell plasma membrane, keeping them open. Activation of rhodopsin by light results in the activation of transducin α subunits. These turn on an enzyme called cyclic GMP phosphodiesterase, which breaks down cyclic GMP to GMP (much as cyclic AMP phosphodiesterase breaks down cyclic AMP; see Figure 16–19). The sharp fall in the cytosolic concentration of cyclic GMP reduces the amount of cyclic GMP bound to the cation channels, which therefore close. Closing these channels decreases the influx of Na^+, thereby altering the voltage gradient (membrane potential) across the plasma membrane and, ultimately, the rate of neurotransmitter release, as described in Chapter 12. The *red* arrows indicate the steps at which amplification occurs, with the thickness of the arrow roughly indicating the magnitude of the amplification.

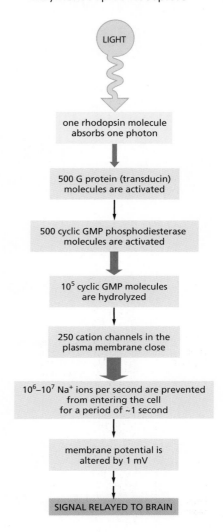

LIGHT

one rhodopsin molecule absorbs one photon

500 G protein (transducin) molecules are activated

500 cyclic GMP phosphodiesterase molecules are activated

10^5 cyclic GMP molecules are hydrolyzed

250 cation channels in the plasma membrane close

$10^6–10^7$ Na^+ ions per second are prevented from entering the cell for a period of ~1 second

membrane potential is altered by 1 mV

SIGNAL RELAYED TO BRAIN

Taste and smell also depend on GPCRs. It seems likely that this mechanism of signal reception, invented early in evolution, has its origins in the basic and universal need of cells to sense and respond to their environment. Of course, GPCRs are not the only receptors that activate intracellular signaling cascades. We now turn to another major class of cell-surface receptors—enzyme-coupled receptors—which play a key part in controlling cell numbers, cell differentiation, and cell movement in multicellular animals, especially during development.

ENZYME-COUPLED RECEPTORS

Like GPCRs, **enzyme-coupled receptors** are transmembrane proteins that display their ligand-binding domains on the outer surface of the plasma membrane (see Figure 16–13C). Instead of associating with a G protein, however, the cytoplasmic domain of the receptor either acts as an enzyme itself or forms a complex with another protein that acts as an enzyme. Enzyme-coupled receptors were discovered through their role in responses to extracellular signal proteins that regulate the growth, proliferation, differentiation, and survival of cells in animal tissues (see Table 16–1, p. 536, for examples). Most of these signal proteins function as local mediators and can act at very low concentrations (about 10^{-9} to 10^{-11} M). Responses to them are typically slow (on the order of hours), and their effects may require many intracellular transduction steps that usually lead to a change in gene expression.

Enzyme-coupled receptors, however, can also mediate direct, rapid reconfigurations of the cytoskeleton, changing the cell's shape and the way that it moves. The extracellular signals that induce such changes are often not diffusible signal proteins, but proteins attached to the surfaces over which a cell is crawling.

The largest class of enzyme-coupled receptors consists of receptors with a cytoplasmic domain that functions as a tyrosine kinase, which phosphorylates particular tyrosines on specific intracellular signaling proteins. These receptors, called **receptor tyrosine kinases (RTKs)**, will be the main focus of this section.

We begin with a discussion of how RTKs are activated in response to extracellular signals. We then consider how activated RTKs transmit the signal along two major intracellular signaling pathways that terminate at various effector proteins in the target cell. Finally, we describe how some

QUESTION 16–6

One important feature of any intracellular signaling pathway is its ability to be turned off. Consider the pathway shown in Figure 16–28. Where would off switches be required? Which ones do you suppose would be the most important?

enzyme-coupled receptors bypass such intracellular signaling cascades and use a more direct mechanism to regulate gene transcription.

Abnormal cell growth, proliferation, differentiation, survival, and migration are fundamental features of a cancer cell, and abnormalities in signaling via RTKs and other enzyme-coupled receptors have a major role in the development of most cancers.

Activated RTKs Recruit a Complex of Intracellular Signaling Proteins

To do its job as a signal transducer, an enzyme-coupled receptor has to switch on the enzyme activity of its intracellular domain (or of an associated enzyme) when an external signal molecule binds to its extracellular domain. Unlike GPCRs, enzyme-coupled receptor proteins usually have only one transmembrane segment, which spans the lipid bilayer as a single α helix. Because a single α helix is poorly suited to transmit a conformational change across the bilayer, enzyme-coupled receptors have a different strategy for transducing the extracellular signal. In many cases, the binding of an extracellular signal molecule causes two receptor molecules to come together in the plasma membrane, forming a dimer. This pairing brings the two intracellular tails of the receptors together and activates their kinase domains, such that each receptor tail phosphorylates the other. In the case of RTKs, the phosphorylations occur on specific tyrosines.

This tyrosine phosphorylation then triggers the assembly of a transient but elaborate intracellular signaling complex on the cytosolic tails of the receptors. The newly phosphorylated tyrosines serve as docking sites for a whole zoo of intracellular signaling proteins—perhaps as many as 10 or 20 different molecules (**Figure 16–29**). Some of these proteins become phosphorylated and activated on binding to the receptors, and they then propagate the signal; others function solely as scaffolds, which couple the receptors to other signaling proteins, thereby helping to build the active signaling complex (see Figure 16–9). All of these docked intracellular signaling proteins possess a specialized *interaction domain*, which recognizes specific phosphorylated tyrosines on the receptor tails. Other

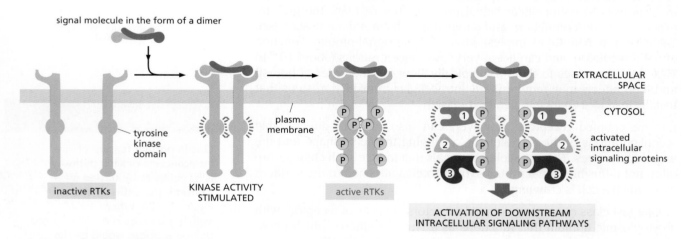

Figure 16–29 Activation of an RTK stimulates the assembly of an intracellular signaling complex. Typically, the binding of a signal molecule to the extracellular domain of an RTK causes two receptor molecules to associate into a dimer. The signal molecule shown here is itself a dimer and thus can physically cross-link two receptor molecules; other signal molecules induce a conformational change in the RTKs, causing the receptors to dimerize (not shown). In either case, dimer formation brings the kinase domain of each cytosolic receptor tail into contact with the other; this activates the kinases to phosphorylate the adjacent tail on several tyrosines. Each phosphorylated tyrosine serves as a specific docking site for a different intracellular signaling protein, which then helps relay the signal to the cell's interior; these proteins contain a specialized interaction domain—in this case, a module called an SH2 domain—that recognizes and binds to specific phosphorylated tyrosines on the cytosolic tail of an activated RTK or on another intracellular signaling protein.

interaction domains allow intracellular signaling proteins to recognize phosphorylated lipids that are produced on the cytosolic side of the plasma membrane in response to certain signals, as we discuss later.

As long as they remain together, the signaling protein complexes assembled on the cytosolic tails of the RTKs can transmit a signal along several routes simultaneously to many destinations in the cell, thus activating and coordinating the numerous biochemical changes that are required to trigger a complex response such as cell proliferation or differentiation. To help terminate the response, the tyrosine phosphorylations are reversed by *tyrosine phosphatases*, which remove the phosphates that were added to the tyrosines of both the RTKs and other intracellular signaling proteins in response to the extracellular signal. In some cases, activated RTKs (as well as some GPCRs) are inactivated in a more brutal way: they are dragged into the interior of the cell by endocytosis and then destroyed by digestion in lysosomes (as discussed in Chapter 15).

Different RTKs recruit different collections of intracellular signaling proteins, producing different effects; however, certain components are used by most RTKs. These include, for example, a phospholipase C that functions in the same way as the phospholipase C activated by GPCRs to trigger the inositol phospholipid signaling pathway discussed earlier (see Figure 16–23). Another intracellular signaling protein that is activated by almost all RTKs is a small GTP-binding protein called Ras, as we discuss next.

Most RTKs Activate the Monomeric GTPase Ras

As we have seen, activated RTKs recruit and activate many kinds of intracellular signaling proteins, leading to the formation of large signaling complexes on the cytosolic tail of the RTK. One of the key members of these signaling complexes is **Ras**—a small GTP-binding protein that is bound by a lipid tail to the cytosolic face of the plasma membrane. Virtually all RTKs activate Ras, including platelet-derived growth factor (PDGF) receptors, which mediate cell proliferation in wound healing, and nerve growth factor (NGF) receptors, which play an important part in the development of certain vertebrate neurons.

The Ras protein is a member of a large family of small GTP-binding proteins, often called **monomeric GTPases** to distinguish them from the trimeric G proteins that we encountered earlier. Ras resembles the α subunit of a G protein and functions as a molecular switch in much the same way. It cycles between two distinct conformational states—active when GTP is bound and inactive when GDP is bound. Interaction with an activating protein called Ras-GEF encourages Ras to exchange its GDP for GTP, thus switching Ras to its activated state (**Figure 16–30**); after a delay, Ras is switched off by a GAP called Ras-GAP (see Figure 16–12), which promotes the hydrolysis of its bound GTP to GDP (Movie 16.7).

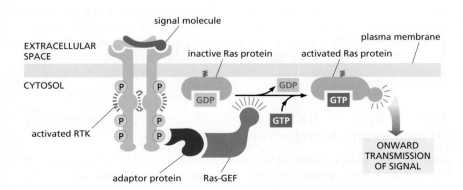

Figure 16–30 RTKs activate Ras. An adaptor protein docks on a particular phosphotyrosine on the activated receptor (the other signaling proteins that would be bound to the receptor, as shown in Figure 16–29, have been omitted for simplicity). The adaptor recruits a Ras guanine nucleotide exchange factor (Ras-GEF) that stimulates Ras to exchange its bound GDP for GTP. The activated Ras protein can now stimulate several downstream signaling pathways, one of which is shown in Figure 16–31. Note that the Ras protein contains a covalently attached lipid group (*red*) that helps anchor the protein to the inside of the plasma membrane.

Figure 16–31 Ras activates a MAP-kinase signaling module. The Ras protein, activated by the process shown in Figure 16–30, activates a three-kinase signaling module, which relays the signal onward. The final kinase in the module, MAP kinase, phosphorylates various downstream signaling or effector proteins.

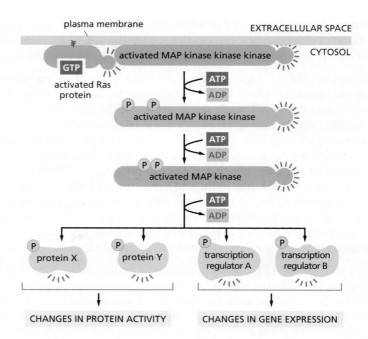

In its active state, Ras initiates a phosphorylation cascade in which a series of serine/threonine kinases phosphorylate and activate one another in sequence, like an intracellular game of dominoes. This relay system, which carries the signal from the plasma membrane to the nucleus, includes a three-kinase module called the **MAP-kinase signaling module**, in honor of the final enzyme in the chain, the mitogen-activated protein kinase, or **MAP kinase**. (As we discuss in Chapter 18, *mitogens* are extracellular signal molecules that stimulate cell proliferation.) In this pathway, outlined in **Figure 16–31**, MAP kinase is phosphorylated and activated by an enzyme called, logically enough, MAP kinase kinase. This protein is itself switched on by a MAP kinase kinase kinase (which is activated by Ras). At the end of the MAP-kinase cascade, MAP kinase phosphorylates various effector proteins, including certain transcription regulators, altering their ability to control gene transcription. The resulting change in the pattern of gene expression may stimulate cell proliferation, promote cell survival, or induce cell differentiation: the precise outcome will depend on which other genes are active in the cell and what other signals the cell receives. How biologists unravel such complex signaling pathways is discussed in **How We Know**, pp. 563–564.

Before Ras was discovered in normal cells, a mutant form of the protein was found in human cancer cells. The mutation inactivates the GTPase activity of Ras, so that the protein cannot shut itself off, promoting uncontrolled cell proliferation and the development of cancer. About 30% of human cancers contain such activating mutations in a *Ras* gene; of the cancers that do not, many have mutations in genes that encode proteins that function in the same signaling pathway as Ras. Many of the genes that encode normal intracellular signaling proteins were initially identified in the hunt for cancer-promoting *oncogenes* (discussed in Chapter 20).

RTKs Activate PI 3-Kinase to Produce Lipid Docking Sites in the Plasma Membrane

Many of the extracellular signal proteins that stimulate animal cells to survive and grow, including signal proteins belonging to the insulin-like

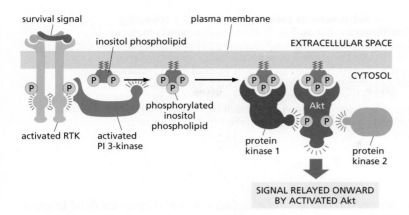

Figure 16–32 Some RTKs activate the PI-3-kinase–Akt signaling pathway.
An extracellular survival signal, such as IGF, activates an RTK, which recruits and activates PI 3-kinase. PI 3-kinase then phosphorylates an inositol phospholipid that is embedded in the cytosolic side of the plasma membrane. The resulting phosphorylated inositol phospholipid attracts intracellular signaling proteins that have a special domain that recognizes it. One of these signaling proteins, Akt, is a protein kinase that is activated at the membrane by phosphorylation mediated by two other protein kinases (here called protein kinases 1 and 2); protein kinase 1 is also recruited by the phosphorylated lipid docking sites. Once activated, Akt is released from the plasma membrane and phosphorylates various downstream proteins on specific serines and threonines (not shown).

growth factor (IGF) family, act through RTKs. One crucially important signaling pathway that these RTKs activate to promote cell growth and survival involves the enzyme **phosphoinositide 3-kinase** (**PI 3-kinase**), which phosphorylates inositol phospholipids in the plasma membrane. These phosphorylated lipids serve as docking sites for specific intracellular signaling proteins, which relocate from the cytosol to the plasma membrane, where they can activate one another. One of the most important of these relocated signaling proteins is the serine/threonine kinase *Akt* (**Figure 16–32**).

Akt, also called protein kinase B (PKB), promotes the growth and survival of many cell types, often by inactivating the signaling proteins it phosphorylates. For example, Akt phosphorylates and inactivates a cytosolic protein called Bad. In its active state, Bad encourages the cell to kill itself by indirectly activating a cell-suicide program called apoptosis (discussed in Chapter 18). Phosphorylation by Akt thus promotes cell survival by inactivating a protein that otherwise promotes cell death (**Figure 16–33**).

In addition to promoting cell survival, the *PI-3-kinase–Akt signaling pathway* stimulates cells to grow in size. It does so by indirectly activating

QUESTION 16–7

Would you expect to activate RTKs by exposing the exterior of cells to antibodies that bind to the respective proteins? Would your answer be different for GPCRs? (Hint: review Panel 4–2, on pp. 140–141, regarding the properties of antibody molecules.)

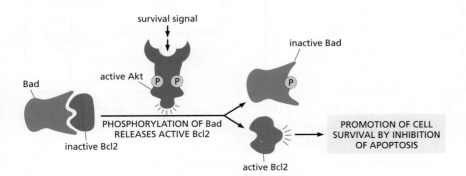

Figure 16–33 Activated Akt promotes cell survival. One way it does so is by phosphorylating and inactivating a protein called Bad. In its unphosphorylated state, Bad promotes apoptosis (a form of cell death) by binding to and inhibiting a protein, called Bcl2, which otherwise suppresses apoptosis. When Bad is phosphorylated by Akt, Bad releases Bcl2, which now blocks apoptosis, thereby promoting cell survival.

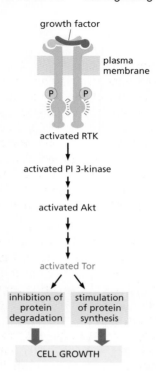

Figure 16–34 Akt stimulates cells to grow in size by activating the serine/threonine kinase Tor. The binding of a growth factor to an RTK activates the PI-3-kinase–Akt signaling pathway (as shown in Figure 16–32). Akt then indirectly activates Tor by phosphorylating and inhibiting a protein that helps to keep Tor shut down (not shown). Tor stimulates protein synthesis and inhibits protein degradation by phosphorylating key proteins in these processes (not shown). The anticancer drug rapamycin slows cell growth by inhibiting Tor. In fact, the Tor protein derives its name from the fact that it is a target of rapamycin.

a large serine/threonine kinase called *Tor*. Tor stimulates cells to grow both by enhancing protein synthesis and by inhibiting protein degradation (**Figure 16–34**). The anticancer drug rapamycin works by inactivating Tor, indicating the importance of this signaling pathway in regulating cell growth and survival—and the consequences of its disregulation in cancer.

The main intracellular signaling cascades activated by GPCRs and RTKs are summarized in **Figure 16–35**. As dauntingly complex as such pathways may seem, the complexity of cell signaling is actually much greater still. First, we have not discussed all of the intracellular signaling pathways that operate in cells. Second, although we depict these signaling pathways as being relatively linear and self-contained, they do not operate entirely independently. We will return to this concept of signal integration at the chapter's conclusion. But first, we take a brief detour to introduce a few important types of signaling systems that we have thus far overlooked.

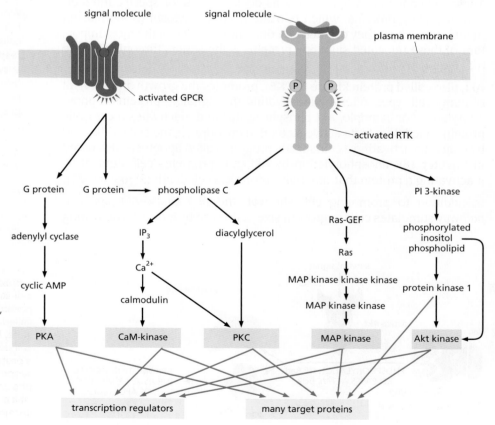

Figure 16–35 Both GPCRs and RTKs activate multiple intracellular signaling pathways. The figure reviews five of these pathways: two leading from GPCRs—through adenylyl cyclase and through phospholipase C—and three leading from RTKs—through phospholipase C, Ras, and PI 3-kinase. Each pathway differs from the others, yet they use some common components to transmit their signals. Because all five eventually activate protein kinases (*gray boxes*), it seems that each is capable in principle of regulating practically any process in the cell.

UNTANGLING CELL SIGNALING PATHWAYS

Intracellular signaling pathways are never mapped out in a single experiment. Although insulin was first isolated from dog pancreas in the early 1920s, the molecular chain of events that links the binding of insulin to its receptor with the activation of the transporter proteins that take up glucose has taken decades to untangle—and is still not completely understood.

Instead, investigators figure out, piece by piece, how all the links in the chain fit together—and how each contributes to the cell's response to an extracellular signal molecule such as the hormone insulin. Here, we discuss the kinds of experiments that allow scientists to identify individual links and, ultimately, to piece together complex signaling pathways.

Close encounters

Most signaling pathways depend on proteins that physically interact with one another. There are several ways to detect such direct contact. One involves using a protein as "bait." For example, to isolate the receptor that binds to insulin, one could attach insulin to a chromatography column. Cells that respond to the hormone are broken open with detergents that disrupt their membranes, releasing the transmembrane receptor proteins (see Figure 11–27). When this slurry is poured over the chromatography column, the proteins that bind to insulin will stick and can later be eluted and identified (see Figure 4–55).

Protein–protein interactions in a signaling pathway can also be identified by *co-immunoprecipitation*. For example, cells exposed to an extracellular signal molecule can be broken open, and antibodies can be used to grab the receptor protein known to recognize the signal molecule (see Panel 4–2, pp. 140–141, and Panel 4–3, pp. 164–165). If the receptor is strongly associated with other proteins, as shown in Figure 16–29, these will be captured as well. In this way, researchers can identify which proteins interact when an extracellular signal molecule stimulates cells.

Once two proteins are known to bind to each other, an investigator can pinpoint which parts of the proteins are required for the interaction using the DNA technology discussed in Chapter 10. For example, to determine which phosphorylated tyrosine on a receptor tyrosine kinase (RTK) is recognized by a certain intracellular signaling protein, a series of mutant receptors can be constructed, each missing a different tyrosine from its cytoplasmic domain (**Figure 16–36**). In this way, the specific tyrosines required for binding can be determined. Similarly, one can determine whether this phosphotyrosine docking site is required for the receptor to transmit a signal to the cell.

Jamming the pathway

Ultimately, one wants to assess what role a particular protein plays in a signaling pathway. A first test may

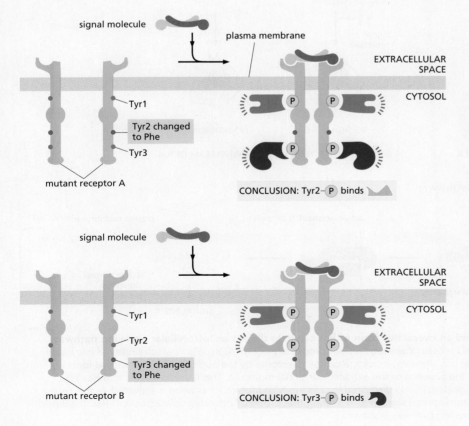

Figure 16–36 Mutant proteins can help to determine exactly where an intracellular signaling molecule binds. As shown in Figure 16–29, on binding their extracellular signal molecule, a pair of RTKs come together and phosphorylate specific tyrosines on each other's cytoplasmic tails. These phosphorylated tyrosines bind different intracellular signaling proteins, which then become activated and pass on the signal. To determine which tyrosine binds to a specific intracellular signaling protein, a series of mutant receptors is constructed. In the mutants shown, tyrosines Tyr2 or Tyr3 have been replaced, one at a time, by phenylalanine (*red*), thereby preventing phosphorylation at that site. As a result, the mutant receptors no longer bind to one of the intracellular signaling proteins shown in Figure 16–29. The effect on the cell's response to the signal can then be determined. It is important that the mutant receptor is tested in a cell that does not have its own normal receptors for the signal molecule.

involve using DNA technology to introduce into cells a gene encoding a constantly active form of the protein, to see if this mimics the effect of the extracellular signal molecule. Consider Ras, for example. The mutant form of Ras involved in human cancers is constantly active because it has lost its ability to hydrolyze the bound GTP that keeps the Ras protein switched on. This continuously active form of Ras can stimulate some cells to proliferate, even in the absence of a proliferation signal.

Conversely, the activity of a specific signaling protein can be inhibited or eliminated. In the case of Ras, for example, one could shut down the expression of the *Ras* gene in cells by RNA interference or CRISPR (see Figure 10–31). Such cells do not proliferate in response to extracellular mitogens, indicating the importance of normal Ras signaling in the proliferative response.

Making mutants

Another powerful strategy that scientists use to determine which proteins participate in cell signaling involves screening tens of thousands of animals—fruit flies or nematode worms, for example (discussed in Chapter 19)—to search for mutants in which a signaling

pathway is not functioning properly. By examining enough mutant animals, many of the genes that encode the proteins involved in a signaling pathway can be identified.

Such classical genetic screens can also help sort out the order in which intracellular signaling proteins act in a pathway. Suppose that a genetic screen uncovers a pair of new proteins, X and Y, involved in the Ras signaling pathway. To determine whether these proteins lie upstream or downstream of Ras, one could create cells that express an inactive, mutant form of each protein, and then ask whether these mutant cells can be "rescued" by the addition of a continuously active form of Ras. If the constantly active Ras overcomes the blockage created by the mutant protein, the protein must operate upstream of Ras in the pathway (**Figure 16–37A**). However, if Ras operates upstream of the protein, a constantly active Ras would be unable to transmit a signal past the obstruction caused by the disabled protein (**Figure 16–37B**). Through such experiments, even the most complex intracellular signaling pathways can be mapped out, one step at a time (**Figure 16–37C**).

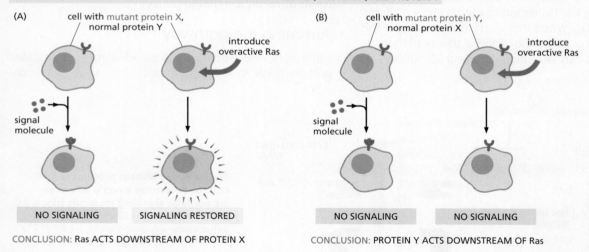

A SIGNALING PATHWAY IS FOUND TO INVOLVE THREE PROTEINS: Ras, PROTEIN X, AND PROTEIN Y

(A) cell with mutant protein X, normal protein Y — introduce overactive Ras

signal molecule

NO SIGNALING   SIGNALING RESTORED

CONCLUSION: Ras ACTS DOWNSTREAM OF PROTEIN X

(B) cell with mutant protein Y, normal protein X — introduce overactive Ras

signal molecule

NO SIGNALING   NO SIGNALING

CONCLUSION: PROTEIN Y ACTS DOWNSTREAM OF Ras

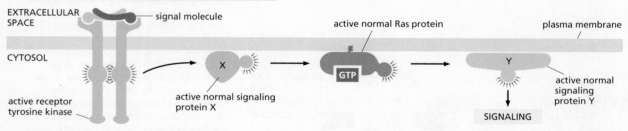

(C) DEDUCED ORDER OF PROTEINS IN SIGNALING PATHWAY

EXTRACELLULAR SPACE — signal molecule

active normal Ras protein

plasma membrane

CYTOSOL

X

GTP

Y

active receptor tyrosine kinase

active normal signaling protein X

active normal signaling protein Y

SIGNALING

Figure 16–37 The use of mutant cell lines and an overactive form of Ras can help dissect an intracellular signaling pathway. In this hypothetical pathway, Ras, protein X, and protein Y are required for proper signaling. (A) In cells in which protein X has been inactivated, signaling does not occur. However, this signaling blockage can be overcome by the addition of an overactive form of Ras, such that the pathway is active even in the absence of the extracellular signal molecule. This result indicates that Ras acts downstream of protein X in the pathway. (B) Signaling is also disrupted in cells in which protein Y has been inactivated. In this case, introduction of an overactive Ras does not restore normal signaling, indicating that protein Y operates downstream of Ras. (C) Based on these results, the deduced order of the signaling pathway is shown.

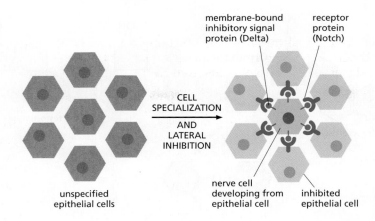

Figure 16–38 Notch signaling controls nerve-cell production in the fruit fly *Drosophila*. The fly nervous system originates in the embryo from a sheet of epithelial cells. Isolated cells in this sheet begin to specialize as neurons (*blue*), while their neighbors remain non-neuronal and maintain the structure of the epithelial sheet. The signals that control this process are transmitted via direct cell–cell contacts: each future neuron delivers an inhibitory signal to the cells next to it, deterring them from specializing as neurons too—a process called lateral inhibition. Both the signal molecule (Delta) and the receptor molecule (Notch) are transmembrane proteins, and the pathway represents a form of contact-dependent signaling (see Figure 16–3D).

Some Receptors Activate a Fast Track to the Nucleus

Not all receptors trigger complex signaling cascades that use multiple components to carry a message to the nucleus. Some take a more direct route to control gene expression. One such receptor is the protein Notch. Notch is a crucially important receptor in all animals, both during development and in adults. Among other things, it controls the development of neural cells in *Drosophila* (**Figure 16–38**).

In this simple signaling pathway, the receptor itself acts as a transcription regulator. When activated by the binding of Delta, a transmembrane signal protein on the surface of a neighboring cell, the Notch receptor is cleaved. This cleavage releases the cytosolic tail of the receptor, which is then free to move to the nucleus, where it helps to activate the appropriate set of Notch-responsive genes (**Figure 16–39**).

Some Extracellular Signal Molecules Cross the Plasma Membrane and Bind to Intracellular Receptors

Another direct route to the nucleus is taken by extracellular signal molecules that rely on intracellular receptor proteins (see Figure 16–4B). These molecules include the **steroid hormones**—*cortisol*, *estradiol*, and *testosterone*—and the thyroid hormones such as *thyroxine* (**Figure 16–40**). All of these hydrophobic molecules pass through the plasma membrane

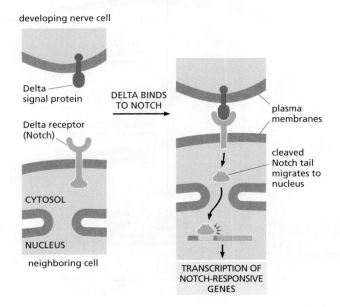

Figure 16–39 The Notch receptor itself is a transcription regulator. When the membrane-bound signal protein Delta binds to its receptor, Notch, on a neighboring cell, the receptor is cleaved by a protease. The released part of the cytosolic tail of Notch migrates to the nucleus, where it activates Notch-responsive genes. One consequence of this signaling process is shown in Figure 16–38.

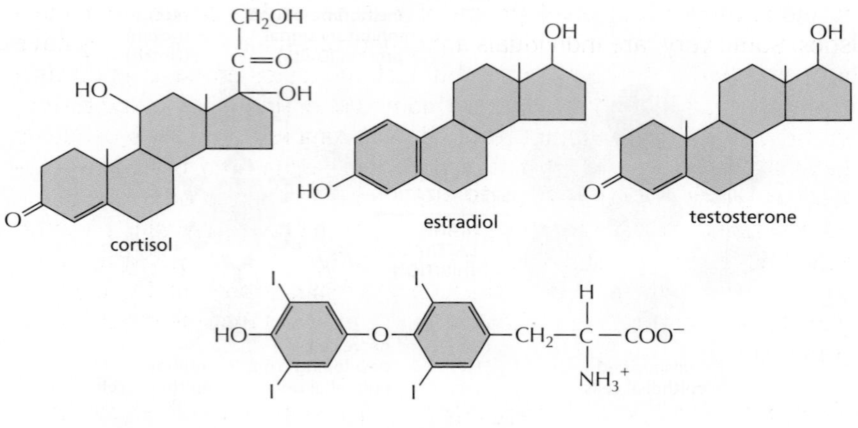

Figure 16–40 Some small, hydrophobic hormones bind to intracellular receptors that act as transcription regulators. Although these signal molecules differ in their chemical structures and functions, they all act by binding to intracellular receptor proteins that act as transcription regulators. Their receptors are not identical, but they are evolutionarily related, belonging to the *nuclear receptor superfamily.* The sites of origin and functions of these hormones are given in Table 16–1 (p. 536).

cortisol

estradiol

testosterone

thyroxine

of the target cell and bind to receptor proteins located in either the cytosol or the nucleus. Regardless of their initial location, these intracellular receptor proteins are referred to as **nuclear receptors** because, when activated by hormone binding, they enter the nucleus, where they regulate the transcription of genes. In unstimulated cells, nuclear receptors are typically present in an inactive form. When a hormone binds, the receptor undergoes a large conformational change that activates the protein, allowing it to promote or inhibit the transcription of specific target genes (**Figure 16–41**). Each hormone binds to a different nuclear receptor, and each receptor acts at a different set of regulatory sites in DNA (discussed in Chapter 8). Moreover, a given hormone usually regulates different sets of genes in different cell types, thereby evoking different physiological responses in different target cells.

Nuclear receptors and the hormones that activate them have essential roles in human physiology (see Table 16–1, p. 536). Loss of these signaling systems can have dramatic consequences, as illustrated by the effects of mutations that eliminate the receptor for the male sex hormone testosterone. Testosterone in humans shapes the formation of the external genitalia and influences brain development in the fetus; at puberty, the

Figure 16–41 The steroid hormone cortisol acts by activating a transcription regulator. Cortisol is one of the hormones produced by the adrenal glands in response to stress. It crosses the plasma membrane of a target cell and binds to its receptor protein, which is located in the cytosol. The receptor–hormone complex is then transported into the nucleus via the nuclear pores. Cortisol binding activates the receptor protein, which is then able to bind to specific regulatory sequences in DNA and activate (or repress, not shown) the transcription of specific target genes. Whereas the receptors for cortisol and some other steroid hormones are located in the cytosol, those for other steroid hormones and for thyroid hormones are already bound to DNA in the nucleus even in the absence of hormone.

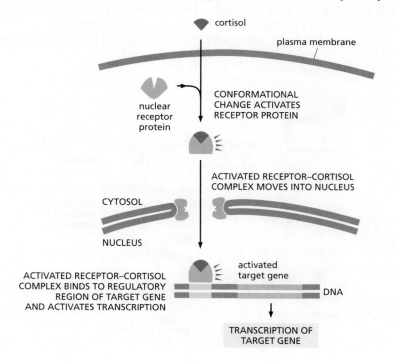

hormone triggers the development of male secondary sexual characteristics. Some very rare individuals are genetically male—that is, they have both an X and a Y chromosome—but lack the testosterone receptor as a result of a mutation in the corresponding gene; thus, they make testosterone, but their cells cannot respond to it. As a result, these individuals develop as females, which is the path that sexual and brain development would take if no male or female hormones were produced. Such a sex reversal demonstrates the crucial role of the testosterone receptor in sexual development, and it also shows that the receptor is required not just in one cell type to mediate one effect of testosterone, but in many cell types to help produce the whole range of features that distinguish men from women.

Plants Make Use of Receptors and Signaling Strategies That Differ from Those Used by Animals

Plants and animals have been evolving independently for more than a billion years, the last common ancestor being a single-celled eukaryote that most likely lived on its own. Because these kingdoms diverged so long ago—when it was still "every cell for itself"—each has evolved its own molecular solutions to the complex problem of becoming multicellular. Thus the mechanisms for cell–cell communication in plants and animals are in some ways quite different. At the same time, however, plants and animals started with a common set of eukaryotic genes—including some used by single-celled organisms to communicate among themselves—so their signaling systems also show some similarities.

Like animals, plants make extensive use of transmembrane cell-surface receptors—especially enzyme-coupled receptors. The spindly weed *Arabidopsis thaliana* (see Figure 1–33) has hundreds of genes encoding **receptor serine/threonine kinases**. These are, however, structurally distinct from the receptor serine/threonine kinases found in animal cells (which we do not discuss in this chapter). The plant receptors are thought to play an important part in a large variety of cell signaling processes, including those governing plant growth, development, and disease resistance. In contrast to animal cells, plant cells seem not to use RTKs, steroid-hormone-type nuclear receptors, or cyclic AMP, and they seem to use few GPCRs.

One of the best-studied signaling systems in plants mediates the response of cells to ethylene—a gaseous hormone that regulates a diverse array of developmental processes, including seed germination and fruit ripening. Tomato growers use ethylene to ripen their fruit, even after it has been picked. Although ethylene receptors are not evolutionarily related to any of the classes of receptor proteins that we have discussed so far, they function as enzyme-coupled receptors. Surprisingly, it is the empty receptor that is active: in the absence of ethylene, the empty receptor activates an associated protein kinase that ultimately shuts off the ethylene-responsive genes in the nucleus; when ethylene is present, the receptor and kinase are inactive, and the ethylene-responsive genes are transcribed (**Figure 16–42**). This strategy, whereby signals act to relieve transcriptional inhibition, is commonly used in plants.

Protein Kinase Networks Integrate Information to Control Complex Cell Behaviors

Whether part of a plant or an animal, a cell receives messages from many sources, and it must integrate this information to generate an appropriate response: to live or die, to divide, to differentiate, to change shape, to move, to send out a chemical message of its own, and so on (see Figure

Figure 16–42 The ethylene signaling pathway turns on genes by relieving inhibition. (A) In the absence of ethylene, the receptor directly activates an associated protein kinase, which then indirectly promotes the destruction of the transcription regulator that switches on ethylene-responsive genes. As a result, the genes remain turned off. (B) In the presence of ethylene, the receptor and kinase are both inactive, and the transcription regulator remains intact and stimulates the transcription of the ethylene-responsive genes. The kinase that ethylene receptors interact with is a serine/threonine kinase that is closely related to the MAP kinase kinase kinase found in animal cells (see Figure 16–31). Note that the ethylene receptor is located in the endoplasmic reticulum; because ethylene is hydrophobic, it passes easily into the cell interior to reach its receptor.

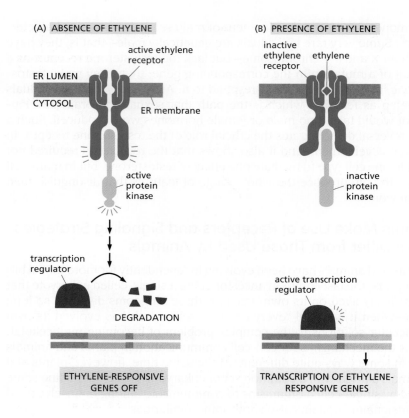

16–6, Movie 16.8, and Movie 16.9). This integration is made possible by connections and interactions that occur between different signaling pathways. Such cross-talk allows the cell to bring together multiple streams of information and react to a rich combination of signals.

The most extensive links among the pathways are mediated by the protein kinases present in each. These kinases often phosphorylate, and hence regulate, components in other signaling pathways, in addition to components in their own pathway (see Figure 16–35). To give an idea of the scale of the complexity, genome sequencing studies suggest that about 2% of our ~19,000 protein-coding genes code for protein kinases; moreover, hundreds of distinct types of protein kinases are thought to be present in a single mammalian cell.

Many intracellular signaling proteins have several potential phosphorylation sites, each of which can be phosphorylated by a different protein kinase. These proteins can thus act as integrating devices. Information received from different intracellular signaling pathways can converge on such proteins, which then convert a multicomponent input to a single outgoing signal (Figure 16–43, and see Figure 16–9). These integrating proteins, in turn, can deliver a signal to many downstream targets. In this way, the intracellular signaling system may act like a network of nerve cells in the brain—or like a collection of microprocessors in a computer—interpreting complex information and generating complex responses.

Our understanding of these intricate networks is still evolving: we are still discovering new links in the chains, new signaling partners, new connections, and even new pathways. Unraveling the intracellular signaling pathways—in both animals and plants—is one of the most active areas of research in cell biology, and new discoveries are being made every day. Genome sequencing projects continue to provide long lists of components involved in signal transduction in a large variety of organisms. Yet even if we could identify every single component in this elaborate

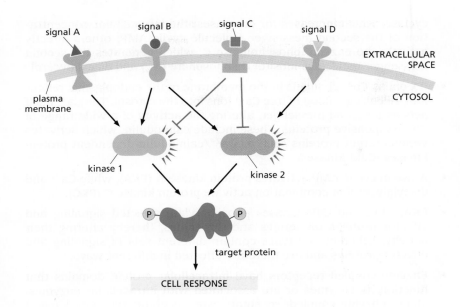

Figure 16–43 Intracellular signaling proteins serve to integrate incoming signals. Extracellular signals A, B, C, and D activate different receptors in the plasma membrane. The receptors act upon two protein kinases, which they either activate (*black* arrow) or inhibit (*red* crossbar). The kinases phosphorylate the same target protein and, when it is fully phosphorylated, this target protein triggers a cell response.

It can be seen that signal molecule B activates both protein kinases and therefore produces a strong output response. Signals A and D each activate a different kinase and therefore produce a response only if they are simultaneously present. Signal molecule C inhibits the cell response and will compete with the other signal molecules. The net outcome will depend both on the numbers of signaling molecules and the strengths of their connections. In a real cell, these parameters would be determined by evolution.

network of signaling pathways, it will remain a major challenge to figure out exactly how they all work together to allow cells—and organisms—to integrate the diverse array of information that inundates them constantly and to respond in a way that enhances their ability to adapt and survive.

ESSENTIAL CONCEPTS

- Cells in multicellular organisms communicate through a huge variety of extracellular chemical signals.

- In animals, hormones are carried in the blood to distant target cells, but most other extracellular signal molecules act over only a short distance. Neighboring cells often communicate through direct cell–cell contact.

- For an extracellular signal molecule to influence a target cell it must interact with a receptor protein on or in the target cell. Each receptor protein recognizes a particular signal molecule.

- Most extracellular signal molecules bind to cell-surface receptor proteins that convert (transduce) the extracellular signal into different intracellular signals, which are usually organized into signaling pathways.

- There are three main classes of cell-surface receptors: (1) ion-channel-coupled receptors, (2) G-protein-coupled receptors (GPCRs), and (3) enzyme-coupled receptors.

- GPCRs and enzyme-coupled receptors respond to extracellular signals by activating one or more intracellular signaling pathways, which, in turn, activate effector proteins that alter the behavior of the cell.

- Turning off signaling pathways is as important as turning them on. Each activated component in a signaling pathway must be subsequently inactivated or removed for the pathway to function again.

- GPCRs activate trimeric GTP-binding proteins called G proteins; these act as molecular switches, transmitting the signal onward for a short period before switching themselves off by hydrolyzing their bound GTP to GDP.

- G proteins directly regulate ion channels or enzymes in the plasma membrane. Some directly activate (or inactivate) the enzyme adenylyl cyclase, which increases (or decreases) the intracellular concentration of the second messenger molecule cyclic AMP; others directly activate the enzyme phospholipase C, which generates the second messenger molecules inositol trisphosphate (IP$_3$) and diacylglycerol.

- IP$_3$ opens Ca^{2+} channels in the membrane of the endoplasmic reticulum, releasing a flood of free Ca^{2+} ions into the cytosol. The Ca^{2+} itself acts as a second messenger, altering the activity of a wide range of Ca^{2+}-responsive proteins. These include calmodulin, which activates various target proteins such as Ca^{2+}/calmodulin-dependent protein kinases (CaM-kinases).

- A rise in cyclic AMP activates protein kinase A (PKA), while Ca^{2+} and diacylglycerol in combination activate protein kinase C (PKC).

- PKA, PKC, and CaM-kinases phosphorylate selected signaling and effector proteins on serines and threonines, thereby altering their activity. Different cell types contain different sets of signaling and effector proteins and are therefore affected in different ways.

- Enzyme-coupled receptors have intracellular protein domains that function as enzymes or are associated with intracellular enzymes. Many enzyme-coupled receptors are receptor tyrosine kinases (RTKs), which phosphorylate themselves and selected intracellular signaling proteins on tyrosines. The phosphotyrosines on RTKs then serve as docking sites for various intracellular signaling proteins.

- Most RTKs activate the monomeric GTPase Ras, which, in turn, activates a three-protein MAP-kinase signaling module that helps relay the signal from the plasma membrane to the nucleus.

- Ras mutations stimulate cell proliferation by keeping Ras (and, consequently, the Ras–MAP kinase signaling pathway) constantly active and are a common feature of many human cancers.

- Some RTKs stimulate cell growth and cell survival by activating PI 3-kinase, which phosphorylates specific inositol phospholipids in the cytosolic leaflet of the plasma membrane lipid bilayer. This inositol phosphorylation creates lipid docking sites that attract specific signaling proteins from the cytosol, including the protein kinase Akt, which becomes active and relays the signal onward.

- Other receptors, such as Notch, have a direct pathway to the nucleus. When activated, part of the receptor migrates from the plasma membrane to the nucleus, where it regulates the transcription of specific genes.

- Some extracellular signal molecules, such as steroid hormones and nitric oxide, are small or hydrophobic enough to cross the plasma membrane and activate intracellular proteins, which are usually either transcription regulators or enzymes.

- Plants, like animals, use enzyme-coupled cell-surface receptors to recognize the extracellular signal molecules that control their growth and development; these receptors often act by relieving the transcriptional repression of specific genes.

- Different intracellular signaling pathways interact, enabling each cell type to produce the appropriate response to a combination of extracellular signals. In the absence of such signals, most animal cells have been programmed to kill themselves by undergoing apoptosis.

- We are far from understanding how a cell integrates all of the many extracellular signals that bombard it to generate an appropriate response.

KEY TERMS

adaptation	GTP-binding protein	phosphoinositide 3-kinase
adenylyl cyclase	hormone	(PI 3-kinase)
Ca^{2+}/calmodulin-dependent	inositol 1,4,5-trisphosphate	phospholipase C
protein kinase (CaM-kinase)	(IP_3)	protein kinase
calmodulin	inositol phospholipid	protein kinase C (PKC)
cell signaling	intracellular signaling pathway	protein phosphatase
cyclic AMP	ion-channel-coupled receptor	Ras
cyclic-AMP-dependent	local mediator	receptor
protein kinase (PKA)	MAP kinase	receptor serine/threonine kinase
diacylglycerol (DAG)	MAP-kinase signaling module	receptor tyrosine kinase (RTK)
enzyme-coupled receptor	molecular switch	serine/threonine kinase
extracellular signal molecule	monomeric GTPase	signal transduction
G protein	neurotransmitter	steroid hormone
G-protein-coupled receptor	nitric oxide (NO)	tyrosine kinase
(GPCR)	nuclear receptor	

QUESTIONS

QUESTION 16–8

Which of the following statements are correct? Explain your answers.

A. The extracellular signal molecule acetylcholine has different effects on different cell types in an animal and often binds to different cell-surface receptor molecules on different cell types.

B. After acetylcholine is secreted from cells, it is long-lived, because it has to reach target cells all over the body.

C. Both the GTP-bound α subunits and nucleotide-free βγ complexes—but not GDP-bound, fully assembled G proteins—can activate other molecules downstream of GPCRs.

D. IP_3 is produced directly by cleavage of an inositol phospholipid without incorporation of an additional phosphate group.

E. Calmodulin regulates the intracellular Ca^{2+} concentration.

F. Different signals originating from the plasma membrane can be integrated by cross-talk between different signaling pathways inside the cell.

G. Tyrosine phosphorylation serves to build binding sites for other proteins to bind to RTKs.

QUESTION 16–9

The Ras protein functions as a molecular switch that is set to its "on" state by other proteins that cause it to release its bound GDP and bind GTP. A GTPase-activating protein helps reset the switch to the "off" state by inducing Ras to hydrolyze its bound GTP to GDP much more rapidly than it would without this encouragement. Thus, Ras works like a light switch that one person turns on and another turns off. You are studying a mutant cell that lacks the GTPase-activating protein. What abnormalities would you expect to find in the way in which Ras activity responds to extracellular signals?

QUESTION 16–10

A. Compare and contrast signaling by neurons, which secrete neurotransmitters at synapses, with signaling carried out by endocrine cells, which secrete hormones into the blood.

B. Discuss the relative advantages of the two mechanisms.

QUESTION 16–11

Two intracellular molecules, X and Y, are both normally synthesized at a constant rate of 1000 molecules per second per cell. Molecule X is broken down slowly: each molecule of X survives on average for 100 seconds. Molecule Y is broken down 10 times faster: each molecule of Y survives on average for 10 seconds.

A. Calculate how many molecules of X and Y the cell contains at any time.

B. If the rates of synthesis of both X and Y are suddenly increased tenfold to 10,000 molecules per second per cell—without any change in their degradation rates—how many molecules of X and Y will there be after one second?

C. Which molecule would be preferred for rapid signaling?

QUESTION 16–12

In a series of experiments, genes that code for mutant forms of an RTK are introduced into cells. The cells also express their own normal form of the receptor from their normal gene, although the mutant genes are constructed so that the mutant RTK is expressed at considerably higher concentration than the normal RTK. What would be the consequences of introducing a mutant gene that codes for an RTK (A) lacking its extracellular domain, or (B) lacking its intracellular domain?

QUESTION 16–13

Discuss the following statement: "Membrane proteins that span the membrane many times can undergo a conformational change upon ligand binding that can be sensed on the other side of the membrane. Thus, individual protein molecules can transmit a signal across a membrane. In contrast, individual single-span membrane proteins cannot transmit a conformational change across the membrane but require oligomerization."

QUESTION 16–14

What are the similarities and differences between the reactions that lead to the activation of G proteins and the reactions that lead to the activation of Ras?

QUESTION 16–15

Why do you suppose cells use Ca^{2+} (which is kept by Ca^{2+} pumps at a cytosolic concentration of 10^{-7} M) for intracellular signaling and not another ion such as Na^+ (which is kept by the Na^+ pump at a cytosolic concentration of 10^{-3} M)?

QUESTION 16–16

It seems counterintuitive that a cell, having a perfectly abundant supply of nutrients available, would commit suicide if not constantly stimulated by signals from other cells (see Figure 16–6). What do you suppose might be the advantages of such regulation?

QUESTION 16–17

The contraction of the myosin–actin system in cardiac muscle cells is triggered by a rise in intracellular Ca^{2+}. Cardiac muscle cells have specialized Ca^{2+} channels—called ryanodine receptors because of their sensitivity to the drug ryanodine—that are embedded in the membrane of the sarcoplasmic reticulum, a specialized form of the endoplasmic reticulum. In contrast to the IP_3-gated Ca^{2+} channels in the endoplasmic reticulum shown in Figure 16–23, the signaling molecule that opens ryanodine receptors is Ca^{2+} itself. Discuss the consequences of this feature of ryanodine channels for cardiac muscle cell contraction.

QUESTION 16–18

Two protein kinases, K1 and K2, function in an intracellular signaling pathway. If either kinase contains a mutation that permanently inactivates its function, no response is seen in cells when an extracellular signal is received. A different mutation in K1 makes it permanently active, so that in cells containing that mutation, a response is observed even in the absence of an extracellular signal. You characterize a double-mutant cell that contains K2 with the inactivating mutation and K1 with the activating mutation. You observe that the response is seen even in the absence of an extracellular signal. In the normal signaling pathway, does K1 activate K2 or does K2 activate K1? Explain your answer.

QUESTION 16–19

A. Trace the steps of a long and indirect signaling pathway from a cell-surface receptor to a change in gene expression in the nucleus.

B. Compare this pathway with an example of a short and direct pathway from the cell surface to the nucleus.

QUESTION 16–20

How does PI 3-kinase activate the Akt kinase after activation of an RTK?

QUESTION 16–21

Consider the structure of cholesterol, a small, hydrophobic molecule with a sterol backbone similar to that of three of the hormones shown in Figure 16–40, but possessing fewer polar groups such as –OH, =O, and –COO⁻. If cholesterol were not normally found in cell membranes, could it be used effectively as a hormone if an appropriate intracellular receptor evolved?

QUESTION 16–22

The signaling mechanisms used by a steroid-hormone-type nuclear receptor and by an ion-channel-coupled receptor are relatively simple as they have few components. Can they lead to an amplification of the initial signal, and, if so, how?

QUESTION 16–23

If some cell-surface receptors, including Notch, can rapidly signal to the nucleus by activating latent transcription regulators at the plasma membrane, why do most cell-surface receptors use long, indirect signaling cascades to influence gene transcription in the nucleus?

QUESTION 16–24

Animal cells and plant cells have some very different intracellular signaling mechanisms but also share some common mechanisms. Why do you think this is so?

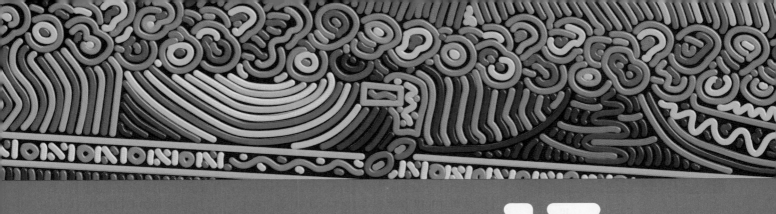

Cytoskeleton

The ability of eukaryotic cells to organize the many components in their interior, adopt a variety of shapes, interact mechanically with the environment, and carry out coordinated movements depends on the **cytoskeleton**—an intricate network of protein filaments that extends throughout the cytoplasm (**Figure 17–1**). This filamentous architecture helps to support the large volume of cytoplasm, a function that is particularly important in animal cells, which have no cell walls. Although some cytoskeletal components are present in bacteria, the cytoskeleton is most prominent in the large and structurally complex eukaryotic cell.

Unlike our own bony skeleton, however, the cytoskeleton is a highly dynamic structure that is continuously reorganized as a cell changes shape, divides, and responds to its environment. The cytoskeleton is not only the "bones" of a cell but its "muscles" too, and it is directly responsible for large-scale movements, including the crawling of cells along a surface, the contraction of muscle cells, and the changes in cell shape that take place as an embryo develops. Without the cytoskeleton, wounds would never heal, muscles would not contract, and sperm would never reach the egg.

While the interior of the eukaryotic cell is dynamic, it is also highly organized, with organelles that carry out specialized functions concentrated in different areas and linked by transport systems (discussed in Chapter 15). It is the cytoskeleton that controls the location of the organelles and provides the machinery for transport between them. A cytoskeletal machine is also responsible for the segregation of chromosomes into two daughter cells at cell division and for pinching apart those two new cells, as we discuss in Chapter 18.

INTERMEDIATE FILAMENTS

MICROTUBULES

ACTIN FILAMENTS

MUSCLE CONTRACTION

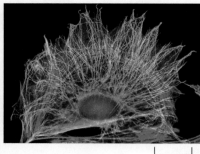

10 μm

Figure 17–1 The cytoskeleton gives a cell its shape and allows the cell to organize its internal components and to move. An animal cell in culture has been labeled to show two of its major cytoskeletal systems, the microtubules (*green*) and the actin filaments (*red*). Where the two filaments overlap, they appear *yellow*. The DNA in the nucleus is labeled in *blue*. (Courtesy of Albert Tousson.)

The cytoskeleton is built on a framework of three types of protein filaments: *intermediate filaments*, *microtubules*, and *actin filaments*. Each type of filament has distinct mechanical properties and is formed from a different protein subunit. A family of fibrous proteins forms the intermediate filaments; globular *tubulin* subunits form microtubules; and globular *actin* subunits form actin filaments (Figure 17–2). In each case, thousands of these subunits assemble into fine threads that sometimes extend across the entire cell.

In this chapter, we consider the structure and function of each of these protein filament networks. We begin with intermediate filaments, which provide cells with mechanical strength. We then see how microtubules organize the cytoplasm of eukaryotic cells and form the hairlike, motile appendages that enable cells like protozoa and sperm to swim. We next consider how the actin cytoskeleton supports the cell surface and allows fibroblasts and other cells to crawl. Finally, we discuss how the actin cytoskeleton enables our muscles to contract.

Figure 17–2 The three types of protein filaments that form the cytoskeleton differ in their composition, mechanical properties, and roles inside the cell. They are shown here in epithelial cells, but they are all found in almost all animal cells.

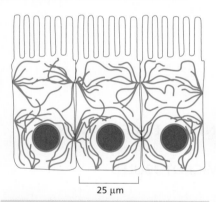

25 μm

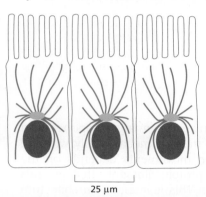

25 μm

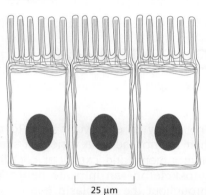

25 μm

| INTERMEDIATE FILAMENTS | MICROTUBULES | ACTIN FILAMENTS |

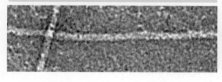

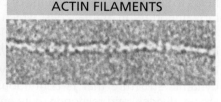

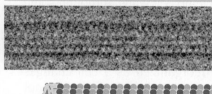

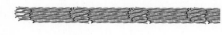

25 nm

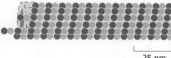

25 nm

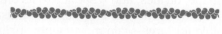

25 nm

Intermediate filaments are ropelike fibers with a diameter of about 10 nm; they are made of fibrous intermediate filament proteins. One type of intermediate filament forms a meshwork called the nuclear lamina just beneath the inner nuclear membrane. Other types extend across the cytoplasm, giving cells mechanical strength and distributing the mechanical stresses in an epithelial tissue by spanning the cytoplasm from one cell–cell junction to another. Intermediate filaments are very flexible and have great tensile strength. They deform under stress but do not rupture. (L. Norlen et al. *Exper. Cell Res.* 313:2217–2227, 2007. With permission from Elsevier.)

Microtubules are hollow cylinders made of the protein tubulin. They are long and straight and typically have one end attached to a single microtubule-organizing center called a *centrosome*. With an outer diameter of 25 nm, microtubules are more rigid than actin filaments or intermediate filaments, and they rupture when stretched. (Micrograph courtesy of Richard Wade.)

Actin filaments (also known as *microfilaments*) are helical polymers of the protein actin. They are flexible structures, with a diameter of about 7 nm, that are organized into a variety of linear bundles, two-dimensional networks, and three-dimensional gels. Although actin filaments are dispersed throughout the cell, they are most highly concentrated in the *cortex*, the layer of cytoplasm just beneath the plasma membrane. (Micrograph courtesy of Roger Craig.)

INTERMEDIATE FILAMENTS

Intermediate filaments have great strength, and their main function is to enable cells to withstand the mechanical stress that occurs when cells are stretched. The filaments are called "intermediate" because, in the smooth muscle cells where they were first discovered, their diameter (about 10 nm) is between that of the thinner actin filaments and the thicker *myosin filaments*. Intermediate filaments are the toughest and most durable of the cytoskeletal filaments: when cells are treated with concentrated salt solutions and nonionic detergents, the intermediate filaments survive, while most of the rest of the cytoskeleton is destroyed.

Intermediate filaments are found in the cytoplasm of most animal cells. They typically form a network throughout the cytoplasm, surrounding the nucleus and extending out to the cell periphery. There, they are often anchored to the plasma membrane at cell–cell junctions called *desmosomes* (discussed in Chapter 20), where the plasma membrane is connected to that of another cell (Figure 17–3). Intermediate filaments are also found within the nucleus of animal cells. There, they form a meshwork called the *nuclear lamina*, which underlies and strengthens the nuclear envelope. In this section, we see how the structure and assembly of intermediate filaments makes them particularly suited to strengthening cells and protecting them from tearing.

Intermediate Filaments Are Strong and Ropelike

An intermediate filament is like a rope in which many long strands are twisted together to provide tensile strength—an ability to withstand tension without breaking (Movie 17.1). The strands of this cable are made of intermediate filament proteins, fibrous subunits each containing a central elongated rod domain with distinct unstructured domains at either

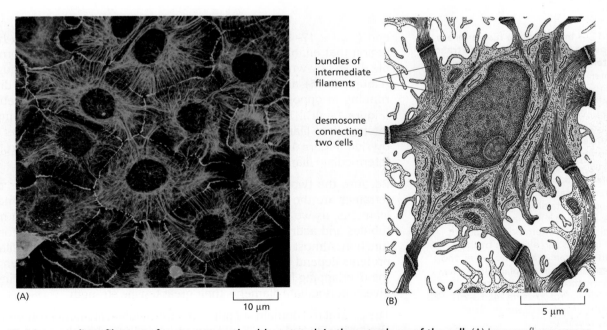

(A)

10 μm

bundles of
intermediate
filaments

desmosome
connecting
two cells

(B)

5 μm

Figure 17–3 Intermediate filaments form a strong, durable network in the cytoplasm of the cell. (A) Immunofluorescence micrograph of a sheet of epithelial cells in culture stained to show the lacelike network of intermediate keratin filaments (*blue*), which surround the nuclei and extend through the cytoplasm of the cells. The filaments in each cell are indirectly connected to those of neighboring cells through the desmosomes, establishing a continuous mechanical link from cell to cell throughout the epithelial sheet. A second protein (*red*) has been stained to show the locations of the cell boundaries. (B) Drawing from an electron micrograph of a section of a skin cell, showing the bundles of intermediate filaments that traverse the cytoplasm and are inserted at desmosomes. (A, from K.J. Green and C.A. Gaudry, *Nat. Rev. Mol. Cell. Biol.* 1:208–216, 2000. With permission from Macmillan Publishers Ltd; B, from R.V. Krstić, *Ultrastructure of the Mammalian Cell: An Atlas.* Berlin: Springer, 1979. With permission from Springer-Verlag.)

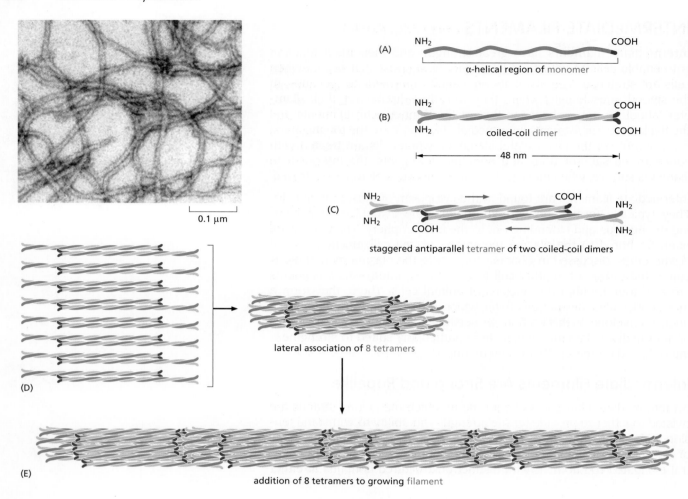

(A) α-helical region of monomer

NH₂ — COOH

(B) coiled-coil dimer

NH₂ — COOH
NH₂ — COOH

48 nm

(C) staggered antiparallel tetramer of two coiled-coil dimers

NH₂ — COOH
NH₂ — COOH
— NH₂
COOH — NH₂

(D) lateral association of 8 tetramers

(E) addition of 8 tetramers to growing filament

0.1 μm

Figure 17–4 Intermediate filaments are like ropes made of long, twisted strands of protein. (A) The intermediate filament monomer consists of an α-helical central rod domain shown with unstructured terminal domains at either end (not shown). The C-terminal end of the monomer is marked in *dark blue* to make its position within the assembled filament. (B) Pairs of monomers associate to form a dimer, and (C) two dimers then line up to form a staggered, antiparallel tetramer. (D) Tetramers can pack together into a helical array containing eight tetramer strands; (E) these in turn assemble into the final ropelike intermediate filament. These filaments can elongate by the addition of tetramer arrays to either end. An electron micrograph of intermediate filaments is shown on the upper left. (U. Aebi et al. *Protoplasma* 145:73–81, 1988. With permission from Springer Science and Business Media.)

end (**Figure 17–4A**). The rod domain consists of an extended α-helical region that enables pairs of intermediate filament proteins to form stable dimers by wrapping around each other in a coiled-coil configuration (**Figure 17–4B**), as described in Chapter 4. Two of these coiled-coil dimers, running in opposite directions, associate to form a staggered tetramer (**Figure 17–4C**). These dimers and tetramers are the soluble subunits of intermediate filaments. The tetramers associate with each other side-by-side (**Figure 17–4D**) and then assemble to generate the final ropelike intermediate filament (**Figure 17–4E**).

Because the two dimers point in opposite directions, both ends of the tetramer are the same, as are the two ends of assembled intermediate filaments; as we will see, this distinguishes these filaments from microtubules and actin filaments, whose structural polarity is crucial for their function. Almost all of the interactions between the intermediate filament proteins depend on noncovalent bonding; it is the combined strength of the overlapping lateral interactions along the length of the proteins that gives intermediate filaments their great tensile strength.

The central rod domains of different intermediate filament proteins are all similar in size and amino acid sequence, so that when they pack together they always form filaments of similar diameter and internal structure. By contrast, the terminal head and tail domains vary greatly in both size and amino acid sequence from one type of intermediate filament protein to another. These unstructured domains are exposed on the surface of the filament, where they allow it to interact with specific components in the cytoplasm.

Intermediate Filaments Strengthen Cells Against Mechanical Stress

Intermediate filaments are particularly prominent in the cytoplasm of cells that are subject to mechanical stress. They are present in large numbers, for example, along the length of nerve cell axons, providing essential internal reinforcement to these extremely long and fine cell extensions. They are also abundant in muscle cells and in epithelial cells such as those of the skin. In all these cells, intermediate filaments distribute the effects of locally applied forces, thereby keeping cells and their membranes from tearing in response to mechanical shear. A similar principle is used to strengthen composite materials such as fiberglass or reinforced concrete, in which tension-bearing linear elements such as carbon fibers (in fiberglass) or steel bars (in concrete) are embedded in a space-filling matrix to give the material strength.

Intermediate filaments can be grouped into four classes: (1) *keratin filaments* in epithelial cells; (2) *vimentin* and *vimentin-related filaments* in connective-tissue cells, muscle cells, and supporting cells of the nervous system (glial cells); (3) *neurofilaments* in nerve cells; and (4) *nuclear lamins*, which strengthen the nuclear envelope. The first three filament types are found in the cytoplasm, whereas the fourth is found in the nucleus (Figure 17–5). Filaments of each class are formed by polymerization of their corresponding intermediate filament subunits.

The **keratin filaments** are the most diverse class of intermediate filament. Every kind of epithelium in the vertebrate body—whether in the tongue, the cornea, or the lining of the gut—has its own distinctive mixture of keratin proteins. Specialized keratins also occur in hair, feathers, and claws. In each case, the keratin filaments are formed from a mixture of different keratin subunits. Keratin filaments typically span the interiors of epithelial cells from one side of the cell to the other, and filaments in adjacent epithelial cells are indirectly connected through desmosomes (see Figure 17–3B). The ends of the keratin filaments are anchored to the desmosomes, and the filaments associate laterally with other cell components through the globular head and tail domains that project from their surface. These strong cables, formed by the filaments throughout the epithelial sheet, distribute the stress that occurs when the skin is stretched. The importance of this function is illustrated by the rare human genetic disease *epidermolysis bullosa simplex*, in which mutations in the keratin genes interfere with the formation of keratin filaments in the epidermis. As a result, the skin is highly vulnerable to mechanical injury, and even a gentle pressure can rupture its cells, causing the skin to blister. The disease can be reproduced in transgenic mice expressing a mutant keratin gene in their skin (Figure 17–6).

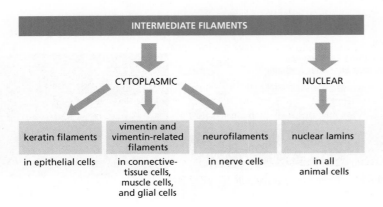

Figure 17–5 **Intermediate filaments are divided into four major classes.** These classes can include numerous subtypes. Humans, for example, have more than 50 keratin genes.

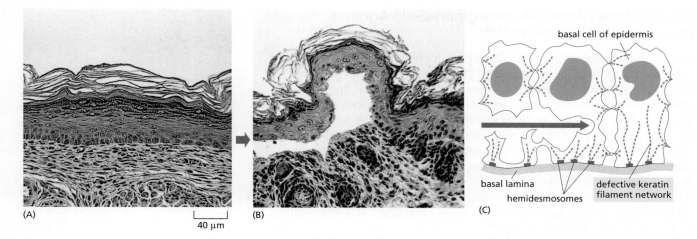

(A)

(B)

(C)

basal cell of epidermis

basal lamina

hemidesmosomes

defective keratin filament network

40 μm

Figure 17–6 A mutant form of keratin makes skin more prone to blistering. A mutant gene encoding a truncated keratin protein was introduced into a mouse. The defective protein assembles with the normal keratins and thereby disrupts the keratin filament network in the skin. (A) Light micrograph of a cross section of normal skin, which is resistant to mechanical pressure. (B) Cross section of skin from a mutant mouse showing the formation of a blister, which results from the rupturing of cells in the basal layer of the mutant epidermis (short *red* arrow). (C) A sketch of three cells in the basal layer of the mutant epidermis. As indicated by the *red arrow*, the cells rupture between the nucleus and the hemidesmosomes that connect the cells—via their keratin filaments—to the underlying basal lamina. (From P.A. Coulombe et al., *J. Cell Biol.* 115:1661–1674, 1991. With permission from The Rockefeller University Press.)

Defects in neurofilaments can also lead to disease. *Neurofilaments* are intermediate filaments that are found along the axons of vertebrate neurons, where they provide strength and stability to the long axons that nerve cells use to transmit information. The neurodegenerative disease amyotrophic lateral sclerosis (ALS, also known as Lou Gehrig's disease) is associated with an abnormal accumulation of neurofilaments in the cell bodies and axons of motor neurons. This accretion may precipitate the axon degeneration and muscle weakness seen in these patients.

The Nuclear Envelope Is Supported by a Meshwork of Intermediate Filaments

Whereas cytoplasmic intermediate filaments form ropelike structures, the intermediate filaments lining and strengthening the inside surface of the inner nuclear membrane are organized as a two-dimensional meshwork (**Figure 17–7**). As mentioned earlier, the intermediate filaments that form this tough **nuclear lamina** are constructed from a class of intermediate filament proteins called *lamins* (not to be confused with laminin, which is an extracellular matrix protein). The nuclear lamina disassembles and re-forms at each cell division, when the nuclear envelope breaks down during mitosis and then re-forms in each daughter cell (discussed in Chapter 18).

The collapse and reassembly of the nuclear lamina is controlled by the phosphorylation and dephosphorylation of the lamins. Phosphorylation of lamins by protein kinases (discussed in Chapter 4) weakens the interactions between the lamin tetramers and causes the filaments to fall apart. Dephosphorylation by protein phosphatases at the end of mitosis allows the lamins to reassemble (see Figure 18–30).

Figure 17–7 Intermediate filaments support and strengthen the nuclear envelope. (A) Schematic cross section through the nuclear envelope. The intermediate filaments of the nuclear lamina line the inner face of the nuclear envelope and are thought to provide attachment sites for the chromosomes. (B) Electron micrograph of a portion of the nuclear lamina from a frog egg. The lamina is formed from a lattice of intermediate filaments composed of lamins. The nuclear lamina in other cell types is not always as regularly organized as the one shown here. (B, from U. Aebi et al., *Nature* 323:560–564, 1986. With permission from Macmillan Publishers Ltd.)

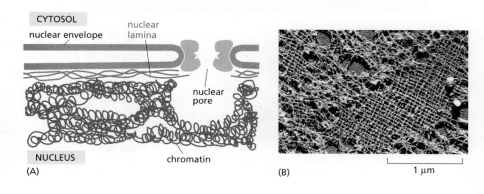

CYTOSOL

nuclear envelope

nuclear lamina

nuclear pore

NUCLEUS

chromatin

(A)

(B)

1 μm

Figure 17–8 **Defects in a nuclear lamin can cause a rare class of premature aging disorders called progeria.** (A) In a normal cell, the protein lamin A (*green*) is assembled into a uniform nuclear lamina inside the nuclear envelope. (B) In a cell with a lamin A mutant that is found in patients with progeria, the nuclear lamina is defective, resulting in structural defects in the nuclear envelope. (C) Children with progeria begin to show features of advanced aging early in life. (A and B, from P. Taimen et al., *Proc. Natl Acad. Sci. USA* 106:20788–20793, 2009. With permission from National Academy of Sciences; C, courtesy of The Progeria Research Foundation, www.progeriaresearch.org.)

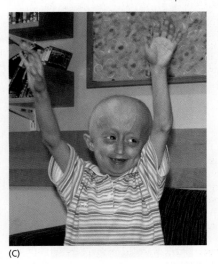

(A)   (B)   10 μm

(C)

Defects in a particular nuclear lamin are associated with certain types of *progeria*—rare disorders that cause affected individuals to age prematurely. Children with progeria have wrinkled skin, lose their teeth and hair, and often develop severe cardiovascular disease by the time they reach their teens (Figure 17–8). How the loss of a nuclear lamin could lead to this devastating condition is not yet clear, but it may be that the resulting nuclear instability leads to impaired cell division, increased cell death, a diminished capacity for tissue repair, or some combination of these. Because the nuclear lamina also helps properly position chromosomes, defects in lamins might also lead to altered chromosome movement and, ultimately, changes in gene expression.

Linker Proteins Connect Cytoskeletal Filaments and Bridge the Nuclear Envelope

Many intermediate filaments are further stabilized and reinforced by accessory proteins, such as *plectin*, that cross-link the filaments into bundles and connect them to microtubules, to actin filaments, and to adhesive structures in desmosomes (Figure 17–9). Mutations in the gene for plectin cause a devastating human disease that combines features of epidermolysis bullosa simplex (caused by disruption of skin keratin), muscular dystrophy (caused by disruption of intermediate filaments in muscle), and neurodegeneration (caused by disruption of neurofilaments). Mice lacking a functional plectin gene die within a few days of birth, with blistered skin and abnormal skeletal and heart muscle. Thus, although plectin may not be necessary for the initial formation of intermediate filaments, its cross-linking action is required to provide cells with the strength they need to withstand mechanical stress.

Plectin and other proteins also interact with protein complexes that link the cytoplasmic cytoskeleton to structures in the nuclear interior, including chromosomes and the nuclear lamina (Figure 17–10). These bridges, which span the nuclear envelope, mechanically couple the nucleus to the cytoskeleton, and they are involved in many processes, including the movement and positioning of the nucleus within the cell interior and the overall organization of the cytoskeleton.

QUESTION 17–1

Which of the following types of cells would you expect to contain a high density of intermediate filaments in their cytoplasm? Explain your answers.
A. *Amoeba proteus* (a free-living amoeba)
B. Skin epithelial cell
C. Smooth muscle cell in the digestive tract
D. *Escherichia coli*
E. Nerve cell in the spinal cord
F. Sperm cell
G. Plant cell

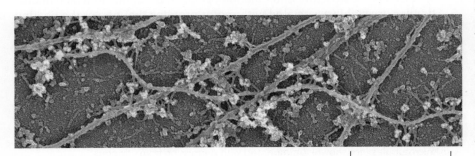

0.5 μm

Figure 17–9 **Plectin aids in the bundling of intermediate filaments and links these filaments to other cytoskeletal protein networks.** In this scanning electron micrograph of the cytoskeletal protein network from cultured fibroblasts, the actin filaments have been removed, and the plectin, intermediate filaments, and microtubules have been artificially colored. Note how the plectin (*orange*) links an intermediate filament (*blue*) to microtubules (*green*). The *yellow dots* are gold particles linked to antibodies that recognize plectin. (From T.M. Svitkina, A.B. Verkhovsky, and G.G. Borisy, *J. Cell Biol.* 135:991–1007, 1996. With permission from The Rockefeller University Press.)

Figure 17–10 Protein complexes bridge the nucleus and cytoplasm through the nuclear envelope. The cytoplasmic cytoskeleton is connected across the nuclear envelope to the nuclear lamina or chromosomes through sets of linker proteins of the SUN (*orange*) and KASH (*purple*) families.

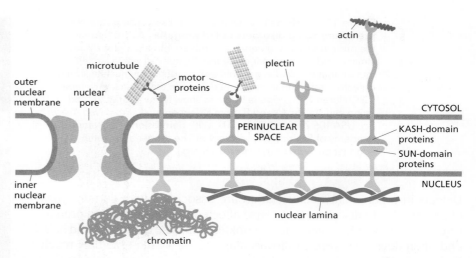

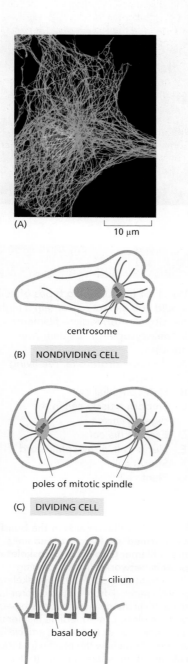

(A)

├── 10 µm

(B)   NONDIVIDING CELL

centrosome

(C)   DIVIDING CELL

poles of mitotic spindle

(D)   CILIATED CELL

cilium

basal body

MICROTUBULES

Microtubules have a crucial organizing role in all eukaryotic cells. These long and relatively stiff, hollow tubes of protein can rapidly disassemble in one location and reassemble in another. In a typical animal cell, microtubules grow out from a small structure near the center of the cell called the *centrosome* (**Figure 17–11A and B**). Extending out toward the cell periphery, they create a system of tracks within the cell, along which vesicles, organelles, and other cell components can be transported. These cytoplasmic microtubules are the part of the cytoskeleton mainly responsible for transporting and positioning membrane-enclosed organelles within the cell and for guiding the intracellular transport of various cytosolic macromolecules.

When a cell enters mitosis, the cytoplasmic microtubules disassemble and then reassemble into an intricate structure called the *mitotic spindle*. As we discuss in Chapter 18, the mitotic spindle provides the machinery that will segregate the chromosomes equally into the two daughter cells just before a cell divides (**Figure 17–11C**). Microtubules can also form stable structures, such as rhythmically beating *cilia* and *flagella* (**Figure 17–11D**). These hairlike structures extend from the surface of many eukaryotic cells, which use them either to swim or to sweep fluid over their surface. The core of a eukaryotic cilium or flagellum consists of a highly organized and stable bundle of microtubules. (Bacterial flagella have an entirely different structure and allow the cells to swim by a very different mechanism.)

In this section, we first consider the structure and assembly of microtubules. We then discuss their role in organizing the cytoplasm—an ability that depends on their association with accessory proteins, especially the *motor proteins* that propel organelles along cytoskeletal tracks. Finally, we discuss the structure and function of cilia and flagella, in which microtubules are stably associated with motor proteins that power the beating of these mobile appendages.

Figure 17–11 Microtubules usually grow out from an organizing center. (A) Fluorescence micrograph of a cytoplasmic array of microtubules in a cultured fibroblast. Unlike intermediate filaments, microtubules (*green*) extend from organizing centers such as (B) a centrosome, (C) the two poles of a mitotic spindle, or (D) the basal body of a cilium. They can also grow from fragments of existing microtubules (not shown). (A, reprinted with permission from Olympus Corporation of the Americas Scientific Solutions Group.)

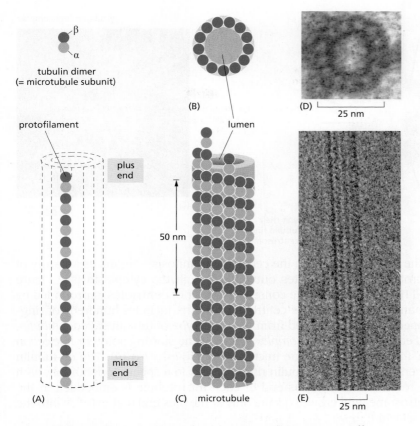

Figure 17–12 Microtubules are hollow tubes made of globular tubulin subunits. (A) One tubulin subunit (an αβ dimer) and one protofilament are shown schematically, together with their position within a microtubule. Note that the tubulin dimers in the protofilament are all arranged with the same orientation. (B and C) Schematic diagrams of a microtubule, showing how tubulin dimers pack together in the microtubule wall. At the top, 13 β-tubulin molecules are shown in cross section. Below this, a side view of a short section of a microtubule shows how the dimers are aligned in the same orientation in all the protofilaments; thus, the microtubule has a definite structural polarity—with a designated plus and a minus end. (D) Electron micrograph of a cross section of a microtubule with its ring of 13 distinct subunits, each of which corresponds to a separate tubulin dimer. (E) Electron micrograph of a microtubule viewed lengthwise. (D, courtesy of Richard Linck; E, courtesy of Richard Wade.)

Microtubules Are Hollow Tubes with Structurally Distinct Ends

Microtubules are built from subunits—molecules of **tubulin**—each of which is a dimer composed of two very similar globular proteins called α-tubulin and β-tubulin, bound tightly together by noncovalent interactions. The tubulin dimers stack together, again by noncovalent bonding, to form the wall of the hollow, cylindrical microtubule. This tubelike structure is made of 13 parallel protofilaments, each a linear chain of tubulin dimers with α- and β-tubulin alternating along its length (**Figure 17–12**). Each protofilament has a structural **polarity**, with α-tubulin exposed at one end and β-tubulin at the other, and this polarity is the same for all the protofilaments in the microfilament. Thus the microtubule as a whole has a structural polarity: the end with β-tubulin showing is called its *plus end*, and the opposite end, which contains exposed α-tubulin, is called the *minus end*.

In a concentrated solution of pure tubulin in a test tube, tubulin dimers will add to either end of a growing microtubule. However, they add more rapidly to the plus end than to the minus end, which is why the ends were originally named this way—not because they are electrically charged. The polarity of the microtubule—the fact that its structure has a definite direction, with the two ends being chemically and functionally distinct—is crucial, both for the assembly of microtubules and for their role once they are formed. If microtubules had no polarity, they could not, for example, guide directional intracellular transport.

The Centrosome Is the Major Microtubule-organizing Center in Animal Cells

Inside cells, microtubules grow from specialized organizing centers that control the location, number, and orientation of the microtubules. In most animal cells, for example, the **centrosome**—which is typically close

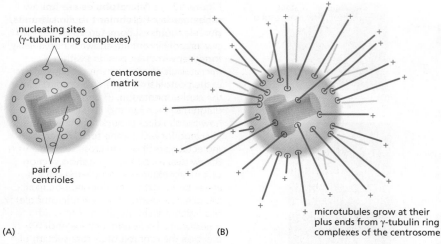

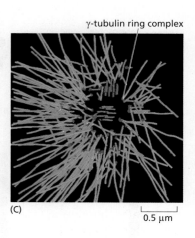

γ-tubulin ring complex

(C)

0.5 μm

nucleating sites
(γ-tubulin ring complexes)

centrosome
matrix

pair of
centrioles

(A)

(B)

+ microtubules grow at their
plus ends from γ-tubulin ring
complexes of the centrosome

Figure 17–13 Tubulin polymerizes from nucleation sites on a centrosome.
(A) Schematic drawing showing that an animal cell centrosome consists of an amorphous matrix of various proteins, including the γ-tubulin rings (*red*) that nucleate microtubule growth, surrounding a pair of centrioles, oriented at right angles to each other. Each member of the centriole pair is made up of a cylindrical array of short microtubules. (B) Diagram of a centrosome with attached microtubules. The minus end of each microtubule is embedded in the centrosome, having grown from a γ-tubulin ring complex, whereas the plus end of each microtubule extends into the cytoplasm. (C) An image of a centrosome, reconstructed from serial sections of a *Caenorhabditis elegans* cell, showing a dense thicket of microtubules (*green*) emanating from γ-tubulin ring complexes (*red*). A pair of centrioles, themselves made of short microtubules (*blue*), can be seen at the center. (C, from E.T. O'Toole et al., *J. Cell Biol.* 163:451–456, 2003. With permission from The Rockefeller University Press.)

to the cell nucleus when the cell is not in mitosis—organizes an array of microtubules that radiates outward through the cytoplasm (see Figure 17–11B). The centrosome consists of a pair of **centrioles**, surrounded by a matrix of proteins. The centrosome matrix includes hundreds of ring-shaped structures formed from a special type of tubulin called *γ-tubulin*, and each *γ-tubulin ring complex* serves as the starting point, or *nucleation site*, for the growth of one microtubule (**Figure 17–13A**). The αβ-tubulin dimers add to each γ-tubulin ring complex in a specific orientation, with the result that the minus end of each microtubule is embedded in the centrosome, and growth occurs only at the plus end that extends into the cytoplasm (**Figure 17–13B and C**).

The paired centrioles at the center of an animal cell centrosome are curious structures. Each centriole, sitting perpendicular to its partner, is made of a cylindrical array of short microtubules (see Figure 17–13C). Yet centrioles have no role in the nucleation of microtubules from the centrosome: the γ-tubulin ring complex alone is sufficient. Thus, their function remains something of a mystery, especially as most plant cells lack them. Centrioles do, however, act as the organizing centers for the microtubules in cilia and flagella, where they are called *basal bodies* (see Figure 17–11D), as we discuss later.

Why do microtubules need nucleating sites such as those provided by the γ-tubulin rings in the centrosome? The answer is that it is much harder to start a new microtubule from scratch, by first assembling a ring of αβ-tubulin dimers, than it is to add such dimers to a preexisting γ-tubulin ring complex. Although purified αβ-tubulin dimers at a high concentration can polymerize into microtubules spontaneously *in vitro*, the concentration of free αβ-tubulin in a living cell is too low to drive the difficult first step of assembling the initial ring of a new microtubule. By providing organizing centers at specific sites, and keeping the concentration of free αβ-tubulin dimers low, cells can control more precisely where microtubules form.

Microtubules Display Dynamic Instability

Once a microtubule has been nucleated, it typically grows outward from the organizing center for many minutes by the addition of αβ-tubulin dimers to its free plus end. Then, without warning, the microtubule can suddenly undergo a transition that causes it to shrink rapidly by losing tubulin dimers from its plus end (**Movie 17.2**). The microtubule may shrink partially and then, no less suddenly, start growing again, or it may disappear completely, to be replaced by a new microtubule that grows from the same γ-tubulin ring complex (**Figure 17–14**).

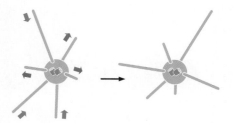

Figure 17–14 Each microtubule grows and shrinks independently of its neighbors. The array of microtubules anchored in a centrosome is continually changing, as some microtubules grow (*red* arrows) and others shrink (*blue* arrows).

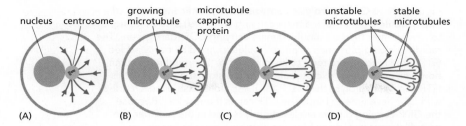

nucleus centrosome growing microtubule microtubule capping protein unstable microtubules stable microtubules

(A)   (B)   (C)   (D)

This remarkable behavior—switching back and forth between polymerization and depolymerization—is known as **dynamic instability**. It allows microtubules to undergo rapid remodeling, and is crucial for their function. In a normal cell, the centrosome (or other organizing center) is continually shooting out new microtubules in different directions in an exploratory fashion, many of which then retract. A microtubule growing out from the centrosome can, however, be prevented from disassembling if its plus end is stabilized by attachment to another molecule or cell structure so as to prevent its depolymerization. If stabilized by attachment to a structure in a more distant region of the cell, the microtubule will establish a relatively stable link between that structure and the centrosome (**Figure 17–15**). The centrosome can thus be compared to a fisherman casting a line: if there is no bite at the end of the line, the line is quickly withdrawn, and a new cast is made; but, if a fish bites, the line remains in place, tethering the fish to the fisherman. This simple strategy of random exploration and selective stabilization enables the centrosome and other nucleating centers to set up a highly organized system of microtubules in selected parts of the cell. The same strategy is used to position organelles relative to one another.

Dynamic Instability Is Driven by GTP Hydrolysis

The dynamic instability of microtubules stems from the intrinsic capacity of tubulin dimers to hydrolyze GTP. This energetically favorable reaction, which generates GDP and inorganic phosphate, is similar to the hydrolysis of ATP (see Figure 3–30).

Each free tubulin dimer contains one GTP molecule tightly bound to β-tubulin, which hydrolyzes the GTP to GDP shortly after the dimer is added to a growing microtubule. The GDP produced by this hydrolysis remains tightly bound to the β-tubulin. When polymerization is proceeding rapidly, tubulin dimers add to the end of the microtubule faster than the GTP they carry is hydrolyzed. As a result, the end of a rapidly growing microtubule is composed entirely of GTP-tubulin dimers, which form a "*GTP cap*." GTP-associated dimers bind more strongly to their neighbors in the microtubule than do dimers that bear GDP, and they pack together more efficiently. Thus the microtubule will continue to grow (**Figure 17–16A**).

Because of the randomness of chemical processes, however, it will occasionally happen that the tubulin dimers at the free end of the microtubule will hydrolyze their GTP before the next dimers are added, so that the free ends of protofilaments are now composed of GDP-tubulin. These GDP-bearing dimers associate less tightly, tipping the balance in favor of disassembly (**Figure 17–16B**). Because the rest of the microtubule is composed of GDP-tubulin, once depolymerization has started, it will tend to continue; the microtubule starts to shrink rapidly and continuously and may even disappear.

The GDP-tubulin that is freed as the microtubule depolymerizes joins the pool of unpolymerized tubulin already in the cytosol. In a typical fibroblast, for example, about half of the tubulin in the cell is in microtubules,

Figure 17–15 Microtubules can be stabilized by attachment to capping proteins. A newly formed microtubule will persist only if both its ends are protected from depolymerization. In cells, the minus ends of microtubules are generally protected by the organizing centers from which the microtubules grow. The plus ends are initially free but can be stabilized by binding to specific capping proteins. (A) Here, for example, a nonpolarized cell is depicted with new microtubules growing from a centrosome in many directions, before shrinking back randomly. (B) If a plus end happens to encounter a capping protein in a specific region of the cell cortex, that microtubule will be stabilized. (C and D) Selective stabilization at one end of the cell will bias the orientation of the microtubule array, such that an organized system of microtubules will be set up selectively in one part of the cell.

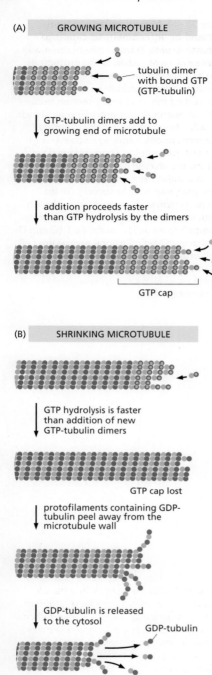

(A)   GROWING MICROTUBULE

tubulin dimer with bound GTP (GTP-tubulin)

GTP-tubulin dimers add to growing end of microtubule

addition proceeds faster than GTP hydrolysis by the dimers

GTP cap

(B)   SHRINKING MICROTUBULE

GTP hydrolysis is faster than addition of new GTP-tubulin dimers

GTP cap lost

protofilaments containing GDP-tubulin peel away from the microtubule wall

GDP-tubulin is released to the cytosol

GDP-tubulin

Figure 17–16 GTP hydrolysis controls the dynamic instability of microtubules. (A) Tubulin dimers carrying GTP (*red*) bind more tightly to one another than do tubulin dimers carrying GDP (*dark green*). The rapidly growing plus ends of microtubules, capped by newly added GTP-tubulin, therefore tend to keep growing. (B) From time to time, however, especially if microtubule growth is slow, the dimers in this GTP cap will hydrolyze their GTP to GDP before fresh dimers loaded with GTP have time to bind. The GTP cap is thereby lost. Because the GDP-carrying dimers are less tightly bound in the polymer, the protofilaments peel away from the plus end, and the dimers are released, causing the microtubule to shrink (Movie 17.3).

while the remainder is free in the cytosol, where it is available for microtubule growth. Tubulin dimers joining this cytosolic pool rapidly exchange their bound GDP for GTP, thereby becoming competent to add to another growing microtubule.

Microtubule Dynamics Can Be Modified by Drugs

Drugs that prevent the polymerization or depolymerization of tubulin dimers can have a rapid and profound effect on the organization of microtubules—and thereby on the behavior of the cell. Consider the mitotic spindle, the microtubule-based apparatus that guides the chromosomes during mitosis (see Figure 17–11C). If a cell in mitosis is exposed to the drug *colchicine*, which binds tightly to free tubulin dimers and prevents their polymerization into microtubules, the mitotic spindle rapidly disappears, and the cell stalls in the middle of mitosis, unable to partition the chromosomes into two groups. This observation, and others like it, demonstrates that the mitotic spindle is normally maintained by a balanced addition and loss of tubulin subunits: when tubulin addition is blocked by colchicine, tubulin loss continues until the spindle disappears.

The drug *Taxol* has the opposite effect on microtubule growth. It binds tightly to microtubules and prevents them from losing subunits. Because new subunits can still be added, the microtubules can grow but cannot shrink. Despite this difference in the mechanism of action, Taxol has the same overall effect as colchicine—arresting dividing cells in mitosis. These experiments show that for the mitotic spindle to function, microtubules must be able to assemble and disassemble. We discuss the behavior of the spindle in more detail in Chapter 18, when we consider mitosis.

The inactivation or destruction of the mitotic spindle eventually kills dividing cells. Because cancer cells divide in a less controlled way than do normal cells of the body, they can sometimes be destroyed preferentially by drugs that either stabilize or destabilize microtubules. Such *antimitotic drugs*, which include colchicine and Taxol, are used to treat human cancers (Table 17–1). As we discuss shortly, there are also drugs that affect the polymerization of actin filaments.

Microtubules Organize the Cell Interior

Cells are able to modify the dynamic instability of their microtubules for particular purposes. As cells enter mitosis, for example, microtubules

TABLE 17–1 DRUGS THAT AFFECT MICROTUBULES	
Microtubule-specific Drugs	**Action**
Taxol	Binds and stabilizes microtubules
Colchicine, colcemid	Binds tubulin dimers and prevents their polymerization
Vinblastine, vincristine	Binds tubulin dimers and prevents their polymerization

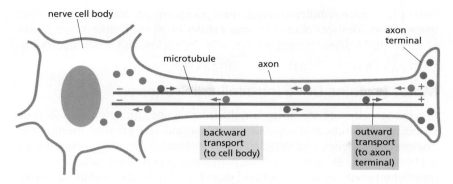

nerve cell body

microtubule

axon

axon terminal

backward transport (to cell body)

outward transport (to axon terminal)

Figure 17–17 Microtubules guide the transport of organelles, vesicles, and macromolecules in both directions along a nerve cell axon. All of the microtubules in the axon point in the same direction, with their plus ends toward the axon terminal. The oriented microtubules serve as tracks for the directional transport of materials synthesized in the cell body but required at the axon terminal. For an axon passing from your spinal cord to a muscle in your shoulder, the journey takes about two days. In addition to this outward traffic (*red* circles), which is driven by one set of motor proteins, there is traffic in the reverse direction (*blue* circles), which is driven by another set of motor proteins. The backward traffic includes worn-out mitochondria and materials ingested by the axon terminals.

become more dynamic, switching between growing and shrinking much more frequently than cytoplasmic microtubules normally do. This change enables microtubules to disassemble rapidly and then reassemble into the mitotic spindle. On the other hand, when a cell has differentiated into a specialized cell type, the dynamic instability of its microtubules is often suppressed by proteins that bind to the ends or the sides of the microtubules and protect them against disassembly. The stabilized microtubules then serve to maintain the organization of the differentiated cell.

Most differentiated animal cells are *polarized*; that is, one end of the cell is structurally or functionally different from the other. Nerve cells, for example, put out an axon from one end of the cell and dendrites from the other (see Figure 12–30). Cells specialized for secretion have their Golgi apparatus positioned toward the site of secretion, and so on. The cell's polarity is a reflection of the polarized systems of microtubules in its interior, which help to position organelles in their required location within the cell and to guide the streams of vesicular and macromolecular traffic moving between one part of the cell and another. In the nerve cell, for example, all the microtubules in the axon point in the same direction, with their plus ends toward the axon terminals; along these oriented tracks, the cell is able to transport organelles, membrane vesicles, and macromolecules—either from the cell body to the axon terminals or in the opposite direction (**Figure 17–17**).

Although some of the traffic along axons travels at speeds in excess of 10 cm per day (**Figure 17–18**), it could still take a week or more for materials to reach the end of a long axon in larger animals. Nonetheless, movement guided by microtubules is immeasurably faster and more efficient than movement driven by free diffusion. A protein molecule traveling by free diffusion could take years to reach the end of a long axon—if it arrived at all (see Question 17–12).

The microtubules in living cells do not act alone. Their activity, like those of other cytoskeletal filaments, depends on a large variety of accessory proteins that bind to them. Some of these **microtubule-associated proteins** stabilize microtubules against disassembly, for example, while

Figure 17–18 Organelles can move rapidly and unidirectionally in a nerve cell axon. In this series of video-enhanced images of a flattened area of an invertebrate nerve axon, numerous membrane vesicles and mitochondria are present, many of which can be seen to move. The white circle provides a fixed frame of reference. These images were recorded at intervals of 400 milliseconds. The two vesicles in the circle are moving along microtubules toward the axon terminal. (Courtesy of P. Forscher.)

mitochondrion

vesicles

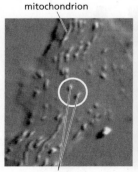
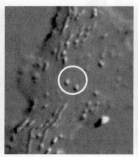
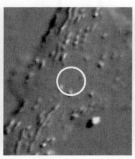
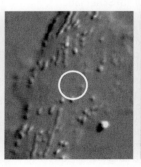
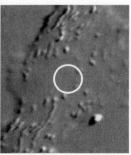

5 μm

QUESTION 17–3

Dynamic instability causes microtubules either to grow or to shrink rapidly. Consider an individual microtubule that is in its shrinking phase.

A. What must happen at the end of the microtubule in order for it to stop shrinking and to start growing again?

B. How would a change in the tubulin concentration affect this switch?

C. What would happen if only GDP, but no GTP, were present in the solution?

D. What would happen if the solution contained an analog of GTP that cannot be hydrolyzed?

others link microtubules to other cell components, including the other types of cytoskeletal filaments (see Figure 17–9). Still others are motor proteins that actively transport organelles, vesicles, and other macromolecules along microtubules, as we discuss next.

Motor Proteins Drive Intracellular Transport

If a living cell is observed in a light microscope, its cytoplasm is seen to be in continual motion. Mitochondria and the smaller membrane-enclosed organelles and vesicles travel in small, jerky steps—moving for a short period, stopping, and then moving again. This *saltatory movement* is much more sustained and directional than the continual, small, Brownian movements caused by random thermal motions. Saltatory movements can occur along either microtubules or actin filaments. In both cases, the movements are driven by **motor proteins**, which use the energy derived from repeated cycles of ATP hydrolysis to travel steadily along the microtubule or actin filament in a single direction (see Figure 4–50). Because the motor proteins also attach to other cell components, they can transport this cargo along the filaments.

The motor proteins that move along cytoplasmic microtubules, such as those in the axon of a nerve cell, belong to two families: the **kinesins** generally move toward the plus end of a microtubule (outward from the cell body in Figure 17–17); the **dyneins** move toward the minus end (toward the cell body in Figure 17–17). Kinesins and cytoplasmic dyneins are generally dimers that have two globular ATP-binding heads and a single tail (**Figure 17–19A**); members of a second class of dyneins, the ciliary dyneins, have a different structure and will be discussed later. The heads of kinesin and cytoplasmic dynein interact with microtubules in a stereospecific manner, so that the motor protein will attach to a microtubule in only one direction. The tail of a motor protein generally binds stably to some cell component, such as a vesicle or an organelle, and thereby determines the type of cargo that the motor protein can transport (**Figure 17–20**). The globular heads of kinesin and dynein are enzymes with ATP-hydrolyzing (ATPase) activity. This reaction provides the energy for driving a directed series of conformational changes in the head that enable the motor protein to move along the microtubule by a cycle of binding, release, and rebinding to the microtubule (**Figure 17–19B** and see Figure 4–50). For a discussion of the discovery and study of motor proteins, see **How We Know**, pp. 588–589.

Figure 17–19 Motor proteins move along microtubules using their globular heads. (A) Kinesins and cytoplasmic dyneins are microtubule motor proteins that generally move in opposite directions along a microtubule. Most kinesins move toward the plus end of a microtubule, whereas dyneins move toward the minus end (Movie 17.4). Each of these proteins (drawn here roughly to scale) is a dimer composed of two identical subunits. Each dimer has two globular heads at one end, which bind and hydrolyze ATP and interact with microtubules, and a single tail at the other end, which interacts with cargo, either directly or indirectly through adaptor proteins (see Figure 17–20). (B) Schematic diagram of a kinesin motor protein "walking" hand-over-hand along a filament. The two heads use the energy of ATP binding and hydrolysis to move in one direction along the filament (ATP in *red*, ADP in *pink*). As shown here, ATP hydrolysis and phosphate release by the rear motor head loosens its attachment to the microtubule. ADP release and ATP binding by the front motor head then cause a dramatic conformational change that flips the rear motor head to the front, thereby completing a single step. (See also Figure 17–23B.)

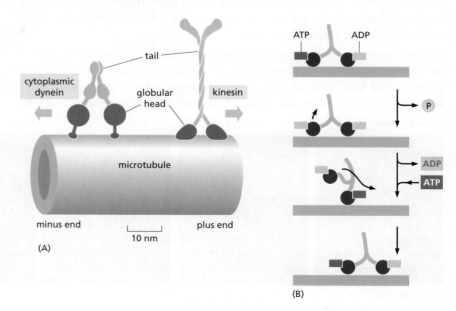

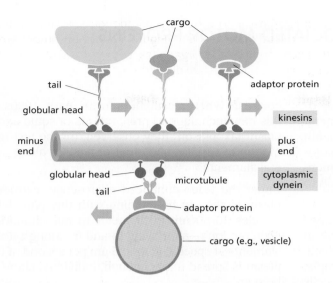

Figure 17–20 Different motor proteins transport different types of cargo along microtubules. The transport of cargo toward the plus end of a microtubule is carried out by different types of kinesin motors, each of which is thought to transport a specific set of vesicles, organelles, or molecules. In some cases, the tail of the kinesin binds directly to the cargo, while in other cases, different adaptor proteins allow the same type of kinesin to carry different cargos. Transport toward the minus end is mediated by cytoplasmic dynein, which generally uses adaptor proteins to interact with its selected cargo.

Microtubules and Motor Proteins Position Organelles in the Cytoplasm

Microtubules and motor proteins play an important part in positioning organelles within a eukaryotic cell. In most animal cells, for example, the tubules of the endoplasmic reticulum (ER) reach almost to the edge of the cell (Movie 17.5), whereas the Golgi apparatus is located in the cell interior, near the centrosome (Figure 17–21A). The ER extends out from its points of connection with the nuclear envelope along microtubules, which reach from the centrally located centrosome out to the plasma membrane. As a cell grows, kinesins attached to the outside of the ER membrane (via adaptor proteins) pull the ER outward along microtubules, stretching it like a net (Figure 17–21B). Cytoplasmic *dyneins* attached to

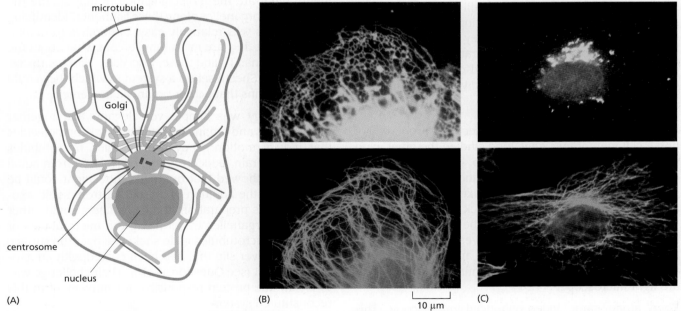

Figure 17–21 Microtubules help position organelles in a eukaryotic cell. (A) Schematic diagram of a cell showing the typical arrangement of cytoplasmic microtubules (*green*), endoplasmic reticulum (*blue*), and Golgi apparatus (*yellow*). The nucleus is shown in *brown*, and the centrosome in *light green*. (B) One part of a cell in culture stained with antibodies to the endoplasmic reticulum (*blue*, upper panel) and to microtubules (*green*, lower panel). Kinesin motor proteins pull the endoplasmic reticulum outward along the microtubules. (C) A different cell in culture stained with antibodies to the Golgi apparatus (*yellow*, upper panel) and to microtubules (*green*, lower panel). In this case, cytoplasmic dyneins pull the Golgi apparatus inward along the microtubules to its position near the centrosome, which is not visible but is located on the Golgi side of the nucleus. (B, courtesy of Mark Terasaki, Lan Bo Chen, and Keigi Fujiwara; C, courtesy of Viki Allan and Thomas Kreis.)

HOW WE KNOW

PURSUING MICROTUBULE-ASSOCIATED MOTOR PROTEINS

The movement of organelles throughout the cell cytoplasm has been a subject of observation, measurement, and speculation since the middle of the nineteenth century. But it was not until the mid-1980s that biologists identified the molecules that drive this movement of organelles and vesicles from one part of the cell to another.

Why the lag between observation and understanding? The problem was in the proteins—or, more precisely, in the difficulty of studying them in isolation outside the cell. To investigate the activity of an enzyme, for example, biochemists first purify the protein: they break open cells or tissues and separate the enzyme from other molecular components (see Panels 4–4 and 4–5, pp. 166–167). They can then study the enzyme in a test tube (*in vitro*), controlling its exposure to substrates, inhibitors, ATP, and so on. Unfortunately, this approach did not seem to work for studies of the motile machinery that underlies intracellular transport. It is not possible to break open a cell and pull out an intact, fully active transport system, free of extraneous material, that continues to carry mitochondria and vesicles from place to place.

That problem was solved by technical advances in two separate fields. First, improvements in microscopy allowed biologists to see that an operational transport system (with extraneous material still attached) could be squeezed from the right kind of living cell. At the same time, biochemists realized that they could assemble a working transport system from scratch—using purified cytoskeletal filaments, motors, and cargo—outside the cell. One such breakthrough started with a squid.

Teeming cytoplasm

Neuroscientists interested in the electrical properties of nerve cell membranes have long studied the giant axon from squid (see How We Know, pp. 412–413). Because of its large size, researchers found that they could squeeze the cytoplasm from the axon like toothpaste, and then study how ions move back and forth through various channels in the empty, tubelike plasma membrane (see Figure 12–33). These investigators discarded the extruded cytoplasmic jelly, as it appeared to be inert (and thus uninteresting) when examined under a standard light microscope.

Then along came video-enhanced microscopy. This type of microscopy, developed by Shinya Inoué, Robert Allen, and others, allows one to detect structures that are smaller than the resolving power of standard light microscopes, which is only about 0.2 μm, or 200 nm (see Panel 1–1, pp. 12–13). The resulting images are captured by a video camera and then enhanced by computer processing to reduce the background and heighten contrast. When researchers in the early 1980s applied this new technique to preparations of squid axon cytoplasm (axoplasm), they observed, for the first time, the motion of vesicles and other organelles along cytoskeletal filaments.

Under the video-enhanced microscope, extruded axoplasm is seen to be teeming with tiny particles—from vesicles 30–50 nm in diameter to mitochondria some 5000 nm long—all moving to and fro along cytoskeletal filaments at speeds of up to 5 μm per second. If the axoplasm is spread thinly enough, individual filaments can be seen.

The movement continues for hours, allowing researchers to manipulate the preparation and study the effects. Ray Lasek and Scott Brady discovered, for example, that the organelle movement requires ATP. Substitution of ATP analogs, such as AMP-PNP, which resemble ATP but cannot be hydrolyzed (and thus provide no energy), inhibit the translocation.

Snaking tubes

More work was needed to identify the individual components that comprise the transport system in squid axoplasm. What kind of filaments support this movement? What are the molecular motors that shuttle the vesicles and organelles along these filaments? Identifying the filaments was relatively easy: antibodies to tubulin revealed that they are microtubules. But what about the motor proteins? To find these, Ron Vale, Thomas Reese, and Michael Sheetz set up a system in which they could fish for proteins that power organelle movement.

Their strategy was simple yet elegant: add together microtubules and organelles and then look for molecules that induce motion. They used purified microtubules from squid brain, added organelles isolated from squid axons, and showed that organelle movement could be triggered by the addition of an extract from squid axoplasm. In this preparation, the researchers could either watch the organelles travel along the microtubules or watch the microtubules glide snakelike over the surface of a glass cover slip that had been coated with an axoplasm extract (see Question 17–18). Their challenge was to isolate the protein responsible for movement in this reconstituted system.

To do that, Vale and his colleagues took advantage of the earlier work with the ATP analog AMP-PNP. Although this analog inhibits the movement of vesicles along microtubules, it still allows organelles to attach to the microtubule filaments. So the researchers incubated the axoplasm extract with microtubules and organelles in the presence of AMP-PNP; they then pulled out the

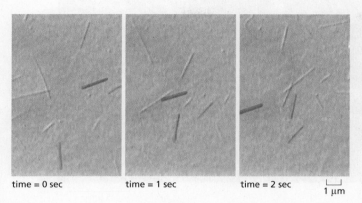

Figure 17–22 Kinesin causes microtubule gliding *in vitro*. In an *in vitro* motility assay, purified kinesin is mixed with microtubules in the presence of ATP. When a drop of the mixture is placed on a glass slide and examined by video-enhanced microscopy, individual microtubules (artificially colored) can be seen gliding over the slide. They are driven by kinesin molecules, which attach to the glass slide by their tails. Images were recorded at 1-second intervals. The microtubules moved at about 1–2 μm/sec. (Courtesy of Nick Carter and Rob Cross.)

time = 0 sec   time = 1 sec   time = 2 sec   ⊢—⊣ 1 μm

microtubules with what they hoped were the motor proteins still attached. Vale and his team then added ATP to release the attached proteins, and they found a 110-kilodalton polypeptide that could stimulate the gliding of microtubules along a glass cover slip (**Figure 17–22**). They dubbed the molecule kinesin (from the Greek *kinein*, "to move").

Similar *in vitro* motility assays have been instrumental in the study of other motor proteins—such as myosins, which move along actin filaments, as we discuss later. Subsequent studies showed that kinesin moves along microtubules from the minus end to the plus end; they also identified many other motor proteins of the kinesin family.

Lights, camera, action

Combining such assays with ever more refined microscopic techniques, researchers can now monitor the movement of individual motor proteins along single microtubules, even in living cells.

Observation of kinesin molecules, labeled with a fluorescent marker protein, revealed that this motor protein marches along microtubules processively—that is, each molecule takes multiple "steps" along the filament (100 or so) before falling off. The length of each step is 8 nm, which corresponds to the spacing of individual tubulin dimers along the microtubule. Combining these observations with assays of ATP hydrolysis, researchers have confirmed that one molecule of ATP is hydrolyzed per step. Kinesin can move in a processive manner because it has two heads. This enables it to walk toward the plus end of the microtubule in a "hand-over-hand" fashion, each head repetitively binding and releasing the filament as it swings past the bound head in front (**Figure 17–23**). Such studies now allow us to follow the footsteps of these fascinating and industrious proteins—step by molecular step.

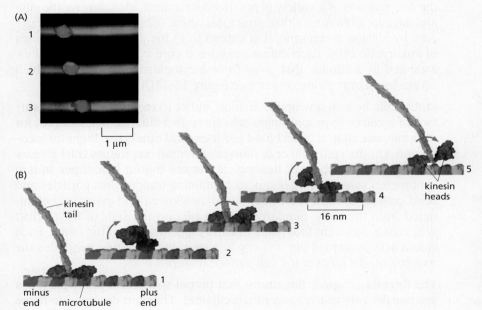

(A)

(B)

kinesin tail

minus end   microtubule   plus end

kinesin heads

Figure 17–23 A single molecule of kinesin moves along a microtubule. (A) Three frames, separated by intervals of 1 second, record the movement of an individual, fluorescently labeled kinesin molecule (*red*) along a microtubule (*green*); the labeled kinesin moves at a speed of 0.3 μm/sec. (B) A series of molecular models of the two heads of a kinesin molecule, showing how they are thought to walk processively (*left* to *right*) along a microtubule in a series of 8-nm steps in which one head swings past the other (Movie 17.6). (A and B, courtesy of Ron Vale.)

Figure 17–24 **Many hairlike cilia project from the surface of the epithelial cells that line the human respiratory tract.** In this scanning electron micrograph, thick tufts of cilia can be seen extended from these ciliated cells, which are interspersed with the dome-shaped surfaces of nonciliated epithelial cells. (Reproduced from R.G. Kessel and R.H. Kardon, *Tissues and Organs.* San Francisco: W.H. Freeman & Co., 1979.)

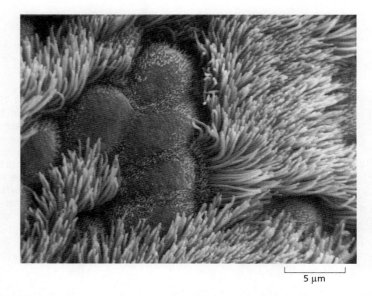

5 µm

the Golgi membranes pull the Golgi apparatus along microtubules in the opposite direction, inward toward the nucleus (**Figure 17–21C**). In this way, the regional differences in these internal membranes—crucial for their respective functions—are created and maintained.

When cells are treated with colchicine—a drug that promotes microtubule disassembly—both the ER and the Golgi apparatus change their location dramatically. The ER, which is physically connected to the nuclear envelope, collapses around the nucleus; the Golgi apparatus, which is not attached to any other organelle, fragments into small vesicles, which then disperse throughout the cytoplasm. When the colchicine is removed, the organelles return to their original positions, dragged by motor proteins moving along the re-formed microtubules.

Cilia and Flagella Contain Stable Microtubules Moved by Dynein

We mentioned earlier that many microtubules in cells are stabilized through their association with other proteins and therefore do not show dynamic instability. Cells use such stable microtubules as stiff supports in the construction of a variety of polarized structures, including motile cilia and flagella. **Cilia** are hairlike structures about 0.25 µm in diameter, covered by plasma membrane, that extend from the surface of many kinds of eukaryotic cells. Each cilium contains a core of stable microtubules, arranged in a bundle, that grow from a cytoplasmic *basal body*, which serves as an organizing center (see Figure 17–11D).

Motile cilia beat in a whiplike fashion, either to move fluid over the surface of a cell or to propel single cells through a fluid. Some protozoa, for example, use cilia to collect food particles, and others use them for locomotion. On the epithelial cells lining the human respiratory tract (**Figure 17–24**), huge numbers of beating cilia (more than a billion per square centimeter) sweep layers of mucus containing trapped dust particles and dead cells up toward the throat, to be swallowed and eventually eliminated from the body. Similarly, beating cilia on the cells of the oviduct wall create a current that helps to carry eggs away from the ovary. Each cilium acts as a small oar, moving in a repeated cycle that generates the movement of fluid over the cell surface (**Figure 17–25**).

The **flagella** (singular **flagellum**) that propel sperm and many protozoa are usually very much longer than cilia are. They are designed to move

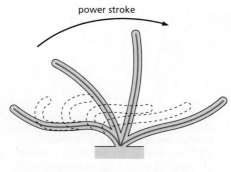

power stroke

Figure 17–25 **A cilium beats by performing a repetitive cycle of movements, consisting of a power stroke followed by a recovery stroke.** In the fast power stroke, the cilium is fully extended and fluid is driven over the surface of the cell; in the slower recovery stroke, the cilium curls back into position with minimal disturbance to the surrounding fluid. Each cycle typically requires 0.1–0.2 second and generates a force parallel to the cell surface.

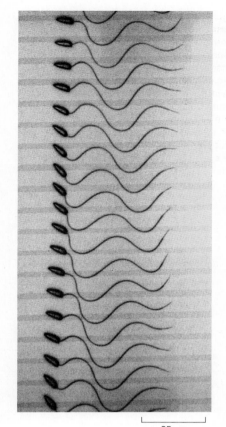

25 μm

the entire cell, rather than moving fluid across the cell surface. Flagella propagate regular waves along their length, propelling the attached cell along (**Figure 17–26**).

Despite these slight differences in operation, cilia and flagella share a similar internal structure. The microtubules in both cilia and flagella are arranged in an elaborate and distinctive pattern, which was one of the most striking revelations of early electron microscopy. A cross section through a cilium shows nine doublet microtubules arranged in a ring around a pair of single microtubules (**Figure 17–27A**). This "9 + 2" array is characteristic of almost all eukaryotic cilia and flagella—from those of protozoa to those in humans.

The movement of a cilium or a flagellum is produced by bending that takes place as its microtubules slide against each other. The microtubules are associated with numerous accessory proteins (**Figure 17–27B**), which project at regular positions along the length of the microtubule bundle. Some of these proteins serve as cross-links to hold the bundle of microtubules together; others generate the force that causes the cilium or flagellum to bend.

The most important of the accessory proteins is the motor protein *ciliary dynein*, which generates the bending motion of the structure. Ciliary dynein is attached by its tail to one microtubule in each outer doublet, while its globular heads interact with the adjacent microtubule to generate a sliding force between the two microtubules. Because of the multiple links that hold the adjacent microtubule doublets together, the sliding force between adjacent microtubules is converted to a bending motion (**Figure 17–28**). Other ciliary components, including the central pair, inner sheath, and radial spokes, control dynein activity, leading to the complex wave forms seen in cilia and flagella.

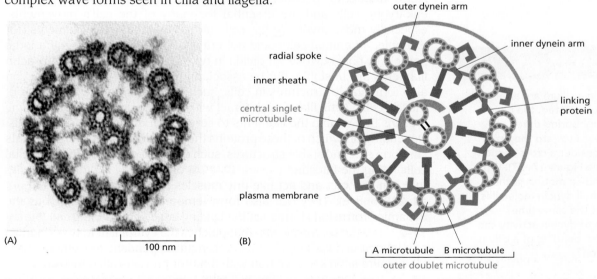

Figure 17–27 Microtubules in a cilium or flagellum are arranged in a "9 + 2" array. (A) Electron micrograph of a flagellum of the unicellular alga *Chlamydomonas* shown in cross section, illustrating the distinctive 9 + 2 arrangement of microtubules. (B) Diagram of the flagellum in cross section. The nine outer microtubules (each a special paired structure) carry two rows of dynein molecules. The heads of each dynein molecule appear in this view like arms reaching toward the adjacent doublet microtubule. In a living cilium, these dynein heads periodically make contact with the adjacent doublet microtubule and move along it, thereby producing the force for ciliary beating. The various other links and projections shown are proteins that serve to hold the bundle of microtubules together and to convert the sliding force produced by dyneins into bending, as illustrated in Figure 17–28. (A, courtesy of Lewis Tilney.)

Figure 17–28 The movement of dynein causes the flagellum to bend. (A) If the outer doublet microtubules and their associated dynein molecules are freed from other components of a sperm flagellum and then exposed to ATP, the doublets slide against each other, telescope-fashion, due to the repetitive action of their associated dyneins. (B) In an intact flagellum, however, the doublets are tied to each other by flexible protein links so that the action of the system produces bending rather than sliding.

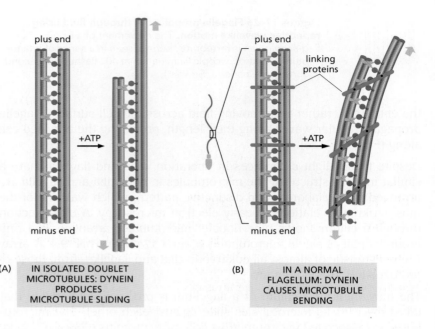

(A) IN ISOLATED DOUBLET MICROTUBULES: DYNEIN PRODUCES MICROTUBULE SLIDING

(B) IN A NORMAL FLAGELLUM: DYNEIN CAUSES MICROTUBULE BENDING

In humans, hereditary defects in ciliary dynein cause Kartagener's syndrome. Men with this disorder are infertile because their sperm are nonmotile, and they have an increased susceptibility to bronchial infections because the cilia that line their respiratory tract are paralyzed and thus unable to clear bacteria and debris from the lungs.

Many animal cells that lack beating cilia contain a single, nonmotile *primary cilium*. This appendage is much shorter than a beating cilium and functions as an antenna for sensing certain extracellular signal molecules.

ACTIN FILAMENTS

Actin filaments, polymers of the protein actin, are present in most eukaryotic cells and are essential for many of the cell's movements, especially those involving the cell surface. Without actin filaments, for example, an animal cell could not crawl along a surface, engulf a large particle by phagocytosis, or divide in two. Like microtubules, many actin filaments are unstable, but by associating with other proteins they can also form stable structures in cells, such as the contractile apparatus of muscle cells. Actin filaments interact with a large number of *actin-binding proteins* that enable the filaments to serve a variety of functions in cells. Depending on which of these proteins they associate with, actin filaments can form stiff and stable structures, such as the *microvilli* on the epithelial cells lining the intestine (**Figure 17–29A**) or the *small contractile bundles* that can contract and act like tiny muscles in most animal cells (**Figure 17–29B and E**). They can also form temporary structures, such as the dynamic protrusions formed at the leading edge of a crawling cell (**Figure 17–29C**) or the *contractile ring* that pinches the cytoplasm in two when an animal cell divides (**Figure 17–29D**). Actin-dependent movements usually require actin's association with a motor protein called myosin.

In this section, we see how the arrangements of actin filaments in a cell depend on the types of actin-binding proteins present. Even though actin filaments and microtubules are formed from unrelated types of subunit proteins, we will see that the principles by which they assemble and disassemble, control cell structure, and work with motor proteins to bring about movement are strikingly similar.

QUESTION 17–4

Dynein arms in a cilium are arranged so that, when activated, the heads push their neighboring outer doublet outward toward the tip of the cilium. Consider a cross section of a cilium (see Figure 17–27). Why would no bending motion of the cilium result if all dynein molecules were active at the same time? What pattern of dynein activity can account for the bending of a cilium in one direction?

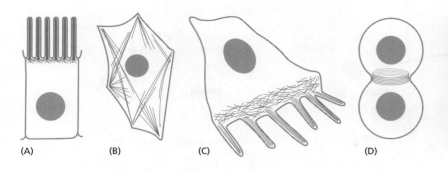 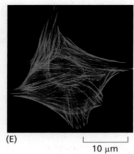

(A)   (B)   (C)   (D)   (E)

⊢————⊣
10 µm

Actin Filaments Are Thin and Flexible

Actin filaments appear in electron micrographs as threads about 7 nm in diameter. Each filament is a twisted chain of identical globular actin monomers, all of which "point" in the same direction along the axis of the chain. Like a microtubule, therefore, an actin filament has a structural polarity, with a plus end and a minus end (**Figure 17–30**).

Actin filaments are thinner, more flexible, and usually shorter than microtubules. There are, however, many more of them, so that the total length of all of the actin filaments in a cell is generally many times greater than the total length of all of the microtubules. Unlike intermediate filaments and microtubules, actin filaments rarely occur in isolation in the cell; they are generally found in cross-linked bundles and networks, which are much stronger than the individual filaments.

Actin and Tubulin Polymerize by Similar Mechanisms

Like microtubles, actin filaments can grow by the addition of monomers at either end but their rate of growth is faster at the plus end than at the minus end. A naked actin filament, like a microtubule without associated proteins, is inherently unstable, and it can disassemble from both ends. In living cells, free actin monomers carry a tightly bound nucleoside triphosphate, in this case ATP. The actin monomer hydrolyzes its bound ATP to ADP soon after it is incorporated into the filament. As with the hydrolysis

Figure 17–29 Actin filaments allow animal cells to adopt a variety of shapes and perform a variety of functions. The actin filaments in four different structures are shown here in *red*: (A) microvilli; (B) contractile bundles in the cytoplasm; (C) fingerlike *filopodia* protruding from the leading edge of a moving cell; and (D) contractile ring during cell division. (E) Micrograph of a cell in which contractile bundles of actin, like those in (B), are stained with fluorescently labeled phalloidin, a molecule that binds specifically to actin filaments (see Table 17–2, p. 594). (E, courtesy of Nikon ® MicroscopyU.)

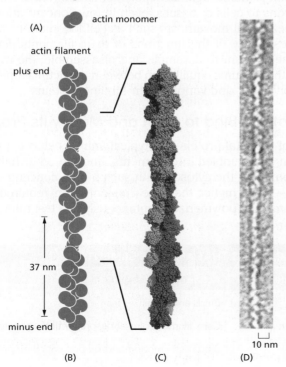

(A) actin monomer

actin filament

plus end

37 nm

minus end

(B)   (C)   (D)

⊢⊣
10 nm

Figure 17–30 Actin filaments are thin, flexible protein threads. (A) The subunit of each actin filament is an actin monomer. A cleft in the monomer provides a binding site for ATP or ADP. (B) Arrangement of actin monomers in an actin filament. Each filament may be thought of as a two-stranded helix with a twist repeating every 37 nm. Multiple, lateral interactions between the two strands prevent the strands from separating. (C) Close-up view showing the extensive interactions between the two strands of the actin filament. (D) Electron micrograph of a negatively stained actin filament. (D, courtesy of Roger Craig.)

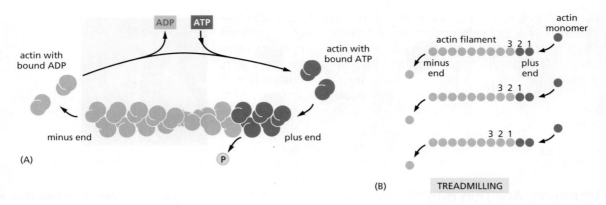

Figure 17–31 Actin filaments can undergo treadmilling. (A) Actin monomers in the cytosol carry ATP, which is hydrolyzed to ADP soon after assembly into a growing filament. The ADP molecules remain trapped within the actin filament, unable to exchange with ATP until the actin monomer that carries them dissociates from the filament. When ATP-actin (*dark red*) adds to the plus end of an actin filament at the same rate that ADP-actin (*light red*) is lost from the minus end, treadmilling occurs. (B) When the rates of addition and loss are equal, the filament stays the same length—although individual actin monomers (three of which are numbered here) move through the filament from the plus to the minus end.

QUESTION 17–5

The formation of actin filaments in the cytosol is controlled by actin-binding proteins. Some actin-binding proteins significantly increase the rate at which the formation of an actin filament is initiated. Suggest a mechanism by which they might do this.

---

of GTP to GDP in a microtubule, hydrolysis of ATP to ADP in an actin filament reduces the strength of binding between the monomers, thereby decreasing the stability of the polymer. Thus in both cases, nucleotide hydrolysis promotes depolymerization, helping the cell to disassemble its microtubules and actin filaments after they have formed.

If the concentration of free actin monomers is very high, an actin filament will grow rapidly, adding monomers at both ends. At intermediate concentrations of free actin, however, something interesting takes place. Actin monomers add to the plus end at a rate faster than the bound ATP can be hydrolyzed, so the plus end grows. At the minus end, by contrast, ATP is hydrolyzed faster than new monomers can be added; because ADP-actin destabilizes the structure, the filament loses subunits from its minus end at the same time as it adds them to the plus end (**Figure 17–31A**). Individual monomers thus move through the filament from the plus to the minus end, a behavior called *treadmilling*. When the rates of addition and loss are equal, the filament remains the same size (**Figure 17–31B**).

Actin filament function can be perturbed experimentally by certain toxins produced by fungi or marine sponges. Some, such as *cytochalasin* and *latrunculin*, prevent actin polymerization; others, such as *phalloidin*, stabilize actin filaments against depolymerization (**Table 17–2**). Addition of these toxins to cells or tissues, even in low concentrations, instantaneously freezes cell movements such as cell locomotion. Thus, as with microtubules, many of the functions of actin filaments depend on the ability of the filament to assemble and disassemble, the rates of which depend on the dynamic equilibrium between the actin filaments, the pool of actin monomers, and various actin-binding proteins.

Many Proteins Bind to Actin and Modify Its Properties

About 5% of the total protein in a typical animal cell is actin; about half of this actin is assembled into filaments, and the other half remains as actin monomers in the cytosol. With such a high concentration of actin monomers—much higher than the concentration required for purified actin monomers to polymerize spontaneously in a test tube—what, then,

TABLE 17–2 DRUGS THAT AFFECT FILAMENTS	
Actin-specific Drugs	**Action**
Phalloidin	Binds and stabilizes filaments
Cytochalasin	Caps filament plus ends, preventing polymerization there
Latrunculin	Binds actin monomers and prevents their polymerization

keeps the actin monomers in cells from polymerizing totally into filaments? The answer is that cells contain small proteins, such as *thymosin* and *profilin*, that bind to actin monomers in the cytosol, preventing them from adding to the ends of actin filaments. By keeping actin monomers in reserve until they are required, these proteins play a crucial role in regulating actin polymerization. When actin filaments are needed, other actin-binding proteins such as *formins* and *actin-related proteins* (*ARPs*) promote actin polymerization.

There are a great many **actin-binding proteins** in cells. Most of these bind to assembled actin filaments and control their behavior (**Figure 17–32**). Actin-bundling proteins, for example, hold actin filaments together in parallel bundles in microvilli; others cross-link actin filaments together in a gel-like meshwork within the *cell cortex*—the specialized layer of actin-filament-rich cytoplasm just beneath the plasma membrane. Filament-severing proteins fragment actin filaments into shorter lengths and thus can convert an actin gel to a more fluid state. Actin filaments can also associate with myosin motor proteins to form contractile bundles, as in muscle cells. And they often form tracks along which myosin motor proteins transport organelles, a function that is especially conspicuous in plant cells.

In the remainder of this chapter, we consider some characteristic structures that actin filaments can form, and we discuss how different types

Figure 17–32 Actin-binding proteins control the behavior of actin filaments in vertebrate cells. Actin is shown in *red*, and the actin-binding proteins are shown in *green*.

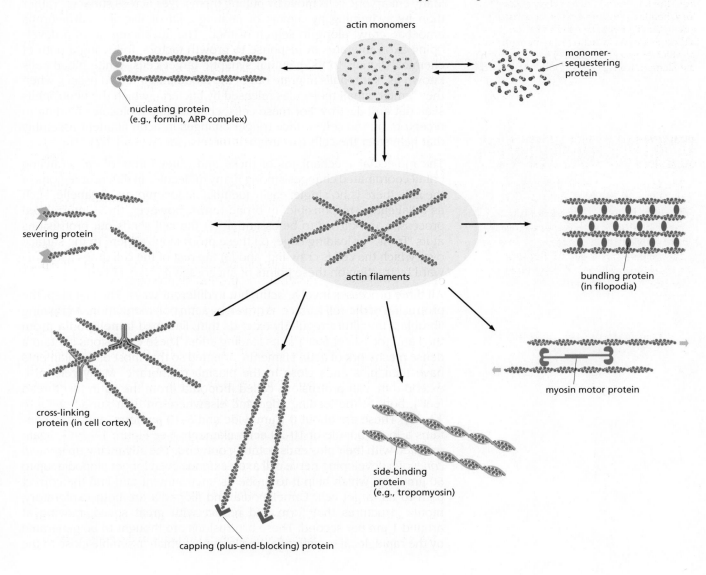

actin monomers

monomer-sequestering protein

nucleating protein
(e.g., formin, ARP complex)

severing protein

actin filaments

bundling protein
(in filopodia)

myosin motor protein

cross-linking
protein (in cell cortex)

side-binding
protein
(e.g., tropomyosin)

capping (plus-end-blocking) protein

of actin-binding proteins are involved in their assembly. We begin with the cell cortex and its role in cell shape and movement, and we conclude with the contractile apparatus of muscle cells.

A Cortex Rich in Actin Filaments Underlies the Plasma Membrane of Most Eukaryotic Cells

Although actin is found throughout the cytoplasm of a eukaryotic cell, in many cells it is highly concentrated in a layer just beneath the plasma membrane. In this region, called the **cell cortex**, actin filaments are linked by actin-binding proteins into a meshwork that supports the plasma membrane and gives it mechanical strength. In human red blood cells, for example, a simple and regular network of fibrous proteins—including actin and spectrin filaments—attaches to the plasma membrane, providing the support necessary for the cells to maintain their simple discoid shape (see Figure 11–29). In other animal cells, the cortex includes a much denser network of actin filaments that are cross-linked into a three-dimensional meshwork. The rearrangements of actin filaments within the cortex provide much of the molecular basis for changes in both cell shape and cell locomotion.

Cell Crawling Depends on Cortical Actin

Many eukaryotic cells move by pulling themselves across surfaces, rather than by swimming by means of beating cilia or flagella. Carnivorous amoebae crawl along in search of food. The advancing tip of a developing axon migrates in response to growth factors, following a path of chemical signals to its eventual synaptic target cells. White blood cells known as *neutrophils* migrate out of the blood into infected tissues when they "smell" small molecules released by bacteria, which the neutrophils seek out and destroy. For these cells, chemotactic molecules binding to receptors on the cell surface trigger changes in actin filament assembly that help steer the cells toward their targets (see Movie 17.7).

The molecular mechanisms of these and other forms of cell crawling entail coordinated changes among many molecules in different regions of the cell; there is no single, easily identifiable locomotory organelle, such as a flagellum, responsible. In broad terms, however, three interrelated processes are known to be essential: (1) the cell sends out protrusions at its "front," or leading edge; (2) these protrusions adhere to the surface over which the cell is crawling; and (3) the rest of the cell drags itself forward by traction on these points of anchorage (Figure 17–33).

All three processes involve actin, but in different ways. The first step, the protrusion of the cell surface, is driven by actin polymerization. A crawling fibroblast in culture regularly extends thin, flattened **lamellipodia** (from the Latin for "sheet feet") at its leading edge. These extensions contain a dense meshwork of actin filaments, oriented so that most of the filaments have their plus ends close to the plasma membrane. Many cells also extend thin, stiff protrusions called **filopodia** (from the Latin for "thread feet"), both at the leading edge and elsewhere on their surface (Figure 17–34). These are about 0.1 μm wide and 5–10 μm long, and each contains a loose bundle of 10–20 actin filaments (see Figure 17–29C), again oriented with their plus ends pointing outward. The advancing tip (*growth cone*) of a developing nerve cell axon extends even longer filopodia, up to 50 μm long, which help it to probe its environment and find the correct path to its target cell. Lamellipodia and filopodia are both exploratory, motile structures that form and retract with great speed, moving at around 1 μm per second. These protrusions are thought to be generated by the rapid, local growth of actin filaments, which assemble close to the

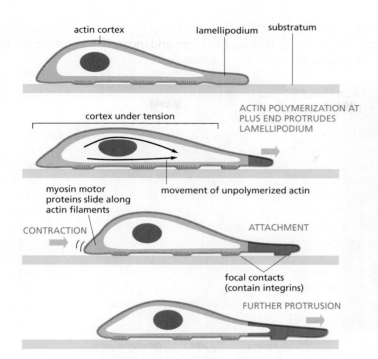

<figure>**Figure 17–33 Forces generated in the actin-filament-rich cortex help move a cell forward.** Actin polymerization at the leading edge of the cell *pushes* the plasma membrane forward (protrusion) and forms new regions of actin cortex, shown here in *red*. New points of anchorage are made between the bottom of the cell and the surface (substratum) on which the cell is crawling (attachment). Contraction at the rear of the cell—mediated by myosin motor proteins moving along actin filaments—then draws the body of the cell forward. New anchorage points are established at the front, and old ones are released at the back, as the cell crawls forward. The same cycle is repeated over and over again, moving the cell forward in a stepwise fashion.</figure>

plasma membrane and elongate by the addition of actin monomers at their plus ends. In this way, the filaments push out the membrane without tearing it.

When the lamellipodia and filopodia touch down on a favorable surface, they stick: transmembrane proteins in their plasma membrane, known as *integrins* (discussed in Chapter 20), adhere to molecules either in the extracellular matrix or on the surface of a neighboring cell over which the moving cell is slithering. Meanwhile, on the intracellular face of the crawling cell's plasma membrane, integrins capture actin filaments in the cortex, thereby creating a robust anchorage for the crawling cell (see Figures 17–33 and 20–14C). To use this anchorage to drag its body forward, the cell calls on the help of myosin motor proteins, which *slide along actin filaments*, as we discuss shortly.

## QUESTION 17–6

Suppose that the actin molecules in a cultured skin cell have been randomly labeled in such a way that 1 in 10,000 molecules carries a fluorescent marker. What would you expect to see if you examined the lamellipodium (leading edge) of this cell through a fluorescence microscope? Assume that your microscope is sensitive enough to detect single fluorescent molecules.

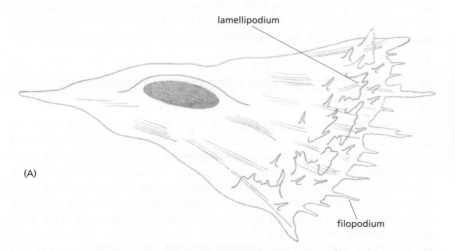

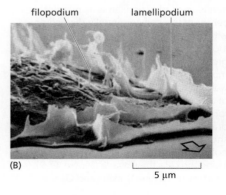

Figure 17–34 Actin filaments allow animal cells to migrate. (A) Schematic drawing of a fibroblast, showing flattened lamellipodia and fine filopodia projecting from its surface, especially in the regions of the leading edge. (B) Scanning electron micrograph showing lamellipodia and filopodia at the leading edge of a human fibroblast migrating in culture; the arrow shows the direction of cell movement. As the cell moves forward, the lamellipodia that fail to attach to the substratum are swept backward over the upper surface of the cell— a movement referred to as ruffling. (B, courtesy of Julian Heath.)

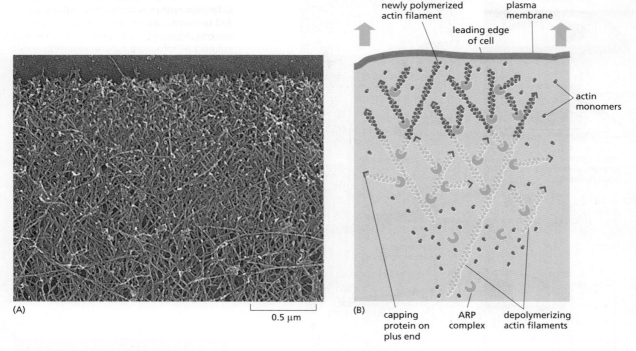

Figure 17–35 A web of polymerizing actin filaments pushes the leading edge of a lamellipodium forward. (A) A highly motile keratocyte from frog skin was fixed, dried, and shadowed with platinum, and examined in an electron microscope. Actin filaments form a dense network, with the fast-growing plus ends of the filaments terminating at the leading margin of the lamellipodium (top of figure; Movie 17.8). (B) Drawing showing how the nucleation of new actin filaments (*pink*) is mediated by ARP complexes (*light green*) attached to the sides of preexisting actin filaments. The resulting branching structure pushes the plasma membrane forward. The plus ends of the actin filaments become protected from depolymerizing by capping proteins (*dark green*), while the minus ends of actin filaments nearer the center of the cell continually disassemble with the help of depolymerizing proteins (not shown). Because of this directional growth and disassembly, individual actin monomers move through this branched web in a rearward direction, while the web of actin as a whole undergoes a continual forward movement. This actin network is drawn to a different scale than the network shown in (A). Some pathogenic bacteria polymerize tails of actin filaments to move inside the cells they invade (Movie 17.9). (A, courtesy of Tatyana Svitkina and Gary Borisy.)

Actin-binding Proteins Influence the Type of Protrusions Formed at the Leading Edge

The formation and growth of actin filaments at the leading edge of a cell are assisted by various actin-binding proteins. The actin-related proteins—or ARPs—mentioned earlier promote the formation of a web of branched actin filaments in lamellipodia. ARPs form complexes that bind to the sides of existing actin filaments and nucleate the formation of new filaments, which grow out at an angle to produce side branches. With the aid of additional actin-binding proteins, this web undergoes continual assembly at the leading edge and disassembly further back, pushing the lamellipodium forward (Figure 17–35).

The other kind of cell protrusion, the filopodium, depends on *formin*, a nucleating protein that attaches to the growing plus ends of actin filaments and promotes the addition of new monomers to form straight, unbranched filaments. Formins are also used elsewhere to assemble unbranched filaments, such as in the contractile ring that pinches a dividing animal cell in two.

Extracellular Signals Can Alter the Arrangement of Actin Filaments

Actin-binding proteins control the location, organization, and behavior of actin filaments. The activities of these proteins are, in turn, controlled by extracellular signal molecules, allowing the cell to rearrange its actin cytoskeleton in response to its environment. These extracellular signals act through a variety of cell-surface receptor proteins, which activate various intracellular signaling pathways. Many of these pathways converge on a group of closely related *monomeric GTPases* that are part of the **Rho protein family**. As discussed in Chapter 16, monomeric GTPases behave as molecular switches that control intracellular processes by cycling between an active GTP-bound state and an inactive GDP-bound state (see Figure 16–11B).

In the case of the actin cytoskeleton, different Rho family members alter the organization of actin filaments in different ways. For example, one

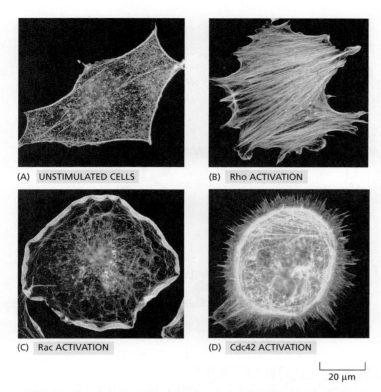

(A) UNSTIMULATED CELLS

(B) Rho ACTIVATION

(C) Rac ACTIVATION

(D) Cdc42 ACTIVATION

20 µm

Figure 17–36 Activation of Rho-family GTPases can have a dramatic effect on the organization of actin filaments in fibroblasts. In these micrographs, actin is stained with fluorescently labeled phalloidin (see Table 17–2, p. 594). (A) Unstimulated fibroblasts have actin filaments primarily in the cortex. (B) Microinjection of an activated form of Rho promotes the rapid assembly of bundles of long, unbranched actin filaments; because myosin is associated with these bundles, they are contractile. (C) Microinjection of an activated form of Rac, a GTP-binding protein similar to Rho, causes the formation of an enormous lamellipodium that extends from the entire circumference of the cell. (D) Microinjection of an activated form of Cdc42, another Rho family member, stimulates the protrusion of a forest of filopodia at the cell periphery. (Courtesy of Catherine Nobes.)

Rho family member triggers the bundling of actin filaments and activation of the formin proteins that promote the formation of filopodia. Another Rho GTPase might stimulate ARP complexes at the cell's leading edge, promoting the formation of lamellipodia and membrane ruffling. Finally, activation of the founding member of the Rho family drives the bundling of actin filaments with myosin motor proteins and the clustering of cell-surface integrins, actions that promote cell crawling (see Figure 17–33). Examples of these dramatic, Rho-driven cytoskeletal rearrangements are shown in **Figure 17–36**.

Actin Associates with Myosin to Form Contractile Structures

Perhaps the most familiar of all the actin-binding proteins is **myosin**. Myosins belong to a family of motor proteins that bind to and hydrolyze ATP, which provides the energy for their movement along actin filaments toward the plus end. Myosin, like actin, was first discovered in skeletal muscle, and much of what we know about the interaction of these two proteins was learned from studies of muscle. There are numerous types of myosins in cells, of which the *myosin-I* and *myosin-II* subfamilies are the most abundant.

Myosin-I molecules, which are present in all cell types, have a head domain and a tail (**Figure 17–37A**). The head domain binds to an actin filament and has the ATP-hydrolyzing motor activity that enables it to move along the filament in a repetitive cycle of binding, detachment, and rebinding (Movie 17.10). The tail varies among the different types of myosin-I and determines what type of cargo the myosin will carry. For example, the tail may bind to a particular type of vesicle and propel it through the cell along actin filament tracks (**Figure 17–37B**), or it may bind to the plasma membrane and pull it into a different shape (**Figure 17–36C**).

Myosin-II is structurally and mechanistically more complex than myosin-I. Muscle cells make use of a specialized form of myosin-II to drive muscle contraction, as we discuss next.

Figure 17–37 **Myosin-I is the simplest myosin.** (A) Myosin-I has a single globular head that attaches to an actin filament and a tail that attaches to another molecule or organelle in the cell. (B) This arrangement allows the head domain to move a vesicle relative to an actin filament, which in this case is anchored to the plasma membrane. (C) Myosin-I can also bind to an actin filament in the cell cortex, ultimately pulling the plasma membrane into a new shape. Note that the head group always walks toward the plus end of the actin filament.

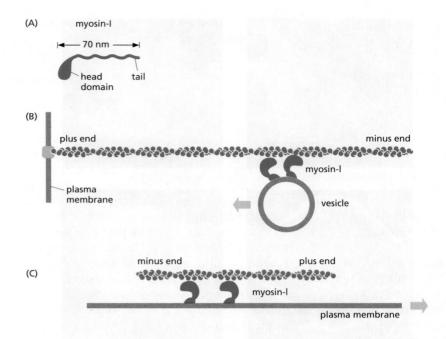

MUSCLE CONTRACTION

Muscle contraction is the best understood of animal cell movements. In vertebrates, running, walking, swimming, and flying all depend on the ability of *skeletal muscle* to contract strongly and move various bones. Involuntary movements such as heart pumping and gut peristalsis depend on *cardiac muscle* and *smooth muscle*, respectively, which are formed from muscle cells that differ in structure from skeletal muscle but use actin and myosin in a similar way to contract. Much of our understanding of the mechanisms of cell movement originated from studies of muscle cell contraction. In this section, we discuss how actin and myosin interact to produce this contraction.

Muscle Contraction Depends on Interacting Filaments of Actin and Myosin

Muscle myosin belongs to the **myosin-II** subfamily of myosins. These proteins are dimers, with two globular ATPase heads at one end and a single coiled-coil tail at the other (**Figure 17–38A**). Clusters of myosin-II molecules bind to each other through their coiled-coil tails, forming a bipolar **myosin filament** from which the heads project (**Figure 17–38B**).

Figure 17–38 **Myosin-II molecules can associate with one another to form myosin filaments.** (A) A molecule of myosin-II contains two identical heavy chains, each with a globular head and an extended tail. (It also contains two light chains bound to each head, but these are not shown.) The tails of the two heavy chains form a single coiled-coil tail. (B) The coiled-coil tails of myosin-II molecules associate with one another to form a bipolar myosin filament in which the heads project outward from the middle in opposite directions. The bare region in the middle of the filament consists of tails only.

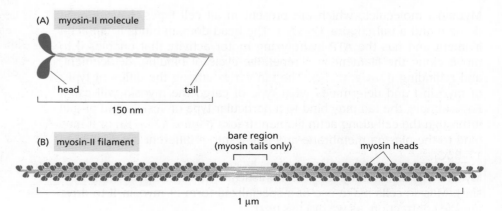

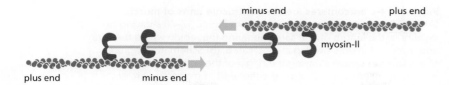

The myosin filament is like a double-headed arrow, with the two sets of myosin heads pointing outward, away from the middle. One set binds to actin filaments in one orientation and moves the filaments one way; the other set binds to other actin filaments in the opposite orientation and moves the filaments in the opposite direction. As a result, a myosin filament slides sets of oppositely oriented actin filaments past one another (Figure 17–39). Thus, if actin filaments and myosin filaments are organized together in a bundle, the bundle can generate a strong contractile force. This is seen most clearly in muscle contraction, but it also occurs in the much smaller *contractile bundles* of actin filaments and myosin-II filaments (see Figure 17–29B) that assemble transiently in nonmuscle cells, and in the *contractile ring* that pinches a dividing cell in two by contracting and pulling inward on the plasma membrane (see Figure 17–29D).

Actin Filaments Slide Against Myosin Filaments During Muscle Contraction

In most animals, *skeletal muscle fibers* are huge, multinucleated individual cells formed by the fusion of many separate smaller cells. The nuclei of the contributing cells are retained in the muscle fiber and lie just beneath the plasma membrane. The bulk of the cytoplasm is made up of **myofibrils**, the contractile elements of the muscle cell. These cylindrical structures are 1–2 μm in diameter and may be as long as the muscle cell itself (Figure 17–40A).

A myofibril consists of a chain of identical tiny contractile units, or **sarcomeres**. Each sarcomere is about 2.5 μm long, and the repeating pattern of sarcomeres gives the vertebrate myofibril a striped appearance (Figure 17–40B). Sarcomeres are highly organized assemblies of two types of filaments—actin filaments and myosin filaments composed

Figure 17–39 A small, bipolar myosin-II filament can slide two actin filaments of opposite orientation past each other. Similar sliding movement mediates the contraction of interacting actin and myosin-II filaments in both muscle and nonmuscle cells. As with myosin-I, a myosin-II head group walks toward the plus end of the actin filament with which it interacts. Note that multiple myosin molecules are required to generate movement: when one myosin head releases the filament to reposition itself, other myosins must remain attached so the structure does not fall apart.

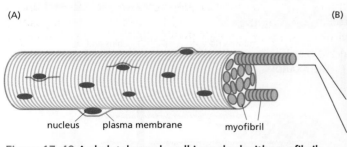

(A)

nucleus   plasma membrane   myofibril

(B)

sarcomere ~2.5 μm   sarcomere   two myofibrils

Figure 17–40 A skeletal muscle cell is packed with myofibrils. (A) In an adult human, these huge, multinucleated cells (also called muscle fibers) are typically 50 μm in diameter, and they can be several centimeters long. They contain numerous myofibrils, in which actin filaments and myosin-II filaments are arranged in a highly organized structure, giving each myofibril—and skeletal muscle cell—a striated or striped appearance; for this reason, skeletal muscle is also called striated muscle. (B) Low-magnification electron micrograph of a longitudinal section through a skeletal muscle cell of a rabbit, showing that each myofibril consists of a repeating chain of sarcomeres, the contractile units of the myofibrils. (B, courtesy of Roger Craig.)

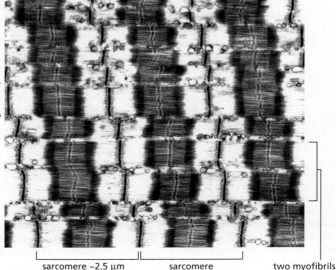

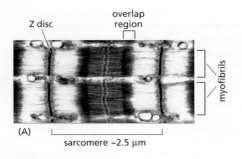

Z disc

overlap region

myofibrils

(A)

sarcomere ~2.5 μm

thin filament (actin)   thick filament (myosin-II)

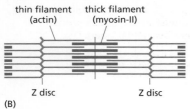

Z disc   Z disc

(B)

Figure 17–41 Sarcomeres are the contractile units of muscle.
(A) Detail of the electron micrograph from Figure 17–40 showing two myofibrils; the length of one sarcomere and the region where the actin and myosin filaments overlap are indicated. (B) Schematic diagram of a single sarcomere showing the origin of the light and dark bands seen in the microscope. Z discs at either end of the sarcomere are attachment points for the plus ends of actin filaments. The centrally located thick filaments (*green*) are each composed of many myosin-II molecules. The thin vertical line running down the center of the thick filament bundle in (A) corresponds to the bare regions of the myosin filaments, as seen in Figure 17–38B. (A, courtesy of Roger Craig.)

of a muscle-specific form of myosin-II. The myosin filaments (the *thick filaments*) are centrally positioned in each sarcomere, whereas the more slender actin filaments (the *thin filaments*) extend inward from each end of the sarcomere, where they are anchored by their plus ends to a structure known as the *Z disc*. The minus ends of the actin filaments overlap the ends of the myosin filaments (**Figure 17–41**).

The contraction of a muscle cell is caused by a simultaneous shortening of all the cell's sarcomeres, which is caused by the actin filaments sliding past the myosin filaments, with no change in the length of either type of filament (**Figure 17–42**). The sliding motion is generated by myosin heads that project from the sides of the myosin filament and interact with adjacent actin filaments (see Figure 17–39). When a muscle is stimulated to contract, the myosin heads start to walk along the actin filament in repeated cycles of attachment and detachment. During each cycle, a myosin head binds and hydrolyzes one molecule of ATP. This causes a series of conformational changes that move the tip of the head by about 5 nm along the actin filament toward the plus end. This movement, repeated with each round of ATP hydrolysis, propels the myosin molecule unidirectionally along the actin filament (**Figure 17–43**). In so doing, the myosin heads pull against the actin filament, causing it to slide against

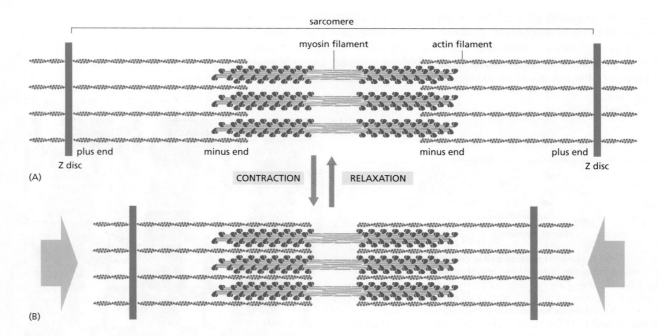

Figure 17–42 Muscles contract by a sliding-filament mechanism. (A) The myosin and actin filaments of a sarcomere overlap with the same relative polarity on either side of the midline. Recall that actin filaments are anchored by their plus ends to the Z disc and that myosin filaments are bipolar. (B) During contraction, the actin and myosin filaments slide past each other. Although the filaments themselves remain the same length, the sarcomere to which they belong shortens. The sliding motion is driven by the myosin heads walking toward the plus ends of the adjacent actin filaments (Movie 17.11).

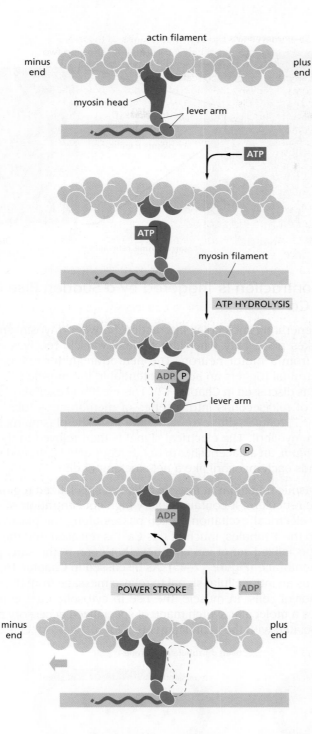

ATP

ATP HYDROLYSIS

P

POWER STROKE   ADP

ATTACHED   At the start of the cycle shown in this figure, a myosin head lacking a bound ATP or ADP is attached tightly to an actin filament in a *rigor* configuration (so named because it is responsible for *rigor mortis*, the rigidity of death). In an actively contracting muscle, this state is very short-lived, being rapidly terminated by the binding of a molecule of ATP to the myosin head.

RELEASED   A molecule of ATP binds to the large cleft on the "back" of the myosin head (that is, on the side furthest from the actin filament) and immediately causes a slight change in the conformation of the domains that make up the actin-binding site. This reduces the affinity of the head for actin and allows it to let go of the filament. (The space drawn here between the head and actin emphasizes this change, although in reality the head probably remains very close to the actin.)

COCKED   The cleft closes like a clam shell around the ATP molecule, triggering a large shape change that causes the head to be displaced along the actin filament by a distance of about 5 nm. Hydrolysis of ATP occurs, but the ADP and inorganic phosphate (P) produced remain tightly bound to the myosin head. Dotted lines show the position of myosin head prior to ATP hydrolysis.

FORCE-GENERATING   Weak binding of the myosin head to a new site on the actin filament causes release of the inorganic phosphate produced by ATP hydrolysis. This release triggers the power stroke—the force-generating change in shape during which the head regains its original conformation. In the course of the power stroke, the head loses its bound ADP, thereby returning to the start of a new cycle.

ATTACHED   At the end of the cycle, the myosin head is again bound tightly to the actin filament in a rigor configuration. Note that the head has moved to a new position on the actin filament, which has slid to the left along the myosin filament.

the myosin filament. The concerted action of many myosin heads pulling the actin and myosin filaments past each other causes the sarcomere to contract. After a contraction is completed, the myosin heads all lose contact with the actin filaments, and the muscle relaxes.

A myosin filament has about 300 myosin heads. Each myosin head can attach and detach from actin about five times per second, allowing the myosin and actin filaments to slide past one another at speeds of up to 15 µm per second. This speed is sufficient to take a sarcomere from a fully extended state (3 µm) to a fully contracted state (2 µm) in less than one-tenth of a second. All of the sarcomeres of a muscle are coupled together and are triggered simultaneously by the signaling system we describe next, so the entire muscle contracts almost instantaneously.

Figure 17–43 The head of a myosin-II molecule walks along an actin filament through an ATP-dependent cycle of conformational changes. Two actin monomers are highlighted to make the movement of the actin filament easier to see. Movie 17.12 shows actin and myosin in action. (Based on I. Rayment et al., *Science* 261:50–58, 1993.)

Figure 17–44 T tubules and the sarcoplasmic reticulum surround each myofibril. (A) Drawing of the two membrane systems that relay the signal to contract from the muscle cell plasma membrane to all of the myofibrils in the muscle cell (see Figure 17–40). (B) Electron micrograph showing a cross section of a T tubule and the adjacent sarcoplasmic reticulum compartments. (B, courtesy of Clara Franzini-Armstrong.)

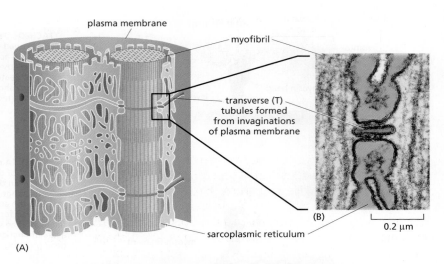

(A)

Muscle Contraction Is Triggered by a Sudden Rise in Cytosolic Ca²⁺

The force-generating molecular interaction between myosin and actin filaments takes place only when the skeletal muscle receives a signal to contract from a motor neuron. The neurotransmitter released from the nerve terminal triggers an action potential in the muscle cell plasma membrane (as discussed in Chapter 12). This electrical excitation spreads in a matter of milliseconds into a series of membranous tubes, called *transverse* (or *T*) *tubules*, that extend inward from the plasma membrane around each myofibril. The electrical signal is then relayed to the *sarcoplasmic reticulum*, an adjacent sheath of interconnected flattened vesicles that surrounds each myofibril like a net stocking (**Figure 17–44**).

The sarcoplasmic reticulum in muscle cells is a specialized region of the endoplasmic reticulum. It contains a very high concentration of Ca^{2+}. In response to electrical excitation, which passes along the plasma membrane and to the T tubules, much of this Ca^{2+} is released into the cytosol through a specialized set of ion channels that open in the sarcoplasmic reticulum membrane (**Figure 17–45**). As discussed in Chapter 16, Ca^{2+} is widely used as an intracellular signal to relay a message from the exterior to the interior of cells. In muscle, the rise in cytosolic Ca^{2+} concentration activates a molecular switch made of specialized accessory proteins closely associated with the actin filaments (**Figure 17–46A**). One of these

QUESTION 17–9

Compare the structure of intermediate filaments with that of the myosin-II filaments in skeletal muscle cells. What are the major similarities? What are the major differences? How do the differences in structure relate to their function?

Figure 17–45 Skeletal muscle contraction is triggered by the release of Ca²⁺ from the sarcoplasmic reticulum into the cytosol. This schematic diagram shows how a Ca²⁺-release channel in the sarcoplasmic reticulum membrane is opened by a physical linkage to a voltage-gated Ca²⁺ channel in the T-tubule membrane. The T-tubule membrane and sarcoplasmic reticulum membrane are drawn in the same orientation shown in the micrograph in Figure 17–44B.

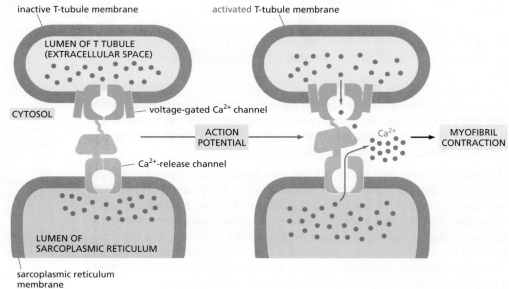

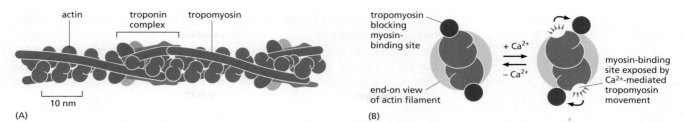

proteins is *tropomyosin*, a rigid, rod-shaped molecule that binds in the groove of the actin helix, where it prevents the myosin heads from associating with the actin filament. The other is *troponin*, a protein complex that includes a Ca^{2+}-sensitive protein associated with the end of a tropomyosin molecule. When the concentration of Ca^{2+} in the cytosol rises, Ca^{2+} binds to troponin and induces a change in its shape. This in turn causes the tropomyosin molecules to shift their positions slightly, allowing myosin heads to bind to the actin filaments, initiating contraction (**Figure 17–46B**).

Because the signal from the plasma membrane is passed within milliseconds (via the T tubules and sarcoplasmic reticulum) to every sarcomere in the cell, all the myofibrils in the cell contract at the same time. The increase in Ca^{2+} in the cytosol is transient because, when the nerve signal terminates, the Ca^{2+} is rapidly pumped back into the sarcoplasmic reticulum by abundant Ca^{2+} pumps in its membrane (discussed in Chapter 12). As soon as the Ca^{2+} concentration returns to the resting level, troponin and tropomyosin molecules move back to their original positions. This reconfiguration once again blocks myosin binding to actin filaments, thereby ending the contraction.

Different Types of Muscle Cells Perform Different Functions

The highly specialized contractile machinery in muscle cells is thought to have evolved from the simpler contractile bundles of myosin and actin filaments found in all eukaryotic cells. The myosin-II in nonmuscle cells is also activated by a rise in cytosolic Ca^{2+}, but the mechanism of activation is different from that of the muscle-specific myosin-II. An increase in Ca^{2+} leads to the phosphorylation of nonmuscle myosin-II, which alters the myosin conformation and enables it to interact with actin. A similar activation mechanism operates in *smooth muscle*, which is present in the walls of the stomach, intestine, uterus, and arteries, and in many other structures that undergo slow and sustained involuntary contractions. This mode of myosin activation is relatively slow, because time is needed for enzyme molecules to diffuse to the myosin heads and carry out the phosphorylation and subsequent dephosphorylation. However, this mechanism has the advantage that—unlike the mechanism used by skeletal muscle cells—it can be activated by a variety of extracellular signals: thus smooth muscle, for example, is triggered to contract by epinephrine, serotonin, prostaglandins, and several other signal molecules.

In addition to skeletal and smooth muscle, other forms of muscle each perform a specific mechanical function. Heart—or *cardiac*—muscle, for instance, drives the circulation of blood. The heart contracts autonomously for the entire life of the organism—some 3 billion (3×10^9) times in an average human lifetime. Even subtle abnormalities in the actin or myosin of heart muscle can lead to serious disease. For example, mutations in the genes that encode cardiac myosin-II or other proteins in the sarcomere cause familial hypertrophic cardiomyopathy, a hereditary disorder responsible for sudden death in young athletes.

Figure 17–46 Skeletal muscle contraction is controlled by tropomyosin and troponin complexes. (A) An actin filament in muscle showing the positions of tropomyosin and troponin complexes along the filament. Every tropomyosin molecule has seven evenly spaced regions with a similar amino acid sequence, each of which is thought to bind to an actin monomer in the filament. (B) This cross section of the muscle actin filament reveals how Ca^{2+} binding to the troponin complex (not shown) leads to movement of tropomyosin away from the myosin-binding site.

QUESTION 17–10

A. Note that in Figure 17–46, troponin molecules are evenly spaced along an actin filament, with one troponin found every seventh actin molecule. How do you suppose troponin molecules can be positioned this regularly? What does this tell you about the binding of troponin to actin filaments?
B. What do you suppose would happen if you mixed actin filaments with (i) troponin alone, (ii) tropomyosin alone, or (iii) troponin plus tropomyosin, and then added myosin? Would the effects be dependent on Ca^{2+}?

The contraction of muscle cells represents a highly specialized use of the basic components of the eukaryotic cytoskeleton. In the following chapter, we discuss the crucial roles of the cytoskeleton in perhaps the most fundamental cell movements of all: the segregation of newly replicated chromosomes and the formation of two daughter cells during the process of cell division.

ESSENTIAL CONCEPTS

- The cytoplasm of a eukaryotic cell is supported and organized by a cytoskeleton of intermediate filaments, microtubules, and actin filaments.

- Intermediate filaments are stable, ropelike polymers—built from fibrous protein subunits—that give cells mechanical strength. Some intermediate filaments form the nuclear lamina that supports and strengthens the nuclear envelope; others are distributed throughout the cytoplasm.

- Microtubules are stiff, hollow tubes formed by globular tubulin dimers. They are polarized structures, with a slow-growing minus end and a fast-growing plus end.

- Microtubules grow out from organizing centers such as the centrosome, in which the minus ends remain embedded.

- Many microtubules display dynamic instability, alternating rapidly between growth and shrinkage. Shrinkage is promoted by the hydrolysis of the GTP that is tightly bound to tubulin dimers, reducing the affinity of the dimers for their neighbors and thereby promoting microtubule disassembly.

- Microtubules can be stabilized by localized proteins that capture the plus ends, thereby helping to position the microtubules and harness them for specific functions.

- Kinesins and dyneins are microtubule-associated motor proteins that use the energy of ATP hydrolysis to move unidirectionally along microtubules. They carry specific organelles, vesicles, and other types of cargo to particular locations in the cell.

- Eukaryotic cilia and flagella contain a bundle of stable microtubules. Their rhythmic beating is caused by bending of the microtubules, driven by the ciliary dynein motor protein.

- Actin filaments are helical polymers of globular actin monomers. They are more flexible than microtubules and are generally found in bundles or networks.

- Like microtubules, actin filaments are polarized, with a fast-growing plus end and a slow-growing minus end. Their assembly and disassembly are controlled by the hydrolysis of ATP tightly bound to each actin monomer and by various actin-binding proteins.

- The varied arrangements and functions of actin filaments in cells stem from the diversity of actin-binding proteins, which can control actin polymerization, cross-link actin filaments into loose networks or stiff bundles, attach actin filaments to membranes, or move two adjacent filaments relative to each other.

- A concentrated network of actin filaments underneath the plasma membrane forms the bulk of the cell cortex, which is responsible for the shape and movement of the cell surface, including the movements involved when a cell crawls along a surface.

- Myosins are motor proteins that use the energy of ATP hydrolysis to move along actin filaments. In nonmuscle cells, myosin-I can carry organelles or vesicles along actin-filament tracks, and myosin-II can cause adjacent actin filaments to slide past each other in contractile bundles.

- In skeletal muscle cells, repeating arrays of overlapping filaments of actin and myosin-II form highly ordered myofibrils, which contract as these filaments slide past each other.

- Muscle contraction is initiated by a sudden rise in cytosolic Ca^{2+}, which delivers a signal to the myofibrils via Ca^{2+}-binding proteins associated with the actin filaments.

KEY TERMS

actin-binding protein	lamellipodium
actin filament	microtubule
cell cortex	microtubule-associated protein
centriole	motor protein
centrosome	myofibril
cilium	myosin
cytoskeleton	myosin-I
dynamic instability	myosin-II
dynein	myosin filament
filopodium	nuclear lamina
flagellum	polarity
intermediate filament	Rho protein family
keratin filament	sarcomere
kinesin	tubulin

QUESTIONS

QUESTION 17–11

Which of the following statements are correct? Explain your answers.

A. Kinesin moves endoplasmic reticulum (ER) membranes along microtubules so that the network of ER tubules becomes stretched throughout the cell.

B. Without actin, cells can form a functional mitotic spindle and pull their chromosomes apart but cannot divide.

C. Lamellipodia and filopodia are "feelers" that a cell extends to find anchor points on the substratum that it will then crawl over.

D. GTP is hydrolyzed by tubulin to cause the bending of flagella.

E. Cells having an intermediate-filament network that cannot be depolymerized would die.

F. The plus ends of microtubules grow faster because they have a larger GTP cap.

G. The transverse tubules in muscle cells are an extension of the plasma membrane, with which they are continuous; similarly, the sarcoplasmic reticulum is an extension of the endoplasmic reticulum.

H. Activation of myosin movement on actin filaments is triggered by the phosphorylation of troponin in some situations and by Ca^{2+} binding to troponin in others.

QUESTION 17–12

The average time taken for a molecule or an organelle to diffuse a distance of x cm is given by the formula

$$t = x^2/2D$$

where t is the time in seconds and D is a constant called the diffusion coefficient for the molecule or particle. Using the above formula, calculate the time it would take for a small molecule, a protein, and a membrane vesicle to diffuse from one side to another of a cell 10 μm across. Typical diffusion coefficients in units of cm^2/sec are: small molecule, 5×10^{-6}; protein molecule, 5×10^{-7}; vesicle, 5×10^{-8}. How long would a membrane vesicle take to reach the end of an axon 10 cm long by free diffusion? How long would it take if it was transported along microtubules at 1 μm/sec?

QUESTION 17–13

Why do eukaryotic cells, and especially animal cells, have such large and complex cytoskeletons? List the differences between animal cells and bacteria that depend on the eukaryotic cytoskeleton.

QUESTION 17–14

Examine the structure of an intermediate filament shown in Figure 17–4. Does the filament have a unique polarity—that is, could you distinguish one end from the other by chemical or other means? Explain your answer.

QUESTION 17–15

There are no known motor proteins that move on intermediate filaments. Suggest an explanation for this.

QUESTION 17–16

When cells enter mitosis, their existing array of cytoplasmic microtubules has to be rapidly broken down and replaced with the mitotic spindle that forms to pull the chromosomes into the daughter cells. The enzyme katanin, named after Japanese samurai swords, is activated during the onset of mitosis, and chops microtubules into short pieces. What do you suppose is the fate of the microtubule fragments created by katanin? Explain your answer.

QUESTION 17–17

The drug Taxol, extracted from the bark of yew trees, has an opposite effect to the drug colchicine, an alkaloid from autumn crocus. Taxol binds tightly to microtubules and stabilizes them; when added to cells, it causes much of the free tubulin to assemble into microtubules. In contrast, colchicine prevents microtubule formation. Taxol is just as pernicious to dividing cells as colchicine, and both are used as anticancer drugs. Based on your knowledge of microtubule dynamics, suggest why both drugs are toxic to dividing cells despite their opposite actions.

QUESTION 17–18

A useful technique for studying microtubule motors is to attach them by their tails to a glass cover slip (which can be accomplished quite easily because the tails stick avidly to a clean glass surface) and then allow them to settle. Microtubules may then be viewed in a light microscope as they are propelled over the surface of the cover slip by the heads of the motor proteins. Because the motor proteins attach at random orientations to the cover slip, however, how can they generate coordinated movement of individual microtubules rather than engaging in a tug-of-war? In which direction will microtubules crawl on a "bed" of kinesin molecules (i.e., will they move plus-end first or minus-end first)?

QUESTION 17–19

A typical time course of polymerization of purified tubulin to form microtubules is shown in Figure Q17–19.

A. Explain the different parts of the curve (labeled A, B, and C). Draw a diagram that shows the behavior of tubulin subunits in each of the three phases.

B. How would the curve in the figure change if centrosomes were added at the outset?

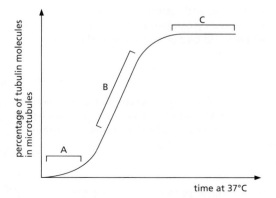

Figure Q17–19

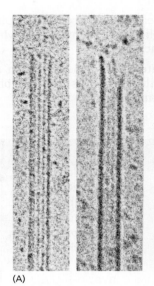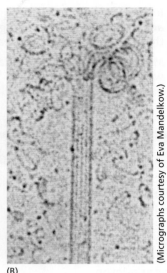

(A)   (B)

(Micrographs courtesy of Eva Mandelkow.)

Figure Q17–20

QUESTION 17–20

The electron micrographs shown in Figure Q17–20A were obtained from a population of microtubules that were growing rapidly. Figure Q17–20B was obtained from microtubules undergoing "catastrophic" shrinking. Comment on any differences between A and B, and suggest likely explanations for the differences that you observe.

QUESTION 17–21

The locomotion of fibroblasts in culture is immediately halted by the drug cytochalasin, whereas colchicine causes fibroblasts to cease to move directionally and to begin extending lamellipodia in seemingly random directions. Injection of fibroblasts with antibodies to the intermediate filament protein vimentin has no discernible effect on their migration. What do these observations suggest to you about the involvement of the three different cytoskeletal filaments in fibroblast locomotion?

QUESTION 17–22

Complete the following sentence accurately, explaining your reason for accepting or rejecting each of the four phrases (more than one can be correct). The role of calcium in muscle contraction is:

A. to detach myosin heads from actin.

B. to spread the action potential from the plasma membrane to the contractile machinery.

C. to bind to troponin, cause it to move tropomyosin, and thereby expose actin filaments to myosin heads.

D. to maintain the structure of the myosin filament.

QUESTION 17–23

Which of the following changes takes place when a skeletal muscle contracts?

A. Z discs move farther apart.

B. Actin filaments contract.

C. Myosin filaments contract.

D. Sarcomeres become shorter.

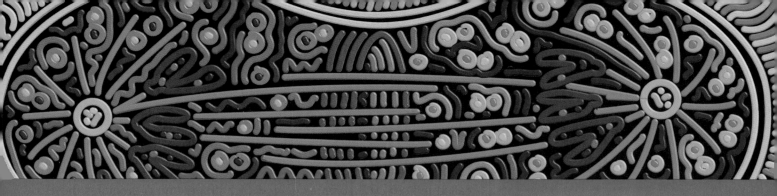

The Cell-Division Cycle

"Where a cell arises, there must be a previous cell, just as animals can only arise from animals and plants from plants." This statement, which appears in a book written by German pathologist Rudolf Virchow in 1858, carries with it a profound message for the continuity of life. If every cell comes from a previous cell, then all living organisms—from a unicellular bacterium to a multicellular mammal—are products of repeated rounds of cell growth and division, stretching back to the beginnings of life more than 3 billion years ago.

A cell reproduces by carrying out an orderly sequence of events in which it duplicates its contents and then divides in two. This cycle of duplication and division, known as the **cell cycle**, is the essential mechanism by which all living things reproduce. The details of the cell cycle vary from organism to organism and at different times in an individual organism's life. In unicellular organisms, such as bacteria and yeasts, each cell division produces a complete new organism, whereas many rounds of cell division are required to make a new multicellular organism from a fertilized egg. Certain features of the cell cycle, however, are universal, as they allow every cell to perform the fundamental task of copying and passing on its genetic information to the next generation of cells.

To explain how cells reproduce, we have to consider three major questions: (1) How do cells duplicate their contents—including the chromosomes, which carry the genetic information? (2) How do they partition the duplicated contents and split in two? (3) How do they coordinate all the steps and machinery required for these two processes? The first question is considered elsewhere in this book: in Chapter 6, we discuss how DNA is replicated, and in Chapters 7, 11, 15, and 17, we describe how the eukaryotic cell manufactures its numerous other components, such as proteins, membranes, organelles, and cytoskeletal filaments. In this chapter, we tackle the second and third questions: how a eukaryotic cell distributes—or *segregates*—its duplicated contents to produce two genetically identical daughter cells, and how it coordinates the various steps of this reproductive cycle.

We begin with an overview of the events that take place during a typical cell cycle. We then describe the complex system of regulatory proteins called the *cell-cycle control system*, which orders and coordinates these events to ensure that they occur in the correct sequence. We next discuss in detail the major stages of the cell cycle, in which the chromosomes are duplicated and then segregated into the two daughter cells. At the end of the chapter, we consider how animals use extracellular signals to control the survival, growth, and division of their cells. These signaling systems allow an animal to regulate the size and number of its cells—and, ultimately, the size and form of the organism itself.

OVERVIEW OF THE CELL CYCLE

The most basic function of the cell cycle is to duplicate accurately the vast amount of DNA in the chromosomes and then to segregate the DNA into genetically identical daughter cells such that each cell receives a complete copy of the entire genome (Figure 18–1). In most cases, a cell also duplicates its other macromolecules and organelles and doubles in size before it reproduces; otherwise, each time a cell divided, it would get smaller and smaller. Thus, to maintain their size, proliferating cells coordinate their growth with their division. We return to the topic of cell-size control later in the chapter; here, we focus on cell division.

The duration of the cell cycle varies greatly from one cell type to another. In an early frog embryo, cells divide every 30 minutes, whereas a mammalian fibroblast in culture divides about once a day (Table 18–1). In this section, we describe briefly the sequence of events that occur in proliferating mammalian cells. We then introduce the cell-cycle control system that ensures that the various events of the cycle take place in the correct sequence and at the correct time.

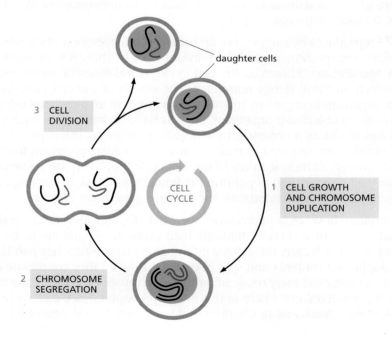

Figure 18–1 **Cells reproduce by duplicating their contents and dividing in two in a process called the cell cycle.** For simplicity, we use a hypothetical eukaryotic cell—which has only one copy each of two different chromosomes—to illustrate how each cell cycle produces two genetically identical daughter cells. Each daughter cell can divide again by going through another cell cycle, and so on for generation after generation.

TABLE 18–1 SOME EUKARYOTIC CELL-CYCLE DURATIONS	
Cell Type	Duration of Cell Cycle
Early fly embryo cells	8 minutes
Early frog embryo cells	30 minutes
Mammalian intestinal epithelial cells	~12 hours
Mammalian fibroblasts in culture	~20 hours

The Eukaryotic Cell Cycle Usually Includes Four Phases

Seen in a microscope, the two most dramatic events in the cell cycle are when the nucleus divides, a process called *mitosis*, and when the cell itself then splits in two, a process called *cytokinesis*. These two processes together constitute the **M phase** of the cycle. In a typical mammalian cell, the whole of M phase takes about an hour, which is only a small fraction of the total cell-cycle time (see Table 18–1).

The period between one M phase and the next is called **interphase**. Viewed with a microscope, it appears, deceptively, as an uneventful interlude during which the cell simply increases in size. Interphase, however, is a very busy time for a proliferating cell, and it encompasses the remaining three phases of the cell cycle. During **S phase** (S = synthesis), the cell replicates its DNA. S phase is flanked by two "gap" phases—called **G_1 phase** and **G_2 phase**—during which the cell continues to grow (**Figure 18–2**). During these gap phases, the cell monitors both its internal state and external environment. This monitoring ensures that conditions are suitable for reproduction and that preparations are complete before the cell commits to the major upheavals of S phase (which follows G_1) and mitosis (following G_2). At particular points in G_1 and G_2, the cell decides whether to proceed to the next phase or pause to allow more time to prepare.

During all of interphase, a cell generally continues to transcribe genes, synthesize proteins, and grow in mass. Together with S phase, G_1 and G_2 provide the time needed for the cell to enlarge and to duplicate its cytoplasmic organelles. If interphase lasted only long enough for DNA replication, the cell would not have time to double its mass before it divided and would consequently shrink with each division. Indeed, in some special circumstances that is exactly what happens. In an early frog embryo, for example, the first cell divisions after fertilization (called *cleavage divisions*) serve to subdivide the giant egg cell into many smaller cells

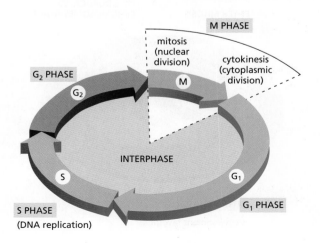

Figure 18–2 **The eukaryotic cell cycle usually occurs in four phases.** The cell grows continuously during interphase, which consists of three phases: G_1, S, and G_2. DNA replication is confined to S phase. G_1 is the gap between M phase and S phase, and G_2 is the gap between S phase and M phase. During M phase, the nucleus divides in a process called mitosis; then the cytoplasm divides, in a process called cytokinesis. In this figure—and in subsequent figures in the chapter—the lengths of the various phases are not drawn to scale: M phase, for example, is typically much shorter and G_1 much longer than shown.

QUESTION 18–2

A population of proliferating cells is stained with a dye that becomes fluorescent when it binds to DNA, so that the amount of fluorescence is directly proportional to the amount of DNA in each cell. To measure the amount of DNA in each cell, the cells are then passed through a flow cytometer, an instrument that measures the amount of fluorescence in individual cells. The number of cells with a given DNA content is plotted on the graph below.

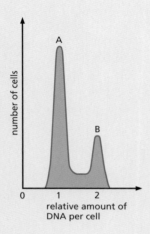

Indicate on the graph where you would expect to find cells that are in G_1, S, G_2, and mitosis. Which is the longest phase of the cell cycle in this population of cells?

as quickly as possible (see Table 18–1). In such embryonic cell cycles, the G_1 and G_2 phases are drastically shortened, and the cells do not grow before they divide.

A Cell-Cycle Control System Triggers the Major Processes of the Cell Cycle

To ensure that they replicate all their DNA and organelles, and divide in an orderly manner, eukaryotic cells possess a complex network of regulatory proteins known as the *cell-cycle control system*. This system guarantees that the events of the cell cycle—DNA replication, mitosis, and so on—occur in a set sequence and that each process has been completed before the next one begins. To accomplish this organizational feat, the control system is itself regulated at certain critical points of the cycle by feedback from the process currently being performed. Without such feedback, an interruption or a delay in any of the processes could be disastrous. All of the nuclear DNA, for example, must be replicated before the nucleus begins to divide, which means that a complete S phase must precede M phase. If DNA synthesis is slowed down or stalled, mitosis and cell division must also be delayed. Similarly, if DNA is damaged, the cycle must be put on hold in G_1, S, or G_2 so that the cell can repair the damage, either before DNA replication is started or completed or before the cell enters M phase. The cell-cycle control system achieves all of this by employing a set of molecular brakes, sometimes called *checkpoints*, to pause the cycle at certain transition points. In this way, the control system does not trigger the next step in the cycle unless the cell is properly prepared.

The cell-cycle control system regulates progression through the cell cycle at three main transition points (**Figure 18–3**). At the transition from G_1 to S phase, the control system confirms that the environment is favorable for proliferation before committing to DNA replication. Cell proliferation in animals requires both sufficient nutrients and specific signal molecules in the extracellular environment; if these extracellular conditions are unfavorable, cells can delay progress through G_1 and may even enter a specialized resting state known as G_0 (G zero). At the transition from G_2 to M phase, the control system confirms that the DNA is undamaged and fully replicated, ensuring that the cell does not enter mitosis unless its DNA is intact. Finally, during mitosis, the cell-cycle control machinery

Figure 18–3 The cell-cycle control system ensures that key processes in the cycle occur in the proper sequence. The cell-cycle control system is shown as a controller arm that rotates clockwise, triggering essential processes when it reaches particular transition points on the outer dial. These processes include DNA replication in S phase and the segregation of duplicated chromosomes in mitosis. The control system can transiently halt the cycle at specific transition points—in G_1, G_2, and M phase—if extracellular or intracellular conditions are unfavorable.

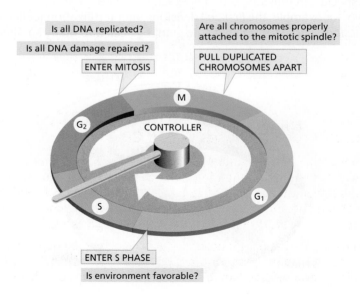

ensures that the duplicated chromosomes are properly attached to a cytoskeletal machine, called the *mitotic spindle*, before the spindle pulls the chromosomes apart and segregates them into the two daughter cells.

In animals, the transition from G_1 to S phase is especially important as a point in the cell cycle where the control system is regulated. Signals from other cells stimulate cell proliferation when more cells are needed—and block it when they are not. The cell-cycle control system therefore plays a central part in the regulation of cell numbers in the tissues of the body; if the control system malfunctions such that cell division is excessive, cancer can result. We discuss later how extracellular signals influence the decisions made at the G_1-to-S transition.

Cell-Cycle Control Is Similar in All Eukaryotes

Some features of the cell cycle, including the time required to complete certain events, vary greatly from one cell type to another, even within the same organism. The basic organization of the cycle, however, is essentially the same in all eukaryotic cells, and all eukaryotes appear to use similar machinery and control mechanisms to drive and regulate cell-cycle events. The proteins of the cell-cycle control system first appeared more than a billion years ago, and they have been so well conserved over the course of evolution that many of them function perfectly when transferred from a human cell to a yeast (see How We Know, pp. 30–31).

Because of this similarity, biologists can study the cell cycle and its regulation in a variety of organisms and use the findings from all of them to assemble a unified picture of how the cycle works. Many discoveries about the cell cycle have come from a systematic search for mutations that inactivate essential components of the cell-cycle control system in yeasts. Likewise, studies of both cultured mammalian cells and the embryos of frogs and sea urchins have been critical for examining the molecular mechanisms that underlie the cycle and its control in multicellular organisms like ourselves.

THE CELL-CYCLE CONTROL SYSTEM

Two types of machinery are involved in cell division: one manufactures the new components of the growing cell, and another hauls the components into their correct places and partitions them appropriately when the cell divides in two. The **cell-cycle control system** switches all this machinery on and off at the correct times, thereby coordinating the various steps of the cycle. The core of the cell-cycle control system is a series of molecular switches that operate in a defined sequence and orchestrate the main events of the cycle, including DNA replication and the segregation of duplicated chromosomes. In this section, we review the protein components of the control system and discuss how they work together to trigger the different phases of the cycle.

The Cell-Cycle Control System Depends on Cyclically Activated Protein Kinases Called Cdks

The cell-cycle control system governs the cell-cycle machinery by cyclically activating and then inactivating the key proteins and protein complexes that initiate or regulate DNA replication, mitosis, and cytokinesis. This regulation is carried out largely through the phosphorylation and dephosphorylation of proteins involved in these essential processes.

As discussed in Chapter 4, phosphorylation followed by dephosphorylation is one of the most common ways by which cells switch the activity of a protein on and off (see Figure 4–46), and the cell-cycle control system

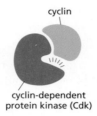

cyclin

cyclin-dependent
protein kinase (Cdk)

Figure 18–4 Progression through the cell cycle depends on cyclin-dependent protein kinases (Cdks). A Cdk must bind a regulatory protein called a cyclin before it can become enzymatically active. This activation also requires an activating phosphorylation of the Cdk (not shown, but see Movie 18.1). Once activated, a cyclin–Cdk complex phosphorylates key proteins in the cell that are required to initiate particular steps in the cell cycle. The cyclin also helps direct the Cdk to the target proteins that the Cdk phosphorylates.

uses this mechanism extensively and repeatedly. The phosphorylation reactions that control the cell cycle are carried out by a specific set of protein kinases, while dephosphorylation is performed by a set of protein phosphatases.

The protein kinases at the core of the cell-cycle control system are present in proliferating cells throughout the cell cycle. They are activated, however, only at appropriate times in the cycle, after which they are quickly inactivated. Thus, the activity of each of these kinases rises and falls in a cyclical fashion. Some of these protein kinases, for example, become active toward the end of G_1 phase and are responsible for driving the cell into S phase; another kinase becomes active just before M phase and drives the cell into mitosis.

Switching these kinases on and off at the appropriate times is partly the responsibility of another set of proteins in the control system—the **cyclins**. Cyclins have no enzymatic activity themselves, but they must bind to the cell-cycle kinases before the kinases can become enzymatically active. The kinases of the cell-cycle control system are therefore known as **cyclin-dependent protein kinases**, or **Cdks** (Figure 18–4). Cyclins are so-named because, unlike the Cdks, their concentrations vary in a cyclical fashion during the cell cycle. The cyclical changes in cyclin concentrations help drive the cyclic assembly and activation of the cyclin–Cdk complexes. Once activated, cyclin–Cdk complexes help trigger various cell-cycle events, such as entry into S phase or M phase (Figure 18–5). We discuss how the Cdks and cyclins were discovered in How We Know, pp. 615–616.

Different Cyclin–Cdk Complexes Trigger Different Steps in the Cell Cycle

There are several types of cyclins and, in most eukaryotes, several types of Cdks involved in cell-cycle control. Different cyclin–Cdk complexes trigger different steps of the cell cycle. As shown in Figure 18–5, the cyclin that acts in G_2 to trigger entry into M phase is called **M cyclin**, and the active complex it forms with its Cdk is called **M-Cdk**. Other cyclins, called **S cyclins** and **G_1/S cyclins**, bind to a distinct Cdk protein late in G_1 to form **S-Cdk** and **G_1/S-Cdk**, respectively; these cyclin–Cdk complexes help launch S phase. The rise and fall of S cyclin and M cyclin concentrations

Figure 18–5 The accumulation of cyclins helps regulate the activity of Cdks. The formation of active cyclin–Cdk complexes drives various cell-cycle events, including entry into S phase or M phase. The figure shows the changes in cyclin concentration and Cdk protein kinase activity responsible for controlling entry into M phase. Increasing concentration of the relevant cyclin (called M cyclin) helps direct the formation of the active cyclin–Cdk complex (M-Cdk) that drives entry into M phase. Although the enzymatic activity of each type of cyclin–Cdk complex rises and falls during the course of the cell cycle, the concentration of the Cdk component does not (not shown).

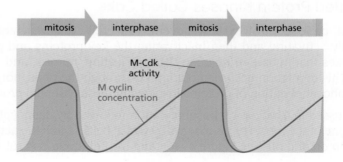

mitosis | interphase | mitosis | interphase

M-Cdk
activity

M cyclin
concentration

DISCOVERY OF CYCLINS AND Cdks

For many years, cell biologists watched the "puppet show" of DNA synthesis, mitosis, and cytokinesis but had no idea what was behind the curtain, controlling these events. The cell-cycle control system was simply a "black box" inside the cell. It was not even clear whether there was a separate control system, or whether the cell-cycle machinery somehow controlled itself. A breakthrough came with the identification of the key proteins of the control system and the realization that they are distinct from the components of the cell-cycle machinery—the enzymes and other proteins that perform the essential processes of DNA replication, chromosome segregation, and so on.

The first components of the cell-cycle control system to be discovered were the cyclins and cyclin-dependent protein kinases (Cdks) that drive cells into M phase. They were found in studies of cell division conducted on animal eggs.

Back to the egg

The fertilized eggs of many animals are especially suitable for biochemical studies of the cell cycle because they are exceptionally large and divide rapidly. An egg of the frog *Xenopus*, for example, is just over 1 mm in diameter (**Figure 18–6**). After fertilization, it divides rapidly to partition the egg into many smaller cells. These rapid cell cycles consist mainly of repeated S and M phases, with very short or no G_1 or G_2 phases between them. There is no new gene transcription: all of the mRNAs and most of the proteins required for this early stage of embryonic development are already packed into the very large egg during its development as an oocyte in the ovary of the mother. In these early division cycles (*cleavage divisions*), no cell growth occurs, and all the cells of the embryo divide synchronously, growing smaller and smaller with each division (**Movie 18.2**).

Because of the synchrony, it is possible to prepare an extract from frog eggs that is representative of the cell-cycle stage at which the extract is made. The biological activity of such an extract can then be tested by injecting it into a *Xenopus* oocyte (the immature precursor of the unfertilized egg) and observing, microscopically, its effects on cell-cycle behavior. The *Xenopus* oocyte is an especially convenient test system for detecting an activity that drives cells into M phase, because of its large size, and because it has completed DNA replication and is suspended at a stage in the meiotic cell cycle (discussed in Chapter 19) that is equivalent to the G_2 phase of a mitotic cell cycle.

Give us an M

In such experiments, Yoshio Masui and colleagues found that an extract from an M-phase egg instantly drives the oocyte into M phase, whereas cytoplasm from a cleaving egg at other phases of the cycle does not. When they first made this discovery, they did not know the molecules or the mechanism responsible, so they referred to the unidentified agent as *maturation promoting factor*, or MPF (**Figure 18–7**). By testing cytoplasm from different stages of the cell cycle, Masui and colleagues found that MPF activity oscillates dramatically during the course of each cell cycle: it increased rapidly just before the start of mitosis and fell rapidly to zero toward the end of mitosis (see Figure 18–5). This oscillation made MPF a strong candidate for a component involved in cell-cycle control.

When MPF was finally purified, it was found to contain a protein kinase that was required for its activity. But the kinase portion of MPF did not act alone. It had to have a specific protein (now known to be M cyclin) bound to it in order to function. M cyclin was discovered in a different type of experiment, involving clam eggs.

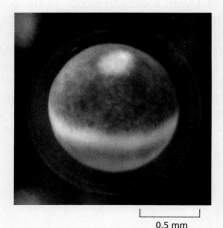

0.5 mm

Figure 18–6 A mature *Xenopus* egg provides a convenient system for studying the cell cycle. (Courtesy of Tony Mills.)

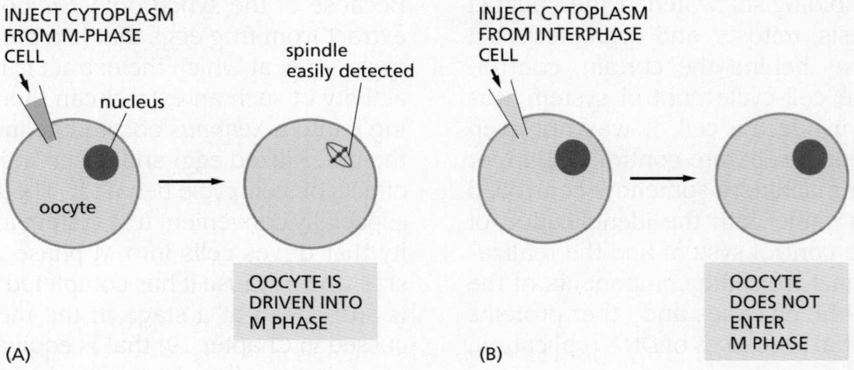

Figure 18–7 MPF activity was discovered by injecting *Xenopus* egg cytoplasm into *Xenopus* oocytes. (A) A *Xenopus* oocyte is injected with cytoplasm taken from a *Xenopus* egg in M phase. The cell extract drives the oocyte into M phase of the first meiotic division (a process called maturation), causing the large nucleus to break down and a spindle to form. (B) When the cytoplasm is instead taken from a cleaving egg in interphase, it does not cause the oocyte to enter M phase. Thus, the extract in (A) must contain some activity—a maturation promoting factor (MPF)—that triggers entry into M phase.

Fishing in clams

M cyclin was initially identified by Tim Hunt as a protein whose concentration rose gradually during interphase and then fell rapidly to zero as cleaving clam eggs went through M phase (see Figure 18–5). The protein repeated this performance in each cell cycle. Its role in cell-cycle control, however, was initially obscure. The breakthrough occurred when cyclin was found to be a component of MPF and to be required for MPF activity. Thus, MPF, which we now call M-Cdk, is a protein complex containing two subunits—a regulatory subunit, M cyclin, and a catalytic subunit, the mitotic Cdk. After the components of M-Cdk were identified, other types of cyclins and Cdks were isolated, whose concentrations or activities, respectively, rose and fell at other stages in the cell cycle.

All in the family

While biochemists were identifying the proteins that regulate the cell cycles of frog and clam embryos, yeast geneticists—led by Lee Hartwell, studying baker's yeast (*Saccharomyces cerevisiae*), and Paul Nurse,

studying fission yeast (*S. pombe*)—were taking a genetic approach to dissecting the cell-cycle control system. By studying mutants that get stuck or misbehave at specific points in the cell cycle, these researchers were able to identify many genes responsible for cell-cycle control. Some of these genes turned out to encode cyclin or Cdk proteins, which were unmistakably similar—in both amino acid sequence and function—to their counterparts in frogs and clams. Similar genes were soon identified in human cells.

Many of the cell-cycle control genes have changed so little during evolution that the human version of the gene will function perfectly well in a yeast cell. For example, Nurse and colleagues were the first to show that a yeast with a defective copy of the gene encoding its only Cdk fails to divide, but it divides normally if a copy of the appropriate human gene is artificially introduced into the defective cell. Surely, even Darwin would have been astonished at such clear evidence that humans and yeasts are cousins. Despite a billion years of divergent evolution, all eukaryotic cells—whether yeast, animal, or plant—use essentially the same molecules to control the events of their cell cycle.

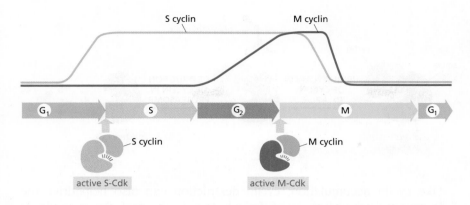

Figure 18–8 Distinct Cdks associate with different cyclins to trigger the different events of the cell cycle. For simplicity, only two types of cyclin–Cdk complexes are shown: one that triggers S phase and one that triggers M phase.

are shown in **Figure 18–8**. Another group of cyclins, called **G_1 cyclins**, act earlier in G_1 and bind to other Cdk proteins to form **G_1-Cdks**, which help drive the cell through G_1 toward S phase. We see later that the formation of these G_1-Cdks in animal cells usually depends on extracellular signal molecules that stimulate cells to divide. The names of the main cyclins and their Cdks are listed in **Table 18–2**.

Each of these cyclin–Cdk complexes phosphorylates a different set of target proteins in the cell. G_1/S-Cdks, for example, phosphorylate regulatory proteins that activate transcription of genes required for DNA replication. By activating different sets of target proteins, each type of complex triggers a different transition step in the cell cycle.

Cyclin Concentrations Are Regulated by Transcription and by Proteolysis

As discussed in Chapter 7, the concentration of a given protein in the cell is determined by the rate at which the protein is synthesized and the rate at which it is degraded. Over the course of the cell cycle, the concentration of each type of cyclin rises gradually and then falls abruptly (see Figure 18–8). The gradual increase in cyclin concentration stems from continued transcription of cyclin genes and synthesis of cyclin proteins, whereas the rapid fall in cyclin concentration is precipitated by a full-scale targeted destruction of the protein.

The abrupt degradation of M and S cyclins partway through M phase depends on a large enzyme called—for reasons that will become clear later—the **anaphase-promoting complex** or cyclosome (**APC/C**). This complex tags these cyclins with a chain of ubiquitin. As discussed in Chapter 7, proteins marked in this way are directed to proteasomes where they are rapidly degraded (see Figure 7–43). The ubiquitylation and degradation of the cyclin returns its Cdk to an inactive state (**Figure 18–9**).

TABLE 18–2 THE MAJOR CYCLINS AND CDKS OF VERTEBRATES		
Cyclin–Cdk Complex	**Cyclin**	**Cdk Partner**
G_1-Cdk	cyclin D*	Cdk4, Cdk6
G_1/S-Cdk	cyclin E	Cdk2
S-Cdk	cyclin A	Cdk2
M-Cdk	cyclin B	Cdk1

*There are three forms of cyclin D in mammals (cyclins D1, D2, and D3).

Figure 18–9 The activity of some Cdks is regulated by cyclin degradation. Ubiquitylation of S or M cyclin by APC/C marks the protein for destruction in proteasomes (as discussed in Chapter 7). The loss of cyclin renders its Cdk partner inactive.

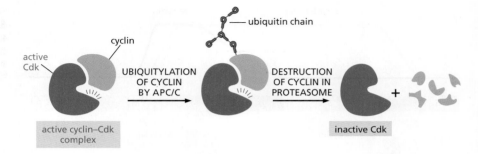

Like cyclin accumulation, cyclin destruction can also help drive the transition from one phase of the cell cycle to the next. For example, M cyclin degradation—and the resulting inactivation of M-Cdk—leads to the molecular events that take the cell out of mitosis.

The Activity of Cyclin–Cdk Complexes Depends on Phosphorylation and Dephosphorylation

The appearance and disappearance of cyclin proteins play an important part in regulating Cdk activity during the cell cycle, but there is more to the story: although cyclin concentrations increase gradually, the activity of the associated cyclin–Cdk complexes tends to switch on abruptly at the appropriate time in the cell cycle (see Figure 18–5). What triggers the abrupt activation of these complexes? It turns out that the cyclin–Cdk complex contains inhibitory phosphates, and to become active, the Cdk must be dephosphorylated by a specific protein phosphatase (**Figure 18–10**). Thus protein kinases and phosphatases act together to regulate the activity of specific cyclin–Cdk complexes and help control progression through the cell cycle.

Cdk Activity Can Be Blocked by Cdk Inhibitor Proteins

In addition to phosphorylation and dephosphorylation, the activity of Cdks can also be modulated by the binding of **Cdk inhibitor proteins**. The cell-cycle control system uses these inhibitors to block the assembly or activity of certain cyclin–Cdk complexes. Some Cdk inhibitor proteins, for example, help maintain Cdks in an inactive state during the G_1 phase of the cycle, thus delaying progression into S phase (**Figure 18–11**). Pausing at this transition point in G_1 gives the cell more time to grow, or allows it to wait until extracellular conditions are favorable for division.

The Cell-Cycle Control System Can Pause the Cycle in Various Ways

As mentioned earlier, the cell-cycle control system can transiently delay progress through the cycle at various transition points to ensure that the major events of the cycle occur only when the cell is fully prepared (see

Figure 18–10 For M-Cdk to be active, inhibitory phosphates must be removed. As soon as the M cyclin–Cdk complex is formed, it is phosphorylated at two adjacent sites by an inhibitory protein kinase called Wee1. This modification keeps M-Cdk in an inactive state until these phosphates are removed by an activating protein phosphatase called Cdc25. It is still not clear how the timing of the critical Cdc25 phosphatase triggering step shown here is controlled.

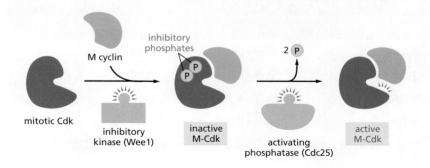

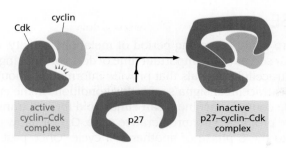

Figure 18–11 The activity of a Cdk can be blocked by the binding of a Cdk inhibitor. In this instance, the inhibitor protein (called p27) binds to an activated cyclin–Cdk complex. Its attachment prevents the Cdk from phosphorylating target proteins required for progress through G_1 into S phase.

Figure 18–3). At these transitions, the control system monitors the cell's internal state and the conditions in its environment, before allowing the cell to continue through the cycle. For example, it allows entry into S phase only if environmental conditions are appropriate; it triggers mitosis only after the DNA has been completely replicated; and it initiates chromosome segregation only after the duplicated chromosomes are correctly aligned on the mitotic spindle.

To accomplish these feats, the control system uses a combination of the mechanisms we have described. At the G_1-to-S transition, it uses Cdk inhibitors to keep cells from entering S phase and replicating their DNA (see Figure 18–11). At the G_2-to-M transition, it suppresses the activation of M-Cdk by inhibiting the phosphatase required to activate the Cdk (see Figure 18–10). And it can delay the exit from mitosis by inhibiting the activation of APC/C, thus preventing the degradation of M cyclin (see Figure 18–9).

These mechanisms, summarized in **Figure 18–12**, allow the cell to make "decisions" about whether to progress through the cell cycle or to arrest in the current phase and await more favorable conditions. In the next section, we take a closer look at how the cell-cycle control system decides whether a cell in G_1 should commit to divide.

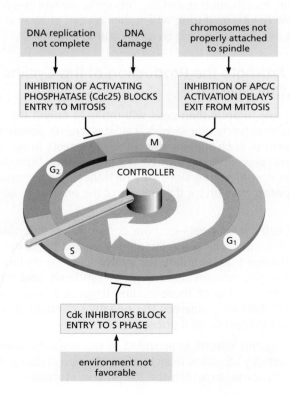

Figure 18–12 The cell-cycle control system uses various mechanisms to pause the cycle at specific transition points.

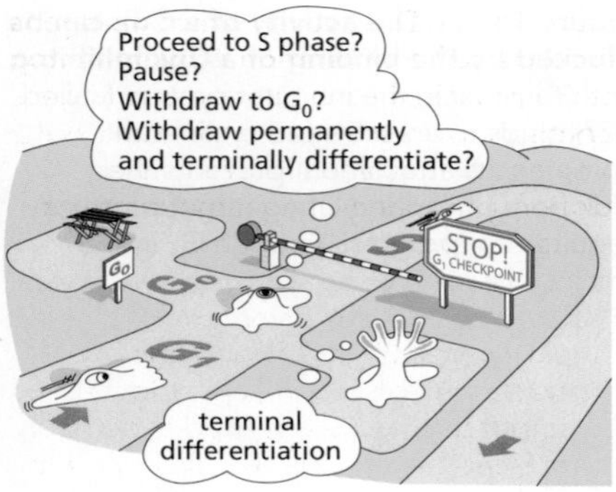

Figure 18–13 The transition from G₁ to S phase offers the cell a crossroad. The cell can commit to completing another cell cycle, pause temporarily until conditions are right, or withdraw from the cell cycle altogether—either temporarily in G₀, or permanently in the case of terminally differentiated cells.

G₁ PHASE

In addition to being a bustling period of metabolic activity, cell growth, and repair, G₁ serves as an important time of decision-making for the cell. Based on intracellular signals that provide information about the size of the cell and extracellular signals reflecting conditions in the environment, the cell-cycle control machinery can either hold the cell transiently in G₁ (or in a more prolonged nonproliferative state, G₀), or allow it to prepare for entry into the S phase of another cell cycle. Once past this critical G₁-to-S transition, a cell usually continues all the way through the rest of the cell cycle. In yeasts, the G₁-to-S transition is therefore sometimes called Start, because passing it represents a commitment to complete a full cell cycle (Figure 18–13).

In this section, we consider how the cell-cycle control system decides whether to proceed to S phase and commit to another cell cycle—and what happens once the decision is made. The molecular mechanisms involved are especially important, as defects in them can lead to unrestrained cell proliferation and cancer.

Cdks Are Stably Inactivated in G₁

During early M phase, when mitosis begins, the cell is awash with active cyclin–Cdk complexes. Those S-Cdks and M-Cdks must be disabled by the end of M phase to allow the cell to complete division and to prevent it from initiating another round of division without spending any time in G₁.

To usher a cell from the upheaval of M phase to the relative tranquility of G₁, the cell-cycle control machinery must inactivate its inventory of S-Cdk and M-Cdk. It does so in several ways: by eliminating all of the existing cyclins, by blocking the synthesis of new ones, and by deploying Cdk inhibitor proteins to muffle the activity of any remaining cyclin–Cdk complexes. The use of multiple mechanisms makes this system of suppression robust, ensuring that essentially all Cdk activity is shut down. This wholesale inactivation resets the cell-cycle control system and generates a stable G₁ phase, during which the cell can grow and monitor its environment before committing to a new round of division.

Mitogens Promote the Production of the Cyclins That Stimulate Cell Division

As a general rule, mammalian cells will multiply only if they are stimulated to do so by extracellular signals, called *mitogens*, produced by other cells. If deprived of such signals, the cell cycle arrests in G₁; if the cell is deprived of mitogens for long enough, it will withdraw from the cell cycle and enter a nonproliferating state, in which the cell can remain for days or weeks, months, or even for the lifetime of the organism, as we discuss shortly.

Escape from cell-cycle arrest—or from certain nonproliferating states—requires the accumulation of cyclins. Mitogens act by switching on cell signaling pathways that stimulate the synthesis of G₁ cyclins, G₁/S cyclins, and other proteins involved in DNA synthesis and chromosome duplication. The buildup of these cyclins triggers a wave of G₁/S-Cdk activity, which ultimately relieves the negative controls that otherwise block progression from G₁ to S phase.

One crucial negative control is provided by the *Retinoblastoma (Rb) protein*. Rb was initially identified from studies of a rare childhood eye tumor called retinoblastoma, in which the Rb protein is missing or defective.

QUESTION 18–3

Why do you suppose cells have evolved a special G₀ phase to exit from the cell cycle, rather than just stopping in G₁ and not moving on to S phase?

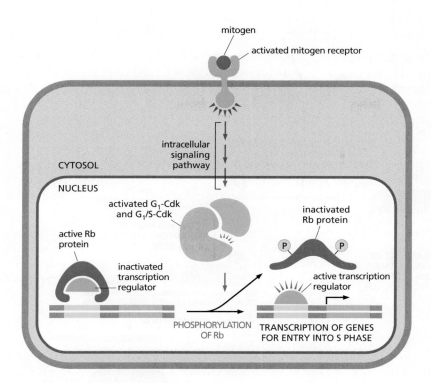

Figure 18–14 One way in which mitogens stimulate cell proliferation is by inhibiting the Rb protein. In the absence of mitogens, dephosphorylated Rb protein holds specific transcription regulators in an inactive state. Mitogens binding to cell-surface receptors activate intracellular signaling pathways that lead to the formation and activation of G_1-Cdk and G_1/S-Cdk complexes. These complexes phosphorylate, and thereby inactivate, the Rb protein, releasing the transcription regulators needed to activate the transcription of genes required for entry into S phase.

Rb is abundant in the nuclei of all vertebrate cells, where it binds to particular transcription regulators and prevents them from turning on the genes required for cell proliferation. Mitogens release the Rb brake by triggering the activation of G_1-Cdks and G_1/S-Cdks. These complexes phosphorylate the Rb protein, altering its conformation so that it releases its bound transcription regulators, which are then free to activate the genes required for entry into S phase (**Figure 18–14**).

DNA Damage Can Temporarily Halt Progression Through G₁

The cell-cycle control system uses several distinct mechanisms to halt progress through the cell cycle if DNA is damaged, and it can do so at various transition points. The mechanism that operates at the G_1-to-S transition, which prevents the cell from replicating damaged DNA, is especially well understood. DNA damage in G_1 causes an increase in both the concentration and activity of a protein called **p53**, which is a transcription regulator that activates the gene encoding a Cdk inhibitor protein called p21. The p21 protein binds to G_1/S-Cdk and S-Cdk, preventing them from driving the cell into S phase (**Figure 18–15**). The arrest of the cell cycle in G_1 gives the cell time to repair the damaged DNA before replicating it. If the DNA damage is too severe to be repaired, p53 can induce the cell to kill itself through *apoptosis*, a form of programmed cell death we discuss later. If p53 is missing or defective, the unrestrained replication of damaged DNA leads to a high rate of mutation and the generation of cells that tend to become cancerous. In fact, mutations in the *p53* gene are found in about half of all human cancers (Movie 18.3).

Cells Can Delay Division for Prolonged Periods by Entering Specialized Nondividing States

As mentioned earlier, cells can delay progress through the cell cycle at specific transition points, to wait for suitable conditions or to repair

Figure 18–15 **DNA damage can arrest the cell cycle in G$_1$.** When DNA is damaged, specific protein kinases respond by both activating the p53 protein and halting its otherwise rapid degradation. Activated p53 protein thus accumulates and stimulates the transcription of the gene that encodes the Cdk inhibitor protein p21. The p21 protein binds to G$_1$/S-Cdk and S-Cdk and inactivates them, so that the cell cycle arrests in G$_1$.

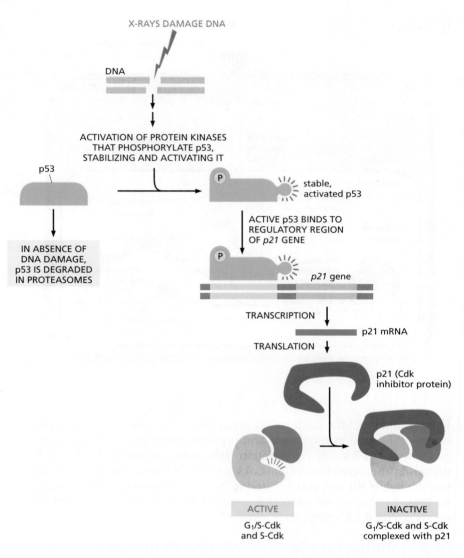

X-RAYS DAMAGE DNA

DNA

ACTIVATION OF PROTEIN KINASES THAT PHOSPHORYLATE p53, STABILIZING AND ACTIVATING IT

p53

IN ABSENCE OF DNA DAMAGE, p53 IS DEGRADED IN PROTEASOMES

stable, activated p53

ACTIVE p53 BINDS TO REGULATORY REGION OF *p21* GENE

p21 gene

TRANSCRIPTION

p21 mRNA

TRANSLATION

p21 (Cdk inhibitor protein)

ACTIVE
G$_1$/S-Cdk and S-Cdk

INACTIVE
G$_1$/S-Cdk and S-Cdk complexed with p21

QUESTION 18–4

What might be the consequences if a cell replicated damaged DNA before repairing it?

damaged DNA. They can also withdraw from the cell cycle for prolonged periods—either temporarily or permanently.

The most radical decision that the cell-cycle control system can make is to withdraw the cell from the cell cycle permanently. This decision has a special importance in multicellular organisms. Many cells in the human body permanently stop dividing when they differentiate. In such *terminally differentiated* cells, such as nerve or muscle cells, the cell-cycle control system is dismantled completely and genes encoding the relevant cyclins and Cdks are irreversibly shut down.

In the absence of appropriate signals, other cell types withdraw from the cell cycle only temporarily, entering an arrested state called G$_0$. They retain the ability to reassemble the cell-cycle control system quickly and to divide again. Most liver cells, for example, are in G$_0$, but they can be stimulated to proliferate if the liver is damaged.

Much of the diversity in cell-division rates in the adult body lies in the variation in the time that cells spend in G$_0$ or in G$_1$. Some cell types, including liver cells, normally divide only once every year or two, whereas certain epithelial cells in the gut divide more than twice a day to renew the lining of the gut continually. Many of our cells fall somewhere in between: they can divide if the need arises but normally do so infrequently.

S PHASE

Before a cell divides, it must replicate its DNA. As we discuss in Chapter 6, this replication must occur with extreme accuracy to minimize the risk of mutations in the next cell generation. Of equal importance, every nucleotide in the genome must be copied once—and only once—to prevent the damaging effects of gene amplification. In this section, we consider the elegant molecular mechanisms by which the cell-cycle control system initiates DNA replication and, at the same time, prevents replication from happening more than once per cell cycle.

S-Cdk Initiates DNA Replication and Blocks Re-Replication

Like any monumental task, configuring chromosomes for replication requires a certain amount of preparation. For eukaryotic cells, this preparation begins early in G_1, when DNA is made replication-ready by the recruitment of proteins to the sites along each chromosome where replication will begin. These nucleotide sequences, called *origins of replication*, serve as landing pads for the proteins and protein complexes that control and carry out DNA synthesis, as discussed in Chapter 6.

One of these protein complexes, called the *origin recognition complex (ORC)*, remains perched on the replication origins throughout the cell cycle. To prepare the DNA for replication, the ORC recruits a protein called Cdc6, whose concentration rises early in G_1. Together, these proteins load the DNA helicases that will ultimately open up the double helix at the origin of replication. Once this *prereplicative complex* is in place, the replication origin is loaded and ready to "fire."

The signal to commence replication comes from S-Cdk, the cyclin–Cdk complex that triggers S phase. S-Cdk is assembled and activated at the end of G_1. During S phase, S-Cdk activates the DNA helicases in the prereplicative complex and promotes the assembly of the rest of the proteins that form the *replication fork* (see Figure 6–20). In doing so, S-Cdk essentially "pulls the trigger" that initiates DNA replication (**Figure 18–16**).

In addition to triggering the initiation of DNA synthesis at a replication origin, S-Cdk also helps prevent re-replication. It does so by phosphorylating both Cdc6 and the ORC. Phosphorylation inactivates these proteins and helps prevent the reassembly of the prereplicative complex. These safeguards help ensure that DNA replication cannot be reinitiated later in the same cell cycle. When Cdks are inactivated in the next G_1 phase, the ORC and Cdc6 are reactivated, thereby allowing origins to be prepared for the following S phase.

Incomplete Replication Can Arrest the Cell Cycle in G_2

Earlier, we described how DNA damage can signal the cell-cycle control system to delay progress through the G_1-to-S transition, preventing the cell from replicating damaged DNA. But what if errors occur during DNA replication—or if replication is delayed? How does the cell keep from dividing with DNA that is incorrectly or incompletely replicated?

To address these issues, the cell-cycle control system uses a mechanism that can delay entry into M phase. As we saw in Figure 18–10, the activity of M-Cdk is inhibited by phosphorylation at particular sites. For the cell to progress into mitosis, these inhibitory phosphates must be removed by an activating protein phosphatase called Cdc25. If DNA replication stalls, the appearance of single-stranded DNA at the replication fork triggers a DNA damage response. Part of this response includes the inhibition of the phosphatase Cdc25, which prevents the removal of the inhibitory

Figure 18–16 The initiation of DNA replication takes place in two steps. During G$_1$, Cdc6 binds to the ORC, and together these proteins load a pair of DNA helicases on the DNA to form the prereplicative complex. At the start of S phase, S-Cdk triggers the firing of this loaded replication origin by guiding the assembly of the DNA polymerase (*green*) and other proteins (not shown) that initiate DNA synthesis at the replication fork (discussed in Chapter 6). S-Cdk also blocks re-replication by phosphorylating Cdc6 (not shown) and the ORC. This phosphorylation keeps these proteins inactive and prevents the reassembly of the prereplicative complex until the Cdks are turned off in the next G$_1$.

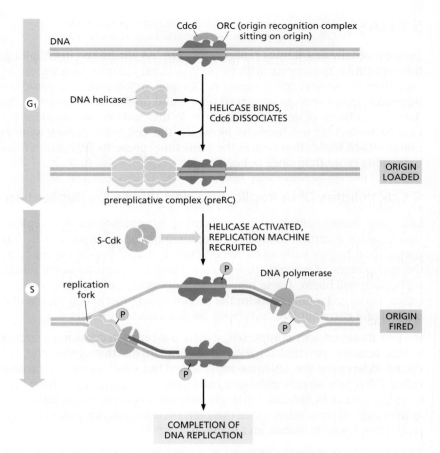

phosphates from M-Cdk. As a result, M-Cdk remains inactive and M phase is delayed until DNA replication is complete and any DNA damage is repaired.

Once a cell has successfully replicated its DNA in S phase, and progressed through G$_2$, it is ready to enter M phase. During this relatively brief period, the cell will accomplish a remarkable reconfiguration, dividing its nucleus (mitosis) and then its cytoplasm (cytokinesis; see Figure 18–2). In the next three sections, we describe the events that occur during M phase. We first present a brief overview of M phase as a whole and then discuss, in sequence, the mechanics of mitosis and of cytokinesis, with a focus on animal cells.

M PHASE

Although M phase (which includes mitosis plus cytokinesis) takes place over a relatively short amount of time—about one hour in a mammalian cell—it is by far the most dramatic phase of the cell cycle. During this brief period, the cell reorganizes virtually all of its components and distributes them equally into the two daughter cells. The earlier phases of the cell cycle, in effect, set the stage for the drama of M phase.

The central problem for a cell in M phase is to accurately segregate the chromosomes that were duplicated in the preceding S phase, so that each new daughter cell receives an identical copy of the genome. With minor variations, all eukaryotes solve this problem in a similar way: they assemble two specialized cytoskeletal machines—one that pulls the duplicated chromosomes apart (during mitosis) and another that divides the cytoplasm into two halves (during cytokinesis). We begin our discussion of M phase with an overview of how the cell sets the processes of M phase in motion.

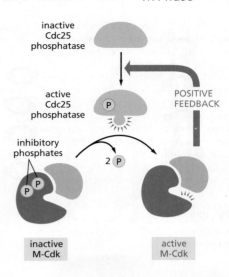

Figure 18–17 Activated M-Cdk indirectly activates more M-Cdk, creating a positive feedback loop. Once activated, M-Cdk phosphorylates, and thereby activates, more Cdk-activating phosphatase (Cdc25). This phosphatase can now activate more M-Cdk by removing the inhibitory phosphate groups from the Cdk subunit.

M-Cdk Drives Entry into Mitosis

One of the most remarkable features of the cell-cycle control system is that a single protein complex, M-Cdk, brings about all the diverse and intricate rearrangements that occur in the early stages of mitosis. Among its many duties, M-Cdk helps prepare the duplicated chromosomes for segregation and induces the assembly of the mitotic spindle—the machinery that will pull the duplicated chromosomes apart.

M-Cdk complexes accumulate throughout G_2. But this stockpile is not switched on until the end of G_2, when the activating phosphatase Cdc25 removes the inhibitory phosphates holding M-Cdk activity in check. This act of activation is self-reinforcing: once activated, each M-Cdk complex can indirectly turn on additional M-Cdk complexes—by phosphorylating and activating more Cdc25 (**Figure 18–17**). Activated M-Cdk also shuts down the inhibitory kinase Wee1 (see Figure 18–10), further promoting the production of activated M-Cdk. The overall consequence is that, once M-Cdk activation begins, it ignites an explosive increase in M-Cdk activity that drives the cell abruptly—and irreversibly—from G_2 into M phase.

The same M-Cdk complexes that drive entry into mitosis also help set the stage for its exit. Activated M-Cdk turns on APC/C, which—after a period of delay—directs the destruction of M cyclin and, ultimately, the inactivation of M-Cdk.

Cohesins and Condensins Help Configure Duplicated Chromosomes for Separation

To ensure that duplicated chromosomes will be properly separated during mitosis, two related protein complexes help cells manage and keep track of the replicated DNA. The first complexes come into play during S phase. When a chromosome is duplicated, the two copies remain tightly bound together. These identical copies—called **sister chromatids**—each contain a single, double-stranded molecule of DNA, along with its associated proteins. The sisters are held together by protein complexes called **cohesins**, which assemble along the length of each chromatid as the DNA is replicated. This cohesion between sister chromatids is crucial for proper chromosome segregation, and it is broken completely only in late mitosis to allow the sisters to be pulled apart by the mitotic spindle. Defects in sister-chromatid cohesion lead to major errors in chromosome segregation. In humans, such mis-segregation can lead to abnormal numbers of chromosomes, resulting in genetic imbalances that are usually deleterious or even lethal.

When the cell enters M phase, the duplicated chromosomes condense, becoming visible under the microscope. Protein complexes called **condensins** help carry out this **chromosome condensation**, which reduces mitotic chromosomes to compact bodies that can be more easily segregated within the crowded confines of the dividing cell. The assembly of condensin complexes onto the DNA is triggered by the phosphorylation of condensins by M-Cdk.

Cohesins and condensins are structurally related, and both are thought to form ring structures around chromosomal DNA. However, whereas cohesins encircle the two sister chromatids, tying them together (**Figure 18–18A**), condensins assemble along each individual sister chromatid,

QUESTION 18–5

A small amount of cytoplasm isolated from a mitotic cell is injected into an unfertilized frog oocyte, causing the oocyte to enter M phase (see Figure 18–7A). A sample of the injected oocyte's cytoplasm is then taken and injected into a second oocyte, causing this cell also to enter M phase. The process is repeated many times until, essentially, none of the original protein sample remains, and yet, cytoplasm taken from the last in the series of injected oocytes is still able to trigger entry into M phase with undiminished efficiency. Explain this remarkable observation.

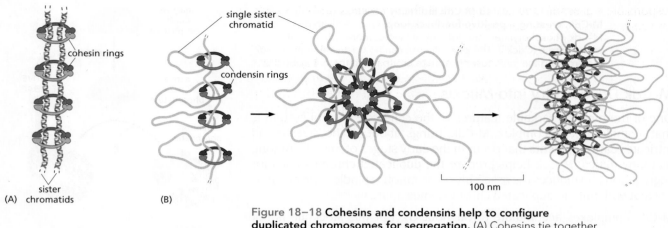

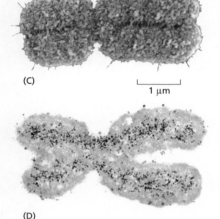

Figure 18–18 **Cohesins and condensins help to configure duplicated chromosomes for segregation.** (A) Cohesins tie together the two adjacent sister chromatids in each duplicated chromosome. They are thought to form large protein rings that surround the sister chromatids, preventing them from coming apart, until the rings are broken late in mitosis. (B) Condensins help coil each sister chromatid (in other words, each DNA double helix) into a smaller, more compact structure that can be more easily segregated during mitosis. These cartoons illustrate one way that condensins might package chromatids; the exact mechanism is not known. (C) A scanning electron micrograph of a condensed, duplicated mitotic chromosome, consisting of two sister chromatids joined along their length. The constricted region (*arrow*) is the centromere, where each chromatid will attach to the mitotic spindle, which pulls the sister chromatids apart toward the end of mitosis. (D) An electron micrograph of a duplicated mitotic chromosome in which condensin is labelled with antibodies attached to tiny gold particles (*dark* dots), showing that condensins are found mainly in the central core of the chromosome. This centralized location of condensins is also represented in the cartoon model shown in (B). (C, courtesy of Terry D. Allen; D, adapted from N. Kireeva et al., *J. Cell Biol.* 166:775–785, 2004. With permission from Rockefeller University Press.)

helping each of these double helices to coil up into a more compact form (**Figure 18–18B–D**). Together, these proteins help configure replicated chromosomes for mitosis.

Different Cytoskeletal Assemblies Carry Out Mitosis and Cytokinesis

After the duplicated chromosomes have condensed, a pair of complex cytoskeletal machines assemble in sequence to carry out the two mechanical processes that occur in M phase. The mitotic spindle carries out nuclear division (mitosis), and, in animal cells and many unicellular eukaryotes, the *contractile ring* carries out cytoplasmic division (cytokinesis) (**Figure 18–19**). Both structures disassemble rapidly after they have performed their tasks.

The mitotic spindle is composed of microtubules and the various proteins that interact with them, including microtubule-associated motor proteins (discussed in Chapter 17). In all eukaryotic cells, the mitotic spindle is

Figure 18–19 **Two transient cytoskeletal structures mediate M phase in animal cells.** The mitotic spindle assembles first to separate the duplicated chromosomes. Then, the contractile ring assembles to divide the cell in two. Whereas the mitotic spindle is based on microtubules, the contractile ring is based on actin and myosin. Plant cells use a very different mechanism to divide the cytoplasm, as we discuss later.

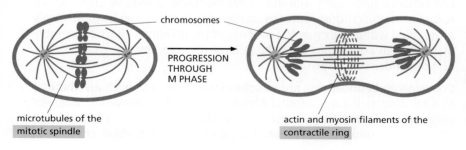

responsible for separating the duplicated chromosomes and allocating one copy of each chromosome to each daughter cell.

The *contractile ring* consists mainly of actin and myosin filaments arranged in a ring around the equator of the cell (see Chapter 17). It starts to assemble just beneath the plasma membrane toward the end of mitosis. As the ring contracts, it pulls the membrane inward, thereby dividing the cell in two (see Figure 18–19). We discuss later how plant cells, which have a cell wall to contend with, divide their cytoplasm by a very different mechanism.

M Phase Occurs in Stages

Although M phase proceeds as a continuous sequence of events, it is traditionally divided into a series of stages. The first five stages of M phase—prophase, prometaphase, metaphase, anaphase, and telophase—constitute **mitosis**, which was originally defined as the period in which the chromosomes are visible in the microscope (because they have become condensed). *Cytokinesis*, which constitutes the final stage of M phase, begins before mitosis ends. The stages of M phase are summarized in Panel 18–1 (pp. 628–629). Together, they form a dynamic sequence in which several independent cycles—involving the chromosomes, cytoskeleton, and centrosomes—are coordinated to produce two genetically identical daughter cells (Movie 18.4 and Movie 18.5).

MITOSIS

Before nuclear division, or mitosis, begins, each chromosome has been duplicated and consists of two identical sister chromatids, held together along their length by cohesin proteins (see Figure 18–18A). During mitosis, the cohesin proteins are removed, the sister chromatids split apart, and the chromosomes are pulled to opposite poles of the cell by the mitotic spindle (Figure 18–20). In this section, we examine how the mitotic spindle assembles and functions. We discuss how the dynamic instability of microtubules and the activity of microtubule-associated motor proteins contribute to both the assembly of the spindle and its ability to segregate the duplicated chromosomes. We then consider the mechanism that operates during mitosis to ensure the synchronous separation of these chromosomes. Finally, we discuss how the daughter nuclei form.

Centrosomes Duplicate to Help Form the Two Poles of the Mitotic Spindle

Before M phase begins, two critical events must be completed: DNA must be fully replicated, and, in animal cells, the centrosome must be duplicated. The **centrosome** is the principal *microtubule-organizing center* in animal cells (see Figure 17–13). Duplication is necessary for the centrosome to be able to help form the two poles of the mitotic spindle and so that each daughter cell will receive its own centrosome.

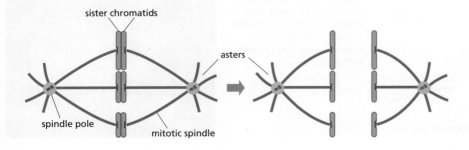

Figure 18–20 Sister chromatids separate at the beginning of anaphase. The mitotic spindle then pulls the separated sisters to opposite poles of the cell.

CELL DIVISION AND THE CELL CYCLE

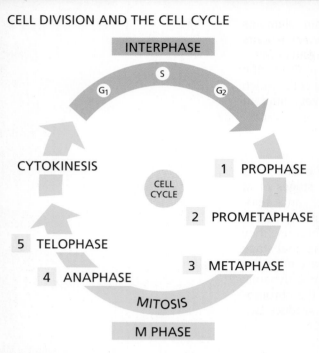

INTERPHASE

S

G₁   G₂

CYTOKINESIS

CELL CYCLE

1 PROPHASE

2 PROMETAPHASE

5 TELOPHASE

3 METAPHASE

4 ANAPHASE

MITOSIS

M PHASE

The division of a cell into two daughters occurs in the M phase of the cell cycle. M phase consists of nuclear division, or mitosis, and cytoplasmic division, or cytokinesis. In this figure, M phase has been greatly expanded for clarity. Mitosis is itself divided into five stages, and these, together with cytokinesis, are described in this panel.

INTERPHASE

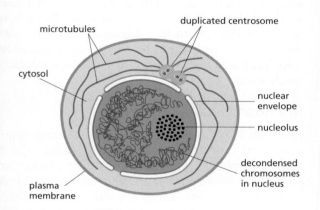

microtubules

duplicated centrosome

cytosol

nuclear envelope

nucleolus

decondensed chromosomes in nucleus

plasma membrane

During interphase, the cell increases in size. The DNA of the chromosomes is replicated, and the centrosome is duplicated.

In the light micrographs of dividing animal cells shown in this panel, chromosomes are stained *orange* and microtubules are *green*.

(Courtesy of Julie Canman and Ted Salmon.)

1 PROPHASE

MITOSIS

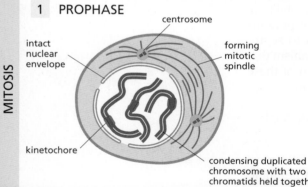

centrosome

intact nuclear envelope

forming mitotic spindle

kinetochore

condensing duplicated chromosome with two sister chromatids held together along their length

At prophase, the duplicated chromosomes, each consisting of two closely associated sister chromatids, condense. Outside the nucleus, the mitotic spindle assembles between the two centrosomes, which have begun to move apart. For simplicity, only three chromosomes are drawn.

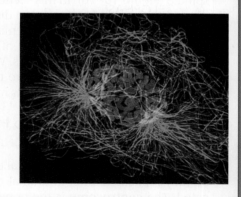

2 PROMETAPHASE

MITOSIS

spindle pole

fragments of nuclear envelope

kinetochore microtubule

chromosome in motion

Prometaphase starts abruptly with the breakdown of the nuclear envelope. Chromosomes can now attach to spindle microtubules via their kinetochores and undergo active movement.

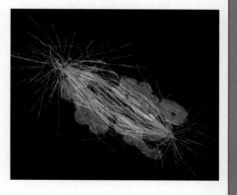

3 METAPHASE

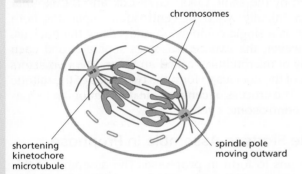

spindle pole

astral microtubule

kinetochore microtubule

spindle pole

kinetochores of all chromosomes aligned in a plane midway between the two spindle poles

At metaphase, the chromosomes are aligned at the equator of the spindle, midway between the spindle poles. The kinetochore microtubules on each sister chromatid attach to opposite poles of the spindle.

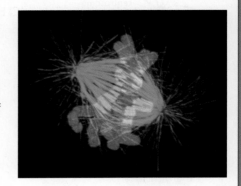

4 ANAPHASE

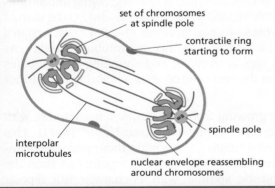

chromosomes

shortening kinetochore microtubule

spindle pole moving outward

At anaphase, the sister chromatids synchronously separate and are pulled slowly toward the spindle pole to which they are attached. The kinetochore microtubules get shorter, and the spindle poles also move apart, both contributing to chromosome segregation.

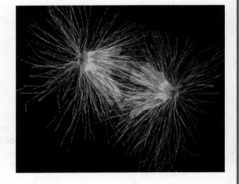

5 TELOPHASE

set of chromosomes at spindle pole

contractile ring starting to form

interpolar microtubules

spindle pole

nuclear envelope reassembling around chromosomes

During telophase, the two sets of chromosomes arrive at the poles of the spindle. A new nuclear envelope reassembles around each set, completing the formation of two nuclei and marking the end of mitosis. The division of the cytoplasm begins with the assembly of the contractile ring.

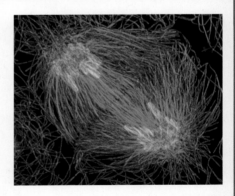

CYTOKINESIS

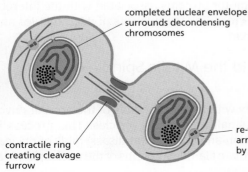

completed nuclear envelope surrounds decondensing chromosomes

contractile ring creating cleavage furrow

re-formation of interphase array of microtubules nucleated by the centrosome

During cytokinesis of an animal cell, the cytoplasm is divided in two by a contractile ring of actin and myosin filaments, which pinches the cell into two daughters, each with one nucleus.

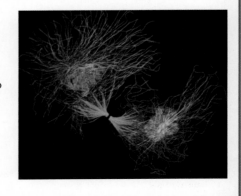

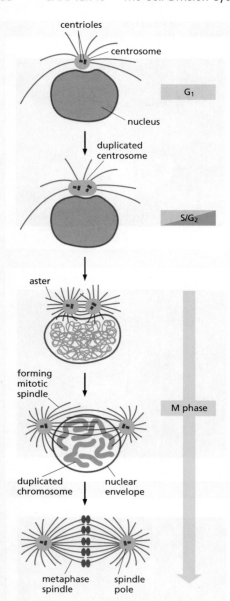

Figure 18–21 The centrosome in an interphase cell duplicates to form the two poles of a mitotic spindle. Most animal cells contain a single centrosome, which consists of a pair of centrioles (*gray*) embedded in a matrix of proteins (*light green*). The volume of the centrosome matrix is exaggerated in this diagram for clarity. Although the centrioles are made of a cylindrical array of short microtubules, they do not participate in the nucleation of microtubules from the centrosome (see Figure 17–13). Centrosome duplication begins at the start of S phase and is complete by the end of G_2. Initially, the two centrosomes remain together, but, in early M phase, they separate, and each nucleates its own aster of microtubules. The centrosomes then move apart, and the microtubules that interact between the two asters elongate preferentially to form a bipolar mitotic spindle, with an aster at each pole. When the nuclear envelope breaks down, the spindle microtubules are able to interact with the duplicated chromosomes.

Centrosome duplication begins at the same time as DNA replication and the process is triggered by the same Cdks—G_1/S-Cdk and S-Cdk—that initiate DNA replication. Initially, when the centrosome duplicates, both copies remain together as a single complex on one side of the nucleus. As mitosis begins, however, the two centrosomes separate, and each nucleates a radial array of microtubules called an **aster**. The two asters move to opposite sides of the nucleus to form the two poles of the mitotic spindle (**Figure 18–21**). The process of centrosome duplication and separation is known as the **centrosome cycle**.

The Mitotic Spindle Starts to Assemble in Prophase

The mitotic spindle begins to form in **prophase**. The assembly of this highly dynamic structure depends on the remarkable properties of microtubules. As discussed in Chapter 17, microtubules continuously polymerize and depolymerize by the addition and loss of their tubulin subunits, and individual filaments alternate between growing and shrinking—a process called *dynamic instability* (see Figure 17–14). At the start of mitosis, dynamic stability rises—in part because M-Cdk phosphorylates microtubule-associated proteins that influence microtubule stability. As a result, during prophase, rapidly growing and shrinking microtubules extend in all directions from the two centrosomes, exploring the interior of the cell.

Some of the microtubules growing from one centrosome interact with the microtubules from the other centrosome (see Figure 18–21). This interaction stabilizes the microtubules, preventing them from depolymerizing, and it joins the two sets of microtubules together to form the basic framework of the **mitotic spindle**, with its characteristic bipolar shape (Movie 18.6). The two centrosomes that give rise to these microtubules are now called **spindle poles**, and the interacting microtubules are called interpolar microtubules (**Figure 18–22**). The assembly of the spindle is driven, in part, by motor proteins associated with the interpolar microtubules that help to cross-link the two sets of microtubules and push the two centrosomes apart.

Chromosomes Attach to the Mitotic Spindle at Prometaphase

Prometaphase starts abruptly with the disassembly of the nuclear envelope, which breaks up into small membrane vesicles. This process is triggered by the phosphorylation and consequent disassembly of nuclear pore proteins and the intermediate filament proteins of the nuclear lamina,

Figure 18–22 A bipolar mitotic spindle is formed by the selective stabilization of interacting microtubules. New microtubules grow out in random directions from the two centrosomes. The two ends of a microtubule (by convention, called the plus and the minus ends) have different properties, and it is the minus end that is anchored in the centrosome (discussed in Chapter 17). The free plus ends are dynamically unstable and switch suddenly from uniform growth (outward-pointing *red* arrows) to rapid shrinkage (inward-pointing *blue* arrows). When two microtubules from opposite centrosomes interact in an overlap zone, motor proteins and other microtubule-associated proteins cross-link the microtubules together (*black* dots) in a way that stabilizes the plus ends by decreasing the probability of their depolymerization.

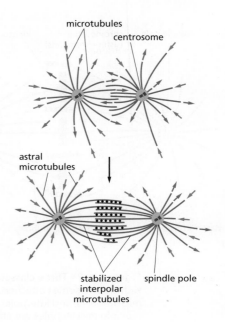

the network of fibrous proteins that underlies and stabilizes the nuclear envelope (see Figure 17–7). The spindle microtubules, which have been lying in wait outside the nucleus, now gain access to the duplicated chromosomes and capture each and everyone (see Panel 18–1, pp. 628–629).

Spindle microtubules attach to the chromosomes at their **kinetochores**, protein complexes that assemble on the centromere of each condensed chromosome during late prophase (**Figure 18–23**). Kinetochores recognize the special DNA sequence that forms a chromosome's centromere: if this sequence is altered, kinetochores fail to assemble and, consequently, the chromosomes fail to segregate properly during mitosis.

Once the nuclear envelope has broken down, a randomly probing microtubule encountering a kinetochore will bind to it, thereby capturing that chromosome and linking it to a spindle pole (see Panel 18–1, pp. 628–629). Of course, each duplicated chromosome has two kinetochores—one on each sister chromatid. Because these sister kinetochores face in opposite directions, they tend to attach to microtubules from opposite poles of

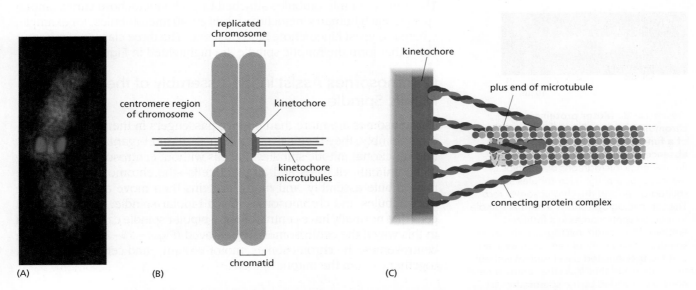

Figure 18–23 Kinetochores attach chromosomes to the mitotic spindle. (A) A fluorescence micrograph of a duplicated mitotic chromosome. The kinetochores are stained *red* with fluorescent antibodies that recognize kinetochore proteins. These antibodies come from patients with scleroderma (a disease that causes progressive overproduction of connective tissue in skin and other organs), who, for unknown reasons, produce antibodies against their own kinetochore proteins. (B) Schematic drawing of a mitotic chromosome showing its two sister chromatids attached to kinetochore microtubules, which bind to the kinetochore at their plus ends. Each kinetochore forms a plaque on the surface of the centromere. (C) Each microtubule is attached to the kinetochore via interactions with multiple copies of an elongated connecting protein complex (*blue*). These complexes bind to the sides of the microtubule near its plus end, allowing the microtubule to grow or shrink while remaining attached to the kinetochore. (A, from R.P. Zinkowski et al., *J. Cell Biol.* 113:1091–1110, 1991. With permission from The Rockefeller University Press.)

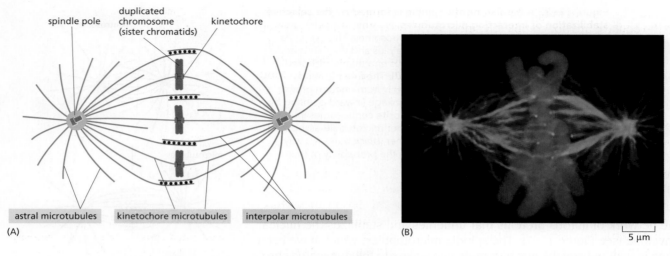

spindle pole

duplicated chromosome (sister chromatids)

kinetochore

astral microtubules

kinetochore microtubules

interpolar microtubules

(A)

(B)

5 µm

Figure 18–24 Three classes of microtubules make up the mitotic spindle. (A) Schematic drawing of a spindle with chromosomes attached, showing the three types of spindle microtubules: astral microtubules, kinetochore microtubules, and interpolar microtubules. In reality, the chromosomes are much larger than shown, and usually multiple microtubules are attached to each kinetochore. (B) Fluorescence micrograph of duplicated chromosomes aligned at the center of the mitotic spindle. In this image, kinetochores are *red* dots, microtubules are *green*, and chromosomes are *blue*. (B, from A. Desai, *Curr. Biol.* 10:R508, 2000. With permission from Elsevier.)

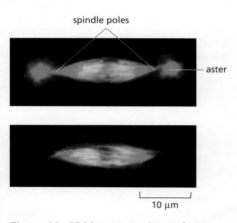

spindle poles

aster

10 µm

Figure 18–25 Motor proteins and chromosomes can direct the assembly of a functional bipolar spindle in the absence of centrosomes. In these fluorescence micrographs of embryos of the insect *Sciara*, the microtubules are stained *green* and the chromosomes *red*. The top micrograph shows a normal spindle formed by centrosomes in a fertilized embryo. The bottom micrograph shows a spindle formed without centrosomes in an embryo that initiated development without fertilization and thus lacks the centrosome normally provided by the sperm when it fertilizes the egg. Note that the spindle with centrosomes has an aster at each pole, whereas the spindle formed without centrosomes does not. As shown, both types of spindles are able to segregate chromosomes. (From B. de Saint Phalle and W. Sullivan, *J. Cell Biol.* 141:1383–1391, 1998. With permission from The Rockefeller University Press.)

the spindle; thus, each duplicated chromosome becomes linked to both spindle poles. The attachment to opposite poles, called **bi-orientation**, generates tension on the kinetochores, which are being pulled in opposite directions. This tension signals to the sister kinetochores that they are attached correctly and are ready to be separated (Movie 18.7). The cell-cycle control system monitors this tension to ensure correct chromosome attachment (see Figure 18–3), a safeguard we discuss in detail shortly.

The number of microtubules attached to each kinetochore varies among species: each human kinetochore binds 20–40 microtubules, for example, whereas a yeast kinetochore binds just one. The three classes of microtubules that form the mitotic spindle are highlighted in Figure 18–24.

Chromosomes Assist in the Assembly of the Mitotic Spindle

Chromosomes are more than passive passengers in the process of spindle assembly: they themselves can stabilize and organize microtubules into functional mitotic spindles. In cells without centrosomes—including some animal cell types and all plant cells—the chromosomes nucleate microtubule assembly, and motor proteins then move and arrange the microtubules and chromosomes into a bipolar spindle. Even in animal cells that normally have centrosomes, a bipolar spindle can still be formed in this way if the centrosomes are removed (Figure 18–25). In cells with centrosomes, the chromosomes, motor proteins, and centrosomes work together to form the mitotic spindle.

Chromosomes Line Up at the Spindle Equator at Metaphase

During prometaphase, the duplicated chromosomes, now attached to the mitotic spindle, begin to move about, as if jerked first this way and then that. Eventually, they align at the equator of the spindle, halfway between the two spindle poles, thereby forming the *metaphase plate*. This event defines the beginning of **metaphase** (see Figure 18–24B and

Figure 18–26). Although the forces that act to bring the chromosomes to the equator are not completely understood, both the continual growth and shrinkage of the microtubules and the action of microtubule motor proteins are required. A continuous balanced addition and loss of tubulin subunits is also required to maintain the metaphase spindle: when tubulin addition to the ends of microtubules is blocked by the drug colchicine, tubulin loss continues until the metaphase spindle disappears.

The chromosomes gathered at the equator of the metaphase spindle oscillate back and forth, continually adjusting their positions, indicating that the tug-of-war between the microtubules attached to opposite poles of the spindle continues to operate after the chromosomes are all aligned. If the kinetochore attachments on one side of a duplicated chromosome are artificially severed with a laser beam during metaphase, the entire chromosome immediately moves toward the pole to which it remains attached. Similarly, if the attachment between sister chromatids is cut, the two chromosomes separate and move toward opposite poles. These experiments show that the duplicated chromosomes are not simply deposited at the metaphase plate. They are suspended there under tension. In anaphase, that tension will pull the sister chromatids apart.

Proteolysis Triggers Sister-Chromatid Separation at Anaphase

Anaphase begins abruptly with the breakage of the cohesin linkages that hold together the sister chromatids in a duplicated chromosome (see Figure 18–18A). This release allows each chromosome to be pulled toward the spindle pole to which it is attached (**Figure 18–27**). The movement segregates the two identical sets of chromosomes to opposite ends of the spindle (see Panel 18–1, pp. 628–629).

The cohesin linkage is destroyed by a protease called *separase*. Before anaphase begins, this protease is held in an inactive state by an inhibitory protein called *securin*. At the beginning of anaphase, securin is targeted for destruction by APC/C—the same protein complex, discussed earlier, that marks M cyclin for degradation. Once securin has been removed, separase is then free to sever the cohesin linkages (**Figure 18–28**).

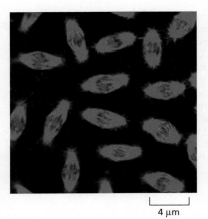

4 µm

Figure 18–26 During metaphase, duplicated chromosomes gather halfway between the two spindle poles. This fluorescence micrograph shows multiple mitotic spindles at metaphase in a fruit fly (*Drosophila*) embryo. The microtubules are stained *green*, and the chromosomes are stained *blue*. At this stage of *Drosophila* development, there are multiple nuclei in one large cytoplasmic compartment, and all of the nuclei divide synchronously, which is why all of the nuclei shown here are at the same metaphase stage of the cell cycle (Movie 18.8). Metaphase spindles are usually pictured in two dimensions, as they are here; when viewed in three dimensions, however, the chromosomes are seen to be gathered at a platelike region at the equator of the spindle—the so-called metaphase plate. (Courtesy of William Sullivan.)

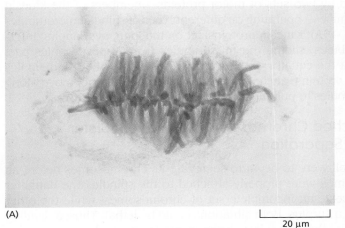

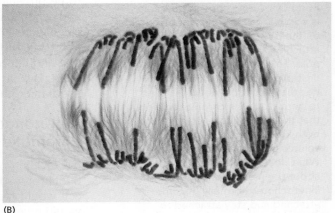

(A)   20 µm   (B)

Figure 18–27 Sister chromatids separate at anaphase. In the transition from (A) metaphase to (B) anaphase, the sister chromatids of duplicated chromosomes (stained *blue*) suddenly separate, allowing the chromosomes to move toward opposite poles, as seen in these plant cells stained with gold-labeled antibodies to label the microtubules (*red*). Plant cells generally do not have centrosomes and therefore have less sharply defined spindle poles than do animal cells (see also Figure 18–35); nonetheless, spindle poles are present here at the top and bottom of each micrograph, although they cannot be seen. (Courtesy of Andrew Bajer.)

Figure 18–28 APC/C triggers the separation of sister chromatids by promoting the destruction of cohesins. APC/C indirectly triggers the cleavage of the cohesins that hold sister chromatids together. It catalyzes the ubiquitylation and destruction of an inhibitory protein called securin, which blocks the activation of a proteolytic enzyme called separase. When freed from securin, separase cleaves the cohesin complexes, allowing the mitotic spindle to pull the sister chromatids apart.

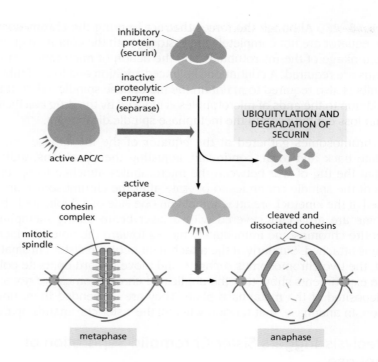

QUESTION 18–6

If fine glass needles are used to manipulate a chromosome inside a living cell during early M phase, it is possible to trick the kinetochores on the two sister chromatids into attaching to the same spindle pole. This arrangement is normally unstable, but the attachments can be stabilized if the needle is used to gently pull the chromosome so that the microtubules attached to both kinetochores (via the same spindle pole) are under tension. What does this suggest to you about the mechanism by which kinetochores normally become attached and stay attached to microtubules from opposite spindle poles? Is the finding consistent with the possibility that a kinetochore is programmed to attach to microtubules from a particular spindle pole? Explain your answers.

Chromosomes Segregate During Anaphase

Once the sister chromatids separate, they all move toward the spindle poles at the same speed, which is typically about 1 µm per minute. The movement is the consequence of two independent and overlapping processes that rely on different parts of the mitotic spindle. In anaphase A, the kinetochore microtubules shorten and the attached chromosomes move poleward. In anaphase B, the spindle poles themselves move apart, further segregating the two sets of chromosomes (**Figure 18–29**).

The driving force for the movements of anaphase A is thought to be provided mainly by the loss of tubulin subunits from both ends of the kinetochore microtubules. The driving forces in anaphase B are thought to be provided by two sets of motor proteins—members of the kinesin and dynein families—operating on different types of spindle microtubules (see Figure 17–19A). Kinesin proteins act on the long, overlapping interpolar microtubules, sliding the microtubules from opposite poles past one another at the equator of the spindle and pushing the spindle poles apart. Dynein proteins, anchored to the plasma membrane, move along astral microtubules to pull the poles apart (see Figure 18–29B).

An Unattached Chromosome Will Prevent Sister-Chromatid Separation

If a dividing cell were to begin to segregate its chromosomes before all the chromosomes were properly attached to the spindle, one daughter cell would receive an incomplete set of chromosomes, while the other would receive a surplus. Both situations could be lethal. Thus, a dividing cell must ensure that every last chromosome is attached properly to the spindle before it completes mitosis. To monitor chromosome attachment, the cell makes use of a negative signal: the kinetochores of unattached chromosomes send a "stop" signal to the cell-cycle control system. This signal inhibits further progress through mitosis by blocking the activation of APC/C (see Figure 18–28). Without active APC/C, the sister chromatids

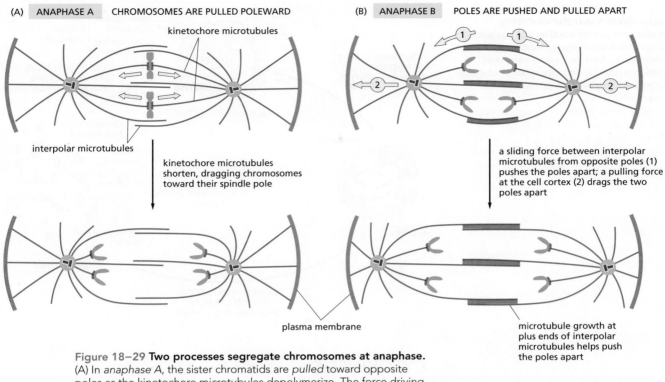

(A) **ANAPHASE A**   CHROMOSOMES ARE PULLED POLEWARD

kinetochore microtubules

interpolar microtubules

kinetochore microtubules shorten, dragging chromosomes toward their spindle pole

(B) **ANAPHASE B**   POLES ARE PUSHED AND PULLED APART

a sliding force between interpolar microtubules from opposite poles (1) pushes the poles apart; a pulling force at the cell cortex (2) drags the two poles apart

plasma membrane

microtubule growth at plus ends of interpolar microtubules helps push the poles apart

Figure 18–29 **Two processes segregate chromosomes at anaphase.** (A) In *anaphase A*, the sister chromatids are *pulled* toward opposite poles as the kinetochore microtubules depolymerize. The force driving this movement is generated mainly at the kinetochore. (B) In *anaphase B*, the two spindle poles move apart as the result of two separate forces: (1) the elongation and sliding of the interpolar microtubules past one another *pushes* the two poles apart, and (2) forces exerted on the outward-pointing astral microtubules at each spindle pole *pull* the poles away from each other, toward the cell cortex. Both forces are thought to depend on the action of motor proteins associated with the microtubules.

remain glued together. Thus, none of the duplicated chromosomes can be pulled apart until every chromosome has been positioned correctly on the mitotic spindle. The absence of APC/C also prevents the destruction of cyclins (see Figure 18–9), so that Cdks remain active—thus prolonging mitosis. This *spindle assembly checkpoint* thereby controls the onset of anaphase, as well as the exit from mitosis, as mentioned earlier (see Figure 18–12).

The Nuclear Envelope Re-forms at Telophase

By the end of anaphase, the chromosomes have separated into two equal groups, one at each pole of the spindle. During **telophase**, the final stage of mitosis, the mitotic spindle disassembles, and a nuclear envelope reassembles around each group of chromosomes to form the two daughter nuclei (Movie 18.9 and Movie 18.10). Vesicles of nuclear membrane associate with the clustered chromosomes and then fuse to re-form the nuclear envelope (see Panel 18–1, pp. 628–629). During this process, the nuclear pore proteins and nuclear lamins that were phosphorylated during prometaphase are now dephosphorylated, which allows them to reassemble and rebuild the nuclear envelope and lamina (Figure 18–30). Once the nuclear envelope has been re-established, the pores restore the localization of cytosolic and nuclear proteins and the condensed chromosomes decondense into their interphase state. A new nucleus has been created, and mitosis is complete. All that remains is for the cell to complete its division into two separate daughter cells.

Figure 18–30 The nuclear envelope breaks down and re-forms during mitosis. The phosphorylation of nuclear pore proteins and lamins helps trigger the disassembly of the nuclear envelope at prometaphase. Dephosphorylation of these proteins at telophase helps reverse the process.

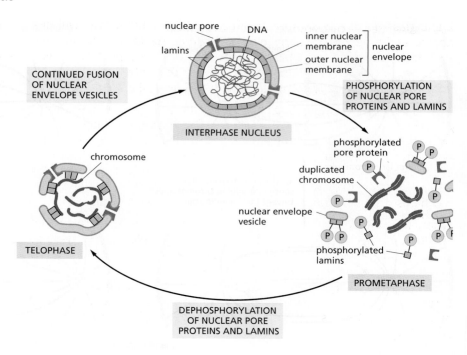

CONTINUED FUSION OF NUCLEAR ENVELOPE VESICLES

nuclear pore

lamins

DNA

inner nuclear membrane
outer nuclear membrane

nuclear envelope

PHOSPHORYLATION OF NUCLEAR PORE PROTEINS AND LAMINS

INTERPHASE NUCLEUS

chromosome

phosphorylated pore protein

duplicated chromosome

nuclear envelope vesicle

phosphorylated lamins

TELOPHASE

PROMETAPHASE

DEPHOSPHORYLATION OF NUCLEAR PORE PROTEINS AND LAMINS

CYTOKINESIS

Cytokinesis, the process by which the cytoplasm is cleaved in two, completes M phase. It usually begins in anaphase but is not completed until after the two daughter nuclei have re-formed in telophase. Whereas mitosis depends on a transient microtubule-based structure, the mitotic spindle, cytokinesis in animal cells depends on a transient structure based on actin and myosin filaments, the *contractile ring* (see Figure 18–19). Both the plane of cleavage and the timing of cytokinesis, however, are determined by the mitotic spindle.

The Mitotic Spindle Determines the Plane of Cytoplasmic Cleavage

The first visible sign of cytokinesis in animal cells is a puckering and furrowing of the plasma membrane that occurs during anaphase (**Figure 18–31**). The furrowing invariably occurs along a plane that runs perpendicular to the long axis of the mitotic spindle. This positioning ensures that the *cleavage furrow* cuts between the two groups of segregated chromosomes, so that each daughter cell receives an identical and complete set of chromosomes. If the mitotic spindle is deliberately displaced (using

QUESTION 18–7

Consider the events that lead to the formation of the new nucleus at telophase. How do nuclear and cytosolic proteins become properly re-sorted so that the new nucleus contains nuclear proteins but not cytosolic proteins?

Figure 18–31 The cleavage furrow is formed by the action of the contractile ring underneath the plasma membrane. In these scanning electron micrographs of a dividing fertilized frog egg, the cleavage furrow is unusually well defined. (A) Low-magnification view of the egg surface. (B) A higher-magnification view of the cleavage furrow. (From H.W. Beams and R.G. Kessel, *Am. Sci.* 64:279–290, 1976. With permission of Sigma Xi.)

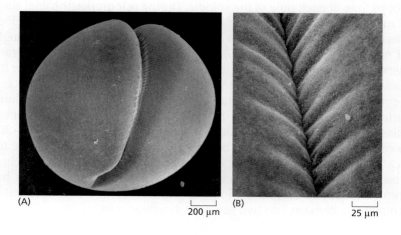

(A) 200 μm (B) 25 μm

a fine glass needle) as soon as the furrow appears, the furrow will disappear and a new one will develop at a site corresponding to the new spindle location and orientation. Once the furrowing process is well under way, however, cleavage proceeds even if the mitotic spindle is artificially sucked out of the cell or depolymerized using the drug colchicine.

How does the mitotic spindle dictate the position of the cleavage furrow? The mechanism is still uncertain, but it appears that, during anaphase, the overlapping interpolar microtubules that form the *central spindle* recruit and activate proteins that signal to the cell cortex to initiate the assembly of the contractile ring at a position midway between the spindle poles (**Figure 18–32**). Because these signals originate during anaphase, this mechanism also contributes to the timing of cytokinesis in late mitosis.

When the mitotic spindle is located centrally in the cell—the usual situation in most dividing cells—the two daughter cells will be of equal size. During embryonic development, however, there are some instances in which the dividing cell moves its mitotic spindle to an asymmetrical position, and, consequently, the furrow creates two daughter cells that differ in size. In most of these *asymmetric divisions*, the daughters also differ in the molecules they inherit, and they usually develop into different cell types.

The Contractile Ring of Animal Cells Is Made of Actin and Myosin Filaments

The **contractile ring** is composed mainly of an overlapping array of actin filaments and myosin filaments (**Figure 18–33**). It assembles at anaphase and is attached to membrane-associated proteins on the cytosolic face of the plasma membrane. Once assembled, the contractile ring is capable of exerting a force strong enough to bend a fine glass needle inserted into the cell before cytokinesis. Much of this force is generated by the sliding of the actin filaments against the myosin filaments. Unlike the stable association of actin and myosin filaments in muscle fibers, however, the contractile ring is a dynamic and transient structure: it assembles to carry out cytokinesis, gradually becomes smaller as cytokinesis progresses, and disassembles completely once the cell has been cleaved in two.

Cell division in many animal cells is accompanied by large changes in cell shape and a decrease in the adherence of the cell to its neighbors, to the extracellular matrix, or to both. These changes result, in part, from the reorganization of actin and myosin filaments in the cell cortex, only one aspect of which is the assembly of the contractile ring. Mammalian fibroblasts in culture, for example, spread out flat during interphase, as a result of the strong adhesive contacts they make with the surface they are growing on—called the *substratum*. As the cells enter M phase, however, they round up. This change in shape takes place, in part, because some of the plasma membrane proteins responsible for attaching the cells to the substratum—the *integrins* (discussed in Chapter 20)—become phosphor-ylated and thus weaken their grip. Once cytokinesis is complete, the daughter cells reestablish their strong contacts with the substratum and

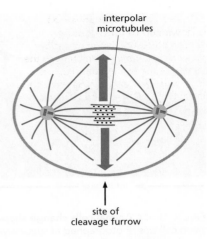

Figure 18–32 Position of the cleavage furrow is dictated by the central spindle. In this model, the interpolar microtubules recruit proteins that generate a signal (*red arrows*) that activates a protein called RhoA in the cell cortex. RhoA, a member of the Rho family of GTPases discussed in Chapter 17, controls the assembly and contraction of the contractile ring midway between the spindle poles.

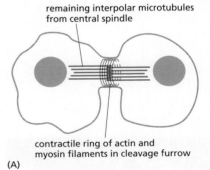

(A)

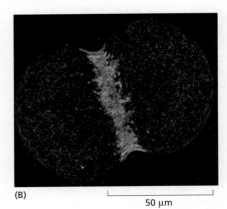

(B)

Figure 18–33 The contractile ring divides the cell in two. (A) Schematic diagram of the midregion of a dividing cell showing the contractile ring beneath the plasma membrane and the remains of the two sets of interpolar microtubules. (B) In this dividing sea urchin embryo, the contractile ring is revealed by staining with a fluorescently labeled antibody that binds to myosin. (B, courtesy of George von Dassow.)

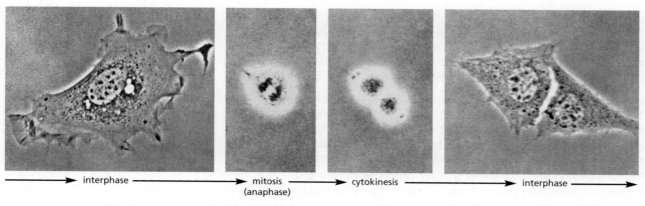

interphase ⟶ mitosis ⟶ cytokinesis ⟶ interphase ⟶
(anaphase)

Figure 18–34 Animal cells change shape during M phase. In these micrographs of a mouse fibroblast dividing in culture, the same cell was photographed at successive times. Note how the cell becomes smaller and rounded as it enters mitosis; the two daughter cells then flatten out again after cytokinesis is complete. (Courtesy of Guenter Albrecht-Buehler.)

flatten out again (Figure 18–34). When cells divide in an animal tissue, this cycle of attachment and detachment presumably allows the cells to rearrange their contacts with neighboring cells and with the extracellular matrix, so that the new cells produced by cell division can be accommodated within the tissue.

Cytokinesis in Plant Cells Involves the Formation of a New Cell Wall

The mechanism of cytokinesis in higher plants is entirely different from that in animal cells, presumably because plant cells are surrounded by a tough cell wall (discussed in Chapter 20). The two daughter cells are separated not by the action of a contractile ring at the cell surface but instead by the construction of a new wall that forms inside the dividing cell. The positioning of this new wall precisely determines the position of the two daughter cells relative to neighboring cells. Thus, the planes of cell division, together with cell enlargement, determine the final form of the plant.

The new cell wall starts to assemble in the cytoplasm between the two sets of segregated chromosomes at the start of telophase. The assembly process is guided by a structure called the **phragmoplast**, which is formed by the remains of the interpolar microtubules at the equator of the old mitotic spindle. Small membrane-enclosed vesicles, largely derived from the Golgi apparatus and filled with polysaccharides and glycoproteins required for the cell wall matrix, are transported along the microtubules to the phragmoplast. Here, they fuse to form a disclike, membrane-enclosed structure, which expands outward by further vesicle fusion until it reaches the plasma membrane and original cell wall, thereby dividing the cell in two (Figure 18–35). Later, cellulose microfibrils are laid down within the matrix to complete the construction of the new cell wall.

Membrane-enclosed Organelles Must Be Distributed to Daughter Cells When a Cell Divides

Organelles such as mitochondria and chloroplasts cannot assemble spontaneously from their individual components; they arise only from the growth and division of the preexisting organelles. Likewise, endoplasmic reticulum (ER) and Golgi apparatus also derive from preexisting organelle fragments. How, then, are these various membrane-enclosed organelles segregated when the cell divides so that each daughter gets its share?

QUESTION 18–8

Draw a detailed view of the formation of the new cell wall that separates the two daughter cells when a plant cell divides (see Figure 18–35). In particular, show where the membrane proteins of the Golgi-derived vesicles end up, indicating what happens to the part of a protein in the Golgi vesicle membrane that is exposed to the interior of the Golgi vesicle. (Refer to Chapter 11 if you need a reminder of membrane structure.)

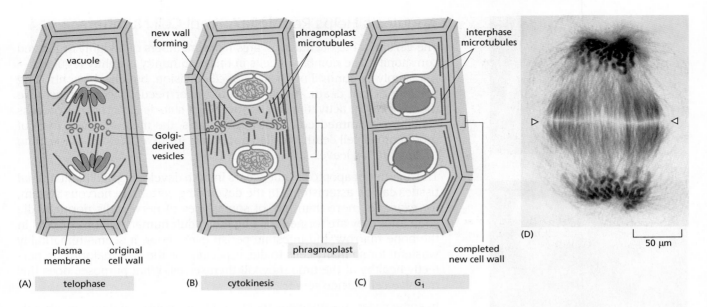

(A)   telophase   (B)   cytokinesis   (C)   G₁   (D)

vacuole — new wall forming — phragmoplast microtubules — Golgi-derived vesicles — interphase microtubules — plasma membrane — original cell wall — phragmoplast — completed new cell wall — 50 μm

Mitochondria and chloroplasts are usually present in large numbers and will be safely inherited if, on average, their numbers simply double once each cell cycle. The ER in interphase cells is continuous with the nuclear membrane and is organized by the microtubule cytoskeleton (see Figure 17–21). Upon entry into M phase, the reorganization of the microtubules releases the ER; in most cells, the released ER remains intact during mitosis and is cut in two during cytokinesis. The Golgi apparatus fragments during mitosis; the fragments associate with the spindle microtubules via motor proteins, thereby hitching a ride into the daughter cells as the spindle elongates in anaphase. Other components of the cell—including the other membrane-enclosed organelles, ribosomes, and all of the soluble proteins—are inherited randomly when the cell divides.

Having discussed how cells divide, we now turn to the general problem of how the size of an animal or an organ is determined, which leads us to consider how cell number and cell size are controlled.

CONTROL OF CELL NUMBERS AND CELL SIZE

A fertilized mouse egg and a fertilized human egg are similar in size—about 100 μm in diameter. Yet an adult mouse is much smaller than an adult human. What are the differences between the control of cell behavior in humans and mice that generate such big differences in size? The same fundamental question can be asked about each organ and tissue in an individual's body. What adjustment of cell behavior explains the length of an elephant's trunk or the size of its brain or its liver? These questions are largely unanswered, but it is at least possible to say what the ingredients of an answer must be. Three fundamental processes largely determine organ and body size: cell growth, cell division, and cell death. Each of these processes, in turn, depends on programs intrinsic to the individual cell, regulated by signals from other cells in the body.

In this section, we first consider how organisms eliminate unwanted cells by a form of programmed cell death called *apoptosis*. We then discuss how extracellular signals balance cell death, cell growth, and cell division—thereby helping control the size of an animal and its organs. We conclude the section with a brief discussion of the extracellular signals that control these three processes.

Figure 18–35 Cytokinesis in a plant cell is guided by a specialized microtubule-based structure called the phragmoplast. (A) At the beginning of telophase, after the chromosomes have segregated, a new cell wall starts to assemble inside the cell at the equator of the old spindle. (B) The interpolar microtubules of the mitotic spindle remaining at telophase form the *phragmoplast* and guide vesicles, derived from the Golgi apparatus, toward the equator of the spindle. The vesicles, which are filled with cell wall material, fuse to form the growing new cell wall that grows outward to reach the plasma membrane and original cell wall. (C) The preexisting plasma membrane and the membrane surrounding the new cell wall then fuse, completely separating the two daughter cells. (D) A light micrograph of a plant cell in telophase is shown at a stage corresponding to (A). The cell has been stained to show both the microtubules and the two sets of chromosomes segregated at the two poles of the spindle. The location of the growing new cell wall is indicated by the arrowheads. (D, courtesy of Andrew Bajer.)

QUESTION 18–9

The Golgi apparatus is thought to be partitioned into the daughter cells at cell division by a random distribution of fragments that are created at mitosis. Explain why random partitioning of chromosomes would not work.

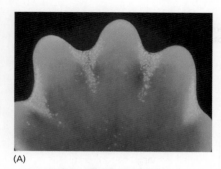

(A)

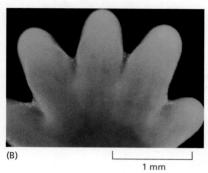

(B)

|—————————————|
1 mm

Figure 18–36 Apoptosis in the developing mouse paw sculpts the digits. (A) The paw in this mouse embryo has been stained with a dye that specifically labels cells that have undergone apoptosis. The apoptotic cells appear as *bright green dots* between the developing digits. (B) This cell death eliminates the tissue between the developing digits, as seen in the paw shown one day later. Here, few, if any, apoptotic cells can be seen—demonstrating how quickly apoptotic cells can be cleared from a tissue. (From W. Wood et al., *Development* 127:5245–5252, 2000. With permission from The Company of Biologists Ltd.)

Apoptosis Helps Regulate Animal Cell Numbers

The cells of a multicellular organism are members of a highly organized community. The number of cells in this community is tightly regulated—not simply by controlling the rate of cell division, but also by controlling the rate of cell death. If cells are no longer needed, they can remove themselves by activating an intracellular suicide program—a process called **programmed cell death**. In animals, the most common form of programmed cell death is called **apoptosis** (from a Greek word meaning "falling off," as leaves fall from a tree).

The amount of apoptosis that occurs in both developing and adult animal tissues can be astonishing. In the developing vertebrate nervous system, for example, more than half of some types of nerve cells normally die soon after they are formed. In a healthy adult human, billions of cells in the bone marrow and intestine perish every hour. It seems remarkably wasteful for so many cells to die, especially as the vast majority are perfectly healthy at the time they kill themselves. What purposes does this massive cell suicide serve?

In some cases, the answers are clear. Mouse paws—and our own hands and feet—are sculpted by apoptosis during embryonic development: they start out as spadelike structures, and the individual fingers and toes separate because the cells between them die (**Figure 18–36**). In other cases, cells die when the structure they form is no longer needed. When a tadpole changes into a frog at metamorphosis, the cells in its tail die, and the tail, which is not needed in the adult frog, disappears (**Figure 18–37**). In these cases, the unneeded cells die largely through apoptosis.

In adult tissues, cell death usually balances cell division, unless the tissue is growing or shrinking. If part of the liver is removed in an adult rat, for example, liver cells proliferate to make up the loss. Conversely, if a rat is treated with the drug phenobarbital, which stimulates liver cell division, the liver enlarges. However, when the phenobarbital treatment is stopped, apoptosis in the liver greatly increases until the organ has returned to its original size, usually within a week or so. Thus, the liver is kept at a constant size through regulation of both the rate of cell death and the rate of cell birth.

Apoptosis Is Mediated by an Intracellular Proteolytic Cascade

Cells that die as a result of acute injury typically swell and burst, spewing their contents across their neighbors, a process called *cell necrosis* (**Figure 18–38A**). This eruption triggers a potentially damaging inflammatory response. By contrast, a cell that undergoes apoptosis dies neatly, without damaging its neighbors. A cell in the throes of apoptosis may develop irregular bulges—or *blebs*—on its surface; but it then shrinks and condenses (**Figure 18–38B**). The cytoskeleton collapses, the nuclear envelope disassembles, and the nuclear DNA breaks up into fragments (**Movie 18.11**). Most importantly, the cell surface is altered in such a manner that it immediately attracts phagocytic cells, usually specialized

Figure 18–37 As a tadpole changes into a frog, the cells in its tail are induced to undergo apoptosis. All of the changes that occur during metamorphosis, including the induction of apoptosis in the tadpole tail, are stimulated by an increase in thyroid hormone in the blood.

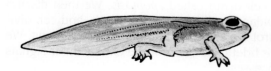
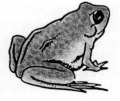

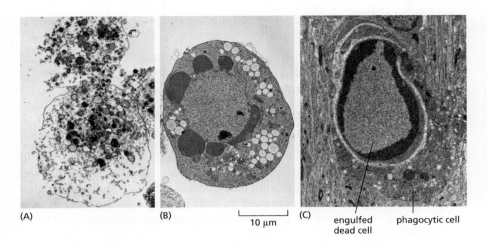

(A)

(B)

10 μm

(C) engulfed dead cell · phagocytic cell

Figure 18–38 Cells undergoing apoptosis die quickly and cleanly. Electron micrographs showing cells that have died (A) by necrosis or (B and C) by apoptosis. The cells in (A) and (B) died in a culture dish, whereas the cell in (C) died in a developing tissue and has been engulfed by a phagocytic cell. Note that the cell in (A) seems to have exploded, whereas those in (B) and (C) have condensed but seem relatively intact. The large vacuoles seen in the cytoplasm of the cell in (B) are a variable feature of apoptosis. (Courtesy of Julia Burne.)

phagocytic cells called macrophages (see Figure 15–32B). These cells engulf the apoptotic cell before its contents can leak out (**Figure 18–38C**). This rapid removal of the dying cell avoids the damaging consequences of cell necrosis, and it also allows the organic components of the apoptotic cell to be recycled by the cell that ingests it.

The molecular machinery responsible for apoptosis, which seems to be similar in most animal cells, involves a family of proteases called **caspases**. These enzymes are made as inactive precursors, called *procaspases*, which are activated in response to signals that induce apoptosis. Two types of caspases work together to take a cell apart. *Initiator caspases* cleave, and thereby activate, downstream *executioner caspases*, which dismember numerous key proteins in the cell (**Figure 18–39**). One executioner caspase, for example, targets the lamin proteins that form the nuclear lamina underlying the nuclear envelope (see Figure 18–30); this cleavage causes the irreversible breakdown of the nuclear lamina, which allows nucleases to enter the nucleus and break down the DNA.

QUESTION 18–10

Why do you think apoptosis occurs by a different mechanism from the cell death that occurs in cell necrosis? What might be the consequences if apoptosis were not achieved in so neat and orderly a fashion, whereby the cell destroys itself from within and avoids leakage of its contents into the extracellular space?

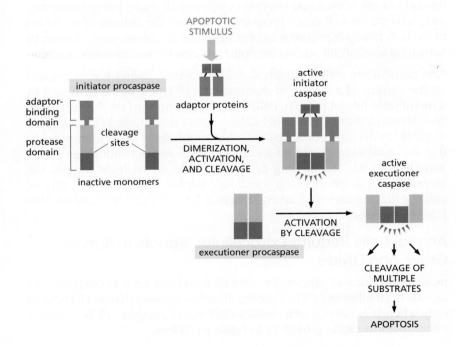

Figure 18–39 Apoptosis is mediated by an intracellular proteolytic cascade. An initiator caspase is first made as an inactive monomer called a procaspase. An apoptotic signal triggers the assembly of adaptor proteins that bring together a pair of initiator caspases, which are thereby activated, leading to cleavage of a specific site in their protease domains. Executioner caspases are initially formed as inactive dimers. Upon cleavage by an initiator caspase, the executioner caspase dimer undergoes an activating conformational change. The executioner caspases then cleave a variety of key proteins, leading to apoptosis.

In this way, the cell dismantles itself quickly and cleanly, and its corpse is rapidly taken up and digested by another cell.

Activation of the apoptotic program, like entry into a new stage of the cell cycle, is usually triggered in an all-or-none fashion: once a cell reaches a critical point along the path to destruction, it cannot turn back.

The Intrinsic Apoptotic Death Program Is Regulated by the Bcl2 Family of Intracellular Proteins

All nucleated animal cells contain the seeds of their own destruction: in these cells, inactive procaspases lie waiting for a signal to destroy the cell. It is therefore not surprising that caspase activity is tightly regulated to ensure that the death program is held in check until it is needed—for example, to eliminate cells that are superfluous, mislocated, or badly damaged.

The main proteins that regulate the activation of caspases are members of the **Bcl2 family** of intracellular proteins. Some members of this protein family promote caspase activation and cell death, whereas others inhibit these processes. Two of the most important death-inducing family members are proteins called *Bax* and *Bak*. These proteins—which are activated in response to DNA damage or other insults—promote cell death by inducing the release of the electron-transport protein cytochrome *c* from mitochondria into the cytosol. Other members of the Bcl2 family (including Bcl2 itself) inhibit apoptosis by preventing Bax and Bak from releasing cytochrome *c*. The balance between the activities of pro-apoptotic and anti-apoptotic members of the Bcl2 family largely determines whether a cell lives or dies by apoptosis.

The cytochrome *c* molecules released from mitochondria activate initiator procaspases—and induce cell death—by promoting the assembly of a large, seven-armed, pinwheel-like protein complex called an apoptosome. The apoptosome then recruits and activates a particular initiator procaspase, which then triggers a caspase cascade that leads to apoptosis (Figure 18–40).

Apoptotic Signals Can Also Come from Other Cells

Sometimes the signal to commit suicide is not generated internally, but instead comes from a neighboring cell. Some of these extracellular signals activate the cell death program by altering the activity of members of the Bcl2 family of proteins. Others stimulate apoptosis more directly by activating a set of cell-surface receptor proteins known as *death receptors*.

One particularly well-understood death receptor, called *Fas*, is present on the surface of a variety of mammalian cell types. Fas is activated by a membrane-bound protein, called *Fas ligand*, present on the surface of specialized immune cells called *killer lymphocytes*. These killer cells help regulate immune responses by inducing apoptosis in other immune cells that are unwanted or are no longer needed—and activating Fas is one way they do so. The binding of Fas ligand to its receptor triggers the assembly of a death-inducing signaling complex, which includes specific initiator procaspases that, when activated, launch a caspase cascade that leads to cell death.

Animal Cells Require Extracellular Signals to Survive, Grow, and Divide

In a multicellular organism, the fate of individual cells is controlled by signals from other cells. Such communication ensures that a cell survives only when it is needed and divides only when another cell is required, either to allow tissue growth or to replace cell loss.

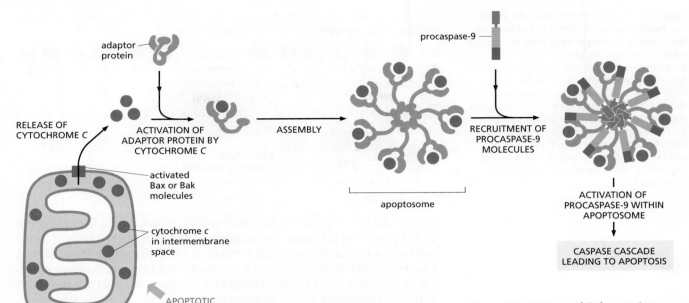

RELEASE OF CYTOCHROME C

ACTIVATION OF ADAPTOR PROTEIN BY CYTOCHROME C

ASSEMBLY

RECRUITMENT OF PROCASPASE-9 MOLECULES

ACTIVATION OF PROCASPASE-9 WITHIN APOPTOSOME

CASPASE CASCADE LEADING TO APOPTOSIS

adaptor protein

procaspase-9

activated Bax or Bak molecules

cytochrome c in intermembrane space

APOPTOTIC STIMULUS

mitochondrion

apoptosome

Figure 18–40 Bax and Bak can trigger apoptosis by releasing cytochrome c from mitochondria. When Bak or Bax proteins are activated by an apoptotic stimulus, they aggregate in the outer mitochondrial membrane, leading to the release of cytochrome c into the cytosol by an unknown mechanism. Additional proteins in the mitochondrial intermembrane space are released at the same time—not shown. Cytochrome c then binds to an adaptor protein, causing it to assemble into a seven-armed complex called the apoptosome. This complex then recruits seven molecules of a specific initiator procaspase (procaspase-9). The procaspase-9 proteins become activated within the apoptosome and then go on to activate executioner procaspases in the cytosol (as shown in Figure 18–39), leading to a caspase cascade and apoptosis.

Most of the extracellular signal molecules that influence cell survival, cell growth, and cell division are either soluble proteins secreted by other cells or proteins that are bound to the surface of other cells or to the extracellular matrix. Although most act positively to stimulate one or more of these cell processes, some act negatively to inhibit a particular process. The positively acting signal proteins can be classified, on the basis of their function, into three major categories:

1. **Survival factors** promote cell survival, largely by suppressing apoptosis.
2. **Mitogens** stimulate cell division, primarily by overcoming the intracellular braking mechanisms that block entry into the cell cycle in late G_1.
3. **Growth factors** stimulate cell growth (an increase in cell size and mass) by promoting the synthesis and inhibiting the degradation of proteins and other macromolecules.

These categories are not mutually exclusive, as many signal molecules have more than one of these functions. Unfortunately, the term "growth factor" is often used as a catch-all phrase to describe a protein with any of these functions. Indeed, the phrase "cell growth" is frequently used inappropriately to mean an increase in cell number, which is more correctly termed "cell proliferation."

In the following three sections, we examine each of these types of signal molecules in turn.

Survival Factors Suppress Apoptosis

Animal cells need signals from other cells just to survive. If deprived of such survival factors, cells activate a caspase-dependent intracellular suicide program and die by apoptosis. This requirement for signals from other cells helps ensure that cells survive only when and where they are needed. Many types of nerve cells, for example, are produced in excess in the developing nervous system and then compete for limited amounts of survival factors that are secreted by the target cells they contact. Those

Figure 18–41 Cell death can help adjust the number of developing nerve cells to the number of target cells they contact. If more nerve cells are produced than can be supported by the limited amount of survival factor released by the target cells, some cells will receive insufficient amounts of survival factor to keep their suicide program suppressed and will undergo apoptosis. This strategy of overproduction followed by culling can help ensure that all target cells are contacted by nerve cells and that the "extra" nerve cells are automatically eliminated.

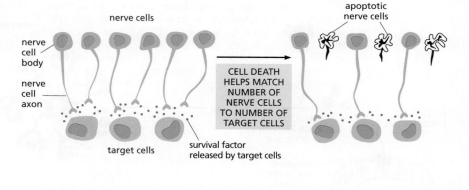

nerve cells that receive enough survival factor live, while the others die by apoptosis. In this way, the number of surviving nerve cells is automatically adjusted to match the number of cells with which they connect (Figure 18–41). A similar dependence on survival signals from neighboring cells is thought to help control cell numbers in other tissues, both during development and in adulthood.

Survival factors usually act through cell-surface receptors. Once activated, the receptors turn on intracellular signaling pathways that keep the apoptotic death program suppressed, usually by regulating members of the Bcl2 family of proteins. Some survival factors, for example, increase the production of Bcl2, a protein that suppresses apoptosis (Figure 18–42).

Mitogens Stimulate Cell Division by Promoting Entry into S Phase

Most mitogens are secreted signal proteins that bind to cell-surface receptors. When activated by mitogen binding, these receptors initiate various intracellular signaling pathways (discussed in Chapter 16) that stimulate cell division. As we saw earlier, these signaling pathways act mainly by releasing the molecular brakes that block the transition from the G_1 phase of the cell cycle into S phase (see Figure 18–14).

Most mitogens have been identified and characterized by their effects on cells in culture. One of the first mitogens identified in this way was *platelet-derived growth factor*, or *PDGF*, the effects of which are typical of many others discovered since. When blood clots form (in a wound, for example), blood platelets incorporated in the clots are stimulated to release PDGF. PDGF then binds to receptor tyrosine kinases (discussed in Chapter 16) in surviving cells at the wound site, stimulating these cells to proliferate and help heal the wound. In a similar way, if part of the liver is lost through surgery or acute injury, a mitogen called *hepatocyte growth factor* helps stimulate the surviving liver cells to proliferate.

Growth Factors Stimulate Cells to Grow

The growth of an organ—or an entire organism—depends as much on cell growth as it does on cell division. If cells divided without growing, they would get progressively smaller, and there would be no increase in total cell mass. In single-celled organisms such as yeasts, both cell growth and cell division require only nutrients. In animals, by contrast, both cell growth and cell division depend on signals from other cells. Cell growth, unlike cell division, does not depend on the cell-cycle control system. Indeed, many animal cells, including nerve cells and most muscle cells, do most of their growing after they have terminally differentiated and permanently stopped dividing.

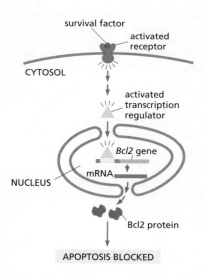

Figure 18–42 Survival factors often suppress apoptosis by regulating Bcl2 family members. In this case, the survival factor binds to cell-surface receptors that activate an intracellular signaling pathway, which in turn activates a transcription regulator in the cytosol. This protein moves to the nucleus, where it activates the gene encoding Bcl2, a protein that inhibits apoptosis (see also Figure 16–33).

Figure 18–43 Extracellular growth factors increase the synthesis and decrease the degradation of macromolecules. Binding of a growth factor to a receptor tyrosine kinase (RTK, a class of cell-surface receptor described in Chapter 16) initiates an intracellular signaling pathway that leads to activation of a protein kinase called Tor, which acts through multiple targets to stimulate protein synthesis and inhibit protein degradation (see also Figure 16–34). This action leads to a net increase in macromolecules and thereby cell growth.

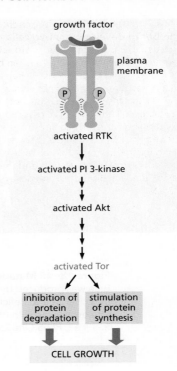

Like most survival factors and mitogens, most extracellular growth factors bind to cell-surface receptors that activate intracellular signaling pathways. These pathways lead to the accumulation of proteins and other macromolecules. Growth factors both increase the rate of synthesis of these molecules and decrease their rate of degradation (**Figure 18–43**).

Some extracellular signal proteins, including PDGF, can act as both growth factors and mitogens, stimulating both cell growth and progression through the cell cycle. Such proteins help ensure that cells maintain their appropriate size as they proliferate.

Compared to cell division, there has been surprisingly little study of how cell size is controlled in animals. As a result, it remains a mystery how different cell types in the same animal grow to be so different in size (**Figure 18–44**).

Some Extracellular Signal Proteins Inhibit Cell Survival, Division, or Growth

The extracellular signal proteins that promote survival, growth, and cell division act positively to increase the size of organs and organisms. Some extracellular signal proteins, however, act to oppose these positive regulators and thereby inhibit tissue growth. *Myostatin*, for example, is a secreted signal protein that normally inhibits the growth and proliferation of the precursor cells (myoblasts) that fuse to form skeletal muscle cells during mammalian development. When the gene that encodes myostatin is deleted in mice, their muscles grow to be several times larger than normal, because both the number and the size of muscle cells is increased. Remarkably, two breeds of cattle that were bred for large muscles turned out to have mutations in the gene encoding myostatin (**Figure 18–45**).

Cancers are similarly the products of mutations that set cells free from the normal "social" controls operating on cell survival, growth, and proliferation. Because cancer cells are generally less dependent than normal cells on signals from other cells, they can out-survive, outgrow, and out-divide their normal neighbors, producing tumors that can kill their host (see Chapter 20).

In our discussions of cell division, we have focused entirely on the ordinary divisions that produce two daughter cells, each with a full and identical complement of the parent cell's genetic material. There is, however, a different and highly specialized type of cell division called meiosis, which is required for sexual reproduction in eukaryotes. In the next chapter, we describe the special features of meiosis and how they underlie the genetic principles that define the laws of inheritance.

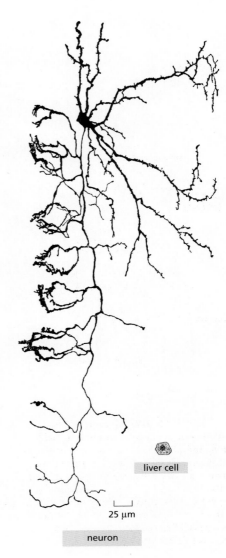

Figure 18–44 The cells in an animal can differ greatly in size. The neuron and liver cell shown here are drawn at the same scale. A neuron grows progressively larger after it has terminally differentiated and permanently stopped dividing. (Neuron adapted from S. Ramón y Cajal, Histologie du Système Nerveux de l'Homme et de Vertébrés, 1909–1911. Paris: Maloine; reprinted, Madrid: C.S.I.C., 1972.)

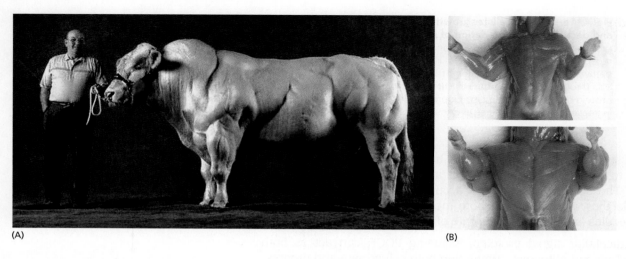

(A)   (B)

Figure 18–45 Mutation of the *myostatin* gene leads to a dramatic increase in muscle mass. (A) This Belgian Blue was produced by cattle breeders and was only later found to have a mutation in the *myostatin* gene. (B) Mice purposely made deficient in the same gene also have remarkably big muscles. A normal mouse is shown at the top for comparison with the muscular mutant shown at the bottom. (A, Yann Arthus-Bertrand/Getty Images; B, from S.-J. Lee, *PLoS One* 2:e789, 2007.)

ESSENTIAL CONCEPTS

- The eukaryotic cell cycle consists of several distinct phases. In interphase, the cell grows and the nuclear DNA is replicated; in M phase, the nucleus divides (mitosis) followed by the cytoplasm (cytokinesis).

- In most cells, interphase consists of an S phase when DNA is duplicated plus two gap phases: G_1 and G_2. These gap phases give proliferating cells more time to grow and prepare for S phase and M phase.

- The cell-cycle control system coordinates events of the cell cycle by sequentially and cyclically switching on and off the appropriate parts of the cell-cycle machinery.

- The cell-cycle control system depends on cyclin-dependent protein kinases (Cdks), which are cyclically activated by the binding of cyclin proteins and by phosphorylation and dephosphorylation; when activated, Cdks phosphorylate key proteins in the cell.

- Different cyclin–Cdk complexes trigger different steps of the cell cycle: G_1-Cdk drives the cell through G_1; G_1/S-Cdk and S-Cdk drive it into S phase; and M-Cdk drives it into mitosis.

- The control system also uses protein complexes, such as APC/C, to trigger the destruction of specific cell-cycle regulators at particular stages of the cycle.

- The cell-cycle control system can halt the cycle at specific transition points to ensure that intracellular and extracellular conditions are favorable and that each step is completed before the next is started. Some of these control mechanisms rely on Cdk inhibitors that block the activity of one or more cyclin–Cdk complexes.

- S-Cdk initiates DNA replication during S phase and helps ensure that the genome is copied only once. The cell-cycle control system can delay cell-cycle progression during G_1 or S phase to prevent cells from replicating damaged DNA. It can also delay the start of M phase to ensure that DNA replication is complete.

- Centrosomes duplicate during S phase and separate during G_2. Some of the microtubules that grow out of the duplicated centrosomes interact to form the mitotic spindle.

- When the nuclear envelope breaks down, the spindle microtubules capture the duplicated chromosomes and pull them in opposite directions, positioning the chromosomes at the equator of the metaphase spindle.

- The sudden separation of sister chromatids at anaphase allows the chromosomes to be pulled to opposite poles; this movement is driven by the depolymerization of spindle microtubules and by microtubule-associated motor proteins.

- A nuclear envelope re-forms around the two sets of segregated chromosomes to form two new nuclei, thereby completing mitosis.

- In animal cells, cytokinesis is mediated by a contractile ring of actin filaments and myosin filaments, which assembles midway between the spindle poles; in plant cells, by contrast, a new cell wall forms inside the parent cell to divide the cytoplasm in two.

- In animals, extracellular signals regulate cell numbers by controlling cell survival, cell growth, and cell proliferation.

- Most animal cells require survival signals from other cells to avoid apoptosis—a form of cell suicide mediated by a proteolytic caspase cascade; this strategy helps ensure that cells survive only when and where they are needed.

- Animal cells proliferate only if stimulated by extracellular mitogens produced by other cells; mitogens release the normal intracellular brakes that block progression from G_1 or G_0 into S phase.

- For an organism or an organ to grow, cells must grow as well as divide; animal cell growth depends on extracellular growth factors that stimulate protein synthesis and inhibit protein degradation.

- Some extracellular signal molecules inhibit rather than promote cell survival, cell growth, or cell division.

- Cancer cells fail to obey these normal "social" controls on cell behavior and therefore outgrow, out-divide, and out-survive their normal neighbors.

KEY TERMS

anaphase	condensin	metaphase
anaphase-promoting complex (APC/C)	contractile ring	mitogen
apoptosis	cyclin	mitosis
aster	cytokinesis	mitotic spindle
Bcl2 family	G_1-Cdk	p53
bi-orientation	G_1 cyclin	phragmoplast
caspase	G_1 phase	programmed cell death
Cdk (cyclin-dependent protein kinase)	G_2 phase	prometaphase
Cdk inhibitor protein	G_1/S-Cdk	prophase
cell cycle	G_1/S cyclin	S-Cdk
cell-cycle control system	growth factor	S cyclin
centrosome	interphase	S phase
centrosome cycle	kinetochore	sister chromatid
chromosome condensation	M-Cdk	spindle pole
cohesin	M cyclin	survival factor
	M phase	telophase

QUESTIONS

QUESTION 18–11

Roughly, how long would it take a single fertilized human egg to make a cluster of cells weighing 70 kg by repeated divisions, if each cell weighs 1 nanogram just after cell division and each cell cycle takes 24 hours? Why does it take very much longer than this to make a 70 kg adult human?

QUESTION 18–12

The shortest eukaryotic cell cycles of all—shorter even than those of many bacteria—occur in many early animal embryos. These so-called cleavage divisions take place without any significant increase in the weight of the embryo. How can this be? Which phase of the cell cycle would you expect to be most reduced?

QUESTION 18–13

One important biological effect of a large dose of ionizing radiation is to halt cell division.

A. How does this occur?

B. What happens if a cell has a mutation that prevents it from halting cell division after being irradiated?

C. What might be the effects of such a mutation if the cell is not irradiated?

D. An adult human who has reached maturity will die within a few days of receiving a radiation dose large enough to stop cell division. What does that tell you (other than that one should avoid large doses of radiation)?

QUESTION 18–14

If cells are grown in a culture medium containing radioactive thymidine, the thymidine will be covalently incorporated into the cell's DNA during S phase. The radioactive DNA can be detected in the nuclei of individual cells by autoradiography: radioactive cells will activate a photographic emulsion and be labeled by black dots when looked at under a microscope. Consider a simple experiment in which cells are radioactively labeled by this method for only a short period (about 30 minutes). The radioactive thymidine medium is then replaced with one containing unlabeled thymidine, and the cells are grown for some additional time. At different time points after replacement of the medium, cells are examined in a microscope. The fraction of cells in mitosis (which can be easily recognized because the cells have rounded up and their chromosomes are condensed) that have radioactive DNA in their nuclei is then determined and plotted as a function of time after the labeling with radioactive thymidine (Figure Q18–14).

A. Would all cells (including cells at all phases of the cell cycle) be expected to contain radioactive DNA after the labeling procedure?

B. Initially, there are no mitotic cells that contain radioactive DNA (see Figure Q18–14). Why is this?

C. Explain the rise and fall and then rise again of the curve.

D. Estimate the length of the G_2 phase from this graph.

QUESTION 18–15

One of the functions of M-Cdk is to cause a precipitous drop in M cyclin concentration halfway through M phase. Describe the consequences of this sudden decrease and suggest possible mechanisms by which it might occur.

QUESTION 18–16

Figure 18–5 shows the rise of M cyclin concentration and the rise of M-Cdk activity in cells as they progress through the cell cycle. It is remarkable that the M cyclin concentration rises slowly and steadily, whereas M-Cdk activity increases suddenly. How do you think this difference arises?

QUESTION 18–17

What is the order in which the following events occur during cell division?

A. anaphase

B. metaphase

C. prometaphase

D. telophase

E. mitosis

F. prophase

Where does cytokinesis fit in?

QUESTION 18–18

The lifetime of a microtubule in a mammalian cell, between its formation by polymerization and its spontaneous disappearance by depolymerization, varies with the stage of the cell cycle. For an actively proliferating cell, the average lifetime is 5 minutes in interphase and 15 seconds in mitosis. If the average length of a microtubule in interphase is 20 μm, how long will it be during mitosis, assuming that the rates of microtubule elongation due to the addition of tubulin subunits in the two phases are the same?

QUESTION 18–19

The balance between plus-end directed and minus-end directed motor proteins that bind to interpolar microtubules in the overlap region of the mitotic spindle is thought to

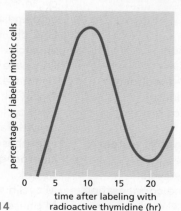

Figure Q18–14

help determine the length of the spindle. How might each type of motor protein contribute to the determination of spindle length?

QUESTION 18–20

Sketch the principal stages of mitosis, using Panel 18–1 (pp. 628–629) as a guide. Color one sister chromatid and follow it through mitosis and cytokinesis. What event commits this chromatid to a particular daughter cell? Once initially committed, can its fate be reversed? What may influence this commitment?

QUESTION 18–21

The polar movement of chromosomes during anaphase A is associated with microtubule shortening. In particular, microtubules depolymerize at the ends at which they are attached to the kinetochores. Sketch a model that explains how a microtubule can shorten and generate force yet remain firmly attached to the chromosome.

QUESTION 18–22

Rarely, both sister chromatids of a replicated chromosome end up in one daughter cell. How might this happen? What could be the consequences of such a mitotic error?

QUESTION 18–23

Which of the following statements are correct? Explain your answers.

A. Centrosomes are replicated before M phase begins.

B. Two sister chromatids arise by replication of the DNA of the same chromosome and remain paired as they line up on the metaphase plate.

C. Interpolar microtubules attach end-to-end and are therefore continuous from one spindle pole to the other.

D. Microtubule polymerization and depolymerization and microtubule motor proteins are all required for DNA replication.

E. Microtubules nucleate at the centromeres and then connect to the kinetochores, which are structures at the centrosome regions of chromosomes.

QUESTION 18–24

An antibody that binds to myosin prevents the movement of myosin molecules along actin filaments (the interaction between actin and myosin is described in Chapter 17). How do you suppose the antibody exerts this effect? What might be the result of injecting this antibody into cells (A) on the movement of chromosomes at anaphase or (B) on cytokinesis? Explain your answers.

QUESTION 18–25

Look carefully at the electron micrographs in Figure 18–38. Describe the differences between the cell that died by necrosis and those that died by apoptosis. How do the pictures confirm the differences between the two processes? Explain your answer.

QUESTION 18–26

Which of the following statements are correct? Explain your answers.

A. Cells do not pass from G_1 into M phase of the cell cycle unless there are sufficient nutrients to complete an entire cell cycle.

B. Apoptosis is mediated by special intracellular proteases, one of which cleaves nuclear lamins.

C. Developing neurons compete for limited amounts of survival factors.

D. Some vertebrate cell-cycle control proteins function when expressed in yeast cells.

E. The enzymatic activity of a Cdk protein is determined both by the presence of a bound cyclin and by the phosphorylation state of the Cdk.

QUESTION 18–27

Compare the rules of cell behavior in an animal with the rules that govern human behavior in society. What would happen to an animal if its cells behaved as people normally behave in our society? Could the rules that govern cell behavior be applied to human societies?

QUESTION 18–28

In his highly classified research laboratory, Dr. Lawrence M. is charged with the task of developing a strain of dog-sized rats to be deployed behind enemy lines. In your opinion, which of the following strategies should Dr. M. pursue to increase the size of rats?

A. Block all apoptosis.

B. Block p53 function.

C. Overproduce growth factors, mitogens, or survival factors.

Explain the likely consequences of each option.

QUESTION 18–29

PDGF is encoded by a gene that can cause cancer when expressed inappropriately. Why do cancers not arise at wounds in which PDGF is released from platelets?

QUESTION 18–30

What do you suppose happens in mutant cells that

A. cannot degrade M cyclin?

B. always express high levels of p21?

C. cannot phosphorylate Rb?

QUESTION 18–31

Liver cells proliferate excessively both in patients with chronic alcoholism and in patients with liver cancer. What are the differences in the mechanisms by which cell proliferation is induced in these diseases?

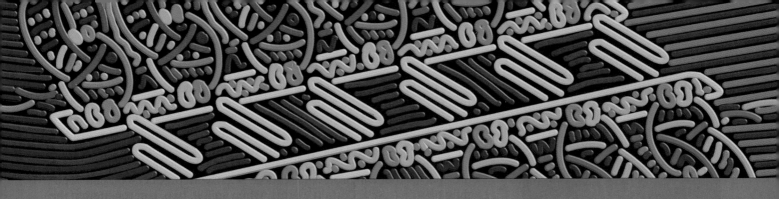

Sexual Reproduction and Genetics

Individual cells reproduce by replicating their DNA and dividing in two. This basic process of cell proliferation occurs in all living species—in the cells of multicellular organisms and in free-living cells such as bacteria and yeasts—and it allows each cell to pass on its genetic information to future generations.

Yet reproduction in a multicellular organism—in a fish or a fly, a person or a plant—is a much more complicated affair. It entails elaborate developmental cycles, in which all of the organism's cells, tissues, and organs must be generated afresh from a single cell. This starter cell is no ordinary cell. It has a very peculiar origin: for most animal and plant species, the single cell from which an organism arises is produced by the union of a pair of cells that hail from two completely separate individuals—a mother and a father. As a result of this cell fusion—a central event in *sexual reproduction*—two genomes merge to form the genome of a new individual. The mechanisms that govern genetic inheritance in sexually reproducing organisms are therefore different, and more complex, than those that operate in organisms that pass on their genetic information asexually—by a straightforward cell division or by budding off a brand new individual.

In this chapter, we explore the cell biology of sexual reproduction. We discuss what organisms gain from sex, and we describe how they do it. We examine the reproductive cells produced by males and females, and we explore the specialized form of division, called *meiosis*, that generates them. We discuss how Gregor Mendel, a nineteenth-century Austrian monk, deduced the basic logic of genetic inheritance by studying the progeny of pea plants. Finally, we describe how scientists can exploit the genetics of sexual reproduction to gain insights into human biology, human origins, and the molecular underpinnings of human disease.

THE BENEFITS OF SEX

MEIOSIS AND FERTILIZATION

MENDEL AND THE LAWS OF INHERITANCE

GENETICS AS AN EXPERIMENTAL TOOL

EXPLORING HUMAN GENETICS

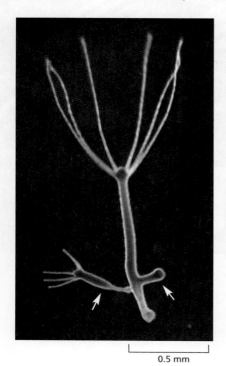

0.5 mm

Figure 19–1 A hydra reproduces by budding. This form of asexual reproduction involves the production of buds (*arrows*), which eventually pinch off to form progeny that are genetically identical to their parent. (Courtesy of Amata Hornbruch.)

THE BENEFITS OF SEX

Most of the creatures we see around us reproduce sexually. However, many organisms, especially those invisible to the naked eye, can produce offspring without resorting to sex. Most bacteria and other single-celled organisms multiply by simple cell division. Many plants also reproduce asexually, forming multicellular offshoots that later detach from the parent to make new independent plants. Even in the animal kingdom, there are species that can procreate without sex. Hydra produce young by budding (**Figure 19–1**). Certain worms, when split in two, can regenerate the "missing halves" to form two complete individuals. And in some species of insects, lizards, and even birds, the females can lay eggs that develop *parthenogenetically*—without the help of males, sperm, or fertilization—into healthy daughters that can also reproduce the same way.

But while such forms of **asexual reproduction** are simple and direct, they give rise to offspring that are genetically identical to the parent organism. **Sexual reproduction**, on the other hand, involves the mixing of DNA from two individuals to produce offspring that are genetically distinct from one another and from both their parents. In this section, we outline briefly the cellular mechanisms that make this mode of reproduction possible. Sexual reproduction apparently has great advantages, as the vast majority of plants and animals on Earth have adopted it.

Sexual Reproduction Involves both Diploid and Haploid Cells

Organisms that reproduce sexually are generally **diploid**: their cells contain two sets of chromosomes—one inherited from each parent. The *maternal* chromosome set and the *paternal* chromosome set are very similar, except for their *sex chromosomes*, which, in many species, distinguish males from females. In humans, for example, the Y chromosome carries genes that specify the development of a male. Males inherit a Y chromosome from their father and an X chromosome from their mother; females inherit one X chromosome from each parent. Aside from these sex chromosomes, the maternal and paternal versions of every chromosome—called the maternal and paternal **homologs**, or homologous chromosomes—carry the same set of genes. Each diploid cell, therefore, carries two copies of every gene (except for those found on the sex chromosomes, which may be present in only one copy).

Unlike the majority of cells in a diploid organism, the specialized cells that carry out the central process in sexual reproduction—the **gametes**—are **haploid**: they each contain only one set of chromosomes. For most organisms, the males and females produce different types of gametes. In animals, one is large and nonmotile and is referred to as the *egg*; the other is small and motile and is referred to as the *sperm* (**Figure 19–2**). These two dissimilar haploid gametes join together to regenerate a diploid cell, called the fertilized egg, or *zygote*, which has homologous chromosomes from both the mother and father. The zygote thus produced develops into a new individual with a diploid set of chromosomes that is distinct from that of either parent (**Figure 19–3**).

For almost all multicellular animals, including vertebrates, most of the life cycle is spent in the diploid state. The haploid cells exist only briefly and are highly specialized for their function as genetic ambassadors. These haploid gametes are generated from diploid precursor cells by a specialized form of reductive division called *meiosis*. This precursor cell lineage is called the **germ line**. The cells forming the rest of the animal's body—the **somatic cells**—ultimately leave no progeny of their own (**Figure 19–4** and see Figure 9–3). They exist, in effect, only to help the cells of the germ line survive and propagate.

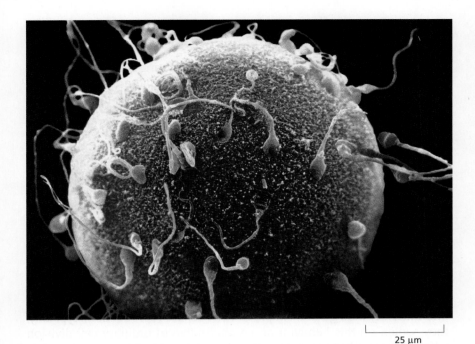

Figure 19–2 Despite their tremendous difference in size, sperm and egg contribute equally to the genetic character of the offspring. This difference in size between male and female gametes (in which eggs contain a large quantity of cytoplasm, whereas sperm contain almost none) is consistent with the fact that the cytoplasm is not the basis of inheritance. If it were, the female's contribution to the makeup of the offspring would be much greater than the male's. Shown here is a scanning electron micrograph of an egg with human sperm bound to its surface. Although many sperm are bound to the egg, only one will fertilize it. (David M. Philips/Science Source.)

25 μm

The sexual reproductive cycle thus involves an alternation of haploid cells, each carrying a single set of chromosomes, with generations of diploid cells, each carrying two sets of chromosomes. One benefit of this arrangement is that it allows sexually reproducing organisms to produce offspring that are genetically diverse, as we discuss next.

Sexual Reproduction Generates Genetic Diversity

Sexual reproduction produces novel chromosome combinations. During meiosis, the maternal and paternal chromosome sets in the diploid germ-line cells are partitioned into the single chromosome sets of the gametes. Each gamete will receive a mixture of maternal homologs and paternal homologs; when the genomes of two gametes combine during fertilization, they produce a zygote with a unique chromosomal complement.

If the maternal and paternal homologs carry the same genes, why should such chromosomal reassortment matter? One answer is that although the set of genes on each homolog is the same, the paternal and maternal version of each gene is not. Genes occur in variant versions, called **alleles**, with slightly different DNA sequences. For any given gene, many different alleles may be present in the "gene pool" of a species. The existence of these variant alleles means that the two copies of any given gene in a particular individual are likely to be somewhat different from each other—and from those carried by other individuals. What makes individuals within a species genetically unique is the inheritance of different combinations of alleles. And with its cycles of diploidy, meiosis, haploidy, and cell fusion, sex breaks up old combinations of alleles and generates new ones.

Sexual reproduction also generates genetic diversity through a second mechanism—*homologous recombination*. We discuss this process, which scrambles the genetic information on each chromosome during meiosis, a bit later.

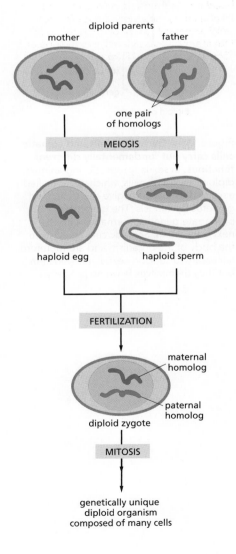

Figure 19–3 Sexual reproduction involves both haploid and diploid cells. Sperm and egg are produced by meiosis of diploid germ-line cells. During fertilization, a haploid egg and a haploid sperm fuse to form a diploid zygote. For simplicity, only one chromosome is shown for each gamete, and the sperm cell has been greatly enlarged. Human gametes have 23 chromosomes, and the egg is much larger than the sperm (see, for example, Figure 19–2).

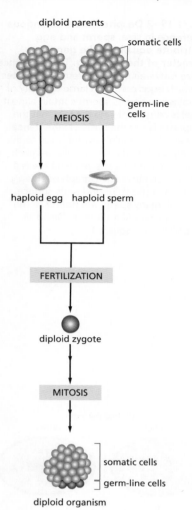

Figure 19–4 Germ-line cells and somatic cells carry out fundamentally different functions. In sexually reproducing animals, diploid germ-line cells, which are specified early in development, give rise to haploid gametes by meiosis. The gametes propagate genetic information into the next generation. Somatic cells (*gray*) form the body of the organism and are therefore necessary to support sexual reproduction, but they themselves leave no progeny.

Sexual Reproduction Gives Organisms a Competitive Advantage in a Changing Environment

The processes that generate genetic diversity during meiosis operate at random, and so the collection of alleles an individual receives from each parent is just as likely to represent a combination that is inferior as it is an improvement. Why, then, should the ability to try out new genetic combinations give organisms that reproduce sexually an evolutionary advantage over those that "breed true" through an asexual process? This question continues to perplex evolutionary geneticists, but one advantage seems to be that reshuffling genetic information through sexual reproduction can help a species survive in an unpredictably variable environment. If two parents produce many offspring with a wide variety of gene combinations, they increase the odds that at least one of their progeny will have a combination of features necessary for survival in a variety of environmental conditions. They are more likely, for example, to survive infections by bacteria, viruses, and parasites, which themselves continually change in a never-ending evolutionary battle. This genetic gamble may explain why even unicellular organisms, such as yeasts, intermittently indulge in a simple form of sexual reproduction. Typically, they switch on this behavior as an alternative to ordinary cell division when times are hard and starvation looms. Yeasts with a genetic defect that makes them unable to reproduce sexually show a reduced ability to adapt when they are subjected to harsh conditions.

Sexual reproduction may also be advantageous for another reason. In any population, new mutations continually occur, giving rise to new alleles—and many of these new mutations may be harmful. Sexual reproduction can speed up the elimination of these deleterious alleles and help to prevent them from accumulating in the population. By mating with only the fittest males, females select for good combinations of alleles and allow bad combinations to be lost from the population more efficiently than they would otherwise be.

Whatever its advantages, sex has clearly been favored by evolution. In the following section, we review the central features of this popular form of reproduction, beginning with meiosis, the process by which gametes are formed.

MEIOSIS AND FERTILIZATION

Our modern understanding of the fundamental cycle of events involved in sexual reproduction grew out of discoveries made in the late 1800s, when biologists noted that the fertilized eggs of a parasitic roundworm contain four chromosomes, whereas the worm's gametes (sperm and eggs) contain only two. Gametes must be therefore produced by a special kind of "reductive" division in which the number of chromosomes is precisely halved (see Figure 19–3). The term **meiosis** was coined to describe this form of cell division; it comes from a Greek word meaning "diminution," or "lessening."

From these early experiments on roundworms and other species, it became clear that the behavior of the chromosomes, which at that time were simply microscopic bodies of unknown function, matched the pattern of inheritance, in which the two parents make equal contributions to the character of the progeny despite the enormous difference in size between egg and sperm (see Figure 19–2). These observations were among the first clues that chromosomes contain the material of heredity. The study of sexual reproduction and meiosis therefore has a central place in the history of cell biology.

In this section, we describe the cell biology of sexual reproduction from a modern point of view, focusing on the elaborate dance of chromosomes that occurs when a cell undertakes meiosis. We take a close look at how homologous chromosomes pair, recombine, and are segregated during meiosis, thereby shuffling the maternal and paternal genes into novel combinations. We also discuss what happens when meiosis goes awry. Finally, we consider briefly the process of fertilization, through which gametes come together to form a new, genetically distinct individual.

Meiosis Involves One Round of DNA Replication Followed by Two Rounds of Nuclear Division

Before a diploid cell divides by mitosis, it duplicates all of its chromosomes. This duplication allows a full set of chromosomes—including a complete maternal set plus a complete paternal set—to be transmitted to each daughter cell (discussed in Chapter 18). Although meiosis ultimately halves this diploid chromosome complement—producing haploid gametes that carry only a single set of chromosomes—it, too, begins with a round of chromosome duplication. The subsequent reduction in chromosome number occurs because this single round of duplication is followed by two successive rounds of nuclear division, without further DNA replication (**Figure 19–5**).

It seems like it would be simpler and more direct if meiosis instead took place by a modified form of mitotic cell division in which DNA replication (S phase) were omitted completely; a single round of division could then, in theory, produce two haploid cells directly. But, for reasons that are still unclear, this is not the way meiosis works.

Meiosis begins in specialized germ-line cells that reside in the ovaries or testes. Like somatic cells, these germ-line cells are diploid; each contains two copies of every chromosome—a paternal homolog, inherited from the individual's father, and a maternal homolog, inherited from the mother. In the first step of meiosis, all of these chromosomes are duplicated, and the resulting copies remain closely attached to each other, as they would during an ordinary mitosis (see Chapter 18).

The next phase of the process, however, is unique to meiosis. During this phase, called meiotic prophase, each duplicated paternal chromosome locates and then attaches itself along its entire length to the corresponding duplicated maternal homolog. This process, called **pairing**, is of fundamental importance in meiosis, as it allows the segregation of homologous chromosome pairs during the first meiotic division (meiosis I).

The two duplicated chromosomes within each homolog are then separated during the second meiotic division (meiosis II), producing four haploid nuclei. Because chromosome segregation during meiosis I and II is random, each haploid gamete will receive a different mixture of maternal and paternal chromosomes.

Thus, meiosis produces four nuclei that are genetically dissimilar and that contain exactly half as many chromosomes as the original parent

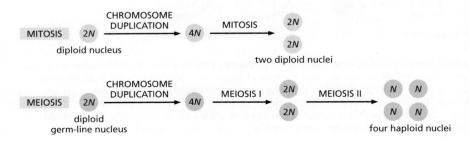

Figure 19–5 **Mitosis and meiosis both begin with a round of chromosome duplication.** In mitosis, chromosome duplication is followed by a single round of cell division to yield two diploid nuclei. In meiosis, chromosome duplication in a diploid germ-line cell is followed by two rounds of division, without further DNA replication, to produce four haploid nuclei. N represents the number of chromosomes in the haploid nucleus.

germ-line cell. Mitosis, in contrast, produces two genetically identical diploid nuclei. **Figure 19–6** summarizes the molecular events that distinguish these two types of division—differences we now discuss in greater detail, beginning with the meiosis-specific pairing of maternal and paternal chromosomes.

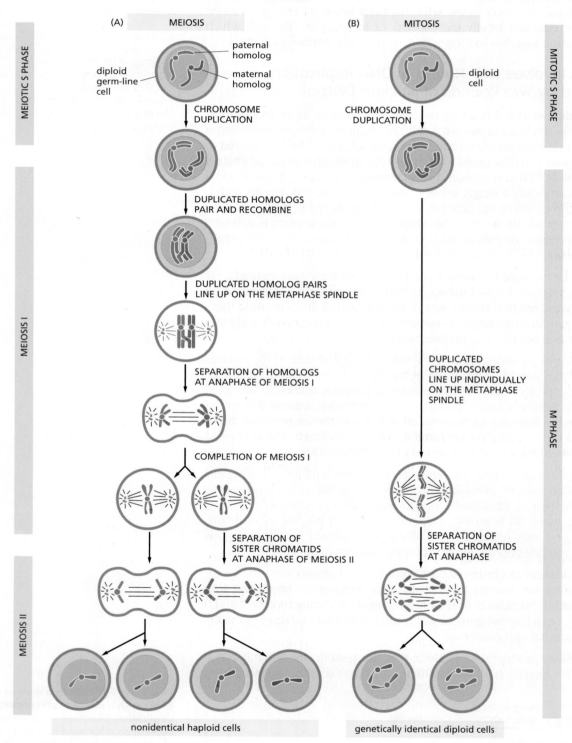

Figure 19–6 Meiosis generates four nonidentical haploid nuclei, whereas mitosis produces two identical diploid nuclei. As in Figure 19–3, only one pair of homologous chromosomes is shown. (A) In meiosis, chromosome duplication is followed by two meiotic divisions to produce haploid nuclei. Each diploid nucleus that enters meiosis therefore produces four haploid nuclei, which are then packaged into haploid gametes by specialized forms of cytokinesis. (B) In mitosis, each diploid nucleus produces two diploid nuclei, which are packaged by cytokinesis into two diploid cells. Although mitosis and meiosis II are similar processes that are usually accomplished within hours, meiosis I can last days, months, or even years, because of the time required for homolog pairing before meiosis I.

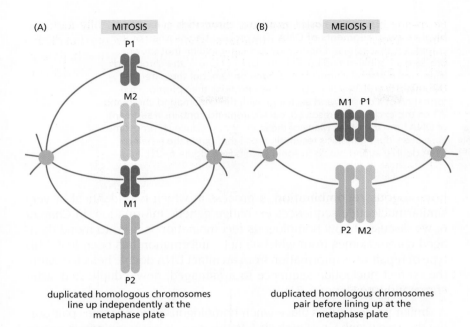

(A) MITOSIS

(B) MEIOSIS I

duplicated homologous chromosomes line up independently at the metaphase plate

duplicated homologous chromosomes pair before lining up at the metaphase plate

Figure 19–7 During meiosis I, duplicated homologous chromosomes pair before lining up on the meiotic spindle. (A) In mitosis, the individual duplicated maternal (M) and paternal (P) chromosomes line up independently at the metaphase plate; each consists of a pair of sister chromatids, which will separate just before the cell divides. (B) By contrast, in meiosis, duplicated maternal and paternal homologs pair before lining up at the metaphase plate. The maternal and paternal homologs separate during the first meiotic division, and the sister chromatids separate during meiosis II. The mitotic and meiotic spindles are shown in *green*.

Duplicated Homologous Chromosomes Pair During Meiotic Prophase

Before a eukaryotic cell divides—by either meiosis or mitosis—it first duplicates all of its chromosomes. The twin copies of each duplicated chromosome, called **sister chromatids**, are tightly linked along their length. The way these duplicated chromosomes are handled subsequently, however, differs between meiosis and mitosis. In mitosis, as we discuss in Chapter 18, the duplicated chromosomes line up, single file, at the metaphase plate (**Figure 19–7A**). They are then segregated into the two daughter nuclei.

In meiosis, however, the need to halve the number of chromosomes introduces an extra demand on the cell-division machinery. The germ-line cell must keep track of the maternal and paternal homologs—to ensure that each of the four haploid cells produced by meiosis will receive a single sister chromatid from each chromosome set. Meiosis therefore begins with a complex and time-consuming process called pairing, in which duplicated homologs are brought together during a stage called meiotic prophase (or prophase I). It is these pairs of duplicated homologs that line up at the metaphase plate in meiosis I (**Figure 19–7B**). Each pairing forms a structure called a **bivalent**, in which all four sister chromatids stick together until the cell is ready to divide (**Figure 19–8**). The maternal and paternal homologs will separate during meiosis I, and the individual sister chromatids will separate during meiosis II.

How the homologs (and the two sex chromosomes) recognize each other during pairing is still not fully understood. In many organisms, the initial association depends on an interaction between matching maternal and paternal DNA sequences at numerous sites that are widely dispersed along the homologous chromosomes. Once formed, bivalents are very stable: they remain associated throughout meiotic prophase, a stage that in some organisms can last for years.

Crossing-Over Occurs Between the Duplicated Maternal and Paternal Chromosomes in Each Bivalent

The picture of meiosis we have just painted is greatly simplified, in that it leaves out a crucial feature. In sexually reproducing organisms, the pairing of the maternal and paternal chromosomes is accompanied by

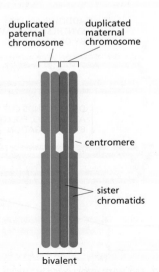

duplicated paternal chromosome

duplicated maternal chromosome

centromere

sister chromatids

bivalent

Figure 19–8 Duplicated maternal and paternal chromosomes pair during meiosis I to form bivalents. Each bivalent contains four sister chromatids.

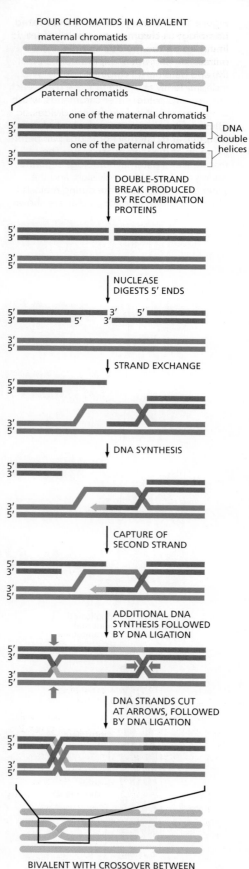

FOUR CHROMATIDS IN A BIVALENT

maternal chromatids

paternal chromatids

one of the maternal chromatids

5′
3′
— DNA
double
helices
one of the paternal chromatids
3′
5′

DOUBLE-STRAND
BREAK PRODUCED
BY RECOMBINATION
PROTEINS

NUCLEASE
DIGESTS 5′ ENDS

STRAND EXCHANGE

DNA SYNTHESIS

CAPTURE OF
SECOND STRAND

ADDITIONAL DNA
SYNTHESIS FOLLOWED
BY DNA LIGATION

DNA STRANDS CUT
AT ARROWS, FOLLOWED
BY DNA LIGATION

BIVALENT WITH CROSSOVER BETWEEN
TWO NON-SISTER CHROMATIDS

Figure 19–9 During meiosis I, non-sister chromatids in each bivalent swap segments of DNA. The process begins when protein complexes that carry out homologous recombination (not shown) produce a double-strand break in the DNA of one of the chromatids. (Here, the maternal chromatid has been broken, but the paternal chromatid is equally vulnerable.) These proteins then promote the formation of a cross-strand exchange with the undamaged chromatid. When this exchange is resolved, each chromatid contains a segment of DNA from the other. Many of the steps that produce chromosome crossovers during meiosis resemble those that guide the repair of DNA double-strand breaks in somatic cells (see Figure 6–31).

homologous recombination, a process in which two identical or very similar nucleotide sequences exchange genetic information. In Chapter 6, we discussed how homologous recombination is used to mend damaged chromosomes from which genetic information has been lost. This type of repair uses information from an intact DNA double helix to restore the correct nucleotide sequence to a damaged, newly duplicated sister chromatid (see Figure 6–31).

A similar process takes place when homologous chromosomes pair during the long prophase of meiosis I. In this case, the recombination occurs between the non-sister chromatids in each bivalent, rather than between the identical sister chromatids within each duplicated chromosome. In the process, the maternal and paternal homologs can physically swap homologous chromosomal segments, an event called **crossing-over** (**Figure 19–9**).

Crossing-over is a complex, multistep process that is facilitated by the formation of a *synaptonemal complex*. As the duplicated homologs pair, this elaborate protein complex helps to hold the bivalent together and align the homologs so that strand exchange can readily occur between the non-sister chromatids (**Figure 19–10**). Each of the chromatids in a duplicated homolog (that is, each of these very long DNA double helices) can form a crossover with either (or both) of the chromatids from the other chromosome in the bivalent.

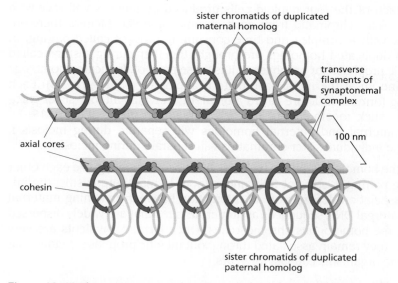

sister chromatids of duplicated
maternal homolog

transverse
filaments of
synaptonemal
complex

100 nm

axial cores

cohesin

sister chromatids of duplicated
paternal homolog

Figure 19–10 The synaptonemal complex helps to align the duplicated homolog pairs. The sister chromatids in the maternal (*red*) and paternal (*blue*) homologs are held together by a protein complex called the axial core (*gray*), which interacts with the cohesins (*green*) that link the sisters together (see Figure 18–18). When the duplicated homologs pair, the axial cores associated with each are pulled closely together in a zipperlike fashion by a set of rod-shaped transverse filaments (*yellow*), forming the synaptonemal complex.

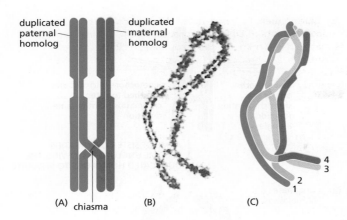

Figure 19–11 Crossover events create chiasmata between non-sister chromatids in each bivalent. (A) Schematic set of paired homologs in which one crossover event has occurred, creating a single chiasma. (B) Micrograph of a grasshopper bivalent with three chiasmata. (C) Schematic of the three crossovers between the paired homologs in (B). Each sister chromatid is numbered. (B, courtesy of Bernard John.)

By the time meiotic prophase ends, the synaptonemal complex has disassembled, allowing the homologs to separate along most of their length. But each bivalent remains held together by at least one **chiasma** (plural **chiasmata**), a structure named after the Greek letter chi, χ, which is shaped like a cross. Each chiasma corresponds to a crossover between two non-sister chromatids (**Figure 19–11A**). Most bivalents contain more than one chiasma, indicating that multiple crossovers occur between homologous chromosomes (**Figure 19–11B and C**). In human oocytes—the cells that give rise to the egg—an average of two to three crossover events occur within each bivalent (**Figure 19–12**).

Crossovers that take place during meiosis are a major source of genetic variation in sexually reproducing species. By scrambling the genetic constitution of each of the chromosomes in the gamete, crossing-over helps to produce individuals with novel assortments of alleles. But crossing-over also has a second important role in meiosis: it helps ensure that the maternal and paternal homologs will segregate from one another correctly at the first meiotic division, as we discuss next.

Chromosome Pairing and Crossing-Over Ensure the Proper Segregation of Homologs

In most organisms, crossing-over during meiosis is required for the correct segregation of the two duplicated homologs into separate daughter nuclei. The chiasmata created by crossover events keep the maternal and paternal homologs bundled together until the spindle separates them during meiotic anaphase I. Before anaphase I, the two poles of the spindle pull on the duplicated homologs in opposite directions, and the

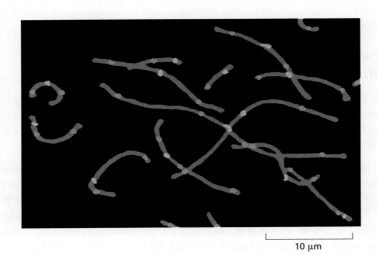

10 µm

Figure 19–12 Multiple crossovers can occur between the duplicated homologous chromosomes in a bivalent. Fluorescence micrograph shows a spread of chromosomes from a human oocyte (egg-cell precursor) at the stage where both maternal and paternal homologs are still tightly associated: each single long thread (stained *red*) is a bivalent, containing four sister chromatids. Sites of crossing-over between the chromatids within each bivalent are marked by the presence of a protein (stained *green*) that is a key component of the meiotic recombination machinery. *Blue* staining marks the positions of centromeres (see Figure 19–8). (From C. Tease et al., *Am. J. Hum. Genet.* 70: 1469–1479, 2002.)

Figure 19–13 Chiasmata help ensure proper segregation of duplicated homologs during the first meiotic division. (A) In metaphase of meiosis I, chiasmata created by crossing-over hold the maternal and paternal homologs together. At this stage, cohesin proteins keep the sister chromatids glued together along their entire length (see Figure 19–10). The kinetochores of sister chromatids function as a single unit in meiosis I, and microtubules that attach to them point toward the same spindle pole. (B) At anaphase of meiosis I, the cohesins holding the arms of the sister chromatids together are suddenly degraded, allowing the homologs to be separated. Cohesins at the centromere continue to hold the sister chromatids together as the homologs are pulled apart.

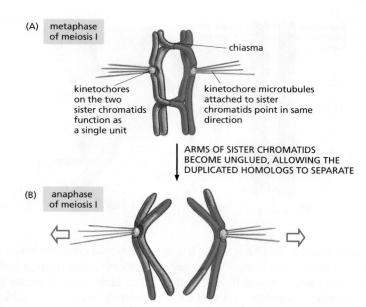

(A) metaphase of meiosis I

chiasma

kinetochores on the two sister chromatids function as a single unit

kinetochore microtubules attached to sister chromatids point in same direction

ARMS OF SISTER CHROMATIDS BECOME UNGLUED, ALLOWING THE DUPLICATED HOMOLOGS TO SEPARATE

(B) anaphase of meiosis I

chiasmata resist this pulling (Figure 19–13A). In so doing, the chiasmata help to position and stabilize bivalents at the metaphase plate.

In addition to the chiasmata, which hold the maternal and paternal homologs together, *cohesin* proteins (described in Chapter 18) keep the sister chromatids glued together along their entire length at meiosis I (see Figure 19–10). At the start of anaphase I, the cohesin proteins that hold the chromosome arms together are suddenly degraded. This release allows the arms to separate and the recombined homologs to be pulled apart (Figure 19–13B). If the arms were not released in this way, the duplicated maternal and paternal homologs would remain tethered to one another by the homologous DNA segments they had exchanged and would not separate during anaphase I.

The Second Meiotic Division Produces Haploid Daughter Nuclei

To separate the sister chromatids and produce cells with a haploid amount of DNA, a second round of division, meiosis II, follows soon after the first—without further DNA replication or any significant interphase period. A meiotic spindle forms, and the kinetochores on each pair of sister chromatids now attach to kinetochore microtubules that point in opposite directions, as they would in an ordinary mitotic division. At anaphase of meiosis II, the remaining, meiosis-specific cohesins—located at the centromere—are degraded, and the sister chromatids are pulled apart (Figure 19–14). The entire process is shown in Movie 19.1.

Haploid Gametes Contain Reassorted Genetic Information

Even though they share the same parents, no two siblings are genetically the same (unless they are identical twins). These genetic differences are initiated long before sperm meets egg, when meiosis I produces two kinds of randomizing genetic reassortment.

First, as we have seen, the maternal and paternal chromosomes are shuffled and dealt out randomly during meiosis I. Although the chromosomes are carefully distributed so that each gamete receives one and only one copy of each chromosome, the choice between the maternal or paternal homolog is made by chance, like the flip of a coin. Thus, each gamete contains the maternal versions of some chromosomes and the paternal

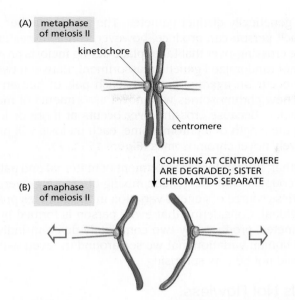

kinetochore

centromere

COHESINS AT CENTROMERE
ARE DEGRADED; SISTER
CHROMATIDS SEPARATE

(B) anaphase
of meiosis II

Figure 19–14 In meiosis II, as in mitosis, the kinetochores on each sister chromatid function independently, allowing the two sister chromatids to be pulled to opposite poles. (A) In metaphase of meiosis II, the kinetochores of the sister chromatids point in opposite directions. (B) At anaphase of meiosis II, the cohesins holding the sister chromatids together at the centromere are degraded, allowing kinetochore microtubules to pull the sister chromatids to opposite poles.

versions of others (**Figure 19–15A**). This random assortment depends solely on the way each bivalent happens to be positioned when it lines up on the spindle during metaphase of meiosis I. Whether the maternal or paternal homolog is captured by the microtubules from one pole or the other depends on which way the bivalent is facing when the microtubules connect to its kinetochore (see Figure 19–13). Because the orientation of each bivalent at the moment of capture is completely random, the assortment of maternal and paternal chromosomes is random as well.

Thanks to this random reassortment of maternal and paternal homologs, an individual could in principle produce 2^n genetically different gametes, where n is the haploid number of chromosomes. With 23 chromosomes to choose from, each human, for example, could in theory produce 2^{23}—or

QUESTION 19–1

Why do you think that organisms do not use the first steps of meiosis (up to and including meiotic division I) for the ordinary mitotic division of somatic cells?

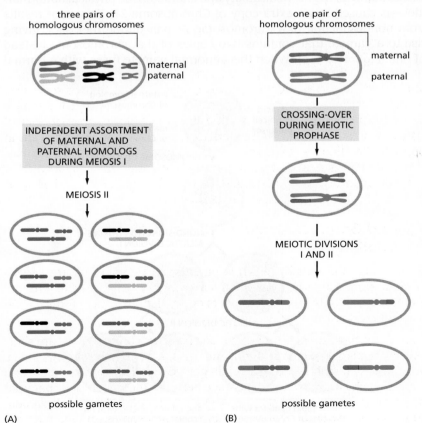

three pairs of
homologous chromosomes

maternal
paternal

INDEPENDENT ASSORTMENT
OF MATERNAL AND
PATERNAL HOMOLOGS
DURING MEIOSIS I

MEIOSIS II

possible gametes

(A)

one pair of
homologous chromosomes

maternal

paternal

CROSSING-OVER
DURING MEIOTIC
PROPHASE

MEIOTIC DIVISIONS
I AND II

possible gametes

(B)

Figure 19–15 Two kinds of genetic reassortment generate new chromosome combinations during meiosis. (A) The independent assortment of the maternal and paternal homologs during meiosis produces 2^n different haploid gametes for an organism with n chromosomes. Here $n = 3$, and there are 2^3, or 8, different possible gametes. For simplicity, chromosome crossing-over is not shown here. (B) Crossing-over during meiotic prophase exchanges segments of DNA between homologous chromosomes and thereby reassorts genes on each individual chromosome. For simplicity, only a single pair of homologous chromosomes is shown. Both independent chromosome assortment and crossing-over occur during every meiosis.

8.4×10^6—genetically distinct gametes. The actual number of different gametes each person can produce, however, is much greater than that, because the crossing-over that takes place during meiosis provides a second source of randomized genetic reassortment. Between two and three crossovers occur on average between each pair of human homologs, generating new chromosomes with novel assortments of maternal and paternal alleles. Because crossing-over occurs at more or less random sites along the length of a chromosome, each meiosis will produce four sets of entirely novel chromosomes (Figure 19–15B).

Taken together, the random reassortment of maternal and paternal chromosomes, coupled with the genetic mixing of crossing-over, provides a nearly limitless source of genetic variation in the gametes produced by a single individual. Considering that every person is formed by the fusion of such gametes, produced by two completely different individuals, the richness of human variation that we see around us, even within a single family, should not be very surprising.

Meiosis Is Not Flawless

The sorting of chromosomes that takes place during meiosis is a remarkable feat of molecular bookkeeping: in humans, each meiosis requires that the starting cell keep track of 92 chromosomes (23 pairs, each of which has duplicated), handing out one complete set to each gamete. Not surprisingly, mistakes can occur in the distribution of chromosomes during this elaborate process.

Occasionally, homologs fail to separate properly—a phenomenon known as *nondisjunction*. As a result, some of the haploid cells that are produced lack a particular chromosome, while others have more than one copy. Upon fertilization, such gametes form abnormal embryos, most of which die. Some, however, survive. *Down syndrome*, for example—a disorder associated with cognitive disability and characteristic physical abnormalities—is caused by an extra copy of Chromosome 21. This error results from nondisjunction of a Chromosome 21 pair during meiosis I, giving rise to a gamete that contains two copies of that chromosome instead of one (Figure 19–16). When this abnormal gamete fuses with a normal

---

QUESTION 19–2

Ignoring the effects of chromosome crossovers, an individual human can in principle produce $2^{23} = 8.4 \times 10^6$ genetically different gametes. How many of these possibilities can be "sampled" in the average life of (A) a female and (B) a male, given that women produce one egg a month during their fertile years, whereas men can make hundreds of millions of sperm each day?

Figure 19–16 Errors in chromosome segregation during meiosis can result in gametes with incorrect numbers of chromosomes. In this example, the duplicated maternal and paternal copies of Chromosome 21 fail to separate normally during the first meiotic division. As a result, two of the gametes receive no copy of the chromosome, while the other two gametes receive two copies. For simplicity, only Chromosome 21 is shown. Gametes that receive an incorrect number of chromosomes are called *aneuploid* gametes. If one of them participates in the fertilization process, the resulting zygote will also have an abnormal number of chromosomes. A child that receives three copies of Chromosome 21 will have Down syndrome.

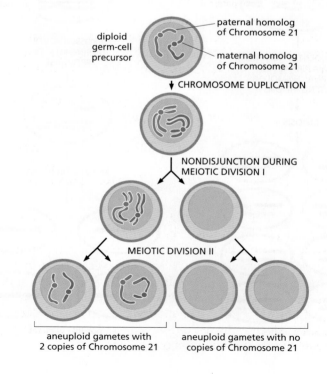

gamete at fertilization, the resulting embryo contains three copies of Chromosome 21 instead of two. This chromosome imbalance produces an extra dose of the proteins encoded by Chromosome 21 and thereby interferes with the proper development of the embryo and normal functions in the adult.

The frequency of chromosome mis-segregation during the production of human gametes is remarkably high, particularly in females: nondisjunction occurs in about 10% of the meioses in human oocytes, giving rise to eggs that contain the wrong number of chromosomes (a condition called *aneuploidy*). Aneuploidy occurs less often in human sperm, perhaps because sperm development is subjected to more stringent quality control than egg development. If meiosis goes wrong in male cells, a cell-cycle checkpoint mechanism is activated, arresting meiosis and leading to cell death by apoptosis. Regardless of whether the segregation error occurs in the sperm or the egg, nondisjunction is thought to be one reason for the high rate of miscarriages—spontaneous early pregnancy losses—in humans.

Fertilization Reconstitutes a Complete Diploid Genome

Having seen how chromosomes are parceled out during meiosis to form haploid germ cells, we now briefly consider how they are reunited in the process of **fertilization** to form a new cell with a diploid set of chromosomes.

Of the 300 million human sperm ejaculated during sexual intercourse, only about 200 reach the site of fertilization in the oviduct. Sperm are attracted to an ovulated egg by chemical signals released by both the egg and the supporting cells that surround it. Once a sperm finds the egg, it must migrate through a protective layer of cells and then bind to, and tunnel through, the egg coat, called the *zona pellucida*. Finally, the sperm must bind to and fuse with the underlying egg plasma membrane (**Figure 19–17**). Although fertilization normally occurs by this process of sperm–egg fusion, it can also be achieved artificially by injecting the sperm directly into the egg cytoplasm; this is often done in infertility clinics when there is a problem with natural sperm–egg fusion.

Although many sperm may bind to an egg (see Figure 19–2), only one normally fuses with the egg plasma membrane and introduces its DNA into the egg cytoplasm. The control of this step is especially important because it ensures that the fertilized egg—also called a **zygote**—will contain two, and only two, sets of chromosomes. Several mechanisms prevent multiple sperm from entering an egg. In one mechanism, the first successful sperm triggers the release of a wave of Ca^{2+} ions in the egg cytoplasm. This flood of Ca^{2+} in turn triggers the secretion of enzymes that cause a "hardening" of the zona pellucida, which prevents "runner up" sperm from penetrating the egg. The Ca^{2+} wave also helps trigger the development of the egg. To watch a fertilization-induced calcium wave, see Movie 19.2.

The process of fertilization is not complete, however, until the two haploid nuclei (called *pronuclei*) come together and combine their chromosomes into a single diploid nucleus. Soon after the pronuclei fuse, the diploid cell begins to divide, forming a ball of cells that—through repeated rounds of cell division and differentiation—will give rise to an embryo and, eventually, an adult organism. Fertilization marks the beginning of one of the most remarkable phenomena in all of biology—the process by which a single-celled zygote initiates the developmental program that directs the formation of a new individual.

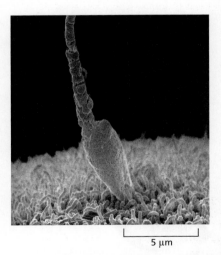

5 μm

Figure 19–17 A sperm binds to the plasma membrane of an egg. Shown here is a scanning electron micrograph of a human sperm coming in contact with a hamster egg. The egg has been stripped of its zona pellucida, exposing the plasma membrane, which is covered in fingerlike microvilli. Such uncoated hamster eggs were sometimes used in infertility clinics to assess whether a man's sperm were capable of penetrating an egg. The zygotes resulting from this test do not develop. (David M. Phillips/ The Population Council/Science Source.)

MENDEL AND THE LAWS OF INHERITANCE

In organisms that reproduce asexually, the genetic material of the parent is transmitted faithfully to its progeny. The resulting offspring are thus genetically identical to a single parent. Before Mendel started working with peas, some biologists suspected that inheritance might work that way in humans (Figure 19–18).

Although children resemble their parents, they are not carbon copies of either the mother or the father. Thanks to the mechanisms of meiosis just described, sex breaks up existing collections of genetic information, shuffles alleles into new combinations, and produces offspring that tend to exhibit a mixture of traits derived from both parents, as well as novel ones. The ability to track characteristics that show some variation from one generation to the next enabled geneticists to begin to decipher the rules that govern heredity in sexually reproducing organisms.

The simplest traits to follow are those that are easy to see or to measure. In humans, these include the tendency to sneeze when exposed to bright sun, whether a person's earlobes are attached or pendulous, or the ability to detect certain odors or flavors (Figure 19–19). Of course, the laws of inheritance were not worked out by studying people with pendulous earlobes, but by following traits in organisms that are easy to breed and that produce large numbers of offspring. Gregor Mendel, the father of genetics, focused on peas. But similar breeding experiments can be performed in fruit flies, worms, dogs, cats, or any other plant or animal that possesses characteristics of interest, because the same basic laws of inheritance apply to all sexually reproducing organisms, from peas to people.

In this section, we describe the logic of genetic inheritance in sexually reproducing organisms. We see how the behavior of chromosomes during meiosis—their segregation into gametes that then unite at random to form genetically unique offspring—explains the experimentally derived laws of inheritance. But first, we discuss how Mendel, breeding peas in his monastery garden, discovered these laws more than 150 years ago.

Mendel Studied Traits That Are Inherited in a Discrete Fashion

Mendel chose to study pea plants because they are easy to cultivate in large numbers and could be raised in a small space—such as an abbey garden. He controlled which plants mated with which by removing sperm (pollen) from one plant and brushing it onto the female structures of another. This careful cross-pollination ensured that Mendel could be certain of the parentage of every pea plant he examined.

Perhaps more important for Mendel's purposes, pea plants were available in many varieties. For example, one variety has purple flowers, another has white. One variety produces seeds (peas) with smooth skin, another produces peas that are wrinkled. Mendel chose to follow seven traits—including flower color and pea shape—that were distinct, easily observable, and, most importantly, inherited in a discrete fashion: for example, the plants have either purple flowers or white flowers—nothing in-between (Figure 19–20).

Mendel Disproved the Alternative Theories of Inheritance

The breeding experiments that Mendel performed were straightforward. He started with stocks of genetically pure, "true-breeding" plants—those that produce offspring of the same variety when allowed to self-fertilize.

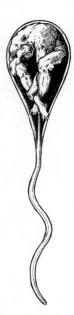

Figure 19–18 One disproven theory of inheritance suggested that genetic traits are passed down solely from the father. In support of this particular theory of uniparental inheritance, some early microscopists fancied they could see a small, perfectly formed human crouched inside the head of each sperm.

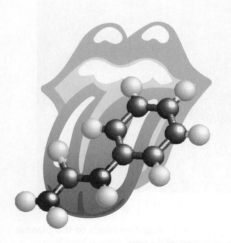

Figure 19–19 Some people taste it, some people don't. The ability to taste the chemical phenylthiocarbamide (PTC) is governed by a single gene. Although geneticists have known since the 1930s that the inability to taste PTC is inherited, it was not until 2003 that researchers identified the responsible gene, which encodes a bitter-taste receptor. Nontasters produce a PTC receptor protein with amino acid substitutions that are thought to reduce the receptor's activity.

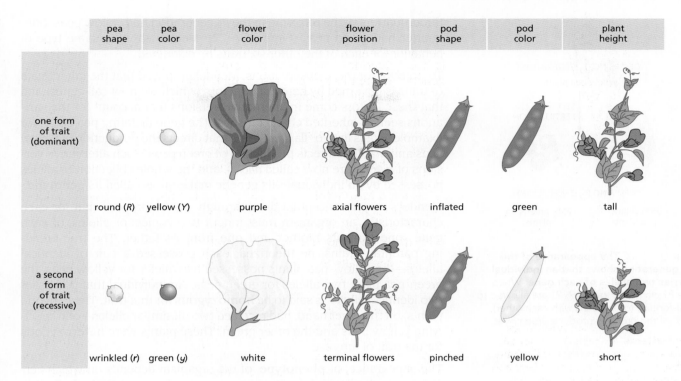

pea shape	pea color	flower color	flower position	pod shape	pod color	plant height

round (*R*)	yellow (*Y*)	purple	axial flowers	inflated	green	tall

one form of trait (dominant)

a second form of trait (recessive)

wrinkled (*r*)	green (*y*)	white	terminal flowers	pinched	yellow	short

If he followed pea color, for example, he used plants with yellow peas that always produced offspring with yellow peas, and plants with green peas that always produced offspring with green peas.

Mendel's predecessors had focused on organisms that varied in multiple traits. These investigators often wound up trying to characterize offspring whose appearance differed in such a complex way that they could not easily be compared with their parents. But Mendel took the unique approach of studying each trait one at a time. In a typical experiment, he would cross-pollinate two of his true-breeding varieties. He then recorded the inheritance of the chosen trait in the next generation. For example, Mendel crossed plants producing yellow peas with plants producing green peas and discovered that the resulting hybrid offspring, called the first filial, or *F₁*, generation, all had yellow peas (**Figure 19–21**). He obtained a similar result for every trait he followed: the F₁ hybrids all resembled only one of their two parents.

Had Mendel stopped there—observing only the F₁ generation—he might have developed some mistaken ideas about the nature of heredity: these results appear to support the theory of uniparental inheritance, which states that the appearance of the offspring will match one parent or the other. Fortunately, Mendel took his breeding experiments to the next step: he crossed the F₁ plants with one another (or allowed them to self-fertilize) and examined the results.

Mendel's Experiments Revealed the Existence of Dominant and Recessive Alleles

One look at the offspring of Mendel's initial cross-fertilization experiments, such as those shown in Figure 19–21, raises an obvious question: what happened to the trait that disappeared in the F₁ generation? Did the plants bearing green peas, for example, fail to make a genetic contribution to their offspring? To find out, Mendel allowed the F₁ plants to self-fertilize. If the trait for green peas had been lost, then the F₁ plants would produce only plants with yellow peas in the next, F₂, generation. Instead, he found that the "disappearing trait" returned: although

Figure 19–20 Mendel studied seven traits that are inherited in a discrete fashion. For each trait, the plants display either one variation or the other, with nothing in-between. As we will see shortly, one form of each trait is dominant, whereas the other is recessive.

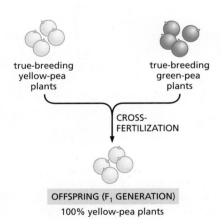

true-breeding yellow-pea plants

true-breeding green-pea plants

CROSS-FERTILIZATION

OFFSPRING (F₁ GENERATION)
100% yellow-pea plants

Figure 19–21 True-breeding varieties, when cross-fertilized with each other, produce hybrid offspring that resemble one parent. In this case, true-breeding green-pea plants, crossed with true-breeding yellow-pea plants, always produce offspring with yellow peas.

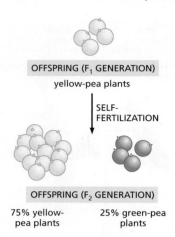

OFFSPRING (F₁ GENERATION)
yellow-pea plants

SELF-
FERTILIZATION

OFFSPRING (F₂ GENERATION)

75% yellow-
pea plants

25% green-pea
plants

Figure 19–22 The appearance of the F₂ generation shows that an individual carries two alleles of each gene. When the F₁ plants in Figure 19–21 are allowed to self-fertilize (or are bred with each other), 25% of the progeny produce green peas.

three-quarters of the offspring in the F₂ generation had yellow peas, one-quarter had green peas (**Figure 19–22**). Mendel saw the same type of behavior for each of the other six traits he examined.

To account for these observations, Mendel proposed that the inheritance of traits is governed by hereditary factors (which we now call genes) and that these factors come in alternative versions that account for the variations seen in inherited characteristics. The gene dictating pea color, for example, exists in two "flavors"—one that directs the production of yellow peas and one that directs production of green peas. Such alternative versions of a gene are now called *alleles*, and the whole collection of alleles possessed by an individual—its genetic makeup—is called its **genotype**.

Mendel's major conceptual breakthrough was to propose that for each characteristic, an organism must inherit two copies, or alleles, of each gene—one from its mother and one from its father. The true-breeding parental strains, he theorized, each possessed a pair of identical alleles—the yellow-pea plants possessed two alleles for yellow peas, the green-pea plant two alleles for green peas. An individual that possesses two identical alleles is said to be **homozygous** for that trait. The F₁ hybrid plants, on the other hand, had received two dissimilar alleles—one specifying yellow peas and the other green. These plants were **heterozygous** for the trait of interest.

The appearance, or **phenotype**, of the organism depends on which versions of each allele it inherits. To explain the disappearance of a trait in the F₁ generation—and its reappearance in the F₂ generation—Mendel supposed that for any pair of alleles, one allele is *dominant* and the other is *recessive*, or hidden. The dominant allele, whenever it is present, would dictate the plant's phenotype. In the case of pea color, the allele that specifies yellow peas is dominant; the green-pea allele is recessive.

One important consequence of heterozygosity, and of dominance and recessiveness, is that not all of the alleles that an individual carries can be detected in its phenotype. Humans have about 24,000 genes, and each of us is heterozygous for a very large number of these. Thus, we all carry a great deal of genetic information that remains hidden in our personal phenotype but that can turn up in future generations.

Each Gamete Carries a Single Allele for Each Character

Mendel's theory—that for every gene, an individual inherits one copy from its mother and one copy from its father—raised some logistical issues. If an organism has two copies of every gene, how does it pass only one copy of each to its progeny? And how do these gene sets come together again in the resulting offspring?

Mendel postulated that when sperm and eggs are formed, the two copies of each gene present in the parent separate so that each gamete receives only one allele for each trait. For his pea plants, each egg (ovum) and each sperm (pollen) receives only one allele for pea color (either yellow or green), one allele for pea shape (round or wrinkled), one allele for flower color (purple or white), and so on. During fertilization, sperm carrying one or other allele unites with an egg carrying one or other allele to produce a fertilized egg or zygote with two alleles. Which sperm unites with which egg at fertilization—thus, which alleles the zygote will receive—is entirely a matter of chance.

This principle of heredity is laid out in Mendel's first law, the **law of segregation**. It states that the two alleles for each trait separate (or segregate) during gamete formation and then unite at random—one from each parent—at fertilization. According to this law, the F₁ hybrid plants

Figure 19–23 **Parent plants produce gametes that each contain one allele for each trait; the phenotype of the offspring depends on which combination of alleles it receives.** Here we see both the genotype and phenotype of the pea plants that were bred in the experiments illustrated in Figures 19–21 and 19–22. The true-breeding yellow-pea plants produce only *Y*-bearing gametes; the true-breeding green plants produce only *y* gametes. The F_1 offspring of a cross between these parents all produce yellow peas, and they have the genotype *Yy*. When these hybrid plants are bred with each other, 75% of the offspring have yellow peas, 25% have green. The gray box at the bottom, called a Punnett square after a British mathematician who was a follower of Mendel, allows one to track the segregation of alleles during gamete formation and to predict the outcomes of breeding experiments like the one outlined in Figure 19–22. According to the system established by Mendel, capital letters indicate a dominant allele and lowercase letters a recessive allele.

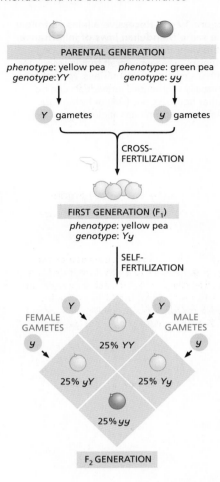

with yellow peas will produce two classes of gametes: half the gametes will get a yellow-pea allele and half will get a green-pea allele. When the hybrid plants self-pollinate, these two classes of gametes will unite at random. Thus, four different combinations of alleles can come together in the F_2 offspring (**Figure 19–23**). One-quarter of the F_2 plants will receive two alleles specifying green peas; these plants will produce green peas. One-quarter of the plants will receive two yellow-pea alleles and will produce yellow peas. But one-half of the plants will inherit one allele for yellow peas and one allele for green. Because the yellow allele is dominant, these plants—like their heterozygous F_1 parents—will all produce yellow peas. All told, three-quarters of the offspring will have yellow peas and one-quarter will have green peas. Thus Mendel's law of segregation explains the 3:1 ratio that he observed in the F_2 generation.

Mendel's Law of Segregation Applies to All Sexually Reproducing Organisms

Mendel's law of segregation explained the data for every trait he examined in pea plants, and he replicated his basic findings with corn and beans. But his rules governing inheritance are not limited to plants: they apply to all sexually reproducing organisms (**Figure 19–24**).

Consider a phenotype in humans that reflects the action of a single gene. The major form of *albinism*—Type II albinism—is a rare condition that is inherited in a recessive manner in many animals, including humans. Like the pea plants that produce green seeds, albinos are homozygous recessive: their genotype is *aa*. The dominant allele of the gene (denoted *A*) encodes an enzyme involved in making melanin, the pigment responsible for most of the brown and black color present in hair, skin, and the

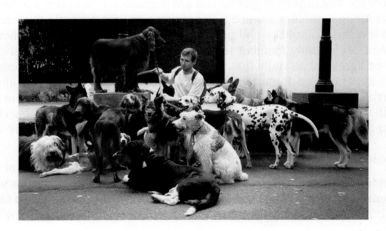

Figure 19–24 **Mendel's law of segregation applies to all sexually reproducing organisms.** Dogs are bred specifically to enhance certain phenotypic traits, including a diverse range of body size, coat color, head shape, snout length, ear position, and fur patterns. Scientists have been conducting genetic analyses on scores of dog breeds to search for the alleles that underlie these common canine characteristics. A single growth factor gene has been linked to body size, and three additional genes have been shown to account for coat length, curliness, and the presence or absence of "furnishings"—bushy eyebrows and beards—in almost all dog breeds. (By Ester Inbar, available from http://commons.wikimedia.org/wiki/User:ST.)

Figure 19–25 Recessive alleles all follow the same Mendelian laws of inheritance. Here we trace the inheritance of Type II albinism, a recessive trait that is associated with a single gene in humans. Note that normally pigmented individuals can be either homozygous (*AA*) or heterozygous (*Aa*) for the dominant allele *A*.

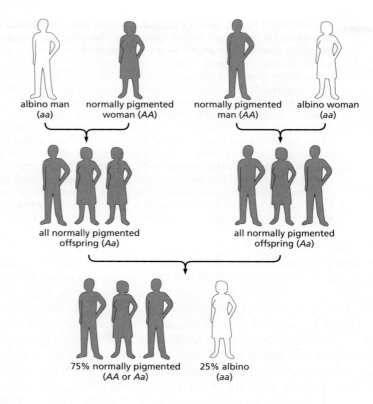

retina of the eye. Because the recessive allele codes for a version of this enzyme that is only weakly active or completely inactive, albinos have white hair, white skin, and pupils that look pink because a lack of melanin in the eye allows the red color of the hemoglobin in blood vessels in the retina to be visible.

The trait for albinism is inherited in the same manner as any other recessive trait, including Mendel's green peas. If a man who is homozygous for the recessive albinism allele (genotype *aa*) has children with a woman who has the same genotype, all of their children will be albino (*aa*). However, if a homozygous nonalbino man (*AA*) marries and has children with an albino woman (*aa*), their children will all be heterozygous (*Aa*) and normally pigmented (**Figure 19–25**). If two nonalbino individuals with an *Aa* genotype start a family, each of their children would have a 25% chance of being an albino (*aa*).

Of course, humans generally don't have families large enough to guarantee perfect Mendelian ratios. (Mendel arrived at his ratios by breeding and counting thousands of pea plants for most of his crosses.) Geneticists that follow the inheritance of specific traits in humans get around this problem by working with large numbers of families—or with several generations of a few large families—and preparing **pedigrees** that show the phenotype of each family member for the relevant trait. **Figure 19–26** shows the pedigree for a family that harbors a recessive allele for deafness. It also illustrates an important practical consequence of Mendel's laws: marriages between related individuals—called consanguineous (from the Latin *sanguis*, "blood")—create a greatly increased risk of producing children that are homozygous for a deleterious recessive mutation.

Alleles for Different Traits Segregate Independently

Mendel deliberately simplified the problem of heredity by starting with breeding experiments that focused on the inheritance of one trait at a time, called *monohybrid crosses*. He then turned his attention to multihybrid

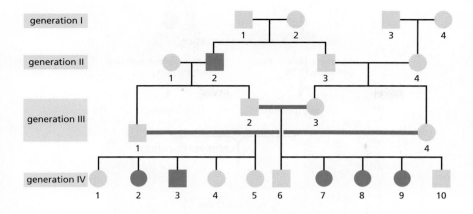

generation I

generation II

generation III

generation IV

Figure 19–26 A pedigree shows the risks of first-cousin marriages. Shown here is an actual pedigree for a family that harbors a rare recessive mutation causing deafness. According to convention, *squares* represent males, *circles* are females. Here, family members that show the deaf phenotype are indicated by a *blue* symbol, those that do not by a *gray* symbol. A *black* horizontal line connecting a male and female represents a mating between unrelated individuals, and a *red* horizontal line represents a mating between blood relatives. The offspring of each mating are shown underneath, in order of their birth from left to right.

Individuals within each generation are labeled sequentially from left to right for purposes of identification. In the third generation in this pedigree, for example, individual 2, a man who is not deaf, marries his first cousin, individual 3, who is also not deaf. Three out of their five children (individuals 7, 8, and 9 in the fourth generation) are deaf. Meanwhile, individual 1, the brother of 2, also marries a first cousin, individual 4, the sister of 3. Two out of their five children are deaf. (Adapted from Z.M. Ahmed et al., *BMC Med. Genet.* 5:24, 2004. With permission from BMC Medical Genetics.)

crosses, examining the simultaneous inheritance of two or more apparently unrelated traits.

In the simplest situation, a *dihybrid cross*, Mendel followed the inheritance of two traits at once: for example, pea color and pea shape. In the case of pea color, we have already seen that yellow is dominant over green; for pea shape, round is dominant over wrinkled (see Figure 19–20). What would happen when plants that differ in both of these characters are crossed? Again, Mendel started with true-breeding parental strains: the dominant strain produced yellow round peas (its genotype is *YYRR*), the recessive strain produced green wrinkled peas (*yyrr*). One possibility is that the two characters, pea color and shape, would be transmitted from parents to offspring as a linked package. In other words, plants would always produce either yellow round peas or green wrinkled ones. The other possibility is that pea color and shape would be inherited independently, which means that at some point plants bearing a novel mix of traits—yellow wrinkled peas or green round peas—would arise.

The F_1 generation of plants all showed the expected phenotype: each produced peas that were yellow and round. But this result would occur whether or not the parental alleles were linked. When the F_1 plants were then allowed to self-fertilize, the results were clear: the two alleles for seed color segregated independently from the two alleles for seed shape, producing four different pea phenotypes: yellow-round, yellow-wrinkled, green-round, and green-wrinkled (Figure 19–27). Mendel tried his seven pea characters in various pairwise combinations and always observed a characteristic 9:3:3:1 phenotypic ratio in the F_2 generation. The independent segregation of each pair of alleles during gamete formation is Mendel's second law—the **law of independent assortment**.

The Behavior of Chromosomes During Meiosis Underlies Mendel's Laws of Inheritance

So far we have discussed alleles and genes as if they are disembodied entities. We now know that Mendel's "factors"—the things we call genes—are carried on chromosomes that are parceled out during the formation of gametes and then brought together in novel combinations in the zygote at fertilization. Chromosomes therefore provide the physical basis for Mendel's laws, and their behavior during meiosis and fertilization—which we discussed earlier—explains these laws perfectly.

During meiosis, the maternal and paternal homologs—and the genes that they contain—pair and then separate from each other as they are parceled out into gametes. These maternal and paternal chromosome copies will possess different variants—or alleles—of many of the genes they carry. Take, for example, a pea plant that is heterozygous for the yellow-pea

Figure 19–27 A dihybrid (two traits) cross demonstrates that alleles can segregate independently. Alleles that segregate independently are packaged into gametes in all possible combinations. So the *Y* allele is equally likely to be packaged with the *R* or *r* allele during gamete formation; and the same holds true for the *y* allele. Thus four classes of gametes are produced in roughly equal numbers: *YR, Yr, yR,* and *yr.* When these gametes are allowed to combine at random to produce the F$_2$ generation, the resulting pea phenotypes are yellow-round, yellow-wrinkled, green-round, and green-wrinkled in a ratio of 9:3:3:1.

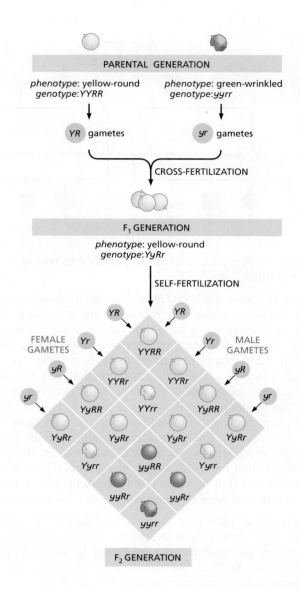

gene (*Yy*). During meiosis, the chromosomes bearing the *Y* and *y* alleles will be separated, producing two types of haploid gametes—ones that contain a *Y* allele and others that contain a *y*. In a plant that self-fertilizes, these haploid gametes come together to produce the diploid individuals of the next generation—which may be *YY, Yy,* or *yy.* Together, the meiotic mechanisms that distribute the alleles into gametes and the combining of gametes at fertilization provide the physical foundation for Mendel's law of segregation.

But what about independent assortment of multiple traits? Because each pair of duplicated homologs attaches to the spindle and lines up at the metaphase plate independently during meiosis, each gamete will inherit a random mixture of paternal and maternal chromosomes (see Figure 19–15A). Thus the alleles of genes on different chromosomes will segregate independently.

Consider a pea plant that is heterozygous for both seed color (*Yy*) and seed shape (*Rr*). The homolog pair carrying the color alleles will attach to the meiotic spindle with a certain orientation: whether the *Y*-bearing homolog or its *y*-bearing counterpart is captured by the microtubules from one pole or the other depends on which way the bivalent happens to be facing at the moment of attachment (**Figure 19–28**). The same

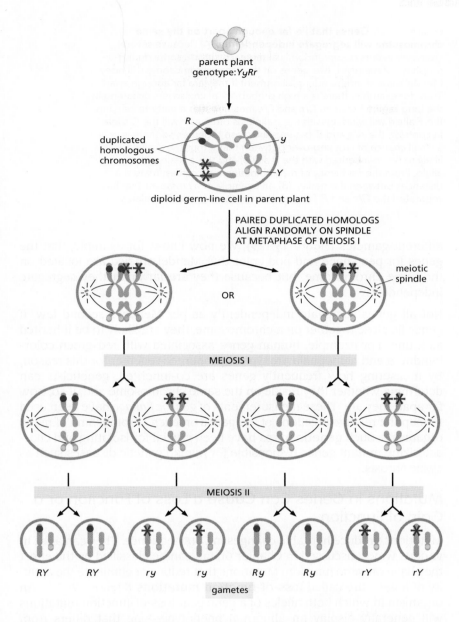

gametes

Figure 19–28 The separation of duplicated homologous chromosomes during meiosis explains Mendel's laws of segregation and independent assortment. Here we show independent assortment of the alleles for seed color, yellow (*Y*) and green (*y*), and for seed shape, round (*R*) and wrinkled (*r*), as an example of how two genes on different chromosomes segregate independently. Although crossovers are not shown, they would not affect the independent assortment of these traits, as the two genes lie on different chromosomes.

is true for the homolog pair carrying the alleles for seed shape. Thus, whether the final gamete receives the *YR*, *Yr*, *yR*, or *yr* allele combination depends entirely on which way the two homolog pairs were facing when they were captured by the meiotic spindle; each outcome has the same degree of randomness as the tossing of a coin.

Genes That Lie on the Same Chromosome Can Segregate Independently by Crossing-Over

Mendel studied seven traits, each of which is controlled by a separate gene. It turns out that most of these genes are located on different chromosomes, which readily explains the independent segregation he observed. But the independent segregation of different traits does not necessarily require that the responsible genes lie on different chromosomes. If two genes are far enough away from each other on the same chromosome, they will also sort independently, because of the crossing-over that occurs during meiosis. As we discussed earlier, when duplicated homologs pair to form bivalents, the maternal and paternal homologs always undergo crossing-over. This genetic exchange can separate alleles that were formerly together on the same chromosome, causing them to segregate into

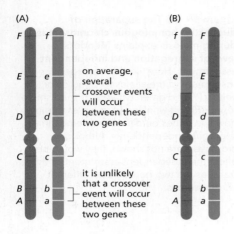

(A)

on average, several crossover events will occur between these two genes

it is unlikely that a crossover event will occur between these two genes

(B)

Figure 19–29 Genes that lie far enough apart on the same chromosome will segregate independently. (A) Because several crossover events occur randomly along each chromosome during prophase of meiosis I, two genes on the same chromosome will obey Mendel's law of independent assortment if they are far enough apart. Thus, for example, there is a high probability of crossovers occurring in the long region between *C/c* and *F/f*, meaning that a gamete carrying the *F* allele will wind up with the *c* allele as often as it will the *C* allele. In contrast, the *A/a* and *B/b* genes are close together, so there is only a small chance of crossing-over between them: thus the *A* allele is likely to be co-inherited with the *B* allele, and the *a* allele with the *b* allele. From the frequency of recombination, one can estimate the distances between the genes. (B) An example of a crossover that has separated the *C/c* and *F/f* alleles, but not the *A/a* and *B/b* alleles.

different gametes (Figure 19–29). We now know, for example, that the genes for pea shape and pod color that Mendel studied are located on the same chromosome, but because they are far apart they segregate independently.

Not all genes segregate independently as per Mendel's second law. If genes lie close together on a chromosome, they are likely to be inherited as a unit. For example, human genes associated with red–green color-blindness and hemophilia are typically inherited together for this reason. By measuring how frequently genes are co-inherited, geneticists can determine whether they reside on the same chromosome and, if so, how far apart they are. These measurements of *genetic linkage* have been used to map the relative positions of the genes on each chromosome of many organisms. Such **genetic maps** have been crucial for isolating and characterizing mutant genes responsible for human genetic diseases such as cystic fibrosis.

Mutations in Genes Can Cause a Loss of Function or a Gain of Function

Mutations produce heritable changes in DNA sequence. They can arise in various ways (discussed in Chapter 6) and can be classified by the effect they have on gene function. Mutations that reduce or eliminate the activity of a gene are called **loss-of-function mutations** (Figure 19–30). An organism in which both alleles of a gene bear loss-of-function mutations will generally display an abnormal phenotype—one that differs from the most commonly occurring phenotype (although the difference may sometimes be subtle and hard to detect). By contrast, the heterozygote, which possesses one mutant allele and one normal, "wild-type" allele, generally makes enough active gene product to function normally and retain a normal phenotype. Thus loss-of-function mutations are usually recessive, because—for most genes—decreasing the normal amount of gene product by 50% has little impact.

In the case of Mendel's peas, the gene that dictates seed shape codes for an enzyme that helps convert sugars into branched starch molecules. The dominant, wild-type allele, *R*, produces an active enzyme; the recessive,

Figure 19–30 Mutations in protein-coding genes can affect the protein product in a variety of ways. (A) In this example, the normal or "wild-type" protein has a specific function, denoted by the *red* rays. (B) Various loss-of-function mutations decrease or eliminate this activity. (C) Gain-of-function mutations boost this activity, as shown, or lead to an increase in the amount of the normal protein (not shown).

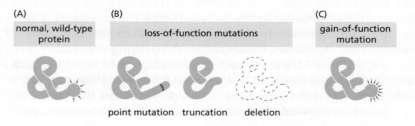

(A) normal, wild-type protein

(B) loss-of-function mutations

point mutation   truncation   deletion

(C) gain-of-function mutation

mutant allele, *r*, does not. Because they lack this enzyme, plants that are homozygous for the *r* allele contain more sugar and less starch than plants that possess the dominant *R* allele, which gives their peas a wrinkled appearance. The sweet peas available in the supermarket are often wrinkled mutants of the same type that Mendel studied.

Although most loss-of-function mutations are recessive, some can be dominant. Take, for example, a mutation that causes a protein to misfold. In a heterozygote, 50% of the proteins produced would be misfolded and inactive, while the other 50% would function normally. However, the misfolded form of the protein could go on to form aggregates that cause severe problems for the cell (see Figure 4–19). Because of its widespread impact, this particular loss-of-function mutation would be dominant.

Mutations that increase the activity of a gene or its product, or result in the gene being expressed in inappropriate circumstances, are called **gain-of-function mutations** (see Figure 19–30). Such mutations are usually dominant. For example, as we saw in Chapter 16, certain mutations in the *Ras* gene generate a form of the protein that is always active. Because the normal Ras protein is involved in controlling cell proliferation, the mutant protein drives cells to multiply inappropriately, even in the absence of signals that are normally required to stimulate cell division—thereby promoting the development of cancer. About 30% of all human cancers contain such dominant, gain-of-function mutations in the *Ras* gene.

Each of Us Carries Many Potentially Harmful Recessive Mutations

As we saw in Chapter 9, mutations that occur in the germ line provide the fodder for evolution. They can alter the fitness of an organism, making it either less or more likely for the individual to survive and leave progeny. Natural selection determines whether these mutations are preserved: those that confer a selective advantage on an organism tend to be perpetuated, whereas those that compromise an organism's fitness or ability to procreate tend to be lost.

The great majority of chance mutations are either neutral, with no effect on phenotype, or deleterious. A deleterious mutation that is dominant—one that exerts its negative effects when present even in a single copy—will be eliminated almost as soon as it arises. In extreme cases, if a mutant organism is unable to reproduce, the mutation that causes that failure will be lost from the population when the mutant individual dies. For deleterious mutations that are recessive, things are a little more complicated. When such a mutation first arises, it will generally be present in only a single copy. The organism that carries the mutation can produce just as many progeny as other individuals; some of these progeny will inherit a single copy of the mutation, and they too will appear fit and healthy. But as they and their descendants begin to mate with one another, some individuals will inherit two copies of the mutant allele and display an abnormal phenotype.

If such a homozygous individual fails to reproduce, two copies of the mutant allele will be lost from the population. Eventually, an equilibrium is reached, where the rate at which new mutations occur in the gene balances the rate at which these mutant alleles are lost through matings that yield abnormal, homozygous mutant individuals. As a consequence, many deleterious recessive mutations are present in heterozygous individuals at a surprisingly high frequency, even though homozygous individuals showing the deleterious phenotype are rare. For example, the most common form of hereditary deafness (due to mutations in a gene

QUESTION 19–3

Imagine that each chromosome undergoes one and only one crossover event on each chromatid during each meiosis. How would the co-inheritance of traits that are determined by genes at opposite ends of the same chromosome compare with the co-inheritance observed for genes on two different chromosomes? How does this compare with the actual situation?

that encodes a gap-junction protein; see Figure 20–28) occurs in about one in 4000 births, but about one in 30 of us are carriers of a loss-of-function mutant allele of the gene.

GENETICS AS AN EXPERIMENTAL TOOL

Unraveling how chromosomes shuttle genetic information from one generation to the next did more than demystify the basis of inheritance: it united the science of genetics with other life sciences, from cell biology and biochemistry to physiology and medicine. **Genetics** provides a powerful way to discover what specific genes do and how variations in those genes underlie the differences between one species and another or between individuals within a species. Such knowledge also has practical benefits, as understanding the genetic and biological basis of diseases can help us to better diagnose, treat, and prevent them.

In this section, we outline the *classical genetic approach* to identifying genes and determining how they influence the phenotype of experimental organisms such as yeast or flies. The process begins with the generation of a very large number of mutants and the identification of those rare individuals that show a phenotype of interest. By analyzing these rare mutant individuals and their progeny, we can track down the genes responsible and work out what these genes normally do—and how mutations that alter their activity affect how an organism looks and behaves.

The Classical Genetic Approach Begins with Random Mutagenesis

Before the advent of DNA technology (discussed in Chapter 10), most genes were identified and characterized by observing the processes disrupted when the gene was mutated. This type of analysis begins with the isolation of mutants that have an interesting or unusual phenotype: fruit flies that have white eyes or curly wings or that become paralyzed when exposed to high temperatures, for example. Working backward from the abnormal phenotype, one then determines the change in DNA that is responsible. This **classical genetic approach**—searching for mutant phenotypes and then isolating the responsible genes—is most easily performed in model organisms that reproduce rapidly and are amenable to genetic manipulation, such as bacteria, yeasts, nematode worms, zebrafish, and fruit flies. A few of the principles behind this classical approach are outlined in **Panel 19–1**, (p. 675).

Although spontaneous mutants with interesting phenotypes can be found by combing through a collection of thousands or millions of organisms, the process can be made much more efficient by generating mutations artificially with agents that damage DNA, called *mutagens*. Different mutagens generate different types of DNA mutations (**Figure 19–31**). Not all mutations will lead to a noticeable change in phenotype. But by treating

Figure 19–31 DNA-damaging agents produce various types of mutations. Some common types of mutation are shown here. Different mutagens each produce a characteristic spectrum of mutations. Other types of mutation involve changes in larger segments of DNA, including deletions, duplications, and chromosomal rearrangements (not shown).

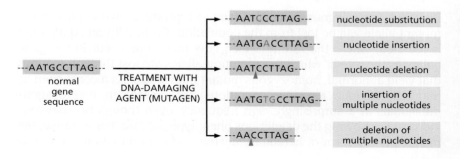

GENES AND PHENOTYPES

Gene: a functional unit of inheritance, corresponding to the segment of DNA coding for a protein or noncoding RNA molecule.

Genome: all of an organism's DNA sequences.

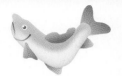

alleles: alternative forms of a gene

Wild type: the common, naturally occurring type

Mutant: differing from the wild type because of a genetic change (a mutation)

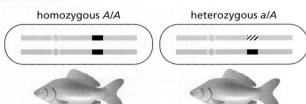

GENOTYPE: the specific set of alleles forming the genome of an individual

PHENOTYPE: the visible or functional characteristics of the individual

homozygous *A/A*   heterozygous *a/A*   homozygous *a/a*

allele *A* is dominant (relative to *a*); allele *a* is recessive (relative to *A*)

In the example above, the phenotype of the heterozygote is the same as that of one of the homozygotes; in cases where it is different from both homozygotes, the two alleles are said to be co-dominant.

MEIOSIS AND GENETIC MAPPING

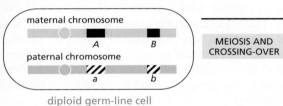

maternal chromosome

A   *B*

paternal chromosome

a   *b*

diploid germ-line cell

genotype $\dfrac{AB}{ab}$

MEIOSIS AND CROSSING-OVER

genotype *Ab*

A   *b*

site of crossing-over

genotype *aB*

a   *B*

haploid gametes (eggs or sperm)

The greater the distance between two loci on a single chromosome, the greater is the chance that they will be separated by crossing-over occurring at a site between them. If two genes are thus reassorted in x% of gametes, they are said to be separated on a chromosome by a genetic map distance of x map units (or x centimorgans).

TWO GENES OR ONE?

Given two mutations that produce the same phenotype, how can we tell whether they are mutations in the same gene? If the mutations are recessive (as they most often are), the answer can be found by a complementation test. In the simplest type of complementation test, an individual who is homozygous for one mutation is mated with an individual who is homozygous for the other. The phenotype of the offspring gives the answer to the question.

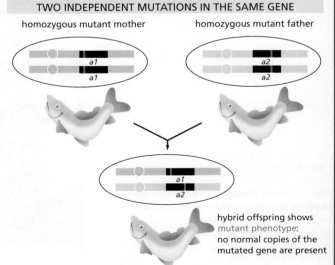

COMPLEMENTATION:
MUTATIONS IN TWO DIFFERENT GENES

homozygous mutant mother   homozygous mutant father

mutation

a
a

b
b

hybrid offspring shows normal phenotype: one normal copy of each gene is present

NONCOMPLEMENTATION:
TWO INDEPENDENT MUTATIONS IN THE SAME GENE

homozygous mutant mother   homozygous mutant father

a1
a1

a2
a2

a1
a2

hybrid offspring shows mutant phenotype: no normal copies of the mutated gene are present large numbers of organisms with mutagens, collections of mutants can be generated quickly, increasing the odds of finding an interesting phenotype, as we discuss next.

Genetic Screens Identify Mutants Deficient in Specific Cell Processes

A **genetic screen** typically involves examining many thousands of mutagenized individuals to find the few that show a specific altered phenotype of interest. To search for genes involved in cell metabolism, for example, one might screen mutagenized bacterial or yeast cells to pick out those that have lost the ability to grow in the absence of a particular amino acid or other nutrient (see Figure 9–5).

Even genes involved in complex phenotypes, such as social behavior, can be identified by genetic screens in multicellular organisms. For example, by screening for worms that feed in clusters (rather than alone, as do wild-type individuals), scientists identified and isolated a gene that affects this "social behavior" (Figure 19–32).

Advances in modern technologies have made it possible to carry out high-throughput genetic screens using large collections of individuals, each of which has a different gene inactivated. Such mutant collections can often be screened using automated robots. For example, investigators have made use of RNA interference (explained in Figure 8–28) to generate a collection of nematode worms in which the activity of every protein-coding gene has been disrupted, with each worm being deficient in just one gene. These collections can be screened rapidly for dramatic changes in phenotype, such as stunted growth, uncoordinated movement, decreased fertility, or impaired embryonic development (Figure 19–33). Using this strategy, the genes needed to produce a particular characteristic can be identified.

Conditional Mutants Permit the Study of Lethal Mutations

Genetic screens are a powerful approach for isolating and characterizing mutations that are compatible with life—those that change the appearance or behavior of an organism without killing it. A problem arises, however, if we wish to study essential genes—those that are absolutely required for fundamental cell processes, such as RNA synthesis or cell division. Defects in these genes are usually lethal, which means that special strategies are needed to isolate and propagate such mutants: if the mutants cannot be bred, their genes cannot be studied.

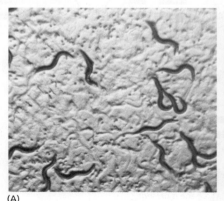
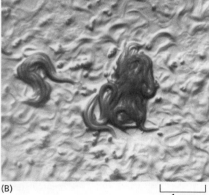

Figure 19–32 **Genetic screens can be used to identify mutations that affect an animal's behavior.** (A) Wild-type *C. elegans* dine alone. (B) Mutant worms engage in social feeding. (Courtesy of Cornelia Bargmann.)

(A)   (B)   └─── 1 mm

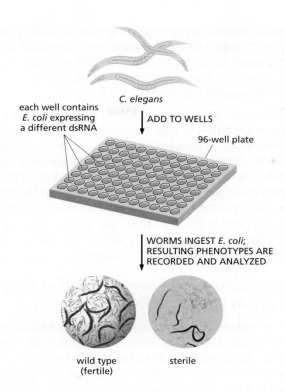

each well contains
E. coli expressing
a different dsRNA

C. elegans

ADD TO WELLS

96-well plate

WORMS INGEST *E. coli*;
RESULTING PHENOTYPES ARE
RECORDED AND ANALYZED

wild type
(fertile)

sterile

Figure 19–33 RNA interference provides a convenient method for conducting genome-wide genetic screens. In this experiment, each well in this 96-well plate is filled with *E. coli* that produce a different double-stranded (ds), interfering RNA. *E. coli* are a standard diet for *C. elegans* raised in the laboratory. Each interfering RNA matches the nucleotide sequence of a single *C. elegans* gene. About 10 worms are added to each well, where they ingest the genetically modified bacteria. The plate is incubated for several days, which gives the RNAs time to bind to and inactivate their target genes—and the worms time to grow, mate, and produce offspring. The plate is then examined in a microscope, which can be controlled robotically, to screen for genes that affect the worms' ability to survive, reproduce, develop, and behave. Because the investigator knows which interfering RNA was added to each well, the gene responsible for any resulting defect can be readily identified. Shown here are wild-type worms alongside a mutant that shows an impaired ability to reproduce. (Adapted from Lehner et al., *Nat. Genet.* 38:896–903, 2006.)

If the organism is diploid—a mouse or a pea plant, say—and the mutant phenotype is recessive, there is a simple solution. Individuals that are heterozygous for the mutation will have a normal phenotype and can be propagated. When they are mated with one another, 25% of the progeny will be homozygous mutants and will show the lethal mutant phenotype; 50% will be heterozygous carriers of the mutation like their parents and can be used to maintain the breeding stock.

But what if the organism is haploid, as is the case for many yeast and bacteria? One way to study lethal mutations in such organisms makes use of *conditional mutants*, in which the protein product of the mutant gene is only defective under certain conditions. For example, in mutants that are *temperature-sensitive*, the protein functions normally within a certain range of temperatures (called the *permissive* temperature) but can be inactivated by a shift to a *nonpermissive temperature* outside this range. Thus the abnormal phenotype can be switched on and off simply by changing the temperature. A cell containing a temperature-sensitive mutation in an essential gene can be propagated at the permissive temperature and then be driven to display its mutant phenotype by a shift to a nonpermissive temperature (**Figure 19–34**).

Many temperature-sensitive bacterial mutants were isolated to identify the genes that encode the bacterial proteins required for DNA replication; investigators treated large populations of bacteria with mutagens and

Figure 19–34 Temperature-sensitive mutants are valuable for identifying the genes and proteins involved in essential cell processes. In this example, yeast cells are treated with a mutagen, spread on a culture plate at a relatively cool temperature, and allowed to proliferate to form colonies. The colonies are then transferred to two identical Petri plates using a technique called replica plating. One of these plates is incubated at a cool temperature, the other at a warmer temperature. Those cells that contain a temperature-sensitive mutation in a gene essential for proliferation can be readily identified, because they form a colony only at the cooler, permissive temperature.

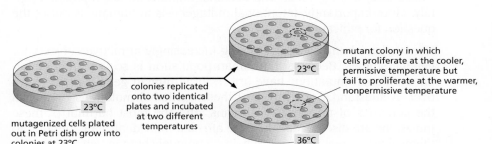

mutagenized cells plated
out in Petri dish grow into
colonies at 23°C

23°C

colonies replicated
onto two identical
plates and incubated
at two different
temperatures

23°C

36°C

mutant colony in which
cells proliferate at the cooler,
permissive temperature but
fail to proliferate at the warmer,
nonpermissive temperature

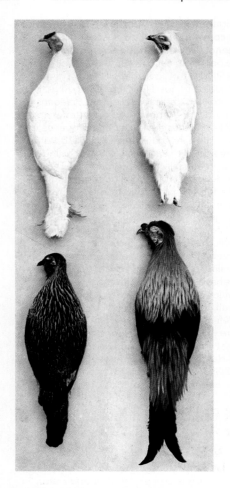

Figure 19–35 A complementation test can reveal that mutations in two different genes are responsible for the same abnormal phenotype. When an albino (white) bird from one strain is bred with an albino from a different strain, the resulting offspring have normal coloration. This restoration of the wild-type plumage implies that the two white breeds lack color because of recessive mutations in different genes. (From W. Bateson, *Mendel's Principles of Heredity,* 1st ed. Cambridge, UK: Cambridge University Press, 1913.)

then screened for cells that stopped making DNA when they were warmed from 30°C to 42°C. Similarly, temperature-sensitive yeast mutants were used to identify many of the proteins involved in regulating the cell cycle (see How We Know, pp. 30–31) and in transporting proteins through the secretory pathway (see Figure 15–28).

The DNA technologies discussed in Chapter 10 have made it possible to construct an entirely different type of conditional mutant—one in which the gene of interest is engineered such that it can be deleted at a particular time in development or in a particular tissue (see Figure 10–30). Essential genes—for example, those whose complete inactivation would cause an organism to die early in development—can be studied in this way because the organism can be allowed to develop past the critical period before the gene is deleted. This strategy is particularly useful for studying genes that are active in many different tissues, as the role they play in each one can be independently assessed.

A Complementation Test Reveals Whether Two Mutations Are in the Same Gene

A large-scale genetic screen can turn up many mutant organisms with the same phenotype. These mutations might affect the same gene or they might affect different genes that function in the same process. How can we distinguish between the two? If the mutations are recessive, a **complementation test** can reveal whether they affect the same or different genes.

In the simplest type of complementation test, an individual that is homozygous for one recessive mutation is mated with an individual that is homozygous for the other mutation. If the two mutations affect the same gene, the offspring will show the mutant phenotype, because they carry only defective copies of the gene in question. If, in contrast, the mutations affect different genes, the resulting offspring will show the normal, wild-type phenotype, because they will have one normal copy (and one mutant copy) of each gene (see Panel 19–1, p. 675).

Whenever the normal phenotype is restored in such a test, the alleles inherited from the two parents are said to complement each other (**Figure 19–35**). For example, complementation tests on mutants identified during genetic screens have revealed that five genes are required for yeast cells to digest the sugar galactose, that 20 genes are needed for *E. coli* to build a functional flagellum, and many hundreds are essential for the normal development of an adult nematode worm from a fertilized egg.

EXPLORING HUMAN GENETICS

Genetic screens in model experimental organisms have been spectacularly successful in identifying genes and relating them to various phenotypes, including many that are conserved between these organisms and humans. But the same approach cannot be used in humans. Unlike flies, worms, yeast, and bacteria, humans do not reproduce rapidly. More importantly, intentional mutagenesis in humans is out of the question for ethical reasons.

Nonetheless, humans are becoming increasingly attractive subjects for genetic studies. Because the human population is so large, spontaneous nonlethal mutations have arisen in all human genes—many times over. A substantial proportion of these nonlethal mutations remain in the genomes of present-day humans, and the most harmful of these mutations are discovered when the affected individuals call attention to themselves by seeking medical help—a uniquely human behavior.

With the recent advances that have enabled the sequencing of entire human genomes rapidly and inexpensively (discussed in Chapter 10), we can now identify such mutations and study their evolution and inheritance in ways that were impossible even a few years ago. By comparing the sequences of tens of thousands of human genomes, we can now identify directly the DNA differences that distinguish one individual from another. In this section, we discuss how analyses of DNA collected from human families and populations all over the world are providing clues about our evolutionary history and about the genes that influence our susceptibility to disease.

Linked Blocks of Polymorphisms Have Been Passed Down from Our Ancestors

As discussed in Chapter 9, when we compare the sequences of multiple human genomes, we find that any two individuals will differ in about 1 nucleotide pair in 1000. Most of these variations are common and relatively harmless. When two sequence variants coexist at the same site and are common in the population, the variants are called **polymorphisms**. The majority of polymorphisms are due to the substitution of a single nucleotide, called **single-nucleotide polymorphisms** or **SNPs** (see Figure 9–38). The rest are due largely to insertions or deletions—called *indels* when the change is small, or *copy number variants* (*CNVs*) when it is large.

Although these common variants can be found throughout the genome, they are not scattered randomly—or even independently. Instead, they tend to travel in groups called **haplotype blocks**—combinations of polymorphisms or other DNA markers that are inherited as a unit.

To understand why such haplotype blocks exist, we need to consider our evolutionary history. It is thought that modern humans expanded from a relatively small population—perhaps around 10,000 individuals—that existed in Africa about 200,000 years ago. Among that small group of our ancestors, some individuals might have carried one set of genetic variants, others a different set. The chromosomes of a present-day human represent a shuffled combination of chromosome segments from different members of this small ancestral group of people. Because only about two thousand generations separate us from them, large segments of these ancestral chromosomes have passed from parent to child, unbroken by the crossover events that occur during meiosis. (Remember, only a few crossovers occur between each set of homologous chromosomes, as shown in Figure 19–12.)

As a result, certain sets of DNA sequences—and their associated polymorphisms—have been inherited in linked groups, with little genetic rearrangement across the generations. These are the haplotype blocks. Like genes that exist in different allelic forms, haplotype blocks also come in a limited number of variants that are common in the human population, each representing a combination of DNA polymorphisms passed down from a particular ancestor long ago.

Polymorphisms Provide Clues to Our Evolutionary History

A detailed examination of haplotype blocks has provided intriguing insights into the history of human populations. Our DNA sequences are constantly being altered by mutation; many of these changes will be neutral, in that they will not affect the reproductive success of the individual. Each of these variants has a chance of becoming common in the population. The more time that has elapsed since the origin of a relatively common polymorphism like a SNP, the smaller should be the haplotype block that surrounds it: that's because, over the course of many generations, crossover events will have had many chances to separate an ancient allele from other variants nearby. Thus by comparing the sizes of haplotype blocks from different human populations, it is possible to estimate how many generations have elapsed since the origin of a specific neutral mutation. By combining such genetic comparisons with archaeological findings, scientists have been able to deduce the most probable routes our ancestors took when they left Africa (see Figure 9–37).

Genome analyses can also be used to estimate when and where humans acquired mutations that have conferred an evolutionary benefit, such as resistance to infection. Such favorable mutations will rapidly accumulate in the population because individuals that carry them will be more likely to survive an epidemic and pass the mutation on to their offspring. A haplotype analysis can be used to "date" the appearance of such a favorable mutation. If it cropped up in the population relatively recently, there will have been fewer opportunities for recombination to break up the DNA sequence around it, so the surrounding haplotype block will be large.

Such is the case for sickle-cell anemia, a disorder caused by a single nucleotide substitution that changes a glutamic acid to a valine in one of the protein subunits of hemoglobin (see Figure 6–32). Although individuals who are homozygous for this allele experience the harmful effects of anemia, heterozygotes who carry one normal and one sickle-cell allele show no ill effects and, in addition, are resistant to malaria. This allele—which confers a benefit under the right set of circumstances—is widespread in Africa, where malaria is rife. A comparison of numerous human genes reveals that the sickle-cell allele is embedded in an unusually large haplotype block, indicating that it arose relatively recently in the African gene pool—probably about 2000 years ago. In this way, analyses of modern human genomes can highlight important events in human evolution, including our initial exposures to specific infections.

Genetic Studies Aid in the Search for the Causes of Human Diseases

Like the wrinkled peas studied by Mendel, our susceptibility to disease is a phenotypic trait—albeit an unfortunate one. Thus, for many diseases, the causes are rooted in our genomes. In some cases, the genetic underpinnings of disease are clear and unequivocal. For example, mutations in specific genes give rise, in a reproducible way, to clearly defined conditions such as congenital deafness, albinism, hemophilia, and sickle-cell anemia. Other times, the genetic connections are more complex. Many of the most common human disorders, such as diabetes or arthritis, involve many genes working together to give rise to the "disease phenotype."

Most diseases are also influenced by environmental factors: availability of nutrition or exposure to toxins, carcinogens, infectious viruses or microorganisms—even to sunlight (see Figure 6–25). Yet even diseases that are clearly environmental in nature, such as infection by specific pathogens can be modified by genetic factors. For example, individuals bearing a sickle-cell allele are resistant to malaria, as we discussed earlier. Others carry an allele that renders them genetically resistant to infection with HIV, the virus that causes AIDS, as we discuss shortly. The ultimate outcome, in terms of disease phenotype, thus depends on an intricate interplay amongst genetic and environmental factors.

Despite these complexities, genetic studies—particularly those that involve a comparison of human genome sequences—are expanding our understanding of the fundamental causes of human disease. In the remainder of this chapter, we explore the genetic underpinnings of disease, and the approaches that investigators use to identify them.

Many Severe, Rare Human Diseases Are Caused by Mutations in Single Genes

About 3000 human diseases are caused by mutations in single genes. These single-gene, or *monogenic*, disorders are sometimes referred to as *Mendelian* because they show a pattern of inheritance that is as simple to trace as that of the wrinkled peas and purple flowers that Mendel studied. Most of these mutations are recessive; individuals who carry only one copy of the mutant allele are largely asymptomatic, while those homozygous for the mutation are severely impaired. For example, individuals with Tay-Sachs disease, which is characterized by seizures, blindness, and neurodegeneration, usually do not survive infancy.

Monogenic disorders also tend to be very rare, affecting only a fraction of one percent of the human population. This low prevalence can be attributed to a number of factors. First, many of these diseases are "early onset," meaning that affected individuals die early in life, often before reproducing. The disease-causing alleles carried by these individuals are thus eliminated from the gene pool. At the same time, because many monogenic disorders are recessive, heterozygous individuals typically lead normal lives and show no signs of the disease. Thus, the disease-causing alleles are never entirely eradicated from the population, and instead persist at a low frequency. The disease then manifests itself only in those rare individuals who inherit two mutant alleles. Monogenic disorders can occur more frequently, however, in families or populations in which the parents are genetically related. Such consanguineous marriages are more likely to produce offspring that are homozygous for the mutant, disease-causing alleles than are marriages between unrelated individuals (**Figure 19–36**).

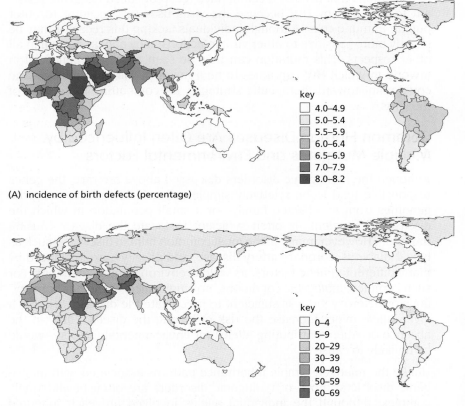

key
- 4.0–4.9
- 5.0–5.4
- 5.5–5.9
- 6.0–6.4
- 6.5–6.9
- 7.0–7.9
- 8.0–8.2

(A) incidence of birth defects (percentage)

key
- 0–4
- 5–9
- 20–29
- 30–39
- 40–49
- 50–59
- 60–69

(B) prevalence of consanguinity (percentage of total marriages between second cousins or closer)

Figure 19–36 The prevalence of consanguineous marriage can increase the likelihood of inheriting disease-causing alleles. A comparison of these two maps indicates the large degree of overlap between the percentage of consanguineous marriages and the incidence of birth defects in countries around the world. (A) The percentage of birth defects is indicated by *blue* shading. Here, a birth defect is defined as any abnormality affecting body structure or function that is present from birth. These include conditions caused by simple, monogenic diseases, as well as environmental factors, such as exposure to chemicals that cause mutations. (B) The proportion of marriages between second cousins or closer is indicated in *orange*. *Gray* shading indicates countries for which data were not available. (Adapted from M.A. Jobling et al., *Human Evolutionary Genetics,* 2nd ed. New York: Garland Science, 2014. With permission from Garland Science.)

Some monogenic diseases are more common in certain populations than in others. In some cases, this prevalence is due to natural selection. The mutant hemoglobin allele that can provide resistance to malaria, for example, is present in higher frequencies in geographic regions where malaria is common. In other cases, the preponderance of a particular mutation is likely due to a founder effect; that is, a subpopulation of humans arose from a small number of individuals, some of which happened to carry a particular mutation. As this subpopulation expanded, the frequency of the mutant allele became higher than it is in the human population as a whole. This appears to be the case for Tay-Sachs disease, which is more prevalent in Ashkenazi Jews.

When we explore the mechanisms by which these rare, single-gene mutations lead to disease, we find that monogenic disorders affect nearly all aspects of cell and molecular biology. Tay-Sachs disease, for example, is caused by loss-of-function mutations in the gene that encodes the enzyme hexosaminidase. Without this enzyme, brain and nerve cells become increasingly damaged, with tragic consequences. Another disease, called cystic fibrosis, arises from mutations in the gene coding for a specialized form of chloride channel. Some of these mutations prevent the channel from opening, while others inhibit its proper folding, which leads to the protein being destroyed. Knowing how a particular mutation affects protein function can point the way toward the most effective treatment. For example, certain drugs can help direct a misfolded channel to its proper place in the plasma membrane and help it to function more effectively. Such treatments can "rescue" mutant proteins and restore enough of their activity to alleviate some of the worst symptoms of cystic fibrosis. Although the consequences of such diseases can be devastating to individuals, families, and communities, their study has provided critical insights into the function of many human genes.

Finally, it should be noted that not all loss-of-function mutations in humans are deleterious. For example, individuals that are homozygous for mutations that destroy a cell-surface receptor called CCR5 are resistant to infection by HIV because the virus uses this receptor to enter human immune cells. Although individuals lacking this receptor may be slightly more sensitive to other viral infections, they appear normal in all other respects. This mutation can thus be seen as largely beneficial in a world in which HIV continues to be a major public health issue—and could point toward therapeutic strategies for combatting the spread of the virus.

Common Human Diseases Are Often Influenced by Multiple Mutations and Environmental Factors

Although the monogenic disorders discussed above are rare, the genes responsible tend to be relatively simple to track down. Analyzing the genomes from an affected family—or a small population in which the disease is prevalent—is often sufficient to locate the disease-causing mutation. However, many of the most common human diseases—such as type 2 diabetes, coronary artery disease, and obesity—are influenced by many different genetic factors, as well as environmental conditions. For such complex, *multigenic* conditions, no single allele—whether homozygous or heterozygous—is sufficient to precipitate the disease. Instead, a given allele might increase the risk of having the disease, but—in the absence of other contributing alleles (or environmental factors)—would be unlikely to cause it.

Unlike the relatively simple inheritance patterns associated with monogenic disorders, those of multigenic disorders are often bewilderingly complex: although the individual alleles involved are each inherited

QUESTION 19–5

In a recent automated analysis, thousands of SNPs across the genome were analyzed in pooled DNA samples from humans who had been sorted into groups according to their age. For the vast majority of these sites, there was no change in the relative frequencies of different variants as these humans aged. Sometimes, albeit rarely, a particular variant at one position was found to decrease in frequency progressively for people over 50 years old. Which of the possible explanations seems most likely?
A. The nucleotide in that SNP at that position is unstable, and mutates with age.
B. Those people born more than 50 years ago came from a population that tended to lack the disappearing SNP variant.
C. The SNP variant alters an important gene product in a way that shortens the human life-span, or is linked to a neighboring allele that has this effect.

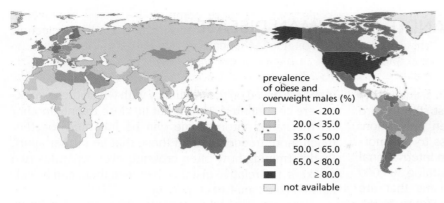

prevalence
of obese and
overweight males (%)

◻ < 20.0
◻ 20.0 < 35.0
◻ 35.0 < 50.0
◻ 50.0 < 65.0
◼ 65.0 < 80.0
◼ ≥ 80.0
◻ not available

Figure 19–37 Complex diseases are widespread geographically and are common in the human population. This map shows the global distribution of overweight and obese males, as determined by an elevated body mass index (a measure of an individual's weight and height). Conditions such as obesity, which depend on complex interactions between genetics and the environment, often occur at frequencies that can be thousands of times higher than those of simple, monogenic disorders. (Adapted from M.A. Jobling et al., *Human Evolutionary Genetics*, 2nd ed. New York: Garland Science, 2014. With permission from Garland Science.)

according to the laws of Mendel, their sheer number greatly complicate the analysis. More importantly, unlike monogenic disorders—which tend to occur early in life—complex, multigenic diseases often occur much later. Because of this delay, many of these disorders do not affect an individual's likelihood of reproducing. As a result, some of the risk-enhancing alleles have become quite common in the population, as they are not eliminated by selection. The resulting disorders can thus affect a large proportion of the population (**Figure 19–37**).

Genome-wide Association Studies Can Aid the Search for Mutations Associated with Disease

Given the complexity of many of the most common human diseases, identifying the associated genes can be a difficult task. One way of uncovering these genetic risk factors involves analyzing the patterns of inherited polymorphisms. Investigators typically collect DNA samples from a large number of people who have the disease and compare them to samples from a group of people who do not. They look for variants—SNPs, for example—that are more common among the people who have the disease. Because DNA sequences that are close together on a chromosome tend to be inherited together, the presence of such SNPs could indicate that these variants themselves—or alleles that lie nearby— increase the risk of the disease (**Figure 19–38**).

Such *genome-wide association studies* (*GWAS*)—which initially focused on SNPs—have been used to search for genes that predispose individuals to common diseases, including diabetes, coronary artery disease, rheumatoid arthritis, and even depression. One such study is described in **How We Know**, pp. 684–685. For many of these conditions, environmental as

healthy controls

individual A
B
C
D
E

affected individuals

individual A
B
C
D
E

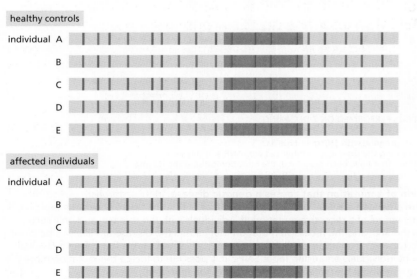

Figure 19–38 Genes that affect the risk of developing a common disease can often be tracked down through linkage to SNPs. Here, the patterns of SNPs are compared between two sets of individuals—a set of healthy controls and a set affected by a particular common disease. A segment of a typical chromosome is shown. For most SNPs in this segment, it is a random matter whether an individual has one SNP variant (*red* vertical bars) or another (*blue* vertical bars); the same randomness is seen both for the control group and for the affected individuals. However, in the part of the chromosome that is shaded in *darker gray*, a bias is seen, such that most normal individuals have the *blue* SNP variants, whereas most affected individuals have the *red* SNP variants. This finding suggests that this region contains, or is very close to, a gene that is involved in the disease. Using carefully selected controls and thousands of affected individuals, this approach can help track down disease-related genes, even when they confer only a slight increase in the risk of developing the disease.

HOW WE KNOW

USING SNPs TO GET A HANDLE ON HUMAN DISEASE

For diseases that have their roots in genetics, finding the gene or genes responsible can be the first step toward improved diagnosis, treatment, and even prevention. The task is not simple, but having access to polymorphisms such as SNPs can help. In 1999, an international group of scientists set out to collect and catalog 300,000 SNPs—the single-nucleotide polymorphisms that are common in the human population (see Figure 9–38). Today, the database has grown to include a catalog of millions upon millions of genetic variations. These SNPs do not only help to define the differences between one individual and another; for geneticists, they also serve as signposts that can point the way toward the genes involved in common human disorders, such as diabetes, obesity, asthma, arthritis, and even gallstones and restless leg syndrome.

Making a map

One way that SNPs have facilitated the search for alleles that predispose to disease is by providing the physical markers needed to construct detailed genetic linkage maps. A genetic linkage map displays the relative locations of genetic markers along each chromosome. Such maps are based on the frequency with which these markers are co-inherited. Those that lie close to one another on the same chromosome will be inherited together much more frequently than those that lie farther apart. By determining how often crossing-over separates two markers, the relative distance between them can be calculated (see Panel 19–1, p. 675).

The same sort of analysis can be used to discover linkage between a SNP and an allele—for example, one that might cause an inherited disease. We simply look for co-inheritance of the SNP with a certain phenotype—in this case, the disease. Finding such a linkage indicates that the mutation responsible for the phenotype is either the SNP itself or, more likely, lies close to the SNP (Figure 19–39). And because we know the exact location in the human genome sequence of every SNP we examine, the linkage tells us the neighborhood in which the causative mutation resides. A more detailed analysis of the DNA in that region—to look for deletions, insertions, or other functionally significant abnormalities in the DNA sequence of affected individuals—can then lead to a precise identification of the critical gene.

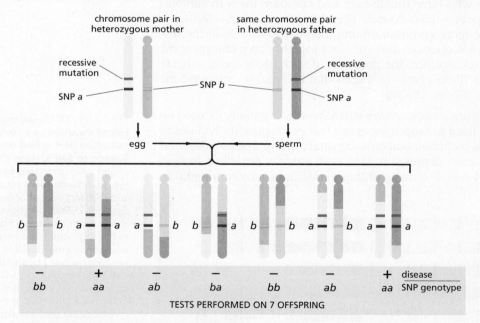

OBSERVATION: Disease is seen only in progeny with SNP genotype *aa*.
CONCLUSION: Recessive mutation causing the disease is co-inherited with SNP *a*. If this same correlation is observed in other families that have been examined, the mutation causing the disease must lie close to SNP *a*.

Figure 19–39 SNP analysis can pin down the location of a mutation that causes a genetic disease. In this approach, one studies the co-inheritance of a specific human phenotype (here a genetic disease) with a particular set of SNPs. The figure shows the logic for the common case of a family in which both parents are carriers of a recessive mutation. If individuals with the disease, and only such individuals, are homozygous for a particular SNP, then the SNP and the recessive mutation that causes the disease are likely to be close together on the same chromosome, as shown here. To prove that an apparent linkage is statistically significant, a few dozen individuals from such families may need to be examined. With more individuals and using more SNPs, it is possible to locate the mutation more precisely. These days it can be just as fast and cheap to use whole-genome sequencing to find the mutation.

Such linkage analyses are usually carried out in families that are particularly prone to a disorder—the larger the family, the better. And the method works best where there is a simple cause-and-effect relationship, such that a particular mutant gene directly and reliably causes the disorder—as is the case, for example, for the mutant gene that causes cystic fibrosis. But most common disorders are not like this. Instead, many factors affect the disease risk—some genetic, some environmental, some just a matter of chance. For such conditions, a different approach is needed to identify risk genes.

Making associations

Genome-wide association studies (GWAS, for short) allow us to discover common genetic variants that affect the risk for a common disease, even if each variant alters susceptibility only slightly. Because mutations that destroy the activity of a key gene are likely to have a disastrous effect on the fitness of the mutant individual, they tend to be eliminated from the population by natural selection and so are rarely seen. Genetic variants that alter a gene's function only slightly, on the other hand, are much more common. By tracking down these common variants, or polymorphisms, we can sniff out some of the genes that contribute to the biology of common diseases.

GWAS rely on genetic markers, such as SNPs, that are located throughout the genome to compare directly the DNA sequences of two populations: individuals who have a particular disease and those who do not. The approach identifies SNPs that are present in the people who have the disease more often than would be expected by chance.

Consider the case of *age-related macular degeneration* (*AMD*), a degenerative disorder of the retina that is a leading cause of blindness in the elderly. To search for genetic variations that are associated with AMD, researchers looked at a panel of just over 100,000 SNPs that spanned the genome. They determined the nucleotide sequence at each of these SNPs in 96 people who had AMD, and 50 who did not. Among the 100,000 SNPs, they discovered that one particular SNP was present significantly more often in the individuals who had the disease (Figure 19–40).

The SNP is located in a gene called *Cfh* (*complement factor H*). But it falls within one of the gene's introns and appears unlikely to have any effect on the protein product. This SNP itself, therefore, did not seem likely to be the cause of the increase in susceptibility to AMD. But it focused the researchers' attention on the *Cfh* gene. So they resequenced the region to look for additional polymorphisms that might also be inherited more often by people with AMD, along with the SNP that they had already identified. They discovered three variants that change the amino acid sequence of the Cfh protein. One substitutes a histidine for a tyrosine at one particular place in the protein, and it was strongly associated with the disease (and almost always coupled with the original SNP that had put the researchers on the track of the *Cfh* gene). Individuals who carried two copies of this risky allele were five to seven times more likely to develop AMD than those who harbored a different allele of the *Cfh* gene.

Several other research teams, using a similar genetic association approach, have also pointed to *Cfh* variants as increasing the likelihood of developing AMD, making it almost certain that the *Cfh* gene has something to do with the biology of the disease. The Cfh protein is part of the complement system, an important component of immunity; the protein helps prevent the system from becoming overactive, a condition that can lead to inflammation and tissue damage. Interestingly, the environmental risk factors associated with the disease—smoking, obesity, and age—also affect inflammation and the activity of the complement system. Thus, whatever the detailed mechanism by which the *Cfh* gene influences the risk of AMD, the finding that complement is critical could lead to new tests for the early diagnosis of the disorder, as well as potential new avenues for treatment.

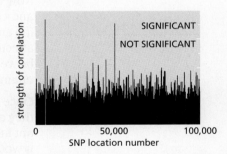

Figure 19–40 Genome-wide association studies identify DNA variations that are significantly more frequent in people with age-related macular degeneration (AMD). In this study, scientists examined more than 100,000 SNPs in each of 146 people. The x-axis of the graph shows the relative position of each SNP in the genome, starting at the left with the SNPs on Chromosome 1. The y-axis shows the strength of each SNP's observed correlation with AMD. The *blue* region indicates a cutoff level for statistical significance, corresponding to a probability of less than 5% of finding that strength of correlation by pure chance anywhere among the whole set of 100,000 tested SNPs. The SNP marked in *red* is the one that led the way to the relevant gene, *Cfh*. The initial association of the other prominent SNP (*black*) with the disease was rendered insignificant when additional sequencing at that site was performed. (Adapted from R.J. Klein et al., *Science* 308:385–389, 2005.)

well as genetic factors play an important part in determining which individuals will develop the disease.

Disappointingly, most of the DNA polymorphisms identified through this strategy increase the risk of disease only slightly. Many of them fall within regulatory DNA sequences and only subtly alter the expression of the genes they control. However, by identifying these "risky alleles," such studies provide insights into the molecular mechanisms underlying these complex disorders, these results are leading to an improved understanding of the molecular basis of common inherited diseases.

We Still Have Much to Learn about the Genetic Basis of Human Variation and Disease

The polymorphisms that have thus far allowed us to track our ancestors and identify genes that increase our risk of disease have to be relatively common to be detected by the methods we have described. Because they arose so long ago in our evolutionary past they are now present, in one form or another, in a substantial portion (1% or more) of the population. Such genetic variants are thought to account for about 90% of the differences between one person's genome and another. But when we try to tie these common alterations to differences in disease susceptibility or other heritable traits, such as height, we find that they do not have as much predictive power as we had anticipated: thus, for example, most confer relatively small increases—less than twofold—in the risk of developing a common disease.

Part of the problem is that many of the mutations that are directly responsible for complex human diseases appeared more recently in our evolutionary history—during a period when the human population underwent an explosive expansion in size, from the few million individuals that existed a mere 10,000 years ago to the 7 billion or so that inhabit the planet today. Because such mutations occur more rarely than the ancient polymorphisms that are common in the human population, they could slip through the type of GWAS approach just described.

Now that the price of DNA sequencing has plummeted, the most efficient and cost-effective way to identify these recent mutations is by sequencing and comparing the genomes of many thousands of individuals—those affected by diseases and those who are not. Such DNA sequencing must be very accurate, so that rare DNA variants in the population can be unambiguously identified (and distinguished from sequencing errors).

Once these variants are identified, the next challenge is to determine how they affect the phenotype of the individuals that carry them. When a variant falls within the coding region of a gene, it is simple to assess whether it would alter the amino acid sequence of the resulting protein. However, as we have seen, many important DNA variants lie outside coding regions. This mechanism could help explain why many alleles have only a small, but statistically significant, effect on the probability of precipitating a particular disease. It is often difficult to predict—from inspection of a genome sequence alone—what the effect of such variants might be; in these cases, additional experiments in cultured cells or animal models are needed to determine the consequences of such a mutation.

As genome sequencing efforts continue, we are discovering many previously unreported genetic variants in people affected by disease—and in apparently healthy individuals. Based on one study, each of us harbors about 100 loss-of-function mutations in protein-coding genes—some of which eliminate the activity of both gene copies. This surprising result means that our genome still holds many secrets, and that we can develop and function as "normal" humans in today's world despite the enormous variations across the human population.

ESSENTIAL CONCEPTS

- Sexual reproduction involves the cyclic alternation of diploid and haploid states: diploid germ-line cells divide by meiosis to form haploid gametes, and the haploid gametes from two individuals fuse at fertilization to form a new diploid cell—the zygote.

- During meiosis, the maternal and paternal homologs are parceled out to gametes such that each gamete receives one copy of each chromosome. Because the segregation of these homologs occurs randomly, and crossing-over occurs between them, many genetically different gametes can be produced from a single individual.

- In addition to enhancing genetic mixing, crossing-over helps ensure the proper segregation of chromosomes during meiosis.

- Although most of the mechanical features of meiosis are similar to those of mitosis, the behavior of the chromosomes is different: meiosis produces four genetically distinct haploid cells by two consecutive cell divisions, whereas mitosis produces two genetically identical diploid cells by a single cell division.

- Mendel unraveled the laws of heredity by studying the inheritance of a handful of discrete traits in pea plants.

- Mendel's law of segregation states that the maternal and paternal alleles for each trait separate from one another during gamete formation and then reunite randomly during fertilization.

- Mendel's law of independent assortment states that, during gamete formation, different pairs of alleles segregate independently of one another.

- The behavior of chromosomes during meiosis explains both of Mendel's laws.

- If two genes are close to each other on a chromosome, they tend to be inherited as a unit; if they are far apart, they will typically be separated by crossing-over. The frequency with which two genes are separated by crossovers can be used to construct a genetic map that shows their order on a chromosome.

- Mutant alleles can be either dominant or recessive. If a single copy of the mutant allele alters the phenotype of an individual that also possesses a wild-type allele, the mutant allele is dominant; if not, it is recessive.

- Complementation tests reveal whether two mutations that produce the same phenotype affect the same gene or different genes.

- Mutant organisms can be generated by treating animals with mutagens, which damage DNA. Such mutants can then be screened to identify phenotypes of interest and, ultimately, to isolate the responsible genes.

- With the possible exception of identical twins, no two human genomes are alike. Each of us carries a unique set of polymorphisms—variations in nucleotide sequence that in some cases contribute to our individual phenotypes.

- Some of the common polymorphisms—including SNPs, indels, and CNVs—provide useful markers for genetic mapping.

- The human genome consists of large haplotype blocks—segments of nucleotide sequence that have been passed down intact from our distant ancestors and, in most individuals, have not yet been broken up by crossovers. The relative sizes of haplotype blocks can give us clues to our evolutionary history and help to identify common disease-associated alleles.

- Many rare, inherited human diseases are due to mutations in a single gene.

- The most common human disorders are due to many genes acting together; DNA sequencing studies are identifying mutations in these genes that increase the risk of developing these diseases.

KEY TERMS

allele	heterozygous
asexual reproduction	homolog
bivalent	homologous recombination
chiasma (plural chiasmata)	homozygous
classical genetic approach	law of independent assortment
complementation test	law of segregation
crossing-over	loss-of-function mutation
diploid	meiosis
fertilization	pairing
gain-of-function mutation	pedigree
gamete	phenotype
genetic map	polymorphism
genetic screen	sexual reproduction
genetics	sister chromatid
genotype	SNP (single-nucleotide
germ line	polymorphism)
haploid	somatic cell
haplotype block	zygote

QUESTIONS

QUESTION 19–6

It is easy to see how deleterious mutations in bacteria, which have a single copy of each gene, are eliminated by natural selection: the affected bacteria die and the mutation is thereby lost from the population. Eukaryotes, however, have two copies of most genes—that is, they are diploid. Often an individual with two normal copies of the gene (homozygous normal) is indistinguishable in phenotype from an individual with one normal copy and one defective copy of the gene (heterozygous). In such cases, natural selection can operate only against an individual with two copies of the defective gene (homozygous defective). Consider the situation in which a defective form of the gene is lethal when homozygous, but without effect when heterozygous. Can such a mutation ever be eliminated from the population by natural selection? Why or why not?

QUESTION 19–7

Which of the following statements are correct? Explain your answers.

A. The egg and sperm cells of animals contain haploid genomes.

B. During meiosis, chromosomes are allocated so that each germ cell obtains one and only one copy of each of the different chromosomes.

C. Mutations that arise during meiosis are not transmitted to the next generation.

QUESTION 19–8

What might cause chromosome nondisjunction, where two copies of the same chromosome end up in the same daughter cell? What could be the consequences of this event occurring (a) in mitosis and (b) in meiosis?

QUESTION 19–9

Why do sister chromatids have to remain paired in division I of meiosis? Does the answer suggest a strategy for washing your socks?

QUESTION 19–10

Distinguish between the following genetic terms:

A. Gene and allele.

B. Homozygous and heterozygous.

C. Genotype and phenotype.

D. Dominant and recessive.

QUESTION 19–11

You have been given three wrinkled peas, which we shall call A, B, and C, each of which you plant to produce a mature pea plant. Each of these three plants, once self-pollinated, produces only wrinkled peas.

A. Given that you know that the wrinkled-pea phenotype is recessive, as a result of a loss-of-function mutation, what can you say about the genotype of each plant?

B. How do you determine if each of the three plants carries a mutation in the same gene or in different genes that produce the phenotype?

QUESTION 19–12

Susan's grandfather was deaf, and passed down a hereditary form of deafness within Susan's family as shown in Figure Q19–12.

A. Is this mutation most likely to be dominant or recessive?

B. Is it carried on a sex chromosome? Why or why not?

C. A complete SNP analysis has been done for all of the 11 grandchildren (4 affected and 7 unaffected). In comparing these 11 SNP results, how long a haplotype block would you expect to find around the critical gene? How might you detect it?

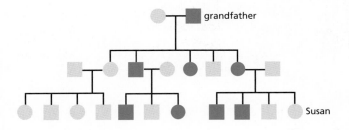

Figure Q19–12

QUESTION 19–13

Given that the mutation causing deafness in the family shown in Figure 19–26 is very rare, what is the most probable genotype of each of the four children in generation II?

QUESTION 19–14

In the pedigree shown in Figure Q19–14, the first born in each of three generations is the only person affected by a dominant genetically inherited disease, D. Your friend concludes that the first child born has a greater chance of inheriting the mutant *D* allele than do later children.

A. According to Mendel's laws, is this conclusion plausible?

B. What is the probability of obtaining this result by chance?

C. What kind of additional data would be needed to test your friend's idea?

D. Is there any way in which your friend's hypothesis might turn out to be right?

Figure Q19–14

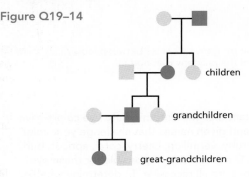
children
grandchildren
great-grandchildren

QUESTION 19–15

Suppose one person in 100 is a carrier of a fatal recessive mutation, such that babies homozygous for the mutation die soon after birth. In a population where there are 1,000,000 births per year, how many babies per year will be born with the lethal homozygous condition?

QUESTION 19–16

Certain mutations are called *dominant-negative mutations*. What do you think this means and how do you suppose these mutations act? Explain the difference between a dominant-negative mutation and a gain-of-function mutation.

QUESTION 19–17

Early genetic studies in *Drosophila* laid the foundation for our current understanding of genes. *Drosophila* geneticists were able to generate mutant flies with a variety of easily observable phenotypic changes. Alterations from the fly's normal brick-red eye color have a venerable history because the very first mutant found by Thomas Hunt Morgan was a white-eyed fly (Figure Q19–17). Since that time, a large

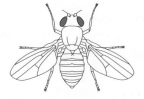

brick-red

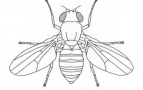

flies with other eye colors

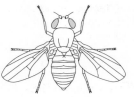

white

Figure Q19–17

TABLE Q19–17 COMPLEMENTATION ANALYSIS OF *Drosophila* EYE-COLOR MUTATIONS

Mutation	white	garnet	ruby	vermilion	cherry	coral	apricot	buff	carnation
white	−	+	+	+	−	−	−	−	+
garnet		−	+	+	+	+	+	+	+
ruby			−	+	+	+	+	+	+
vermilion				−	+	+	+	+	+
cherry					−	−	−	−	+
coral						−	−	−	+
apricot							−	−	+
buff								−	+
carnation									−

+ indicates that progeny of a cross between individuals showing the indicated eye colors are phenotypically normal; − indicates that the eye color of the progeny is abnormal.

number of mutant flies with intermediate eye colors have been isolated and given names that challenge your color sense: garnet, ruby, vermilion, cherry, coral, apricot, buff, and carnation. The mutations responsible for these eye-color phenotypes are all recessive. To determine whether the mutations affected the same or different genes, homozygous flies for each mutation were bred to one another in pairs and the eye colors of their progeny were noted. In Table Q19–17, a + or a − indicates the phenotype of the progeny flies produced by mating the fly listed at the top of the column with the fly listed to the left of the row; brick-red wild-type eyes are shown as + and other colors are indicated as −.

A. How is it that flies with two different eye colors—ruby and white, for example—can give rise to progeny that all have brick-red eyes?

B. Which mutations are alleles of the same gene and which affect different genes?

C. How can different alleles of the same gene give different eye colors?

QUESTION 19–18

What are single-nucleotide polymorphisms (SNPs), and how can they be used to locate a mutant gene by linkage analysis?

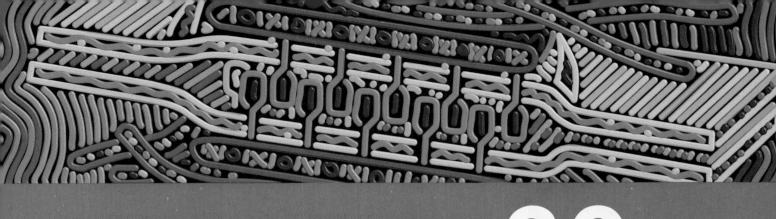

CHAPTER TWENTY

20

Cell Communities: Tissues, Stem Cells, and Cancer

Cells are the building blocks of multicellular organisms. Although this seems a relatively simple statement, it raises deep questions. Cells are not like bricks: they are small and squishy and enclosed in a flimsy membrane less than a hundred-thousandth of a millimeter thick. How, then, can cells be joined together robustly to construct a giraffe's neck, a redwood tree, or muscles that can support an elephant's weight? How are all the different cell types in a plant or an animal produced, and how do they assemble so that each is in its proper place (Figure 20–1)? Most mysterious of all, if cells are the building blocks, where is the builder and where are the architect's plans?

Most of the cells in multicellular organisms are organized into cooperative assemblies called **tissues**, such as the nervous, muscular, epithelial, and connective tissues found in vertebrates; tissues, in turn, are organized into organs, such as heart, lung, brain and kidney (Figure 20–2). In this chapter, we begin by discussing the architecture of tissues from a mechanical point of view. We see that tissues are composed not only of cells, with their internal framework of cytoskeletal filaments (discussed in Chapter 17), but also of **extracellular matrix**, the material that cells secrete around themselves; it is this matrix that gives supportive tissues such as bone or wood their strength. At the same time, cells can also attach to one another directly. Thus, we also discuss the *cell junctions* that link cells together in the flexible epithelial tissues of animals. These junctions transmit forces either from the cytoskeleton of one cell to that of the next, or from the cytoskeleton of a cell to the extracellular matrix.

But there is more to the organization of tissues than mechanics. Just as a building needs plumbing, telephone lines, and other fittings, so an animal tissue requires blood vessels, nerves, and other components formed

EXTRACELLULAR MATRIX AND CONNECTIVE TISSUES

EPITHELIAL SHEETS AND CELL JUNCTIONS

STEM CELLS AND TISSUE RENEWAL

CANCER

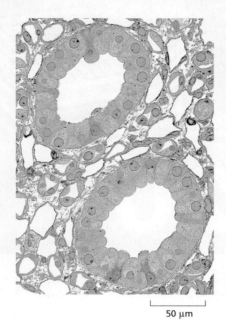

Figure 20–1 Multicellular organisms are built from organized collections of cells. This thin section shows cells in the urine-collecting ducts of a human kidney. Each duct is made of closely packed "principal" cells, which form an epithelial tube, seen here in cross section as rings of cells. The ducts are embedded in an extracellular matrix populated by other types of cells. (Jose Luis Calvo/Shutterstock.)

50 μm

from a variety of specialized cell types. All the tissue components have to be appropriately organized and functionally coordinated, and many of them require continual maintenance and renewal. Cells die and have to be replaced with new cells of the right type, in the right places, and in the right numbers. In the third section of this chapter, we discuss how these processes are organized, as well as the crucial role that *stem cells*—self-renewing, undifferentiated cells—play in the renewal and repair of some tissues.

Disorders of tissue renewal are a major medical concern, and those due to the misbehavior of mutant cells underlie the development of *cancer*. We discuss cancer in the final section of this chapter and of the book as a whole. The study of cancer requires a synthesis of knowledge of cells and tissues at every level, from the molecular biology of DNA repair to the principles of natural selection and the social interactions of cells in tissues. Many fundamental advances in cell biology have been driven by cancer research, and basic cell biology in return continues to deepen our understanding of cancer and provide us with renewed optimism about its treatment.

EXTRACELLULAR MATRIX AND CONNECTIVE TISSUES

Plants and animals have evolved their multicellular organization independently, and their tissues are constructed on different principles. Animals prey on other living things—and often are preyed on by other animals—and for these reasons they must be strong and agile: they must possess tissues capable of rapid movement, and the cells that form those tissues must be able to generate and transmit forces and to change shape quickly. Plants, by contrast, are sedentary: their tissues are more or less rigid, although their cells are weak and fragile if isolated from the stiff supporting matrix that surrounds them.

In plants, the supportive matrix is called the **cell wall**, a boxlike structure that encloses, protects, immobilizes, and shapes each cell (Figure 20–3).

Figure 20–2 Cells are organized into tissues, and tissues often assemble into organs. Simplified drawing of a cross section through part of the wall of the intestine of a mammal. This long, tubelike organ is constructed from epithelial tissues (*red*), connective tissues (*green*), and muscle tissues (*yellow*). Each tissue is an organized assembly of cells, held together by cell–cell adhesions, extracellular matrix, or both.

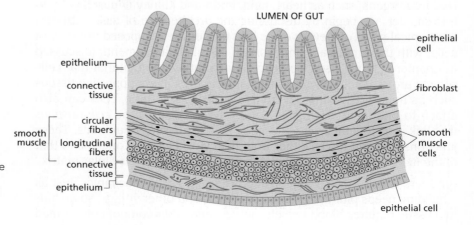

LUMEN OF GUT

epithelium

connective tissue

smooth muscle { circular fibers / longitudinal fibers }

connective tissue

epithelium

epithelial cell

fibroblast

smooth muscle cells

epithelial cell

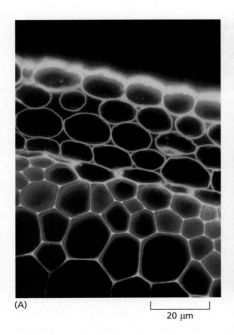

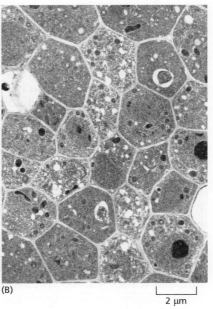

(A) ⊢————————⊣
20 μm

(B) ⊢————————⊣
2 μm

Figure 20–3 Plant tissues are strengthened by cell walls. (A) A cross section of part of the stem of the flowering plant *Arabidopsis* is shown, stained with fluorescent dyes that label two different cell wall polysaccharides—cellulose in *blue*, and pectin in *green*. The cells themselves are unstained and invisible in this preparation. Regions rich in both cellulose and pectin appear white. Pectin predominates in the outer layers of cells, which have only primary cell walls (deposited while the cell is still growing). Cellulose is more plentiful in the inner layers, which have thicker, more rigid secondary cell walls (deposited after cell growth has ceased). (B) Cells and their primary cell walls are clearly seen in this electron micrograph of the young cells in the root of the same plant. These cells are much smaller than those in the stem, as can be seen by the different scale bars in the two micrographs. (Courtesy of Paul Linstead.)

Plant cells themselves synthesize, secrete, and control the composition of this extracellular matrix: a cell wall can be thick and hard, as in wood, or thin and flexible, as in a leaf. But the principle of construction is the same in either case: many tiny boxes are cemented together, with a delicate cell living inside each one. Indeed, as we noted in Chapter 1, it was the close-packed mass of microscopic chambers that Robert Hooke saw in a slice of cork three centuries ago that inspired the term "cell."

Animal tissues are more diverse. Like plant tissues, they consist of both cells and extracellular matrix, but these components are organized in many different ways. In specialized connective tissues, such as bone or tendon, extracellular matrix is plentiful and mechanically all-important; in other tissues, such as muscle or the epidermis of the skin, extracellular matrix is scanty, and the cytoskeletons of the cells themselves carry the mechanical load. We begin this section with a brief discussion of plant cells and tissues before considering those of animals.

Plant Cells Have Tough External Walls

A naked plant cell, artificially stripped of its wall, is a delicate and vulnerable thing. With care, it can be kept alive in culture; but it is easily ruptured, and even a small decrease in the osmotic strength of the culture medium can cause the cell to swell and burst. Its cytoskeleton lacks the tension-bearing intermediate filaments found in animal cells, and as a result, it has virtually no tensile strength. An external wall, therefore, is essential.

The plant cell wall has to be tough, but it does not necessarily have to be rigid. Osmotic swelling of the cell, limited by the resistance of the cell wall, can keep the chamber distended, and a mass of such swollen chambers cemented together forms a semirigid tissue. Such is the state of a crisp lettuce leaf. If water is lacking, the cells shrink and the leaf wilts.

Most newly formed cells in a plant initially make relatively thin *primary cell walls*, which can slowly expand to accommodate cell growth (see Figure 20–3B). The driving force for cell growth is the same as that keeping the lettuce leaf crisp—a swelling pressure, called the *turgor pressure*, that develops as the result of an osmotic imbalance between the interior

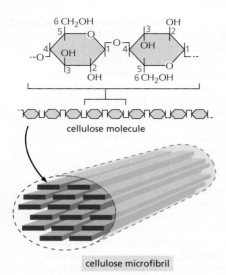

Figure 20–4 A cellulose microfibril is made from a bundle of cellulose molecules. Cellulose molecules are long, unbranched chains of glucose. Each glucose subunit is inverted with respect to its neighbors and joined to them via a β1,4-linkage. The resulting disaccharide repeat occurs hundreds of times in each individual cellulose molecule. About 16 cellulose molecules are held together via hydrogen bonds in a single cellulose microfibril, as shown.

of the plant cell and its surroundings. Once cell growth stops and the wall no longer needs to expand, a more rigid *secondary cell wall* is often produced (see Figure 20–3A)—either by thickening of the primary wall or by deposition of new layers with a different composition underneath the old ones. When plant cells become specialized, they generally produce specially adapted types of walls: waxy, waterproof walls for the surface epidermal cells of a leaf; hard, thick, woody walls for the xylem cells of the stem; and so on.

Cellulose Microfibrils Give the Plant Cell Wall Its Tensile Strength

Like all extracellular matrices, plant cell walls derive their tensile strength from long fibers oriented along the lines of stress. In higher plants, the long fibers are generally made from the polysaccharide *cellulose*, the most abundant organic macromolecule on Earth (**Figure 20–4**). These **cellulose microfibrils** are interwoven with other polysaccharides and some structural proteins, all bonded together to form a complex structure that resists both compression and tension (**Figure 20–5**). In woody tissue, a highly cross-linked network of *lignin* (a complex polymer built from aromatic alcohol groups) is deposited within this matrix to make it more rigid and waterproof.

For a plant cell to grow or change its shape, the cell wall has to stretch or deform. Because the cellulose microfibrils resist stretching, their orientation governs the direction in which the growing cell enlarges: if, for example, they are arranged circumferentially as a corset, the cell will grow more readily in length than in girth (**Figure 20–6**). By controlling the way that it lays down its wall, the plant cell consequently controls its own shape and thus the direction of growth of the tissue to which it belongs.

Cellulose is produced in a radically different way from most other extracellular macromolecules. Instead of being made inside the cell and then exported by exocytosis (discussed in Chapter 15), it is synthesized on the outer surface of the cell by enzyme complexes embedded in the plasma membrane. These complexes transport glucose monomers from the cytosol across the plasma membrane and incorporate them into a set of growing cellulose chains at their points of membrane attachment. The resulting cellulose chains assemble to form a cellulose microfibril (see Figure 20–4).

The paths followed by the membrane-embedded enzyme complexes dictate the orientation in which cellulose is deposited in the cell wall. But

Figure 20–5 A scale model shows a portion of a primary plant cell wall. Cellulose microfibrils (*blue*) provide tensile strength. Other polysaccharides (*red* strands) cross-link the cellulose microfibrils, while the polysaccharide pectin (*green* strands) fills the spaces between the microfibrils, providing resistance to compression. The middle lamella (*yellow*) is rich in pectin and is the layer that cements one cell wall to another.

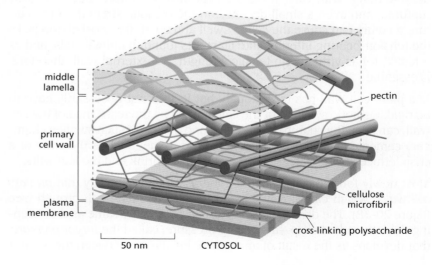

what directs the enzyme complexes? Just beneath the plasma membrane, microtubules are aligned exactly with the cellulose microfibrils outside the cell. The microtubules serve as tracks that help guide the movement of the enzyme complexes (**Figure 20–7**). In this curiously indirect way, the cytoskeleton controls the shape of the plant cell and the modeling of the plant tissues. We will see that animal cells use their cytoskeleton to control tissue architecture in a much more direct manner.

Animal Connective Tissues Consist Largely of Extracellular Matrix

It is traditional to distinguish four major types of tissues in animals: connective, epithelial, nervous, and muscular. But the basic architectural distinction is between connective tissues and the rest. In **connective tissues**, extracellular matrix is abundant and carries the mechanical load. In other tissues, such as epithelia, extracellular matrix is sparse, and the cells are directly joined to one another and carry the mechanical load themselves. We discuss connective tissues first.

Animal connective tissues are enormously varied. They can be tough and flexible like tendons or the dermis of the skin; hard and dense like bone; resilient and shock-absorbing like cartilage; or soft and transparent like the jelly that fills the interior of the eye. In all these examples, the bulk of the tissue is occupied by extracellular matrix, and the cells that produce

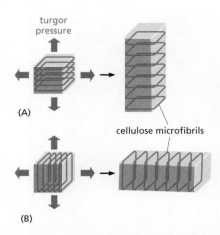

Figure 20–6 The orientation of cellulose microfibrils within the plant cell wall influences the direction in which the cell elongates. The cells in (A) and (B) start off with identical shapes (shown here as *cubes*) but with different orientations of cellulose microfibrils (*blue*) in their walls. Although turgor pressure is uniform in all directions, each cell tends to elongate in a direction perpendicular to the orientation of the microfibrils, which have great tensile strength. The final shape of an organ, such as a shoot, is determined by the direction in which its cells expand.

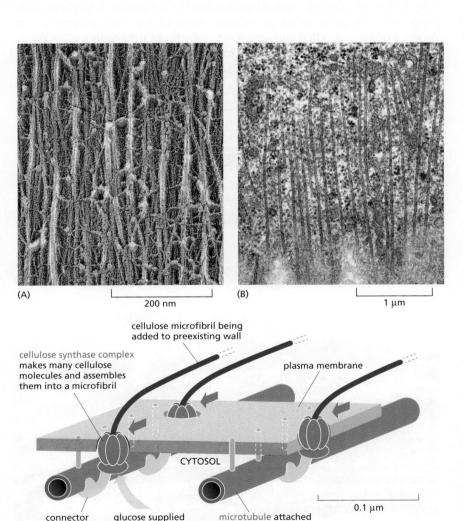

(A) 200 nm (B) 1 μm

cellulose microfibril being added to preexisting wall

cellulose synthase complex makes many cellulose molecules and assembles them into a microfibril

plasma membrane

CYTOSOL

connector protein

glucose supplied from cytosol

microtubule attached to plasma membrane

0.1 μm

(C)

Figure 20–7 Microtubules help direct the deposition of cellulose in the plant cell wall. Electron micrographs show (A) oriented cellulose microfibrils in a plant cell wall and (B) microtubules just beneath a plant cell's plasma membrane. (C) The orientation of the newly deposited extracellular cellulose microfibrils (*dark blue* strands) is determined by the orientation of the underlying intracellular microtubules (*dark green*). The large *cellulose synthase* enzyme complexes (*light blue*) are integral membrane proteins that continuously synthesize cellulose microfibrils on the outer face of the plasma membrane. The distal ends of the stiff microfibrils become integrated into the texture of the cell wall (not shown), and their elongation at the other end pushes the synthase complex along in the plane of the plasma membrane (*blue* arrow). The cortical array of microtubules attached to the plasma membrane by transmembrane proteins (light *green* vertical bars) helps determine the direction in which the microfibrils are laid down. (A, courtesy of Brian Wells and Keith Roberts; B, courtesy of Brian Gunning: from Plant Cell Biology on DVD, Information for Students and a Resource for Teachers. Springer 2009.)

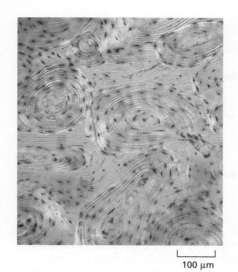

Figure 20–8 Extracellular matrix is plentiful in connective tissue such as bone. This micrograph shows a cross section of bone in which the cells have been lost during preparation. The spaces where the cells had been appear as small, dark, antlike shapes in the bone matrix, which occupies most of the volume of the tissue and provides all its mechanical strength. The alternating light and dark bands are layers of matrix, consisting almost entirely of oriented fibrils of type I collagen (made visible with the help of polarized light). Calcium phosphate crystals (not visible) fill the interstices between the collagen fibrils, strengthening the bone matrix and hardening it like reinforced concrete.

QUESTION 20–1

Cells in the stem of a seedling that is grown in the dark orient their microtubules horizontally. How would you expect this to affect the growth of the plant?

Figure 20–9 Collagen fibrils are organized into bundles. The drawings show the steps of collagen assembly, from individual polypeptide chains to triple-stranded collagen molecules, then to fibrils and, finally, fibers. The electron micrograph shows fully assembled collagen fibers in the connective tissue of embryonic chick skin. The fibrils are bundled into fibers, some running in the plane of the section, others approximately at right angles to it. The cell in the micrograph is a fibroblast, which secretes collagen and other extracellular matrix components. (Photograph from C. Ploetz, E.I. Zycband, and D.E. Birk, *J. Struct. Biol.* 106:73–81, 1991. With permission from Elsevier.)

the matrix are scattered within it like raisins in a pudding (**Figure 20–8**); the tensile strength—whether great or small—is chiefly provided not by a polysaccharide, as it is in the cell wall of plants, but by fibrous proteins, principally collagens. The various types of connective tissues owe their specific characters to the type of collagen that they contain, to its quantity, and, most importantly, to the other molecules that are interwoven with it in varying proportions. These other molecules include the rubbery protein *elastin*, which gives the walls of arteries their resilience as blood pulses through them, as well as a host of specialized polysaccharide molecules, which we discuss shortly.

Collagen Provides Tensile Strength in Animal Connective Tissues

The **collagens** are a family of proteins that come in many varieties. Mammals have over 40 different collagen genes coding for the various collagens that support the structure and function of different tissues. Collagens are the chief proteins in bone, tendon, and skin (leather is pickled collagen), and they constitute 25% of the total protein mass in a mammal—more than any other type of protein. Type I collagen, which is the most abundant, accounts for 90% of the body's collagen.

The characteristic feature of a typical collagen molecule is its long, stiff, triple-stranded helical structure, in which three collagen polypeptide chains are wound around one another in a ropelike superhelix (see Figure 4–29A). Some types of collagen molecules in turn assemble into ordered polymers called *collagen fibrils*, which are thin cables 10–300 nm in diameter and many micrometers long; these can pack together into still thicker *collagen fibers* (**Figure 20–9**). Other types of collagen molecules

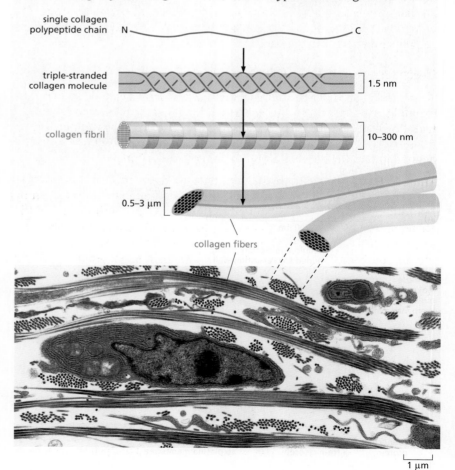

decorate the surface of collagen fibrils and link the fibrils to one another and to other components in the extracellular matrix.

The connective-tissue cells that manufacture and inhabit the extracellular matrix go by various names according to their tissue type: in skin, tendon, and many other connective tissues, they are called **fibroblasts** (see Figure 20–9); in bone, they are called *osteoblasts*. These cells make both the collagen and the other macromolecules of the matrix. Almost all of these molecules are synthesized intracellularly and then secreted in the standard way by exocytosis (discussed in Chapter 15). Outside the cell, they assemble into huge, cohesive aggregates. If assembly were to occur prematurely, before secretion, the cell would become choked with its own products. In the case of collagen, the cells avoid this catastrophe by secreting collagen molecules in a precursor form, called *procollagen*, which has additional peptide extensions at each end that obstruct premature assembly into collagen fibrils. Extracellular enzymes—called procollagen proteinases—cut off these terminal extensions to allow assembly only after the molecules have emerged into the extracellular space (**Figure 20–10**).

Some people have a genetic defect in one of the extracellular proteinases, so that their collagen fibrils do not assemble correctly. As a result, their connective tissues have a lower tensile strength and are extraordinarily stretchable (**Figure 20–11**).

Cells in tissues have to be able to degrade extracellular matrix as well as make it. This ability is essential for tissue growth, repair, and renewal; it is also important where migratory cells, such as macrophages, need to burrow through the thicket of collagen and other matrix polymers. Matrix proteases that cleave extracellular proteins play a part in many disease processes, ranging from arthritis, where they contribute to the breakdown of cartilage in affected joints, to cancer, where they help cancer cells invade normal tissue.

Cells Organize the Collagen They Secrete

To do their job, collagen fibrils must be correctly aligned. In skin, for example, they are woven in a wickerwork pattern, or in alternating layers with different orientations so as to resist tensile stress in multiple directions (**Figure 20–12**). In tendons, which attach muscles to bone, they are aligned in parallel bundles along the major axis of tension.

The connective-tissue cells that produce collagen control this orientation, first by depositing the collagen in an oriented fashion and then by rearranging it. During development of the tissue, fibroblasts work on the collagen they have secreted, crawling over it and pulling on it—helping to compact it into sheets and draw it out into cables. This mechanical role of fibroblasts in shaping collagen matrices has been demonstrated dramatically in cell culture. When fibroblasts are mixed with a meshwork of randomly oriented collagen fibrils that form a gel in a culture dish, the fibroblasts tug on the meshwork, drawing in collagen from their surroundings and compacting it. If two small pieces of embryonic tissue containing fibroblasts are placed far apart on a collagen gel, the

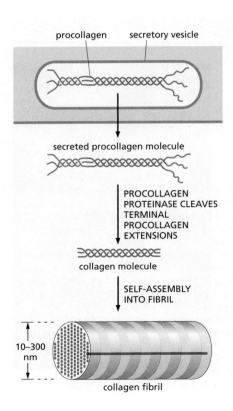

Figure 20–10 Procollagen precursors are cleaved to form mature collagen outside the cell. Collagen is synthesized as a procollagen molecule that has unstructured peptides at either end. These peptides prevent collagen fibrils from assembling inside the fibroblast. When the procollagen is secreted, extracellular procollagen proteinases remove its terminal peptides, producing mature collagen molecules. These molecules can then self-assemble into ordered collagen fibrils (see also Figure 20–9).

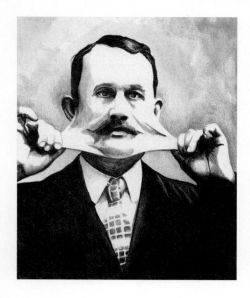

Figure 20–11 **Incorrect collagen assembly can cause the skin to be hyperextensible.** James Morris, "the elastic skin man," from a photograph taken in about 1890. Abnormally stretchable skin is part of a genetic syndrome that results from a defect in collagen assembly. In some individuals, this condition arises from a lack of an enzyme that converts procollagen to collagen; in others, it is caused by a defect in procollagen itself.

intervening collagen becomes organized into a dense band of aligned fibers that connect the two explants (**Figure 20–13**). The fibroblasts migrate out from the explants along the aligned collagen fibers. In this way, the fibroblasts influence the alignment of the collagen fibers, and the collagen fibers in turn affect the distribution of the fibroblasts. Fibroblasts presumably play a similar role in generating long-range order in the extracellular matrix inside the developing body—in helping to create tendons, for example, and the tough, dense layers of connective tissue that ensheathe and bind together most organs. Fibroblast migration is also important for healing wounds (Movie 20.1).

Integrins Couple the Matrix Outside a Cell to the Cytoskeleton Inside It

Cells are able to interact with the collagen in the extracellular matrix thanks to a family of transmembrane receptor proteins called **integrins**. The extracellular domain of an integrin binds to components of the matrix, while its intracellular domain interacts with the cell cytoskeleton. This internal mooring provides a strong and stable point of attachment; without it, integrins would be easily torn from the flimsy lipid bilayer, and cells would be unable to anchor themselves to the matrix.

Integrins do not, however, interact directly with collagen fibers in the extracellular matrix. Instead, another extracellular matrix protein, **fibronectin**, provides a linkage: part of the fibronectin molecule binds to collagen, while another part forms an attachment site for integrins.

When the extracellular domain of the integrin binds to fibronectin, the intracellular domain binds (through a set of adaptor molecules) to an actin filament inside the cell (**Figure 20–14**). For many cells, it is the formation and breakage of these attachments on either end of an integrin molecule that allows the cell to crawl through a tissue, grabbing hold of the matrix at its front end and releasing its grip at the rear (see Figure 17–33). Integrins coordinate these "catch-and-release" maneuvers by undergoing remarkable conformational changes. Binding to a molecule on one side of the plasma membrane causes the integrin molecule to stretch out into an extended, activated state so that it can then latch onto a different molecule on the opposite side—an effect that operates in either direction across the membrane (**Figure 20–15**). Thus, an intracellular signaling molecule can activate the integrin from the cytosolic side, causing it to reach out and grab hold of an extracellular structure. Similarly, binding to an external structure can switch on a variety of intracellular signaling pathways by activating protein kinases that associate with the intracellular end of the integrin. In this way, a cell's external attachments can help regulate its behavior—and even its survival.

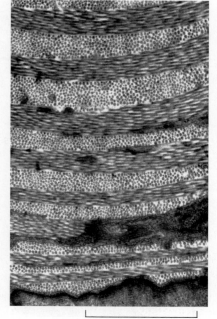

5 μm

Figure 20–12 **Collagen fibrils in the skin of some animals are arranged in a plywoodlike pattern.** The electron micrograph shows a cross section of tadpole skin. Successive layers of fibrils are laid down nearly at right angles to each other (see also Figure 20–9). This arrangement is also found in mature bone and in the cornea, but not in mammalian skin. (Courtesy of Jerome Gross.)

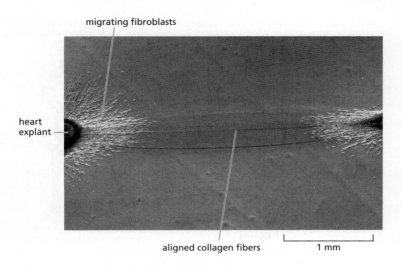

migrating fibroblasts

heart explant

aligned collagen fibers   1 mm

Figure 20–13 Fibroblasts influence the alignment of collagen fibers. This micrograph shows a region between two pieces of embryonic chick heart (rich in fibroblasts and heart muscle cells), which have grown in culture on a collagen gel for four days. A dense tract of aligned collagen fibers has formed between the explants, presumably as a result of the fibroblasts, which have proliferated and migrated out from the explants, tugging on the collagen. Elsewhere in the culture dish, the collagen remains disorganized and unaligned, so that it appears uniformly gray. (From D. Stopak and A.K. Harris, *Dev. Biol.* 90:383–398, 1982. With permission from Elsevier.)

Humans make at least 24 kinds of integrins, each of which recognizes distinct extracellular molecules and has distinct functions, depending on the cell type in which it resides. For example, the integrins on white blood cells (leukocytes) help the cells crawl out of blood vessels at sites of infection so as to deal with marauding microbes. People who lack this type of integrin develop a disease called *leucocyte adhesion deficiency* and suffer from repeated bacterial infections. A different form of integrin is found on blood platelets, and individuals who lack this integrin bleed excessively because their platelets cannot bind to the necessary blood-clotting protein in the extracellular matrix.

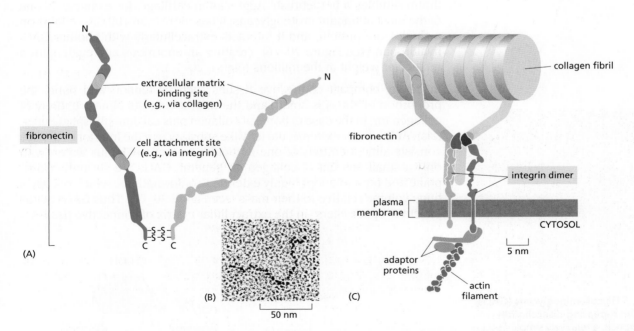

N

extracellular matrix binding site (e.g., via collagen)

N

fibronectin

cell attachment site (e.g., via integrin)

—S—S—
—S—S—
C   C

(A)

(B)

50 nm

collagen fibril

fibronectin

integrin dimer

plasma membrane

CYTOSOL

5 nm

adaptor proteins

actin filament

(C)

Figure 20–14 Fibronectin and transmembrane integrin proteins help attach a cell to the extracellular matrix. Fibronectin molecules bind to collagen fibrils outside the cell. Integrins in the plasma membrane bind to the fibronectin and tether it to the cytoskeleton inside the cell. (A) Diagram and (B) electron micrograph of a molecule of fibronectin. (C) The transmembrane linkage mediated by an integrin protein (*blue* and *green* dimer). The integrin molecule transmits tension across the plasma membrane: it is anchored inside the cell via adaptor proteins to the actin cytoskeleton and externally via fibronectin to other extracellular matrix proteins, such as the collagen fibril shown. The integrin shown here links fibronectin to an actin filament inside the cell. Other integrins can connect different extracellular proteins to the cytoskeleton (usually to actin filaments, but sometimes to intermediate filaments). (B, from J. Engel et al., *J. Mol. Biol.* 150:97–120, 1981. With permission from Elsevier.)

Figure 20–15 An integrin protein switches to an active conformation when it binds to molecules on either side of the plasma membrane. An integrin protein consists of two different subunits, α (*green*) and β (*blue*), both of which can switch between a folded, inactive form and an extended, active form. The switch to the activated state can be triggered by binding to an extracellular matrix molecule (such as fibronectin) or to intracellular adaptor proteins that then link the integrin to the cytoskeleton (see Figure 20–14). In both cases, the conformational change alters the integrin so that its opposite end rapidly forms a counterbalancing attachment to the appropriate structure. In this way, the integrin establishes a reversible mechanical linkage across the plasma membrane. (Based on T. Xiao et al., *Nature* 432:59–67, 2004.)

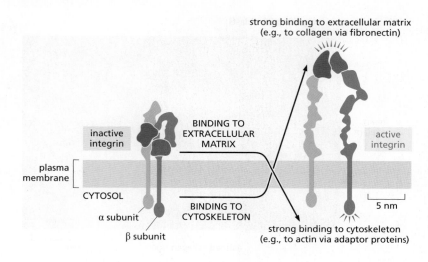

Gels of Polysaccharides and Proteins Fill Spaces and Resist Compression

While collagen provides tensile strength to resist stretching, a completely different group of macromolecules in the extracellular matrix of animal tissues provides the complementary function, resisting compression. These are the **glycosaminoglycans** (GAGs), negatively charged polysaccharide chains made of repeating disaccharide units (Figure 20–16). Chains of GAGs are usually covalently linked to a core protein to form **proteoglycans**, which are extremely diverse in size, shape, and chemistry. Typically, many GAG chains are attached to a single core protein that may, in turn, be linked to another GAG, creating a macromolecule that resembles a bottlebrush. Aggrecan in cartilage, for example, is one of the most abundant proteoglycans; it has more than 100 GAG chains on a single core protein, and it interacts extracellularly with another GAG, hyaluronan (see Figure 20–16), creating an enormous aggregate with a molecular weight in the millions (Figure 20–17).

In dense, compact connective tissues such as tendon and bone, the proportion of GAGs is small, and the matrix consists almost entirely of collagen (or, in the case of bone, of collagen plus calcium phosphate crystals). At the other extreme, the jellylike substance in the interior of the eye consists almost entirely of one particular type of GAG, plus water, with only a small amount of collagen. In general, GAGs are strongly hydrophilic and tend to adopt highly extended conformations, which occupy a huge volume relative to their mass (see Figure 20–17). Thus GAGs act as effective "space fillers" in the extracellular matrix of connective tissues.

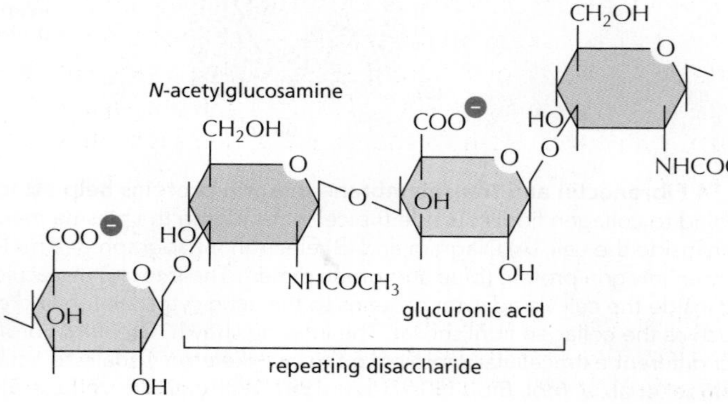

Figure 20–16 Glycosaminoglycans (GAGs) are built from repeating disaccharide units. Hyaluronan, a relatively simple GAG, is shown here. It consists of a single long chain of up to 25,000 repeated disaccharide units, each carrying a negative charge (*red*). As in other GAGs, one of the sugar monomers (*green*) in each disaccharide unit is an amino sugar. Many GAGs have additional negative charges, often from sulfate groups (not shown).

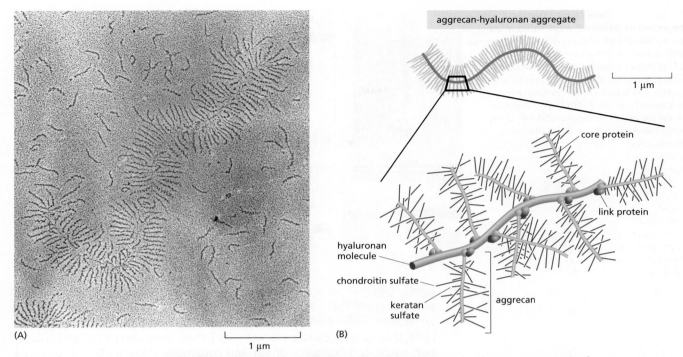

Figure 20–17 Proteoglycans and GAGs can form large aggregates. (A) Electron micrograph of an aggrecan–hyaluronan aggregate from cartilage, spread out on a flat surface. (B) Schematic drawing of the giant aggregate illustrated in (A), showing how it is built up from aggrecan subunits bristling with numerous GAG chains—chondroitin sulfate (long *blue* lines) and keratan sulfate (short *blue* lines)—attached to a core protein (*light green*). These subunits then aggregate via link proteins (*green*) to the GAG hyaluronan (*blue*). The mass of such a complex can be 10^8 daltons or more, and it occupies a volume equivalent to that of a bacterium, which is about 2×10^{-12} cm^3. (A, from J.A. Buckwalter, P.J. Roughley, and L.C. Rosenberg, *Microscopy Research & Technique* 28:398–408, 1994. With permission from John Wiley & Sons.)

Even at very low concentrations, GAGs form hydrophilic gels: their multiple negative charges attract a cloud of cations, such as Na$^+$, that are osmotically active, causing large amounts of water to be sucked into the matrix. This gives rise to a swelling pressure, which is balanced by tension in the collagen fibers interwoven with the GAGs. When the matrix is rich in collagen and large quantities of GAGs are trapped in the mesh, both the swelling pressure and the counterbalancing tension are enormous. Such a matrix is tough, resilient, and resistant to compression. The cartilage matrix that lines the knee joint, for example, has this character: it can support pressures of hundreds of kilograms per square centimeter.

Proteoglycans perform many sophisticated functions in addition to providing hydrated space around cells. They can form gels of varying pore size and charge density that act as filters to regulate the passage of molecules through the extracellular medium. They can bind secreted growth factors and other proteins that serve as extracellular signals for cells. They can block, encourage, or guide cell migration through the matrix. In all these ways, the matrix components influence the behavior of cells, often the same cells that make the matrix—a reciprocal interaction that has important effects on cell differentiation and the arrangement of cells in a tissue. Much remains to be learned about how cells weave the tapestry of matrix molecules and how the chemical messages they deposit in this intricate biochemical fabric are organized and act.

EPITHELIAL SHEETS AND CELL JUNCTIONS

There are more than 200 visibly different cell types in the body of a vertebrate. The majority of these are organized into **epithelia** (singular **epithelium**)—multicellular sheets in which adjacent cells are joined

QUESTION 20–3

Proteoglycans are characterized by the abundance of negative charges on their sugar chains. How would the properties of these molecules differ if the negative charges were not as abundant?

Figure 20–18 Cells can be packed together in different ways to form an epithelial sheet. Micrographs along with drawings show four basic types of epithelia. In each case, the cells are sitting on a thin mat of extracellular matrix, the basal lamina (*yellow*), as discussed shortly. (From D.W. Fawcett, *A Textbook of Histology*, 12th ed. 1994. With permission from Taylor & Francis Books UK.)

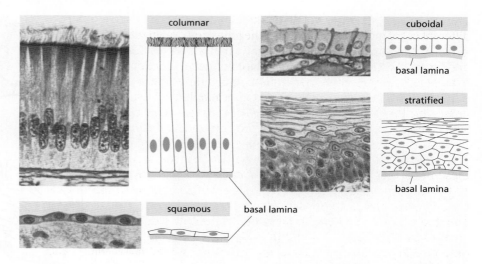

tightly together. In some cases, the sheet is many cells thick, or *stratified*, as in the epidermis (the outer layer of the skin); in other cases, it is a *simple epithelium*, only one cell thick, as in the lining of the gut. The epithelial cells, themselves, can also take many forms. They can be tall and columnar, squat and cuboidal, or flat and squamous (**Figure 20–18**). Within a given sheet, the cells may be all the same type or a mixture of different types. Some epithelia, like the epidermis, act mainly as a protective barrier; others have complex biochemical functions. Some secrete specialized products such as hormones, milk, or tears; others, such as the epithelium lining the gut, absorb nutrients; yet others detect signals, such as light, sensed by the layer of photoreceptors in the retina of the eye, or sound, sensed by the epithelium containing the auditory hair cells in the ear (see Figure 12–28).

Despite these and many other variations, one can recognize a standard set of features that virtually all animal epithelia share. Epithelia cover the external surface of the body and line all its internal cavities, and they must have been an early feature in the evolution of animals. Cells joined together into an epithelial sheet create a barrier, which has the same significance for the multicellular organism that the plasma membrane has for a single cell. It keeps some molecules in, and others out; it takes up nutrients and exports wastes; it contains receptors for environmental signals; and it protects the interior of the organism from invading microorganisms and fluid loss.

The arrangement of cells into epithelia is so commonplace that we sometimes take it for granted. Yet, as we discuss in this section, establishing epithelia requires a collection of specialized structures and molecular devices, which are common to a wide variety of epithelial cell types.

Epithelial Sheets Are Polarized and Rest on a Basal Lamina

An epithelial sheet has two faces: the **apical** surface is free and exposed to the air or to a bodily fluid; the **basal** surface is attached to a sheet of connective tissue called the basal lamina (**Figure 20–19**). The **basal lamina** consists of a thin, tough sheet of extracellular matrix, composed mainly of a specialized type of collagen (type IV collagen) and a protein called *laminin* (**Figure 20–20**). Laminin provides adhesive sites for integrin molecules in the basal plasma membranes of epithelial cells, and it thus serves a linking role like that of fibronectin in other connective tissues.

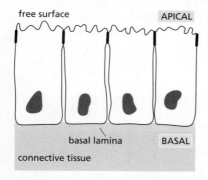

Figure 20–19 A sheet of epithelial cells has an apical and a basal surface. The basal surface sits on a specialized sheet of extracellular matrix called the basal lamina, while the apical surface is free.

The apical and basal faces of an epithelium are different: each contains a different set of molecules that reflect the polarized organization of the individual epithelial cells: each has a top and a bottom, with different properties and functions. This polarity is crucial for epithelial function. Consider, for example, the simple columnar epithelium that lines the small intestine of a mammal. It mainly consists of two intermingled cell types: absorptive cells, which take up nutrients, and goblet cells (so called because of their shape), which secrete the mucus that protects and lubricates the gut lining (Figure 20–21). Both cell types are polarized. The absorptive cells import food molecules from the gut lumen through their apical surface and export these molecules from their basal surface into the underlying tissues. To do this, absorptive cells require different sets of membrane transport proteins in their apical and basal plasma membranes (see Figure 12–17). The goblet cells also have to be polarized, but in a different way: they have to synthesize mucus and then discharge it from their apical end only (see Figure 20–21); their Golgi apparatus, secretory vesicles, and cytoskeleton are all polarized so as to bring this about. For both types of epithelial cells, polarity depends on the junctions that the cells form with one another and with the basal lamina. These cell junctions in turn control the arrangement of an elaborate system of membrane-associated intracellular proteins that create the polarized organization of the cytoplasm, as we discuss next.

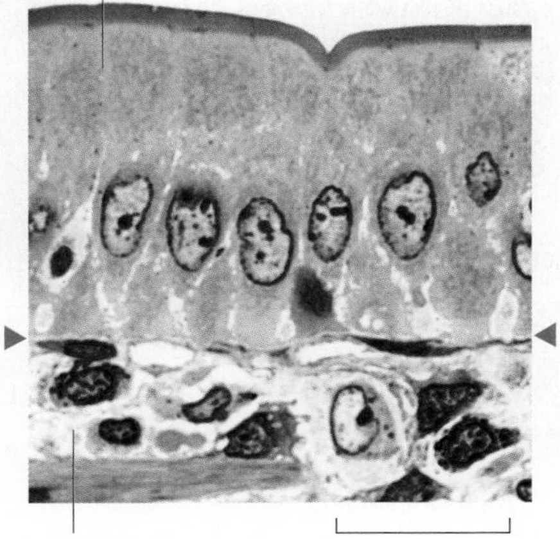

Tight Junctions Make an Epithelium Leakproof and Separate Its Apical and Basolateral Surfaces

Epithelial **cell junctions** can be classified according to their function. Some provide a tight seal to prevent the leakage of molecules across the epithelium through the gaps between its cells; some provide strong mechanical attachments; and some provide for an intimate type of inter-cytosolic exchange. In most epithelia, all these types of junctions are present. As we will see, each type of junction is characterized by its own class of transmembrane proteins.

In vertebrates, the barrier function of epithelial sheets is made possible by **tight junctions**. These junctions seal neighboring cells together so

Figure 20–20 The basal lamina supports a sheet of epithelial cells. Light micrograph of the epithelial sheet that lines the small intestine. The sheet of columnar cells sits on a thin mat-like structure, the basal lamina (*red* arrowheads), which is woven from type IV collagen and laminin proteins. A network of other collagen fibrils and fibers in the underlying connective tissue interacts with the lower face of the lamina. (Jose Luis Calvo/Shutterstock.)

overlying epithelial cells

underlying connective tissue

20 μm

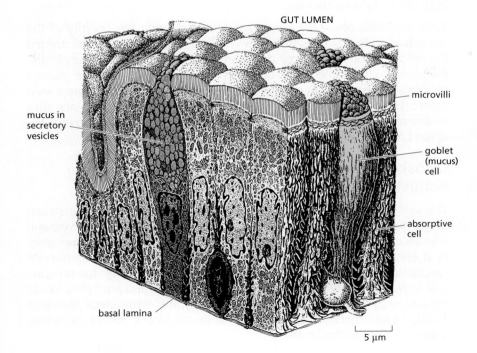

GUT LUMEN

mucus in secretory vesicles

microvilli

goblet (mucus) cell

absorptive cell

basal lamina

5 μm

Figure 20–21 Different types of functionally polarized cell types line the intestine. Absorptive cells, which take up nutrients from the intestine, are mingled in the gut epithelium with goblet cells (*brown*), which secrete mucus into the gut lumen. The absorptive cells are often called *brush-border cells*, because of the brushlike mass of microvilli on their apical surface; the microvilli serve to increase the area of apical plasma membrane for the transport of small molecules into the cell. The goblet cells owe their gobletlike shape to the mass of mucus-containing secretory vesicles that distends the cytoplasm in their apical region. (Adapted from R. Krstić, Human Microscopic Anatomy. Berlin: Springer, 1991. With permission from Springer-Verlag.)

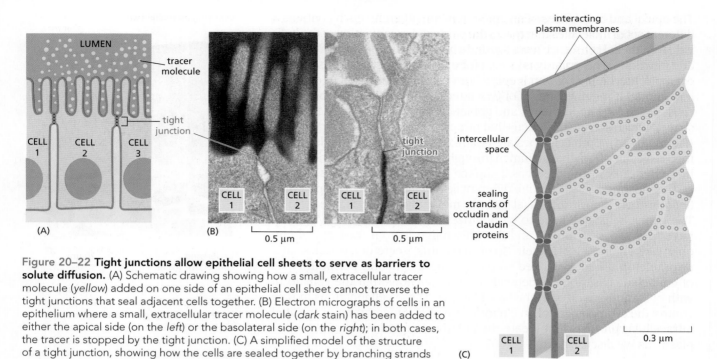

Figure 20–22 Tight junctions allow epithelial cell sheets to serve as barriers to solute diffusion. (A) Schematic drawing showing how a small, extracellular tracer molecule (*yellow*) added on one side of an epithelial cell sheet cannot traverse the tight junctions that seal adjacent cells together. (B) Electron micrographs of cells in an epithelium where a small, extracellular tracer molecule (*dark* stain) has been added to either the apical side (on the *left*) or the basolateral side (on the *right*); in both cases, the tracer is stopped by the tight junction. (C) A simplified model of the structure of a tight junction, showing how the cells are sealed together by branching strands of transmembrane proteins (*green*), called claudins and occludins, in the plasma membranes of the interacting cells. Each type of protein binds to the same type in the apposed membrane (not shown). (B, courtesy of Daniel Friend, by permission of E.L. Bearer.)

that water-soluble molecules cannot easily leak between them. If a small tracer molecule is added to one side of an epithelial cell sheet, it will usually not pass beyond the tight junction (**Figure 20–22A and B**). The tight junction is formed from proteins called *claudins* and *occludins*, which are arranged in strands along the lines of the junction to create the seal (**Figure 20–22C**). Without tight junctions to prevent leakage, the pumping activities of absorptive cells such as those in the gut would be futile, and the composition of the extracellular fluid would become the same on both sides of the epithelium.

Tight junctions also play a key part in maintaining the polarity of the individual epithelial cells in two ways. First, the tight junctions around the apical region of each cell prevent diffusion of proteins in the plasma membrane and so keep the contents of apical domain of the plasma membrane separate—and different—from the basolateral domain (see Figure 11–32). Second, in many epithelia, the tight junctions are sites of assembly for the complexes of intracellular proteins that govern the apico-basal polarity of the cell interior.

Cytoskeleton-linked Junctions Bind Epithelial Cells Robustly to One Another and to the Basal Lamina

The cell junctions that hold an epithelium together by forming strong mechanical attachments are of three main types. *Adherens junctions* and *desmosomes* bind one epithelial cell to another, while *hemidesmosomes* bind epithelial cells to the basal lamina. All of these junctions provide mechanical strength to the epithelium by the same strategy: the proteins that form the junctions span the plasma membrane and are linked inside the cell to cytoskeletal filaments. In this way, the cytoskeletal filaments are tied into a network that extends from cell to cell across the whole expanse of the epithelial sheet.

Adherens junctions and desmosomes are both built around transmembrane proteins that belong to the **cadherin** family: a cadherin molecule in the plasma membrane of one cell binds directly to an identical cadherin molecule in the plasma membrane of its neighbor (Figure 20–23). Such interaction of like-with-like is called *homophilic* binding. In the case of cadherins, binding also requires that Ca^{2+} be present in the extracellular medium—hence the name.

At an **adherens junction**, each cadherin molecule is tethered inside its cell, via several linker proteins, to actin filaments. Often, the adherens junctions form a continuous adhesion belt around each of the interacting epithelial cells; this belt is located near the apical end of the cell, just below the tight junctions (Figure 20–24). Bundles of actin filaments are thus connected from cell to cell across the epithelium. This network of actin filaments also contains myosin filaments and can thus contract, giving the epithelial sheet the capacity to develop tension and to change its shape in remarkable ways. By shrinking the apical surface of an epithelial sheet along one axis, the sheet can roll itself up into a tube (Figure 20–25A and B). Alternatively, by shrinking its apical surface locally along all axes at once, the sheet can invaginate into a cup and eventually create a spherical vesicle by pinching off from the rest of the epithelium (Figure 20–25C). Epithelial movements such as these are crucial during embryonic development, when they create structures such as the neural tube (see Figure 20–25B), which gives rise to the brain and spinal cord, and the lens vesicle, which develops into the lens of the eye (see Figure 20–25C).

At a **desmosome**, a different set of cadherin molecules connects to *keratin filaments*—the intermediate filaments found specifically in epithelial cells (see Figure 17–5). Bundles of ropelike keratin filaments criss-cross the cytoplasm and are "spot-welded" via desmosome junctions to the bundles of keratin filaments in adjacent cells (Figure 20–26). This arrangement confers great tensile strength to the epithelial sheet and is characteristic of tough, exposed epithelia such as the epidermis of the skin.

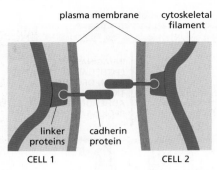

Figure 20–23 Cadherin proteins mediate mechanical attachment of one cell to another. Identical cadherin molecules in the plasma membranes of adjacent cells bind to each other extracellularly; inside the cell, they are attached, via linker proteins, to cytoskeletal filaments—either actin filaments or keratin intermediate filaments. Movie 20.2 shows how, when epithelial cells in culture touch one another, their cadherins become concentrated at the point of attachment, leading to the formation of adherens junctions.

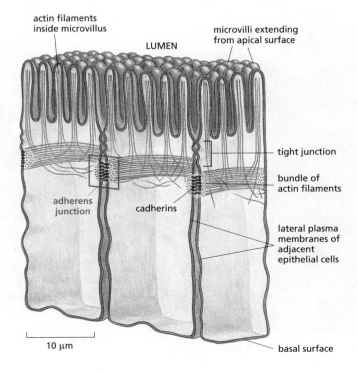

Figure 20–24 Adherens junctions form adhesion belts around epithelial cells in the small intestine. A contractile bundle of actin filaments runs along the cytoplasmic surface of the plasma membrane near the apex of each cell. These bundles are linked to those in adjacent cells via transmembrane cadherin molecules (see Figure 20–23).

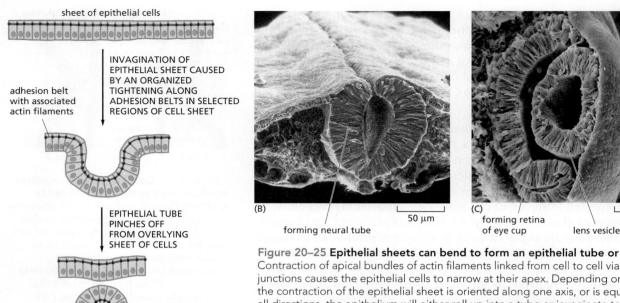

(A)

forming neural tube

(B) 50 μm

forming retina of eye cup   lens vesicle

(C) 50 μm

Figure 20–25 Epithelial sheets can bend to form an epithelial tube or vesicle.
Contraction of apical bundles of actin filaments linked from cell to cell via adherens junctions causes the epithelial cells to narrow at their apex. Depending on whether the contraction of the epithelial sheet is oriented along one axis, or is equal in all directions, the epithelium will either roll up into a tube or invaginate to form a vesicle, respectively. (A) Diagram showing how an apical contraction along one axis of an epithelial sheet can cause the sheet to form a tube. (B) Scanning electron micrograph of a cross section through the trunk of a two-day chick embryo, showing the formation of the neural tube by the process shown in (A). Part of the epithelial sheet that covers the surface of the embryo has thickened and rolled up by apical contraction; the opposing folds are about to fuse, after which the structure will pinch off to form the neural tube. (C) Scanning electron micrograph of a chick embryo showing the formation of the eye cup and lens. A patch of surface epithelium overlying the forming eye cup has become concave and has pinched off as a separate vesicle—the lens vesicle—within the eye cup. This process is driven by an apical narrowing of epithelial cells in all directions. (B, courtesy of Jean-Paul Revel; C, courtesy of K.W. Tosney.)

Blisters are a painful reminder that it is not enough for epidermal cells to be firmly attached to one another: they must also be anchored to the underlying connective tissue. As we noted earlier, the anchorage is mediated by integrins in the cells' basal plasma membranes. The extracellular

Figure 20–26 Desmosomes link the keratin intermediate filaments of one epithelial cell to those of another.
(A) An electron micrograph of a desmosome joining two cells in the epidermis of newt skin, showing the attachment of keratin filaments.
(B) Schematic drawing of a desmosome. On the cytoplasmic surface of each interacting plasma membrane is a dense plaque composed of a mixture of intracellular linker proteins. A bundle of keratin filaments is attached to the surface of each plaque. The cytoplasmic tails of transmembrane cadherin proteins bind to the outer face of each plaque; their extracellular domains interact to hold the cells together. (A, from D.E. Kelly, *J. Cell Biol.* 28:51–72, 1966. With permission from The Rockefeller University Press.)

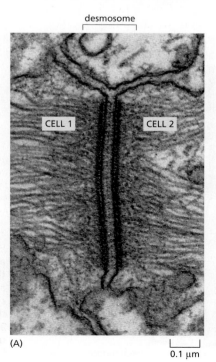

(A) 0.1 μm

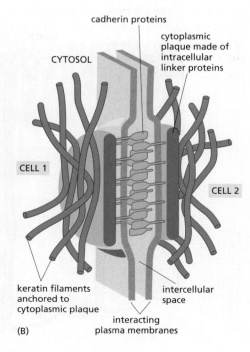

(B)

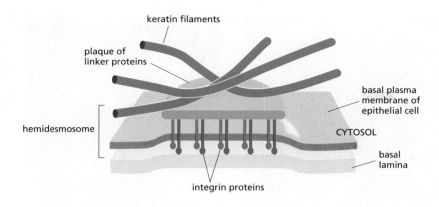

keratin filaments

plaque of
linker proteins

hemidesmosome

basal plasma
membrane of
epithelial cell

CYTOSOL

basal
lamina

integrin proteins

Figure 20–27 Hemidesmosomes anchor the keratin filaments in an epithelial cell to the basal lamina. The linkage is mediated by a transmembrane attachment complex containing integrins, rather than cadherins.

domains of these integrins bind to laminin in the basal lamina; inside the cell, the integrin tails are bound via linker proteins to keratin filaments, creating a structure that looks superficially like half a desmosome. These attachments of epithelial cells to the basal lamina beneath them are therefore called **hemidesmosomes** (Figure 20–27).

Gap Junctions Allow Cytosolic Inorganic Ions and Small Molecules to Pass from Cell to Cell

The final type of epithelial cell junction, found in virtually all epithelia and in many other types of animal tissues, serves a totally different purpose from the junctions discussed so far. In the electron microscope, **gap junctions** appear as regions where the plasma membranes of two cells lie close together and exactly parallel, with a very narrow gap of 2–4 nm between them. The gap, however, is not entirely empty; it is spanned by the protruding ends of many identical, transmembrane protein complexes that reside in the plasma membranes of the two apposed cells. These complexes, called *connexons*, are aligned end-to-end to form narrow, water-filled channels across the interacting membranes (Figure 20–28). The channels allow inorganic ions and small, water-soluble molecules (up to a molecular mass of about 1000 daltons) to move directly from the cytosol of one cell to the cytosol of the other. This flow creates an electrical and a metabolic coupling between the cells. Gap junctions between cardiac muscle cells, for example, provide the electrical coupling that allows electrical waves of excitation to spread synchronously through the heart, triggering the coordinated contraction of the cells that produces each heart beat.

Gap junctions in many tissues can be opened or closed in response to extracellular or intracellular signals. The neurotransmitter dopamine, for

QUESTION 20–4

Analogs of hemidesmosomes are the focal contacts described in Chapter 17, which are also sites where the cell attaches to the extracellular matrix. These junctions are prevalent in fibroblasts but largely absent in epithelial cells. On the other hand, hemidesmosomes are prevalent in epithelial cells but absent in fibroblasts. In focal contact sites, intracellular connections are made to actin filaments, whereas, in hemidesmosomes, connections are made to intermediate filaments. Why do you suppose these two different cell types attach differently to the extracellular matrix?

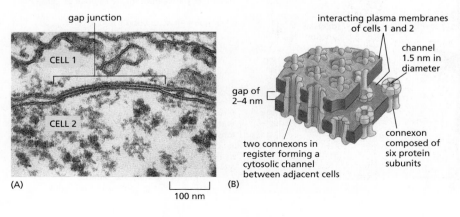

gap junction

CELL 1

CELL 2

(A)

100 nm

interacting plasma membranes
of cells 1 and 2

channel
1.5 nm in
diameter

gap of
2–4 nm

two connexons in
register forming a
cytosolic channel
between adjacent cells

connexon
composed of
six protein
subunits

(B)

Figure 20–28 Gap junctions provide neighboring cells with a direct channel of intercytosolic communication. (A) Electron micrograph of a gap junction between two cells in culture. (B) A model of a gap junction. The drawing shows the interacting plasma membranes of two adjacent cells. The apposed membranes are penetrated by protein assemblies called *connexons* (*green*), each of which is formed from six identical protein subunits. Two connexons join across the intercellular gap to form an aqueous channel connecting the cytosols of the two cells. (A, from N.B. Gilula, in Cell Communication [R.P. Cox, ed.], pp. 1–29. New York: Wiley, 1974. With permission from John Wiley & Sons, Inc.)

Figure 20–29 Extracellular signals can regulate the permeability of gap junctions. (A) A neuron in a rabbit retina (center) was injected with a dye (dark stain) that passes readily through gap junctions. The dye diffuses rapidly from the injected cell to label the surrounding neurons, which are connected by gap junctions. (B) Treatment of the retina with the neurotransmitter dopamine prior to dye injection decreases the permeability of the gap junctions and hampers the spread of the dye. (Courtesy of David Vaney.)

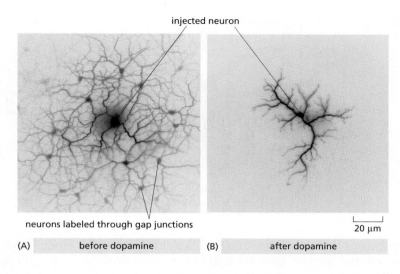

injected neuron

neurons labeled through gap junctions

20 µm

(A)   before dopamine   (B)   after dopamine

QUESTION 20–5

Gap junctions are dynamic structures that, like conventional ion channels, are gated: they can close by a reversible conformational change in response to changes in the cell. The permeability of gap junctions decreases within seconds, for example, when the intracellular Ca^{2+} concentration is raised. Speculate why this form of regulation by Ca^{2+} might be important for the health of a tissue.

Figure 20–30 Several types of cell junctions are found in epithelia in animals. Whereas tight junctions are peculiar to epithelia, the other types also occur, in modified forms, in various nonepithelial tissues.

example, reduces gap-junction communication between certain neurons in the mammalian retina when secreted in response to an increase in light intensity (**Figure 20–29**). This reduction in gap-junction permeability alters the pattern of electrical signaling and helps the retina switch from using rod photoreceptors, which are good detectors of low light levels, to cone photoreceptors, which detect color and fine detail in bright light. The function of gap junctions—and of the other junctions found in animal cells—are summarized in **Figure 20–30**.

Plant tissues lack all the types of cell junctions we have discussed so far, as their cells are held together by their cell walls. Importantly, however, they have a functional counterpart of the gap junction. The cytoplasms of adjacent plant cells are connected via minute communicating channels called **plasmodesmata**, which span the intervening cell walls. In contrast to gap-junction channels, plasmodesmata are cytoplasmic channels lined with plasma membrane (**Figure 20–31**). Thus in plants, the cytoplasm is, in principle, continuous from one cell to the next, allowing the passage of both small and large molecules—including some proteins and regulatory RNAs. The controlled traffic of transcription regulators and regulatory RNAs from one cell to another is important in plant development.

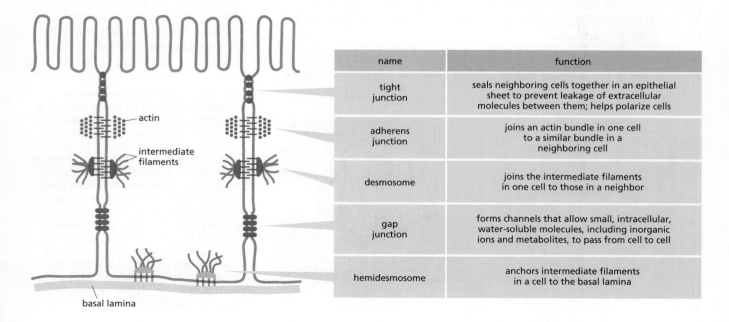

actin

intermediate filaments

basal lamina

name	function
tight junction	seals neighboring cells together in an epithelial sheet to prevent leakage of extracellular molecules between them; helps polarize cells
adherens junction	joins an actin bundle in one cell to a similar bundle in a neighboring cell
desmosome	joins the intermediate filaments in one cell to those in a neighbor
gap junction	forms channels that allow small, intracellular, water-soluble molecules, including inorganic ions and metabolites, to pass from cell to cell
hemidesmosome	anchors intermediate filaments in a cell to the basal lamina

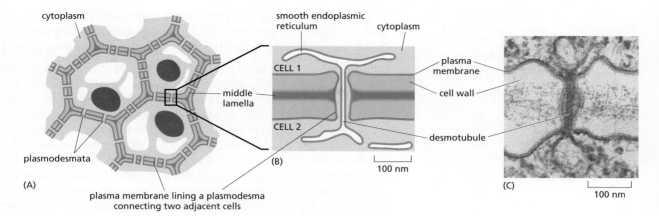

Figure 20–31 The cytoplasms of adjacent plant cells are connected via plasmodesmata. (A) The intercytoplasmic channels of plasmodesmata pierce the plant cell walls and connect the interiors of all cells in a plant. (B) Each plasmodesma is lined with plasma membrane common to the two connected cells. It usually also contains a fine tubular structure, the desmotubule, derived from smooth endoplasmic reticulum. (C) Micrograph of plasmodesmata. (C, courtesy of L.G. Tilney.)

STEM CELLS AND TISSUE RENEWAL

One cannot contemplate the organization of tissues without wondering how these astonishingly patterned structures come into being. This question raises an even more challenging one—a puzzle that is one of the most ancient and fundamental in all of biology: how is a complex multicellular organism generated from a single fertilized egg?

In the process of development, the fertilized egg cell divides repeatedly to give a clone of cells—about 10,000,000,000,000 for a human—essentially all containing the same genome but specialized in different ways. This clone has a remarkable structure. It may take the form of a daisy or an oak tree, a sea urchin, a whale, or a mouse. The structure is determined by the genome that the fertilized egg contains (**Figure 20–32**). The linear sequence of A, G, C, and T nucleotides in the DNA directs the production

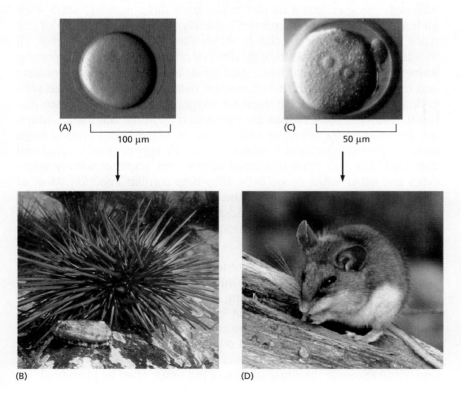

Figure 20–32 The genome of the fertilized egg determines the ultimate structure of the clone of cells that will develop from it. (A and B) A sea-urchin egg gives rise to a sea urchin; (C and D) a mouse egg gives rise to a mouse. (A, courtesy of David McClay; B, courtesy of Alaska Department of Fish and Game; C, courtesy of Patricia Calarco; D, US Department of Agriculture, Agricultural Research Service.)

of a variety of distinct cell types, each expressing different sets of genes and arranged in a precise, intricate, three-dimensional pattern. No one builds these amazing organisms: they self-assemble during development.

Although the final structure of an animal's body may be enormously complex, it is generated by a limited repertoire of cell activities. Examples of all these activities have been discussed in earlier pages of this book. Cells grow, divide, migrate, establish connections with other cells, and die. They form mechanical attachments and generate forces that bend epithelial sheets (see Figure 20–25). They differentiate by switching on or off the production of specific sets of proteins and regulatory RNAs. They produce molecular signals to influence neighboring and distant cells, and they respond to signals that other cells deliver to them. They remember the effects of previous signals they have received, and so progressively become more and more specialized in the characteristics they adopt. The genome, identical in virtually every cell, defines the rules by which these various cell activities are called into play. Through its operation in each cell individually, the genome guides the whole intricate process by which a multicellular organism assembles itself, starting from a fertilized egg. Movie 1.1, Movie 20.3, and Movie 20.4 offer some visual examples of how development unfurls for the embryos of a frog, a fruit fly, and a zebrafish, respectively.

For developmental biologists, the challenge is to explain how genes orchestrate the entire sequence of interlocking events that lead from the egg to the adult organism. We will not attempt to set out an answer to this problem here: we do not have space to do it justice, even though a great deal of the genetic and cell-biological basis of development is now understood. But the same basic activities that combine to create the organism during development continue even in the adult body, where fresh cells are continually generated in precisely controlled patterns. It is this more limited topic that we discuss in this section, focusing on the organization and maintenance of the tissues of adult vertebrates.

Tissues Are Organized Mixtures of Many Cell Types

Although the specialized tissues in our body differ in many ways, they all have certain basic requirements, usually fulfilled by a mixture of cell types, as illustrated for the skin in Figure 20–33. As discussed earlier, all tissues need mechanical strength, which is often supplied by a supporting framework of connective tissue laid down and inhabited by fibroblasts and related cell types. In this connective tissue, blood vessels lined with endothelial cells satisfy the need for oxygen, nutrients, and waste disposal. Likewise, most tissues are innervated by nerve cell axons, which are ensheathed by Schwann cells, some of which wrap around large axons to provide electrical insulation. Macrophages dispose of dead and damaged cells and other unwanted debris, and, together with lymphocytes and other white blood cells, they help combat infection. Most of these cell types originate outside the tissue and invade it, either early in the course of its development (endothelial cells, nerve cell axons, and Schwann cells) or continuously throughout life (macrophages and other cells derived from the blood).

A similar supporting apparatus is required to maintain the principal specialized cells of many tissues: the contractile cells of muscle, the secretory cells of glands, or the blood-forming cells of bone marrow, for example. Almost every tissue is therefore an intricate mixture of many cell types that must remain different from one another while coexisting in the same environment. Moreover, in almost all adult tissues, cells are continually dying and being replaced; throughout this hurly-burly of cell replacement and tissue renewal, the organization of the tissue must be preserved.

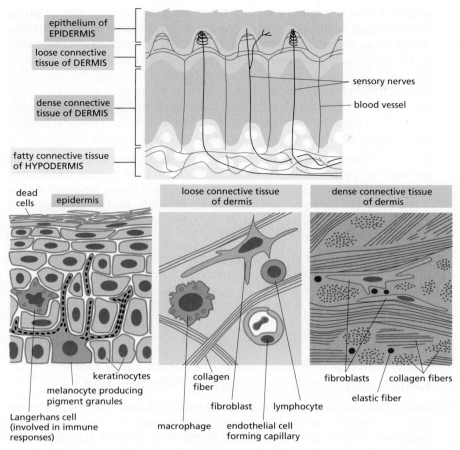

epithelium of
EPIDERMIS

loose connective
tissue of DERMIS

dense connective
tissue of DERMIS

fatty connective tissue
of HYPODERMIS

sensory nerves

blood vessel

dead
cells   epidermis

loose connective tissue
of dermis

dense connective tissue
of dermis

keratinocytes

melanocyte producing
pigment granules

Langerhans cell
(involved in immune
responses)

collagen
fiber

macrophage

fibroblast   lymphocyte

endothelial cell
forming capillary

fibroblasts   collagen fibers

elastic fiber

Figure 20–33 Mammalian skin is made of a mixture of cell types. Schematic diagrams showing the cellular architecture of the main layers of thick skin. Skin can be viewed as a large organ composed of two main tissues: epithelial tissue (the *epidermis*) on the outside, and connective tissue on the inside. The outermost layer of the epidermis consists of flat, dead cells, whose intracellular organelles have disappeared (see Figure 20–36). The underlying connective tissue consists of the tough *dermis* (from which leather is made) and the deeper, fatty *hypodermis*. The dermis and hypodermis are richly supplied with blood vessels and nerves; some of the nerves extend into the epidermis, as shown.

Three main factors contribute to this stability.

1. *Cell communication*: each type of specialized cell continually monitors its environment for signals from other cells and adjusts its behavior accordingly; the proliferation and even the survival of most vertebrate cells depends on such social signals (discussed in Chapters 16 and 18). This communication ensures that new cells are produced and survive only when and where they are required.

2. *Selective cell adhesion*: because different cell types have different cadherins and other cell adhesion molecules in their plasma membrane, they tend to stick selectively, by homophilic binding, to other cells of the same type. They may also form selective attachments to certain other cell types and to specific extracellular matrix components. The selectivity of these cell adhesions keeps cells in their proper positions.

3. *Cell memory*: as discussed in Chapter 8, specialized patterns of gene expression, evoked by signals that acted during embryonic development, are afterward stably maintained, so that cells autonomously preserve their distinctive character and pass it on to their progeny. A fibroblast divides to produce more fibroblasts, an endothelial cell divides to produce more endothelial cells, and so on.

Different Tissues Are Renewed at Different Rates

Human tissues vary enormously in their rate and pattern of *cell turnover*. At one extreme is the intestinal epithelium, in which cells are replaced every three to six days. At the other extreme is nervous tissue, in which most of the nerve cells last a lifetime without replacement. Between these extremes there is a spectrum of different speeds and styles of tissue renewal. Bone (see Figure 20–8) has a turnover time of about ten years, and it involves renewal of the matrix as well as of cells: old bone matrix is slowly eaten away by a set of cells called *osteoclasts*, akin to macrophages, while new matrix is deposited by another set of cells, *osteoblasts*, akin to fibroblasts. New red blood cells are generated continually by blood-forming precursor cells in the bone marrow; they are released into the bloodstream, where they recirculate continually for about 120 days before being removed and destroyed by phagocytic cells in the liver and spleen. In the skin, dead cells in the outer layers of the epidermis are continually flaking off and being replaced from below, so that the epidermis is renewed with a turnover time of about two months. And so on.

Our life depends on these renewal processes, as evidenced by our response to excessive exposure to radiation. In high enough doses, ionizing radiation blocks cell division and thus halts tissue renewal: within a few days, the lining of the intestine, for example, becomes denuded of cells, leading to the devastating diarrhea and water loss characteristic of acute radiation sickness.

Clearly, there have to be elaborate control mechanisms to keep cell production and cell loss in balance in the normal, healthy adult body. Cancers originate through violation of these controls, allowing rare mutant cells in the self-renewing tissues to survive and proliferate prodigiously. To understand cancer, therefore, it is important to understand the normal social controls on cell turnover that cancer perverts.

Stem Cells and Proliferating Precursor Cells Generate a Continuous Supply of Terminally Differentiated Cells

Most of the specialized, **differentiated cells** that need continual replacement are themselves unable to divide. This is true of red blood cells, the epidermal cells in the upper layers of the skin, and the absorptive and goblet cells of the gut epithelium. Such cells are referred to as *terminally differentiated*: they lie at the dead end of their developmental pathway.

The cells that replace the terminally differentiated cells that are lost are generated from a stock of proliferating *precursor cells*, which themselves usually derive from a much smaller number of self-renewing **stem cells**. Stem cells are not differentiated and can divide without limit (or at least for the lifetime of the animal). When a stem cell divides, though, each daughter has a choice: either it can remain a stem cell, or it can embark on a course leading to terminal differentiation, usually via a series of precursor-cell divisions (**Figure 20–34**). The job of the stem cells and precursor cells, therefore, is not to carry out the specialized function of the differentiated cells, but rather to produce cells that will.

Both stem cells and proliferating precursor cells are usually retained in their resident tissue along with their differentiated progeny cells. Stem cells are mostly present in small numbers and often have a nondescript appearance, making them difficult to spot; in some tissues, specific molecular markers can help identify them. Despite being undifferentiated, stem cells and precursor cells are nonetheless developmentally restricted: under normal conditions, they stably express sets of transcription regulators that ensure that their differentiated progeny will be of the appropriate cell types.

QUESTION 20–6

Why does ionizing radiation stop cell division?

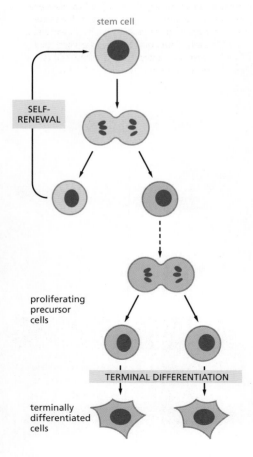

stem cell

SELF-RENEWAL

proliferating precursor cells

TERMINAL DIFFERENTIATION

terminally differentiated cells

Figure 20–34 When a stem cell divides, each daughter can either remain a stem cell (self-renewal) or go on to become terminally differentiated. The terminally differentiated cells usually develop from proliferating precursor cells (sometimes called transit amplifying cells) that divide a limited number of times before they terminally differentiate. Stem-cell divisions can also produce two stem cells or two precursor cells, as long as the pool of stem cells is maintained.

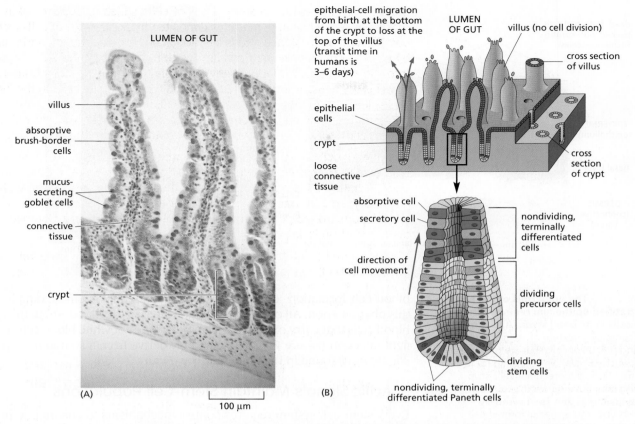

Figure 20–35 Renewal occurs continuously in the epithelial lining of the adult mammalian intestine.
(A) Micrograph of a section of part of the lining of the small intestine showing the villi and crypts. Mucus-secreting goblet cells (stained *purple*) are interspersed among the absorptive brush-border cells in the epithelium covering the villi. Smaller numbers of two other secretory cell types—enteroendocrine cells (not visible here), which secrete gut hormones, and Paneth cells, which secrete antibacterial proteins—are also present and derive from the same stem cells. (B) Drawings showing the pattern of cell turnover and the proliferation of stem cells and precursor cells. The stem cells (*red*) give rise mainly to proliferating precursor cells (*yellow*), which slide continuously upward and terminally differentiate into secretory (*purple*) or absorptive (*blue*) cells, which are shed from the tip of the villus. The stem cells also give rise directly to terminally differentiated Paneth cells (*gray*), which move down to the bottom of the crypt.

The pattern of cell replacement varies from one stem-cell-based tissue to another. In the lining of the small intestine, for example, the absorptive and secretory cells are arranged as a single-layered, simple epithelium covering the surfaces of the fingerlike villi that project into the gut lumen. This epithelium is continuous with the epithelium lining the *crypts*, which descends into the underlying connective tissue (**Figure 20–35A**). The stem cells lie near the bottom of the crypts, where they give rise mostly to proliferating precursor cells, which move upward in the plane of the epithelial sheet. As they move upward, the precursor cells terminally differentiate into absorptive or secretory cells, which are shed into the gut lumen and die when they reach the tips of the villi (**Figure 20–35B**).

A contrasting example is the epidermis, a stratified epithelium. In the epidermis, proliferating stem cells and precursor cells are confined to the basal layer, adhering to the basal lamina. The differentiating cells travel outward from their site of origin in a direction perpendicular to the plane of the cell sheet; terminally differentiated cells and their corpses are eventually shed from the skin surface (**Figure 20–36**).

Often, a single type of stem cell gives rise to several types of differentiated progeny: the stem cells of the intestine, for example, produce absorptive cells, goblet cells, and several other secretory cell types. The process of

QUESTION 20–7

Why do you suppose epithelial cells lining the gut are lost and replaced (renewed) frequently, whereas most neurons last for the lifetime of the organism?

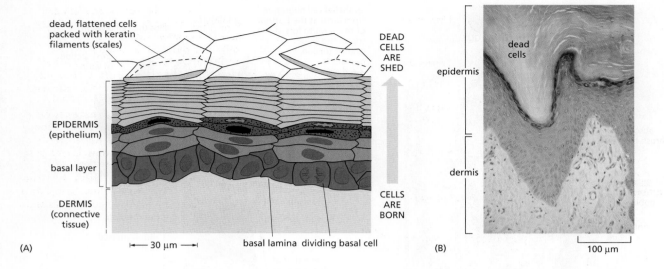

(A)

(B)

Figure 20–36 The epidermis of the skin is a stratified epithelium renewed from stem cells in its basal layer. (A) The basal layer contains a mixture of stem cells and dividing precursor cells that are produced from the stem cells. On emerging from the basal layer, the precursor cells stop dividing and move outward, progressively differentiating as they go. Eventually, the cells undergo a special form of cell death: the nucleus and other organelles disintegrate, and the cell shrinks to the form of a flattened scale, packed with keratin filaments. These scales are ultimately shed from the skin surface. (B) Light micrograph of a cross section through the sole of a human foot, stained with hematoxylin and eosin.

blood-cell formation, or *hemopoiesis*, provides an extreme example of this phenomenon. All of the different cell types in the blood—both the red blood cells that carry oxygen and the many types of white blood cells that fight infection (**Figure 20–37**)—ultimately derive from a shared *hemopoietic stem cell* found in the bone marrow (**Figure 20–38**).

Specific Signals Maintain Stem-Cell Populations

Every stem-cell system requires control mechanisms to ensure that new differentiated cells are generated in the appropriate places and in the right numbers. The controls depend on extracellular signals exchanged between the stem cells, their progeny, and other cell types. These signals, and the intracellular signaling pathways they activate, fall into a surprisingly small number of families, corresponding to half-a-dozen basic signaling mechanisms, some of which are discussed in Chapter 16. These few mechanisms are used again and again—in different combinations—evoking different responses in different contexts in both the embryo and the adult.

Almost all these signaling mechanisms contribute to the task of maintaining the complex organization of a stem-cell system such as that of the intestine. In this system, a class of signal molecules known as the **Wnt proteins** serves to promote the proliferation of the stem cells and precursor cells at the base of each intestinal crypt (**Figure 20–39**). Cells in the crypt produce, in addition, other signals that act at longer range to prevent activation of the Wnt pathway outside the crypts. The crypt cells also exchange yet other signals that control cell diversification, so that some precursor cells differentiate into secretory cells while others become absorptive cells.

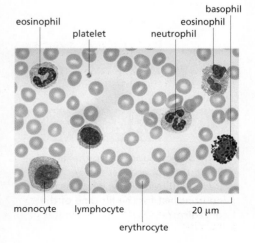

Figure 20–37 Blood contains many circulating cell types, all derived from a single type of stem cell. A sample of blood is smeared onto a glass cover slip, fixed (see Panel 1–1, p. 12), and stained with a dye that mainly stains the nucleus *blue* and cytoplasm *red*. Microscopic examination reveals numerous small erythrocytes (red blood cells), which lack a nucleus and DNA. The nucleated cells are different types of white blood cell: lymphocytes, eosinophils, basophils, neutrophils, and monocytes. Blood smears of this kind are routinely used as a clinical test in hospitals to look for increases or decreases in specific types of blood cells; for example, an increase in specific types of white blood cells could signal infection, inflammatory disorders, or leukemia. (Courtesy of Peter Takizawa.)

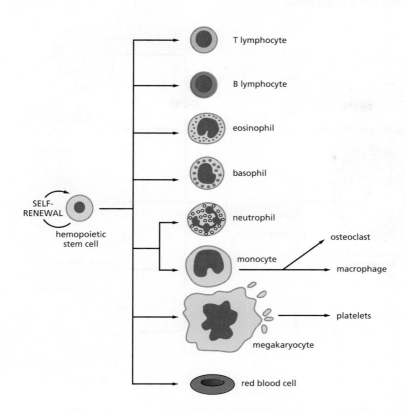

Figure 20–38 **A hemopoietic stem cell divides to generate more stem cells, as well as various types of precursor cells (not shown) that proliferate and differentiate into the mature blood cell types found in the circulation.** Note that monocytes give rise to both macrophages, which are found in many tissues of the body, and osteoclasts, which eat away bone matrix. Megakaryocytes give rise to blood platelets by shedding cell fragments (Movie 20.5). A large number of extracellular signal molecules are known to act at various points in this cell lineage to help control the production of each cell type and to maintain appropriate numbers of precursor cells and stem cells.

Disorders of these signaling mechanisms disrupt the structure of the gut lining. In particular, as we see later, defects in the regulation of Wnt signaling underlie colorectal cancer—the commonest forms of human intestinal cancer.

Stem Cells Can Be Used to Repair Lost or Damaged Tissues

Because stem cells can proliferate indefinitely and produce progeny that differentiate, they provide for both continual renewal of normal tissue and repair of tissue lost through injury. For example, by transfusing a few hemopoietic stem cells into a mouse whose own blood stem cells have been destroyed by irradiation, it is possible to fully repopulate the animal with new blood cells and ultimately rescue it from death by anemia, infection, or both. A similar approach is used in the treatment of human leukemia with irradiation (or cytotoxic drugs) followed by bone marrow transplantation.

Although stem cells taken directly from adult tissues such as bone marrow have already proven their clinical value, another type of stem cell, first identified through experiments in mice, may have even greater potential—both for treating and understanding human disease. It is possible, through cell culture, to derive from early mouse embryos an extraordinary class of stem cells called **embryonic stem cells**, or **ES cells**. Under appropriate conditions, these cells can be kept proliferating indefinitely in culture and yet retain unrestricted developmental potential, and are thus said to be **pluripotent**: if the cells from the culture dish are put back into an early embryo, they can give rise to all the tissues and cell types in the body, including the reproductive germ-line cells. Their descendants in the embryo are able to integrate perfectly into whatever site they come to occupy, adopting the character and behavior that normal cells would show at that site. Such an approach can be used to study gene function: in this case, the ES cells are genetically manipulated—to inactivate a gene or insert a modified one—prior to being returned to an embryo (see

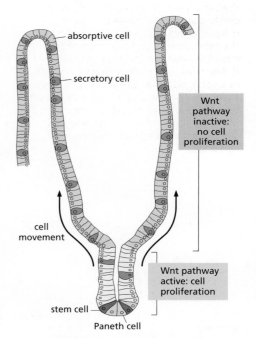

Figure 20–39 **The Wnt signaling pathway maintains the proliferation of the stem cells and precursor cells in the intestinal crypt.** The Wnt proteins are secreted by cells in and around the crypt base, especially by the Paneth cells—a subclass of terminally differentiated secretory cells that are generated from the gut stem cells. Newly formed Paneth cells, which move down to the crypt bottom instead of up to the tip of the villus, have a dual function: they secrete antimicrobial peptides to keep infection at bay, and at the same time they provide the signals to sustain the stem-cell population.

Figure 20–40 Mouse ES cells can be induced to differentiate into specific cell types in culture. ES cells are harvested from the inner cell mass of an early mouse embryo and can be maintained indefinitely as pluripotent stem cells in culture. If they are allowed to aggregate (not shown) and are then exposed to the appropriate extracellular signal molecules, in the correct sequence and at the right time, these cells can be induced to differentiate into specific cell types of interest (Movie 20.6). (Based on data from E. Fuchs and J.A. Segré, *Cell* 100:143–155, 2000.)

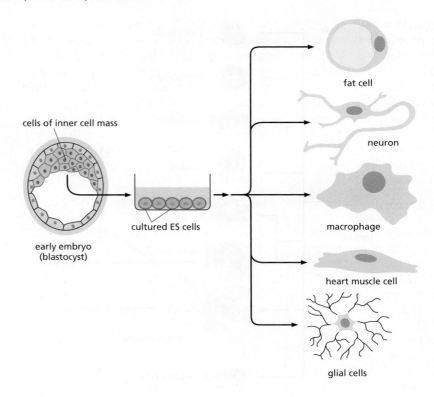

cells of inner cell mass

early embryo
(blastocyst)

cultured ES cells

fat cell

neuron

macrophage

heart muscle cell

glial cells

Figure 10–28). ES cells can also be induced, by the appropriate extracellular signal molecules, to differentiate in culture into a large variety of cell types (Figure 20–40).

Cells with properties similar to those of mouse ES cells can also be derived from early human embryos, and these cells can be induced to differentiate into a variety of cell types as illustrated in Figure 20–40. In principle, human ES cells provide a potentially inexhaustible supply of cells that might be used for the replacement or repair of mature human tissues that are damaged. For example, experiments in mice suggest that it should be possible to use cells derived from human ES cells to replace the skeletal muscle fibers that degenerate in victims of muscular dystrophy, the nerve cells that die in patients with Parkinson's disease, the insulin-secreting cells that are destroyed by the immune system in type 1 diabetics, and the cardiac muscle cells that die during a heart attack. Perhaps one day it might even become possible to grow entire organs from human ES cells by a recapitulation of embryonic development, as we discuss shortly.

There are, however, many hurdles to be cleared before such dreams can become reality. One major problem concerns immune rejection: if the transplanted cells are genetically different from the cells of the patient into whom they are grafted, they are likely to be rejected and destroyed by the immune system. Beyond the practical scientific difficulties, there have been ethical concerns about the use of human embryos to produce human ES cells. One way around both of these problems is to generate human pluripotent cells in another way, as we now discuss.

Induced Pluripotent Stem Cells Provide a Convenient Source of Human ES-like Cells

It is now possible to produce pluripotent stem cells without the use of embryos. Differentiated cells can be taken from an adult mouse or human tissue, grown in culture, and reprogrammed into an ES-like state by artificially driving the expression of a set of three or four transcription regulators, including Oct4, Sox2, and Klf4. This treatment is sufficient to permanently convert fibroblasts into cells with practically all the properties of ES cells, including the ability to proliferate indefinitely, differentiate in diverse ways, and, in the case of mouse cells, contribute to the formation of any tissue. These ES-like cells are called **induced pluripotent stem cells** (**iPS cells**). The drawbacks to this approach include a low conversion rate—only a small proportion of the fibroblasts make the switch to become iPS cells—and concerns over the safety of implanting cells with such an abnormal developmental history into humans. Much work remains to be done before this approach can be used to treat human diseases effectively and ethically.

Better ways of producing human iPS cells are continually being developed. In the meantime, human ES cells, and especially human iPS cells, are proving to be valuable in other ways. They can be used to generate large, homogeneous populations of differentiated human cells of specific types in culture; these can be used to test for potential toxic or beneficial effects of candidate drugs. Moreover, it is possible to generate iPS cells from patients who suffer from a genetic disease and to use these iPS cells to produce affected, differentiated cell types, which can then be studied to learn more about the disease mechanism and to search for potential treatments. An example is Timothy syndrome, a rare genetic disease caused by mutations in a gene that encodes a specific type of Ca^{2+} channel. The altered channel fails to close properly after opening, leading to multiple defects, including abnormal heart rhythm and, in some individuals, autism. The iPS cells produced from such individuals have been coaxed to differentiate in culture into neurons and heart muscle cells, which are now being used to study the physiological consequences of the Ca^{2+} channel abnormality and to hunt for drugs that can correct the defects.

In addition, experiments on pluripotent ES and iPS cells themselves are providing insights into some of the many unsolved mysteries of developmental and stem-cell biology, including the molecular mechanisms that maintain pluripotency and those that restrict specific developmental fates.

Mouse and Human Pluripotent Stem Cells Can Form Organoids in Culture

Remarkably, under appropriate conditions, mouse or human ES cells and iPS cells can proliferate, differentiate, and self-assemble in culture to form miniature, three-dimensional organs called **organoids**, which closely resemble the normal organ in its organization. An early striking example is shown in **Figure 20–41**, where a developing eye-like structure

Figure 20–41 Cultured ES cells can give rise to a three-dimensional organoid. (A) Schematic drawing shows how, under appropriate conditions, mouse or human pluripotent cells in culture can proliferate, differentiate, and self-assemble to form a three-dimensional, eye-like structure (an optic cup), which includes a multilayered retina similar in organization to the one that forms during normal eye development *in vivo*. (B) Fluorescence micrograph of an optic cup formed by human ES cells in culture. The structure includes a developing retina containing multiple layers of neural cells (stained *green*) and an underlying layer of pigmented epithelium, the apical surface of which is stained *red*. All nuclei are stained *blue*. (A, adapted from M. Eiraku and Y. Sasai, *Curr. Opin. Neurobiol.* 22:768–777, 2012; B, adapted from T. Nakano et al., *Cell Stem Cell* 10:771–785, 2012.)

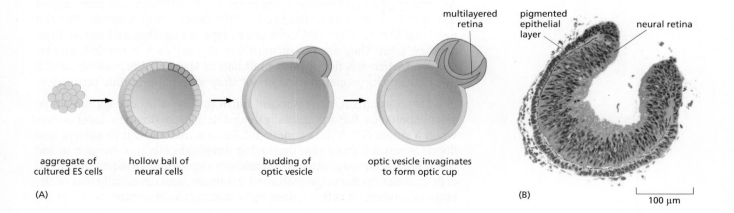

aggregate of cultured ES cells — hollow ball of neural cells — budding of optic vesicle — optic vesicle invaginates to form optic cup

multilayered retina

pigmented epithelial layer

neural retina

100 µm

(A)   (B)

is formed from human ES cells, including a multilayered retina similar in organization to that seen in the developing human eye *in vivo*.

Mouse and human iPS cells, and precursor cells derived from them, have now been used to form organoids that resemble a variety of developing organs, including the human brain, arguably the most complex and sophisticated structure on Earth. Such organoids provide powerful models for studying organ development in a culture dish, where one can identify and manipulate the genes involved and explore the roles of cell–cell interactions in ways not possible in an intact organism. In addition, organoids can be used to investigate how developmental pathways can be derailed by disease. For example, brain organoids have been produced using human iPS cells derived from an individual with microcephaly, a condition characterized by severely stunted brain growth and development. Careful analysis of these developing brain organoids revealed that the microcephaly in this case was probably caused by the premature cessation of proliferation and differentiation of the brain precursor cells, resulting in a decreased production of brain cells.

The development of iPS cells and organoid technology has opened up an entirely new way to study human development and disease. It also opens up promising avenues for treatment.

CANCER

Humans pay a price for having tissues that can renew and repair themselves. The delicately balanced mechanisms that control these processes can break down, leading to catastrophic disruption of tissue structure. Foremost among the diseases of tissue renewal is **cancer**, which stands alongside infection, malnutrition, war, and heart disease as a major cause of death in human populations. In Europe and North America, for example, at least one in five of us will die of cancer.

Cancer arises from violations of the basic rules of social cell behavior. To make sense of the origins and progression of the disease, and to devise treatments, we have to draw upon almost every part of our knowledge of how cells work and interact in tissues. In this section, we examine the causes and mechanisms of cancer, the types of cell misbehavior that contribute to its progress, and the ways in which we hope to use our understanding to defeat these misbehaving cells and, hence, the disease. Although there are many types of cancer, each with distinct properties, we will refer to them collectively by the umbrella term "cancer," as they are united by certain common principles and abnormalities.

Cancer Cells Proliferate Excessively and Migrate Inappropriately

As tissues grow and renew themselves, each individual cell must adjust its behavior according to the needs of the organism as a whole. The cell must divide only when new cells of that type are needed, and refrain from dividing when they are not; it must live as long as it is needed, and be removed when it is not; it must maintain its specialized character; and it must occupy its proper place and not stray into inappropriate territories.

In a large organism, no significant harm is done if an occasional single cell misbehaves. But a potentially devastating breakdown of order occurs when a single cell suffers genetic alterations that allow it to survive and divide when it should not, producing daughter cells that behave in the same antisocial way. Such a relentlessly expanding clone of abnormal cells can disrupt the organization of the tissue, and eventually that of the body as a whole. It is this catastrophe that occurs in cancer.

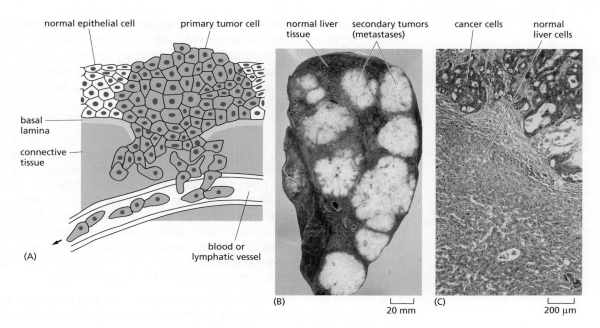

normal epithelial cell   primary tumor cell   normal liver tissue   secondary tumors (metastases)   cancer cells   normal liver cells

basal lamina

connective tissue

(A)

blood or lymphatic vessel

(B)   20 mm

(C)   200 μm

Cancer cells are defined by two heritable properties: they and their progeny (1) proliferate in defiance of the normal constraints and (2) invade and colonize territories normally reserved for other cells (Movie 20.7). It is the combination of these socially deviant features that creates the lethal danger. Cells that have the first property but not the second proliferate excessively but remain clustered together in a single mass, forming a tumor. Such a tumor is said to be *benign*, and it can usually be removed cleanly and completely by surgery. A tumor is cancerous only if its cells have the ability to invade surrounding tissue, in which case the tumor is said to be *malignant*. Malignant tumor cells with this invasive property often break loose from the primary tumor and enter the bloodstream or lymphatic vessels, from where they form secondary tumors, or **metastases**, at other sites in the body (Figure 20–42). The more widely the cancer spreads, the harder it is to eradicate.

Epidemiological Studies Identify Preventable Causes of Cancer

Prevention is always better than cure, but to prevent cancer we need to know what causes it. Do factors in our environment or features of our way of life trigger the disease and help it to progress? If so, what are they? Answers to these questions come mainly from *epidemiology*—the statistical analysis of human populations in search of factors that correlate with disease incidence. This approach has provided strong evidence that the environment plays an important part in the causation of most cases of human cancer. The types of cancers that are common, for example, vary from country to country, and studies of migrants show that it is usually where people live, rather than where they were born, that governs their cancer risk.

Although it is still hard to discover which specific factors in the environment or lifestyle are significant, and many remain unknown, some have been precisely identified. For example, it was noted long ago that cervical cancer, which arises in the epithelium lining the cervix (neck) of the uterus, was much more common in women who were sexually active than in those who were not, suggesting a cause related to sexual activity. We now know that most cases of cervical cancer depend on infection of

Figure 20–42 Cancers invade surrounding tissues and often metastasize to distant sites. (A) To give rise to a colony in a new site—called a secondary tumor or metastasis—the cells of a primary tumor in an epithelium must typically cross the protective barrier provided by the basal lamina (*yellow*), migrate through connective tissue (*blue*), and get into either blood or lymphatic vessels. They then have to exit from the bloodstream or lymph and settle, survive, and proliferate in a new location (not shown). (B) Secondary tumors in a human liver, originating from a primary tumor in the colon. (C) Higher-magnification view of one of the secondary tumors, stained differently to show the contrast between the normal liver cells and the cancer cells. (B and C, courtesy of Peter Isaacson.)

the cervical epithelium with certain subtypes of a common virus called *human papillomavirus*. These viruses are transmitted through sexual intercourse and can sometimes, if one is unlucky, provoke uncontrolled proliferation of the infected cells. Knowing this, we can attempt to prevent the cancer by preventing the infection—for example, by vaccination against the relevant papillomaviruses. Such a vaccine is now available, conferring a high level of protection if given to young people before they become sexually active.

In the great majority of human cancers, however, viruses do not appear to play a part: as we will see, cancer is not an infectious disease. But epidemiology reveals that other factors increase the risk of cancer. Obesity is one such factor. Smoking tobacco is another: tobacco smoke is not only responsible for the great majority of lung cancer cases, but it also raises the incidence of several other cancers, such as those of the bladder. By stopping the use of tobacco, we could prevent about 30% of all cancer deaths. No other single policy or treatment is known that would have such a dramatic impact on the number of cancer deaths.

As we will explain, although environmental factors affect the incidence of cancer and are critical for some forms of the disease, it would be wrong to conclude that they are the only cause of cancers. No matter how hard we try, healthy living alone will not reduce our risk of cancer to zero.

Cancers Develop by an Accumulation of Somatic Mutations

Cancer is fundamentally a genetic disease: it arises as a consequence of pathological changes in the information carried by DNA. It differs from other genetic diseases in that the mutations underlying cancer are mainly *somatic mutations*—those that occur in individual somatic cells of the body—as opposed to germ-line mutations, which are handed down via the germ cells from which the entire multicellular organism develops.

Most of the identified agents known to contribute to the causation of cancer, including ionizing radiation and most chemical carcinogens, are mutagens: they cause changes in the nucleotide sequence of DNA. But even in an environment that is free of tobacco smoke, radioactivity, and all the other external mutagens that worry us, mutations will occur spontaneously as a result of the fundamental limitations on the accuracy of DNA replication and DNA repair (discussed in Chapter 6). In fact, environmental carcinogens other than tobacco smoke probably account for only a small fraction of the mutations responsible for cancer, and elimination of all these external risk factors would still leave us prone to the disease.

Although DNA is replicated and repaired with great accuracy, an average of one mistake slips by for every 10^9 or 10^{10} nucleotides copied, as we discuss in Chapter 6. This means that spontaneous mutations occur at an estimated rate of about 10^{-6} or 10^{-7} mutations per gene per cell division, even without encouragement by external mutagens. About 10^{16} cell divisions take place in a human body in the course of an average lifetime; thus, every single gene is likely to have acquired a mutation on more than 10^9 separate occasions in any individual. From this point of view, the problem of cancer seems to be not why it occurs, but why it occurs so infrequently.

The explanation is that most mutations do not contribute to cancer—even though they may happen to be found in a cancer cell; these mutations are called *passenger mutations*. At the same time, for those mutations that do promote cancer, a single mutation is generally not sufficient. Precisely how many of these *cancer-critical*, or *driver*, *mutations* are required is still a matter of debate, but for most full-blown cancers it could be at least

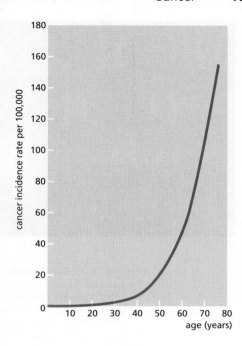

Figure 20–43 Cancer incidence increases dramatically with age. The number of newly diagnosed cases of cancer of the colon in women in England and Wales in one year is plotted as a function of age at diagnosis. Colon cancer, like most human cancers, is caused by the accumulation of multiple mutations. Because cells are continually experiencing accidental changes to their DNA—which accumulate and are passed on to progeny cells when the mutated cells divide—the chance that a cell will become cancerous increases greatly with age. (Data from C. Muir et al., Cancer Incidence in Five Continents, Vol. V. Lyon: International Agency for Research on Cancer, 1987.)

10—and, as we will see, they have to affect the right type of gene. These mutations do not all occur at once but occur sequentially, usually over a period of many years.

Cancer, therefore, is most often a disease of old age, because it takes a long time for an individual clone of cells—those derived from a common founder—to accumulate a sufficient number of cancer-critical mutations (Figure 20–43). Many human cancer cells are able to speed up this acquisition of mutations because they are also genetically unstable. This **genetic instability** results from mutations that interfere with the accurate replication and maintenance of the genome and thereby increase the rate at which mutations accumulate. Sometimes, the increased mutation rate may result from a defect in one of the many proteins needed to repair damaged DNA or to correct errors in DNA replication. Sometimes, there may be a defect in the cell-cycle checkpoint mechanisms that normally prevent a cell with damaged DNA from attempting to divide before the damage has been fully repaired (discussed in Chapter 18). Sometimes, there may be a fault in the machinery of mitosis, which can lead to chromosomal damage, loss, or gain; an abnormal chromosome number can then, itself, increase mitotic errors. These potential sources of genetic instability are summarized in Table 20–1.

Genetic instability can produce chromosome breaks and rearrangements—even complete chromosome duplications. Such gross abnormalities can often be seen in a karyotype of the cancer cell (Figure 20–44).

Cancer Cells Evolve, Acquiring an Increasing Competitive Advantage

The mutations that lead to cancer do not cripple the mutant cells. On the contrary, they give these cells a competitive advantage over their neighbors. It is this advantage enjoyed by the mutant cells that leads to disaster for the organism as a whole. As an initial population of mutant cells grows, it slowly evolves: new chance mutations occur, some of which are favored by natural selection because they enhance cell proliferation, cell survival, or both. This process of random mutation followed by selection culminates in the genesis of cancer cells that run riot within the population of cells that form the body, upsetting its regular structure (Figure 20–45).

Certain environmental or lifestyle factors, such as obesity, may further favor the development of cancer by altering the selection pressures that operate in tissues. A glut of circulating nutrients, or abnormal increases in hormones, survival factors, mitogens, or growth factors, for example, may help cells with dangerous mutations to survive, grow, and proliferate. Eventually, cells emerge that have all the abnormalities required for full-blown cancer.

To be successful, a cancer cell must acquire a whole range of abnormal properties—a collection of subversive behaviors. A proliferating

TABLE 20–1 A VARIETY OF FACTORS CAN CONTRIBUTE TO GENETIC INSTABILITY
Defects in DNA replication
Defects in DNA repair
Defects in cell-cycle checkpoint mechanisms
Mistakes in mitosis
Abnormal chromosome numbers

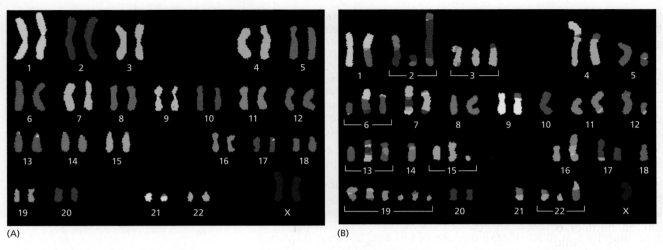

(A)   (B)

Figure 20–44 Cancer cells often have highly abnormal chromosomes, reflecting genetic instability. Shown here are karyotypes displaying the chromosomes of (A) a normal human cell and (B) a breast cancer cell. The chromosomes are "painted" with a combination of fluorescent stains that give each chromosome a different color. The breast cancer karyotype shows multiple translocations, including two instances of a translocation of material from chromosome 6 (*red*) to chromosome 4 (*light blue*), one of which also includes a piece of chromosome 1 (*yellow*). Whereas the normal cell contains 46 chromosomes, the breast cancer cell has 51; several of its chromosomes are missing, and it has an extra copy of a handful of chromosomes—along with 6 copies of chromosome 19. Such abnormalities in chromosome number can cause chromosome-segregation errors when the cell divides, so that the degree of genetic disruption goes from bad to worse over time (see Table 20–1). (Courtesy of Mira Grigorova and Paul Edwards.)

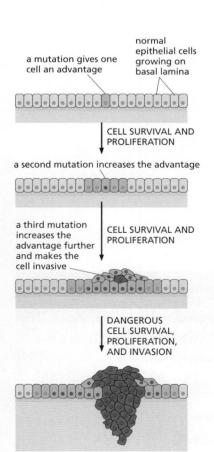

precursor cell in the epithelial lining of the gut, for example, must undergo changes that permit it to carry on dividing when it would normally stop (see Figure 20–35). That cell and its progeny must also be able to avoid cell death, displace their normal neighbors, and attract a blood supply to nourish continued tumor growth (Movie 20.9). For the tumor cells to then become invasive, they must be able to detach from the epithelial sheet and digest their way through the basal lamina into the underlying connective tissue. To spread to other organs and form metastases, they must be able to get in, and then out, of blood or lymph vessels and settle, survive, and proliferate in new sites (see Figure 20–42).

Different cancers display different combinations of properties. Nevertheless, we can draw up a general list of characteristics that distinguish cancer cells from normal cells.

1. Cancer cells have a reduced dependence on signals from other cells for their survival, growth, and division. Often, this is because they contain mutations in components of the cell signaling pathways that normally respond to such stimuli. An activating mutation in a *Ras* gene (discussed in Chapter 16), for instance, can cause an intracellular signal for proliferation even in the absence of the extracellular cue that would normally be needed to turn Ras on—like a faulty doorbell that rings even when nobody is pressing the button.

Figure 20–45 Tumors evolve by repeated rounds of mutation, proliferation, and natural selection. The final outcome is a fully malignant tumor. At each step, a single cell undergoes a mutation that enhances its ability to proliferate, or survive, or both, so that its progeny become a dominant clone in the tumor. Proliferation of this clone then hastens occurrence of the next step of tumor progression by increasing the size of the cell population at risk of undergoing an additional mutation. Some cancers contain multiple malignant clones, each with its own collection of mutations, in addition to a common set of mutations that reflect the tumor's origin from a founding mutant cell (not shown).

2. Cancer cells can survive levels of stress and internal derangement that would cause normal cells to kill themselves by apoptosis. This avoidance of cell suicide is often the result of mutations in genes that regulate the intracellular death program responsible for apoptosis (discussed in Chapter 18). For example, about 50% of all human cancers have an inactivating mutation in the *p53* gene. The p53 protein normally acts as part of a DNA damage response that causes cells with DNA damage to either cease dividing (see Figure 18–15) or die by apoptosis. Chromosome breakage, for example, if not repaired, will generally cause a cell to commit suicide; but if the cell is defective in p53, it may survive and divide, creating highly abnormal daughter cells that have the potential for further mischief (Movie 20.8).

3. Unlike most normal human cells, cancer cells can often proliferate indefinitely. Most normal human somatic cells will only divide a limited number of times in culture, after which they permanently stop; this cessation of proliferation—called *cell senescence*—occurs, at least in part, because many cells in the adult organism lose the ability to produce the enzyme *telomerase*. The telomeres at the ends of their chromosomes thus become progressively shorter with each cell division (see Figure 6–22). In cultured cells, this erosion of telomerase sequences can activate a DNA damage response that permanently halts cell proliferation. Cancer cells typically break through this proliferation barrier by reactivating production of telomerase, enabling them to maintain telomere length indefinitely.

4. Most cancer cells are genetically unstable, with a greatly increased mutation rate and an abnormal number of chromosomes (see Table 20–1 and Figure 20–44).

5. Cancer cells are abnormally invasive, at least partly because they often lack certain cell adhesion molecules, such as cadherins, that help hold normal cells in their proper place.

6. Cancer cells are abnormally avid for nutrients, which they use to generate much of their ATP by glycolysis in the cell cytosol. This process is less efficient than producing ATP by oxidative phosphorylation in the mitochondria, but is useful for fast-growing tumors in which cells in the interior are often oxygen-deprived.

7. Cancer cells can survive and proliferate in abnormal locations, whereas most normal cells die when misplaced. This colonization of unfamiliar territory may result from the ability of cancer cells to produce their own extracellular survival signals and to suppress their apoptosis program (as described in #2, above).

8. As cancer cells evolve, they secrete signals that influence the behavior of cells in the surrounding connective tissue, thereby modifying the tumor's microenvironment. Cells in the remodeled microenvironment, in return, produce signals that support the survival and proliferation of the cancer cells, which renders the microenvironment even more hospitable for tumor growth.

To understand these abnormal properties of cancer cells, we have to identify the mutations responsible.

Two Main Classes of Genes Are Critical for Cancer: Oncogenes and Tumor Suppressor Genes

Investigators have made use of a variety of approaches to track down the genes and mutations that are critical for cancer—from studying viruses that cause cancer in chickens to following families in which a particular cancer occurs unusually often. Though many of the most important of these genes have now been identified, the hunt for others continues.

For many of the cancer-critical genes, the most dangerous mutations are ones that render the encoded protein hyperactive. These *gain-of-function*

QUESTION 20–8

About 10^{16} cell divisions take place in a human body during a lifetime, yet an adult human body consists of only about 10^{13} cells. How can you reconcile these apparently conflicting two numbers?

Figure 20–46 **Genes that are critical for cancer are classified as proto-oncogenes or tumor suppressor genes, according to whether the dangerous mutations are dominant or recessive.** (A) Oncogenes act in a dominant manner: a gain-of-function mutation in a single copy of the proto-oncogene can drive a cell toward cancer. (B) Loss-of-function mutations in tumor suppressor genes generally act in a recessive manner: the function of both copies of the gene must be lost to drive a cell toward cancer. In this diagram, normal genes are represented by *light blue* squares, activating mutations by *red* rays, and inactivating mutations by hollow *red* squares.

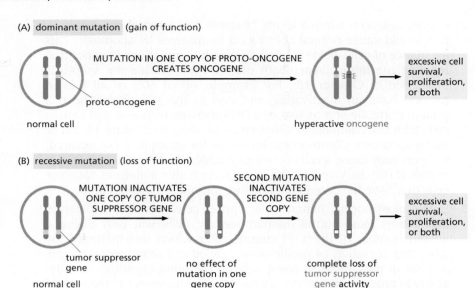

mutations have a dominant effect: only one gene copy needs to be mutated to promote the development of cancer. The resulting mutant gene is called an **oncogene**, and the corresponding normal form of the gene is called a **proto-oncogene** (Figure 20–46A). Figure 20–47 shows a variety of ways in which a proto-oncogene can be converted into its corresponding oncogene.

For other cancer-critical genes, the danger lies in mutations that destroy their activity. These *loss-of-function mutations* are generally recessive: both copies of the gene must be lost or inactivated to contribute to cancer development; the normal gene is called a **tumor suppressor gene** (Figure 20–46B). In addition to such genetic alterations, tumor suppressor genes can also be silenced by *epigenetic changes*, which alter gene expression without changing the gene's nucleotide sequence (as discussed in Chapter 8). Epigenetic changes are thought to silence some tumor suppressor genes in most human cancers. Figure 20–48 highlights a few of the ways in which the activity of a tumor suppressor gene can be lost.

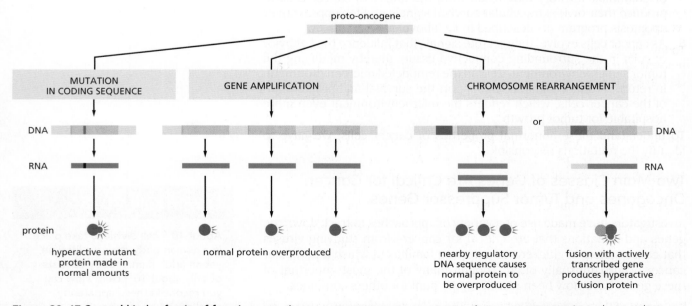

Figure 20–47 **Several kinds of gain-of-function mutations can convert a proto-oncogene into an oncogene.** In each case, the change leads to an increase in the gene's function.

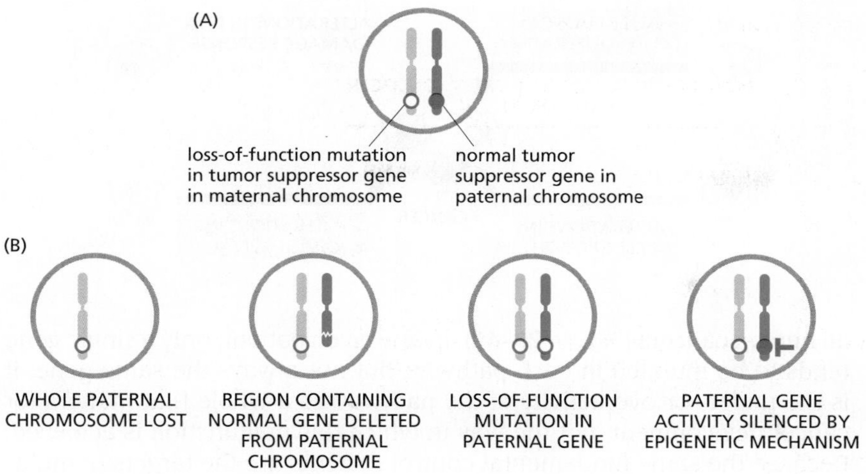

(A)

loss-of-function mutation
in tumor suppressor gene
in maternal chromosome

normal tumor
suppressor gene in
paternal chromosome

(B)

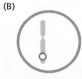

WHOLE PATERNAL
CHROMOSOME LOST

REGION CONTAINING
NORMAL GENE DELETED
FROM PATERNAL
CHROMOSOME

LOSS-OF-FUNCTION
MUTATION IN
PATERNAL GENE

PATERNAL GENE
ACTIVITY SILENCED BY
EPIGENETIC MECHANISM

Figure 20–48 Several kinds of genetic events can eliminate the activity of a tumor suppressor gene. Note that both copies of such a gene must be lost to eliminate its function. (A) A cell in which the maternal copy of the tumor suppressor gene is inactive because of a loss-of-function mutation; this cell is one step away from a complete loss of this tumor-suppressor function. (B) Cells in which the paternal copy of the gene is also inactivated in different ways, as shown.

Proto-oncogenes and tumor suppressor genes code for proteins of many different types, contributing to the many kinds of misbehavior that cancer cells display. Some of these proteins are involved in signaling pathways that regulate cell survival, cell growth, cell division, or some combination of these. Others take part in DNA repair, help mediate the DNA damage response, modify chromatin, or help regulate the cell cycle or apoptosis. Still others (such as cadherins) are involved in cell adhesion or other properties critical for metastasis, or have roles that we do not yet properly understand.

Cancer-critical Mutations Cluster in a Few Fundamental Pathways

From the point of view of a cancer cell, proto-oncogenes and tumor suppressor genes—and the mutations that affect them—are flip sides of the same coin. Activation of a proto-oncogene and inactivation of a tumor suppressor gene can both promote the development of cancer. And both types of mutations contribute to the development of most cancers. In classifying cancer-critical genes, it seems that the type of mutation—gain-of-function or loss-of-function—matters less than the pathway in which it acts.

Today, rapid, low-cost DNA sequencing is providing an unprecedented amount of information about the mutations that drive a variety of cancers. We can now compare the complete genome sequences of the cancer cells from a patient's tumor to the genome sequence of the noncancerous cells in the same individual—or of cancer cells that have spread to another location in the body. By putting together such data from many different patients, we can begin to draw up exhaustive lists of the genes that are critical for specific classes of cancer. And by analyzing data from a single patient, we can deduce the "family tree" of his or her cancer cells, showing how the progeny of the original founder cell have evolved and diversified as they multiplied and metastasized to different sites.

One remarkable finding has been that many of the driver mutations in individual tumors affect genes that fall into a small number of key regulatory pathways: those that govern cell proliferation, cell growth, cell survival, and the cell's response to DNA damage and stress. For example, in almost every case of glioblastoma—the most common type of human brain cancer—mutations disrupt all four of these fundamental pathways, and the same pathways are subverted, in one way or another, in almost

Figure 20–49 A small number of key regulatory pathways are perturbed in almost all human cancers. These pathways regulate cell proliferation, cell growth, cell survival, and the cell's response to DNA damage or stress.

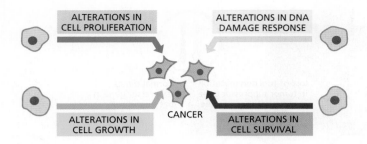

all human cancers (Figure 20–49). In any given patient, only a single gene tends to be mutated in each pathway, but not always the same gene: it is the under- or overactivity of the pathway as a whole that matters for cancer development, not the way in which this malfunction is achieved. Because the same fundamental control systems are the targets of mutation in so wide a variety of cancers, it seems that their misregulation must be crucial to most cancers' success.

Colorectal Cancer Illustrates How Loss of a Tumor Suppressor Gene Can Lead to Cancer

Colorectal cancer provides one well-studied example of how a tumor suppressor gene can be identified and its role in tumor growth determined. Colorectal cancer arises from the epithelium lining the colon and rectum; most cases are seen in old people and do not have any discernible hereditary cause. A small proportion of cases, however, occurs in families that are exceptionally prone to the disease and show an unusually early onset. In one set of such "predisposed" families, the affected individuals develop colorectal cancer in early adult life, and the onset of their disease is foreshadowed by the development of hundreds or thousands of little tumors, called polyps, in the epithelial lining of the colon and rectum.

By studying these families, investigators traced the development of the polyps to a deletion or inactivation of a tumor suppressor gene called *APC*—for *Adenomatous Polyposis Coli*. (Note that the protein encoded by this gene is different from the anaphase-promoting complex, abbreviated APC/C, discussed in Chapter 18.) Affected individuals inherit one mutant copy of the gene and one normal copy. Although one normal gene copy is enough for normal cell behavior, all the cells of these individuals are only one mutational step away from total loss of the gene's function (as compared to two steps away for a person who inherits two normal copies of the gene). The individual tumors arise from cells that have undergone a somatic mutation that inactivates the remaining good copy of *APC* (see Figure 20–46B). Not surprisingly, the disease strikes these individuals at an earlier age than it does in individuals with two good copies of *APC*.

But what about the great majority of colorectal cancer patients, who do not have the hereditary condition or any significant family history of cancer? When their tumors are analyzed, it turns out that in more than 60% of cases, although both copies of *APC* are present in the adjacent normal tissue, the tumor cells themselves have lost or inactivated both copies of this gene (see Figure 20-48B).

All these findings clearly identify *APC* as a tumor suppressor gene and, knowing its sequence and mutant phenotype, one can begin to decipher how its loss helps to initiate the development of cancer. As explained in **How We Know** (pp. 730–731), the *APC* gene was found to encode an inhibitory protein that normally restricts the activation of the Wnt signaling pathway, which is involved in stimulating cell proliferation in the

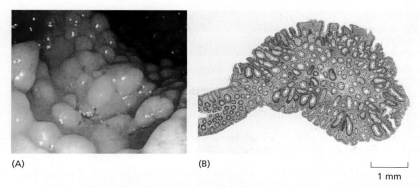

(A)   (B)

1 mm

Figure 20–50 Colorectal cancer often begins with the inactivation of both copies of the tumor suppressor gene *APC*, leading to growth of a polyp. (A) Thousands of small polyps, and a few much larger ones, are seen in the lining of the colon of a patient with an inherited *APC* mutation (whereas individuals without an *APC* mutation might have one or two polyps). Such polyps arise from cells in which both copies of *APC* are inactivated. Through additional mutations in other tumor suppressor genes or proto-oncogenes, some of the larger polyps will progress to become invasive cancers, unless the tissue is removed surgically. (B) Cross section of one such polyp; note the excessive quantities of deeply infolded epithelium, corresponding to crypts full of abnormal, proliferating cells (Movie 20.10). (A, courtesy of Kevin Monahan; B, David Litman/Shutterstock.)

crypts of the gut lining, as described earlier (see Figure 20–39). When *APC* function is lost, the pathway is hyperactive and epithelial cells proliferate to excess, generating a polyp (**Figure 20–50**). Within this growing mass of tissue, further driver mutations occur, sometimes resulting in invasive cancer (**Figure 20–51**).

The effect of mutations in a variety of tumor suppressor genes and proto-oncogenes, including those involved in colorectal cancer, is presented in **Table 20–2**.

An Understanding of Cancer Cell Biology Opens the Way to New Treatments

The nature of the defects that promote the survival, proliferation, and spread of cancer cells makes the development of effective treatment strategies particularly challenging. Because cancer cells are highly mutable, they can rapidly evolve resistance to treatments used to exterminate them. Moreover, because mutations arise randomly, every case of cancer is likely to have its own unique combination of genes mutated. Even within an individual patient, tumor cells do not all contain the same genetic lesions. Thus, no single treatment is likely to work in every patient, or even for every cancer cell within the same patient. Finally, the fact that cancers generally are not detected until the primary tumor has reached a diameter of 1 cm or more—by which time it consists of hundreds of millions of cells that are already genetically diverse and often have already begun to metastasize (**Figure 20–52**)—makes treatment even harder still.

Figure 20–51 A polyp in the epithelial lining of the colon or rectum, caused by loss of both copies of the *APC* gene, can progress to cancer by accumulation of additional driver mutations. The diagram shows a sequence of random driver mutations that might underlie a typical case of colorectal cancer. After the initial mutation, all subsequent driver mutations arise in a single cell that has already acquired the previous driver mutations. A sequence of events such as that shown here would usually be spread over 10 to 20 years or more. Though most colorectal cancers are thought to begin with the sequential loss or inactivation of both copies of the *APC* tumor suppressor gene, the subsequent sequence of driver mutations is quite variable; indeed, most polyps never progress to cancer.

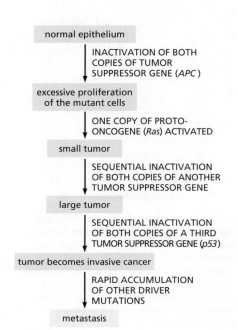

TABLE 20–2 EXAMPLES OF CANCER-CRITICAL GENES

Gene	Class	Effect of Mutation
Ras	Proto-oncogene	Activating mutations in *Ras* render the Ras protein continuously active, promoting cell proliferation (discussed in Chapter 16)
β-catenin	Proto-oncogene	Activating mutations in *β-catenin* make the β-catenin protein resistant to degradation, promoting cell proliferation (see How We Know, pp. 730–731)
p53	Tumor suppressor gene	Inactivation of both copies of *p53* allows cancer cells to continue to survive and divide, even in the presence of damaged DNA (discussed in Chapter 18)
APC	Tumor suppressor gene	Inactivation of both copies of *APC* promotes excessive proliferation of cells in the intestinal crypt (see Figure 20–52 and How We Know, pp. 730–731)
Brca1 and *Brca2*	Tumor suppressor genes	Inactivation of both copies of *Brca1* or *Brca2* allows cancer cells to continue to survive and divide in the presence of massively damaged DNA (discussed below).

Yet, in spite of these difficulties, an increasing number of cancers are being treated effectively. Surgery remains a highly effective tactic, and surgical techniques are continually improving: in many cases, if a cancer has not spread far, it can often be cured by simply removing it. Where surgery fails, the intrinsic peculiarities of cancer cells can be used against them. Lack of normal cell-cycle control mechanisms, for example, may help make cancer cells particularly vulnerable to DNA damage: whereas a normal cell will halt its proliferation until such damage is repaired, a cancer cell may charge ahead regardless, producing daughter cells that may die because they inherit too many unrepaired breakages in their chromosomes. Presumably for this reason, cancer cells can often be killed by doses of radiotherapy or DNA-damaging chemotherapy that leave most normal cells relatively unharmed.

Surgery, radiation, and chemotherapy are long-established treatments, but many novel approaches are also being enthusiastically pursued. In some cases, as with loss of a normal response to DNA damage, the very feature that helps to make the cancer cell dangerous also makes it vulnerable, enabling doctors to kill it with a properly targeted treatment. Some cancers of the breast and ovary, for example, owe their genetic instability to the lack of a tumor suppressor protein (either Brca1 or Brca2) that aids in the accurate repair of double-strand breaks in DNA (discussed in Chapter 6); the cancer cells survive by relying on alternative types of DNA repair mechanisms. Drugs that inhibit one of these alternative DNA repair mechanisms specifically destroy the cancer cells by raising their genetic instability to such a level that the cells die from chromosome fragmentation when they attempt to divide. Normal cells, which possess an intact double-strand break repair mechanism, remain relatively unaffected.

Another set of strategies aims to use the immune system to kill the tumor cells. Antibodies that recognize tumor-specific cell-surface molecules can be produced *in vitro* and injected into the patient to mark the tumor cells for destruction. Other antibodies, aimed at the patient's immune cells rather than the cancer cells, can promote the elimination of cancer cells by neutralizing the inhibitory cell-surface proteins that keep the killer lymphocytes of the immune system (discussed in Chapter 18) in check. Such "checkpoint inhibitor" antibodies, which unleash a killer cell attack on cancer cells, are proving to be remarkably effective in the treatment of certain cancers, such as melanomas, even after they have metastasized (**Figure 20–53**).

In some cancers, the products of specific oncogenes can be targeted directly so as to block their action, causing the cancer cells to die. In

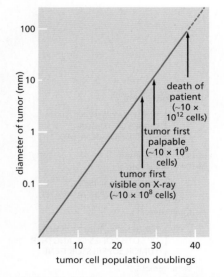

Figure 20–52 A tumor is generally not diagnosed until it has grown to contain hundreds of millions of cells. Here, the growth of a typical tumor is plotted on a logarithmic scale. Years may elapse before the tumor becomes noticeable. The time it takes for the number of cells in a typical breast tumor to double, for example, is about 100 days.

Figure 20–53 Anti-immune-checkpoint antibodies release a killer cell attack on cancer cells. The antibodies disinhibit the killer cells that recognize the novel parts of the proteins encoded by the mutant oncogenes of the cancer cells. A patient with advanced metastatic melanoma received treatment with such an antibody called ipilimumab. After 16 weeks of treatment, the tumors were noticeably smaller, and by week 72 they had essentially been eliminated. (From A. Hoos et al., *J. Natl Cancer Inst.* 102:1388–1397, 2010.)

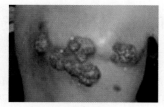

week 12

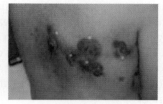

week 16

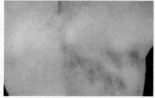

week 72

chronic myeloid leukemia (CML), the misbehavior of the cancer cells depends on a mutant intracellular signaling protein (a tyrosine kinase) that causes the cells to proliferate and survive when they should not. A small drug molecule, called imatinib (trade name Gleevec), blocks the activity of this hyperactive mutant kinase. The results have been a dramatic success: in many patients, the abnormal proliferation and survival of the leukemic cells are strongly inhibited, providing many years of symptom-free patient survival. The same drug is also effective in some other cancers that depend on similar oncogenes.

With these examples before us, we can hope that our modern understanding of the molecular biology of cancer will soon allow us to devise effective rational treatments for even more forms of cancer. At the same time, cancer research has taught us many important lessons about basic cell biology. The applications of that knowledge go far beyond the treatment of cancer, giving us insight into the way that cells and organisms develop and operate.

ESSENTIAL CONCEPTS

- Tissues are composed of cells and extracellular matrix.

- In plants, each cell surrounds itself with extracellular matrix in the form of a cell wall, which is made chiefly of cellulose and other polysaccharides.

- An osmotic swelling pressure on plant cell walls keeps plant tissue turgid.

- Cellulose microfibrils in the plant cell wall confer tensile strength, while other cell-wall polysaccharides resist compression.

- The orientation in which the cellulose microfibrils are deposited in the cell wall controls the orientation of plant cell growth.

- Animal connective tissues provide mechanical support to organs and limbs; these tissues consist mainly of extracellular matrix, which is secreted by a sparse scattering of embedded cells.

- In the extracellular matrix of animals, tensile strength is provided by the fibrous collagen proteins, while glycosaminoglycans (GAGs), covalently linked to proteins to form proteoglycans, act as space-fillers and provide resistance to compression.

- Transmembrane integrin proteins link extracellular matrix proteins such as collagen and fibronectin to the intracellular cytoskeleton of cells that contact the matrix.

- Cells are connected to one another via cell junctions in epithelial sheets that line all external and internal surfaces of the animal body.

- Cell adhesion proteins of the cadherin family span the epithelial cell plasma membrane and bind to identical cadherins in adjacent epithelial cells.

- At an adherens junction, the cadherins are linked to intracellular actin filaments; at a desmosome junction, they are linked to intracellular keratin intermediate filaments.

MAKING SENSE OF THE GENES THAT ARE CRITICAL FOR CANCER

The search for genes that are critical for cancer sometimes begins with a family that shows an inherited predisposition to a particular form of the disease. *APC*—a tumor suppressor gene that is frequently deleted or inactivated in colorectal cancer—was tracked down by searching for genetic defects in such families prone to the disease. But identifying the gene is only half the battle. The next step is determining what the normal gene does in a normal cell—and why alterations in the gene promote cancer.

Guilt by association

Determining what a gene—or its encoded product—does inside a cell is not a simple task. Imagine isolating an uncharacterized protein and being told that it acts as a protein kinase. That information does not reveal how the protein functions in the context of a living cell. What proteins does the kinase phosphorylate? In which tissues is it active? What role does it have in the growth, development, or physiology of the organism? A great deal of additional information is required to understand the biological context in which the kinase acts.

Most proteins do not function in isolation: they interact with other proteins in the cell. Thus one way to begin to decipher a protein's biological role is to identify its binding partners. If an uncharacterized protein interacts with a protein whose role in the cell is understood, the function of the unknown protein is likely to be in some way related. The simplest method for identifying proteins that bind tightly to one another is co-immunoprecipitation (see Panel 4–2, pp. 140–141). In this technique, an antibody is used to capture and precipitate a specific target protein from an extract prepared by breaking open cells; if this target protein is associated tightly with another protein, the partner protein will precipitate as well. This is the approach that was taken to characterize the *Adenomatous Polyposis Coli* gene product, APC.

Two groups of researchers used antibodies against APC to isolate the protein from extracts prepared from cultured human cells. The antibodies captured APC along with a second protein. When the researchers examined the amino acid sequence of this partner, they recognized the protein as β-catenin.

The discovery that APC interacts with β-catenin initially led to some wrong guesses about the role of APC in colorectal cancer. In mammals, β-catenin was known primarily for its role at adherens junctions, where it serves as a linker to connect membrane-spanning cadherin proteins to the intracellular actin cytoskeleton (see, for example, Figure 20–23). Thus, for some time, scientists thought that APC might be involved in cell adhesion. But within a few years, it emerged that β-catenin also has another, completely different function. It is this unexpected function that turned out to be the one that is relevant for understanding APC's role in cancer.

Wingless flies

Not long before the discovery that APC binds to β-catenin, developmental biologists working on the fruit fly *Drosophila* had noticed that the human β-catenin protein is very similar in amino acid sequence to a *Drosophila* protein called Armadillo. Armadillo was known to be a key protein in a signaling pathway that has important roles in normal development in flies. The pathway is activated by the Wnt family of extracellular signal proteins, the founding member of which was called *Wingless*, after its mutant phenotype in flies. Wnt proteins bind to receptors on the surface of a cell, switching on an intracellular signaling pathway that ultimately leads to the activation of a set of genes that influence cell growth, division, and differentiation. Mutations in any of the proteins in this pathway lead to developmental errors that disrupt the basic body plan of the fly. The least devastating mutations cause flies to develop without wings; most mutations, however, result in the death of the embryo. In either case, the damage is done through effects on gene expression. This strongly suggested that Armadillo, and hence its vertebrate homolog β-catenin, were not just involved in cell adhesion, but somehow mediated the control of gene expression through the Wnt signaling pathway.

Although the Wnt signaling pathway was discovered and studied intensively in fruit flies, it was later found to control many aspects of development in vertebrates, including mice and humans. Indeed, some of the proteins in the Wnt pathway function almost interchangeably in *Drosophila* and vertebrates. The direct link between β-catenin and gene expression became clear from work in mammalian cells. Just as APC could be used as "bait" to catch its partner β-catenin by immunoprecipitation, so β-catenin could be used as bait to catch the next protein in the signaling pathway. This was found to be a transcription regulator called LEF-1/TCF, or TCF for short. It too was found to have a *Drosophila* counterpart in the Wnt pathway, and a combination of *Drosophila* genetics and mammalian cell biology revealed how the gene control mechanism works.

Wnt transmits its signal by promoting the accumulation of "free" β-catenin (or, in flies, Armadillo)—that is, of β-catenin that is not locked up in cell junctions. This free protein migrates from the cytoplasm into the nucleus. There it binds to the TCF transcription regulator, creating a complex that activates transcription of various Wnt-responsive genes, including genes whose products stimulate cell proliferation (**Figure 20–54**).

It turns out that APC regulates the activity of this pathway by facilitating degradation of β-catenin and thereby preventing it from activating TCF in cells where no Wnt signal has been received (see Figure 20–54A). Loss of APC allows the concentration of β-catenin to rise, so that TCF is activated and Wnt-responsive genes are turned on even in the absence of a Wnt signal. But how does this promote the development of colorectal cancer? To find out, researchers turned to mice that lack TCF4, a member of the TCF gene family that is specifically expressed in the gut epithelial lining.

Tales from the crypt

Although it may seem counterintuitive, one of the most direct ways of finding out what a gene normally does is to see what happens to the organism when that gene is missing. If one can pinpoint the processes that are disrupted or compromised, one can begin to decipher the gene's function.

With this in mind, researchers generated "knockout" mice in which the gene encoding TCF4 was disrupted. The mutation is lethal: mice lacking TCF4 die shortly after birth. But the dying animals showed an interesting abnormality in their intestines. The intestinal crypts, which contain the stem cells responsible for the renewal of the gut lining (see Figure 20–35), had completely failed to develop. The researchers concluded that TCF4 is normally required for maintaining the pool of proliferating gut stem cells.

When APC is missing, we see the other side of the coin: without APC to promote its degradation, β-catenin accumulates in excessive quantities, binds to the TCF4 transcription regulator, and thereby overactivates the TCF4-responsive genes. This drives the formation of polyps by promoting the inappropriate proliferation of gut stem cells and precursor cells. Differentiated progeny cells continue to be produced and discarded into the gut lumen, but the crypt cell population grows too fast for this disposal mechanism to keep pace. The result is crypt enlargement and a steady increase in the number of crypts. The growing mass of tissue bulges out into the gut lumen as a polyp (see Figure 20–50 and Movie 20.9). A number of additional mutations are needed, however, to convert this benign tumor into an invasive cancer (see Figure 20–51).

More than 60% of human colorectal tumors harbor mutations in the *APC* gene. Interestingly, among the minority class of tumors that retain functional APC, about a quarter have activating mutations in β-catenin instead. These mutations tend to make the β-catenin protein more resistant to degradation and thus produce the same effect as loss of APC. In fact, mutations that enhance the activity of β-catenin have been found in a wide variety of other tumor types, including melanomas, stomach cancers, and liver cancers. Thus, the genes that encode proteins that act in the Wnt signaling pathway provide multiple targets for mutations that can spur the development of cancer.

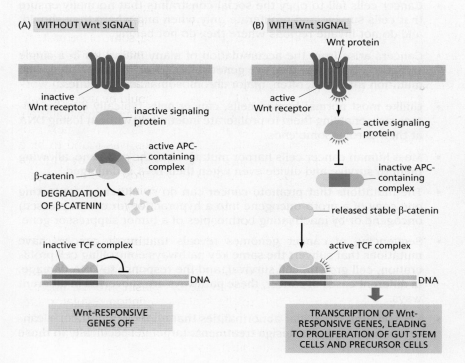

Figure 20–54 **The APC protein keeps the Wnt signaling pathway inactive when the cell is not exposed to a secreted Wnt signal protein.** (A) It does this by promoting degradation of the signaling molecule β-catenin. (B) In the presence of Wnt (or in the absence of active APC), free β-catenin becomes plentiful and combines with the transcription regulator TCF to drive transcription of Wnt-responsive genes and, ultimately, the proliferation of stem cells and precursor cells in the intestinal crypt (see Figure 20–39). In the colon, mutations that inactivate APC initiate tumors by causing excessive activation of the Wnt signaling pathway.

- During development, the actin bundles at the adherens junctions that connect cells in an epithelial sheet can contract, helping the epithelium to bend and pinch off, forming an epithelial tube or vesicle.

- Hemidesmosomes attach the basal face of an epithelial cell to the basal lamina, a specialized sheet of extracellular matrix; the attachment is mediated by transmembrane integrin proteins, which are linked to intracellular keratin filaments.

- Tight junctions seal one epithelial cell to the next, barring the diffusion of water-soluble molecules across the epithelium.

- Gap junctions form channels that allow the direct passage of inorganic ions and small, hydrophilic molecules from cell to cell; in plants, plasmodesmata form a different type of channel, which traverses the cell walls, is lined by plasma membrane, and allows both small and large molecules to pass from cell to cell.

- Most tissues in vertebrates are complex mixtures of cell types that are subject to continual turnover.

- Most tissues of an adult animal are maintained and renewed by the same basic cell processes that generated them in the embryo: cell proliferation, movement, differentiation, and death. As in the embryo, these processes are controlled by intercellular communication, selective cell–cell adhesion, and cell memory.

- In many tissues, nondividing, terminally differentiated cells are generated from stem cells, usually via proliferating precursor cells.

- Embryonic stem cells (ES cells) can proliferate indefinitely in culture and remain capable of differentiating into any cell type in the body— that is, they are pluripotent.

- Induced pluripotent stem cells (iPS cells), which resemble ES cells, can be generated from the cells of adult mammalian tissues, including those of human, through the artificial expression of a small set of transcription regulators.

- Pluripotent stem cells can be induced to form specific cell types and even small organs (organoids) in suitable culture conditions, providing powerful models for studying human development and genetic diseases.

- Cancer cells fail to obey the social constraints that normally ensure that cells survive and proliferate only when and where they should, and do not invade regions where they do not belong.

- Cancers arise from the accumulation of many mutations in a single somatic cell lineage; they are genetically unstable, having increased mutation rates and, often, major chromosomal abnormalities.

- Unlike most normal human cells, cancer cells typically express telomerase, enabling them to proliferate indefinitely without losing DNA at their chromosome ends.

- Most human cancer cells harbor mutations in the *p53* gene, allowing them to survive and divide even when their DNA is damaged.

- The mutations that promote cancer can do so either by converting one copy of a proto-oncogene into a hyperactive (or overexpressed) oncogene or by inactivating both copies of a tumor suppressor gene.

- Sequencing of cancer genomes reveals that most cancers have mutations that subvert the same key pathways controlling cell proliferation, cell growth, cell survival, and the response to DNA damage. In different cases of cancer, these pathways are subverted in different ways.

- Knowing the molecular abnormalities that underlie a particular cancer, one can begin to design treatments targeted specifically to those abnormalities.

KEY TERMS

adherens junction	genetic instability
apical	glycosaminoglycan (GAG)
basal	hemidesmosome
basal lamina	induced pluripotent stem (iPS) cell
cadherin	integrin
cancer	metastasis
cell junction	oncogene
cell wall	organoid
cellulose microfibril	plasmodesma
collagen	(plural plasmodesmata)
connective tissue	pluripotent
desmosome	proteoglycan
differentiated cell	proto-oncogene
embryonic stem (ES) cell	stem cell
epithelium (plural epithelia)	tight junction
extracellular matrix	tissue
fibroblast	tumor suppressor gene
fibronectin	Wnt protein
gap junction	

QUESTIONS

QUESTION 20–9

Which of the following statements are correct? Explain your answers.

A. Gap junctions connect the cytoskeleton of one cell to that of a neighboring cell or to the extracellular matrix.

B. A wilted plant leaf can be likened to a deflated bicycle tire.

C. Because of their rigid structure, proteoglycans can withstand a large amount of compressive force.

D. The basal lamina is a specialized layer of extracellular matrix to which sheets of epithelial cells are attached.

E. Epidermal cells in the skin are continually shed and are renewed every few weeks; for a tattoo to be long-lasting, it is therefore necessary to deposit pigment below the epidermis.

F. Although stem cells are not differentiated, they are specialized in the sense that they give rise only to specific cell types.

QUESTION 20–10

Which of the following substances would you expect to spread from one cell to the next through (a) gap junctions and (b) plasmodesmata: glutamic acid, mRNA, cyclic AMP, Ca^{2+}, proteins, and plasma membrane phospholipids?

QUESTION 20–11

Discuss the following statement: "If plant cells contained intermediate filaments to provide the cells with tensile strength, their cell walls would be dispensable."

QUESTION 20–12

Through the exchange of small metabolites and ions, gap junctions provide metabolic and electrical coupling between cells. Why, then, do you suppose that neurons communicate primarily through chemical synapses (as shown in Figure 12–40) rather than through gap junctions?

QUESTION 20–13

Gelatin is primarily composed of collagen, which is responsible for the remarkable tensile strength of connective tissue. It is the basic ingredient of jello; yet, as you probably experienced many times yourself while consuming the strawberry-flavored variety, jello has virtually no tensile strength. Why?

QUESTION 20–14

"The structure of an organism is determined by the genome that the fertilized egg contains." What is the evidence on which this statement is based? Indeed, a friend challenges you and suggests that you replace the DNA of a stork's egg with human DNA to see if a human baby results. How would you answer him?

QUESTION 20–15

Leukemias—that is, cancers arising through mutations that cause excessive production of white blood cells—have an earlier average age of onset than other cancers. Propose an explanation for why this might be the case.

QUESTION 20–16

Carefully consider the graph in Figure 20–43, which shows

the number of cases of colon cancer diagnosed per 100,000 women per year as a function of age. Why is this graph so steep and curved, if mutations occur with a similar frequency throughout a person's life-span?

QUESTION 20–17

Heavy smokers or industrial workers exposed for a limited time to a chemical carcinogen that induces mutations in DNA do not usually begin to develop cancers characteristic of their habit or occupation until 10, 20, or even more years after the exposure. Suggest an explanation for this long delay.

QUESTION 20–18

High levels of the female sex hormone estrogen increase the risk of some forms of cancer. Thus, some early types of contraceptive pills containing high concentrations of estrogen were eventually withdrawn from use because this was found to increase the risk of cancer of the lining of the uterus. Male transsexuals who use estrogen preparations to give themselves a female appearance have an increased risk of breast cancer. High levels of androgens (male sex hormones) increase the risk of some other forms of cancer, such as cancer of the prostate. Can one infer that estrogens and androgens are mutagenic?

QUESTION 20–19

Is cancer hereditary?

Answers

Chapter 1

ANSWER 1–1   Trying to define life in terms of properties is an elusive business, as suggested by this scoring exercise (Table A1–1). Vacuum cleaners are highly organized objects, and take matter and energy from the environment and transform the energy into motion, responding to stimuli from the operator as they do so. On the other hand, they cannot reproduce themselves, or grow and develop—but then neither can old animals. Potatoes are not particularly responsive to stimuli, and so on. It is curious that standard definitions of life usually do not mention that living organisms on Earth are largely made of organic molecules—that is, life is carbon based. As we now know, the key types of "informational macromolecules"—DNA, RNA, and protein—are the same in every living species.

TABLE A1–1 PLAUSIBLE "LIFE" SCORES FOR A VACUUM CLEANER, A POTATO, AND A HUMAN

Characteristic	Vacuum Cleaner	Potato	Human
1. Organization	Yes	Yes	Yes
2. Homeostasis	Yes	Yes	Yes
3. Reproduction	No	Yes	Yes
4. Development	No	Yes	Yes
5. Energy	Yes	Yes	Yes
6. Responsiveness	Yes	No	Yes
7. Adaptation	No	Yes	Yes

ANSWER 1–2   Most random changes to the shoe design would result in objectionable defects: shoes with multiple heels, with no soles, or with awkward sizes would obviously not sell and would therefore be selected against by market forces. Other changes would be neutral, such as minor variations in color or in size. A minority of changes, however, might result in more desirable shoes: deep scratches in a previously flat sole, for example, might create shoes that would perform better in wet conditions; the loss of high heels might produce shoes that are more comfortable (and less dangerous). The example illustrates that random changes can lead to significant improvements if the number of trials is large enough and selective pressures are imposed.

ANSWER 1–3   It is extremely unlikely that you created a new organism in this experiment. Far more probably, a spore from the air landed in your broth, germinated, and gave rise to the cells you observed. In the middle of the nineteenth century, Louis Pasteur invented a clever apparatus to disprove the then widely accepted belief that life could arise spontaneously. He showed that sealed flasks containing a nutrient broth that could support microbial growth never grew anything if properly heat-sterilized first. He overcame the objections of those who pointed out the lack of oxygen, or who suggested that his heat sterilization killed the life-generating principle, by using a special flask with a slender "swan's neck," which was designed to prevent spores carried in the air from contaminating the culture (Figure A1–3). The heat-sterilized nutrient broth in these flasks never showed any signs of life; however, it was capable of supporting life, as could be demonstrated by washing some of the "dust" from the neck of the flask into the broth.

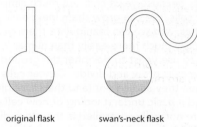

original flask   swan's-neck flask

Figure A1–3

ANSWER 1–4 6×10^{39} (= 6×10^{27} g/10^{-12} g) bacteria would have the same mass as the Earth. And 6×10^{39} = $2^{t/20}$, according to the equation describing exponential growth. Solving this equation for t results in t = 2642 minutes (or 44 hours). This represents only 132 generation times(!), whereas 5×10^{14} bacterial generation times have passed during the last 3.5 billion years. Obviously, the total mass of bacteria on this planet is nowhere close to the mass of the Earth. This illustrates that exponential growth can occur only for very few generations—that is, for minuscule periods of time compared with evolution. In any realistic scenario, food supplies very quickly become limiting.

This simple calculation shows us that the ability to grow and divide quickly when food is ample is only one factor in the survival of a species. Food is generally scarce, and individuals of the same species have to compete with one another for the limited resources. Natural selection favors mutants that either win the competition or find ways to exploit food sources that their neighbors are unable to use.

ANSWER 1–5   By engulfing substances such as food particles, eukaryotic cells can sequester them and feed on them efficiently. Bacteria, in contrast, have no way of capturing lumps of food; they can export substances that help break down food substances in the environment, but the products of this labor must then be shared with other organisms in the same neighborhood.

ANSWER 1–6   Conventional light microscopy is much easier to use and requires much simpler instruments. Objects that are 1 μm in size can easily be resolved; the lower limit of resolution is 0.2 μm, which is a theoretical limit imposed by the wavelength of visible light. Visible light is nondestructive and passes readily through water, making it possible to observe living cells. Electron microscopy, on the other hand, is much more complicated, both in the nature of the instrument and in the preparation of the sample (which needs to be extremely thinly sliced, stained with an electron-dense heavy metal, and completely dehydrated). Living cells cannot be observed in an electron microscope. The resolution of electron microscopy is much higher, however, and biological objects as small as 1 nm can be resolved. To see any structural detail, microtubules, mitochondria, and bacteria would need to be analyzed either by electron microscopy or by using specific dyes to make them visible by confocal or super-resolution fluorescence microscopy (although no form of fluorescence microscopy can match the resolution of an electron microscope).

ANSWER 1–7   Because the basic workings of all cells are so similar, a great deal has been learned from studying model systems. Brewer's yeast is a good model for eukaryotic cells because yeast cells are much simpler than human cancer cells. We can grow them inexpensively and in vast quantities, and we can manipulate them genetically and biochemically much more easily than human cells. This allows us to use yeast to decipher the ground rules governing how cells grow and divide. Cancer cells grow and divide when they should not (and therefore give rise to tumors), and a basic understanding of how cell growth and division are normally controlled is therefore directly relevant to the cancer problem. Indeed, the National Cancer Institute, the American Cancer Society, and many other institutions that are devoted to finding a cure for cancer strongly support basic research on various aspects of cell growth and division in different model systems, including yeast.

ANSWER 1–8   Check your answers using the Glossary and Panel 1–2 (p. 25).

ANSWER 1–9

A. False. The hereditary information is encoded in the cell's DNA, which in turn specifies its proteins (via RNA).
B. True. Bacteria do not have a nucleus.
C. False. Plants, like animals, are composed of eukaryotic cells, but unlike animal cells, they contain chloroplasts as cytoplasmic organelles. The chloroplasts are thought to be evolutionarily derived from engulfed photosynthetic bacteria.
D. True. The number of chromosomes varies from one organism to another, but is constant in all nucleated cells (except germ cells) within the same multicellular organism.
E. False. The cytosol is the cytoplasm excluding all membrane-enclosed organelles.
F. True. The nuclear envelope is a double membrane, and mitochondria are surrounded by both an inner and an outer membrane.
G. False. Protozoans are single-celled organisms and therefore do not have different tissues or cell types. They have a complex structure, however, that has highly specialized parts.
H. Somewhat true. Peroxisomes and lysosomes contain enzymes that catalyze the breakdown of substances produced in the cytosol or taken up by the cell. One can argue, however, that many of these substances are degraded to generate food molecules, and as such are certainly not "unwanted."

ANSWER 1–10   In this plant cell, A is the nucleus, B is a vacuole, C is the cell wall, and D is a chloroplast. The scale bar is about 10 μm, the width of the nucleus.

ANSWER 1–11   The three major filaments are actin filaments, intermediate filaments, and microtubules. Actin filaments are involved in rapid cell movement, and are the most abundant filaments in a muscle cell; intermediate filaments provide mechanical stability and are the most abundant filaments in epidermal cells of the skin; and microtubules function as "railroad tracks" for many intracellular movements and are responsible for the separation of chromosomes during cell division. Other functions of all these filaments are discussed in Chapter 17.

ANSWER 1–12   It takes only 20 hours (i.e., less than a day) before mutant cells become more abundant in the culture. Using the equation provided in the question, we see that the number of the original ("wild-type") bacterial cells at time t minutes after the mutation occurred is $10^6 \times 2^{t/20}$. The number of mutant cells at time t is $1 \times 2^{t/15}$. To find out when the mutant cells "overtake" the wild-type cells, we simply have to make these two numbers equal to each other (i.e., $10^6 \times 2^{t/20} = 2^{t/15}$). Taking the logarithm to base 10 of both sides of this equation and solving it for t results in $t = 1200$ minutes (or 20 hours). At this time, the culture contains 2×10^{24} cells ($10^6 \times 2^{60} + 1 \times 2^{80}$). Incidentally, 2×10^{24} bacterial cells, each weighing 10^{-12} g, would weigh 2×10^{12} g (= 2×10^9 kg, or 2 million tons!). This can only have been a thought experiment.

ANSWER 1–13   Bacteria continually acquire mutations in their DNA. In the population of cells exposed to the poison, one or a few cells may already harbor a mutation that makes them resistant to the action of the poison. Antibiotics that are poisonous to bacteria because they bind to certain bacterial proteins, for example, would not work if the proteins have a slightly changed surface so that binding occurs more weakly or not at all. These mutant bacteria would continue dividing rapidly while their cousins are slowed down. The antibiotic-resistant bacteria would soon become the predominant species in the culture.

ANSWER 1–14 $10^{13} = 2^{(t/1)}$. Therefore, it would take only 43 days [$t = 13/\log(2)$]. This explains why some cancers can progress extremely rapidly. Many cancer cells divide much more slowly, however, and many die because of their internal abnormalities or because they do not have a sufficient blood supply, and so the actual progression of cancer is usually slower.

ANSWER 1–15   Living cells evolved from nonliving matter, but they grow and replicate. Like the material they originated from, they are governed by the laws of physics, thermodynamics, and chemistry. Thus, for example, they cannot create energy *de novo* or build ordered structures without the expenditure of free energy. We can understand virtually all cellular events, such as metabolism, catalysis, membrane assembly, and DNA replication, as complicated chemical reactions that can be experimentally reproduced, manipulated, and studied in test tubes.

Despite this fundamental reducibility, a living cell is more than the sum of its parts. We cannot randomly mix proteins, nucleic acids, and other chemicals together in a test tube, for example, and make a cell. The cell functions by virtue of its organized structure, and this is a product of its evolutionary history. Cells always come from preexisting cells, and the division of a mother cell passes both chemical constituents and structures to its daughters. The plasma membrane, for example, never has to form *de novo*, but grows by expansion of a preexisting membrane; there will always be a ribosome, in part made up of proteins, whose function it is to make more proteins, including those that build more ribosomes.

ANSWER 1–16   In a multicellular organism, different cells take on specialized functions and cooperate with one another, so that any one cell type does not have to perform all activities for itself. Through such division of labor, multicellular organisms are able to exploit food sources that are inaccessible to single-celled organisms. A plant, for example, can reach the soil with its roots to take up water and nutrients, while at the same time, its leaves above ground can harvest light energy and CO_2 from the air. By protecting its reproductive cells with other specialized cells, the multicellular organism can develop new ways to survive in harsh environments or to fight off predators. When food runs out, it may be able to preserve its reproductive cells by allowing them to draw upon resources stored by their companions—or even to cannibalize relatives (a common process, in fact).

ANSWER 1–17   The volume and the surface area are 5.24×10^{-19} m^3 and 3.14×10^{-12} m^2 for the bacterial cell, and 1.77×10^{-15} m^3 and 7.07×10^{-10} m^2 for the animal cell, respectively. From these numbers, the surface-to-volume ratios are 6×10^6 m^{-1} and 4×10^5 m^{-1}, respectively. In other words, although the animal cell has a 3375-fold larger volume, its membrane surface is increased only 225-fold. If internal membranes are included in the calculation, however, the surface-to-volume ratios of both cells are about equal. Thus, because of their internal membranes, eukaryotic cells can grow bigger and still maintain a sufficiently large area of membrane, which—as we discuss in more detail in later chapters—is required for many essential cell functions.

ANSWER 1–18   There are many lines of evidence for a common ancestor cell. Analyses of modern-day living cells show an amazing degree of similarity in the basic components that make up the inner workings of otherwise vastly different cells. Many metabolic pathways, for example, are conserved from one cell type to another, and the organic compounds that make up polynucleotides (DNA and RNA) and proteins are the same in all living cells, even though it is easy to imagine that a different choice of compounds (e.g., amino acids with different side chains) would have worked just as well. Similarly, it is not uncommon to find that important proteins have closely similar detailed structures in prokaryotic and eukaryotic cells. Theoretically, there would be many different ways to build proteins that could perform the same functions. The evidence overwhelmingly shows that most important processes were "invented" only once and then became fine-tuned during evolution to suit the particular needs of specialized cells and specific organisms.

It seems highly unlikely, however, that the first cell survived to become the primordial founder cell of today's living world. As evolution is not a directed process with purposeful progression, it is more likely that there were a vast number of unsuccessful trial cells that replicated for a while and then became extinct because they could not adapt to changes in the environment or could not survive in competition with other trial cells. We can therefore speculate that the primordial ancestor cell was a "lucky" cell that ended up in a relatively stable environment in which it had a chance to replicate and evolve.

ANSWER 1–19   A quick inspection might reveal the characteristic beating of cilia on the cell surface; their presence would tell you that the cell was eukaryotic (prokaryote flagella have entirely different structures and motions compared to eukaryote cilia and flagella). If you don't see them—and you are quite likely not to—you will have to look for other distinguishing features. If you are lucky, you might see the cell divide. Watch it then with the right optics, and you might be able to see condensed mitotic chromosomes, which again would tell you that it was a eukaryote. Fix the cell and stain it with a dye for DNA: if the DNA is contained in a well-defined nucleus, the cell is a eukaryote; if you cannot see a well-defined nucleus, the cell may be a prokaryote. Alternatively, stain it with fluorescent antibodies that bind actin or tubulin (proteins that are highly conserved in eukaryotes but absent in bacteria). Embed it, section it, and look with an electron microscope: can you see organelles such as mitochondria inside your cell? Try staining it with Gram stain, which is specific for molecules in the cell wall of some classes of bacteria. But all these tests might fail, leaving you still uncertain. For a definitive answer, you could attempt to analyze the sequences of the DNA and RNA molecules that it contains, using the sophisticated methods we describe more fully in Chapter 10. If the nucleic acid sequences encode molecules that are highly conserved in eukaryotes, such as those that form the core components of the nuclear pore, you can be sure your cell is a eukaryote. If there are no eukaryote-specific sequences, you should still be able to distinguish whether you are looking at a bacterium or an archaeon. If you can't detect any DNA or RNA, you are probably looking not at a cell but at a piece of dirt.

Chapter 2

ANSWER 2–1   The chances are excellent because of the enormous size of Avogadro's number. The original cup contained one mole of water, or 6×10^{23} molecules, and the volume of the world's oceans, converted to cubic centimeters, is 1.5×10^{24} cm^3. After mixing, there should be on average 0.4 of a "Greek" water molecule per cm^3 ($6 \times 10^{23}/1.5 \times 10^{24}$), or 7.2 molecules in 18 g of Pacific Ocean.

ANSWER 2–2
A. The atomic number is 6; the atomic weight is 12 (= 6 protons + 6 neutrons).
B. The number of electrons is 6 (= the number of protons).
C. The first shell can accommodate two and the second shell eight electrons. Carbon therefore needs four additional electrons (or would have to give up four electrons) to obtain a full outermost shell. Carbon is most stable when it shares four additional electrons with other atoms (including other carbon atoms) by forming four covalent bonds.

D. Carbon-14 has two additional neutrons in its nucleus. Because the chemical properties of an atom are determined by its electrons, carbon-14 is chemically identical to carbon-12.

ANSWER 2–3   The statement is correct. Both ionic and covalent bonds are based on the same principles: an exchange of electrons. In polar covalent bonds, the electrons are shared unequally between the interacting atoms. In ionic bonds, the electrons are completely lost by one atom and gained by the other. And at the other end of the spectrum, electrons can be shared equally between two interacting atoms to form a nonpolar covalent bond. There are bonds of every conceivable intermediate state, and for borderline cases it becomes arbitrary whether a bond is described as a very polar covalent bond or an ionic bond.

ANSWER 2–4   The statement is correct. The hydrogen–oxygen bond in water molecules is polar, so the oxygen atom carries a more negative charge than the hydrogen atoms. These partial negative charges are attracted to the positively charged sodium ions, but are repelled from the negatively charged chloride ions.

ANSWER 2–5

A. Hydronium (H_3O^+) ions result from water dissociating into protons and hydroxyl ions, each proton binding to a water molecule to form a hydronium ion ($2H_2O \rightarrow H_2O + H^+ + OH^- \rightarrow H_3O^+ + OH^-$). At neutral pH—that is, in the absence of an acid providing more H_3O^+ ions or a base providing more OH^- ions—the concentrations of H_3O^+ ions and OH^- ions are equal. We know that at neutrality the pH = 7.0, and therefore the H^+ concentration is 10^{-7} M. The H^+ concentration equals the H_3O^+ concentration.

B. To calculate the ratio of H_3O^+ ions to H_2O molecules, we need to know the concentration of water molecules. The molecular weight of water is 18 (i.e., 18 g/mole), and 1 liter of water weighs 1 kg. Therefore, the concentration of water is 55.6 M (= 1000 [g/L]/[18 g/mole]), and the ratio of H_3O^+ ions to H_2O molecules is 1.8×10^{-9} (= $10^{-7}/55.6$); that is, only two water molecules in a billion are dissociated at neutral pH.

ANSWER 2–6   The synthesis of a macromolecule with a unique structure requires that in each position only one stereoisomer is used. Changing one amino acid from its L- to its D-form would result in a different protein. Thus, if for each amino acid a random mixture of the D- and L-forms were used to build a protein, its amino acid sequence could not specify a single structure, but many different structures (2^N different structures) would be formed (where N is the number of amino acids in the protein).

Why L-amino acids were selected in evolution as the exclusive building blocks of proteins is a mystery; we could easily imagine a cell in which certain (or even all) amino acids were used in the D-forms to build proteins, as long as these particular stereoisomers were used exclusively.

ANSWER 2–7   The term "polarity" has two different meanings. In one meaning, polarity refers to a directional asymmetry—for example, in linear polymers such as polypeptides, which have an N-terminus and a C-terminus; or nucleic acids, which have a 3′ and a 5′ end. Because bonds form only between the amino and the carboxyl groups of the amino acids in a polypeptide, and between the 3′ and the 5′ ends of nucleotides, nucleic acids and polypeptides always have two different ends, which give the chains a defined chemical polarity.

In the other meaning, polarity refers to a separation of electric charge in a bond or molecule. This kind of polarity promotes hydrogen-bonding to water molecules, and because the water solubility, or hydrophilicity, of a molecule depends upon its being polar in this sense, the term "polar" also indicates water solubility.

ANSWER 2–8   A major advantage of condensation reactions is that they are readily reversible by hydrolysis (and water is readily available in the cell). This allows cells to break down their macromolecules (or macromolecules of other organisms that were ingested as food) and to recover the subunits intact so that they can be "recycled;" that is, used to build new macromolecules.

ANSWER 2–9   Many of the functions that macromolecules perform rely on their ability to associate and dissociate readily. This chemical flexibility allows cells, for example, to remodel their interior when they move or divide, and to transport components from one organelle to another. Covalent bonds would be too strong and too permanent for such a purpose, requiring a specific enzyme to break each kind of bond.

ANSWER 2–10

A. True. All nuclei are made of positively charged protons and uncharged neutrons; the only exception is the hydrogen nucleus, which consists of only one proton.

B. False. Atoms are electrically neutral. The number of positively charged protons is always balanced by an equal number of negatively charged electrons.

C. True—but only for the cell nucleus (see Chapter 1), not for the atomic nucleus discussed in this chapter.

D. False. Elements can have different isotopes, which differ only in their number of neutrons.

E. True. In certain isotopes, the large number of neutrons destabilizes the nucleus, which decomposes in a process called radioactive decay.

F. True. Examples include granules of glycogen, a polymer of glucose, found in liver cells; and fat droplets, made of aggregated triacylglycerols, found in fat cells.

G. True. Individually, these bonds are weak and readily broken by thermal motion, but because interactions between two macromolecules involve a large number of such bonds, the overall binding can be quite strong; and because hydrogen bonds form only between correctly positioned groups on the interacting macromolecules, they are very specific.

ANSWER 2–11

A. One cellulose molecule has a molecular weight of $n \times (12[C] + 2 \times 1[H] + 16[O])$. We do not know n, but we can determine the ratio with which the individual elements contribute to the weight of cellulose. The contribution of carbon atoms is 40% [= $12/(12 + 2 + 16) \times 100\%$]. Therefore, 2 g (40% of 5 g) of carbon atoms are contained in the cellulose that makes up this page. The atomic weight of carbon is 12 g/mole, and there are 6×10^{23} atoms or molecules in a mole. Therefore, 10^{23} carbon atoms [= (2 g/12 [g/mole]) × 6×10^{23} (molecules/mole)] make up this page.

B. The volume of the page is 4×10^{-6} m³ (= 21.2 cm × 27.6 cm × 0.07 mm), which is the same as the volume of a cube with a side length of 1.6 cm (= $\sqrt[3]{4 \times 10^{-6}}$ m³). Because we know from part A that the page contains 10^{23} carbon atoms, geometry tells us that there could be about 4.6×10^7 carbon atoms (= $\sqrt[3]{10^{23}}$) lined up along each side of this cube. Therefore, in cellulose, about 200,000 carbon atoms [= $(4.6 \times 10^7) \times (0.07 \times 10^{-3}$ m)/ 1.6×10^{-2} m] span the thickness of the page.

C. If tightly stacked, 350,000 carbon atoms with a 0.2-nm diameter would span the 0.07-mm thickness of the page.

D. The 1.7-fold difference in the two calculations reflects (1) that carbon is not the only atom in cellulose and (2) that paper is not an atomic lattice of precisely arranged molecules (as a diamond would be for precisely arranged carbon atoms), but a random meshwork of fibers containing many voids.

ANSWER 2–12

A. The occupancies of the three innermost electron levels are 2, 8, 8.

B.
helium	already has full outer electron shell
oxygen	gain 2
carbon	gain 4 or lose 4
sodium	lose 1
chlorine	gain 1

C. Helium, with its fully occupied outer electron shell, is chemically unreactive. Sodium and chlorine, on the other hand, are extremely reactive and readily form stable Na^+ and Cl^- ions that form ionic bonds, as in table salt.

ANSWER 2–13   Whether a substance is a liquid or a gas at a given temperature depends on the attractive forces between its molecules. H_2S is a gas at room temperature and H_2O is a liquid because the hydrogen bonds that hold H_2O molecules together do not form between H_2S molecules. A sulfur atom is much larger than an oxygen atom, and because of its larger size, the outermost electrons are not as strongly attracted to the nucleus of the sulfur atom as they are in an oxygen atom. Consequently, the hydrogen–sulfur bond is much less polar than the hydrogen–oxygen bond. Because of the reduced polarity, the sulfur in an H_2S molecule is not strongly attracted to the hydrogen atoms in an adjacent H_2S molecule, and the hydrogen bonds that are so predominant in water do not form.

ANSWER 2–14   The reactions are diagrammed in Figure A2–14, where R_1 and R_2 are amino acid side chains.

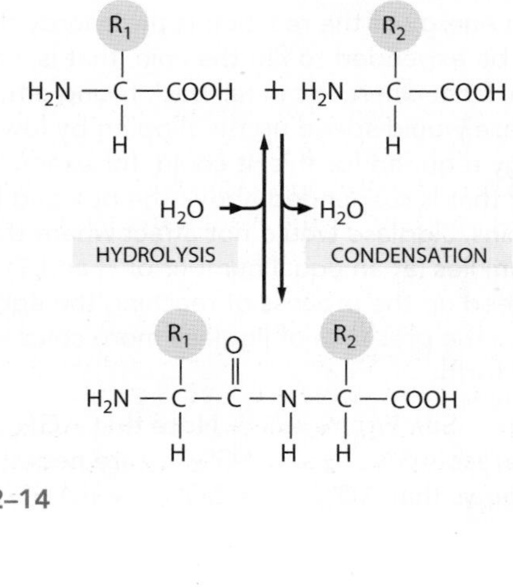

Figure A2–14

ANSWER 2–15

A. False. The properties of a protein depend on both the amino acids it contains and the order in which they are linked together. The diversity of proteins is due to the almost unlimited number of ways in which 20 different amino acids can be combined in a linear sequence.

B. False. Lipids assemble into bilayers by noncovalent bonds. A membrane is therefore not a macromolecule.

C. True. The backbone of nucleic acids is made up of alternating ribose (or deoxyribose in DNA) and phosphate groups. Ribose and deoxyribose are sugars.

D. True. About half of the 20 naturally occurring amino acids have hydrophobic side chains. In folded proteins, many of these side chains face toward the inside of the folded-up proteins, because they are repelled from water.

E. True. Hydrophobic hydrocarbon tails contain only nonpolar covalent bonds. Thus, they cannot participate in hydrogen-bonding and are repelled from water. We consider the underlying principles in more detail in Chapter 11.

F. False. RNA contains the four listed bases, but DNA contains T instead of U. T and U are very much alike, however, and differ only by a single methyl group.

ANSWER 2–16

A. (a) 400 (= 20^2); (b) 8000 (= 20^3); (c) 160,000 (= 20^4).

B. A protein with a molecular mass of 4800 daltons is made of about 40 amino acids; thus there are 1.1×10^{52} (= 20^{40}) different ways to make such a protein. Each individual protein molecule weighs 8×10^{-21} g (= $4800/6 \times 10^{23}$); thus a mixture of one molecule each weighs 9×10^{31} g (= 8×10^{-21} g × 1.1×10^{52}), which is 15,000 times the total weight of the planet Earth, weighing 6×10^{24} kg. You would need a very large container indeed.

C. Given that most cellular proteins are even larger than the one used in this example, it is clear that only a minuscule fraction of the total possible amino acid sequences is used in living cells.

ANSWER 2–17   Because all living cells are made up of chemicals, and because all chemical reactions (whether in living cells or in test tubes) follow the same rules, an understanding of basic chemical principles is fundamentally important to the understanding of biology. In the course of this book, we will frequently refer back to these principles, on which all of the more complicated pathways and reactions that occur in cells are based.

ANSWER 2–18

A. Hydrogen bonds require specific groups to interact; one is always a hydrogen atom linked by a polar covalent bond to an oxygen or a nitrogen, and the other is usually a nitrogen or an oxygen atom. Van der Waals attractions are weaker and occur between any two atoms that are in close enough proximity. Both hydrogen bonds and van der Waals attractions are short-range interactions that come into play only when two molecules are already close. Both types of bonds can therefore be thought of as a means of "fine-tuning" an interaction; that is, helping to position two molecules correctly with respect to each other once they have been brought together by diffusion.

B. Van der Waals attractions would form in all three examples. Hydrogen bonds would form in (c) only.

ANSWER 2–19   Noncovalent bonds form between the subunits of macromolecules—e.g., the side chains of amino acids in a polypeptide chain—and cause the polymer chain to assume a unique shape. These interactions include hydrogen bonds, ionic bonds, van der Waals attractions, and hydrophobic forces. Because these interactions are weak, they can be broken with relative ease; thus, most macromolecules can be unfolded by heating, which increases thermal motion.

ANSWER 2–20   Amphipathic molecules have both a hydrophilic and a hydrophobic end. Their hydrophilic ends can hydrogen-bond to water, but their hydrophobic ends are repelled from water because they interfere with the water structure. Consequently, the hydrophobic ends of amphipathic molecules tend to be exposed to air at air–water interfaces, or will always cluster together to minimize their contact with water molecules—both at this interface and in the interior of an aqueous solution. (See Figure A2–20.)

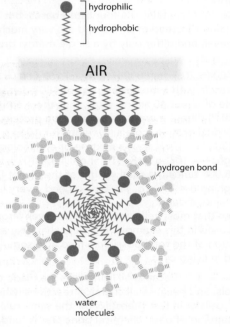

Figure A2–20

ANSWER 2–21

A, B. (A) and (B) are both correct formulas of the amino acid phenylalanine. In formula (B), phenylalanine is shown in the ionized form that exists in solution in water, where the basic amino group is protonated and the acidic carboxylic group is deprotonated.
C. Incorrect. This structure of a peptide bond is missing a hydrogen atom bound to the nitrogen.
D. Incorrect. This formula of an adenine base features one double bond too many, creating a five-valent carbon atom and a four-valent nitrogen atom.
E. Incorrect. In this formula of a nucleoside triphosphate, there should be two additional oxygen atoms, one between each of the phosphorus atoms.
F. This is the correct formula of ethanol.
G. Incorrect. Water does not hydrogen-bond to hydrogens bonded to carbon. The lack of the capacity to hydrogen-

bond makes hydrocarbon chains hydrophobic; that is, water-hating.
H. Incorrect. Na and Cl form an ionic bond, Na^+Cl^-, but a covalent bond is drawn.
I. Incorrect. The oxygen atom attracts electrons more than the carbon atom; the polarity of the two bonds should therefore be reversed.
J. This structure of glucose is correct.
K. Almost correct. It is more accurate to show that only one hydrogen is lost from the $-NH_2$ group and the $-OH$ group is lost from the $-COOH$ group.

Chapter 3

ANSWER 3–1   The equation represents the "bottom line" of photosynthesis, which occurs as a large set of individual reactions that are catalyzed by many individual enzymes. Because sugars are more complicated molecules than CO_2 and H_2O, the reaction generates a more ordered state inside the cell. As demanded by the second law of thermodynamics, this increase in order must be accompanied by a greater increase in disorder, which occurs because heat is generated at many steps on the long pathway leading to the products summarized in this equation.

ANSWER 3–2   Oxidation is defined as removal of electrons, and reduction represents a gain of electrons. Therefore, (A) is an oxidation and (B) is a reduction. The *red* carbon atom in (C) remains largely unchanged; the neighboring carbon atom, however, loses a hydrogen atom (i.e., an electron and a proton) and hence becomes oxidized. The *red* carbon atom in (D) becomes oxidized because it loses a hydrogen atom, whereas the *red* carbon atom in (E) becomes reduced because it gains a hydrogen atom.

ANSWER 3–3
A. Both states of the coin, H and T, have an equal probability. There is therefore no driving force—that is, no energy difference—that would favor H turning to T, or vice versa. Therefore, $\Delta G° = 0$ for this reaction. However, a reaction proceeds if H and T coins are not present in the box in equal numbers. In this case, the concentration difference between H and T creates a driving force and $\Delta G \neq 0$; when the reaction reaches equilibrium—that is, when there are equal numbers of H and T—$\Delta G = 0$.
B. The amount of shaking corresponds to the temperature, as it results in the "thermal" motion of the coins. The activation energy of the reaction is the energy that needs to be expended to flip the coin, that is, to stand it on its rim, from where it can fall back facing either side up. Jigglase would speed up the flipping by lowering the energy required for this; it could, for example, be a magnet that is suspended above the box and helps lift the coins. Jigglase would not affect where the equilibrium lies (at an equal number of H and T), but it would speed up the process of reaching the equilibrium, because in the presence of jigglase more coins would flip back and forth.

ANSWER 3–4   See Figure A3–4. Note that $\Delta G°_{X \to Y}$ is positive, whereas $\Delta G°_{Y \to Z}$ and $\Delta G°_{X \to Z}$ are negative. The graph also shows that $\Delta G°_{X \to Z} = \Delta G°_{X \to Y} + \Delta G°_{Y \to Z}$.

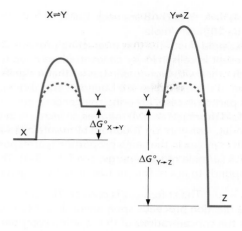

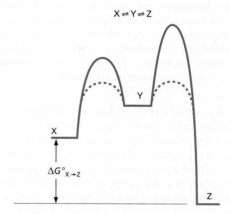

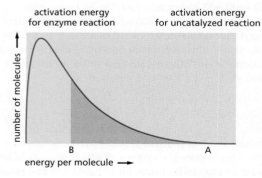

Figure A3–4

We do not know from the information given in Figure 3–12 how high the activation-energy barriers are; they are therefore drawn to an arbitrary height (solid lines). The activation energies would be lowered by enzymes that catalyze these reactions, thereby speeding up the reaction rates (dotted lines), but the enzymes would not change the $\Delta G°$ values.

ANSWER 3–5 The reaction rates might be limited by: (1) the concentration of the substrate—that is, how often a molecule of CO_2 collides with the active site on the enzyme; (2) how many of these collisions are energetic enough to lead to a reaction; and (3) how fast the enzyme can release the products of the reaction and therefore be free to bind more CO_2. The diagram in Figure A3–5 shows that the

enzyme lowers the activation-energy barrier, so that more CO_2 molecules have sufficient energy to undergo the reaction. The area under the curve from point A to infinite energy or from point B to infinite energy indicates the total number of molecules that will react without or with the enzyme, respectively. Although not drawn to scale, the ratio of these two areas should be 10^7.

ANSWER 3–6 All reactions are reversible. If the compound AB can dissociate to produce A and B, then it must also be possible for A and B to associate to form AB. Which of the two reactions predominates depends on the equilibrium constant of the reaction and the concentrations of A, B, and AB (as discussed in Figure 3–19). Presumably, when this enzyme was isolated, its activity was detected by supplying A and B in relatively large amounts and measuring the amount of AB generated. But suppose, however, that in the cell there is a large concentration of AB, in which case the enzyme would actually catalyze AB → A + B. (This question is based on an actual example in which an enzyme was isolated and named according to the reaction in one direction, but was later shown to catalyze the reverse reaction in living cells.)

ANSWER 3–7

A. The rocks in Figure 3–29B provide the energy to lift the bucket of water. (i) In the reaction X + ATP → Y + ADP + P_i, ATP hydrolysis is driving the reaction; thus ATP corresponds to the rocks on top of the cliff. (ii) The broken debris in Figure 3–29B corresponds to ADP and P_i, the products of ATP hydrolysis. (iii) and (iv) In the reaction, ATP hydrolysis is coupled to the conversion of X to Y. X, therefore, is the starting material, the bucket on the ground, which is converted to Y, the bucket at its highest point.

B. (i) The rocks hitting the ground would be the futile hydrolysis of ATP—for example, in the absence of an enzyme that uses the energy released by the ATP hydrolysis to drive an otherwise unfavorable reaction; in this case, the energy stored in the phosphoanhydride bond of ATP would be lost as heat. (ii) The energy stored in Y could be used to drive another reaction. If Y represented the activated form of amino acid X, for example, it could undergo a condensation reaction to form a peptide bond during protein synthesis.

ANSWER 3–8 The free energy ΔG derived from ATP hydrolysis depends on both the $\Delta G°$ and the concentrations of the substrate and products. For example, for a particular set of concentrations, one might have

$$\Delta G = -50 \text{ kJ/mole} = -30.5 \text{ kJ/mole} + 2.58 \ln \frac{[\text{ADP}] \times [P_i]}{[\text{ATP}]}$$

ΔG is smaller than $\Delta G°$, largely because the ATP concentration in cells is high (in the millimolar range) and the ADP concentration is low (in the 10 μM range). The concentration term of this equation is therefore smaller than 1 and its logarithm is a negative number.

$\Delta G°$ is a constant for the reaction and will not vary with reaction conditions. ΔG, in contrast, depends on the concentrations of ATP, ADP, and phosphate, which can be somewhat different between cells.

ANSWER 3–9 Reactions B, D, and E all require coupling to other, energetically favorable reactions. In each case, higher-order structures are formed that are more complicated and have higher-energy bonds than the starting materials. In contrast, reaction A is a catabolic reaction that leads to compounds in a lower energy state and will occur spontaneously. The nucleoside triphosphates in reaction C contain enough energy to drive DNA synthesis (see Figure 3–42).

ANSWER 3–10

A. Nearly true, but strictly speaking, false. Because enzymes enhance the rate but do not change the equilibrium point of a reaction, a reaction will always occur in the absence of the enzyme, though often at a minuscule rate. Moreover, competing reactions may use up the substrate more quickly, thus further impeding the desired reaction. Thus, in practical terms, without an enzyme, some reactions may never occur to an appreciable extent.

B. False. High-energy electrons are more easily transferred; that is, they are more loosely bound to the donor molecule. This does not mean that they move any faster.

C. True. Hydrolysis of an ATP molecule to form AMP also produces a pyrophosphate (PP_i) molecule, which in turn is hydrolyzed into two phosphate molecules. This second reaction releases almost the same amount of energy as the initial hydrolysis of ATP, thereby approximately doubling the energy total yield.

D. True. Oxidation is the removal of electrons, which reduces the diameter of the carbon atom.

E. True. ATP, for example, can donate both chemical-bond energy and a phosphate group.

F. False. Living cells have a particular kind of chemistry in which most oxidations are energy-releasing events; under different conditions, however, such as in a hydrogen-containing atmosphere, reductions would be energy-releasing events.

G. False. All cells, including those of cold- and warm-blooded animals, radiate comparable amounts of heat as a consequence of their metabolic reactions. For bacterial cells, for example, this becomes apparent when a compost pile heats up.

H. False. The equilibrium constant of the reaction $X \leftrightarrow Y$ remains unchanged. If Y is removed by a second reaction, more X is converted to Y so that the ratio of X to Y remains constant.

ANSWER 3–11   The free-energy difference ($\Delta G°$) between Y and X due to three hydrogen bonds is –12.6 kJ/mole. (Note that the free energy of Y is lower than that of X, because energy would need to be expended to break the bonds to convert Y to X. The value for $\Delta G°$ for the transition $X \rightarrow Y$ is therefore negative.) The equilibrium constant for the reaction is therefore about 100 (from Table 3–1, p. 96); that is, there are about 100 times more molecules of Y than of X at equilibrium. An additional three hydrogen bonds would increase $\Delta G°$ to –25.2 kcal/mole and increase the equilibrium constant about another 100-fold to 10^4. Thus, relatively small differences in energy can have a major effect on equilibria.

ANSWER 3–12

A. The equilibrium constant is defined as $K = [AB]/([A] \times [B])$. The square brackets indicate the concentration. Thus, if A, B, and AB are each 1 µM (10^{-6} M), K will be 10^6 liters/mole [= $10^{-6}/(10^{-6} \times 10^{-6})$].

B. Similarly, if A, B, and AB are each 1 nM (10^{-9} M), then K will be 10^9 liters/mole.

C. This example illustrates that interacting proteins that are present in cells in lower concentrations need to bind to each other with higher affinities so that a significant fraction of the molecules are bound at equilibrium. In this particular case, lowering the concentration by 1000-fold (from µM to nM) requires an increase in the equilibrium constant by 1000-fold to maintain the AB protein complex in the same proportion (corresponding to –17.8 kJ/mole of free energy; see Table 3–1). This corresponds to about four or five extra hydrogen bonds.

ANSWER 3–13   The statement is correct. The criterion for whether a reaction proceeds spontaneously is ΔG, not $\Delta G°$, and takes the concentrations of the reacting components into account. A reaction with a negative $\Delta G°$, for example, would not proceed spontaneously under conditions where there is a large enough excess of products; that is, more than at equilibrium. Conversely, a reaction with a positive $\Delta G°$ might spontaneously go forward under conditions where there is a huge excess of substrate.

ANSWER 3–14

A. A maximum of 57 ATP molecules (= 2867/50) corresponds to the total energy released by the complete oxidation of glucose to CO_2 and H_2O.

B. The overall efficiency of ATP production would be about 53%, calculated as the number of actually produced ATP molecules (30) divided by the number of ATP molecules that could be obtained if all the energy stored in a glucose molecule could be harvested as chemical energy in ATP (57).

C. During the oxidation of 1 mole of glucose, 1347 kJ (the remaining 47% of the available 2867 kJ in one mole of glucose that is not stored as chemical energy in ATP) would be released as heat. This amount of energy would heat your body by 4.3°C (1347 kJ × 0.24 = 323 kcal; 323 kcal/75 kg = 4.3). This is a significant amount of heat, considering that 4°C of elevated temperature would be a quite incapacitating fever and that 1 mole (180 g) of glucose is no more than two cups of sugar.

D. If the energy yield were only 20%, then instead of 47% in part (C) above, 80% of the available energy would be released as heat and would need to be dissipated by your body. The heat production would be more than 1.7-fold higher than normal, and your body would certainly overheat.

E. The chemical formula of ATP is $C_{10}H_{12}O_{13}N_5P_3$, and its molecular weight is therefore 503 g/mole. Your resting body therefore hydrolyzes about 80 moles (= 40 kg/0.503 kg/mole) of ATP in 24 hours (this corresponds to about 4200 kJ of liberated chemical energy). Because every mole of glucose yields 30 moles of ATP, this amount of energy could be produced by oxidation of 480 g glucose (= 180 g/mole × 80 moles/30).

ANSWER 3–15   This scientist is definitely a fake. The 57 ATP molecules would store about 2850 kJ (= 57 × 50 kJ) of chemical energy, which implies that the efficiency of ATP production from glucose would have been greater than 99%. This impossible degree of efficiency would leave virtually no energy to be released as heat, and this release is required according to the laws of thermodynamics.

ANSWER 3–16

A. From Table 3–1 (p. 96) we know that a free-energy difference of 17.8 kJ/mole corresponds to an equilibrium constant of 10^{-3}; that is, $[A^*]/[A] = 10^{-3}$. The concentration of A* is therefore 1000-fold lower than that of A at equilibrium.

B. The ratio of A to A* would be unchanged. Lowering the activation-energy barrier with an enzyme would accelerate the rate of the reaction; that is, it would allow more molecules in a given time period to convert from $A \rightarrow A^*$ and from $A^* \rightarrow A$, but it would not affect the ratio of A to A* at equilibrium.

ANSWER 3–17

A. The mutant mushroom would probably be safe to eat. ATP hydrolysis can provide approximately –50 kJ/mole of energy. This amount of energy shifts the equilibrium point of a reaction by an enormous factor: about 10^8-fold. (From Table 3–1, p. 96, we see that –23.8 kJ/mole corresponds to an equilibrium constant of 10^4; thus, –50 kJ/mole corresponds to about 10^8. Note that, for coupled reactions, energies are additive, whereas equilibrium constants are multiplied.) Therefore, if the energy of ATP hydrolysis cannot be utilized by the enzyme, 10^8-fold less poison is made. This example illustrates that coupling a reaction to the hydrolysis of an activated carrier molecule can shift the equilibrium point drastically.

B. It would be risky to consume this mutant mushroom. Slowing down the reaction rate would not affect its equilibrium point, and if the reaction were allowed to proceed for a long enough time, the mushroom would likely be loaded with poison. It is possible that the reaction would not reach equilibrium, but it would not be advisable to take a chance.

ANSWER 3–18

Enzyme A is beneficial. It allows the interconversion of two energy-carrier molecules, both of which are required as the triphosphate form for many metabolic reactions. Any ADP that is formed is quickly converted to ATP, and thus the cell maintains a high ATP/ADP ratio. Because of enzyme A, called nucleotide phosphokinase, some of the ATP is used to keep the GTP/GDP ratio similarly high.

Enzyme B would be highly detrimental to the cell. Cells use NAD^+ as an electron acceptor in catabolic reactions and must maintain high concentrations of this form of the carrier, as it is used in reactions that break down glucose to make ATP. In contrast, NADPH is used as an electron donor in biosynthetic reactions and is kept at a high concentration in the cells so as to allow the synthesis of nucleotides, fatty acids, and other essential molecules. Because enzyme B would deplete the cell's reserves of both NAD^+ and NADPH, it would decrease the rates of both catabolic and biosynthetic reactions.

ANSWER 3–19

Because enzymes are catalysts, enzyme reactions have to be thermodynamically feasible; the enzyme only lowers the activation-energy barrier that otherwise slows the rate with which the reaction occurs. Heat confers more kinetic energy to substrates so that a higher fraction of them can surmount the normal activation-energy barrier. Many substrates, however, have many different ways in which they could react, and all of these potential pathways will be enhanced by heat. An enzyme, by contrast, acts selectively to facilitate only one particular pathway that, in evolution, was selected to be useful for the cell. Heat, therefore, cannot substitute for enzyme function, and chicken soup must exert its claimed beneficial effects by other mechanisms, which remain to be discovered.

Chapter 4

ANSWER 4–1

Urea is a very small organic molecule that functions both as an efficient hydrogen-bond donor (through its NH_2 groups) and as an efficient hydrogen-bond acceptor (through its C=O group). As such, it can squeeze between hydrogen bonds that stabilize protein molecules and thus destabilize protein structures. In addition, the nonpolar side chains of a protein are held together in the interior of the folded structure because they would disrupt the structure of water if they were exposed. At high concentrations of urea, the hydrogen-bonded network of water molecules becomes disrupted so that these hydrophobic forces are significantly diminished. Proteins unfold in urea as a consequence of its effect on these two forces.

ANSWER 4–2

The amino acid sequence consists of alternating nonpolar and charged or polar amino acids. The resulting strand in a β sheet would therefore be polar on one side and hydrophobic on the other. Such a strand would probably be surrounded on either side by similar strands that together form a β sheet with a hydrophobic face and a polar face. In a protein, such a β sheet (called "amphipathic," from the Greek *amphi*, "of both kinds," and *pathos*, "passion," because of its two surfaces with such different properties) would be positioned so that the hydrophobic side would face the protein's interior and the polar side would be on its surface, exposed to the water outside.

ANSWER 4–3

Mutations that are beneficial to an organism are selected in evolution because they confer a reproductive or survival advantage to the organism. Examples might be a more efficient utilization of a food source, enhanced resistance to environmental insults, or an improved ability to attract a mate for sexual reproduction. In contrast, useless proteins are detrimental to organisms, as the metabolic energy required to make them is a wasted cost. If such mutant proteins were made in excess, the synthesis of normal proteins would suffer because the synthetic capacity of the cell is limited. In more severe cases, a mutant protein could interfere with the normal workings of the cell; a mutant enzyme that still binds an activated carrier molecule but does not catalyze a reaction, for example, may compete for a limited amount of this carrier and therefore inhibit normal processes. Natural selection therefore provides a strong driving force that eliminates both useless and harmful proteins.

ANSWER 4–4

Strong reducing agents that break all of the S–S bonds would cause all of the keratin filaments to separate. Individual hairs would be weakened and fragment. Indeed, strong reducing agents are used commercially in hair-removal creams sold by your local pharmacist. However, mild reducing agents are used in treatments that either straighten or curl hair, the latter requiring hair curlers. (See Figure A4–4.)

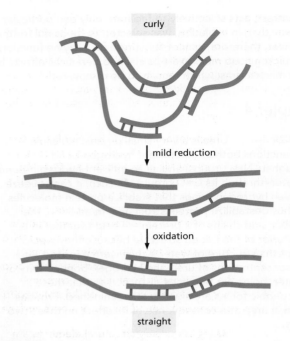

Figure A4–4

ANSWER 4–5   See Figure A4–5.

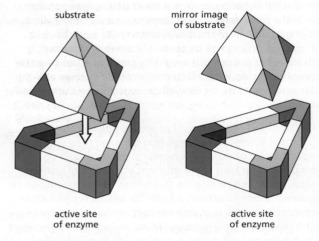

Figure A4–5

ANSWER 4–6

A. Feedback inhibition from Z that affects the reaction B → C would increase the flow through the B → X → Y → Z pathway, because the conversion of B to C is inhibited. Thus, the more Z there is, the more production of Z would be stimulated. This is likely to result in an uncontrolled "runaway" amplification of this pathway.

B. Feedback inhibition from Z affecting Y → Z would only inhibit the production of Z. In this scheme, however, X and Y would still be made at normal rates, even though both of these intermediates are no longer needed at this level. This pathway is therefore less efficient than the one shown in Figure 4–42.

C. If Z is a positive regulator of the step B → X, then the more Z there is, the more B will be converted to X and therefore shunted into the pathway producing more Z.

This would result in a runaway amplification similar to that described for (A).

D. If Z is a positive regulator of the step B → C, then accumulation of Z leads to a redirection of the pathway to make more C. This is a second possible way, in addition to that shown in the figure, to balance the distribution of compounds into the two branches of the pathway.

ANSWER 4–7   Both nucleotide binding and phosphorylation can induce allosteric changes in proteins. These can have a multitude of consequences, such as altered enzyme activity, drastic shape changes, and changes in affinity for other proteins or small molecules. Both mechanisms are quite versatile. An advantage of nucleotide binding is the fast rate with which a small nucleotide can diffuse to the protein; the shape changes that accompany the function of motor proteins, for example, require quick nucleotide replenishment. If the different conformational states of a motor protein were controlled by phosphorylation, for example, a protein kinase would either need to diffuse into position at each step, a much slower process, or be associated permanently with each motor protein. One advantage of phosphorylation is that it requires only a single amino acid on the protein's surface, rather than a specific binding site. Phosphates can therefore be added to many different side chains on the same protein (as long as protein kinases with the proper specificities exist), thereby vastly increasing the complexity of regulation that can be achieved for a single protein.

ANSWER 4–8   In working together in a complex, all three proteins contribute to the specificity (by binding to the safe and key directly). They help position one another correctly, and provide the mechanical bracing that allows them to perform a task that they could not perform individually (the key is grasped by two of the proteins, for example). Moreover, their functions are generally coordinated in time (for instance, the binding of ATP to one subunit is likely to require that ATP has already been hydrolyzed to ADP by another).

ANSWER 4–9   The α helix is right-handed. The three strands that form the large β sheet are antiparallel. There are no knots in the polypeptide chain, presumably because a knot would interfere with the folding of the protein into its three-dimensional conformation after protein synthesis.

ANSWER 4–10

A. True. Only a few amino acid side chains contribute to the active site. The rest of the protein is required to maintain the polypeptide chain in the correct conformation, provide additional binding sites for regulatory purposes, and localize the protein in the cell.

B. True. Some enzymes form covalent intermediates with their substrates (see middle panels of Figure 4–39); however, in all cases, the enzyme is restored to its original structure after the reaction.

C. False. β sheets can, in principle, contain any number of strands because the two strands that form the rims of the sheet are available for hydrogen-bonding to other strands. (β sheets in known proteins contain from 2 to 16 strands.)

D. False. It is true that the specificity of an antibody molecule is exclusively contained in polypeptide loops on its surface; however, these loops are contributed by both the folded light and heavy chains (see Figure 4–33).

E. False. The possible linear arrangements of amino acids that lead to a stably folded protein domain are so few that most new proteins evolve by alteration of old ones.

F. True. Allosteric enzymes generally bind one or more molecules that function as regulators at sites that are distinct from the active site.

G. False. Although single noncovalent bonds are weak, many such bonds acting together are major contributors to the three-dimensional structure of macromolecules.

H. False. Affinity chromatography separates specific macromolecules because of their interactions with specific ligands, not because of their charge.

I. False. The larger an organelle is, the more centrifugal force it experiences and the faster it sediments, despite an increased frictional resistance from the fluid through which it moves.

ANSWER 4–11   In an α helix and in the central strands of a β sheet, all of the N–H and C=O groups in the polypeptide backbone are engaged in hydrogen bonds. This gives considerable stability to these secondary structural elements, and it allows them to form in many different proteins.

ANSWER 4–12   No. It would not have the same or even a similar structure, because the peptide bond has a polarity. Looking at two sequential amino acids in a polypeptide chain, the amino acid that is closer to the N-terminal end contributes the carboxyl group and the other amino acid contributes the amino group to the peptide bond that links the two amino acids. Changing their order would put the side chains into different positions with respect to the peptide backbone and therefore change the way the polypeptide folds.

ANSWER 4–13   As it takes 3.6 amino acids to complete a turn of an α helix, this sequence of 14 amino acids would make close to 4 full turns. It is remarkable because its polar and hydrophobic amino acids are spaced so that all the polar ones are on one side of the α helix and all the hydrophobic ones are on the other. It is therefore likely that such an amphipathic α helix is exposed on the protein surface with its hydrophobic side facing the protein's interior. In addition, two such helices might wrap around each other as shown in Figure 4–16.

ANSWER 4–14

A. ES represents the enzyme–substrate complex.

B. Enzyme and substrate are in equilibrium between their free and bound states; once bound to the enzyme, a substrate molecule may either dissociate again (hence the bidirectional arrows) or be converted to product. As the substrate is converted to product (with the concomitant release of free energy), however, a reaction usually proceeds strongly in the forward direction, as indicated by the unidirectional arrow.

C. The enzyme is a catalyst and is therefore liberated in an unchanged form after the reaction; thus, E appears at both ends of the equation.

D. Often, the product of a reaction resembles the substrate sufficiently that it can also bind to the enzyme. Any enzyme molecules that are bound to the product

(i.e., are part of an EP complex) are unavailable for catalysis; excess P therefore can inhibit the reaction by lowering the concentration of free E.

E. Compound X would act as an inhibitor of the reaction and work similarly by forming an EX complex. However, since P has to be made before it can inhibit the reaction, it takes longer to act than X, which is present from the beginning of the reaction.

ANSWER 4–15   The polar amino acids Ser, Ser-P, Lys, Gln, His, and Glu are more likely to be found on a protein's surface, and the hydrophobic amino acids Leu, Phe, Val, Ile, and Met are more likely to be found in its interior. The oxidation of two cysteine side chains to form a disulfide bond eliminates their potential to form hydrogen bonds and therefore makes them even more hydrophobic; thus disulfide bonds are usually found in the interior of proteins. Irrespective of the nature of their side chains, the most N-terminal amino acid and the most C-terminal amino acid each contain a charged group (the amino and carboxyl groups, respectively, that mark the ends of the polypeptide chain) and hence are usually found on the protein's surface.

ANSWER 4–16   Many secondary structural elements are not stable in isolation but are stabilized by other parts of the polypeptide chain. Hydrophobic regions of fragments, which would normally be hidden in the inside of a folded protein, would be exposed to water molecules in an aqueous solution; such fragments would tend to aggregate nonspecifically, and not have a defined structure, and they would be inactive for ligand binding, even if they contained all of the amino acids that would normally contribute to the ligand-binding site. A protein domain, in contrast, is considered a folding unit, and fragments of a polypeptide chain that correspond to intact domains are often able to fold correctly. Thus, separated protein domains often retain their activities, such as ligand binding, if the binding site is contained entirely within the domain. Thus the most likely place in which the polypeptide chain of the protein in Figure 4–20 could be severed to give rise to stable fragments is at the boundary between the two domains (i.e., at the loop between the two α helices at the bottom right of the structure shown).

ANSWER 4–17   Because of the lack of secondary structure, the C-terminal region of neurofilament proteins undergoes continual Brownian motion. The high density of negatively charged phosphate groups means that the C-terminals also experience repulsive interactions, which cause them to stand out from the surface of the neurofilament like the bristles of a brush. In electron micrographs of a cross section of an axon, the region occupied by the extended C-terminals appears as a clear zone around each neurofilament, from which organelles and other neurofilaments are excluded.

ANSWER 4–18   The heat-inactivation of the enzyme suggests that the mutation causes the enzyme to have a less stable structure. For example, a hydrogen bond that is normally formed between two amino acid side chains might no longer be formed because the mutation replaces one of these amino acids with a different one that cannot participate in the bond. Lacking such a bond that normally helps to keep the polypeptide chain folded properly, the protein partially or completely unfolds at a temperature at which it would normally be stable. Polypeptide chains that denature when the temperature is raised often aggregate, and they rarely refold into active proteins when the temperature is decreased.

ANSWER 4–19   The motor protein in the illustration can move just as easily to the left as to the right and so will not move steadily in one direction. However, if just one of the steps is coupled to ATP hydrolysis (for example, by making detachment of one foot dependent on binding of ATP and coupling the reattachment to hydrolysis of the bound ATP), then the protein will show unidirectional movement that requires the continued consumption of ATP. Note that, in principle, it does not matter which step is coupled to ATP hydrolysis (Figure A4–19).

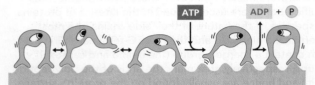

Figure A4–19

ANSWER 4–20   The slower migration of small molecules through a gel-filtration column occurs because smaller molecules have access to many more spaces in the porous beads that are packed into the column than do larger molecules. However, it is important that the flow rate through the column is slow enough to give the smaller molecules sufficient time to diffuse into the spaces inside the beads. At very rapid flow rates, all molecules will move rapidly around the beads, so that large and small molecules will now tend to exit together from the column.

ANSWER 4–21   The α helix in the figure is right-handed, whereas the coiled-coil is left-handed. The reversal occurs because of the staggered positions of hydrophobic side chains in the α helix.

ANSWER 4–22   The atoms at the binding sites of proteins must be precisely located to fit the molecules that they bind. Their location in turn requires the precise positioning of many of the amino acids and their side chains in the core of the protein, distant from the binding site itself. Thus, even a small change in this core can disrupt protein function by altering the conformation at a binding site far away.

ANSWER 4–23
A. When [S] << K_M, the term (K_M + [S]) approaches K_M. Therefore, the equation is simplified to rate = V_{max}[S]/K_M. Therefore, the rate is proportional to [S].
B. When [S] = K_M, the term [S]/(K_M + [S]) equals ½. Therefore, the reaction rate is half of the maximal rate V_{max}.
C. If [S] >> K_M, the term (K_M + [S]) approaches [S]. Therefore, [S]/(K_M + [S]) equals 1 and the reaction occurs at its maximal rate V_{max}.

ANSWER 4–24   The substrate concentration is 1 mM. This value can be obtained by substituting values into the equation, but it is simpler to note that the desired rate (50 μmole/sec) is exactly half of the maximum rate, V_{max}, where the substrate concentration is typically equal to the K_M. The two plots requested are shown in Figure A4–24.

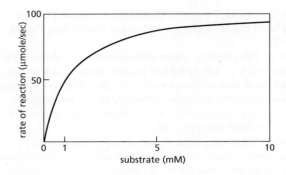

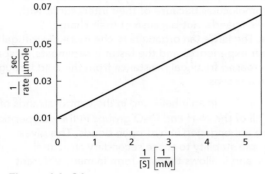

Figure A4–24

A plot of 1/rate versus 1/[S] is a straight line because rearranging the standard equation yields the equation given in Question 4–26B.

ANSWER 4–25   If [S] is very much smaller than K_M, the active site of the enzyme is mostly unoccupied. If [S] is very much greater than K_M, the reaction rate is limited by the enzyme concentration (because most of the catalytic sites are fully occupied).

ANSWER 4–26
A,B. The data in the boxes have been used to plot the *red* curve and *red* line in Figure A4–26. From the plotted data, the K_M is 1 μM and the V_{max} is 2 μmole/min. Note that the data are much easier to interpret in the linear plot, because the curve in (A) approaches, but never reaches, V_{max}.
C. It is important that only a small quantity of product is made, because otherwise the rate of reaction would decrease as the substrate was depleted and product accumulated. Thus the measured rates would be lower than they should be.
D. If the K_M increases, then the concentration of substrate needed to give a half-maximal rate is increased. As more substrate is needed to produce the same rate, the enzyme-catalyzed reaction has been inhibited by the phosphorylation. The expected data plots for the phosphorylated enzyme are the *green* curve and the *green* line in Figure A4–26.

Chapter 5

ANSWER 5–1
A. False. The polarity of a DNA strand commonly refers to the orientation of its sugar–phosphate backbone, one end of which contains a phosphate group and the other a hydroxyl group.

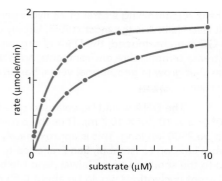

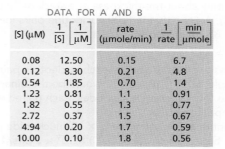

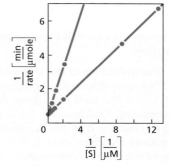

Figure A4–26

B. True. G-C base pairs are held together by three hydrogen bonds, whereas A-T base pairs are held together by only two.

ANSWER 5–2   Histone octamers occupy about 9% of volume of the nucleus. The volume of the nucleus is

$$V = 4/3 \times 3.14 \times (3 \times 10^3 \text{ nm})^3$$

$$V = 1.13 \times 10^{11} \text{ nm}^3$$

The volume of the histone octamers is

$$V = 3.14 \times (4.5 \text{ nm})^2 \times (5 \text{ nm}) \times (32 \times 10^6)$$

$$V = 1.02 \times 10^{10} \text{ nm}^3$$

The ratio of the volume of histone octamers to the nuclear volume is 0.09; thus, histone octamers occupy about 9% of the nuclear volume. Because the DNA also occupies about 9% of the nuclear volume, together they occupy about 18% of the volume of the nucleus.

ANSWER 5–3   In contrast to most proteins, which accumulate amino acid changes over evolutionary time, the functions of histone proteins must involve nearly all of their amino acids, so that a change in any position would be deleterious to the cell.

ANSWER 5–4   Men have only one copy of the X chromosome in their cells; a defective gene carried on it therefore has no backup copy. Women, on the other hand, have two copies of the X chromosome in their cells, one inherited from each parent, so a defective copy of the gene on one X chromosome can generally be compensated for by a normal copy on the other chromosome. This is the case with regard to the gene that causes color blindness. However, during female development, one X chromosome in each cell is inactivated by compaction into heterochromatin, shutting down gene expression from that chromosome (see Figure 5–28). This inactivation occurs at random in each cell to one or the other of the two X chromosomes, and therefore some cells of the woman will express the mutant copy of the gene, whereas others will express the normal copy. This process results in a retina in which, on average, only every other cone cell is color-sensitive, and women carrying the mutant gene on one X chromosome therefore see colored objects with reduced resolution.

A woman who is color-blind must have two defective copies of this gene, one inherited from each parent. Her father must therefore carry the mutation on his X chromosome; because this is his only copy of the gene, he would be color-blind. Her mother could carry the defective gene on either or both of her X chromosomes: if she carried it on both, she would be color-blind; if she carried it on one, she would have color vision but reduced resolution, as described above. Several different types of inherited color blindness are found in the human population; this question applies to only one type.

ANSWER 5–5

A. The complementary strand reads
   5'-**TGATTGTGGACAAAAATCC**-3'. Paired DNA strands have opposite polarity, and the convention is to write a single-stranded DNA sequence in the 5'-to-3' direction.

B. The DNA is made of four nucleotides (100% = 13% A + x% T + y% G + z% C). Because A pairs with T, the two nucleotides are represented in equimolar proportions in DNA. Therefore, the bacterial DNA in question contains 13% thymine. This leaves 74% [= 100% − (13% + 13%)] for G and C, which also form base pairs and hence are equimolar. Thus $y = z = 74/2 = 37$% of each.

C. A single-stranded DNA molecule that is N nucleotides long can have any one of 4^N possible sequences.

D. To specify a unique sequence that is N nucleotides long, 4^N has to be larger than 3×10^6. Thus, $4^N > 3 \times 10^6$, solved for N, gives $N > \ln(3 \times 10^6)/\ln(4) = 10.7$. Thus, on average, a sequence of only 11 nucleotides in length is unique in the genome. Performing the same calculation for the genome size of an animal cell yields a minimal stretch of 16 nucleotides. This shows that a relatively short sequence can mark a unique position in the genome and is sufficient, for example, to serve as an identity tag for one specific gene.

ANSWER 5–6   If the wrong bases were frequently incorporated during DNA replication, genetic information could not be inherited accurately. Life, as we know it, could not exist. Although the bases can form hydrogen-bonded pairs as indicated, these do not fit into the structure of the double helix. The angle at which the A base is attached to the sugar–phosphate backbone is vastly different in the A-C pair compared with A-T, and the spacing between the two sugar–phosphate strands is considerably increased in the A-G pair, where two large purine rings interact. Consequently, it is energetically unfavorable to incorporate a wrong base in DNA, and such errors occur only very rarely.

ANSWER 5–7

A. The bases V, W, X, and Y can form a DNA-like double-helical molecule with virtually identical properties to those of bona fide DNA. V would always pair with X, and W with Y. Therefore, the macromolecule could be derived from a living organism that uses the same principles to replicate its genome as those used by organisms on Earth. In principle, different bases, such as V, W, X, and Y, could have been selected during evolution on Earth as building blocks for DNA. (Similarly, there are many more conceivable amino acid side chains than the set of 20 selected in evolution that make up all proteins.)

B. None of the bases V, W, X, or Y can replace A, T, G, or C. To preserve the distance between the two sugar–phosphate strands in a double helix, a pyrimidine always has to pair with a purine (see, for example, Figure 5–4). Thus, the eight possible combinations would be V-A, V-G, W-A, W-G, X-C, X-T, Y-C, and Y-T. Because of the positions of hydrogen-bond acceptors and hydrogen-bond donor groups, however, no stable base pairs would form in any of these combinations, as shown for the pairing of V and A in Figure A5–7, where only a single hydrogen bond could form.

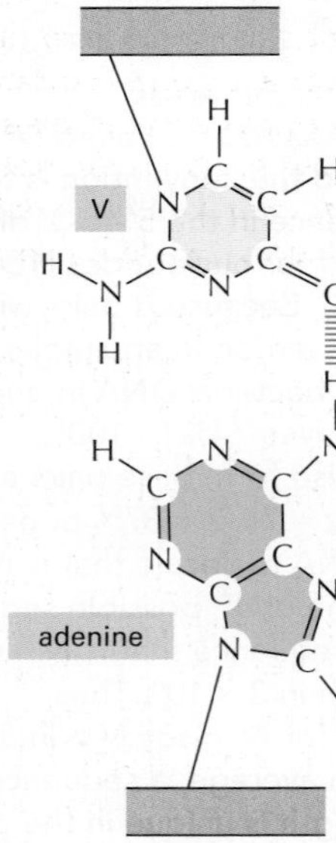

Figure A5–7

ANSWER 5–8 As the two strands are held together by hydrogen bonds between the bases, the stability of a DNA double helix is largely dependent on the number of hydrogen bonds that can be formed. Thus two parameters determine the stability: the number of nucleotide pairs and the number of hydrogen bonds that each nucleotide pair contributes. As shown in Figure 5–4, an A-T pair contributes two hydrogen bonds, whereas a G-C pair contributes three hydrogen bonds. Therefore, helix C (containing a total of 34 hydrogen bonds) would melt at the lowest temperature, helix B (containing a total of 65 hydrogen bonds) would melt

next, and helix A (containing a total of 78 hydrogen bonds) would melt last. Helix A is the most stable, largely owing to its high GC content. Indeed, the DNA of organisms that grow in extreme temperature environments, such as certain prokaryotes that grow in geothermal vents, has an unusually high GC content.

ANSWER 5–9 The DNA would be enlarged by a factor of 2.5×10^6 ($= 5 \times 10^{-3}/2 \times 10^{-9}$ m). Thus the extension cord would be 2500 km long. This is approximately the distance from London to Istanbul, San Francisco to Kansas City, Tokyo to the southern tip of Taiwan, and Melbourne to Cairns. Adjacent nucleotides would be about 0.85 mm apart (which is only about the thickness of a stack of 12 pages of this book). A gene that is 1000 nucleotide pairs long would be about 85 cm in length.

ANSWER 5–10

A. It takes two bits to specify each nucleotide pair (for example, 00, 01, 10, and 11 would be the binary codes for the four different nucleotides, each paired with its appropriate partner).

B. The entire human genome (3×10^9 nucleotide pairs) could be stored on two CDs ($3 \times 10^9 \times 2$ bits$/4.8 \times 10^9$ bits).

ANSWER 5–11

A. True.

B. False. Nucleosome core particles are approximately 11 nm in diameter.

ANSWER 5–12 The definitions of the terms can be found in the Glossary. DNA assembles with specialized proteins to form *chromatin*. At a first level of packing, *histones* form the core of *nucleosomes*. A nucleosome includes the DNA wrapped around this histone core plus a segment of linker DNA. Between nuclear divisions—that is, in interphase—the *chromatin* of the *interphase chromosomes* is in a relatively extended form in the nucleus, although some regions of it, the *heterochromatin*, remain densely packed and are transcriptionally inactive. During nuclear division—that is, in mitosis—replicated chromosomes become condensed into *mitotic chromosomes*, which are transcriptionally inactive and are designed to be readily distributed between the two daughter cells.

ANSWER 5–13 Colonies are clumps of cells that originate from a single founder cell and grow outward as the cells divide again and again. In the lower colony of Figure Q5–13, the *Ade2* gene is inactivated when placed near a telomere, but apparently it can become spontaneously activated in a few cells, which then turn white. Once activated in a cell, the *Ade2* gene continues to be active in the descendants of that cell, resulting in clumps of white cells (the white sectors) in the colony. This result shows both that the inactivation of a gene positioned close to a telomere can be reversed and that this change is passed on to further generations. This change in *Ade2* expression probably results from a spontaneous decondensation of the chromatin structure around the gene.

ANSWER 5–14 In the electron micrographs, one can detect chromatin regions of two different densities; the densely stained regions correspond to heterochromatin, while less condensed chromatin is more lightly stained. The chromatin in (A) is mostly in the form of condensed, transcriptionally inactive heterochromatin, whereas most of the chromatin in (B) is decondensed and therefore potentially transcriptionally active. The nucleus in (A) is from a reticulocyte, a red blood cell precursor, which is largely devoted to making a single protein, hemoglobin. The nucleus in (B) is from a lymphocyte, which is active in transcribing many different genes.

ANSWER 5–15   Helix (A) is right-handed. Helix (C) is left-handed. Helix (B) has one right-handed strand and one left-handed strand. There are several ways to tell the handedness of a helix. For a vertically oriented helix, like the ones in Figure Q5–15, if the strands in front point up to the right, the helix is right-handed; if they point up to the left, the helix is left-handed. Once you are comfortable identifying the handedness of a helix, you will be amused to note that nearly 50% of the "DNA" helices shown in advertisements are left-handed, as are a surprisingly high number of the ones shown in books. Amazingly, a version of Helix (B) was used in advertisements for a prominent international conference, celebrating the 30-year anniversary of the discovery of the DNA helix.

ANSWER 5–16   The packing ratio within a nucleosome core is 4.5 [(147 bp × 0.34 nm/bp)/(11 nm) = 4.5]. If there is an additional 54 bp of linker DNA, then the packing ratio for "beads-on-a-string" DNA is 2.3 [(201 bp × 0.34 nm/bp)/ (11 nm + {54 bp × 0.34 nm/bp}) = 2.3]. This first level of packing represents only 0.023% (2.3/10,000) of the total condensation that occurs at mitosis.

Chapter 6

ANSWER 6–1

A. The distance between replication forks 4 and 5 is about 280 nm, corresponding to 824 nucleotides (= 280/0.34). These two replication forks would collide in about 8 seconds. Forks 7 and 8 move away from each other and would therefore never collide.

B. The total length of DNA shown in the electron micrograph is about 1.5 μm, corresponding to 4400 nucleotides. This is only about 0.002% [= (4400/1.8 × 10^8) × 100%] of the total DNA in a fly cell.

ANSWER 6–2   Although the process may seem wasteful, it is not possible to proofread during the initial stages of primer synthesis. To start a new primer on a piece of single-stranded DNA, one nucleotide needs to be put in place and then linked to a second, and then to a third, and so on. Even if these first nucleotides were perfectly matched to the template strand, they would bind with very low affinity, and it would consequently be difficult for a hypothetical primase with proofreading activity to distinguish the correct from incorrect bases; the enzyme would therefore stall. The task of the primase is to "just polymerize nucleotides that bind reasonably well to the template without worrying too much about accuracy." Later, these sequences are removed and replaced by DNA polymerase, which uses newly synthesized, adjacent DNA—which has already been proofread—as its primer.

ANSWER 6–3

A. Without DNA polymerase, no replication can take place at all. RNA primers will be laid down at the origin of replication.

B. DNA ligase links the DNA fragments that are produced on the lagging strand. In the absence of ligase, the newly replicated DNA strands will remain as fragments, but no nucleotides will be missing.

C. Without the sliding clamp, the DNA polymerase will frequently fall off the DNA template. In principle, it can rebind and continue, but the continual falling off and rebinding will be so time-consuming that the cell will be unable to divide.

D. In the absence of RNA-excision enzymes, the RNA fragments will remain covalently attached to the newly replicated DNA fragments. No ligation will take place, because the DNA ligase will not link DNA to RNA. The lagging strand will therefore consist of fragments composed of both RNA and DNA.

E. Without DNA helicase, the DNA polymerase will stall because it cannot separate the strands of the template DNA ahead of it. Little or no new DNA will be synthesized.

F. In the absence of primase, RNA primers cannot be made on either the leading or the lagging strand. DNA replication therefore cannot begin.

ANSWER 6–4   DNA damage by deamination and depurination reactions occurs spontaneously. This type of damage is not the result of replication errors and is therefore equally likely to occur on either strand. If DNA repair enzymes recognized such damage only on newly synthesized DNA strands, half of the defects would go uncorrected. The statement is therefore incorrect.

ANSWER 6–5   If the old strand were "repaired" using the new strand that contains a replication error as the template, then the error would become a permanent mutation in the genome. The old information would be erased in the process. Therefore, if repair enzymes did not distinguish between the two strands, there would be only a 50% chance that any given replication error would be corrected.

ANSWER 6–6   You cannot transform an individual from one species into another species simply by introducing random changes into the DNA. It is exceedingly unlikely that the 5000 mutations that would accumulate every day in the absence of the DNA repair enzyme would be in the very positions where human and chimpanzee DNA sequences are different. It is very likely that, at such a high mutation frequency, many essential genes would be inactivated, leading to cell death. Furthermore, your body is made up of about 10^13 cells. For you to turn into an ape, not just one but many of these cells would need to be changed. And even then, many of these changes would have to occur during development to effect changes in your body plan (making your arms longer than your legs, for example).

ANSWER 6–7

A. False. Identical DNA polymerase molecules catalyze DNA synthesis on the leading and lagging strands of a bacterial replication fork. The replication fork is asymmetrical because the lagging strand is made in pieces while the leading strand is synthesized continuously.

B. False. Okazaki fragments initially contain both RNA primers and DNA, but only the RNA primers are removed by RNA nucleases.

C. True. With proofreading, DNA polymerase has an error rate of one mistake in 10^7 nucleotides polymerized; 99% of its errors are corrected by DNA mismatch repair enzymes, bringing the final error rate to one in 10^9.

D. True. Mutations would accumulate rapidly, inactivating many genes.

E. True. If a damaged nucleotide also occurred naturally in DNA, the repair enzyme would have no way of identifying the damage. It would therefore have only a 50% chance of fixing the right strand.

F. True. Usually, multiple mutations of specific types need to accumulate in a somatic cell lineage to produce a cancer. A mutation in a gene that codes for a DNA repair enzyme can make a cell more liable to accumulate these mutations, thereby accelerating the onset of cancer.

ANSWER 6–8   With a single origin of replication, which launches two DNA polymerases in opposite directions on the DNA, each moving at 100 nucleotides per second, the number of nucleotides replicated in 24 hours will be 1.73×10^7 (= $2 \times 100 \times 24 \times 60 \times 60$). To replicate all the 6×10^9 nucleotides of DNA in the cell in this time, therefore, will require at least 348 (= $6 \times 10^9/1.73 \times 10^7$) origins of replication. The estimated 10,000 origins of replication in the human genome are therefore more than sufficient to satisfy this minimum requirement.

ANSWER 6–9

A. Dideoxycytidine triphosphate (ddCTP) is identical to dCTP, except it lacks the 3′-hydroxyl group on the sugar ring. ddCTP is recognized by DNA polymerase as dCTP and becomes incorporated into DNA; because it lacks the crucial 3′-hydroxyl group, however, its addition to a growing DNA strand creates a dead end to which no further nucleotides can be added. Thus, if ddCTP is added in large excess, new DNA strands will be synthesized until the first G (the nucleotide complementary to C) is encountered on the template strand. ddCTP will then be incorporated instead of C, and no further extension of this strand will occur. This strategy is exploited by a drug, 3′-azido-3′-deoxythymidine (AZT), that is now commonly used in HIV-infected patients to treat AIDS. AZT is converted in cells to the triphosphate form and is incorporated into the growing viral DNA. Because the drug lacks a 3′-hydroxyl group, it blocks further DNA synthesis and replication of the virus. AZT inhibits viral replication preferentially because reverse transcriptase has a higher affinity for the drug than for thymidine triphosphate; human cellular DNA polymerases do not show this preference and therefore still function in the presence of the drug.

B. If ddCTP is added at about 10% of the concentration of the available dCTP, there is a 1 in 10 chance of its being incorporated whenever a G is encountered on the template strand. Thus a population of DNA fragments will be synthesized, and from their lengths one can deduce where the G nucleotides are located on the template strand. This strategy forms the basis of methods used to determine the sequence of nucleotides in a stretch of DNA (discussed in Chapter 10).

C. Dideoxycytidine monophosphate (ddCMP) lacks the 5′-triphosphate group as well as the 3′-hydroxyl group of the sugar ring. It therefore cannot provide the energy that drives the polymerization reaction of nucleotides into DNA and therefore will not be incorporated into the replicating DNA. Addition of this compound should thus not affect DNA replication.

ANSWER 6–10   See Figure A6–10.

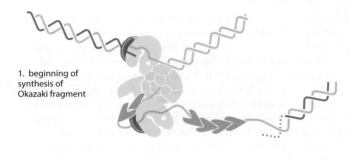

1. beginning of synthesis of Okazaki fragment

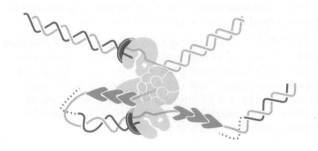

2. midpoint of synthesis of Okazaki fragment

Figure A6–10

ANSWER 6–11   The two strands of the bacterial chromosome contain 6×10^6 nucleotides in total. During the polymerization of nucleoside triphosphates into DNA, two phosphoanhydride bonds are broken for each nucleotide added: the nucleoside triphosphate is hydrolyzed to produce the nucleoside monophosphate added to the growing DNA strand, and the released pyrophosphate is hydrolyzed to phosphate. Therefore, 1.2×10^7 high-energy bonds are hydrolyzed during each round of bacterial DNA replication. This requires 4×10^5 (= $1.2 \times 10^7/30$) glucose molecules, which weigh 1.2×10^{-16} g [= (4×10^5 molecules) $\times$ (180 g/mole)/(6×10^{23} molecules/mole)], which is 0.01% of the total weight of the cell.

ANSWER 6–12   The statement is correct. If the DNA in somatic cells is not sufficiently stable (that is, if it accumulates mutations too rapidly), the organism dies (of cancer, for example), and because this may often happen before the organism can reproduce, the species will die out. If the DNA in reproductive cells is not sufficiently stable, many mutations will accumulate and be passed on to future generations, so that the species will not be maintained.

ANSWER 6–13   As shown in Figure A6–13, thymine and uracil lack amino groups and therefore cannot be deaminated. Deamination of adenine and guanine produces purine rings that are not found in conventional nucleic acids. In contrast, deamination of cytosine produces uracil. Therefore, if uracil were a naturally occurring base in DNA

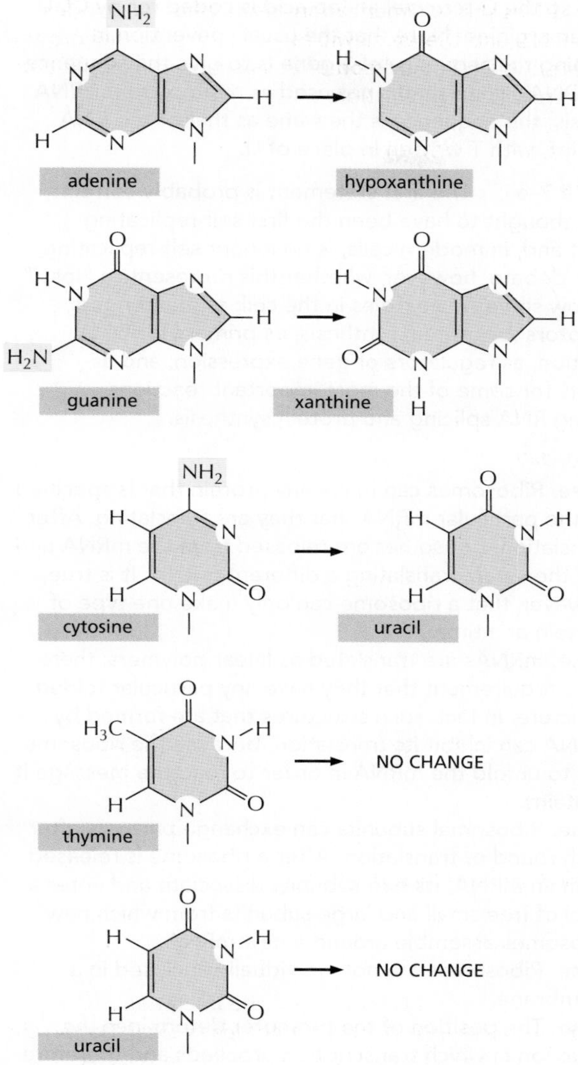

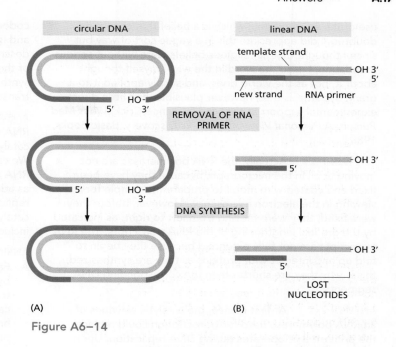

Figure A6–14

(as it is in RNA), repair enzymes could not distinguish whether a uracil is the appropriate base or whether it arose through spontaneous deamination of cytosine. This dilemma is not encountered, however, because thymine, rather than uracil, is used in DNA. Therefore, if a uracil base is found in DNA, it can be automatically recognized as a damaged base and then excised and replaced by cytosine.

ANSWER 6–14

A. DNA polymerase requires a 3'-OH to synthesize DNA; without telomeres and telomerase, the ends of linear chromosomes would shrink during each round of DNA replication. For bacterial chromosomes, which have no ends, the problem does not arise; there will always be a 3'-OH group available to prime the DNA polymerase that replaces the RNA primer with DNA (Figure A6–14). Telomeres and telomerase prevent the shrinking of chromosomes because they extend the 3' end of the template DNA strand (see Figure 6–23). This extension of the lagging-strand template provides the "space" to begin the final Okazaki fragments.

B. As shown in Figure A6–14A, telomeres and telomerase are still needed even if the last fragment of the lagging

strand were initiated by primase at the very 3' end of chromosomal DNA, inasmuch as the RNA primer must be removed.

ANSWER 6–15

A. If the single origin of replication were located exactly in the center of the chromosome, it would take more than 8 days to replicate the DNA [= 75×10^6 nucleotides/(100 nucleotides/sec)]. The rate of replication would therefore severely limit the rate of cell division. If the origin were located at one end, the time required to replicate the chromosome would be approximately double this.

B. A chromosome end that is not "capped" with a telomere would lose nucleotides during each round of DNA replication and would gradually shrink. Eventually, essential genes would be lost, and the chromosome's ends might be recognized by the DNA damage-response mechanisms, which would stop cell division or induce cell death.

C. Without centromeres, which attach mitotic chromosomes to the mitotic spindle, the two new chromosomes that result from chromosome duplication would not be partitioned accurately between the two daughter cells. Therefore, many daughter cells would die, because they would not receive a full set of chromosomes.

Chapter 7

ANSWER 7–1   Perhaps the best answer was given by Francis Crick himself, who coined the term in the mid-1950s: "I called this idea the central dogma for two reasons, I suspect. I had already used the obvious word hypothesis in the sequence hypothesis, which proposes that genetic information is encoded in the sequence of the DNA bases, and in addition I wanted to suggest that this new assumption was more central and more powerful…. As it turned out, the use of the word dogma caused more trouble than it was worth. Many years later Jacques Monod pointed out to me that I did not appear to understand the correct

Figure A6–13

use of the word dogma, which is a belief that cannot be doubted. I did appreciate this in a vague sort of way but since I thought that all religious beliefs were without serious foundation, I used the word in the way I myself thought about it, not as the world does, and simply applied it to a grand hypothesis that, however plausible, had little direct experimental support at the time." (Francis Crick, *What Mad Pursuit: A Personal View of Scientific Discovery*. Basic Books, 1988.)

ANSWER 7–2   Actually, the RNA polymerases are not moving at all in the micrograph, because they have been fixed and coated with metal to prepare the sample for viewing in the electron microscope. However, before they were fixed, they were moving from left to right, as indicated by the gradual lengthening of the RNA transcripts. The RNA transcripts are not fully extended because they begin to fold up and interact with proteins as they are synthesized; this is why they are shorter than the corresponding DNA segments.

ANSWER 7–3   At first glance, the catalytic activities of an RNA polymerase used for transcription could replace the primase that operates during DNA replication. Upon further reflection, however, there would be some serious problems. (1) The RNA polymerase used to make primers would need to initiate every few hundred bases, which is much more often than promoters are spaced on the DNA. Initiation would therefore need to occur in a promoter-independent fashion or many more promoters would have to be present in the DNA, both of which would be problematic for the synthesis of mRNA. In addition, RNA polymerase normally begins transcription on double-stranded DNA, whereas the DNA replication primers are synthesized using single-stranded DNA. (2) Similarly, the RNA primers used in DNA replication are much shorter than mRNAs. The RNA polymerase would therefore need to terminate much more frequently than during transcription. Termination would need to occur spontaneously (i.e., without requiring a terminator sequence in the DNA) or else many more terminators would need to be present. Again, both of these scenarios would be problematic for mRNA production. Although it might be possible to overcome this problem if special control proteins became attached to RNA polymerase during replication, the problem has been solved by the evolution of separate enzymes with specialized properties. Some small DNA viruses, however, do utilize the host RNA polymerase to make RNA primers for their replication.

ANSWER 7–4   This experiment demonstrates that, once an amino acid has been coupled to a tRNA, the ribosome will trust the tRNA and "blindly" incorporate that amino acid into the position according to the match between the codon and anticodon. We can therefore conclude that a significant part of the correct reading of the genetic code—that is, the matching of a codon in an mRNA with the correct amino acid—is performed by the synthetase enzymes that correctly match tRNAs and amino acids.

ANSWER 7–5   The mRNA will have a 5′-to-3′ polarity, opposite to that of the DNA strand that serves as the template. Thus the mRNA sequence will read 5′-GAAAAAAGCCGUUAA-3′. The N-terminal amino acid coded for by GAA is glutamic acid. UAA specifies a stop

codon, so the C-terminal amino acid is coded for by CGU and is an arginine. Note that the usual convention in describing the sequence of a gene is to give the sequence of the DNA strand that is not used as a template for RNA synthesis; this sequence is the same as that of the RNA transcript, with T written in place of U.

ANSWER 7–6   The first statement is probably correct: RNA is thought to have been the first self-replicating catalyst and, in modern cells, is no longer self-replicating. We can debate, however, whether this represents a "loss." RNA now serves many roles in the cell: as messengers, as adaptors for protein synthesis, as primers for DNA replication, as regulators of gene expression, and as catalysts for some of the most important reactions, including RNA splicing and protein synthesis.

ANSWER 7–7
A. False. Ribosomes can make any protein that is specified by the particular mRNA that they are translating. After translation, ribosomes are released from the mRNA and can then start translating a different mRNA. It is true, however, that a ribosome can only make one type of protein at a time.
B. False. mRNAs are translated as linear polymers; there is no requirement that they have any particular folded structure. In fact, such structures that are formed by mRNA can inhibit its translation, because the ribosome has to unfold the mRNA in order to read the message it contains.
C. False. Ribosomal subunits can exchange partners after each round of translation. After a ribosome is released from an mRNA, its two subunits dissociate and enter a pool of free small and large subunits from which new ribosomes assemble around a new mRNA.
D. False. Ribosomes are not individually enclosed in a membrane.
E. False. The position of the promoter determines the direction in which transcription proceeds and therefore which of the two DNA strands is used as the template. Transcription of the other strand would produce an mRNA with a completely different (and in most cases meaningless) sequence.
F. False. RNA contains uracil but not thymine.
G. False. The level of a protein depends on its rate of synthesis and degradation but not on its catalytic activity.

ANSWER 7–8   Because the deletion in the Lacheinmal mRNA is internal, it likely arose from incorrect splicing of the pre-mRNA. The simplest interpretation is that the *Lacheinmal* gene contains a 173-nucleotide-long exon (labeled "E2" in Figure A7–8), and that this exon is lost ("skipped") during the processing of the mutant precursor mRNA (pre-mRNA). This could occur, for example, if the mutation changed the 3′ splice site in the preceding intron ("I1") so that it was no longer recognized by the splicing machinery (a change in the CAG sequence shown in Figure 7–20 could do this). The snRNP would search for the next available 3′ splice site, which is found at the 3′ end of the next intron ("I2"), and the splicing reaction would therefore remove E2 together with I1 and I2, resulting in a shortened mRNA. The mRNA is then translated into a defective protein, resulting in the Lacheinmal deficiency.

Because 173 nucleotides do not amount to an integral

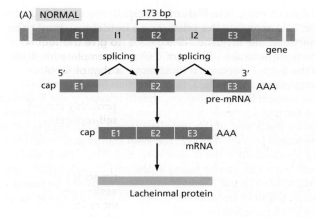

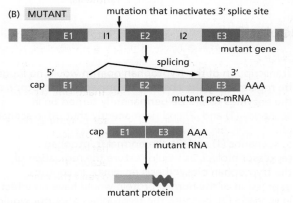

Figure A7–8

number of codons, the lack of this exon in the mRNA will shift the reading frame at the splice junction. Therefore, the Lacheinmal protein would be made correctly only through exon E1. As the ribosome begins translating sequences in exon E3, it will be in the wrong reading frame and will therefore will produce a protein sequence that is unrelated to the Lacheinmal sequence normally encoded by exon E3. Most likely, the ribosome will soon encounter a stop codon, which would be expected to occur on average about once in every 21 codons (there are 3 stop codons in the 64 codons of the genetic code).

ANSWER 7–9   Sequence 1 and sequence 4 both code for the peptide Arg-Gly-Asp. Because the genetic code is redundant, different nucleotide sequences can encode the same amino acid sequence.

ANSWER 7–10

A. Incorrect. The bonds are not covalent, and their formation does not require an input of energy.

B. Correct. The aminoacyl-tRNA enters the ribosome at the A site and forms hydrogen bonds with the codon in the mRNA.

C. Correct. As the ribosome moves along the mRNA, the tRNAs that have donated their amino acid to the growing polypeptide chain are ejected from the ribosome and the mRNA. The ejection takes place two cycles after the tRNA first enters the ribosome (see Figure 7–37).

ANSWER 7–11   *Replication.* Dictionary definition: the creation of an exact copy; molecular biology definition: the act of copying a DNA sequence. *Transcription.* Dictionary definition: the act of writing out a copy, especially from one

physical form to another; molecular biology definition: the act of copying the information stored in DNA into RNA. *Translation.* Dictionary definition: the act of putting words into a different language; molecular biology definition: the act of polymerizing amino acids into a defined linear sequence using the information provided by the linear sequence of nucleotides in mRNA. (Note that "translation" is also used in a quite different sense, both in ordinary language and in scientific contexts, to mean a movement from one place to another.)

ANSWER 7–12   With four different nucleotides to choose from, a code of two nucleotides could specify 16 different amino acids (= 4^2), and a triplet code in which the position of the nucleotides is not important could specify 20 different amino acids (= 4 possibilities of 3 of the same bases + 12 possibilities of 2 bases the same and one different + 4 possibilities of 3 different bases). In both cases, these maximal amino acid numbers would need to be reduced by at least 1 because of the need to specify translation stop codons. It is relatively easy to envision how a doublet code could be translated by a mechanism similar to that used in our world by providing tRNAs with only two relevant bases in the anticodon loop. It is more difficult to envision how the nucleotide composition of a stretch of three nucleotides could be translated without regard to their order, because base-pairing can then no longer be used: AUG, for example, will not base-pair with the same anticodon as UGA.

ANSWER 7–13   It is likely that in early cells the matching between codons and amino acids was less accurate than it is in present-day cells. The feature of the genetic code described in the question may have allowed early cells to tolerate this inaccuracy by allowing a blurred relationship between sets of roughly similar codons and roughly similar amino acids. One can easily imagine how the matching between codons and amino acids could have become more accurate, step by step, as the translation machinery evolved into that found in modern cells.

ANSWER 7–14   The codon for Trp is 5′-UGG-3′. Thus a normal tRNA^{Trp} contains the sequence 5′-CCA-3′ as its anticodon (see Figure 7–33). If this tRNA contains a mutation so that its anticodon is changed to UCA, it will recognize a UGA codon and lead to the incorporation of a tryptophan instead of causing translation to stop. Many other protein-encoding sequences, however, contain UGA codons as their natural stop sites, and these stops would also be affected by the mutant tRNA. Depending on the competition between the altered tRNA and the normal translation release factors (Figure 7–41), some of these proteins would be made with additional amino acids at their C-terminal end. The additional lengths would depend on the number of codons before the ribosomes encounter a non-UGA stop codon in the mRNA in the reading frame in which the protein is translated.

ANSWER 7–15   One effective way of driving a reaction to completion is to remove one of the products, so that the reverse reaction cannot occur. ATP contains two high-energy bonds that link the three phosphate groups. In the reaction shown, PP$_i$ is released, consisting of two phosphate groups linked by one of these high-energy bonds. Thus PP$_i$ can be hydrolyzed with a considerable gain of free energy, and thereby can be efficiently removed. This happens rapidly in cells, and reactions that produce and further hydrolyze PP_i are therefore virtually irreversible (see Figure 3–41).

ANSWER 7–16

A. A titin molecule is made of 25,000 (3,000,000/120) amino acids. It therefore takes about 3.5 hours $[(25,000/2) \times (1/60) \times (1/60)]$ to synthesize a single molecule of titin in muscle cells.

B. Because of its large size, the probability of making a titin molecule without any mistakes is only 0.08 $[= (1 - 10^{-4})^{25,000}]$; that is, only 8 in 100 titin molecules synthesized are free of mistakes. In contrast, over 97% of newly synthesized proteins of average size are made correctly.

C. The error rate limits the sizes of proteins that can be synthesized accurately. If a eukaryotic ribosomal protein were synthesized as a single molecule, a large portion (87%) of this hypothetical giant ribosomal protein would be expected to contain at least one mistake. It is therefore more advantageous to make ribosomal proteins individually, because in this way only a small proportion of each type of protein will be defective, and these few bad molecules can be individually eliminated by proteolysis to ensure that there are no defects in the ribosome as a whole.

D. To calculate the time it takes to transcribe a titin mRNA, you would need to know the size of its gene, which is likely to contain many introns. Transcription of the exons alone (25,000 × 3 = 75,000 nucleotides) requires about 42 minutes $[(75,000/30) \times (1/60)]$. Because introns can be quite large, the time required to transcribe the entire gene is likely to be considerably longer.

ANSWER 7–17

Mutations of the type described in (B) and (D) are often the most harmful. In both cases, the reading frame would be changed, and because this frameshift occurs near the beginning or in the middle of the coding sequence, much of the protein will contain a nonsensical and/or truncated sequence of amino acids. In contrast, a reading-frame shift that occurs toward the end of the coding sequence, as described in (A), will result in a largely correct protein that may be functional. Deletion of three consecutive nucleotides, as described in (C), leads to the deletion of an amino acid but does not alter the reading frame. The deleted amino acid may or may not be important for the folding or activity of the protein; in many cases, such mutations are silent—that is, they have no or only minor consequences for the organism. Substitution of one nucleotide for another, as in (E), is often completely harmless. In some cases, it will not change the amino acid sequence of the protein; in other cases, it will change a single amino acid; at worst, it may create a new stop codon, giving rise to a truncated protein.

ANSWER 7–18

The RNA transcripts that are growing from the DNA template like bristles on a bottlebrush tend to be shorter at the left-hand side of each gene and longer on the right-hand side. Because RNA polymerase synthesizes in the 5′-to-3′ direction it must move along the DNA template strand in the 3′-to-5′ direction (see Figure 7–7). The longest RNAs, therefore, should appear at the 5′ end of the template strand—when transcription is nearly complete. Hence the 3′ end of the template strand is toward the left of the image (Figure A7–18). The RNA transcripts, meanwhile, are synthesized in the 5′-to-3′ direction. Thus, the 5′ end of each transcript can be found at the end of each bristle (see Figure A7–18); the 3′ end of each transcript can be found within the RNA polymerase molecules that dot the spine of the DNA template molecule.

Chapter 8

ANSWER 8–1

A. Transcription of the tryptophan operon would no longer be regulated by the absence or presence of tryptophan; the enzymes would be permanently turned on in scenarios (1) and (2) and permanently shut off in scenario (3).

B. In scenarios (1) and (2), the normal tryptophan repressor molecules would restore the regulation of the tryptophan biosynthesis enzymes. In contrast, expression of the normal protein would have no effect in scenario (3), because the tryptophan operator would remain occupied by the mutant protein, even in the presence of tryptophan.

ANSWER 8–2

Contacts can form between the protein and the edges of the base pairs that are exposed in the major groove of the DNA (Figure A8–2). These sequence-specific contacts can include hydrogen bonds with the highlighted oxygen, nitrogen, and hydrogen atoms, as well as hydrophobic interactions with the methyl group on thymine (*yellow*). Note that the arrangement of hydrogen-bond donors (*blue*) and hydrogen-bond acceptors (*red*) of a T-A pair is different from that of a C-G pair. Similarly, the arrangements of hydrogen-bond donors and hydrogen-bond acceptors of A-T and G-C pairs are different from one another and from the two pairs shown in the figure. These differences allow recognition of specific DNA sequences via the major groove. In addition to the contacts shown in the figure, electrostatic attractions between the positively charged amino acid side chains of the protein and the negatively charged phosphate groups in the DNA backbone usually stabilize DNA–protein interactions. Finally, some DNA-binding proteins also contact bases from the minor

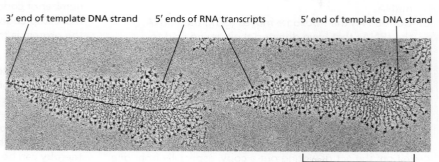

3′ end of template DNA strand   5′ ends of RNA transcripts   5′ end of template DNA strand

Figure A7–18

1 µm

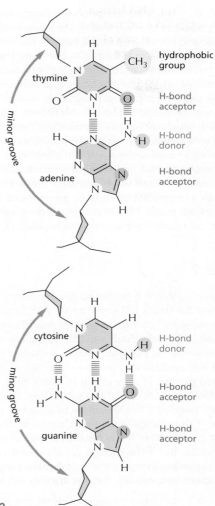

Figure A8–2

groove (see Figure 8–4). The minor groove, however, contains fewer features that distinguish one base from another than does the major groove.

ANSWER 8–3   Bending proteins can help to bring distant DNA regions together that normally would contact each other only inefficiently (Figure A8–3). Such proteins are found in both prokaryotes and eukaryotes and are involved in many examples of transcriptional regulation.

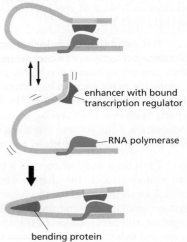

Figure A8–3   bending protein

ANSWER 8–4

A. UV light throws the switch from the prophage to the lytic state: when cI protein is destroyed, Cro is made and turns off the further production of cI. The virus produces coat proteins, and new virus particles are made.

B. When the UV light is switched off, the virus remains in the lytic state. Thus, cI and Cro form a transcription switch that "memorizes" its previous setting.

C. This switch makes sense in the viral life cycle: UV light tends to damage the bacterial DNA (see Figure 6–25), thereby rendering the bacterium an unreliable host for the virus. A prophage will therefore switch to the lytic state and leave the "sinking ship" in search of new host cells to infect.

ANSWER 8–5

A. True. Prokaryotic mRNAs are often transcripts of entire operons. Ribosomes can initiate translation at the internal AUG start sites of these "polycistronic" mRNAs (see Figures 7–40 and 8–6).

B. True. The major groove of double-stranded DNA is sufficiently wide to allow a protein surface, such as one face of an α helix, access to the base pairs. The sequence of H-bond donors and acceptors in the major groove can then be "read" by the protein to determine the sequence of the DNA (see Figure A8–2).

C. True. It is advantageous to exert control at the earliest possible point in a pathway. This conserves metabolic energy because unnecessary products are not made.

ANSWER 8–6   From our knowledge of enhancers, one would expect their function to be relatively independent of their distance from the promoter—possibly weakening as this distance increases. The surprising feature of the data (which have been adapted from an actual experiment) is the periodicity: the enhancer is maximally active at certain distances from the promoter (50, 60, or 70 nucleotides), but almost inactive at intermediate distances (55 or 65 nucleotides). The periodicity of 10 suggests that the mystery can be explained by considering the structure of double-helical DNA, which has 10 base pairs per turn. Thus, placing an enhancer on the side of the DNA opposite to that of the promoter (Figure A8–6) would make it more difficult for the activator that binds to it to interact with the proteins bound at the promoter. At longer distances, there is more DNA to absorb the twist, and the effect is diminished.

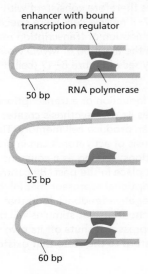

Figure A8–6   60 bp

ANSWER 8–7   The affinity of the dimeric λ repressor for its binding site depends on the interactions made by each of the two DNA-binding domains. A single DNA-binding domain can make only half the contacts and therefore provide just half the binding energy compared with the dimer. Although cleavage of the repressor does not change the concentration of binding domains, the affinity that each repressor monomer has for DNA is sufficiently weak that the repressors do not remain bound. As a result, the genes for lytic growth are turned on.

ANSWER 8–8   The function of these *Arg* genes is to encode the enzymes that synthesize arginine. When arginine is abundant, expression of these genes should be turned off. If ArgR acts as a gene repressor (which it does in reality), then binding of arginine should increase its affinity for its regulatory sites, allowing it to bind and shut off gene expression. If ArgR acted as a gene activator instead, then the binding of arginine would be predicted to reduce its affinity for its regulatory DNA, preventing its binding and thereby shutting off expression of the *Arg* genes.

ANSWER 8–9   The results of this experiment favor DNA looping, which should not be affected by the protein bridge (so long as it allowed the DNA to bend, which it does). The scanning or entry-site model, however, is predicted to be affected by the nature of the linkage between the enhancer and the promoter. If the proteins enter at the enhancer and scan to the promoter, they would have to traverse the protein linkage. If such proteins are geared to scan on DNA, they would likely have difficulty scanning across such a barrier.

ANSWER 8–10   The most definitive result is one showing that a single differentiated cell taken from a specialized tissue can re-create a whole organism. This proves that the cell must contain all the information required to produce a whole organism, including all of its specialized cell types. Experiments of this type are summarized in Figure 8–2.

ANSWER 8–11   In principle, you could create 16 different cell types with 4 different transcription regulators (all the 8 cell types shown in Figure 8–17, plus another 8 created by adding an additional transcription regulator). MyoD by itself is sufficient to induce muscle-specific gene expression only in certain cell types, such as some kinds of fibroblasts. The action of MyoD is therefore consistent with the model shown in Figure 8–17: if muscle cells were specified, for example, by the combination of transcription regulators 1, 3, and MyoD, then the addition of MyoD would convert only two of the cell types of Figure 8–17 (cells F and H) to muscle.

ANSWER 8–12   The induction of a transcriptional activator protein that stimulates its own synthesis creates a positive feedback loop that can produce cell memory. The continued self-stimulated synthesis of activator A can in principle last for many cell generations, serving as a constant reminder of an event that took place in the past. By contrast, the induction of a transcriptional repressor that inhibits its own synthesis creates a negative feedback loop that ensures that the response to the transient stimulus will be similarly transient. Because repressor R shuts off its own synthesis, the cell will quickly return to the state that existed before the signal.

ANSWER 8–13   Many transcription regulators are continually made in the cell; that is, their expression is constitutive and the activity of the protein is controlled by signals from inside or outside the cell (e.g., the availability of nutrients, as for the tryptophan repressor, or by hormones, as for the glucocorticoid receptor). In this way, the transcriptional program is adjusted to the physiological needs of the cell. Moreover, a given transcription regulator usually controls the expression of many different genes. Transcription regulators are often used in various combinations and can affect each other's activity, thereby further increasing the possibilities for regulation with a limited set of proteins. Nevertheless, most cells devote a large fraction of their genomes to the control of transcription: about 10% of protein-coding genes in eukaryotic cells code for transcription regulators.

Chapter 9

ANSWER 9–1   When it comes to genetic information, a balance must be struck between stability and change. If the mutation rate were too high, a species would eventually die out because all its individuals would accumulate mutations in genes essential for survival. And for a species to be successful—in evolutionary terms—individual members must have a good genetic memory; that is, there must be high fidelity in DNA replication. At the same time, occasional changes are needed if the species is to adapt to changing conditions. If the change leads to an improvement, it will persist by selection; if it is neutral, it may or may not accumulate; but if the change proves disastrous, the individual organism that was the unfortunate subject of nature's experiment will die, but the species will survive.

ANSWER 9–2   In single-celled organisms, the genome is the germ line and any modification is passed on to the next generation. By contrast, in multicellular organisms, most of the cells are somatic cells and make no contribution to the next generation; thus, modification of those cells by horizontal gene transfer would have no consequence for the next generation. The germ-line cells are usually sequestered in the interior of multicellular organisms, minimizing their contact with foreign cells, viruses, and DNA, thus insulating the species from the effects of horizontal gene transfer. Nevertheless, horizontal gene transfer is possible for multicellular organisms. For example, the genomes of some insect species contain DNA that was horizontally transferred from bacteria that infect them.

ANSWER 9–3   It is extremely unlikely that any gene came into existence perfectly optimized for its function. Ribosomal RNA sequences have been highly conserved because this molecule plays such an important role in protein synthesis in the cell. Nonetheless, the environment an organism finds itself in is changeable, so no gene can be optimal indefinitely. Thus we find there are indeed significant differences in ribosomal RNAs among species.

ANSWER 9–4   Each time another copy of a transposon is inserted into a chromosome, the change can be either neutral, beneficial, or detrimental for the organism. Because individuals that accumulate detrimental insertions would be selected against, the proliferation of transposons is controlled by natural selection. If a transposon arose that proliferated uncontrollably, it is unlikely that a viable host organism could be maintained. For this reason, most transposons move only rarely. Many transposons, for example, synthesize only infrequent bursts of very small amounts of the transposase that is required for their movement.

ANSWER 9–5   Viruses cannot exist as free-living organisms: they have no internal metabolism, and cannot reproduce themselves. They thus have none of the attributes that one normally associates with life. Indeed, they can even be crystallized. Only inside cells can they redirect normal cellular biosynthetic activities to the task of making more copies of themselves. Thus, the only aspect of "living" that viruses display is their capacity to direct their own reproduction once inside a cell.

ANSWER 9–6   Although they can harm individuals, mobile genetic elements do provide opportunities for homologous recombination events, thereby causing genomic rearrangements. They could insert into genes, possibly obliterating splicing signals and thereby changing the protein produced by the gene. They could also insert into the regulatory DNA sequences of a gene, where insertion between an enhancer and a transcription start site could block the function of the enhancer and therefore reduce the level of expression of a gene. In addition, the mobile genetic element could itself contain an enhancer and thereby change the time and place in the organism where the gene is expressed.

ANSWER 9–7   With their ability to facilitate genetic recombination, mobile genetic elements have almost certainly played an important part in the evolution of modern-day organisms. They can facilitate gene duplication and the creation of new genes via exon shuffling, and they can change the way in which existing genes are expressed. Although the transposition of a mobile genetic element can be harmful for an individual organism—if, for example, it disrupts the activity of a critical gene—these agents of genetic change may well be beneficial to the species as a whole.

ANSWER 9–8   About 7.6% of each gene is converted to mRNA [(5.4 exons/gene × 266 nucleotide pairs/exon)/(19,000 nucleotide pairs/gene) = 7.6%]. Protein-coding genes occupy about 28% of Chromosome 22 [(700 genes × 19,000 nucleotide pairs/gene)/(48 × 10^6 nucleotide pairs) = 27.7%]. However, over 90% of this DNA is made of introns.

ANSWER 9–9   This statement is probably true. For example, nearly half our DNA is composed of defunct mobile genetic elements. And only about 10% of the human genome appears to be under positive selection. However, it is possible that future research will uncover functions for some portion of our DNA that now seems unimportant.

ANSWER 9–10   The HoxD cluster is packed with complex and extensive regulatory DNA sequences that direct each of its genes to be expressed at the correct time and place during development. Insertions of mobile genetic elements into the HoxD cluster were probably selected against because they would disrupt proper regulation of these genes.

ANSWER 9–11

A. The exons in the human β-globin gene correspond to the positions of sequence similarity (in this case identity) with the cDNA, which is a direct copy of the mRNA and thus contains no introns. The introns correspond to the regions between the exons. The positions of the introns and exons in the human β-globin gene are indicated in Figure A9–11A. Also shown (in open bars) are sequences present in the mature β-globin mRNA (and in the gene) that are not translated into protein.

B. From the positions of the exons, as defined in Figure A9–11A, it is clear that the first two exons of the human β-globin gene have counterparts, with similar sequence, in the mouse β-globin gene (Figure A9–11B). However, only the first half of the third exon of the human β-globin gene is similar to the mouse β-globin gene. The similar portion of the third exon contains sequences that encode protein, whereas the portion that is different represents the 3′ untranslated region of the gene. Because this portion of the gene does not encode protein (nor does it contain extensive regulatory DNA sequences), its sequence is probably not constrained and the mouse and human sequences have drifted apart.

C. The human and mouse β-globin genes are also similar at their 5′ ends, as indicated by the cluster of points along the same diagonal as the first exon (Figure A9–11B). These sequences correspond to the regulatory DNA sequences upstream of the start sites for transcription. Functional sequences, which are under selective pressure, diverge much more slowly than sequences without function.

D. The diagon plot shows that the first intron, although it is not conserved in sequence, it is nearly the same length in the human and mouse genes; however, the length of

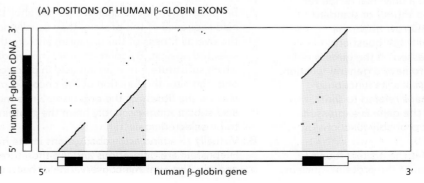

(A) POSITIONS OF HUMAN β-GLOBIN EXONS

human β-globin cDNA   5′ — 3′

human β-globin gene   5′ — 3′

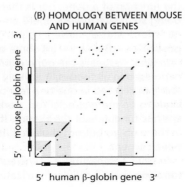

(B) HOMOLOGY BETWEEN MOUSE AND HUMAN GENES

mouse β-globin gene   5′ — 3′

5′ human β-globin gene 3′

Figure A9–11

the second intron is noticeably different (Figure A9–11B). If the introns were the same length, the line segments that represent sequence similarity would fall on the same diagonal. The easiest way to test for the colinearity of the line segments is to tilt the page and sight along the diagonal. It is impossible to tell from this comparison if the change in length is due to a shortening of the mouse intron or to a lengthening of the human intron, or some combination of those possibilities.

ANSWER 9–12   Computer algorithms that search for exons are complex, as you might imagine. To identify unknown genes, these programs combine statistical information derived from known genes, such as:

1. An exon that encodes protein will have an open reading frame. If the amino acid sequence specified by this open reading frame matches a protein sequence in any database, there is a high likelihood that it is an authentic exon.
2. The reading frames of adjacent exons in the same gene will match up when the intron sequences are omitted.
3. Internal exons (excluding the first and the last) will have splicing signals at each end; most of the time (~98%) these will be AG at the 5′ ends of the exons and GT at the 3′ ends.
4. The multiple codons for most individual amino acids are not used with equal frequency. This so-called coding bias, which varies from one species to the next, can be factored in to aid in the recognition of true exons.
5. Exons and introns have characteristic length distributions. The median length of exons in human genes is about 120 nucleotide pairs. Introns tend to be much larger: a median length of about 2 kb in genomic regions of 30–40% GC content, and a median length of about 500 nucleotide pairs in regions above 50% GC.
6. The initiation codon for protein synthesis (nearly always an ATG) has a statistical association with adjacent nucleotides that seem to enhance its recognition by translation factors.
7. The terminal exon will have a signal (most commonly AATAAA) for cleavage and polyadenylation close to its 3′ end.

The statistical nature of these features, coupled with the low frequency of coding information in the genome (1.5% for humans) and the high frequency of alternative splicing (estimated to occur in 95% of human genes), makes it difficult for an algorithm to correctly identify all exons. As shown in Figure 9–36, these bioinformatic approaches are usually coupled with direct experimental data, such as those obtained from full-genome RNA sequencing (RNA-Seq).

ANSWER 9–13   It is often not a simple matter to determine the function of a gene, nor is there a universal recipe for doing so. Nevertheless, there are a variety of standard questions whose answers help to narrow down the possibilities. Below we list some of these questions.

In what tissues is the gene expressed? If the gene is expressed in all tissues, it is likely to have a general function. If it is expressed in one or a few tissues, its function is likely to be more specialized, perhaps related to the specific functions of the tissues. If the gene is expressed in the embryo but not the adult, it probably functions in development.

In what compartment of the cell is the protein found? Knowing the subcellular localization of the protein—nucleus,

plasma membrane, mitochondria, etc.—can also help to rule out or support potential functions. For example, a protein that is localized to the plasma membrane is likely to be a transporter, a receptor or other component of a signaling pathway, a cell adhesion molecule, etc.

What are the effects of mutations in the gene? Mutations that eliminate or modify the function of the gene product can provide important clues to function. For example, if the gene product is critical at a certain time during development, mutant embryos will often die at that stage or develop obvious abnormalities.

With what other proteins does the encoded protein interact? In carrying out their function, proteins often interact with other proteins involved in the same or closely related processes. If an interacting protein can be identified, and if its function is already known (through previous research or through the searching of databases), the range of possible functions can often be narrowed.

Can mutations in other genes alter effects of mutation in the unknown gene? Searching for such mutations can be a very powerful approach to investigating gene function, especially in organisms such as bacteria and yeast, which have simple genetic systems. Although much more difficult to perform in the mouse, this type of approach can nonetheless be used. The rationale for this strategy is analogous to that of looking for interacting proteins: genes that interact genetically—so that the double-mutant phenotype is more selective than either of the individual mutants—are often involved in the same process or in closely related processes. Identification of such an interacting gene (and knowledge of its function) would provide an important clue to the function of the unknown gene.

Addressing each of these questions requires specialized experimental expertise and a substantial time commitment from the investigator. It is no wonder that progress is made much more rapidly when a clue to a gene's function can be found simply by identifying a similar gene of known function in the database. As more and more genes are studied, this strategy will become increasingly successful.

ANSWER 9–14   In a long, random sequence of DNA, each of the 64 different codons will occur with equal frequency. Because 3 of the 64 are stop codons, they will be expected to occur on average every 21 codons (64/3 = 21.3).

ANSWER 9–15   All of these mechanisms contribute to the evolution of new protein-coding genes. A, C, D, and E were discussed in the text. Recent studies indicate that certain short protein-coding genes arose from previously untranslated regions of genomes, so choice B is also correct.

ANSWER 9–16

A. Because synonymous changes do not alter the amino acid sequence of the protein, they usually do not affect the overall fitness of the organism and are therefore not selected against. By contrast, nonsynonymous changes, which substitute a new amino acid in place of the original one, can alter the function of the encoded protein and change the fitness of the organism. Since most amino acid substitutions probably harm the protein, they tend to be selected against.
B. Virtually all amino acid substitutions in the histone H3 protein are deleterious and are therefore selected against. The extreme conservation of histone H3 argues

that its function is very tightly constrained, probably because of extensive interactions with other proteins and with DNA.

C. Histone H3 is clearly not in a "privileged" site in the genome because it undergoes synonymous nucleotide changes at about the same rate as other genes.

ANSWER 9–17

A. The data embodied in the phylogenetic tree (Figure Q9–17) refutes the hypothesis that plant hemoglobin genes were acquired by horizontal transfer from animals. Looking at the more familiar parts of the tree, we see that the hemoglobins of vertebrates (fish to human) have approximately the same phylogenetic relationships as do the species themselves. Plant hemoglobins also form a distinct group that displays accepted evolutionary relationships, with barley, a monocot, diverging before bean, alfalfa, and lotus, which are all dicots (and legumes). The basic hemoglobin gene, therefore, was in place long ago in evolution. The phylogenetic tree of Figure Q9–17 indicates that the hemoglobin genes in modern plant and animal species were inherited from a common ancestor.

B. Had the plant hemoglobin genes arisen by horizontal transfer from a nematode, then the plant sequences would have clustered with the nematode sequences in the phylogenetic tree in Figure Q9–17.

ANSWER 9–18   In each human lineage, new mutations will be introduced at a rate of 10^{-10} alterations per nucleotide per cell generation, and the differences between two human lineages will accumulate at twice this rate. To accumulate 10^{-3} differences per nucleotide will thus take $10^{-3}/(2 \times 10^{-10})$ cell generations, corresponding to $(1/200) \times 10^{-3}/(2 \times 10^{-10}) = 25,000$ human generations, or 750,000 years. In reality, we are not descended from one pair of genetically identical ancestral humans; rather, it is likely that we are descended from a relatively small founder population of humans who were already genetically diverse. More sophisticated analysis suggests that this founder population existed about 200,000 years ago.

ANSWER 9–19   The virus that causes AIDS in humans, HIV, is a retrovirus, and thus synthesizes DNA from an RNA template using reverse transcriptase. This leads to frequent mutation of the viral genome. In fact, people who are HIV-positive often carry many different genetic variants of HIV that are distinct from the original virus that infected them. This posed a problem in treating the infection: drugs that block essential viral enzymes would work only temporarily, because new strains of the virus resistant to these drugs arose rapidly by mutation. Today's strategy employs multiple drugs simultaneously, which greatly decreases the likelihood that a fully resistant mutant virus could arise.

Like reverse transcriptases, RNA replicases (enzymes that synthesize RNA using RNA as a template) do not proofread. Thus, RNA viruses that replicate their RNA genomes directly (that is, without using DNA as an intermediate) also mutate frequently. In such a virus, this tends to produce changes in the coat proteins that cause the mutated virus to appear "new" to our immune systems; the virus is therefore not suppressed by immunity that has arisen to the previous version. This is part of the explanation for the new strains of the influenza (flu) virus and the common cold virus that regularly appear.

Chapter 10

ANSWER 10–1   The presence of a mutation in a gene does not necessarily mean that the protein expressed from it is defective. For example, the mutation could change one codon into another that still specifies the same amino acid, and so does not change the amino acid sequence of the protein. Or, the mutation may cause a change from one amino acid to another in the protein, but in a position that is not important for the folding or function of the protein. In assessing the likelihood that such a mutation might cause a defective protein, information on the known β-globin mutations that are found in humans is essential. You would therefore want to know the precise nucleotide change in your mutant gene, and whether this change has any known or predictable consequences for the function of the encoded protein. If your mate has two normal copies of the globin gene, 50% of your children would be carriers of your mutant gene.

ANSWER 10–2

A. Digestion with EcoRI produces two products:

```
5'-AAGAATTGCGG    AATTCGGGCCTTAAGCGCCGCGTCGAGGCCTTAAA-3'
3'-TTCTTAACGCCTTAA    GCCCGGAATTCGCGGCGCAGCTCCGGAATTT-5'
```

B. Digestion with HaeIII produces three products:

```
5'-AAGAATTGCGGAATTCGGG    CCTTAAGCGCCGCGTCGAGG    CCTTAAA-3'
3'-TTCTTAACGCCTTAAGCCC    GGAATTCGCGGCGCAGCTCC    GGAATTT-5'
```

C. The sequence lacks a HindIII cleavage site.

D. Digestion with all three enzymes therefore produces:

```
5'-AAGAATTGCGG    AATTCGGG    CCTTAAGCGCCGCGTCGAGG    CCTTAAA-3'
3'-TTCTTAACGCCTTAA    GCCC    GGAATTCGCGGCGCAGCTCC    GGAATTT-5'
```

ANSWER 10–3   Protein biochemistry is still very important because it provides the link between the amino acid sequence (which can be deduced from DNA sequences) and the functional properties of the protein. We are still not able to infallibly predict the folding of a polypeptide chain from its amino acid sequence, and in most cases information regarding the function of the protein, such as its catalytic activity, cannot be deduced from the gene sequence alone. Instead, such information must be obtained experimentally by analyzing the properties of proteins biochemically. Furthermore, the structural information that can be deduced from DNA sequences is necessarily incomplete. We cannot, for example, accurately predict covalent modifications of the protein, proteolytic processing, the presence of tightly bound small molecules, or the association of the protein with other subunits. Moreover, we cannot accurately predict the effects these modifications might have on the activity of the protein.

ANSWER 10–4

A. After an additional round of amplification there will be 2 gray, 4 green, 4 red, and 22 yellow-outlined fragments; after a second additional round there will be 2 gray, 5 green, 5 red, and 52 yellow-outlined fragments. Thus the DNA fragments outlined in yellow increase exponentially and will eventually overrun the other reaction products. Their length is determined by the DNA sequence that spans the distance between the two primers plus the length of the primers.

B. The mass of one DNA molecule 500 nucleotide pairs long is 5.5×10^{-19} g [= $2 \times 500 \times 330$ (g/mole)/6×10^{23} (molecules/mole)]. Ignoring the complexities of the first few steps of the amplification reaction (which produce longer products that eventually make an insignificant contribution to the total DNA amplified), this amount of product approximately doubles for every amplification step. Therefore, 100×10^{-9} g $= 2^N \times 5.5 \times 10^{-19}$ g, where N is the number of amplification steps of the reaction. Solving this equation for $N = \log(1.81 \times 10^{11})/\log(2)$ gives $N = 37.4$. Thus, only about 40 cycles of PCR amplification are sufficient to amplify DNA from a single molecule to a quantity that can be readily handled and analyzed biochemically. This whole procedure is automated and takes only a few hours in the laboratory.

ANSWER 10–5   If the ratio of dideoxyribonucleoside triphosphates to deoxyribonucleoside triphosphates is increased, DNA polymerization will be terminated more frequently and thus shorter DNA strands will be produced. Such conditions are favorable for determining nucleotide sequences that are close to the DNA primer used in the reaction. In contrast, decreasing the ratio of dideoxyribonucleoside triphosphates to deoxyribonucleoside triphosphates will produce longer DNA fragments, thus allowing one to determine nucleotide sequences more distant from the primer.

ANSWER 10–6   Although several explanations are possible, the simplest is that the DNA probe has hybridized predominantly with its corresponding mRNA, which is typically present in many more copies per cell than is the gene. The different extents of hybridization probably reflect different levels of gene expression. Perhaps each of the different cell types that make up the tissue expresses the gene at a different level.

ANSWER 10–7   Like the vast majority of mammalian genes, the attractase gene likely contains introns. Bacteria do not have the splicing machinery required to remove introns, and therefore the correct protein would not be expressed from the gene. For expression of most mammalian genes in bacterial cells, a cDNA version of the gene must be used.

ANSWER 10–8

A. False. Restriction sites are found at random throughout the genome, within as well as between genes.

B. True. DNA bears a negative charge at each phosphate, giving DNA an overall negative charge.

C. False. Clones isolated from cDNA libraries do not contain promoter sequences. These sequences are not transcribed and are therefore not part of the mRNAs that are used as the templates to make cDNAs.

D. True. Each polymerization reaction produces double-stranded DNA that must, at each cycle, be denatured to allow new primers to hybridize so that the DNA strand can be copied again.

E. False. Digestion of genomic DNA with restriction enzymes that recognize four-nucleotide sequences produces fragments that are on average 256 nucleotides

long. However, the actual lengths of the fragments produced will vary considerably on both sides of the average.

F. True. Reverse transcriptase is first needed to copy the mRNA into single-stranded DNA, and DNA polymerase is then required to make the second DNA strand.

G. True. Using a sufficient number of STRs, individuals can be uniquely "fingerprinted" (see Figure 10–15).

H. True. If cells of the tissue do not transcribe the gene of interest, it will not be represented in a cDNA library prepared from this tissue. However, it will be represented in a genomic library prepared from the same tissue.

ANSWER 10–9

A. The DNA sequence, from its 5′ end to its 3′ end, is read starting from the bottom of the gel, where the smallest DNA fragments migrate. Each band results from the incorporation of the appropriate dideoxyribonucleoside triphosphate, and as expected there are no two bands that have the same mobility. This allows one to determine the DNA sequence by reading off the bands in strict order, proceeding upward from the bottom of the gel, and assigning the correct nucleotide according to which lane the band is in.

   The nucleotide sequence of the top strand (Figure A10–9A) was obtained directly from the data of Figure Q10–9, and the bottom strand was deduced from the complementary base-pairing rules.

B. The DNA sequence can then be translated into an amino acid sequence using the genetic code. However, there are two strands of DNA that could be transcribed into RNA and three possible reading frames for each strand. Thus there are six amino acid sequences that can in principle be encoded by this stretch of DNA. Of the three reading frames possible from the top strand, only one is not interrupted by a stop codon (underlined in the DNA sequence and represented by *yellow* blocks in the three amino acid sequences in Figure A10–9B).

   From the bottom strand, two of the three reading frames also have stop codons (not shown). The third frame gives the following sequence:
   `SerAlaLeuGlySerSerGluAsnArgProArgThrProAlaArg`
   `ThrGlyCysProValTyr`
   It is not possible from the information given to tell which of the two open reading frames corresponds to the actual protein encoded by this stretch of DNA. What additional experiment could distinguish between these two possibilities?

ANSWER 10–10

A. Cleavage of human genomic DNA with HaeIII would generate about 11×10^6 different fragments [$= 3 \times 10^9/4^4$] and with EcoRI about 730,000 different fragments [$= 3 \times 10^9/4^6$]. There will also be some

(A) 5′ TATAAACTGGACAACCAGTTCGAGCTGGTGTTCGTGGTCGGTTTTCAGAAGATCCTAACGCTGACG 3′
     3′ ATATTTGACCTGTTGGTCAAGCTCGACCACAAGCACCAGCCAAAAGTCTTCTAGGATTGCGACTGC 5′

(B)   top strand of DNA
     5′ TATAAACTGGACAACCAGTTCGAGCTGGTGTTCGTGGTCGGTTTTCAGAAGATCCTAACGCTGACG 3′
   1 TyrLysLeuAspAsnGlnPheGluLeuValPheValValGlyPheGlnLysIleLeuThrLeuThr
   2 IleAsnTrpThrThrSerSerSerTrpCysSerTrpSerValPheArgArgSer ▪▪ Arg ▪▪ Ar
   3   ▪▪ ThrGlyGlnProValArgAlaGlyValArgGlyArgPheSerGluAspProAsnAlaAsp

Figure A10–9

additional fragments generated because the maternal and paternal chromosomes are very similar but not identical in DNA sequence.

B. A set of overlapping DNA fragments will be generated. Libraries constructed from sets of overlapping fragments are valuable because they can be used to order cloned sequences in relation to their original order in the genome and thus obtain the DNA sequence of a long stretch of DNA (see Figure 10–20).

ANSWER 10–11 By comparison with the positions of the size markers, we find that EcoRI treatment gives two fragments of 4 kb and 6 kb; HindIII treatment gives one fragment of 10 kb; and treatment with EcoRI + HindIII gives three fragments of 6 kb, 3 kb, and 1 kb. This gives a total length of 10 kb calculated as the sum of the fragments in each lane. Thus the original DNA molecule must be 10 kb (10,000 nucleotide pairs) long. Because treatment with HindIII gives a fragment 10 kb long it could be that the original DNA is a linear molecule with no cutting site for HindIII. But we can rule that out by the results of the EcoRI + HindIII digestion. We know that EcoRI cleavage alone produces two fragments of 6 kb and 4 kb, and in the double digest this 4-kb fragment is further cleaved by HindIII into a 3-kb and a 1-kb fragment. The DNA therefore contains a single HindIII cleavage site, and thus it must be circular, as a single fragment of 10 kb is produced when it is cut with HindIII alone. Arranging the cutting sites on a circular DNA to give the appropriate sizes of fragments produces the map illustrated in Figure A10–11.

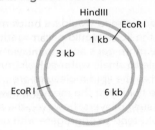

Figure A10–11

ANSWER 10–12

A. Infants 2 and 8 have identical STR patterns and therefore must be identical twins. Infants 3 and 6 also have identical STR patterns and must also be identical twins. The other two sets of twins must be fraternal twins because their STR patterns are not identical. Fraternal twins, like any pair of siblings born to the same parents, will have roughly half their genome in common. Thus, roughly half the STR polymorphisms in fraternal twins will be identical. Using this criterion, you can identify infants 1 and 7 as fraternal twins and infants 4 and 5 as fraternal twins.

B. You can match infants to their parents by using the same sort of analysis of STR polymorphisms. Every band present in the analysis of an infant should have a matching band in one or the other of the parents, and, on average, each infant will share half of its polymorphisms with each parent. Thus, the degree of match between each child and each parent will be approximately the same as that between fraternal twins.

ANSWER 10–13 Mutant bacteria that do not produce ice-protein have probably arisen many times in nature.

However, bacteria that produce ice-protein have a slight growth advantage over bacteria that do not, so it would be difficult to find such mutants in the wild. Recombinant DNA technology makes these mutants much easier to obtain. In this case, the consequences, both advantageous and disadvantageous, of using a genetically modified organism are therefore nearly indistinguishable from those of a natural mutant. Indeed, bacterial and yeast strains have been selected for centuries for desirable genetic traits that make them suitable for industrial-scale applications such as cheese and wine production. The possibilities of recombinant DNA technology are endless, however, and as with any technology, there is a risk of unforeseen consequences. Recombinant DNA experimentation, therefore, is regulated, and the risks of individual projects are carefully assessed by review panels before permissions are granted. The state of our knowledge is sufficiently advanced that the consequences of some changes, such as the disruption of a bacterial gene in the example above, can be predicted with reasonable certainty. Other applications, such as germ-line gene therapy to correct human disease, may have far more complex outcomes, and it will take many more years of research and ethical debate to determine whether such treatments will eventually be used.

Chapter 11

ANSWER 11–1 Water is a liquid, and the hydrogen bonds that form between water molecules are not static; they are continually broken and remade again by thermal motion. When a water molecule happens to be next to a hydrophobic molecule, it is more restricted in motion and has fewer neighbors with which it can interact, because it cannot form any hydrogen bonds in the direction of the hydrophobic molecule. It will therefore form hydrogen bonds to the more limited number of water molecules in its proximity. Bonding to fewer partners results in a more ordered water structure, which represents the cagelike structure in Figure 11–9. This structure has been likened to ice, although it is a more transient, less organized, and less extensive network than even a tiny ice crystal. The formation of any ordered structure decreases the entropy of the system and is thus energetically unfavorable (discussed in Chapter 3).

ANSWER 11–2 (B) is the correct analogy for lipid bilayer assembly because exclusion from water rather than attractive forces between the lipid molecules is involved. If the lipid molecules formed bonds with one another, the bilayer would be less fluid, and might even become rigid, depending on the strength of the interaction.

ANSWER 11–3 The fluidity of the bilayer is strictly confined to one plane: lipid molecules can diffuse laterally in their own monolayer but do not readily flip from one monolayer to the other. Lipid molecules inserted into one monolayer therefore remain in it unless they are actively transferred to the other monolayer by a transporter such as a scramblase or a flippase.

ANSWER 11–4 In both an α helix and a β barrel, the polar peptide bonds of the polypeptide backbone can be completely shielded from the hydrophobic environment of the lipid bilayer by the hydrophobic amino acid side chains.

Internal hydrogen bonds between the peptide bonds stabilize the α helix and β barrel.

ANSWER 11–5   The sulfate group in SDS is charged and therefore hydrophilic. The OH group and the C–O–C groups in Triton X-100 are polar; they can also form hydrogen bonds with water molecules and are therefore hydrophilic. In contrast, the red portions of the detergents are either hydrocarbon chains or aromatic rings, neither of which has polar groups that could form hydrogen bonds with water molecules; they are therefore hydrophobic. (One example of a tripeptide with hydrophobic side chains is shown in Figure A11–5.)

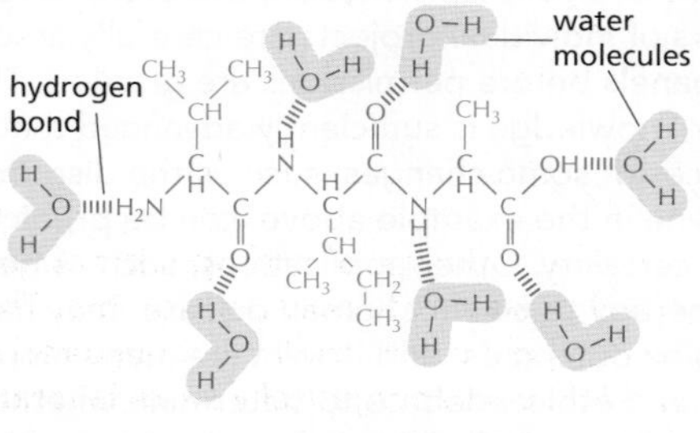

valine   isoleucine   alanine

Figure A11–5

ANSWER 11–6   Some of the transmembrane proteins are anchored to the spectrin filaments of the cell cortex. These molecules are not free to rotate or diffuse within the plane of the membrane. There is an excess of transmembrane proteins over the available attachment sites in the cortex, however, so some of the transmembrane protein molecules are not anchored. These proteins are free to rotate and diffuse within the plane of the membrane. Indeed, measurements of protein mobility show that there are two populations of each transmembrane protein, corresponding to those proteins that are anchored and those that are not.

ANSWER 11–7   The different ways in which membrane proteins can be restricted to different regions of the membrane are summarized in Figure 11–31. The mobility of the membrane proteins is drastically reduced if they are bound to other proteins such as those of the cell cortex or the extracellular matrix. Some membrane proteins are confined to membrane domains by barriers, such as tight junctions. The fluidity of the lipid bilayer is not significantly affected by the anchoring of membrane proteins; the sea of lipid molecules flows around anchored membrane proteins like water around the posts of a pier.

ANSWER 11–8   All of the statements are correct.
A. The lipid bilayer is fluid because its lipid can undergo these motions.
B. The lipid bilayer is fluid because its lipid can undergo these motions.
C. Such exchanges require the action of a transporter.
D. Hydrogen bonds are formed and broken by thermal motion.
E. Glycolipids are mostly restricted to the monolayer of membranes that faces away from the cytosol. Some special glycolipids, such as phosphatidylinositol (discussed in Chapter 16), are found specifically in the cytosolic monolayer.

F. The reduction of double bonds (by hydrogenation) allows the resulting saturated lipid molecules to pack more tightly against one another and therefore increases viscosity—that is, it turns oil into margarine.
G. Examples include the many membrane enzymes involved in signaling (discussed in Chapter 16).
H. Polysaccharides are the main constituents of mucus and slime; the carbohydrate coat of a cell, which is made up of polysaccharides and oligosaccharides, is a very important lubricant, particularly for cells that line blood vessels or circulate in the bloodstream.

ANSWER 11–9   In a two-dimensional fluid, the molecules are free to move only in one plane; the molecules in a normal fluid, in contrast, can move in three dimensions.

ANSWER 11–10
A. You would have a detergent. The diameter of the lipid head would be much larger than that of the hydrocarbon tail, so that the shape of the molecule would be a cone rather than a cylinder and the molecules would aggregate to form micelles rather than bilayers.
B. The lipid bilayers formed would be much more fluid. The bilayers would also be less stable, as the shorter hydrocarbon tails would be less hydrophobic, so the forces that drive the formation of the bilayer would be reduced.
C. The lipid bilayers formed would be much less fluid. Whereas a normal lipid bilayer has the viscosity of olive oil, a bilayer made of the same lipids but with saturated hydrocarbon tails would have the consistency of bacon fat.
D. The lipid bilayers formed would be much more fluid. Also, because the lipids would pack together less well, there would be more gaps and the bilayer would be more permeable to small, water-soluble molecules.
E. If we assume that the lipid molecules are completely intermixed, the fluidity of the membrane would be unchanged. In such bilayers, however, the saturated lipid molecules would tend to aggregate with one another because they can pack so much more tightly and would therefore form patches of much-reduced fluidity. The bilayer would not, therefore, have uniform properties over its surface. Because in membrane lipid molecules, one saturated and one unsaturated hydrocarbon tail are typically linked to the same hydrophilic head, such segregation does not occur in cell membranes.
F. The lipid bilayers formed would have virtually unchanged properties. Each lipid molecule would now span the entire membrane, with one of its two head groups exposed at each surface. Such lipid molecules are found in the membranes of thermophilic bacteria, which can live at temperatures approaching boiling water. Their bilayers do not come apart at elevated temperatures, as usual bilayers do, because the original two monolayers are now covalently linked into a single membrane.

ANSWER 11–11   Phospholipid molecules are approximately cylindrical in shape. Detergent molecules, by contrast, are conical or wedge-shaped. A phospholipid molecule with only one hydrocarbon tail, for example, would be a detergent. To make a phospholipid molecule into a detergent, you would have to make its hydrophilic head larger or remove one of its tails so that it could form a micelle. Detergent molecules also usually have shorter hydrocarbon tails than lipid molecules. This makes them slightly water-soluble, so that detergent molecules leave and reenter micelles frequently in aqueous solution. Because of this, some monomeric detergent molecules are always present in aqueous solution and therefore can enter the lipid bilayer of a cell membrane to solubilize the proteins (see Figure 11–27).

ANSWER 11–12
A. There are about 4000 lipid molecules, each 0.5 nm wide, between one end of the bacterial cell and the other. So if a lipid molecule at one end moved directly in a straight line it would require only 4×10^{-4} sec (= 4000 $\times 10^{-7}$) to reach the other end. In reality, however, the lipid molecule would move in a random path, so that it would take considerably longer. We can calculate the approximate time required from the equation: $t = x^2/2D$, where x is the average distance moved, t is the time taken, and D is a constant called the diffusion coefficient. Inserting step values $x = 0.5$ nm and $t = 10^{-7}$ sec, we obtain $D = 1.25 \times 10^{-8}$ cm^2/sec. Using this value in the same equation but with distance $x = 2 \times 10^{-4}$ cm (= µm) gives the time taken $t = 0.16$ seconds.
B. Similarly, if a 4-cm-diameter ping-pong ball exchanged partners every 10^{-7} seconds and moved in a linear fashion, it would reach the opposite wall in 1.5×10^{-5} sec, traveling at 1,440,000 km/hr. [But a random walk would take longer. Using the equation above, we calculate the constant D in this case to be 8×10^7 cm^2/sec and the time required to travel 6 m about 2 msec (= $600^2/1.6 \times 10^8$).]

ANSWER 11–13 Transmembrane proteins anchor the plasma membrane to the underlying cell cortex, strengthening the membrane so that it can withstand the forces on it when the red blood cell is pumped through small blood vessels. Transmembrane proteins also transport nutrients and ions across the plasma membrane.

ANSWER 11–14 The hydrophilic faces of the five membrane-spanning α helices, each contributed by a different subunit, are thought to come together to form a pore across the lipid bilayer that is lined with the hydrophilic amino acid side chains (Figure A11–14). Ions can pass through this hydrophilic pore without coming into contact with the lipid tails of the bilayer. The hydrophobic side chains interact with the hydrophobic lipid tails.

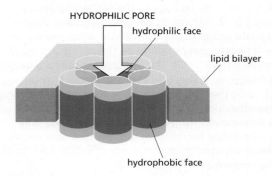

HYDROPHILIC PORE
hydrophilic face
lipid bilayer
hydrophobic face

Figure A11–14

ANSWER 11–15 There are about 100 lipid molecules (i.e., phospholipid + cholesterol) for every protein molecule in the membrane [(2/50,000)/(1/800 + 1/386)]. A similar protein/lipid ratio is seen in many cell membranes.

ANSWER 11–16 Membrane fusion does not alter the orientation of the membrane proteins with their attached color tags: the portion of each transmembrane protein that is exposed to the cytosol always remains exposed to the cytosol, and the portion exposed to the outside always remains exposed to the outside (Figure A11–16). At 0°C, the fluidity of the membrane is reduced, and the mixing of the membrane proteins is significantly slowed.

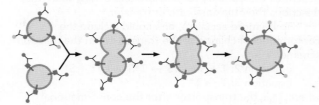

Figure A11–16

ANSWER 11–17 The exposure of hydrophobic amino acid side chains to water is energetically unfavorable. There are two ways that such side chains can be sequestered away from water to achieve an energetically more favorable state. First, they can form transmembrane segments that span a lipid bilayer. This requires about 20 of them to be located sequentially in a polypeptide chain. Second, the hydrophobic amino acid side chains can be sequestered in the interior of the folded polypeptide chain. This is one of the major forces that lock the polypeptide chain into a unique three-dimensional structure. In either case, the hydrophobic forces in the lipid bilayer or in the interior of a protein are based on the same principles.

ANSWER 11–18 (A) Antarctic fish live at subzero temperatures and are cold-blooded. To keep their membranes fluid at these temperatures, they have a high percentage of unsaturated phospholipids.

ANSWER 11–19 Sequence B is most likely to form a transmembrane helix. It is composed primarily of hydrophobic amino acids, and therefore can be stably integrated into a lipid bilayer. In contrast, sequence A contains many polar amino acids (S, T, N, Q), and sequence C contains many charged amino acids (K, R, H, E, D), which would be energetically disfavored in the hydrophobic interior of the lipid bilayer.

ANSWER 11–20 Triacylglycerol is an entirely hydrophobic molecule. Without a hydrophilic portion, it is unable to form favorable interactions with water. Thus, triacylglycerol would be unlikely to become part of a lipid bilayer. Instead, such purely hydrophobic molecules cluster together to limit their contact with surrounding water molecules (see Figure 11–9). In this way, triacylglycerols—which are major components of animal fats and plant oils—coalesce into fat droplets in an aqueous environment, including those in fat cells and plant seeds.

Chapter 12

ANSWER 12–1
A. The movement of a solute mediated by a transporter can be described by a strictly analogous equation:
equation 1: T + S ↔ TS → T + S*
where S is the solute, S* is the solute on the other

side of the membrane (i.e., although it is still the same molecule, it is now located in a different environment), and T is the transporter.

B. This equation is useful because it describes a binding step followed by a delivery step. The mathematical treatment of this equation would be very similar to that described for enzymes (see Figure 4–35); thus transporters are characterized by a K_m value that describes their affinity for a solute and a V_{max} value that describes their maximal rate of transfer.

   To be more accurate, one could include the conformational change of the transporter in the reaction scheme:

   equation 2: $T + S \leftrightarrow TS \leftrightarrow T{*}S{*} \rightarrow T{*} + S{*}$
   equation 3: $T \leftrightarrow T{*}$

   where $T{*}$ is the transporter after the conformational change that exposes its solute-binding site on the other side of the membrane. This account requires a second equation (3) that allows the transporter to return to its starting conformation.

C. The equations do not describe the behavior of channels because solutes passing through channels do not bind to them in the way that a substrate binds to an enzyme.

ANSWER 12–2   If the Na$^+$ pump is not working at full capacity because it is partially inhibited by ouabain or digitalis, the electrochemical gradient of Na$^+$ that the pump generates is less steep than that in untreated cells. Consequently, the Ca^{2+}–Na$^+$ antiport works less efficiently, and Ca^{2+} is removed from the cell more slowly. When the next cycle of muscle contraction begins, there is still an elevated level of Ca^{2+} left in the cytosol. The entry of the same number of Ca^{2+} ions into the cell therefore leads to a higher Ca^{2+} concentration than in untreated cells, which in turn leads to a stronger and longer-lasting muscle contraction. Because the Na$^+$ pump fulfills essential functions in all animal cells, both to maintain osmotic balance and to generate the Na$^+$ gradient used to power many transporters, the drugs are deadly poisons if too much is taken.

ANSWER 12–3

A. Each of the rectangular peaks corresponds to the opening of a single channel that allows a small current to pass. You note from the recording that the channels present in the patch of membrane open and close frequently. Each channel remains open for a very short, somewhat variable time, averaging about 5 milliseconds. When open, the channels allow a small current with a unique amplitude (4 pA; one picoampere = 10^{-12} A) to pass. In one instance, the current doubles, indicating that two channels in the same membrane patch opened simultaneously.

B. If acetylcholine is omitted or is added to the solution outside the pipette, you would measure only the baseline current. Acetylcholine must bind to the extracellular portion of the acetylcholine receptor in the membrane patch to allow the channel to open frequently enough to detect changes in the currents; in the membrane patch shown in Figure 12–25B, only the cytoplasmic side of the receptor is exposed to the solution outside the microelectrode.

ANSWER 12–4   The equilibrium potential of K$^+$ is –90 mV [= 62 mV log$_{10}$ (5 mM/140 mM)], and that of Na$^+$ is +72 mV [= 62 mV log$_{10}$ (145 mM/10 mM)]. The K$^+$ leak channels are the main ion channels open in the plasma membrane of a resting cell, and they allow K$^+$ to come to equilibrium; the membrane potential of the cell is therefore close to –90 mV. When Na$^+$ channels open, Na$^+$ rushes in, and, as a result, the membrane potential reverses its polarity to a value nearer to +72 mV, the equilibrium value for Na$^+$. Upon closure of the Na$^+$ channels, the K$^+$ leak channels allow K$^+$, now no longer at equilibrium, to exit from the cell until the membrane potential is restored to the equilibrium value for K$^+$, about –90 mV.

ANSWER 12–5   When the resting membrane potential of an axon (inside negative) rises to a threshold value, voltage-gated Na$^+$ channels in the immediate neighborhood open and allow an influx of Na$^+$. This depolarizes the membrane further, causing more voltage-gated Na$^+$ channels to open, including those in the adjacent plasma membrane. This creates a wave of depolarization that spreads rapidly along the axon, called the action potential. Because Na$^+$ channels become inactivated soon after they open, the outward flow of K$^+$ through voltage-gated K$^+$ channels and K$^+$ leak channels is rapidly able to restore the original resting membrane potential. (96 words)

ANSWER 12–6   If the number of functional acetylcholine receptors is reduced by the antibodies, the neurotransmitter (acetylcholine) that is released from the nerve terminals cannot (or can only weakly) stimulate the muscle to contract.

ANSWER 12–7   Although the concentration of Cl$^-$ outside cells is much higher than inside, when transmitter-gated Cl$^-$ channels open in the plasma membrane of a postsynaptic neuron in response to an inhibitory neurotransmitter, very little Cl$^-$ enters the cell. This is because the driving force for the influx of Cl$^-$ across the membrane is close to zero at the resting membrane potential, which opposes the influx. If, however, the excitatory neurotransmitter opens Na$^+$ channels in the postsynaptic membrane at the same time that an inhibitory neurotransmitter opens Cl$^-$ channels, the resulting depolarization caused by the Na$^+$ influx will cause Cl$^-$ to move into the cell through the open Cl$^-$ channels, neutralizing the effect of the Na$^+$ influx. In this way, inhibitory neurotransmitters suppress the production of an action potential by making the target cell membrane much harder to depolarize.

ANSWER 12–8   By analogy to the Na$^+$ pump shown in Figure 12–12, ATP might be hydrolyzed and donate a phosphate group to the transporter when—and only when—it has the solute bound on the cytosolic face of the membrane (step 1 $\rightarrow$ 2). The attachment of the phosphate would trigger an immediate conformational change (step 2 $\rightarrow$ 3), thereby capturing the solute and exposing it to the other side of the membrane. The phosphate would be removed from the protein when—and only when—the solute had dissociated, and the now empty, nonphosphorylated transporter would switch back to the starting conformation (step 3 $\rightarrow$ 4) (Figure A12–8).

ANSWER 12–9

A. False. The plasma membrane contains transport proteins that confer selective permeability to many but not all charged molecules. In contrast, a pure lipid bilayer lacking proteins is highly impermeable to all charged molecules.

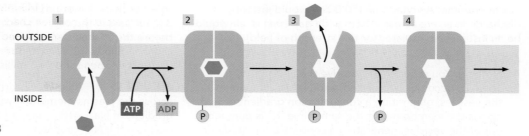

Figure A12–8

B. False. Channels do not have binding pockets for the solute that passes through them. Selectivity of a channel is achieved by the size of the internal pore and by charged regions at the entrance of the pore that attract or repel ions of the appropriate charge.

C. False. Transporters are slower. They have enzyme-like properties; that is, they bind solutes and need to undergo conformational changes during their functional cycle. This limits the maximal rate of transport to about 1000 solute molecules per second, whereas channels can pass up to 1,000,000 solute molecules per second.

D. True. The bacteriorhodopsin of some photosynthetic bacteria pumps H^+ out of the cell using energy captured from visible light.

E. True. Most animal cells contain K^+ leak channels in their plasma membrane that are predominantly open. The K^+ concentration inside the cell still remains higher than outside because the membrane potential is negative and therefore inhibits the positively charged K^+ from leaking out. K^+ is also continually pumped into the cell by the Na^+ pump.

F. False. A symport binds two different solutes on the same side of the membrane. Turning it around would not change it into an antiport, which must also bind two different solutes but on opposing sides of the membrane.

G. False. The peak of an action potential corresponds to a transient shift of the membrane potential from a negative to a positive value. The influx of Na^+ causes the membrane potential first to move toward zero and then to reverse, rendering the cell positively charged on its inside. Eventually, the resting potential is restored by an efflux of K^+ through voltage-gated K^+ channels and K^+ leak channels.

ANSWER 12–10   The permeabilities are N_2 (small and nonpolar) > ethanol (small and slightly polar) > water (small and polar) > glucose (large and polar) > Ca^{2+} (small and charged) > RNA (very large and charged).

ANSWER 12–11

A. Both couple the movement of two different solutes across a cell membrane. Symports transport both solutes in the same direction, whereas antiports transport the solutes in opposite directions.

B. Both are mediated by membrane transport proteins. Passive transport of a solute occurs downhill, in the direction of its concentration or electrochemical gradient, whereas active transport occurs uphill and therefore needs an energy source. Active transport can be mediated by transporters but not by channels, whereas passive transport can be mediated by either.

C. Both terms describe gradients across a membrane. The membrane potential refers to the voltage gradient; the

electrochemical gradient is a composite of the voltage gradient and the concentration gradient of a specific charged solute (ion). The membrane potential is defined independently of the solute of interest, whereas an electrochemical gradient refers to the particular solute.

D. A pump is a specialized transporter that uses energy to transport a solute uphill—against an electrochemical gradient for a charged solute or a concentration gradient for an uncharged solute.

E. Both transmit electrical signals, by means of electrons in wires and by ion movements across the plasma membrane in axons. Wires are made of copper, axons are not. The signal passing down an axon does not diminish in strength because it is self-amplifying, whereas the signal in a wire decreases over distance (by leakage of current across the insulating sheath).

F. Both affect the osmotic pressure in a cell. An ion is a solute that bears a charge.

ANSWER 12–12   A bridge allows vehicles to pass over water in a steady stream; the entrance can be designed to exclude, for example, oversized trucks, and it can be intermittently closed to traffic by a gate. By analogy, gated channels allow ions to pass across a cell membrane, imposing size and charge restrictions.

A ferry, in contrast, loads vehicles on one side of the body of water, crosses, and unloads on the other side—a slower process. During loading, particular vehicles could be selected from the waiting line because they fit particularly well on the car deck. By analogy, transporters bind solutes on one side of the membrane and then, after a conformational movement, release them on the other side. Specific binding selects the molecules to be transported. As in the case of coupled transport, sometimes you have to wait until the ferry is full before you can go.

ANSWER 12–13   Acetylcholine is being transported into the vesicles by an H^+–acetylcholine antiport in the vesicle membrane. The H^+ gradient that drives the uptake is generated by an ATP-driven H^+ pump in the vesicle membrane, which pumps H^+ into the vesicle (hence the dependence of the reaction on ATP). Raising the pH of the solution surrounding the vesicles decreases the H^+ concentration of the solution, thereby increasing the outward gradient across the vesicle membrane, explaining the enhanced rate of acetylcholine uptake.

ANSWER 12–14   The voltage gradient across the membrane is about 150,000 V/cm (70×10^{-3} V/4.5×10^{-7} cm). This extremely powerful electric field is close to the limit at which insulating materials—such as the lipid bilayer—break down and cease to act as insulators. The large field indicates what a large amount of energy can be stored in electrical gradients across the membrane, as well as the extreme electrical forces that proteins can experience in a membrane. A voltage of 150,000 V would instantly discharge in an arc across a 1-cm-wide gap (that is, air would be an insufficient insulator for this strength of field).

ANSWER 12–15

A. Nothing. You require ATP to drive the Na^+ pump.

B. The ATP becomes hydrolyzed, and Na^+ is pumped into the vesicles, generating a concentration gradient of Na^+ across the membrane. At the same time, K^+ is pumped out of the vesicles, generating a concentration gradient of K^+ of opposite polarity. When all the K^+ is pumped out of the vesicle or the ATP runs out, the pump would stop.

C. The pump would initiate a transport cycle and then cease. Because all reaction steps must occur strictly sequentially, dephosphorylation and the accompanying conformational switch cannot occur in the absence of K^+. The Na^+ pump will therefore become stuck in the phosphorylated state, waiting indefinitely for a potassium ion. The number of sodium ions transported would be minuscule, because each pump molecule would have functioned only a single time. Similar experiments, leaving out individual ions and analyzing the consequences, were used to determine the sequence of steps by which the Na^+ pump works.

D. ATP would become hydrolyzed, and Na^+ and K^+ would be pumped across the membrane as described in (B). However, the pump molecules that sit in the membrane in the reverse orientation would be completely inactive (i.e., they would not—as one might have erroneously assumed—pump ions in the opposite direction) because ATP would not have access to the site on these molecules where phosphorylation occurs, which is normally exposed to the cytosol. ATP is highly charged and cannot cross membranes without the help of specific transporters.

E. ATP becomes hydrolyzed, and Na^+ and K^+ are pumped across the membrane, as described in (B). K^+, however, immediately flows back into the vesicles through the K^+ leak channels. K^+ moves down the K^+ concentration gradient formed by the action of the Na^+ pump. With each K^+ that moves into the vesicle through a leak channel, a positive charge is moved across the membrane, generating a membrane potential that is positive on the inside of the vesicles. Eventually, K^+ will stop flowing through the leak channels when the membrane potential balances the K^+ concentration gradient. The scenario described here is a slight oversimplification: the Na^+ pump in mammalian cells actually moves three sodium ions out of cells for each two potassium ions that it pumps, thereby driving an electric current across the membrane and making a small additional contribution to the resting membrane potential (which therefore corresponds only approximately to a state of equilibrium for K^+ moving via K^+ leak channels).

ANSWER 12–16   Ion channels can be ligand-gated, voltage-gated, or mechanically- (stress-) gated.

ANSWER 12–17   The cell has a volume of 10^{-12} liters (= 10^{-15} m^3) and thus contains 6×10^4 calcium ions (= 6×10^{23} molecules/mole $\times$ 100 $\times$ 10^{-9} moles/liter $\times$ 10^{-12} liters). Therefore, to raise the intracellular Ca^{2+} concentration fiftyfold, another 2,940,000 calcium ions have

to enter the cell (note that at 5 µM concentration there are 3×10^6 ions in the cell, of which 60,000 are already present before the channels are opened). Because each of the 1000 channels allows 10^6 ions to pass per second, each channel has to stay open for only 3 milliseconds.

ANSWER 12–18   Animal cells drive most transport processes across the plasma membrane with the electrochemical gradient of Na^+. ATP is needed to fuel the Na^+ pump to maintain the Na^+ gradient.

ANSWER 12–19

A. If H^+ is pumped across the membrane into the endosomes, an electrochemical gradient of H^+ results, composed of both an H^+ concentration gradient and a membrane potential, with the interior of the vesicle positive. Both of these components add to the energy that is stored in the gradient and that must be supplied to generate it. The electrochemical gradient will limit the transfer of more H^+. If, however, the membrane also contains Cl^- channels, the negatively charged Cl^- in the cytosol will flow into the endosomes and diminish their membrane potential. It therefore becomes energetically less expensive to pump more H^+ across the membrane, and the interior of the endosomes can become more acidic.

B. No. As explained in (A), some acidification would still occur in their absence.

ANSWER 12–20

A. See Figure A12–20.

B. The transport rates of compound A are proportional to its concentration, indicating that compound A can diffuse through membranes on its own. Compound A is likely to be ethanol, because it is a small and relatively nonpolar molecule that can diffuse readily through the lipid bilayer (see Figure 12–2). In contrast, the transport rates of compound B saturate at high concentrations, indicating that compound B is transported across the membrane by some sort of membrane transport protein. Transport rates cannot increase beyond a maximal rate at which this protein can function. Compound B is likely to be acetate, because it is a charged molecule that could not cross the membrane without the help of a membrane transport protein.

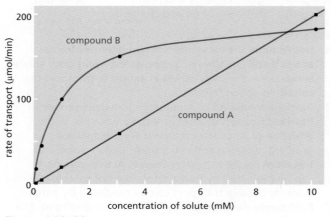

Figure A12–20

ANSWER 12–21 The membrane potential and the high extracellular Na^+ concentration provide a large inward electrochemical driving force and a large reservoir of Na^+ ions, so that mostly Na^+ ions enter the cell as acetylcholine receptors open. Ca^{2+} ions will also enter the cell, but their influx is much more limited because of their lower extracellular concentration. (Most of the Ca^{2+} that enters the cytosol to stimulate muscle contraction is released from intracellular stores, as we discuss in Chapter 17). Because of the high intracellular K^+ concentration and the opposing direction of the membrane potential, there will be little if any movement of K^+ ions upon opening of a cation channel.

ANSWER 12–22 The diversity of neurotransmitter-gated ion channels raises the hope of developing new drugs specific for each channel type. Each of the diverse subtypes of these channels is expressed in a narrow subset of neurons. This narrow range of expression should make it possible, in principle, to discover or design drugs that affect particular receptor subtypes present in a selected set of neurons, thus targeting particular brain functions with greater specificity.

Chapter 13

ANSWER 13–1 To keep glycolysis going, cells need to regenerate NAD^+ from NADH. In the absence of oxygen, there is no efficient way to do this without fermentation. Without regenerated NAD^+, step 6 of glycolysis [the oxidation of glyceraldehyde 3-phosphate to 1,3-bisphosphoglycerate (Panel 13–1, pp. 436–437)] could not occur, and the product glyceraldehyde 3-phosphate would accumulate. The same thing would happen in cells unable to make either lactate or ethanol: neither would be able to regenerate NAD^+, and so glycolysis would be blocked at the same step.

ANSWER 13–2 Arsenate instead of phosphate becomes attached in step 6 of glycolysis to form 1-arseno-3-phosphoglycerate (Figure A13–2). Because of its sensitivity to hydrolysis in water, the high-energy bond is destroyed before the molecule that contains it can diffuse to reach the next enzyme. The product of the hydrolysis, 3-phosphoglycerate, is the same product normally formed in step 7 by the action of phosphoglycerate kinase. But because hydrolysis occurs nonenzymatically, the energy liberated by breaking the high-energy bond cannot be captured to generate ATP. In Figure 13–7, therefore, the reaction corresponding to the downward-pointing arrow in step 7 would still occur, but the wheel that provides the coupling to ATP synthesis is missing. Arsenate wastes metabolic energy by uncoupling many phosphotransfer reactions by the same mechanism, which is why it is so poisonous.

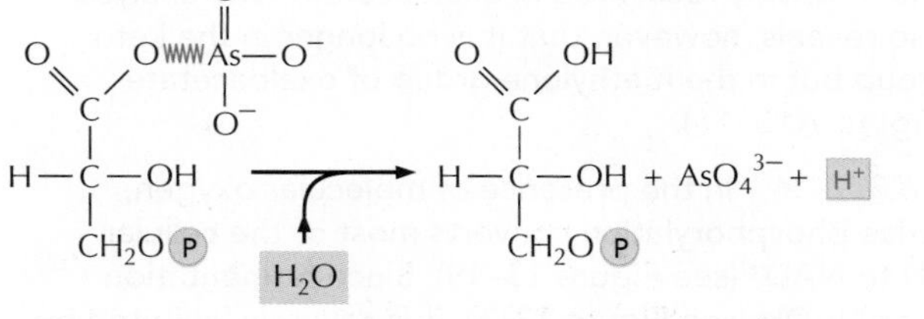

Figure A13–2

ANSWER 13–3 The oxidation of fatty acids breaks the carbon chain down into two-carbon units at a time (acetyl groups that had become attached to CoA). Conversely, during biogenesis, fatty acids are constructed by linking together acetyl groups. Most fatty acids therefore have an even number of carbon atoms.

ANSWER 13–4 Because the function of the citric acid cycle is to harvest the energy released during the oxidation, it is advantageous to break the overall reaction into as many steps as possible (see Figure 13–1). Using a two-carbon compound (acetyl CoA), the available chemistry would be much more limited, and it would be impossible to generate as many intermediates.

ANSWER 13–5 It is true that oxygen atoms are returned to the atmosphere as part of CO_2 during the oxidative degradation of glucose (see Figure 13–3). The CO_2 released from the cells, however, does not contain the specific oxygen atoms consumed as part of the oxidative phosphorylation process; these are converted into water. One can show this directly by incubating living cells in an atmosphere that includes molecular oxygen containing the ^{18}O isotope of oxygen instead of the naturally abundant isotope, ^{16}O. In such an experiment, one finds that all the CO_2 released from cells contains only ^{16}O. Therefore, the oxygen atoms in the released CO_2 molecules do not come directly from the atmosphere but from organic molecules that the cell has first made and then oxidized as fuel (see top of first page of Panel 13–2, pp. 442–443).

ANSWER 13–6 The cycle continues because intermediates are replenished as necessary by reactions leading into the citric acid cycle (instead of away from it). One of the most important reactions of this kind is the conversion of pyruvate to oxaloacetate by the enzyme pyruvate carboxylase:

pyruvate + CO_2 + ATP + H_2O → oxaloacetate + ADP + P_i + $2H^+$

This reaction feeds oxaloacetate into the citric acid cycle. It is one of the many examples of how metabolic pathways are carefully coordinated to work together to maintain appropriate concentrations of all metabolites required by the cell (see Figure A13–6).

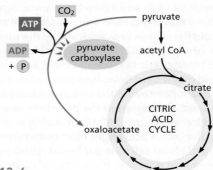

Figure A13–6

ANSWER 13–7 The carbon atoms in sugar molecules are already partially oxidized. In contrast, only the very first carbon atom in the acyl chains of fatty acids is oxidized. Thus, two carbon atoms from glucose are lost as CO_2 during the conversion of pyruvate to acetyl CoA (see Figure 13–3), leaving only four carbons to enter the citric acid cycle, where most of the energy is captured. In contrast, all carbon atoms of a fatty acid are converted into acetyl CoA (see Figure 13–11).

ANSWER 13–8

A. False. If this were the case, the reaction would be useless for the cell. No chemical energy would be harvested in a useful form (e.g., ATP) to be used for metabolic processes. (The cells would certainly be warm, though!)

B. False. No energy-conversion process can be 100% efficient. Recall that entropy in the universe always has to increase, and for most reactions this occurs by releasing heat.

C. True. The carbon atoms in glucose are in a reduced state compared with those in CO_2, in which they are fully oxidized.

D. False. The final steps of oxidative phosphorylation do indeed produce some water (see Figure 13–3). But water is so abundant in the biosphere that this is no more than "a drop in the ocean."

E. True. If it had occurred in only one step, then all the energy would be released at once and it would be impossible to harness it efficiently to drive other reactions, such as the synthesis of ATP.

F. False. Molecular oxygen (O_2) is used only in the very last step of the reaction (see Figure 13–3).

G. True. Plants convert CO_2 into sugars by harvesting the energy of light in photosynthesis. O_2 is produced in the process and released into the atmosphere by plant cells.

H. True. Anaerobically growing cells use glycolysis to oxidize sugars to pyruvate: animal cells convert the pyruvate into lactate, and no CO_2 is produced; yeast cells, however, convert the pyruvate into ethanol and CO_2. It is this CO_2 gas released from yeast cells during fermentation that makes bread dough rise and that carbonates beer and champagne.

ANSWER 13–9   Darwin exhaled the carbon atom, which therefore must be the carbon atom of a CO_2 molecule. After spending some time in the atmosphere, the CO_2 molecule must have entered a plant cell, where it became "fixed" by photosynthesis and converted into part of a sugar molecule. While it is certain that these early steps must have happened this way, there are many different paths from there that the carbon atom could have taken. The sugar could have been broken down by the plant cell into pyruvate or acetyl CoA, for example, which then could have entered biosynthetic reactions to build an amino acid. The amino acid might have been incorporated into a plant protein. You might have eaten the delicious leaves of the plant in your salad, and digested the protein in your gut to produce amino acids again. After circulating in your bloodstream, the amino acid might have been taken up by a developing red blood cell to make its own protein, such as the hemoglobin in question. If we wish, of course, we can make our food-chain scenario more complicated. The plant, for example, might have been eaten by an animal that in turn was consumed by you during a lunch break. Moreover, because Darwin died more than 100 years ago, the carbon atom could have traveled such a route many times. In each round, however, it would have started again as fully oxidized CO_2 gas and entered the living world through photosynthesis in a plant.

ANSWER 13–10   Yeast cells proliferate much better aerobically. Under anaerobic conditions they cannot perform oxidative phosphorylation and therefore have to produce all their ATP by glycolysis, which is less efficient. Whereas one glucose molecule yields a net gain of two ATP molecules by glycolysis, the additional use of the citric acid cycle and oxidative phosphorylation boosts the energy yield up to about 30 ATP molecules. The citric acid cycle depends on O_2 because it needs NAD^+ to continue running.

ANSWER 13–11   The amount of free energy stored in the phosphate bond in creatine phosphate is larger than that of the anhydride bonds in ATP. Hydrolysis of creatine phosphate can therefore be directly coupled to the production of ATP.

$$\text{creatine phosphate} + \text{ADP} \rightarrow \text{creatine} + \text{ATP}$$

The $\Delta G°$ for this reaction is –12.6 kJ/mole, indicating that it proceeds rapidly to the right, as written.

ANSWER 13–12   The extreme conservation of glycolysis is some of the evidence that all present-day cells are derived from a single founder cell, as discussed in Chapter 1. The elegant reactions of glycolysis would therefore have evolved only once, and then they would have been inherited as organisms evolved. The later invention of oxidative phosphorylation allowed organisms to capture 15 times more energy from fuel molecules than is possible by glycolysis alone. This remarkable efficiency is close to the theoretical limit and hence virtually eliminates the opportunity for further improvements. Thus, the generation of alternative pathways would result in no obvious reproductive advantage that would have been selected in evolution.

ANSWER 13–13   If one glucose molecule produces 30 ATPs, then to generate 10^9 ATP molecules will require $1 \times 10^9/30 = 3.3 \times 10^7$ glucose molecules and $6 \times 3.3 \times 10^7 = 2 \times 10^8$ molecules of oxygen. Thus, in one minute, the cell will consume $2 \times 10^8/(6 \times 10^{23})$ or 3.3×10^{-16} moles of oxygen, which would occupy $3.3 \times 10^{-16} \times 22.4 = 7.4 \times 10^{-15}$ liters in gaseous form. The volume of the cell is 10^{-15} cubic meters [$= (10^{-5})^3$], which is 10^{-12} liter. The cell therefore consumes an amount of O_2 gas equivalent to about 0.7% of the cell volume every minute, or an amount of O_2 gas equivalent to the cell volume in 2 hours and 15 minutes.

ANSWER 13–14   The reactions each have negative ΔG values and are therefore energetically favorable (see Figure A13–14 for energy diagrams).

ANSWER 13–15

A. Pyruvate is converted to acetyl CoA, and the labeled ^{14}C atom is released as $^{14}CO_2$ gas (see Figure 13–10).

B. By following the ^{14}C-labeled atom through every reaction in the citric acid cycle, shown in Panel 13–2 (pp. 442–443), you find that the added ^{14}C label would be quantitatively recovered in oxaloacetate. The analysis also reveals, however, that it is no longer in the keto group but in the methylene group of oxaloacetate (Figure A13–15).

ANSWER 13–16   In the presence of molecular oxygen, oxidative phosphorylation converts most of the cellular NADH to NAD^+ (see Figure 13–19). Since fermentation requires NADH (see Figure 13–6), it is severely inhibited by the availability of oxygen gas.

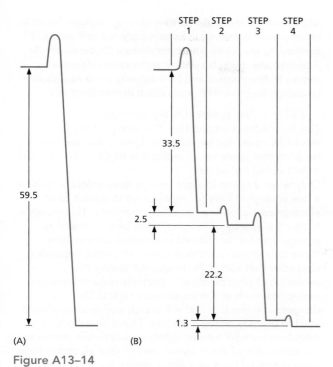

Figure A13–14

COO⁻ COO⁻ structures (not transcribed as text)

radioactive
oxaloacetate
added to
the extract

radioactive
oxaloacetate
isolated after
one turn of
citric acid cycle

Figure A13–15

Chapter 14

ANSWER 14–1 By making membranes permeable to protons, DNP collapses—or, at very small concentrations, diminishes—the proton gradient across the inner mitochondrial membrane. Cells continue to oxidize food molecules to feed high-energy electrons into the electron-transport chain, but H⁺ ions pumped across the membrane flow back across that membrane in a futile cycle. As a result, the energy of the electrons cannot be tapped to drive ATP synthesis, and instead is released as heat. Patients who have been given small doses of DNP lose weight because their fat reserves are used more rapidly to feed the electron-transport chain, and the whole process simply "wastes" energy as heat. A similar mechanism of heat production is used naturally in a specialized tissue composed of brown fat cells, which is abundant in newborn humans and in hibernating animals. These cells are packed with mitochondria that leak part of their H⁺ gradient futilely back across the membrane for the sole purpose of warming up the organism. These cells are brown because they are packed with mitochondria, which contain high concentrations of pigmented proteins such as cytochromes.

ANSWER 14–2 The inner mitochondrial membrane is the site of oxidative phosphorylation, and it produces most of the cell's ATP. Cristae are portions of the mitochondrial inner membrane that are folded inward. Mitochondria that have a higher density of cristae have a larger area of inner membrane and therefore a greater capacity to carry out oxidative phosphorylation. Heart muscle expends a lot of energy during its continuous contractions, whereas skin cells have a smaller energy demand. An increased density of cristae therefore increases the ATP-production capacity of the heart muscle cell. This is a remarkable example of how cells adjust the abundance of their individual components according to need.

ANSWER 14–3
A. The DNP collapses the electrochemical proton gradient completely. H⁺ ions that are pumped to one side of the membrane flow back freely, and therefore no energy to drive ATP synthesis can be stored across the membrane.
B. An electrochemical gradient is made up of two components: a concentration gradient and an electrical potential. If the membrane is made permeable to K⁺ with nigericin, K⁺ will be driven into the matrix by the electrical potential of the inner membrane (negative inside, positive outside). The influx of positively charged K⁺ will abolish the membrane's electrical potential. In contrast, the concentration component of the H⁺ gradient (the pH difference) is unaffected by nigericin. Therefore, only part of the driving force that makes it energetically favorable for H⁺ ions to flow back into the matrix is lost.

ANSWER 14–4
A. Such a turbine running in reverse is an electrically driven water pump, which is analogous to what the ATP synthase becomes when it uses the energy of ATP hydrolysis to pump protons against their electrochemical gradient across the inner mitochondrial membrane.
B. The ATP synthase should stall when the energy that it can draw from the proton gradient is just equal to the ΔG required to make ATP; at this equilibrium point there will be neither net ATP synthesis nor net ATP consumption.
C. As the cell uses up ATP, the ATP/ADP ratio in the matrix falls below the equilibrium point just described, and ATP synthase uses the energy stored in the proton gradient to synthesize ATP in order to restore the original ATP/ADP ratio. Conversely, when the electrochemical proton gradient drops below that at the equilibrium point, ATP synthase uses ATP in the matrix to restore this gradient.

ANSWER 14–5 An electron pair, when passing from NADH to O₂ through the three respiratory complexes, causes 10 H⁺ to be pumped across the membrane. Four H⁺ are needed to make each ATP: three for synthesis from ADP and one for ATP export to the cytosol. Therefore, 2.5 ATP molecules are synthesized from each NADH molecule.

ANSWER 14–6 One can describe four essential roles for the proteins in the process. First, the chemical environment provided by a protein's amino acid side chains sets the redox potential of each Fe ion such that electrons can be passed in a defined order from one component to the next, giving up their energy in small steps and becoming more firmly bound as they proceed. Second, the proteins position the Fe ions so that the electrons can move efficiently between them. Third, the proteins prevent electrons from skipping an intermediate step; thus, as we have learned for other enzymes (discussed in Chapter 4), they channel the electron flow along a defined path. Fourth, the proteins couple the movement of the electrons down their energy ladder to the pumping of protons across the membrane, thereby harnessing the energy that is released and storing it in a proton gradient that is then used for ATP production.

ANSWER 14–7   It would not be productive to use the same carrier in two steps. If ubiquinone, for example, could transfer electrons directly to the cytochrome c oxidase, the cytochrome c reductase complex would often be skipped when electrons are collected from NADH dehydrogenase. Given the large difference in redox potential between ubiquinone and cytochrome c oxidase, a large amount of energy would be released as heat and thus be wasted. Electron transfer directly between NADH dehydrogenase and cytochrome c would similarly allow the cytochrome c reductase complex to be bypassed.

ANSWER 14–8   Protons pumped across the inner mitochondrial membrane into the intermembrane space equilibrate with the cytosol, which functions as a huge H^+ sink. Both the mitochondrial matrix and the cytosol support many metabolic reactions that require a pH around neutrality. The H^+ concentration difference, ΔpH, that can be achieved between the mitochondrial matrix and the cytosol is therefore relatively small (less than one pH unit). Much of the energy stored in the mitochondrial electrochemical proton gradient is instead due to the membrane potential (see Figure 14–15). In contrast, chloroplasts have a smaller, dedicated compartment into which H^+ ions are pumped. Much higher concentration differences can be achieved (up to a thousandfold, or 3 pH units), and much of the energy stored in the thylakoid H^+ gradient is due to the H^+ concentration difference between the thylakoid space and the stroma.

ANSWER 14–9   NADH and NADPH differ by the presence of a single phosphate group. That phosphate gives NADPH a slightly different shape from NADH, which allows these molecules to be recognized by different enzymes, and thus to deliver their electrons to different destinations. Such a division of labor is useful because NADPH tends to be involved in biosynthetic reactions, where high-energy electrons are used to produce energy-rich biological molecules. NADH, on the other hand, is involved in reactions that oxidize energy-rich food molecules to produce ATP. Inside the cell, the ratio of NAD^+ to NADH is kept high, whereas the ratio of $NADP^+$ to NADPH is kept low. This provides plenty of NAD^+ to act as an oxidizing agent and plenty of NADPH to act as a reducing agent—as required for their special roles in catabolism and anabolism, respectively.

ANSWER 14–10
A. Photosynthesis produces sugars, most importantly sucrose, that are transported from the photosynthetic cells through the sap to root cells. There, the sugars are oxidized by glycolysis in the root cell cytoplasm and by oxidative phosphorylation in the root cell mitochondria to produce ATP, as well as being used as the building blocks for many other metabolites.

B. Mitochondria are required even during daylight hours in chloroplast-containing cells to supply the cell with ATP derived by oxidative phosphorylation. Glyceraldehyde 3-phosphate made by photosynthesis in chloroplasts moves to the cytosol and is eventually used as a source of energy to drive ATP production in mitochondria.

ANSWER 14–11   All statements are correct.
A. This is a necessary condition. If it were not true, electrons could not be removed from water and the reaction that splits water molecules ($H_2O \rightarrow 2H^+ + \frac{1}{2}O_2 + 2e^-$) would not occur.
B. Only when excited by light energy does chlorophyll have a low enough affinity for an electron to pass it to an electron carrier with a low electron affinity. This transfer allows the energy of the photon to be harnessed as energy that can be utilized in chemical conversions.
C. It can be argued that this is one of the most important obstacles that had to be overcome during the evolution of photosynthesis: partially reduced oxygen molecules, such as the superoxide radical O_2^-, are dangerously reactive and will attack and destroy almost any biologically active molecule. These intermediates therefore have to remain tightly bound to the metals in the active site of the enzyme until all four electrons have been removed from two water molecules. This requires the sequential capture of four photons by the same reaction center.

ANSWER 14–12
A. True. NAD^+ and quinones are examples of compounds that do not have metal ions but can participate in electron transfer.
B. False. The potential is due to protons (H^+) that are pumped across the membrane from the matrix to the intermembrane space. Electrons remain bound to electron carriers in the inner mitochondrial membrane.
C. True. Both components add to the driving force that makes it energetically favorable for H^+ to flow back into the matrix.
D. True. Both move rapidly in the plane of the membrane.
E. False. Not only do plants need mitochondria to make ATP in cells that do not have chloroplasts, such as root cells, but mitochondria make most of the cytosolic ATP in all plant cells.
F. True. Chlorophyll's physiological function requires it to absorb light; heme just happens to be a colored compound from which blood derives its red color.
G. False. Chlorophyll absorbs light and transfers energy in the form of an energized electron, whereas the iron in heme is a simple electron carrier.
H. False. Most of the dry weight of a tree comes from carbon derived from the CO_2 that has been fixed during photosynthesis.

ANSWER 14–13   It takes three protons. The precise value of the ΔG for ATP synthesis depends on the concentrations of ATP, ADP, and P_i (as described in Chapter 3). The higher the ratio of the concentration of ATP to ADP, the more energy it takes to make additional ATP. The lower value of 46 kJ/mole therefore applies to conditions where cells have expended a lot of energy and have therefore decreased the normal ATP/ADP ratio.

ANSWER 14–14   If no O_2 is available, all components of the mitochondrial electron-transport chain will accumulate in their *reduced* form. This is the case because electrons derived from NADH enter the chain but cannot be transferred to O_2. The electron-transport chain therefore stalls with all of its components in the reduced form. If O_2 is suddenly added again, the electron carriers in cytochrome *c* oxidase will become *oxidized before* those in NADH dehydrogenase. This is true because, after O_2 addition, cytochrome *c* oxidase will donate its electrons directly to O_2, thereby becoming oxidized. A wave of increasing oxidation then passes backward with time from cytochrome *c* oxidase through the components of the electron-transport chain, as each component regains the opportunity to pass on its electrons to downstream components.

ANSWER 14–15   As oxidized ubiquinone becomes reduced, it picks up two electrons but also two protons from water (Figure 14–21). Upon oxidation, these protons are released. If reduction occurs on one side of the membrane and oxidation at the other side, a proton is pumped across the membrane for each electron transported. Electron transport by ubiquinone thereby contributes directly to the generation of the H^+ gradient.

ANSWER 14–16   Photosynthetic bacteria and plant cells use the electrons derived in the reaction $2H_2O \rightarrow 4e^- + 4H^+ + O_2$ to reduce $NADP^+$ to NADPH, which is then used to produce useful metabolites. If the electrons were used instead to produce H_2 in addition to O_2, the cells would lose any benefit they derive from carrying out the reaction, because the electrons could not take part in metabolically useful reactions.

ANSWER 14–17

A. The switch in solutions creates a pH gradient across the thylakoid membrane. The flow of H^+ ions down the electrochemical proton gradient drives ATP synthase, which converts ADP to ATP.
B. No light is needed, because the H^+ gradient is established artificially without a need for the light-driven electron-transport chain.
C. Nothing. The H^+ gradient would be in the wrong direction; ATP synthase would not work.
D. The experiment provided early supporting evidence for the chemiosmotic model by showing that an H^+ gradient alone is sufficient to drive ATP synthesis (see How We Know, pp. 476–477).

ANSWER 14–18

A. When the vesicles are exposed to light, H^+ ions (derived from H_2O) pumped into the vesicles by the bacteriorhodopsin flow back out through the ATP synthase, causing ATP to be made in the solution surrounding the vesicles.
B. If the vesicles are leaky, no H^+ gradient can form and thus ATP synthase cannot work.
C. Using components from widely divergent organisms can be a very powerful experimental tool. Because the two proteins come from such different sources, it is very unlikely that they form a direct functional interaction. The experiment therefore strongly suggests that electron transport and ATP synthesis are separate events. This approach is therefore a valid one.

ANSWER 14–19   The redox potential of $FADH_2$ is too low to transfer electrons to the NADH dehydrogenase complex, but high enough to transfer electrons to ubiquinone (Figure

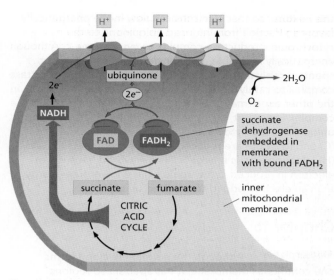

Figure A14–19

14–22). Therefore, electrons from $FADH_2$ can enter the electron-transport chain only at this step (Figure A14–19). Because the NADH dehydrogenase complex is bypassed, fewer H^+ ions are pumped across the membrane and less ATP is made. This example shows the versatility of the electron-transport chain. The ability to use vastly different sources of electrons from the environment to feed electron transport is thought to have been an essential feature in the early evolution of life.

ANSWER 14–20   If these bacteria used a proton gradient to make their ATP in a fashion analogous to that in other bacteria (that is, fewer protons inside than outside), they would need to raise their cytoplasmic pH even higher than that of their environment (pH 10). Cells with a cytoplasmic pH greater than 10 would not be viable. These bacteria must therefore use gradients of ions other than H^+, such as Na^+ gradients, in the chemiosmotic coupling between electron transport and an ATP synthase.

ANSWER 14–21   Statements A and B are accurate. Statement C is incorrect, because the chemical reactions that are carried out in each cycle are completely different, even though the net effect is the same as that expected for simple reversal.

ANSWER 14–22   This experiment would suggest a two-step model for ATP synthase function. According to this model, the flow of protons through the base of the synthase drives rotation of the head, which in turn causes ATP synthesis. In their experiment, the authors have succeeded in uncoupling these two steps. If rotating the head mechanically is sufficient to produce ATP in the absence of any applied proton gradient, the ATP synthase is a protein machine that indeed functions like a "molecular turbine." This would be a very exciting experiment indeed, because it would directly demonstrate the relationship between mechanical movement and enzymatic activity. There is no doubt that it should be published and that it would become a "classic."

ANSWER 14–23   Only under condition (E) is electron transfer observed, with cytochrome *c* becoming reduced. A portion of the electron-transport chain has been reconstituted in this mixture, so that electrons can flow in the energetically favored direction from reduced ubiquinone to the cytochrome *c* reductase complex to cytochrome *c*. Although energetically favorable, the transfer in (A) cannot occur spontaneously in the absence of the cytochrome *c* reductase complex to catalyze this reaction. No electron flow occurs in the other experiments, whether the cytochrome *c* reductase complex is present or not: in experiments (B) and (F), both ubiquinone and cytochrome *c* are oxidized; in experiments (C) and (G), both are reduced; and in experiments (D) and (H), electron flow is energetically disfavored because an electron in reduced cytochrome *c* has a lower free energy than an electron added to oxidized ubiquinone.

Chapter 15

ANSWER 15–1   Although the nuclear envelope forms one continuous membrane, it has specialized regions that contain special proteins and have a characteristic appearance. One such specialized region is the inner nuclear membrane. Membrane proteins can indeed diffuse between the inner and outer nuclear membranes, at the connections formed around the nuclear pores. Those proteins with particular functions in the inner membrane, however, are usually anchored there by their interaction with other components such as chromosomes and the nuclear lamina (a protein meshwork underlying the inner nuclear membrane that helps give structural integrity to the nuclear envelope).

ANSWER 15–2   Eukaryotic gene expression is more complicated than prokaryotic gene expression. In particular, prokaryotic cells do not have introns that interrupt the coding sequences of their genes, so that an mRNA can be translated immediately after it is transcribed, without a need for further processing (discussed in Chapter 7). In fact, in prokaryotic cells, ribosomes start translating most mRNAs before transcription is finished. This would have disastrous consequences in eukaryotic cells, because most RNA transcripts have to be spliced before they can be translated. The nuclear envelope separates the transcription and translation processes in space and time: a primary RNA transcript is held in the nucleus until it is properly processed to form an mRNA, and only then is it allowed to leave the nucleus so that ribosomes can translate it.

ANSWER 15–3   An mRNA molecule is attached to the ER membrane by the ribosomes translating it. This ribosome population, however, is not static; the mRNA is continuously moved through the ribosome. Those ribosomes that have finished translation dissociate from the 3′ end of the mRNA and from the ER membrane, but the mRNA itself remains bound by other ribosomes, newly recruited from the cytosolic pool, that have attached to the 5′ end of the mRNA and are still translating the mRNA. Depending on its length, there are about 10–20 ribosomes attached to each membrane-bound mRNA molecule.

ANSWER 15–4
A. The internal signal sequence functions as a membrane anchor, as shown in Figure 15–17. Because there is no stop-transfer sequence, however, the C-terminal end of the protein continues to be translocated into the ER lumen. The resulting protein therefore has its N-terminal domain in the cytosol, followed by a single

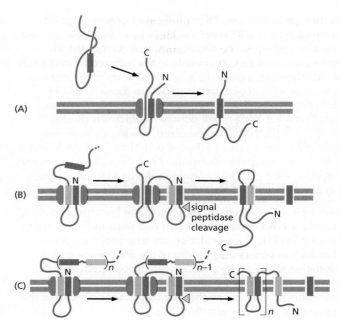

Figure A15–4

transmembrane segment, and a C-terminal domain in the ER lumen (Figure A15–4A).
B. The N-terminal signal sequence initiates translocation of the N-terminal domain of the protein until translocation is stopped by the stop-transfer sequence. A cytosolic domain is synthesized until the start-transfer sequence initiates translocation again. The situation now resembles that described in (A), and the C-terminal domain of the protein is translocated into the lumen of the ER. The resulting protein therefore spans the membrane twice. Both its N-terminal and C-terminal domains are in the ER lumen, and a loop domain between the two transmembrane regions is exposed in the cytosol (Figure A15–4B).
C. It would need a cleaved signal sequence, followed by an internal stop-transfer sequence, followed by pairs of start- and stop-transfer sequences (Figure A15–4C).
These examples demonstrate that complex protein topologies can be achieved by simple variations and combinations of the two basic mechanisms shown in Figures 15–16 and 15–17.

ANSWER 15–5
A. Clathrin coats cannot assemble in the absence of adaptins that link the clathrin to the membrane. At high clathrin concentrations and under the appropriate ionic conditions, clathrin cages assemble in solution, but they are empty shells, lacking other proteins, and they contain no membrane. This shows that the information to form clathrin baskets is contained in the clathrin molecules themselves, which are therefore able to self-assemble.
B. Without clathrin, adaptins still bind to receptors in the membrane, but no clathrin coat can form and thus no clathrin-coated pits or vesicles are produced.
C. Deeply invaginated clathrin-coated pits form on the membrane, but they do not pinch off to form closed vesicles (see Figure A15–21B).

D. Prokaryotic cells do not perform endocytosis. A prokaryotic cell therefore does not contain any receptors with appropriate cytosolic tails that could mediate adaptin binding. Therefore, no clathrin can bind and no clathrin coats can assemble.

ANSWER 15–6   The preassembled sugar chain allows better quality control. The assembled oligosaccharide chains can be checked for accuracy before they are added to the protein; if a mistake were made in adding sugars individually to the protein, the whole protein would have to be discarded. Because far more energy is used in building a protein than in building a short oligosaccharide chain, this is a much more economical strategy. The difficulty of modifying oligosaccharides precisely becomes apparent as the protein moves to the cell surface: although sugar chains are continually modified by enzymes in various compartments of the secretory pathway, these modifications are often incomplete and result in considerable heterogeneity of the glycoproteins that leave the cell. This heterogeneity is largely due to the restricted access that the enzymes have to the sugar trees attached to the surface of proteins. The heterogeneity also explains why glycoproteins are more difficult to study and purify than nonglycosylated proteins.

ANSWER 15–7   Aggregates of the secretory proteins would form in the ER, just as they do in the *trans* Golgi network. As the aggregation is specific for secretory proteins, ER proteins would be excluded from the aggregates. The aggregates would eventually be degraded.

ANSWER 15–8   Transferrin without Fe bound does not interact with its receptor and circulates in the bloodstream until it catches an Fe ion. Once iron is bound, the iron–transferrin complex can bind to the transferrin receptor on the surface of a cell and be endocytosed. Under the acidic conditions of the endosome, the transferrin releases its iron, but the transferrin remains bound to the transferrin receptor, which is recycled back to the cell surface, where it encounters the neutral pH environment of the blood. The neutral pH causes the receptor to release the transferrin into the circulation, where it can pick up another Fe ion to repeat the cycle. The iron released in the endosome, like the LDL in Figure 15–33, moves on to lysosomes, from where it is transported into the cytosol.

   The system allows cells to take up iron efficiently even though the concentration of iron in the blood is extremely low. The iron bound to transferrin is concentrated at the cell surface by binding to transferrin receptors; it becomes further concentrated in clathrin-coated pits, which collect the transferrin receptors. In this way, transferrin cycles between the blood and endosomes, delivering the iron that cells need to grow.

ANSWER 15–9

A. True.
B. False. The signal sequences that direct proteins to the ER contain a core of eight or more hydrophobic amino acids. The sequence shown here contains many hydrophilic amino acid side chains, including the charged amino acids His, Arg, Asp, and Lys, and the uncharged hydrophilic amino acids Gln and Ser.
C. True. Otherwise they could not dock at the correct target membrane or recruit a fusion complex to a docking site.
D. True.
E. True. Lysosomal proteins are selected in the *trans* Golgi network and packaged into transport vesicles that deliver them to the late endosome. If not selected, they would enter by default into transport vesicles that move constitutively to the cell surface.
F. False. Lysosomes also digest internal organelles by autophagy.
G. False. Mitochondria do not participate in vesicular transport, and therefore *N*-linked glycoproteins, which are exclusively assembled in the ER, cannot be transported to mitochondria.
H. False. The outer nuclear membrane is continuous with the ER and all proteins made by ribosomes bound there end up in the ER lumen.

ANSWER 15–10   They must contain a nuclear localization signal as well. Proteins with nuclear export signals shuttle between the nucleus and the cytosol. An example is the A1 protein, which binds to mRNAs in the nucleus and guides them through the nuclear pores. Once in the cytosol, a nuclear localization signal ensures that the A1 protein is re-imported so that it can participate in the export of further mRNAs.

ANSWER 15–11   Influenza virus enters cells by endocytosis and is delivered to endosomes, where it encounters an acidic pH that activates its fusion protein. The viral membrane then fuses with the membrane of the endosome, releasing the viral genome into the cytosol (Figure A15–11). NH_3 is a small molecule that readily penetrates membranes. Thus, it can enter all intracellular compartments, including endosomes, by diffusion. Once in a compartment that has an acidic pH, NH_3 binds H^+ to form NH_4^+, which is a charged ion and therefore cannot cross the membrane by diffusion. NH_4^+ ions therefore accumulate in acidic compartments, raising their pH. When the pH of the endosome is raised, viruses are still endocytosed, but because the viral fusion protein cannot be activated, the virus cannot enter the cytosol. Remember this the next time you have the flu and have access to a stable.

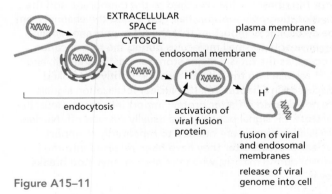

Figure A15–11

ANSWER 15–12

A. The problem is that vesicles having two different kinds of v-SNAREs in their membrane could dock on either of two different membranes.
B. The answer to this puzzle is currently not known, but we can predict that cells must have ways of turning the docking ability of SNAREs on and off. This may be achieved through other proteins that are, for example,

co-packaged in the ER with SNAREs into transport vesicles and facilitate the interactions of the correct v-SNARE with the t-SNARE in the *cis* Golgi network.

ANSWER 15–13   Synaptic transmission involves the release of neurotransmitters by exocytosis. During this event, the membrane of the synaptic vesicle fuses with the plasma membrane of the nerve terminals. To make new synaptic vesicles, membrane must be retrieved from the plasma membrane by endocytosis. This endocytosis step is blocked if dynamin is defective, as the protein is required to pinch off the clathrin-coated endocytic vesicles.

ANSWER 15–14   The first two sentences are correct. The third is not. It should read: "Because the contents of the lumen of the ER, or any other compartment in the secretory or endocytic pathways, never mix with the cytosol, proteins that enter these pathways will never need to be imported again."

ANSWER 15–15   The protein is translocated into the ER. Its ER signal sequence is recognized as soon as it emerges from the ribosome. The ribosome then becomes bound to the ER membrane, and the growing polypeptide chain is transferred through the ER translocation channel. The nuclear localization sequence is therefore never exposed to the cytosol. It will never encounter nuclear import receptors, and the protein will not enter the nucleus.

ANSWER 15–16   (1) Proteins are imported into the nucleus after they have been synthesized, folded, and, if appropriate, assembled into complexes. In contrast, unfolded polypeptide chains are translocated into the ER as they are being made by the ribosomes. Ribosomes are assembled in the nucleus yet function in the cytosol, and the enzyme complexes that catalyze RNA transcription and splicing are assembled in the cytosol yet function in the nucleus. Thus, both ribosomes and these enzyme complexes need to be transported through the nuclear pores intact. (2) Nuclear pores are gates, which are always open to small molecules; in contrast, translocation channels in the ER membrane are normally closed, and open only after the ribosome has attached to the membrane and the translocating polypeptide chain has sealed the channel from the cytosol. It is important that the ER membrane remain impermeable to small molecules during the translocation process, as the ER is a major store for Ca^{2+} in the cell, and Ca^{2+} release into the cytosol must be tightly controlled (discussed in Chapter 16). (3) Nuclear localization signals are not cleaved off after protein import into the nucleus; in contrast, ER signal peptides are usually cleaved off. Nuclear localization signals are needed to repeatedly re-import nuclear proteins after they have been released into the cytosol during mitosis, when the nuclear envelope breaks down.

ANSWER 15–17   The transient intermixing of nuclear and cytosolic contents during mitosis supports the idea that the nuclear interior and the cytosol are indeed evolutionarily related. In fact, one can consider the nucleus as a subcompartment of the cytosol that has become surrounded by the nuclear envelope, with access only through the nuclear pores.

ANSWER 15–18   The actual explanation is that the single amino acid change causes the protein to misfold slightly

so that, although it is still active as a protease inhibitor, it is prevented by chaperone proteins in the ER from exiting this organelle. It therefore accumulates in the ER lumen and is eventually degraded. Alternative interpretations might have been that (1) the mutation affects the stability of the protein in the bloodstream so that it is degraded much faster in the blood than the normal protein, or (2) the mutation inactivates the ER signal sequence and prevents the protein from entering the ER. (3) Another explanation could have been that the mutation altered the sequence to create an ER retention signal, which would have retained the mutant protein in the ER. One could distinguish between these possibilities by using fluorescently tagged antibodies against the protein or by expressing the protein as a fusion with GFP to follow its transport in the cells (see How We Know, pp. 520–521).

ANSWER 15–19   Critique: "Dr. Outonalimb proposes to study the biosynthesis of forgettin, a protein of significant interest. The main hypothesis on which this proposal is based, however, requires further support. In particular, it is questionable whether forgettin is indeed a secreted protein, as proposed. ER signal sequences are normally found at the N-terminus. C-terminal hydrophobic sequences will be exposed outside the ribosome only after protein synthesis has already terminated and can therefore not be recognized by an SRP during translation. It is therefore unlikely that forgettin will be translocated by an SRP-dependent mechanism; it is more likely that it will remain in the cytosol. Dr. Outonalimb should take these considerations into account when submitting a revised application."

ANSWER 15–20   The Golgi apparatus may have evolved from specialized patches of ER membrane. These regions of the ER might have pinched off, forming a new compartment (Figure A15–20), which still communicates with the ER by vesicular transport. For the newly evolved Golgi compartment to be useful, transport vesicles would also have to have evolved.

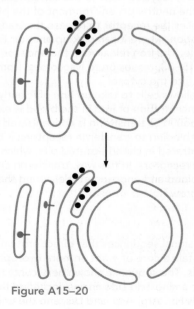

Figure A15–20

ANSWER 15–21   This is a chicken-and-egg question. In fact, the situation never arises in present-day cells, although it must have posed a considerable problem for the first cells that evolved. New cell membranes are made by expansion of existing membranes, and the ER is never made de novo. There will always be an existing piece of ER with translocation channels to integrate new translocation channels. Inheritance is therefore not limited to the propagation of the genome; a cell's organelles must also be passed from generation to generation. In fact, the ER translocation channels can be traced back to structurally related translocation channels in the prokaryotic plasma membrane.

ANSWER 15–22

A. Extracellular space
B. Cytosol
C. Plasma membrane
D. Clathrin coat
E. Membrane of deeply invaginated, clathrin-coated pit
F. Captured cargo particles
G. Lumen of deeply invaginated, clathrin-coated pit

ANSWER 15–23 A single, incomplete round of nuclear import would occur. Because nuclear transport is fueled by GTP hydrolysis, under conditions of insufficient energy, GTP would be used up and no Ran-GTP would be available to unload the cargo protein from its nuclear import receptor upon arrival in the nucleus (see Figure 15–10). Unable to release its cargo, the nuclear import receptor would be stuck at the nuclear pore and not return to the cytosol. Because the nuclear cargo protein is not released, it would not be functional, and no further import could occur.

Chapter 16

ANSWER 16–1 Most paracrine signaling molecules are very short-lived after they are released from a signaling cell: they are either degraded by extracellular enzymes or are rapidly taken up by neighboring target cells. In addition, some become attached to the extracellular matrix and are thus prevented from diffusing too far.

ANSWER 16–2 The protein could be an enzyme that produces a large number of small intracellular signaling molecules such as cyclic AMP or cyclic GMP. Or, it could be an enzyme that modifies a large number of intracellular target proteins—for example, by phosphorylation.

ANSWER 16–3 The mutant G protein would be almost continuously activated, because GDP would dissociate spontaneously, allowing GTP to bind even in the absence of an activated GPCR. The consequences for the cell would therefore be similar to those caused by cholera toxin, which modifies the α subunit of G_s so that it cannot hydrolyze GTP to shut itself off. In contrast to the cholera toxin case, however, the mutant G protein would not stay permanently activated: it would switch itself off normally, but then it would instantly become activated again as the GDP dissociated and GTP re-bound.

ANSWER 16–4 Rapid breakdown keeps the intracellular cyclic AMP concentrations low. The lower the cAMP levels are, the larger and faster the increase achieved upon activation of adenylyl cyclase, which makes new cyclic AMP. If you have $100 in the bank and you deposit another $100, you have doubled your wealth; if you have only $10 to start with and you deposit $100, you have increased your wealth tenfold, a much larger proportional increase resulting from the same deposit.

ANSWER 16–5 Recall that the plasma membrane constitutes a rather small area compared with the total membrane surfaces in a cell (discussed in Chapter 15). The endoplasmic reticulum is especially abundant and spans the entire volume of the cell as a vast network of membrane tubes and sheets. The Ca^{2+} stored in the endoplasmic reticulum can therefore be released throughout the cytosol. This is important because the rapid clearing of Ca^{2+} ions from the cytosol by Ca^{2+} pumps prevents Ca^{2+} from diffusing any significant distance in the cytosol.

ANSWER 16–6 Each reaction involved in the amplification scheme must be turned off to reset the signaling pathway to a resting level. Each of these off switches is equally important.

ANSWER 16–7 Because each antibody has two antigen-binding sites, it can cross-link the receptors and cause them to cluster on the cell surface. This clustering is likely to activate RTKs, which are usually activated by dimerization. For RTKs, clustering allows the individual kinase domains of the receptors to phosphorylate adjacent receptors in the cluster. The activation of GPCRs is more complicated, because the ligand has to induce a particular conformational change; only very special antibodies mimic receptor ligands sufficiently well to induce the conformational change that activates a GPCR.

ANSWER 16–8

A. True. Acetylcholine, for example, slows the beating of heart muscle cells by binding to a GPCR, and stimulates the contraction of skeletal muscle cells by binding to a different acetylcholine receptor, which is an ion-channel-coupled receptor.
B. False. Acetylcholine is short-lived and exerts its effects locally. Indeed, the consequences of prolonging its lifetime can be disastrous. Compounds that inhibit the enzyme acetylcholinesterase, which normally breaks down acetylcholine at a nerve–muscle synapse, are extremely toxic: for example, the nerve gas sarin, used in chemical warfare, is an acetylcholinesterase inhibitor.
C. True. Nucleotide-free $\beta\gamma$ complexes can activate ion channels, and GTP-bound α subunits can activate enzymes. The GDP-bound form of trimeric G proteins is the inactive state.
D. True. The inositol phospholipid that is cleaved to produce IP_3 contains three phosphate groups, one of which links the sugar to the diacylglycerol lipid. IP_3 is generated by a simple hydrolysis reaction (see Figure 16–23).
E. False. Calmodulin senses but does not regulate intracellular Ca^{2+} levels.
F. True. See Figure 16–35.
G. True. See Figure 16–29.

ANSWER 16–9

1. You would expect a high background level of Ras activity, because Ras cannot be turned off efficiently.
2. Because many Ras molecules are already GTP-bound, Ras activity in response to an extracellular signal would be greater than normal, but this activity would be liable to saturate when all Ras molecules are converted to the GTP-bound form.

3. The response to a signal would be much less rapid, because the signal-dependent increase in GTP-bound Ras would occur over an elevated background of preexisting GTP-bound Ras.

4. The increase in Ras activity in response to a signal would also be prolonged compared to the response in normal cells.

ANSWER 16–10

A. Both types of signaling can occur over a long range: neurons can send action potentials along very long axons (think of the axons in the neck of a giraffe, for example), and hormones are carried via the bloodstream throughout the organism. Because neurons secrete large amounts of neurotransmitters at a synapse, a small, well-defined space between two cells, the concentrations of these signal molecules are high; neurotransmitter receptors, therefore, need to bind to neurotransmitters with only low affinity. Hormones, in contrast, are vastly diluted in the bloodstream, where they circulate at often minuscule concentrations; hormone receptors therefore generally bind their hormone with extremely high affinity.

B. Whereas neuronal signaling is a private affair, with one neuron talking to a select group of target cells through specific synaptic connections, endocrine signaling is a public announcement, with any target cell with appropriate receptors able to respond to the hormone in the blood. Neuronal signaling is very fast, limited only by the speed of propagation of the action potential and the workings of the synapse, whereas endocrine signaling is slower, limited by blood flow and diffusion over larger distances.

ANSWER 16–11

A. There are 100,000 molecules of X and 10,000 molecules of Y in the cell (= rate of synthesis × average lifetime).

B. After one second, the concentration of X will have increased by 10,000 molecules per cell. The concentration of X, therefore, one second after its synthesis is increased, is about 110,000 molecules per cell—which is a 10% increase over the concentration of X before the boost of its synthesis. The concentration of Y will also increase by 10,000 molecules per cell, which, in contrast to X, represents a full twofold increase in its concentration (for simplicity, we can neglect the breakdown in this estimation because X and Y are relatively stable during the one-second stimulation).

C. Because of its larger proportional increase, Y is the preferred signaling molecule. This calculation illustrates the surprising but important principle that the time it takes to switch a signal on is determined by the lifetime of the signaling molecule.

ANSWER 16–12

A. The mutant RTK lacking its extracellular ligand-binding domain is inactive. It cannot bind extracellular signals, and its presence has no consequences for the function of the normal RTK (Figure A16–12A). If the mutant receptors are present at extremely high levels, however, they might dimerize in the absence of the extracellular signal molecule, causing activation of signaling.

B. The mutant RTK lacking its intracellular domain is also inactive, but its presence will block signaling by the normal receptors. When a signal molecule binds to

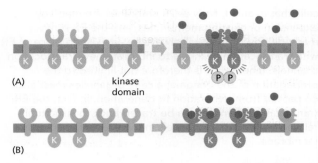

Figure A16–12

either receptor, it will induce their dimerization. Two normal receptors have to come together to activate each other by phosphorylation. In the presence of an excess of mutant receptors, however, normal receptors will usually form mixed dimers, in which their intracellular domain cannot be activated because their partner is a mutant and lacks a kinase domain (Figure A16–12B).

ANSWER 16–13   The statement is largely correct. Upon ligand binding, transmembrane helices of multispanning receptors, like the GPCRs, shift and rearrange with respect to one another (Figure A16–13A). This conformational change is sensed on the cytosolic side of the membrane because of a change in the arrangement of the cytoplasmic loops. A single transmembrane segment is not sufficient to transmit a signal across the membrane directly; no rearrangements in the membrane are possible upon ligand binding. Thus, upon ligand binding, single-span receptors such as most RTKs tend to dimerize, thereby bringing their intracellular kinase domains into proximity so that they can cross-phosphorylate and activate each other (Figure A16–13B).

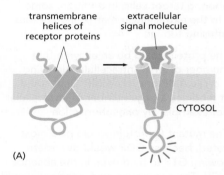

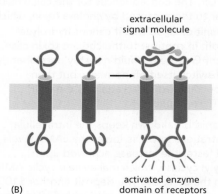

Figure A16–13

ANSWER 16–14   Activation in both cases depends on proteins that catalyze GDP–GTP exchange on the G protein or Ras protein. Whereas activated GPCRs perform this function directly for G proteins, enzyme-linked receptors assemble multiple signaling proteins into a signaling complex when the receptors are activated by phosphorylation; one of these proteins is an adaptor protein that recruits a guanine nucleotide exchange factor that fulfills this function for Ras.

ANSWER 16–15   Because the cytosolic concentration of Ca^{2+} is so low, an influx of relatively few Ca^{2+} ions leads to large changes in its cytosolic concentration. Thus, a tenfold increase in cytosolic Ca^{2+} can be achieved by raising its concentration into the micromolar range, which would require far fewer ions than would be required to change significantly the cytosolic concentration of a more abundant ion such as Na^+. In muscle, a greater than tenfold change in cytosolic Ca^{2+} concentration can be achieved in microseconds by releasing Ca^{2+} from the sarcoplasmic reticulum, a task that would be difficult to accomplish if changes in the millimolar range were required.

ANSWER 16–16   In a multicellular organism such as an animal, it is important that cells survive only when and where they are needed. Having cells depend on signals from other cells may be a simple way of ensuring this. A misplaced cell, for example, would probably fail to get the survival signals it needs (as its neighbors would be inappropriate) and would therefore kill itself. This strategy can also help regulate cell numbers: if cell type A depends on a survival signal from cell type B, the number of B cells could control the number of A cells by making a limited amount of the survival signal, so that only a certain number of A cells could survive. There is indeed evidence that such a mechanism does operate to help regulate cell numbers—in both developing and adult tissues (see Figure 18–41).

ANSWER 16–17 Ca^{2+}-activated Ca^{2+} channels create a positive feedback loop: the more Ca^{2+} that is released, the more Ca^{2+} channels that open. The Ca^{2+} signal in the cytosol is therefore propagated explosively throughout the cardiac muscle cell, thereby ensuring that all myosin–actin filaments contract almost synchronously.

ANSWER 16–18   K2 activates K1. If K1 is permanently activated, a response is observed regardless of the status of K2. If the order were reversed, K1 would need to activate K2, which cannot occur because in our example K2 contains an inactivating mutation.

ANSWER 16–19

A. Three examples of extended signaling pathways to the nucleus are: (1) extracellular signal → RTK → adaptor protein → Ras-activating protein → MAP kinase kinase kinase → MAP kinase kinase → MAP kinase → transcription regulator; (2) extracellular signal → GPCR → G protein → phospholipase C → IP_3 → Ca^{2+} → calmodulin → CaM-kinase → transcription regulator; (3) extracellular signal → GPCR → G protein → adenylyl cyclase → cyclic AMP → PKA → transcription regulator.

B. An example of a direct signaling pathway to the nucleus is Delta → Notch → cleaved Notch tail → transcription.

ANSWER 16–20   When PI 3-kinase is activated by an activated RTK, it phosphorylates a specific inositol phospholipid in the plasma membrane. The resulting phosphorylated inositol phospholipid then recruits to the plasma membrane both Akt and another protein kinase that helps phosphorylate and activate Akt. A third kinase that is permanently associated with the membrane also helps activate Akt (see Figure 16–32).

ANSWER 16–21   Polar groups are hydrophilic, so cholesterol, with only one polar –OH group, would be too hydrophobic to be an effective hormone by itself. Because it is virtually insoluble in water, it could not move readily as a messenger from one cell to another via the extracellular fluid, unless carried by specific proteins.

ANSWER 16–22   In the case of the steroid-hormone receptor, a one-to-one complex of steroid and receptor binds to DNA to activate or inactivate gene transcription; there is thus no amplification between ligand binding and transcriptional regulation. Amplification occurs later, because transcription of a gene gives rise to many mRNAs, each of which is translated to give many copies of the protein it encodes (discussed in Chapter 7). For the ion-channel-coupled receptor, a single ion channel will let through thousands of ions in the time it remains open; this serves as the amplification step in this type of signaling system.

ANSWER 16–23   The more steps there are in an intracellular signaling pathway, the more places the cell has to regulate the pathway, amplify the signal, integrate signals from different pathways, and spread the signal along divergent paths (see Figure 16–9).

ANSWER 16–24   Animals and plants are thought to have evolved multicellularity independently, and therefore will be expected to have evolved some distinct signaling mechanisms for their cells to communicate with one another. On the other hand, animal and plant cells are thought to have evolved from a common eukaryotic ancestor cell, and so plants and animals would be expected to share some intracellular signaling mechanisms that the common ancestor cell used to respond to its environment.

Chapter 17

ANSWER 17–1   Cells that migrate rapidly from one place to another, such as amoebae (A) and sperm cells (F), do not in general need intermediate filaments in their cytoplasm, since they do not develop or sustain large tensile forces. Plant cells (G) are pushed and pulled by the forces of wind and water, but they resist these forces by means of their rigid cell walls rather than by their cytoskeleton. Epithelial cells (B), smooth muscle cells (C), and the long axons of nerve cells (E) are all rich in cytoplasmic intermediate filaments, which prevent them from rupturing as they are stretched and compressed by the movements of their surrounding tissues. All of the above eukaryotic cells possess intermediate filaments in their nuclear lamina. Bacteria, such as *Escherichia coli* (D), have none whatsoever.

ANSWER 17–2   Two tubulin dimers have a lower affinity for each other (because of a more limited number of interaction sites) than a tubulin dimer has for the end of a microtubule (where there are multiple possible interaction sites, both end-to-end for tubulin dimers adding to a protofilament, and side-to-side for the tubulin dimers interacting with tubulin subunits in adjacent protofilaments forming the ringlike cross section). Thus, to initiate a microtubule from scratch, enough tubulin dimers have to come together, and remain bound to one another for long enough, for other tubulin molecules to add to them. Only when a number of tubulin dimers have already assembled will the binding of the next subunit be favored. The formation of these initial "nucleating sites" is therefore rare and does not occur spontaneously at cellular concentrations of tubulin. Centrosomes contain preassembled rings of γ-tubulin (in which the γ-tubulin subunits are held together in much tighter side-to-side interactions than αβ-tubulin can form) to which αβ-tubulin dimers can bind. The binding conditions of αβ-tubulin dimers resemble those of adding to the end of an assembled microtubule. The γ-tubulin rings in the centrosome can therefore be thought of as permanently preassembled nucleation sites.

ANSWER 17–3

A. The microtubule is shrinking because it has lost its GTP cap; that is the tubulin subunits at its end are all in their GDP-bound form. GTP-loaded tubulin subunits from solution will still add to this end, but they will be short-lived—either because they hydrolyze their GTP or because they fall off as the microtubule rim around them disassembles. If, however, sufficient GTP-loaded subunits are added quickly enough to cover up the GDP-containing tubulin subunits at the microtubule end, a new GTP cap can form and regrowth is favored.

B. The rate of addition of GTP-tubulin will be greater at higher tubulin concentrations. The frequency with which shrinking microtubules switch to the growing mode will therefore increase with increasing tubulin concentration. The consequence of this regulation is that the system is self-balancing: the more microtubules shrink (resulting in a higher concentration of free tubulin), the more frequently microtubules will start to grow again. Conversely, the more microtubules grow, the lower the concentration of free tubulin will become and the rate of GTP-tubulin addition will slow down; at some point, GTP hydrolysis will catch up with new GTP-tubulin addition, the GTP cap will be destroyed, and the microtubule will switch to the shrinking mode.

C. If only GDP were present, microtubules would continue to shrink and eventually disappear, because tubulin dimers with GDP have very low affinity for each other and will not add stably to microtubules.

D. If GTP is present but cannot be hydrolyzed, microtubules will continue to grow until all free tubulin subunits have been used up.

ANSWER 17–4   If all the dynein arms were equally active, there could be no significant relative motion of one microtubule to the other as required for bending. (Think of a circle of nine weightlifters, each trying to lift his neighbor off the ground: if they all succeeded, the group would levitate!). Thus, a few ciliary dynein molecules must be activated selectively on one side of the cilium. As they move their neighboring microtubules toward the tip of the cilium, the cilium bends away from the side containing the activated dyneins.

ANSWER 17–5   Any actin-binding protein that stabilizes complexes of two or more actin monomers without blocking the ends required for filament growth will facilitate the initiation of a new filament (nucleation).

ANSWER 17–6   Only fluorescent actin molecules assembled into filaments are visible, because unpolymerized actin molecules diffuse so rapidly that they produce a dim, uniform background. Since, in your experiment, so few actin molecules are labeled (1:10,000), there should be at most one labeled actin monomer per filament (see Figure 17–30). The lamellipodium as a whole has many actin filaments, some of which overlap, and it therefore shows a random, speckled pattern of actin molecules, each marking a different filament. This technique (called "speckle fluorescence") can be used to follow the movement of polymerized actin in a migrating cell. If you watch this pattern with time, you will see that individual fluorescent spots move steadily back from the leading edge toward the interior of the cell, a movement that occurs whether or not the cell is actually migrating. Rearward movement takes place because actin monomers are added to filaments at the plus end and are lost from the minus end (where they are depolymerized) (see Figure 17–35B). In effect, actin monomers "move through" the actin filaments, a phenomenon termed "treadmilling." Treadmilling has been demonstrated to occur in isolated actin filaments in solution and also in dynamic microtubules, such as those within a mitotic spindle.

ANSWER 17–7   Cells contain actin-binding proteins that bundle and cross-link actin filaments (see Figure 17–32). The filaments extending the lamellipodia and filopodia are firmly anchored in the filamentous meshwork of the cell cortex, thus providing the mechanical anchorage required for the growing rodlike filaments to deform the cell membrane.

ANSWER 17–8   Although the subunits are indeed held together by noncovalent bonds that are individually weak, there are a very large number of them, distributed among a very large number of filaments. As a result, the stress a human being exerts by lifting a heavy object is dispersed over so many subunits that their interaction strength is not exceeded. By analogy, a single thread of silk is not nearly strong enough to hold a human, but a rope woven of such fibers is.

ANSWER 17–9   Both filaments are composed of subunits in the form of protein dimers that are held together by coiled-coil interactions. Moreover, in both cases, the dimers polymerize through their coiled-coil domains into filaments. Whereas intermediate filament dimers assemble head-to-head, however, and thereby create a filament that has no polarity, all myosin molecules in the same half of the myosin filament are oriented with their heads pointing in the same direction. This polarity is necessary for them to be able to develop a contractile force in muscle.

ANSWER 17–10

A. Successive actin molecules in an actin filament are identical in position and conformation. After a first protein (such as troponin) has bound to the actin filament, there would be no way in which a second protein could recognize every seventh monomer in a naked actin filament. Tropomyosin, however, binds along the length of an actin filament, spanning precisely seven monomers, and thus provides a molecular "ruler" that measures the length of seven actin monomers. Troponin becomes localized by binding to the evenly spaced ends of tropomyosin molecules.

B. Calcium ions influence force generation in the actin–myosin system only if both troponin (to bind the calcium ions) and tropomyosin (to transmit the information to the actin filament that troponin has bound calcium) are present. (i) Troponin cannot bind to actin without tropomyosin. The actin filament would be permanently exposed to the myosin, and the system would be continuously active, independently of whether calcium ions were present or not (a muscle cell would therefore be continuously contracted with no possibility of regulation). (ii) Tropomyosin would bind to actin and block binding of myosin completely; the system would be permanently inactive, no matter whether calcium ions were present, because tropomyosin is not affected by calcium. (iii) The system will contract in response to calcium ions.

ANSWER 17–11

A. True. A continual outward movement of ER is required; in the absence of microtubules, the ER collapses toward the center of the cell.

B. True. Actin is needed to make the contractile ring that causes the physical cleavage between the two daughter cells, whereas the mitotic spindle that partitions the chromosomes is composed of microtubules.

C. True. Both extensions are associated with transmembrane proteins that protrude from the plasma membrane and enable the cell to form new anchor points on the substratum.

D. False. To cause bending, ATP is hydrolyzed by the dynein motor proteins that are attached to the outer microtubules in the flagellum.

E. False. Cells could not divide without rearranging their intermediate filaments, but many terminally differentiated and long-lived cells, such as nerve cells, have stable intermediate filaments that are not known to depolymerize.

F. False. The rate of growth is independent of the size of the GTP cap. The plus and minus ends have different growth rates because they have physically distinct binding sites for the incoming tubulin subunits; the rate of addition of tubulin subunits differs at the two ends.

G. True. Both are nice examples of how the same membrane can have regions that are highly specialized for a particular function.

H. False. Myosin movement is activated by the phosphorylation of myosin, or by calcium binding to troponin.

ANSWER 17–12   The average time taken for a small molecule (such as ATP) to diffuse a distance of 10 µm is given by the calculation

$$(10^{-3})^2 / (2 \times 5 \times 10^{-6}) = 0.1 \text{ seconds}$$

Similarly, a protein takes 1 second and a vesicle 10 seconds on average to travel 10 µm. A vesicle would require on average 10^9 seconds, or more than 30 years, to diffuse to the end of a 10 cm axon. Motorized transport at 1 µm/sec would require 10^5 seconds, or 28 hours. These calculations make it clear why kinesin and other motor proteins evolved to carry molecules and organelles along microtubules.

ANSWER 17–13   (1) Animal cells are much larger and more diversely shaped than bacteria, and they do not have a cell wall. Cytoskeletal elements are required to provide mechanical strength and shape in the absence of a cell wall. (2) Animal cells, and all other eukaryotic cells, have a nucleus that is shaped and held in place in the cell by intermediate filaments; the nuclear lamins attached to the inner nuclear membrane support and shape the nuclear membrane, and a meshwork of intermediate filaments surrounds the nucleus and spans the cytosol. (3) Animal cells can move by a process that requires a change in cell shape. Actin filaments and myosin motor proteins are required for these activities. (4) Animal cells have a much larger genome than bacteria; this genome is fragmented into many chromosomes. For cell division, chromosomes need to be accurately distributed to the daughter cells, requiring the function of the microtubules that form the mitotic spindle. (5) Animal cells have internal organelles. Their localization in the cell is dependent on motor proteins that move them along microtubules. A remarkable example is the long-distance travel of membrane-enclosed vesicles (organelles) along microtubules in an axon that can be up to 1 m long in the case of the nerve cells that extend from your spinal cord to your feet.

ANSWER 17–14   The ends of an intermediate filament are indistinguishable from each other, because the filaments are built by the assembly of symmetrical tetramers made from two coiled-coil dimers. In contrast to microtubules and actin filaments, intermediate filaments therefore have no polarity.

ANSWER 17–15   Intermediate filaments have no polarity; their ends are chemically indistinguishable. It would therefore be difficult to envision how a hypothetical motor protein that bound to the middle of the filament could sense a defined direction. Such a motor protein would be equally likely to attach to the filament facing one end or the other.

ANSWER 17–16   Katanin breaks microtubules along their length, and at positions remote from their GTP caps. The fragments that form therefore contain GDP-tubulin at their exposed ends and rapidly depolymerize. Katanin thus provides a very quick means of destroying existing microtubules.

ANSWER 17–17   Cell division depends on the ability of microtubules both to polymerize and to depolymerize. This is most obvious when one considers that the formation of the mitotic spindle requires the prior depolymerization of other microtubules to free up the tubulin required to build the spindle. This rearrangement is not possible in Taxol-treated cells, whereas in colchicine-treated cells, division is blocked because a spindle cannot be assembled. On a less obvious but no less important level, both drugs block the dynamic instability of microtubules and would therefore interfere with the workings of the mitotic spindle, even if one could be properly assembled.

ANSWER 17–18   Motor proteins are unidirectional in their action; kinesin always moves toward the plus end of a microtubule and dynein toward the minus end. Thus if kinesin molecules are attached to glass, only those individual motors that have the correct orientation in relation to the microtubule that settles on them can attach to the microtubule and exert force on it to propel it forward. Since kinesin moves toward the plus end of the microtubule, the microtubule will always crawl minus-end first over the cover slip.

ANSWER 17–19

A. Phase A corresponds to a lag phase, during which tubulin dimers assemble to form nucleation centers (Figure A17–19A). Nucleation is followed by a rapid rise (phase B) to a plateau value as tubulin dimers add to the ends of the elongating microtubules (Figure A17–19B). At phase C, equilibrium is reached, with some microtubules in the population growing while others are rapidly shrinking (Figure A17–19C). The concentration of free tubulin is constant at this point because polymerization and depolymerization are balanced (see also Question 17–3, p. 586).

B. The addition of centrosomes introduces nucleation sites that eliminate the lag phase A, as shown by the *red* curve in Figure A17–19D. The rate of microtubule growth (i.e., the slope of the curve in the elongation phase B) and the equilibrium level of free tubulin remain unchanged, because the presence of centrosomes does not affect the rates of polymerization and depolymerization.

ANSWER 17–20   The ends of the shrinking microtubule are visibly frayed, and the individual protofilaments appear to come apart and curl as the end depolymerizes. This micrograph therefore suggests that the GTP cap (which is lost from shrinking microtubules) holds the protofilaments properly aligned with each other, perhaps by strengthening the side-to-side interactions between αβ-tubulin subunits when they are in their GTP-bound form.

ANSWER 17–21   Cytochalasin interferes with actin filament formation, and its effect on the cell demonstrates the importance of actin to cell locomotion. The experiment with colchicine shows that microtubules are required to give a cell a polarity that then determines which end becomes the leading edge (see Figure 17–15). In the absence of microtubules, cells still go through the motions normally associated with cell movement, such as the extension of lamellipodia, but in the absence of cell polarity these are futile exercises because they happen indiscriminately in all directions. Antibodies bind tightly to the antigen (in this

case vimentin) to which they were raised (see Panel 4–2, pp. 140–141). When bound, an antibody can interfere with the function of the antigen by preventing it from interacting properly with other cell components. The antibody injection experiment therefore suggests that intermediate filaments are not required for the maintenance of cell polarity or for the motile machinery.

ANSWER 17–22   Either (B) or (C) would complete the sentence correctly. The direct result of the action potential in the plasma membrane is the release of Ca^{2+} into the cytosol from the sarcoplasmic reticulum; muscle cells are triggered to contract by this rapid rise in cytosolic Ca^{2+}. Calcium ions at high concentrations bind to troponin, which in turn causes tropomyosin to move to expose myosin-binding sites on the actin filaments. (A) and (D) would be wrong because Ca^{2+} has no effect on the detachment of the myosin head from actin, which is the result of ATP hydrolysis. Nor does it have any role in maintaining the structure of the myosin filament.

ANSWER 17–23   Only (D) is correct. Upon contraction, the Z discs move closer together, and neither actin nor myosin filaments contract (see Figures 17–41 and 17–42).

Chapter 18

ANSWER 18–1   Because all cells arise by division of another cell, this statement is correct, assuming that "first cell division" refers to the division of the successful founder cell from which all life as we know it has derived. There were probably many other unsuccessful attempts to start the chain of life.

ANSWER 18–2   Cells in peak B contain twice as much DNA as those in peak A, indicating that they contain replicated DNA, whereas the cells in peak A contain unreplicated DNA. Peak A therefore contains cells that are in G_1, and peak B contains cells that are in G_2 and mitosis. Cells in S phase have begun but not finished DNA synthesis; they therefore have various intermediate amounts of DNA and are found in the region between the two peaks. Most cells are in G_1, indicating that it is the longest phase of the cell cycle (see Figure 18–2).

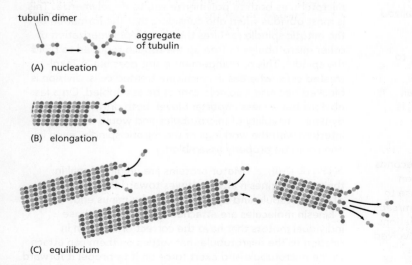

(A) nucleation

(B) elongation

(C) equilibrium

Figure A17–19

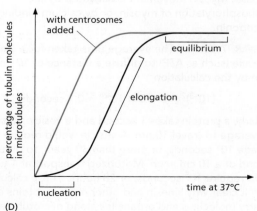

(D)

ANSWER 18–3   For multicellular organisms, the control of cell division is extremely important. Individual cells must not proliferate unless it is to the benefit of the whole organism. The G_0 state offers protection from aberrant activation of cell division because the cell-cycle control system is largely dismantled. If, on the other hand, a cell just paused in G_1, it would still contain all of the cell-cycle control system and could readily be induced to divide. The cell would also have to remake the "decision" not to divide almost continuously. To re-enter the cell cycle from G_0, a cell has to resynthesize all of the components that have disappeared.

ANSWER 18–4   The cell would replicate its damaged DNA and therefore would introduce mutations to the two daughter cells when the cell divides. Such mutations could increase the chances that the progeny of the affected daughter cells would eventually become cancer cells.

ANSWER 18–5   Before injection, the frog oocytes must contain inactive M-Cdk. Upon injection of the M-phase cytoplasm, the small amount of the active M-Cdk in the injected cytoplasm activates the inactive M-Cdk by switching on the activating phosphatase (Cdc25), which removes the inhibitory phosphate groups from the inactive M-Cdk (see Figure 18–17). An extract of the second oocyte, now in M phase itself, will therefore contain as much active M-Cdk as the original cytoplasmic extract, and so on.

ANSWER 18–6   The experiment shows that kinetochores are not preassigned to one or other spindle pole; microtubules attach to the kinetochores that they are able to reach. For the chromosome to remain attached to a microtubule, however, tension has to be exerted. Tension is normally achieved by the opposing pulling forces from opposite spindle poles. The requirement for such tension ensures that if two sister kinetochores ever become attached to the same spindle pole, so that tension is not generated, one or both of the connections would be lost, and microtubules from the opposing spindle pole would have another chance to attach properly.

ANSWER 18–7   Recall from Figure 18–30 that the new nuclear envelope reassembles on the surface of the chromosomes. The close apposition of the envelope to the chromosomes prevents cytosolic proteins from being trapped between the chromosomes and the envelope. Nuclear proteins are then selectively imported through the nuclear pores, causing the nucleus to expand while maintaining its characteristic protein composition.

ANSWER 18–8   The membranes of the Golgi vesicles fuse to form part of the plasma membranes of the two daughter cells. The interiors of the vesicles, which are filled with cell wall material, become the new cell wall matrix separating the two daughter cells. Proteins in the membranes of the Golgi vesicles thus become plasma membrane proteins. Those parts of the proteins that were exposed to the lumen of the Golgi vesicle will end up exposed to the new cell wall (Figure A18–8).

ANSWER 18–9   In a eukaryotic organism, the genetic information that the organism needs to survive and reproduce is distributed between multiple chromosomes. It is therefore crucial that each daughter cell receives a copy of each chromosome when a cell divides; if a daughter cell receives too few or too many chromosomes, the effects are usually deleterious or even lethal. Only two copies of each chromosome are produced by chromosome replication in mitosis. If the cell were to randomly distribute the chromosomes when it divided, it would be very unlikely that each daughter cell would receive precisely one copy of each chromosome. In contrast, the Golgi apparatus fragments into tiny vesicles that are all alike, and by random distribution it is very likely that each daughter cell will receive an approximately equal number of them.

ANSWER 18–10   As apoptosis occurs on a large scale in both developing and adult tissues, it must not trigger alarm reactions that are normally associated with cell injury. Tissue injury, for example, leads to the release of signal molecules that stimulate the proliferation of surrounding cells so that the wound heals. It also causes the release of signals that can cause a destructive inflammatory reaction. Moreover, the release of intracellular contents could elicit an immune response against molecules that are normally not encountered by the immune system. Such reactions would be self-defeating if they occurred in response to the massive cell death that occurs in normal development.

ANSWER 18–11   Because the cell population is increasing exponentially, doubling its weight at every cell division, the weight of the cell cluster after N cell divisions is $2^N \times 10^{-9}$ g. Therefore, 70 kg (70×10^3 g) = $2^N \times 10^{-9}$ g, or $2^N = 7 \times 10^{13}$. Taking the logarithm of both sides allows you to solve the equation for N. Therefore, $N = \ln(7 \times 10^{13}) / \ln 2 = 46$; that is it would take only 46 days if cells proliferated exponentially. Cell division in animals is tightly controlled, however, and most cells in the human body stop dividing when they become highly specialized. The example demonstrates that exponential cell proliferation occurs only for very brief periods, even during embryonic development.

ANSWER 18–12   The egg cells of many animals are big and contain stores of enough cell components to last for many cell divisions. The daughter cells that form during the first cell divisions after fertilization are progressively smaller in size and thus can be formed without a need for new protein or RNA synthesis. Whereas normally dividing cells would grow continuously in G_1, G_2, and S phases, until their size doubled, there is no cell growth in these early cleavage divisions, and both G_1 and G_2 are virtually absent. As G_1 is usually longer than G_2 and S phase, G_1 is the most drastically reduced phase in these divisions.

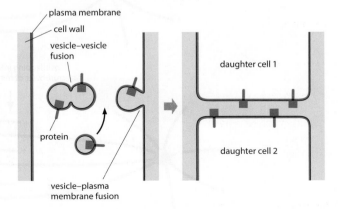

Figure A18–8

ANSWER 18–13

A. Radiation leads to DNA damage, which activates a regulatory mechanism (mediated by p53 and p21; see Figure 18–15) that arrests the cell cycle until the DNA has been repaired.

B. The cell will replicate damaged DNA and thereby introduce mutations in the daughter cells when the cell divides.

C. The cell will be able to divide normally, but it will be prone to mutations, because some DNA damage always occurs as the result of natural irradiation caused, for example, by cosmic rays. The mechanism mediated by p53 is mainly required as a safeguard against the devastating effects of accumulating DNA damage; this mechanism is not required for the natural progression of the cell cycle in undamaged cells.

D. Cell division in humans is an ongoing process that does not cease upon reaching maturity, and it is required for survival. Blood cells and epithelial cells in the skin or lining the gut, for example, are being constantly produced by cell division to meet the body's needs; each day, your body produces about 10^{11} new red blood cells alone.

ANSWER 18–14

A. Only the cells that were in the S phase of their cell cycle (i.e., those cells making DNA) during the 30-minute labeling period contain any radioactive DNA.

B. Initially, mitotic cells contain no radioactive DNA because these cells were not engaged in DNA synthesis during the labeling period. Indeed, it takes about two hours before the first labeled mitotic cells appear.

C. The initial rise of the curve corresponds to cells that were just finishing DNA replication when the radioactive thymidine was added. The curve rises as more labeled cells enter mitosis; the peak corresponds to those cells that had just started S phase when the radioactive thymidine was added. The labeled cells then exit from mitosis, and are replaced by unlabeled mitotic cells, which were not yet in S phase during the labeling period. After 20 hours, the curve starts rising again, because the labeled cells enter their second round of mitosis.

D. The initial two-hour lag before any labeled mitotic cells appear corresponds to the G_2 phase, which is the time between the end of S phase and the beginning of mitosis. The first labeled cells seen in mitosis were those that were just finishing S phase (DNA synthesis) when the radioactive thymidine was added.

ANSWER 18–15   Loss of M cyclin leads to inactivation of M-Cdk. As a result, the M-Cdk target proteins become dephosphorylated by phosphatases, and the cells exit from mitosis: they disassemble the mitotic spindle, reassemble the nuclear envelope, decondense their chromosomes, and so on. The M cyclin is degraded by ubiquitin-dependent destruction in proteasomes, and the activation of M-Cdk leads to the activation of APC/C, which ubiquitylates the cyclin, but with a substantial delay. As discussed in Chapter 7, ubiquitylation tags proteins for degradation in proteasomes.

ANSWER 18–16   M cyclin accumulates gradually as it is steadily synthesized. As it accumulates, it will tend to form complexes with the mitotic Cdk molecules that are present. The Cdk in these complexes is inhibited by phosphorylation (see Figure 18–10). After a certain threshold level has been reached, M-Cdk is activated by the phosphatase Cdc25. Once activated, M-Cdk acts to enhance the activity of the activating phosphatase; this positive feedback leads to the complete activation of M-Cdk (see Figure 18–17). Thus, M cyclin accumulation acts like a slow-burning fuse, which eventually helps trigger the explosive self-activation of M-Cdk. The precipitous destruction of M cyclin terminates M-Cdk activity, and a new round of M cyclin accumulation begins.

ANSWER 18–17   The order is F, C, B, A, D. Together, these five steps are referred to as mitosis (E). Cytokinesis is the last step in M phase, which overlaps with anaphase and telophase. Mitosis and cytokinesis are both part of M phase.

ANSWER 18–18   If the growth rate of microtubules is the same in mitotic and in interphase cells, their length is proportional to their lifetime. Thus, the average length of microtubules in mitosis is 1 μm (= 20 μm × 15 s/300 s).

ANSWER 18–19   As shown in Figure A18–19, the

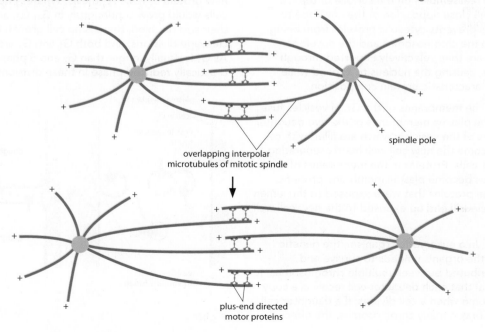

overlapping interpolar microtubules of mitotic spindle

spindle pole

plus-end directed motor proteins

Figure A18–19

overlapping interpolar microtubules from opposite poles of the spindle have their plus ends pointing in opposite directions. Plus-end directed motor proteins cross-link adjacent, antiparallel microtubules together and tend to move the microtubules in the direction that will push the two poles of the spindle apart, as shown in the figure. Minus-end directed motor proteins also cross-link adjacent, antiparallel microtubules together but move in the opposite direction, tending to pull the spindle poles together (not shown).

ANSWER 18–20 The sister chromatid becomes committed when a microtubule from one of the spindle poles attaches to the kinetochore of the chromatid. Microtubule attachment is still reversible until a second microtubule from the other spindle pole attaches to the kinetochore of its partner sister chromatid, so that the duplicated chromosome is now put under mechanical tension by pulling forces from both poles. The tension ensures that both microtubules remain attached to the chromosome. The position of a chromatid in the cell at the time that the nuclear envelope breaks down will influence which spindle pole it will be pulled to, as its kinetochore is most likely to become attached to the spindle pole toward which it is facing.

ANSWER 18–21 It is still not certain what drives the poleward movement of chromosomes during anaphase. In principle, two possible models could explain it (**Figure A18–21**). In the model shown in (A), microtubule motor proteins associated with the kinetochore dash toward the minus end of the depolymerizing microtubule, dragging the chromosome toward the pole. Although this model is appealingly simple, there is little evidence that motor proteins are required for chromosome movement during anaphase. Instead, current experimental evidence greatly supports the model outlined in (B). In this model, chromosome movement is driven by kinetochore proteins that cling to the sides of the depolymerizing microtubule (see Figure 18–23). These proteins frequently detach from—and reattach to—the kinetochore microtubule. As tubulin subunits continue to dissociate, the kinetochore must slide poleward to maintain its grip on the retreating end of the shrinking microtubule.

ANSWER 18–22 Both sister chromatids could end up in the same daughter cell for any of a number of reasons. (1) If the microtubules or their connections with a kinetochore were to break during anaphase, both sister chromatids could be drawn to the same pole, and hence into the same daughter cell. (2) If microtubules from the same spindle pole attached to both kinetochores, the chromosome would be pulled to the same pole. (3) If the cohesins that link sister chromatids were not degraded, the pair of chromatids might be pulled to the same pole. (4) If a duplicated chromosome never engaged microtubules and was left out of the spindle, it would also end up in one daughter cell.

Some of these errors in the mitotic process would be expected to activate a checkpoint mechanism that delays the onset of anaphase until all chromosomes are attached properly to both poles of the spindle. This "spindle assembly checkpoint" mechanism should allow most chromosome-attachment errors to be corrected, which is one reason why such errors are rare. The consequences of both sister chromatids ending up in one daughter cell are usually dire. One daughter cell would contain only one copy of all the genes carried on that chromosome and the other daughter cell would contain three copies. The altered gene dosage, leading to correspondingly changed amounts of the mRNAs and proteins produced, is often detrimental to the cell. In addition, there is the possibility that the single copy of the chromosome may contain a defective gene with a critical function, which would normally be taken care of by the good copy of the gene on the other chromosome that is now missing.

ANSWER 18–23

A. True. Centrosomes replicate during interphase, before M phase begins.
B. True. Sister chromatids separate completely only at the start of anaphase.
C. False. The ends of interpolar microtubules overlap and attach to one another via proteins (including motor proteins) that bridge between the microtubules.
D. False. Microtubules and their motor proteins play no role in DNA replication.
E. False. To be a correct statement, the terms "centromere" and "centrosome" must be switched.

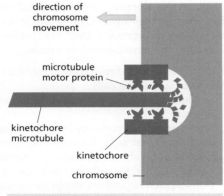

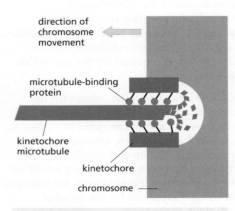

Figure A18–21   (A)   (B)

ANSWER 18–24   Antibodies bind tightly to the antigen (in this case myosin) to which they were raised. When bound, an antibody can interfere with the function of the antigen by preventing it from interacting properly with other cell components. (A) The movement of chromosomes at anaphase depends on microtubules and their motor proteins and does not depend on actin or myosin. Injection of an anti-myosin antibody into a cell will therefore have no effect on chromosome movement during anaphase. (B) Cytokinesis, on the other hand, depends on the assembly and contraction of a ring of actin and myosin filaments, which forms the cleavage furrow that splits the cell in two. Injection of an anti-myosin antibody will therefore block cytokinesis.

ANSWER 18–25   The plasma membrane of the cell that died by necrosis in Figure 18–38A is ruptured; a clear break is visible, for example, at a position corresponding to the 12 o'clock mark on a watch. The cell's contents, mostly membranous and cytoskeletal debris, are seen spilling into the surroundings through these breaks. The cytosol stains lightly, because most soluble cell components were lost before the cell was fixed. In contrast, the cell that underwent apoptosis in Figure 18–38B is surrounded by an intact membrane, and its cytosol is densely stained, indicating a normal concentration of cell components. The cell's interior is remarkably different from a normal cell, however. Particularly characteristic are the large "blobs" that extrude from the nucleus, probably as the result of the breakdown of the nuclear lamina. The cytosol also contains many large, round, membrane-enclosed vesicles of unknown origin, which are not normally seen in healthy cells. The pictures visually confirm the notion that necrosis involves cell lysis, whereas cells undergoing apoptosis remain relatively intact until they are phagocytosed and digested by another cell.

ANSWER 18–26
A. False. There is no G_1 to M phase transition. The statement is correct, however, for the G_1 to S phase transition, in which cells commit themselves to a division cycle.
B. True. Apoptosis is an active process carried out by special proteases (caspases).
C. True. This mechanism is thought to adjust the number of neurons to the number of specific target cells to which the neurons connect.
D. True. An amazing evolutionary conservation!
E. True. Association of a Cdk protein with a cyclin is required for its activity (hence its name <u>c</u>yclin-<u>d</u>ependent <u>k</u>inase). Furthermore, dephosphorylation at specific sites on the Cdk protein is required for the cyclin–Cdk complex to be active.

ANSWER 18–27   Cells in an animal must behave for the good of the organism as a whole—to a much greater extent than people generally act for the good of society as a whole. In the context of an organism, unsocial behavior would lead to a loss of organization and possibly to cancer. Many of the rules that cells have to obey would be unacceptable in a human society. Most people, for example, would be reluctant to kill themselves for the good of society, yet our cells do it all the time.

ANSWER 18–28   The most likely approach to success (if that is what the goal should be called) is plan C, which should

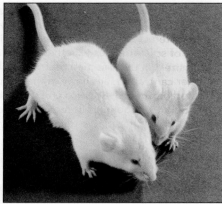

Figure A18–28   Courtesy of Ralph Brinster

result in an increase in cell numbers. The problem is, of course, that cell numbers of each tissue must be increased similarly to maintain balanced proportions in the organism, yet different cells respond to different growth factors. As shown in Figure A18–28, however, the approach has indeed met with limited success. A mouse producing very large quantities of growth hormone (*left*)—which acts to stimulate the production of a secreted protein that acts as a survival factor, growth factor, or mitogen, depending on the cell type—grows to almost twice the size of a normal mouse (*right*). To achieve this twofold change in size, however, growth hormone was massively overproduced (about fiftyfold). And note that the mouse did not even attain the size of a rat, let alone a dog.

The other two approaches have conceptual problems:
A. Blocking all apoptosis would lead to defects in development, as rat development requires the selective death of many cells. It is unlikely that a viable animal would be obtained.
B. Blocking p53 function would eliminate an important mechanism in the cell cycle that detects DNA damage and stops the cycle so that the cell can repair the damage; removing p53 would increase mutation rates and lead to cancer. Indeed, mice without p53 usually develop normally but die of cancer at a young age.

ANSWER 18–29   The on-demand, limited release of PDGF at a wound site triggers cell division of neighboring cells for a limited amount of time, until the PDGF is degraded. This is different from the continuous release of PDGF from mutant cells, where PDGF is made in an uncontrolled way at high levels. Moreover, the mutant cells that make PDGF often express their own PDGF receptor inappropriately, so that they can stimulate their own proliferation, thereby promoting the development of cancer.

ANSWER 18–30   All three types of mutant cells would be unable to divide. The cells:
A. would enter mitosis but would not be able to exit mitosis.
B. would arrest permanently in G_1 because the cyclin–Cdk complexes that act in G_1 would be inactivated.
C. would not be able to activate the transcription of genes required for cell division because the required transcription regulators would be constantly inhibited by unphosphorylated Rb.

ANSWER 18–31   In alcoholism, liver cells proliferate because the organ is overburdened and becomes damaged by the large amounts of alcohol that have to be metabolized. This need for more liver cells activates the control mechanisms that normally regulate cell proliferation. Unless badly damaged and full of scar tissue, the liver will usually shrink back to a normal size after the patient stops drinking excessively. In liver cancer, in contrast, mutations abolish normal cell proliferation control and, as a result, cells divide and keep on dividing in an uncontrolled manner, which is usually fatal.

Chapter 19

ANSWER 19–1 After the first meiotic division, each nucleus has a diploid amount of DNA; however, that DNA effectively contains only a haploid set of chromosomes (albeit in two copies), representing only one or other homolog of each type of chromosome (although some mixing will have occurred during crossing-over). Because the maternal and paternal chromosomes of a pair will carry different versions of many of the genes, these daughter cells will not be genetically identical; each one will, however, have lost either the paternal or the maternal version of each chromosome. In contrast, somatic cells dividing by mitosis inherit a diploid set of chromosomes, and all daughter cells are genetically identical and inherit both maternal and paternal gene copies. The role of gametes produced by meiosis is to mix and reassort gene pools during sexual reproduction, and thus it is a definite advantage for each of them to have a slightly different genetic constitution. The role of somatic cells on the other hand is to build an organism that contains the same genes in all its cells and retains in each cell both maternal and paternal genetic information.

ANSWER 19–2 A typical human female produces fewer than 1000 mature eggs in her lifetime (12 per year over about 40 years); this is less than one-tenth of a percent of the possible gametes, excluding the effects of meiotic crossing-over. A typical human male produces billions of sperm during a lifetime, so in principle, every possible chromosome combination is sampled many times.

ANSWER 19–3 For simplicity, consider the situation where a father carries genes for two dominant traits, M and N, on one of his two copies of human Chromosome 1. If these two genes were located at opposite ends of this chromosome, and there was one and only one crossover event per chromosome as postulated in the question, half of his children would express trait M and the other half would express trait N—with no child resembling the father in carrying both traits. This is very different from the actual situation, where there are multiple crossover events per chromosome, causing the traits M and N to be inherited as if they were on separate chromosomes. By constructing a Punnett square like that in Figure 19–27, one can see that in this latter, more realistic case, we would actually expect one-fourth of the children of this father to inherit both traits, one-fourth to inherit trait M only, one-fourth to inherit trait N only, and one-fourth to inherit neither trait.

ANSWER 19–4 Inbreeding tends to give rise to individuals who are homozygous for many genes. To see why, consider the extreme case where the consanguineous relationship takes the form of brother–sister inbreeding (as among the Pharaohs of ancient Egypt): because the parents are closely related, there is a high probability that the maternal and paternal alleles inherited by the offspring will be the same. Inbreeding continued over many generations gives rise to individuals who are homozygous for almost every gene. Because of the randomness of the mechanism of inheritance, some deleterious alleles will become prevalent in the descendants. If the gene is important, individuals that inherit two defective copies will be unhealthy—often severely so. In another, separate inbred population, the same thing will happen, but chances are a different set of deleterious alleles will become prevalent. When individuals from the two separate inbred populations mate, their offspring will inherit deleterious alleles of genes A, B, and C, for example, from the mother, but functional alleles of those genes from the father; conversely, they will inherit deleterious alleles of genes D, E, and F from the father, but functional alleles of those genes from the mother. Because most deleterious mutations are recessive, the hybrid offspring—who are heterozygous for these genes—will thus escape the deleterious effects.

ANSWER 19–5 Although any one of the three explanations could in principle account for the observed result, A and B can be ruled out as being implausible.

A. There is no precedent for any instability in DNA so great as to be detectable in such a SNP analysis; in any case, the hypothesis would predict a steady decrease in the frequency of the SNP with age, not a drop in frequency that begins only at age 50.

B. Human genes change only very slowly over time (unless a massive population migration brings an influx of individuals who are genetically different). People born 50 years ago will be, on average, virtually the same genetically as the population being born today.

C. This hypothesis is correct. A SNP with these properties has been used to discover a gene that appears to cause a substantial increase in the probability of death from cardiac abnormalities.

ANSWER 19–6 Natural selection alone is not sufficient to eliminate recessive lethal genes from the population. Consider the following line of reasoning. Homozygous defective individuals can arise only as the offspring of a mating between two heterozygous individuals. By the rules of Mendelian genetics, offspring of such a mating will be in the ratio of 1 homozygous normal: 2 heterozygous: 1 homozygous defective. Thus, statistically, heterozygous individuals should always be more numerous than the homozygous, defective individuals. And although natural selection effectively eliminates the defective genes in homozygous individuals through death, it cannot act to eliminate the defective genes in heterozygous individuals because they do not affect the phenotype. Natural selection will keep the frequency of the defective gene low in the population, but, in the absence of any other effect, there will always be a reservoir of defective genes in the heterozygous individuals.

At low frequencies of the defective gene, another important factor—chance—comes into play. Chance variation can increase or decrease the frequency of heterozygous individuals (and thereby the frequency of the defective gene). By chance, the offspring of a mating between heterozygotes could all be normal, which would eliminate the defective gene from that lineage. Increases in the frequency of a deleterious gene are opposed by natural selection; however, decreases are unopposed and can, by chance, lead to elimination of the defective gene from the population. On the other hand, new mutations are continually occurring, albeit at a low rate, creating fresh copies of the deleterious recessive allele. In a large population, a balance will be struck between the creation of new copies of the allele in this way, and their elimination through the death of homozygotes.

ANSWER 19–7

A. True.

B. True.

C. False. Mutations that occur during meiosis can be propagated, unless they give rise to nonviable gametes.

ANSWER 19–8   In mitosis, two copies of the same chromosome can end up in the same daughter cell if one of the microtubule connections breaks before sister chromatids are separated. Alternatively, microtubules from the same spindle pole could attach to both kinetochores of the chromosome. As a consequence, one daughter cell would receive only one copy of all the genes carried on that chromosome, and the other daughter cell would receive three copies. The imbalance of the genes on this chromosome compared with the genes on all the other chromosomes would produce imbalanced levels of protein which, in most cases, is detrimental to the cell. If the mistake happens during meiosis, in the process of gamete formation, it will be propagated in all cells of the organism. A form of mental retardation called Down syndrome, for example, is due to the presence of three copies of Chromosome 21 in all of the nucleated cells in the body.

ANSWER 19–9   Meiosis begins with DNA replication, producing a tetraploid cell containing four copies of each chromosome. These four copies have to be distributed equally during the two sequential meiotic divisions into four haploid cells. Sister chromatids remain paired so that (1) the cells resulting from the first division receive two complete sets of chromosomes and (2) the chromosomes can be evenly distributed again in the second meiotic division. If the sister chromatids did not remain paired, it would not be possible in the second division to distinguish which chromatids belong together, and it would therefore be difficult to ensure that precisely one copy of each chromatid is pulled into each daughter cell. Keeping two sister chromatids paired in the first meiotic division is therefore an easy way to keep track of which chromatids belong together.

This biological principle suggests that you might consider clamping your socks together in matching pairs before putting them into the laundry. In this way, the cumbersome process of sorting them out afterward—and the seemingly inevitable mistakes that occur during that process—could be avoided.

ANSWER 19–10

A. A gene is a stretch of DNA that codes for a protein or functional RNA. An allele is an alternative form of a gene. Within the population, there are often several "normal" alleles, whose functions are indistinguishable. In addition, there may be many rare alleles that are defective to varying degrees. An individual, however, normally carries a maximum of two alleles of each gene.

B. An individual is said to be homozygous if the two alleles of a gene are the same. An individual is said to be heterozygous if the two alleles of a gene are different. An individual can be heterozygous for gene A and homozygous for gene B.

C. The genotype is the specific set of alleles present in the genome of an individual. In practice, for organisms studied in a laboratory, the genotype is usually specified as a list of the known differences between the individual and the wild type, which is the standard, naturally occurring type. The phenotype is a description of the visible characteristics of the individual. In practice, the phenotype is usually a list of the differences in visible characteristics between the individual and the wild type.

D. An allele A is dominant (relative to a second allele a) if the presence of even a single copy of A is enough to affect the phenotype; that is, if heterozygotes (with genotype Aa) appear different from aa homozygotes. An allele a is recessive (relative to a second allele A) if the presence of a single copy makes no difference to the phenotype, so that Aa individuals look just like AA individuals. If the phenotype of the heterozygous individual differs from the phenotypes of individuals that are homozygous for either allele, the alleles are said to be co-dominant.

ANSWER 19–11

A. Since the pea plant is diploid, any true-breeding plant must carry two mutant copies of the same gene—both of which have lost their function.

B. If each plant carries a mutation in a different gene, this will be revealed by complementation tests (see Panel 19–1, p. 675). When plant A is crossed with plant B, all of the F_1 plants will produce only round peas. And the same result will be obtained when plant B is crossed with plant C, or when plant A is crossed with plant C. In contrast, a cross between any two true-breeding plants that carry loss-of-function mutations in the same gene should produce only plants with wrinkled peas. This is true if the mutations themselves lie in different parts of the gene.

ANSWER 19–12

A. The mutation is likely to be dominant, because roughly half of the progeny born to an affected parent—in each of three marriages to hearing partners—are deaf, and it is unlikely that all these hearing partners were heterozygous carriers of the mutation.

B. The mutation is not present on a sex chromosome. If it were, either only the female progeny should be affected (expected if the mutation arose in a gene on the grandfather's X chromosome), or only the male progeny should be affected (expected if the mutation arose in a gene on the grandfather's Y chromosome). In fact, the pedigree reveals that both males and females have inherited the mutant form of the gene.

C. Suppose that the mutation was present on one of the two copies of the grandfather's Chromosome 12. Each of these copies of Chromosome 12 would be expected to carry a different pattern of SNPs, since one of them was inherited from his father and the other was inherited from his mother. Each of the copies of Chromosome 12 that was passed to his grandchildren will have gone through two meioses—one meiosis per generation. Because two or three crossover events occur per chromosome during a meiosis, each chromosome inherited by a grandchild will have been subjected to about five crossovers since it left the grandfather, dividing it into six segments. An identical pattern of SNPs should surround whatever gene causes the deafness in each of the four affected grandchildren; moreover, this SNP pattern should be clearly different from that surrounding the same gene in each of the seven grandchildren who are normal. These SNPs would form an unusually long haplotype block—one that extends for about one-sixth of the length of Chromosome 12. (One-quarter of the DNA of each grandchild will have been inherited from the grandfather, in roughly 70 segments of this length scattered among the grandchild's 46 chromosomes.)

ANSWER 19–13   Individual 1 might be either heterozygous (+/–) or homozygous for the normal allele (+/+). Individual 2 must be homozygous for the recessive deafness allele (–/–). (Both his parents must have been heterozygous because they produced a deaf son.) Individual 3 is almost certainly heterozygous (+/–) and responsible for transmitting the mutant allele to his children and grandchildren. Given that the mutant allele is rare, individual 4 is most probably homozygous for the normal allele (+/+).

ANSWER 19–14   Your friend is wrong.

A. Mendel's laws, and the clear understanding that we now have concerning the mechanisms that produce them, rule out many false ideas concerning human heredity. One of them is that a first-born child has a different chance of inheriting particular traits from its parents than its siblings.

B. The probability of this type of pedigree arising by chance is one-fourth for each generation, or one in 64 for the three generations shown.

C. Data from an enlarged sampling of family members, or from more generations, would quickly reveal that the regular pattern observed in this particular pedigree arose by chance.

D. If statistical tests showed that the pattern was not due to chance, it would suggest that some process of selection was involved: for example, parents who had had a first child that was affected might regularly opt for screening of subsequent pregnancies and selectively terminate those pregnancies in which the fetus was found to be affected. Fewer second children would then be born with the abnormality.

ANSWER 19–15   Each carrier is a heterozygote, and 50% of his sperm or her eggs will carry the lethal allele. When two carriers marry, there is therefore a 25% chance that any baby will inherit the lethal allele from both parents and so will show the fatal phenotype. Because one person in 100 is a carrier, one partnership in 10,000 (100 × 100) will be a partnership of carriers (assuming that people choose their partners at random). Other things being equal, one baby in 40,000 will then be born with the defect, or 25 babies per year out of a total of a million babies born.

ANSWER 19–16   A dominant-negative mutation gives rise to a mutant gene product that interferes with the function of the normal gene product, causing a loss-of-function phenotype even in the presence of a normal copy of the gene. For example, if a protein forms a hexamer, and the mutant protein can interact with the normal subunits and inhibit the function of the hexamer, the mutation will be dominant. This ability of a single defective allele to determine the phenotype is the reason why such an allele is dominant. A gain-of-function mutation increases the activity of the gene or makes it active in inappropriate circumstances. The change in activity often has a phenotypic consequence, which is why such mutations are usually dominant.

ANSWER 19–17

A. As outlined in Figure A19–17, if flies that are defective in different genes mate, their progeny will have one normal gene. In the case of a mating between a ruby-

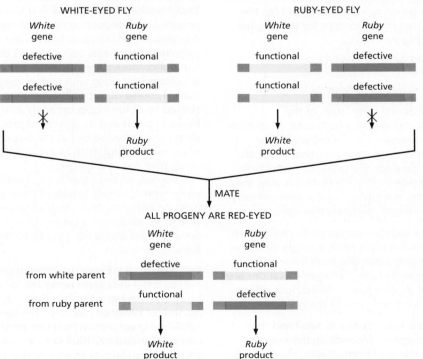

Figure A19–17

eyed fly and a white-eyed fly, every progeny fly will inherit one functional copy of the *White* gene from one parent and one functional copy of the *Ruby* gene from the other parent. Note that the normal white allele produces brick-red eyes and the mutated form of the gene produces white eyes. Because each of the mutant alleles is recessive to the corresponding wild-type allele, the progeny will have the wild-type phenotype—brick-red eyes.

B. Garnet, ruby, vermilion, and carnation complement one another and the various alleles of the *White* gene (that is, when these mutant flies are mated with each other, they produce flies with a normal eye color); thus each of these mutants defines a separate gene. In contrast, white, cherry, coral, apricot, and buff do not complement each other; thus, they must be alleles of the same gene, which has been named the *White* gene. Thus, these nine different eye-color mutants define five different genes.

C. Different alleles of the same gene, like the five alleles of the *White* gene, often have different phenotypes. Different mutations compromise the function of the gene product to different extents, depending on the location of the mutation. Alleles that do not produce any functional product (null alleles), even if they result from different DNA sequence changes, do have the same phenotype.

ANSWER 19–18   SNPs are single-nucleotide differences between individuals for which two or more variants are each found at high frequency in the population. In the human population, SNPs occur roughly once per 1000 nucleotides of sequence. Many have been identified and mapped in various organisms, including millions in the human genome. SNPs, which are detected by sequencing, serve as physical markers whose genomic locations are known. By tracking a mutant gene through different matings, and correlating the presence of the gene with the co-inheritance of particular SNP variants, one can narrow down the potential location of a gene to a chromosomal region that may contain only a few genes. These candidate genes can then be tested for the presence of a mutation that could account for the original mutant phenotype (see Figure 19–38).

Chapter 20

ANSWER 20–1   The horizontal orientation of the microtubules will be associated with a horizontal orientation of cellulose microfibrils deposited in the cell walls. The growth of the cells will therefore be in a vertical direction, expanding the distance between the cellulose microfibrils without stretching them (see Figure 20–6). In this way, the stem will rapidly elongate; in a typical natural environment, this will hasten emergence from darkness into light.

ANSWER 20–2   As three collagen polypeptide chains have to come together to form the triple helix, a single defective polypeptide chain will impair assembly, even if normal chains are present at the same time. Collagen mutations are therefore dominant; that is, they have a deleterious effect even in the presence of a normal copy of the gene.

ANSWER 20–3   The remarkable ability to swell and thus occupy a large volume of space depends on the negative charges. These attract a cloud of positive ions, chiefly Na^+, which by osmosis draw in large amounts of water, thus giving proteoglycans their unique properties. With fewer negative charges, proteoglycans will attract less water and occupy less space. By contrast, uncharged polysaccharides such as cellulose, starch, and glycogen (all composed entirely of glucose subunits) are easily compacted into fibers or granules.

ANSWER 20–4   Focal contacts are common in connective tissue, where fibroblasts exert traction forces on the extracellular matrix, and in cell culture, where cell crawling is observed. The forces for pulling on the matrix or for crawling are generated by the actin cytoskeleton. In mature epithelia, focal contacts are presumably rare because the cells are largely fixed in place and have no need to crawl over the basal lamina or actively pull on it.

ANSWER 20–5   Suppose a cell is damaged so that its plasma membrane becomes leaky. Ions present in high concentration in the extracellular fluid, such as Na^+ and Ca^{2+}, then rush into the cell, and valuable metabolites leak out. If the cell were to remain connected to its healthy neighbors by open gap junctions, these cells too would suffer from the damage. But the influx of Ca^{2+} into the sick cell causes its gap junctions to close immediately, effectively isolating the cell and preventing damage from spreading in this way.

ANSWER 20–6   Ionizing (high-energy) radiation tears through matter, knocking electrons out of their orbits and breaking chemical bonds. In particular, it creates breaks and other damage in DNA, and thus causes cells to arrest in the cell cycle to allow time to repair the damaged DNA before proceeding to cell division (discussed in Chapter 18). If the damage is so severe that it cannot be repaired, cells usually kill themselves by undergoing apoptosis.

ANSWER 20–7   Cells in the gut epithelium are exposed to a quite hostile environment, containing digestive enzymes and many other substances that vary drastically from day to day depending on the food intake of the organism. These epithelial cells form a first line of defense against potentially hazardous compounds and mutagens that we consume or are ubiquitous in our environment. Rapid turnover of epithelial cells protects the organism from harmful consequences, as wounded and sick epithelial cells are discarded (along with undamaged ones during the normal course of gut epithelium renewal). If an epithelial cell started to divide inappropriately as the result of a mutation, for example, it and its unwanted progeny would most often simply be discarded by natural disposal from the tip of the villus: even though such mutations must occur often, they rarely give rise to a cancer.

A neuron, on the other hand, lives in a highly protected environment, largely insulated from the outside world. Its function depends on a complex system of connections with other neurons—a system that is created during development and is not easy to reconstruct if the neuron subsequently dies.

ANSWER 20–8   Every cell division generates one additional cell; so if the cells were never lost or discarded from the body, the number of cells in the body should equal the number of divisions plus one. The number of divisions is 1000-fold greater than the number of cells because, in the course of a lifetime, 1000 cells are discarded by mechanisms such as apoptosis for every cell that is retained in the body.

ANSWER 20–9

A. False. Gap junctions are not connected to the cytoskeleton; they form cell–cell channels that allow small molecules to pass from one cell to another.

B. True. Upon wilting, the turgor pressure in the plant cell is reduced, and consequently the cell walls, having tensile but little compressive strength, like a deflated rubber tire, no longer provide rigidity.

C. False. Proteoglycans can withstand a large amount of compressive force but do not have a rigid structure. Their space-filling properties and ability to resist compression result from their tendency to absorb large amounts of water.

D. True.

E. True.

F. True. Stem cells stably express control genes that ensure that their daughter cells can only develop into certain differentiated cell types.

ANSWER 20–10 Small cytosolic molecules, such as glutamic acid, cyclic AMP, and Ca^{2+} ions, pass readily through both gap junctions and plasmodesmata. Some proteins and mRNAs can pass through plasmodesmata, but all such macromolecules are excluded from gap junctions. Plasma membrane phospholipids diffuse in the plane of the membrane through plasmodesmata because the plasma membranes and smooth ER membranes of adjacent cells are continuous through these junctions. This traffic is not possible through gap junctions, because the membranes of the connected cells remain separate.

ANSWER 20–11 Plants are exposed to extreme changes in the environment, which often are accompanied by huge fluctuations in the osmotic properties of their surroundings. An intermediate-filament network as we know it from animal cells would not be able to provide full osmotic support for cells: the sparse, rivetlike attachment points would not be able to prevent the membrane from bursting in response to a huge osmotic pressure applied from the inside of the cell.

ANSWER 20–12 Action potentials can, in fact, be passed from cell to cell through gap junctions. Indeed, heart muscle cells contract synchronously by this mechanism. This way of passing the signal from cell to cell is rather limited, however. As we discuss in Chapter 12, synapses are far more sophisticated and allow signals to be modulated and integrated with other signals received by the cell. Thus, gap junctions are like simple soldered joints between electrical components, while synapses are like complex relay devices, enabling systems of neurons to perform computations.

ANSWER 20–13 To make jello, gelatin is boiled in water, which denatures the collagen fibers. Upon cooling, the disordered fibers form a tangled mess that solidifies into a gel. This gel actually resembles the collagen as it is initially secreted by fibroblasts. It is not until the fibers have been aligned, bundled, and cross-linked that they acquire their ability to resist tensile forces.

ANSWER 20–14 The evidence that DNA is the blueprint that specifies all the structural characteristics of an organism is based on observations that small changes in the DNA by mutation can result in large changes in the organism. Although DNA provides the plans that specify structure, these plans need to be executed during development. This requires a suitable environment (a human baby would not fit into a stork's egg shell), suitable nourishment, suitable molecular tools present in the egg (such as the appropriate transcription regulators required for early embryo development), suitable spatial organization (such as the asymmetries in the egg cell required to allow for appropriate cell differentiation during the early cell divisions), and so on. Thus inheritance is not restricted to the passing on of the organism's DNA, because development requires appropriate conditions to be set up by the parent. Nevertheless, when all these conditions are met, the plans that are archived in the genome will determine the structure of the organism to be built.

ANSWER 20–15 White blood cells circulate in the bloodstream and migrate into and out of tissues in performance of their normal function of defending the body against infection: they are therefore naturally invasive. Once mutations have occurred to upset the normal controls on production of these cells, there is no need for additional mutations to enable the cells to spread through the body. Thus, the number of mutations that have to accumulate to give rise to leukemia is smaller than for other types of cancer.

ANSWER 20–16 The shape of the curve reflects the need for multiple driver mutations to accumulate in a cell before a cancer results. If a single driver mutation were sufficient, the graph would be a straight horizontal line: the likelihood of occurrence of a particular mutation, and therefore of cancer, would be the same at any age. If two driver mutations were required, the graph would be a straight line sloping upward from the origin: the second mutation has an equal chance of occurring at any time, but will tip the cell into cancerous behavior only if the first mutation has already occurred in the same cell lineage; and the likelihood that the first mutation has already occurred will be proportional to the age of the individual. The steeply curved graph shown in the figure goes up approximately as the fifth power of the age, and this indicates that far more than two driver mutations have to accumulate before cancer sets in. It is not easy to say precisely how many, because of the complex ways in which cancers develop. Successive mutations can alter cell numbers and cell behavior, and thereby change both the probability of subsequent mutations and the selection pressures that drive the evolution of a cancer.

ANSWER 20–17 During exposure to the carcinogen, mutations are induced, but the number of relevant (driver) mutations in any one cell is usually not enough to convert it directly into a cancer cell. Over the years, the cells that have become predisposed to cancer through the induced mutations accumulate progressively more mutations. Eventually, one of the mutant cells will turn into a cancer cell. The long delay between exposure and cancer has made it extremely difficult to hold cigarette manufacturers or producers of industrial carcinogens legally responsible for the damage that is caused by their products.

ANSWER 20–18 By definition, a carcinogen is any substance that promotes the occurrence of one or more types of cancer. The sex hormones can therefore be classified as naturally occurring carcinogens. Although most carcinogens act by directly causing mutations, carcinogenic effects are also often exerted in other ways. The sex hormones increase both the rate of cell division and the survival of cells, thereby increasing cell numbers in hormone-sensitive organs such as breast, uterus, and prostate. The increase in cell division boosts the mutation rate per cell, because mutations, regardless of environmental factors, are spontaneously generated in the course of DNA replication and chromosome segregation. The increase in cell numbers increases the total pool of cells at risk. In these and possibly other ways, the hormones can favor the development of cancer, even though they do not directly cause mutations.

ANSWER 20–19 The short answer is no—cancer in general is not a hereditary disease. It arises from new mutations occurring in our own somatic cells, rather than from mutations we inherit from our parents. In some rare types of cancer, however, there is a strong heritable risk factor, so that parents and their children both show the same predisposition to a specific form of the disease. This occurs, for example, in families carrying a mutation that knocks out one of the two copies of the tumor suppressor gene *APC*; the children then inherit a propensity to colorectal cancer. Much weaker heritable tendencies are also seen in several other cancers, including breast cancer, but the genes responsible for these effects are still mostly unknown.

Glossary

acetyl CoA

Activated carrier that donates the carbon atoms in its readily transferable acetyl group to many metabolic reactions, including the citric acid cycle and fatty acid biosynthesis; the acetyl group is linked to coenzyme A (CoA) by a thioester bond that releases a large amount of energy when hydrolyzed.

acid

A molecule that releases a proton when dissolved in water; this dissociation generates hydronium (H_3O^+) ions, thereby lowering the pH.

actin filament

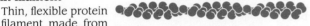

Thin, flexible protein filament made from a chain of globular actin molecules; a major constituent of all eukaryotic cells, this cytoskeletal element is essential for cell movement and for the contraction of muscle cells.

actin-binding protein

Protein that interacts with actin monomers or filaments to control the assembly, structure, and behavior of actin filaments and networks.

action potential

Traveling wave of electrical excitation caused by rapid, transient, self-propagating depolarization of the plasma membrane in a neuron or other excitable cell; also called a nerve impulse.

activated carrier

A small molecule that stores energy or chemical groups in a form that can be donated to many different metabolic reactions. Examples include ATP, acetyl CoA, and NADH.

activation energy

The energy that must be acquired by a molecule to undergo a chemical reaction.

active site

Region on the surface of an enzyme that binds to a substrate molecule and catalyzes its chemical transformation.

active transport

The movement of a solute across a membrane against its electrochemical gradient; requires an input of energy, such as that provided by ATP hydrolysis.

adaptation

Adjustment of sensitivity following repeated stimulation; allows a cell or organism to register small changes in a signal despite a high background level of stimulation.

adenylyl cyclase

Enzyme that catalyzes the formation of cyclic AMP from ATP; an important component in some intracellular signaling pathways.

adherens junction

Cell junction that helps hold together epithelial cells in a sheet of epithelium; actin filaments inside the cell attach to its cytoplasmic face.

ADP

Nucleoside diphosphate produced by hydrolysis of the terminal phosphate of ATP. (*See* Figure 3–31.)

allele

An alternative form of a gene; for a given gene, many alleles may exist in the gene pool of the species.

allosteric

Describes a protein that can exist in multiple conformations depending on the binding of a molecule (ligand) at a site other than the catalytic site; such changes from one conformation to another often alter the protein's activity or ligand affinity.

alpha helix (α helix)

Folding pattern, common in many proteins, in which a single polypeptide chain twists around itself to form a rigid cylinder stabilized by hydrogen bonds between every fourth amino acid.

alternative splicing

The production of different mRNAs (and proteins) from the same gene by splicing its RNA transcripts in different ways.

Alu sequence

Family of mobile genetic elements that comprises about 10% of the human genome; this short, repetitive sequence is no longer mobile on its own, but requires enzymes encoded by other elements to transpose.

amino acid

Small organic molecule containing both an amino group and a carboxyl group; it serves as the building block of proteins.

amino acid sequence

The order of the amino acid subunits in a protein chain. Sometimes called the primary structure of a protein.

aminoacyl-tRNA synthetase

During protein synthesis, an enzyme that attaches the correct amino acid to a tRNA molecule to form a "charged" aminoacyl-tRNA.

amphipathic

Having both hydrophobic and hydrophilic regions, as in a phospholipid or a detergent molecule.

anabolic pathway

Series of enzyme-catalyzed reactions by which large biological molecules are synthesized from smaller subunits; usually requires an input of energy.

anabolism

Set of metabolic pathways by which large molecules are made from smaller ones.

anaphase

Stage of mitosis during which the two sets of chromosomes separate and are pulled toward opposite ends of the dividing cell.

anaphase-promoting complex (APC/C)

A protein complex that triggers the separation of sister chromatids and orchestrates the carefully timed destruction of proteins that control progress through the cell cycle; the complex catalyzes the ubiquitylation of its targets.

antenna complex

In chloroplasts and photosynthetic bacteria, the part of the membrane-bound photosystem that captures energy from sunlight; contains an array of proteins that bind hundreds of chlorophyll molecules and other photosensitive pigments.

antibody
Protein produced by B lymphocytes in response to a foreign molecule or invading organism. Binds to the foreign molecule or cell extremely tightly, thereby inactivating it or marking it for destruction.

anticodon
Set of three consecutive nucleotides in a transfer RNA molecule that recognizes, through base-pairing, the three-nucleotide codon on a messenger RNA molecule; this interaction helps to deliver the correct amino acid to a growing polypeptide chain.

antigen
Molecule or fragment of a molecule that is recognized by an antibody.

antiport
Type of coupled transporter that transfers two different ions or small molecules across a membrane in opposite directions, either simultaneously or in sequence.

apical
Describes the top or the tip of a cell, structure, or organ; in an epithelial cell, for example, this surface is opposite the base, or basal surface.

apoptosis
A tightly controlled form of programmed cell death that allows excess cells to be eliminated from an adult or developing organism.

archaeon
Microscopic organism that is a member of one of the two divisions of prokaryotes; often found in hostile environments such as hot springs or concentrated brine. (*See also* **bacterium**.)

asexual reproduction
Mode of reproduction in which offspring arise from a single parent, producing an individual genetically identical to that parent; includes budding, binary fission, and parthenogenesis.

aster
Star-shaped array of microtubules emanating from a centrosome or from a pole of a mitotic spindle.

atom
The smallest particle of an element that still retains its distinctive chemical properties; consists of a positively charged nucleus surrounded by a cloud of negatively charged electrons.

atomic weight
The mass of an atom relative to the mass of a hydrogen atom; equal to the number of protons plus the number of neutrons that the atom contains.

ATP
Activated carrier that serves as the principal carrier of energy in cells; a nucleoside triphosphate composed of adenine, ribose, and three phosphate groups. (*See* Figure 2–26.)

ATP synthase
Abundant membrane-associated enzyme complex that catalyzes the formation of ATP from ADP and inorganic phosphate during oxidative phosphorylation and photosynthesis.

autophagy
Mechanism by which a cell "eats itself," digesting molecules and organelles that are damaged or obsolete.

Avogadro's number
The number of molecules in a mole, the quantity of a substance equal to its molecular weight in grams; approximately 6×10^{23}.

axon
Long, thin extension that conducts electrical signals away from a nerve cell body toward remote target cells.

bacteriorhodopsin
Pigmented protein found in abundance in the plasma membrane of the salt-loving archaeon Halobacterium halobium; pumps protons out of the cell, fueled by light energy.

bacterium
Microscopic organism that is a member of one of the two divisions of prokaryotes; some species cause disease. The term is sometimes used to refer to any prokaryotic microorganism, although the world of prokaryotes also includes archaea, which are only distantly related to each other. (*See also* **archaeon**.)

basal
Situated near the base; opposite of apical.

basal lamina
Thin mat of extracellular matrix, secreted by epithelial cells, upon which these cells sit.

base
Molecule that accepts a proton when dissolved in water; also used to refer to the nitrogen-containing purines or pyrimidines in DNA and RNA.

base pair
Two complementary nucleotides in an RNA or a DNA molecule that are held together by hydrogen bonds—normally G with C, and A with T or U.

Bcl2 family
Related group of intracellular proteins that regulates apoptosis; some family members promote cell death, others inhibit it.

beta sheet (β sheet)
Folding pattern found in many proteins in which neighboring regions of the polypeptide chain associate side-by-side with each other through hydrogen bonds to give a rigid, flattened structure.

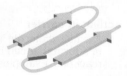

bi-orientation
The symmetrical attachment of a sister-chromatid pair on the mitotic spindle, such that one chromatid in the duplicated chromosome is attached to one spindle pole and the other is attached to the opposite pole.

binding site
Region on the surface of a protein, typically a cavity or groove, that interacts with another molecule (a ligand) through the formation of multiple noncovalent bonds.

biosynthesis
An enzyme-catalyzed process by which complex molecules are formed from simpler substances by living cells; also called anabolism.

bivalent
Structure formed when a duplicated chromosome pairs with its homolog at the beginning of meiosis; contains four sister chromatids.

buffer
Mixture of weak acids and bases that maintains the pH of a solution by releasing and taking up protons.

C-terminus
The end of a polypeptide chain that carries a free carboxyl group (–COOH).

Ca²⁺ pump (or Ca²⁺ ATPase)
An active transporter that uses energy supplied by ATP hydrolysis to actively expel Ca^{2+} from the cell cytosol.

Ca²⁺/calmodulin-dependent protein kinase (CaM-kinase)
Enzyme that phosphorylates target proteins in response to an increase in Ca^{2+} ion concentration through its interaction with the Ca^{2+}-binding protein calmodulin.

cadherin
A member of a family of Ca^{2+}-dependent proteins that mediates the attachment of one cell to another in animal tissues.

calmodulin
Small Ca^{2+}-binding protein that modifies the activity of many target proteins in response to changes in Ca^{2+} concentration.

cancer
Disease caused by abnormal and uncontrolled cell proliferation, followed by invasion and colonization of body sites normally reserved for other cells.

carbon fixation
Process by which green plants and other photosynthetic organisms incorporate carbon atoms from atmospheric carbon dioxide into sugars. The second stage of photosynthesis.

caspase
One of a family of proteases that, when activated, mediates the destruction of the cell by apoptosis.

catabolism
Set of enzyme-catalyzed reactions by which complex molecules are degraded to simpler ones with release of energy; intermediates in these reactions are sometimes called catabolites.

catalyst
Substance that accelerates a chemical reaction by lowering its activation energy; enzymes perform this role in cells.

Cdk (cyclin-dependent protein kinase)
Enzyme that, when complexed with a regulatory cyclin protein, can trigger various events in the cell-division cycle by phosphorylating specific target proteins.

Cdk inhibitor protein
Regulatory protein that blocks the assembly or activity of cyclin–Cdk complexes, delaying progression primarily through the G_1 and S phases of the cell cycle.

cDNA library
Collection of DNA fragments synthesized using all of the mRNAs present in a particular type of cell as a template.

cell
The basic unit from which a living organism is made; an aqueous solution of chemicals, enclosed by a membrane, that has an ability to self-replicate.

cell cortex
Specialized layer of cytoplasm on the inner face of the plasma membrane. In animal cells, it is rich in actin filaments that govern cell shape and drive cell movement.

cell cycle
The orderly sequence of events by which a cell duplicates its contents and divides into two.

cell junction
Specialized region of connection between two cells or between a cell and the extracellular matrix.

cell memory
The ability of differentiated cells and their descendants to maintain their identity.

cell respiration
Process by which cells harvest the energy stored in food molecules; usually accompanied by the uptake of O_2 and the release of CO_2.

cell signaling
The molecular mechanisms by which cells detect and respond to external stimuli and send messages to other cells.

cell wall
Mechanically strong fibrous layer deposited outside the plasma membrane of some cells. Prominent in most plants, bacteria, algae, and fungi, but not present in most animal cells.

cell-cycle control system
Network of regulatory proteins that govern the orderly progression of a eukaryotic cell through the stages of cell division.

cellulose microfibril
Long, thin polysaccharide fiber that helps strengthen plant cell walls.

centriole
Cylindrical array of microtubules usually found in pairs at the center of a centrosome in animal cells. Also found at the base of cilia and flagella, where they are called basal bodies.

centromere
Specialized DNA sequence that allows duplicated chromosomes to be separated during M phase; can be seen as the constricted region of a mitotic chromosome.

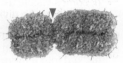

centrosome
Microtubule-organizing center that sits near the nucleus in an animal cell; during the cell cycle, this structure duplicates to form the two poles of the mitotic spindle.

centrosome cycle
Process by which the centrosome duplicates (during interphase) and the two new centrosomes separate (at the beginning of mitosis) to form the poles of the mitotic spindle.

channel
A protein that forms a hydrophilic pore across a membrane, through which selected small molecules or ions can passively diffuse.

chemical bond
A sharing or transfer of electrons that holds two atoms together. (*See also* **covalent bond** and **noncovalent bond**.)

chemical group
A combination of atoms, such as a hydroxyl group (–OH) or an amino group ($-NH_2$), with distinct chemical and physical properties that influence the behavior of the molecule in which it resides.

chemiosmotic coupling
Mechanism that uses the energy stored in a transmembrane proton gradient to drive an energy-requiring process, such as the synthesis of ATP by ATP synthase or the transport of a molecule across a membrane.

chiasma (plural chiasmata)
X-shaped connection between paired homologous chromosomes during meiosis; represents a site of crossing-over between two non-sister chromatids.

chlorophyll
Light-absorbing green pigment that plays a central part in photosynthesis.

chloroplast
Specialized organelle in algae and plants that contains chlorophyll and serves as the site for photosynthesis.

cholesterol

Short, rigid lipid molecule present in large amounts in the plasma membranes of animal cells, where it makes the lipid bilayer less flexible.

chromatin

Complex of DNA and proteins that makes up the chromosomes in a eukaryotic cell.

chromatin-remodeling complex

Enzyme (typically multisubunit) that uses the energy of ATP hydrolysis to alter the arrangement of nucleosomes in eukaryotic chromosomes, changing the accessibility of the underlying DNA to other proteins.

chromatography

Technique used to separate the individual molecules in a complex mixture on the basis of their size, charge, or their ability to bind to a particular chemical group. In a common form of the technique, the mixture is run through a column filled with a material that binds the desired molecule, and it is then eluted from the column with a solvent gradient.

chromosome

Long, threadlike structure composed of DNA and proteins that carries the genetic information of an organism; becomes visible as a distinct entity when a plant or animal cell prepares to divide.

chromosome condensation

Process by which a duplicated chromosome becomes packed into a more compact structure prior to cell division.

cilium

Hairlike structure made of microtubules found on the surface of many eukaryotic cells; when present in large numbers, its rhythmic beating can drive the movement of fluid over the cell surface, as in the epithelium of the lungs.

citric acid cycle

Series of reactions that generate large amounts of NADH by oxidizing acetyl groups derived from food molecules to CO_2. In eukaryotic cells, this central metabolic pathway takes place in the mitochondrial matrix.

classical genetic approach

Experimental techniques used to isolate the genes responsible for an interesting phenotype.

clathrin

Protein that makes up the coat of a type of transport vesicle that buds from either the Golgi apparatus (on the outward secretory pathway) or from the plasma membrane (on the inward endocytic pathway).

coated vesicle

Small membrane-enclosed sac that wears a distinctive layer of proteins on its cytosolic surface. It is formed by pinching-off of a protein-coated region of cell membrane.

codon

Group of three consecutive nucleotides that specifies a particular amino acid or that starts or stops protein synthesis; applies to the nucleotides in an mRNA or in a coding sequence of DNA.

coenzyme

Small molecule that binds tightly to an enzyme and helps it to catalyze a reaction.

cohesin

Protein complex that holds sister chromatids together after DNA has been replicated in the cell cycle.

coiled-coil

Stable, rodlike protein structure formed when two or more α helices twist repeatedly around each other.

collagen

Triple-stranded, fibrous protein that is a major component of the extracellular matrix and connective tissues; it is the main protein in animal tissues, and different forms can be found in skin, tendon, bone, cartilage, and blood vessels.

combinatorial control

Describes the way in which groups of transcription regulators work together to regulate the expression of a single gene.

complementary

Describes two molecular surfaces that fit together closely and form noncovalent bonds with each other. Examples include complementary base pairs, such as A and T, and the two complementary strands of a DNA molecule.

complementary DNA (cDNA)

DNA molecule synthesized from an mRNA molecule and therefore lacking the introns that are present in genomic DNA.

complementation test

Genetic experiment that determines whether two mutations that are associated with the same phenotype lie in the same gene or in different genes.

condensation reaction

Chemical reaction in which a covalent bond is formed between two molecules as water is expelled; used to build polymers, such as proteins, polysaccharides, and nucleic acids.

condensin

Protein complex that helps configure duplicated chromosomes for segregation by making them more compact.

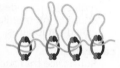

conformation

Precise, three-dimensional shape of a protein or other macromolecule, based on the spatial location of its atoms in relation to one another.

connective tissue

Tissues such as bone, tendons, and the dermis of the skin, in which extracellular matrix makes up the bulk of the tissue and carries the mechanical load.

conserved synteny

The preservation of gene order in the genomes of different species.

contractile ring

Structure made of actin and myosin filaments that forms a belt around a dividing cell, pinching it in two.

coupled reaction

Linked pair of chemical reactions in which free energy released by one reaction serves to drive the other reaction.

covalent bond

Stable chemical link between two atoms produced by sharing one or more pairs of electrons.

CRISPR

System for gene editing based on a bacterial enzyme that uses a guide RNA molecule to search for and modify specific nucleotide sequences in the genome.

crossing-over

Process whereby two homologous chromosomes break at corresponding sites and rejoin to produce two recombined chromosomes that have physically exchanged segments of DNA.

cryoelectron microscopy (cryo-EM)

Technique for observing the detailed structure of a macromolecule at very low temperatures after freezing native structures in ice.

cyclic AMP
Small intracellular signaling molecule generated from ATP in response to hormonal stimulation of cell-surface receptors.

cyclic-AMP-dependent protein kinase (PKA)
Enzyme that phosphorylates target proteins in response to a rise in intracellular cyclic AMP concentration.

cyclin
Regulatory protein whose concentration rises and falls at specific times during the eukaryotic cell cycle; cyclins help control progression from one stage of the cell cycle to the next by binding to cyclin-dependent protein kinases (Cdks).

cytochrome
A family of membrane-bound, colored, heme-containing proteins that transfer electrons during cellular respiration and photosynthesis.

cytochrome _c_ oxidase
Protein complex that serves as the final electron carrier in the respiratory chain; removes electrons from cytochrome _c_ and passes them to O_2 to produce H_2O.

cytokinesis
Process by which the cytoplasm of a plant or animal cell divides in two to form individual daughter cells.

cytoplasm
Contents of a cell that are contained within its plasma membrane but, in the case of eukaryotic cells, outside the nucleus.

cytoskeleton
System of protein filaments in the cytoplasm of a eukaryotic cell that gives the cell shape and the capacity for directed movement. Its most abundant components are actin filaments, microtubules, and intermediate filaments.

cytosol
Contents of the main compartment of the cytoplasm, excluding membrane-enclosed organelles such as endoplasmic reticulum and mitochondria. The cell fraction remaining after membranes, cytoskeletal components, and other organelles have been removed.

dendrite
Short, branching structure that extends from the surface of a nerve cell and receives signals from other neurons.

deoxyribonucleic acid (DNA)
Double-stranded polynucleotide formed from two separate chains of covalently linked deoxyribonucleotide units. It serves as the cell's store of genetic information that is transmitted from generation to generation.

depolarization
A shift in the membrane potential, making it less negative on the inside of the cell.

desmosome
Specialized cell–cell junction, usually formed between two epithelial cells, that serves to connect the ropelike keratin filaments of the adjoining cells, providing tensile strength.

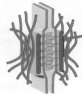

detergent
Soapy substance used to solubilize lipids and membrane proteins.

diacylglycerol (DAG)
Small messenger molecule produced by the cleavage of membrane inositol phospholipids in response to extracellular signals. Helps activate protein kinase C.

dideoxy (Sanger) sequencing
The standard method of determining the nucleotide sequence of DNA; utilizes DNA polymerase and a set of chain-terminating nucleotides.

differentiated cell
Cell that has undergone a coordinated change in gene expression, enabling it to perform a specialized function.

differentiation
Process by which a pluripotent cell undergoes a progressive, coordinated change to a more specialized cell type, brought about by large-scale changes in gene expression.

diffusion
Process by which molecules and small particles move from one location to another by random, thermally driven motion.

diploid
Describes a cell or organism containing two sets of homologous chromosomes, one inherited from each parent. (_See also_ **haploid**.)

disulfide bond
Covalent cross-link formed between the sulfhydryl groups on two cysteine side chains; often used to reinforce a secreted protein's structure or to join two different proteins together.

DNA
Double-stranded polynucleotide formed from two separate chains of covalently linked deoxyribonucleotide units. It serves as the cell's store of genetic information that is transmitted from generation to generation.

DNA cloning
Production of many identical copies of a DNA sequence.

DNA library
Collection of cloned DNA molecules, representing either an entire genome (genomic library) or copies of the mRNA produced by a cell (cDNA library).

DNA ligase
Enzyme that seals nicks that arise in the backbone of a DNA molecule; in the laboratory, can be used to join together two DNA fragments.

DNA methylation
The enzymatic addition of methyl groups to cytosine bases in DNA; this covalent modification generally turns off genes by attracting proteins that block gene expression.

DNA polymerase
Enzyme that catalyzes the synthesis of a DNA molecule from a DNA template using deoxyribonucleoside triphosphate precursors.

DNA repair
Collective term for the enzymatic processes that correct damage to DNA.

DNA replication
The process by which a copy of a DNA molecule is made.

double helix
The typical structure of a DNA molecule in which the two complementary polynucleotide strands are wound around each other with base-pairing between the strands.

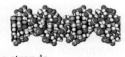

dynamic instability
The rapid switching between growth and shrinkage shown by microtubules.

dynein
Motor protein that uses the energy of ATP hydrolysis to move toward the minus end of a microtubule. One form of the protein is responsible for the bending of cilia.

electrochemical gradient
Driving force that determines which way an ion will move across a membrane; consists of the combined influence of the ion's concentration gradient and the membrane potential.

electron
Negatively charged subatomic particle that occupies space around an atomic nucleus (e^-).

electron microscope
Instrument that illuminates a specimen using beams of electrons to reveal and magnify the structures of very small objects, such as organelles and large molecules.

electron-transport chain
A series of membrane-embedded electron carrier molecules that facilitate the movement of electrons from a higher to a lower energy level, as in oxidative phosphorylation and photosynthesis.

electronegativity
The tendency of an atom to attract electrons.

electrophoresis
Technique for separating a mixture of proteins or DNA fragments by placing them on a polymer gel and subjecting them to an electric field. The molecules migrate through the gel at different speeds depending on their size and net charge.

electrostatic attraction
Force that draws together oppositely charged atoms. Examples include ionic bonds and the attractions between molecules containing polar covalent bonds.

embryonic stem (ES) cell
An undifferentiated cell type derived from the inner cell mass of an early mammalian embryo and capable of differentiating to give rise to any of the specialized cell types in the adult body.

endocytosis
Process by which cells take in materials through an invagination of the plasma membrane, which surrounds the ingested material in a membrane-enclosed vesicle. (*See also* **pinocytosis** and **phagocytosis**.)

endomembrane system
Interconnected network of membrane-enclosed organelles in a eukaryotic cell; includes the endoplasmic reticulum, Golgi apparatus, lysosomes, peroxisomes, and endosomes.

endoplasmic reticulum (ER)
Labyrinthine membrane-enclosed compartment in the cytoplasm of eukaryotic cells where lipids and proteins are made.

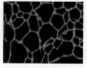

endosome
Membrane-enclosed compartment of a eukaryotic cell through which material ingested by endocytosis passes on its way to lysosomes.

entropy
Thermodynamic quantity that measures the degree of disorder in a system.

enzyme
A protein that catalyzes a specific chemical reaction.

enzyme-coupled receptor
Transmembrane protein that, when stimulated by the binding of a ligand, activates an intracellular enzyme (either a separate enzyme or part of the receptor itself).

epigenetic inheritance
The transmission of a heritable pattern of gene expression from one cell to its progeny that does not involve altering the nucleotide sequence of the DNA.

epithelium (plural epithelia)
Sheet of cells covering an external surface or lining an internal body cavity.

equilibrium
State in which the forward and reverse rates of a chemical reaction are equal so that no net chemical change occurs.

equilibrium constant, *K*
For a reversible chemical reaction, the ratio of substrate to product when the rates of the forward and reverse reactions are equal.

euchromatin
One of the two main states in which chromatin exists within an interphase cell. Prevalent in gene-rich areas, its less compact structure allows access for proteins involved in transcription. (*See also* **heterochromatin**.)

eukaryote
An organism whose cells have a distinct nucleus and cytoplasm.

evolution
Process of gradual modification and adaptation that occurs in living organisms over generations.

exocytosis
Process by which most molecules are secreted from a eukaryotic cell. These molecules are packaged in membrane-enclosed vesicles that fuse with the plasma membrane, releasing their contents to the outside.

exon
Segment of a eukaryotic gene that is transcribed into RNA and dictates the amino acid sequence of part of a protein.

exon shuffling
Mechanism for the evolution of new genes; in the process, coding sequences from different genes are brought together to generate a protein with a new combination of domains.

extracellular matrix
Complex network of polysaccharides (such as glycosaminoglycans or cellulose) and proteins (such as collagen) secreted by cells. A structural component of tissues that also influences their development and physiology.

extracellular signal molecule
Any molecule present outside the cell that can elicit a response inside the cell when the molecule binds to a receptor.

FAD
A molecule that accepts electrons and hydrogen atoms from an electron donor; see **FADH₂**.

FADH₂
A high-energy electron carrier produced by reduction of FAD during the breakdown of molecules derived from food, including fatty acids and acetyl CoA.

fat
Type of lipid used by living cells to store metabolic energy. Mainly composed of triacylglycerols. (*See* Panel 2–5, pp. 74–75.)

fat droplet
Large cluster of hydrophobic fats or oils that forms inside the cells.

fatty acid
Molecule that consists of a carboxylic acid attached to a long hydrocarbon chain.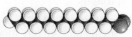
Used as a major source of energy during metabolism and as a starting point for the synthesis of phospholipids.

feedback inhibition
A form of metabolic control in which the end product of

a chain of enzymatic reactions reduces the activity of an enzyme early in the pathway.

feedback regulation
Process whereby enzymes are either positively or negatively regulated in response to the levels of metabolites that are not their substrates.

fermentation
The breakdown of organic molecules without the involvement of molecular oxygen. This form of oxidation yields less energy than aerobic cell respiration.

fertilization
The fusion of two gametes—sperm and egg—to produce a new individual organism.

fibroblast
Cell type that produces the collagen-rich extracellular matrix in connective tissues such as skin and tendon. Proliferates readily in wounded tissue and in tissue culture.

fibronectin
Extracellular matrix protein that helps cells attach to the matrix by acting as a "linker" that binds to a cell-surface integrin molecule on one end and to a matrix component, such as collagen, on the other.

fibrous protein
A protein with an elongated, rodlike shape, such as collagen or a keratin filament.

filopodium
Long, thin, actin-containing extension on the surface of an animal cell. Sometimes has an exploratory function, as in a growth cone.

flagellum
Long, whiplike structure capable of propelling a cell through a fluid medium with its rhythmic beating. Eukaryotic flagella are longer versions of cilia; bacterial flagella are completely different, being smaller and simpler in construction.

fluorescence microscope
Instrument used to visualize a specimen that has been labeled with a fluorescent dye; samples are illuminated with a wavelength of light that excites the dye, causing it to fluoresce.

free energy, G
Energy that can be harnessed to do work, such as driving a chemical reaction.

free-energy change, ΔG
"Delta G": in a chemical reaction, the difference in free energy between reactant and product molecules. A large negative value of ΔG indicates that the reaction has a strong tendency to occur. (*See also* **standard free-energy change**.)

G protein
A membrane-bound GTP-binding protein involved in intracellular signaling; composed of three subunits, this intermediary is usually activated by the binding of a hormone or other ligand to a transmembrane receptor.

G-protein-coupled receptor (GPCR)
Cell-surface receptor that associates with an intracellular trimeric GTP-binding protein (G protein) after activation by an extracellular ligand. These receptors are embedded in the membrane by seven transmembrane α helices.

G₁ cyclin
Regulatory protein that helps drive a cell through the first gap phase of the cell cycle and toward S phase.

G₁ phase
Gap 1 phase of the eukaryotic cell cycle; falls between the end of cytokinesis and the start of DNA synthesis.

G₁-Cdk
Protein complex whose activity drives the cell through the first gap phase of the cell cycle; consists of a G₁ cyclin plus a cyclin-dependent protein kinase (Cdk).

G₁/S cyclin
Regulatory protein that helps to launch the S phase of the cell cycle.

G₁/S-Cdk
Protein complex whose activity triggers entry into S phase of the cell cycle; consists of a G₁/S cyclin plus a cyclin-dependent protein kinase (Cdk).

G₂ phase
Gap 2 phase of the eukaryotic cell cycle; falls between the end of DNA synthesis and the beginning of mitosis.

gain-of-function mutation
Genetic change that increases the activity of a gene or makes it active in inappropriate circumstances; such mutations are usually dominant.

gamete
Cell type in a diploid organism that carries only one set of chromosomes and is specialized for sexual reproduction. A sperm or an egg; also called a germ cell.

gamete
Cell type in a diploid organism that carries only one set of chromosomes and is specialized for sexual reproduction. A sperm or an egg; also called a germ cell.

gap junction
In animal tissues, specialized connection between juxtaposed cells through which ions and small molecules can pass from one cell to the other.

GDP
Nucleoside diphosphate that is produced by the hydrolysis of the terminal phosphate of GTP, a reaction that also produces inorganic phosphate.

gene
Unit of heredity containing the instructions that dictate the characteristics or phenotype of an organism; in molecular terms, a segment of DNA that directs the production of a particular protein or functional RNA molecule.

gene duplication and divergence
A process by which new genes can form; involves the accidental generation of an additional copy of a stretch of DNA containing one or more genes, followed by an accumulation of mutations that over time can alter the function or expression of either the original or its copy.

gene expression
The process by which a gene makes a product that is useful to the cell or organism by directing the synthesis of a protein or an RNA molecule with a characteristic activity.

gene family
A set of related genes that has arisen through a process of gene duplication and divergence.

gene knockout
A genetically engineered animal in which a specific gene has been inactivated.

general transcription factors
Proteins that assemble on the promoters of eukaryotic genes near the start site of transcription and load the RNA polymerase in the correct position.

genetic code
Set of rules by which the information contained in the nucleotide sequence of a gene and its corresponding RNA

molecule is translated into the amino acid sequence of a protein.

genetic instability
An increased rate of mutation often caused by defects in the systems that govern the accurate replication and maintenance of the genome; the resulting mutations sometimes drive the evolution of cancer.

genetic map
A graphic representation of the order of genes in chromosomes spaced according to the amount of recombination that occurs between them.

genetic screen
Experimental technique used to search through a collection of mutants for a particular phenotype.

genetics
The study of genes, heredity, and the variation that gives rise to differences between one living organism and another.

genome
The total genetic information carried by all the chromosomes of a cell or organism; in humans, the total number of nucleotide pairs in the 22 autosomes plus the X and Y chromosomes.

genomic library
Collection of cloned DNA molecules that represents the entire genome of a cell.

genotype
The genetic makeup of a cell or organism, including which alleles (gene variants) it carries.

germ line
The lineage of reproductive cells that contributes to the formation of a new generation of organisms, as distinct from somatic cells, which form the body and leave no descendants in the next generation.

globular protein
Any protein in which the polypeptide chain folds into a compact, rounded shape. Includes most enzymes.

gluconeogenesis
Set of enzyme-catalyzed reactions by which glucose is synthesized from small organic molecules such as pyruvate, lactate, or amino acids; in effect, the reverse of glycolysis.

glucose
Six-carbon sugar that plays a major role in the metabolism of living cells. Stored in polymeric form as glycogen in animal cells and as starch in plant cells. (*See* Panel 2–4, pp. 72–73.)

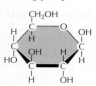

glycocalyx
Protective layer of carbohydrates on the outside surface of the plasma membrane formed by the sugar residues of membrane glycoproteins, proteoglycans, and glycolipids.

glycogen
Branched polymer composed exclusively of glucose units used to store energy in animal cells. Granules of this material are especially abundant in liver and muscle cells.

glycolysis
Series of enzyme-catalyzed oxidation reactions in which sugars are partially degraded and their energy is captured by the activated carriers ATP and NADH. (Literally, "sugar splitting.")

glycosaminoglycan (GAG)
Polysaccharide chain that can form a gel that acts as a "space filler" in the extracellular matrix of connective tissues; helps animal tissues resist compression.

Golgi apparatus
Membrane-enclosed organelle in eukaryotic cells that modifies the proteins and lipids made in the endoplasmic reticulum and sorts them for transport to other sites.

gradient-driven pump
A protein that uses energy stored in the electrochemical gradient of ions to actively transport a solute across a membrane.

green fluorescent protein (GFP)
Fluorescent protein, isolated from a jellyfish, that is used experimentally as a marker for monitoring the location and movement of proteins in living cells.

growth factor
Extracellular signal molecule that stimulates a cell to increase in size and mass. Examples include epidermal growth factor (EGF) and platelet-derived growth factor (PDGF).

GTP
Nucleoside triphosphate used in the synthesis of RNA and DNA. Like the closely related ATP, serves as an activated carrier in some energy-transfer reactions. Also has a special role in microtubule assembly, protein synthesis, and cell signaling.

GTP-binding protein
Intracellular signaling protein whose activity is determined by its association with either GTP or GDP. Includes both trimeric G proteins and monomeric GTPases, such as Ras.

H⁺ pump
A protein or protein complex that uses energy supplied by ATP hydrolysis, an ion gradient, or light to actively move protons across a membrane.

haploid
Describes a cell or organism with only one set of chromosomes, such as a sperm cell or a bacterium. (*See also* **diploid**.)

haplotype block
A combination of alleles or other DNA markers that has been inherited as a unit, undisturbed by genetic recombination, across many generations.

helix
An elongated structure whose subunits twist in a regular fashion around a central axis, like a spiral staircase.

hemidesmosome
Structure that anchors epithelial cells to the basal lamina beneath them.

heterochromatin
Highly condensed region of an interphase chromosome; generally gene-poor and transcriptionally inactive. (*See also* **euchromatin**.)

heterozygous
Possessing dissimilar alleles for a given gene.

histone
One of a small group of abundant, highly conserved proteins around which DNA wraps to form nucleosomes, structures that represent the most fundamental level of chromatin packing.

histone-modifying enzyme
Enzyme that catalyzes the covalent addition of a small molecule, such as a methyl or acetate group, to a specific amino acid side chain on a histone.

homolog
A gene, chromosome, or any structure that has a close similarity to another as a result of common ancestry.

homologous

Describes genes, chromosomes, or any structures that are similar because of their common evolutionary origin. Can also refer to similarities between protein sequences or nucleic acid sequences.

homologous gene—*see* **homologous.**

homologous recombination

Mechanism by which double-strand breaks in a DNA molecule can be repaired flawlessly; uses an undamaged, duplicated, or homologous chromosome to guide the repair. During meiosis, the mechanism results in an exchange of genetic information between the maternal and paternal homologs.

homozygous

Possessing identical alleles for a given gene.

horizontal gene transfer

Process by which DNA is passed from the genome of one organism to that of another, even to an individual from another species. This contrasts with "vertical" gene transfer, which refers to the transfer of genetic information from parent to progeny.

hormone

Extracellular signal molecule that is secreted and transported via the bloodstream (in animals) or the sap (in plants) to target tissues on which it exerts a specific effect.

hybridization

Experimental technique in which two complementary nucleic acid strands come together and form hydrogen bonds to produce a double helix; used to detect specific nucleotide sequences in either DNA or RNA.

hydrogen bond

A weak noncovalent interaction between a positively charged hydrogen atom in one molecule and a negatively charged atom, such as nitrogen or oxygen, in another; hydrogen bonds are key to the structure and properties of water.

hydrolysis

Chemical reaction that involves cleavage of a covalent bond with the accompanying consumption of water (its –H being added to one product of the cleavage and its –OH to the other); the reverse of a condensation reaction.

hydronium ion

The form taken by a proton (H^+) in aqueous solution.

hydrophilic

Molecule or part of a molecule that readily forms hydrogen bonds with water, allowing it to readily dissolve; literally, "water loving."

hydrophobic

Nonpolar, uncharged molecule or part of a molecule that forms no hydrogen bonds with water molecules and therefore does not dissolve; literally, "water fearing."

hydrophobic force

A noncovalent interaction that forces together the hydrophobic portions of dissolved molecules to minimize their disruption of the hydrogen-bonded network of water; causes membrane phospholipids to self-assemble into a bilayer and helps to fold proteins into a compact, globular shape.

***in situ* hybridization**

Technique in which a single-stranded RNA or DNA probe is used to locate a complementary nucleotide sequence in a chromosome, cell, or tissue; used to diagnose genetic disorders or to track gene expression.

induced pluripotent stem (iPS) cell

Somatic cell that has been reprogrammed to resemble and behave like a pluripotent embryonic stem (ES) cell through the artificial introduction of a set of genes encoding particular transcription regulators.

initiator tRNA

Special tRNA that initiates the translation of an mRNA in a ribosome. It always carries the amino acid methionine.

inorganic

Not composed of carbon atoms.

inositol 1,4,5-trisphosphate (IP₃)

Small intracellular signaling molecule that triggers the release of Ca^{2+} from the endoplasmic reticulum into the cytosol; produced when a signal molecule activates a membrane-bound protein called phospholipase C.

inositol phospholipid

Minor lipid component of plasma membranes that plays a part in signal transduction in eukaryotic cells; cleavage yields two small messenger molecules, IP₃ and diacylglycerol.

integrin

One of a family of transmembrane proteins present on cell surfaces that enable cells to make and break attachments to the extracellular matrix, allowing them to crawl through a tissue.

intermediate filament

Fibrous cytoskeletal element, about 10 nm in diameter, that forms ropelike networks in animal cells; helps cells resist tension applied from outside.

interphase

Long period of the cell cycle between one mitosis and the next. Includes G_1 phase, S phase, and G_2 phase.

intracellular condensate

A large aggregate of phase-separated macromolecules that creates a region with a special biochemistry without the use of an encapsulating membrane.

intracellular signaling pathway

A set of proteins and small-molecule second messengers that interact with each other to relay a signal from the cell membrane to its final destination in the cytoplasm or nucleus.

intrinsically disordered sequence

Region in a polypeptide chain that lacks a definite structure.

intron

Noncoding sequence within a eukaryotic gene that is transcribed into an RNA molecule but is then excised by RNA splicing to produce an mRNA.

ion

An atom carrying an electrical charge, either positive or negative.

ion channel

Transmembrane protein that forms a pore across the lipid bilayer through which specific inorganic ions can diffuse down their electrochemical gradients.

ion-channel-coupled receptor

Transmembrane receptor protein or protein complex that opens in response to the binding of a ligand to its external face, allowing the passage of a specific inorganic ion.

ionic bond

Interaction formed when one atom donates electrons to another; this transfer of electrons causes both atoms to become electrically charged.

iron–sulfur center
Tightly bound metal complex that carries electrons in proteins that operate early in the electron-transport chain; has a relatively weak affinity for electrons.

K+ leak channel
Ion channel permeable to K+ that randomly flickers between an open and closed state; largely responsible for the resting membrane potential in animal cells.

karyotype
An ordered display of the full set of chromosomes of a cell, arranged with respect to size, shape, and number.

keratin filament
Class of intermediate filament abundant in epithelial cells, where it provides tensile strength; main structural component of hair, feathers, and claws.

kinesin
A large family of motor proteins that uses the energy of ATP hydrolysis to move toward the plus end of a microtubule.

kinetochore
Protein complex that assembles on the centromere of a condensed mitotic chromosome; the site to which spindle microtubules attach.

L1 element
Type of retrotransposon that constitutes 15% of the human genome; also called LINE-1.

lagging strand
At a replication fork, the DNA strand that is made discontinuously in short fragments that are later joined together to form one continuous new strand.

lamellipodium
Dynamic sheetlike extension on the surface of an animal cell, especially one migrating over a surface.

law of independent assortment
Principle that, during gamete formation, the alleles for different traits segregate independently of one another; Mendel's second law of inheritance.

law of segregation
Principle that the maternal and paternal alleles for a trait separate from one another during gamete formation and then reunite during fertilization; Mendel's first law of inheritance.

leading strand
At a replication fork, the DNA strand that is made by continuous synthesis in the 5′-to-3′ direction.

ligand
General term for a small molecule that binds to a specific site on a macromolecule.

ligand-gated channel
An ion channel that is stimulated to open by the binding of a small molecule such as a neurotransmitter.

light reactions
In photosynthesis, the set of reactions that converts the energy of sunlight into chemical energy in the form of ATP and NADPH (stage 1 of photosynthesis).

lipid
An organic molecule that is insoluble in water but dissolves readily in nonpolar organic solvents; typically contains long hydrocarbon chains or multiple rings. One class, the phospholipids, forms the structural basis for biological membranes.

lipid bilayer
Thin pair of closely juxtaposed sheets, composed mainly of phospholipid molecules, that forms the structural basis for all cell membranes.

local mediator
Secreted signal molecule that acts at a short range on adjacent cells.

long noncoding RNA
Class of RNA molecules more than 200 nucleotides in length that does not encode proteins. Often used to regulate gene expression.

loss-of-function mutation
A genetic alteration that reduces or eliminates the activity of a gene. Such mutations are usually recessive: the organism can function normally as long as it retains at least one normal copy of the affected gene.

lysosome
Membrane-enclosed organelle that breaks down worn-out proteins and organelles and other waste materials, as well as molecules taken up by endocytosis; contains digestive enzymes that are typically most active at the acid pH found inside these organelles.

lysozyme
Enzyme that severs the polysaccharide chains that form the cell walls of bacteria; found in many secretions including saliva and tears, where it serves as an antibiotic.

M cyclin
Regulatory protein that binds to mitotic Cdk to form M-Cdk, the protein complex that triggers the M phase of the cell cycle.

M phase
Period of the eukaryotic cell cycle during which the nucleus and cytoplasm divide.

M-Cdk
Protein complex that triggers the M phase of the cell cycle; consists of an M cyclin plus a mitotic cyclin-dependent protein kinase (Cdk).

macromolecule
Polymer built from covalently linked subunits; includes proteins, nucleic acids, and polysaccharides with a molecular mass greater than a few thousand daltons.

MAP kinase
Mitogen-activated protein kinase. Signaling molecule that is the final kinase in a three-kinase sequence called the MAP-kinase signaling module.

MAP-kinase signaling module
Set of three functionally interlinked protein kinases that allows cells to respond to extracellular signal molecules that stimulate proliferation; includes a mitogen-activated protein kinase (MAP kinase), a MAP kinase kinase, and a MAP kinase kinase kinase.

mass spectrometry
Sensitive technique that enables the determination of the exact mass of all of the molecules in a complex mixture.

matrix
Large internal compartment within a mitochondrion.

mechanically-gated channel
An ion channel that allows the passage of select ions across a membrane in response to a physical perturbation.

meiosis
Specialized type of cell division by which eggs and sperm cells are made. Two successive nuclear divisions with only one round of DNA replication generate four haploid cells from an initial diploid cell.

membrane domain
Functionally and structurally specialized region in the

membrane of a cell or organelle; typically characterized by the presence of specific proteins.

membrane potential

Voltage difference across a membrane due to a slight excess of positive ions on one side and of negative ions on the other.

membrane protein

A protein associated with the lipid bilayer of a cell membrane.

membrane transport protein

Any transmembrane protein that provides a passageway for the movement of select substances across a cell membrane.

membrane-enclosed organelle

Any organelle in a eukaryotic cell that is surrounded by a lipid bilayer—for example, the endoplasmic reticulum, Golgi apparatus, and lysosome.

messenger RNA (mRNA)

RNA molecule that specifies the amino acid sequence of a protein.

metabolism

The sum total of the chemical reactions that take place in the cells of a living organism.

metaphase

Stage of mitosis in which chromosomes are properly attached to the mitotic spindle at its equator but have not yet segregated toward opposite poles.

metastasis

The spread of cancer cells from the initial site of the tumor to form secondary tumors at other sites in the body.

Michaelis constant (K_M)

The concentration of substrate at which an enzyme works at half its maximum velocity; serves as a measure of how tightly the substrate is bound.

micrometer

Unit of length equal to one millionth (10^{-6}) of a meter or 10^{-4} centimeter.

microRNA (miRNA)

Small noncoding RNA that controls gene expression by base-pairing with a specific mRNA to regulate its stability and its translation.

microscope

Instrument for viewing extremely small objects. Some use a focused beam of visible light and are used to examine cells and organelles. Others use a beam of electrons and can be used to examine objects as small as individual molecules.

microtubule

Long, stiff, cylindrical structure composed of the protein tubulin. Used by eukaryotic cells to organize their cytoplasm and guide the intracellular transport of macromolecules and organelles.

microtubule-associated protein

Accessory protein that binds to microtubules; can stabilize microtubule filaments, link them to other cell structures, or transport various components along their length.

mismatch repair

Mechanism for recognizing and correcting incorrectly paired nucleotides—those that are noncomplementary.

mitochondrion

Membrane-enclosed organelle, about the size of a bacterium, that carries out oxidative phosphorylation and produces most of the ATP in eukaryotic cells.

mitogen

An extracellular signal molecule that stimulates cell proliferation.

mitosis

Division of the nucleus of a eukaryotic cell.

mitotic spindle

Array of microtubules and associated molecules that forms between the opposite poles of a eukaryotic cell during mitosis and pulls duplicated chromosome sets apart.

mobile genetic element

Short segment of DNA that can move, sometimes through an RNA intermediate, from one location in a genome to another; an important source of genetic variation in most genomes. Also called a transposon.

model organism

A living thing selected for intensive study as a representative of a large group of species. Examples include the mouse (representing mammals), the yeast *Saccharomyces cerevisiae* (representing a unicellular eukaryote), and *Escherichia coli* (representing bacteria).

molecular switch

Intracellular signaling protein that toggles between an active and inactive state in response to receiving a signal.

molecular weight

Sum of the atomic weights of the atoms in a molecule; as a ratio of molecular masses, it is a number without units.

molecule

Group of atoms joined together by covalent bonds.

monomer

Small molecule that can be linked to others of a similar type to form a larger molecule (polymer).

monomeric GTPase

Small, single-subunit GTP-binding protein. Proteins of this family, such as Ras and Rho, are part of many different signaling pathways.

motor protein

Protein such as myosin or kinesin that uses energy derived from the hydrolysis of a tightly bound ATP molecule to propel itself along a protein filament or polymeric molecule.

mutation

A randomly produced, permanent change in the nucleotide sequence of DNA.

myofibril

Long, cylindrical structure that constitutes the contractile element of a muscle cell; constructed of arrays of highly organized bundles of actin, myosin, and other accessory proteins.

myosin

Type of motor protein that uses ATP to drive movements along actin filaments. One subtype interacts with actin to form the thick contractile bundles of skeletal muscle.

myosin filament

Polymer composed of interacting molecules of myosin-II; interaction with actin promotes contraction in muscle and nonmuscle cells.

myosin-I

Simplest type of myosin, present in all cells; consists of a single actin-binding head and a tail that can attach to other molecules or organelles.

myosin-II

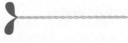

Type of myosin that exists as a dimer with two actin-binding heads and a coiled-coil tail; can associate to form long myosin filaments.

N-terminus
The end of a polypeptide chain that carries a free α-amino group.

Na+ pump (or **Na+-K+ ATPase**)
Transporter found in the plasma membrane of most animal cells that actively pumps Na+ out of the cell and K+ in using the energy derived from ATP hydrolysis.

NAD+
A molecule that accepts a hydride ion (H−) from a donor molecule, thereby producing the activated carrier NADH. Widely used in the energy-producing breakdown of sugar molecules. (*See* Figure 3–34.)

NADH
Activated carrier of electrons that is widely used in the energy-producing breakdown of sugar molecules. (*See* Figure 3–34.)

NADP+
Molecule that accepts a hydride ion (H−) from a donor molecule, thereby producing the activated carrier NADPH; widely used as an electron donor in biosynthetic pathways.

NADPH
Activated carrier closely related to NADH and used as an electron donor in biosynthetic pathways. In the process it is oxidized to NADP+.

Nernst equation
An equation that relates the concentrations of an inorganic ion on the two sides of a permeable membrane to the membrane potential at which there would be no net movement of the ion across the membrane.

nerve terminal
Structure at the end of an axon that signals to another neuron or target cell.

neuron
An electrically excitable cell that integrates and transmits information as part of the nervous system; a nerve cell.

neurotransmitter
Small signaling molecule secreted by a nerve cell at a synapse to transmit information to a postsynaptic cell. Examples include acetylcholine, glutamate, GABA, and glycine.

nitric oxide (NO)
Locally acting gaseous signal molecule that diffuses across cell membranes to affect the activity of intracellular proteins.

nitrogen fixation
Conversion of nitrogen gas from the atmosphere into nitrogen-containing molecules by soil bacteria and cyanobacteria; requires a great deal of energy.

noncovalent bond
Chemical association that does not involve the sharing of electrons; singly they are relatively weak, but they can sum together to produce strong, highly specific interactions between molecules. Examples are hydrogen bonds and van der Waals attractions.

nonhomologous end joining
An error-prone mechanism for repairing double-strand breaks in DNA by rejoining the two broken ends; often results in a loss of information at the site of repair.

nuclear envelope
Double membrane surrounding the nucleus. Consists of outer and inner membranes, perforated by nuclear pores.

nuclear lamina
Fibrous layer on the inner surface of the inner nuclear membrane formed as a network of intermediate filaments made from nuclear lamins.

nuclear magnetic resonance (NMR) spectroscopy
Technique used for determining the three-dimensional structure of a protein in solution.

nuclear pore
Channel through which selected large molecules move between the nucleus and the cytoplasm.

nuclear receptor
Protein inside a eukaryotic cell that, on binding to a signal molecule, enters the nucleus and regulates transcription.

nucleolus
Large structure within the nucleus where ribosomal RNA is transcribed and ribosomal subunits are assembled.

nucleosome
Beadlike structural unit of a eukaryotic chromosome composed of a short length of DNA wrapped around an octameric core of histone proteins; includes a nucleosomal core particle (DNA plus histone protein) along with a segment of linker DNA that ties the core particles together.

nucleotide
Basic building block of the nucleic acids, DNA and RNA; a nucleoside linked to a phosphate.

nucleus
In biology, refers to the prominent, rounded structure that contains the DNA of a eukaryotic cell. In chemistry, refers to the dense, positively charged center of an atom.

Okazaki fragment
Short length of DNA, including an RNA primer, produced on the lagging strand during DNA replication. Following primer removal, adjacent fragments are rapidly joined together by DNA ligase to form a continuous DNA strand.

oncogene
A gene that, when activated, can potentially make a cell cancerous. Typically a mutant form of a normal gene (proto-oncogene) involved in the control of cell growth or division.

open reading frame (ORF)
Long sequence of nucleotides that contains no stop codon; used to identify potential protein-coding sequences in DNA.

optogenetics
Technique that uses light to control the activity of neurons into which light-gated ion channels have been artificially introduced.

organelle
A discrete structure or subcompartment of a eukaryotic cell that is specialized to carry out a particular function. Examples include mitochondria and the Golgi apparatus.

organic molecule
Chemical compound that contains carbon and hydrogen.

organoid
A miniature, three-dimensional collection of tissues formed from the proliferation, differentiation, and self-assembly of pluripotent cells in culture.

osmosis
Passive movement of water across a cell membrane from a region where the concentration of water is high (because the concentration of solutes is low) to a region where the concentration of water is low (and the concentration of solutes is high).

oxidation
Removal of electrons from an atom, as occurs during the addition of oxygen to a carbon atom or when a hydrogen is removed from a carbon atom; can also refer to a partial shift of electrons between atoms linked by a covalent bond.

oxidative phosphorylation
Membrane-based process in bacteria and mitochondria in which ATP formation is driven by the transfer of electrons from food molecules to molecular oxygen.

p53
Transcription regulator that controls the cell's response to DNA damage, preventing the cell from entering S phase until the damage has been repaired or inducing the cell to commit suicide if the damage is too extensive; mutations in the gene encoding this protein are found in many human cancers.

pairing
In meiosis, the process by which a pair of duplicated homologous chromosomes attach to one another to form a structure containing four sister chromatids.

passive transport
The spontaneous movement of a solute down its concentration gradient across a cell membrane via a membrane transport protein, such as a channel or a transporter.

patch-clamp recording
Technique used to monitor the activity of ion channels in a membrane; involves the formation of a tight seal between the tip of a glass electrode and a small region of cell membrane, and manipulation of the membrane potential by varying the concentrations of ions in the electrode.

pedigree
Chart showing the line of descent, or ancestry, of an individual organism.

peptide bond
Covalent chemical bond between the carbonyl group of one amino acid and the amino group of a second amino acid. (*See* Panel 2–6, pp. 76–77.)

peroxisome
Small membrane-enclosed organelle that contains enzymes that degrade lipids and destroy toxins.

pH scale
Concentration of hydrogen ions in a solution, expressed as a logarithm. An acidic solution with pH 3 will contain 10^{-3} M hydrogen ions.

phagocytic cell
A cell such as a macrophage or neutrophil that is specialized to take up particles and microorganisms by phagocytosis.

phagocytosis
The process by which particulate material is engulfed ("eaten") by a cell. Prominent in predatory cells, such as *Amoeba proteus*, and in cells of the vertebrate immune system, such as macrophages.

phenotype
The observable characteristics of a cell or organism.

phosphatidylcholine
Common phospholipid present in abundance in most cell membranes; uses choline attached to a phosphate as its head group.

phosphoinositide 3-kinase (PI 3-kinase)
Enzyme that phosphorylates inositol phospholipids in the plasma membrane, which generates docking sites for intracellular signaling proteins that promote cell growth and survival.

phospholipase C
Enzyme associated with the plasma membrane that generates two small messenger molecules in response to activation.

phospholipid
A major type of lipid molecule in many cell membranes. Generally composed of two fatty acid tails linked to one of a variety of phosphate-containing polar groups.

photosynthesis
The process by which plants, algae, and some bacteria use the energy of sunlight to drive the synthesis of organic molecules from carbon dioxide and water.

photosystem
Large multiprotein complex containing chlorophyll that captures light energy and converts it into chemical-bond energy; consists of a set of antenna complexes and a reaction center.

phragmoplast
In a dividing plant cell, structure made of microtubules and membrane vesicles that guides the formation of a new cell wall.

phylogenetic tree
Diagram or "family tree" showing the evolutionary relationships among groups of organisms or proteins.

pinocytosis
Type of endocytosis in which soluble materials are taken up from the environment and incorporated into vesicles for digestion. (Literally, "cell drinking.")

plasma membrane
The protein-containing lipid bilayer that surrounds a living cell.

plasmid
Small, circular DNA molecule that replicates independently of the genome. Used extensively as a vector for DNA cloning.

plasmodesma (plural plasmodesmata)
Cell–cell junction that connects one plant cell to the next; consists of a channel of cytoplasm lined by membrane.

pluripotent
Capable of giving rise to any type of cell or tissue.

point mutation
Change in a single nucleotide pair in a DNA sequence.

polar
In chemistry, describes a molecule or bond in which electrons are distributed unevenly.

polarity
An inherent asymmetry that allows one end of an object to be distinguished from another; can refer to a molecule, a polymer (such as an actin filament), or even a cell (for example, an epithelial cell that lines the mammalian small intestine).

polyadenylation
The addition of multiple adenine nucleotides to the 3′ end of a newly synthesized mRNA molecule.

polymer
Long molecule made by covalently linking multiple identical or similar subunits (monomers).

polymerase chain reaction (PCR)
Technique for amplifying selected regions of DNA by multiple cycles of DNA synthesis; can produce billions of copies of a given sequence in a matter of hours.

polymorphism
DNA sequence for which two or more variants are present at high frequency in the general population.

polypeptide backbone
Repeating sequence of the atoms (–N–C–C–) that form the

core of a protein molecule and to which the amino acid side chains are attached.

polypeptide, polypeptide chain
Linear polymer composed of multiple amino acids. Proteins are composed of one or more long polypeptide chains.

positive feedback loop
An important form of regulation in which the end product of a reaction or pathway stimulates continued production or activity; controls a variety of biological processes, including enzyme activity, cell signaling, and gene expression.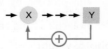

post-transcriptional control
Regulation of gene expression that occurs after transcription of the gene has begun; examples include RNA splicing and translational control.

primary structure
The amino acid sequence of a protein.

primase
An RNA polymerase that uses DNA as a template to produce an RNA fragment that serves as a primer for DNA synthesis.

programmed cell death
A tightly controlled form of cell suicide that allows cells that are unneeded or unwanted to be eliminated from an adult or developing organism; the major form is called apoptosis.

prokaryote
Major category of living cells distinguished by the absence of a nucleus; includes the archaea and the eubacteria (commonly called bacteria).

prometaphase
Stage of mitosis in which the nuclear envelope breaks down and duplicated chromosomes are captured by the spindle microtubules; precedes metaphase.

promoter
DNA sequence that initiates gene transcription; includes sequences recognized by RNA polymerase and its accessory proteins.

promoter
DNA sequence that initiates gene transcription; includes sequences recognized by RNA polymerase and its accessory proteins.

proofreading
The process by which DNA polymerase corrects its own errors as it moves along DNA.

prophase
First stage of mitosis, during which the duplicated chromosomes condense and the mitotic spindle forms.

protease
Enzyme that degrades proteins by hydrolyzing their peptide bonds.

proteasome
Large protein machine that degrades proteins that are damaged, misfolded, or no longer needed by the cell; its target proteins are marked for destruction primarily by the attachment of a short chain of ubiquitin.

protein
Macromolecule built from amino acids that provides cells with their shape and structure and performs most of their activities.

protein domain
Segment of a polypeptide chain that can fold into a compact, stable structure and that often carries out a specific function.

protein family
A group of polypeptides that share a similar amino acid sequence or three-dimensional structure, reflecting a common evolutionary origin. Individual members often have related but distinct functions, such as kinases that phosphorylate different target proteins.

protein kinase
Enzyme that catalyzes the transfer of a phosphate group from ATP to a specific amino acid side chain on a target protein.

protein kinase C (PKC)
Enzyme that phosphorylates target proteins in response to a rise in diacylglycerol and Ca^{2+} ions.

protein machine
Assembly of protein molecules that operates as a cooperative unit to perform a complex series of biological activities, such as replicating DNA.

protein phosphatase
Enzyme that catalyzes the removal of a phosphate group from a protein, often with high specificity for the phosphorylated site.

protein phosphorylation
The covalent addition of a phosphate group to a side chain of a protein, catalyzed by a protein kinase; serves as a form of regulation that usually alters the activity or properties of the target protein.

proteoglycan
Molecule consisting of one or more glycosaminoglycan chains attached to a core protein; these aggregates can form gels that regulate the passage of molecules through the extracellular medium and guide cell migration.

proto-oncogene
Gene that when mutated or overexpressed can transform a normal cell into a cancerous one.

proton
Positively charged particle found in the nucleus of every atom; also, another name for a hydrogen ion (H^+).

protozoan
A free-living, nonphotosynthetic, single-celled, motile eukaryote.

pump
Transporter that uses a source of energy, such as ATP hydrolysis or sunlight, to actively move a solute across a membrane against its electrochemical gradient.

purifying selection
Preservation of a specific nucleotide sequence by the elimination of individuals carrying mutations that interfere with its functions.

pyruvate
Three-carbon metabolite that is the end product of the glycolytic breakdown of glucose; provides a crucial link to the citric acid cycle and many biosynthetic pathways.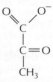

quaternary structure
Complete structure formed by multiple, interacting polypeptide chains that form a larger protein molecule.

quinone
Small, lipid-soluble, mobile electron carrier molecule that functions in the respiratory and photosynthetic electron-transport chains. (*See* Figure 14–21.)

Rab protein
One of a family of small GTP-binding proteins present on the surfaces of transport vesicles and organelles that serves

as a molecular marker to help ensure that transport vesicles fuse only with the correct membrane.

Ras
One of a large family of small GTP-binding proteins (the monomeric GTPases) that helps relay signals from cell-surface receptors to the nucleus. Many human cancers contain an overactive mutant form of the protein.

reaction center
In photosynthetic membranes, a protein complex that contains a special pair of chlorophyll molecules; it performs the photochemical reactions that convert the energy of photons (light) into high-energy electrons for transport down the photosynthetic electron-transport chain.

reading frame
One of the three possible ways in which a set of successive nucleotide triplets can be translated into protein, depending on which nucleotide serves as the starting point.

receptor
Protein that recognizes and responds to a specific signal molecule.

receptor serine/threonine kinase
Enzyme-coupled receptor that phosphorylates target proteins on serine or threonine.

receptor tyrosine kinase (RTK)
Enzyme-coupled receptor in which the intracellular domain has a tyrosine kinase activity, which is activated by ligand binding to the receptor's extracellular domain.

receptor-mediated endocytosis
Mechanism of selective uptake of material by animal cells in which a macromolecule binds to a receptor in the plasma membrane and enters the cell in a clathrin-coated vesicle.

recombinant DNA
A DNA molecule that is composed of DNA sequences from different sources.

redox pair
Two molecules that can be interconverted by the gain or loss of an electron; for example, NADH and NAD^+.

redox potential
A measure of the tendency of a given redox pair to donate or accept electrons.

redox reaction
A reaction in which electrons are transferred from one chemical species to another. An oxidation–reduction reaction.

reduction
Addition of electrons to an atom, as occurs during the addition of hydrogen to a carbon atom or the removal of oxygen from it; can also refer to a partial shift of electrons between atoms linked by a covalent bond.

regulatory DNA sequence
DNA sequence to which a transcription regulator binds to determine when, where, and in what quantities a gene is to be transcribed into RNA.

regulatory RNA
RNA molecule that plays a role in controlling gene expression.

replication fork
Y-shaped junction at the site where DNA is being replicated.

replication origin
Nucleotide sequence at which DNA replication is initiated.

reporter gene
Gene encoding a protein whose activity is easy to monitor experimentally; used to study the expression pattern of a target gene or the localization of its protein product.

respiratory enzyme complex
Set of proteins in the inner mitochondrial membrane that facilitates the transfer of high-energy electrons from NADH to water while pumping protons into the intermembrane space.

resting membrane potential
Voltage difference across the plasma membrane when a cell is not stimulated.

restriction enzyme
Enzyme that can cleave a DNA molecule at a specific, short sequence of nucleotides. Extensively used in recombinant DNA technology.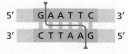

retrotransposon
Type of mobile genetic element that moves by being first transcribed into an RNA copy that is reconverted to DNA by reverse transcriptase and inserted elsewhere in the chromosomes.

retrovirus
RNA-containing virus that replicates in a cell by first making a double-stranded DNA intermediate that becomes integrated into the cell's chromosome.

reverse transcriptase
Enzyme that makes a double-stranded DNA copy from a single-stranded RNA template molecule. Present in retroviruses and as part of the transposition machinery of retrotransposons.

Rho protein family
Family of small, monomeric GTPases that controls the organization of the actin cytoskeleton.

ribosomal RNA (rRNA)
RNA molecule that forms the structural and catalytic core of the ribosome.

ribosome
Large macromolecular complex, composed of RNAs and proteins, that translates a messenger RNA into a polypeptide chain.

ribozyme
An RNA molecule with catalytic activity.

RNA
Molecule produced by the transcription of DNA; usually single-stranded, it is a polynucleotide composed of covalently linked ribonucleotide subunits. Serves a variety of informational, structural, catalytic, and regulatory functions in cells.

RNA (ribonucleic acid)
Molecule produced by the transcription of DNA; usually single-stranded, it is a polynucleotide composed of covalently linked ribonucleotide subunits. Serves a variety of informational, structural, catalytic, and regulatory functions in cells.

RNA capping
The modification of the 5′ end of a maturing RNA transcript by the addition of an atypical nucleotide.

RNA interference (RNAi)
Cellular mechanism activated by double-stranded RNA molecules that results in the destruction of RNAs containing a similar nucleotide sequence. It is widely exploited as an experimental tool for preventing the expression of selected genes (gene silencing).

RNA polymerase
Enzyme that catalyzes the synthesis of an RNA molecule

from a DNA template using ribonucleoside triphosphate precursors.

RNA processing
Broad term for the modifications that a precursor mRNA undergoes as it matures into an mRNA. It typically includes 5′ capping, RNA splicing, and 3′ polyadenylation.

RNA splicing
Process in which intron sequences are excised from RNA molecules in the nucleus during the formation of a mature messenger RNA.

RNA transcript
RNA molecule produced by transcription that is complementary to one strand of DNA.

RNA world
Hypothetical period in Earth's early history in which life-forms were thought to use RNA both to store genetic information and to catalyze chemical reactions.

RNA-Seq
Sequencing technique used to determine directly the nucleotide sequence of a collection of RNAs.

rough endoplasmic reticulum
Region of the endoplasmic reticulum associated with ribosomes and involved in the synthesis of secreted and membrane-bound proteins.

S cyclin
Regulatory protein that helps to launch the S phase of the cell cycle.

S phase
Period during a eukaryotic cell cycle in which DNA is synthesized.

S-Cdk
Protein complex whose activity initiates DNA replication; consists of an S cyclin plus a cyclin-dependent protein kinase (Cdk).

sarcomere
Highly organized assembly of actin and myosin filaments that serves as the contractile unit of a myofibril in a muscle cell.

saturated
Describes an organic molecule that contains a full complement of hydrogen; in other words, no double or triple carbon–carbon bonds.

scaffold protein
Protein with multiple binding sites for other macromolecules, holding them in a way that speeds up their functional interactions.

secondary structure
Regular local folding pattern of a polymeric molecule. In proteins, it refers to α helices and β sheets.

secretion
Production and release of a substance from a cell.

secretory vesicle
Membrane-enclosed organelle in which molecules destined for secretion are stored prior to release.

sequence
The linear order of monomers in a large molecule—for example, amino acids in a protein or nucleotides in DNA; encodes information that specifies a macromolecule's precise biological function.

serine/threonine kinase
Enzyme that phosphorylates target proteins on serines or threonines.

sexual reproduction
Mode of reproduction in which the genomes of two individuals are mixed to produce an individual that is genetically distinct from its parents.

side chain
Portion of an amino acid not involved in forming peptide bonds; its chemical identity gives each amino acid unique properties.

signal sequence
Amino acid sequence that directs a protein to a specific location in the cell, such as the nucleus or mitochondria.

signal transduction
Conversion of an impulse or stimulus from one physical or chemical form to another. In cell biology, the process by which a cell responds to an extracellular signal.

single-nucleotide polymorphism (SNP)
Form of genetic variation in which one portion of the population differs from another in terms of which nucleotide is found at a particular position in the genome.

sister chromatid
Copy of a chromosome, produced by DNA replication, that remains bound to the other copy.

small interfering RNA (siRNA)
Short length of RNA produced from double-stranded RNA during the process of RNA interference. It base-pairs with identical sequences in other RNAs, leading to the inactivation or destruction of the target RNA.

small nuclear RNA (snRNA)
RNA molecule of around 200 nucleotides that participates in RNA splicing.

SNARE
One of a family of membrane proteins responsible for the selective fusion of vesicles with a target membrane inside the cell.

SNP (single-nucleotide polymorphism)
Form of genetic variation in which one portion of the population differs from another in terms of which nucleotide is found at a particular position in the genome.

somatic cell
Any cell that forms part of the body of a plant or animal that is not a germ cell or germ-line precursor.

spindle pole
Centrosome from which microtubules radiate to form the mitotic spindle.

spliceosome
Large assembly of RNA and protein molecules that splices introns out of pre-mRNA in the nucleus of eukaryotic cells.

standard free-energy change, $\Delta G°$
The free-energy change measured at a defined concentration, temperature, and pressure. (*See also* **free-energy change**.)

starch
Polysaccharide composed exclusively of glucose units, used as an energy store in plant cells.

stem cell
Relatively undifferentiated, self-renewing cell that produces daughter cells that can either differentiate into more specialized cell types or can retain the developmental potential of the parent cell.

steroid hormone
Hydrophobic signal molecule related to cholesterol; can pass through the plasma membrane to interact with intracellular receptors that affect gene expression in the target cell. Examples include estrogen and testosterone.

stroma

In a chloroplast, the large interior space that contains the enzymes needed to incorporate CO_2 into sugars during the carbon-fixation stage of photosynthesis; equivalent to the matrix of a mitochondrion.

substrate

A molecule on which an enzyme acts to catalyze a chemical reaction.

substrate

A molecule on which an enzyme acts to catalyze a chemical reaction.

subunit

A monomer that forms part of a larger molecule, such as an amino acid residue in a protein or a nucleotide residue in a nucleic acid. Can also refer to a complete molecule that forms part of a larger molecule. Many proteins, for example, are composed of multiple polypeptide chains, each of which is called a protein subunit.

sugar

A substance made of carbon, hydrogen, and oxygen with the general formula $(CH_2O)_n$. A carbohydrate or saccharide. The "sugar" of everyday use is sucrose, a sweet-tasting disaccharide made of glucose and fructose.

survival factor

Extracellular signal molecule that must be present to suppress apoptosis.

symport

A transporter that transfers two different solutes across a cell membrane in the same direction.

synapse

Specialized junction where a nerve cell communicates with another cell (such as a nerve cell, muscle cell, or gland cell), usually via a neurotransmitter secreted by the nerve cell.

synaptic vesicle

Small membrane-enclosed sac filled with neurotransmitter that releases its contents by exocytosis at a synapse.

telomerase

Enzyme that elongates telomeres, synthesizing the repetitive nucleotide sequences found at the ends of eukaryotic chromosomes.

telomere

Repetitive nucleotide sequence that caps the ends of linear chromosomes. Counteracts the tendency of the chromosome otherwise to shorten with each round of replication.

telophase

Final stage of mitosis in which the two sets of separated chromosomes decondense and become enclosed by a nuclear envelope.

template

A molecular structure that serves as a pattern for the production of other molecules. For example, one strand of DNA directs the synthesis of the complementary DNA strand.

tertiary structure

Complete three-dimensional structure of a fully folded protein.

tethering protein

Filamentous transmembrane protein involved in the docking of transport vesicles to target membranes.

thylakoid

In a chloroplast, the flattened, disclike sac whose membranes contain the proteins and pigments that convert light energy into chemical-bond energy during photosynthesis.

tight junction

Cell–cell junction that seals adjacent epithelial cells together, preventing the passage of most dissolved molecules from one side of the epithelial sheet to the other.

tissue

Cooperative assembly of cells and matrix woven together to form a distinctive multicellular fabric with a specific function.

transcription

Process in which RNA polymerase uses one strand of DNA as a template to synthesize a complementary RNA sequence.

transcription regulator

Protein that binds specifically to a regulatory DNA sequence to switch a gene either on or off.

transcriptional activator

A protein that binds to a specific regulatory region of DNA to stimulate transcription of an adjacent gene.

transcriptional repressor

A protein that binds to a specific regulatory region of DNA to prevent transcription of an adjacent gene.

transfer RNA (tRNA)

Small RNA molecule that serves as an adaptor that "reads" a codon in mRNA and adds the correct amino acid to the growing polypeptide chain.

transformation

Process by which cells take up DNA molecules from their surroundings and then express genes present on that DNA.

transgenic organism

A plant or animal that has stably incorporated into its genome one or more genes derived from another cell or organism.

transition state

Transient structure that forms during the course of a chemical reaction; in this configuration, a molecule has the highest free energy; it is no longer the substrate, but is not yet the product.

translation

Process by which the sequence of nucleotides in a messenger RNA molecule directs the incorporation of amino acids into protein.

translation initiation factor

Protein that promotes the proper association of ribosomes with mRNA and is required for the initiation of protein synthesis.

transmitter-gated ion channel

Transmembrane receptor protein or protein complex that opens in response to the binding of a neurotransmitter, allowing the passage of a specific inorganic ion; its activation can trigger an action potential in a postsynaptic cell.

transport vesicle

Membrane vesicle that carries proteins from one intracellular compartment to another—for example, from the endoplasmic reticulum to the Golgi apparatus.

transporter

Membrane transport protein that moves a solute across a cell membrane by undergoing a series of conformational changes.

transposon

General name for short segments of DNA that can move from one location to another in the genome. Also known as mobile genetic elements.

tubulin
Protein from which microtubules are made.

tumor suppressor gene
A gene that in a normal tissue cell inhibits cancerous behavior. Loss or inactivation of both copies of such a gene from a diploid cell can cause it to behave as a cancer cell.

turnover number
The maximum number of substrate molecules that an enzyme can convert into product per second.

tyrosine kinase
Enzyme that phosphorylates target proteins on tyrosines.

unfolded protein response (UPR)
Molecular program triggered by the accumulation of misfolded proteins in the endoplasmic reticulum. Allows cells to expand the endoplasmic reticulum and produce more of the molecular machinery needed to restore proper protein folding and processing.

unsaturated
Describes an organic molecule that contains one or more double or triple bonds between its carbon atoms.

van der Waals attraction
Weak noncovalent interaction, due to fluctuating electrical charges, that comes into play between two atoms within a short distance of each other.

vesicular transport
Movement of material between organelles in the eukaryotic cell via membrane-enclosed vesicles.

virus
Particle consisting of nucleic acid (RNA or DNA) enclosed in a protein coat and capable of replicating within a host cell and spreading from cell to cell.

V_{max}
The maximum rate of an enzymatic reaction, reached when the active sites of all of the enzyme molecules in a sample are fully occupied by substrate.

voltage-gated channel
Channel protein that permits the passage of selected ions, such as Na^+, across a membrane in response to changes in the membrane potential. Found primarily in electrically excitable cells such as nerve and muscle cells.

voltage-gated Na^+ channel
Protein in the plasma membrane of electrically excitable cells that opens in response to membrane depolarization, allowing Na^+ to enter the cell. It is responsible for action potentials in these cells.

Wnt protein
Member of a family of extracellular signal molecules that regulates cell proliferation and migration during embryonic development and that maintains stem cells in a proliferative state.

x-ray crystallography
Technique used to determine the three-dimensional structure of a protein molecule by analyzing the diffraction pattern produced when a beam of x-rays is passed through an ordered array of the protein.

zygote
Diploid cell produced by fusion of a male and a female gamete. A fertilized egg.

Index

Note: The index covers the text and figure captions but not the marginal or end-of-chapter questions. The suffixes F and T after a page reference indicate relevant figures or tables on pages where no text treatment has been indexed.

H